Color Atlas of
Cardiovascular Disease

System requirements:

- **Operating System—Windows Vista or above**
- **Web Browser—Google Chrome, Mozilla Firefox, Internet Explorer 9 and above**
- **Essential plugins—Java & Flash Player**
  - If you are experiencing problems viewing content, please check that your system has Java enabled.
  - If the video clips do not appear, your system may require Flash Player or require an update to Flash Player settings. To learn more about Flash Player settings, please click on the link in the "Help" section of the DVD.
  - You can test Java and Flash Player by using the associated links available in the "Help" section of the DVD.

Please note that this CD/DVD will only play in a computer or laptop and will not work properly in a DVD player.

This CD/DVD come with an "Autorun" function; it may take a few seconds to load on your computer. If the content does not load, please follow the steps listed below to access the contents manually:

- Click on "My Computer".
- Select the CD/DVD drive and Click "Open/Explore". A list of available files will appear.
- Find and double click the file "launch.html".

For more information about troubleshooting, please click on http://support.microsoft.com/kb/330135.

BOOK COVER IMAGE CREDITS

Left image: 4D velocity mapping MRI pathline visualization of cardiac blood flow in the heart and great vessels. Image courtesy of Dr Michael Markl. Image from Markl M, et al. Comprehensive 4D velocity (3 dimensional, 3 directionally encoded, time resolved velocity acquisition) mapping of the heart and great vessels by cardiovascular magnetic resonance. Journal of Cardiovascular Magnetic Resonance 2011;(13):7.

Top right image: Gross pathological features of constrictive pericarditis. Image courtesy of Dr William D Edwards, Mayo Clinic. Image and legend text from Khandaker MH and Nishimura RA. Pericardial disease. In Chatterjee K, et al. (ed). Cardiology—an illustrated textbook. Jaypee Brothers Medical Publishers (P) Ltd., New Delhi, India.

Middle right image: Gross pathology specimen of calcific aortic stenosis. Image adapted from Armed Forces Institute of Pathology.

Bottom right image: Volume rendered CT angiogram demonstrating separate origins from the left coronary sinus of the left anterior descending and left circumflex coronary arteries. Image from Oyama-Manae N, et al. Non-coronary cardiac findings and pitfalls in coronary computed tomography angiography. J Clin Imaging Sci 2011;1:51. http://www.clinicalimagingscience.org.

Color Atlas of
Cardiovascular Disease

Editor

Glenn N Levine MD FAHA FACC
Professor of Medicine
Baylor College of Medicine
Director, Cardiac Care Unit
Michael E DeBakey VA Medical Center
Houston, Texas, USA

JAYPEE *The Health Sciences Publisher*
New Delhi | London | Philadelphia | Panama

Jaypee Brothers Medical Publishers (P) Ltd

Headquarters
Jaypee Brothers Medical Publishers (P) Ltd.
4838/24, Ansari Road, Daryaganj
New Delhi 110 002, India
Phone: +91-11-43574357
Fax: +91-11-43574314
E-mail: jaypee@jaypeebrothers.com

Overseas Offices
J.P. Medical Ltd.
83, Victoria Street, London
SW1H 0HW (UK)
Phone: +44-20 3170 8910
Fax: +44(0)20 3008 6180
E-mail: info@jpmedpub.com

Jaypee-Highlights Medical Publishers Inc.
City of Knowledge, Bld. 237, Clayton
Panama City, Panama
Phone: +1 507-301-0496
Fax: +1 507-301-0499
E-mail: cservice@jphmedical.com

Jaypee Medical Inc.
The Bourse
111, South Independence Mall East
Suite 835, Philadelphia, PA 19106, USA
Phone: +1 267-519-9789
E-mail: jpmed.us@gmail.com

Jaypee Brothers Medical Publishers (P) Ltd.
17/1-B, Babar Road, Block-B, Shaymali
Mohammadpur, Dhaka-1207
Bangladesh
Mobile: +08801912003485
E-mail: jaypeedhaka@gmail.com

Jaypee Brothers Medical Publishers (P) Ltd.
Bhotahity, Kathmandu, Nepal
Phone: +977-9741283608
E-mail: kathmandu@jaypeebrothers.com

Website: www.jaypeebrothers.com
Website: www.jaypeedigital.com

Inquiries for bulk sales may be solicited at: jaypee@jaypeebrothers.com

Color Atlas of Cardiovascular Disease

First Edition: **2015**

ISBN: 978-93-5152-244-7

Printed at Replika Press Pvt. Ltd.

Dedicated to

All those who devote their lives to the
diagnosis and treatment of cardiovascular disease,
and hence to the betterment of one's fellow man and woman.

"Cure sometimes, treat often, comfort always"

—Hippocrates

Contributors

Hamid Afshar MD
Assistant Professor
Department of Medicine
Baylor College of Medicine
Houston, Texas, USA

Philippe R Akhrass MD FACP
Clinical Assistant Instructor
Division of Cardiovascular Medicine
SUNY Downstate Medical Center
Brooklyn, New York, USA

Khaled Albouaini MSc MD MRCP(UK)
Consultant Cardiologist
Department of Cardiology
Royal Liverpool University Hospital
Liverpool, UK

Nandan S Anavekar MBBCh
Assistant Professor of Medicine
Department of Cardiovascular
Diseases and Radiology
Mayo Clinic
Rochester, Minnesota, USA

Ivan Anderson MD
Fellow
Division of Cardiovascular Medicine
University of California, Davis
Sacramento, California, USA

Faisal G Bakaeen MD FACS
Chief of Cardiovascular Surgery
MEDVAMC
Associate Professor
Department of Surgery
Baylor College of Medicine
Houston, Texas, USA

Luc M Beauchesne MD FRCPC FACC
Associate Professor
Division of Cardiology
University of Ottawa Heart Institute
Ottawa, Ontario, Canada

Carlos F Bechara MD MS FACS RPVI
Assistant Professor of Surgery
Department of Vascular and
Endovascular Surgery
Baylor College of Medicine
Houston, Texas, USA

Alvin S Blaustein MD
Associate Professor of Medicine
Cardiology Section
Baylor College of Medicine
Michael E DeBakey VA Medical Center
Houston, Texas, USA

Elijah H Bolin MD
Fellow
Pediatric Cardiology
Baylor College of Medicine
Houston, Texas, USA

Jamieson M Bourque MD
Assistant Professor
Medicine and Radiology
University of Virginia
Charlottesville, Virginia, USA

Biykem Bozkurt MD PhD
The Mary and Gordon Cain Chair and
Professor of Medicine
Baylor College of Medicine
Director, Winters Center for Heart
Failure Research
Medical Care Line Executive and Chief
Section of Cardiology
Michael E DeBakey VA Medicial Center
Houston, Texas, USA

Alan C Braverman MD
Alumni Endowed Professor in
Cardiovascular Diseases
Professor of Medicine
Cardiovascular Division
Department of Medicine
Washington University School of
Medicine
St Louis, Missouri, USA

Gerd Brunner MS PhD
Assistant Professor
Department of Medicine
Baylor College of Medicine
Houston, Texas, USA

Adam S Budzikowski MD PhD FHRS
Assistant Professor
Division of Cardiovascular
Medicine—EP Section
SUNY Downstate Medical Center
Brooklyn, New York, USA

Blase A Carabello MD
Professor of Medicine
Icahn School of Medicine
Chairman, Mount Sinai Beth Israel
Department of Cardiology
New York, New York, USA

Kanu Chatterjee MBBS FRCP FACC FAC MACP
Professor of Medicine
Department of Medicine
University of Iowa
Iowa City, Iowa, USA

Melvin D Cheitlin MD MACC
Professor of Medicine
University of California, San Francisco
San Francisco, California, USA

Yeon Hyeon Choe MD
Professor in Cardiothoracic Imaging
Department of Radiology
Samsung Medical Center
Sungkyunkwan University
School of Medicine
Seoul, Korea

Heidi M Connolly MD
Professor
Division of Cardiovascular
Diseases, Mayo Clinic
Rochester, Minnesota, USA

Lorraine D Cornwell MD
Assistant Professor
Department of Surgery
Baylor College of Medicine
Houston, Texas, USA

Joseph A Dearani MD
Professor
Department of Surgery
Mayo Clinic
Rochester, Minnesota, USA

Ali E Denktas MD
Associate Professor of Medicine
Baylor College of Medicine
Director, Cardiac Catheterization
Laboratory,
Michael E. DeBakey VA Medical Center
Houston, TX, USA

Carole J Dennie MD FRCPC
Professor
Department of Radiology
University of Ottawa
Ottawa, Ontario, Canada

Anita Deswal MD MPH
Associate Professor
Baylor College of Medicine
Associate Chief
Section of Cardiology
Michael E. DeBakey VA Medical Center
Houston, TX, USA

Marc W Deyell MD MSc (EPI)
Assistant Professor
Division of Cardiology
University of British Columbia
Vancouver, British Columbia, Canada

Unnati H Doshi MD MPH
Clinical Fellow
Department of Pediatric Cardiology
University of Texas Medical School at Houston
Houston, Texas, USA

David M Dudzinski MD JD
Division of Cardiology
Massachusetts General Hospital
Harvard Medical School
Boston, Massachusetts, USA

William D Edwards MD FACC
Professor of Pathology
Department of Laboratory Medicine and Pathology
Mayo Clinic
Rochester, Minnesota, USA

Christopher R Ellis MD FACC
Assistant Professor
Cardiac Electrophysiology
Department of Medicine
Vanderbilt University School of Medicine/VHVI
Nashville, Tennessee, USA

Luis H Eraso MD
Assistant Professor of Medicine and Surgery
Jefferson Medical College
Thomas Jefferson University
Philadelphia, Pennsylvania, USA

Lothar Faber MD
Professor
Department of Cardiology
Heart and Diabetes Centre North-Rhine Westphalia
University Clinic of the Ruhr-University Bochum
Bad Oeynhausen, Germany

Gregory K Feld MD
Professor of Medicine
Department of Medicine
Division of Cardiology
Electrophysiology Program
University of California, San Diego
San Diego, California, USA

Michael E Field MD
Assistant Professor
Director, Cardiac Arrhythmia Service
Division of Cardiology
University of Wisconsin
Madison, Wisconsin, USA

Kevin C Floyd MD
Assistant Professor
Department of Medicine
University of Massachusetts
Worcester, Massachusetts, USA

Arul D Furtado MD
Cardiac Surgery Fellow
Division of Cardiothoracic Surgery
Department of Surgery
Emory University School of Medicine
Atlanta, Georgia, USA

Taki Galanis MD
Assistant Professor
Department of Surgery
Jefferson Medical College
Philadelphia, Pennsylvania, USA

Sanjay Ganapathi MD DM
Assistant Professor
Department of Cardiology
Sree Chitra Tirunal Institute for Medical Sciences and Technology
Trivandrum, Kerala, India

Brian Ghoshhajra MD MBA
Instructor
Department of Radiology
Harvard University
Boston, Massachusetts, USA

Salil Ginde MD
Assistant Professor
Department of Pediatrics—Cardiology
Medical College of Wisconsin
Milawaukee, Wisconsin, USA

Irakli Giorgberidze MD
Assistant Professor of Medicine
Department of Medicine
Cardiology Section
Michael E DeBakey VA Medical Center
Baylor College of Medicine
Houston, Texas, USA

Ramil Goel MD
Fellow
Department of Cardiac Electrophysiology
University of Michigan
Ann Arbor, Michigan, USA

Lorena Gonzalez MD RPVI
Department of Vascular and Endovascular Surgery
Baylor College of Medicine
Houston, Texas, USA

Ambarish Gopal MD FACC FSCCT
Consultant, Cardiovascular Disease and Interventional Cardiology
Medical Director, Cardiovascular CT and Transcatheter Heart Valve Program
Heart Hospital Baylor Plano
Baylor Scott and White Healthcare System
Plano, Texas, USA

Aaron W Grossman MD PhD
Fellow in Vascular and Interventional Neurology
Department of Neurology
University of Cincinnati
Cincinnati, Ohio, USA

T Sloane Guy MD
Assistant Professor
Department of Surgery
Temple University
Philadelphia, Pennsylvania, USA

Sivadasanpillai Harikrishnan MD
Additional Professor in Cardiology
Department of Cardiology
Sree Chitra Tirunal Institute for Medical Sciences and Technology
Trivandrum, Kerala, India

Ravi S Hira MD
Cardiovascular Disease Fellow
Cardiology Division
Department of Medicine
Baylor College of Medicine
Houston, Texas, USA

Brian D Hoit MD
Professor of Medicine and
Physiology and Biophysics
Department of Medicine
Case Western Reserve University
University Hospitals Case Medical Center
Harrington Heart Vascular Institute
Cleveland, Ohio, USA

Phillip A Horwitz MD
Associate Professor of Medicine
Department of Internal Medicine
University of Iowa Carver College of Medicine
Iowa City, Iowa, USA

Eric M Isselbacher MD
Co-Director, Thoracic Aortic Center
Massachusetts General Hospital
Associate Professor of Medicine
Harvard Medical School
Boston, Massachusetts, USA

Sebastian A Iturra MD
Fellow
Department Cardiothoracic Surgery
Emory University
Atlanta, Georgia, USA

Hiroyuki Iwano MD PhD
Postdoctoral Research Fellow
Division of Cardiology
University of Mississippi Medical Center
Jackson, Mississippi, USA

Michael R Jaff DO
Professor
Department of Medicine
Harvard Medical School
Boston, Massachusetts, USA

Trevor L Jenkins MD
Assistant Professor of Medicine
Division of Cardiovascular Medicine
Case Western Reserve University
University Hospitals Case
Medical Center
Cleveland, Ohio, USA

Hani Jneid MD FACC FAHA FSCAI
Assistant Professor
Division of Cardiology
Baylor College of Medicine
Houston, Texas, USA

Susan M Joseph MD
Assistant Professor of Medicine
Department of Internal Medicine
Division of Cardiology
Washington University School of Medicine
St Louis, Missouri, USA

Christine H Attenhofer Jost MD
Professor
Cardiovascular Center
Klinik Im Park
Zurich, Switzerland

Arvindh N Kanagasundram MD
Assistant Professor
Cardiac Electrophysiology
Vanderbilt Heart and Vascular Institute
Nashville, Tennessee, USA

Mohammad A Kashem MD PhD
Assistant Professor of Surgery (Adjunct)
Division of Cardiovascular Surgery
Department of Surgery
Temple University School of Medicine
Philadelphia, Pennsylvania, USA

Demosthenes G Katritsis MD
Director
Department of Cardiology
Athens Euroclinic
Athens, Greece

George D Katritsis
Medical Student
Faculty of Medicine
University of Bristol
Bristol, UK

Ann Kavanaugh-McHugh MD
Associate Professor
Thomas P Graham Jr
Division of Pediatric Cardiology
Monroe Carell Jr
Children's Hospital at Vanderbilt
Vanderbilt University
Nashville, Tennessee, USA

Thomas A Kent MD
Professor and Director of Stroke
Research and Education
Department of Neurology
Baylor College of Medicine
Michael E DeBakey VA Medical Center
Stroke Program
Houston, Texas, USA

Kiran K Khush MD MAS
Assistant Professor
Department of Medicine
Stanford University
Stanford, California, USA

Eun Young Kim MD
Assistant Professor in
Cardiothoracic Imaging
Department of Radiology
Gachon University Gil Hospital
Incheon, Korea

Jin T Kim MD
Assistant Professor of Radiology
Department of Radiology
Baylor College of Medicine
Houston, Texas, USA

Christopher M Kramer MD
Ruth C Heede Professor of Cardiology
Departments of Medicine and
Radiology
University of Virginia Health System
Charlottesville, Virginia, USA

Richard A Lange MD MBA
Professor
Department of Medicine
University of Texas Health Science Center
San Antonio, Texas, USA

Kory J Lavine MD PhD
Instructor of Medicine
Department of Internal Medicine
Division of Cardiology
Washington University School of Medicine
St Louis, Missouri, USA

Glenn N Levine MD FAHA FACC
Professor of Medicine
Baylor College of Medicine
Director, Cardiac Care Unit
Michael E DeBakey VA Medical Center
Houston, Texas, USA

William C Little MD
Professor of Medicine
Department of Medicine
University of Mississippi Medical Center
Jackson, Mississippi, USA

Michael J Mack MD FACC
Medical Director
Cardiovascular Services
Baylor Scott and White Health
Dallas, Texas, USA

Peace C Madueme MD
Assistant Professor
Heart Institute
Cincinnati Children's Hospital Medical Center
Cincinnati, Ohio, USA

Jothiharan Mahenthiran MBBB MRCP FACC
Clinical Associate Professor of Medicine/Cardiology
Marian University, Indianapolis
Director, Advanced Cardiac Imaging
Community Heart and Vascular Hospital
Indianapolis, Indiana, USA

Sharyl R Martini MD PhD
Assistant Professor
Department of Neurology
Baylor College of Medicine
Houston, Texas, USA

Paula Martins MD
Pediatric Cardiologist
Pediatric Hospital of Coimbra
Coimbra Hospital and University Centre
Coimbra, Portugal

Thomas J McGarry MD
Electrophysiology Fellow
Department of Medicine
Division of Cardiology
Electrophysiology Program
University of California
San Diego, California, USA

Geno J Merli MD
Professor of Medicine and Surgery
Department of Medicine
Jefferson Medical College
Philadelphia, Pennsylvania, USA

Farouk Mookadam MD FRCPC FACC MSc (HRM)
Professor, College of Medicine Mayo
Consultant, Cardiovascular Diseases
Mayo Clinic
Scottsdale, Arizona, USA

Ryan Allen Moore MD
Pediatric Cardiology Fellow
The Heart Institute, Cincinnati Children's Hospital Medical Center
Cincinnati, Ohio, USA

Gareth J Morgan MD MRCPCH
Department of Pediatric Cardiology
Evelina Children's Hospital
Guys and St Thomas Trust
London, UK

Darra T Murphy MB BCh BAO MRCPI
Department of Radiology
St Paul's Hospital
Vancouver, British Columbia, Canada

Vijay Nambi MD PhD
Staff Cardiologist
Michael E DeBakey VA Medical Center
Assistant Professor of Medicine
Baylor College of Medicine
Houston, Texas, USA

Patrick W O'Leary MD
Consultant
Division of Pediatric Cardiology
Professor of Pediatrics
Department of Pediatrics
Mayo Clinic
Rochester, Minnesota, USA

Jae K Oh MD
Professor
Division of Cardiovascular Diseases
Mayo Clinic
Rochester, Minnesota, USA

A Afsin Oktay MD
Chief Resident
Department of Internal Medicine
Presence Saint Francis Hospital
Evanston, Illinois, USA

Shuab Omer MD
Assistant Professor
Division of Cardiothoracic Surgery
Baylor College of Medicine
Houston, Texas, USA

David Paniagua MD FACC FSCAI
Assistant Professor of Medicine
Department of Cardiology
Baylor College of Medicine
Michael E DeBakey VA Medical Center
Houston, Texas, USA

David A Parra MD
Assistant Professor
Department of Pediatrics
Monroe Carrell Jr
Children's Hospital at Vanderbilt
Nashville, Tennessee, USA

Pravin V Patil MD
Assistant Professor of Medicine
Section of Cardiology
Department of Internal Medicine
Temple University School of Medicine
Philadelphia, Pennsylvania, USA

Daniel J Penny MD
Professor
Department of Pediatrics
Baylor College of Medicine
Houston, Texas, USA

George T Pisimisis MD RPVI FACS
Assistant Professor of Surgery
Michael E DeBakey VA Medical Center
Department of Surgery
Division of Vascular Surgery and Endovascular Therapy
Baylor College of Medicine
Houston, Texas, USA

Yashashwi Pokharel MD MSCR
Fellow
The Lipid and Atherosclerosis Program
Cardiovascular Disease Prevention Center
Baylor College of Medicine
Houston, Texas, USA

Christian Prinz MD
Department of Cardiology
University of Leuven
Leuven, Belgium

Allison M Pritchett MD
Assistant Professor
Department of Medicine
Baylor College of Medicine
Houston, Texas, USA

Min Pu MD PhD
Professor
Department of Internal Medicine/Cardiology
Wake Forest University
Winston-Salem, North Carolina, USA

Shakeel Ahmed Qureshi FRCP
Professor
Department of Pediatric Cardiology
Evelina Children's Hospital
Guys and St Thomas Trust
London, UK

Rekha Raju MBChB
Fellow
Department of Radiology
St Paul's Hospital
Vancouver, British Columbia, Canada

P Syamasundar Rao MD FAAP FACC FSCAI
Professor
Pediatrics and Medicine
Director
Pediatric Cardiology Fellowship Programs
Emeritus Chief of Pediatric Cardiology
University of Texas-Houston Medical School
Houston, Texas, USA

Jason H Rogers MD
Professor
Division of Cardiovascular Medicine
University of California
Davis Medical Center
Sacramento, California, USA

Lawrence S Rosenthal PhD MD
Professor
Department of Medicine
University of Massachusetts Memorial Medical Center
Worcester, Massachusetts, USA

James D Rossen MD
Professor
Departments of Internal Medicine and Neurosurgery
University of Iowa College of Medicine
Iowa City, Iowa, USA

Sanjiv J Shah MD
Associate Professor of Medicine
Division of Cardiology
Department of Medicine
Northwestern University Feinberg School of Medicine
Chicago, Illinois, USA

Tina Shah MD
Assistant Professor
Department of Cardiology
Baylor College of Medicine
Houston, Texas, USA

Ahmad Y Sheikh MD
Clinical Assistant Professor
Department of Cardiothoracic Surgery
Stanford University
Stanford, California, USA

Ajay V Srivastava MD
Advanced Heart Failure/Transplant Fellow
Department of Cardiovascular Medicine
Stanford University
Stanford, California, USA

Komandoor Srivathsan MD
Assistant Professor of Medicine
Department of Medicine
Mayo Clinic, College of Medicine
Phoenix, Arizona, USA

Faisal F Syed BSc (Hons) MBChB MRCP
Assistant Professor
Division of Cardiovascular Diseases
Mayo Clinic
Rochester, Minnesota, USA

Vinod H Thourani MD
Associate Professor of Cardiothoracic Surgery
Department of Surgery
Emory University
Atlanta, Georgia, USA

Philip C Ursell MD
Professor of Clinical Pathology
Department of Pathology
University of California, San Francisco
San Francisco, California, USA

Pradeep Vaideeswar MD
Professor, Additional
Department of Pathology
Cardiovascular and Thoracic Division
Seth GS Medical College and KEM Hospital
Mumbai, Maharashtra, India

John P Veinot MD
Professor
Department of Pathology and Laboratory Medicine
University of Ottawa
Ottawa, Ontario, Canada

Gruschen R Veldtman MBChB FRCP
Professor of Pediatrics
Department of Pediatric Cardiology
University of Cincinnati
Cincinnati, Ohio, USA

Salim S Virani MD PhD
Staff Cardiologist and Investigator
Michael E DeBakey VA Medical Center
Assistant Professor
Section of Cardiovascular Research
Department of Medicine
Baylor College of Medicine
Houston, Texas, USA

Gary D Webb MD
Director
Adolescent and Adult Congenital Heart Disease Program
Cincinnati Children's Hospital Medical Center
Cincinnati, Ohio, USA

Ido Weinberg MD MSC
Instructor
Department of Medicine
Cardiology Division
Harvard Medical School
Boston, Massachusetts, USA

Steven D Zangwill MD
Professor
Department of Pediatrics, Cardiology
Medical College of Wisconsin
Milawaukee, Wisconsin, USA

Preface

Color Atlas of Cardiovascular Disease is a novel twenty-first century print and electronic media endeavor which integrates traditional and cutting-edge multimedia images and videos, gross and microscopic pathology digital photographs, scores of specially created schematic figures, dozens of summary tables and flow diagrams, and comprehensive yet concise text, in order to educate the reader, both visually and through the written word, on normal and abnormal cardiovascular anatomy, function, and pathology.

The book contains over 3,000 multimedia images and dozens of videos, including all standard cardiovascular tests and imaging results such as 12-lead electrocardiography, electrophysiological studies and mapping, treadmill testing, 2D and Doppler echocardiography, peripheral ultrasound, cardiac SPECT, coronary angiography and IVUS, cardiac CT, coronary CT angiography, cardiovascular MRI and MRA, and PET CT, as well as novel and cutting-edge images such as strain and 3D echocardiography, 4D MRI, electroanatomic imaging, optical coherence tomography, and ECG isochrones mapping.

Over one hundred and fifty national and international cardiovascular experts, representing almost every continent and part of the world, have contributed to the 8 sections and 58 chapters in the book. Hundreds of other investigators, academicians, and practitioners shared images that were used in this book.

Color Atlas of Cardiovascular Disease covers the gamut of cardiovascular disease, including coronary artery disease and acute coronary syndromes, coronary revascularization, valvular and structural heart disease, heart failure and cardiomyopathies, pericardial disease, conduction abnormalities and arrhythmias, congenital heart disease, cardiac tumors, hyperlipidemia, peripheral vascular disease, stroke and cerebrovascular disease, renovascular disease, diseases of the aorta, and venous thromboembolism. Dozens of well established and emerging device-based therapies are illustrated and discussed, including PCI, CABG, ablation therapy, stent grafts, peripheral bypass, endarterectomy, arrhythmia ablation, septal closure devices, atrial appendage occluders, and TAVR. Both American and European practice guidelines for the management of specific cardiovascular diseases are summarized and discussed.

My hope is that this book will prove interesting, educational, and clinically relevant and useful to healthcare professionals of all levels of training and expertise, including medical students, medical, neurology and surgical residents, medical and surgical nurses, pathologists, allied health care professionals, and established and experienced cardiologists, surgeons, and others who already have expertise in the diagnosis and treatment of cardiovascular disease. The ultimate goal we all share, of course, is to improve the care of patients with cardiovascular disease in the area where we live, in our country, and worldwide, and if this book contributes to this goal in even the smallest of ways, then it has been an endeavor well worth pursuing.

Glenn N Levine

Acknowledgments

This *Color Atlas of Cardiovascular Disease* would not be possible without the efforts of all the national and international experts who were willing to contribute chapters to the book. A special thanks also goes out to the hundreds of persons who were willing to allow us to use their images and videos in this book, and to all those who published their manuscripts under Creative Commons licenses, which allows the sharing of published images for educational purposes, as long as the image creators are fully acknowledged (which we have so done in this book).

I would also like to thank Marco Ulloa (Development Editor), Joe Rusko (Publisher), and Sh Jitendar P Vij, Group Chairman of Jaypee Brothers Medical Publishers (P) Ltd., as well as the entire publishing team at Jaypee Brothers Medical Publishers (P) Ltd., New Delhi, India.

A heartfelt acknowledge must also go out to my 3 dogs, all adopted from animal rescue organizations, who were at my feet (or on my lap) giving me moral support during the many late weeknights and long weekends I spent working on this book.

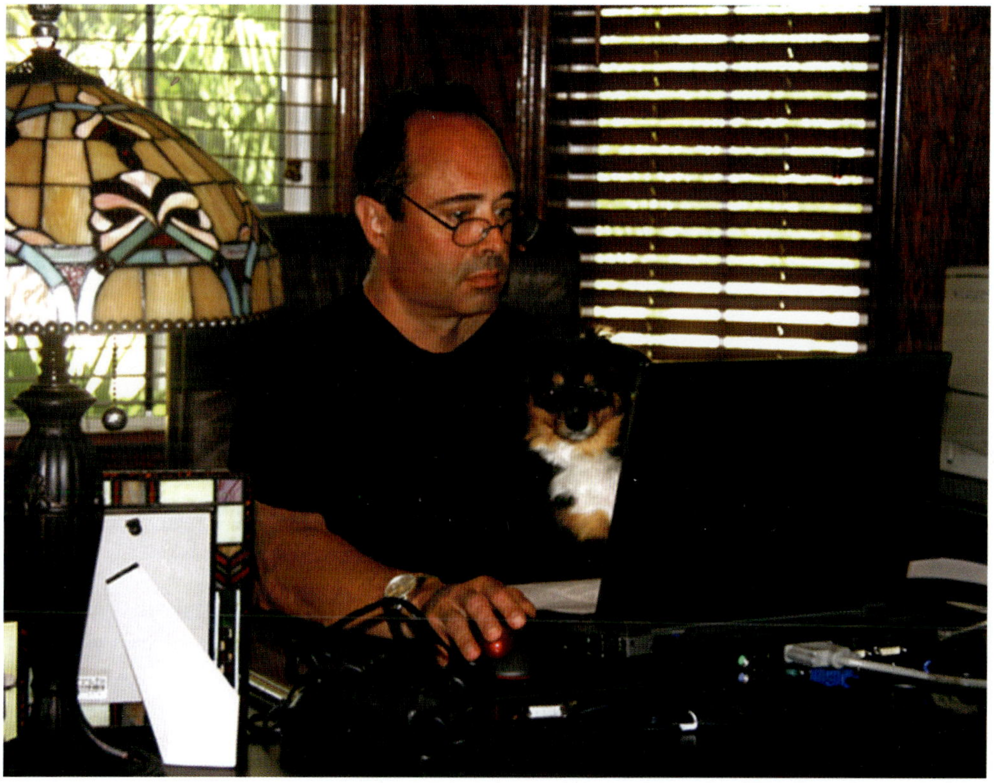

Contents

Section 1: Coronary Artery Disease

Section 2: Valvular Heart Disease

Section 3: Heart Failure and Cardiomyopathy

Section 4: Arrhythmias

Section 5: Pericardial Disease

Section 6: Congenital Heart Disease

Section 7: Peripheral Vascular Disease

Section 8: Miscellaneous Cardiovascular Disease

Video Legends

SECTION 1

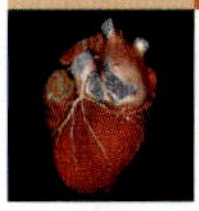

Coronary Artery Disease

1. Normal Coronary and Venous Anatomy

Video 1.1: CT 3D volume-rendered image showing the course of the coronary arteries.

Video 1.2: Right anterior oblique cranial angiogram showing the left anterior descending (LAD). The LAD gives off septal branches which supply the superior interventricular septum and gives off diagonal branches which supply a portion of the anterior and anterolateral walls.

Video 1.3: Right anterior oblique caudal angiogram showing the left circumflex artery and several obtuse marginal branches of the left circumflex artery.

Video 1.4: AP angiogram of the right coronary artery.

2. Coronary Artery Anomalies

Video 2.1: Angiogram of a mid left anterior descending (LAD) myocardial bridge. (Video courtesy of Glenn N Levine).

5. Stable Ischemic Heart Disease

Video 5.1A: Right anterior oblique projection angiogram showing a discrete tight stenosis in the mid to distal segment of a large "wrap around" left anterior descending artery.

Video 5.1B: Angiogram showing diffuse coronary artery disease of the left anterior descending (LAD) artery in a diabetic patient with stable ischemic heart disease. The catheter is subselectively engaged in the LAD so the left circumflex artery is not well visualized.

Video 5.2: Angiogram showing discrete stenosis in a segment of a large branching obtuse marginal artery in a patient with stable ischemic heart disease.

Video 5.3: Angiogram showing a discrete moderate stenosis of the right coronary artery (RCA) before the take-off of the PDA in a patient with stable ischemic heart disease. Several posterolateral branches of the RCA are also visualized.

6. Acute Coronary Syndromes

Video 6.1: Angiogram obtained in a patient undergoing primary percutaneous coronary intervention of the right coronary artery for an inferior wall myocardial infarction. After the guidewire is passed, the shown angiogram demonstrates a large, complex, filling defect, which is due to thrombus formation that has resulted from plaque rupture.

Videos 6.2A to E: Primary percutaneous coronary intervention of an occluded mid left anterior descending (LAD) artery in a patient with acute anterior wall myocardial infarction. (A) Initial angiogram showing complete occlusion at the level of the mid LAD. (B) Guidewire passed across occlusion, resulting in some restoration of blood flow. A residual stenotic lesion is visible. (C) A coronary stent being positioned at the site of residual stenosis. (D) Inflation of the balloon and deployment of the coronary stent. (E) Post-stent deployment angiogram showing the treated stenosis and TIMI 3 flow throughout the coronary artery.

Videos 6.3 to 6.7: Examples of apical thrombi that developed in patients with transmural infarctions and apical akinesis.

7. Percutaneous Coronary Intervention

Videos 7.1A to D: Example of primary stenting in a patient with chronic stable angina. (A) Initial angiogram shows a moderate mid left anterior descending (LAD) stenosis. (B) Guide wire across the mid-LAD stenosis and a coronary stent positioned at the site of the stenosis. (C) Balloon inflation and stent deployment. (D) Post-stent deployment angiogram showing 0% residual stenosis.

Videos 7.2A to E: Primary percutaneous coronary interventions of an occluded mid left anterior descending (LAD) artery in a patient with acute anterior wall myocardial infarction. (A) Initial angiogram showing complete occlusion at the level of the mid LAD. (B) Guide wire passed across occlusion, resulting in some restoration of blood flow. A residual stenotic lesion is visible. (C) A coronary stent being positioned at the site of residual stenosis. (D) Inflation of the balloon and deployment of the coronary stent. (E) Post-stent deployment angiogram showing the treated stenosis and TIMI 3 flow throughout the coronary artery.

Videos 7.3A to G: Primary percutaneous coronary interventions of an occluded left circumflex artery. (A) Angiogram showing a subtotally occluded left circumflex artery with TIMI grade 1 flow. Contrast is visible just distal to the culprit lesion from a previous contrast injection. A late-filing large obtuse marginal (OM) branch is visible. (B) Guide wire passed across the lesion and balloon positioned at the site of subtotal occlusion. (C) Balloon inflation. (D) Post-balloon inflation angiogram showing some improvement in blood flow to TIMI grade 2 and a residual stenosis. (E) Positioning of a long coronary stent. (F) Deployment of the coronary stent. (G) Final coronary angiogram showing the treated culprit lesion and restoration of TIMI grade 3 blood flow.

8. Coronary Artery Bypass Graft Surgery

Video 8.1: Left internal mammary artery (LIMA) to left anterior descending (LAD).

Video 8.2: Saphenous vein graft (SVG) to obtuse marginal (OM) branch.

Video 8.3: Saphenous vein graft (SVG) to posterior descending artery (PDA).

Video 8.4: Saphenous vein graft (SVG) occluded.

SECTION 2

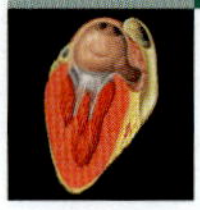

Valvular Heart Disease

9. Normal Valve Anatomy and Function

Video 9.1: Apical four chamber TTE showing a mitral valve with good coaptation.

Video 9.2: Parasternal short-axis showing a trileaflet aortic valve (center of image). The tricuspid valve is visible at the 9 O'clock position in the image. The pulmonic valve, which is usually not well visualized, is imaged at the 2 O'clock position.

Video 9.3: Parasternal long-axis TTE showing a normal aortic valve.

10. Aortic Stenosis

Videos 10.1 to 10.3: Parasternal long-axis transthoracic echocardiography (TTE) of heavily calcified and stenotic aortic valves. Note the markedly decreased excursion of the aortic valve leaflets during systole. Videos (Video courtesy of Glenn N Levine, MD).

Video 10.4: MRI of a stenotic bicuspid aortic valve. (Video courtesy of Scott D Flamm, MD).

11. Aortic Regurgitation

Video 11.1: Parasternal long axis echocardiographic image demonstrating severe AI (Video courtesy of Glenn N. Levine, MD).

Video 11.2: Color Doppler imaging in the parasternal long axis view showing mild AI due to a dilated aortic annulus (Video courtesy of Glenn N. Levine, MD).

Videos 11.3A and B: Severe aortic regurgitation due to a flail right aortic leaflet. (A) 2D video and (B) Corresponding color. Doppler video (Video courtesy of Glenn N. Levine, MD).

Video 11.4: Five-chamber view showing AI in a patient with heavily calcified aortic leaflets (Video courtesy of Glenn N. Levine, MD).

Video 11.5: MRI demonstrating aortic regurgitation in a patient with a dilated aortic annulus and proximal ascending aorta (Video courtesy of Scott D. Flamm, MD).

12. Mitral Stenosis and Percutaneous Mitral Valvotomy

Video 12.1: Parasternal long axis transthoracic echocardiography (TTE) showing mitral stenosis (MS) in a patient with rheumatic heart disease. The anterior mitral leaflet (AML) forms a "hockey stick" as it tries to open during ventricular diastole. Note also aortic stenosis is present in this patient. (Video courtesy of Levine GN, MD).

Video 12.2: Parasternal short axis transthoracic echocardiography (TTE) of a patient with mitral stenosis (MS). A "fish mouth" appearance of the stenotic mitral valve (MV) is present.

Video 12.3: Transesophageal echocardiography (TEE) of a patient showing mitral stenosis (MS).

13. Mitral Regurgitation

Video 13.1: Parasternal long axis transthoracic echocardiography (TTE) showing mild mitral regurgitation (MR) in a patient with myxomatous mitral leaflets.

Videos 13.2A and B: Transesophageal echocardiography (TEE) study showing (A) endocarditis of mitral valve and (B) resulting mitral regurgitation.

Video 13.3: Transesophageal echocardiography (TEE) showing endocarditis of the mitral valve and resulting regurgitation.

Video 13.4: Apical 4 chamber transthoracic echocardiography (TTE) showing severe, somewhat eccentric, mitral regurgitation (MR). Tethering of the posterior mitral leaflet is contributing to the MR.

Videos 13.5A and B: Transesophageal echocardiography (TEE) study showing (A) a restricted posterior mitral leaflet with (B) resulting mitral regurgitation.

Video 13.6: Mitral regurgitation due to mitral valve prolapse.

Video 13.7: Transesophageal echocardiography (TEE) showing mitral regurgitation due to a flail mitral leaflet.

Video 13.8: Transesophageal echocardiography (TEE) showing a flail A1 scallop with resulting mitral regurgitation (MR).

Video 13.9: Functional mitral regurgitation (MR) in a patient with dilated cardiomyopathy and a dilated mitral annulus.

14. Mitral Valve Prolapse

Video 14.1: Parasternal long-axis TTE showing mitral valve prolapse. During systole both the anterior and posterior mitral leaflets are seen prolapsing into the left atrium. Video courtesy of Glenn N. Levine, MD. (TTE: Transthoracic echocardiogram).

Video 14.2: Zoomed parasternal long-axis TTE demonstrating mitral valve prolapse (MVP). (TTE: Transthoracic echocardiogram).

Video 14.3: TEE showing mitral regurgitation in a patient with mitral valve prolapse. (TEE: Transesophageal echocardiography).

Video 14.4: Left ventriculography performed in the right anterior oblique projection with a straight pigtail catheter (end-systole) demonstrating prolapse of a posteromedial scallop (arrow).

Video 14.5: 2-Dimensional transesophageal echocardiography (TEE) of mitral valve prolapse demonstrating Barlow's disease with thickened leaflets and bileaflet prolapse

Video 14.6: 2-Dimensional transesophageal echocardiography (TEE) of mitral valve prolapse. Fibroelastic deficiency with thin leaflets and focal scallop prolapse (arrow).

Video 14.7: Real-time full volume (wide-angle) 3-dimensional transesophageal echocardiography of MVP.

Video 14.8: Real-time 3D zoom/live 3D (narrow-angle) 3-dimensional transesophageal echocardiography demonstrating a flail P2 leaflet with a ruptured chordae, typical of fibroelastic deficiency.

Video 14.9: Real-time full volume (wide-angle) 3-dimensional transesophageal echocardiography utilizing a simultaneous display of a multiplanar reformat in orthogonal planes and a 3D volume rendering of the region of interest (flail P2 scallop).

Video 14.10: Real-time 3D zoom/live 3D (narrow-angle) 3-dimensional transesophageal echocardiography demonstrating multi-scallop prolapse A1, P1 and P2 shown in from a left atrial view.

Video 14.11: Intraoperative video. Totally endoscopic robotic repair of the mitral valve. Following resection of the prolapsing P2 leaflet, the mitral valve has been sutured. Suturing of the annuloplasty ring prosthesis with the robotic arms is underway.

15. Right-Sided Valvular Heart Disease

Video 15.1: Non-standard RV inflow view demonstrating severe tricuspid regurgitation in the patient pictured in Fig. 15.7.

Video 15.2: Additional non-standard RV inflow view demonstrating severe tricuspid regurgitation.

Video 15.3: 4-chamber view similar to Fig 15.7B demonstrating severe tricuspid regurgitation. In severe tricuspid regurgitation, the rapid normalization of pressures between the right atrium and right ventricle results in a dense, triangular jet as seen in Fig. 15.14 (red arrows).

16. Endocarditis

Video 1: Parasternal long axis TTE showing small vegetations on the aortic valve. Video courtesy of Glenn N. Levine, MD.

Video 2: Transesophageal echocardiography (TEE) videoclip showing complex vegetation on the posterior mitral leaflet. Video courtesy of Alvin Blaustein, MD.

Video 3: Transesophageal echocardiography (TEE) videoclip showing complex vegetation on the mitral valve in a patient with endocarditis. Video courtesy of Alvin Blaustein, MD.

Video 4: TEE videoclip of large, highly mobile vegetation on a prosthetic mitral valve.

Video 5: TEE showing a mobile vegetation on a prosthetic mitral valve in a patient with endocarditis. Video courtesy of Alvin Blaustein, MD.

Video 6: TEE showing a complex and highly mobile vegetation on a prosthetic mitral valve in a patient with endocarditis. Video courtesy of Alvin Blaustein, MD.

Video 7: Large, complex vegetation on a prosthetic mitral valve in a patient with blood-culture documented endocarditis.

Video 8: Color Doppler TEE showing mitral regurgitation as a result of mitral valve endocarditis and valve destruction. Video courtesy of Alvin Blaustein, MD.

17. Transcatheter Aortic Valve Replacement

Video 17.1: Animation of transfemoral transcatheter aortic valve replacement with the Edwards Sapian valve. (Video courtesy of Edwards Lifesciences).

Video 17.2: Fluoroscopy of deployment of a Edwards Sapien valve. (Video courtesy of Edwards Lifesciences).

Video 17.3: Animation of apical transcatheter aortic valve replacement with the Edwards Sapian valve. (Video courtesy of Edwards Lifesciences).

18. Valve Surgery and Prosthetic Heart Valves

Video 18.1: TEE video of a prosthetic aortic valve showing valve dehiscence, visible most prominently from 1 o'clock to 3 o'clock. The sutures are visualized.

Video 18.2: Color Doppler TEE video corresponding to Video 18.1, showing that the valve dehiscence has led to significant paravalvular leak.

SECTION 3

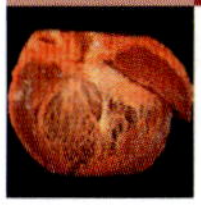

Heart Failure and Cardiomyopathy

20. Systolic Heart Failure and Dilated Cardiomyopathy

Videos 20.1 to 20.3: Representative magnetic resonance imaging (MRI) video clips of left ventricular (LV) noncompaction. (Videos courtesy of Flamm SD, MD).

Video 20.4: Example of noncompaction demonstrated on four chamber magnetic resonance imaging (MRI).

Video 20.5: Example of noncompaction demonstrated on shortaxis magnetic resonance imaging (MRI).

21. Heart Failure with Preserved Ejection Fraction

Video 21.1: Apical 4-chamber transthoracic echocardiography (TTE) showing moderate tricuspid regurgitation.

Video 21.2: Apical 4-chamber transthoracic echocardiography (TTE) showing moderate mitral regurgitation.

Video 21.3: 3-chamber transthoracic echocardiography (TTE) showing moderate aortic insufficiency.

Video 21.4: Short-axis transthoracic echocardiography (TTE) showing prominent "septal bounce" in constrictive pericarditis.

Video 21.5: Apical 4-chamber transthoracic echocardiography (TTE) showing prominent "septal bounce" in constrictive pericarditis.

Video 21.6: MRI of a patient with systemic sclerosis with pericardial effusion and constriction causing heart failure with preserved ejection fraction. The video shows a smallto- moderate sized pericardial effusion, which is resulting in decreased cardiac chamber compliance and ventricular interdependence. There is interventricular septal flattening with inversion of the septum into the left ventricle (LV) during peak inspiration.

Video 21.7: Apical 4-chamber transthoracic echocardiography (TTE) showing small, thickened left ventricle (LV) and right ventricle (RV) with biatrial enlargement in a patient with restrictive cardiomyopathy.

Videos 21.8 to 21.10: Parasternal long-axis (Fig. 21.8), shortaxis (Fig. 21.9) and apical 4-chamber (Fig. 21.10) transthoracic echocardiography (TTE) images of a patient with infiltrative cardiomyopathy. The findings of abnormal myocardia texture and thickened left ventricle (LV) and right ventricle (RV) with biatrial enlargement raise the possibility of infiltrative cardiomyopathy from amyloidosis.

22. Hypertrophic Cardiomyopathy

Video 22.1: Parasternal long-axis TTE showing septal hypertrophy in a patient with HCM. (Video courtesy of Glenn N. Levine, MD).

Video 22.2: Apical 4-chamber TTE of a patient with marked septal hypertrophy and HCM.

Video 22.3: Parasternal long axis transthoracic echocardiography video clip of a patient with HCM showing thickening of the interventricular septum.

Video 22.4: MRI displayed in the 4-chamber view showing apical hypertrophic cardiomyopathy. (Video courtesy of Scott D. Flamm, MD).

Video 22.5: MRI displayed in the 2-chamber view showing apical hypertrophic cardiomyopathy. (Video courtesy of Scott D. Flamm, MD).

Video 22.6: Apical 4-chamber TTE from a patient with apical HCM. (Video courtesy of Glenn N. Levine, MD).

Video 22.7: Apical 2-chamber TTE from a patient with apical HCM. (Video courtesy of Glenn N. Levine, MD).

Videos 22.8A and B: Apical 4-chamber TTE images of a patient with septal hypertrophy and HCM. (A) 2D video shows systolic anterior motion (SAM) of the anterior mitral leaflet during systole. (B) Corresponding color Doppler video clip shows the resulting mitral regurgitation.

Videos 22.9A and B: Parasternal long-axis TTE images showing modest SAM and resulting mitral regurgitation in a patient with HCM and dynamic outflow obstruction. Note also the turbulent blood flow in the left ventricular outflow tract.

Video 22.10: Three-chamber TTE in a patient with HCM demonstrating SAM and resulting severe eccentric MR during Valsalva maneuver. (Video courtesy of Glenn N. Levine, MD).

24. Arrhythmogenic Right Ventricular Cardiomyopathy

Video 24.1: MRI of a patient with arrhythmogenic right ventricular dysplasia demonstrating a dilated right ventricle with markedly depressed systolic function. (Video courtesy of Scott D Flamm, MD).

SECTION 4

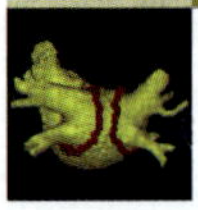

Arrhythmias

29. Atrial Fibrillation

Video 29.1: Transesophageal echocardiography (TEE) video clip showing thrombus in the left atrial appendage.

SECTION 5

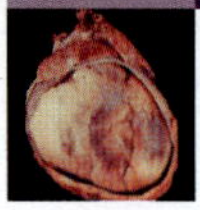

Pericardial Disease

36. Pericarditis

Video 36.1: Parasternal long-axis transthoracic echocardiography (TTE) demonstrating a circumferential pericardial effusion in a patient with pericarditis.

Video 36.2: Pericardial effusion imaged in the parasternal long axis view in a patient with suspected pericarditis.

Video 36.3: Apical 4-chamber transthoracic echocardiography (TTE) in a patient with pericarditis demonstrating a circumferential pericardial effusion.

37. Pericardial Effusion

Video 37.1: Parasternal long-axis TTE demonstrating a large circumferential pericardial effusion.

Video 37.2: Circumferential effusion imaged in the parasternal long-axis view.

Video 37.3: Parasternal long-axis transthoracic echocardiogram videoclip showing pericardial effusion with RV collapse.

Video 37.4: Apical 4-chamber TTE showing pericardial effusion with some inversion and compression of the right atrium.

SECTION 6

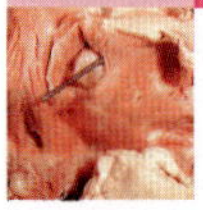

Congenital Heart Disease

39. Patent Foramen Ovale

Video 39.1: Transesophageal echocardiogram (TEE) showing a patent foramen ovale (PFO) with intermittent right to left flow during an agitated saline ("bubble") study. (Video clip courtesy of Glenn N Levine, MD).

Video 39.2: Color Doppler transesophageal echocardiogram (TEE) demonstrating a patent foramen ovale (PFO).

Video 39.3: Color Doppler transesophageal echocardiogram (TEE) showing a patent foramen ovale (PFO) with intermittent left-right flow (intermittent thin blue jet). (Video clip courtesy of Glenn N Levine, MD).

40. Atrial Septal Defects

Video 40.1: Apical four-chamber TTE showing a large secundum ASD. Note that the right atrium and right ventricle are both dilated. Video courtesy of Glenn N. Levine, MD.

Video 40.2: Color Doppler apical four-chamber TTE corresponding to video 40.1, showing left to right flow across a large secundum ASD. Note that the right atrium and right ventricle are dilated, and some tricuspid regurgitation is also present. Video courtesy of Glenn N. Levine, MD.

Video 40.3: Zoomed video of videos 40.1 and 40.2, showing a large secundum ASD with left to right flow. Video courtesy of Glenn N. Levine, MD.

Video 40.4: Subcostal view TTE showing a small restrictive ASD with relatively high velocity left to right flow. Video courtesy of Glenn N. Levine, MD.

41. Ventricular Septal Defect

Videos 41.1 and 41.2: Magnetic resonance imaging (MRI) video clips demonstrating a ventricular septal defect (VSD) with flow from the left ventricle (LV) to the right ventricle (RV). (Videoclips courtesy of Scott D Flamm, MD).

Video 41.3: Five-chamber transthoracic echocardiography (TTE) demonstrating a perimembranous ventricular septal defect (VSD) with flow from the left ventricle (LV) to the right ventricle (RV). (Video courtesy of Glenn N Levine, MD).

Video 41.4: Short-axis transthoracic echocardiography (TTE) demonstrating a perimembranous ventricular septal defect (VSD). (Video courtesy of Glenn N Levine, MD).

42. Ebstein Anomaly

Video 42.1: MRI in the 4-chamber projection demonstrating Ebstein anomoly.

43. Tetralogy of Fallot

Video 43.1: Severe pulmonary regurgitation in a patient with repaired Tetralogy of Fallot (TOF). Blue coloration demonstrates forward flow toward the branch pulmonary arteries and red flow demonstrates regurgitation toward the right ventricle (RV).

46. Aortic Coarctation

Video 46.1: CT demonstrating aortic coarctation. (Video courtesy of Scott D Flamm).

SECTION 7

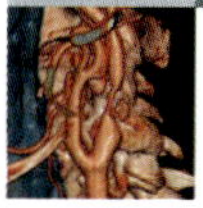

Peripheral Vascular Disease

49. Carotid Artery Disease

Video 49.1: Three-dimensional (3D) computed tomography (CT) reconstruction of the carotid arteries.

51. Aortic Dissection

Video 51.1: Echocardiography videoclip illustrating a dissection flap in a patient with aortic dissection. Color Doppler shows flow only in what in this case is the true lumen.

Video 51.2: Transthoracic echocardiogram demonstrating a dilated aortic root and ascending aorta and acute type A aortic dissection. There is malcoaptation of the aortic valve leaflets due to aortic root and annular dilatation. The intimal flap prolapses across the aortic valve.

Video 51.3: Transthoracic echocardiogram of acute type A aortic dissection with severe aortic regurgitation. Multiple mechanisms are present contributing to aortic regurgitation including dilatation of the aortic root; loss of commissural support of the valve leaflets and intimal flap prolapse across the aortic valve.

Video 51.4: Transesophageal echocardiogram of an acute type B aortic dissection. The mobile intimal flap separates the true lumen (at the top of the image) from the larger false lumen (at the bottom on the image).

SECTION 8

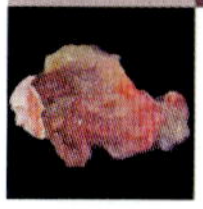

Miscellaneous Cardiovascular Disease

54. Cardiac Tumors

Video 54.1: Magnetic resonance imaging (MRI) demonstrating a left atrial myxoma. (Video courtesy of Scott D Flamm, MD).

57. Stroke

Video 57.1: Transesophageal echocardiogram showing thrombus in the left atrial appendage of a patient with atrial fibrillation and recent stroke. (Videos courtesy of Glenn N Levine).

Videos 57.2 to 57.7: Transthoracic echocardiography videos demonstrating left ventricular apical thrombi in patients with an akinetic apex. (Videos courtesy of Glenn N Levine).

Video 57.8: Transthoracic echocardiography showing vegetations on the posterior mitral leaflet.

Video 57.9: Transthoracic echocardiography showing vegetations on a prosthetic mitral valve.

Video 57.10: Transthoracic echocardiography showing mobile vegetations on a prosthetic mitral valve. (Video courtesy of Glenn N Levine).

Video 57.11: Cardiac MRI showing a left atrial myxoma. (Video courtesy of Scott D Flamm).

Video 57.12: Transthoracic echocardiography showing a patent foramen ovale with intermittent right to left flow during an agitated saline ("bubble") study.

Video 57.13: Color Doppler transthoracic echocardiography demonstrating a patent foramen ovale.

Video 57.14: Transthoracic echocardiography study showing mobile atheroma in the aortic arch. (Video courtesy of Glenn N Levine).

58. Venous Thromboembolism

Videos 58.1 and 58.2: Parasternal short-axis TTE imaging showing a thrombus present in the distal main and proximal right pulmonary artery. (Videos courtesy of Glenn N Levine, MD).

Section 1

Coronary Artery Disease

Chapters

CHAPTER 1

Normal Coronary and Venous Anatomy

Melvin D Cheitlin, Glenn N Levine, Philip C Ursell

INTRODUCTION AND HISTORICAL PERSPECTIVE

The circulatory system and coronary anatomy were described and illustrated many centuries ago (Figs. 1.1 and 1.2). For centuries though, the course, position and variations of the coronary arterial system were of interest only to anatomists and pathologists and of no interest to clinicians. However, with the development of coronary angiography, coronary bypass surgery, and more recently percutaneous coronary intervention, knowledge of the details of coronary arterial anatomy has become essential.

The anatomy of the coronary sinus and venous system is important in retrograde myocardial perfusion in patients who undergo cardiopulmonary bypass, during the placement of a left ventricular pacing wire in patients treated with cardiac resynchronization therapy (CRT), and in some patients undergoing radiofrequency catheter ablation for the treatment of cardiac arrhythmias.

Although coronary arteriography has been the "gold standard" for visualizing the coronary arteries, the development of noninvasive imaging with computed tomography (CT), coronary angiography (Figs. 1.3 and 1.4) and magnetic resonance imaging (MRI) (Figs. 1.5A and B) has markedly improved our ability to define the exact origin and course of the coronary arteries as they spread out across the surface of the heart. Another advance in coronary artery imaging is intravascular ultrasound (IVUS), which allows for visualizing the details of the coronary artery lumen and walls (Figs. 1.6A and B).

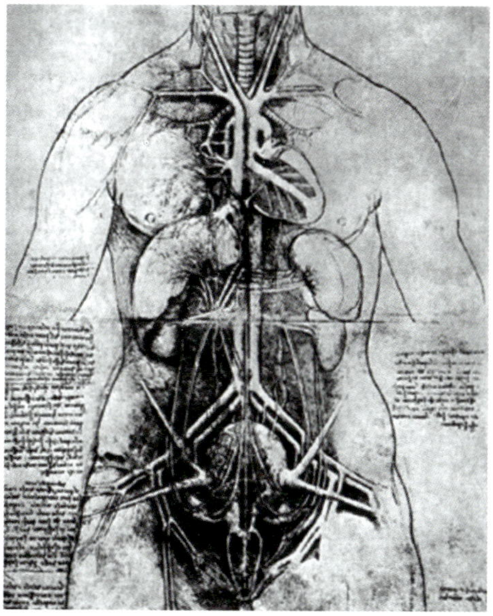

Fig. 1.1: Purported first drawing of the circulatory system by Leonardo da Vinci. (Image from Bansal M, Mehrotra R, Kasliwal RR. The history of acute coronary syndrome. In: Chopra HK, Nanda NC (Eds). Textbook of Cardiology (A Clinical & Historical Perspective). New Delhi, India: Jaypee Brothers Medical Publishers (P) Ltd. 2013).

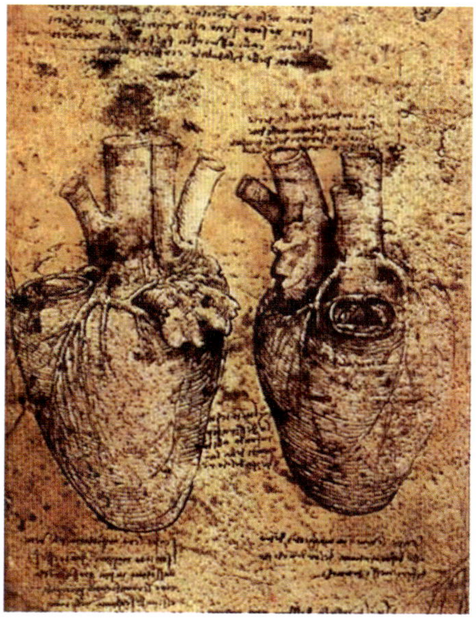

Fig. 1.2: Drawing of the heart and blood vessels by Leonardo da Vinci. (Image from Wikimedia public domain work. Available from http://commons.wikimedia.org/wiki/File:Heart_and_blood_vessels_by_da_Vinci.jpg).

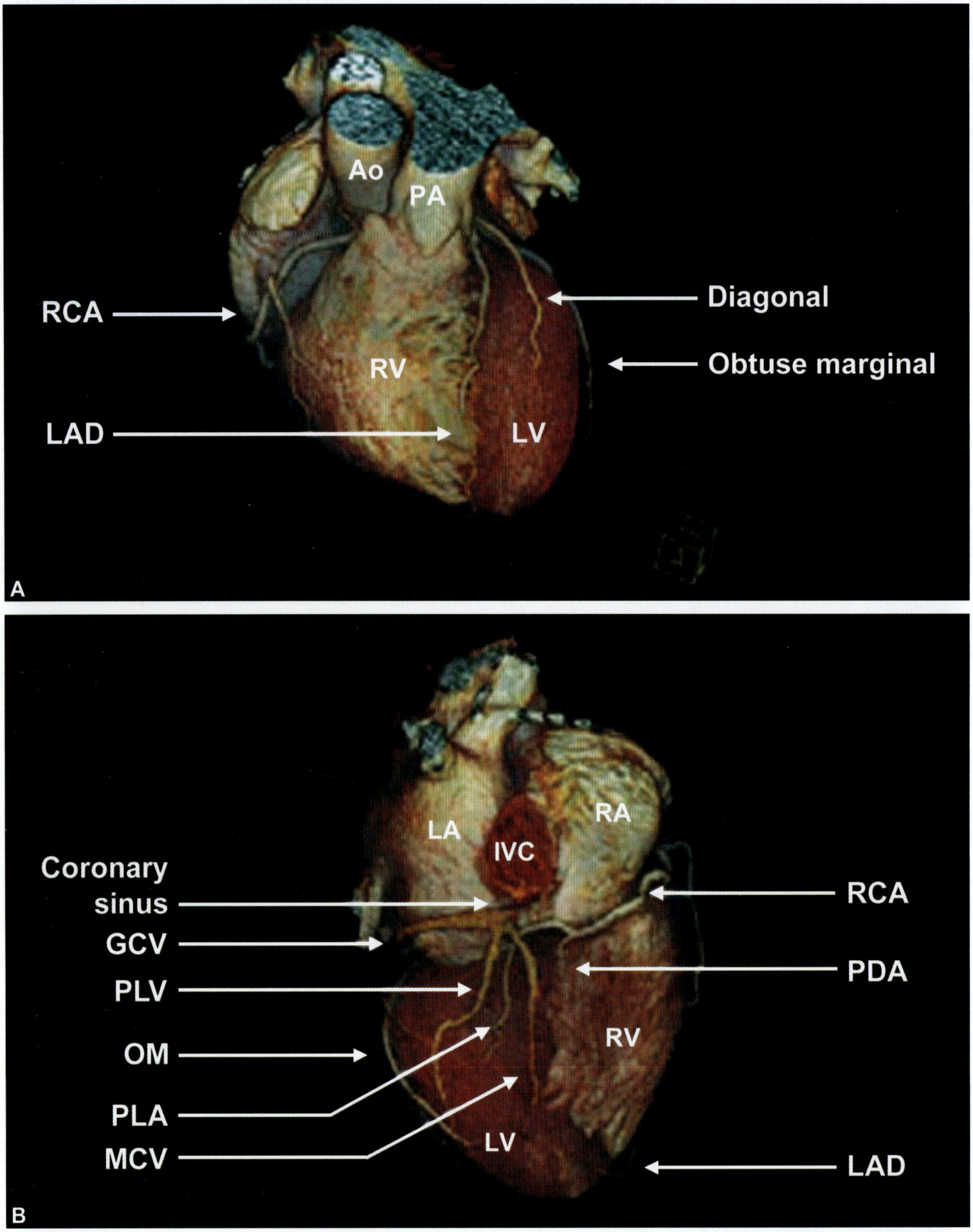

Figs. 1.3A and B: Three-dimensional volume-rendered CT coronary angiography images of the coronary anatomy. (A) Anterior view of the heart. (B) Posterior view of the heart. (Image reproduced with permission from Okere CI, Sigurdsson G. Cardiac computed tomography. In: Chatterjee K, Anderson M, Heistad D, Kerber RE (Eds). Cardiology—An Illustrated Textbook. New Delhi, India: Jaypee Brothers Medical Publishers (P) Ltd. 2012). (Ao: Aorta; PA: Pulmonary artery; GCV: Great cardiac vein; IVC: Inferior vena cava; LA: Left atrium; LV: Left ventricle; RA: Right atrium; RV: Right ventricle; LAD: Left anterior descending artery; MCV: Middle cardiac vein; OM: Obtuse marginal coronary artery; PDA: Posterior descending artery; PLV: Posterolateral vein; PLA: Posterolateral artery; RCA: Right coronary artery).

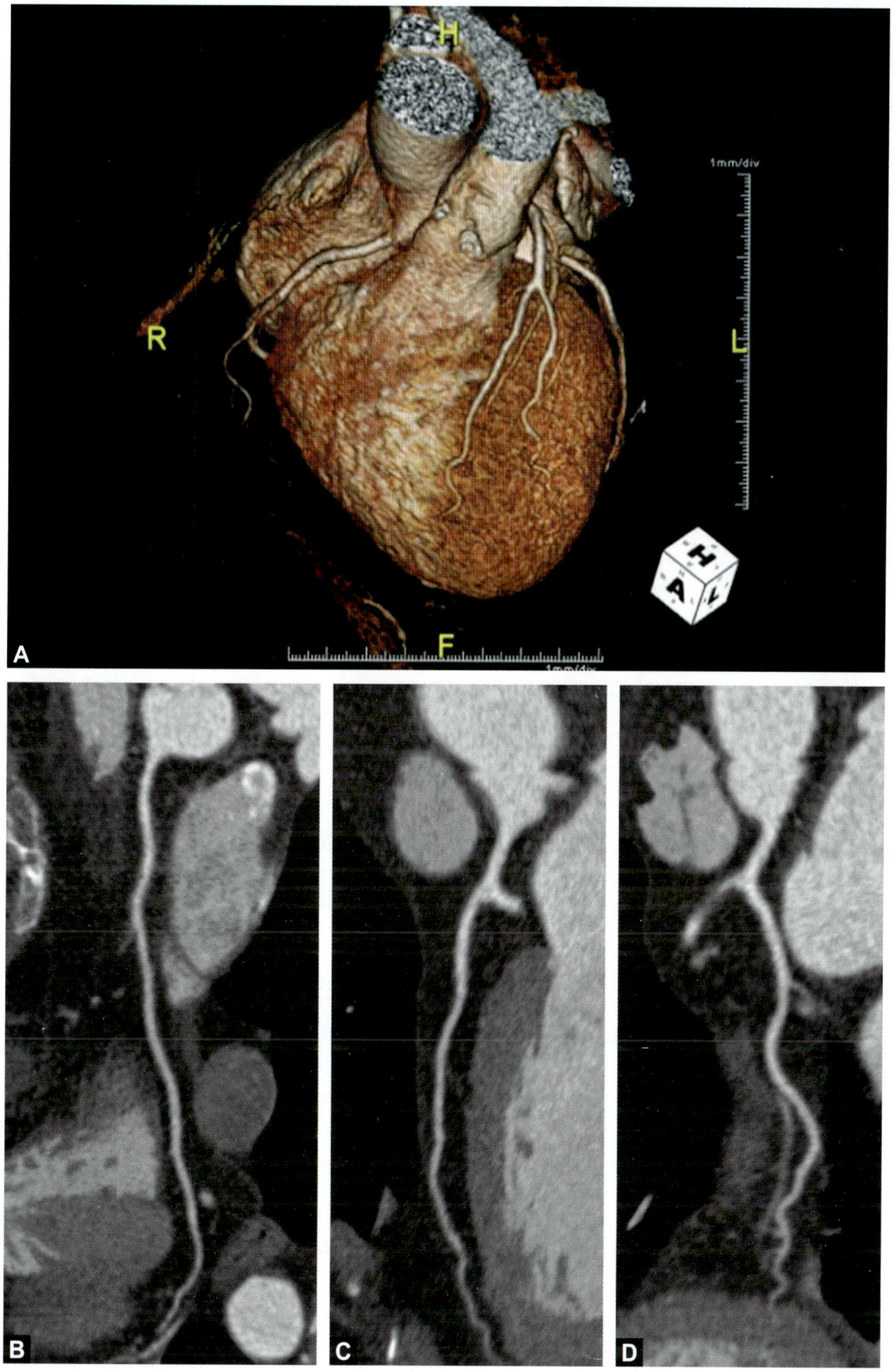

Figs. 1.4A to D: Computed tomography coronary angiography demonstrating normal coronary anatomy. (A) 3D volume-rendered reconstruction of heart and coronary arteries. (B) Right coronary artery. (C) Left anterior descending coronary artery. (D) Left circumflex artery. (Image from Pelgrim GJ, Oudkerk M, Vliegenthart R. Computed tomography imaging of the coronary arteries. In: Baskot BG (Ed). What Should We Know About Prevented, Diagnostic, and Interventional Therapy in Coronary Artery Disease. InTech; 2013, with permission. Available from http://www.intechopen.com/books/what-should-we-know-about-prevented-diagnostic-and-interventional-therapy-in-coronary-artery-disease).

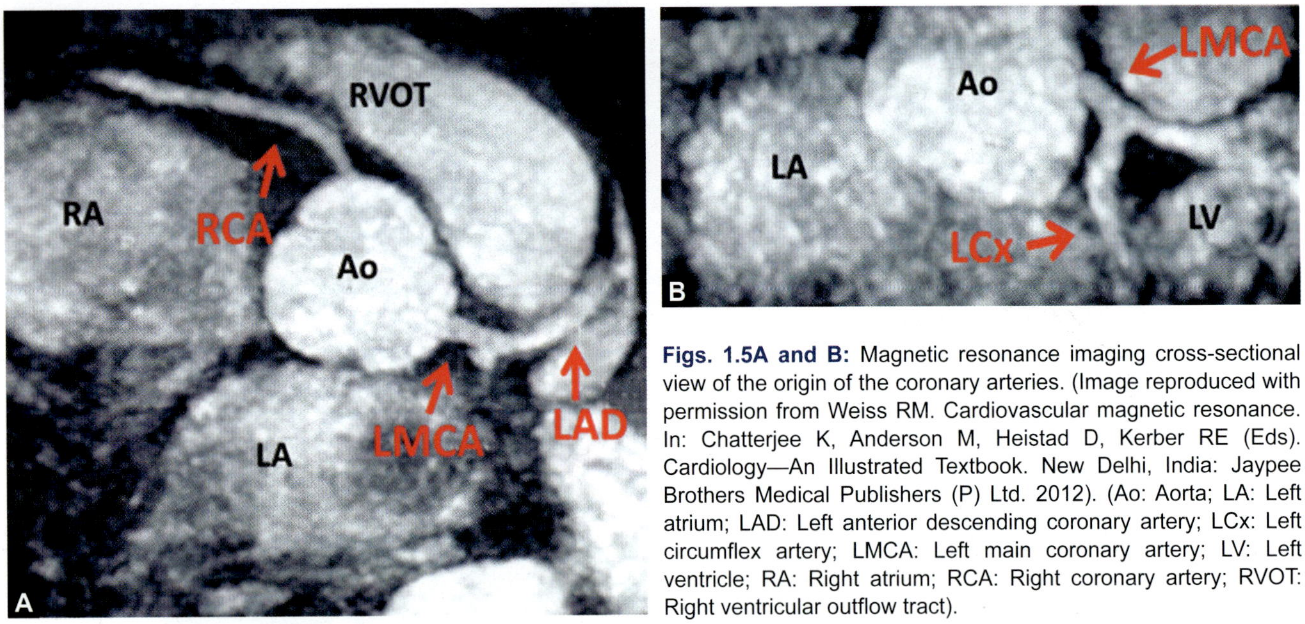

Figs. 1.5A and B: Magnetic resonance imaging cross-sectional view of the origin of the coronary arteries. (Image reproduced with permission from Weiss RM. Cardiovascular magnetic resonance. In: Chatterjee K, Anderson M, Heistad D, Kerber RE (Eds). Cardiology—An Illustrated Textbook. New Delhi, India: Jaypee Brothers Medical Publishers (P) Ltd. 2012). (Ao: Aorta; LA: Left atrium; LAD: Left anterior descending coronary artery; LCx: Left circumflex artery; LMCA: Left main coronary artery; LV: Left ventricle; RA: Right atrium; RCA: Right coronary artery; RVOT: Right ventricular outflow tract).

The coronary arteries arise as the first branches off the aorta and provide the blood supply to the heart (Figs. 1.7 and 1.8 Video 1.1). The descriptions of the course of the coronary arteries and veins over the epicardial surface of the heart (extramural vessels) in this chapter apply to the majority of normal hearts. The coronary arteries that penetrate the myocardium are called intramural vessels, and unlike the extramural coronary arteries, do not become atherosclerotic. In adults, the extramural coronaries are frequently encased in epicardial fat. At times, varying lengths of myocardium called "myocardial bridges" cover portions of the extramural arteries (Figs. 1.9A to F). There are reports that these muscle-encased segments of extramural coronary artery can have clinical significance in that the vessel can be severely compressed during systole, causing myocardial ischemia or even infarction. The regions of the myocardium perfused by the major coronary arteries are illustrated in Figure 1.10.

LEFT MAIN CORONARY ARTERY

The left main coronary artery arises from the left sinus of Valsalva (Figs. 1.11 and 1.12) and passes leftward, posterior to the right ventricular outflow tract and anterior to the left atrial appendage, before bifurcating into the left anterior descending (LAD) and left circumflex coronary arteries. The subjacent position of these arteries to the left atrial appendage is important to electrophysiologists when performing ablations for arrhythmias. The length of the left main coronary artery varies between 0.5 and 2.5 cm. The location of the ostium of the left coronary artery with respect to the sinotubular junction is 48% of the time at the same level; 34% above the sinotubular junction; and 18% below the sinotubular junction. The left main coronary artery is absent in 0.5–1.0% of hearts. The left main coronary artery bifurcates into the LAD and left circumflex artery in approximately two-thirds of patients. In approximately one-third of patients the left main trifurcates and there is a third branch, called the ramus intermedius artery (Fig. 1.13), which supplies the anterolateral left ventricular wall.

LEFT ANTERIOR DESCENDING CORONARY ARTERY (ANTERIOR INTERVENTRICULAR ARTERY)

The LAD artery arises from the left main coronary artery as a direct continuation and passes in the anterior descending interventricular groove distally toward the apex (Figs. 1.14 and 1.15, Video 1.2). It terminates before or at

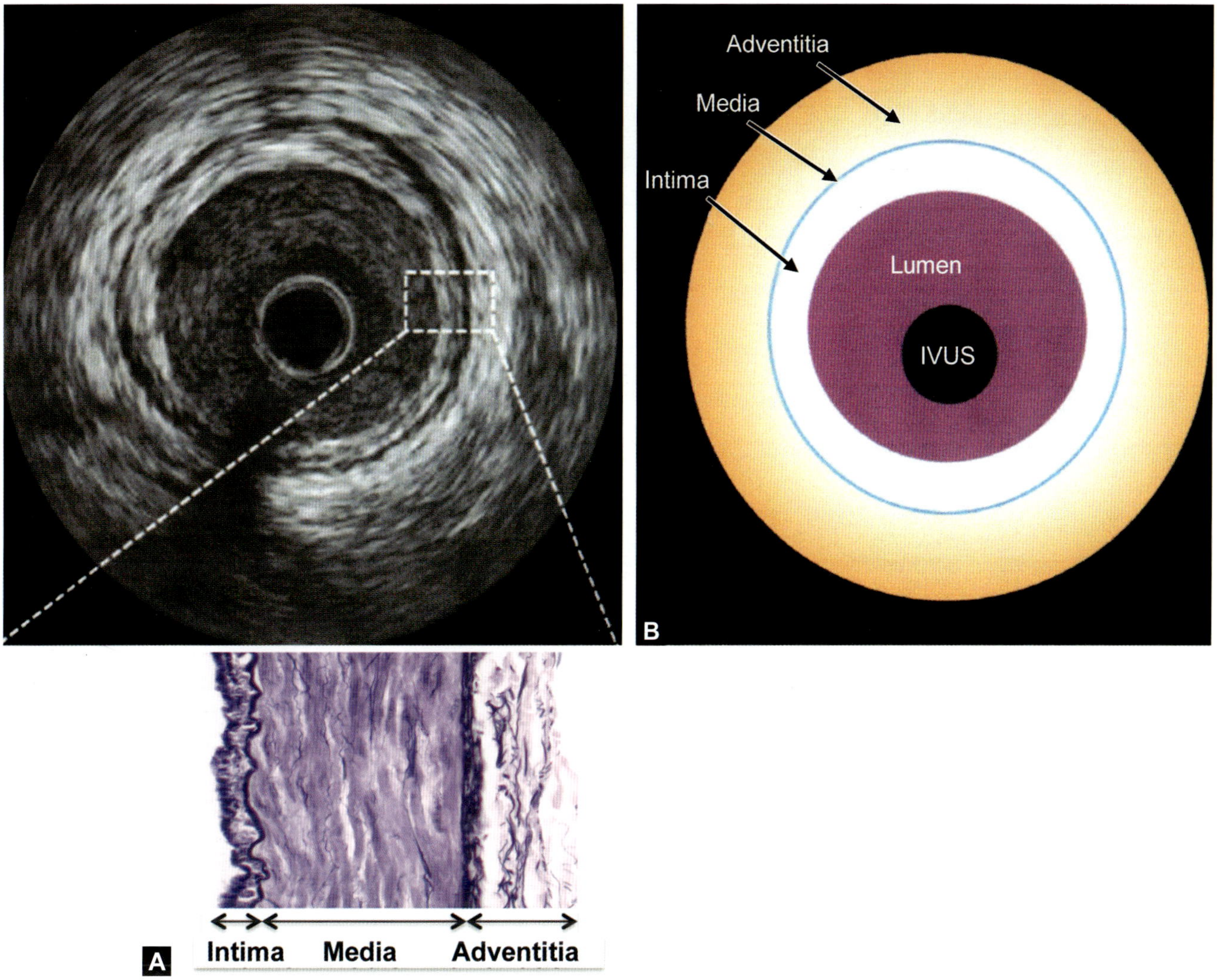

Figs. 1.6A and B: Cross sectional format of a representative coronary intravascular ultrasound (IVUS) image. IVUS is the imaging catheter in the coronary lumen. Histological section with elastic stain shows correlation with intima, media, and adventitia. The media has a lower ultrasound reflectance owing to less collagen and elastin than neighboring layers. Since the intima reflects ultrasound more strongly than the media, there is spillover in the image resulting in slight overestimation of intimal thickness and underestimation of medial thickness. (Adapted with permission from Kume T, Honda Y, Fitzgerald PJ. Intravascular coronary ultrasound and beyond. In: Chatterjee K, Anderson M, Heistad D, Kerber RE (Eds). Cardiology—An Illustrated Textbook. New Delhi, India: Jaypee Brothers Medical Publishers (P) Ltd. 2012, adapted from Figures 3A and B with permission).

the apex in 35% of hearts, and continues around the apex to the inferior interventricular groove of the heart ("wrap around LAD") in 64% of hearts. It has a variable number of secondary branches to the right and left ventricles adjacent to the artery. The right ventricular branches are usually small and not constant in arrangement. Those to the left ventricle are termed diagonal branches. These branches supply the anterolateral wall and the anterior papillary muscle of the left ventricle. Occasionally, shortly after its origin, the LAD divides into two equal parallel vessels that pass in the anterior interventricular groove distally (referred to as a "dual LAD").

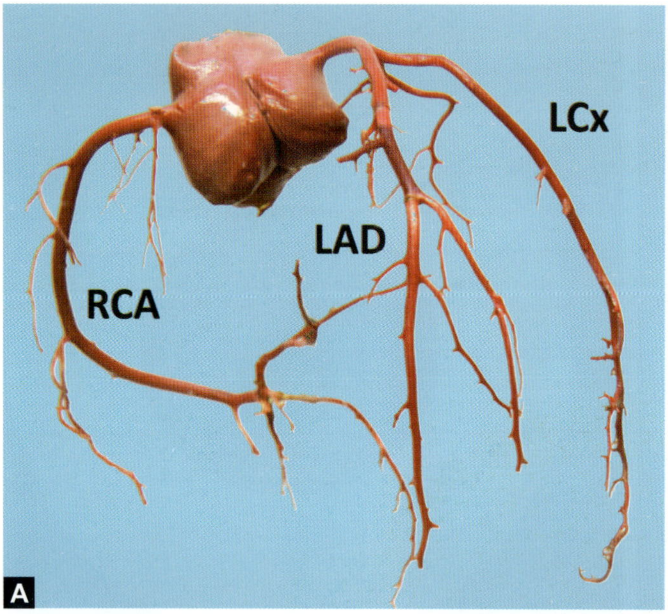

Fig. 1.7A: Three-dimensional image of the coronary arteries. The coronary arteries arise as the first branches off the aorta and provide the blood supply to the heart. (Courtesy of CanStockphoto, Canada).

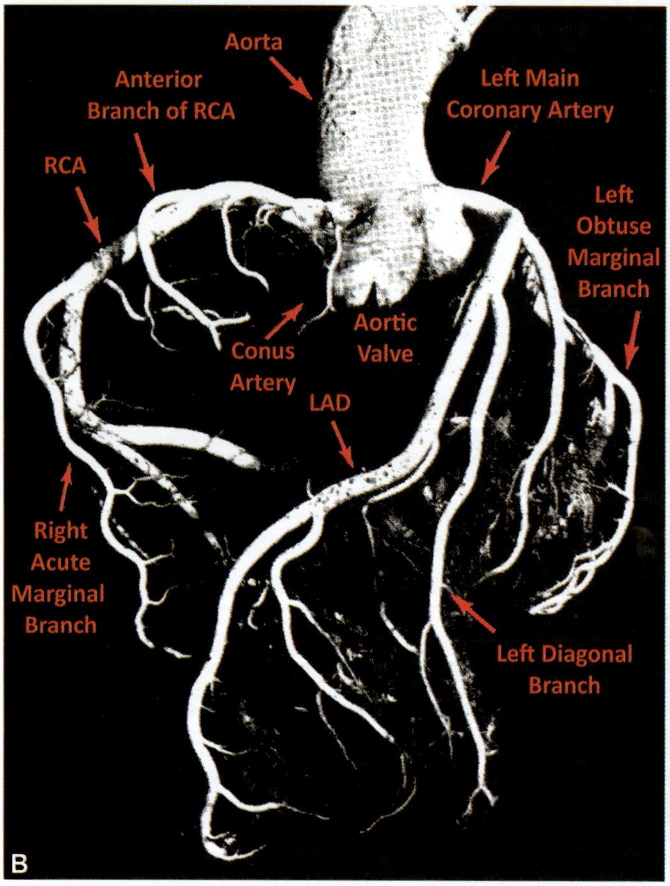

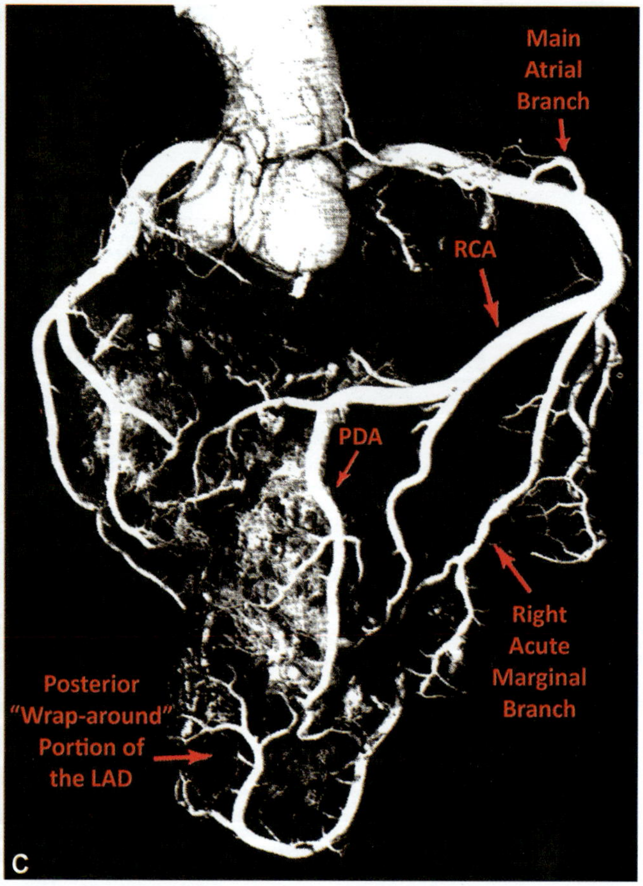

Figs. 1.7B and C: Plaster cast of extramural coronary arteries, (B) anterior view and (C) posterior surface of the heart. (Image modified with permission from Baroldi G, Scomazzoni G. Coronary Circulation in the Normal and the Pathologic Heart. Washington DC: Armed Forces Institute of Pathology, Office of the Surgeon General, Department of the Army; 1965. Part 1, P. 5). (RCA: Right coronary artery; LAD: Left anterior descending artery; PDA: Posterior descending artery; LCx: Left circumflex artery).

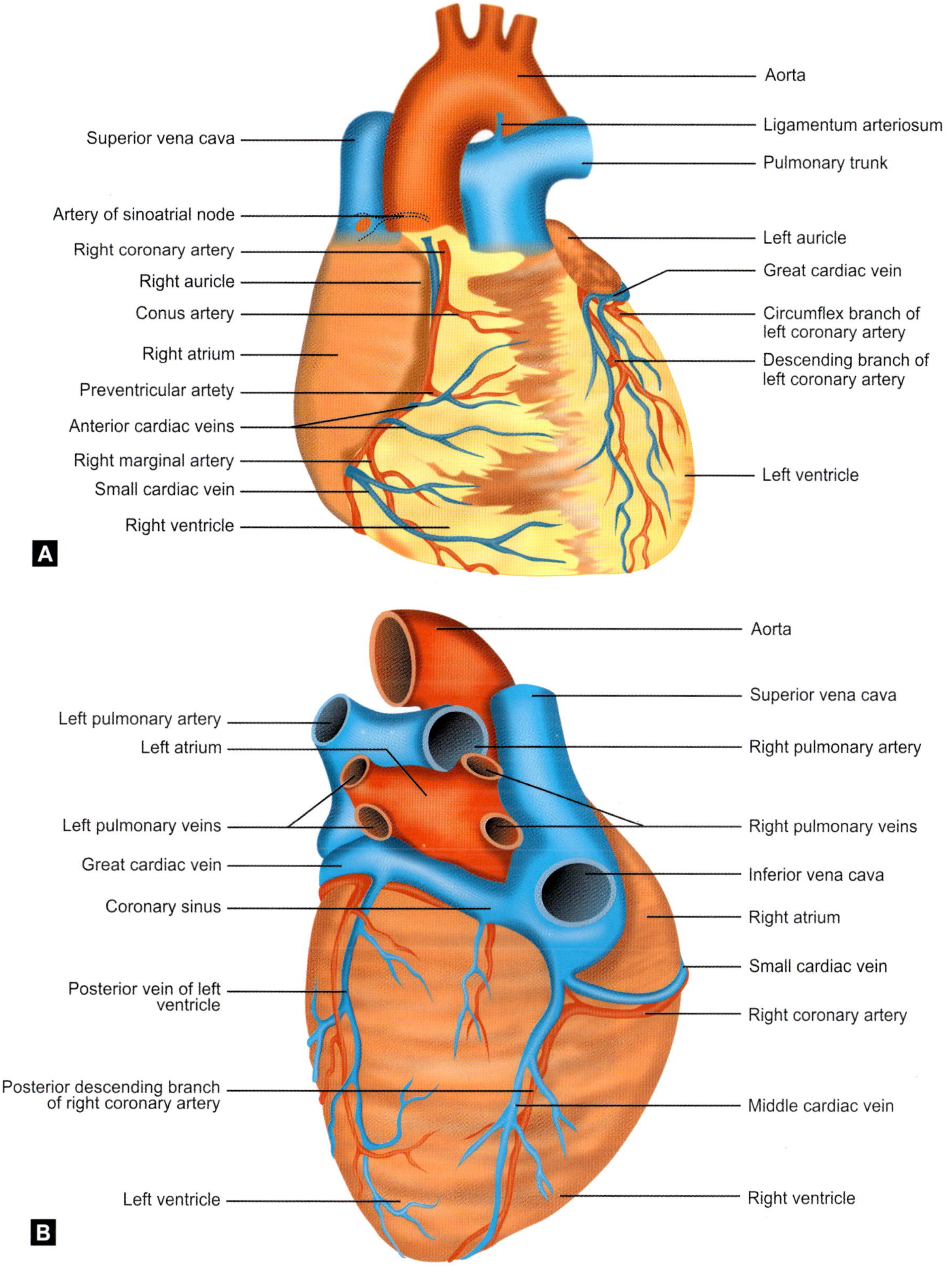

Figs. 1.8A and B: (A) Ventral surface of the heart showing coronary veins and arteries. (B) Dorsocaudal surface of the heart showing coronary veins and arteries. (Image with permission from Cheitlin MD, Ursell PC. Cardiac anatomy. In: Chatterjee K, Anderson M, Heistad D, Kerber RE (Eds). Cardiology—An Illustrated Textbook. New Delhi, India: Jaypee Brothers Medical Publishers (P) Ltd. 2012) Image reproduced with permission from Charles C Thomas Publisher LTD, Springfield Ill.

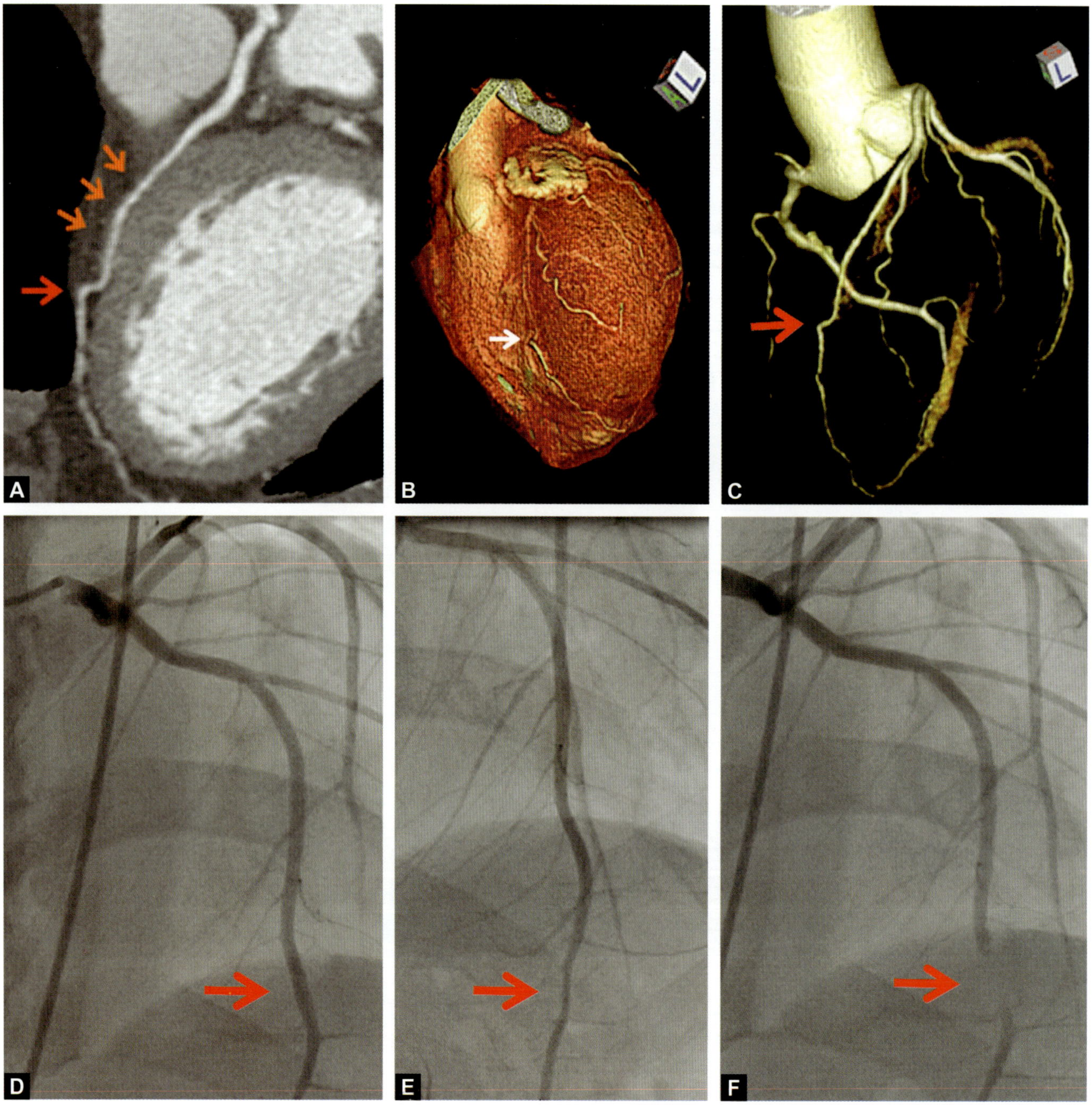

Figs. 1.9A to F: Myocardial bridge involving the mid left anterior descending (LAD) artery demonstrated by CT coronary angiography. (A) Maximum intensity projection (MIP) CT coronary angiogram demonstrating myocardial bridging over the mid LAD (orange arrows). The area where the artery emerges from the myocardium and becomes epicardial is shown with the red arrow. (B) Volume-rendered image of the heart. The point where the LAD becomes epicardial is denoted by the white arrow. (C) 3D reconstruction of the coronary arteries. A clear "step up" of the LAD is visible (red arrow), corresponding to where the LAD becomes epicardial. (Images from Bamoshmoosh M, Marraccini P. Myocardial bridges in the era of non-invasive angiography. In: Baskot BG (Ed). What Should We Know About Prevented, Diagnostic, and Interventional Therapy in Coronary Artery Disease. InTech; 2013, with permission. Available from http://www.intechopen.com/books/what-should-we-know-about-prevented-diagnostic-and-interventional-therapy-in-coronary-artery-disease). (D to F) Still images from a coronary angiogram demonstrating an area of bridging in the distal LAD. In diastole (figure D), the coronary artery at the area where a myocardial bridge exists does not appear to be narrowed. In early systole (figure E), there is clear compression and narrowing of the artery. In later systole (figure F), the artery appears to be completely compressed.

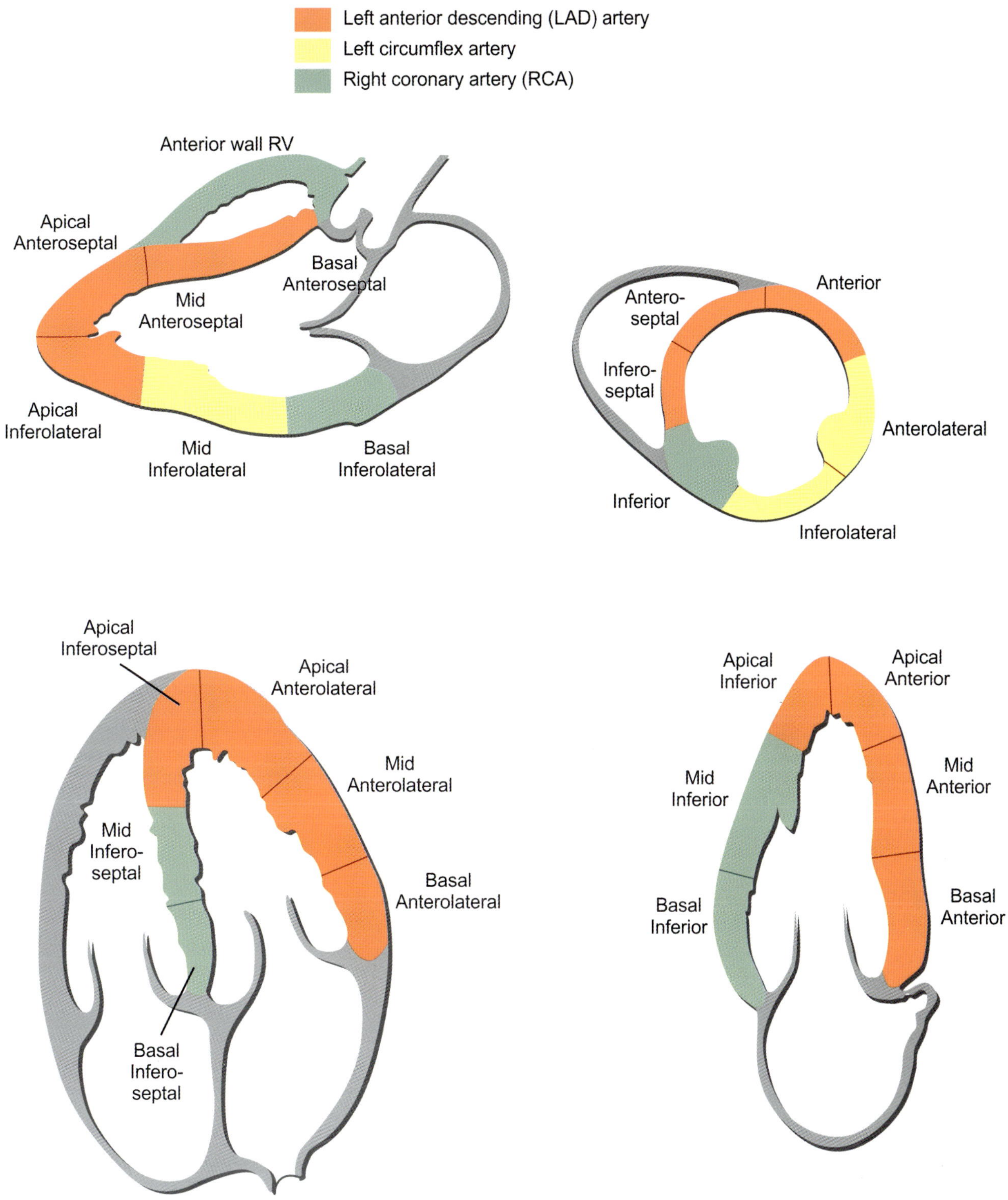

Fig. 1.10: Illustration of the usual regions of the heart perfused by each of the major coronary arteries. (Composite image courtesy of Glenn N Levine, MD).

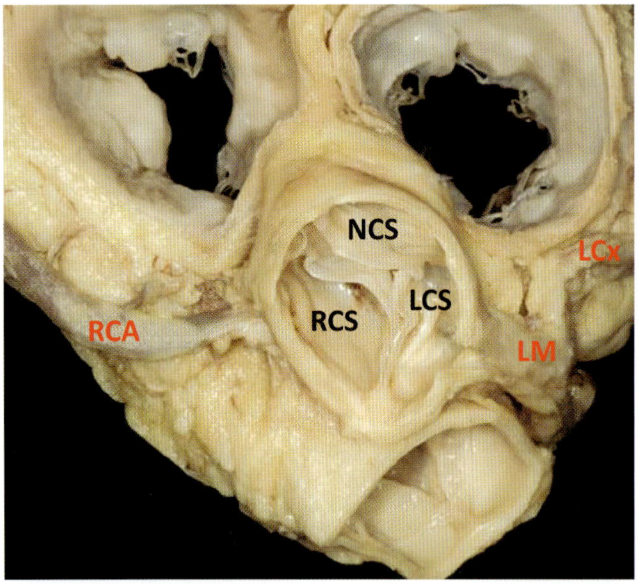

Fig. 1.11: Pathologic specimen demonstrating the origin of the left main coronary artery (LMCA) from the left coronary sinus (LCS). The left circumflex artery (LCx) arises from the left main artery. The right coronary artery (RCA) is seen originating from the right coronary sinus (RCS). (Image modified with permission from Cheitlin MD, Ursell PC. Cardiac anatomy. In: Chatterjee K, Anderson M, Heistad D, Kerber RE (Eds). Cardiology—An Illustrated Textbook. New Delhi, India: Jaypee Brothers Medical Publishers (P) Ltd. 2012). (NCS: Noncoronary sinus).

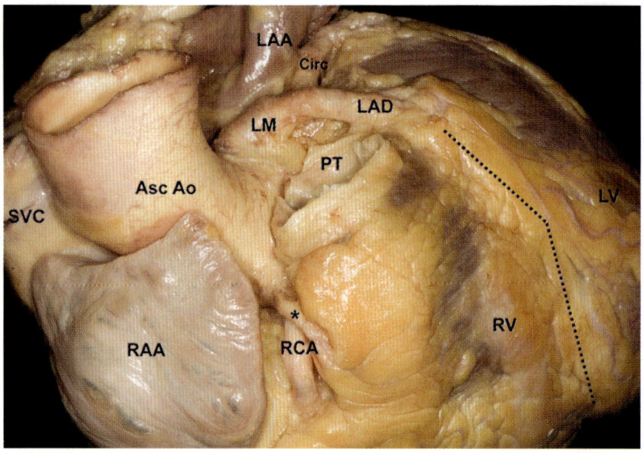

Fig. 1.12: Anterior aspect of the heart showing the origin of the left main coronary artery from the aorta and the course of the coronary arteries. With the parietal pericardium removed, epicardial fat has been partially dissected away to show the proximal courses of the coronary arteries. The pulmonary trunk (PT) is truncated to uncover the origin of the left main coronary artery (LM) from the left side of the aortic root and its relatively short course. With the left atrial appendage (LAA) reflected superiorly, the divergence of the left anterior descending (LAD) and circumflex (Circ) branches is revealed. The left anterior descending branch continues in the anterior interventricular groove (dashed line) that is filled with non-dissected fat that covers the distal portion of artery. The circumflex branch courses under the left atrial appendage in the left atrioventricular groove posteriorly towards the inferior surface of the heart. From the right side of the aortic root, the right coronary artery (RCA) courses in the fat-filled atrioventricular groove towards the heart's inferior surface. A small conal branch (*) of the RCA courses toward the infundibulum. (RAA: Right atrial appendage; SVC: Superior vena cava; Asc Ao: Ascending aorta; RCA: Right coronary artery; RV: Right ventricle; LV: Left ventricle).

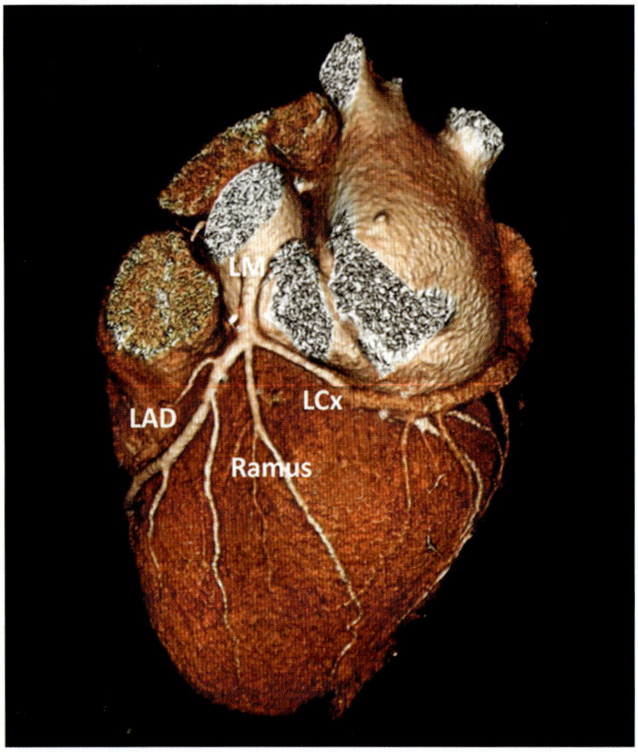

Fig. 1.13: Three-dimensional volume-rendered CT coronary angiogram showing trifurcation of the left main coronary artery (LM) into the left anterior descending artery (LAD), ramus intermedius artery, and left circumflex artery (LCx). (Image adapted from Rabelo DR, Barros MV, Nunes Mdo C, et al. Multislice coronary angiotomography in the assessment of coronary artery anomalous origin. Arq Bras Cardiol. 2012;98(3):266-272).

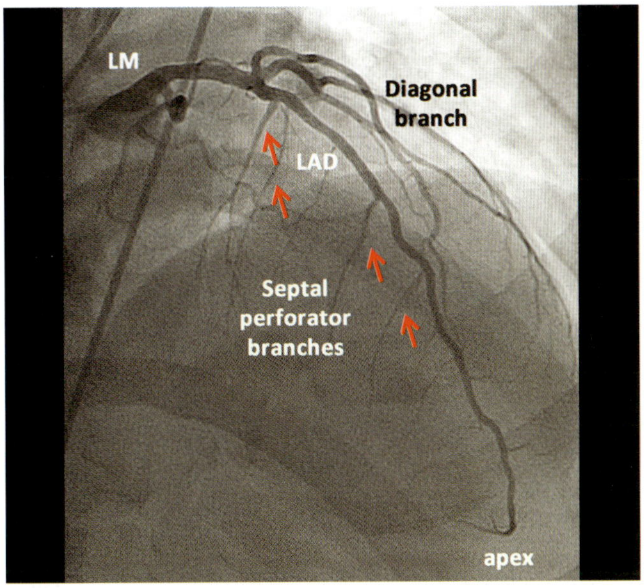

Fig. 1.14: Coronary angiogram of the left anterior descending (LAD) artery. The LAD is seen arising from the left main (LM) coronary artery. The LAD usually gives off several diagonal branches, though in this case it gives off one very large branching diagonal branch. Numerous septal perforators (arrows) arise at right angles from the LAD and penetrate into the interventricular septum. The LAD can be seen wrapping around the apex of the heart.

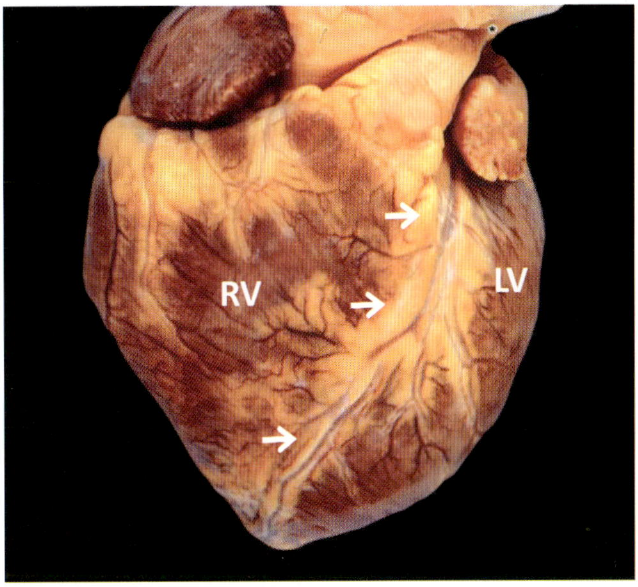

Fig. 1.15: Gross pathology specimen of the heart demonstrating the course of the LAD (arrows), running from base to apex, along the interventricular septum between the left ventricle (LV) and right ventricle (RV). (Image reproduced with permission from Cheitlin MD, Ursell PC. Cardiac anatomy. In: Chatterjee K, Anderson M, Heistad D, Kerber RE (Eds). Cardiology—An Illustrated Textbook. New Delhi, India: Jaypee Brothers Medical Publishers (P) Ltd. 2012).

Shortly after the origin of the LAD there are a number of perforating intramural septal branches (Figs. 1.16A and B), the largest being the most proximal. These perforating septal branches (Fig. 1.17) supply the anterior two-thirds of the interventricular septum, as well as the atrioventricular (His) bundle and the bundle branches of the conduction system. A septal branch may pass along the moderator band and supply the anterior papillary muscle of the right ventricle.

LEFT CIRCUMFLEX CORONARY ARTERY

The left circumflex coronary artery arises at right angles from the left main coronary and proceeds in the left anterior atrioventricular groove, giving off small obtuse marginal branches to the left ventricular lateral wall and the left atrium (Fig. 1.18 and Video 1.3). The left circumflex artery terminates between the obtuse margin and the crux of the heart in 85% of cases, and at or beyond the crux in 15% of hearts. It may also continue down the inferior interventricular groove a variable distance as the posterior descending artery (PDA). Occlusion of the left circumflex artery will result in infarction of the lateral wall of the left ventricle.

There is a constant ventricular branch arising at right angles from the circumflex at the obtuse margin of the heart called the *obtuse marginal coronary artery* that passes distally along the left obtuse margin toward the apex (see Fig. 1.18). The internal diameter of the vessel is 2 mm. In 10% of the hearts, the circumflex does not follow the atrioventricular groove but passes obliquely over the lateral left ventricular wall toward the apex.

RIGHT CORONARY ARTERY

The ostium of the right coronary artery (RCA) is in the right coronary sinus of the aortic valve. The RCA originates at the same level with respect to the sinotubular junction in 70% of hearts, above the level of the sinotubular junction in 20% of hearts, and below the level of the sinotubular junction in 10% of the hearts. The RCA then passes posterior to the right ventricular infundibulum and into the right anterior atrioventricular groove (Figs. 1.19A to C and Video 1.4). In about 10% of the hearts the RCA terminates at or just beyond the acute margin of the heart, but usually it passes around to the inferior atrioventricular groove and then at the crux of the heart, down the inferior interventricular groove as the PDA. In this more common

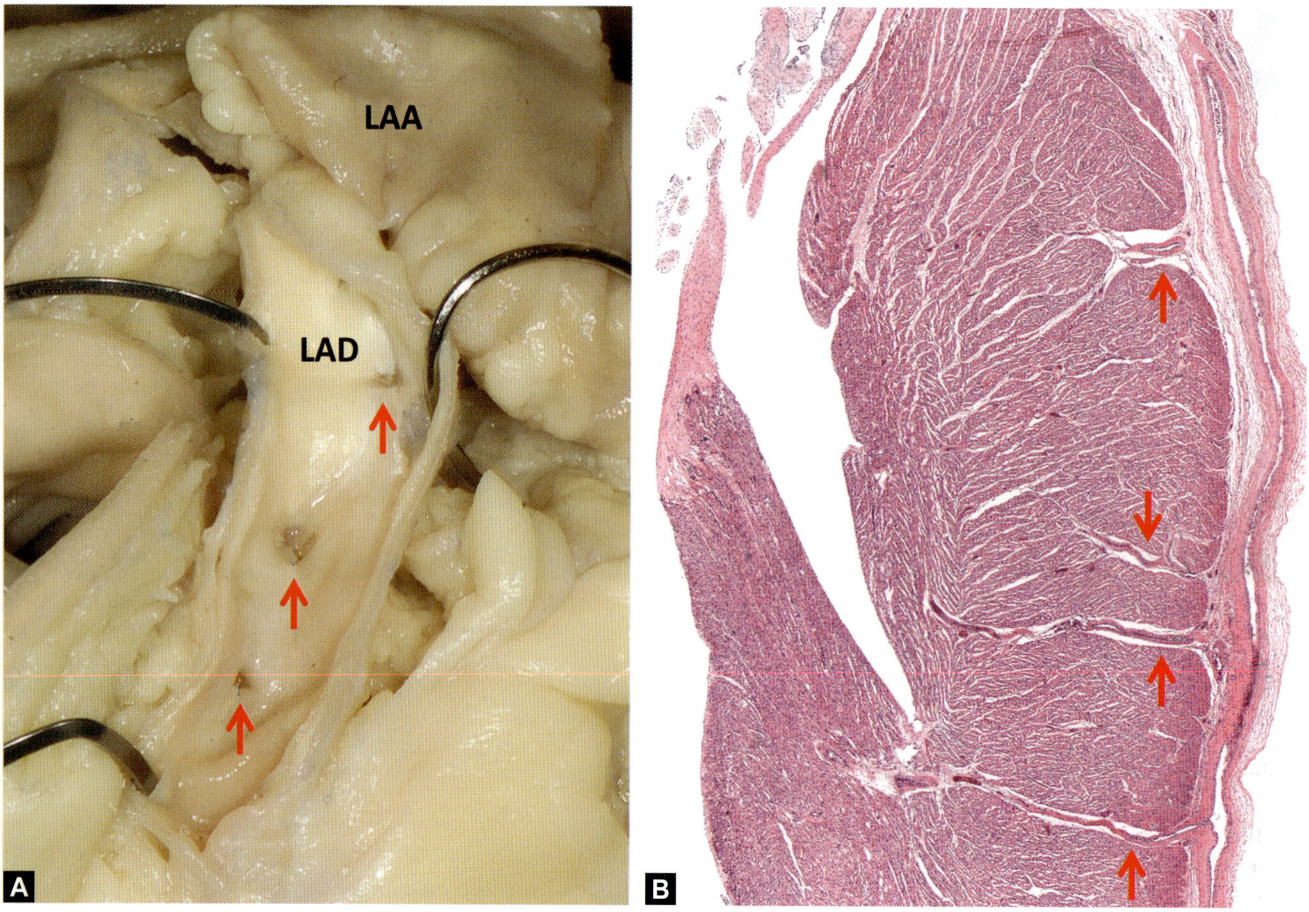

Figs. 1.16A and B: Perforating branches from extramural coronary arteries as intramyocardial resistance arteries. (A) As the left anterior descending (LAD) coronary emerges from under the left atrial appendage (LAA), the proximal portion of the vessel has been opened to show the origins of several septal perforators (arrows). (B) A histological section from an infant shows the perpendicular course of similar resistance arteries (arrows) in the left ventricular free wall. These perforating branches arise at right angles from the extramural coronary arteries.

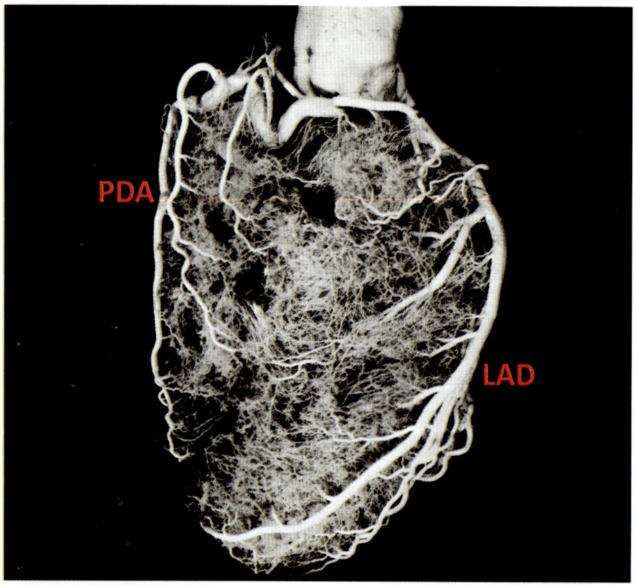

Fig. 1.17: Interventricular septal arterial circulation. Septal perforating arteries arise from the left anterior descending artery (LAD) and the posterior descending artery (PDA) branch, which most commonly arises from the right coronary artery. (With permission from Baroldi G, Scomazzoni G. Coronary Circulation in the Normal and the Pathologic Heart. Washington DC: Armed Forces Institute of Pathology, Office of the Surgeon General, Department of the Army; 1965. Part 1, P. 5).

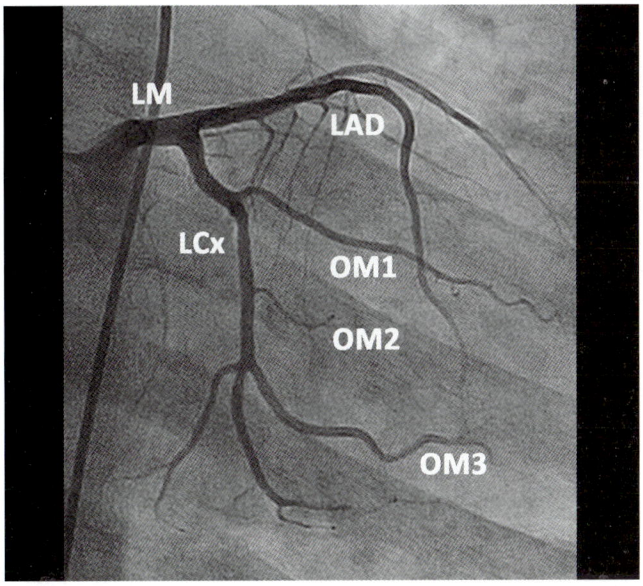

Fig. 1.18: Coronary angiogram showing the left circumflex artery (LCx) arising from the left main coronary artery (LM) and giving off several obtuse marginal (OM) branches. (LAD: Left anterior descending artery).

situation, the heart is said to have a right dominant coronary system. In cases in which the RCA does not give off the PDA but is only a small artery that supplies the right ventricle, the RCA is referred to as a "nondominant" RCA.

The first branch of the right coronary artery, called the conal artery, passes anteromedially to the anterior surface of the right ventricular outflow tract. In 50% of hearts, the conal artery arises from the right coronary sinus from a separate ostium from the right coronary artery.

In most patients, the RCA gives off the sinoatrial (SA) nodal artery, which supplies the SA node. The SA nodal artery originates shortly after the origin of the RCA. In a minority of hearts, the SA nodal artery arises from a continuation of an anterior atrial branch of the circumflex coronary artery.

As the RCA travels around the right ventricle (RV), it gives off at right angles one or two acute marginal arteries (also called RV branches) which supply the anterior wall of the right ventricle. Proximal occlusion of the RCA will compromise blood flow to the RV, and thus approximately one-third of inferior STEMI patients will have some clinical degree of RV infarction.

As the RCA turns at the crux to become the PDA, the atrioventricular nodal artery arises and passes superiorly to supply the atrioventricular (AV) node.

In 65% of hearts the RCA continues past the crux and after giving off the PDA continues on as the posterolateral segment, giving off one or more posterolateral branches, supplying the inferior (or "posterior") wall of the left ventricle. In patients with this anatomy, acute occlusion of the RCA will result in not only inferior wall myocardial infarction (MI) but also what is referred to as posterior wall MI.

POSTERIOR DESCENDING CORONARY ARTERY

In the majority of patients the PDA (more anatomically correct termed the inferior descending artery) is given off by the RCA, and the patient is said to have a "right dominant system". In a minority of patients, the PDA is given off by the left circumflex artery and the patient is said to have a "left dominant system". In 30% of the hearts there are either two parallel inferior descending arteries from the right coronary or one from the right and one from the circumflex coronary artery (Figs. 1.20A and B).

In 50% of the hearts the PDA coronary artery terminates at the left ventricular apex, and in the other half it terminates before it reaches the apex. Whether arising from the distal RCA or the left circumflex coronary artery the PDA supplies the left and right ventricular inferior walls. It also has vertical perforating intramural branches which supply the inferior third of the interventricular septum.

INTRAMURAL CORONARY VASCULATURE

Arising at right angles from the extramural coronary arteries, the perforating branches in the ventricular walls form a complex network of resistance arteries that form a capillary meshwork around myocardial fibers. The perforating arteries vary in their course through the myocardium, branching off at right angles at all levels of the ventricular wall like the tines of a fork (Fig. 1.21). Some proceed to the subendocardium and then spread out parallel to the endocardium of the cardiac chambers. At the subendocardial level there are anastomosing vessels as well as end-arteries. There are also arterioluminal and venoluminal channels connecting terminal intramural arteries with the ventricular and atrial chambers. These channels have different names depending on the connections and histology of the small vessels. The ostia of these vessels can be seen on examination of the endocardial surface of the ventricles and more prominently of the atria. A general name for these vessels that empty into the cardiac chambers is that of Thebesian veins or vessels.

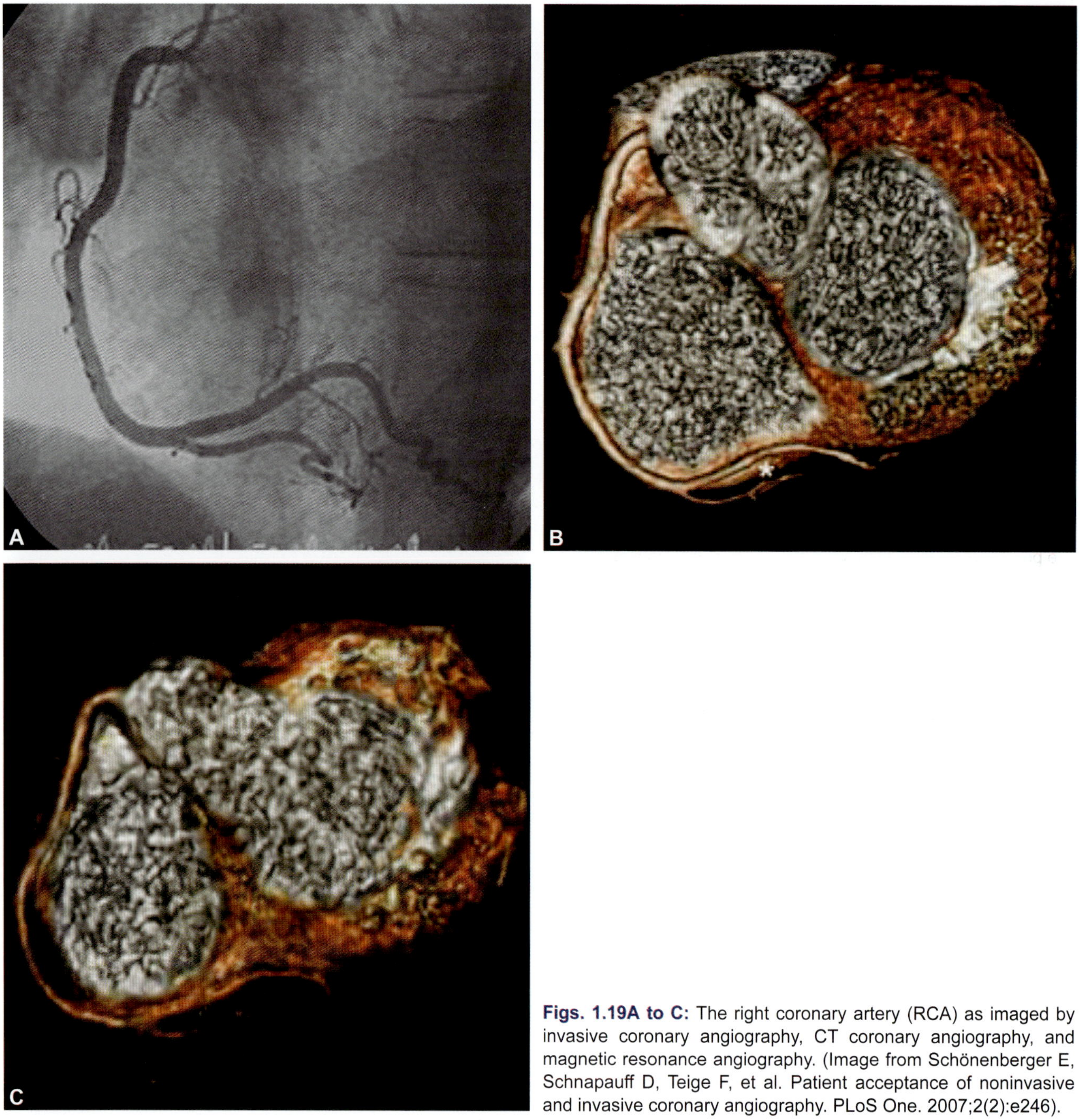

Figs. 1.19A to C: The right coronary artery (RCA) as imaged by invasive coronary angiography, CT coronary angiography, and magnetic resonance angiography. (Image from Schönenberger E, Schnapauff D, Teige F, et al. Patient acceptance of noninvasive and invasive coronary angiography. PLoS One. 2007;2(2):e246).

Collateral or anastomosing subarteriolar arteries of 25–250 μm between coronary arterial systems (Fig. 1.22) have been demonstrated by postmortem coronary contrast injections. Those that connect different branches of the same coronary artery are called homocoronary anastomoses, and those that connect branches of the other two or three coronary arteries, intercoronary anastomoses. These vessels form the basis for collateral circulation that becomes visible on angiography when a major coronary artery becomes obstructed or occluded by atherosclerosis. The homocoronary and intercoronary collaterals are rare in the subepicardium but are found at all other levels of the ventricular wall. This explains why collateral vessels are rarely seen on the epicardial surface of the heart on coronary angiograms.

There are also extracardiac collaterals that connect the coronary arterial system with vessels other than the heart. These collaterals are very small vessels that connect

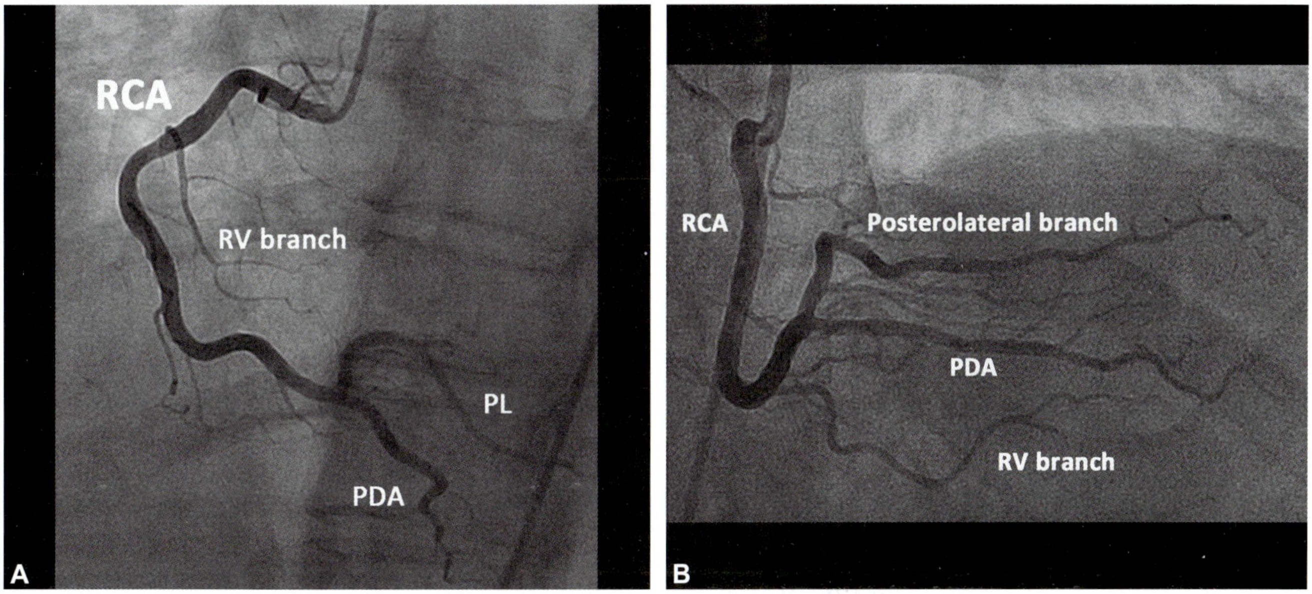

Figs. 1.20A and B: Coronary angiograms of the right coronary artery (RCA) and the posterior descending artery (PDA). The RCA is seen giving off an right ventricular (RV) branch (also called an acute marginal branch), then giving off the PDA. The RCA continues as the posterolateral segment, which gives off a posterolateral (PL) branch.

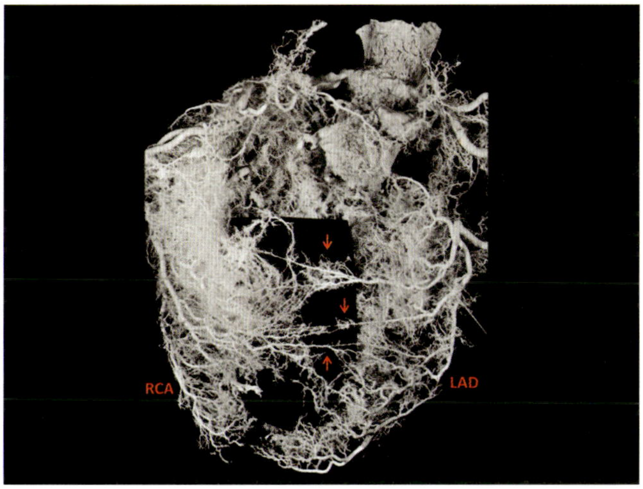

Fig. 1.21: Intercoronary anastomoses: collaterals between branches of the two coronary arteries. Placing a black paper inserted below the collateral vessels highlights slender collateral vessels (arrows) between the right coronary artery (RCA) and the left anterior descending (LAD) coronary artery.

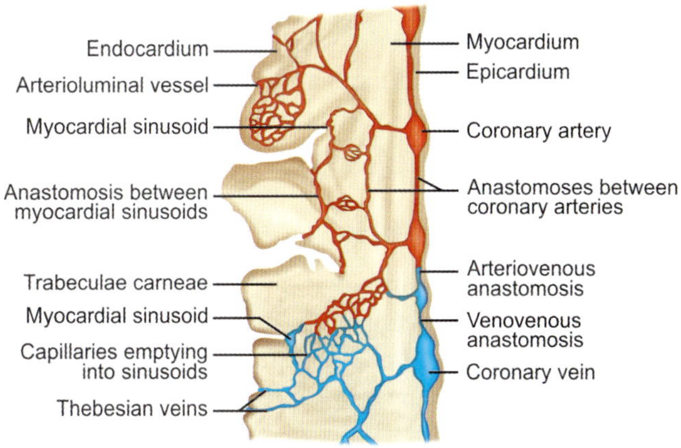

Fig. 1.22: Diagram of the ventricular wall, showing the relationship between the various intramural channels With permission from Chatterjee, et al. Cardiology An Illustrated Textbook, Cheitlin MD and Ursell P. Chapter 1, Figure 24, page 17. New Delhi, India: Jaypee Brothers Medical Publishers (P) Ltd; 2013.

the left circumflex coronary with the vasa vasorum of the aortic root, the pulmonary artery with the bronchial and mediastinal arteries, the atrial branches to the vasa vasorum of the venae cavae, and the atrial branches to the pericardial vessels along the pericardial reflections.

THE CORONARY VENOUS SYSTEM

The coronary venous system (Fig. 1.23) can be divided into two sections: the extramural veins that drain into the coronary sinus as well as the anterior cardiac veins that drain

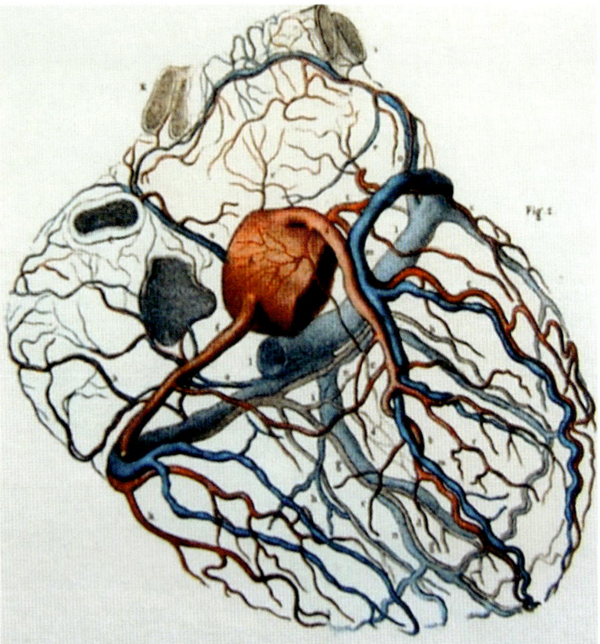

Fig. 1.23: The cardiac venous system and arterial circulation. Illustration by Jean-Baptiste Marc Bourgery. Atlas of human anatomy and surgery. Published 1831.

directly into the right atrial chamber, and the intramural or Thebesian veins that are at every level within the cardiac walls and are arranged parallel to the myocardial fibers. As with other veins, the cardiac veins have both unifoliate (one-leaflet) and bifoliate (two-leaflet) valves.

The Coronary Sinus

Not a proper vein histologically, the coronary sinus (Figs. 1.24A to C) is a muscular conduit that is formed at the confluence of the oblique vein of the left atrium and the great cardiac vein near the obtuse margin of the heart. The coronary sinus then courses in the inferior left atrioventricular groove toward the right atrium and drains most of the left ventricular wall, as well as parts of the left and right atrium. Joining the coronary sinus is the oblique vein of the left atrium that passes between the left atrial appendage and the left pulmonary veins. The proximal end of the oblique vein is a tendon of Marshall, a vestige of the embryonic left anterior cardinal vein. However, if the embryonic vein remains open, it functions as a persistent left superior vena cava draining into the coronary sinus.

As the coronary sinus courses rightward in the inferior left atrioventricular groove, it receives tributary veins from the left and right atria and from the inferior wall of the left ventricle, finally emptying into the right atrial cavity posteroinferiorly. The diameter of the coronary sinus is 6–16 mm and its length varies from 2 cm to 5 cm, depending on the size of the heart. The ostium of the coronary sinus is inferior and medial to the entrance of the inferior vena cava and is guarded in two-thirds of hearts by the usually inconspicuous Thebesian valve. However, at times the valve covers the ostium almost completely, may be fenestrated, and may make it impossible to enter the coronary sinus by catheter.

THE ANTERIOR INTERVENTRICULAR VEIN

A major vein, the *anterior interventricular vein* is the most consistent of the coronary venous system. It originates at or near the left ventricular apex and ascends in the anterior interventricular groove, draining the apex and anterior wall of the left ventricle, the anterior two-thirds of the interventricular septum, and the adjacent right ventricular wall. As it reaches the anterior atrioventricular groove the vein passes leftward between the origin of the pulmonary trunk and the tip of the left atrial appendage. It continues as the great cardiac vein, receiving branches that drain the anterior left atrial wall and superior left ventricle, and then becomes the coronary sinus where the oblique vein of the left atrium enters the coronary sinus.

THE MIDDLE CARDIAC VEIN

The middle cardiac vein (Fig. 1.25), also known as the inferior interventricular vein, drains the diaphragmatic wall of the left ventricle and the posterior third of the interventricular septum. At the inferior aspect of the left ventricular apex, the middle cardiac vein arises from one or two small superficial veins. Enlarging as it courses in the inferior interventricular groove toward the base of the heart, it usually drains into the coronary sinus near that conduit's entrance to the right atrium, and less often directly into the right atrium. From 2–6 veins drain the diaphragmatic and lateral left ventricular wall into the coronary sinus, the most consistent of these being the *inferior left ventricular vein* draining the diaphragmatic lateral wall of the left ventricle and the *obtuse marginal vein* draining the lateral wall of the left ventricle.

THE SMALL CARDIAC VEIN

The small cardiac vein (also known as the right coronary vein) is present in about 70% of hearts. The small cardiac

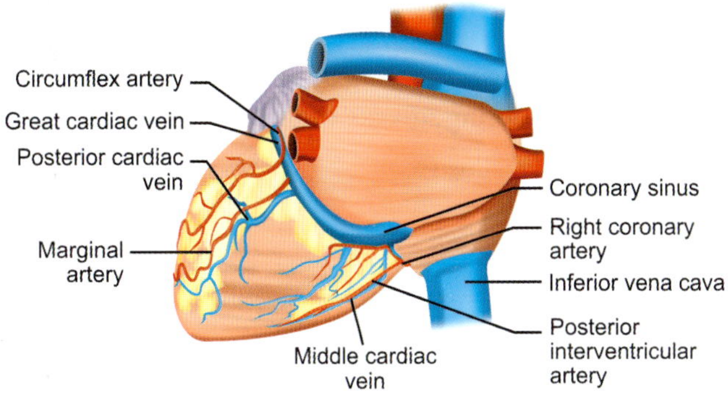

Fig. 1.24A: Schematic illustration of the coronary sinus and cardiac veins, as viewed on the posterior aspect of the heart. (Image created by Bruce Blaus and posted on Wikipedia).

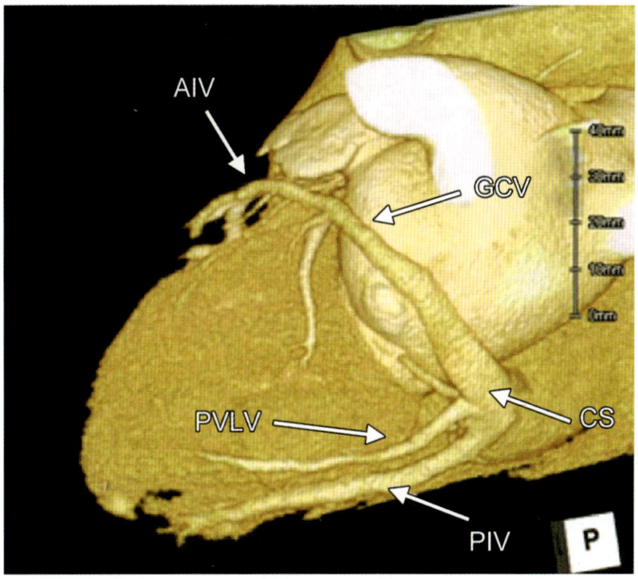

Fig. 1.24B: Cardiac CT venography demonstrating the coronary sinus (CS), great cardiac vein (GCV), posterior interventricular vein (PIV), posterior vein of the left ventricle (PVLV), and anterior interventricular vein (AIV). (Image from Ohta Y, Fujii S, Kakite S, et al. Evaluation of the optimal image reconstruction interval for noninvasive coronary 64-slice computed tomography venography. O J Rad. 2013;3(2):66-72.).

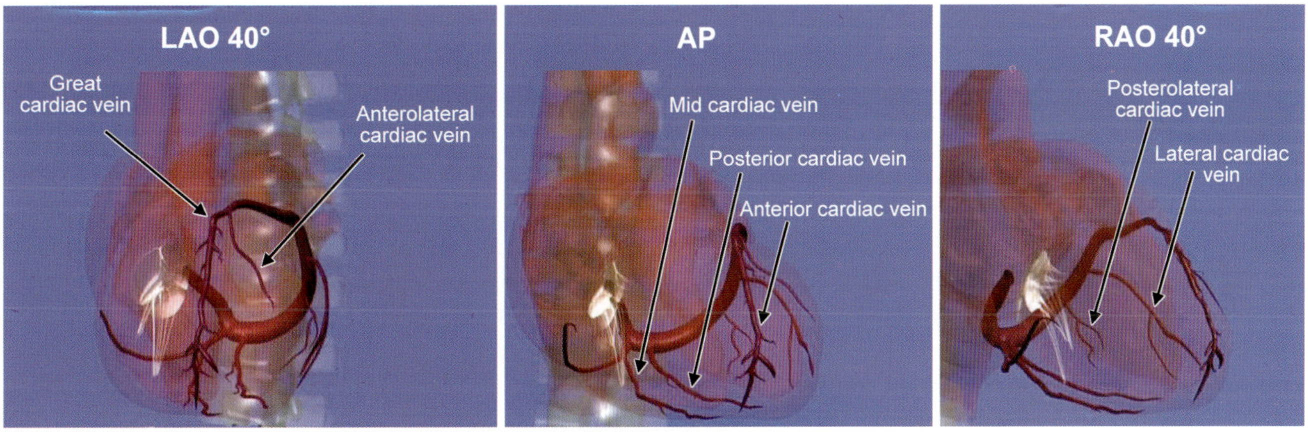

Fig. 1.24C: Schematic illustration of the cardiac venous anatomy viewed from LAO 40°, AP, and RAO 40° angulation. (Image courtesy of Medtronic, Inc.).

vein, when present, runs in the right inferior atrioventricular groove and terminates at the ostial opening of the coronary sinus or directly into the right atrium. It drains most of the walls of the right atrium, and in the absence of the right cardiac veins, the anterior surface of the right ventricle. In some hearts, the small cardiac vein receives the right marginal vein in which case it drains the anterior wall of the right ventricle.

THE ANTERIOR CARDIAC VEINS

The anterior cardiac veins, between 3 and 6 in number, drain most of the anterior and lateral wall of the right ventricle directly into the right atrium. Within this group is the right marginal vein, originating at or near the cardiac apex, and ascending along the acute margin of the heart, draining both the adjacent anterior and diaphragmatic surfaces of the right ventricle.

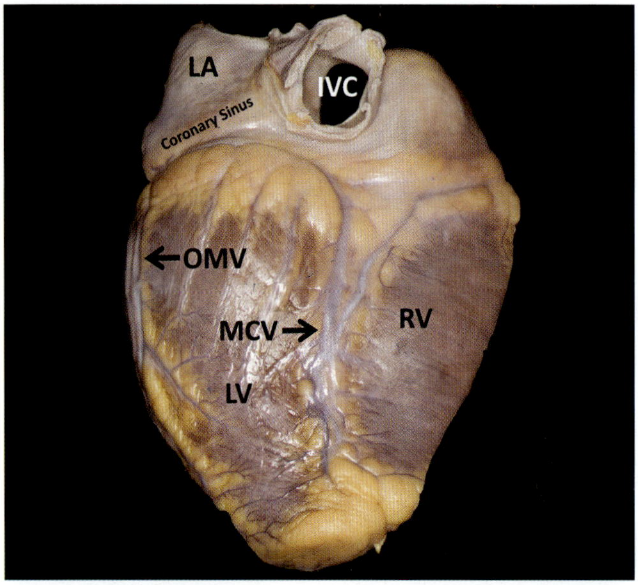

Fig. 1.25: Cardiac veins on the diaphragmatic (inferior) surface of the heart. Cardiac veins run superficial to their corresponding arteries. On the inferior surface of this adult heart the middle cardiac vein (MCV) courses in the interventricular groove towards the base of the heart, where it connects with the coronary sinus. The obtuse marginal vein (OMV) courses along the obtuse margin towards the base of the heart and coronary sinus. (IVC: Inferior vena caval connection with right atrium; LA: Left atrium; LV: Left ventricle; RV: Right ventricle).

VEINS DRAINING THE RIGHT AND LEFT ATRIA

The walls of the right atrium are drained through small, largely intramural, vessels and intramural conduits. They predominantly drain through very small orifices directly into the right atrial cavity and are called Thebesian veins. The large intramyocardial channels, numbering from 1 to 3, are located variably but usually in the posterior and lateral atrial walls, and drain venous blood from the anterior cardiac veins and from the sinoatrial and atrioventricular nodes.

The left atrial veins are small and are divided into three groups. The posterolateral group drains the posterolateral areas of the left atrium through two or three veins, as well as draining the left atrial appendage. Included in the posterolateral group is the oblique vein of the left atrium. Most of the posterolateral groups of veins drain into the coronary sinus. The posterosuperior groups of veins, usually 3 in number, drain the small area of left atrial wall surrounded by the pulmonary venous ostia.

CONCLUSION

Our understanding of cardiovascular anatomy and physiology continues to advance, even in the current age. A detailed knowledge of normal coronary vascular anatomy is important to understanding the heart's circulation. It is critical to deciphering images of the pathologic anatomy in living patients.

VIDEO LEGENDS

Video 1.1: CT 3D volume-rendered image showing the course of the coronary arteries.

Video 1.2: Right anterior oblique cranial angiogram showing the left anterior descending (LAD). The LAD gives off septal branches which supply the superior interventricular septum and gives off diagonal branches which supply a portion of the anterior and anterolateral walls.

Video 1.3: Right anterior oblique caudal angiogram showing the left circumflex artery and several obtuse marginal branches of the left circumflex artery.

Video 1.4: AP angio gram of the right coronary artery.

REFERENCES

Almuwaqqat Z, Tranquilli M, Elefteriades J. Anatomy of main coronary artery location: radial position around the aortic root circumference. Int J Angiol. 2012;21(3):125-8.

Anderson RH, Becker AE. The Heart: Structure in Health and Disease. London: Gower Medical Publishing; 1992. pp. 1.32-1.35.

Baroldi G, Mantero O, Scomazzoni G. The collaterals of the coronary arteries in normal and pathologic hearts. Circ Res. 1956;4(2):223-9.

Fiss DM. Normal coronary anatomy and anatomic variations. Applied Radiol. 2007;36:14-26.

Loukas M, Bilinsky S, Bilinsky E, et al. Cardiac veins: a review of the literature. Clin Anat. 2009;22(1):129-45.

Loukas M, Groat C, Khangura R, et al. The normal and abnormal anatomy of the coronary arteries. Clin Anat. 2009;22(1):114-28.

Młynarski R, Młynarski A, Sosnowski M. Anatomical variants of left circumflex artery, coronary sinus and mitral valve can determine safety of percutaneous mitral annuloplasty. Cardiol J. 2013;20(3):235-40.

Spenser J, Fitch E, Iaizzo PA. Anatomical reconstructions of the human cardiac venous system using contrast-computed tomography of perfusion-fixed specimens. J Vis Exp. 2013;(74). doi: 10.3791/50258.

Trivellato M, Angelini P, Leachman RD. Variations in coronary artery anatomy: Normal versus abnormal. Cardiovasc Dis. 1980;7(4):357-70.

Von Lüdinghausen M. The venous drainage of the human myocardium. Adv Anat Embryol Cell Biol. 2003;168:I-VIII,1-104.

CHAPTER

Coronary Artery Anomalies

2

Shakeel Ahmed Qureshi, Gareth J Morgan

INTRODUCTION

Coronary artery anomalies (Figs. 2.1 and 2.2) are relatively rare among congenital defects, occurring as isolated findings or in association with other common congenital heart defects. In the latter circumstance, they can have a profound impact on the natural and surgical history, and may cause a significant alteration in the course of treatment offered.

CORONARY ARTERY EMBRYOLOGY

Embryological theories of coronary artery development remain under debate. In the last 15–20 years, the mainstream concept of a coronary system, which develops on the epicardial surface and finds its way towards the aortic root, has taken over from the original concept of the coronary arteries budding out from the aorta. The newer model has allowed more logical understanding of the pathological embryogenesis of several of the major coronary anomalies.

NORMAL CORONARY ANATOMY

Significant normal variation exists in the coronary tree with a myriad of variation in branching pattern and regional myocardial supply. We will not attempt to cover these inconsequential variations, but present a brief overview of the normal coronary arterial tree.

The coronary arteries consist of large central epicardial arteries which divide and subdivide, initially on the epicardial surface and then within the myocardium, leading to the arteriolar-capillary bed. The network usually originates as a (1) "left" coronary artery, typically originating from the left posterior aortic sinus, and a (2) "right" coronary artery (RCA), which originates from the right anterior aortic sinus.

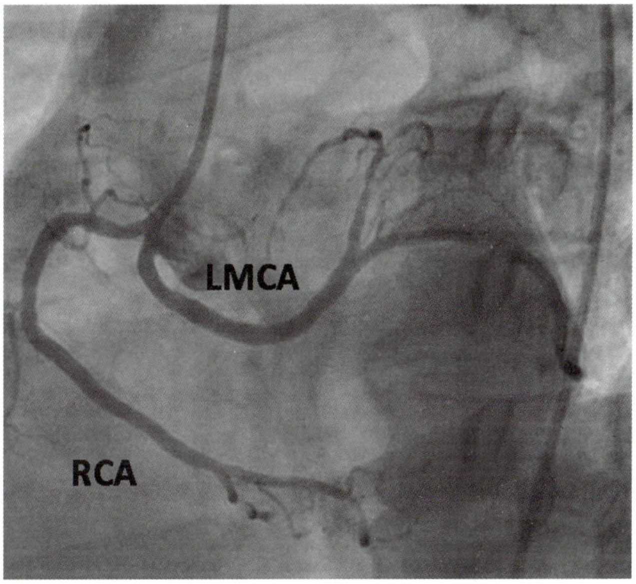

Fig. 2.1: Coronary angiogram showing the left main coronary artery (LMCA) arising from the right coronary cusp. The LMCA takes a retroaortic course. (Image from Charan L, Shiradkar S, Kerkar PG, et al. Stenting of anomalous left main coronary artery stenosis in an adult with a retroaortic course. Cardiol Res Pract. 2011;2011:296946).

The left coronary artery (LCA) (or left main stem) courses laterally, between the left atrial appendage and the pulmonary artery, before dividing into the circumflex artery, which runs under the atrial appendage and into the left atrioventricular groove, and the left anterior descending (LAD) (or anterior interventricular) artery.

The RCA initially courses anteriorly toward the right atrioventricular groove, giving branches which supply the sinoatrial node and the free wall of the right ventricle.

CORONARY DOMINANCE

Around 90% of the population have a "right-dominant" pattern, with the posterior descending coronary artery

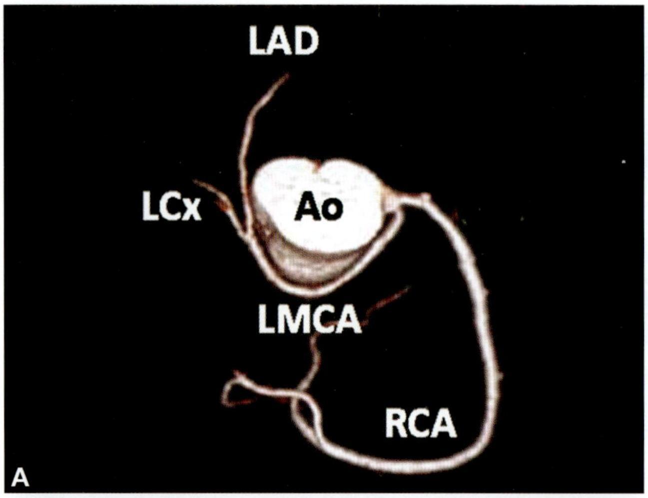

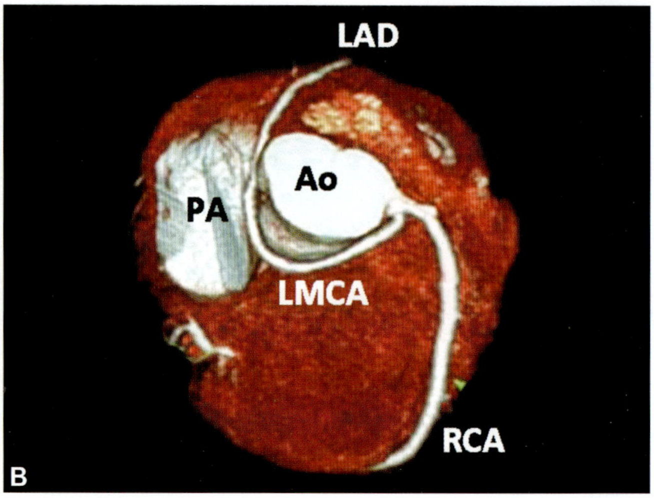

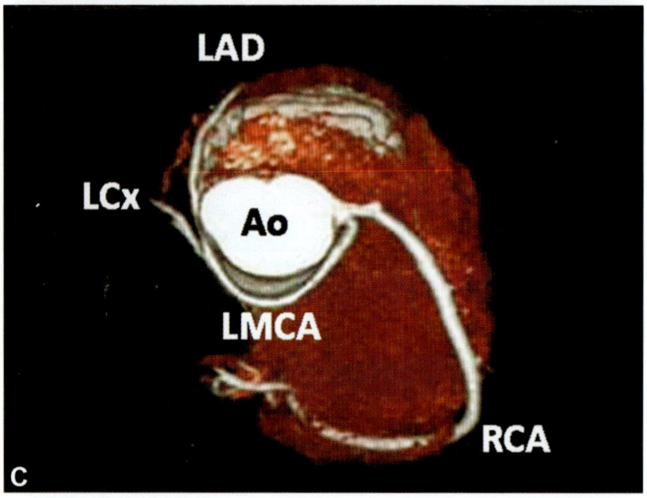

Figs. 2.2A to C: Coronary CT images showing the left main coronary artery (LMCA) originating from the right coronary sinus. The left main can be seen taking an interarterial course, passing between the aorta (Ao) and the pulmonary artery (PA). [Image from Shabestari AA, Akhlaghpoor S, Tayebivaljozi R, et al. Prevalence of congenital coronary artery anomalies and variants in 2697 consecutive patients using 64-detector row coronary CT angiography. Iran J Radiol. 2012;9(3):111-21]. (LAD: Left anterior descending artery; LCx: Left circumflex artery; RCA: Right coronary artery).

(supplying the inferior surface of both ventricles—the posterior ventricular septum, and the atrioventricular node) being an extension of the RCA. In the remaining 10%, the circumflex artery continues in the posterior ventricular groove, in a pattern referred to as "left dominant".

CLASSIFICATION OF CORONARY ANOMALIES

Congenital coronary abnormalities are perhaps best classified according to their morphology and anatomy, outlined in Table 2.1.

Coronary Artery Origins from the Aortic Root but Taking an Abnormal Course or Origin

Coronary artery origins from the aortic root with an abnormal origin or course that are encountered in clinical practice include origin of the left main coronary artery (LMCA) from the right (anterior) sinus, origin of the left circumflex artery (LCx) from the right (anterior) coronary sinus, and origin of the RCA from the left coronary sinus.

Left Main Coronary Artery from Right Anterior Sinus

With prevalence estimated between 0.1% and 0.3% of the general population, this represents a significant number of asymptomatic individuals. After its origin, the LCA takes one of four possible routes back to the left side of the heart (Figs. 2.3 to 2.11):

1. Anteriorly around the pulmonary artery
2. Between the great arteries (interarterial)
3. Within the subpulmonary muscular infundibulum
4. Posteriorly around the aorta (retroaortic).

There may also be an associated proximal intramural course, slit-like opening of the coronary ostium and/or kinking of the coronary artery.

Table 2.1: Classification of coronary anomalies. [Simplified and adapted from Angelini P. Coronary artery anomalies—current clinical issues: definitions, classification, incidence, clinical relevance, and treatment guidelines. Tex Heart Inst J. 2002;29(4):271-8]. (RCA: Right coronary artery; LAD: Left anterior descending; LMCA: Left main coronary artery; LCx: Left circumflex artery).

Anomalies of Origination and Course
I. Anomalous location of coronary artery outside the root 1. Right ventricle 2. Pulmonary artery a. From one of the pulmonary sinuses b. From the pulmonary trunk c. From the left or right branch pulmonary artery 3. Aortic arch or one of its branches II. Anomalous location of coronary artery from the improper sinus 1. RCA that arises from the left anterior sinus, with anomalous course a. Posterior atrioventricular groove or retrocardiac b. Retroaortic c. Between aorta and pulmonary artery d. Intraseptal e. Anterior to pulmonary outflow f. Posteroanterior interventricular groove (wraparound) 2. LAD that arises from right anterior sinus, with anomalous course a. Between aorta and pulmonary artery b. Intraseptal c. Anterior to pulmonary outflow d. Posteroanterior interventricular groove (wraparound) 3. LCx that arises from right anterior sinus, with anomalous course a. Posterior atrioventricular groove b. Retroaortic 4. LMCA that arises from right anterior sinus, with anomalous course a. Posterior atrioventricular groove b. Retroaortic c. Between aorta and pulmonary artery d. Intraseptal e. Anterior to pulmonary outflow f. Posteroanterior interventricular groove 5. Either coronary artery arising from the posterior "non-facing" sinus
Anomalies of Intrinsic Coronary Arterial Anatomy
1. Congenital ostial stenosis or atresia (LMCA, LAD, RCA, LCx) a. Discrete muscular bridge b. Coronary ostial dimple c. Coronary ectasia or aneurysm d. Absent coronary artery e. Coronary hypoplasia f. Intramural coronary artery g. Subendocardial coronary course
Anomalies of Coronary Termination
1. Inadequate arteriolar/capillary ramifications 2. Fistulas from RCA, LMCA, or infundibular artery to: a. Right ventricle b. Right atrium c. Coronary sinus d. Superior vena cava e. Pulmonary artery f. Pulmonary vein g. Left atrium h. Left ventricle i. Multiple, right + left ventricles

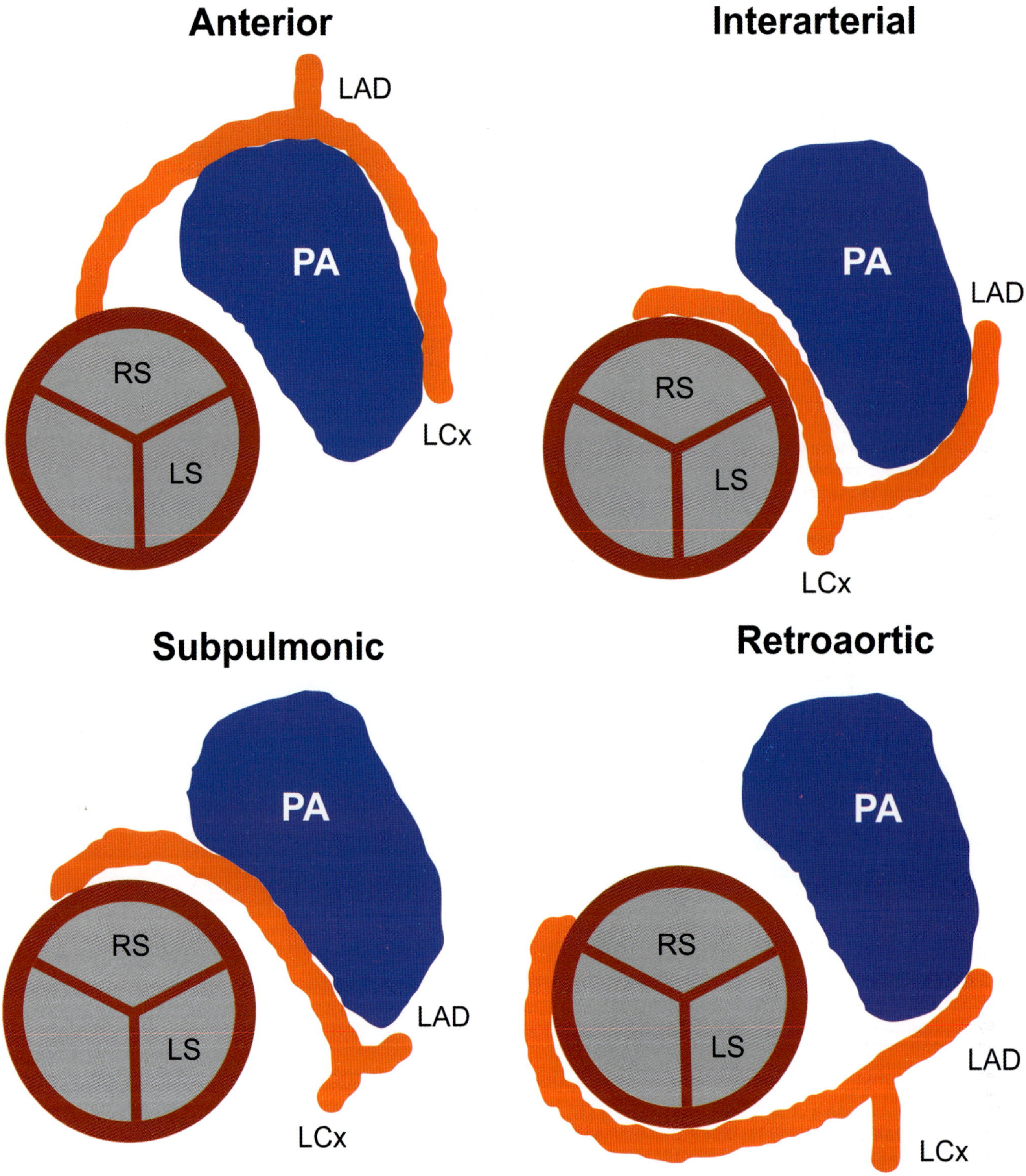

Fig. 2.3: Anatomic representation of the courses of an anomalous left coronary artery arising from the right sinus. [Image and text adapted from Aubry P, Fretay XH, Calvert PA, et al. Proximal anomalous connections of coronary arteries in adults. In: Rao PS (Ed). Congenital Heart Disease—Selected Aspects. In Tech; 2012. Available from http://www.intechopen.com/books/congenital-heart-disease-selected-aspects].

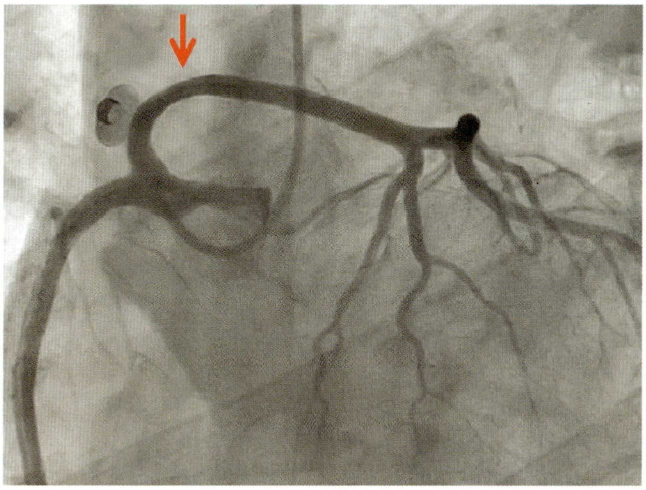

Fig. 2.4: Coronary angiogram showing an anomalous origin of the left main coronary artery (arrow) from the ostium of the right coronary artery. [Image from Aubry P, Fretay XH, Calvert PA, et al. Proximal anomalous connections of coronary arteries in adults. In: Rao PS (Ed). Congenital Heart Disease—Selected Aspects. Intech; 2012. Available from http://www.intechopen.com/books/congenital-heart-disease-selected-aspects].

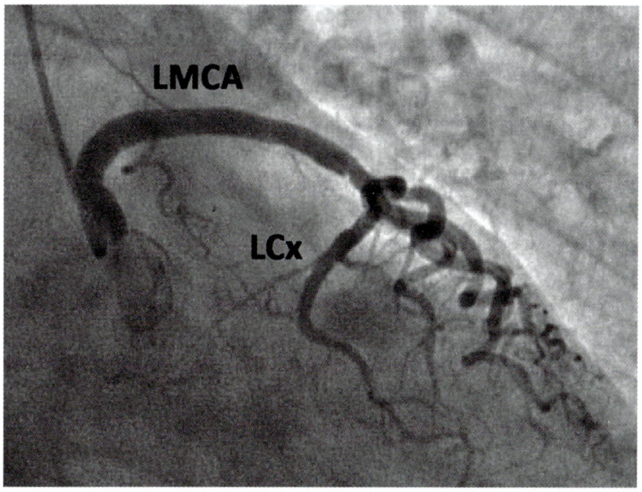

Fig. 2.5: Right anterior oblique (RAO) view coronary angiogram showing a preinfundibular course of a left main coronary artery (LMCA). [Image from Aubry P, Fretay XH, Calvert PA, et al. Proximal anomalous connections of coronary arteries in adults. In: Rao PS (Ed). Congenital Heart Disease—Selected Aspects. Intech; 2012. Available from http://www.intechopen.com/books/congenital-heart-disease-selected-aspects]. (LCx: Left circumflex artery).

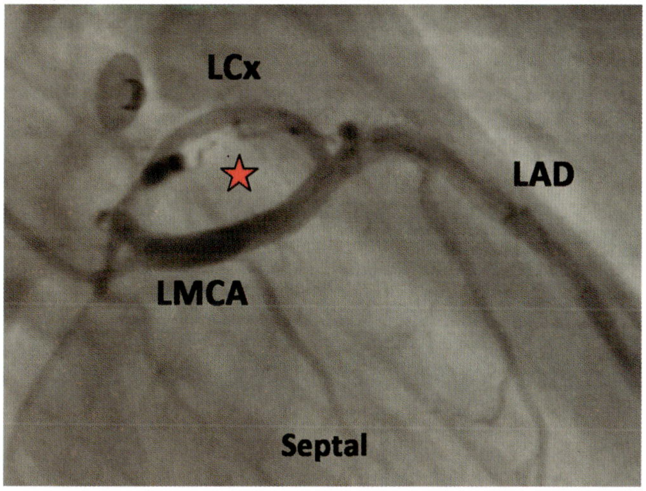

Fig. 2.6: Angiographic view (RAO projection) showing a retroinfundibular course of a left main coronary artery (LMCA) forming an "eye" (star) with the circumflex coronary artery (LCx). Note a septal branch originated from the left main coronary artery. [Image and legend text from Aubry P, Fretay XH, Calvert PA, et al. Proximal anomalous connections of coronary arteries in adults. In: Rao PS (Ed). Congenital Heart Disease—Selected Aspects. Intech; 2012. Available from http://www.intechopen.com/books/congenital-heart-disease-selected-aspects].

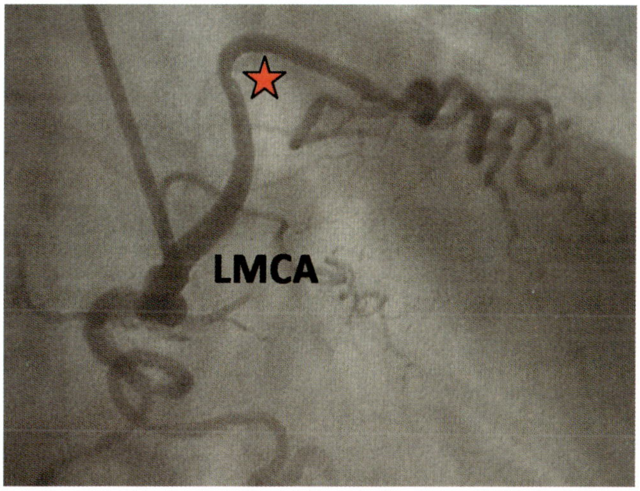

Fig. 2.7: Angiographic view (RAO projection) showing a preaortic course of a left main coronary artery arising from the right sinus with a posterior and upward loop (star). [Image and legend text from Aubry P, Fretay XH, Calvert PA, et al. Proximal anomalous connections of coronary arteries in adults. In: Rao PS (Ed). Congenital Heart Disease—Selected Aspects. Intech; 2012. Available from http://www.intechopen.com/books/congenital-heart-disease-selected-aspects].

This lesion is associated with sudden cardiac death in young adults, particularly in those with an interarterial coronary course. The mechanism of myocardial ischemia probably includes compression of the coronary artery as it passes between the great arteries, aggravated by increased stroke volume and arterial distension during exertion, just as the myocardial oxygen demand is highest. Why comparatively few patients report preceding symptoms of

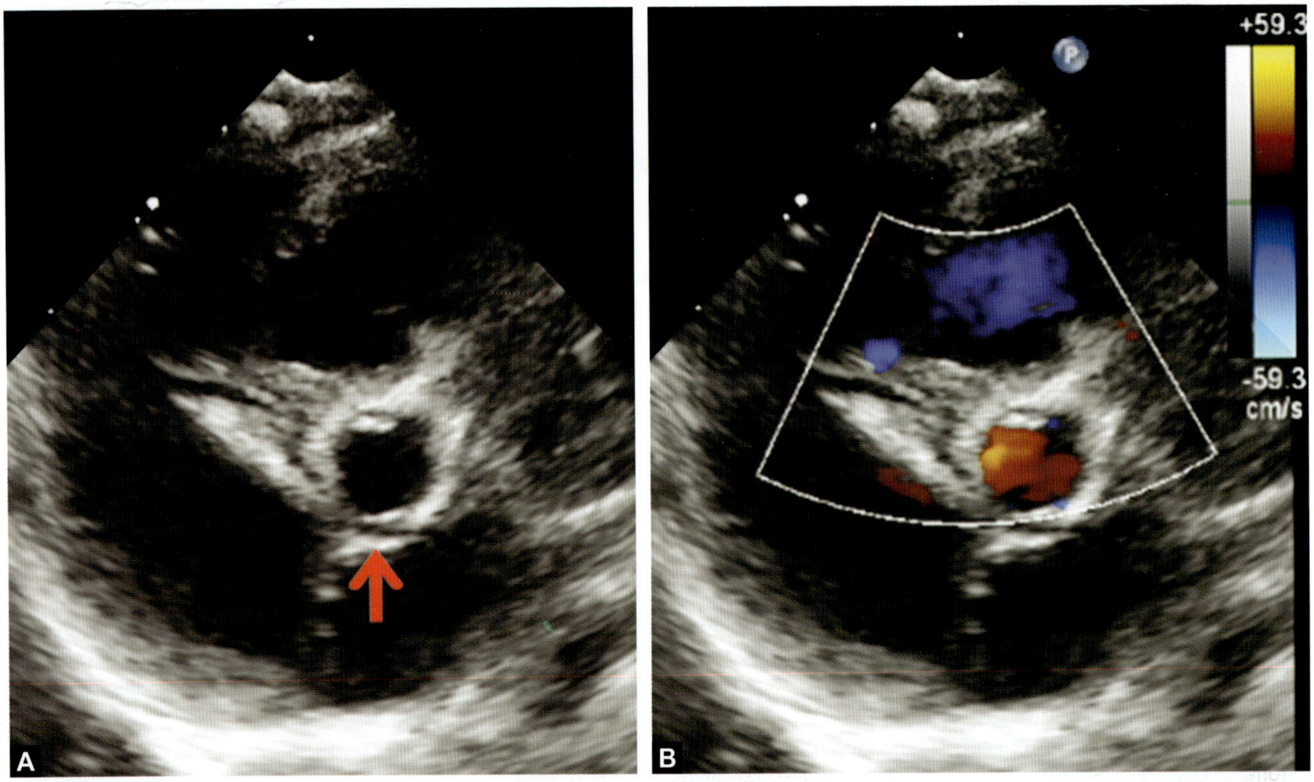

Figs. 2.8A and B: Echocardiogram in the parasternal short-axis demonstrating a retroaortic course of the left coronary artery (arrow), having originated from the right aortic sinus. [Image from Hayes N, Qureshi S. Congenital coronary artery anomalies. In: Vijayalakshmi IB, P Syamasundar Rao, Reema Chugh (Eds). Comprehensive Approach to Congenital Heart Disease. New Delhi, India: Jaypee Brothers Medical Publishers (P) Ltd. 2013].

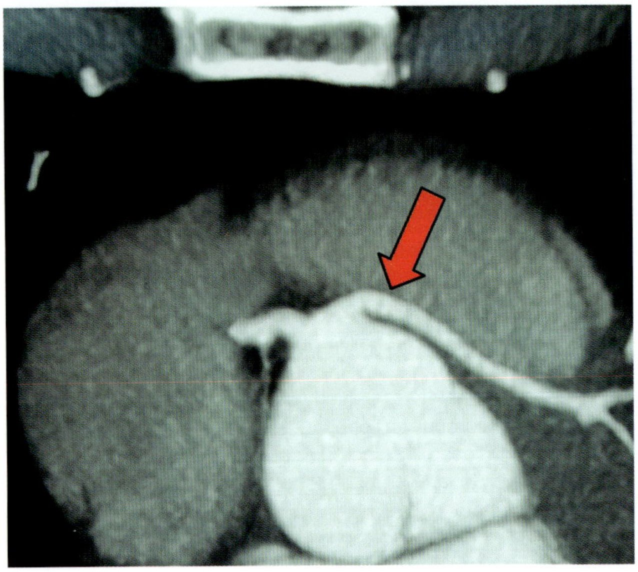

Fig. 2.9: Cardiac CT image demonstrating anomalous origin of the left main coronary artery (arrow) from the right coronary cusp. [Image from Aubry P, Fretay XH, Calvert PA, et al. Proximal anomalous connections of coronary arteries in adults. In: Rao PS (Ed). Congenital Heart Disease—Selected Aspects. Intech; 2012. Available from http://www.intechopen.com/books/congenital-heart-disease-selected-aspects].

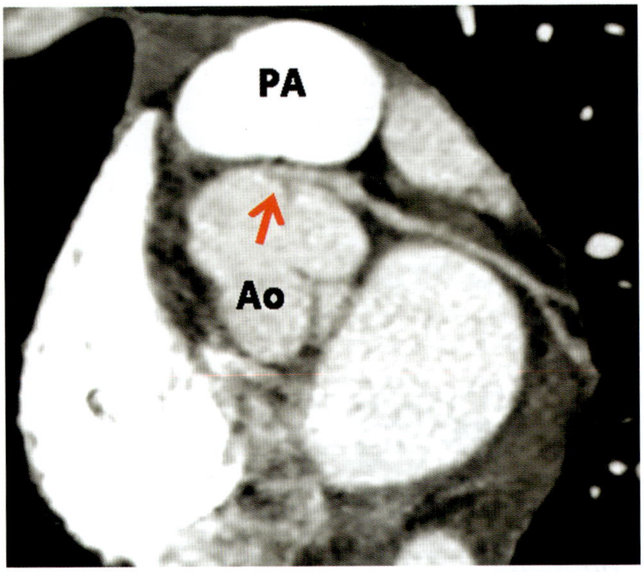

Fig. 2.10: CT coronary angiogram showing the left main coronary artery arising from the right coronary sinus (arrow), near to the commissure. A significant length of the course is therefore interarterial and a short course is intramural at the origin. (Ao: Aorta; PA: Pulmonary artery).

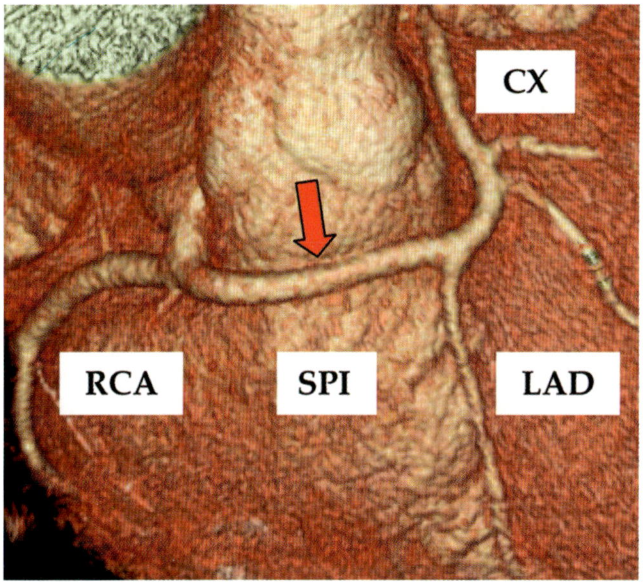

Fig. 2.11: Three-dimensional volume-rendered reconstruction of computed tomography showing an ectopic origin of the left main coronary artery (arrow) arising from the right coronary artery (RCA) with an ectopic course coursing on the subpulmonary infundibulum (SPI). [Image and legend text from Aubry P, Fretay XH, Calvert PA, et al. Proximal anomalous connections of coronary arteries in adults. In: Rao PS (Ed). Congenital Heart Disease—Selected Aspects. Intech; 2012. Available from http://www.intechopen.com/books/congenital-heart-disease-selected-aspects]. (Cx: Circumflex coronary artery, LAD: Left anterior descending coronary artery).

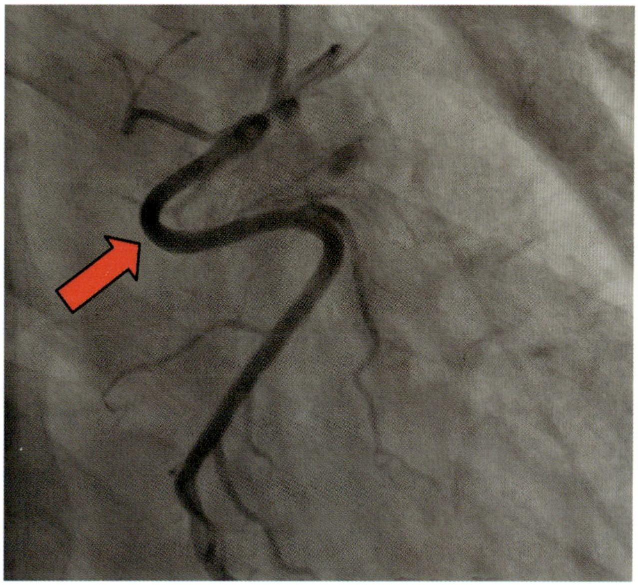

Fig. 2.12: Right anterior oblique (RA) view coronary angiogram showing a retroaortic course of an ectopic left circumflex coronary artery (arrow) arising from the right sinus. [Image from Aubry P, Fretay XH, Calvert PA, et al. Proximal anomalous connections of coronary arteries in adults. In: Rao PS (Ed). Congenital Heart Disease—Selected Aspects. Intech; 2012. Available from http://www.intechopen.com/books/congenital-heart-disease-selected-aspects].

ischemia despite multiple previous episodes of exertion is unclear. If echocardiography cannot exclude the diagnosis, further investigation is undertaken. Cardiac catheterization, CT and MRI have been shown to clearly identify the proximal course of anomalous coronary arteries. Surgery is warranted in symptomatic patients and there is general consensus that asymptomatic patients with high-risk lesions, such as intra-arterial course, ostial narrowing or an intramural segment should also undergo surgery to reduce the risk of sudden death, although patients without these features can be managed conservatively as the risk of coronary insufficiency appears low.

Left Circumflex Artery from the Right Aortic Sinus

The incidence of LCx originating from the right coronary sinus ranges from 0.15% to 0.67% in different series. The LCx usually courses behind the aortic root (Figs. 2.12 to 2.14) and this finding has not been associated with a risk of sudden death.

Right Coronary Artery from the Left Aortic Sinus

Origin of the RCA from the left coronary sinus (Figs. 2.15 to 2.18) is relatively rare. The lower reported incidence of this anomaly may reflect the lower incidence of sudden cardiac death compared with aberrant origin of the LMCA. The aberrant take-off right coronary can follow any of the previously mentioned routes for the LCA. The origin and proximal-most portion of the aberrant RCA often is oblique or "slit-like" (Figs. 2.19 and 2.20). Although mechanisms for myocardial ischemia are presumably the same as for the LCA, patients very rarely complain of symptoms and presentation with sudden cardiac death is extremely unusual, but not unheard of.

Separate Ostia

Infrequently, there is no true LMCA, and the LAD and left circumflex arteries arise from separate ostia from the left coronary sinus (Fig. 2.21). While this finding

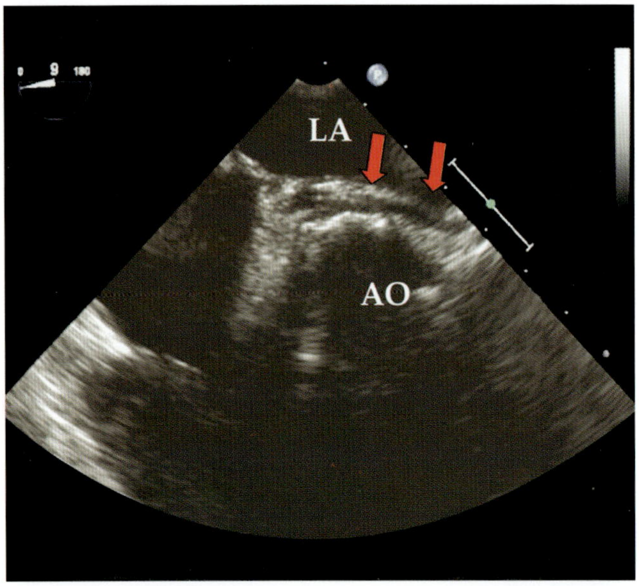

Fig. 2.13: Short-axis transesophageal echocardiogram showing an ectopic left circumflex artery (arrows) taking a retroaortic course and coursing between the left aorta (Ao) and the left atrium (LA). (Image and legend text from Aubry P, Fretay XH, Calvert PA, et al. Proximal anomalous connections of coronary arteries in adults. In: Rao PS (Ed). Congenital Heart Disease—Selected Aspects. Intech; 2012. Available from http://www.intechopen.com/books/congenital-heart-disease-selected-aspects).

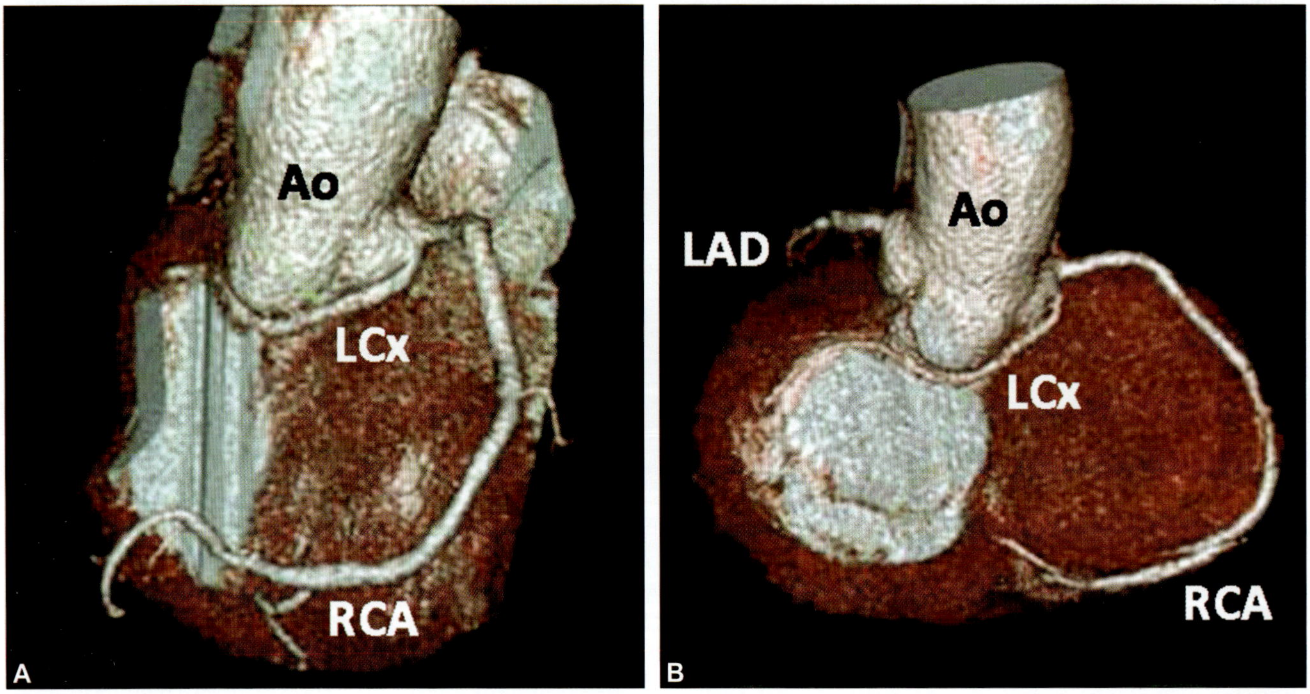

Figs. 2.14A and B: Volume rendered cardiac CT images demonstrating the left circumflex artery (LCx) originating from the right coronary sinus. [Image from Shabestari AA, Akhlaghpoor S, Tayebivaljozi R, et al. Prevalence of congenital coronary artery anomalies and variants in 2697 consecutive patients using 64-detector row coronary CT angiography. Iran J Radiol. 2012;9(3):111-21]. (Ao) Aorta; RCA: Right coronary artery; LAD: Left anterior descending artery).

may make angiography of the arteries more challenging, this is considered a benign finding. Similarly, in a small percentage of patients, there may be separate ostia for the RCA proper and the conus branch.

Single Coronary Artery

An extremely uncommon finding is that of a single coronary artery (Fig. 2.22). Single coronary arteries may originate from either the left or right coronary sinus.

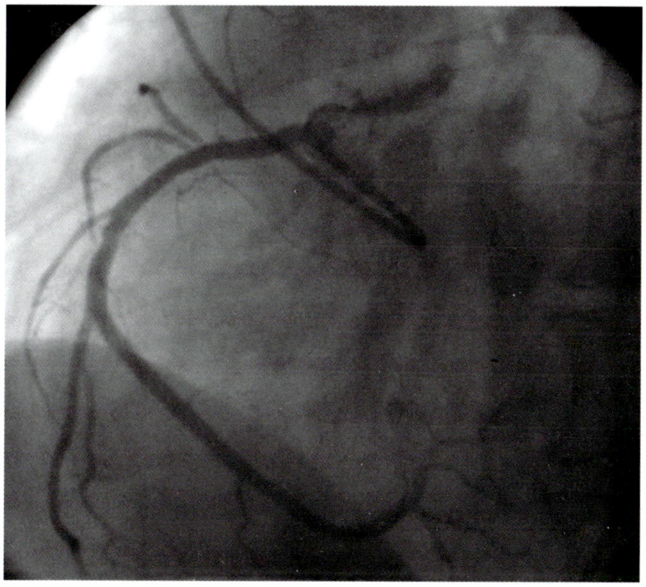

Fig. 2.15: Left anterior oblique angiogram of an anomalous right coronary artery originating from the left sinus of Valsalva and with an interatrial course. (Image from Qin X, Xiong W, Guan E, et al. Coronary anomaly: anomalous right coronary artery originates from the left sinus of Valsalva and coursing between the pulmonary artery and aorta. Clin Interv Aging. 2013;8:1217-20).

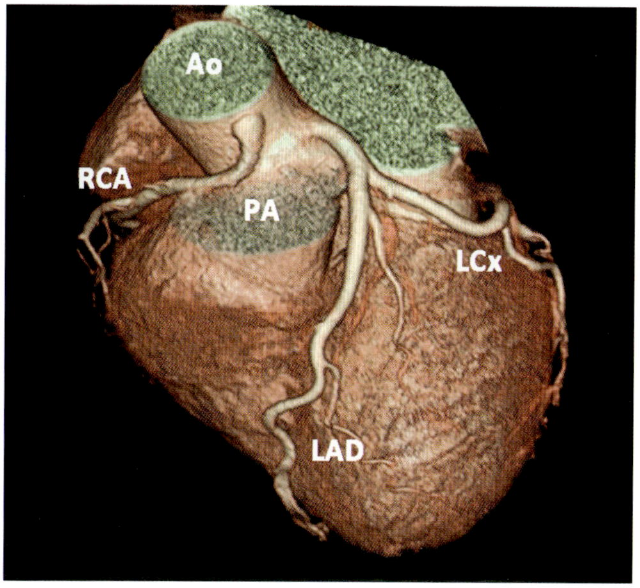

Fig. 2.16: Anomalous and high takeoff of the right coronary artery (RCA) above the sinotubular junction, with an interatrial course between the aorta (Ao) and pulmonary artery (PA). (Image from Oyama-Manabe N, Sugaya T, Yamaguchi T, et al. Non-coronary cardiac findings and pitfalls in coronary computed tomography angiography. J Clin Imaging Sci. 2011;1:51). (LAD: Left anterior descending artery; LCx: Left circumflex artery).

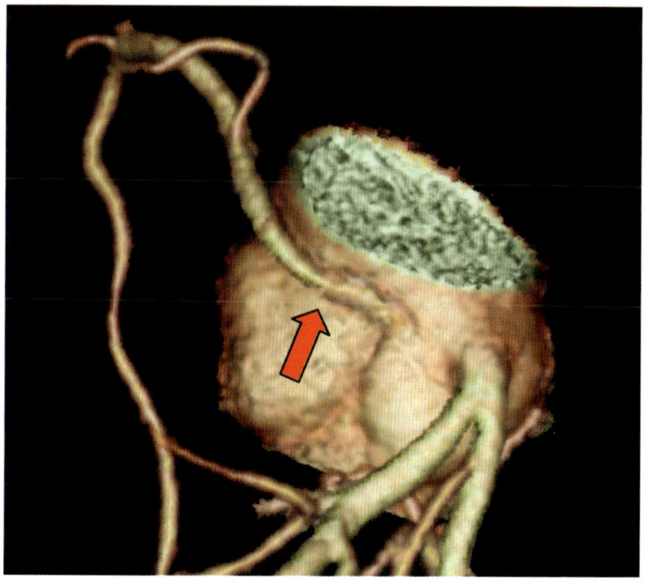

Fig. 2.17: Volume-rendered computed tomography images of an ectopic right coronary artery arising from the left sinus (arrow) with a preaortic course tangential to the aorta. (Image and legend textfrom Aubry P, Fretay XH, Calvert PA, et al. Proximal anomalous connections of coronary arteries in adults. In: Rao PS (Ed). Congenital Heart Disease—Selected Aspects. Intech; 2012. Available from http://www.intechopen.com/books/congenital-heart-disease-selected-aspects).

Abnormalities of Course and Origin

Although it is possible for any of the major coronary arteries to arise from the main pulmonary trunk or one of the branch pulmonary arteries; the classical and most frequently encountered variation is the anomalous left coronary artery from the pulmonary artery (ALCAPA) (Figs. 2.23 to 2.26). Usually the anomalous origin is from the right posterior pulmonary sinus, although it may arise from any position on the main pulmonary artery trunk or from either pulmonary arterial branch. Pathophysiology and presentation depend on the pattern of blood flow in the vessel, which is in turn dependent on the relative pressure in the pulmonary artery and the aorta. The high pulmonary vascular resistance (PVR) of the neonatal period usually ensures sufficient antegrade perfusion (albeit with desaturated blood) to prevent early ischemia. As the PVR falls, so does the coronary perfusion pressure, causing myocardial perfusion to become more dependent on collateralization from the RCA. The rate of change in these physiological parameters determines the stage at which chronic ischemia and resultant ventricular dysfunction produce clinical symptoms. This can be at any

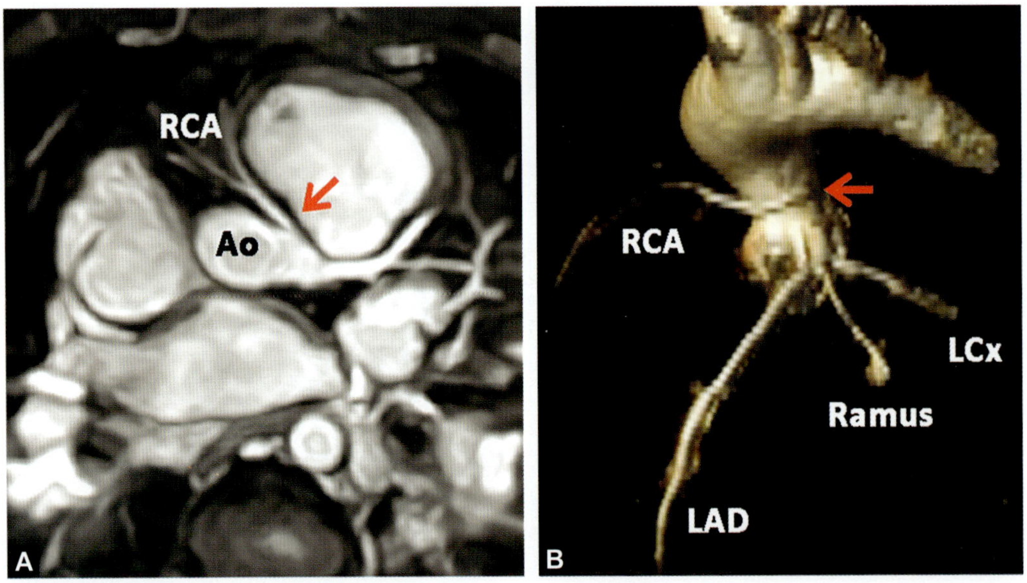

Figs. 2.18A and B: Cardiac MRI images demonstrating origin of the right coronary artery (RCA) (arrows) from a high position of the left aortic sinus. [Image from Hayes N, Qureshi S. Congenital coronary artery anomalies. In: Vijayalakshmi IB, P Syamasundar Rao, Reema Chugh (Eds). Comprehensive Approach to Congenital Heart Disease. New Delhi, India: Jaypee Brothers Medical Publishers (P) Ltd. 2013]. (Ao: Aorta; LAD: Left anterior descending artery; LCx: Left circumflex artery).

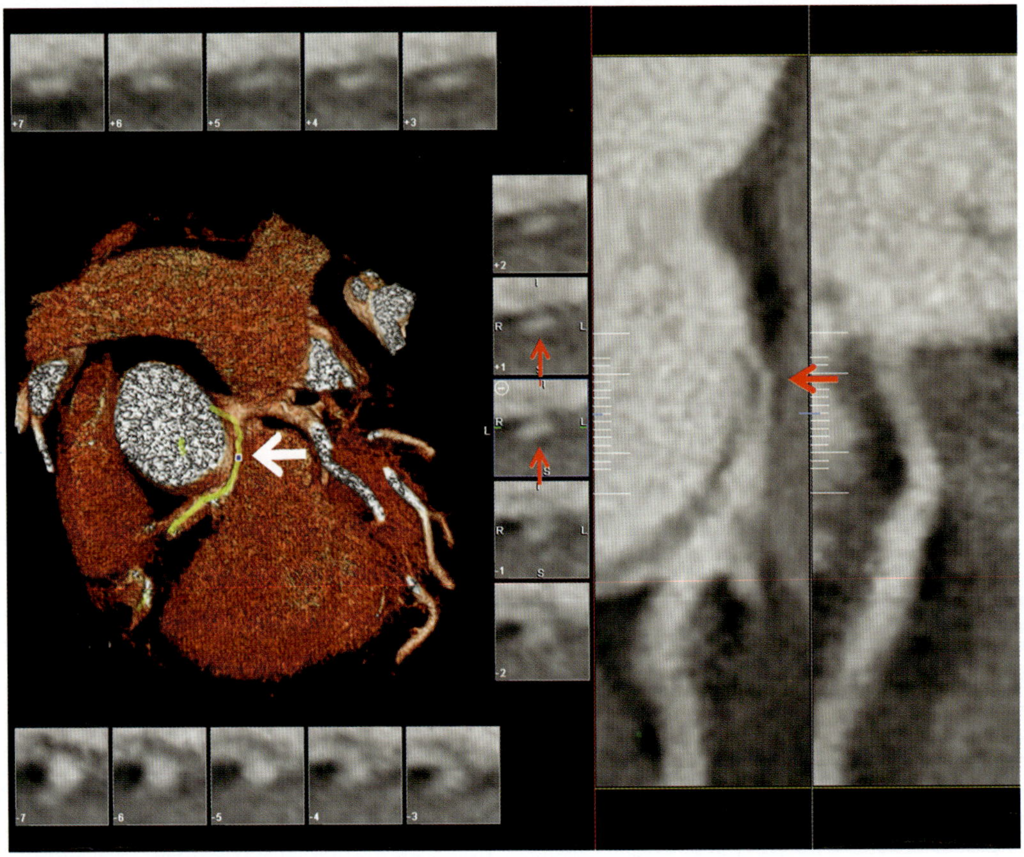

Fig. 2.19: Cardiac CT imaging and analysis of an aberrant right coronary artery (RCA). Left panel shows a 3D volume-rendered analysis, demonstrating anomalous takeoff of the RCA from the left coronary sinus. The path of the RCA is traced with the green line. The ostial and proximal-most portions (red arrows) of the RCA are markedly oblique and "slit-like". The white arrow shows the area of interrogation that corresponds to the red arrows. (Image courtesy of Glenn N Levine).

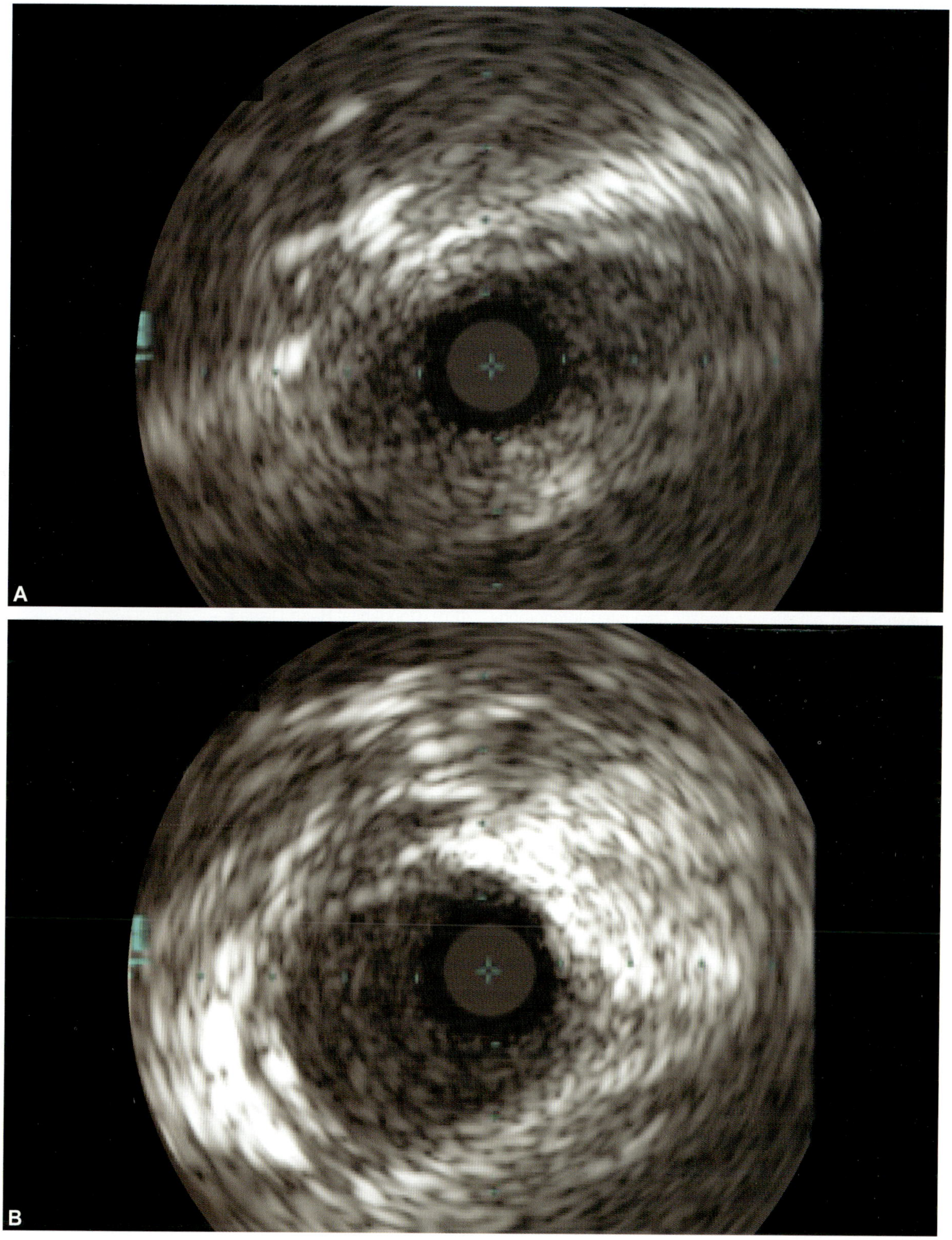

Figs. 2.20A and B: Intravascular ultrasound (IVUS) of a right coronary artery originating from the left coronary sinus. (A) Note how there is an abnormal shape of the intramural segment resulting from a shared media with the aorta, as well as probable incomplete growth of the ectopic vessel in the aortic wall; (B) The extramural segment of the RCA appears normal in shape. [Image and legend text adapted from Aubry P, Fretay XH, Calvert PA, et al. Proximal anomalous connections of coronary arteries in adults. In: Rao PS (Ed). Congenital Heart Disease—Selected Aspects. Intech; 2012. Available from http://www.intechopen.com/books/congenital-heart-disease-selected-aspects].

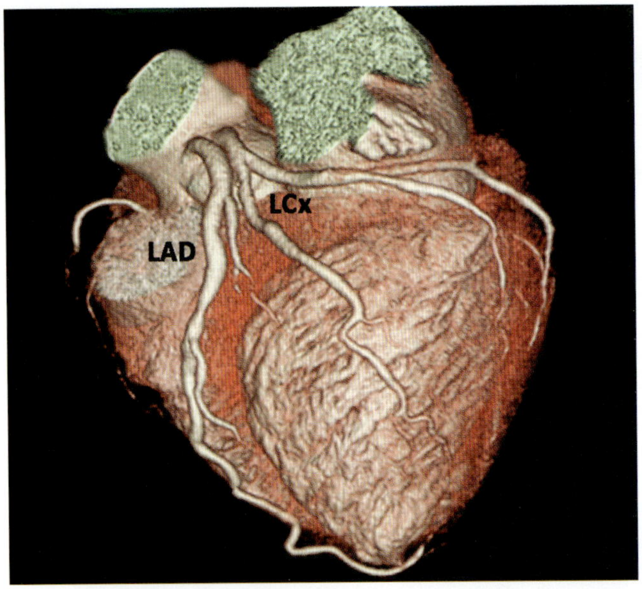

Fig. 2.21: Volume rendered CT angiogram demonstrating separate origins from the left coronary sinus of the left anterior descending (LAD) and left circumflex (LCx) arteries. This finding is considered a normal variant. While it may make coronary angiography more challenging, it is not considered a pathological finding. (Image from Oyama-Manabe N, Sugaya T, Yamaguchi T, et al. Non-coronary cardiac findings and pitfalls in coronary computed tomography angiography. J Clin Imaging Sci. 2011;1:51).

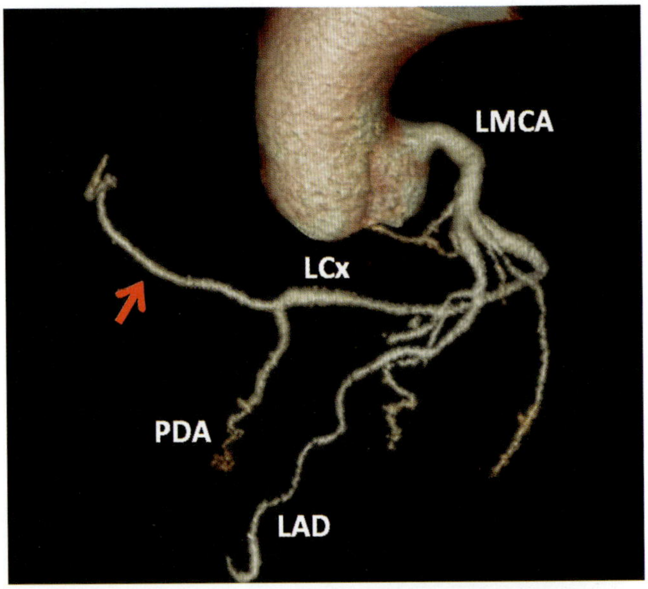

Fig. 2.22: Volume rendered cardiac CT angiogram demonstrating a single coronary artery. Note that the left circumflex artery (LCx) gives off the posterior descending artery (PDA) and then continues into the territory (arrow) normally supplied by the right coronary artery. [Image from Aubry P, Fretay XH, Calvert PA, et al. Proximal anomalous connections of coronary arteries in adults. In: Rao PS (Ed). Congenital Heart Disease—Selected Aspects. Intech; 2012. Available from http://www.intechopen.com/books/congenital-heart-disease-selected-aspects]. (LAD: Left anterior descending artery; LMCA: Left main coronary artery).

stage from infancy to adulthood, and is not infrequently discovered due to an incidental finding of ischemia on an electrocardiogram (Fig. 2.27) or echocardiographic finding of dilated cardiomyopathy with echogenic papillary muscles (Fig. 2.28). Currently, for treatment, most centers choose to re-implant the coronary artery into the aorta to improve ventricular function, even in the absence of signs of reversible ischemia.

A rarer finding than ALCAPA is anomalous right coronary artery from the pulmonary artery (ARCAPA) (Figs. 2.29A to C).

Abnormalities of Intrinsic Coronary Arterial Anatomy

Left Main Coronary Artery Atresia

A rare condition where the left coronary ostium and LMCA are absent (sometimes a remnant fibrous cord is present) with the distal left coronary system filling via collateral flow from the RCA. As with ALCAPA, patients can present in infancy with critical myocardial ischemia, although perhaps due to the lack of pulmonary artery "steal", a much larger proportion of patients may present in later childhood or adulthood with symptoms of myocardial ischemia or occasionally sudden death. Surgical therapy generally consists of internal mammary artery bypass grafting. A less severe form of this is congenital ostial stenosis and hypoplasia of the proximal LCA.

Myocardial Bridging

A myocardial bridge is formed when an area of myocardial muscle overlies a major epicardial coronary artery, producing a tunneled intramyocardial segment of coronary artery (Fig. 2.30). Myocardial bridges are present in approximately one-third of adults, and are reported even more frequently in patients with hypertrophic obstructive cardiomyopathy. The muscle bridge contracts during ventricular systole causing coronary compression (Figs. 2.31A and B and Video 2.1) and reduced coronary flow. Angina, myocardial ischemia, exercise induced

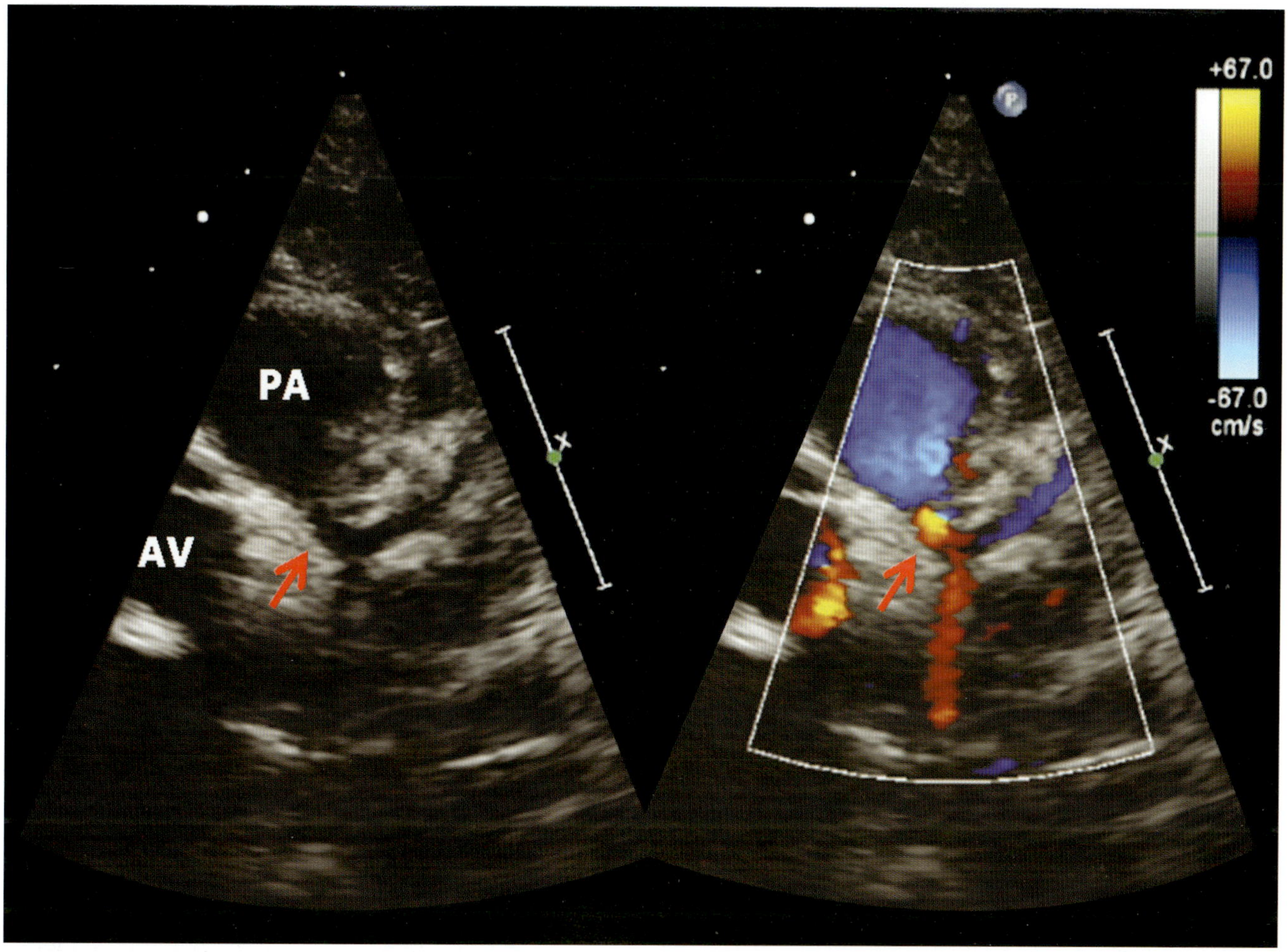

Fig. 2.23: Echocardiogram in parasternal short axis demonstrating the connection of the left coronary artery to the pulmonary artery (PA), with retrograde flow from the coronary artery into the pulmonary artery noted on color flow mapping. [Image from Hayes N, Qureshi S. Congenital coronary artery anomalies. In: Vijayalakshmi IB, P Syamasundar Rao, Reema Chugh (Eds). Comprehensive Approach to Congenital Heart Disease. New Delhi, India: Jaypee Brothers Medical Publishers (P) Ltd. 2013]. (AV: Aortic valve).

arrhythmia and sudden death have all been reported. Medical therapy with beta-blockers or calcium antagonists is used as the first line, although nitrates should be avoided as they may worsen symptoms. Surgical myotomy is reserved for patients with objective evidence of regional ischemia refractive to medical therapy.

Abnormalities of Coronary Termination

Coronary Artery Fistulas

Coronary artery fistulas (Figs. 2.32 to 2.36) are abnormal direct vascular communications between the coronary arteries and cardiac chambers (coronary-cameral fistulas), major veins (coronary-arteriovenous fistulas) or pulmonary arteries (coronary-pulmonary fistulas) with a reported prevalence of 0.13–0.22%. Clinical symptoms depend on the degree of shunting, coronary anatomy and the site of drainage. Presentation may be in infancy with congestive cardiac failure, but most pediatric presentations are with asymptomatic incidental murmurs, classically continuous and louder in diastole. Symptomatic presentation with cardiac symptoms including arrhythmia and myocardial ischemia may be more common in young adults.

Treatment depends on the age of the patient, the size of the fistula and the degree of symptoms. Elective closure of medium to large asymptomatic fistulas should be considered and is usually undertaken via a percutaneous transcatheter route.

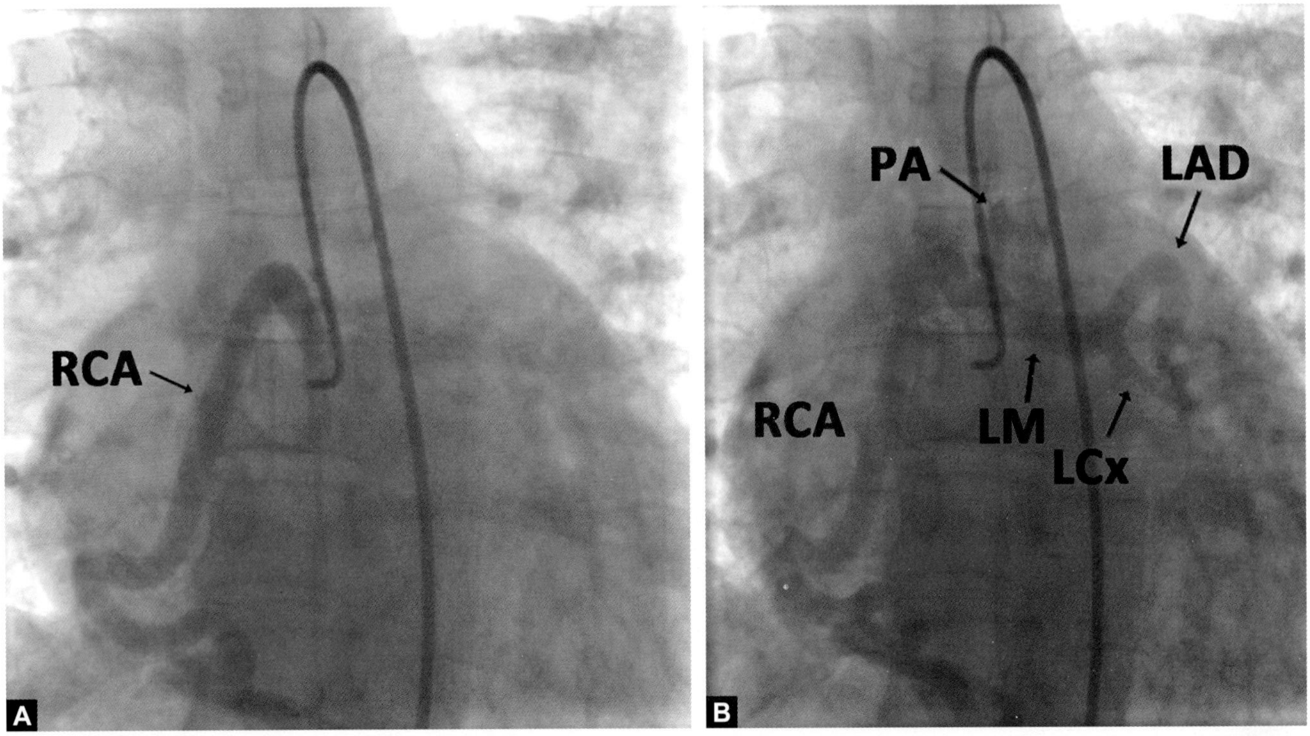

Figs. 2.24A and B: Coronary angiogram in a patient with ALCAPA. Selective injection of the right coronary artery demonstrates a markedly dilated right coronary artery (RCA). Late filling of same injection demonstrates collateral flow to the entire left coronary artery circulation. [Image from Separham A, Aliakbarzadeh P. Anomalous left coronary artery from the pulmonary artery presenting with aborted sudden death in an octogenarian: a case report. J Med Case Rep. 2012;6(1):12]. (PA: Pulmonary artery; LAD: Left anterior descending artery; LCx: Left circumflex artery; LM: Left mainstem).

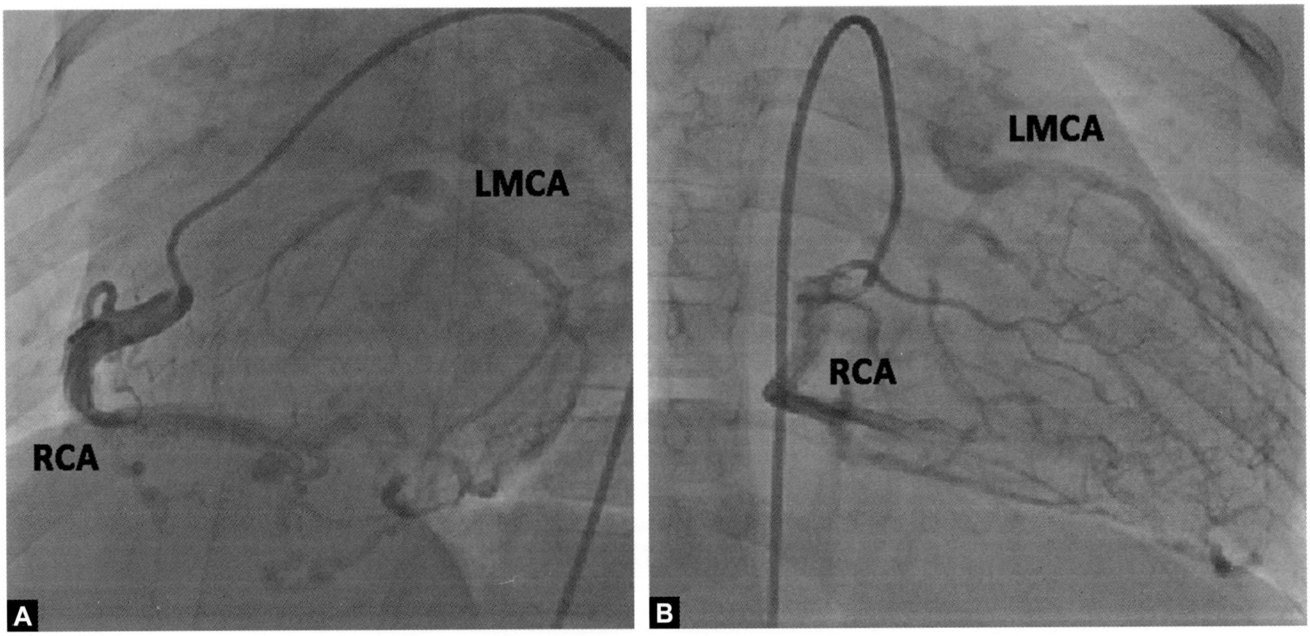

Figs. 2.25A and B: Coronary angiogram in ALCAPA. Selective injection of the right coronary artery (RCA) shows a dilated RCA collateralizing the left coronary circulation. Contrast fills the left main coronary artery (LMCA) retrograde, and a small amount of contrast can be seen entering the pulmonary artery. [Image from Amuthan V, Janarthanan RA, Balasubramanian S, et al. Anomalous origin of left coronary artery from pulmonary artery. In: Amuthan V (Ed). Manual of 3D Echocardiography. New Delhi, India: Jaypee Brothers Medical Publishers (P) Ltd. 2013].

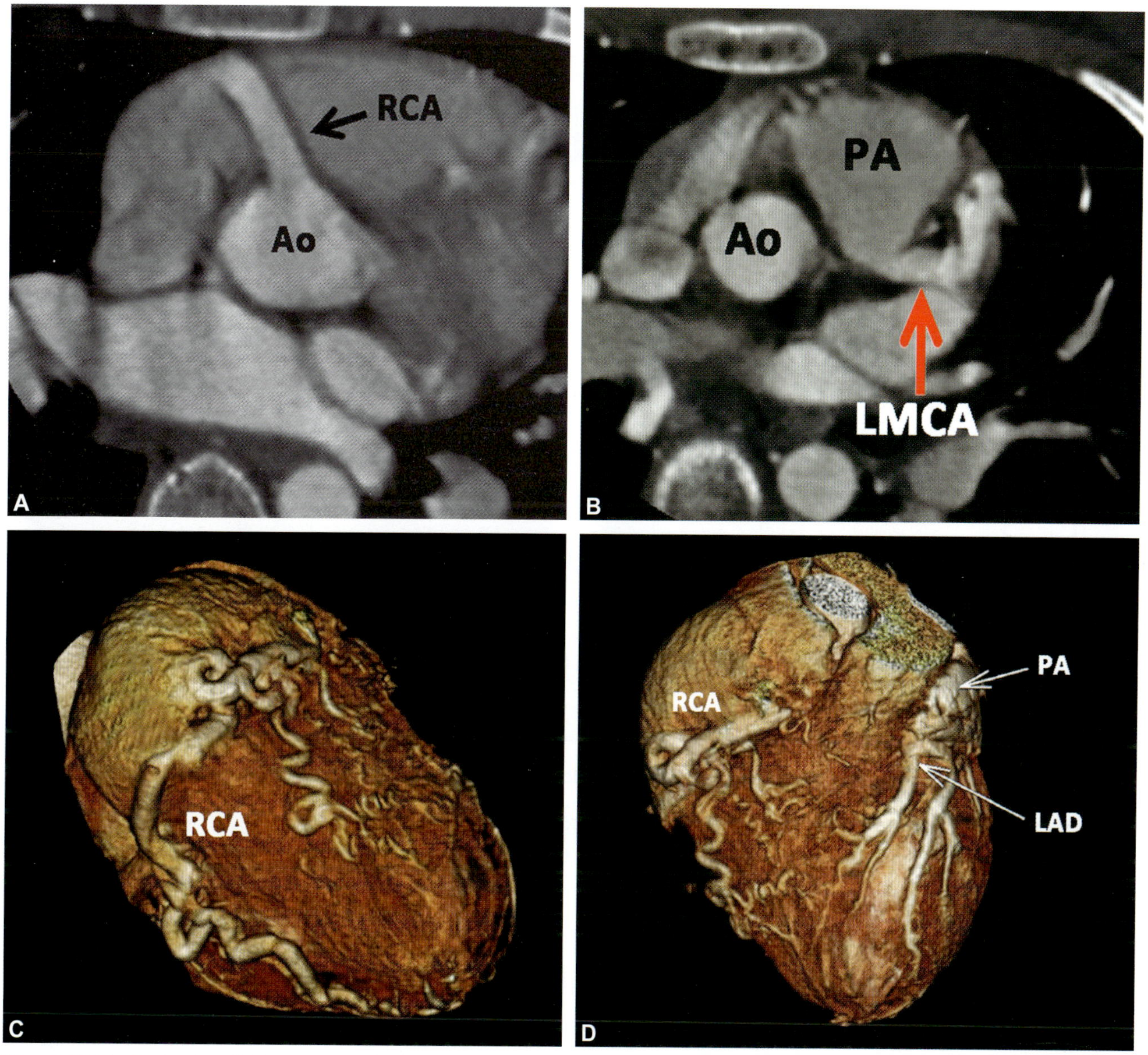

Figs. 2.26A to D: Cardiac CT images of ALCAPA. (A) Multiplanar reformatted images demonstrating a markedly dilated right coronary artery (RCA) originating from the right aortic sinus; (B) CT angiogram demonstrating the left main coronary artery (LMCA) originating from the pulmonary artery (PA) trunk; (C) Volume rendered CT angiogram showing an enormously dilated and tortuous RCA with a large number of collateral vessels; (D) CT angiogram demonstrating numerous collateral arteries from the RCA feeding the left coronary system. The left coronary system can be seen originating from the pulmonary artery. (Image and legend text from Oncel G, Oncel D. Anomalous origin of the left coronary artery from the pulmonary artery: diagnosis with CT angiography. J Clin Imaging Sci. 2013;3:4). (Ao: Aorta; LAD: Left anterior descending).

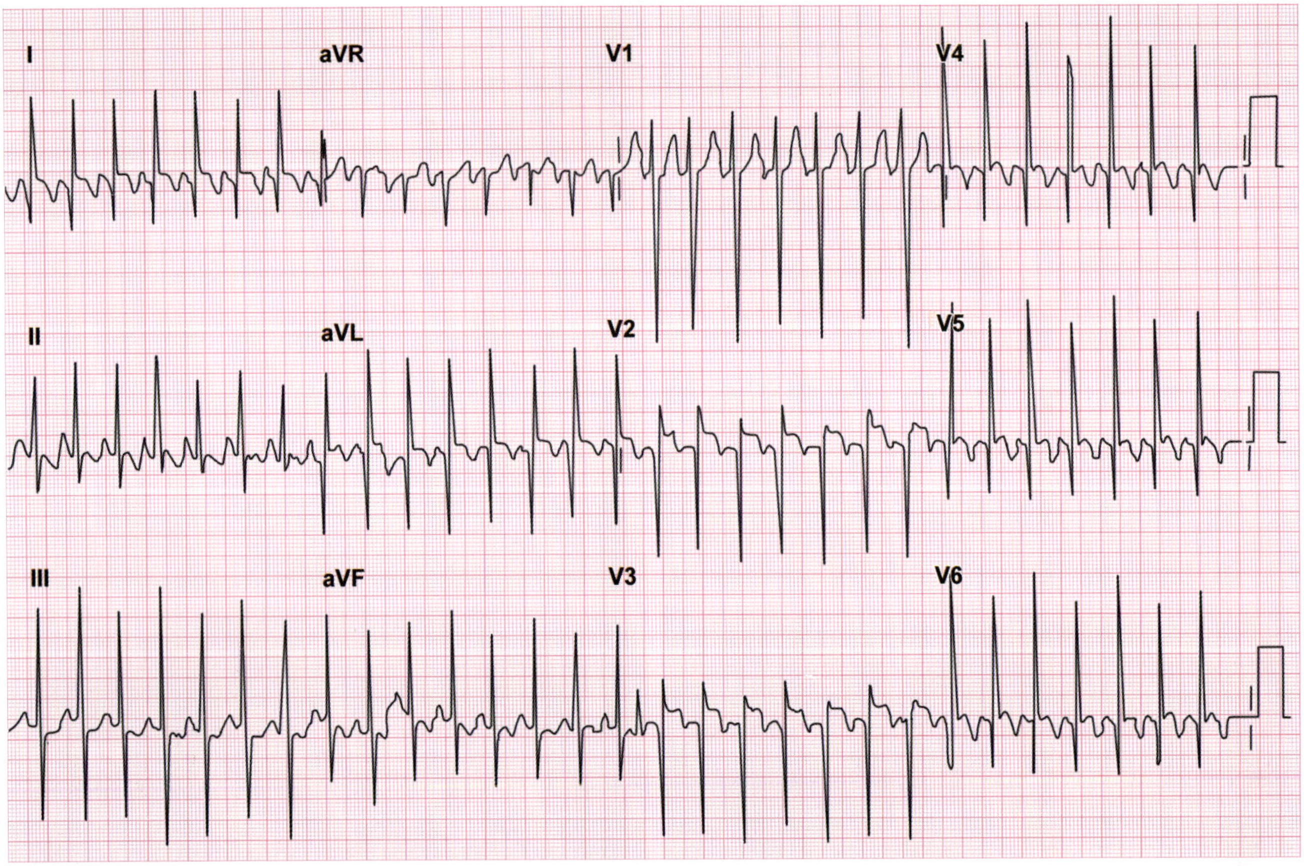

Fig. 2.27: 12 lead ECG in a 6-week-old patient with ALCAPA. Note the pathological Q waves and T wave inversion in I, aVL and V_{4-6}, along with ST elevation in V_{2-3}. The deep Q wave in aVL is nearly pathognomonic. [Image from Hayes N, Qureshi S. Congenital coronary artery anomalies. In: Vijayalakshmi IB, P Syamasundar Rao, Reema Chugh (Eds). Comprehensive Approach to Congenital Heart Disease. New Delhi, India: Jaypee Brothers Medical Publishers (P) Ltd. 2013].

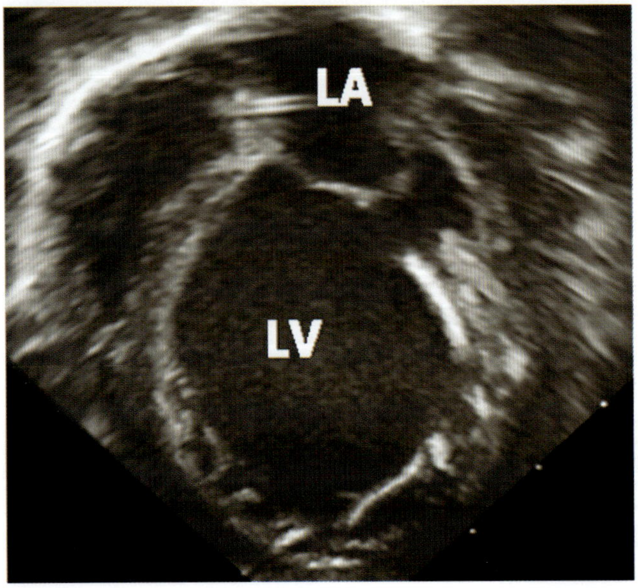

Fig. 2.28: Two-dimensional echocardiogram from the apical four chamber view in a patient with ALCAPA. The left ventricle (LV) is dilated, with severely impaired ventricular function and in particular note the highly echogenic appearance of the papillary muscles secondary to ischaemic fibrosis. A left atrium (LA) line is also seen crossing the atrial septum. [Image from Hayes N, Qureshi S. Congenital coronary artery anomalies. In: Vijayalakshmi IB, P Syamasundar Rao, Reema Chugh (Eds). Comprehensive Approach to Congenital Heart Disease. New Delhi, India: Jaypee Brothers Medical Publishers (P) Ltd. 2013].

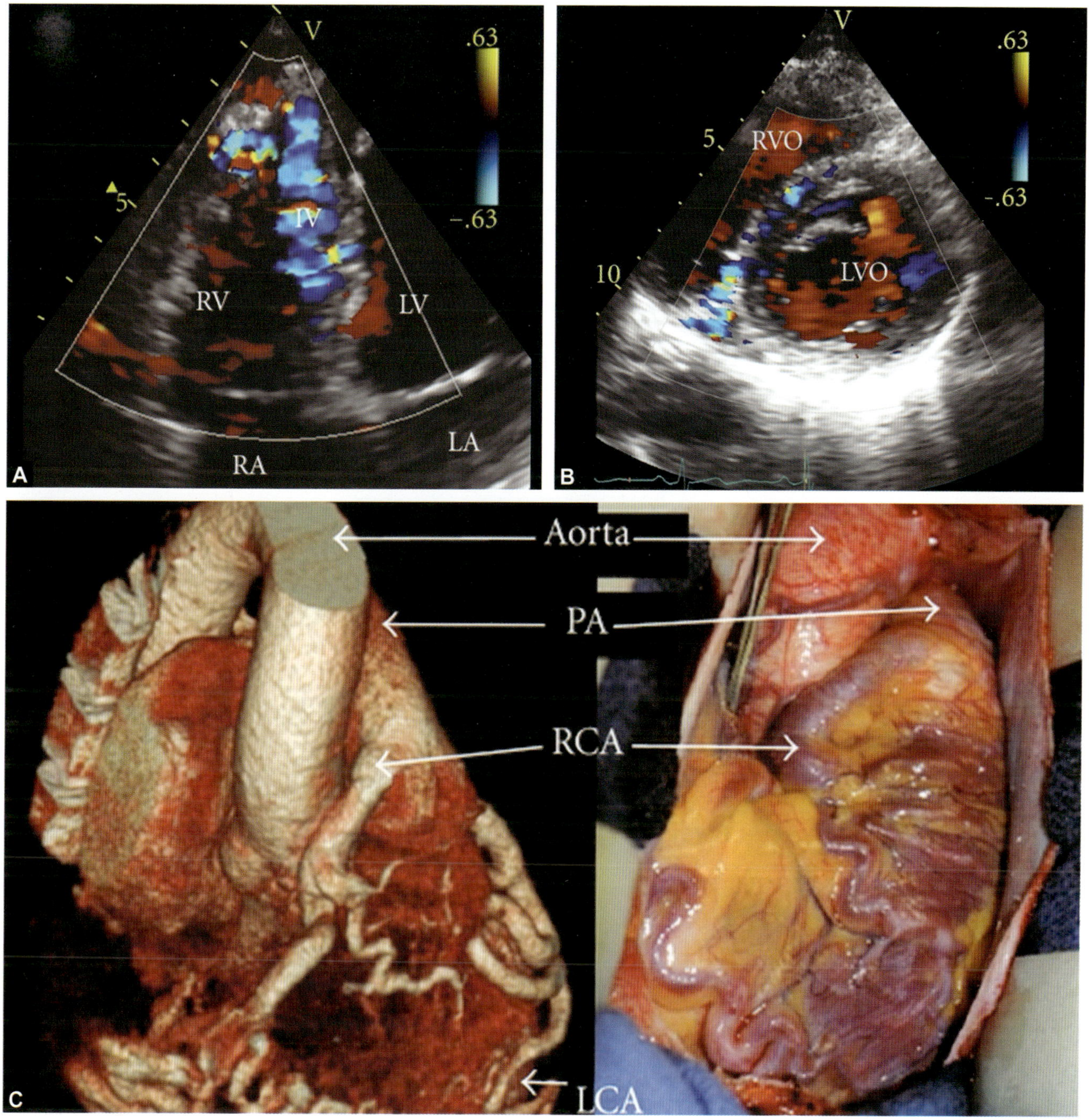

Figs. 2.29A to C: Anomalous origin of the right coronary artery from the pulmonary artery (ARCAPA). (A and B) Transthoracic color flow Doppler (A) four chamber and (B) parasternal short-axis views demonstrating markedly abnormal flow within the interventricular septum, which is due to multiple collateral vessels within the septum. (C) Three-dimensional volume rendered CT scan and intraoperative image demonstrate the right coronary artery originating from the pulmonary artery. [Image from Gilmour J, Kafka H, Ropchan G, et al. Anomalous right coronary artery: a multimodality hunt for the origin. Case Reports in Cardiology. Volume 2011(2011), Article ID 286598. Available from http://dx.doi.org/10.1155/2011/286598]. (RA: Right atrium; RV: Right ventricle; LA: Left atrium; LV: Left ventricle; RVO: Right ventricle oblique; LVO: Left ventricle oblique; PA: Pulmonary artery; RCA: Right coronary artery; LCA: Left coronary artery).

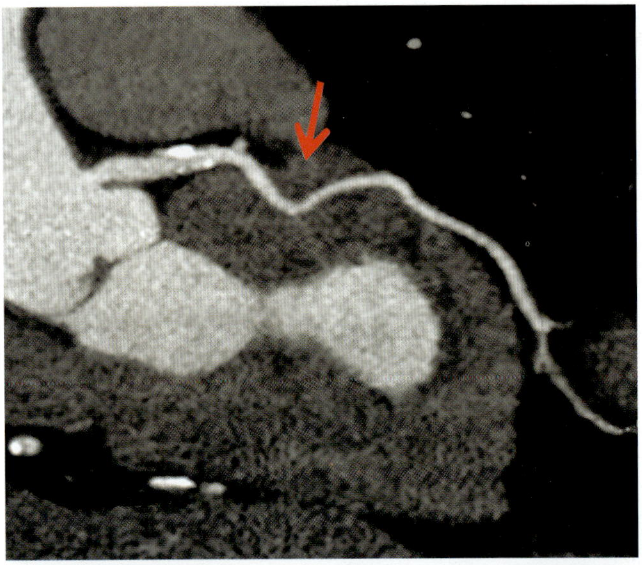

Fig. 2.30: Curved MPR cardiac CT angiogram demonstrating a dramatic coronary bridge (arrow) of the mid left anterior descending (LAD) artery. (Image from Oyama-Manabe N, Sugaya T, Yamaguchi T, et al. Non-coronary cardiac findings and pitfalls in coronary computed tomography angiography. J Clin Imaging Sci. 2011;1:51).

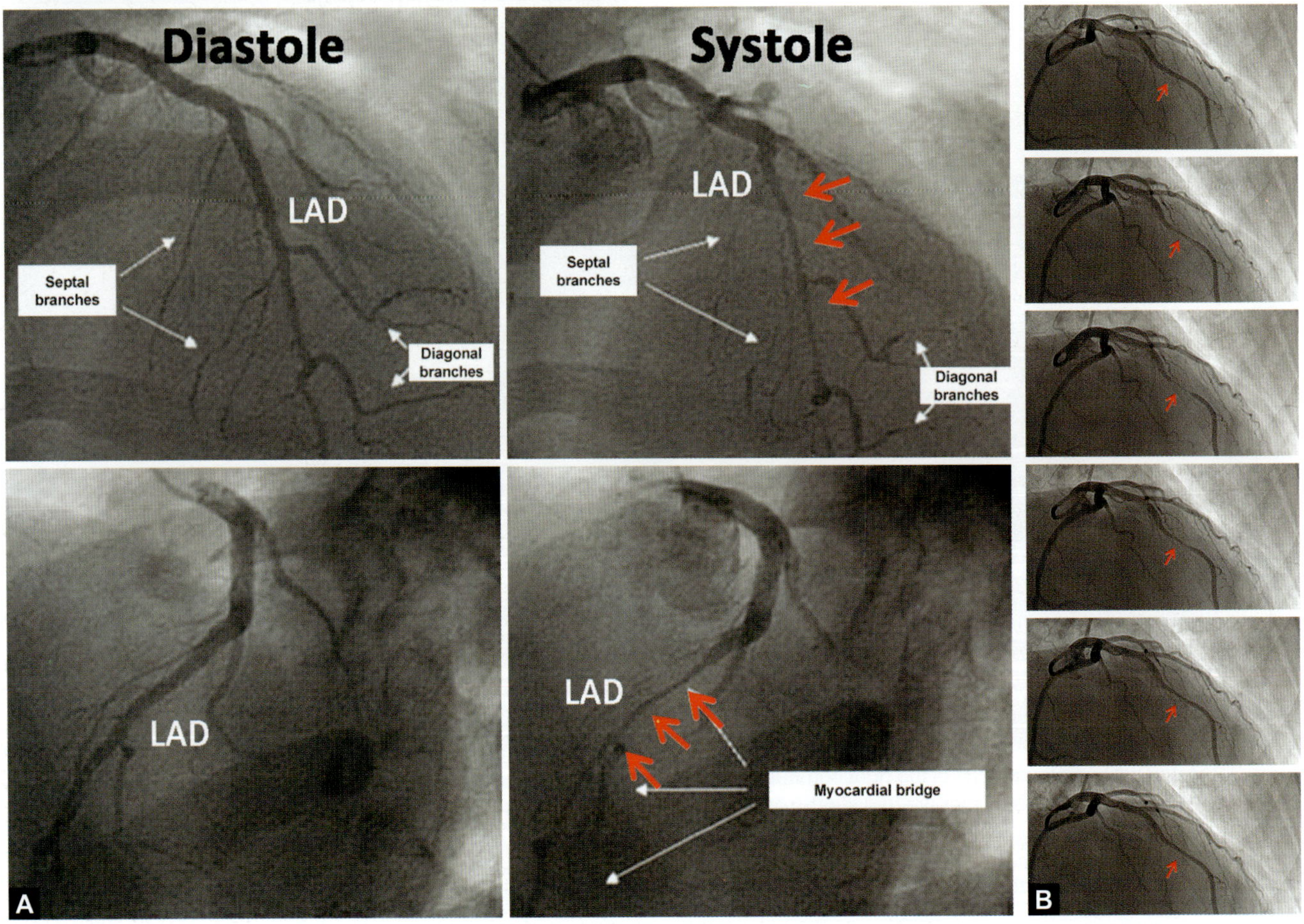

Figs. 2.31A and B: Myocardial bridge causing coronary artery compression. Images of the left anterior descending (LAD) are shown during diastole (left column) and systole (right column), obtained in the right anterior oblique (top row) and left anterior oblique (bottom row) views. Note that there is marked compression a long segment of the mid LAD during systole (red arrows). [Image from Santos Lde M, de Araújo EC, de Sousa LN. Multi-arterial myocardial bridge: uncommon clinical and anatomical presentations. Arq Bras Cardiol. 2007;88(4);e73-5]; (B) Representative cine frames over one full cardiac cycle showing dynamic compression of a mid-LAD myocardial bridge). Video 2.1 shows the corresponding cine of these still images. (Images courtesy of Glenn N Levine).

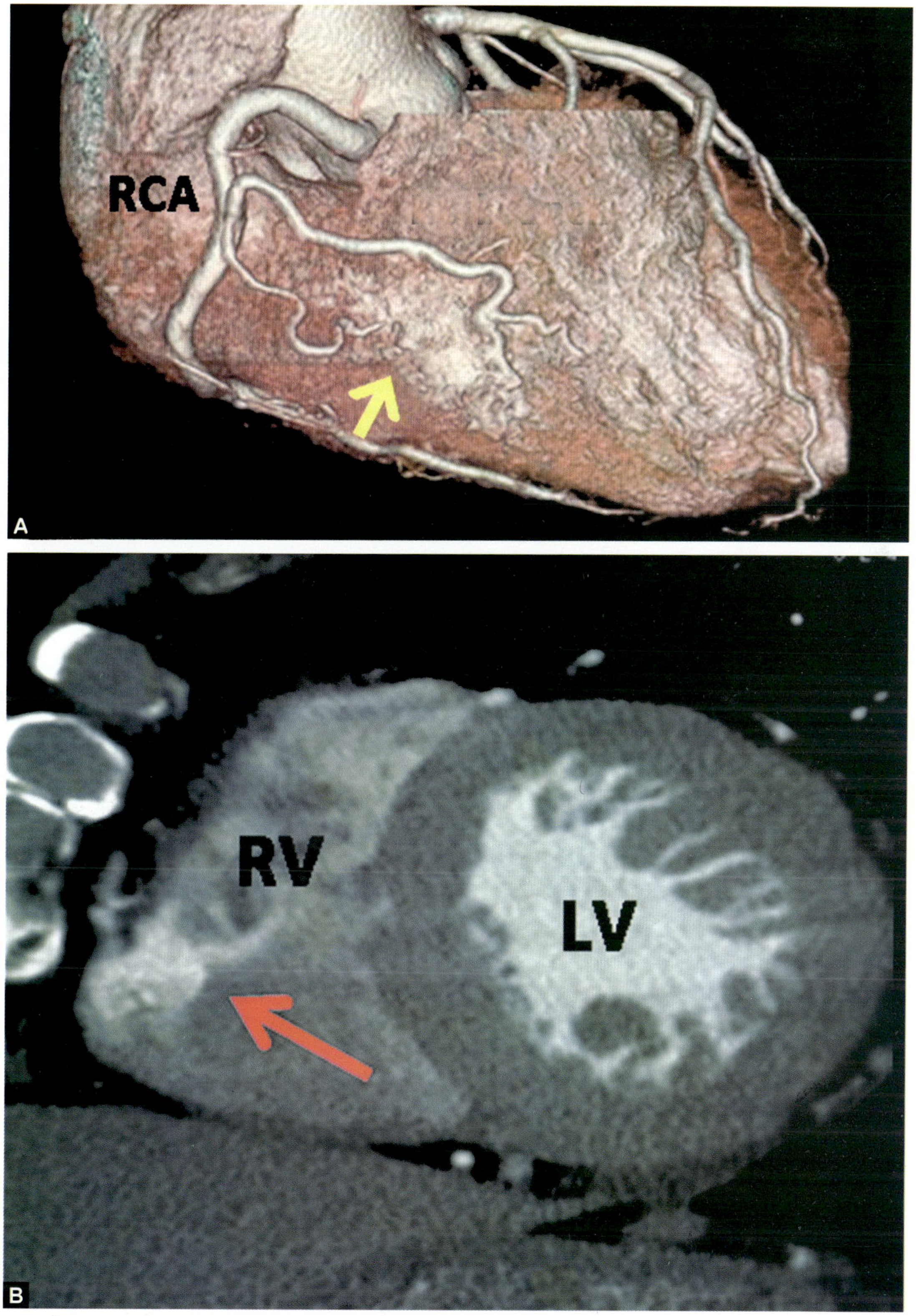

Figs. 2.32A and B: Cardiac CT image of a coronary-right ventricle (RV) fistula. (A) Volume rendered image shows a tortuous right ventricular branch (arrow) from the RCA. (B) Short-axis image of the ventricles shows contrast flow into the right ventricle, due to the RV branch-right ventricular fistula. (Image from Oyama-Manabe N, Sugaya T, Yamaguchi T, et al. Non-coronary cardiac findings and pitfalls in coronary computed tomography angiography. J Clin Imaging Sci. 2011;1:51).

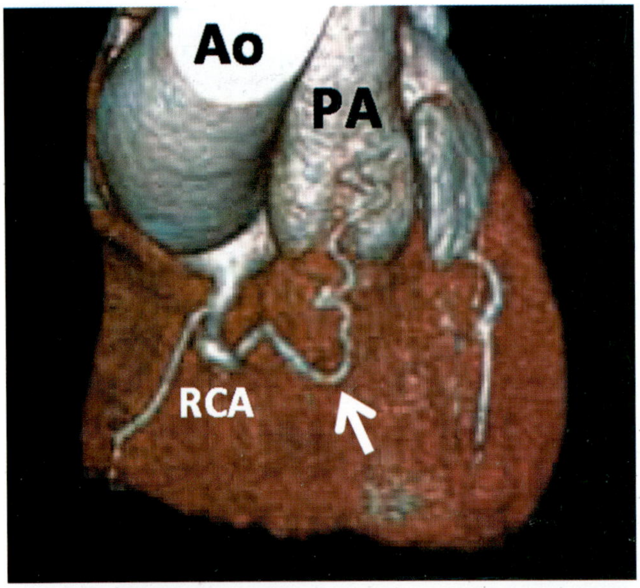

Fig. 2.33: Volume rendered CT image of a coronary-pulmonary artery fistula arising from the right coronary artery. [Image from Shabestari AA, Akhlaghpoor S, Tayebivaljozi R, et al. Prevalence of congenital coronary artery anomalies and variants in 2697 consecutive patients using 64-detector row coronary CT angiography. Iran J Radiol. 2012;9(3):111-21]. (Ao: Aorta; PA: Pulmonary artery; RCA: Right coronary artery).

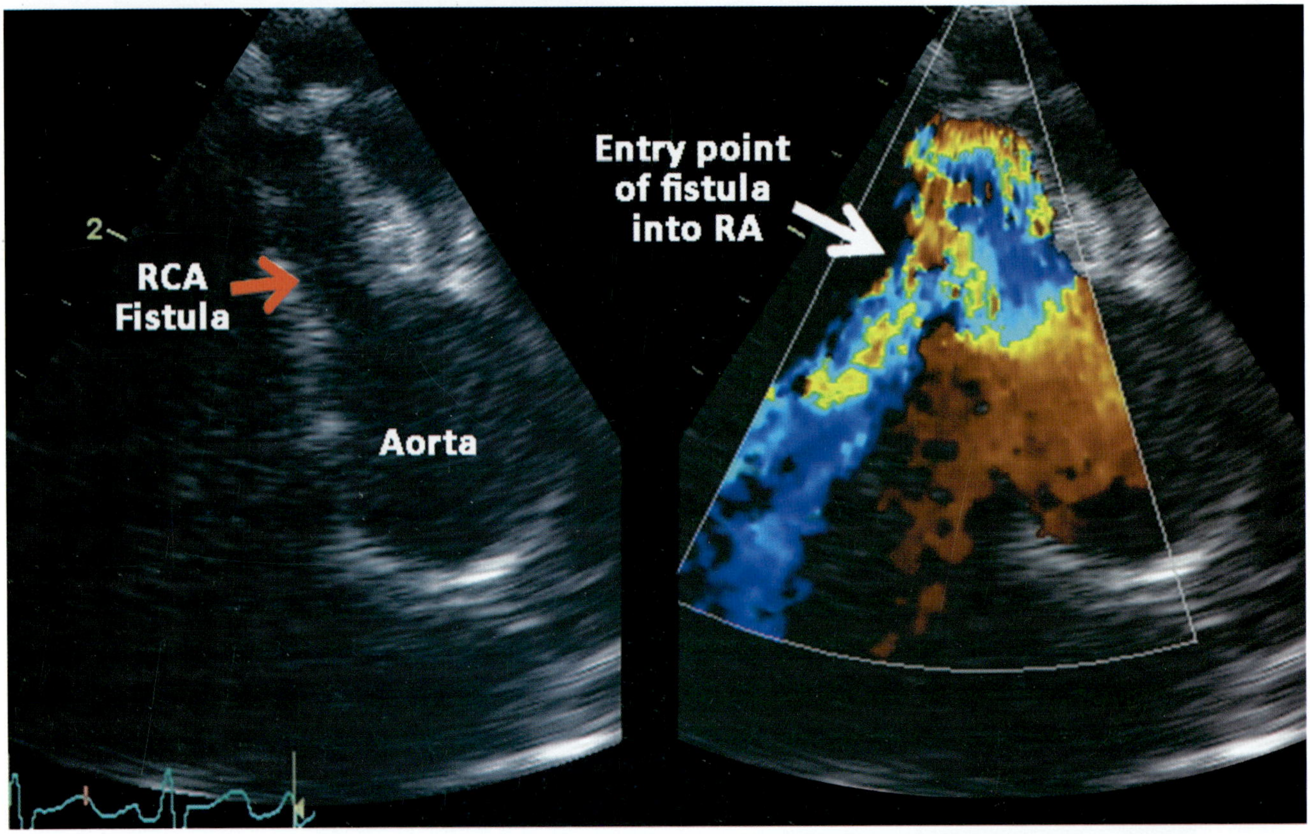

Fig. 2.34: Echocardiogram in an oblique plane demonstrating a dilated proximal right coronary artery (RCA) and large coronary fistula draining to the right atrium (RA). [Image from Hayes N, Qureshi S. Congenital coronary artery anomalies. In: Vijayalakshmi IB, P Syamasundar Rao, Reema Chugh (Eds). Comprehensive Approach to Congenital Heart Disease. New Delhi, India: Jaypee Brothers Medical Publishers (P) Ltd. 2013].

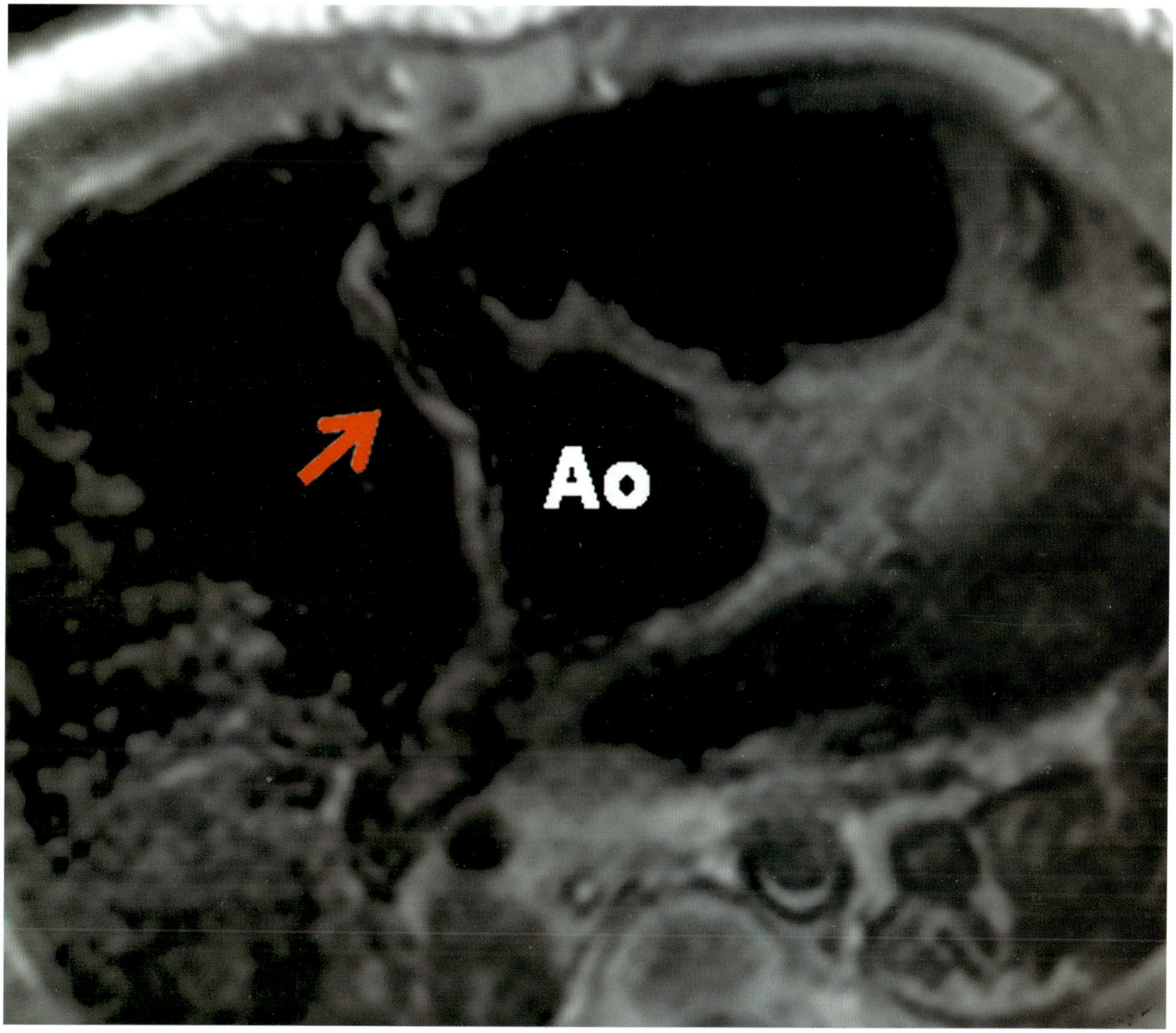

Fig. 2.35: Cardiac MRI in the same patient as Figure 2.34 confirming proximal right coronary artery dilation and fistula draining to the right atrium. [Image from Hayes N, Qureshi S. Congenital coronary artery anomalies. In: Vijayalakshmi IB, P Syamasundar Rao, Reema Chugh (Eds). Comprehensive Approach To Congenital Heart Disease. New Delhi, India: Jaypee Brothers Medical Publishers (P) Ltd. 2013]. (Ao: Aorta).

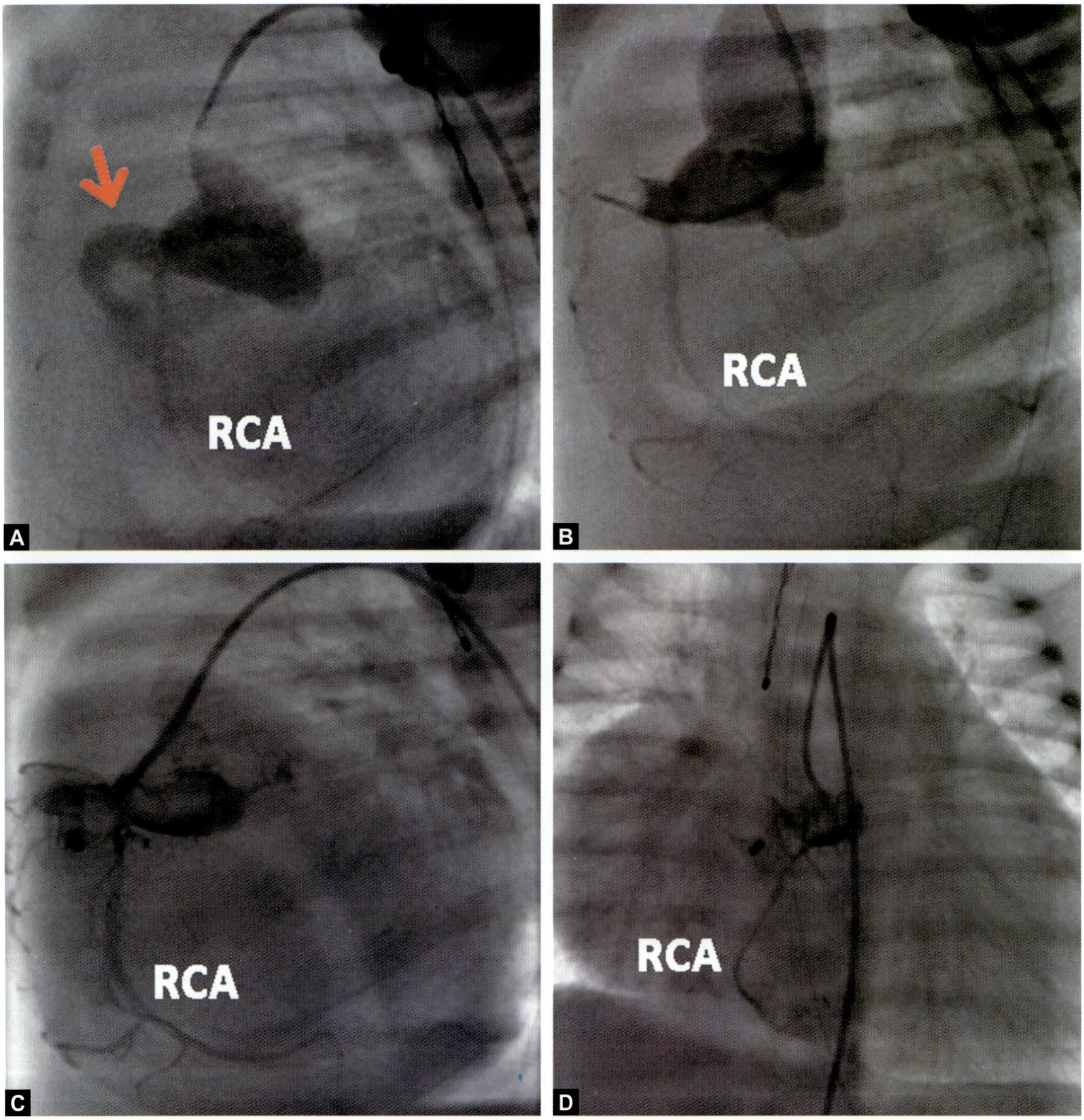

Figs. 2.36A to D: Catheter occlusion of coronary artery fistula. (A) The large fistula (arrow) is delineated on angiography from the right coronary artery (RCA) connecting to the right atrium, with the normal coronary artery seen descending at 6 o'clock. (B) Occlusion of the fistula with a wedge catheter and injection of contrast proximally further delineates the right coronary artery and confirms no important myocardial supply distal to the occlusion. (C and D) Lateral and anteroposterior projections following occlusion of the fistula with an Amplatzer muscular ventricular septal defect occlude. [Image from Hayes N, Qureshi S. Congenital coronary artery anomalies. In: Vijayalakshmi IB, P Syamasundar Rao, Reema Chugh (Eds). Comprehensive Approach to Congenital Heart Disease. New Delhi, India: Jaypee Brothers Medical Publishers (P) Ltd. 2013].

VIDEO LEGEND

Video 2.1: Angiogram of a mid left anterior descending (LAD) myocardial bridge. (Video courtesy of Glenn N Levine).

REFERENCES

Achrafi H. Hypertrophic cardiomyopathy and myocardial bridging. Int J Cardiol. 1992;37(1):111-2.

Alegria JR, Herrmann J, Holmes DR, et al. Myocardial bridging. Eur Heart J. 2005;26(12):1159-68.

Ben Ali W, Metton O, Roubertie F, et al. Anomalous origin of the left coronary artery from the pulmonary artery: late results with special attention to the mitral valve. Eur J Cardiothorac Surg. 2009;36(2):244-8.

Angelini P. Coronary artery anomalies—current clinical issues: definitions, classification, incidence, clinical relevance, and treatment guidelines. Tex Heart Inst J. 2002;29(4):271-8.

Angelini P. Normal and anomalous coronary arteries: definitions and classification. Am Heart J. 1989;117(2):418-34.

Basso C, Maron BJ, Corrado D, et al. Clinical profile of congenital coronary artery anomalies with origin from the wrong aortic sinus leading to sudden death in young competitive athletes. J Am Coll Cardiol. 2000;35(6):1493-501.

Bland EF, White PD, Garland J. Congenital anomalies of the coronary arteries: report of an unusual case associated with cardiac hypertrophy. Am Heart J. 1933;8:787-801.

Brown JW, Ruzmetov M, Parent JJ, et al. Does the degree of preoperative mitral regurgitation predict survival or the need for mitral valve repair or replacement in patients with anomalous origin of the left coronary artery from the pulmonary artery? J Thorac Cardiovasc Surg. 2008;136(3):743-8.

Driscoll DJ, Nihill MR, Mullins CE, et al. Management of symptomatic infants with anomalous origin of the left coronary artery from the pulmonary artery. Am J Cardiol. 1981;47(3):642-8.

Holzer R, Johnson R, Ciotti G, et al. Review of an institutional experience of coronary arterial fistulas in childhood set in context of review of the literature. Cardiol Young. 2004;14(4):380-5.

James TN. Anatomy of the coronary arteries. New York: Hoeber; 1961. pp. 103-6.

Knobel B, Rosman P, Kriwisky M, et al. Sudden death and cerebral anoxia in a young woman with congenital ostial stenosis of the left main coronary artery. Catheter Cardiovasc Interv. 1999;48(1):67-70.

Kottayil BP, Jayakumar K, Dharan BS, et al. Anomalous origin of left coronary artery from pulmonary artery in older children and adults: direct aortic implantation. Ann Thorac Surg. 2011;91(2):549-53.

Lange R, Vogt M, Hörer J, et al. Long-term results of repair of anomalous origin of the left coronary artery from the pulmonary artery. Ann Thorac Surg. 2007;83(4):1463-71.

Latson LA. Coronary artery fistulas: how to manage them. Catheter Cardiovasc Interv. 2007;70(1):110-6.

Liberthson RR, Sagar K, Berkoben JP, et al. Congenital coronary artery fistula. Report of 13 patients, review of the literature and delineation of management. Circulation. 1979;59(5):849-54.

Liberthson RR. Sudden death from cardiac causes in children and young adults. N Engl J Med. 1996;334(16):1039-44.

Loukas M, Groat C, Khangura R, et al. The normal and abnormal anatomy of the coronary arteries. Clin Anat. 2009;22(1):114-28.

Möhlenkamp S, Hort W, Ge J, et al. Update on myocardial bridging. Circulation. 2002;106(20):2616-22.

Morgan G, Caldarone C, Anderson R, et al. Anomalous origin of the left coronary artery from the right pulmonary artery presenting following relief of left heart obstruction: a distinct and predictable clinico-pathological syndrome. Congenit Heart Dis. 2010;5(3):327-30.

Musiani A, Cernigliaro C, Sansa M, et al. Left main coronary artery atresia: literature review and therapeutical considerations. Eur J Cardiothorac Surg. 1997;11(3):505-14.

Post JC, van Rossum AC, Bronzwaer JG, et al. Magnetic resonance angiography of anomalous coronary arteries. A new gold standard for delineating the proximal course? Circulation. 1995;92(11):3163-71.

Roberts WC, Shirani J. The four subtypes of anomalous origin of the left main coronary artery from the right aortic sinus (or from the right coronary artery). Am J Cardiol. 1992;70(1):119-21.

Said SM, Dearani JA, Burkhart HM, et al. Surgical management of congenital coronary arterial anomalies in adults. Cardiol Young. 2010;20 Suppl 3:68-85.

Satran A, Dawn B, Leesar MA. Congenital ostial left main coronary artery stenosis associated with a bicuspid aortic valve in a young woman. J Invasive Cardiol. 2006;18(3):E114-6.

Sharland GK, Tynan M, Qureshi SA. Prenatal detection and progression of right coronary artery to right ventricle fistula. Heart. 1996;76(1):79-81.

Soon KH, Chaitowitz I, Selvanayagam JB, et al. Comparison of fluoroscopic coronary angiography and multi-slice coronary angiography in the characterization of anomalous coronary artery. Int J Cardiol. 2008;130(1):96-8.

CHAPTER

3

Cardiac Stress Tests

Jothiharan Mahenthiran

INTRODUCTION

Cardiac stress testing is an important noninvasive tool for the diagnosis and prognostic risk assessment of patients with suspected or known coronary artery disease (CAD). Stress tests elicit the physiological significance of a high grade (≥70%) lumen stenosis by highlighting the mismatch between coronary blood flow (supply) and myocardial oxygen consumption (demand) as the cause of myocardial ischemia (Fig. 3.1). Since the pioneering work of Robert Arthur Bruce (Fig. 3.2), there have been a dramatic evolution in cardiac stress testing.

Common indications for stress testing are listed on Table 3.1. Cardiac stress testing is generally not indicated as part of screening asymptomatic patients except for a few select sub-groups, such as high-risk occupations (airline pilots) and CAD risk equivalent clinical status (diabetes, high coronary calcium score). Stress testing should be avoided in acutely symptomatic patients, such as those with clear rest (unstable) angina.

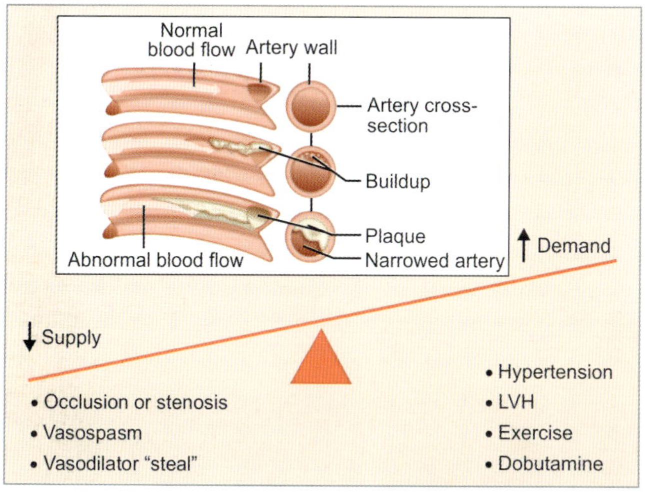

Fig. 3.1: Schematic diagram outlining the principle of stress testing and common causes of imbalance between decreased blood supply and increased myocardial oxygen demand. (LVH: Left ventricular hypertrophy).

Figure 3.3 summarizes the ischemic cascade in patient who develops myocardial ischemia. It is of note that other than frank myocardial necrosis, chest pain is the last manifestation of myocardial ischemia.

STRESS MODALITIES

Cardiac stress testing is generally performed with exercise in most patients who are able to attain adequate cardiac work load. Pharmacological agents are used as an alternate in those who cannot or unable to exercise adequately. Low level exercise can be combined with some pharmacological agents to reduce side effects. Common types of cardiac stress modalities include: symptom-limited exercise electrocardiographic stress; symptom-limited exercise ECG combined with imaging using either echocardiography (stress echo) or radionuclide myocardial perfusion imaging (stress MPI); pharmacological stress test using vasodilator stress agents (adenosine, dipyridamole or A2A receptor agonists such as regadenoson) or inotropic and/or chronotropic agents (dobutamine, dopamine) combined with stress echo or stress MPI or cardiac manetic resonance imaging (CMRI); and alternate rare forms of stress includes rapid pacing, emotional stress and cold pressor.

The choice of stress tests depends on many factors such as but not limited to: the patient's ability and willingness to exercise; resting electrocardiogram (ECG) abnormalities; body habitus; clinical indication(s) for stress testing; the need for obtaining a conclusive test (specificity, sensitivity, positive and negative predictive values); and whether there is a clinical reason to compare a current stress test result with a similar prior stress test result.

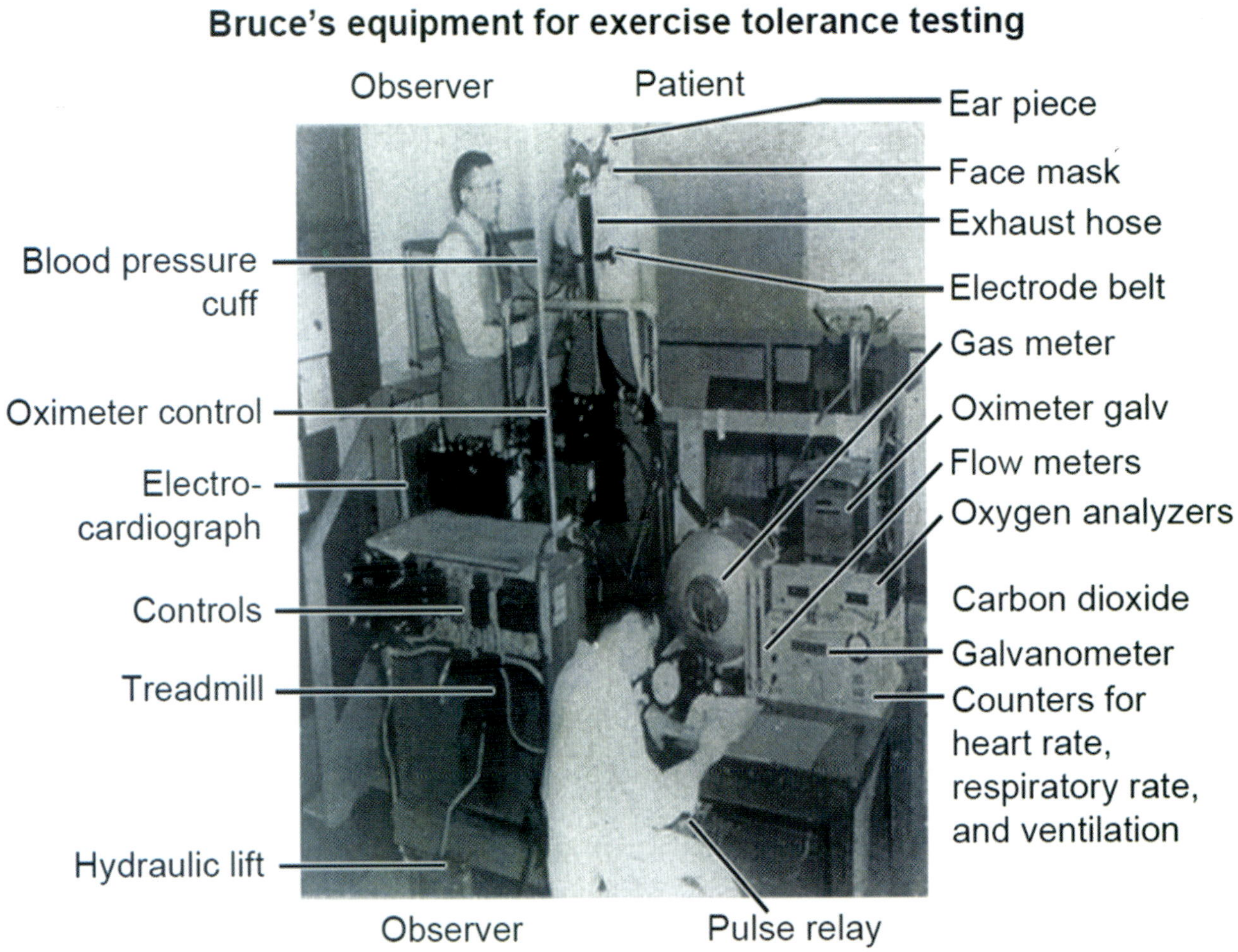

Fig. 3.2: Historic photograph of the arrangement of equipment for Bruce's method of exercise tolerance testing. While one observer remains on the treadmill platform with the patient, records blood pressure, electrocardiogram, symptoms and signs, the other observer seated at the continuous analyzer records the heart rate respiratory rate, ventilation volume, gas concentrations, and oxymeter at 1 minute intervals [Image and figure legend from Upadhyayula S, Kapur KK. History of stress echocardiography. In Chopra HK, Nanda NC (eds). Textbook of Cardiology: A Clinical & Historical Perspective. New Delhi, India: Jaypee Brothers Medical Publishers (P) Ltd.].

Table 3.1: Indications for cardiac stress testing.

• Adult patients with chest pain suspected of angina or angina equivalent symptoms, or abnormal ECG suspicious for coronary artery disease with intermediate or high pre-test probability for atherosclerotic vascular diseases based on gender, age and medical comorbidities
• Low-risk patients with unstable angina symptoms, 8–12 hours after presentation without active ischemic or heart failure signs
• Patients following myocardial infarction after > 48 hours of presentation without active ischemic symptoms or signs for active prescription, prognostic risk stratification or evaluation of medical treatment
• Patients with known CAD or prior coronary revascularization with new or worsening symptoms suggestive of coronary ischemia or heart failure
• Patients with certain valve disease for assessment of functional status, symptoms and/or hemodynamic response with exercise
• Patients with cardiomyopathy or heart failure for exclusion of ischemia, to assess functional capacity and for being considered for heart transplant (with ventilatory gas analysis)
• Prior to selected non-cardiac surgeries as part of further CAD risk stratification
• Patients with selected heart rhythm disorders, congenital heart block, exercise induced arrhythmia and to evaluate response to therapy

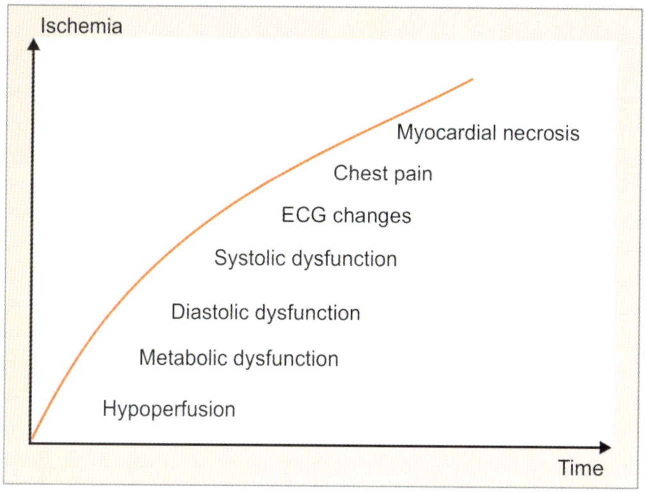

Fig. 3.3: The ischemic cascade. [Image from Lonnebakken MT, Gerdts E. Contrast echocardiography in coronary artery disease. In Baskot B (ed). Coronary Angiography—Advances in Noninvasive Imaging Approach for Evaluation of Coronary Artery Disease. Intechweb.org. CC].

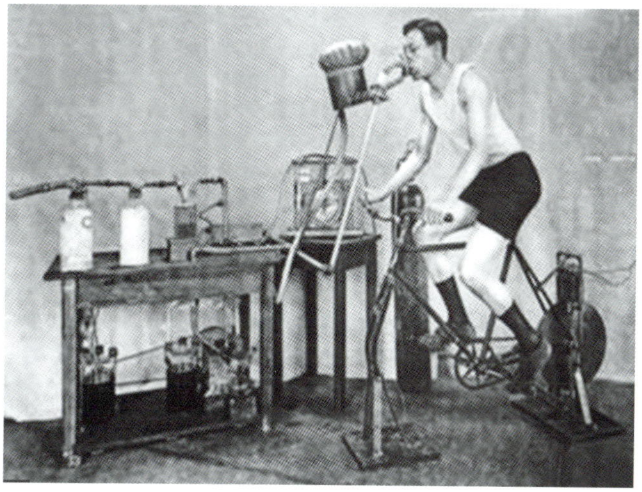

Fig. 3.4: Historic photograph of the original bicycle ergometer used in Benedict's experiments to assess exercise energy metabolism in 1919. [Image and figure legend from Upadhyayula S, Kapur KK. History of stress echocardiography. In Chopra HK, Nanda NC (eds). Textbook of Cardiology: A Clinical & Historical Perspective. New Delhi, India: Jaypee Brothers Medical Publishers (P) Ltd.].

EXERCISE STRESS TESTS

Symptom-limited exercise on a treadmill would be the preferred stress modality in most patients who are able to exercise and have a normal resting ECG. Exercise provides additional information on symptoms, hemodynamic response, rhythm abnormalities and additional incremental prognostic risk assessment. Other modes of exercise include bicycle (supine and upright) and 6-minute walk test. A cardiopulmonary stress testing combines exercise with ventilatory gas exchange analysis (Fig. 3.4). Although numerous exercise protocols have been developed and utilized over time (Fig. 3.5), the most common exercise treadmill test (ETT) protocol currently utilized is the Bruce protocol, in which treadmill elevation grade and speed increase every 3 minutes.

Maximum predicted heart rate (HR) during treadmill testing is predicted by the formula:

$$\text{Maximum Heart Rate (HR) Estimate} = 220 - \text{Age (in years)} \pm 10\text{–}12 \text{ beats/minute}$$

Estimated 85% of this maximum HR is considered diagnostic with exercise stress testing.

Metabolic equivalent (MET) as a measure of exercise capacity refers to a unit of oxygen uptake in a resting person. 1 MET is equivalent to 3.5 mL O_2/Kg/min of the body weight. Measured respiratory oxygen uptake (VO_2) in milliliter O_2/Kg/min divided by 3.5 mL O_2/Kg/min determines the number of METS. This helps to standardize exercise protocols, quantify exercise capacity, and assess prognosis.

Patients with ECG abnormalities such as complete left bundle branch block (LBBB), pre-excitation [Wolff-White Parkinson syndrome (WPW)], left ventricular hypertrophy (LVH) with ST-segment changes greater than 1 mm (0.1 mV), ST-segment depression on resting ECG, current digoxin use, and paced ventricular rhythms are considered to have conditions that preclude diagnostic interpretation of changes in the ST-segment, and should undergo a pharmacological stress exam combined with an imaging modality. A summary of the common contraindications and indications for terminating an exercise stress is listed in Tables 3.2 and 3.3, respectively.

EXERCISE STRESS ECG

The standard configuration of ECG leads during exercise stress testing is shown in Figure 3.6. Peak exercise stress ECG with the development of 1 mm (0.1 mV) or greater junctional point (J-point) depression, as compared to PQ segment as the isoelectric reference, with relatively flat ST-segment slope or 1.0 mm or more horizontal or downsloping ST depression 60–80 msec after the J-point, on three consecutive beats with a stable baseline, is

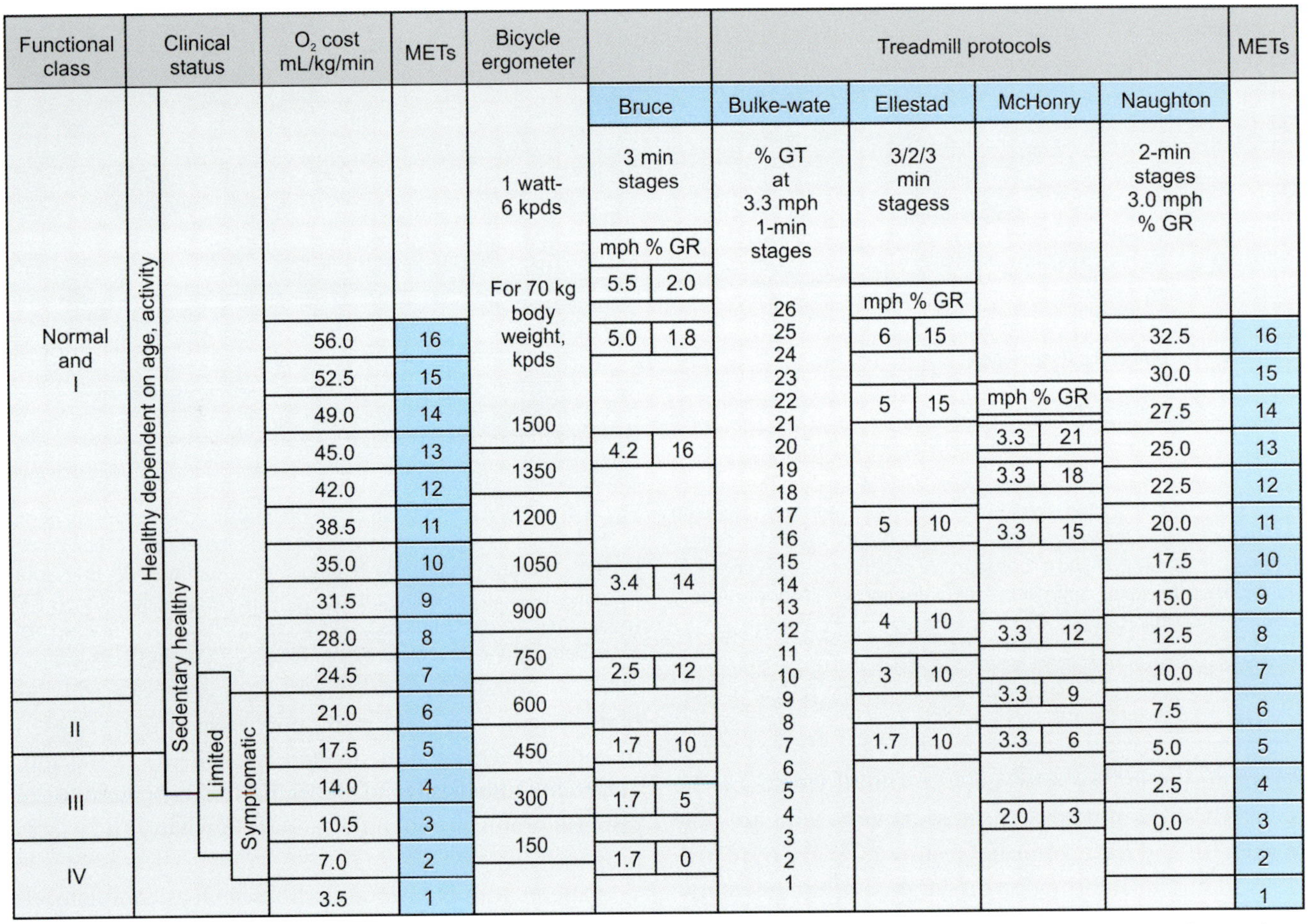

Fig. 3.5: Exercise treadmill testing protocols and their associated metabolic equivalents (METS) at different test stages. [Image from Uveroi A, Froelicher. In Chatterjee K et al. (eds). Cardiology—an Illustrated Textbook. New Delhi, India: Jaypee Brothers Medical Publishers (P) Ltd.].

Table 3.2: Contraindication to cardiac stress testing.

• Acute myocardial infarction of <2 days duration
• High-risk unstable angina
• Decompensated clinical heart failure or arrhythmia
• Advanced atrioventricular heart block
• Symptomatic severe valve disease
• Acute myocarditis or pericarditis
• Uncontrolled accelerated hypertension (>220/110 mm Hg)
• Acute systemic illness (pulmonary embolism, aortic dissection)

are contraindicated in patients with hypersensitivity to the agents, severe bronchospasm-related airway disease, sick sinus syndrome, second degree or higher degree atrioventricular block in the absence of a pacemaker, severe hypotension (systolic < 90 mm Hg), and in acute clinical syndromes as listed in Table 3.2. Several transient systemic

Table 3.3: Indications for terminating exercise testing.

• ST segment elevation (≥1.0 mm) in two contiguous leads without pathological Q-waves other than leads V1 or aVR
• Systolic blood pressure drop >20 mm Hg from baseline despite an increase in workload, especially with other evidence of coronary ischemia
• Patient's desire to stop or increasing nervous system symptoms such as ataxia or near syncope
• Exercise limiting symptoms of severe angina, fatigue or shortness of breath
• Sustained or symptomatic ventricular tachycardia, uncontrolled arrhythmia
• Technical difficulties in monitoring ECG or blood pressure
• Marked ST-segment (>2.5 mm horizontal ST depression) or marked QRS axis shift
• Accelerated hypertensive response (systolic pressure >240 mm Hg and/or diastolic pressure >115 mm Hg)

considered abnormal (Figs. 3.7 to 3.10). The J-point depression with a rapid upsloping ST-segment shift of more than 1 mm (0.1 mV) but less than 1.5 mm is considered a normal variant exercise ECG response (Fig. 3.11).

Greater ST-segment depression (>1.5 mm), early onset, greater number of leads (especially involving leads V4–V6) with ST-segment depression have the greatest diagnostic yield for myocardial ischemia. About 10% of patients would have ST-segment depression seen only during the recovery stages of exercise (Fig. 3.12). This finding has comparable diagnostic accuracy compared to ST depression occurring during exercise. Exercise induced new persistent ST-segment elevation of ≥ 1.0 mm at 60–80 msec after J-point in three consecutive beats with a stable baseline and in the absence of corresponding Q-waves (Fig. 3.13) is a specific marker of transmural ischemia due to high-grade coronary luminal stenosis or coronary spasm. ST-segment elevation in lead aVR during exercise stress testing, particularly if there is also diffuse ST-segment depression in other leads (Fig. 3.14), has been correlated with a greater incidence of significant left main and/or 3-vessel CAD.

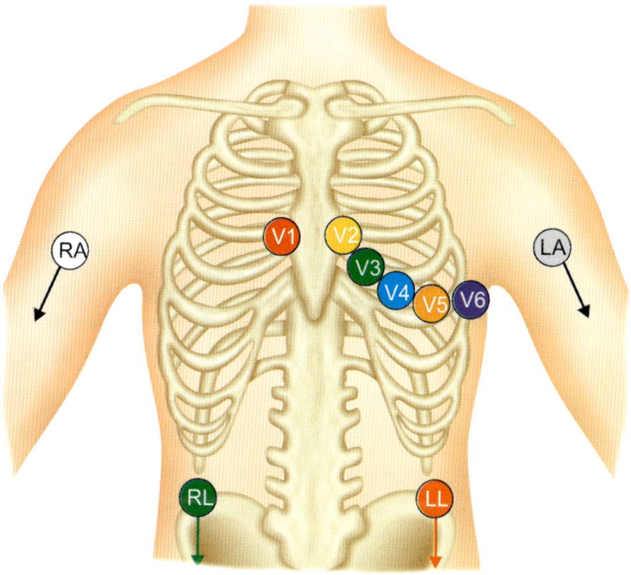

Fig. 3.6: Standard configuration of ECG lead placement during exercise treadmill testing.

Exercise-induced ST-segment depression is a poor localizer and ST-elevation is more specific for the territory of coronary ischemia. Anemia, hyperventilation, LVH, cardiomyopathy, valve disease, hyperglycemia and hypokalemia are some common non-CAD related causes of abnormal ST-segment depression with exercise.

PHARMACOLOGIC STRESS TESTS

Adenosine receptor agonists (adenosine), A2A receptor agonists (regadenoson), and dipyridamole (Persantine) induce coronary arteriolar vasodilation and may induce relative or absolute reduction in blood flow and ischemia in areas of the myocardium subtended by significant coronary stenoses by coronary steal phenomenon. These agents

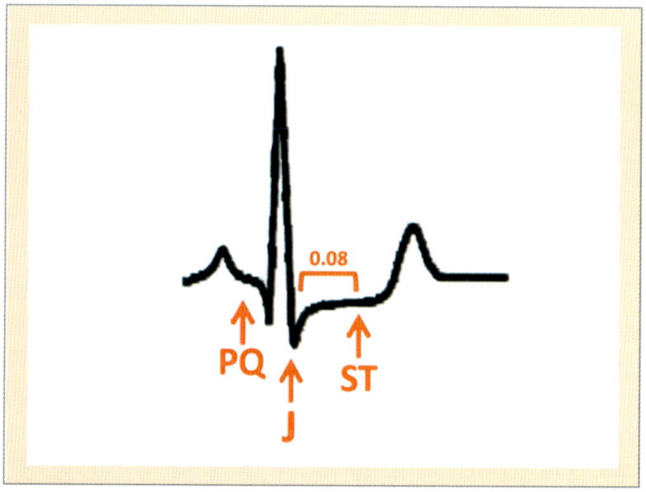

Fig. 3.7: Interpretation of ST-segment changes during treadmill stress testing. ST-segment depression is assessed 0.08 msec after the J-point (0.06 msec during tachycardia). The PQ segment is used as a reference isoelectric point to assess the degree of ST-segment depression.

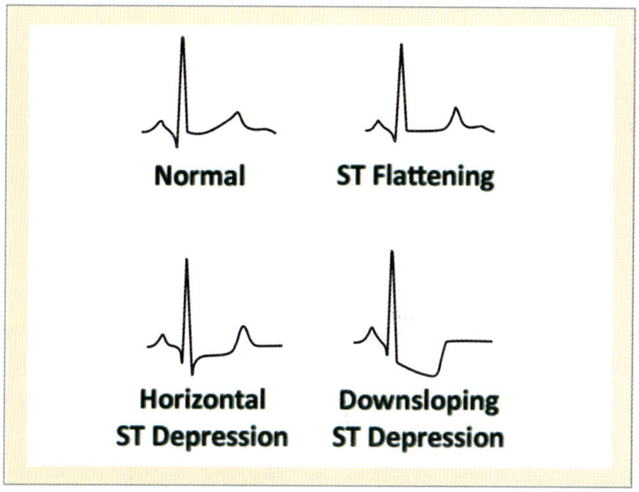

Fig. 3.8: Normal and abnormal ST-segment responses to exercise.

side effects such as headache, nausea, flushing, dizziness, abdominal discomfort, dysgeusia and shortness of breath are commonly reported with these agents. Development of chest discomfort is non-specific for ischemia with these agents. Recent exposure to caffeine, aminophylline or theobromine block the effect of adenosine, and anti-ischemic

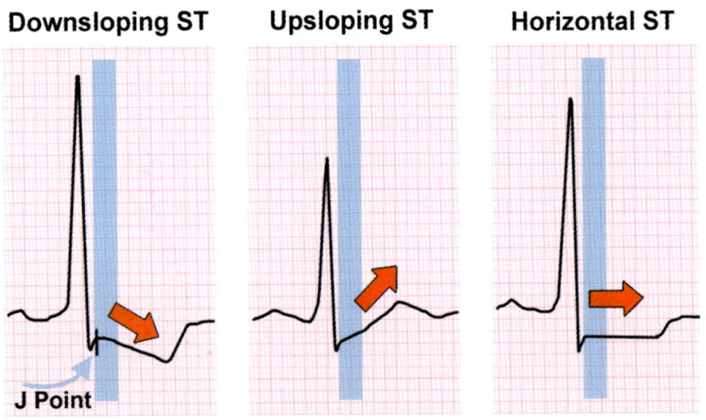

Fig. 3.9: The types of ST-segment depression during exercise stress testing. A downsloping ST-segment is considered more specific for ischemia than an upsloping ST-segment.

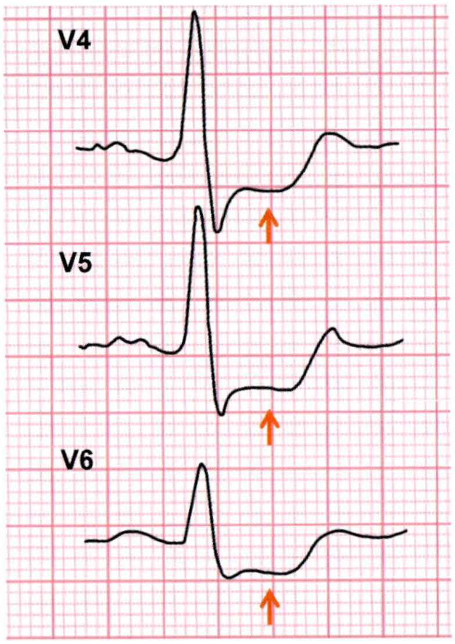

Fig. 3.10: Example of horizontal ST segment during exercise treadmill testing. There is 2–3 mm horizontal ST segment depression in leads V4–V6. [Image adapted from Bhalerao JC. Exercise electrocardiographic testing. In Bhalerao JC (ed). Essentials of Clinical Cardiology. New Delhi, India: Jaypee Brothers Medical Publishers (P) Ltd.].

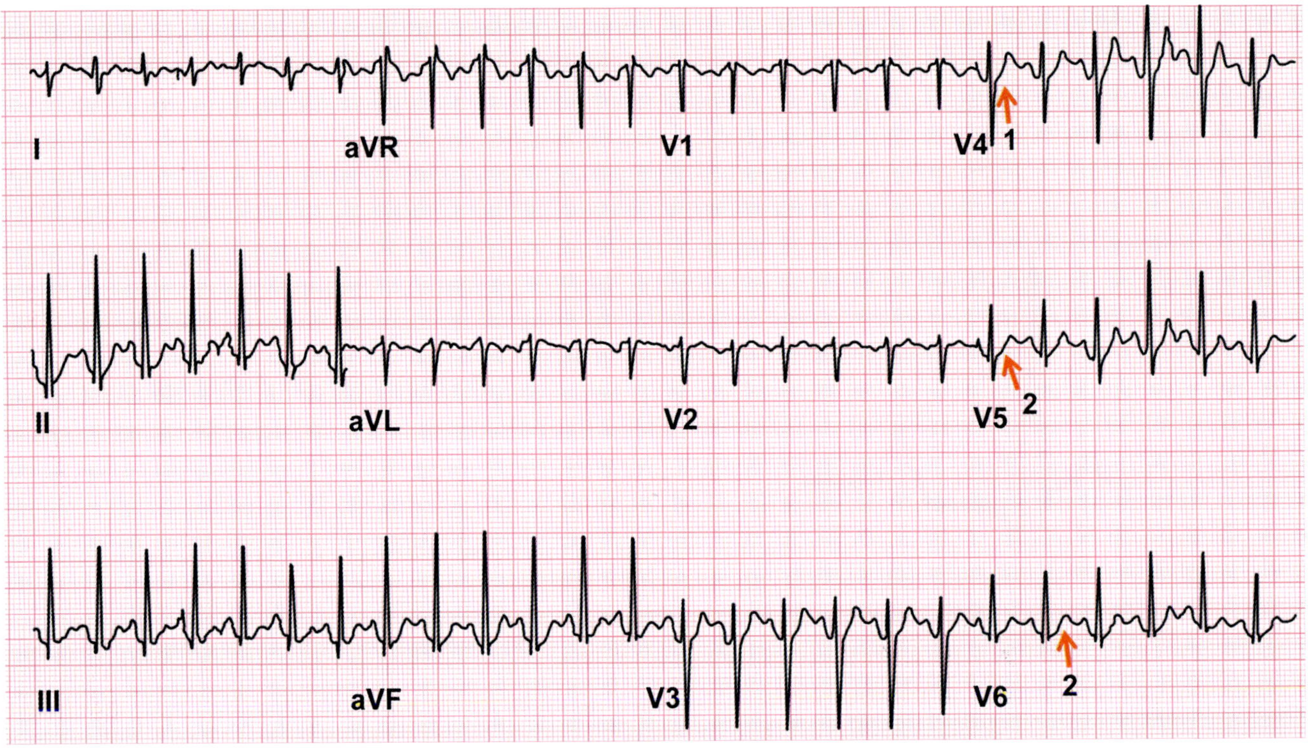

Fig. 3.11: Peak exercise 12-lead ECG with upsloping J-point depression (arrow 1) and < 1.5 mm early upsloping ST-segment depression (arrow 2) is a normal response with exercise.

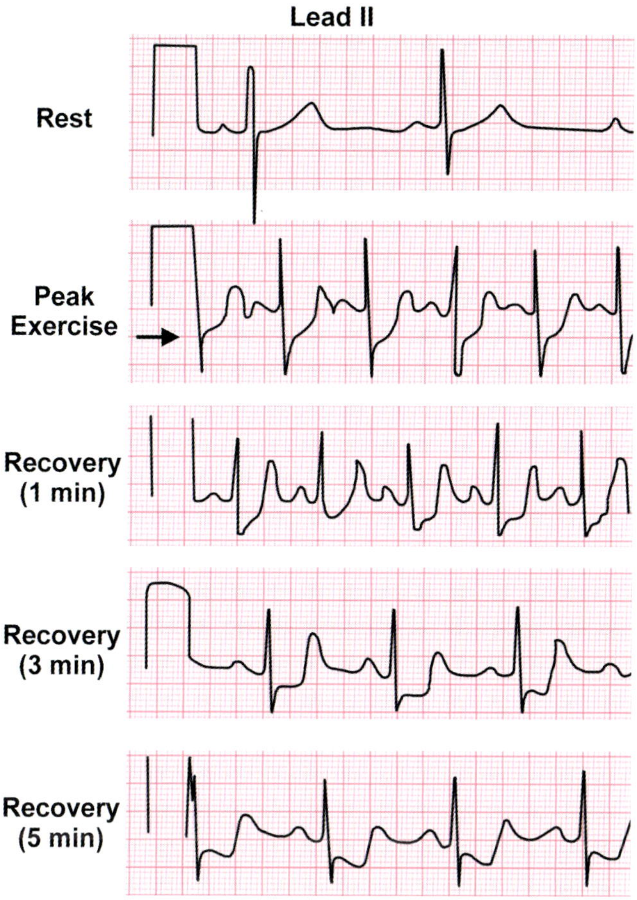

Fig. 3.12: ST-segment depression occurring predominantly during the recovery phase of an exercise treadmill test. This finding has comparable diagnostic accuracy compared to ST-depression occurring during exercise. [Image from Chugh SN. Stress electrocardiography. In Chugh SN (ed). Textbook of Clinical Electrocardiography, 2nd edition. New Delhi, India: Jaypee Brothers Medical Publishers (P) Ltd.].

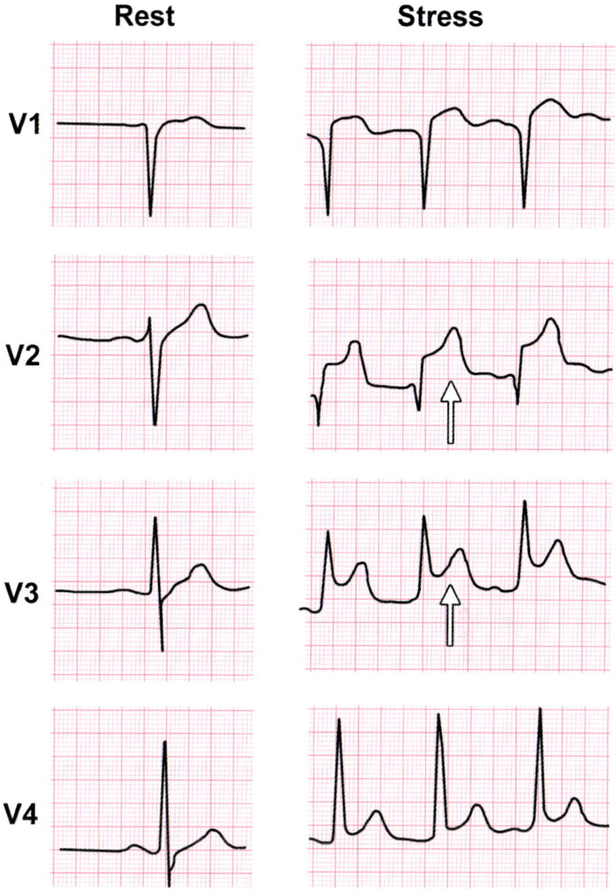

Fig. 3.13: ST-segment elevation, most prominently in leads V2 and V3 (arrows), occurring during an exercise treadmill test. Exercise induced new persistent ST-segment elevation of ≥1.0 mm at 60–80 msec after the J-point occurring in three consecutive beats with a stable baseline and in the absence of corresponding baseline Q-waves is a specific marker of transmural ischemia due to high grade coronary luminal stenosis or coronary spasm. [Image from Chugh SN. Stress electrocardiography. In Chugh SN (ed). Textbook of Clinical Electrocardiography, 2nd edition. New Delhi, India: Jaypee Brothers Medical Publishers (P) Ltd.].

medications may decrease the diagnostic accuracy of such pharmacologic stress testing, and thus it is recommended that patients refrain from ingestion of caffeine-containing products, and hold aminophylline- or theobromine-containing drugs and anti-ischemic medications prior to such testing. Some patients who experience significant chest pain with dipyridamole stress testing may be treated with aminophylline administration to reverse the vasodilating effects of dipyridamole.

The sensitivity of ECG changes with pharmacological agents is low, but rare abnormal ST-segment depression in response to administration of vasodilator agents may be a specific marker of high-grade CAD (Fig. 3.15).

An alternative to vasodilator agents in the performance of stress testing is the use instead of dobutamine. Dobutamine is a synthetic catecholamine that causes ischemia by increased HR and increased myocardial contractility via beta-adrenergic receptor stimulation that results in increased myocardial work load and wall stress. Hypotension, hypertension and rhythm complications are more common with high-dose dobutamine stress testing. Achieving adequate stress peak HR and double product (HR × systolic BP) improves CAD diagnosis. If an adequate HR response is not achieved with dobutamine infusion alone, atropine may be additionally administered in some cases.

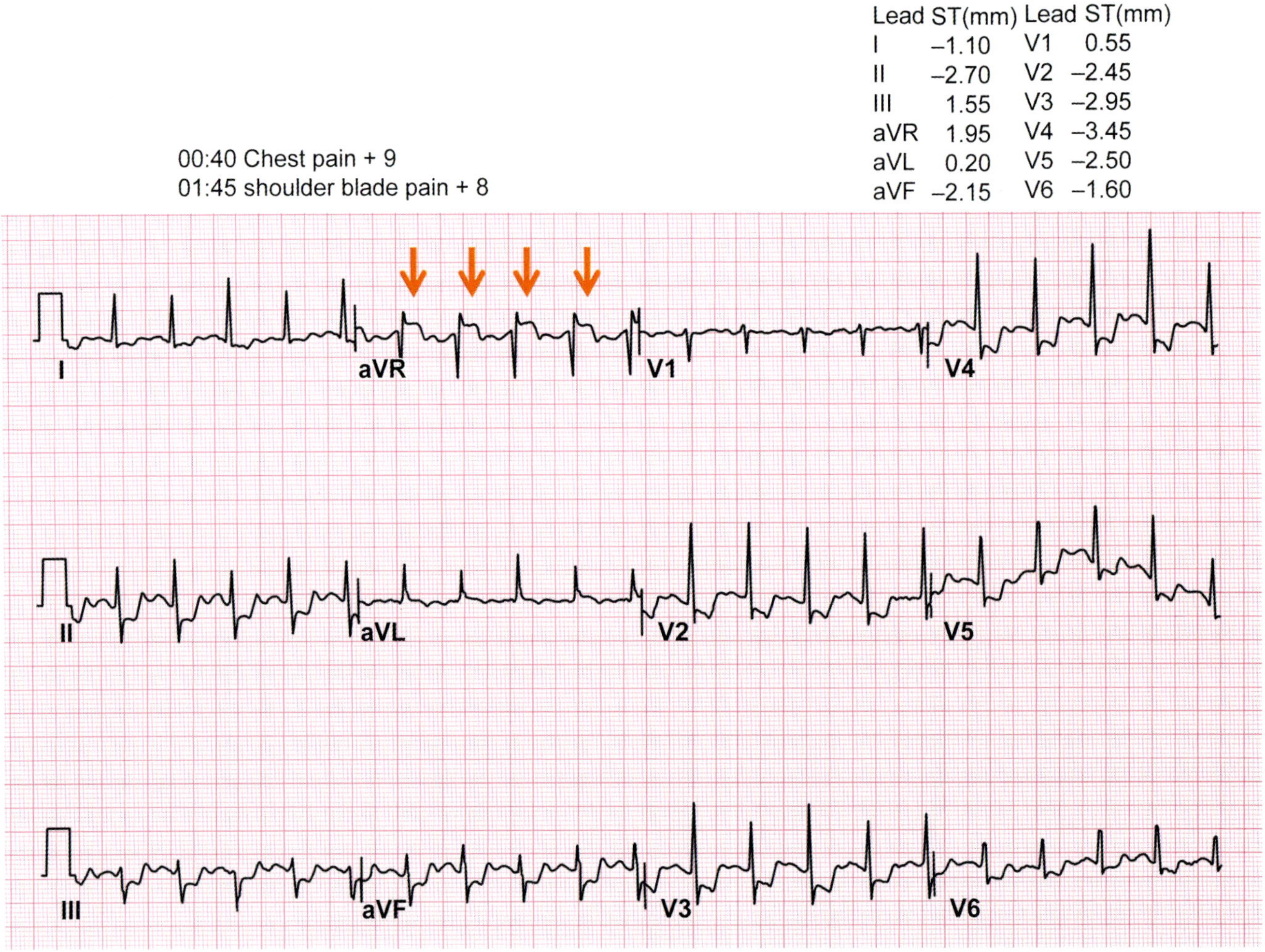

Fig. 3.14: ST-segment elevation in lead aVR (arrows), as well as diffuse marked ST-segment depression in numerous other leads during exercise treadmill testing. These findings are suggestive of the presence of left main or three vessel coronary artery disease.

STRESS ECHOCARDIOGRAPHY

In stress echocardiography, ventricular wall thickening and ventricular contraction are compared between basal conditions and during stress. Both treadmill stress testing and pharmacological-induced stress testing are utilized in clinical practice. Treadmill stress testing has the advantage of being a more "physiological" stress test, though obtaining good quality images immediately after exercise performance can be challenging. The agent most commonly utilized during stress echocardiography is dobutamine. Although the earliest forms of stress testing imaged the heart using M-mode echocardiography (Figs. 3.16A and B), current practice is to image the heart using 2D images obtained in multiple views (usually including apical 4 chamber, apical 2 chamber, and short-axis views). 3D imaging is also being used at some centers.

The current standard for analysis of a normal stress echo is the visual assessment of uniform increase in systolic wall motion, systolic wall thickening and reduction in left ventricular cavity size from rest to stress. Reduction or worsening regional wall motion and/or reduced thickening with increase in corresponding cavity size in systole following stress is indicative of myocardial ischemia (Figs. 3.17 to 3.19).

With exercise (treadmill) stress echocardiography, images are obtained before and after exercise (Fig. 3.17). With dobutamine stress echo, images are obtained during test, low dose dobutamine infusion, high dose dobutamine infusion, and during recovery (Fig. 3.18).

Administration of an echo contrast agent is often used during dobutamine stress echo to improve image quality (Figs. 3.19A to D and 3.20). Myocardial contrast echocardiography with administration of a contrast agent may also

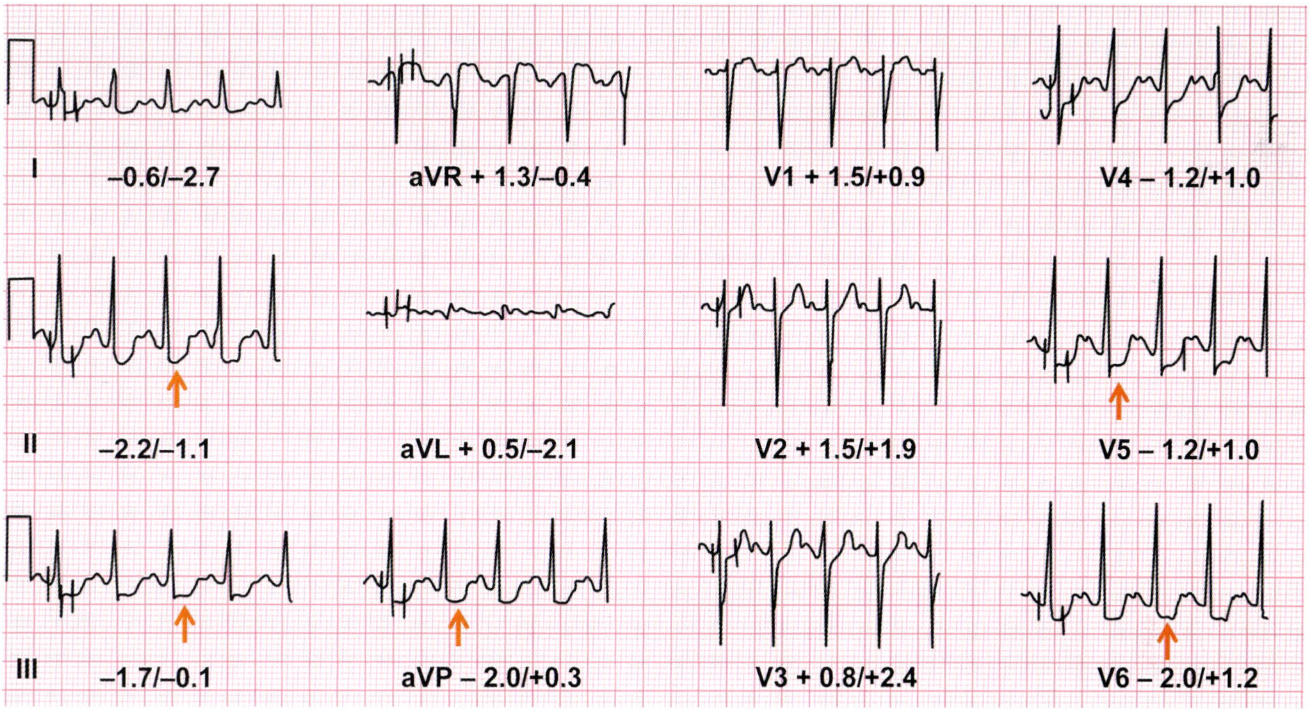

Fig. 3.15: Rare ST-depression (arrows) occurring with dipyridamole administration during a chemical nuclear stress test, suggestive of high grade obstructive CAD. [Image from Mahapa GN. History of nuclear cardiology. In Chopra HK, Nanda NC (eds). Textbook of Cardiology: A Clinical and Historical Perspective. New Delhi, India: Jaypee Brothers Medical Publishers (P) Ltd.].

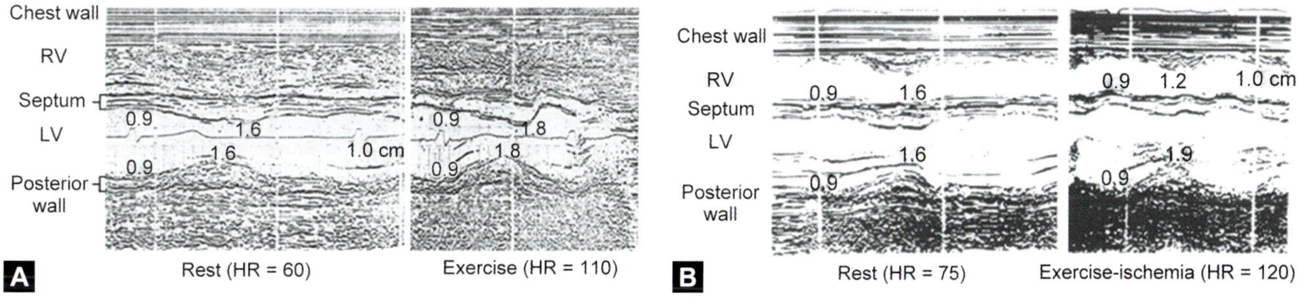

Figs. 3.16A and B: Historical images of M-mode echocardiography during stress testing. (A) M-mode echocardiograms at rest (left) and exercise (right) in a person without any significant coronary artery disease. Systolic thickening of the septal and posterior (inferolateral) walls is the same at rest and increases in both territories with exercise. (B) M-mode echocardiograms at rest (left) and peak exercise (right) from a patient with near total occlusion of the left anterior descending (LAD) artery and normal left circumflex and right coronary arteries. Both septal and posterior wall thickening are the same at rest. In exercise, at the time of ischemia, posterior wall systolic thickening has increased, while septal thickening has decreased, indicative of ischemia. [Image and figure legend from Upadhyayula S, Kapur KK. History of stress echocardiography. In Chopra HK, Nanda NC (eds). Textbook of Cardiology: A Clinical & Historical Perspective. New Delhi, India: Jaypee Brothers Medical Publishers (P) Ltd.].

allow for detection of delayed contrast enhancement in areas of the left ventricle, suggestive of significant coronary stenosis or occlusion in the artery subtending that segment or segments (Fig. 3.21).

Regional wall motion abnormalities are interpreted with respect to the usual coronary artery which subtends the abnormal myocardial segment or segments with the recognition that there is some variability and overlap in the coronary supply of some segments (Fig. 3.22).

Stress echocardiography has a number of advantages as compared to other imaging techniques, including great versatility and providing ancillary information of global left and right ventricular systolic function, diastolic function, valvular function, and hemodynamics, with reliable

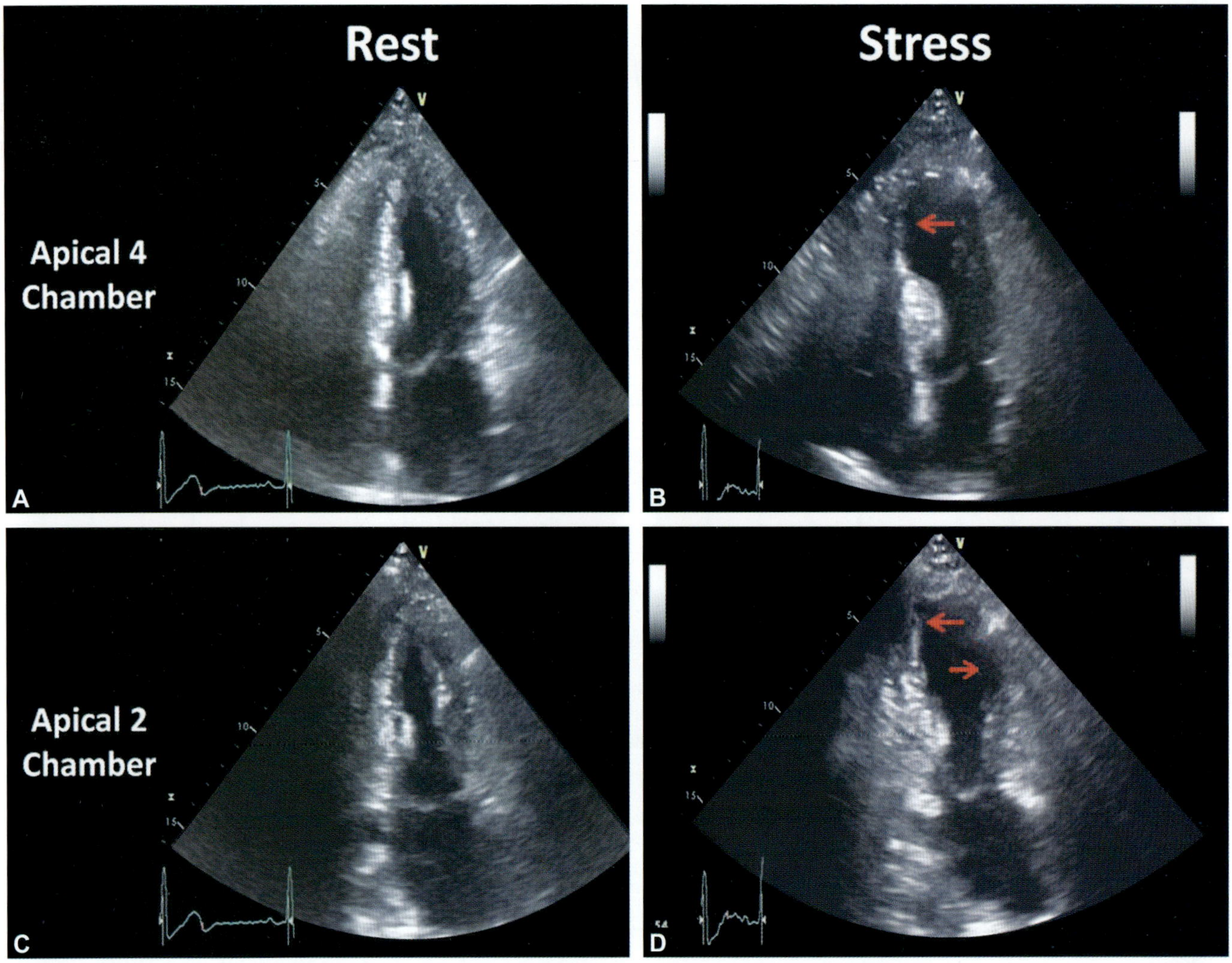

Figs. 3.17A to D: Exercise stress echo test images. Apical four and two chamber stress echo images demonstrate normal systolic wall thickening at rest and reduced systolic thickening, motion and increased cavity size (arrows) in the mid and distal anterior walls, apex, and distal inferoseptal wall immediately postexercise, suggestive of left anterior descending coronary artery (LAD) stenosis (large wrap-around LAD).

accuracy and at a low cost. However, several factors, suboptimal image quality [such as in patients of very large body habitus or with severe chronic obstructive pulmonary disease (COPD)], inadequate achievement of peak stress (such as poor chronotropic response), and subjectivity and variability of image interpretation, may reduce the overall sensitivity of stress echocardiography, especially in patients with less severe CAD. Although some false positive studies may result from challenges in wall motion assessment, a significant proportion of false positive studies are due to myocardial ischemia in the absence of obstructive CAD as seen with LVH, cardiomyopathy, or microvascular disease. False positive studies may result from tethering of myocardial segments from prior myocardial infarction or to less mobile structures such as the mitral annulus, or from dyssynchronous contraction due to LBBB, paced rhythm or right ventricular pathology. To overcome some of the challenges of stress echo interpretation, some centers utilize regional quantitative Doppler-derived stress echo data, such as myocardial strain imaging, to improve detection of ischemia.

RADIONUCLIDE MYOCARDIAL PERFUSION IMAGING STRESS

Myocardial perfusion imaging with radionuclide tracer using single photon emission computed tomography (SPECT) is the most common technique of stress MPI.

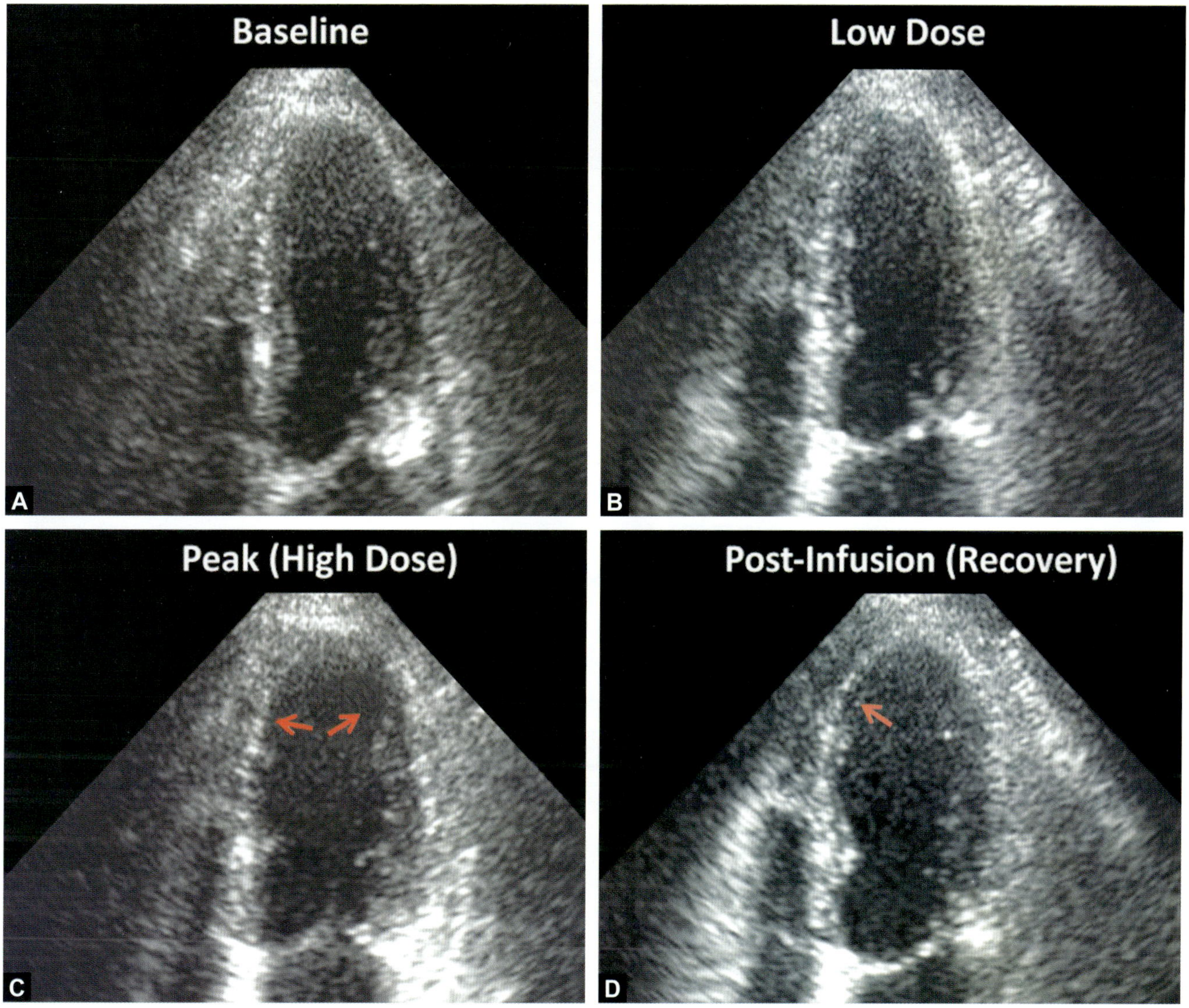

Figs. 3.18A to D: End-systolic images obtained during dobutamine stress echocardiography. Images displayed are the apical four chamber view at baseline, at low dose dobutamine infusion, at peak dobutamine infusion, and postinfusion (recovery). There is reduced wall thickening (arrows) and an increase in cavity size at peak and postinfusion images, consistent with stress-induced ischemia in multiple coronary artery territories, suggestive of the presence of multivessel coronary artery disease.

Common SPECT tracers are thallium (Tl)-201 and technetium (Tc)-99m. Myocardial stress is induced with either exercise testing or with vasodilator therapy (adenosine, dipyridamole or more recently regadenoson). Images obtained around the time of myocardial stress are compared with images obtained under basal conditions. SPECT reconstructed images are typically displayed in the short axis, vertical long and horizontal axis projections. The degree of tracer uptake is related to the amount of blood flow to viable myocardium. The tracer activity can be viewed in gray scale or in various color scale maps, which allow for easier qualitative and quantitative grading of severity of reduced tracer activity in the regions corresponding to the severity of the coronary lumen disease. Display of rest and stress images in a single polar plot diagram representing all left ventricular (LV) segments with automated comparison to an established normal distribution, gender and tracer matched database permits greater degree of quantification of the defect size and severity.

Uniform tracer uptake during basal and stress conditions indicates viable, non-ischemic myocardium throughout (Fig. 3.23). Greater than normal heterogeneous reduction of regional tracer activity following stress

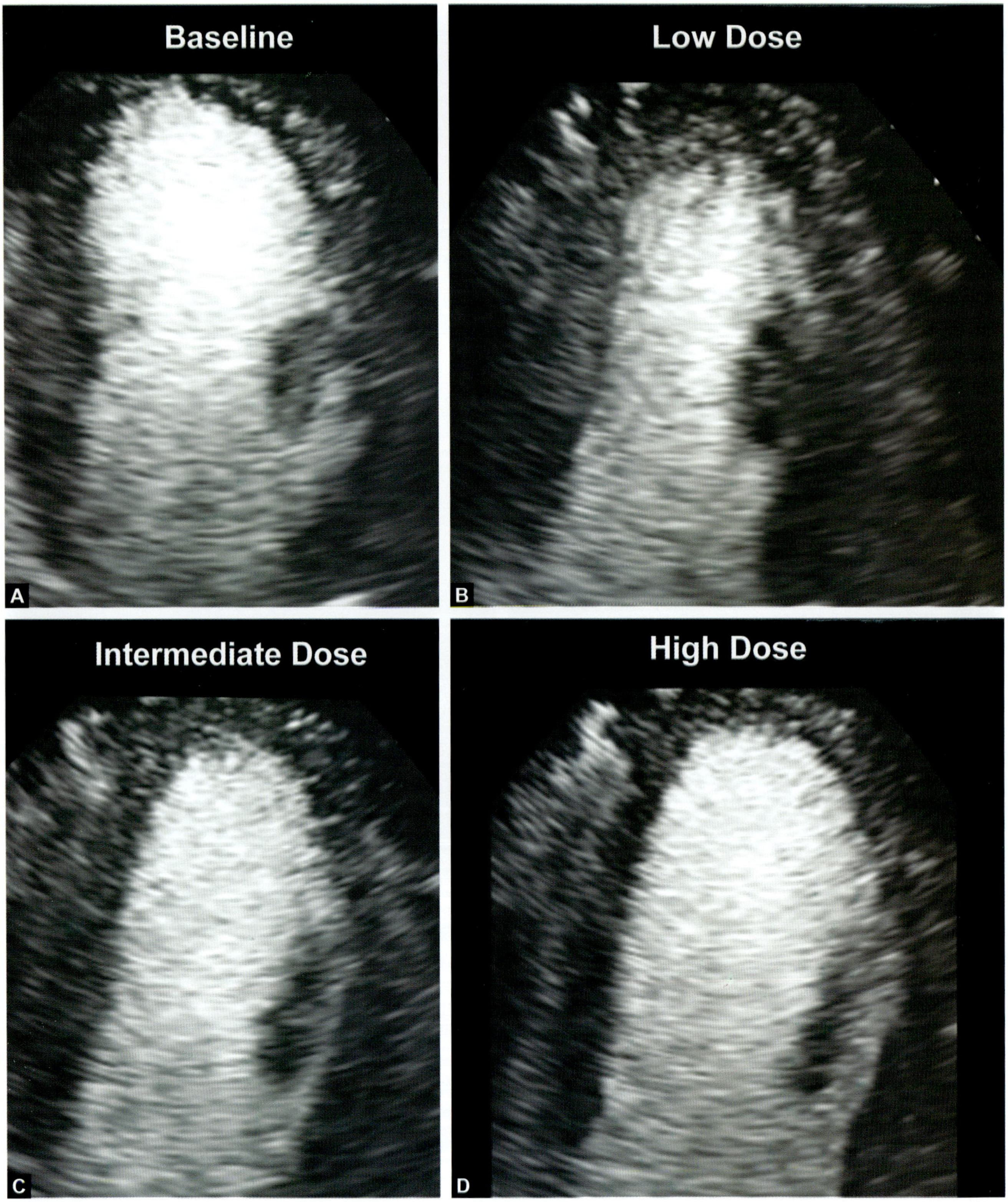

Figs. 3.19A to D: Contrast-enhanced dobutamine stress echocardiography illustrating a biphasic response to progressively higher doses of dobutamine infusion. Left ventricular ejection fraction and wall thickening improves at low dose dobutamine infusion. However, there is a worsening of left ventricular myocardial contractility at higher doses of dobutamine infusion. (Image courtesy of Glenn N Levine, MD).

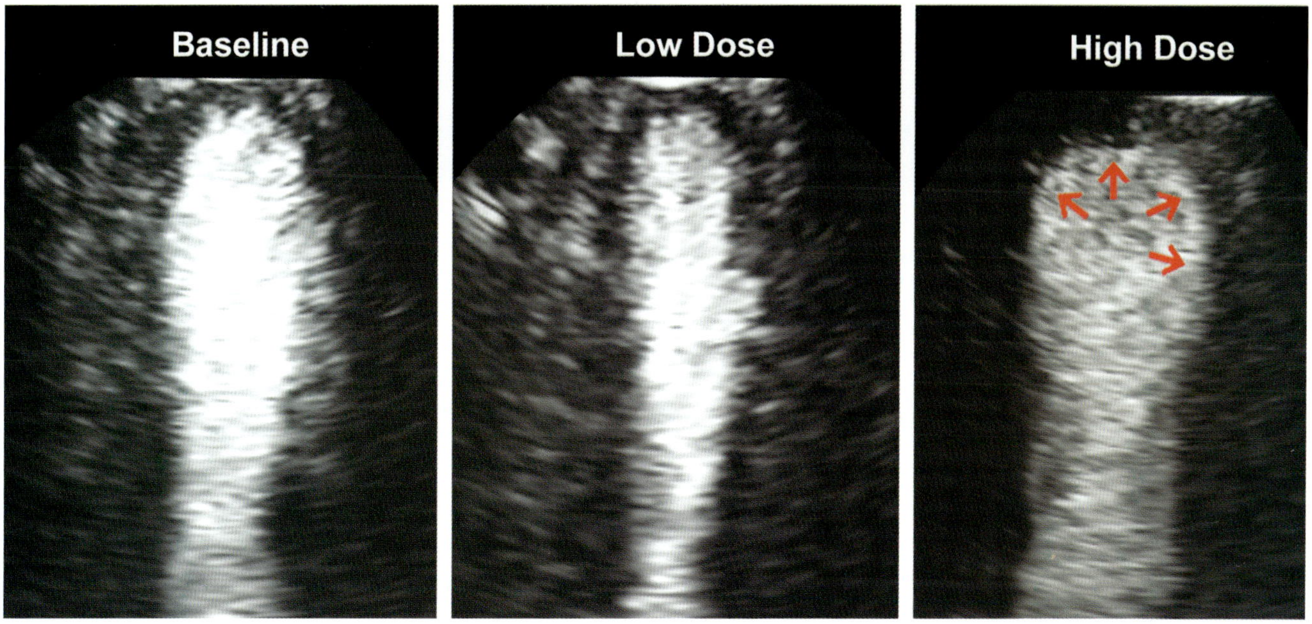

Fig. 3.20: Contrast-enhanced dobutamine stress echo. Two chamber images show increased contractility at low dose dobutamine but marked worsening of contractility with frank dyskinesis of the distal anterior wall and apex (arrows) at high dose dobutamine.

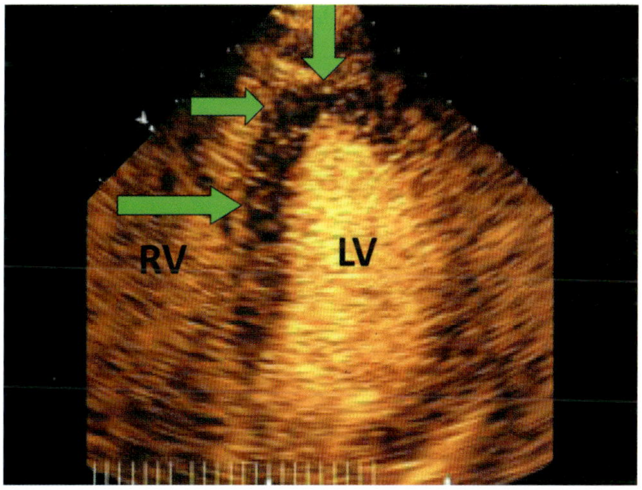

Fig. 3.21: Myocardial contrast echocardiography with low mechanical index demonstrating the delayed contrast enhancement in the distal septum and apex of the left ventricle (arrows) compared to the proximal septum and lateral wall in an apical 4-chamber view. [Image and figure legend from Lonnebakken MT, Gerdts E. Contrast echocardiography in coronary artery disease. In Baskot B (ed). Coronary Angiography—Advances in Noninvasive Imaging Approach for Evaluation of Coronary Artery Disease. Intechweb.org. CC]. (LV: Left ventricle; RV: Right ventricle).

with reversible improved activity at rest on two or more consecutive slices and on more than one orthogonal projection is abnormal for myocardial ischemia (Figs. 3.24 and 3.25). Defects observed during both stress and rest conditions are termed "fixed perfusion defects" and are usually indicative of infarcted myocardium (Figs. 3.25A to D). Occasionally, dedicated viability testing may reveal such areas as potentially viable. ECG-gated images with variation in tracer counts between systole and diastole provide assessment of the regional and global LV function with SPECT (Figs. 3.27 and 3.28).

Stress SPECT MPI exams are affected less by subjective interpretation and patient body size. Exposure to radiation due to radionuclide tracers and soft tissue attenuation, patient motion, and ECG-gating related errors are other limitations with this imaging technique. False positive and false negative nuclear perfusion studies can result from attenuation, inadequate stress, small LV cavity, LV hypertrophy, cardiomyopathy, balanced multivessel ischemia and with the use of anti-ischemic medications such as beta receptor blocker and nitrates. Several attenuation and motion correction hardware and software solutions are commercially available to improve on SPECT image quality and diagnostic accuracy.

Positron emission tomography (PET) MPI stress is an alternate nuclear imaging modality. Commonly three positron-emitting radiotracers nitrogen-13, rubidium-82, and fluorine-18 deoxy-D-glucose are clinically used in cardiac PET studies. The short half-live of rubidium-82 (75 sec) results in low radiation and less attenuation of the

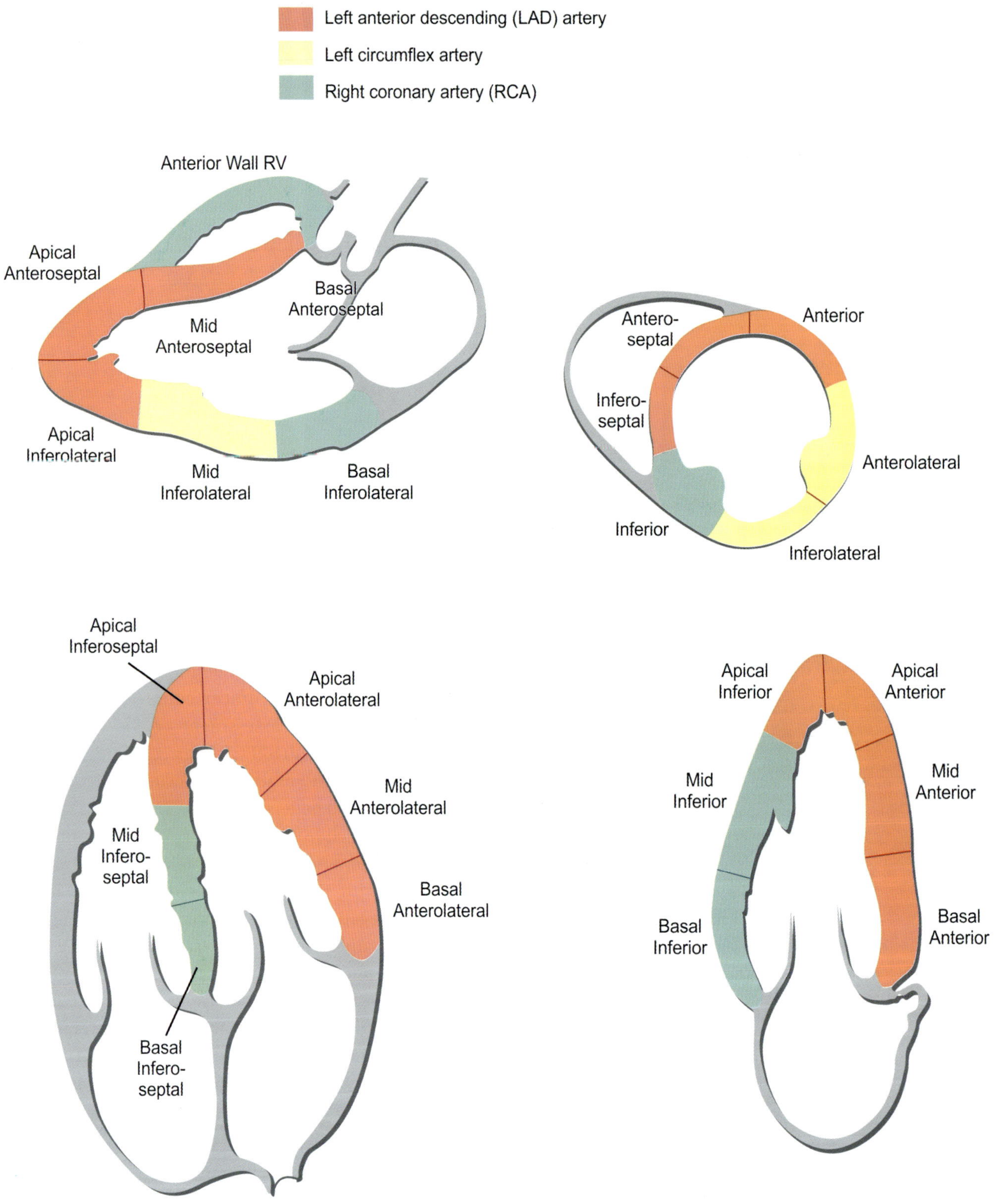

Fig. 3.22: Illustration of the usual regions of the heart perfused by each of the major coronary arteries. In some regions of the heart, there is some variability in the artery that supplies that region. (Image courtesy of Glenn N Levine, MD).

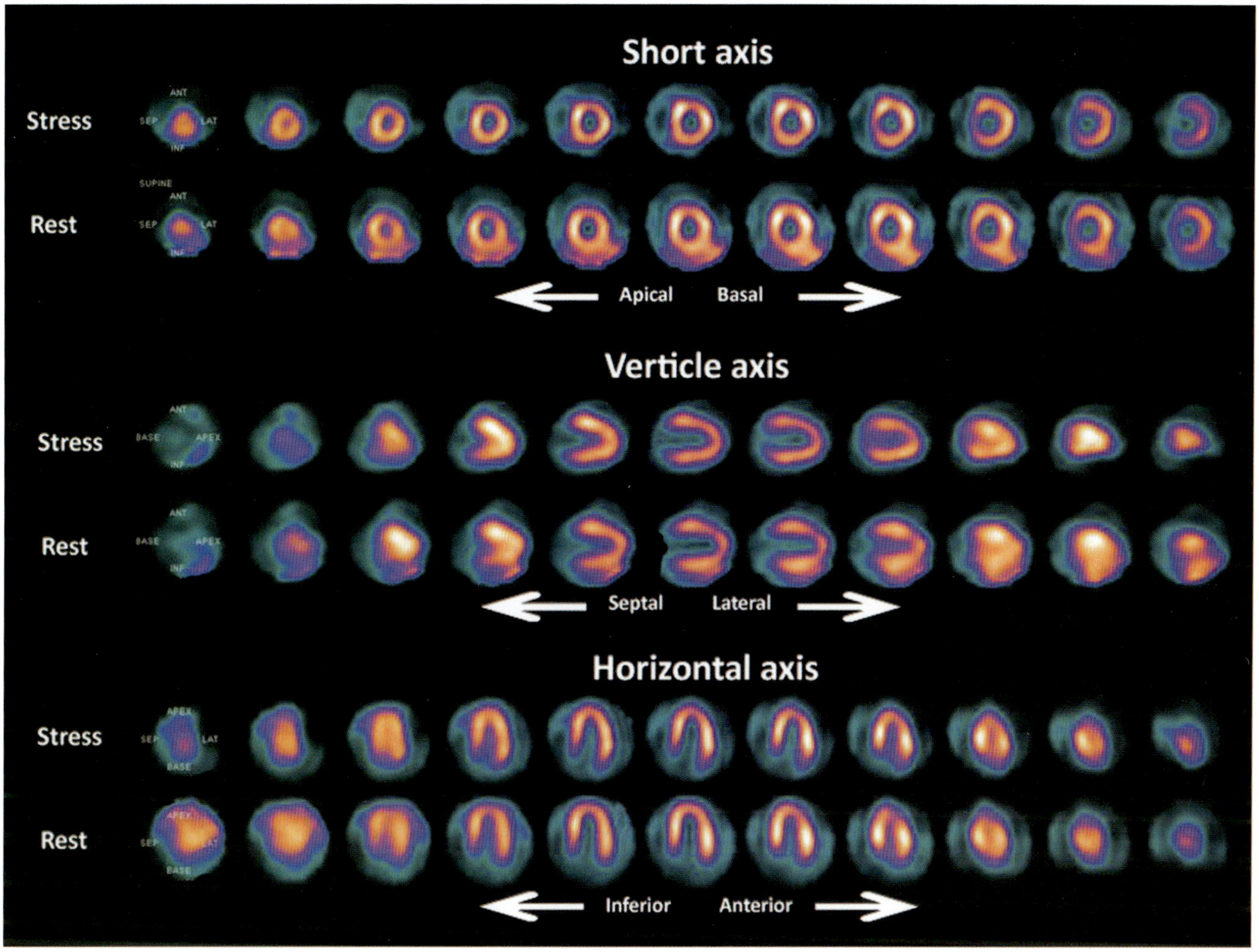

Fig. 3.23: Single photon emission computed tomography (SPECT) images of the left ventricle in short, vertical long and horizontal long-axis with uniform normal tracer uptake following stress (top row for each view) and rest (bottom row for each view). The displayed color is representative of the extent of tracer uptake.

images with improved diagnostic quality (Figs. 3.29A and B). Both rest and stress images can be ECG gated to obtain function analysis and PET imaging has been combined with CT for improved attenuation correction. Image uniformity, improved spatial resolution, less attenuation and shorter scan time are significant advantages of PET over SPECT, making PET imaging an attractive alternative imaging modality in selected patients (e.g. obese patients). In addition, PET imaging also provides the opportunity to assess myocardial viability and coronary blood flow with alternate PET tracers. A number of limitations hamper the use of PET, including greater expense, limited availability, number of artifacts related to acquisition techniques, heart displacement during stress, and the exposure to radiation.

CARDIAC COMPUTED TOMOGRAPHY

Currently, noninvasive, ECG-gated multi-detector computed tomography (CT) technology is capable of obtaining good spatial resolution (~0.6 mm) images of the coronary anatomy. CT coronary angiography also allows for assessment of extent of coronary plaque beyond what can be visualized with a simple luminogram. Although, anatomic detection of CAD with coronary CT angiography is the current dominant clinical use, the technology is capable of assessing global and regional systolic function, myocardial perfusion with stress, and the presence infarct scar (Figs. 3.30 and 3.31). Exposure to iodinated contrast with nephrotoxicity, lack of validated clinical protocols, and exposure to radiation are major limiting factors for CT.

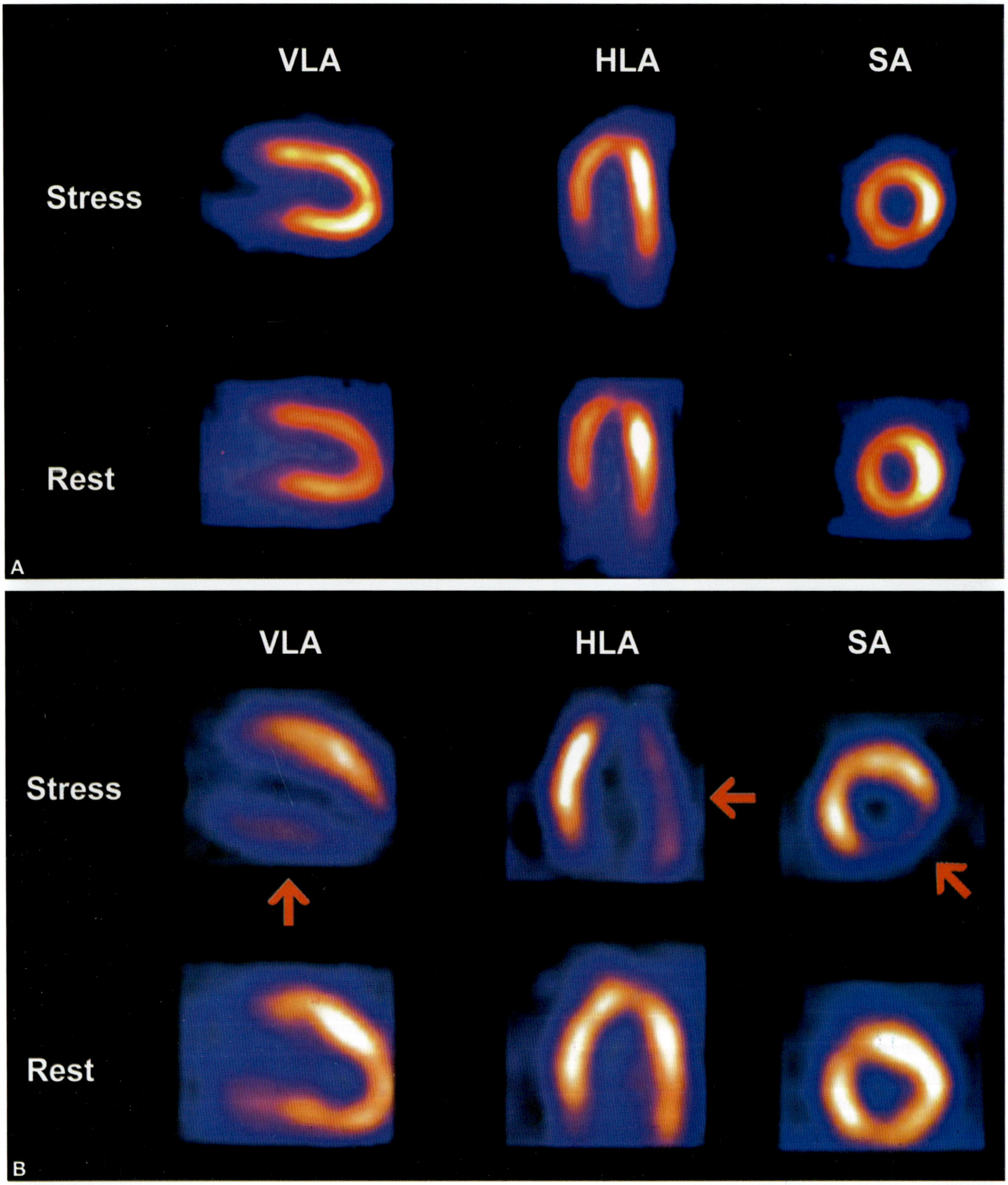

Figs. 3.24A and B: Representative images from cardiac nuclear stress tests. (A) An example of a normal nuclear stress test showing no ischemia or fixed perfusion defect. (B) Stress testing showing reversible inferior ischemia (arrows). [Image from Mehta S. Nuclear imaging in cardiology: an overview. In Bhalerao J (ed). Essentials of Clinical Cardiology. New Delhi, India: Jaypee Brothers Medical Publishers (P) Ltd.]. (VLA: Vertical long-axis; HLA: Horizontal long axis; SA: Short-axis).

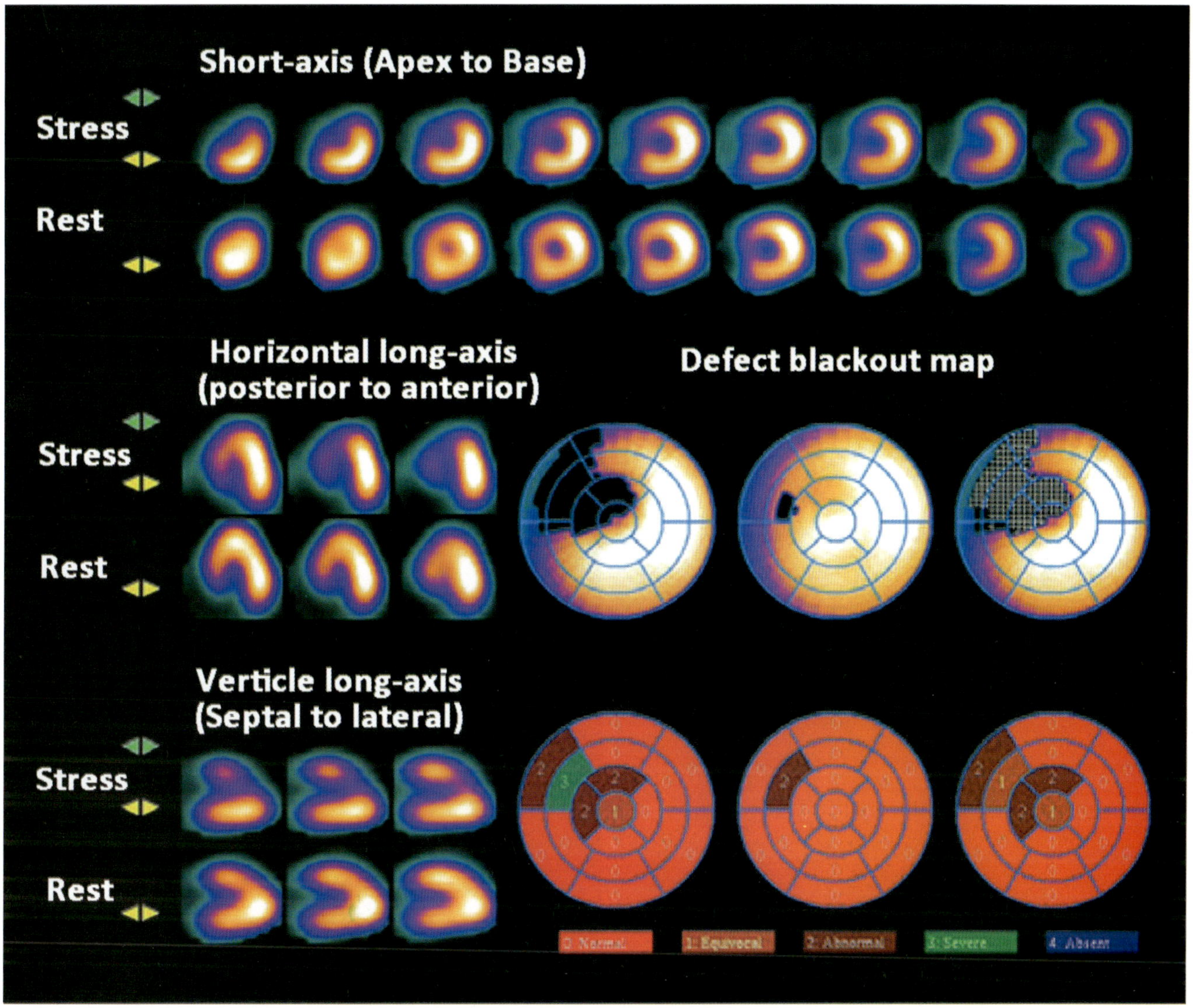

Fig. 3.25: Single photon emission computed tomography (SPECT) color map tracer activity images of the left ventricle in short, vertical long and horizontal long axis with moderately reduced tracer activity of the anteroseptal wall in two or more slices and in two orthogonal planes with reversible improved tracer uptake of the corresponding regions at rest, indicative of stress-induced myocardial ischemia. [Image from Mahapa GN. History of nuclear cardiology. In Chopra HK, Nanda NC (eds). Textbook of Cardiology: A Clinical and Historical Perspective. New Delhi, India: Jaypee Brothers Medical Publishers (P) Ltd.].

CARDIAC MRI STRESS

Use of CMRI imaging with pharmacological stress agents for detecting CAD (Figs. 3.32A and B) has emerged as a potential alternate noninvasive test in the past decade. MRI uses high intensity magnetic fields and radiofrequency to generate three-dimensional, tomographic images with high resolution (~0.8 mm), excellent tissue contrast and ECG-gated cines images. CMRI evaluates the presence of CAD using different techniques including: (1) evaluation of wall motion and thickening during stress by cine; (2) dynamic first pass perfusion imaging, which assess capillary permeability for inducible perfusion defects; (3) anatomical assessment (coronary MR angiography) which provides visualization of the coronary tree; and (4) delayed post-contrast enhancement to detect myocardial infarct scar.

Cardiac magnetic resonance imaging has several advantages that includes highly versatile imaging modality with multiple techniques, greater image resolution, lack of

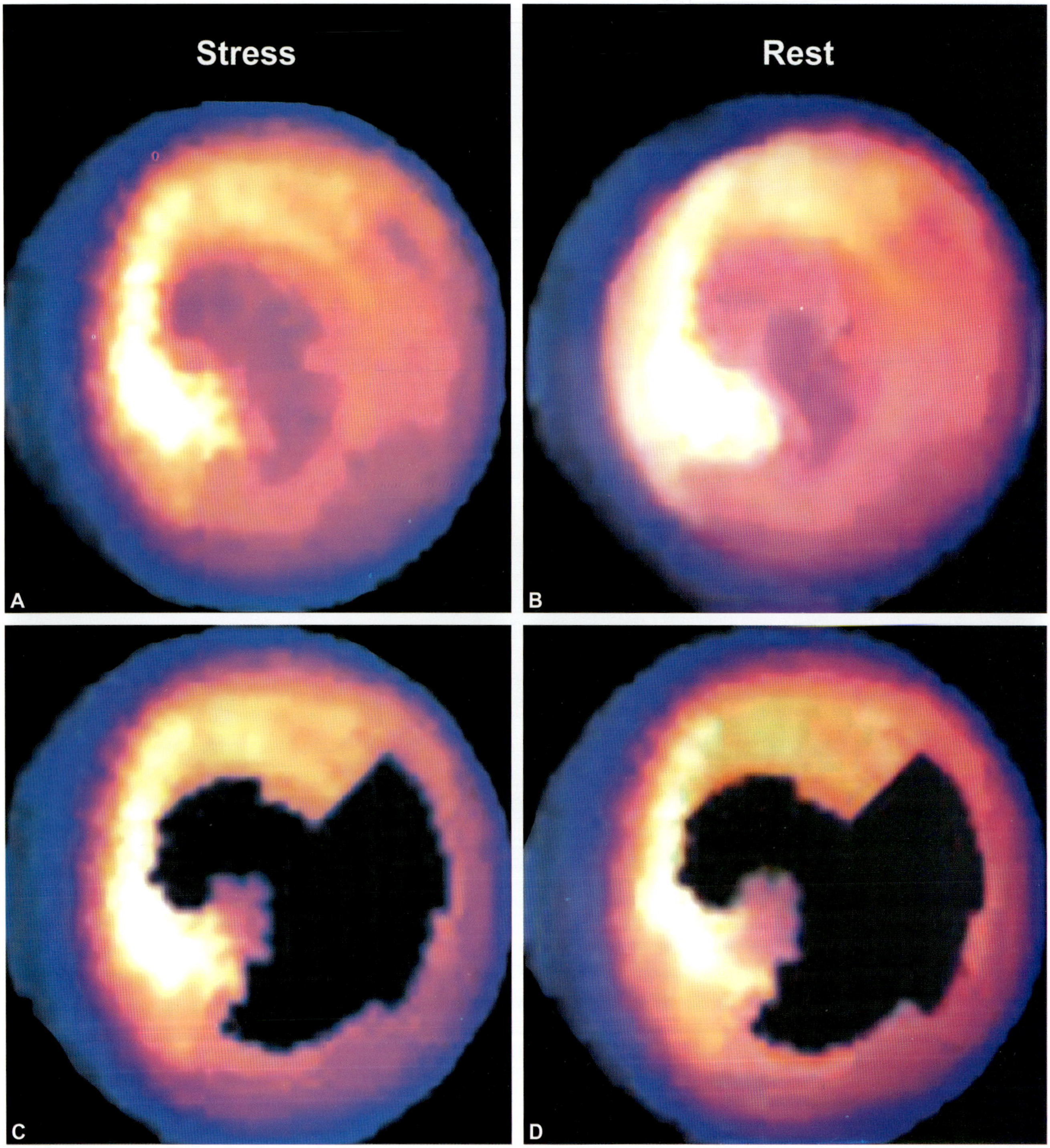

Figs. 3.26A to D: Polar map of "bull's eye" display of a nuclear stress test result demonstrating fixed perfusion defect. [Image from Mehta S Nuclear imaging in cardiology: an overview. In Bhalerao J (ed). Essentials of Clinical Cardiology. New Delhi, India: Jaypee Brothers Medical Publishers (P) Ltd.].

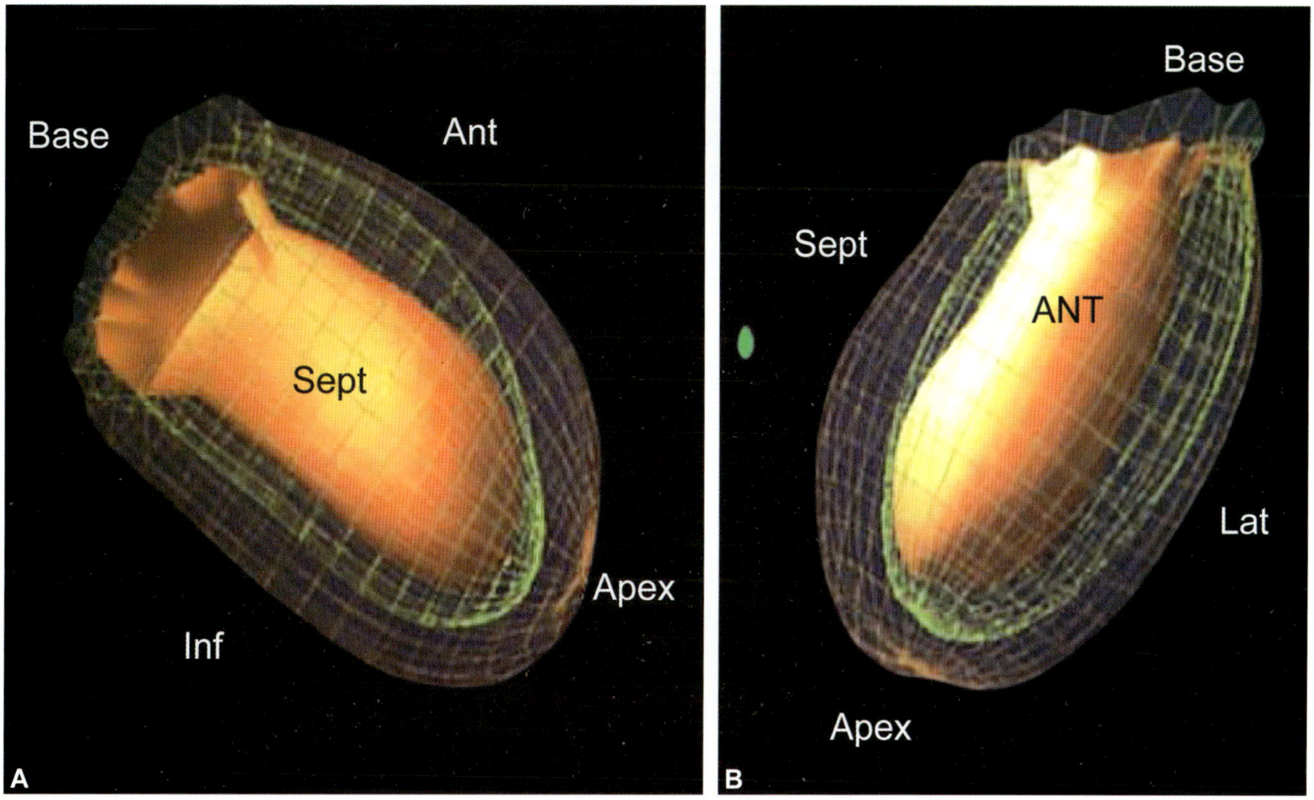

Figs. 3.27A and B: Left ventricular contours derived from gated stress perfusion images. Image shows the epicardial (orange mesh) and endocardial contours at end-diastole (yellow mesh) and end systolic (solid orange region). A septal wall motion abnormality is demonstrated. [Image courtesy of Dr Eli Botvinick, UCSF. [Image reproduced from Mahenthiran J. Cardiac stress testing. In Levine GN (ed). Color Atlas of Clinical Cardiology. New Dehli: Jaypee Brothers Medical Publishers (P) Ltd. 2004].

radiation, greater sensitivity for detecting early subendocardial ischemia, improved quantification of volumes without geometric assumptions of cardiac chambers, images independent of body habitus and anatomical assessment of the coronary tree by angiography (Fig. 3.33). Other major clinical advantage of CMRI is the ability to accurately quantify the anatomic extent of myocardial infarct scar and the presence of viable myocardium by delayed contrast enhancement imaging (Fig. 3.33). Limited availability, claustrophobia, technical limitations, artifacts related to motion, breathing and arrhythmia; and the inability to do it on patients with metallic implants are some of the disadvantages of CMRI.

DIAGNOSIS AND PROGNOSTIC ROLE OF CARDIAC STRESS TESTS

The diagnostic capability of cardiac stress testing for detecting CAD using invasive coronary angiography as the reference gold standard is influenced by the pretest probability of disease based on patient's age, gender, symptoms and atherosclerotic risk factors. The greatest diagnostic power of a stress test is when the pretest probability is intermediate (30–70%). The diagnostic yield is lowest in low-risk (<10%) asymptomatic patients. Exercise testing combined with imaging techniques improves sensitivity of detecting CAD as compared to exercise ECG alone in selected patient populations. The averages of overall sensitivity and specificity of various cardiac stress testing modalities is summarized on Table 3.4. Data pooled from several studies showed that exercise and pharmacological stress imaging had comparable weighted mean sensitivity and specificity for the diagnosis of CAD.

In general, radionuclide MPI is more sensitive and preferred in females, sedentary individuals, diabetic patients, and with pharmacological stress. Radionuclide MPI can also provide a quantitative estimation of ischemic burden. Stress echocardiography and CMRI provides greater

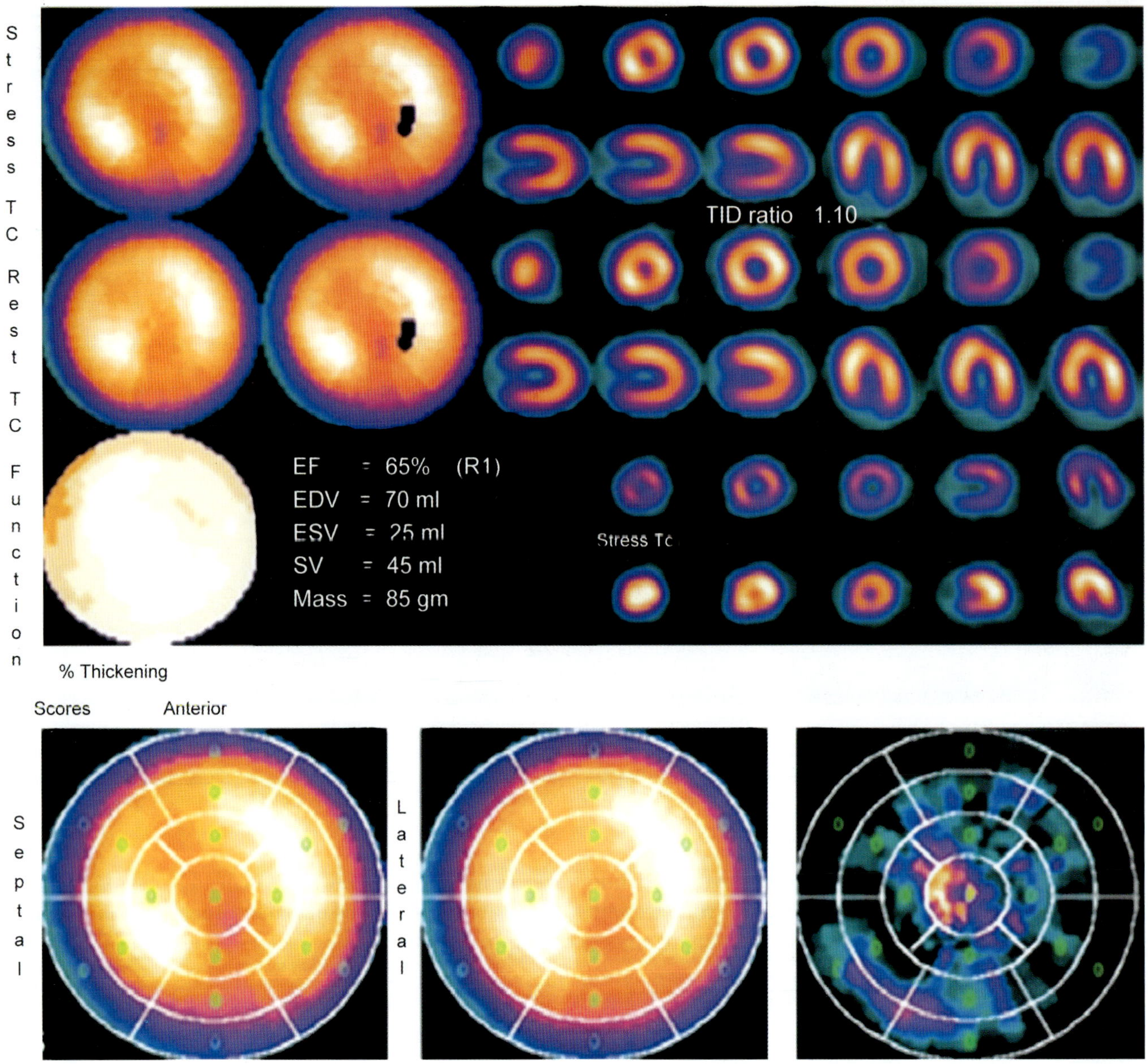

Fig. 3.28: Nuclear stress test stress images demonstrating uniform stress perfusion pattern with normal systolic wall thickening, and normal ejection fraction. [Image from Mahapa GN. History of nuclear cardiology. In Chopra HK, Nanda NC (eds). Textbook of Cardiology: A Clinical and Historical Perspective. New Delhi, India: Jaypee Brothers Medical Publishers (P) Ltd.].

specificity for detecting obstructive coronary disease. Both echocardiography and MRI may be preferred in those with concomitant suspected valve disease or pulmonary hypertension, and in those requiring viability assessment.

There are several large observational studies published that have demonstrated the prognostic use of cardiac stress tests. Inability exercise along with exercise duration (<5 METS), exercise induced hypotension, chronotropic incompetence, HR recovery, sustained ventricular tachycardia and angina at low level of exercise are some variables with adverse prognosis. Duke treadmill score based on exercise duration, symptoms (angina) and exercise ECG STD identifies patients at low, intermediate

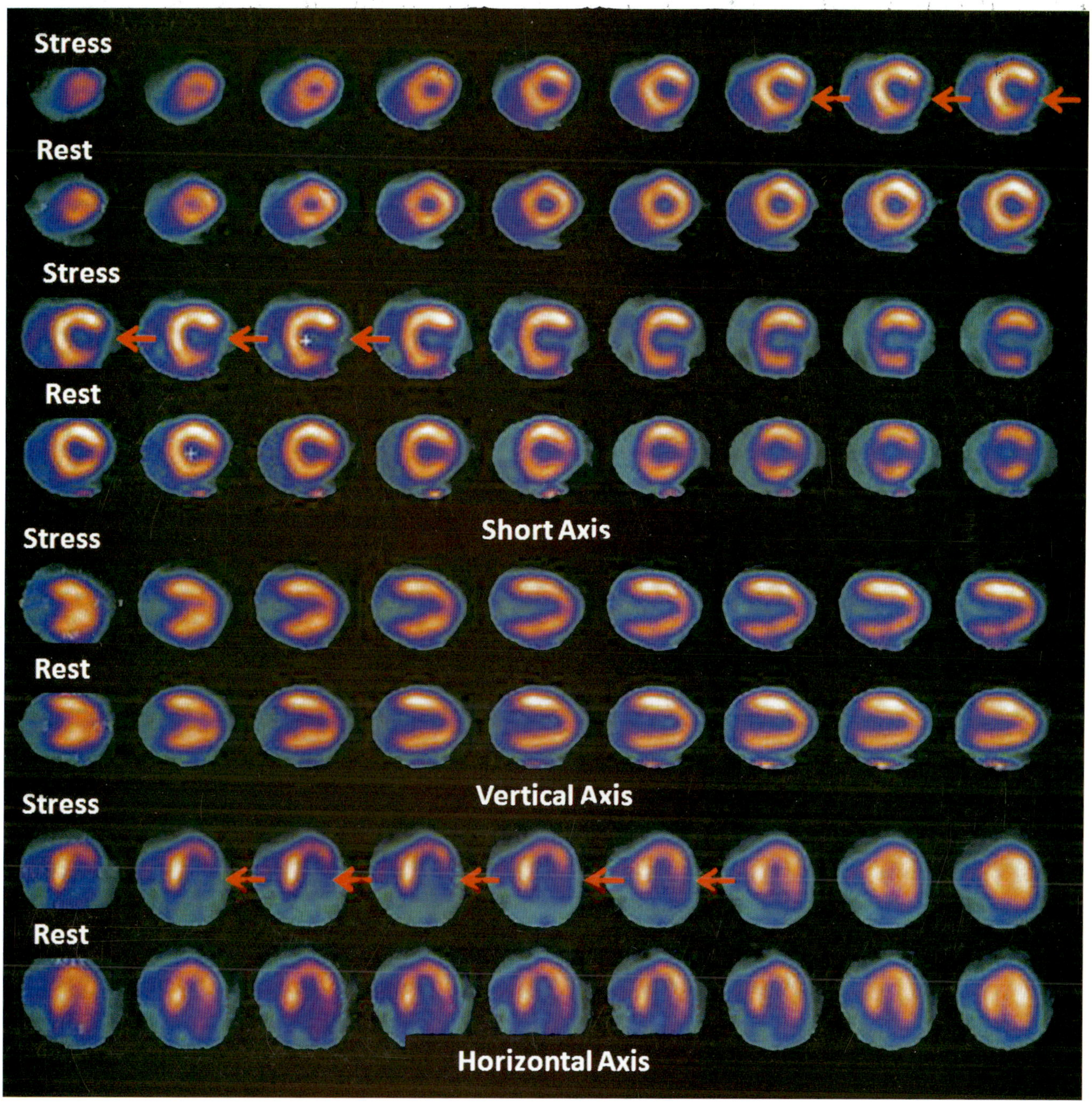

Fig. 3.29A: Rubidium-82 myocardial perfusion PET-CT study with stress and rest images in corresponding short-axis (top), vertical long-axis (middle), and horizontal long-axis (bottom) views showing abnormal moderate reversible reduced tracer uptake (top and bottom row arrows) in the lateral segments (left circumflex territory) consistent with ischemia in an obese male.

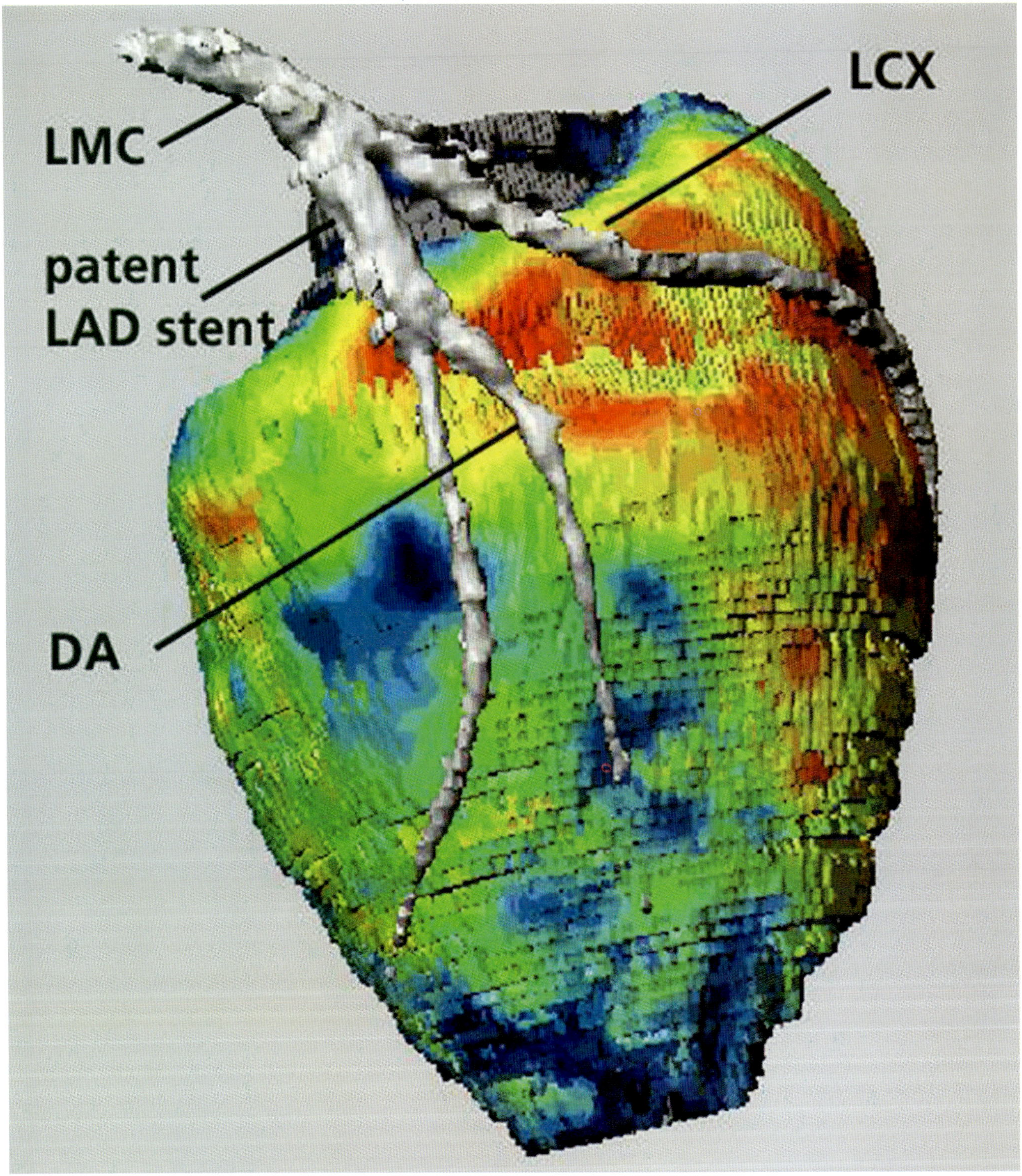

Fig. 3.29B: PET-CT scan. Image shown consists of a coronary angiogram obtained using CT scanning and colored surface of the heart is from ammonia PET stress perfusion imaging. The areas in the distal LAD territory represent reduced stress perfusion. Advances in technology have led to even clearer images than the one shown in this figure. (Image courtesy of Dr Philipp A Kaufmann, University Hospital Zurich). (DA: Diagonal artery branch; LAD: Left anterior descending artery; LCX: Left circumflex artery; LMC: Left main coronary artery).

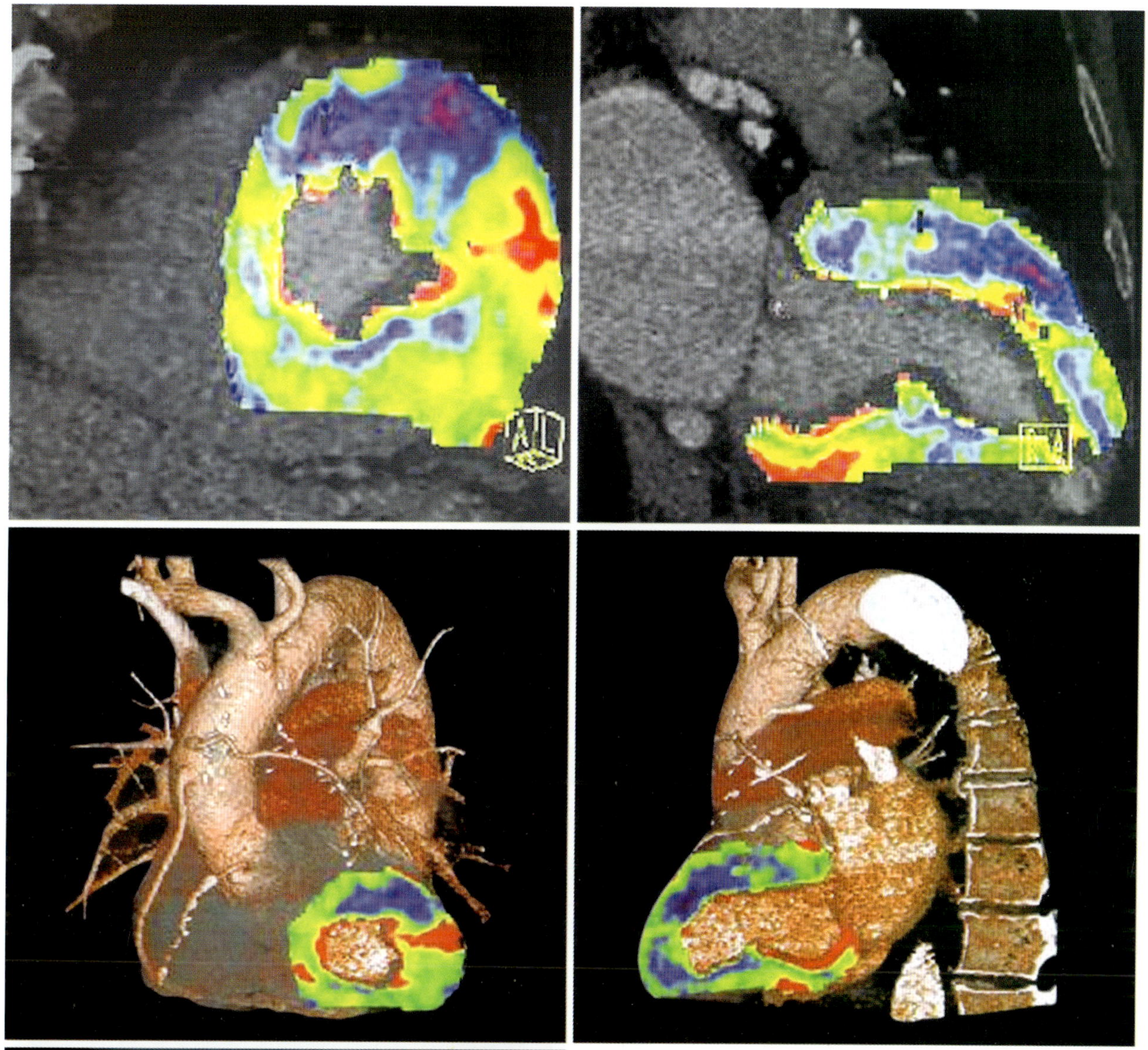

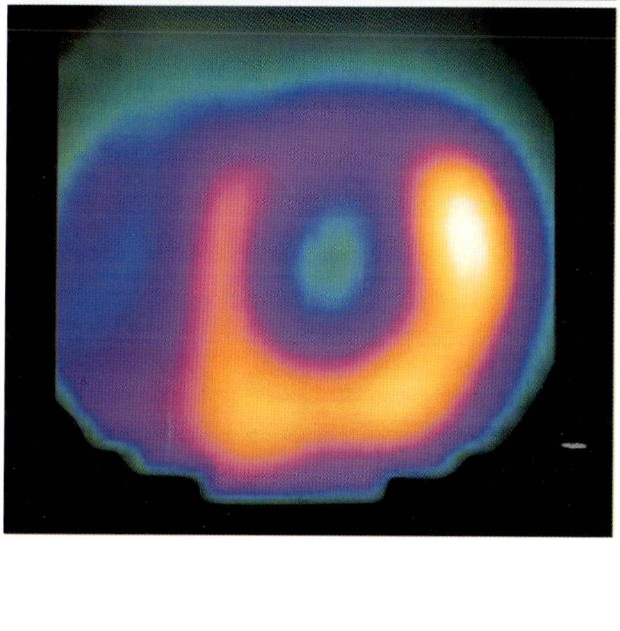

Fig. 3.30A: Color-coded CT myocardial stress perfusion images with superimposed color-coded perfusion maps (A–D) revealing a perfusion deficit of the anterior wall (blue color). The corresponding nuclear stress study image is displaced in panel E. (Image courtesy of U. Joseph Schoepf, MD, FAHA, FSCBT-MR, FNASCI, FSCCT, Medical University of South Carolina. Image from DSCT.com).

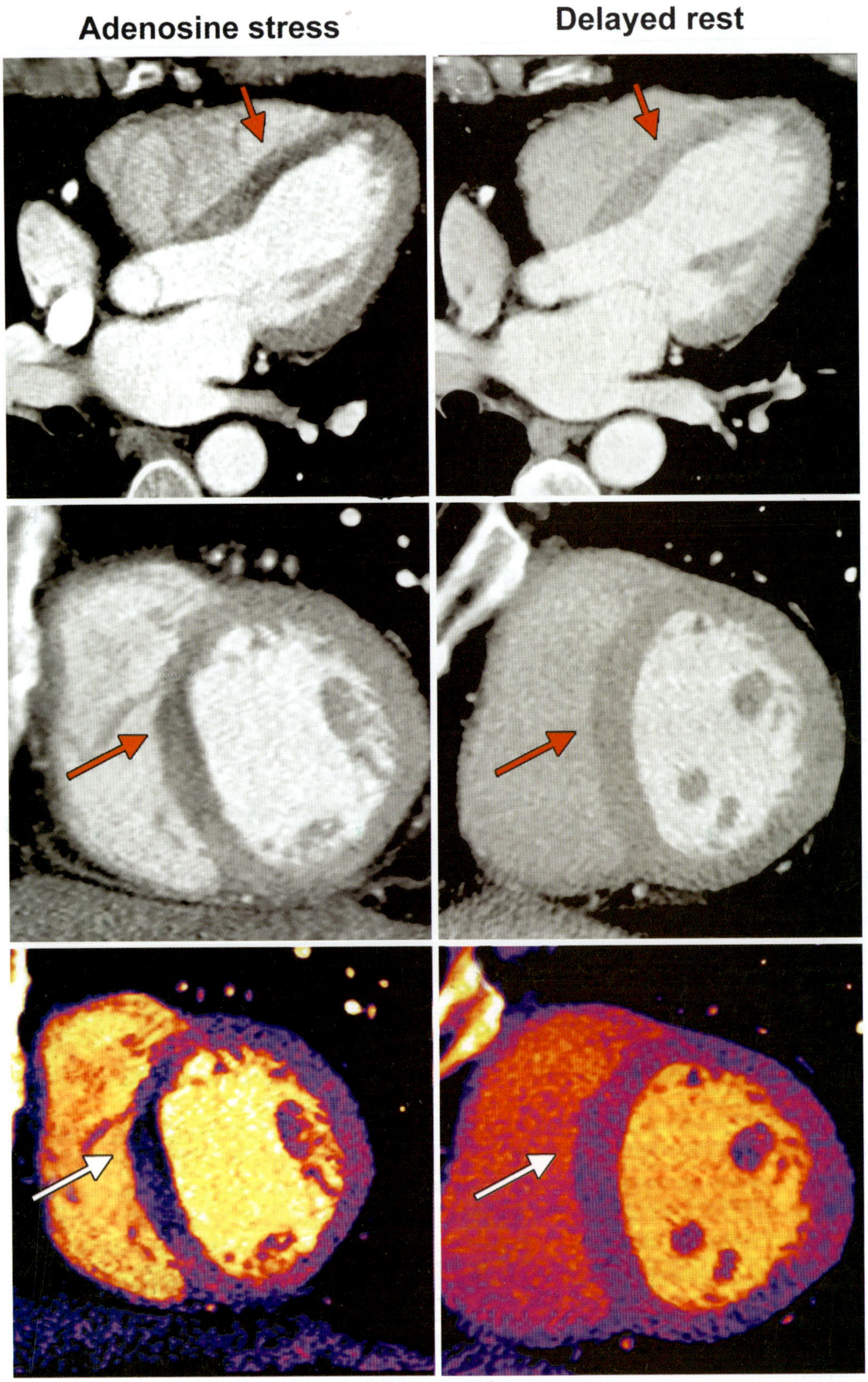

Fig. 3.30B: Cardiac T adenosine myocardial stress perfusion. Images demonstrate an adenosine-stress induced anteroseptal perfusion defect. Delayed rest images no longer demonstrate the defect, indicating an area of reversible ischemia. (Image courtesy of Dr Gudrun Feuchtner, Institute of Diagnostic Radiology).

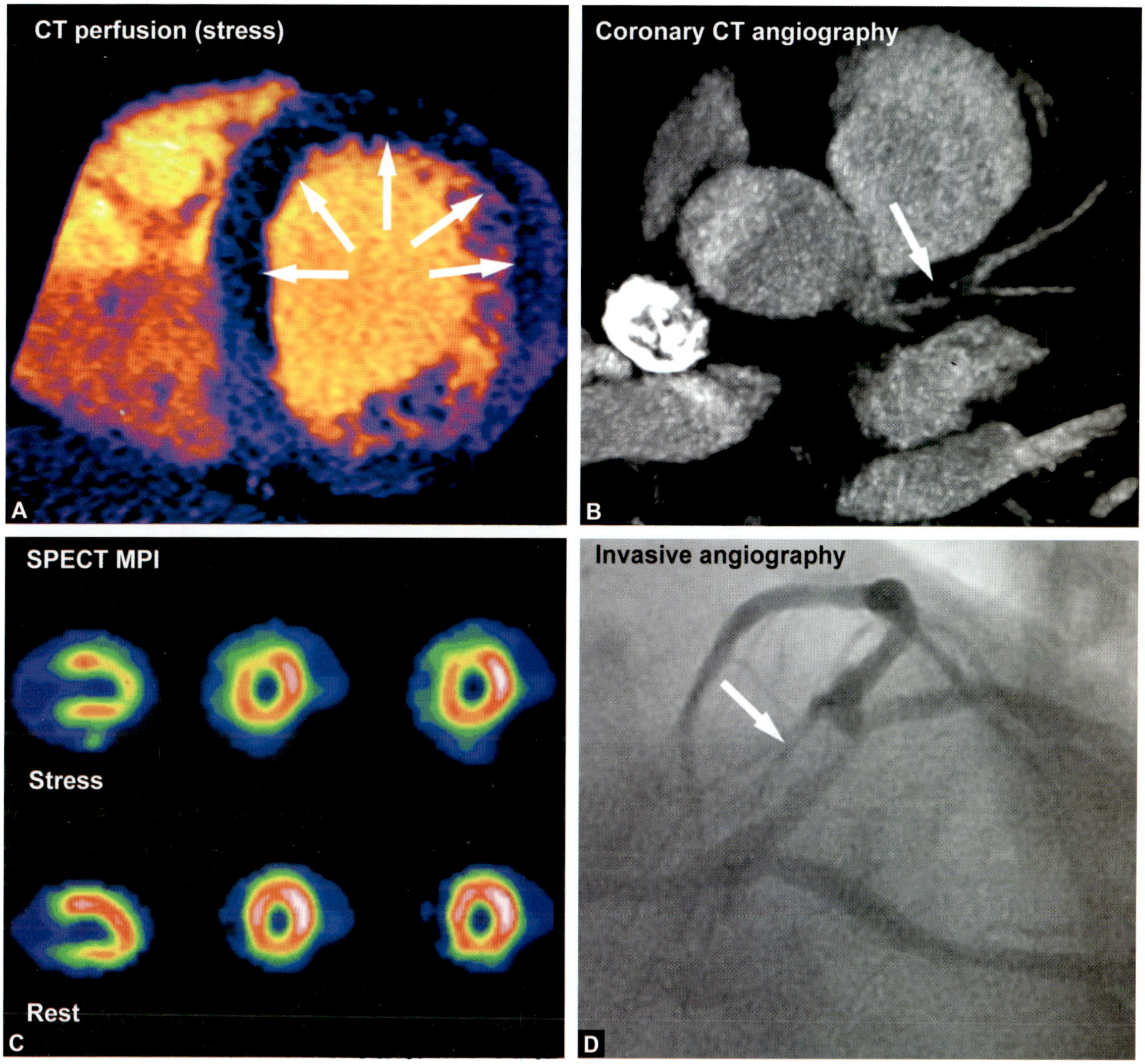

Figs. 3.31A to D: Correlation of CT perfusion imaging, CT coronary angiography, SPECT MPI and coronary angiography. (A) CT perfusion images during adenosine infusion demonstrating a large perfusion defect in the anteroseptal, anterior, and anterolateral walls (arrows); (B) CT coronary angiography demonstrating a large non-calcified plaque in the proximal LAD; (C) Exercise SPECT imaged showing a medium size defect of moderate to severe intensity throughout the mid to distal anterior and anteroseptal walls and the apex; (D) Cardiac catheterization (LAO caudal image) showing severe stenosis in the LAD prior to the takeoff of the first diagonal branch. Image and legend text from Blankstein R et al. Adenosine induced stress myocardial perfusion imaging using dual source computed tomography: a novel technique allowing simultaneous visualization of coronary anatomy and physiology. Published on Cardiovascular Images website (www.mgh-cardiovascularimages.org). [Image from Suhny Abbara MD (editor), with permission].

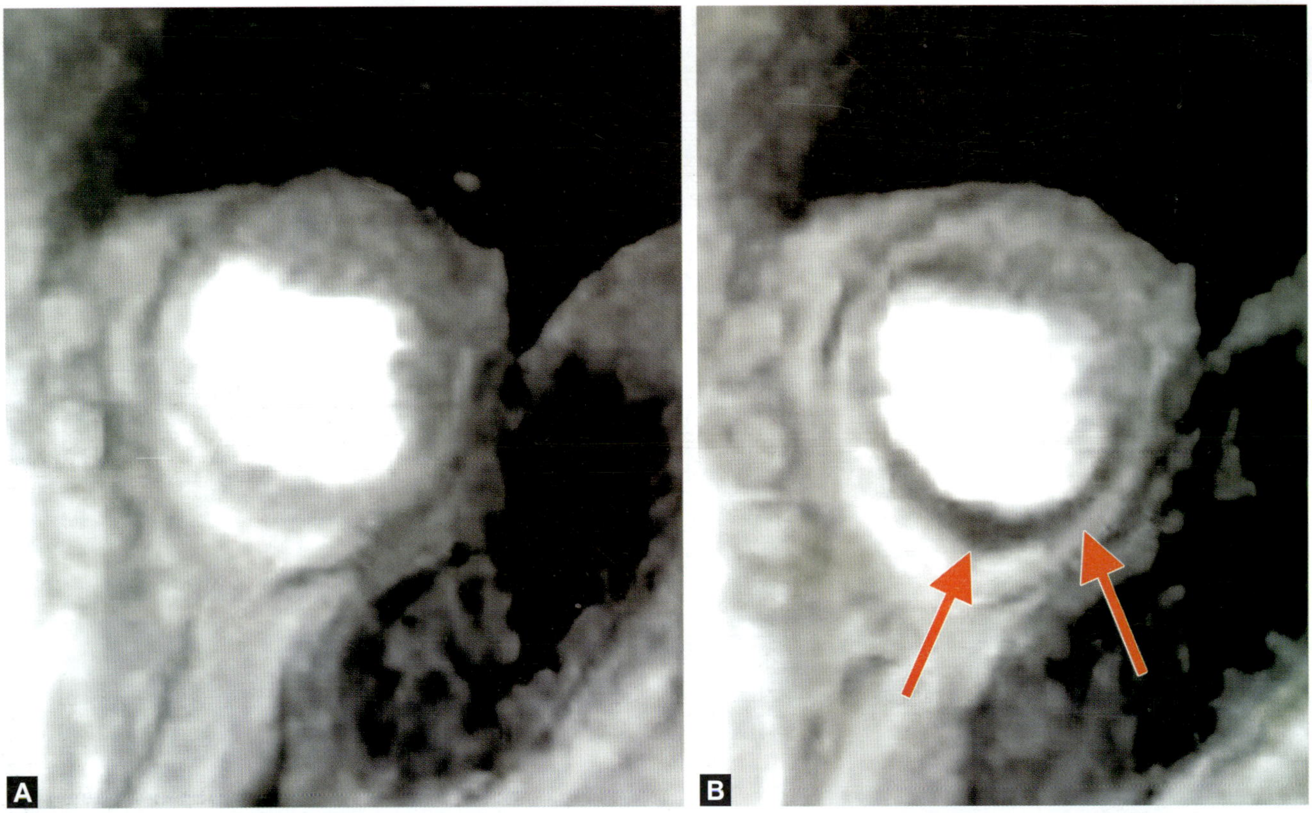

Figs. 3.32A and B: Cardiac magnetic resonance dynamic perfusion images showing normal perfusion at basal conditions (Fig. 3.32A) and stress-induced subendocardial hypoperfusion (non-enhanced, dark appearing areas) of the inferior and inferior lateral regions (Fig. 3.32B, arrows) consistent with inducible ischemia.

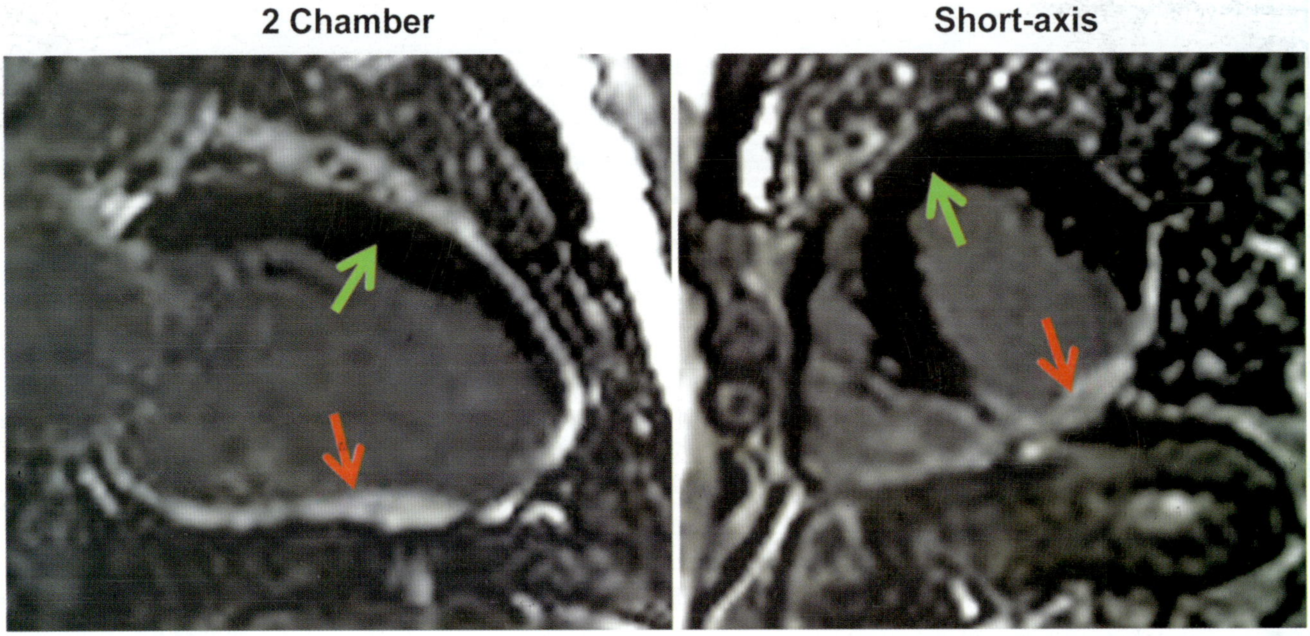

Fig. 3.33: Cardiac magnetic resonance postcontrast late enhancement images of the left ventricle. 2 chamber and short-axis views are shown. There is no enhancement of the anterior wall (dark myocardium, green arrows), indicating viable, non-infarcted myocardium, and clear delayed enhancement (white areas, red arrows) of the inferior wall, indicative of transmural myocardial fibrosis and scar.

and high risk for adverse prognosis. Studies comparing stress echo and SPECT MI have in general found comparable prognostic risk value of both techniques.

Table 3.4: Comparison of diagnostic accuracy of various stress modalities for detection of CAD. (Echo: Echocardiography; SPECT: Single photon computed tomography; PET: Positron emission tomography; MSCT: Multi-slice computed tomography; CMRI: Cardiac magnetic resonance imaging).

Method	*Sensitivity (Range)*	*Specificity (Range)*
Exercise ECG	68% (25–71)	77% (53–81)
Stress echocardiography:		
• Exercise echo	88% (74–97)	79% (64–86)
• Dobutamine echo	81% (61–95)	80% (51–95)
Stress SPECT:		
• Exercise SPECT	88% (86–90)	69% (62–75)
• Adenosine SPECT	90% (89–92)	81% (73–89)
• Dobutamine SPECT	84% (78–89)	75% (71–79)
Stress PET	92% (85–98)	85% (50–100)
Stress CMRI:		
• Wall motion analysis	83% (79–88)	86% (81–91)
• Perfusion imaging	91% (88–94)	81% (77–85)
• Coronary MRA	88% (82–92)	56% (43–68)
MSCT (64-slice)¶	97% (96–99)	91% (87–94)

A normal stress imaging study (stress echo and MPI) in the setting of good exercise capacity identifies patients at low risk (<1% per year risk of myocardial infarction or cardiac death) for the ensuing 12–18 months following the test. Important incremental adverse prognostic markers include ischemia involving >20% of the left ventricle, study results suggesting the presence of multivessel disease, poststress cavity dilation, reduced global LV systolic function, right ventricular dysfunction and increased lung tracer uptake.

CHOICES OF STRESS TESTS AND OPTIMAL SELECTION

A summary comparison of available imaging stress modalities is outlined on Table 3.5. A working algorithm of choices of available cardiac stress modalities and a guide to optimum selection of an appropriate test is outlined on Flow chart 3.1. The local availability, cost and local expertise are other factors that may determine the selection of these tests. A schematic proposed paradigm on approach to these various noninvasive CAD tests based on clinical risk is outlined on Flow chart 3.2.

Table 3.5: Comparison of various stress imaging modalities for detection of coronary artery disease. (ECG: Electrocardiogram; SPECT: Single photon computed tomography; PET: Positron emission tomography; MSCT: Multi-slice computed tomography; CMRI: Cardiac magnetic resonance imaging).

Method	*Availability*	*Feasibility*	*Limitations*	*Portable*	*Versatility*	*Reproducible*	*Axial resolution (mm)*	*Time*
Stress Echo	High	High	Obesity, COPD Subjective	Yes	High Anatomy LV Function Valves Pressures	Medium	1	30–45 min
Stress SPECT	High	High	Radiation Artifacts	No	Medium LV Function	High	6–8	2–4 hours
Stress PET	Low	High	Radiation Cost	No	Medium LV Function	High	2–4	30–60 min
CMRI	Low to Medium	High	Claustrophobia, Arrhythmia Metallic implants	No	High Anatomy LV Function Valves Pressures Viability	High	0.5–1	45–90 min
MSCT	Medium	High	Radiation Renal Injury Arrhythmia	No	Medium Anatomy LV Function	Medium	0.4–0.7	30 min

Flow chart. 3.1: A working algorithm for appropriate selection of cardiac stress tests choices for CAD evaluation based on patient clinical data. (CAD: Coronary artery disease; ECG: Electrocardiogram; Echo: Echocardiography; SPECT: Single photon computed tomography; PET: Positron emission tomography; CMRI: Cardiac magnetic resonance imaging; LBBB: Left bundle branch block; WPW: Wolf-Parkinson-White; LVH: Left ventricular hypertrophy; AF: Atrial fibrillation; V paced: Ventricular paced rhythm; PCI: Percutaneous coronary intervention; CABG: Coronary artery bypass grafting).

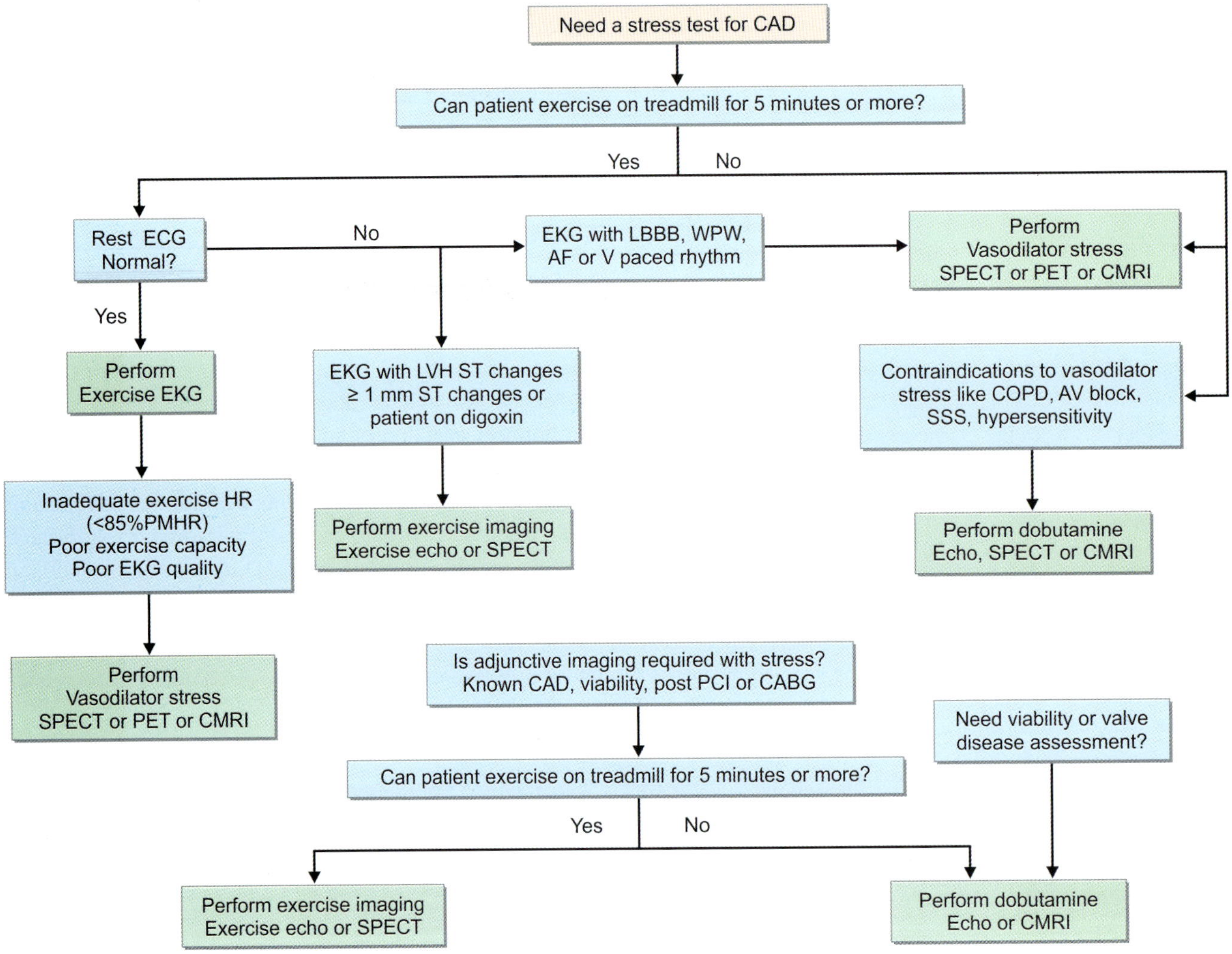

Flow chart. 3.2: Schematic diagram of a proposed testing paradigm for CAD testing with current choices of diagnostic tests based on pre-test probability of CAD and symptoms. In patients at intermediate risk there is a clear overlap in possible testing modalities, and appropriate selection should be based on patient and clinical factors as suggested in Figure 3.31. (CAD: Coronary artery disease; ECG: Electrocardiogram; Echo: Echocardiography; SPECT: Single photon computed tomography; CTA: Computed tomographic angiography; CMRI: Cardiac magnetic resonance imaging).

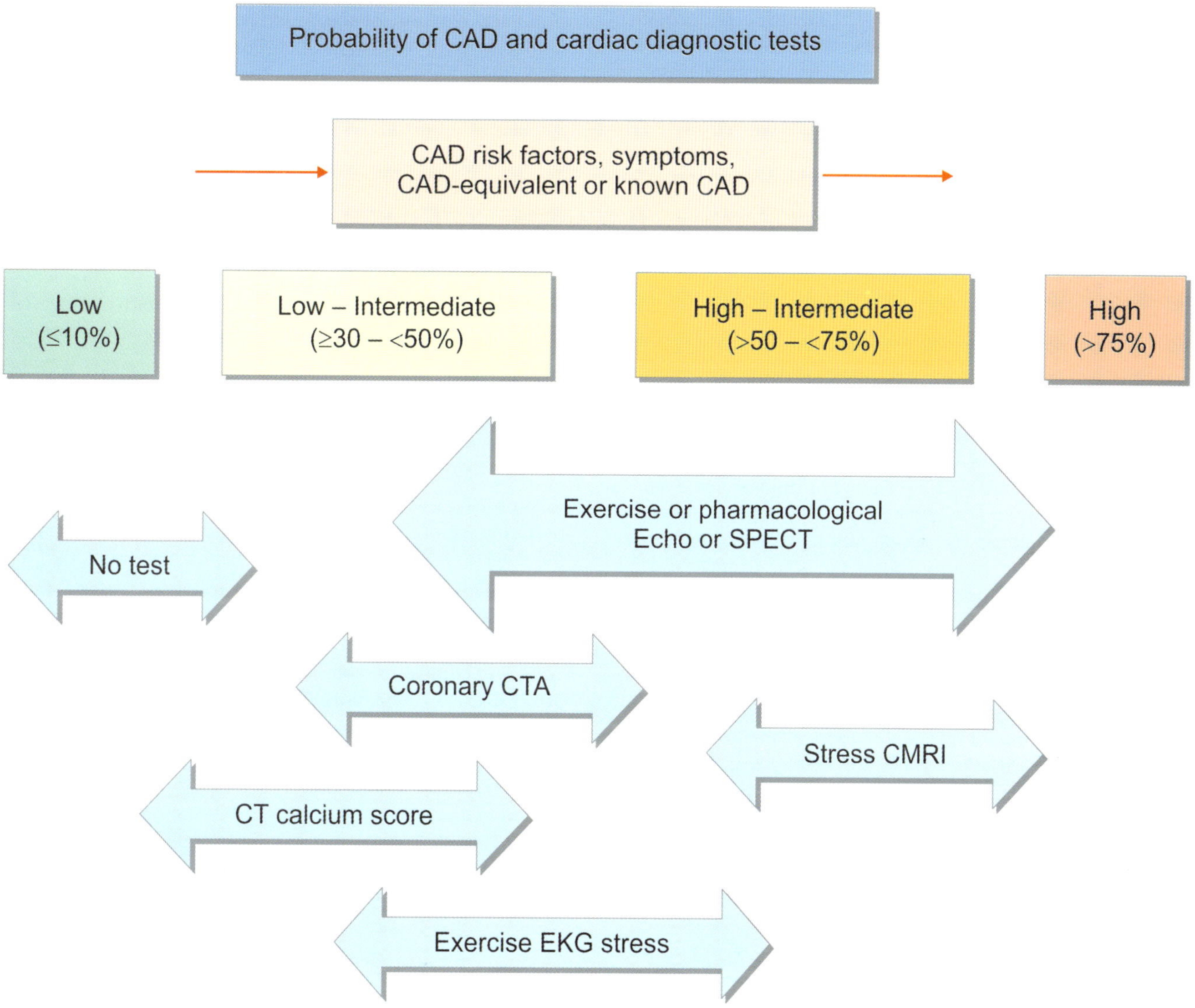

REFERENCES

Bach DS, Muller DW, Gros BJ, et al. False positive dobutamine stress echocardiograms: characterization of clinical, echocardiographic and angiographic findings. J Am Coll Cardiol. 1994;24(4):928-33.

Budoff MJ, Dowe D, Jollis JG, et al. Diagnostic performance of 64-multidetector row coronary computed tomographic angiography for evaluation of coronary artery stenosis in individuals without known coronary artery disease: results from the prospective multicenter ACCURACY (Assessment by Coronary Computed Tomographic Angiography of Individuals Undergoing Invasive Coronary Angiography) Trial. J Am Coll Cardiol. 2008;52(21):1724-32.

Douglas PS, Khandheria B, Stainback RF, et al. ACCF/ASE/ACEP/AHA/ASNC/SCAI/SCCT/SCMR 2008 appropriateness criteria for stress echocardiography. J Am Coll Cardiol. 2008;51:1127-47.

Fletcher GF, Mills WC, Taylor WC. Update on exercise stress testing. Am Fam Physician. 2006;74(10):1749-56.

Gibbons RJ, Balady GJ, Bricker JT, et al. American College of Cardiology/American Heart Association Task Force on Practice Guidelines (Committee to Update the 1997 Exercise Testing Guidelines). ACC/AHA 2002 Guideline update for exercise testing-summary article: a report of the American College of Cardiology/American Heart Association Task Force on Practice Guidelines (Committee to Update the 1997 Exercise Testing Guidelines). Circulation. 2002;106:1883-92.

Hendel RC, Berman DS, Di Carli MF, et al. ACCF/ASNC/ACR/AHA/ASE/SCCT/SCMR/SNM 2009 appropriate use criteria for cardiac radionuclide imaging. J Am Coll Cardiol. 2009;53(23):2201-29.

Henzlova MJ, Cerqueira MD, Mahmarian, et al. Stress protocols and tracers. J Nuc Cardiol. 2006;13(6):e80-90.

Hoque A, Maaieh M, Longaker RA, et al. Exercise echocardiography and thallium-201 single-photon emission computed tomography stress test for 5- and 10-year prognosis of mortality and specific cardiac events. J Am Soc Echocardiogr. 2002;15(11):1326-34.

Jahnke C, Nagel E, Gebker R, et al. Prognostic value of cardiac magnetic resonance stress tests: adenosine stress perfusion and dobutamine stress wall motion imaging. Circulation. 2007;115(13):1769-76.

Klocke FJ, Baird MG, Lorell BH, et al. ACC/AHA/ASNC Guidelines for the clinical use of cardiac radionuclide imaging—executive summary: a report of the American College of Cardiology/American Heart Association Task Force on Practice Guidelines (ACC/AHA/ASNC Committee to Revise the 1995 Guidelines for the Clinical Use of Cardiac Radionuclide Imaging). Circulation. 2003;108(11):1404-18.

Libby P, Bonow RO, et al. Braunwald's Heart Disease. Volume1, 8th edition. Philadelphia: Saunders Elsiver; 2008.

Mark DB, Shaw L, Harrell FE, et al. Prognostic value of treadmill exercise score in outpatients with suspected coronary artery disease. N Eng J Med. 1991;325:849.

Mastouri R, Sawada SG, Mahenthiran J. Current noninvasive imaging techniques for detection of coronary artery disease. Expert Rev Cardiovasc Ther. 2010;8(1):77-91.

Metz LD, Beattie M, Hom R, et al. The prognostic value of normal exercise myocardial perfusion imaging and exercise echocardiography: a meta-analysis. J Am Coll Cardiol. 2007;49(2):227-37.

Nandalur KR, Dwamena BA, Choudhri AF, et al. Diagnostic performance of stress cardiac magnetic resonance imaging in the detection of coronary artery disease: a meta-analysis. J Am Coll Cardiol. 2007;50(14):1343-53.

Olmos LI, Dakik H, Gordon R, et al. Long-term prognostic value of exercise echocardiography compared with exercise 201Tl, ECG, and clinical variables in patients evaluated for coronary artery disease. Circulation. 1998;98(24):2679-86.

Sampson UK, Dorbala S, Limaye A, et al. Diagnostic accuracy of rubidium-82 myocardial perfusion imaging with hybrid positron emission tomography/computed tomography in the detection of coronary artery disease. J Am Coll Cardiol. 2007;49(10):1052-8.

Sawada SG, Segar DS, Ryan T, et al. Catecholamine stress echocardiography. Echocardiography. 1992;9(2):177-88.

CHAPTER

Myocardial Viability Testing 4

Jamieson M Bourque, Christopher M Kramer

INTRODUCTION

Congestive heart failure with reduced left ventricular systolic function due to ischemic heart disease has high morbidity and mortality. Some patients have improved symptoms, function, and prognosis with revascularization, while others receive little benefit. Predicting which patients are likely to improve is critical to maximize the benefit/risk ratio for revascularization.

One cause of impaired systolic function in ischemic heart failure is irreversible myocyte necrosis and replacement with scar. This tissue will not regain function even if normal blood flow is restored. However, some myocytes within these regions remain alive but stunned due to chronic repetitive ischemia, and thus fail to contract. With restoration of blood flow, this viable hibernating myocardium may recover function.

The extent and degree of myocardial viability can be determined through the assessment of myocardial morphology, function, perfusion, and metabolism. Multiple imaging modalities examine these different markers of viability, including nuclear positron emission tomography (PET) and single-photon emission computed tomography (SPECT), dobutamine echocardiography, cardiac magnetic resonance (CMR), and cardiac computed tomography (CT). The sensitivities and specificities of these techniques for the recovery of myocardial function have been compared as shown in Figure 4.1.

SPECT Nuclear Imaging

Single-photon emission computed tomography nuclear imaging is widely available, with an extensive body of research to support its use. SPECT nuclear imaging assesses myocardial tracer uptake, which is dependent on the degree of perfusion and either the integrity of the Na^+/K^+ cell membrane pump (for Thallium-201) or intact mitochondrial function (for Technetium-99m). Protocols examine resting tracer uptake and changes with delayed tracer redistribution or after reinjection. Multiple criteria for viability have been used, but typically uptake of <0.3 (<30%) of the segment with the highest uptake is consistent with nonviable myocardium, 0.3–0.5 (30–50%) is equivocal, and uptake >0.5 (>50%) is consistent with viable myocardium. A typical case is shown in Figure 4.2.

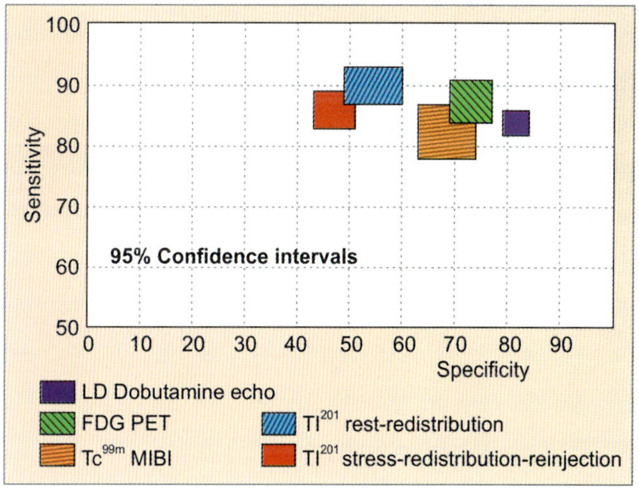

Fig. 4.1: Receiver operating characteristic plot graphing the 95% confidence intervals for viability assessment tools. Positron emission tomography (PET) imaging of fluorine-18-fluorodeoxyglucose (^{18}F-FDG) has the highest overall diagnostic accuracy. Thallium-201 single-photon emission computed tomography (SPECT) has the highest sensitivity but lacks specificity, and dobutamine echocardiography has the highest specificity at the expense of sensitivity. [Figure adapted with permission from Bax JJ, Wijns W, Cornel JH, et al. Accuracy of currently available techniques for prediction of functional recovery after revascularization in patients with left ventricular dysfunction due to chronic coronary artery disease: comparison of pooled data. J Am Coll Cardiol. 1997;30(6):1451-60].

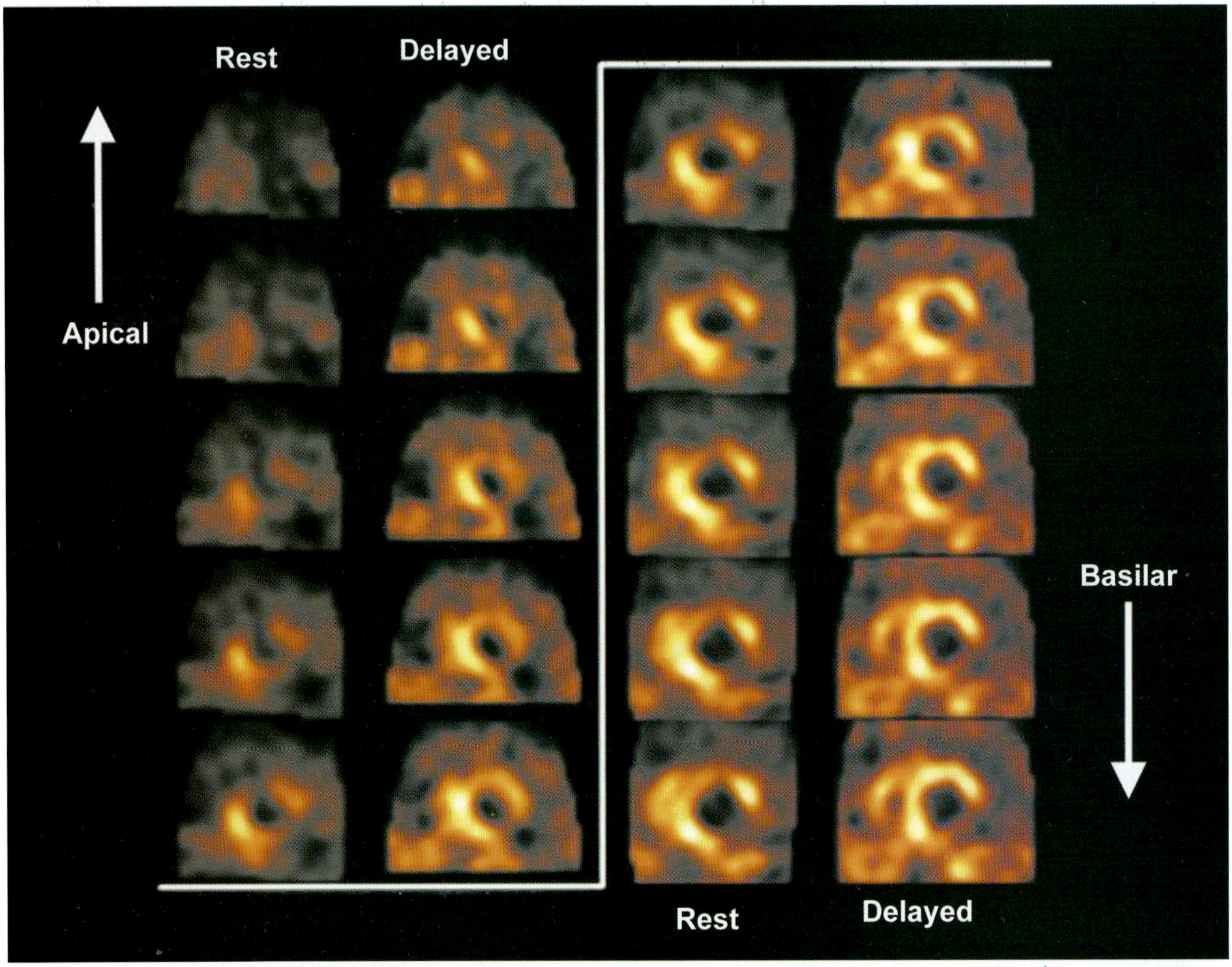

Fig. 4.2: Thallium-201 single-photon emission computed tomography (SPECT) myocardial viability short-axis images. Thallium-201 uptake at rest reveals minimal apical, mid-anterior, and basilar inferolateral uptake. After an 8-hour delay, increased uptake is appreciated in the apex and mid-anterior regions, consistent with myocardial viability. There is poor uptake and minimal increase with redistribution in the basilar inferolateral region, indicating nonviable scar.

PET Viability Imaging

Positron emission tomography viability imaging is typically performed using a perfusion tracer (rubidium-82 or ^{13}N-ammonia) and a metabolic tracer [fluorine-18-fluorodeoxyglucose (^{18}F-FDG)]. FDG is a glucose analog taken up by ischemic cells that have switched from fatty acid to glucose utilization. Areas of perfusion-metabolic mismatch, where there is FDG uptake and poor ^{13}N-ammonia or rubidium-82 uptake, are consistent with viable myocardium (Figs. 4.3 and 4.4). Matched defects demarcate absent perfusion and metabolism and are consistent with scar. A benefit with revascularization has been appreciated with as little as 5–7% mismatch. PET imaging is less widely available and is complicated in diabetic patients due to impaired cellular glucose entry.

Dobutamine Echocardiography

Viability can be assessed by dobutamine echocardiography. Viability is defined by increased regional myocardial thickening, representative of contractile reserve, with dobutamine-mediated inotropic stimulation. A biphasic response, in which function improves with low dose dobutamine due to recruitment of stunned myocardium, and then worsens at peak stress due to progressive ischemia, is highly specific for myocardial viability (Figs. 4.5 and 4.6). This imaging technique is

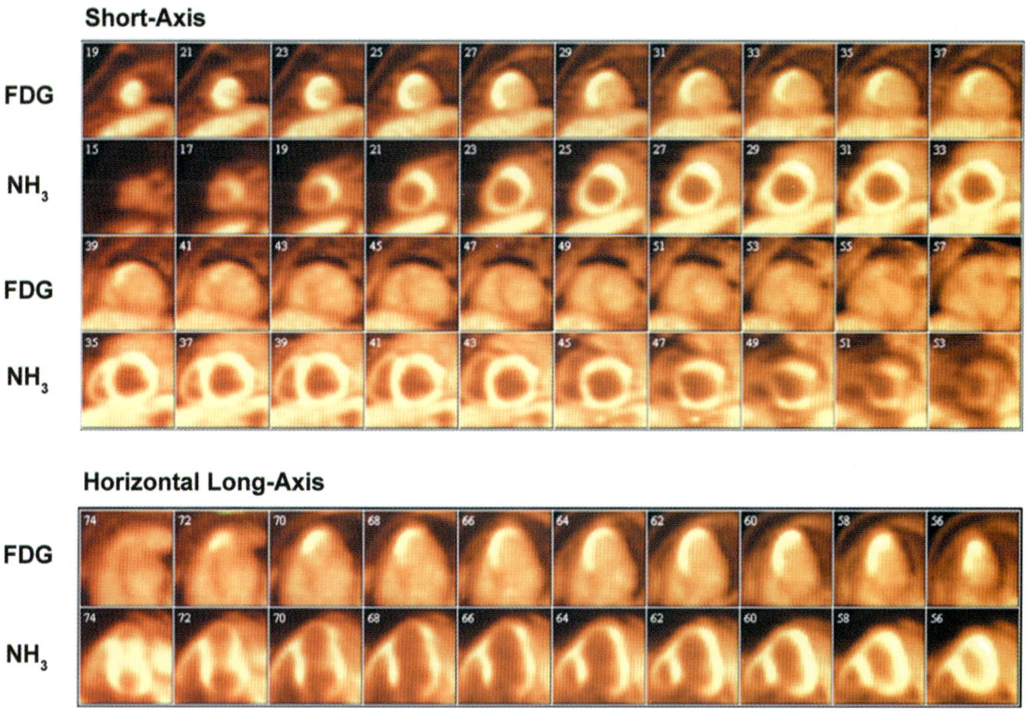

Fig. 4.3: Positron emission tomography (PET) viability images. The ^{13}N-ammonia (NH_3) resting perfusion images reveal a prominent anterior, septal, and apical defect consistent with infarction. The corresponding fluorine-18-fluorodeoxyglucose (^{18}F-FDG) metabolic images show uptake in the ammonia defect area. This perfusion-metabolism mismatch is an indicator of viable myocardium.

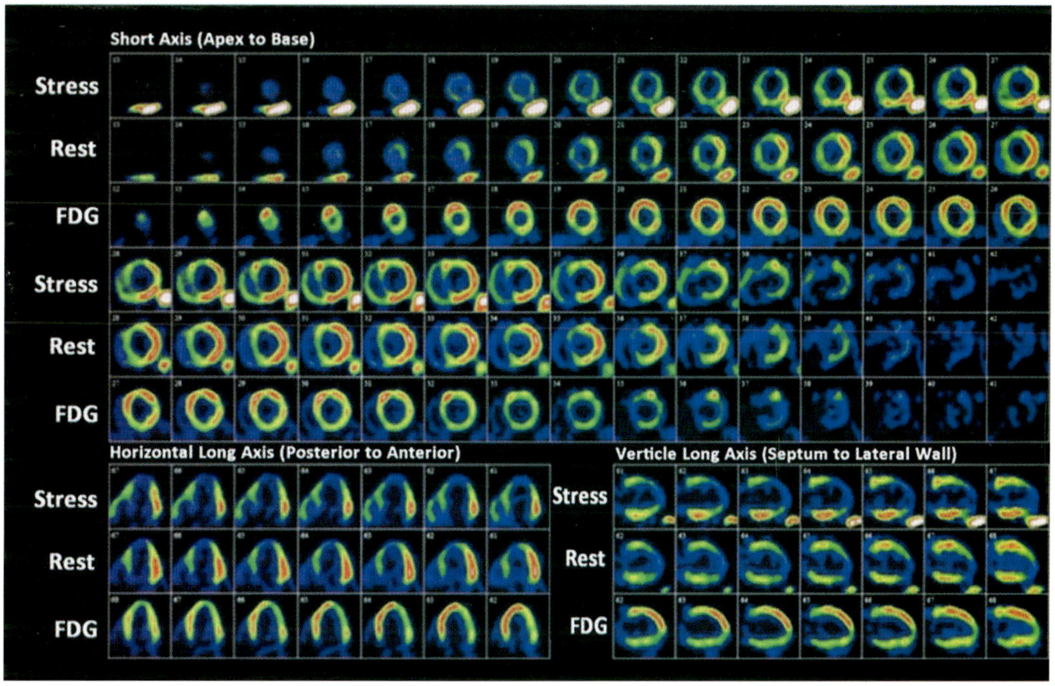

Fig. 4.4: Rubidium-82 stress and fluorine-18-fluorodeoxyglucose (^{18}F-FDG) positron emission tomography (PET) viability imaging. Stress images (rows labeled "stress") demonstrate a moderate to severe reduction in uptake in the anterior wall, apex, distal inferior wall, and septum with minimal improvement on rest (rows labeled "rest"), consistent with mild ischemia, transmural, and nontransmural scar in the left anterior descending (LAD) territory. ^{18}F-FDG images (rows labeled "FDG") demonstrate a mismatch pattern in the mentioned territories, signifying viable myocardium. [Image and legend text from Mylonas I, Beanlands RS. Radionuclide Imaging of Viable Myocardium: Is it underutilized? Curr Cardiovasc Imaging Rep. 2011;4(3):251-61].

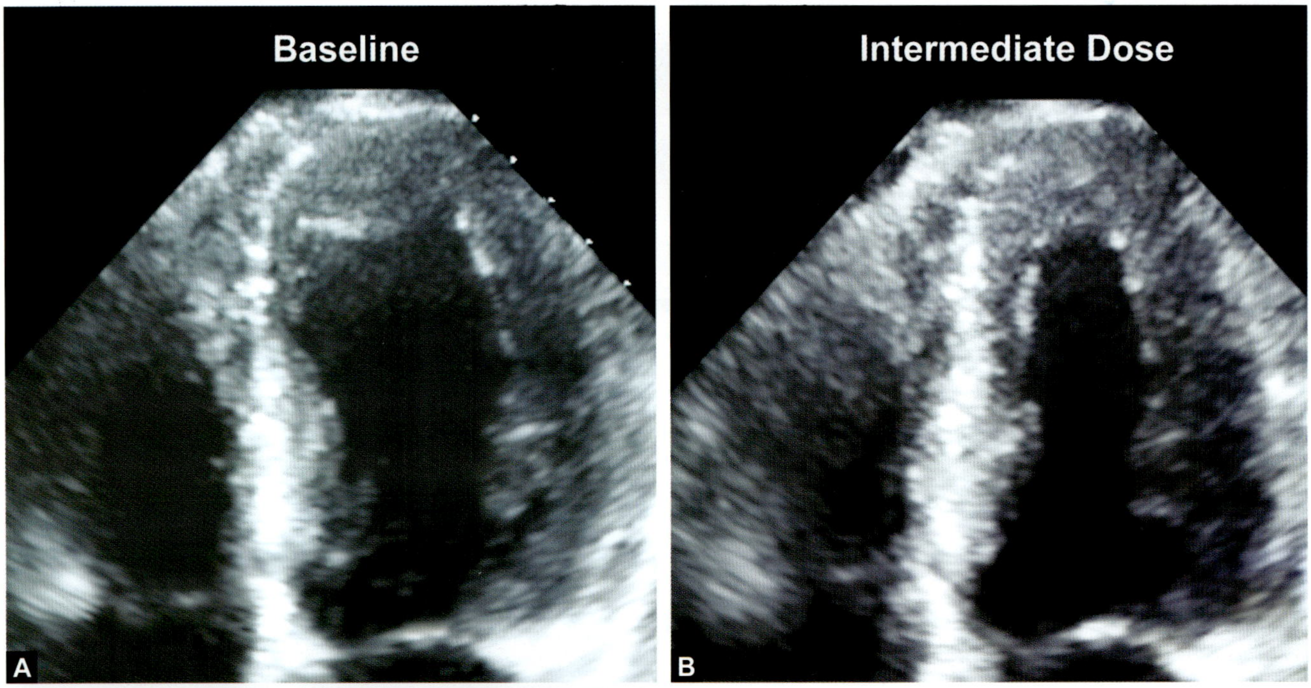

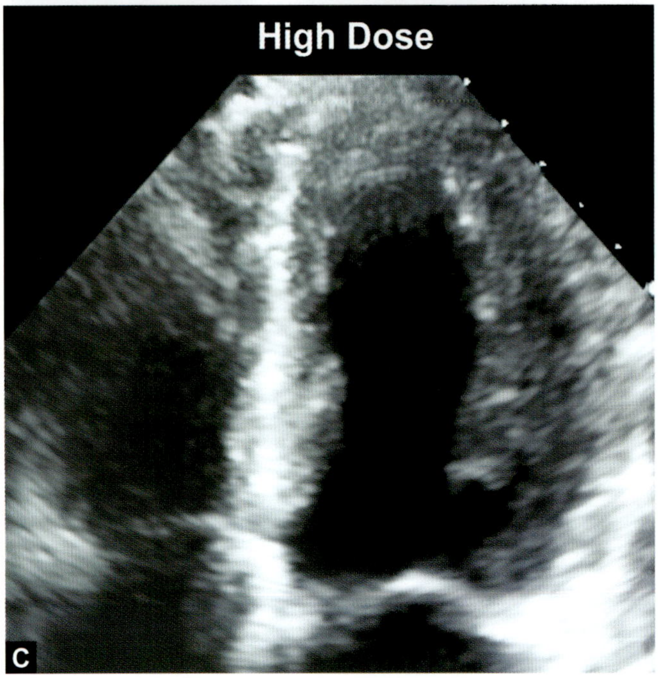

Figs. 4.5A to C: Illustration of a biphasic response during dobutamine stress test. Four-chamber apical images obtained at peak systole show depressed systolic function at baseline, with improvement in systolic function at intermediate dose dobutamine due to recruitment of hibernating myocardium, but worsening of systolic function at high dose dobutamine due to ischemia. This finding suggests the presence of hibernating but viable myocardium subtended by hemodynamically significant coronary artery disease. (Image courtesy of Glenn N Levine, MD).

also readily available in most clinical settings. Other advanced tools such as strain assessment and myocardial contrast echocardiography (Figs. 4.7 and 4.8) remain investigational.

Cardiac Magnetic Resonance

Cardiac magnetic resonance has high spatial resolution that allows precise assessment of regional wall motion and the distribution and transmurality of scar. However, it may be limited by patient ineligibility due to implanted devices, claustrophobia, and stage 4 or 5 chronic kidney disease due to the risk of nephrogenic systemic fibrosis (NSF) with gadolinium administration. CMR viability imaging can be performed by examining contractile reserve, as with dobutamine echocardiography, or through analysis of the distribution of scar. Gadolinium is trapped in

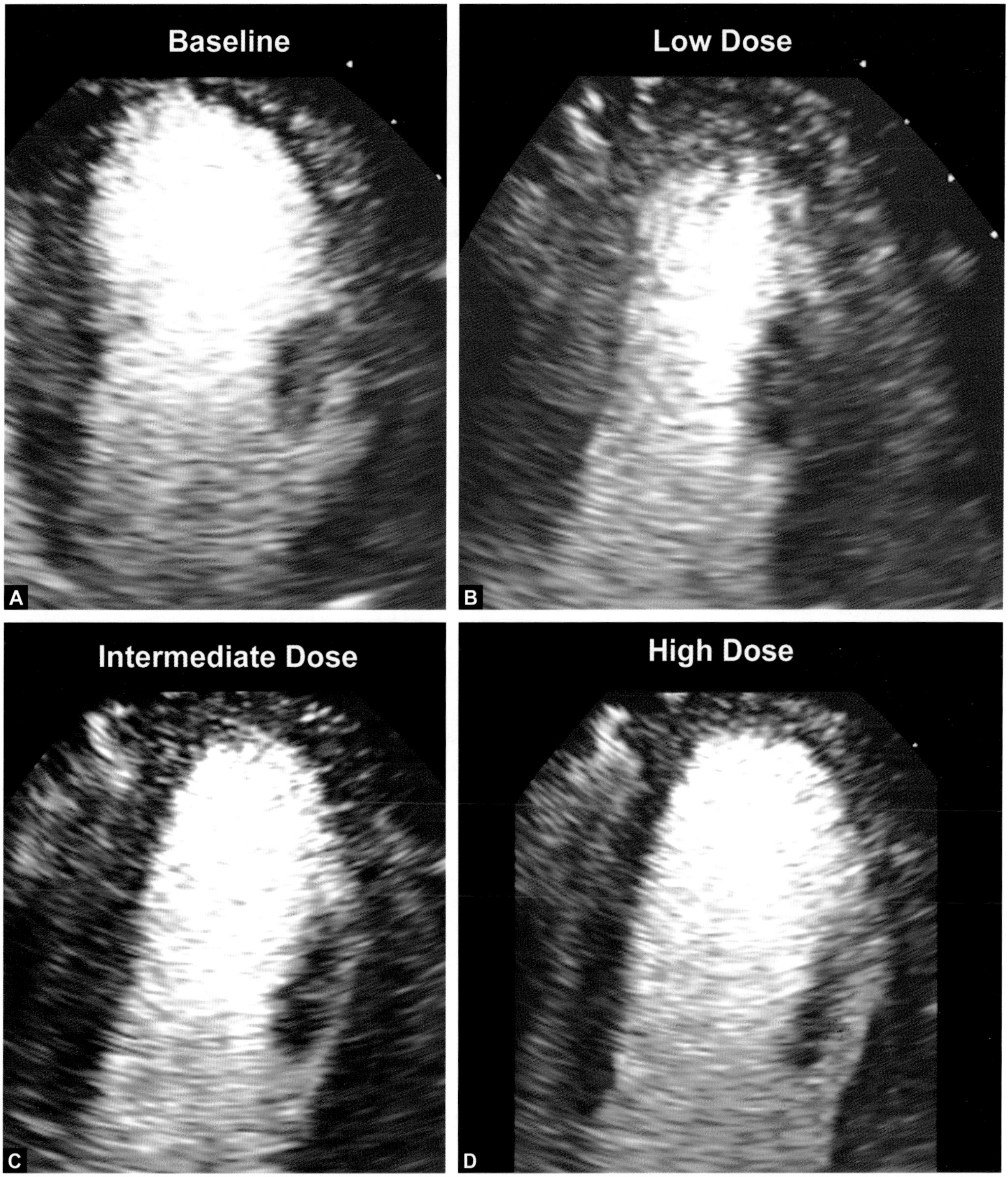

Figs. 4.6A to D: Contrast-enhanced dobutamine stress echocardiography illustrating a biphasic response to progressively higher doses of dobutamine infusion. Left ventricular ejection fraction and wall thickening improve at low dose dobutamine infusion. However, there is a worsening of left ventricular myocardial contractility at higher doses of dobutamine infusion. (Image courtesy of Glenn N Levine, MD).

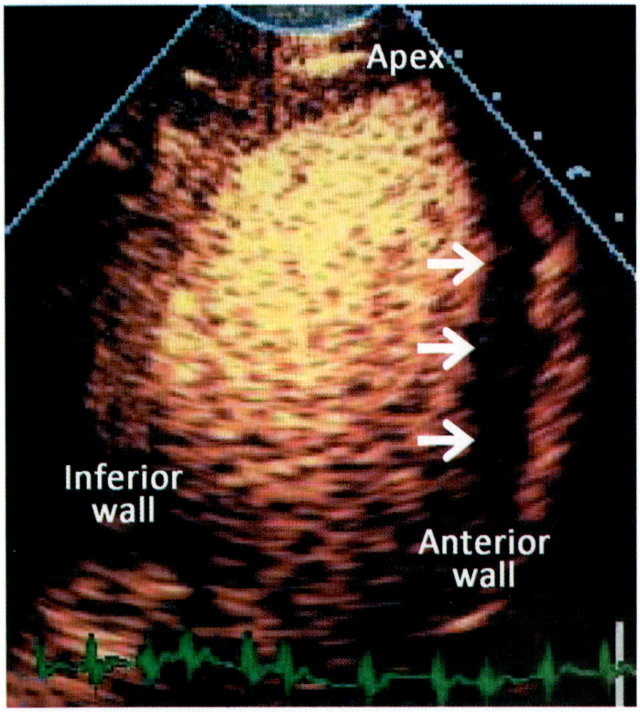

Fig. 4.7: Myocardial contrast echocardiography. Myocardial contrast echocardiographic image obtained in the apical 2-chamber view, 10 beats post-flash, demonstrating absent perfusion in the anterior myocardial wall. Note that the inferior wall and apex are clearly perfused, while the anterior wall remains dark in color (arrows), indicating lack of any perfusion and likely non-viable myocardium. (Image and legend text from Moir S, Marwick TH. Combination of contrast with stress echocardiography: a practical guide to methods and interpretation. Cardiovasc Ultrasound. 2004; 2:15).

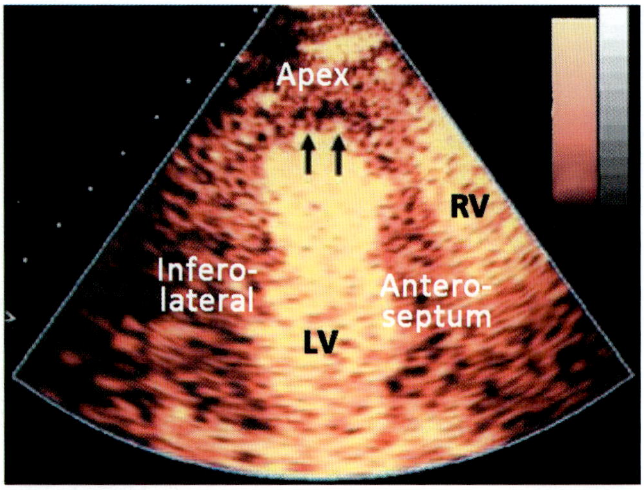

Fig. 4.8: Myocardial perfusion image shows only a small, subendocardial area in the apex (arrows) of non-perfused myocardium, while the remainder of the visualized left ventricle appears perfused. [Image from Ashrafian H, Dwivedi G, Senior R. Assessing myocardial perfusion after myocardial infarction. PLoS Med. 2006;3(3):e131].

nonviable tissue due to increased volume of distribution and delayed washout, leading to late gadolinium enhancement (LGE) (Figs. 4.9 and 4.10). The degree of scar transmurality identifies likelihood of functional recovery (Fig. 4.11), with a finding of < 50% scar in myocardial wall thickness generally considered and indicative of viable myocardium.

Cardiac CT

Cardiovascular CT viability imaging has shown promise, but has lower contrast-to-noise as compared to CMR. Two scans are performed, the first to assess the coronaries and the second delayed scan to examine for contrast accumulation consistent with scar from myocyte loss and increased volume of distribution (Figs. 4.12A and B). It remains an investigational technique.

PROGNOSTIC VALUE OF VIABILITY TESTING

Viability imaging has not only been able to reliably predict recovery in left ventricular function, but it has also been shown in some studies to predict outcomes, including all-cause survival. The strongest prognostic data is in nuclear and dobutamine echocardiography, though there is emerging data in CMR. A meta-analysis including 3,088 patients from 24 studies who underwent SPECT, PET, or dobutamine echocardiography viability testing showed the degree of viability to predict survival and benefit with revascularization (Fig. 4.13). Regarding CMR, Gerber et al. examined 144 patients who underwent CMR viability testing. In one modest-sized study of CMR, the 3-year mortality rates for patients with viable myocardium were lower for those receiving revascularization (13%) compared with medical therapy alone (52%). Patients without viability had an intermediate survival rate (23–29%).

There has been some disagreement in the literature about the benefit of viability testing, however. A substudy of the Surgical Treatment of Ischemic Heart Failure (STICH) trial found no benefit to a strategy of viability testing. This analysis was limited by its observational and nonrandomized design, small group without viability, and failure to include PET and CMR data. A randomized trial of

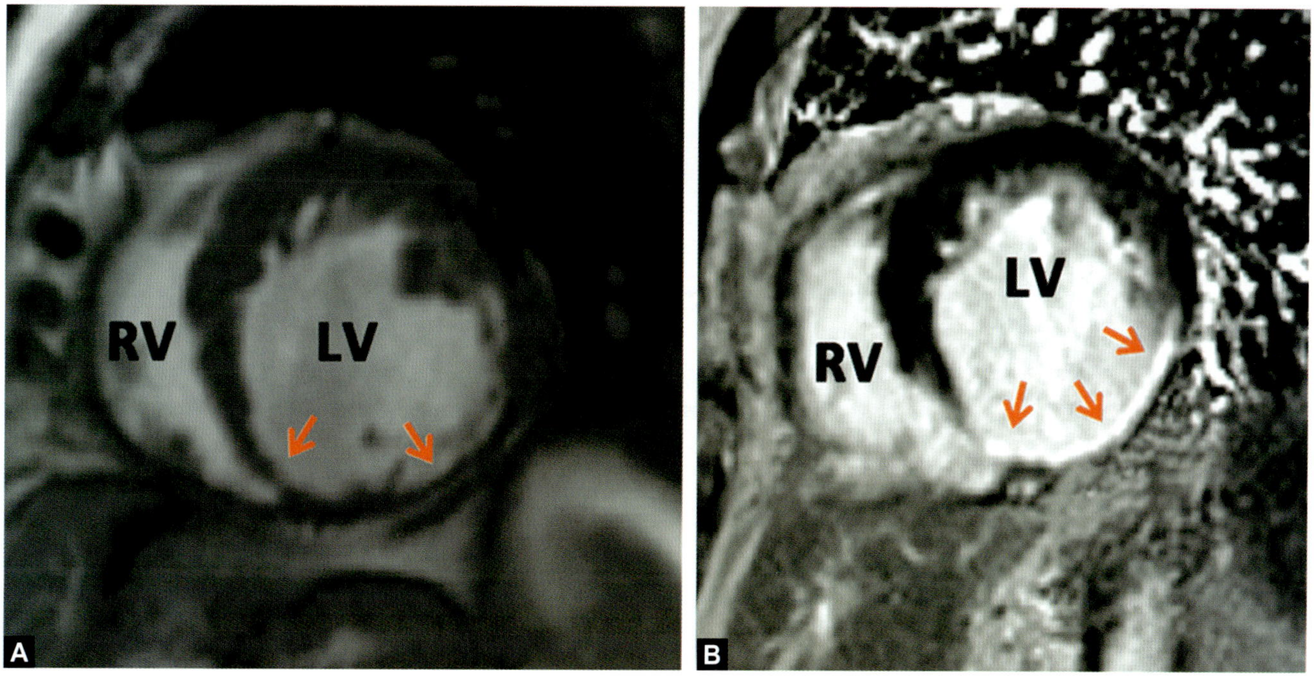

Figs. 4.9A and B: Cardiac magnetic resonance (CMR) viability assessment. Mid-ventricular short-axis cine images are provided in (A) showing inferior and lateral wall thinning and akinesis. Late gadolinium enhancement imaging of the same short-axis slice; (B) reveals an enhancement pattern consistent with transmural infarction. These images suggest the absence of myocardial viability.

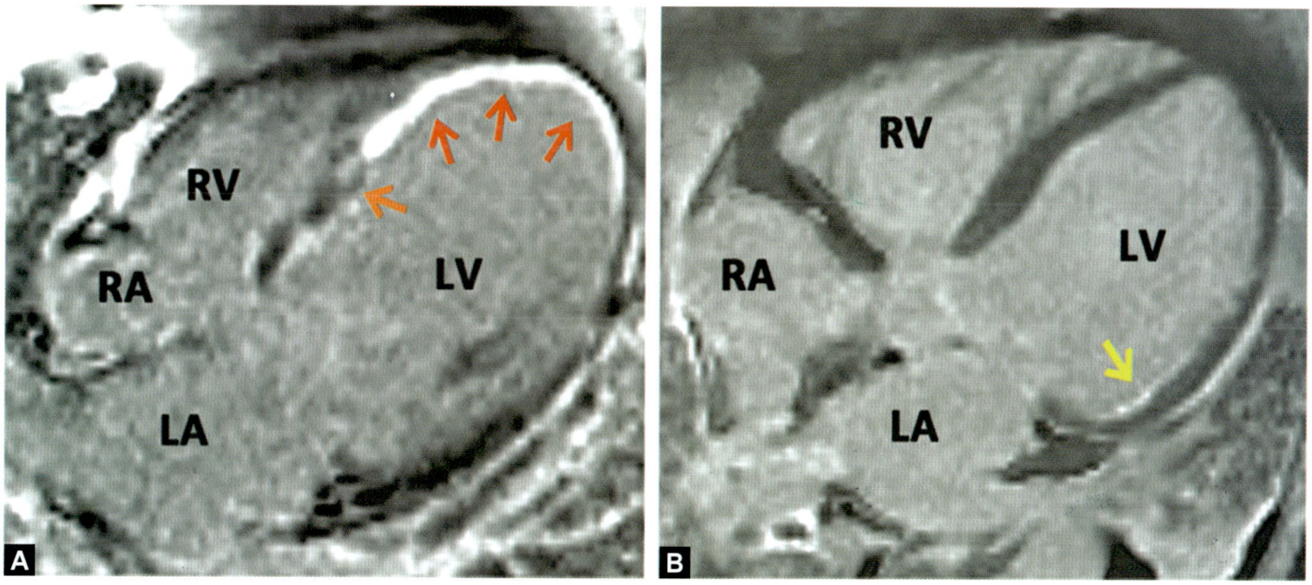

Figs. 4.10A and B: Cardiovascular magnetic resonance late gadolinium enhancement imaging in patients "with dilated cardiomyopathy". (A) Image acquired 10 minutes following administration of gadolinium contrast demonstrates a transmural infarction (red arrows) in the septum and apex, as well as microvascular obstruction in the basal septum (orange arrow). Contractility in this area would not be likely to improve with revascularization; (B) Viability testing in this patient reveals only a small area of subendocardial infarction (yellow arrow) in the basal anterolateral segment. Coronary revascularization is likely to lead to improvement in ejection fraction in this patient with ischemic cardiomyopathy. [Image from Weiss RM. Cardiovascular magnetic resonance. In: Chatterjee K, Anderson M, Heistad D, Kerber RE (Eds). Cardiology: an Illustrated Textbook. New Delhi, India: Jaypee Brothers Medical Publishers (P) Ltd. 2013].

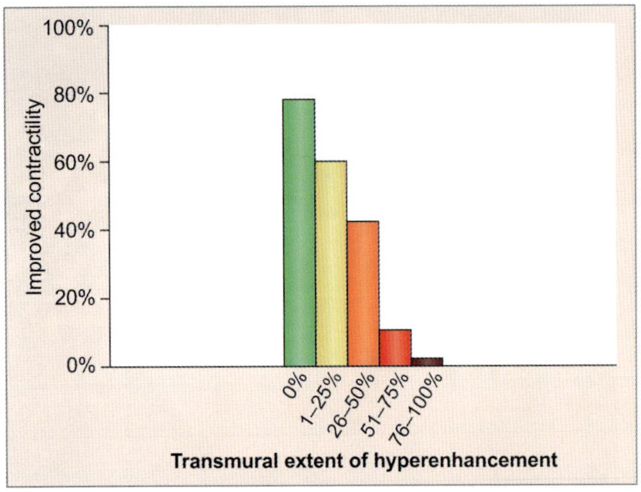

Fig. 4.11: Relationship between the extent of hyperenhancement transmurality (scar extent) and likelihood of improved contractility after revascularization. There is a stepwise decrease in the likelihood of functional improvement as the transmurality of scar increases. Whether improvement will occur with hyperenhancement transmurality between 26–75% is unclear.

a strategy of PET viability imaging [the PET and Recovery Following Revascularization (PARR-2) study] was negative. However, a post-hoc analysis showed a survival benefit when treatment was given based on the recommendation of the PET study (Fig. 4.14). There was also a benefit when data from only the most experienced centers was used (Ottawa-5 Substudy). Although there has been some controversy, the majority of the existing evidence suggests that a strategy of viability testing is useful for prognosis.

Myocardial viability testing using nuclear imaging, dobutamine echocardiography, and CMR imaging have all been classified as "appropriate" in the relevant appropriateness criteria guidelines. Cardiac CT is classified as "uncertain" given the lack of sufficient data. The 2013 American College of Cardiology Foundation/American Heart Association (ACCF/AHA) heart failure guidelines state that it is reasonable to consider viability imaging (class IIa) prior to revascularization in patients with heart failure and coronary artery disease (CAD).

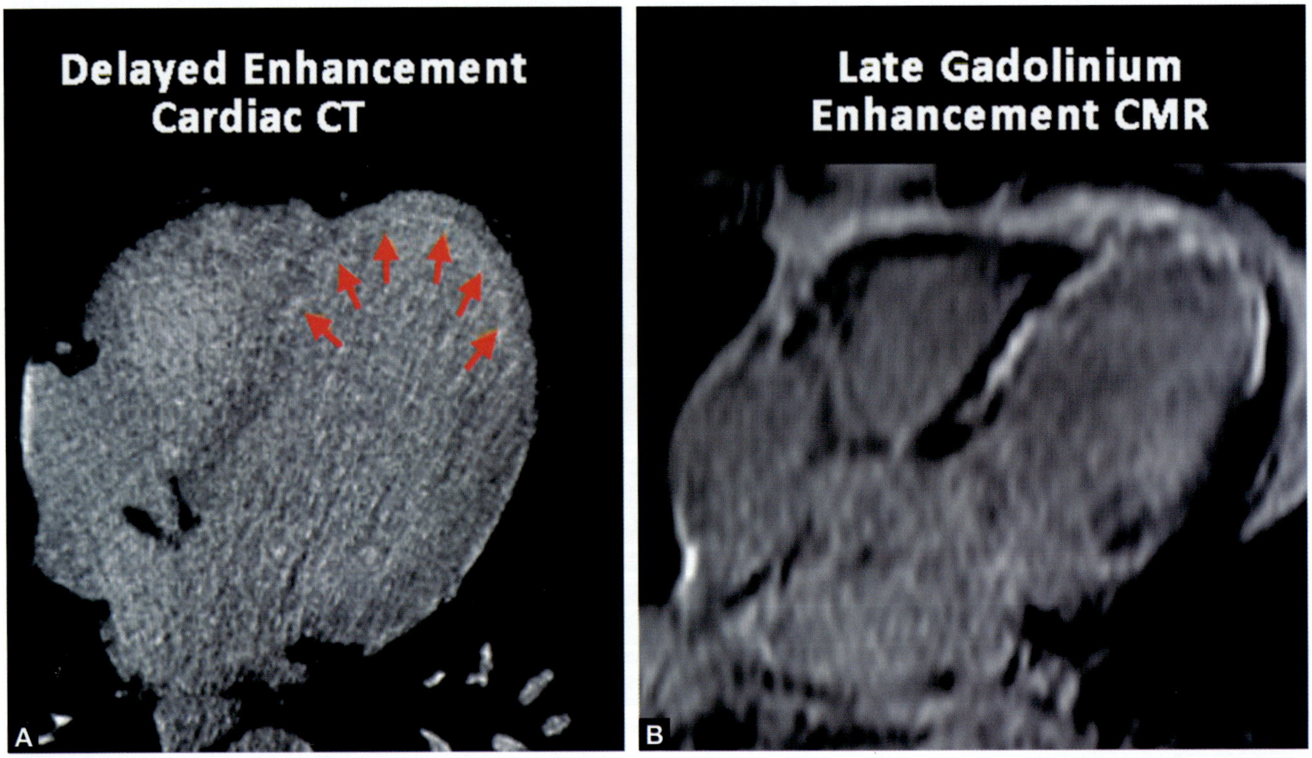

Figs. 4.12A and B: (A) Viability imaging using delayed enhancement cardiac computed tomography (CT). Gated CT imaging 15 minutes post-contrast infusion reveals delayed enhancement of the subendocardium in the left anterior descending (LAD) distribution (arrows); (B) Late gadolinium enhancement cardiac magnetic resonance (CMR) imaging reveals a myocardial infarction in the same distribution. This technique remains experimental. [Adapted with permission from Mendoza DD, Joshi SB, Weissman G, et al. Viability imaging by cardiac computed tomography. J Cardiovasc Comput Tomogr. 2010;4(2):83-91].

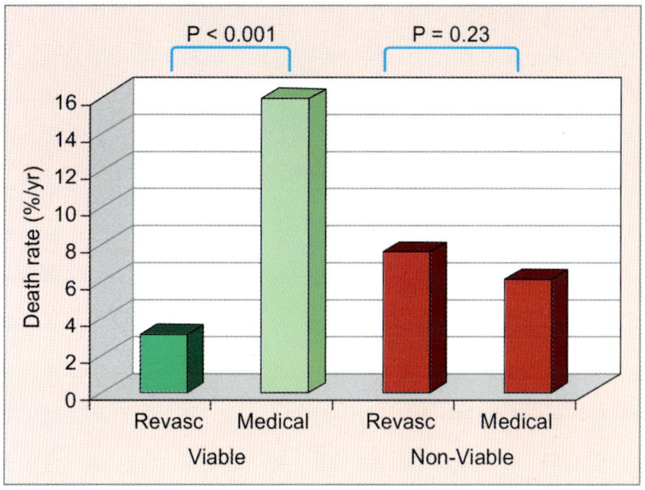

Fig. 4.13: Annual death rates by viability status and treatment received. Patients with viable myocardium who are treated with medical therapy have a 5-fold increase in death rate over those revascularized, who have the lowest event rate. Patients without significant viability have similar intermediate event rates irrespective of treatment received. [Adapted with permission from Allman KC, Shaw LJ, Hachamovitch R, et al. Myocardial viability testing and impact of revascularization on prognosis in patients with coronary artery disease and left ventricular dysfunction: a meta-analysis. J Am Coll Cardiol. 2002;39(7):1151-8].

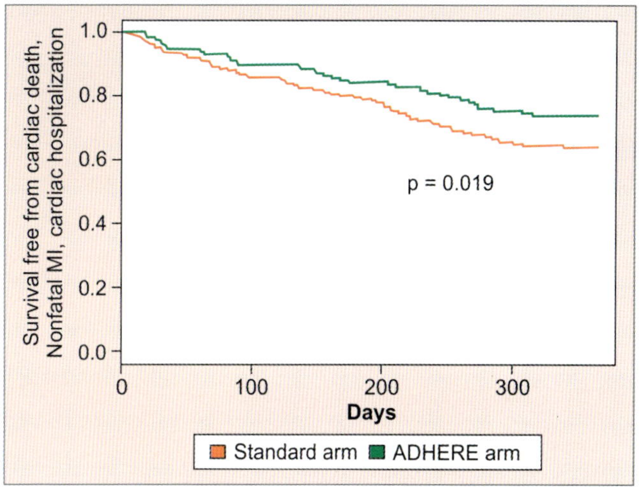

Fig. 4.14: Kaplan-Meier curve of survival free from the composite endpoint of cardiac death, nonfatal myocardial infarction, and cardiac hospitalization in patients adhering to positron emission tomography (PET) viability recommendations for revascularization (ADHERE) versus treatment without viability testing (standard). There was a statistically-significant reduction in composite events in those receiving PET viability imaging. [Adapted with permission from Beanlands RS, Graham N, Huszti E, et al. F-18-Fluorodeoxyglucose positron emission tomography imaging-assisted management of patients with severe left ventricular dysfunction and suspected coronary disease: a randomized, controlled trial (PARR-2). J Am Coll Cardiol. 2007;50(20):2002-12].

REFERENCES

Allman KC. Noninvasive assessment of myocardial viability: current status and future directions. J Nucl Cardiol. 2013;20(6): 618-37.

Allman KC, Shaw LJ, Hachamovitch R, et al. Myocardial viability testing and impact of revascularization on prognosis in patients with coronary artery disease and left ventricular dysfunction: a meta-analysis. J Am Coll Cardiol. 2002;39(7):1151-8.

Bax JJ, Wijns W, Cornel JH, et al. Accuracy of currently available techniques for prediction of functional recovery after revascularization in patients with left ventricular dysfunction due to chronic coronary artery disease: comparison of pooled data. J Am Coll Cardiol. 1997;30(6):1451-60.

Beanlands RS, Graham N, Huszti E, et al. F-18-fluorodeoxyglucose positron emission tomography imaging-assisted management of patients with severe left ventricular dysfunction and suspected coronary disease: a randomized, controlled trial (PARR-2). J Am Coll Cardiol. 2007;50(20):2002-12.

Kim RJ, Wu E, Allen R, et al. The use of contrast-enhanced magnetic resonance imaging to identify reversible myocardial dysfunction. N Engl J Med. 2000;343(20):1445-53.

Yancy CW, Jessup M, Bozkurt B, et al. 2013 ACCF/AHA Guideline for the management of heart failure: a report of the American College of Cardiology Foundation/American Heart Association Task Force on Practice Guidelines. J Am Coll Cardiol. 2013;62 (16):e147-239.

CHAPTER

Stable Ischemic Heart Disease 5

Richard A Lange

PATHOPHYSIOLOGY

Coronary artery disease (CAD) is the result of repetitive vascular injury and the subsequent responses to injury. Traditional risk factors increase an individual's likelihood of developing CAD by potentiating the magnitude of vascular injury or altering the response to it; ~90% of patients with CAD have had or presently have at least one major risk factor (see below).

The coronary artery consists of three layers—the adventitia, media, and intima (Figs. 5.1A and B). Coronary arterial endothelial injury initiates a sequence of events

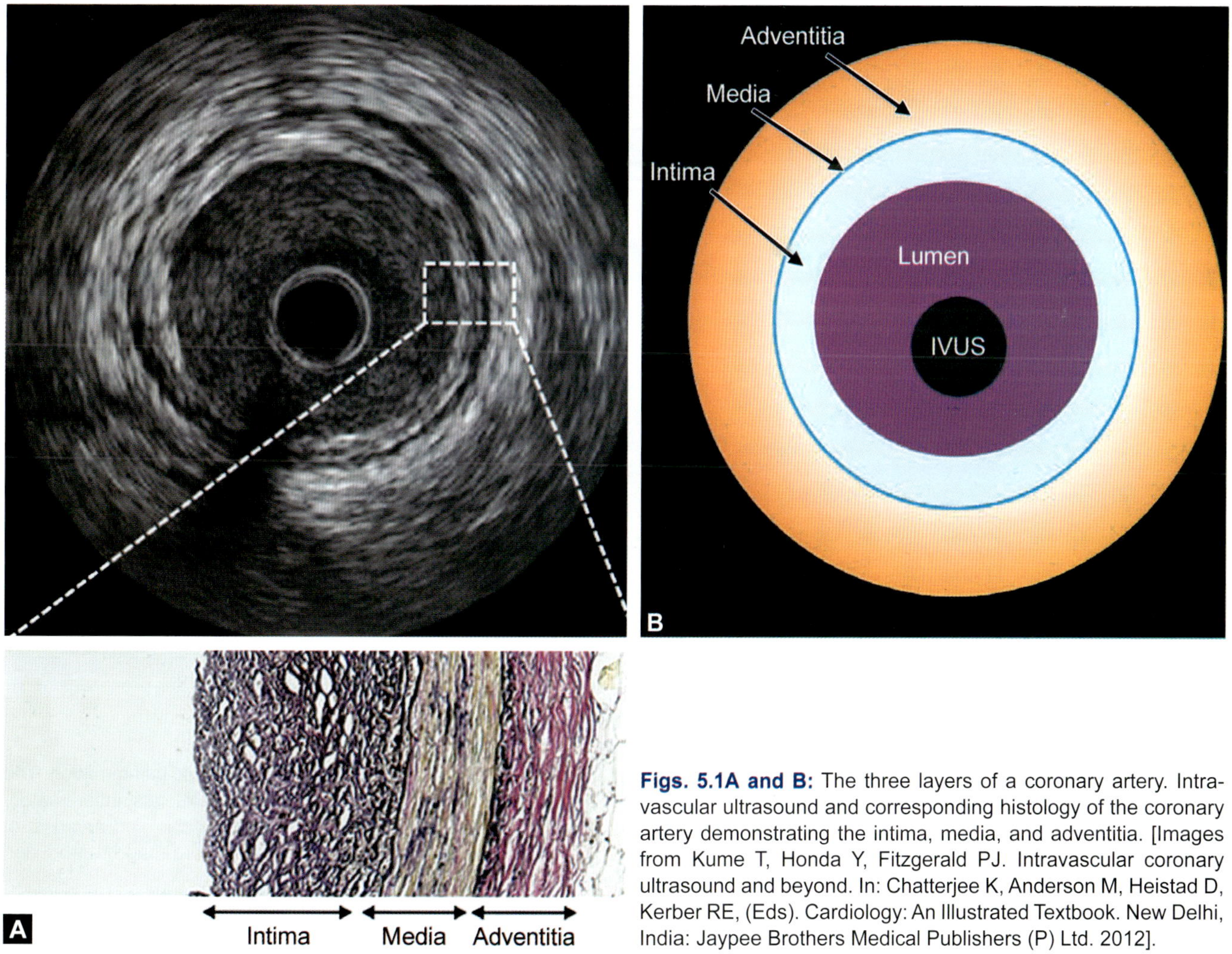

Figs. 5.1A and B: The three layers of a coronary artery. Intravascular ultrasound and corresponding histology of the coronary artery demonstrating the intima, media, and adventitia. [Images from Kume T, Honda Y, Fitzgerald PJ. Intravascular coronary ultrasound and beyond. In: Chatterjee K, Anderson M, Heistad D, Kerber RE, (Eds). Cardiology: An Illustrated Textbook. New Delhi, India: Jaypee Brothers Medical Publishers (P) Ltd. 2012].

similar to chronic inflammation: the injured endothelium elaborates procoagulants, vasoactive molecules, growth factors, and cytokines that attract platelets, inflammatory cells (monocytes and T-cells), and smooth muscle cells (Fig. 5.2). Repetitive injury and repair may result in progressive atherosclerosis and resultant luminal narrowing. Histologically, atherosclerotic plaques are composed of a core of oxidized lipids, inflammatory cells, and cellular debris, which is covered by a fibrous cap derived from smooth muscle cells. These mature plaques (i.e. stable core covered by thick fibrous cap) often are severely obstructive and, therefore, are readily visualized by coronary angiography (Fig. 5.3 and Videos 5.1 to 5.3). Plaques in patients with stable ischemic heart disease (SIHD) consist of variable amounts of fibrotic, calcific, necrotic, and lipid components (Figs. 5.4 and 5.5). Plaques containing a large lipid core and a relatively thin fibrous cap (Figs. 5.6A and B) are more prone to rupture, leading to acute coronary syndrome.

RISK FACTORS

The major modifiable risk factors for atherosclerotic CAD include cigarette smoking, an elevated serum total

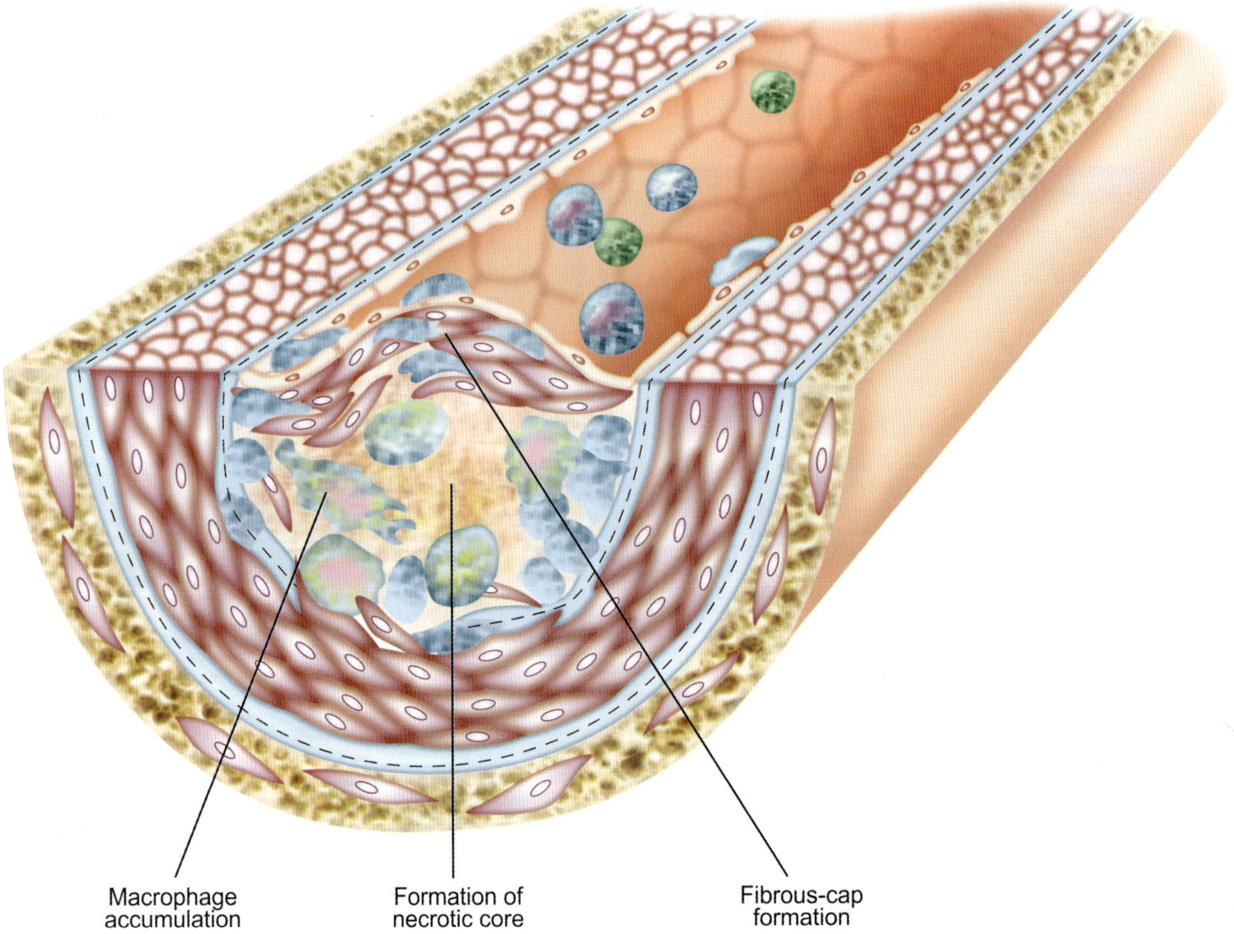

Fig. 5.2: Formation of an atherosclerotic plaque. Atherosclerosis represents a healing response to arterial injury and inflammation. The injured endothelium elaborates procoagulants, vasoactive molecules, growth factors, and cytokines that attract platelets, inflammatory cells (monocytes and T-cells), and smooth muscle cells. The necrotic core represents the results of (1) apoptosis and necrosis of leukocytes, macrophages and smooth muscle cells and (2) lipid accumulation, and it is covered by a fibrous cap. (Image reproduced with permission from Ross R. Atherosclerosis—an inflammatory disease. N Eng J Med. 1999;340:115-26).

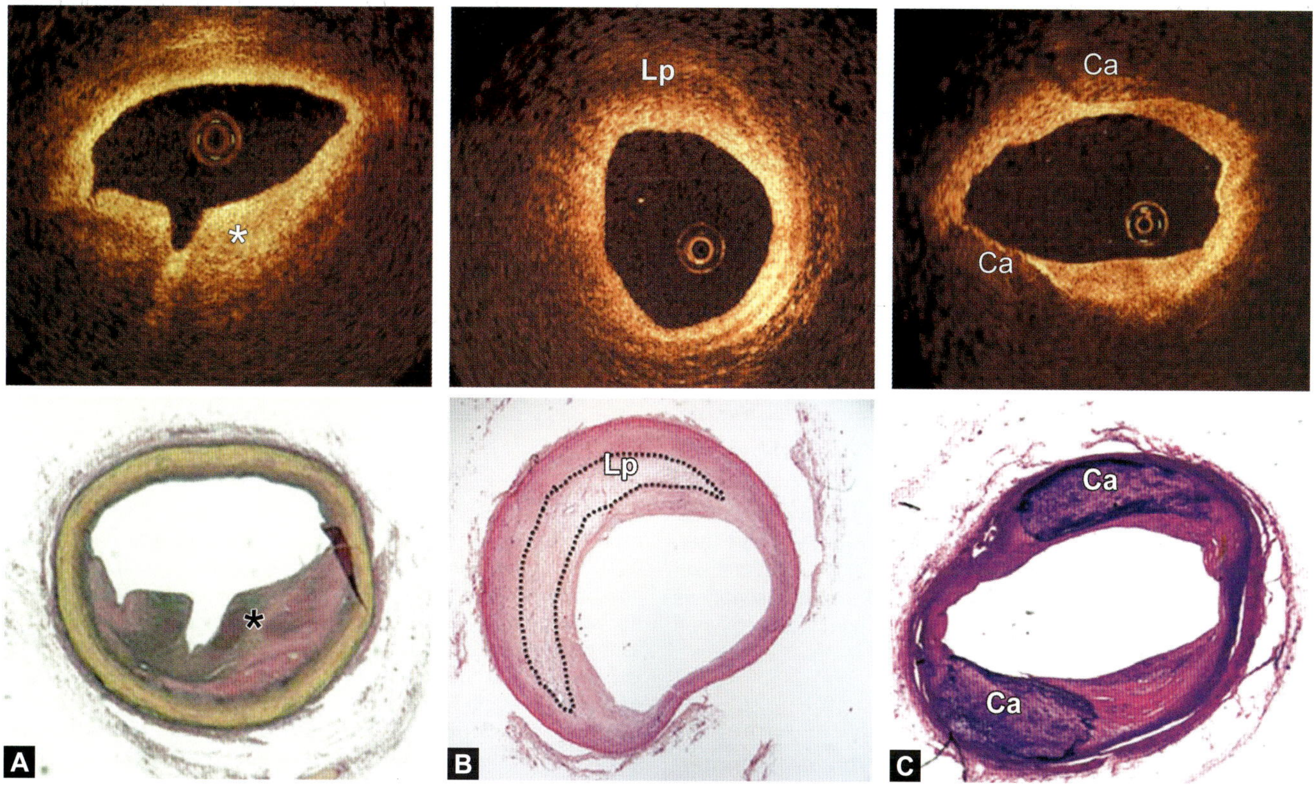

Figs. 5.5A to C: Optical coherence tomography (top) and corresponding histology (bottom) for (A) fibrous, (B) lipid-rich and (C) calcific plaques. [Images from Kume T, Honda Y, Fitzgerald PJ. Intravascular coronary ultrasound and beyond. In: Chatterjee K, Anderson M, Heistad D, Kerber RE, (Eds). Cardiology: An Illustrated Textbook. New Delhi, India: Jaypee Brothers Medical Publishers (P) Ltd. 2012). (Ca: Calcific region; Lp: Lipid-rich region; Asterisk, fibrotic region].

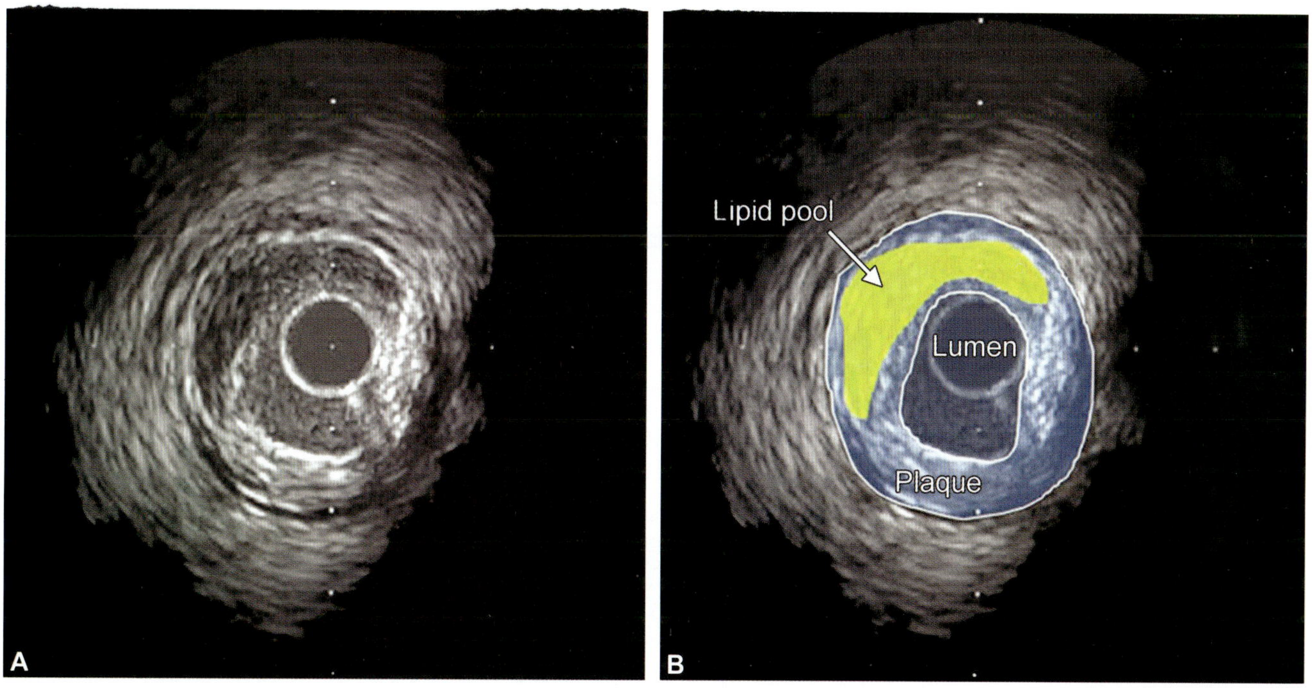

Figs. 5.6A and B: Intravascular ultrasound demonstrating a coronary plaque with a large lipid core and a relatively thin fibrous cap. [Images from Kume T, Honda Y, Fitzgerald PJ. Intravascular coronary ultrasound and beyond. In: Chatterjee K, Anderson M, Heistad D, Kerber RE, (Eds). Cardiology: An Illustrated Textbook. New Delhi, India: Jaypee Brothers Medical Publishers (P) Ltd. 2012].

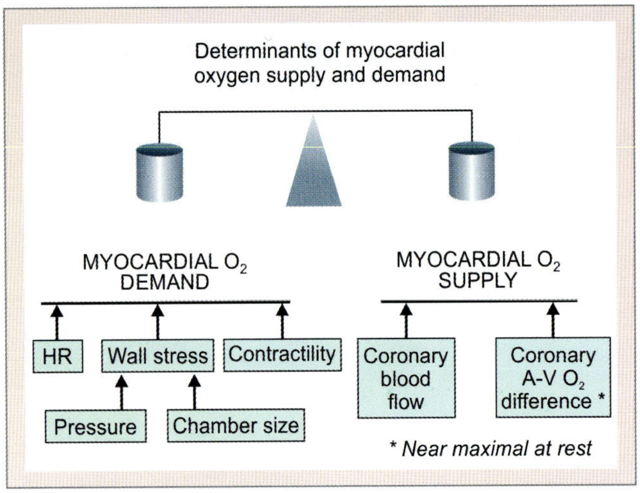

Fig. 5.7: Determinants of myocardial oxygen supply and demands. Myocardial oxygen demands are determined by the heart rate, ventricular wall stress (a reflection of the systolic pressure and chamber size) and contractility. Myocardial oxygen supply is directly related to coronary blood flow, since extraction of oxygen from the blood is near maximal at rest.

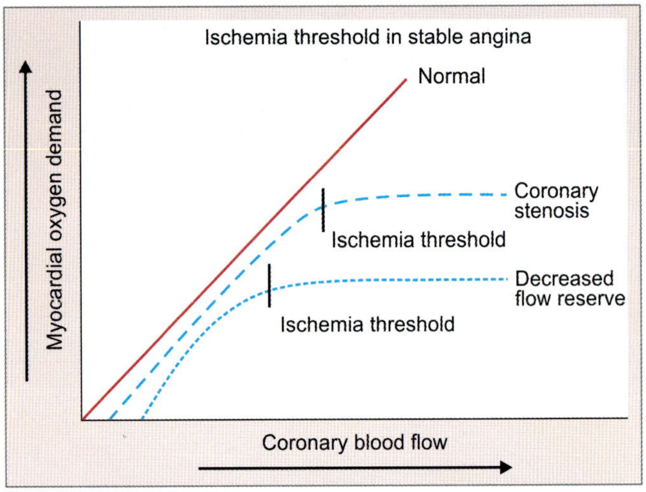

Fig. 5.8: Pathophysiology of myocardial ischemia. With increasing myocardial oxygen demand, there is an increase in coronary blood flow. In the presence of coronary artery stenosis, coronary blood flow cannot increase sufficiently and ischemia is precipitated (ischemia threshold). Due to associated endothelial dysfunction in the presence of atherosclerosis coronary, blood flow reserve is impaired and the threshold occurs at a lower level of oxygen demand. [Image from Chatterjee K. Coronary circulation in physiology and pathology. In: Chatterjee K, Anderson M, Heistad D, Kerber RE, (Eds). Cardiology: An Illustrated Textbook. New Delhi, India: Jaypee Brothers Medical Publishers (P) Ltd. 2012].

pre-test probability of CAD who have an uninterpretable ECG or who are unable to exercise, or who have uninterpretable or equivocal stress test results.

THERAPEUTIC GOALS

In the patient with stable CAD, the goals of medical therapy are to ameliorate angina and/or prevent major cardiovascular (CV) events. The initial approach to all patients should be focused upon eliminating unhealthy behaviors such as smoking and effectively promoting lifestyle changes that reduce CV risk such as maintaining a healthy weight, engaging in physical activity, and adopting a healthy diet.

Antianginal agents improve the myocardial oxygen demand:supply mismatch (Table 5.4). These agents—nitrates, beta-blockers and calcium channel blockers—improve symptoms (i.e. decrease frequency of angina episodes and increase exercise tolerance); however, they have not been shown to improve survival in stable CAD patients. Medical therapies that retard progression (or promote regression) of atherosclerosis, stabilize atherosclerotic plaques, or prevent thrombosis should be administered to decrease the risk of MI and death (Flow chart 5.2). Such therapies include antiplatelet agents, angiotensin converting enzyme inhibitors, and lipid-lowering therapy, with the latter adjusted to achieve target total and LDL serum cholesterol concentration goals.

Table 5.1: Clinical features of typical stable angina.

Location	• Usually retrosternal, can be epigastric or interscapular
Localization	• Usually diffuse, difficult to localize • When very localized (point sign), it is unlikely to be angina
Quality	• Pressure, heaviness, squeezing, indigestion
Radiation	• One or both arms, upper back, neck, epigastrium, shoulder • Lower jaw (radiation to the upper jaw, head, lower back, lower abdomen or lower extremities is not a feature of angina)
Duration	• Usually 1–10 minutes (not a few seconds or hours)
Precipitating factors	• Physical activity, emotional stress, sexual intercourse
Aggravating factors	• Cold weather, heavy meals
Relieving factors	• Cessation of activity, nitroglycerin (if relief is instantaneous it is unlikely to be angina)
Associated symptoms	• Usually none, occasionally dyspnea

Table 5.2: Pretest probability* of coronary artery disease by symptoms, gender and age.

Pretest Probability of Coronary Artery Disease by Symptoms, Gender and Age*					
Age (yrs)	***Gender***	***Typical angina*****	***Atypical angina*****	***Nonanginal chest pain*****	***Asymptomatic***
30–39	Men	Intermediate**	Intermediate	Low	Very low
	Women	Intermediate	Very low	Very low	Very low
40–49	Men	High	Intermediate	Intermediate	Low
	Women	Intermediate	Low	Very low	Very low
50–59	Men	High	Intermediate	Intermediate	Low
	Women	Intermediate	Intermediate	Low	Very low
60–69	Men	High	Intermediate	Intermediate	Low
	Women	High	Intermediate	Intermediate	Low

*Probability: High > 90%; Intermediate = 10–90%; Low < 10%; Very low < 5%

**Typical angina has 3 characteristics: (1) retrosternal chest discomfort of characteristic quality and duration that is (2) provoked by exertion or emotional stress and is (3) relieved by rest or nitroglycerin. Angina is said to be atypical if two of these three are present, whereas noncardiac chest pain has only one or none of these characteristics.

Table 5.3: Canadian Cardiovascular Society functional classification of angina.

Class I
• Ordinary physical activity, such as walking and climbing stairs, does not cause angina • Angina with strenuous or rapid or prolonged exertion at work or recreation
Class II
• Slight limitation of ordinary activity (i.e. walking or climbing stairs rapidly to prevent angina; chest pain with walking uphill; walking or stair climbing after meals, in cold, in wind or when under emotional stress, or only during the few hours after awakening) • Angina with walking more than two blocks on the level and climbing more than one flight of ordinary stairs at a normal pace and in normal conditions
Class III
• Marked limitation of ordinary physical activity • Angina with walking 1–2 blocks on the level and climbing more than one flight in normal conditions
Class IV
• Inability to carry on any physical activity without discomfort—angina syndrome may be present at rest

REVASCULARIZATION

Revascularization should be reserved for individuals with (1) symptoms that interfere with the patient's lifestyle despite optimal medical therapy or (2) coronary anatomic findings that indicate that revascularization would provide a survival benefit. For the patient with medically refractory angina, the optimal method of revascularization—coronary artery bypass grafting (CABG) or percutaneous coronary intervention (PCI)—is selected based on the coronary angiographic findings, the likelihood of success (or complications) of each procedure, and the subject's preferences (Table 5.5).

For most patients with chronic stable angina, survival with optimal medical therapy is similar to that resulting from revascularization; however, revascularization results in improved survival in selected patient subgroups (Table 5.6). In the 1970s and 1980s, randomized trials comparing CABG with medical therapy established that CABG improves survival in patients with (1) significant (>50% luminal narrowing) disease of the left main coronary artery, (2) multivessel CAD and left ventricular ejection fraction < 50%, and (3) multivessel CAD with more than 75% luminal narrowing of the proximal left anterior descending coronary artery. Accordingly, current guidelines recommend revascularization for the patient with any of these anatomic findings regardless of symptoms, unless a contraindication to revascularization is present.

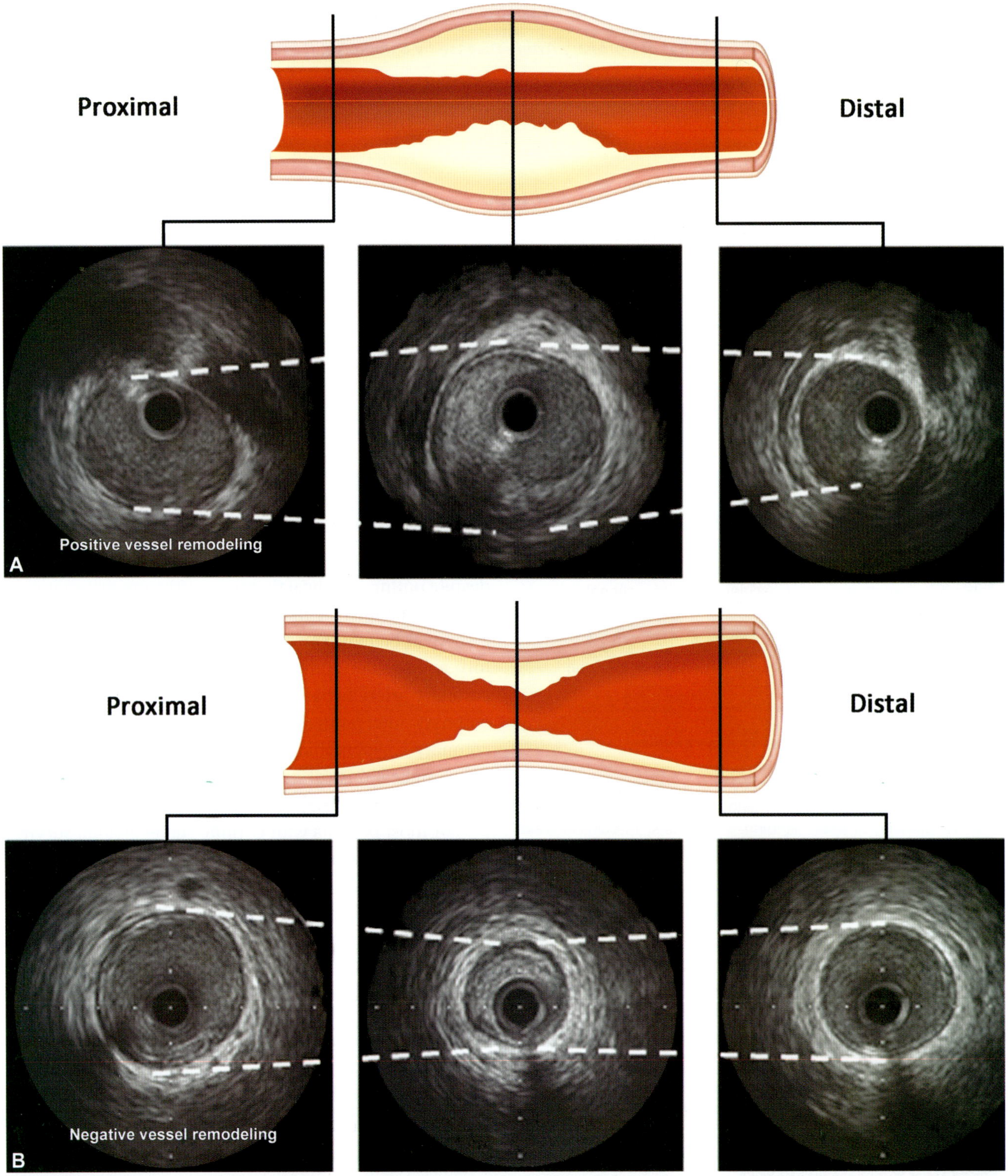

Figs. 5.9A and B: Intravascular ultrasound demonstrating positive and negative vessel remodeling. (A) Positive remodeling with localized expansion of the vessel in the area of plaque accumulation; (B) Negative remodeling (narrowing) in an area of atherosclerosis. [Images from Kume T, Honda Y, Fitzgerald PJ. Intravascular coronary ultrasound and beyond. In: Chatterjee K, Anderson M, Heistad D, Kerber RE, (Eds). Cardiology: An Illustrated Textbook. New Delhi, India: Jaypee Brothers Medical Publishers (P) Ltd. 2012].

Flow chart 5.1: Algorithm for risk assessment of patients with stable ischemic heart disease. Colors correspond to the class of recommendations in the ACCF/AHA guidelines with green being class 1 recommendations and orange being class 2 recommendations. (Figures adapted with permission from Fihn SD, Gardin JM, Abrams J, et al. 2012 ACCF/AHA/ACP/AATS/PCNA/SCAI/STS guideline for the diagnosis and management of patients with stable ischemic heart disease: executive summary: a report of the American College of Cardiology Foundation/American Heart Association task force on practice guidelines, and the American College of Physicians, American Association for Thoracic Surgery, Preventive Cardiovascular Nurses Association, Society for Cardiovascular Angiography and Interventions, and Society of Thoracic Surgeons. J Am Coll Cardiol. 2012;60:e44-164). (CCTA: Computed coronary tomography angiography; CMR: Cardiac magnetic resonance; ECG: Electrocardiogram; Echo: Echocardiography; MPI: Myocardial perfusion imaging; Pharm: Pharmacological).

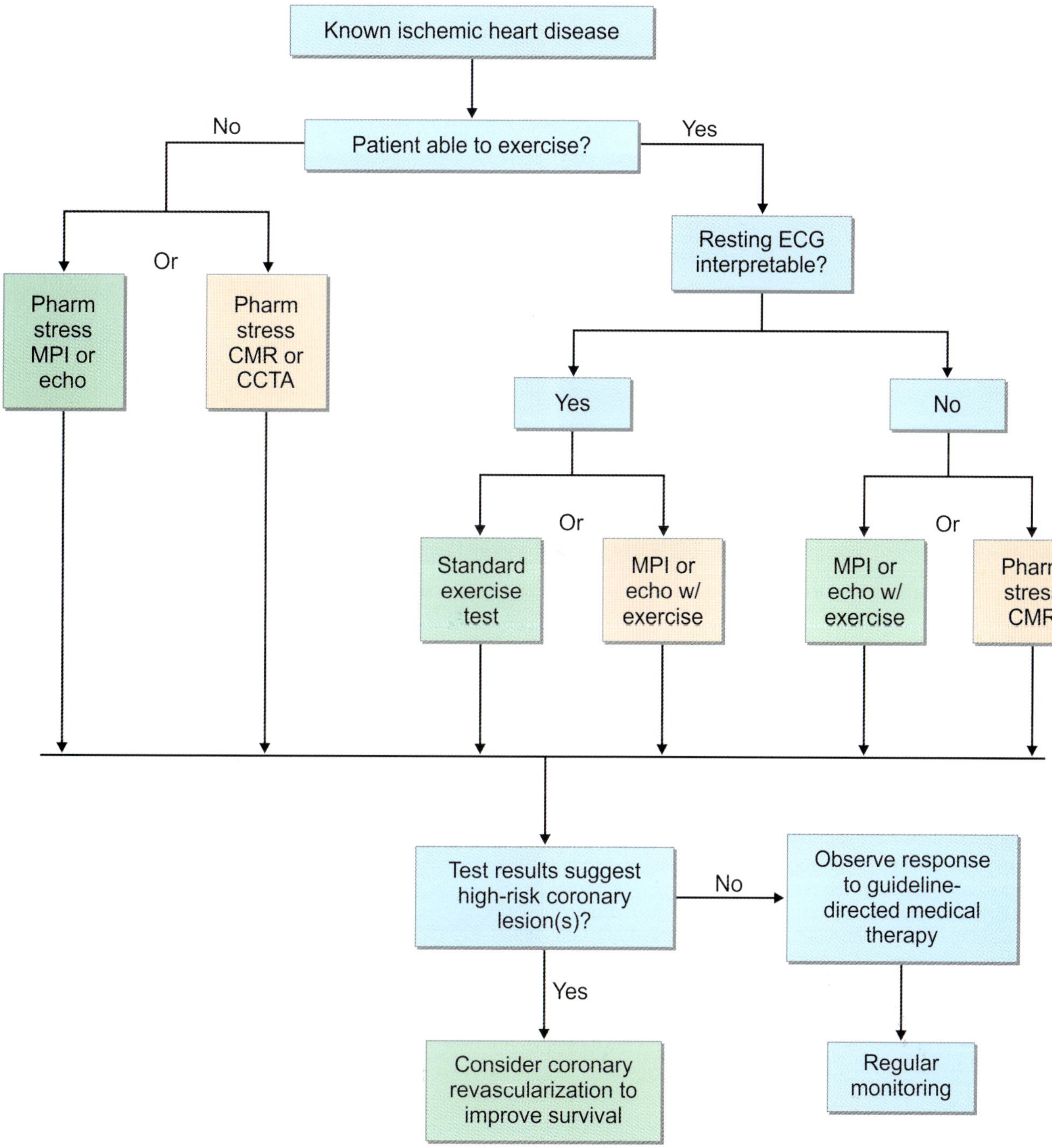

Table 5.4: Effects of antianginal agents on determinants of myocardial oxygen supply and demand.

Medication	***Heart rate***	***Left ventricular contractility***	***Left ventricular wall stress***	***Coronary blood flow***
Beta-blocker	Reduce	Reduce	Reduce	No change
Nitrates	No change	No change	Reduce	Increase
Dihydropyridine calcium channel blockers	No change	No change	Reduce	Increase
Nondihydropyridine calcium channel blockers (Verapamil, Diltiazem)	Reduce	Reduce	Reduce	Increase
Ranolazine	No change	No change	No change	No change

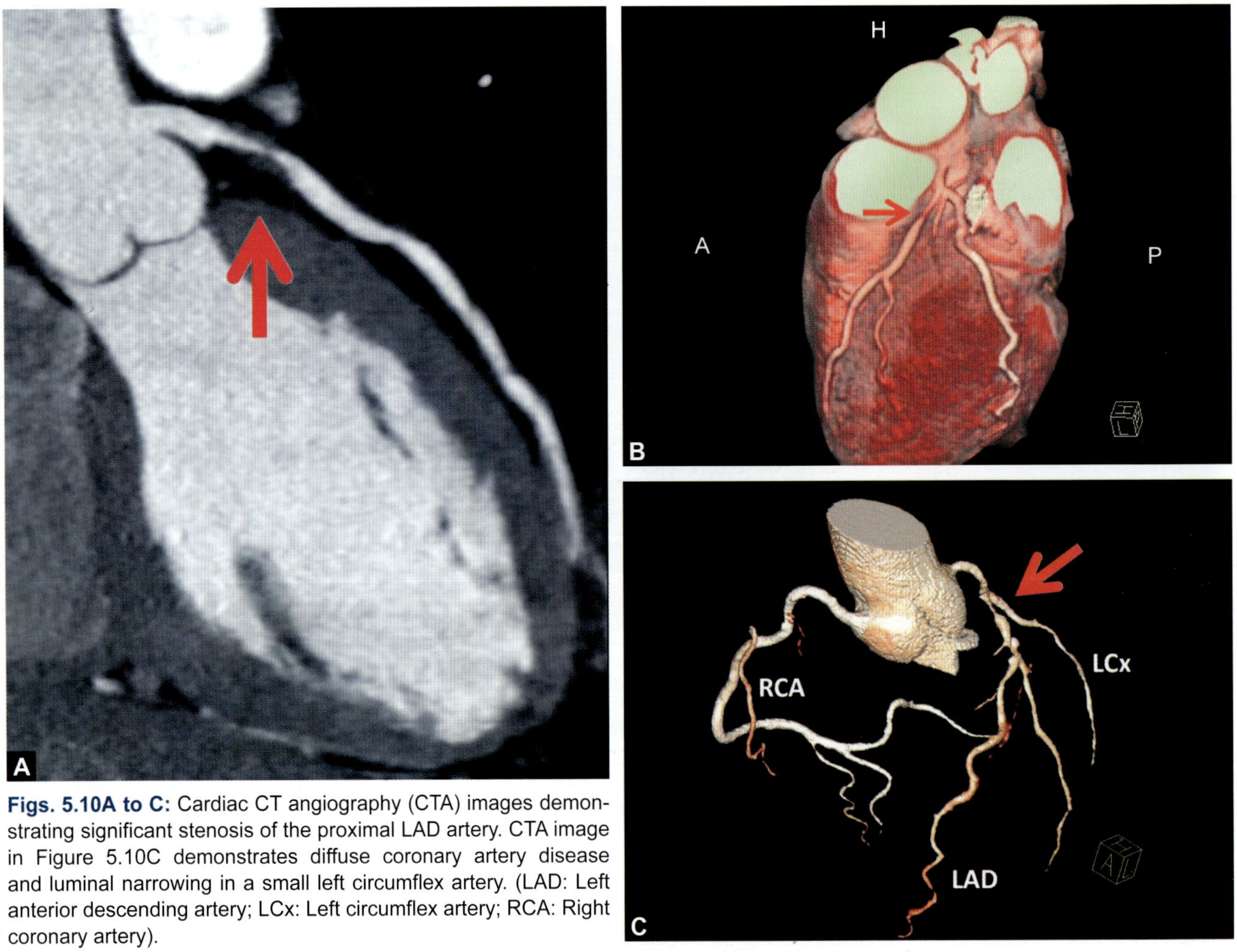

Figs. 5.10A to C: Cardiac CT angiography (CTA) images demonstrating significant stenosis of the proximal LAD artery. CTA image in Figure 5.10C demonstrates diffuse coronary artery disease and luminal narrowing in a small left circumflex artery. (LAD: Left anterior descending artery; LCx: Left circumflex artery; RCA: Right coronary artery).

Flow chart 5.2: Algorithm for guideline-directed medical therapy for patients with stable ischemic heart disease. Colors correspond to the class of recommendations in the ACCF/AHA guidelines with green being class 1 recommendations and orange being class 2 recommendations. (Figure adapted from Fihn SD, Gardin JM, Abrams J, et al. 2012 ACCF/AHA/ACP/AATS/PCNA/SCAI/STS guideline for the diagnosis and management of patients with stable ischemic heart disease: executive summary: a report of the American College of Cardiology Foundation/American Heart Association task force on practice guidelines, and the American College of Physicians, American Association for Thoracic Surgery, Preventive Cardiovascular Nurses Association, Society for Cardiovascular Angiography and Interventions, and Society of Thoracic Surgeons. J Am Coll Cardiol 2012;60:e44-164). (ACEI: Angiotensin-converting enzyme inhibitor; ARB: Angiotensin-receptor blocker; ASA: Aspirin; BP: Blood pressure; CCB: Calcium channel blocker; CKD: Chronic kidney disease; LV: Left ventricular; MI: Myocardial infarction; NTG: Nitroglycerin).

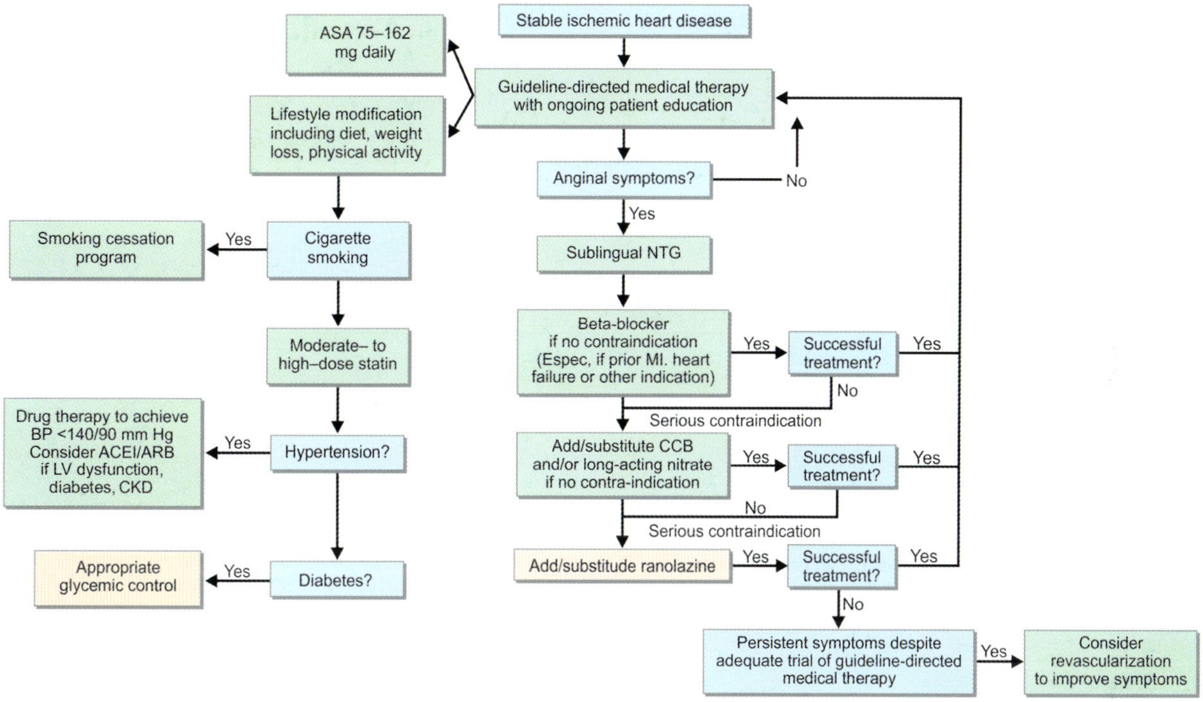

Table 5.5: Revascularization to improve symptoms with significant CAD. Revascularization to improve angina symptoms may be accomplished with CABG or PCI depending upon the coronary anatomy and the patient's preference. (CABG: Coronary artery bypass grafting; COR: Class of recommendation; GDMT: Guideline-directed medical therapy; LAD: Left anterior descending artery; LOE: Level of evidence; PCI: Percutaneous coronary intervention; SYNTAX: SYNergy between PCI with TAXus and cardiac surgery; TMR: Transmyocardial laser revascularization).

Clinical Setting	***COR***	***LOE***
≥1 significant stenoses amenable to revascularization and unacceptable angina despite GDMT	I: CABG I: PCI	A
≥1 significant stenoses and unacceptable angina in whom GDMT cannot be implemented because of medication contraindications, adverse effects, or patient preferences	IIa: CABG IIa: PCI	C
Previous CABG with ≥1 significant stenoses associated with ischemia and unacceptable angina despite GDMT	IIb: CABG	C
	IIa: PCI	C
Complex three-vessel disease (e.g. SYNTAX score >22) with or without involvement of the proximal LAD and a good candidate for CABG	IIa: CABG preferred over PCI	B
No anatomic or physiologic criteria for revascularization	III: Harm–CABG III: Harm–PCI	C

Source: Adapted with permission from Fihn SD, Gardin JM, Abrams J, et al. 2012 ACCF/AHA/ACP/AATS/PCNA/SCAI/STS guideline for the diagnosis and management of patients with stable ischemic heart disease: executive summary: a report of the American College of Cardiology Foundation/American Heart Association task force on practice guidelines, and the American College of Physicians, American Association for Thoracic Surgery, Preventive Cardiovascular Nurses Association, Society for Cardiovascular Angiography and Interventions, and Society of Thoracic Surgeons. J Am Coll Cardiol. 2012;60:e44-164.

Table 5.6: Revascularization to improve survival compared to medical therapy in patients with stable ischemic heart disease. In patients with certain coronary anatomy, survival is improved with coronary revascularization compared to medical therapy. (CABG: Coronary artery bypass grafting; COR: Class of recommendation; LAD: Left anterior descending artery; LIMA: Left internal mammary artery; LOE: Level of evidence; PCI: Percutaneous coronary intervention; SIHD: Stable ischemic heart disease).

	COR	*LOE*
Unprotected left main coronary artery		
CABG	I	B
PCI	*IIa—for SIHD when both of the following are present*: • Anatomic conditions associated with a low risk of PCI procedural complications and high likelihood of good long-term outcome • Clinical characteristics that predict a significantly increased risk of adverse surgical outcomes	B
	IIb—for SIHD when both of the following are present: • Anatomic conditions associated with a low to intermediate risk of PCI procedural complications and intermediate to high likelihood of good long-term outcome • Clinical characteristics that predict an increased risk of adverse surgical outcomes	B
	III: Harm—for SIHD in patients (versus performing CABG) with unfavorable anatomy for PCI and who are good candidates for CABG	B
Three-vessel disease with or without proximal LAD disease*		
CABG	I	B
PCI	IIb—of uncertain benefit	B
Two-vessel disease with proximal LAD disease*		
CABG	I	B
PCI	IIb—of uncertain benefit	B
Two-vessel disease without proximal LAD disease*		
CABG	IIa—with extensive ischemia	B
	IIb—of uncertain benefit without extensive ischemia	C
PCI	IIb—of uncertain benefit	B
Single-vessel proximal LAD disease		
CABG	IIa—with LIMA for long-term benefit	B
PCI	IIb—of uncertain benefit	B
Single-vessel disease without proximal LAD involvement		
CABG	III: Harm	B
PCI	III: Harm	B

*In patients with multivessel disease who also have diabetes; it is reasonable to choose CABG (with LIMA) over PCI (Class IIa/Level of Evidence: B).

Source: Adapted with permission from Fihn SD, Gardin JM, Abrams J, et al. 2012 ACCF/AHA/ACP/AATS/PCNA/SCAI/STS guideline for the diagnosis and management of patients with stable ischemic heart disease: executive summary: a report of the American College of Cardiology Foundation/American Heart Association task force on practice guidelines, and the American College of Physicians, American Association for Thoracic Surgery, Preventive Cardiovascular Nurses Association, Society for Cardiovascular Angiography and Interventions, and Society of Thoracic Surgeons. J Am Coll Cardiol. 2012;60:e44-164.

VIDEO LEGENDS

Video 5.1A: Right anterior oblique projection angiogram showing a discrete tight stenosis in the mid to distal segment of a large "wrap around" left anterior descending artery.

Video 5.1B: Angiogram showing diffuse coronary artery disease of the left anterior descending (LAD) artery in a diabetic patient with stable ischemic heart disease. The catheter is subselectively engaged in the LAD so the left circumflex artery is not well visualized.

Video 5.2: Angiogram showing discrete stenosis in a segment of a large branching obtuse marginal artery in a patient with stable ischemic heart disease.

Video 5.3: Angiogram showing a discrete moderate stenosis of the right coronary artery (RCA) before the take-off of the PDA in a patient with stable ischemic heart disease. Several posterolateral branches of the RCA are also visualized.

REFERENCES

Fihn SD, Abrams J, Berra K, et al. 2012 ACCF/AHA/ACP.AATS/PCNA/SCAI/STS Guideline for the diagnosis and management of patients With stable ischemic heart disease: A report of the American College of Cardiology Foundation/American Heart Association Task Force on Practice Guidelines, and the American College of Physicians, American Association for Thoracic Surgery, Preventive Cardiovascular Nurses Association, Society for Cardiovascular Angiography and Interventions, and Society of Thoracic Surgeons. J Am Coll Cardiol. 2012:60;e44-164.

Hillis LD, Smith PK, Anderson JL, et al. 2011 ACCF/AHA Guideline for coronary artery bypass graft surgery: Executive summary: A report of the American College of Cardiology Foundation/American Heart Association Task Force on Practice Guidelines. J Am Coll Cardiol. 2011;58:2584-614.

Levine GN, Bates ER, Blankenship JC, et al. 2011 ACCF/AHA/SCAI Guideline for percutaneous intervention: executive summary: a report of the American College of Cardiology Foundation/American Heart Association task force on practice guidelines. J Am Coll Cardiol. 2011;58:2550-83.

Taylor AJ, Cerqueira M, Hodgson JM, et al. ACCF/SCCT/ACR/AHA/ASE/ASNC/NASCI/SCAI/SCMR 2010 appropriate use criteria for cardiac computed tomography. A report of the American College of Cardiology Foundation Appropriate Use Criteria Task Force, the Society of Cardiovascular Computed Tomography, the American College of Radiology, the American Heart Association, the American Society of Echocardiography, the American Society of Nuclear Cardiology, the North American Society for Cardiovascular Imaging, the Society for Cardiovascular Angiography and Interventions, and the Society for Cardiovascular Magnetic Resonance. J Am Coll Cardiol. 2010;56(22):1864-94.

CHAPTER

Acute Coronary Syndromes

6

Glenn N Levine, Ali E Denktas

TERMINOLOGY

The term "acute coronary syndrome" (ACS) encompasses the previously named conditions including unstable angina, non-Q wave myocardial infarction (NQMI), non-ST-elevation myocardial infarction (NSTEMI), and ST-segment elevation myocardial infarction (STEMI). ACS denotes the clinical syndrome in which coronary plaque rupture or fissure leads to intracoronary thrombus formation at the site of the atherosclerotic plaque (Figs. 6.1 to 6.5), with transient or persistent partial or complete obstruction of blood flow, leading to myocardial ischemia and in many cases myocardial infarction (MI).

ETIOLOGY OF ACUTE CORONARY SYNDROMES

The initiating event in most cases of ACS is plaque rupture, erosion, or fissure. Coronary atherosclerotic plaques more predisposed to rupture (so called "vulnerable plaques") are those with a large lipid core and thin fibrous caps. These plaques more commonly than not occupy <50% of the arterial lumen. Plaque rupture (or in some cases erosion or fissure) leads to a complex series of events that results in thrombus formation (Fig. 6.6 and Video 6.1). Factors that can precipitate plaque rupture include local inflammation (most commonly in the shoulder of the fibrous cap)

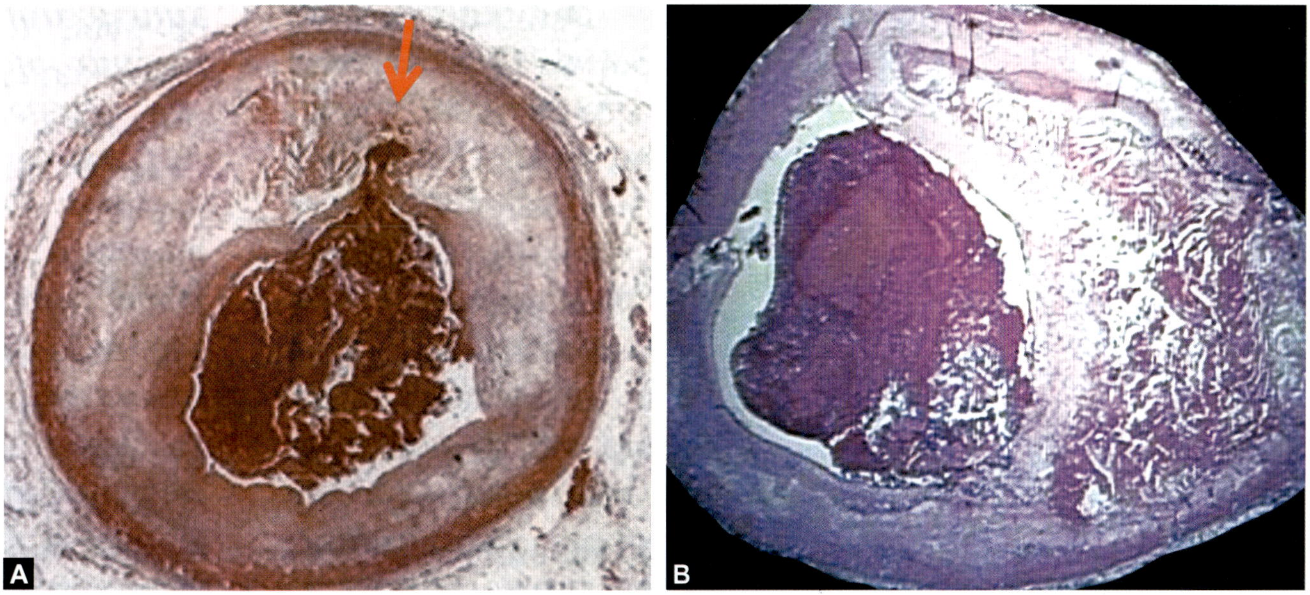

Figs. 6.1A and B: Vulnerable plaque and plaque rupture. (A and B) Pathological specimens of lipid-dense plaques with plaque rupture (arrow) and thrombus formation. (Image 6.1B from Armed Forces Institute of Pathology, Washington, DC, USA).

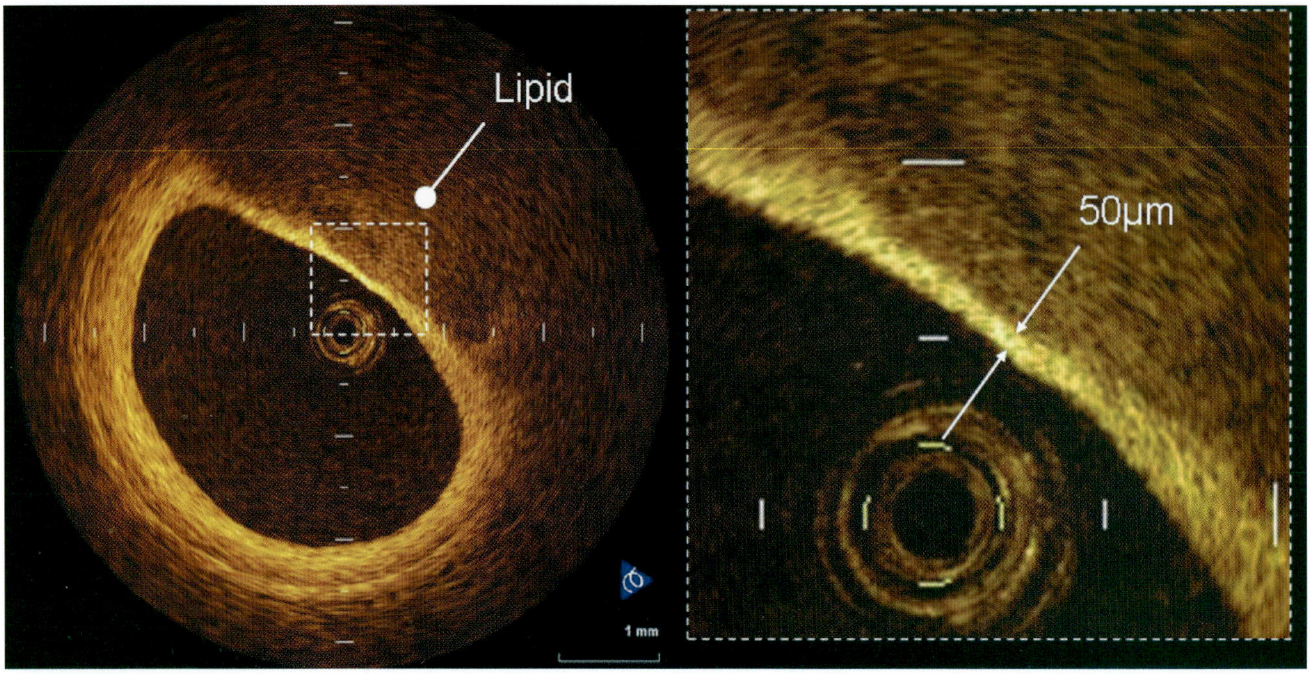

Fig. 6.1C: Optical coherence tomography demonstrating a vulnerable plaque. Plaque consists of a large lipid pool and thin fibrous cap. [Image 6.1C from Kubo T, Akasaka T. Identification of vulnerable plaques with optical coherence tomography. In: Pesek K (Ed). Atherosclerotic Cardiovascular Disease. Shanghai: InTech; 2011].

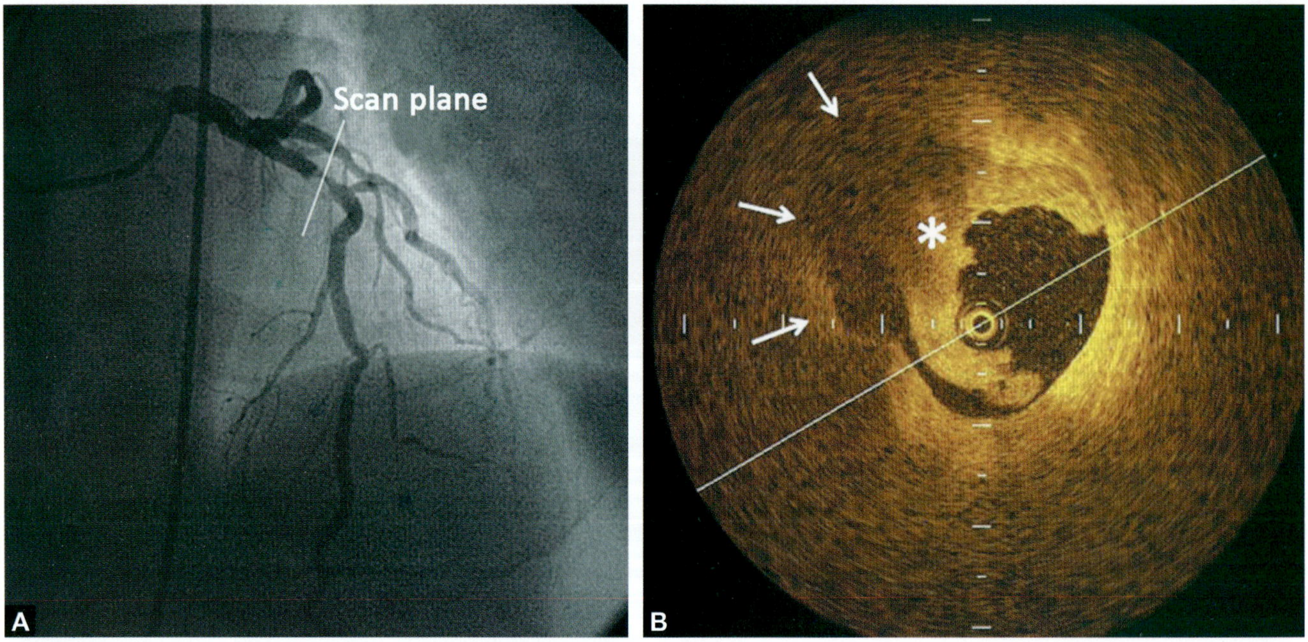

Figs. 6.2A and B: Culprit lesion in the left anterior descending artery (LAD) in a patient with acute coronary syndromes. (A) Coronary angiogram demonstrates significant lumen narrowing at the proximal portion of the LAD; (B) Optical coherence tomography visualizes the protruded thrombus (asterisk) at the site of plaque rupture (arrows). [Images from Kume T, Honda Y, Fitzgerald PJ. Intravascular coronary ultrasound and beyond. In: Chatterjee K, Anderson M, Heistad D, Kerber RE (Eds). Cardiology: An Illustrated Textbook. New Delhi, India: Jaypee Brothers Medical Publishers (P) Ltd. 2012].

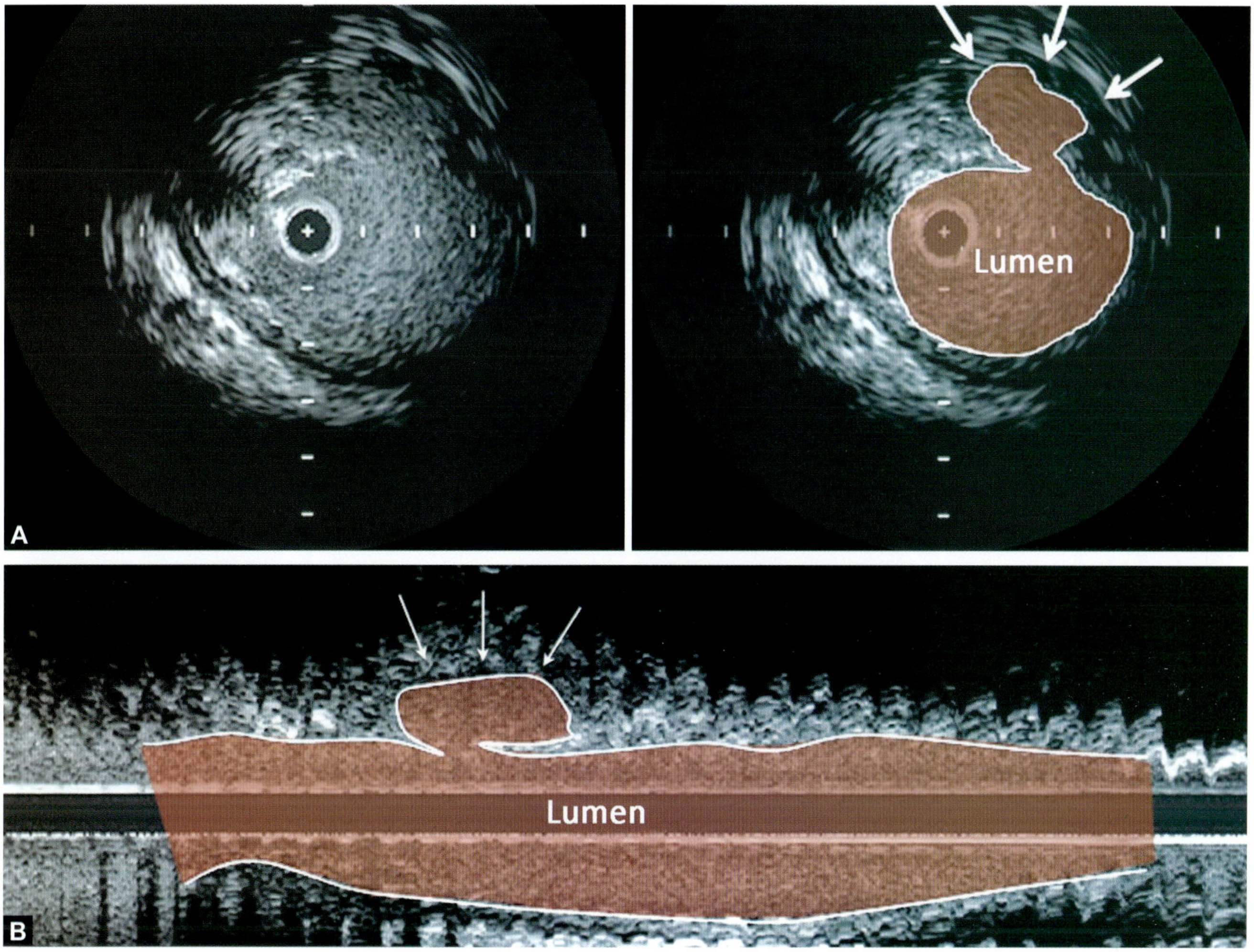

Figs. 6.3A and B: Plaque rupture demonstrated by intravascular ultrasound imaging (IVUS). (A) On the cross-sectional IVUS images, a cavity in contact with the vessel is observed; (B) The longitudinal IVUS image shows a spatial representation of the plaque rupture. The rupture occurs in an eccentric plaque and has a residual thin flap that probably corresponds to a thin fibrous cap. [Images from Kume T, Honda Y, Fitzgerald PJ. Intravascular coronary ultrasound and beyond. In: Chatterjee K, Anderson M, Heistad D, Kerber RE (Eds). Cardiology: An Illustrated Textbook. New Delhi: Jaypee Brothers Medical Publishers (P) Ltd. 2012].

and shear stress forces. With rupture (or fissure) of the plaque, subendothelial factors (e.g. collagen, tissue factor) are exposed to circulating platelets. Platelets bind to the damaged endothelium, become activated, undergo a conformational change, release mediators that lead to further platelet activation, and begin to aggregate (Fig. 6.7). The coagulation cascade is activated, resulting in local thrombin and then fibrin production (Fig. 6.8). The resulting thrombus consists of platelet aggregates, red blood cells, and a fibrin mesh (Fig. 6.9). In addition to epicardial vessel occlusion, distal embolization of thrombotic material and small vessel occlusion can variably contribute to myocardial necrosis and may be the cause of at least some cases of observed troponin elevation in patients with ACS. Focal coronary vasoconstriction may also contribute to and exacerbate the reduction in blood flow from thrombus formation. Less common causes of ACS include coronary vasospasm due to focal endothelial dysfunction (Prinzmetal's angina) or cocaine use, spontaneous coronary dissection (which may occur with vasculitis or in peripartum women), or coronary artery embolism.

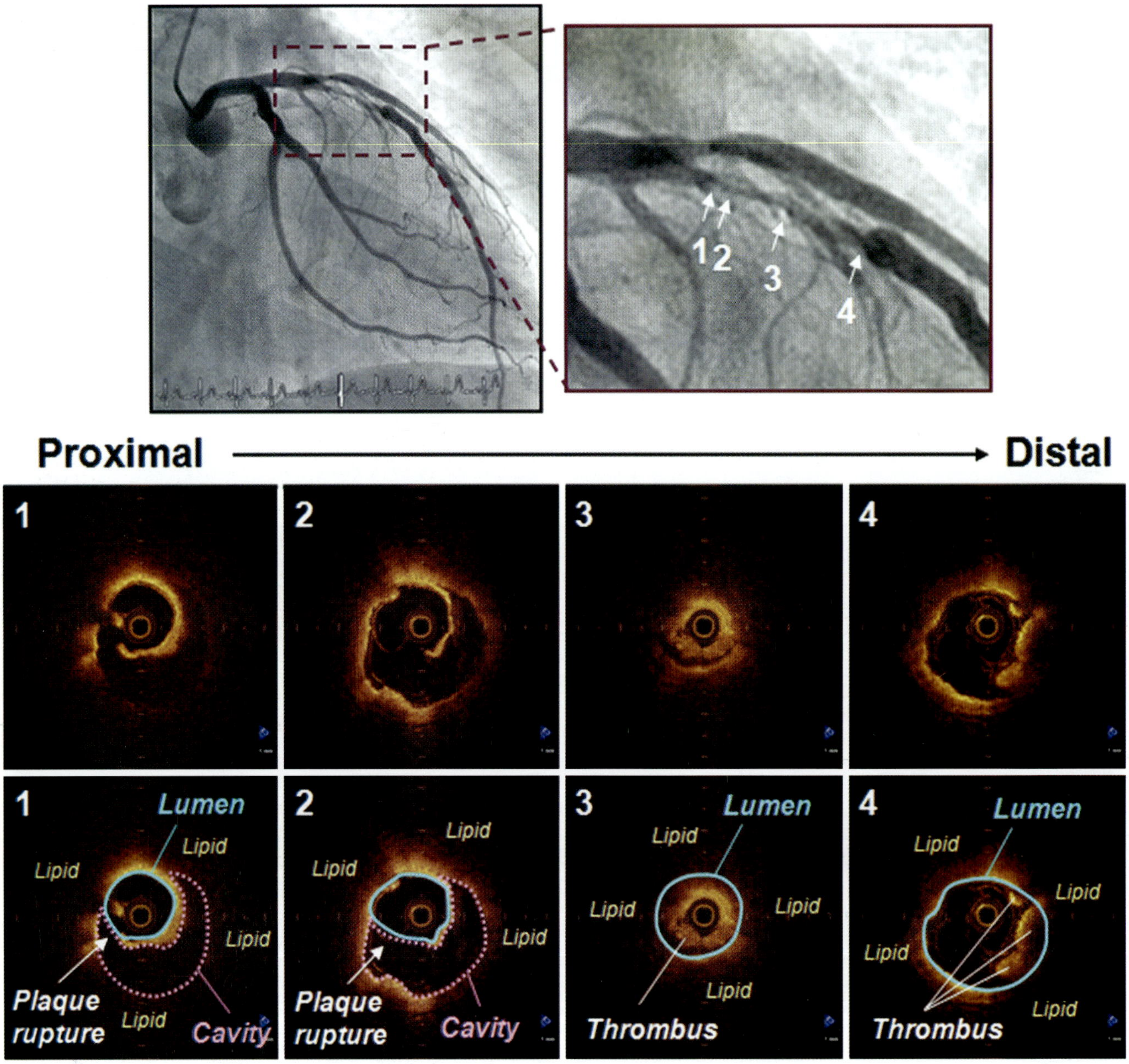

Fig. 6.4: Coronary angiogram and corresponding optical coherence tomography of plaque rupture and thrombus in the proximal left anterior descending artery of a patient with acute coronary syndrome. (Images courtesy of Dr Takashi Kubo. Department of Cardiovascular Medicine, Wakayama Medical University, Wakayama, Japan. Images from Kubo T, Tanaka A, Kitabata H, et al. Optical coherence tomography analysis of clinical and subclinical plaque rupture. J Clinic Experiment Cardiol. 2011;S:1-002).

NON-ST-SEGMENT ELEVATION ACUTE CORONARY SYNDROME

Electrocardiography first evolved during the early 1900s (Fig. 10) and continues to play an important role in the assessment of patients with acute coronary syndromes Patients with ACS are triaged based on whether or not there is ST-segment elevation [or new left bundle branch block (LBBB)] present on the electrocardiogram. Those without ST-segment elevation are classified as having non-ST-segment elevation acute coronary syndrome (NSTE-ACS). Typical ECG findings in patients with NSTE-ACS include ST-segment depression (Fig. 6.11A) and/or T-wave inversion (Fig. 6.11B). Initial treatment of NSTE-ACS patients includes antiplatelet, anticoagulant, and antianginal therapies. Antiplatelet therapy consists of aspirin and at least one additional antiplatelet agent, either an oral P2Y12 inhibitor (clopidogrel or ticagrelor) or

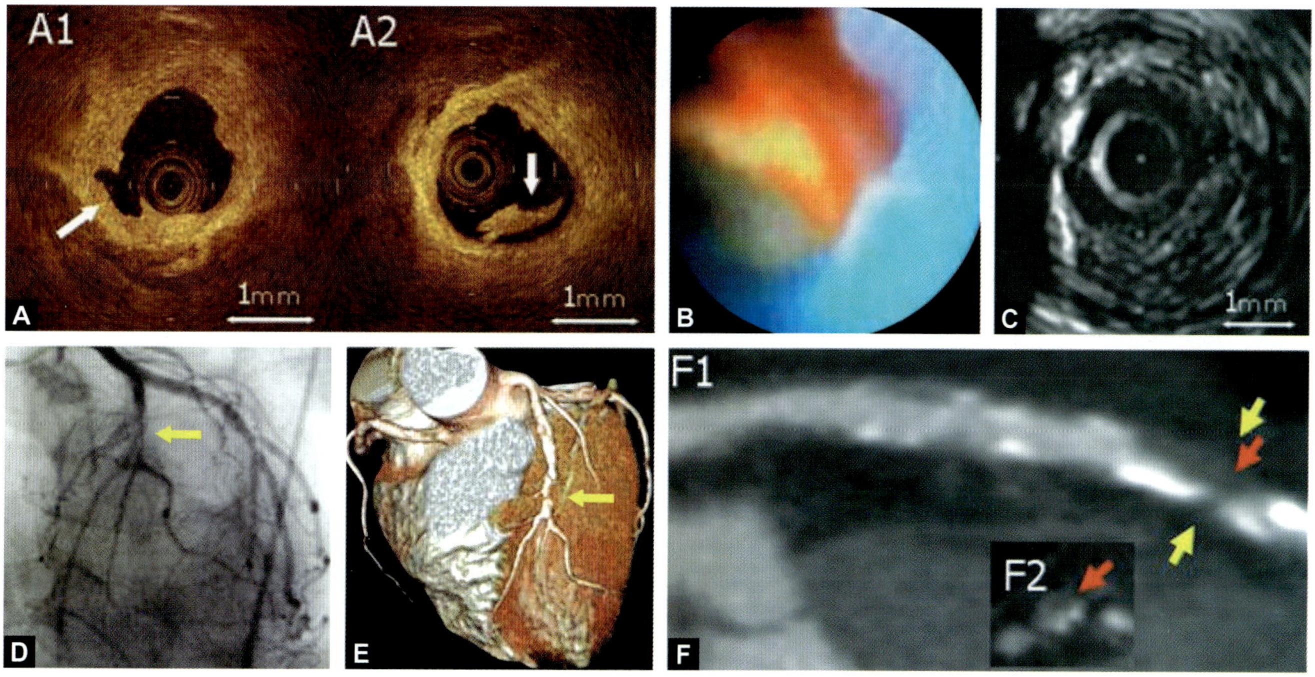

Figs. 6.5A to F: Ruptured fibrous cap of a coronary stenoses leading to thrombus formation in a patient with acute coronary syndrome. (A1 and A2) Optical coherence tomography reveals fibrous cap disruption (white arrow in A1) and thrombus formation in adjacent slices (white arrow in A2); (B) Coronary angioscopy demonstrates yellow plaque and red thrombus formation through the blue coronary angioscopy guide catheter; (C) Intravascular ultrasound shows two focal calcium deposits; (D) Coronary angiography; (E) volume-rendered CT images disclose a significant stenosis in the mid left anterior descending artery (yellow arrows in D and E). (F1) Curved multiplanar reformation CT images reveal positive remodeling associated with focal calcium deposits (yellow arrows in F1). (F2) Curved multiplanar reformation and the cross-sectional images display the presence of soft plaque (red arrow in F1 and F2). (Reproduced with permission from Ozaki Y, Okumura M, Ismail TF, et al. Coronary CT angiographic characteristics of culprit lesions in acute coronary syndromes not related to plaque rupture as defined by optical coherence tomography and angioscopy. Eur Heart J. 2011;43:2814-23).

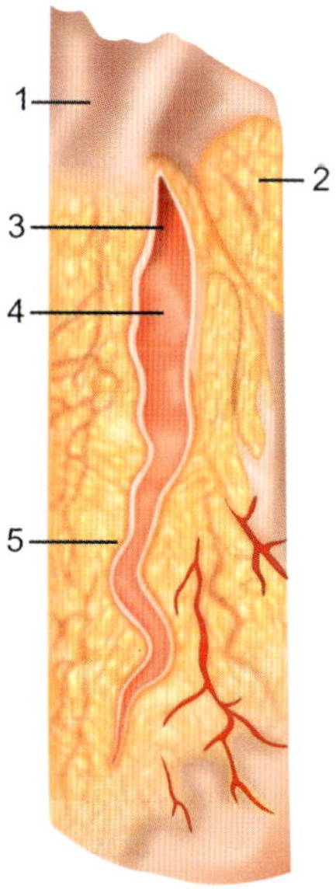

Fig. 6.6A: Early description and illustration of coronary artery occlusion. (Image is from a textbook by Dmochowski published in 1903 demonstrating complete occlusion of the left anterior descending (LAD) artery. Image taken From Skalski J. Myocardial infarction and angina pectoris in the history of medicine on the Polish soil. In: Pesek K (Ed). Atherosclerotic Cardiovascular Disease. Shanghai: InTech China; 2011.

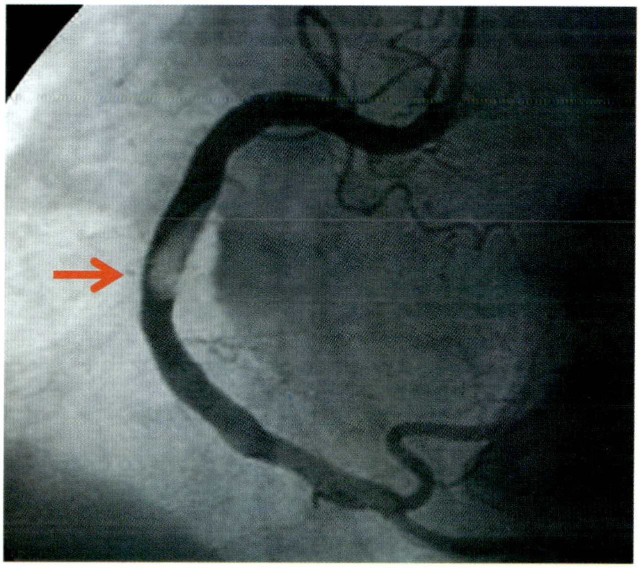

Fig. 6.6B: Coronary angiography demonstrating large filling defect (arrow) due to thrombus formation at the site of plaque rupture in the right coronary artery. (Adapted from Alioglu E, Tuzun N, Sahin F, et al. Non ST-segment elevation myocardial infarction in patients with essential thrombocytopenia. Thromb J. 2009;7:1).

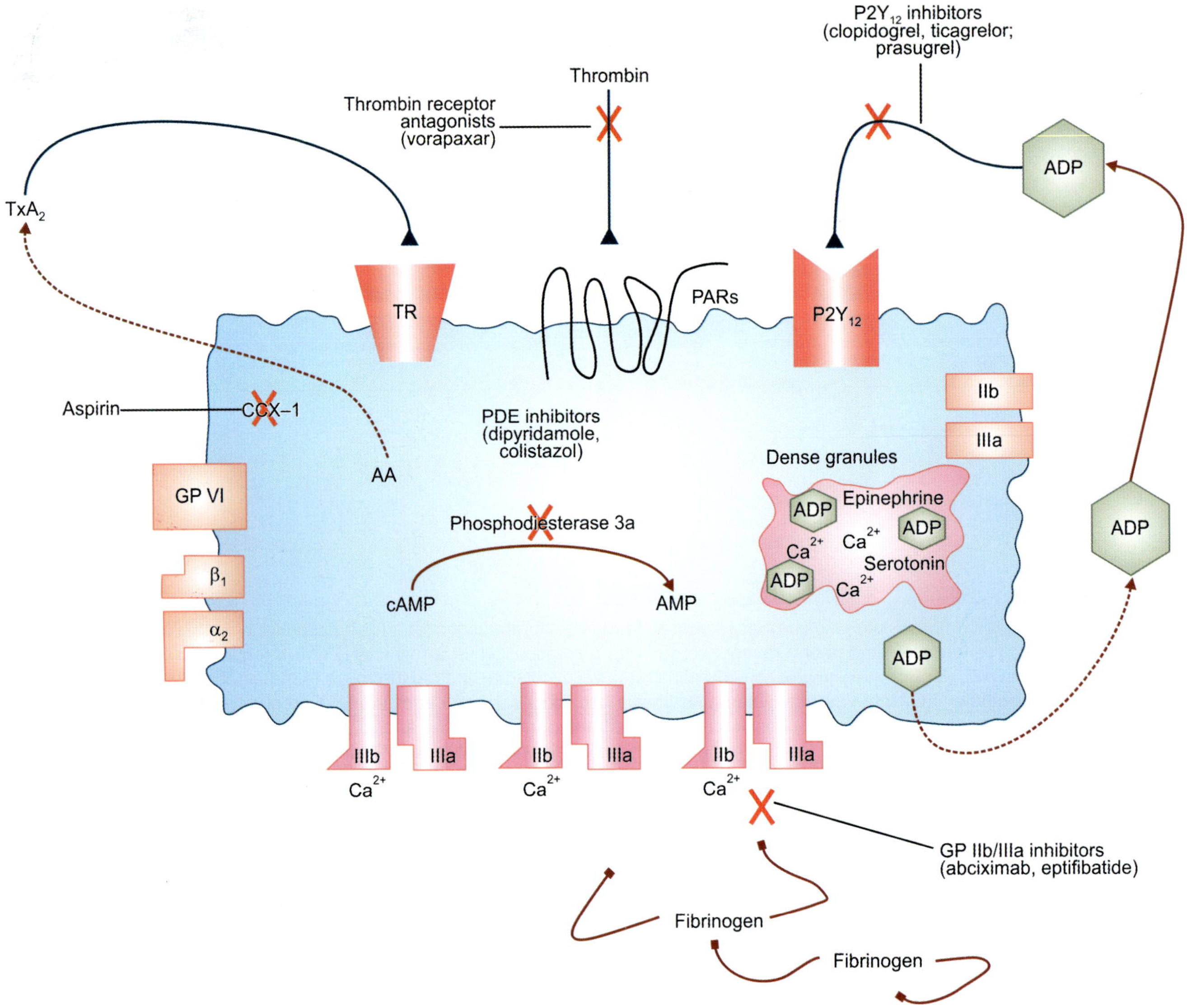

Fig. 6.7: Mechanisms of platelet activation. Proceeding clockwise, the first step in activation is platelet adhesion. After endothelial injury, exposed components of the extracellular matrix and subendothelium, such as collagen and von Willebrand factor (vWF), bind to glycoprotein VI (GP VI) and integrin $\alpha_2\beta_1$ on the platelet surface. Binding arrests platelet movement at sites of injury and begins the sequence of platelet activation through intracellular signal transduction. Platelet activation and recruitment occur through several signaling pathways. The three major pathways are depicted. Thromboxane A_2, generated from arachidonic acid by COX-1, signals through the thromboxane receptor (TR). The ADP, released from platelets, signals through the P2Y12 receptor. Thrombin cleaves the PAR-1 and PAR-4 receptors, leading to intracellular signaling. Of the three, thrombin is the most powerful activating agent. Activation occurs through a number of intracellular pathways in response to thrombin, TxA_2 or ADP signaling. As a result, dense granules are released and conformational changes of GP IIb/IIa occur, making them highly avid for fibrinogen. Other cellular changes, including platelet flattening and exposure of negatively charged phospholipids, also result. The final step is aggregation (4). Divalent fibrinogen molecules bind to the GP IIb/IIIa receptors of adjacent platelets. Given the high density of this receptor on the platelet surface, adjacent platelets become interconnected, forming a platelet plus. [Image from Kohl LP, Weiss E. Antithrombotic and antiplatelet agents. In: Chatterjee K, Anderson M, Heistad D, Kerber RE (Eds). Cardiology: An Illustrated Textbook. New Delhi, India. Jaypee Brothers Medical Publishers (P) Ltd. 2012].

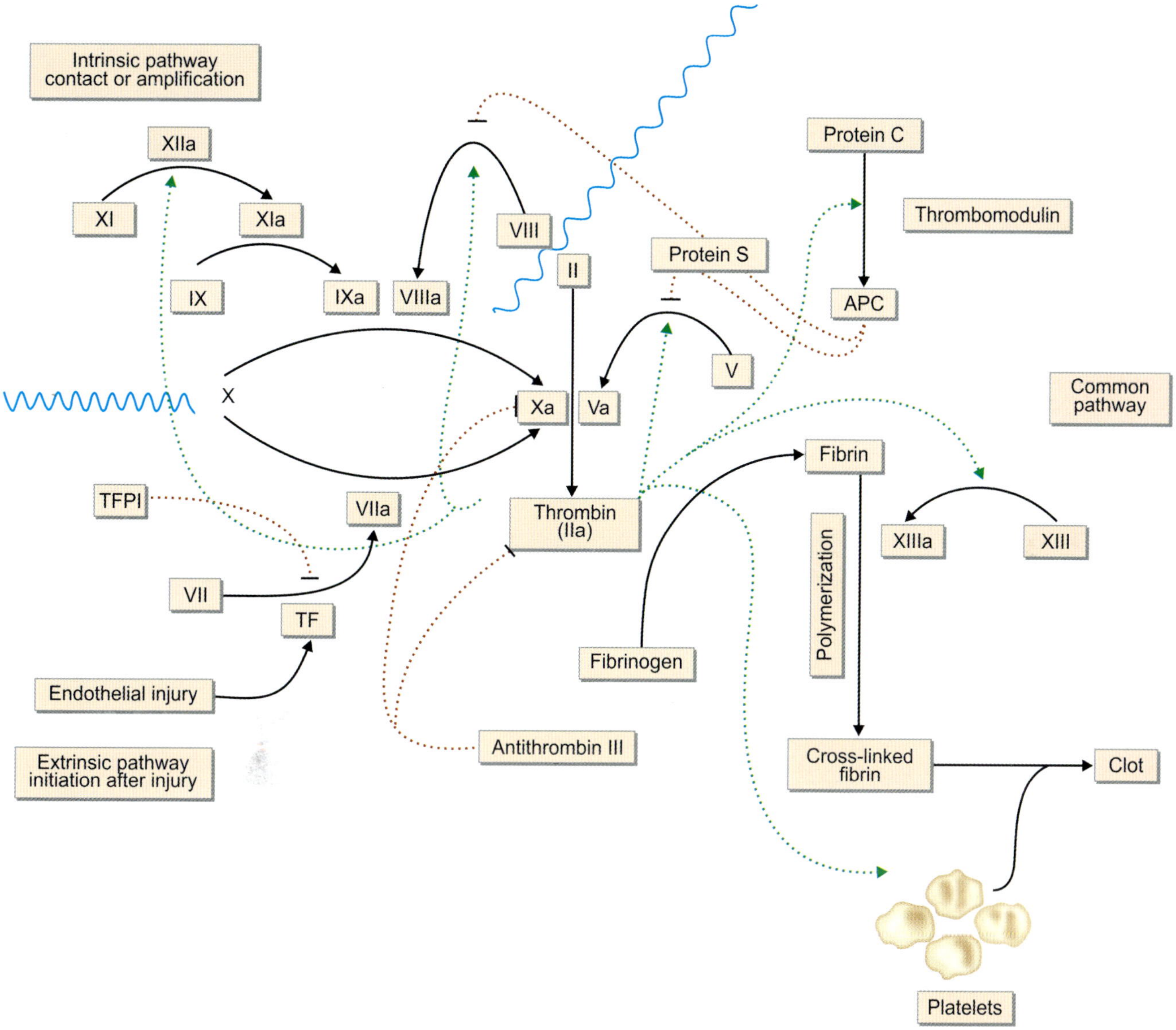

Fig. 6.8: Clotting cascade as currently understood: the intrinsic pathway (upper left) proceeds through factors XI, IX and VIII to activation of factor X. Activation of factor XI can occur through factor XIIa, as occurs after addition of a negatively charged trigger in the aPTT, or through thrombin feedback. After endothelial injury, exposed tissue factor complexes with and activates factor VII via the extrinsic pathway, which activates factor X in turn. The common pathway integrates procoagulant signal and leads to conversion of fibrinogen to fibrin by thrombin. Thrombin and factor Xa, the two principal anticoagulant targets, are components of the common pathway. Green dotted arrows signify action by thrombin as an activating agent. Mechanism of action of antithrombotic molecules are denoted by red dotted lines. [Image from Kohl LP, Weiss E. Antithrombotic and antiplatelet agents. In Chatterjee K, Anderson M, Heistad D, Kerber RE (Eds). Cardiology: An Illustrated Textbook. New Delhi, India: Jaypee Brothers Medical Publishers (P) Ltd. 2012].

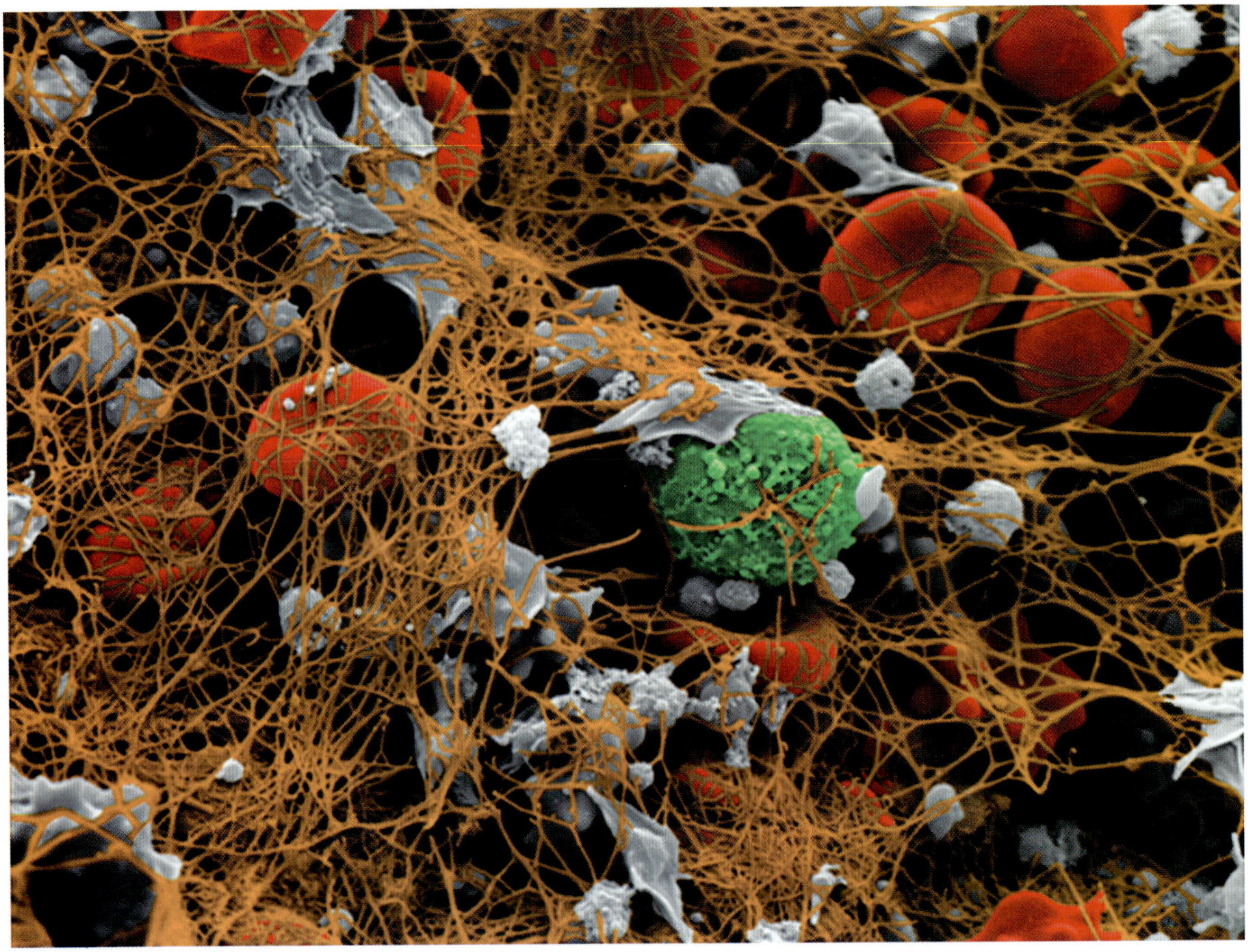

Fig. 6.9: Colorized scanning electron micrograph of a thrombus aspirated from a patient with ST-elevation myocardial infarction. The thrombus is made up of a fibrin meshwork (brown) together with platelets (light gray/purple). Erythrocytes (red) and leukocytes (green) are trapped in the network (Image courtesy of Brown AEX, Nagaswami C, Litvinov RI, and Weisel JW).

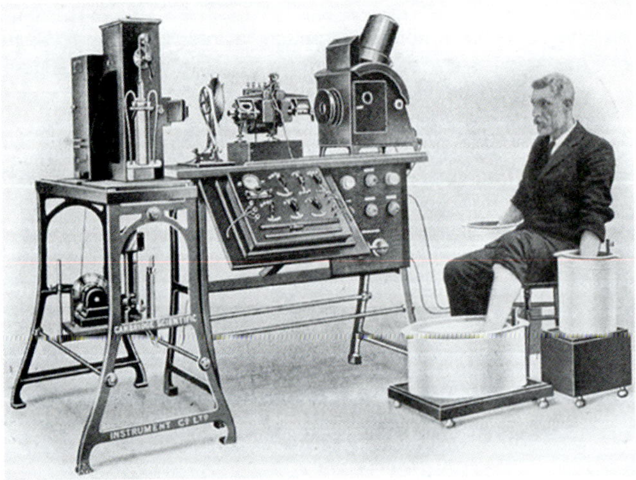

Fig. 6.10: One of the reputed earliest ECG machines. [Image from Bansal M et al. History of acute coronary syndrome. In: Chopra HK and Nanda NC (Ed). Textbook of cardiology—a clinical and historical perspective. New Delhi, India: Jaypee Brothers Medical Publishers (P) Ltd].

an intravenous glycoprotein IIb/IIIa inhibitor (Fig. 6.12). Anticoagulant therapy consists of unfractionated heparin, the low-molecular-weight heparin enoxaparin, the anti-Xa agent fondaparinux, or the direct thrombin inhibitor bivalirudin. Bleeding risk can be estimated using the **C**an **R**apid risk stratification of **U**nstable angina patients **S**uppress **AD**verse outcomes with **E**arly Implementation of the ACC/AHA guidelines (CRUSADE) bleeding risk calculator (Fig. 6.13). Risk can be assessed by measurement of troponin levels, inspection of the ECG, and/or calculation of the thrombolysis in myocardial infarction (TIMI) or Global Registry of Acute Coronary Events (GRACE) risk score (Table 6.1 and Fig. 6.14). Most patients with high-risk features (positive troponin, ST-segment deviation, high TIMI or GRACE risk score) are referred for prompt (within 24–48 hours) catheterization and, when appropriate, revascularization. It is estimated that optimal medical and revascularization (when appropriate) therapy decreases the rates of MI and recurrent ischemia by approximately 20–40% and decreases the rate of death by approximately 10%.

ST-SEGMENT ELEVATION ACUTE CORONARY SYNDROME (STEMI)

Patients with ACS who do have ST-segment elevation (Figs. 6.15A to D) are classified as "STEMI" patients and require emergent treatment, as the majority of such patients have an occluded artery. When not treated with reperfusion therapy, STEMI will usually result in transmural infarction (Figs. 6.16A and B). For several decades, thrombolytic treatment was the primary treatment of such patients. Primary percutaneous coronary intervention (PCI) (Figs. 6.17A to D and Videos 6.2A to E) is now the preferred intervention if primary PCI can be expeditiously performed. Compared to thrombolytic therapy, primary PCI leads to higher rates of infarct artery patency and TIMI 3 flow, and lower rates of recurrent ischemia, reinfarction, emergency revascularization, intracranial hemorrhage, and death. Target system goals for door-to-needle time are within 30 minutes; target system goals for first medical contact to first device activation "door-to-balloon" times are within 90 minutes (120 minutes for patients being transferred from a satellite hospital to a hub hospital for primary PCI). For those being transferred from a non-PCI-capable hospital to a hospital capable of performing primary PCI, the "door-in-door-out" (DIDO) goal is <30 minutes. PCI at the time of primary PCI of non-infarct arteries is associated with a worse outcome and should not in general be performed, unless the patient is in cardiogenic shock and the non-infarct artery stenosis may be contributing to hemodynamic instability.

Complications of STEMI

Cardiogenic shock usually occurs in the setting of STEMI but may occasionally occur in patients with NSTE-ACS. Cardiogenic shock may be caused by extensive left ventricular infarction, right ventricular (RV) infarction (Fig. 6.18), or by mechanical complications such as papillary muscle rupture (leading to severe mitral regurgitation) (Fig. 6.19) or ventricular septal rupture (Figs. 6.20 to 6.22). Clinical RV infarction complicates approximately 1/3 of cases of STEMI due to inferior MI and right coronary artery occlusion.

Free wall rupture (Figs. 6.23A to D) as a result of STEMI usually leads to death. Rarely, with free wall rupture, a pseudoaneurysm (Fig. 6.24) will form and the patient will survive. Transmural anterior and apical MI may predispose to ventricular thrombus formation for several months (Videos 6.3 to 6.7). Long-term complications of STEMI include aneurysm formation (Fig. 6.25), heart failure (discussed in the chapter on Heart Failure), and predisposition to ventricular arrhythmias (discussed in the chapter on Ventricular Tachycardia and Fibrillation and the chapter on ICDs).

OTHER CAUSES OF ACS AND ACS-LIKE SYNDROMES

Although ACS is most commonly due to plaque rupture or fissure, other conditions can result in the development of chest pain, ECG changes, and myocardial ischemia and necrosis. Large coronary aneurysms (Figs. 6.26 to 6.28), such as in patients with a history of Kawasaki disease, may result in in-situ thrombus formation and distal embolization, leading to MI. Takayasu's arteritis may affect the coronary arteries, leading to coronary artery stenosis, occlusion or aneurismal dilation (Figs. 6.29A to C). The coronary arteries and the second most commonly affected vascular bed in patients with polyarteritis nodosa (PAN).

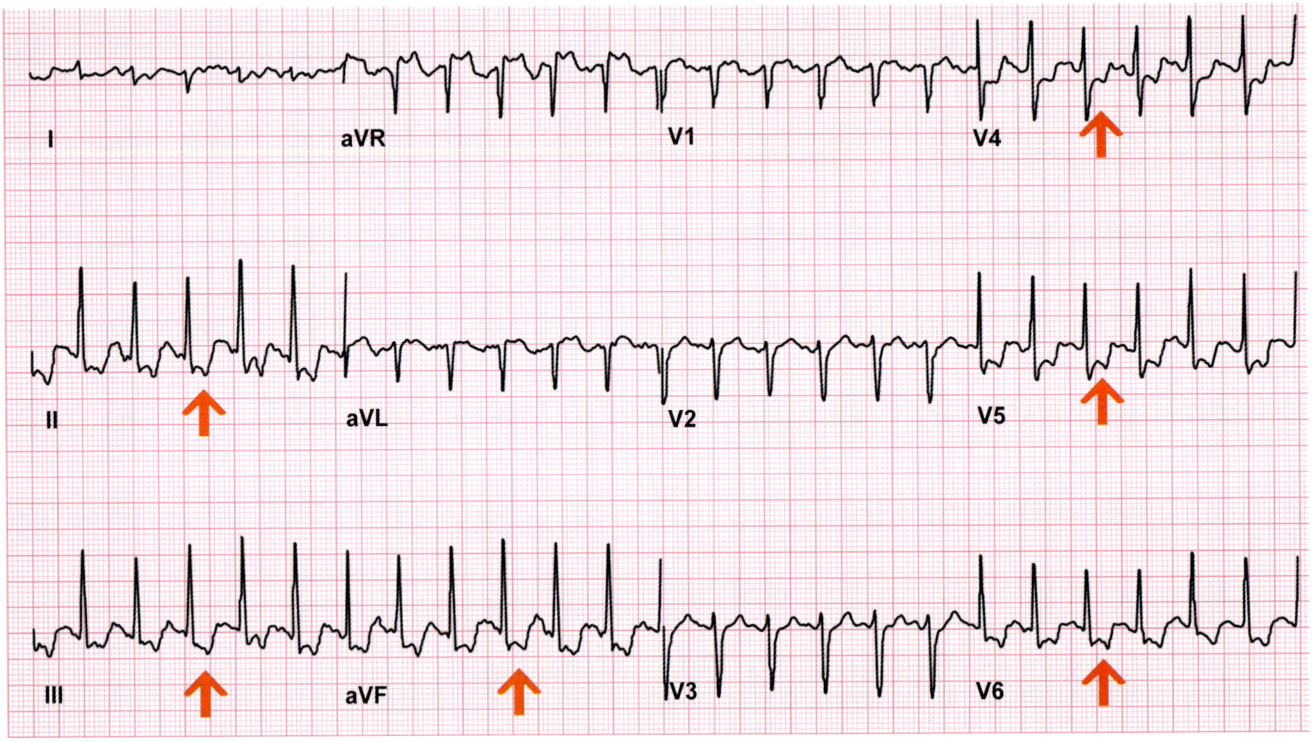

Fig. 6.11A: ECG demonstrating ST-segment depression (arrows) in a patient with non-ST-segment elevation acute coronary syndrome.

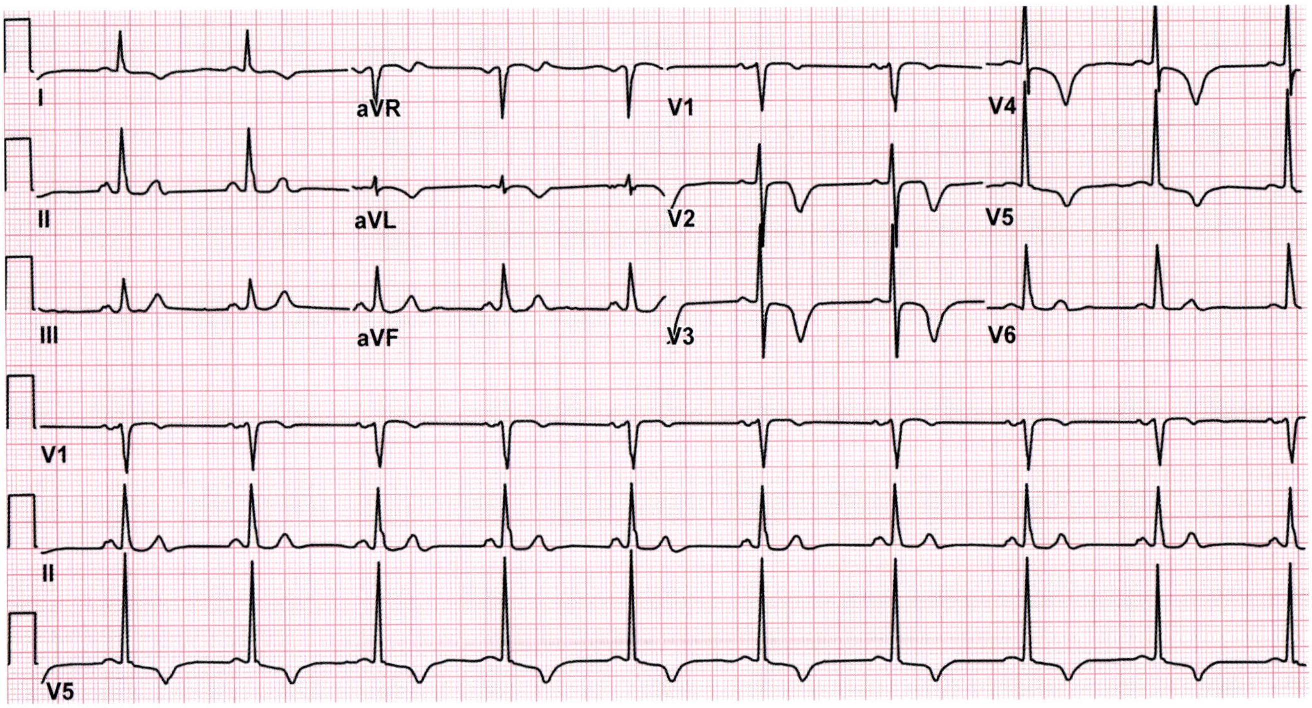

Fig. 6.11B: ECG demonstrating deep symmetric T-wave inversions in the precordial leads in a patient with non-ST-segment elevation acute coronary syndrome.

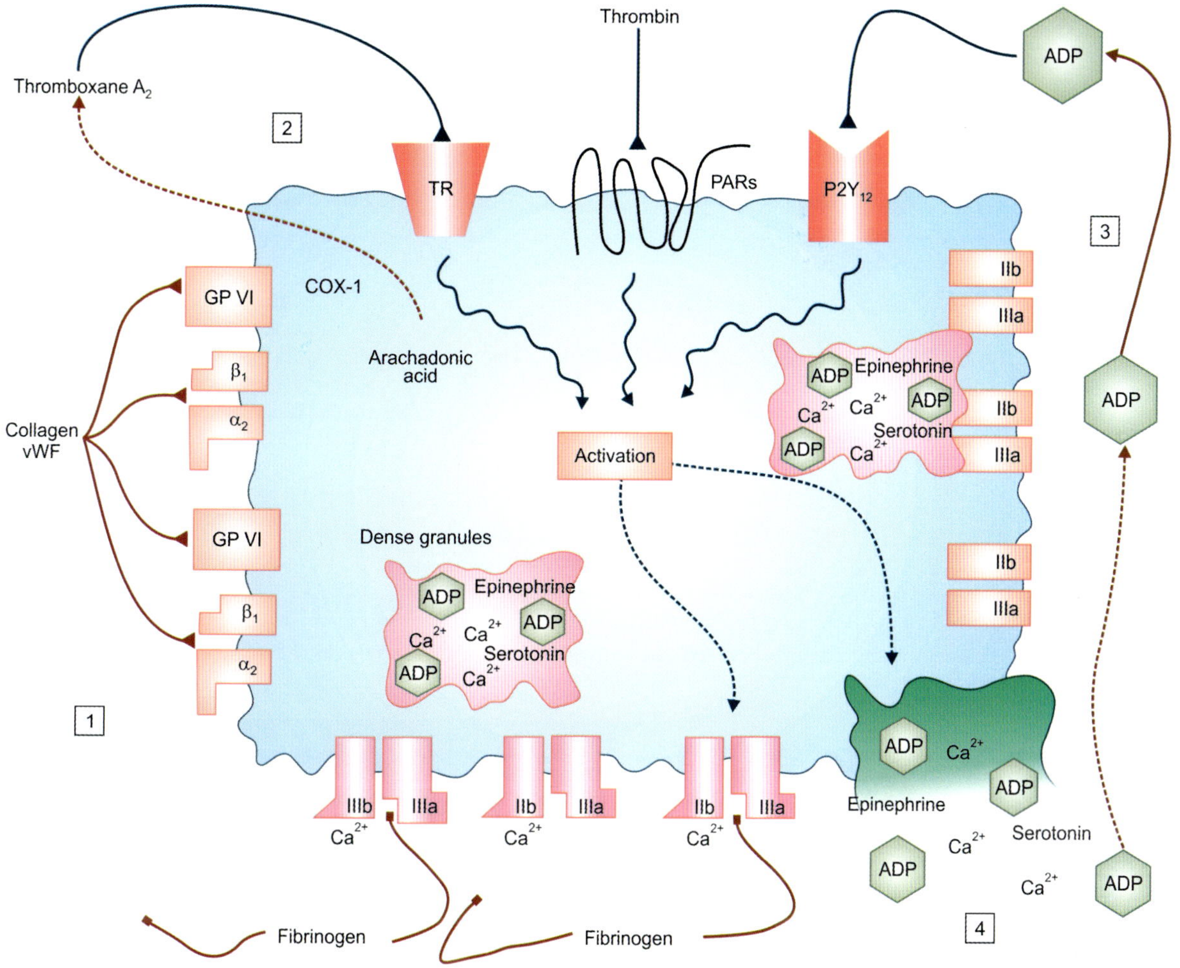

Fig. 6.12: Mechanism of action of oral and intravenous antiplatelet agents. Aspirin is the major inhibitor of the TxA2 pathway. Clopidogrel, ticagrelor, and prasugrel are $P2Y_{12}$ receptor inhibitors. The GP IIb/IIIa inhibitors block fibrinogen binding and thus platelet aggregation. [Image from Kohl LP, Weiss E. Antithrombotic and antiplatelet agents. In: Chatterjee K, Anderson M, Heistad D, Kerber RE (Eds). Cardiology: An Illustrated Textbook. New Delhi: Jaypee Brothers Medical Publishers (P) Ltd. 2012].

Table 6.1: Factors used to calculate the TIMI risk score. (CAD: Coronary artery disease; TIMI: Thrombolysis in myocardial infarction).

Age ≥ 65 years
≥ 3 risk factors for CAD*
Known CAD (stenosis ≥ 50%)
Aspirin use in the past 7 days
Severe angina (≥ 2 episodes within 24 hours)
ST-segment changes ≥ 0.5 mm
Positive cardiac biomarker

*Risk factors for CAD are considered to be diabetes, cigarette smoking, hypertension, hypercholesterolemia, and family history of CAD.

PAN may lead to coronary artery aneurysm formation and to coronary artery thrombosis (Fig. 6.30). Takotsubo cardiomyopathy, also called stress cardiomyopathy, apical ballooning cardiomyopathy, or "broken heart syndrome", is a condition usually associated with severe emotional stress. The classic presentation includes ECG changes (such as anterior ST-segment elevation) and apical dyskinesis (Figs. 6.31 to 6.33). In most patients, LV function recovers in the days to weeks after presentation. Other conditions that can mimic some of the signs and symptoms seen in patients with ACS include pulmonary embolism and aortic dissection, which are discussed in other chapters in this atlas.

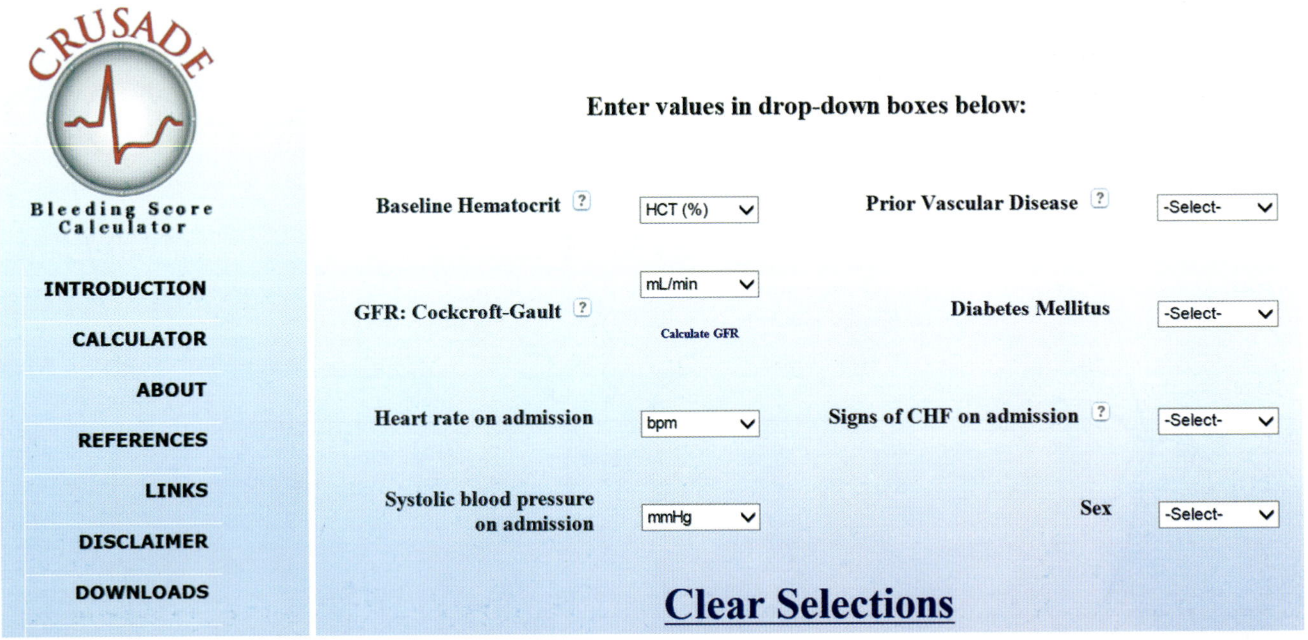

Fig. 6.13: The CRUSADE bleeding score calculator, which can be used to assess bleeding risk in patients with acute coronary syndrome.

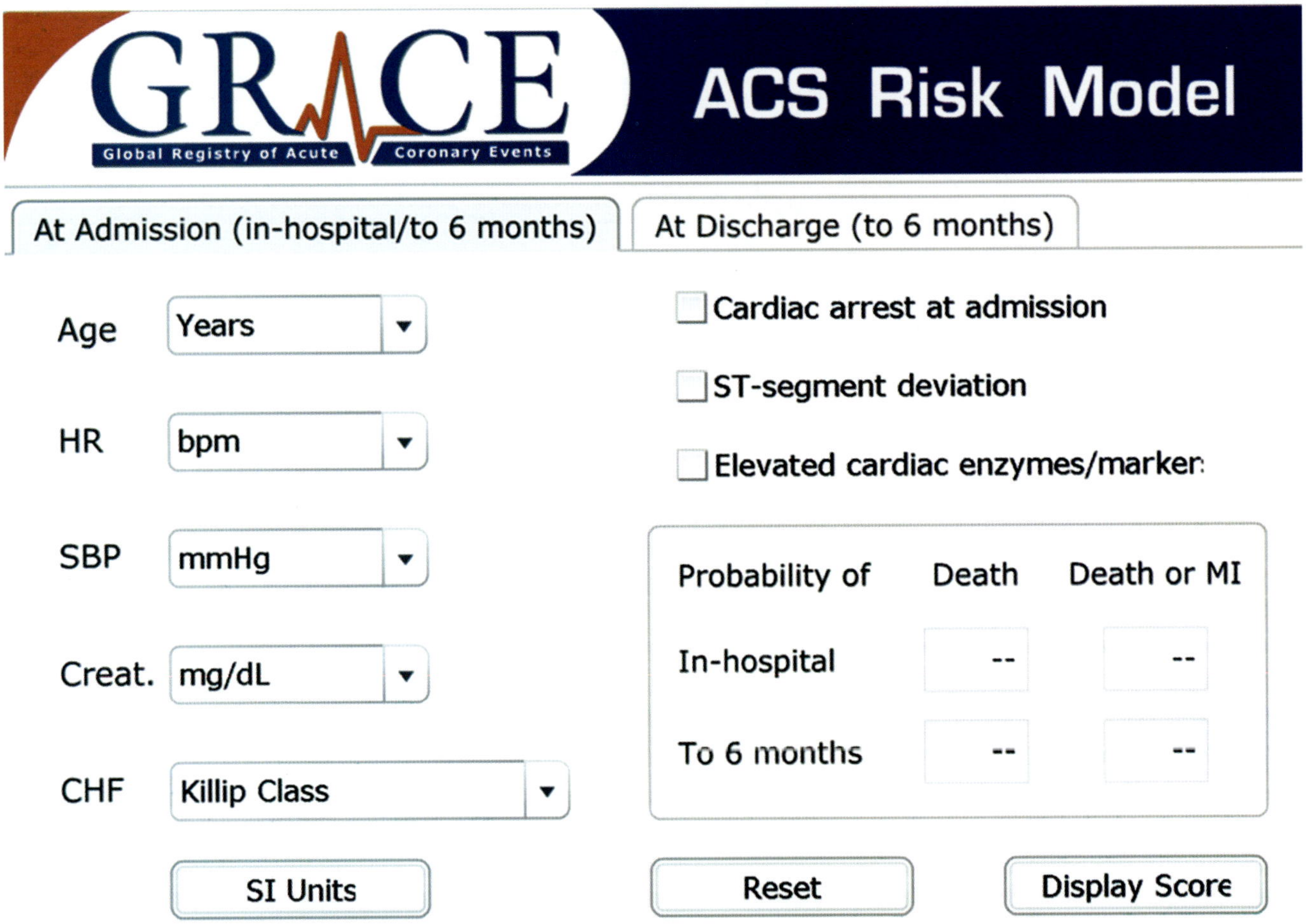

Fig. 6.14: The Global Registry of Acute Coronary Events (GRACE) risk score calculator for patients with acute coronary syndrome.

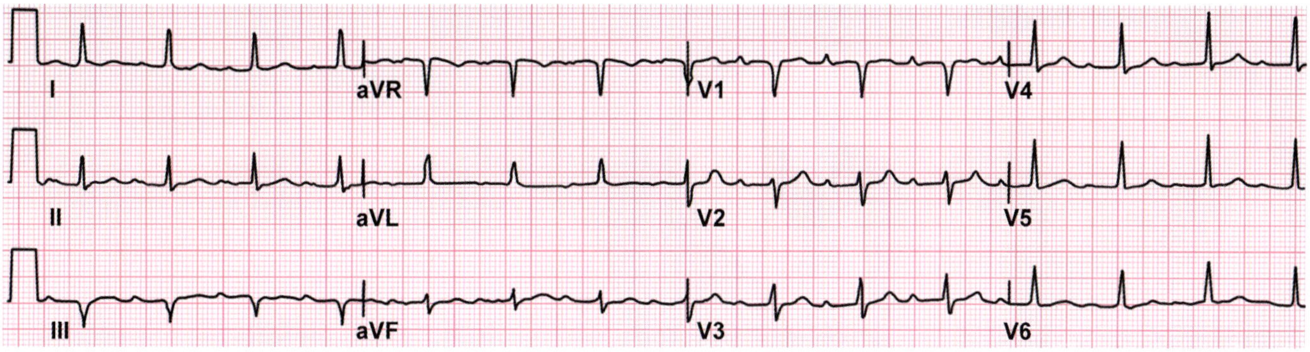

Fig. 6.15A: 12-lead ECGs showing evolution of ST-segment elevation in a patient with inferior wall myocardial infarction. (A) Baseline ECG obtained without chest pain.

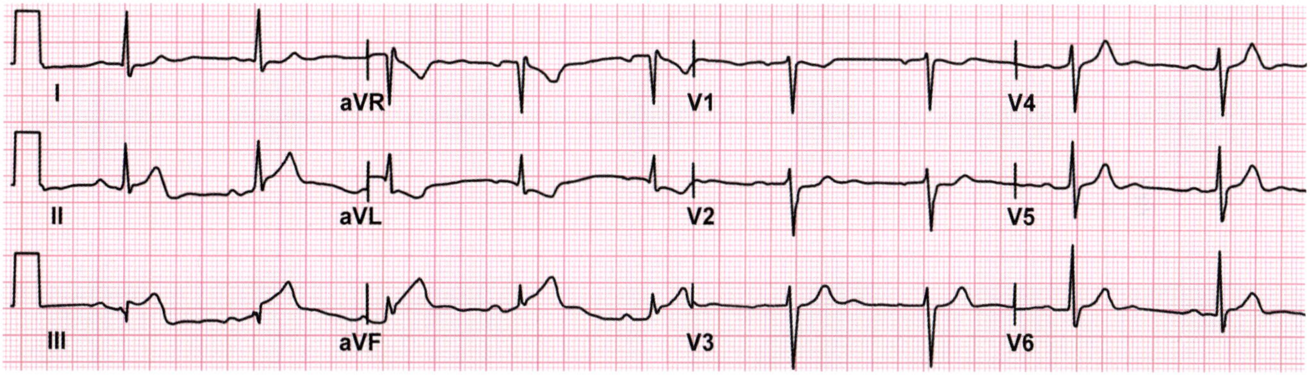

Fig. 6.15B: ECG obtained shortly after the onset of chest pain showing modest ST-segment elevation in the inferior leads (II, III, aVF).

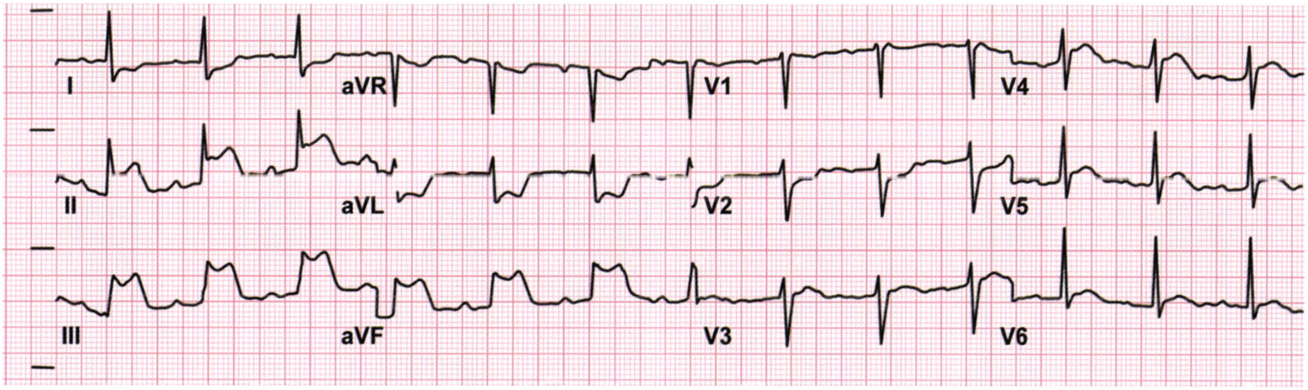

Fig. 6.15C: ECG obtained a short-time afterward showing marked ST-segment elevation in the inferior leads, as well as some ST-elevation in leads V4–V6 and reciprocal ST-depressions in other leads.

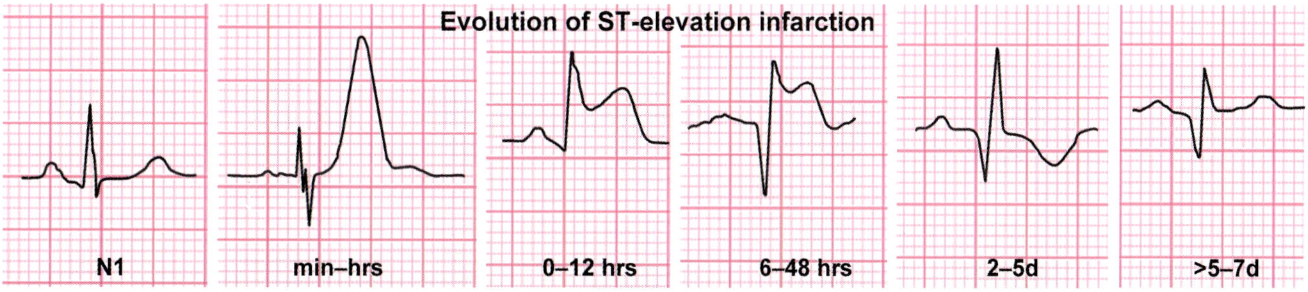

Fig. 6.15D: Time course of the ECG changes in a patient with STEMI. [Image from Wang K. Atlas of Electrocardiography. New Delhi, India: Jaypee Brothers Medical Publishers (P) Ltd. 2013].

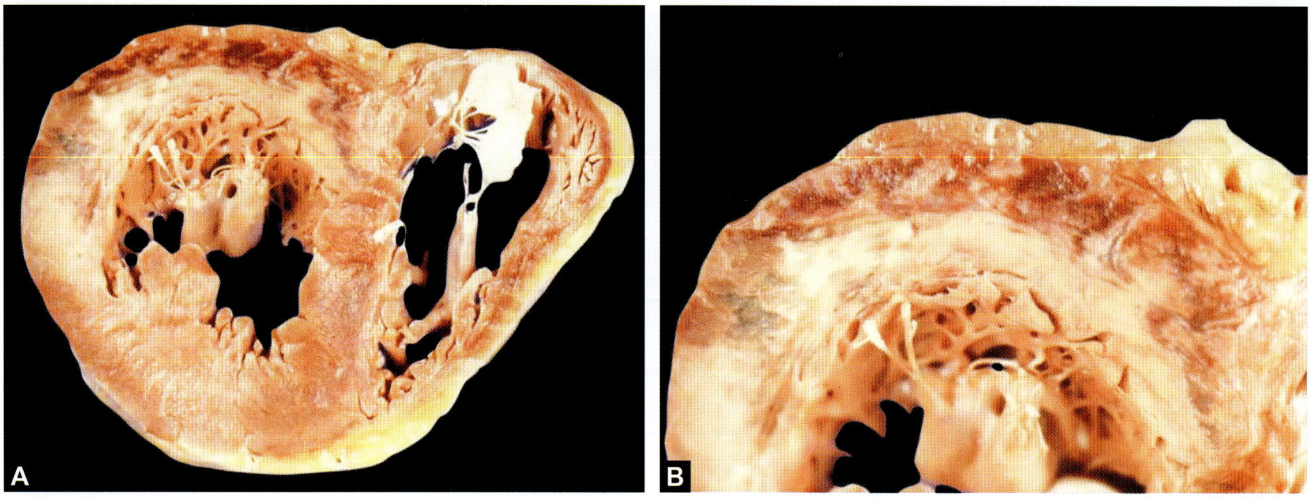

Figs. 6.16A and B: STEMI resulting in transmural myocardial infarction. (A and B) Large transmural infarction. (Reproduced with permission of Munther K Homound and Tufts University. Clinico-Pathological Correlation PowerPoint lecture, Cardiovascular Pathophysiology. Tufts OpenCourseWare; 2005–2013).

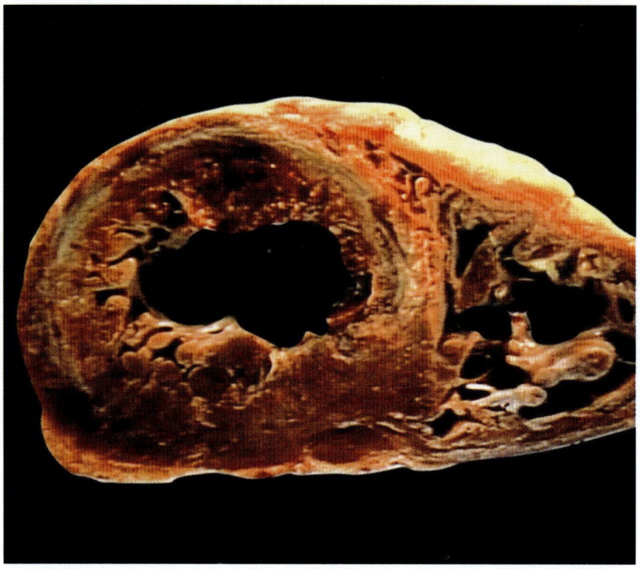

Fig. 6.16C: Gross pathology specimen demonstrating massive recent myocardial infarction. (Courtesy of Armed Forced Institute of Pathology).

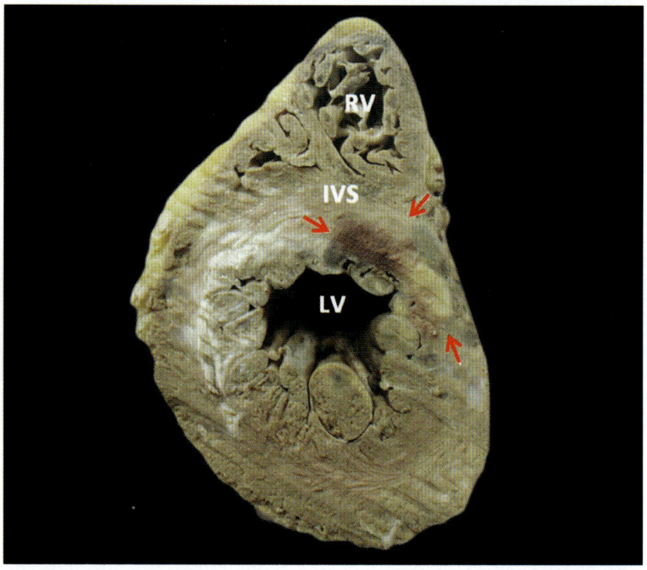

Fig. 6.16D: Gross pathology specimen of recent near transmural myocardial infarction (arrows). Note the white fibrotic area indicative of a more distant prior infarction. [Courtesy of Pradeep Vaideeswar, Professor (Additional), Department of Pathology, Cardiovascular & Thoracic Division, Seth Gordhandas Sunderdas Medical College, Mumbai, India]. (IVC: Interventricular septum; LV: Left ventricle; RV: Right ventricle).

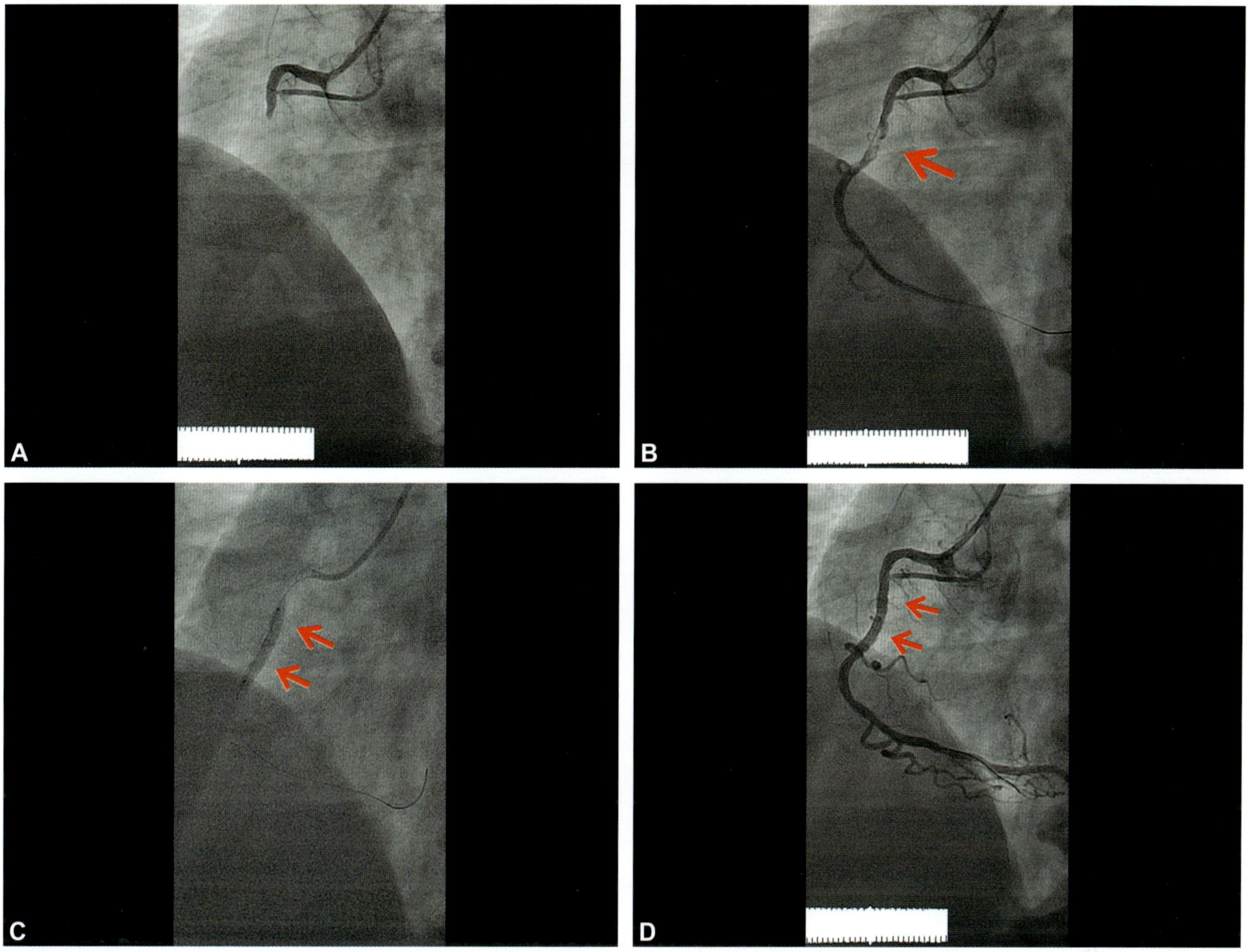

Figs. 6.17A to D: Primary percutaneous coronary intervention. (A) Occluded proximal right coronary artery; (B) Initial wiring of the lesion restores some blood flow and allows visualization of a complex ruptured plaque with thrombus formation (arrow); (C) Balloon dilation and stent deployment (arrows) at the site of the culprit lesion; (D) Final angiogram demonstrating the deployed stent (arrows) and restoration of blood flow.

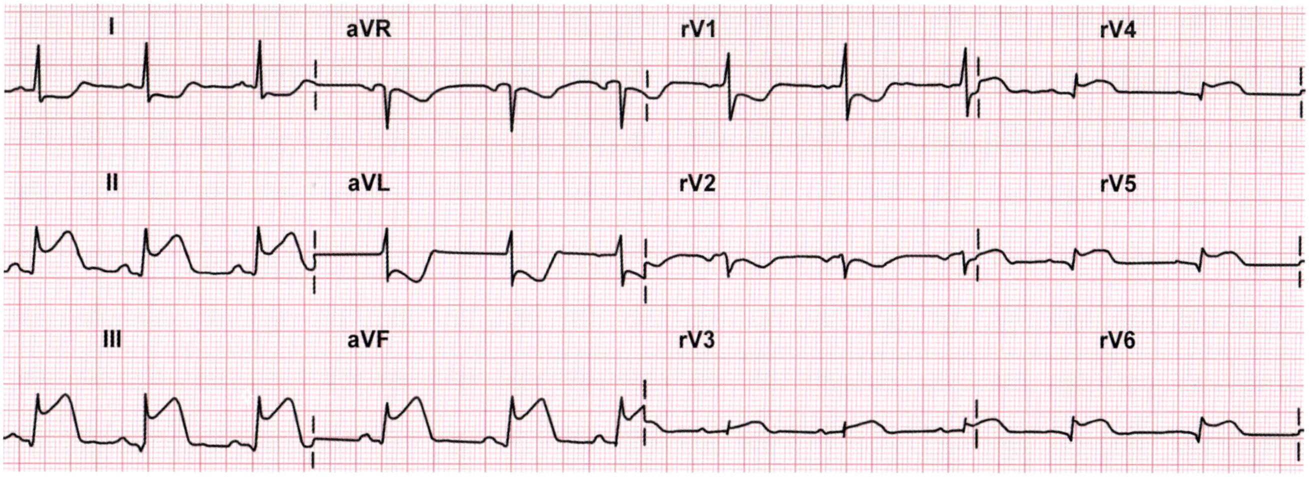

Fig. 6.18: ECG with "right sided leads" in a patient with acute inferior myocardial infarction (IMI). Note the clear ST-elevation in lead rV4, highly suggestive of right ventricular infarction.

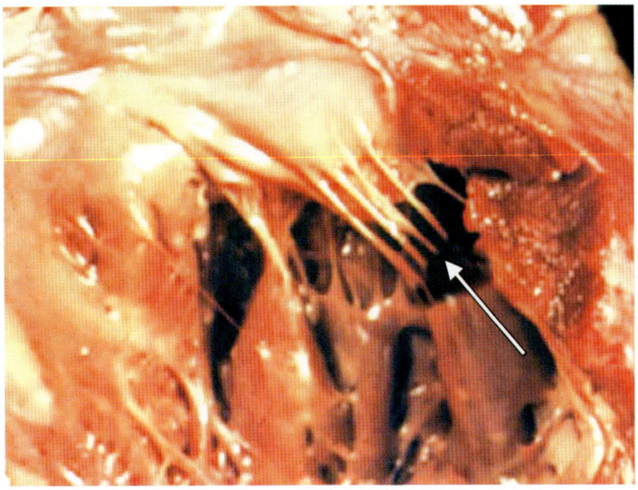

Fig. 6.19: Ruptured papillary muscle in a patient with recent STEMI, resulting in severe mitral regurgitation and cardiogenic shock. [From Shah SK, Ivan E, Michaels AD. Cardiogenic shock in acute coronary syndromes. In: Chatterjee K, Anderson M, Heistad D, Kerber RE (Eds). Cardiology: An Illustrated Textbook. New Delhi, India: Jaypee Brothers Medical Publishers (P) Ltd. 2012].

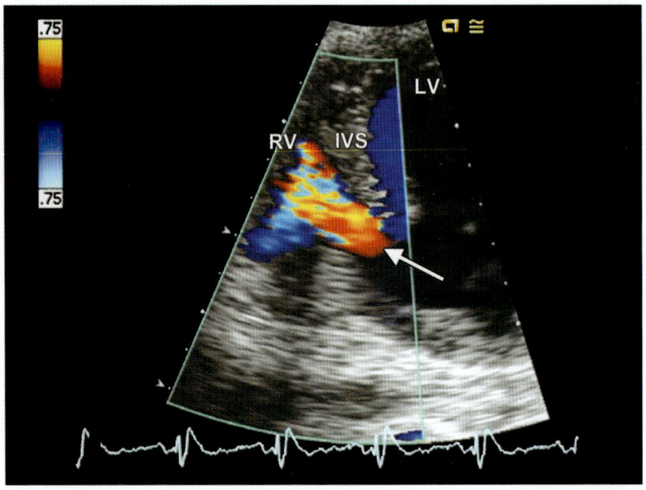

Fig. 6.20: Transesophageal echocardiography showing post-myocardial infarction ventricular septal defect with left-to-right flow (arrow). [Image from Shah SK, Ivan E, Michaels AD. Cardiogenic shock in acute coronary syndromes. In: Chatterjee K, Anderson M, Heistad D, Kerber RE (Eds). Cardiology: An Illustrated Textbook. New Delhi, India: Jaypee Brothers Medical Publishers (P) Ltd. 2012). (IVS: Interventricular septum; LV: Left ventricle; RV: Right ventricle].

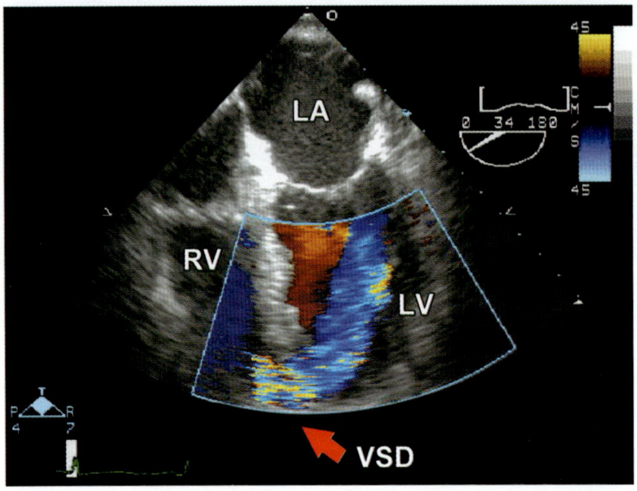

Fig. 6.21: Transesophageal echocardiography color Doppler demonstrating an apical ventricular septal defect with flow from the left ventricle to the right ventricle complicating acute myocardial infarction. [Image from Firstenberg MS, Kissling KT, Nelson K. Management and controversies of postmyocardial infarction ventricular septal defects. In: Firstenberg MS (Ed). Principles and Practice of Cardiothoracic Surgery. Shanghai: InTech China; 2012].

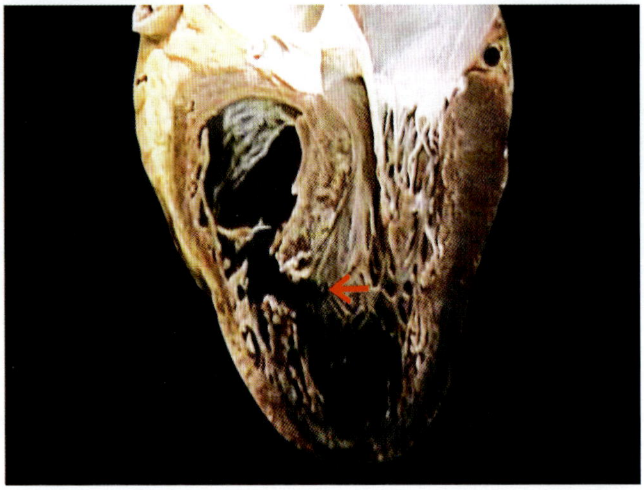

Fig. 6.22: Pathologic example of postmyocardial infarction ventricular septal defect (arrow). (Image from Armed Forces Institute of Pathology, Washington, DC, USA).

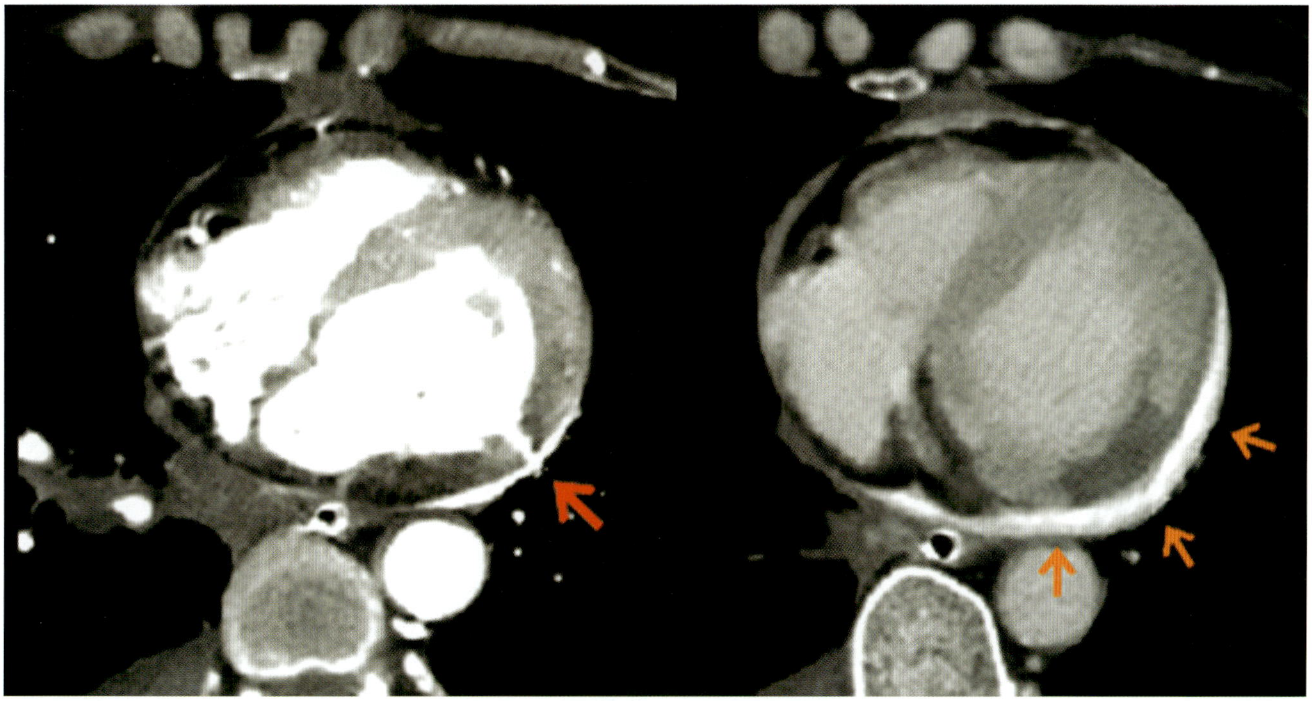

Fig. 6.23A: Cardiac CT examination showing free wall rupture. Initial scan (left panel) shows a small rupture (arrow) in the inferolateral wall of the left ventricle, with the presence of hemopericardium. A delayed image (60 seconds after initial image) shows the hypodense area of infarction in the inferolateral wall and further contrast extravasation, suggesting active bleeding into the pericardial sac. (Images and figure legend adapted from Brenes JA, Keifer T, Karim R, et al. Adjuvant role of CT in the diagnosis of postinfarction left ventricular free-wall rupture. Cardiol Res. 2012;3:284-7).

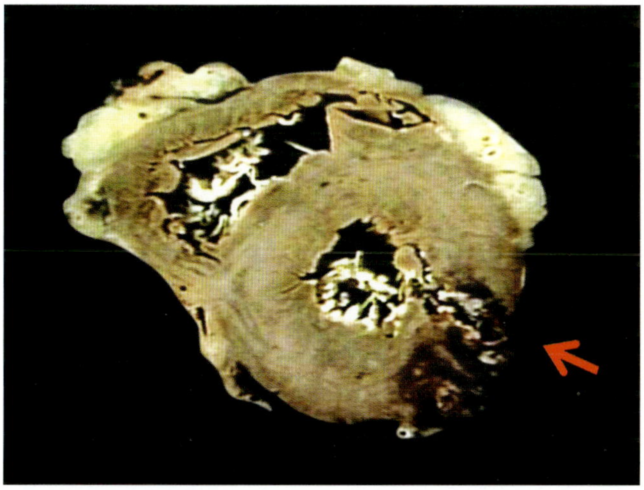

Fig. 6.23B: Pathologic example of postmyocardial infarction LV rupture (arrow). (Image from Armed Forces Institute of Pathology, Washington, DC, USA).

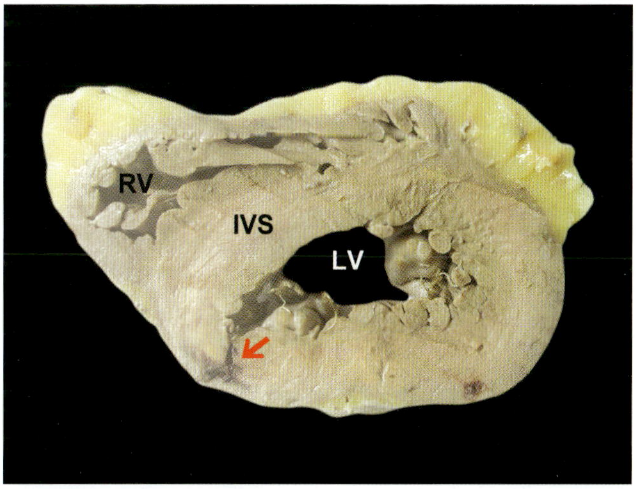

Fig. 6.23C: Free wall rupture of the inferior wall (arrow) in a patient with acute inferior wall myocardial infarction. [Image courtesy of Pradeep Vaideeswar, Professor (Additional), Department of Pathology, Cardiovascular & Thoracic Division, Seth Gordhandas Sunderdas Medical College, Mumbai, India].

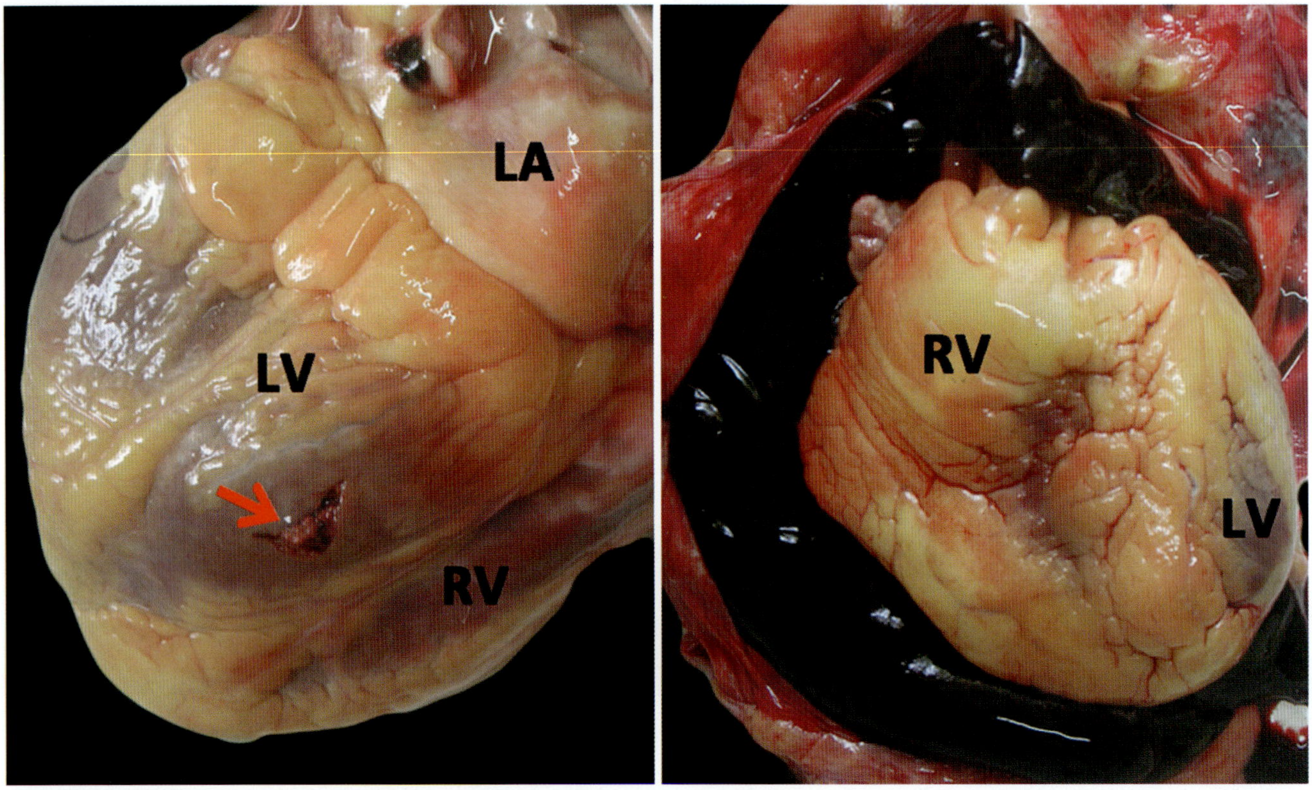

Fig. 6.23D: Free wall rupture and resulting hemopericardium. Left panel shows an area of free wall rupture (arrow) from transmural myocardial infarction. Right panel shows in situ specimen of same heart with hemopericardium. [Image courtesy of Pradeep Vaideeswar, Professor (Additional), Department of Pathology, Cardiovascular & Thoracic Division, Seth Gordhandas Sunderdas Medical College, Mumbai, India].

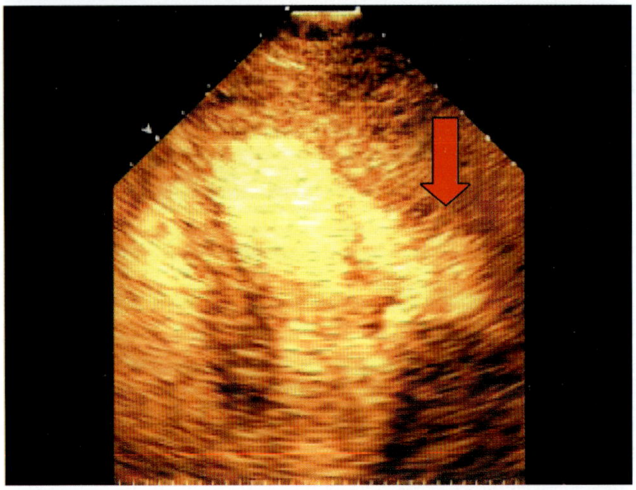

Fig. 6.24: Pseudoaneurysm of the lateral wall (arrow) discovered on contrast-enhanced transthoracic echocardiography. [Image from Lonnebakken MT, Gerdts E. Contrast echocardiography in coronary artery disease. In Baskot B (Ed). Coronary angiography—Advances in Noninvasive Imaging Approach for Evaluation of Coronary Artery Disease. Shanghai: InTech China; 2011].

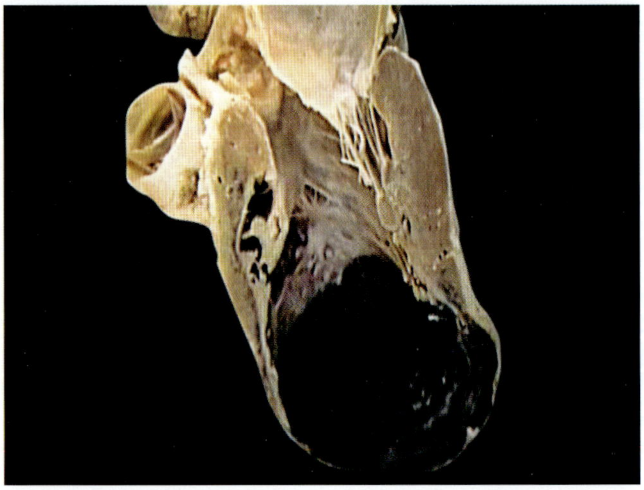

Fig. 6.25: Pathologic example of postmyocardial infarction left ventricular aneurysm.

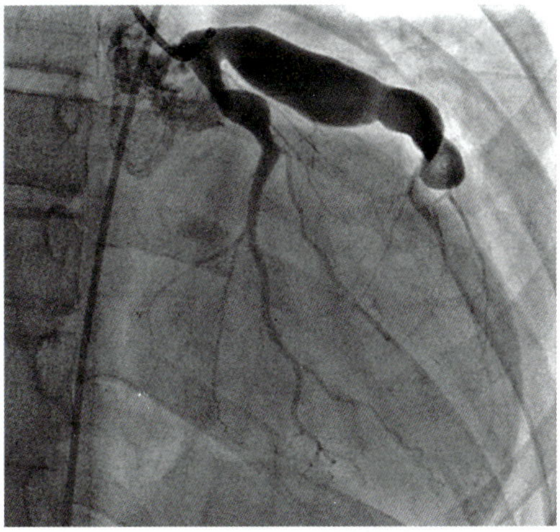

Fig. 6.26: Massive aneurismal dilation of the proximal left circumflex artery in a patient with a history of Kawasaki's Disease. There is also a small aneurysm in the proximal left anterior descending coronary artery. [Image from Yim D, Burgner D, Cheung M, et al. Echocardiography in Kawasaki disease. In Bajraktari G (Ed). Echocardiography—in Specific Disorders. Shanghai: InTech China; 2012].

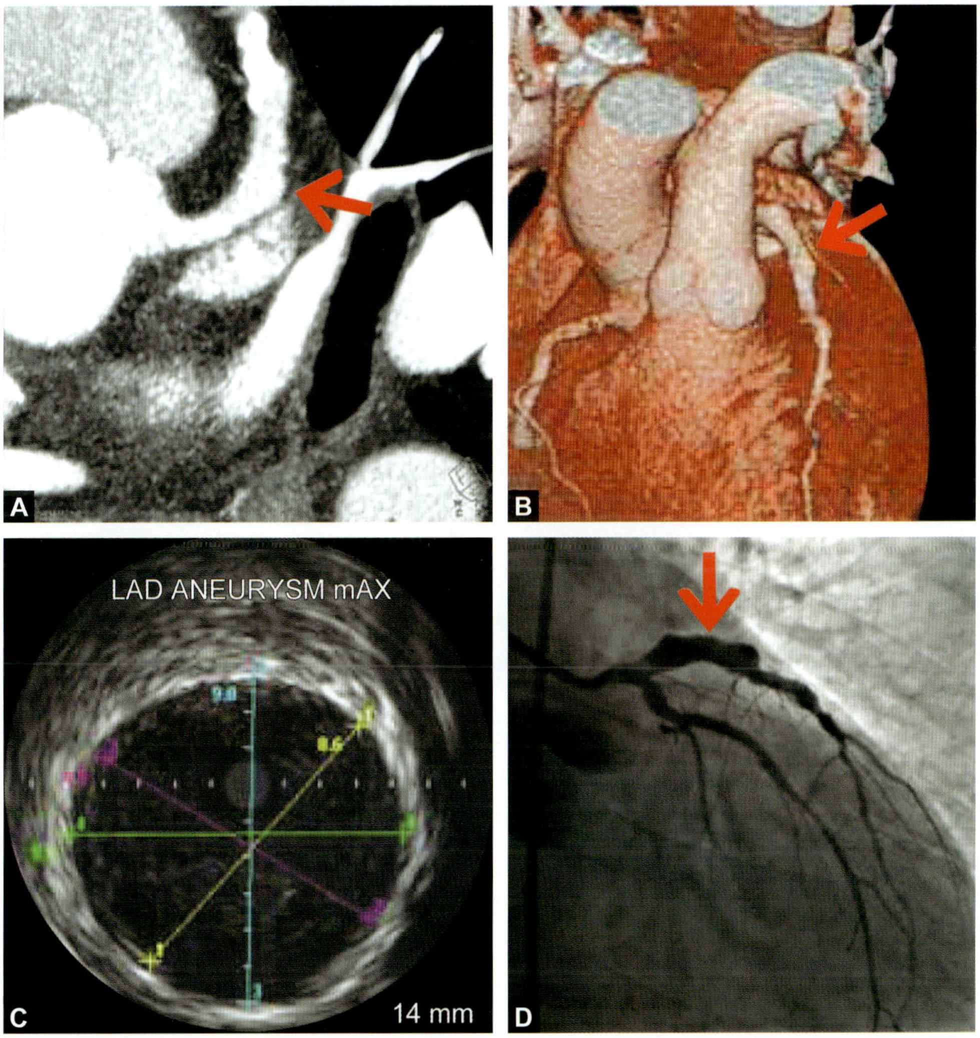

Figs. 6.27A to D: Aneurysm of the proximal left anterior descending coronary artery (LAD) (arrows) in a patient who had recurrent coronary emboli. (A) Maximum intensity projection cardiac CT angiogram; (B) Volume rendered cardiac CT angiogram; (C) Intravascular ultrasound of the proximal LAD demonstrating aneurysm diameter of 8 mm x 9 mm; (D) Coronary angiogram. [Image from Rao S, Thompson RC. Coronary CT angiography as an alternative to invasive coronary angiography. In Baskot B (Ed). Coronary angiography—Advances in Noninvasive Imaging Approach for Evaluation of Coronary Artery Disease. Shanghai: InTech China; 2012].

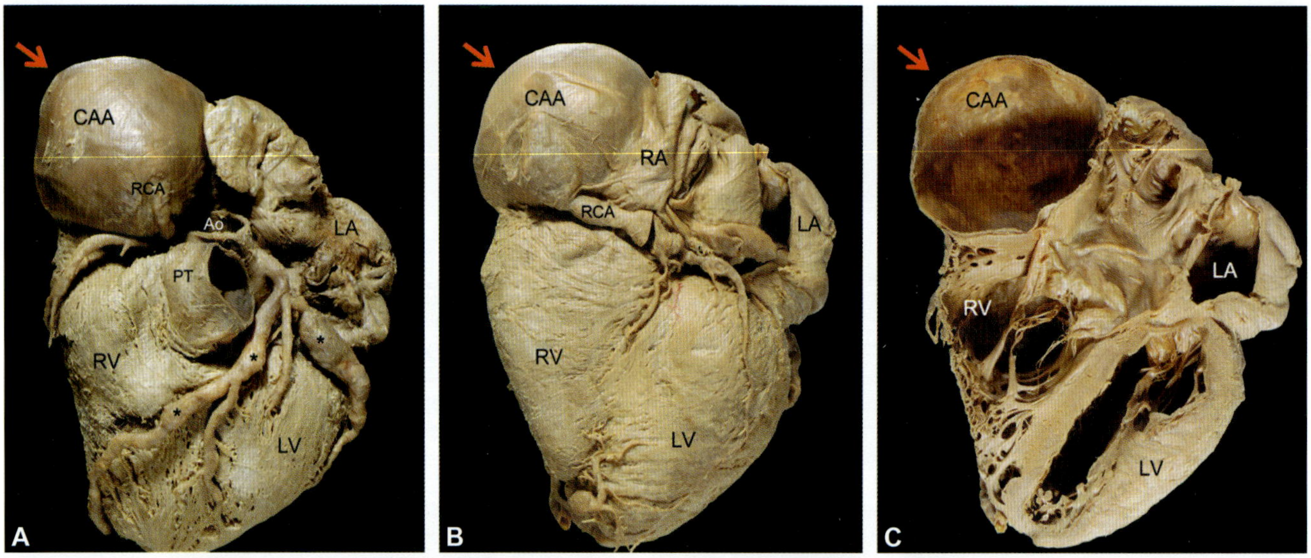

Figs. 6.28A to C: Pathology specimen of a massive proximal right coronary artery aneurysm (arrow). (A) Anterior view of the heart; (B) Posterior view of the heart; (C) Coronal section of the heart. [Image from Mata KM, Fernandes CR, Floriano EM, et al. Coronary artery aneurysms: An update. In: Lakshmanadoss U (Ed). Novel Strategies in Ischemic Heart Disease. Shanghai: InTech China; 2012].

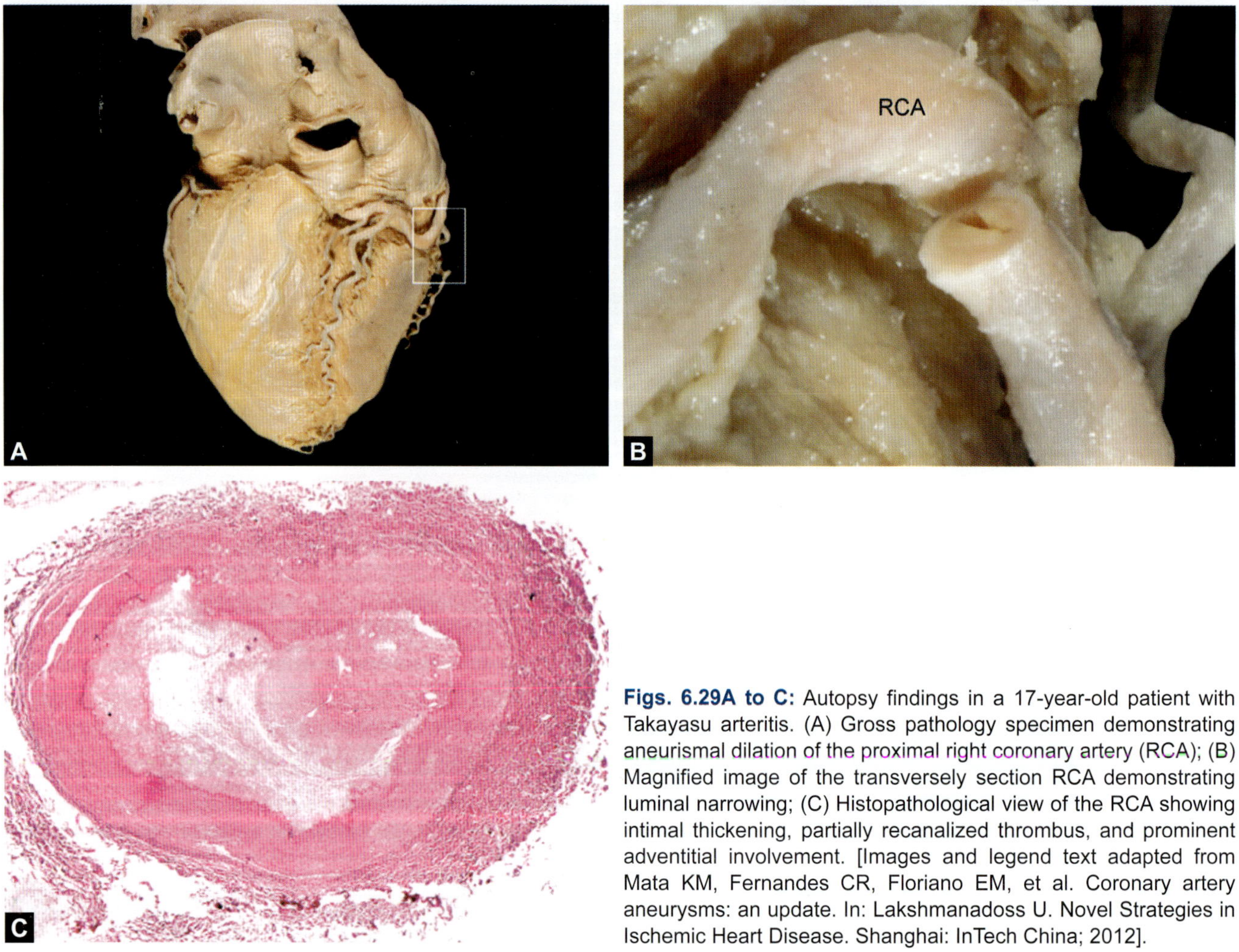

Figs. 6.29A to C: Autopsy findings in a 17-year-old patient with Takayasu arteritis. (A) Gross pathology specimen demonstrating aneurismal dilation of the proximal right coronary artery (RCA); (B) Magnified image of the transversely section RCA demonstrating luminal narrowing; (C) Histopathological view of the RCA showing intimal thickening, partially recanalized thrombus, and prominent adventitial involvement. [Images and legend text adapted from Mata KM, Fernandes CR, Floriano EM, et al. Coronary artery aneurysms: an update. In: Lakshmanadoss U. Novel Strategies in Ischemic Heart Disease. Shanghai: InTech China; 2012].

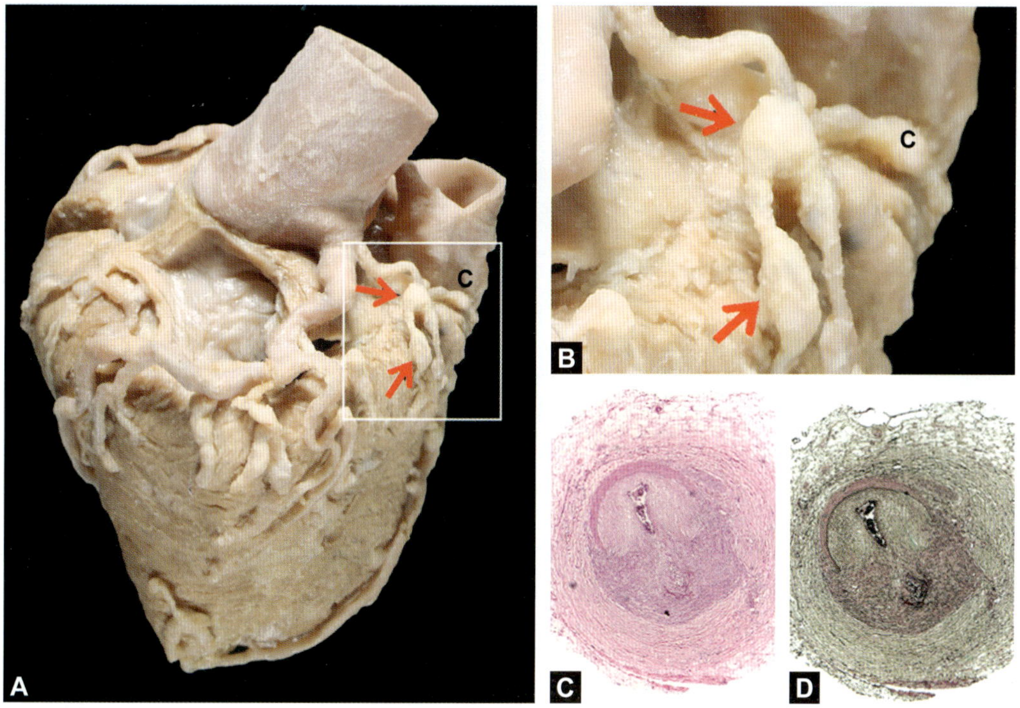

Figs. 6.30A to D: Coronary artery aneurysm and thrombosis in a patient with polyarteritis nodosa (PAN). (A) Right posterolateral view of the heart of 56-year-old woman with systemic PAN demonstrating multiple aneurysms (arrows) in the coronary vasculature; (B) Zoomed image of Figure 6.30A; (C and D) Histopathology of a coronary artery in a patient with PAD demonstrating luminal occlusion due to intimal proliferation, partial disruption of the internal elastic laminae and tunica media, intense inflammatory infiltrate and marked adventitial fibrotic thickening. (Images and legend text from Mata KM, Fernandes CR, Floriano EM, et al. Coronary artery aneurysms: An update. In: Lakshmanadoss U. Novel Strategies in Ischemic Heart Disease. Shanghai: InTech China; 2012).

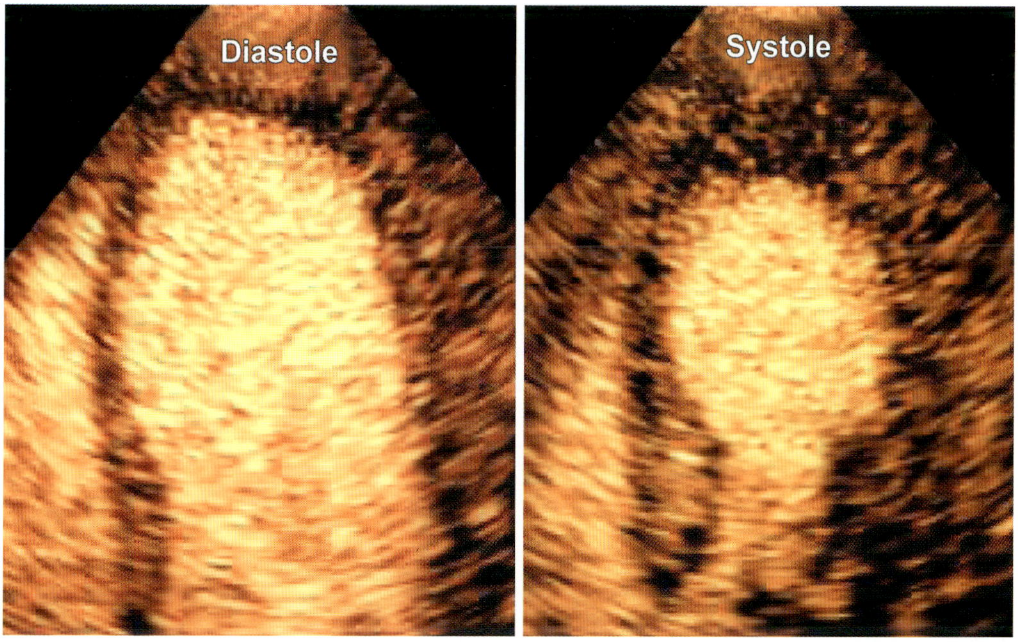

Fig. 6.31: Contrast enhanced transthoracic echocardiography demonstrating aneurysmal systolic bulging (dyskinesis) of the left ventricular apex in a patient with Takotsubo cardiomyopathy. [From Lonnebakken MT, Gerdts E. Contrast echocardiography in coronary artery disease. In: Baskot B (Ed). Coronary Angiography—Advances in Noninvasive Imaging Approach for Evaluation of Coronary Artery Disease. Shanghai: InTech China; 2011].

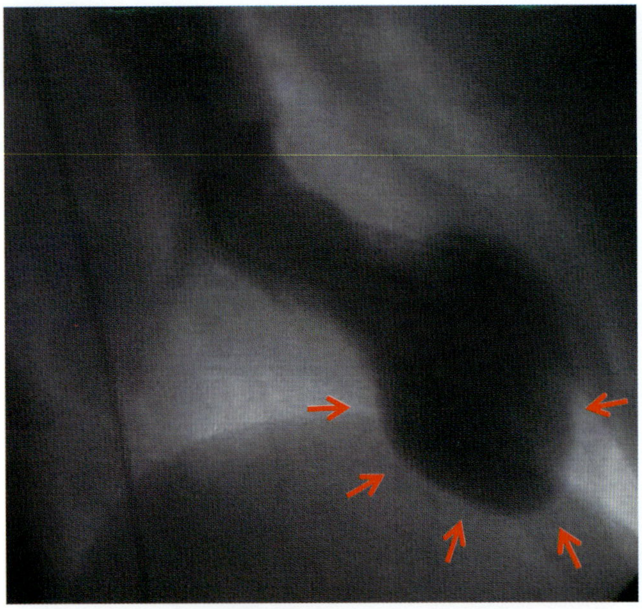

Fig. 6.32: Left ventriculogram demonstrating apical bulging (arrows) in a patient with Takotsubo cardiomyopathy. [Image from Emmanuel M, Julien S, Martinage A, et al. Tako-tsubo cardiomyopathy: A recent clinical syndrome mimicking an acute coronary syndrome. In Baskot B (Ed). Coronary Angiography—The Need for Improvement in Medical and Interventional Therapy. Shanghai: InTech China; 2011].

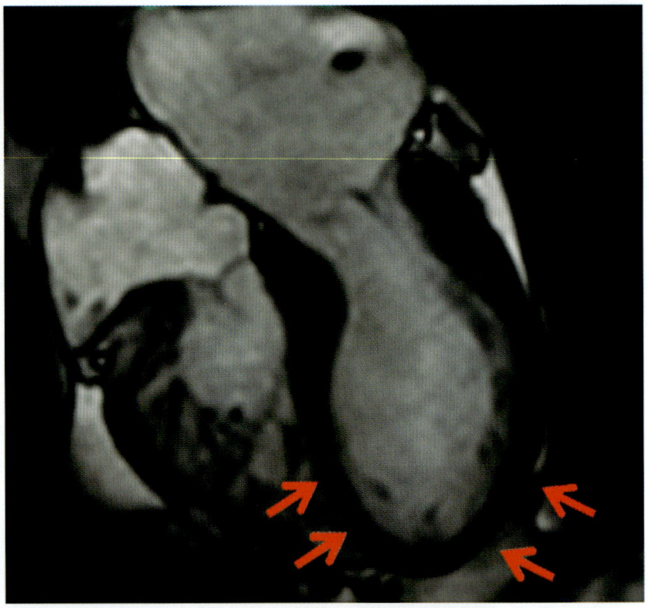

Fig. 6.33: MRI demonstrating apical bulging in a patient with Takotsubo cardiomyopathy. [Image from Olimulder MAGM, Galjee MA, van Es J, et al. The use of contrast-enhanced cardiovascular magnetic resonance imaging in cardiomyopathies. In: Veselka J (Ed) Cardiomyopathies—From Basic Research to Clinical Management. Shanghai: InTech China; 2012].

VIDEO LEGENDS

Video 6.1: Angiogram obtained in a patient undergoing primary percutaneous coronary intervention of the right coronary artery for an inferior wall myocardial infarction. After the guidewire is passed, the shown angiogram demonstrates a large, complex, filling defect, which is due to thrombus formation that has resulted from plaque rupture.

Videos 6.2A to E: Primary percutaneous coronary intervention of an occluded mid left anterior descending (LAD) artery in a patient with acute anterior wall myocardial infarction. (A) Initial angiogram showing complete occlusion at the level of the mid LAD. (B) Guidewire passed across occlusion, resulting in some restoration of blood flow. A residual stenotic lesion is visible. (C) A coronary stent being positioned at the site of residual stenosis. (D) Inflation of the balloon and deployment of the coronary stent. (E) Post-stent deployment angiogram showing the treated stenosis and TIMI 3 flow throughout the coronary artery.

Videos 6.3 to 6.7: Examples of apical thrombi that developed in patients with transmural infarctions and apical akinesis.

REFERENCES

Freiman DG. The structure of thrombi. In: Colman RW, Hirsh J, Marder VJ, Salzman E (Eds). Hemostasis and Thrombosis: Basic Principles and Clinical Practice. Philadelphia: JB Lippincott; 1987. pp. 766-80.

Hillis LD, Lange RA. Optimal management of acute coronary syndromes. N Engl J Med. 2009;360(21):2237-40.

Kohl LP, Weiss E. Antithrombotic and antiplatelet agents. In: Chatterjee K, Anderson M, Heistad D, Kerber RE (Eds). Cardiology: An Illustrated Textbook. New Delhi: Jaypee Brothers Medical Publishers (P) Ltd. 2012.

CHAPTER

Percutaneous Coronary Intervention

7

Glenn N Levine, Hani Jneid, David Paniagua

EVOLUTION OF PERCUTANEOUS CORONARY INTERVENTION

The first percutaneous coronary intervention was performed by Andreas Gruentzig in 1977 (Figs. 7.1 and 7.2). The procedure was performed using a simple balloon catheter with a 5 mm wire affixed to the most proximal portion of the balloon. Since then, there has been enormous evolution in the coronary interventional devices, including balloon catheters (Figs. 7.3 and 7.4), guide wires (Fig. 7.5), and stents (Figs. 7.6A to H). Currently, well over one million percutaneous coronary interventions (PCI) are performed each year.

Balloon angioplasty is a reasonably effective method of coronary stenosis dilation (Figs. 7.7A to C), but is associated with a significant rate of restenosis, as well as a small but real incidence of need for emergency coronary bypass surgery (CABG). Restenosis after balloon angioplasty is due to a combination of intimal hyperplasia and vessel elastic recoil.

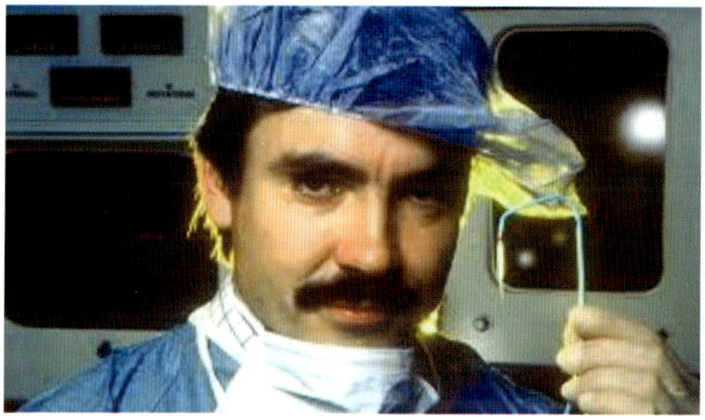

Fig. 7.1: Andreas Gruentzig, the father of percutaneous coronary angioplasty.

The introduction of coronary stents in the 1990s revolutionized the practice of PCI (Figs. 7.8A to C). Coronary stents allow a greater dilation of the vessel and prevent vessel recoil (Fig. 7.9 and Videos 7.1A to D), significantly reducing the rates of angiographic and clinical restenosis. Coronary stents also facilitate the treatment of vessel dissection (Figs. 7.10A and B) and occlusion, dramatically reducing the need for emergency CABG. The degree of intimal hyperplasia after coronary stent implantation is actually greater than the degree of intimal hyperplasia after balloon angioplasty (Figs. 7.11 and 7.12), and although rates of restenosis were decreased with the use of coronary stents, restenosis (termed “in-stent restenosis”) does still occur.

Drug-eluting stents (DES) are coronary stents that are coated with a compound that decreases or inhibits the processes that lead to intimal hyperplasia and in-stent restenosis. Drugs used in DES include sirolimus, paclitaxel, everolimus, biolimus, and numerous other compounds currently in development or clinical testing. Once implanted in to the coronary artery, the DES elutes the antiproliferative compound into the local milieu over the subsequent weeks to months. Compared to non-drug eluting stents (now referred to as “bare metal stents” or “BMS”), DES have lower rates of both angiographic and clinical restenosis (Figs. 7.13A and B).

COMPLICATIONS OF PERCUTANEOUS CORONARY INTERVENTION

Complications of PCI include myocardial infarction, stroke, coronary dissection (Fig. 7.14A), coronary perforation (Figs. 7.14B and C), and vascular and bleeding complications (Figs. 7.15A and B). The risk of need for

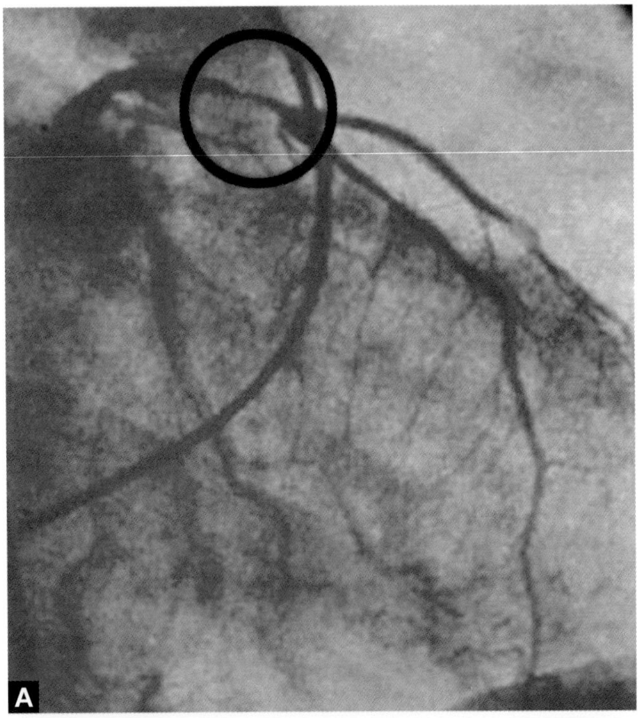

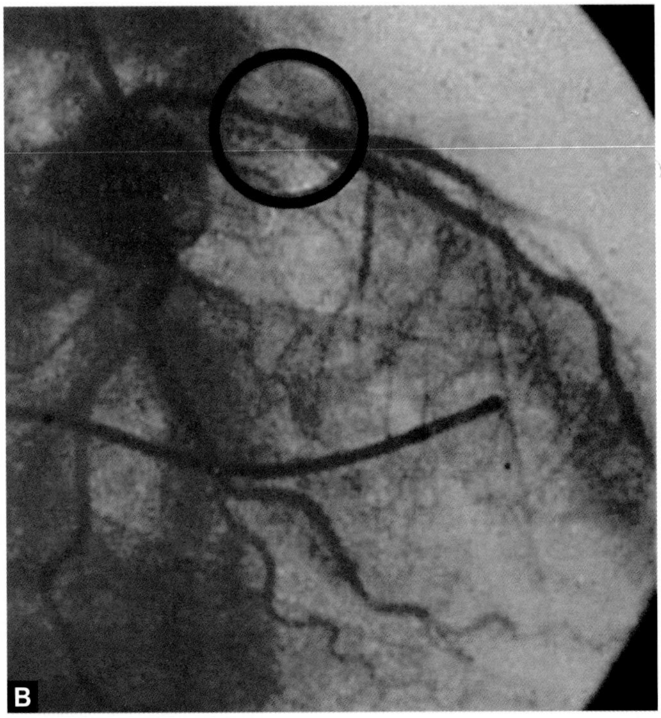

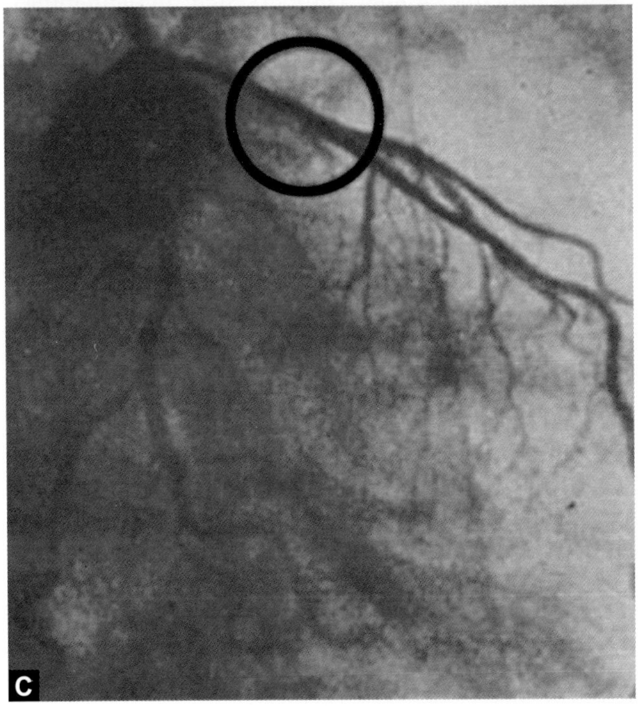

Figs. 7.2A to C: The first percutaneous coronary angioplasty performed by Andreas Gruentzig. (A) Coronary angiography showing a stenosis of the proximal left anterior descending coronary artery; (B) Result after balloon angioplasty; (C) Angiographic result after one month. [Images from Rao SS, Khanna NN. History of peripheral vascular interventions. In: Chopra HK, Nanda NC. Textbook of Cardiology—A Clinical & Historic Perspective. New Delhi, India: Jaypee Brothers Medical Publishers (P) Ltd. 2013].

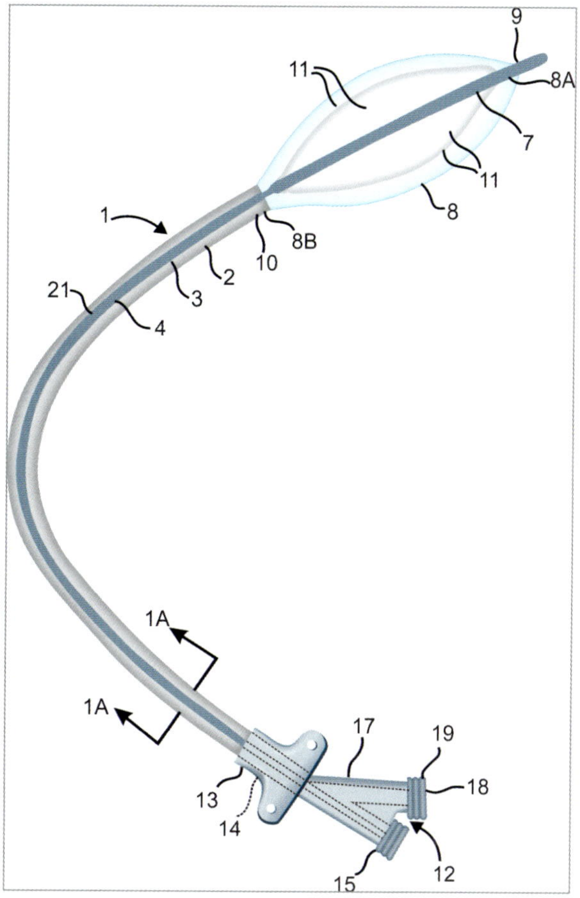

Fig. 7.3: Design of an early coronary balloon catheter.

emergency surgery, which was non-trivial in the era of balloon angioplasty, is extremely low in the era of coronary stenting. Stent thrombosis may occur acutely or months or years after stent implantation. Incomplete stent apposition increases the risk of stent thrombosis (Fig. 7.16).

INDICATIONS FOR PERCUTANEOUS CORONARY INTERVENTION

Guidelines have been established by the American College of Cardiology Foundation (ACCF), American Heart Association (AHA), and the Society for Cardiovascular Angiography and Interventions (SCAI) on the indications for PCI to improve survival and to improve symptoms in patients with stable ischemic heart disease or with acute coronary syndrome (Tables 7.1 to 7.3). Increasingly, PCI in the appropriate clinical setting of unprotected left main coronary artery lesions is becoming an acceptable and increasingly utilized procedure.

ADJUNCTIVE DEVICES USED IN PERCUTANEOUS CORONARY INTERVENTION

Numerous adjunctive devices may be utilized in PCI. Rotablator (Figs. 7.17 and 7.18) is a diamond-tipped burr that rotates at approximately 120,000 RPM and ablates stenotic material in the coronary artery. Rotational atherectomy was initially hoped to decrease the incidence

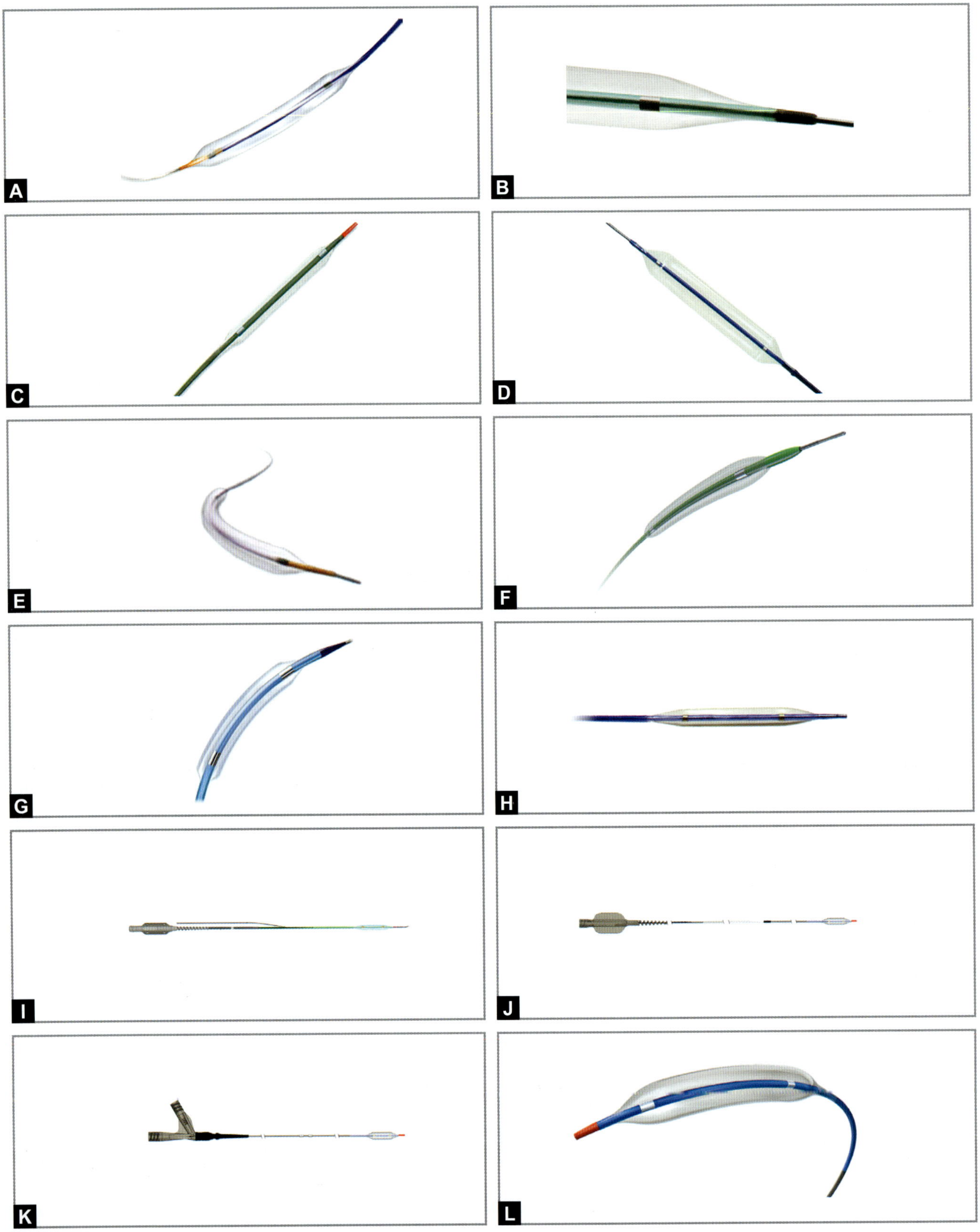

Figs. 7.4A to L: More modern percutaneous balloon catheters.

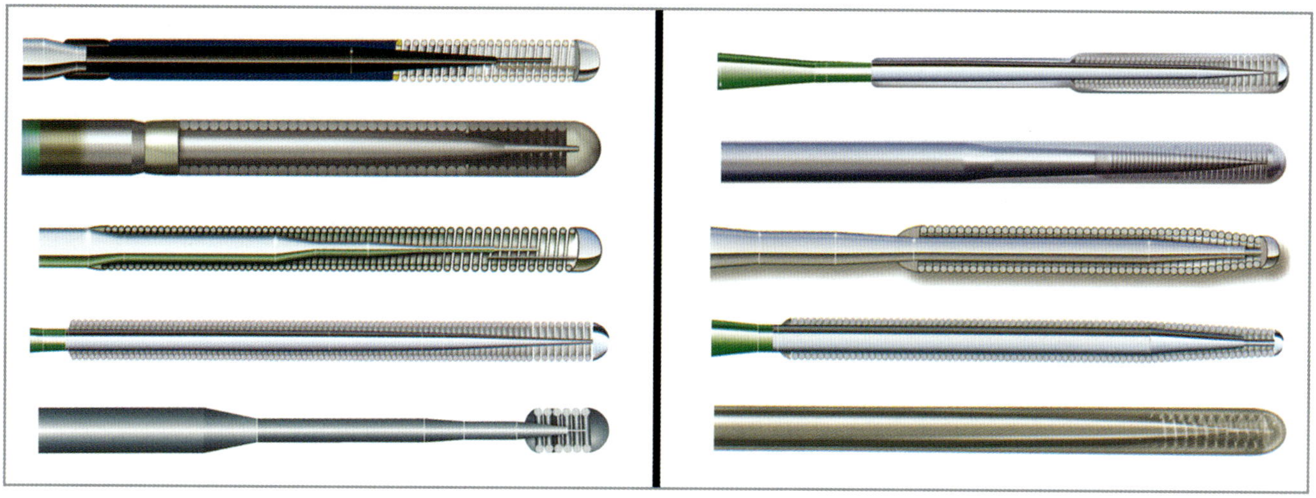

Fig. 7.5: Design of modern guide wires. Guide wires vary in numerous aspects, including degree of stiffness and support, tip design, and whether they are hydrophilic or hydrophobic.

of restenosis, but studies failed to demonstrate any such benefit. In current practice, rotational atherectomy may be utilized as the initial treatment in heavily calcified lesions, in order to facilitate dilation and stenting of the lesion. In the ACCF/AHA/SCAI PCI guidelines, rotational atherectomy is considered a reasonable treatment for fibrotic or heavily calcified lesions that might not be crossed by a balloon catheter or adequately dilated before stent implantation (class IIa recommendation).

Balloon dilation and stenting of degenerated saphenous vein grafts (SVG) results in distal embolization of material in to the downstream native coronary artery, resulting in microvascular obstruction and myocardial infarction. Embolic protection devices (Fig. 7.19) have been shown to decrease the risk of such embolization (Figs. 7.20A and B), and in patients undergoing SVG PCI, such devices decrease the risks of ischemic complications. In the ACCF/AHA/SCAI PCI guidelines, use of an embolic protection device is recommended during SVG PCI when use of such a device is technically feasible (class I recommendation).

Intravascular ultrasound (IVUS) and optical coherence tomography (OCT) allow a more complete assessment of coronary stenosis composition (lipid, calcium, thrombus) and severity. Compared with IVUS, OCT has greater resolution (10–20 micrometers) but more limited depth of imaging (1–1.5 mm). Intravascular imaging is used to assess lesion severity for lesions that are deemed indeterminate or intermediate on coronary angiography. In general, for left main coronary stenoses, a minimal lumen diameter of < 2.8 mm or a minimal lumen area of < 6 mm^2 suggests that the lesion is physiologically significant and revascularization should be considered; a minimal lumen area > 7.5 mm^2 suggests that revascularization may be deferred. Both techniques can be used to assess adequacy of stent deployment during initial stent implantation and can be used in cases of restenosis or thrombosis to assess for issues related to stent deployment. Depending on the specific indication, the use of IVUS is generally given a class IIa or class IIb recommendation in the ACCF/AHA/SCAI PCI guidelines. Examples of how IVUS and OCT can be used to assess stent deployment and complications are illustrated in Figures 7.21 to 7.24. The role of virtual histology (Fig. 7.25) in the treatment of patients with coronary artery disease continues to undergo evaluation.

Primary PCI (Fig. 7.26 and Videos 7.2A to E and 7.3A to G) is the preferred treatment in patients with ST-segment elevation myocardial infarction (STEMI), when primary PCI can be carried out in an expeditious manner by skilled operators and cardiac catheterization laboratory personnel. In patients with STEMI, a significant thrombus burden is often present. Some, but not all, studies of manual aspiration thrombectomy in patients undergoing primary PCI have demonstrated benefit with the use of such devices (Figs. 7.27 and 7.28). In the ACCF/AHA/SCAI PCI guidelines, the use of aspiration thrombectomy is considered reasonable for patients undergoing primary PCI (class IIa recommendation). Studies of rheolytic thrombectomy (Fig. 7.29) in patients undergoing

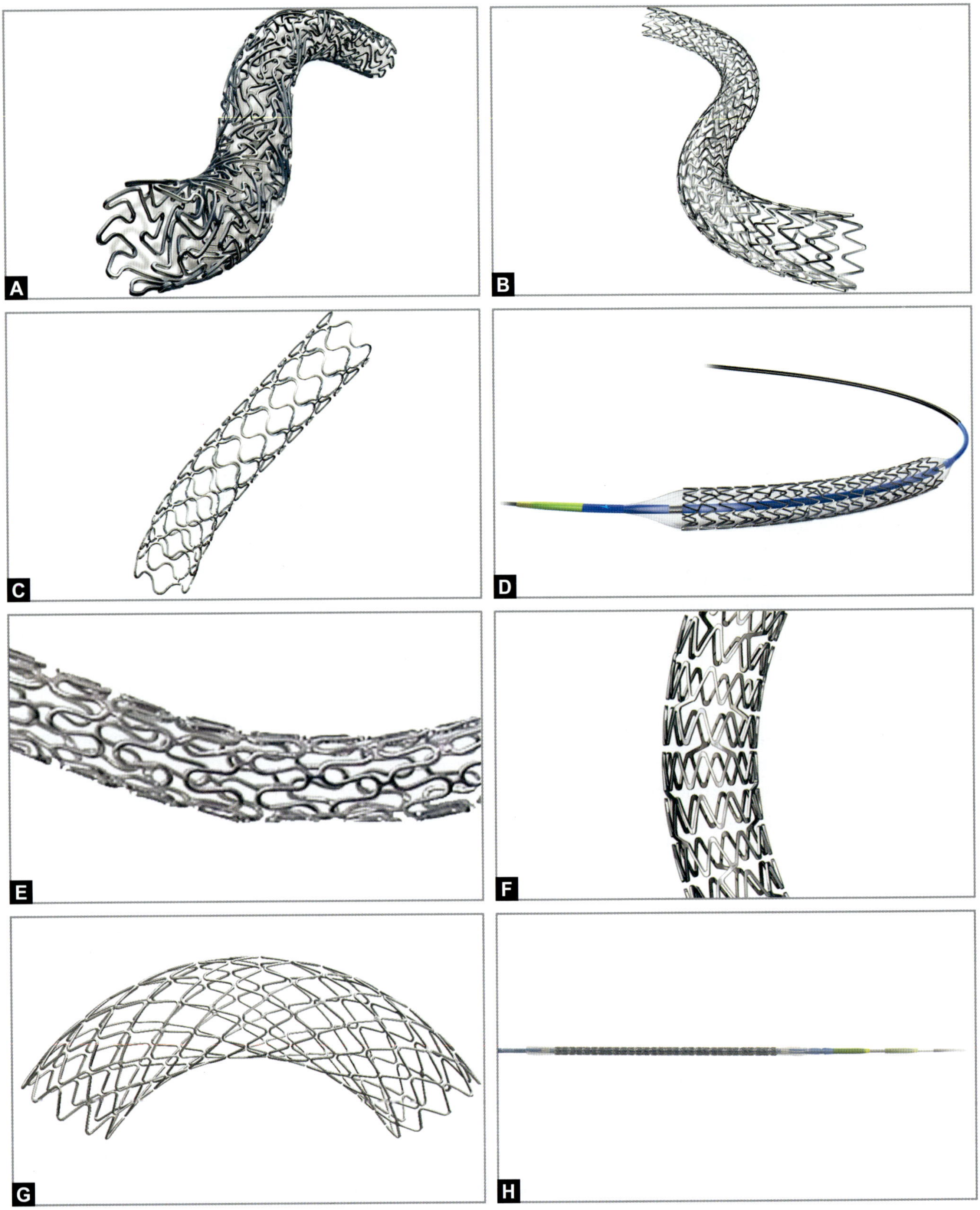

Figs. 7.6A to H: Representative examples of modern stent designs.

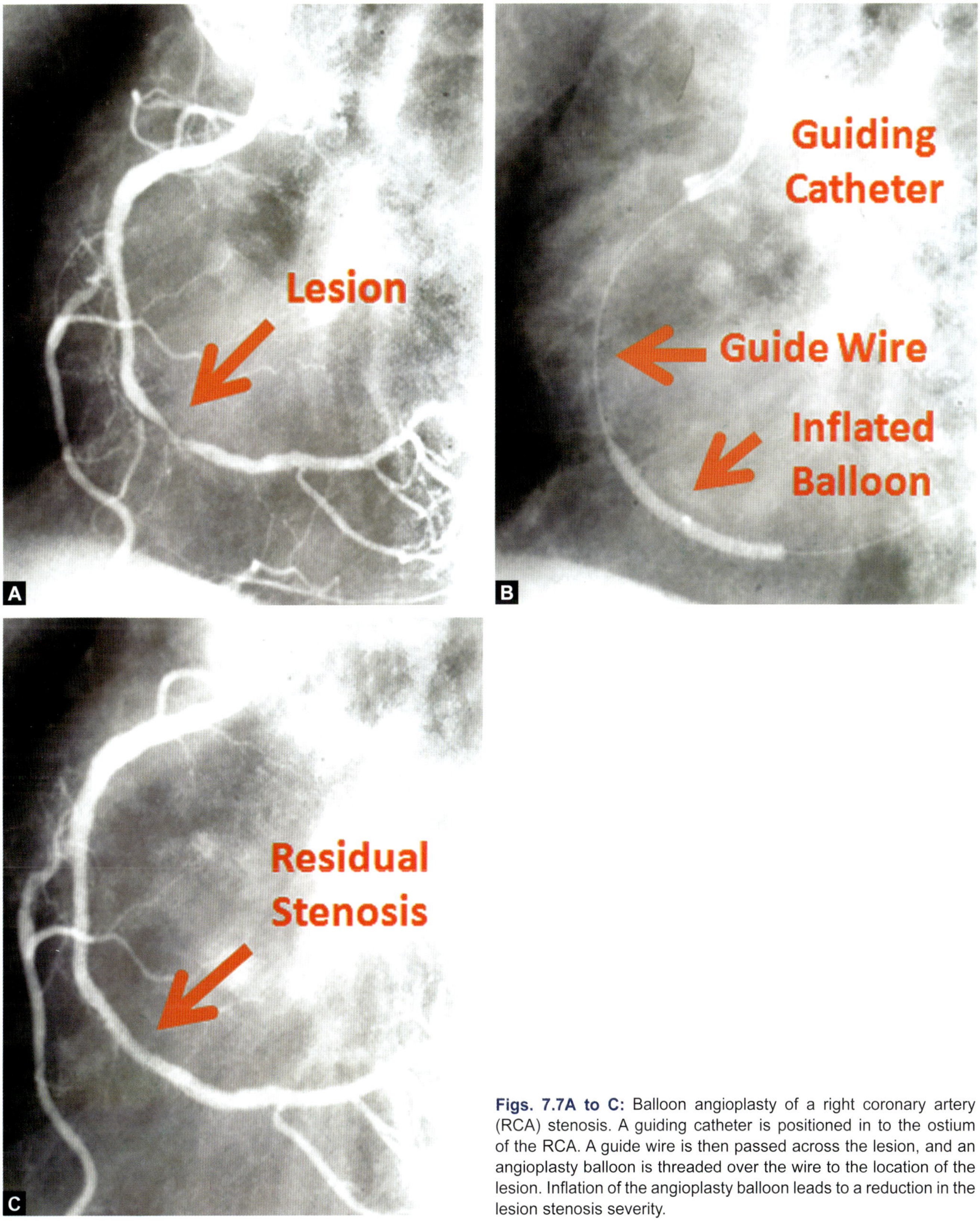

Figs. 7.7A to C: Balloon angioplasty of a right coronary artery (RCA) stenosis. A guiding catheter is positioned in to the ostium of the RCA. A guide wire is then passed across the lesion, and an angioplasty balloon is threaded over the wire to the location of the lesion. Inflation of the angioplasty balloon leads to a reduction in the lesion stenosis severity.

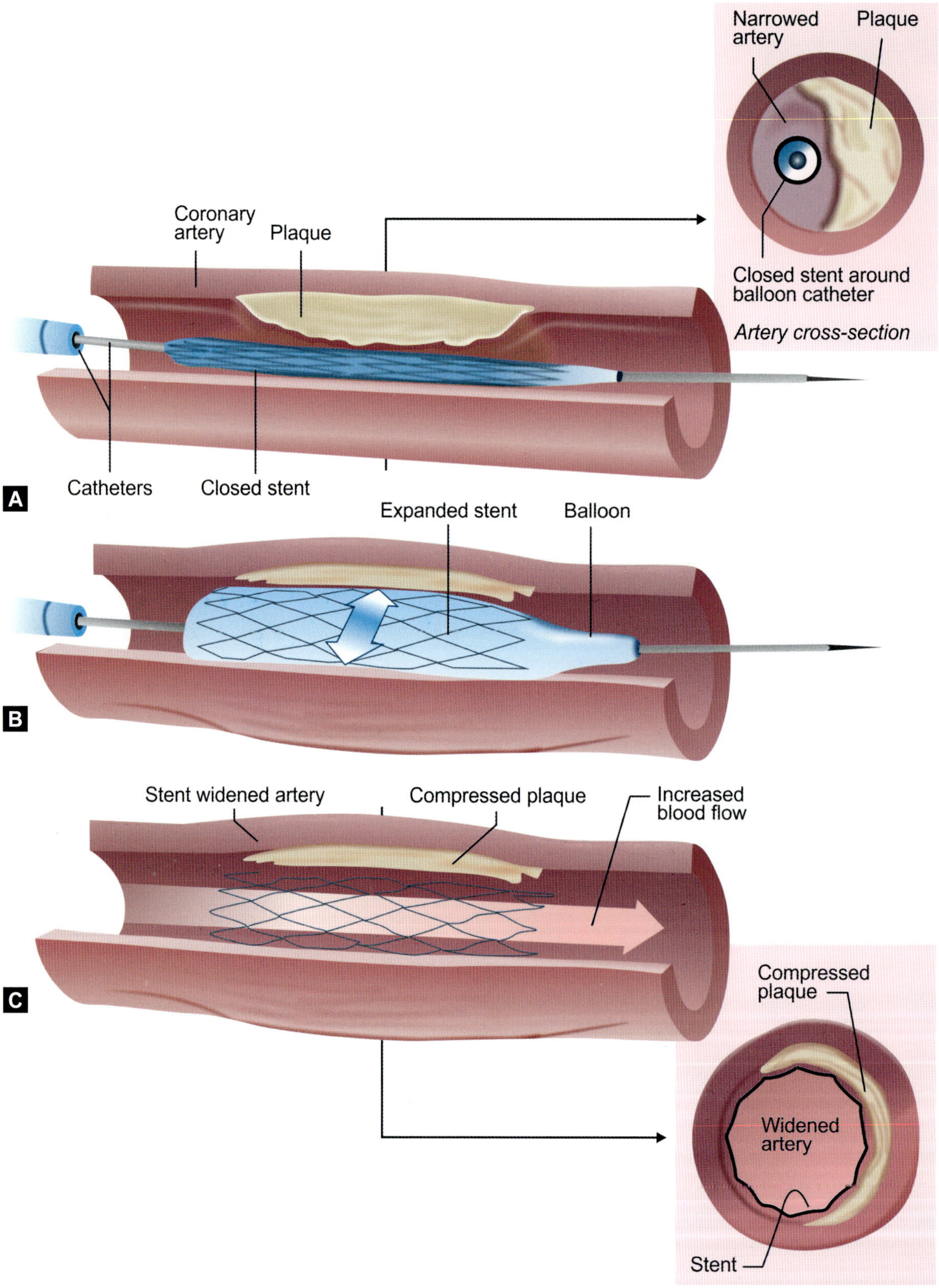

Figs. 7.8A to C: Coronary stenting procedure. (A) The coronary stent, premounted on a balloon catheter, is delivered over a guide wire to the area of stenosis; (B) The balloon is inflated, expanding the stent and embedding it against the wall of the coronary artery; (C) The deployed stent embedded against the coronary artery.

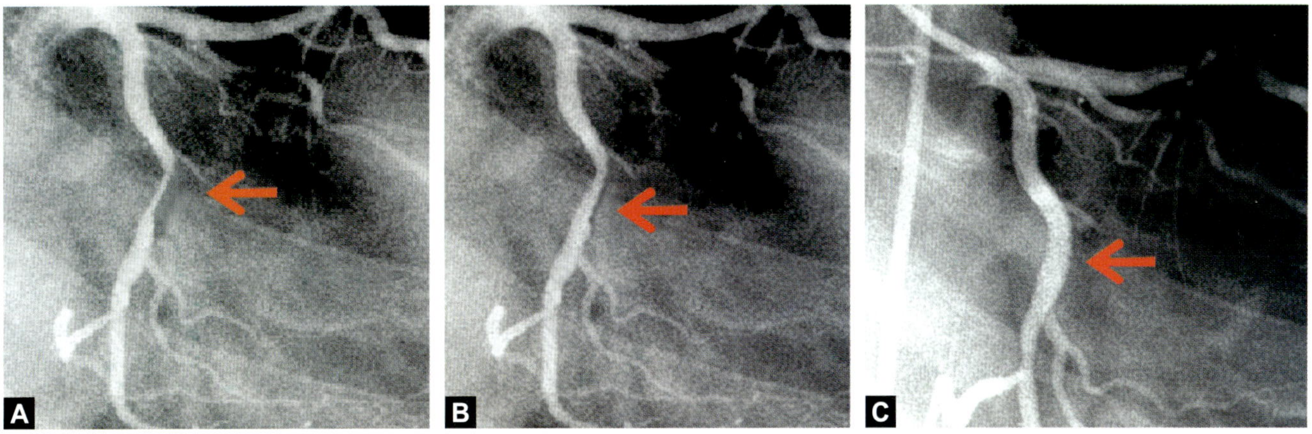

Figs. 7.9A to C: Percutaneous balloon angioplasty and stenting of the left circumflex artery. (A) Stenosis in the left circumflex artery. (B) After balloon angioplasty the degree of stenosis is decreased, but a significant residual lesion remains. (C) After coronary artery stenting, there is no residual stenosis visible on angiography.

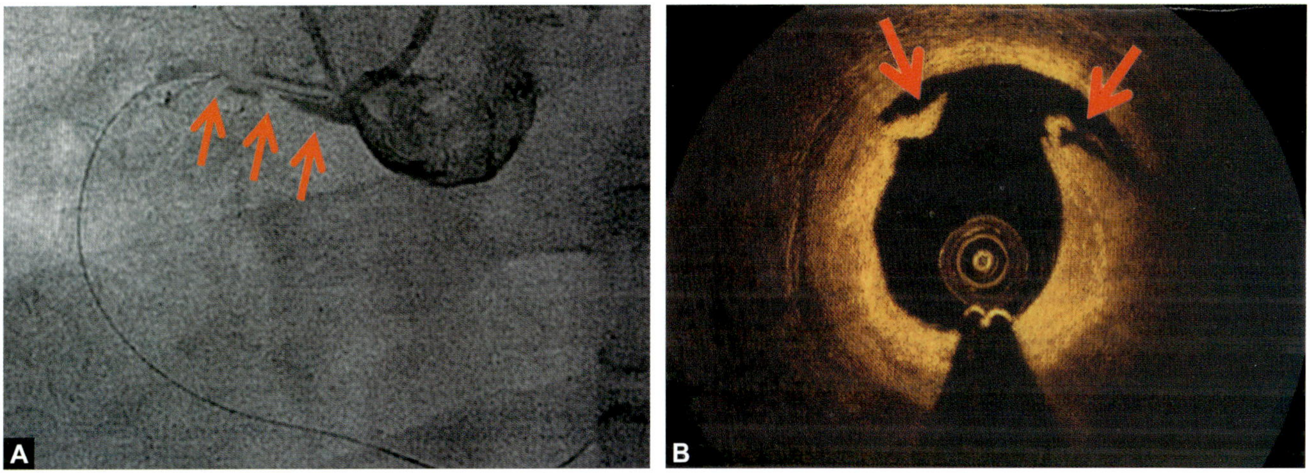

Figs. 7.10A and B: Coronary artery dissection. (A) Coronary angiogram demonstrating marked dissection (arrows) of the right coronary artery after balloon angioplasty. The dissection has resulted in essentially complete occlusion of the vessel; (B) Optical coherence tomography revealing coronary dissection.

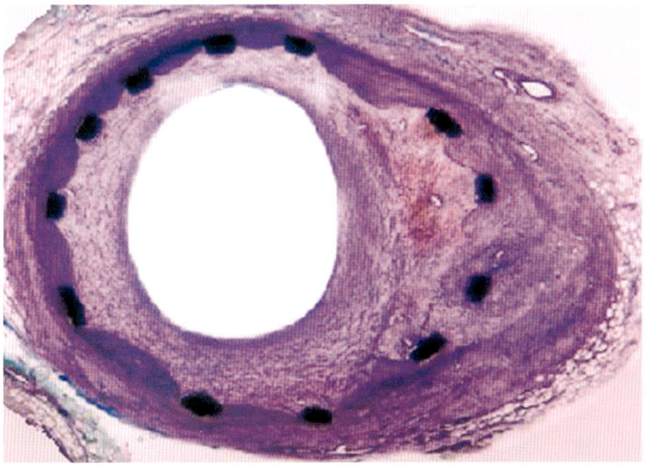

Fig. 7.11: Pathology specimen demonstrating intimal hyperplasia and a modest degree of in-stent restenosis in a patient treated with a bare metal stent.

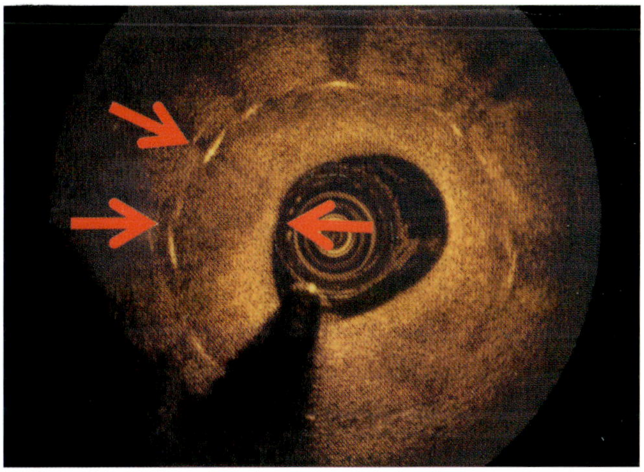

Fig. 7.12: Optical coherence tomography (OCT) demonstrating intimal hyperplasia and modest in-stent restenosis in a patient treated with a bare metal stent. Image courtesy of St. Jude Medical.

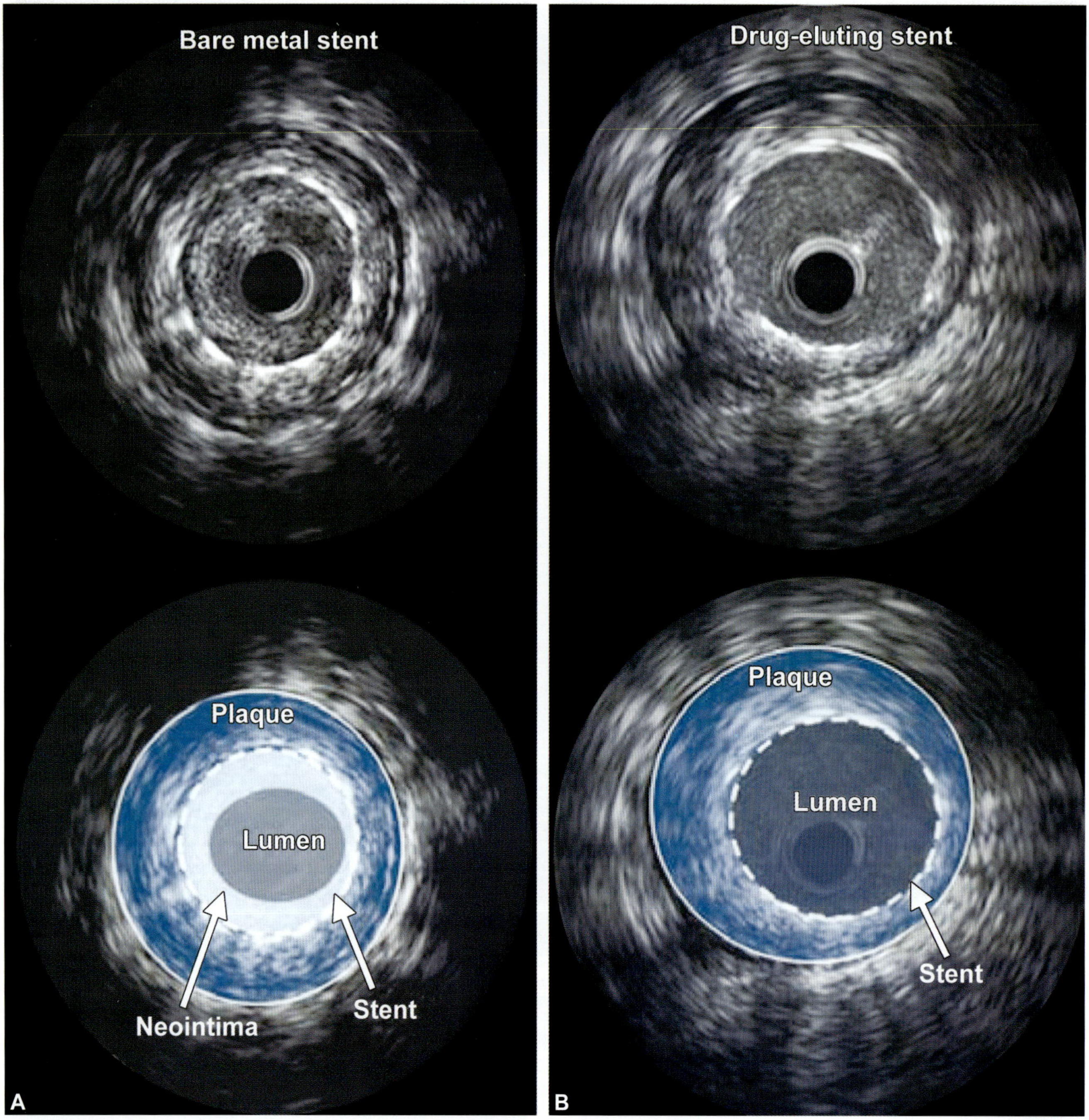

Figs. 7.13A and B: Intravascular ultrasound (IVUS) 8 months after stent deployment. (A) Bare metal stent with significant neointimal proliferation within the stent; (B) Drug-eluting stent with only modest neointimal proliferation and a greater residual luminal area. [Image and legend text from Kume T, Honda Y, Fitzgerald PJ. Intravascular coronary ultrasound and beyond. In: Chatterjee K, Anderson M, Heistad D, Kerber RE (Eds). Cardiology: An Illustrated Textbook. New Delhi: Jaypee Brothers Medical Publishers (P) Ltd. 2012].

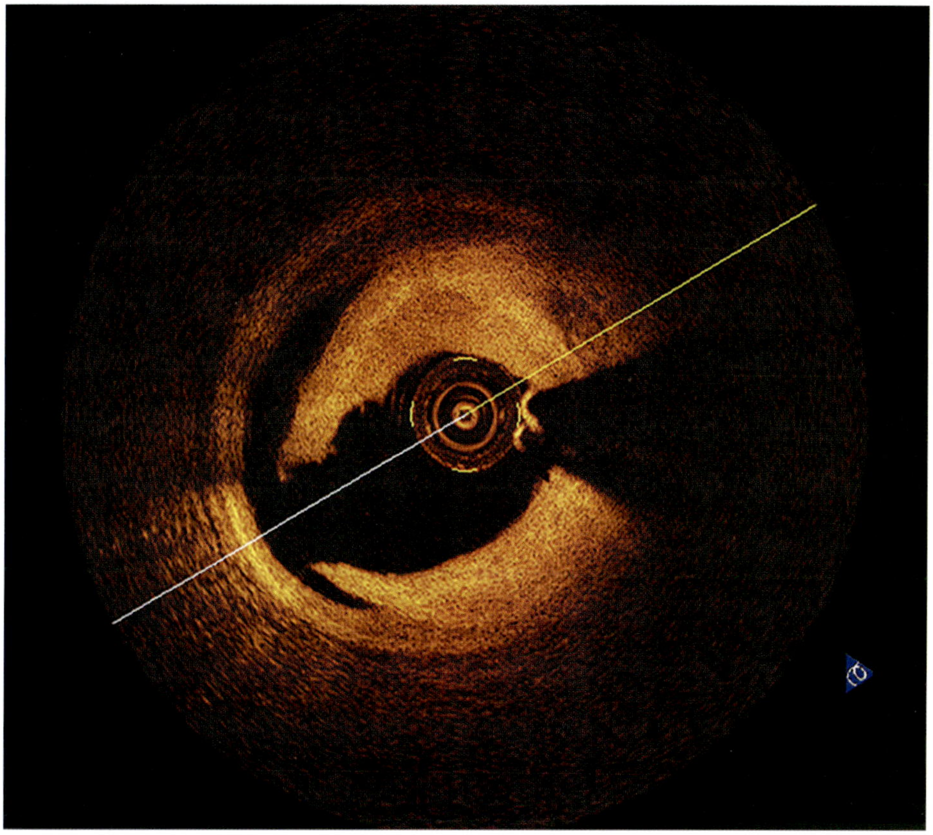

Fig. 7.14A: Optical coherence tomography demonstrating edge dissection after implantation of a coronary stent. (Image courtesy of St. Jude Medical Inc., Little Canada, Minnesota, United States).

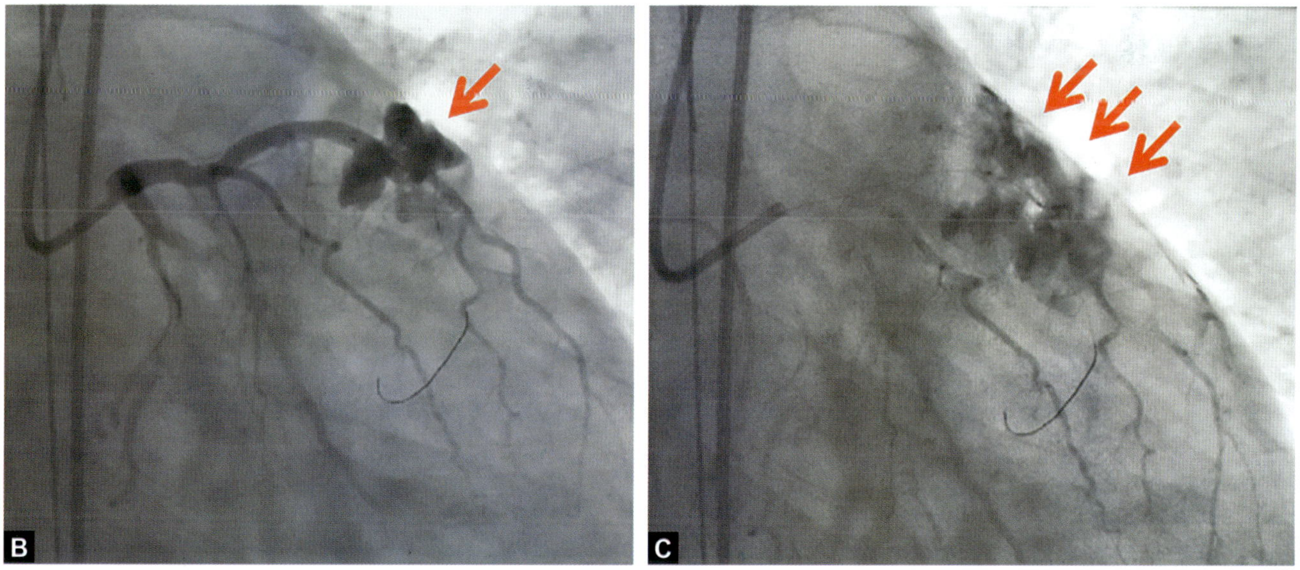

Figs. 7.14B and C: Examples of coronary artery perforation. Arrows indicate area of perforation and subsequent extravascular contrast extravasation. (Images courtesy of Dr Carl Tommaso).

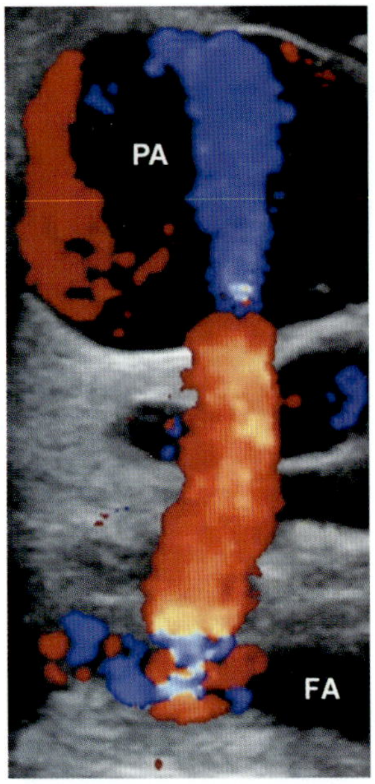

Fig. 7.15A: Ultrasound examination demonstrating a femoral pseudoaneurysm in a patient who has recently undergone percutaneous coronary interventions. [Image from Milne CPE, Lee R, Handa AI. Iatrogenic pseudoaneurysms. In: Yamanouchi E (Ed). Vascular Surgery: Principles and Practice. InTeOp; 2012].

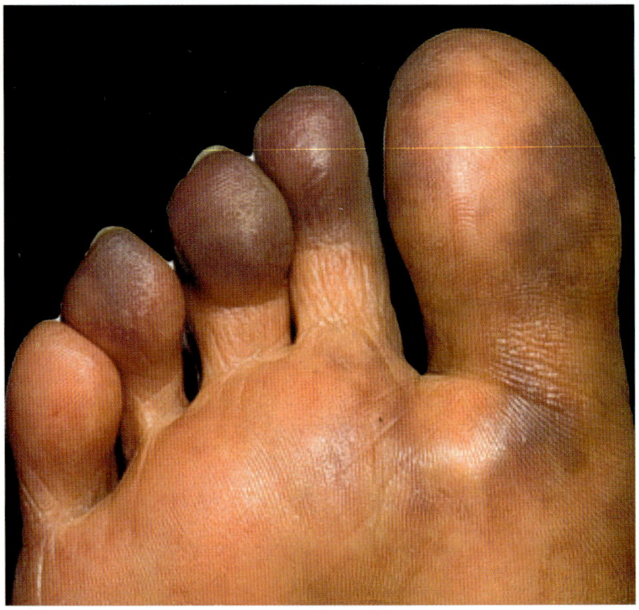

Fig. 7.15B: Blue toe syndrome due to cholesterol emboli from the aorta in a patient treated with coronary stent implantation. [Image from Garcia-Borbolla M. Complications of cardiac catheterization. In: Kirac SF (Ed). Advances in the Diagnosis of Coronary Atherosclerosis. Shanghai: InTech China; 2012].

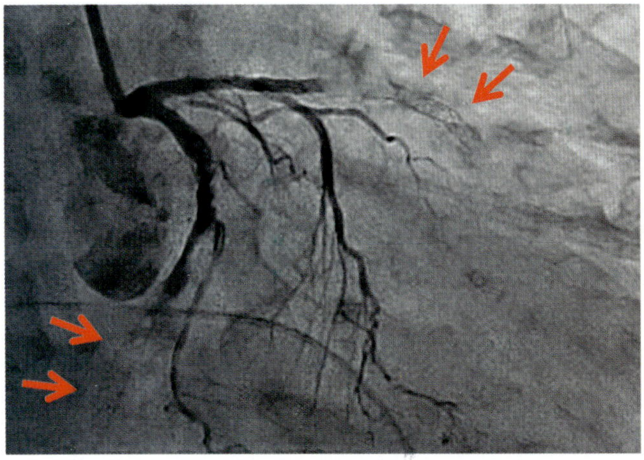

Fig. 7.16: Stent thrombosis (arrows) in both the left anterior descending (LAD) artery and left circumflex artery in a patient who briefly had dual antiplatelet therapy interrupted. [Image from Chen HY. Simultaneous thrombosis of two drug-eluting stents after discontinuation of dual antiplatelet therapy for a day. Cardiol Res. 2012:3(6):281-3].

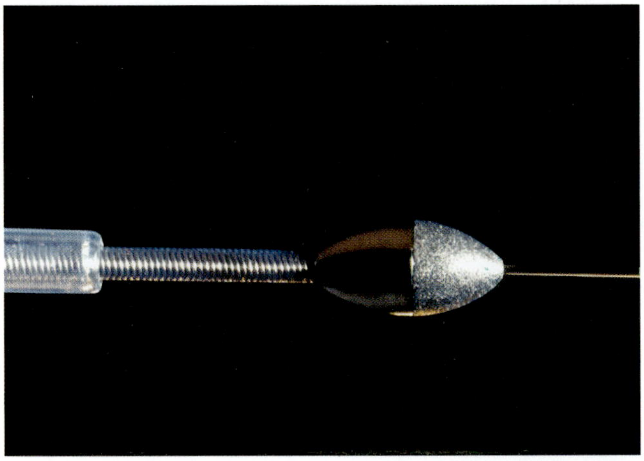

Fig. 7.17: Image of a rotational atherectomy (Rotablator) burr. (Image courtesy of Boston Scientific Corporation).

Table 7.1: ACCF/AHA/SCAI guidelines for unprotected left main percutaneous coronary intervention to improve survival in patients with stable ischemic heart disease and acute coronary syndromes. (LOE: Level of evidence; NSTE-ACS: Non-ST-segment elevation acute coronary syndrome; NSTEMI: Non-ST-segment elevation MI; STS: Society of Thoracic Surgeons; UA: Unstable angina; SIHD: Stable Ischemic Heart Disease; SYNTAX: Synergy between Percutaneous Coronary Intervention with Taxus and Cardiac Surgery).

Class I (is recommended; is beneficial)
• No recommendations
Class IIa (is reasonable)
• For SIHD when low risk of PCI complications and *high* likelihood of good long-term outcome (e.g. SYNTAX score of ≤ 22, ostial or trunk left main CAD), **and** a *significantly increased* CABG risk (e.g. STS-predicted risk of operative mortality ≥ 5%) (LOE = B)
• For UA/NSTEMI (NSTE-ACS) if not a CABG candidate (LOE = B)
• For STEMI when distal coronary flow is <TIMI grade 3 and PCI can be performed more rapidly and safely than CABG (LOE = C)
Class IIb (may be considered)
• For SIHD when *low to intermediate* risk of PCI complications and *intermediate to high* likelihood of good long-term outcome (e.g. SYNTAX score of < 33, bifurcation left main CAD) **and** increased CABG risk (e.g. moderate-severe COPD, disability from prior stroke, prior cardiac surgery, STS-predicted operative mortality > 2%) (LOE = B)
Class III (harmful)
• For SIHD in patients (versus performing CABG) with *unfavorable* anatomy for PCI and who are *good* candidates for CABG (LOE = B)

Table 7.2: ACCF/AHA/SCAI guidelines for percutaneous coronary intervention in patients with stable single or multivessel CAD to improve survival. (LAD: Left anterior descending; LOE: Level of evidence).

Class I (is recommended; is beneficial)
• No recommendations
Class IIa (is reasonable)
• No recommendations
Class IIb (uncertain benefit)
• 2–3 vessel or 1 vessel CAD with proximal LAD disease (LOE = B)
Class III (harmful)
• 1 vessel CAD without proximal LAD disease (LOE = B)
• No anatomic or physiologic criteria for revascularization (LOE = B)

Table 7.3: ACCF/AHA/SCAI guidelines for percutaneous coronary intervention in patients with stable CAD to improve symptoms. (COR: Class of recommendation; LOE: Level of evidence).

Class I (is recommended; is beneficial)
• ≥ 1 significant stenoses amenable to revascularization and unacceptable angina despite GDMT (LOE = A)
Class IIa (is reasonable)
• ≥ 1 significant stenoses and unacceptable angina in whom GDMT cannot be implemented because of medication contraindications, adverse effects, or patient preferences (LOE = C)
• Previous CABG with ≥ 1 significant stenoses associated with ischemia and unacceptable angina despite GDMT (LOE = C)
Class IIb (may be considered, uncertain benefit)
• No recommendations
Class III (harmful)
• No anatomic or physiologic criteria for revascularization (LOE = C)

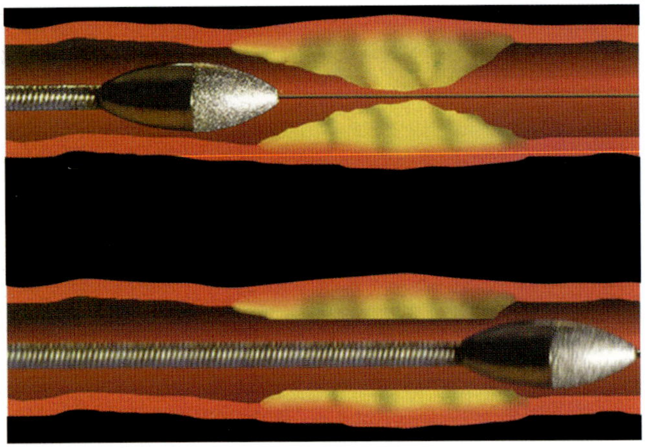

Fig. 7.18: Schematic representation of rotational atherectomy with a Rotablator.

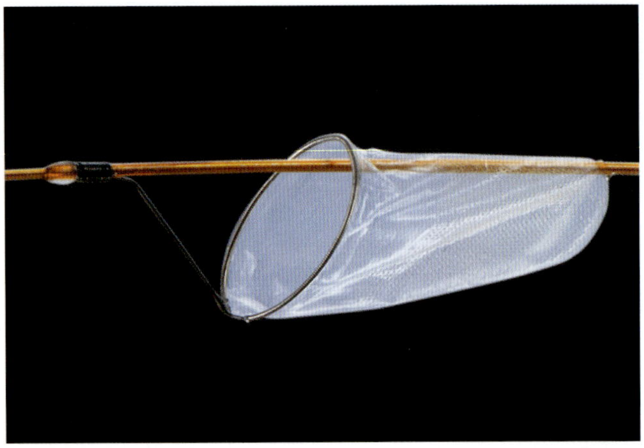

Fig. 7.19: Distal embolization protection device. Embolization protection devices decrease the risk of distal embolization during saphenous vein graft percutaneous coronary interventions. (Image courtesy of Boston Scientific Corporation).

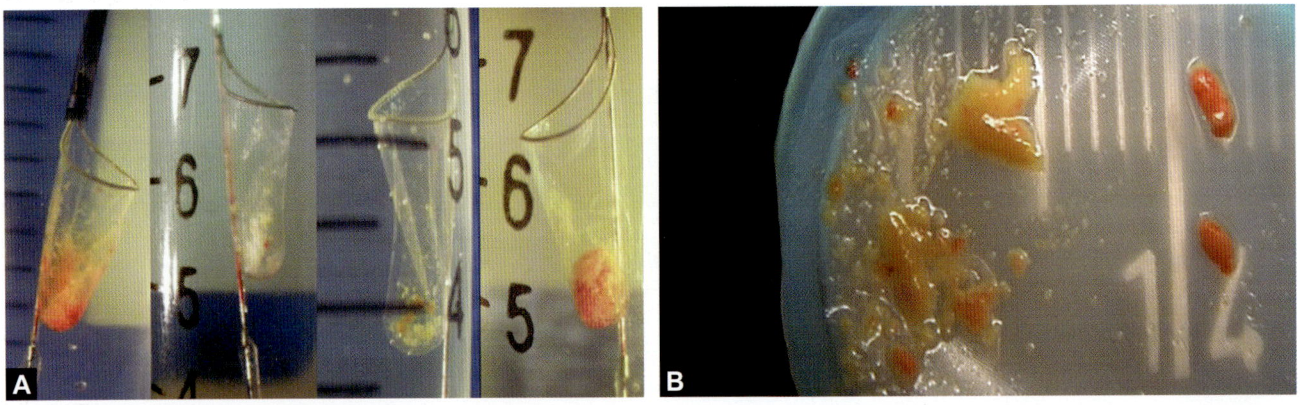

Figs. 7.20A and B: Examples of atheroembolic material captured with the use of distal embolic protection devices during saphenous vein graft percutaneous coronary interventions.

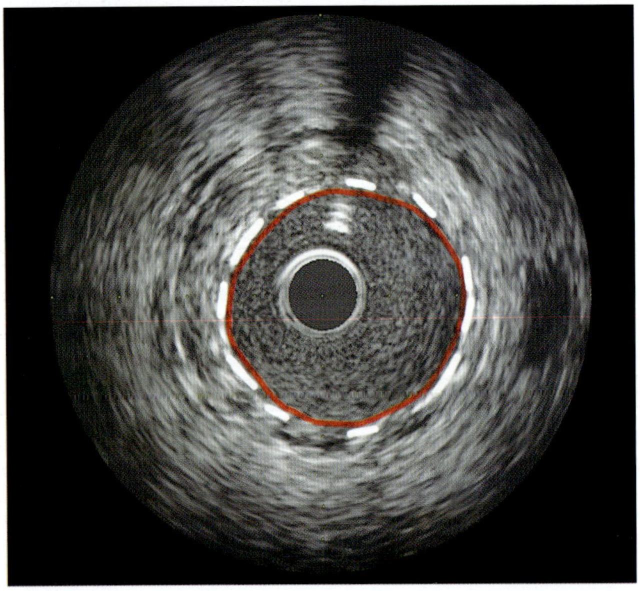

Fig. 7.21: Intravascular ultrasound demonstrates good stent apposition.

primary PCI have not demonstrated benefit, and no recommendations for the use of this device is made in the PCI guidelines.

In patients undergoing high-risk PCI, or in those with hemodynamic instability, PCI may be performed using a percutaneous hemodynamic support device. For several decades, the device that was utilized was an intra-aortic balloon pump (IABP) (Figs. 7.30 to 7.32). Interestingly, the routine use of IABP in high-risk PCI has not been clearly demonstrated to be of benefit. Newer percutaneous hemodynamic support devices include the Impella (Figs. 7.33 and 7.34) and TandemHeart (Fig. 7.35). Both these devices can generate blood flow up to 4–5 liters/minute. ACCF/AHA/SCAI PCI guidelines state that elective insertion of an appropriate hemodynamic support device as an adjunct to PCI may be reasonable in carefully selected high-risk patients.

Fractional flow reserve (FFR) is a technique that compares the pressure in the coronary artery distal to a coronary stenosis with the pressure proximal to a stenosis (Fig. 7.36). The assessment is done during administration of intracoronary or intravenous adenosine, which causes vasodilation of the resistance vessels in the coronary circulation. A drop in the ratio of distal to proximal coronary arterial pressure to less than 0.75–0.80 denotes that the coronary lesion is physiologically significant. The use of

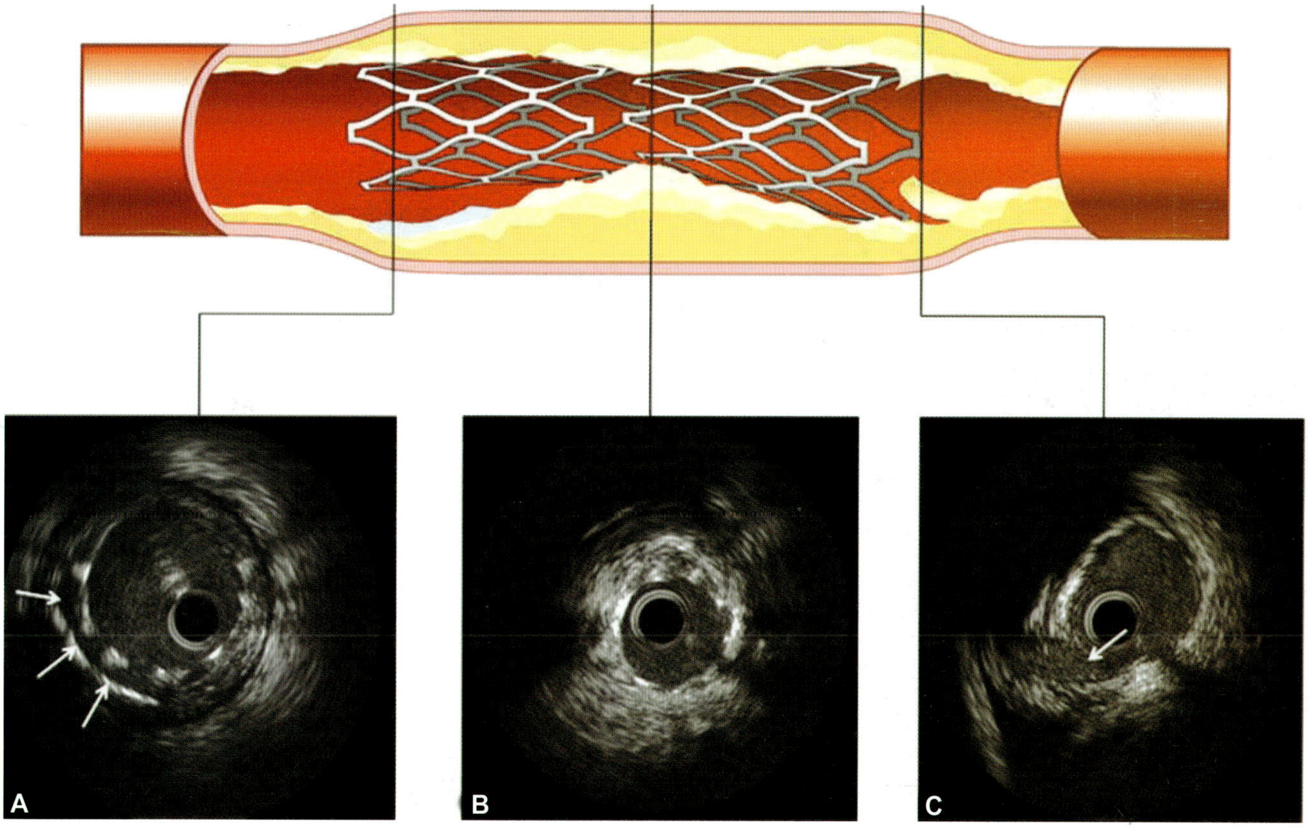

Figs. 22A to C: Intravascular ultrasound-detected problems with stent deployment. (A) Incomplete stent apposition with a gap between a portion of the stent and the vessel wall between 6 O'clock and 10 O'clock; (B) Incomplete stent expansion relative to the ends of the stent and the reference segments; (C) An edge tear or "pocket flap" with plaque disruption at the stent margin. [Images and legend text from Kume T, Honda Y, Fitzgerald PJ. Intravascular coronary ultrasound and beyond. In: Chatterjee K, Anderson M, Heistad D, Kerber RE (Eds). Cardiology: An Illustrated Textbook. New Delhi, India: Jaypee Brothers Medical Publishers (P) Ltd. 2012].

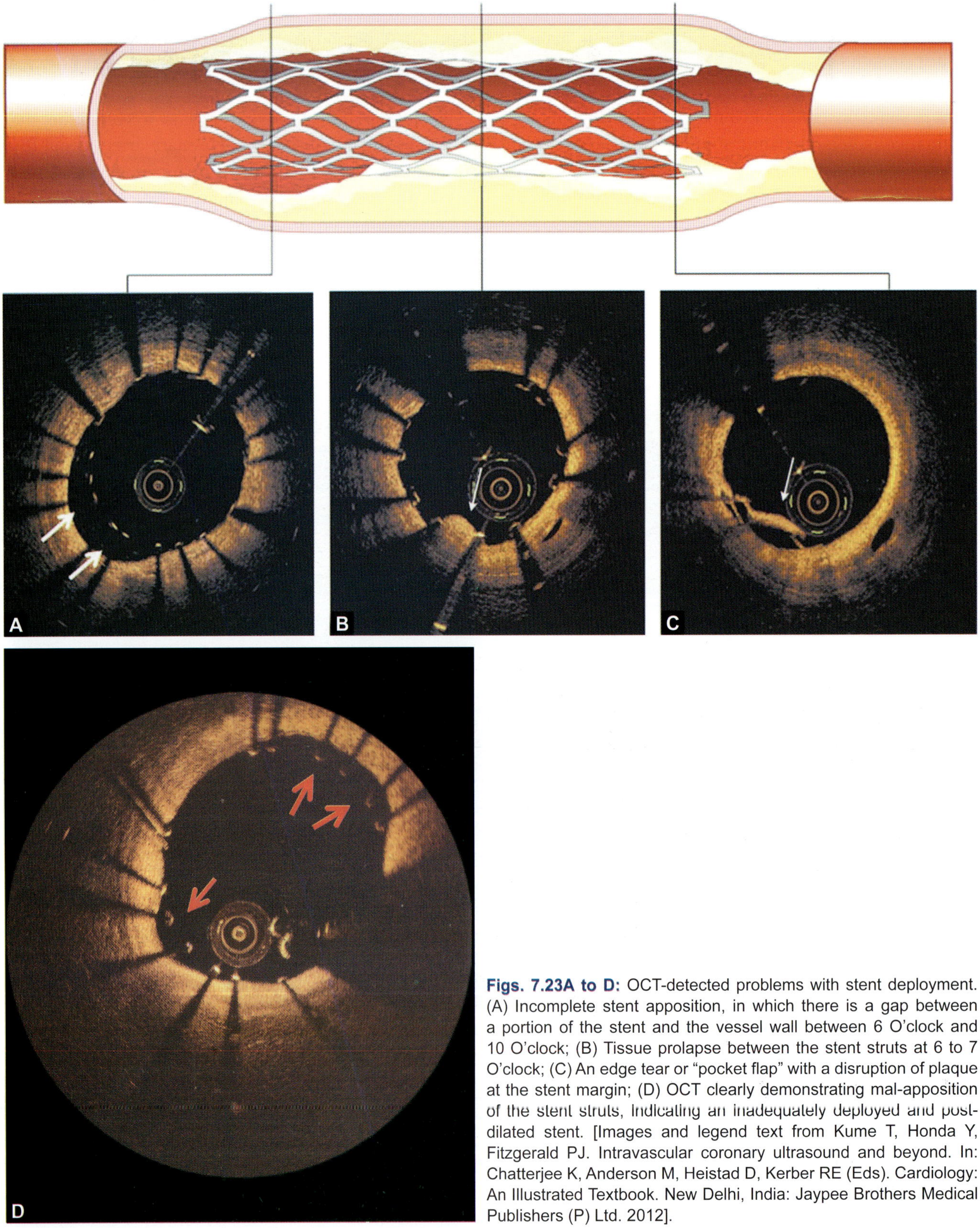

Figs. 7.23A to D: OCT-detected problems with stent deployment. (A) Incomplete stent apposition, in which there is a gap between a portion of the stent and the vessel wall between 6 O'clock and 10 O'clock; (B) Tissue prolapse between the stent struts at 6 to 7 O'clock; (C) An edge tear or "pocket flap" with a disruption of plaque at the stent margin; (D) OCT clearly demonstrating mal-apposition of the stent struts, indicating an inadequately deployed and post-dilated stent. [Images and legend text from Kume T, Honda Y, Fitzgerald PJ. Intravascular coronary ultrasound and beyond. In: Chatterjee K, Anderson M, Heistad D, Kerber RE (Eds). Cardiology: An Illustrated Textbook. New Delhi, India: Jaypee Brothers Medical Publishers (P) Ltd. 2012].

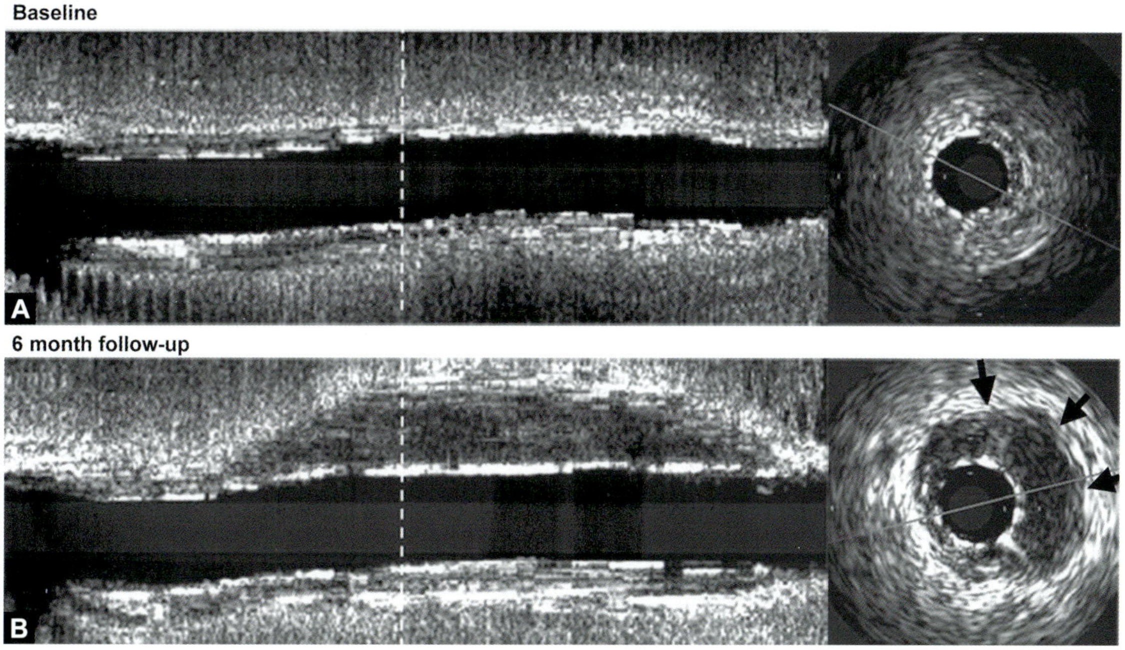

Figs. 7.24A and B: Serial Intravascular ultrasound (IVUS) images demonstrate late-acquired stent apposition. (A) Baseline IVUS shows excellent post-procedure stent apposition in a patient treated with a drug-eluting stent for a mid-LAD stenosis; (B) At 6 months, focal increase in vessel size is observed in the longitudinal IVUS image. The cross sectional IVUS image on the right shows stent struts which are now separated from the vessel wall (arrows). [Images and legend text from Kume T, Honda Y, Fitzgerald PJ. Intravascular coronary ultrasound and beyond. In: Chatterjee K, Anderson M, Heistad D, Kerber RE (Eds). Cardiology: An Illustrated Textbook. New Delhi, India: Jaypee Brothers Medical Publishers (P) Ltd. 2012].

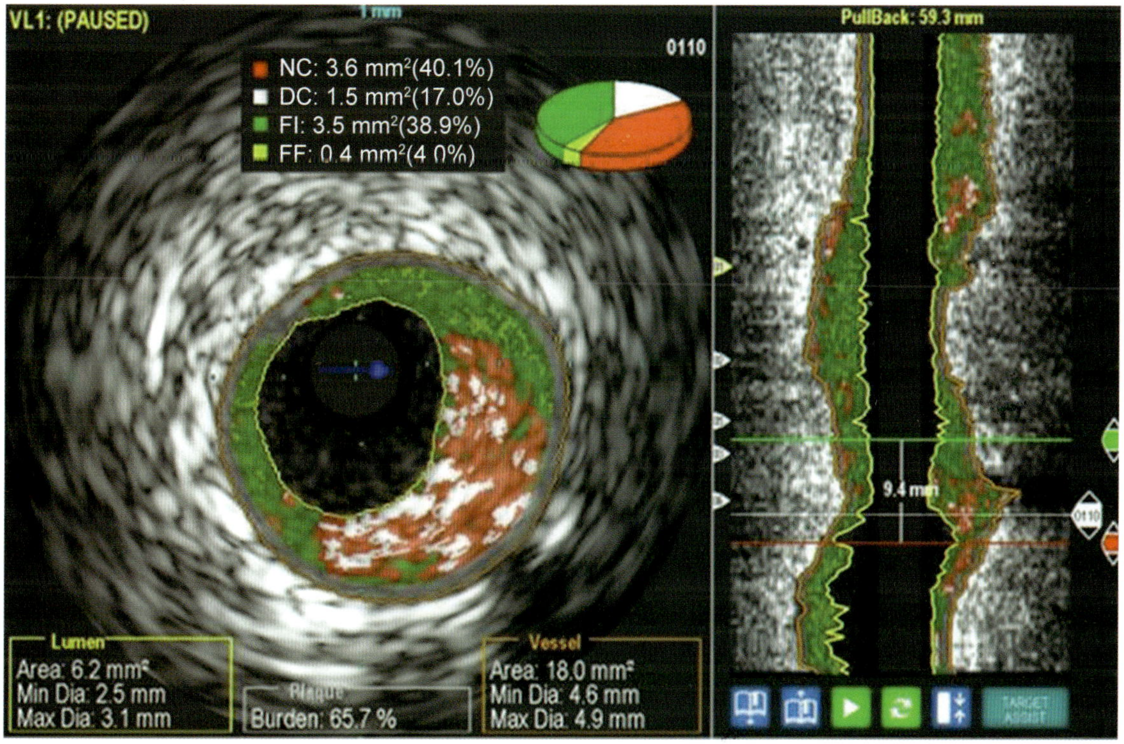

Fig. 7.25: Virtual histology intravascular ultrasound of a coronary artery atheroma. (DC: Dense calcium; FF: Fibrofatty; FI: Fibrous).

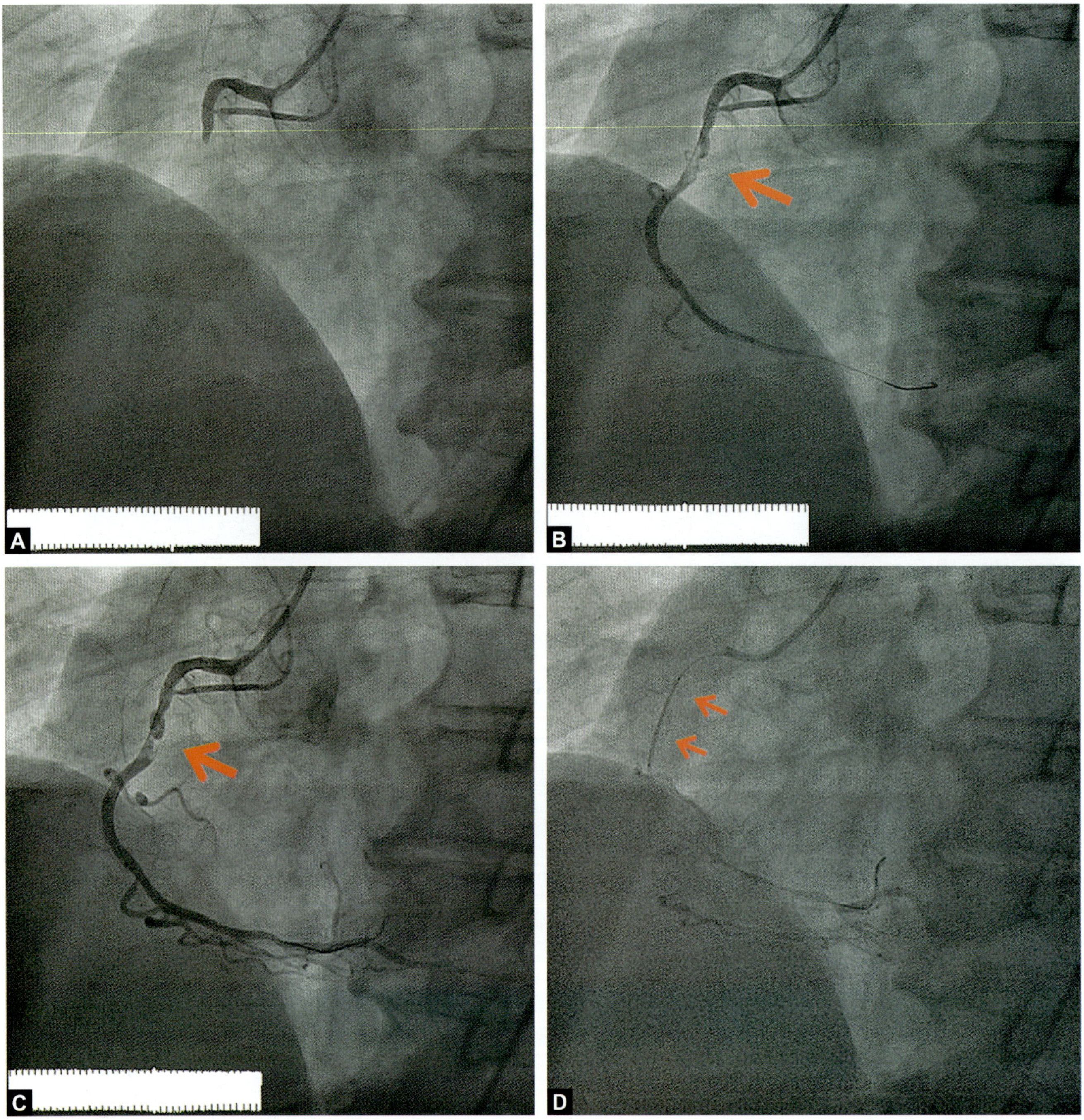

Figs. 7.26A to D: Primary percutaneous coronary interventions of the right coronary artery (RCA) in a patient with STEMI. (A) Initial angiogram showing complete occlusion at the level of the proximal RCA; (B) Angiogram after wiring of the occlusion, which has restored some flow in the artery. A significant thrombus burden is clearly visible (arrow); (C) Angiogram after aspiration thrombectomy, which a modest reduction in thrombus burden (arrow); (D) Placement of the coronary stent (arrows) in the area of the culprit lesion.

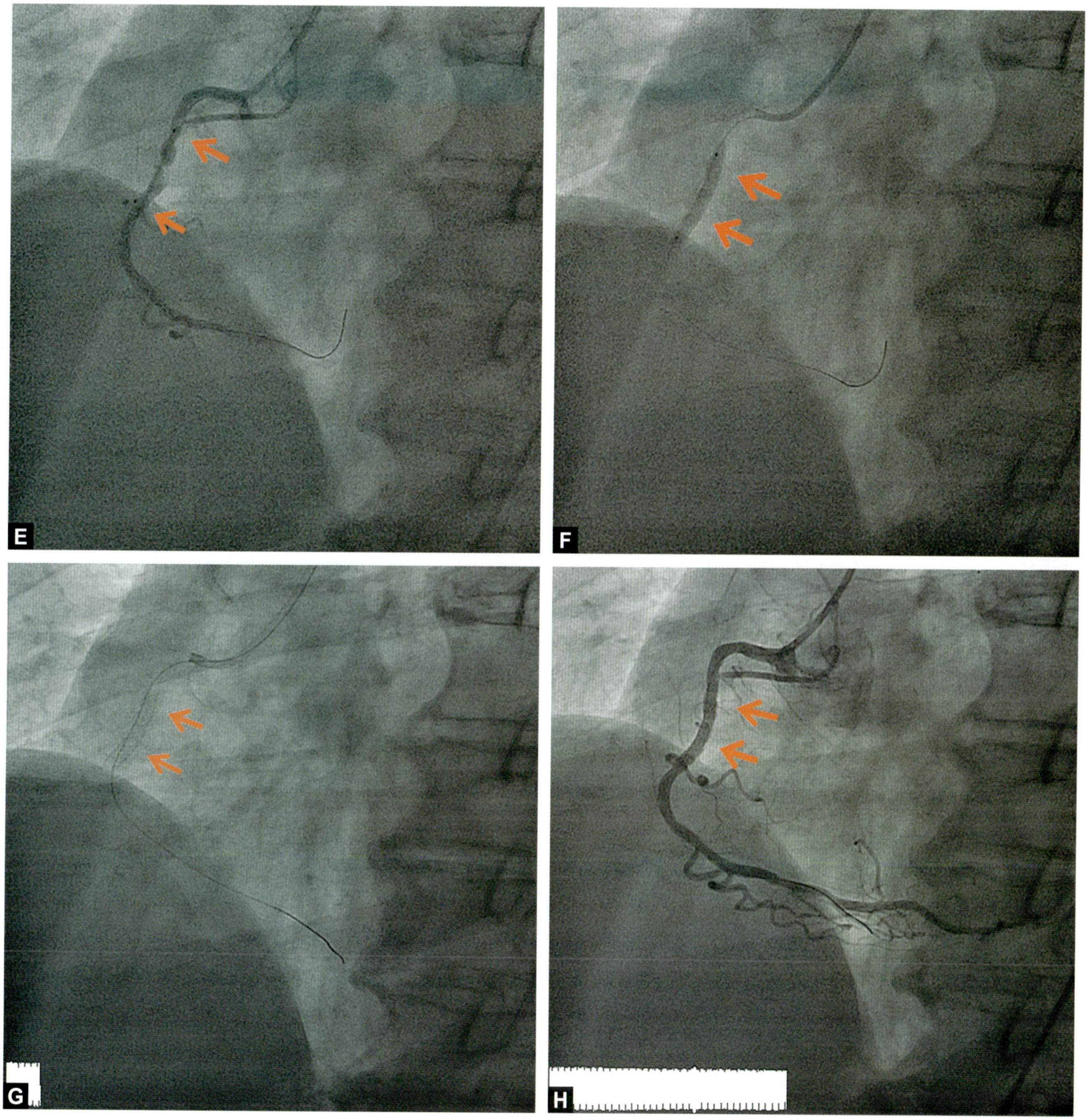

Figs. 7.26E to H: (E) Angiogram confirming correct placement of the coronary stent. Arrows point to the proximal and distal markers of the balloon-mounted stent; (F) Balloon inflation and deployment of the stent; (G) The deployed stent (arrows) is visible; (H) Angiogram showing final result, with 0% residual stenosis after stent deployment (arrows) and good flow throughout the entire RCA.

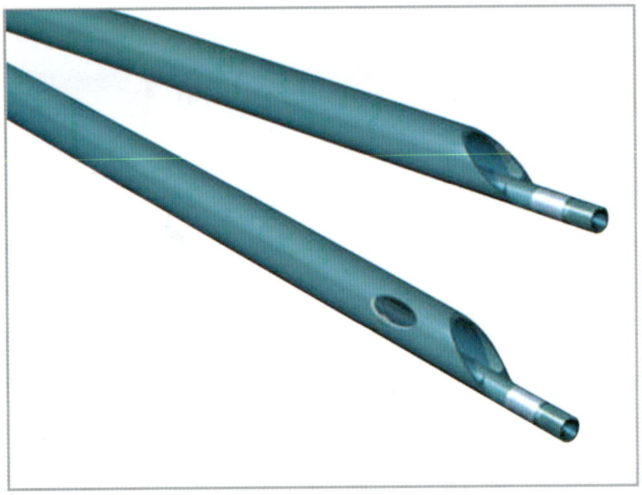

Fig. 7.27: Manual aspiration catheter. (Image courtesy of Boston Scientific Corporation).

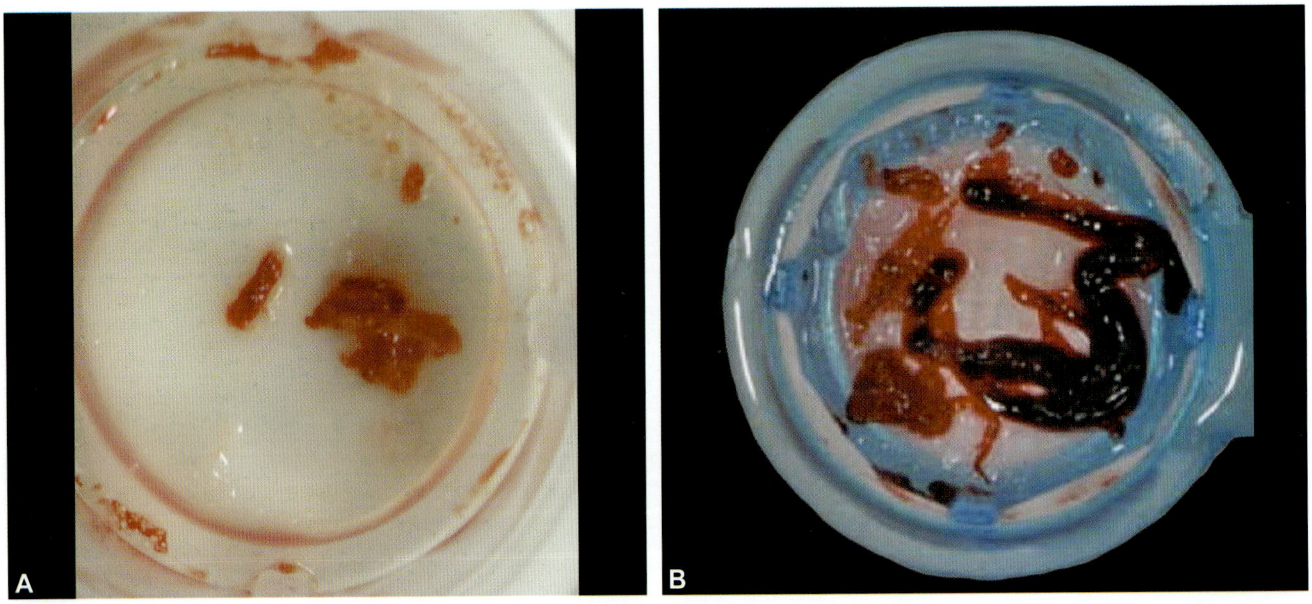

Figs. 7.28A and B: Thrombus aspirated using manual aspiration catheters in patients with STEMI undergoing primary percutaneous coronary interventions. (Image 7.28A courtesy of Dr David Paniagua).

FFR has been demonstrated to allow one to assess if an angiographically intermediate coronary lesion is hemodynamically significant. The use of FFR-guided PCI, when compared with solely angiographically-guided PCI, has been shown in several studies to lead to better long-term outcome. ACCF/AHA/SCAI PCI guidelines state that FFR is reasonable to assess angiographically intermediate coronary lesions (50–70% diameter stenosis) and can be useful

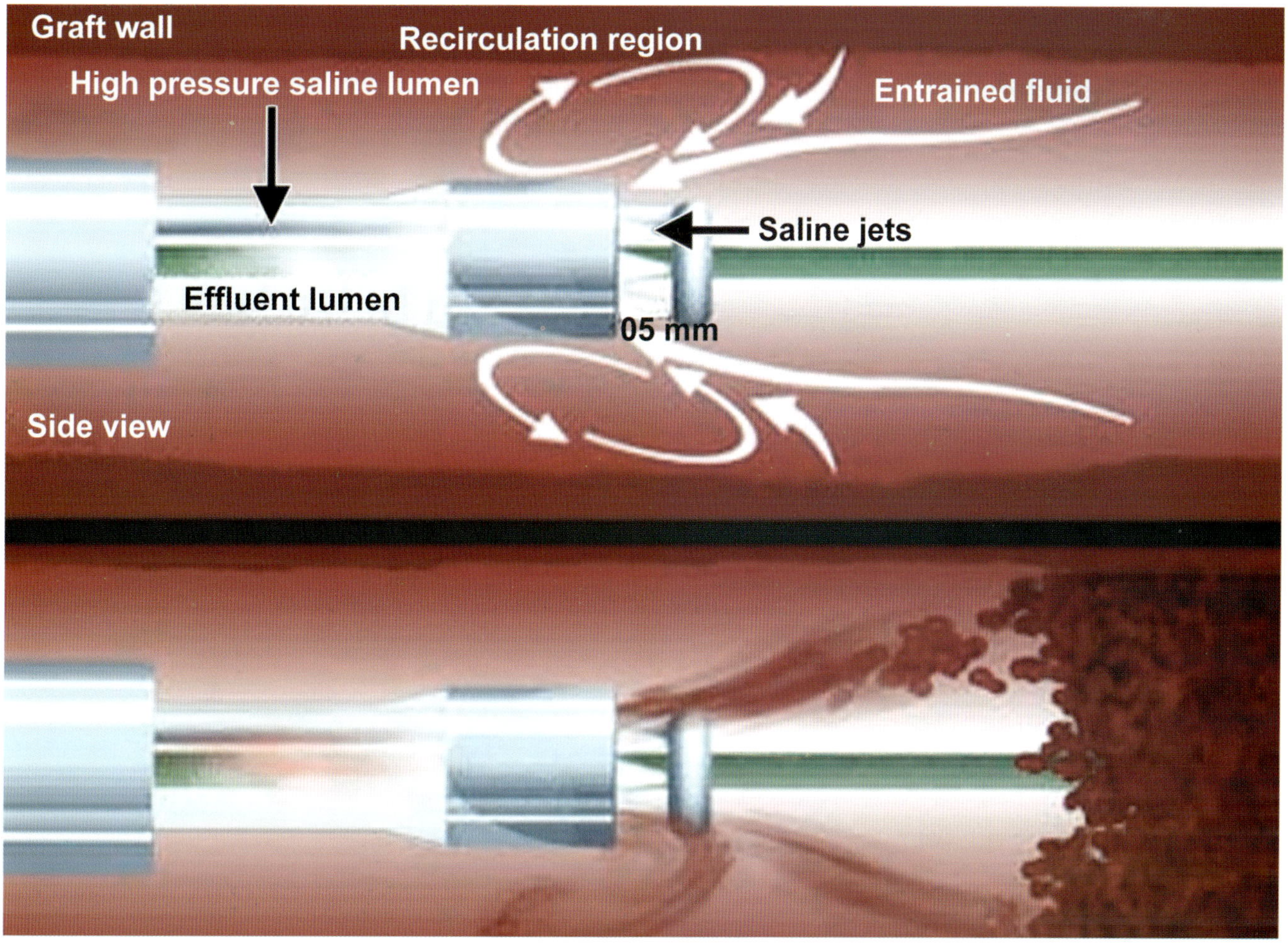

Fig. 7.29: The AngioJet rheolytic thrombectomy device.

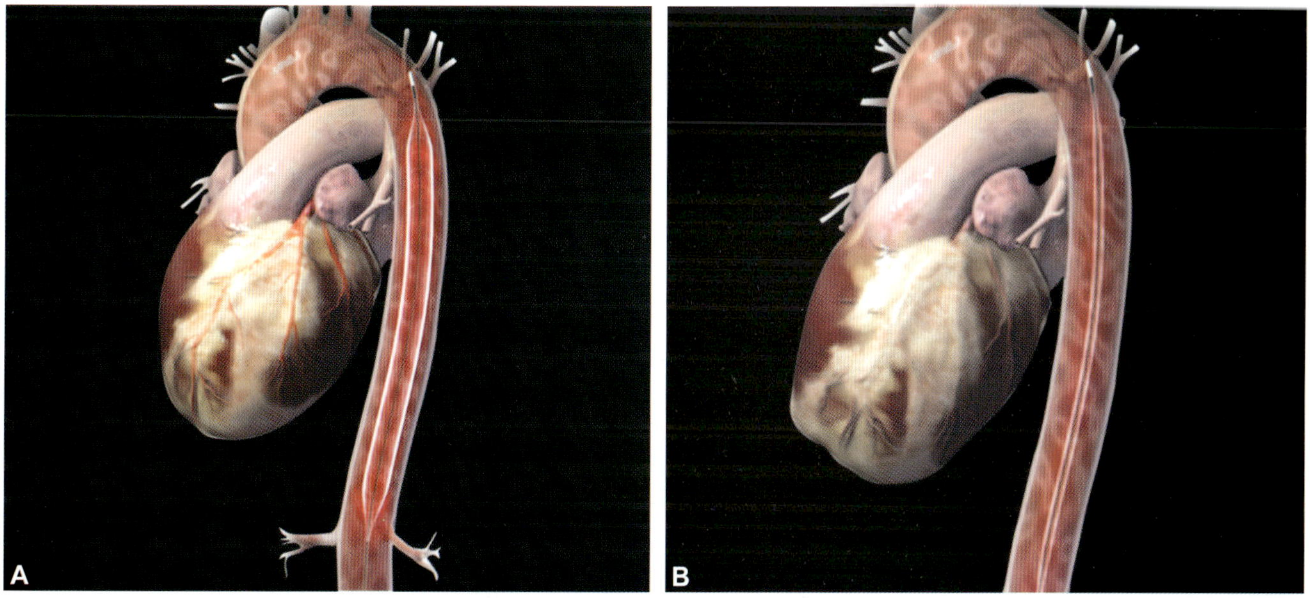

Figs. 7.30A and B: Intra-aortic balloon pump. (A) Inflated; (B) Deflated.

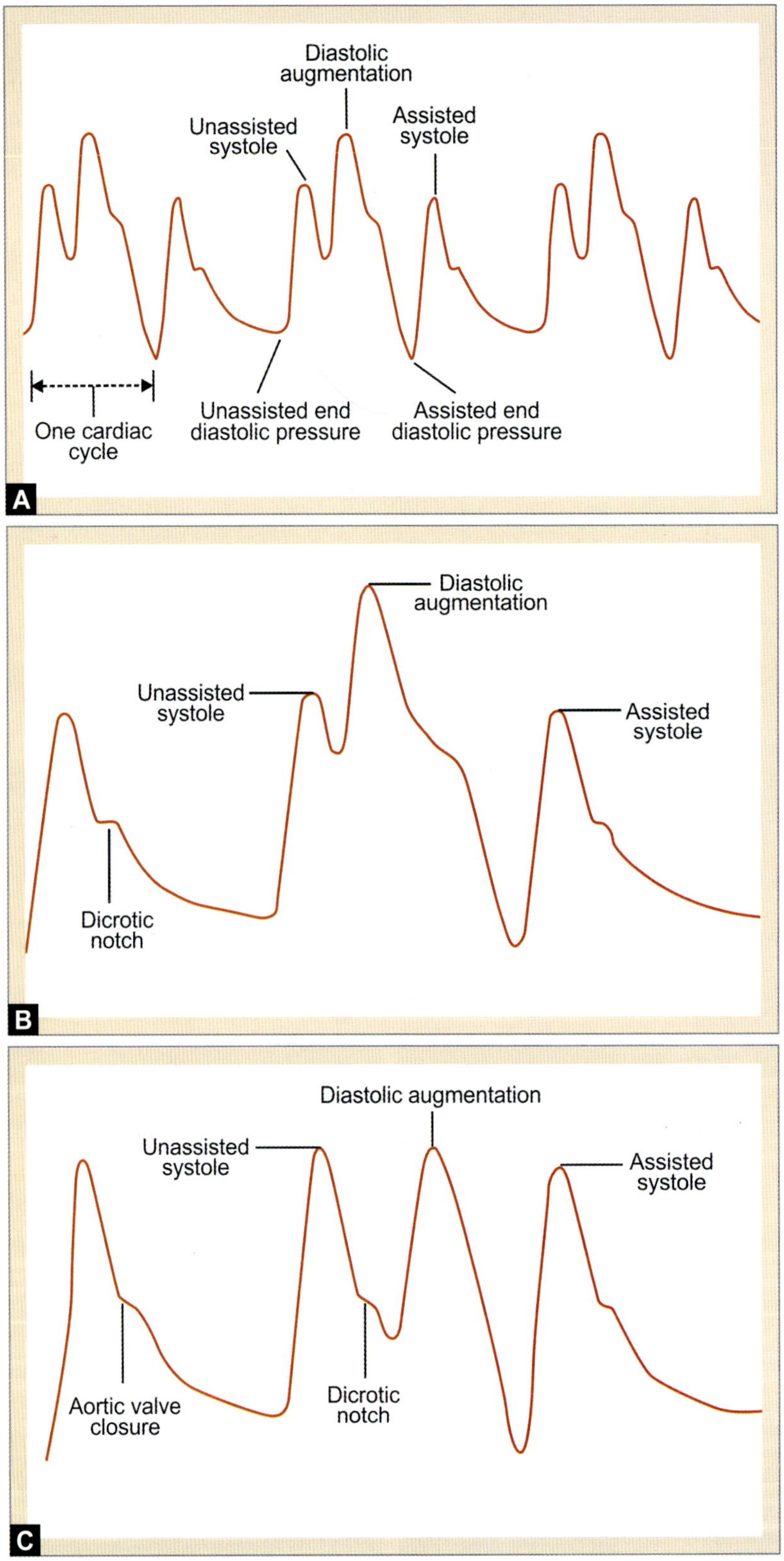

Figs. 7.31A to C: Proper and improper timing of intra-aortic balloon pump inflation and deflation. Correct timing of inflation and deflation is assessed with the device set to 1:2 augmentation (inflating and deflating every other cardiac cycle) (A) Correct timing. The balloon inflates at the dicrotic notch, and deflates just before ventricular systole; (B) Early inflation. The balloon is inflating before the dicrotic notch; (C) Late inflation. The balloon is inflating after the dicrotic notch.

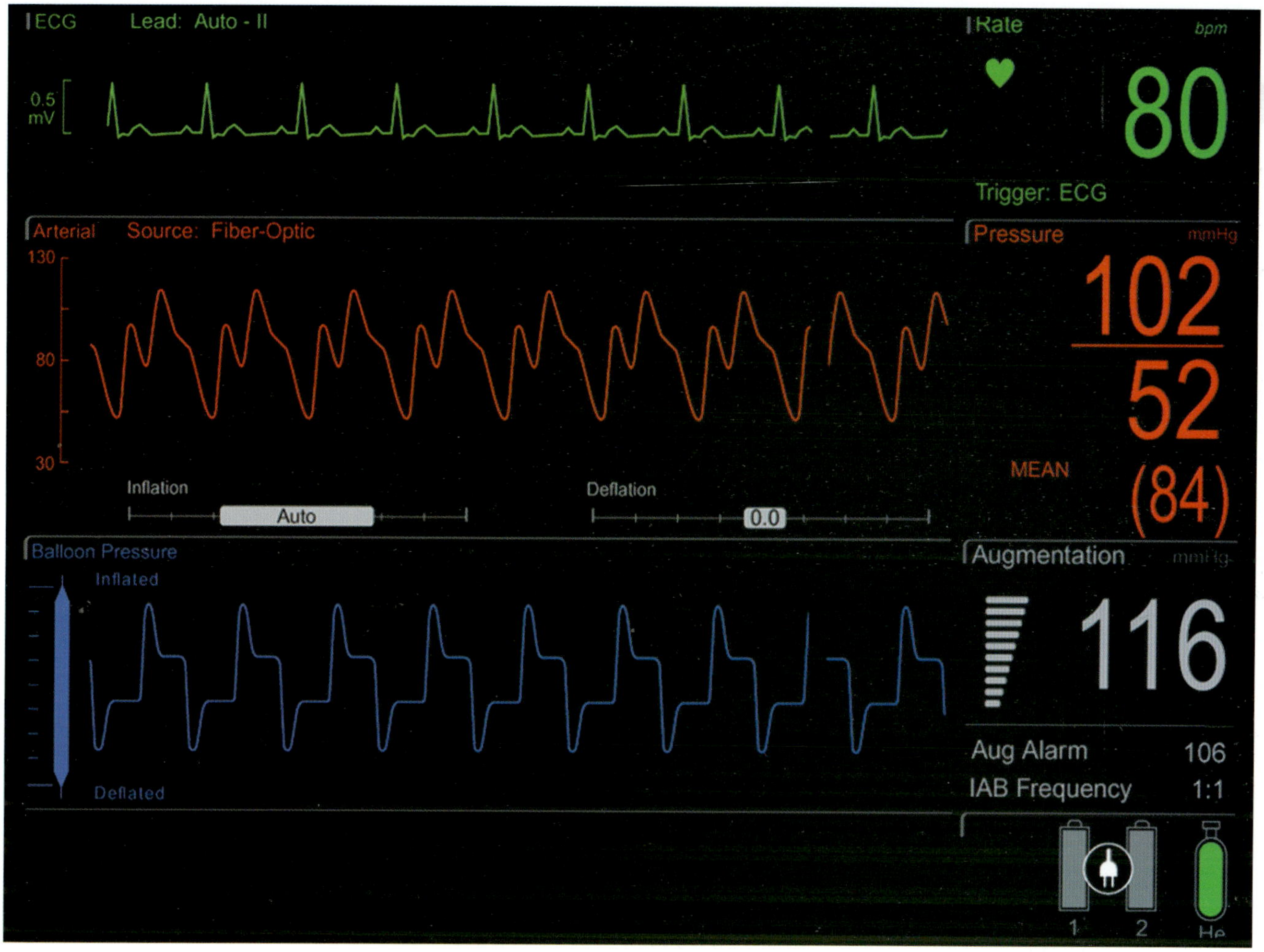

Fig. 7.32: Simultaneous display of the ECG, arterial waveform, and intra-aortic balloon pump (IABP) balloon inflation status in a patient with IABP with 1:1 augmentation (balloon inflation with each cardiac cycle).

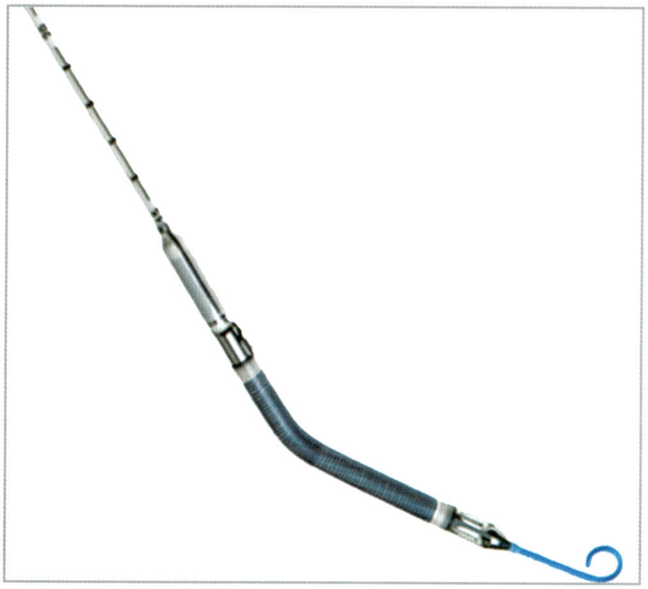

Fig. 7.33: The Impella percutaneous ventricular assist device.

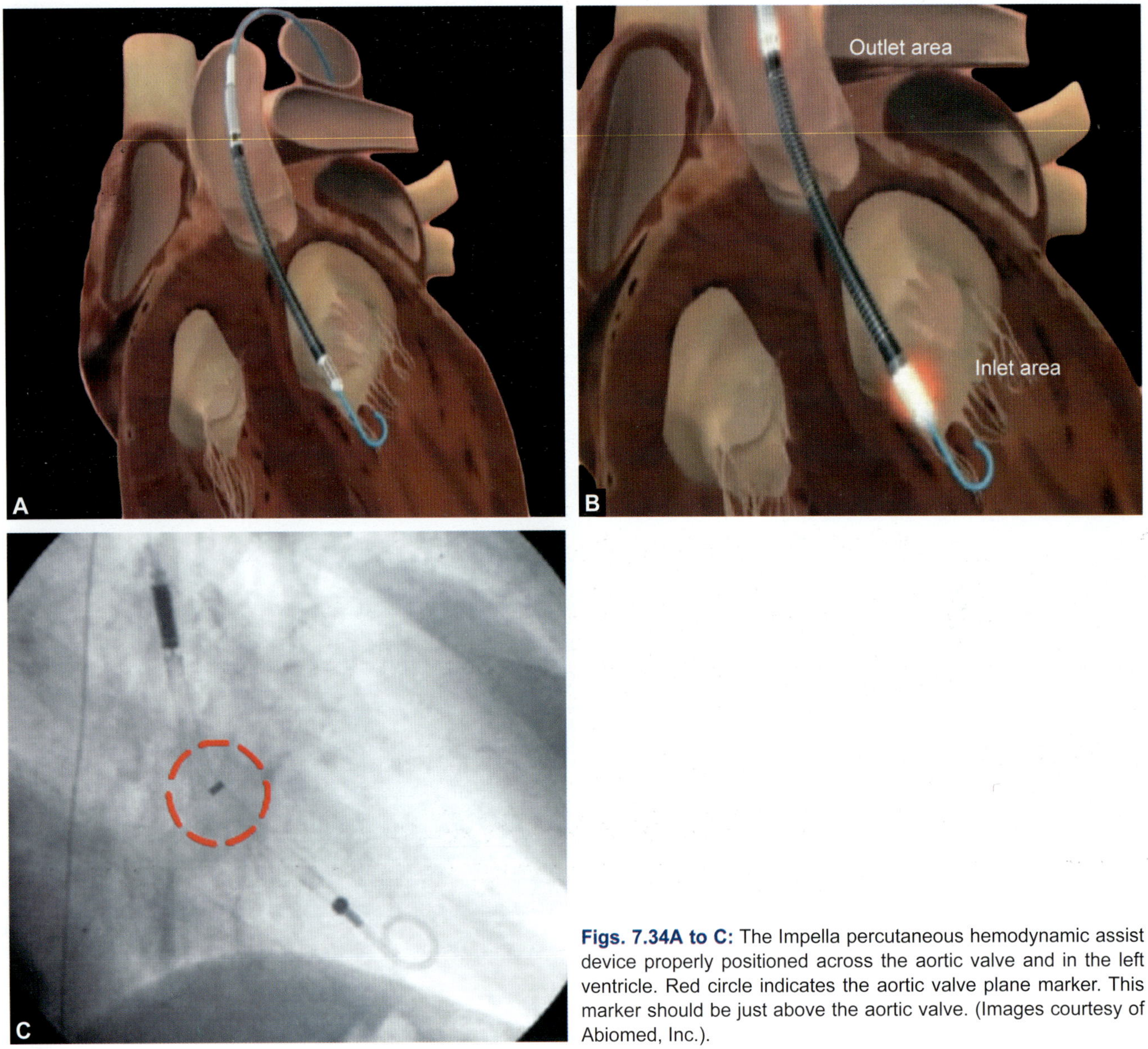

Figs. 7.34A to C: The Impella percutaneous hemodynamic assist device properly positioned across the aortic valve and in the left ventricle. Red circle indicates the aortic valve plane marker. This marker should be just above the aortic valve. (Images courtesy of Abiomed, Inc.).

for guiding revascularization decisions in patients with stable ischemic heart disease (class IIa recommendation).

Vascular closure devices (VSDs, also called arteriotomy closure devices) are often used after the PCI procedure (Figs. 7.37A to D). Although VCDs have not convincingly been shown to decrease vascular and bleeding complications in patients who undergo PCI performed via the femoral artery, they do lead to quicker hemostasis, shorter duration of bed rest, and possibly improved patient comfort.

RADIAL ARTERY PERCUTANEOUS CORONARY INTERVENTION

The radial artery (Figs. 7.38A and B) is being increasingly utilized for arterial access in patients undergoing PCI. Compared to PCI via the femoral artery, radial artery PCI may lead to a lower incidence of vascular and bleeding complications. The Allen test (Figs. 7.39A and B) is performed prior to radial artery PCI to verify adequate distal perfusion via the ulnar artery.

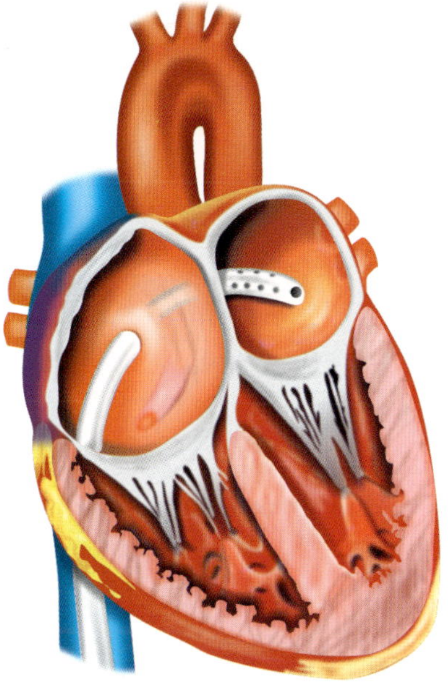

Fig. 7.35: The TandemHeart device. A large catheter is inserted over a wire through the femoral vein, up the inferior vena cava, in to the right atrium, and then across the intra-atrial septum in to the left atrium. Oxygenated blood is withdrawn from the left atrium and then, via a circulating pump and second catheter in the femoral artery, pumped in to the arterial circulation.

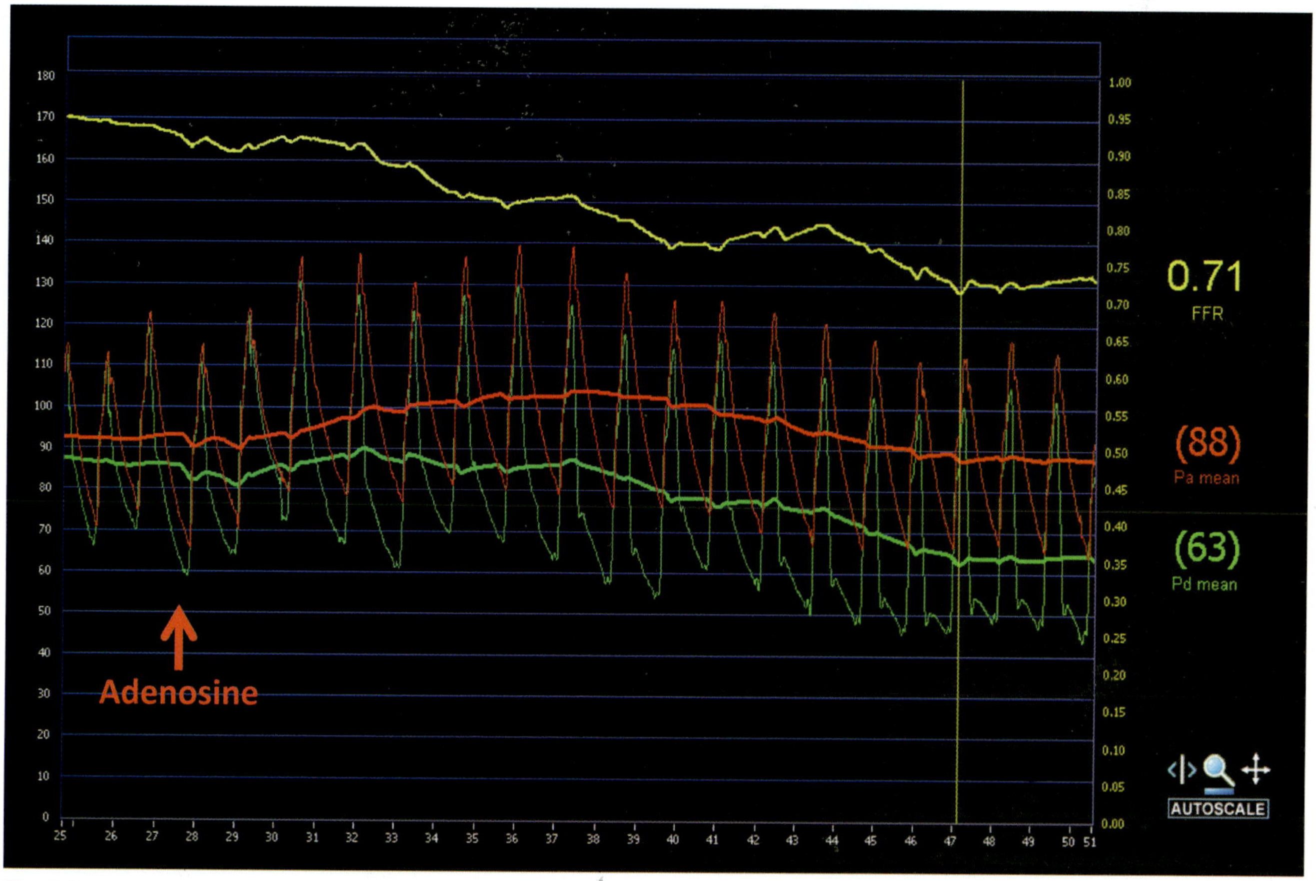

Fig. 7.36: Fractional flow reserve (FFR) study using pressure wire of an angiographically intermediate coronary lesion. Tracings display both the actual and mean pressure tracings, as well as the fractional flow reserve (yellow line, FFR). With adenosine administration, the pressure distal to the lesion (green tracing, Pd) decreases significantly when compared to the arterial pressure proximal to the lesion (red tracing, Pa). [Modified from Incani A, Camuglia AC, Poon KK, et al. Improving the utility of coronary angiography: the use of adjuvant imaging and physiological assessment. In Baskot BG (Ed). What should we know about prevented, diagnostic, and interventional therapy in coronary artery disease. Shanghai: InTech China; 2013].

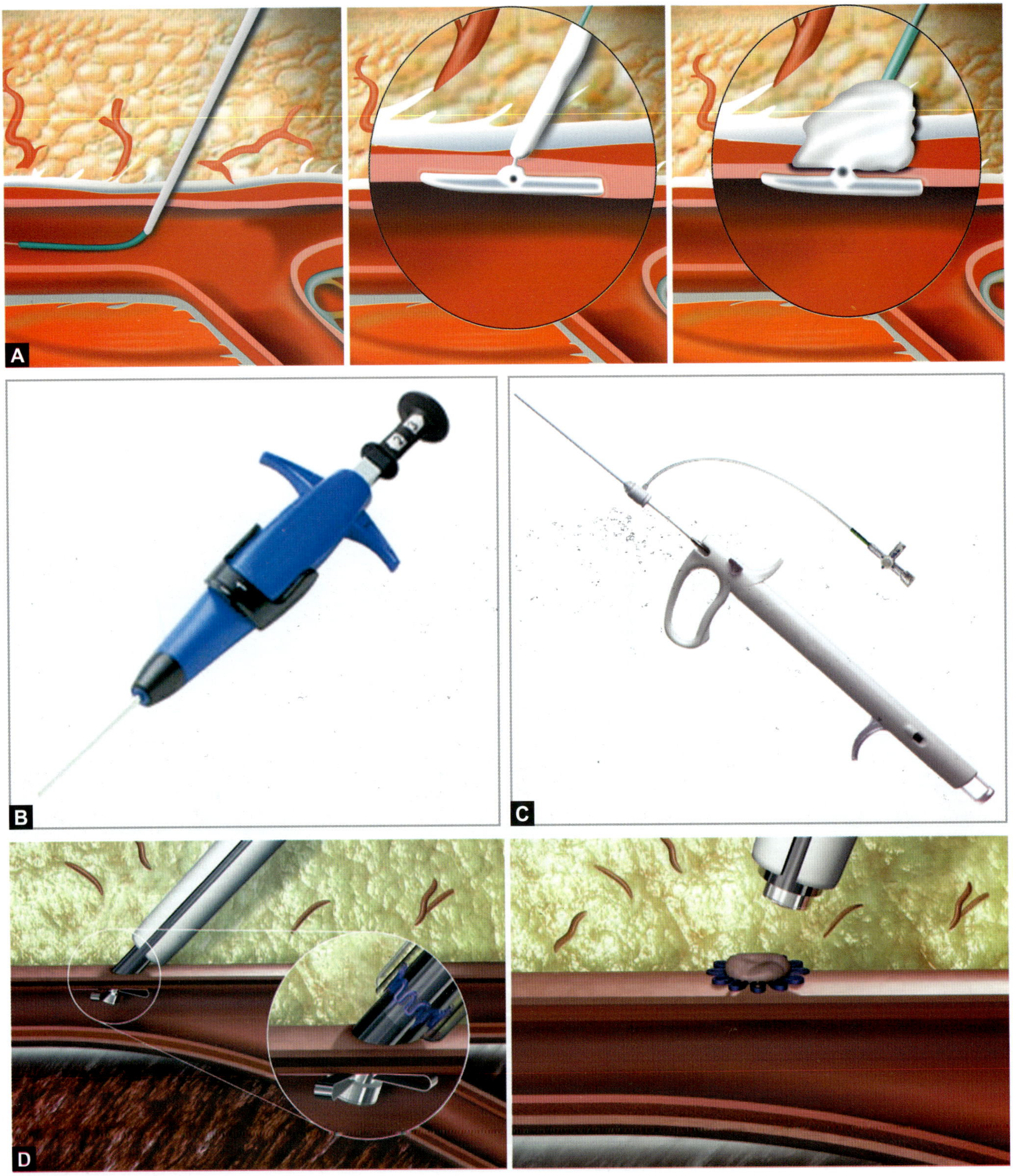

Figs. 7.37A to D: Examples of vascular (arteriotomy) closure devices.

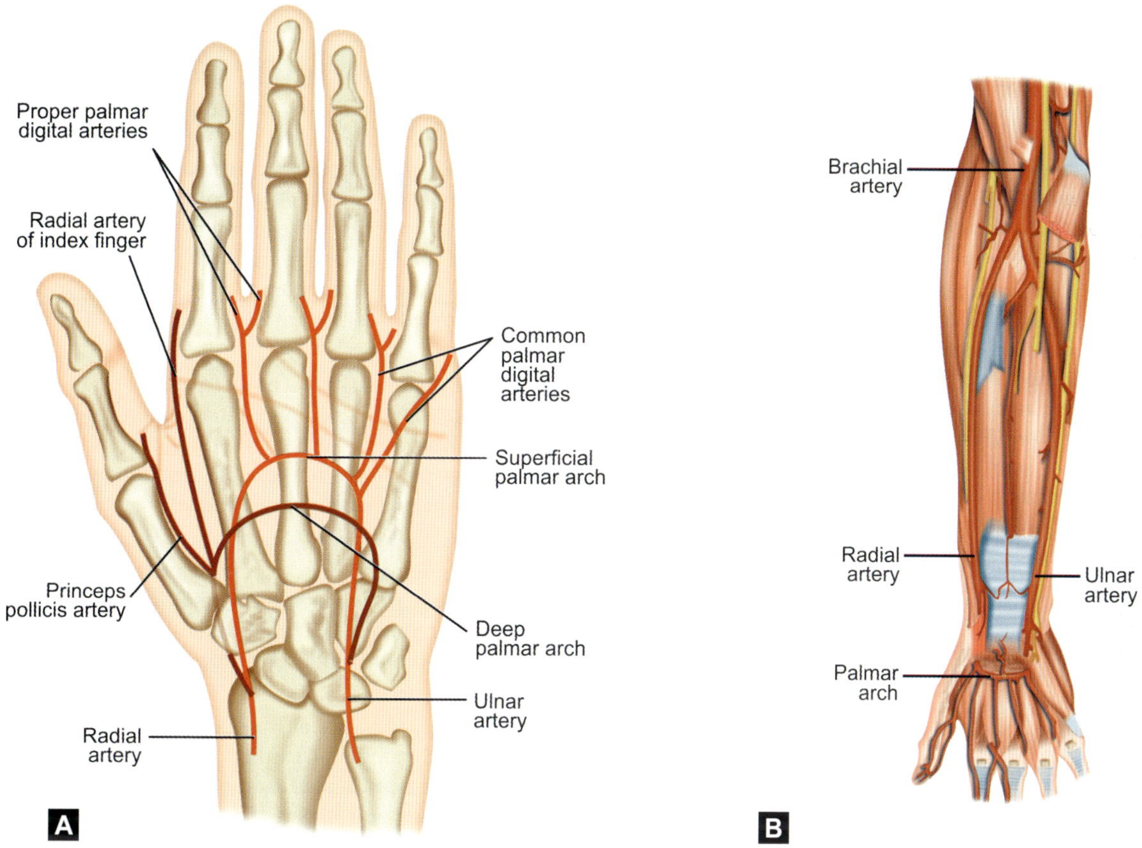

Figs. 7.38A and B: Radial artery anatomy. (A) Circulation in the wrist and hand; (B) Arteries of the arm and wrist.

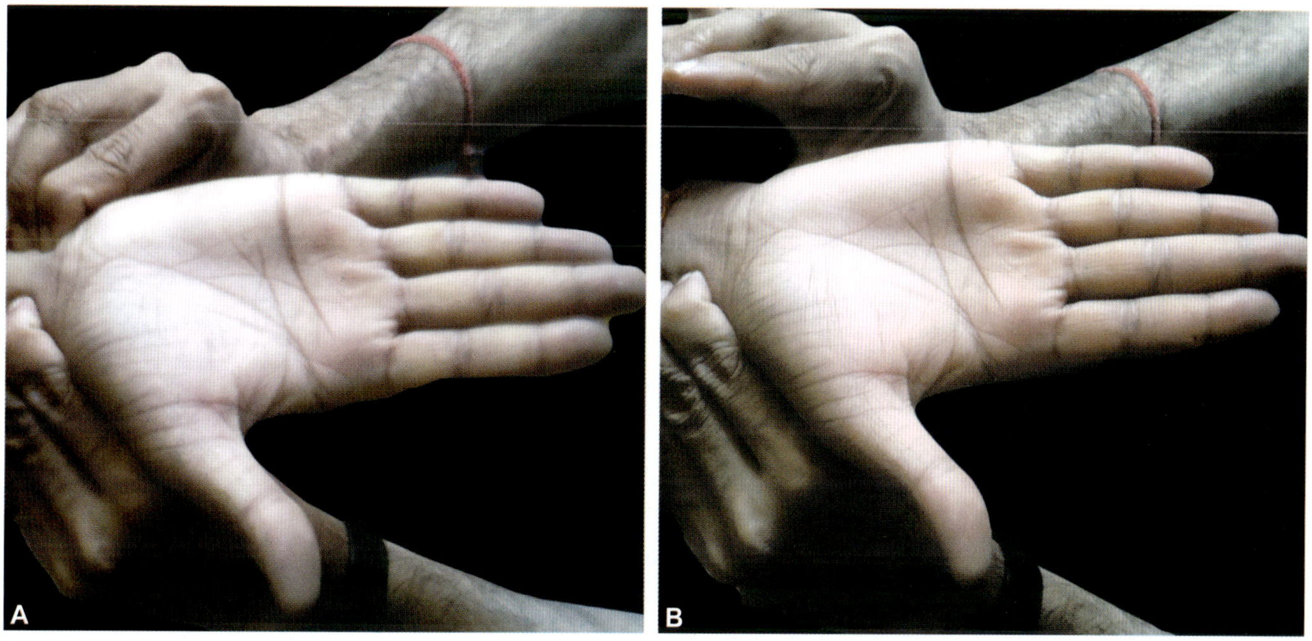

Figs. 7.39A and B: Performance of the Allen test. (A) Simultaneous hand pressure occlusion of the radial and ulnar arteries, with resultant hypoperfusion of the hand; (B) Release of occlusive pressure on the ulnar artery, while continuing occlusive hand pressure on the radial artery, demonstrating adequate perfusion of the hand by the ulnar artery. [Images from Natarajan D. Transradial access for diagnostic coronary angiography and percutaneous coronary interventions: current concepts and future challenges. In Baskot B (Ed). Coronary angiography—The Need for Improvement in Medical and Interventional Therapy. Shanghai: InTech China; 2013].

VIDEO LEGENDS

Videos 7.1A to D: Example of primary stenting in a patient with chronic stable angina. (A) Initial angiogram shows a moderate mid left anterior descending (LAD) stenosis. (B) Guide wire across the mid-LAD stenosis and a coronary stent positioned at the site of the stenosis. (C) Balloon inflation and stent deployment. (D) Post-stent deployment angiogram showing 0% residual stenosis.

Videos 7.2A to E: Primary percutaneous coronary interventions of an occluded mid left anterior descending (LAD) artery in a patient with acute anterior wall myocardial infarction. (A) Initial angiogram showing complete occlusion at the level of the mid LAD. (B) Guide wire passed across occlusion, resulting in some restoration of blood flow. A residual stenotic lesion is visible. (C) A coronary stent being positioned at the site of residual stenosis. (D) Inflation of the balloon and deployment of the coronary stent. (E) Post-stent deployment angiogram showing the treated stenosis and TIMI 3 flow throughout the coronary artery.

Videos 7.3A to G: Primary percutaneous coronary interventions of an occluded left circumflex artery. (A) Angiogram showing a subtotally occluded left circumflex artery with TIMI grade 1 flow. Contrast is visible just distal to the culprit lesion from a previous contrast injection. A late-filing large obtuse marginal (OM) branch is visible. (B) Guide wire passed across the lesion and balloon positioned at the site of subtotal occlusion. (C) Balloon inflation. (D) Post-balloon inflation angiogram showing some improvement in blood flow to TIMI grade 2 and a residual stenosis. (E) Positioning of a long coronary stent. (F) Deployment of the coronary stent. (G) Final coronary angiogram showing the treated culprit lesion and restoration of TIMI grade 3 blood flow.

REFERENCES

Harold JG, Bass TA, Bashore TM, et al. ACCF/AHA/ACP Task force on clinical competence and training members. ACCF/AHA/SCAI 2013 update of the clinical competence statement on coronary artery interventional procedures: a report of the American College of Cardiology Foundation/American Heart Association/American College of Physicians task force on clinical competence and training (Writing Committee to Revise the 2007 Clinical Competence Statement on Cardiac Interventional Procedures). J Am Coll Cardiol. 2013;62(4):357-96.

Levine GN, Bates ER, Blankenship JC, et al. 2011 ACCF/AHA/SCAI Guideline for percutaneous coronary intervention. a report of the American College of Cardiology Foundation/American Heart Association task force on practice guidelines and the society for cardiovascular angiography and interventions. J Am Coll Cardiol. 2011;58(24):e44-122.

Levine GN, Kern MJ, Berger PB, et al. American Heart Association Diagnostic and Interventional Cardiac Catheterization Committee. Management of Patients Undergoing Percutaneous Coronary Revascularization. Ann Intern Med. 2003;139:123-36.

Patel MR, Jneid H, Derdeyn CP, et al. American Heart Association Diagnostic and interventional cardiac catheterization committee of the Council on Clinical Cardiology, Council on Cardiovascular Radiology and Intervention, Council on Peripheral Vascular Disease, Council on Cardiovascular Surgery and Anesthesia, and Stroke Council. Arteriotomy closure devices for cardiovascular procedures: a scientific statement from the American Heart Association. Circulation. 2010;122(18):1882-93.

CHAPTER

Coronary Artery Bypass Graft Surgery

8

Lorraine D Cornwell, Shuab Omer, Faisal G Bakaeen

INTRODUCTION

Coronary artery disease (CAD) is the single largest cause of mortality in Americans, with almost half a million deaths per year. Revascularization for CAD has been shown to improve survival, and guidelines currently recommend coronary artery bypass grafting surgery (CABG) as an important means for revascularization in many patients with CAD, especially in the setting of multivessel disease or with left main involvement. The goals of CABG are to improve symptoms and prolong survival (Tables 8.1 and 8.2).

The era of open heart surgery started in 1954, when Dr John Gibbon first reported on the development of the cardiopulmonary bypass (CPB) machine (Fig. 8.1), which enabled open heart surgery to be performed. The first reported results of CABG in 1969 by René Favaloro and Dudley Johnson initiated the modern era of coronary artery revascularization. CABG quickly became the most common cardiac operation performed, and still dominates the field of cardiac surgery, with approximately 400,000 operations performed each year in the US alone, and an estimated 800,000 operations performed worldwide annually.

Table 8.1: American College of Cardiology Foundation (ACCF)/ American Heart Association (AHA) guideline recommendations for the performance of coronary artery bypass graft surgery (CABG) in patients with stable ischemic coronary artery disease (CAD) to improve survival. (CAD: Coronary artery disease; LAD: Left anterior descending; LOE: Level of evidence; LIMA: Left internal mammary artery; LVEF: Left ventricular ejection fraction; EF: Ejection fraction).

***Class I (is recommended; is beneficial)*:**
• Unprotected left main CAD (LOE=B) • 3-vessel disease with or without proximal LAD artery disease (LOE = B) • 2-vessel disease with proximal LAD artery disease (LOE = B)
***Class IIa (is reasonable)*:**
• 2-vessel CAD without proximal LAD artery disease, with extensive ischemia (LOE = B) • 1-vessel proximal LAD artery disease, with LIMA grafting performed (LOE = B) • LVEF 35–50% (LOE = B)
***Class IIb (uncertain benefit)*:**
• 2-vessel CAD without LAD artery disease, without extensive ischemia (LOE = C) • EF <35% without significant left main CAD (LOE = B)
***Class III (harmful)*:**
• 1-vessel disease without proximal LAD artery involvement (LOE = B) • No anatomic or physiologic criteria for revascularization (LOE = B)

Table 8.2: American College of Cardiology Foundation (ACCF)/ American Heart Association (AHA) guideline recommendations for the performance of coronary artery bypass graft surgery (CABG) in patients with stable ischemic coronary artery disease (CAD) to improve symptoms. (GDMT: Guideline-directed medical therapy; LOE: Level of evidence; CABG: Coronary artery bypass grafting surgery).

***Class I (is recommended; is beneficial)*:**
≥ 1 significant stenoses amenable to revascularization and unacceptable angina despite GDMT (LOE = A)
***Class IIa (is reasonable)*:**
≥ 1 significant stenoses and unacceptable angina in whom GDMT cannot be implemented because of medication contraindications, adverse effects, or patient preferences (LOE = C)
***Class IIb (uncertain benefit)*:**
Previous CABG with ≥ 1 significant stenoses associated with ischemia and unacceptable angina despite GDMT (LOE = C)
***Class III (harmful)*:**
No anatomic of physiologic criteria for revascularization (LOE = C)

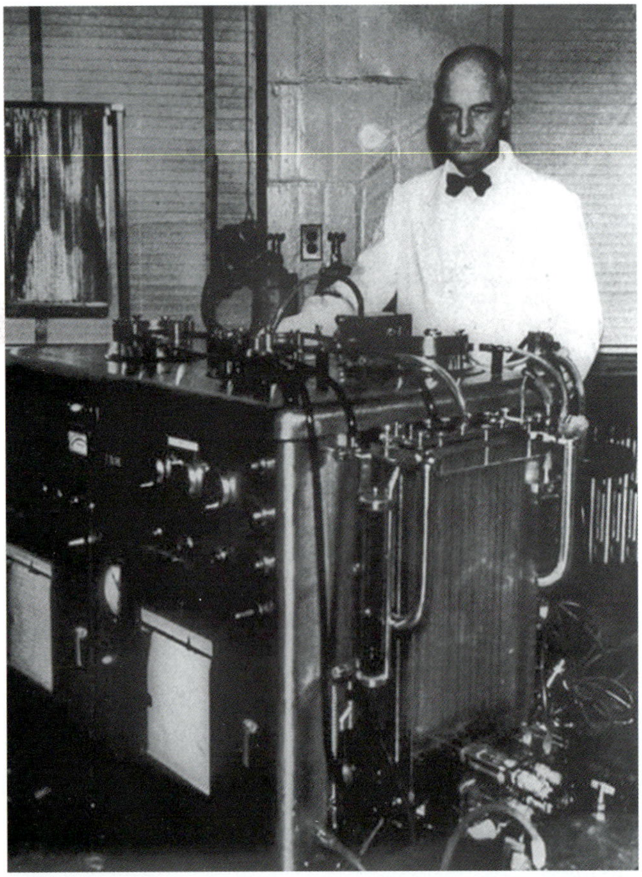

Fig. 8.1: John Gibbons and his heart lung machine. [Image from Maheshwari S, Kiran VS. History of pediatric cardiology: from the "untouchable" heart to the brave new era. In: Chopra HK, Nanda NC (Eds). Textbook of Cardiology: A Clinical and Historical Perspective. New Delhi, India: Jaypee Brothers Medical Publishers (P) Ltd. 2013. pp. 270-82].

Coronary artery bypass grafting surgery (Figs. 8.2 to 8.4) is the most scrutinized procedure currently performed in the US. Outcomes are carefully reported and compared, in both State and National databases. Trends have shown an ongoing reduction in morbidity and mortality rates as experience has been gained and the procedure and technology have evolved, and present-day CABG operations are generally associated with low perioperative morbidity and mortality, despite worsening risk profiles of the patient population presenting for surgery [e.g. older patients, more comorbidities, lower ejection fractions (EFs)]. According to data from the most widely used database, the Society of Thoracic Surgeons (STS) database, overall operative mortality has decreased to an all-time low of approximately 2%. Long-term outcomes in appropriately selected patients are also excellent.

CABG VERSUS MEDICAL THERAPY OR PCI

Several trials [Coronary Artery Surgery Study (CASS), Veterans Affairs (VA) Cooperative Study, and European Cooperative Surgical Study (ECSS)] conducted in the 1980s compared CABG with contemporaneous medical therapy. These trials revealed a survival advantage in patients with significant left main CAD, 3-vessel CAD, and multivessel disease which included proximal left anterior descending (LAD) stenosis. The relative benefit of surgery on survival was found to be greatest in those patients at highest risk of death from the disease itself, as indicated by the severity of angina or ischemia, the number of diseased vessels, and presence of left ventricular (LV) dysfunction. Trials comparing CABG with percutaneous coronary intervention (PCI) (including trials utilizing drug-eluting stents) in patients with 3-vessel coronary disease have found decreased rates of major adverse cardiac and cerebrovascular events (MACCE) and improved survival with CABG. Improved outcomes are seen, especially in those patients with complex 3-vessel disease, diabetes, and low LVEF, and CABG is generally preferred as the mode of coronary revascularization in these patient subgroups. In general, the more extensive and complex the coronary disease, the more likely the patient will benefit from undergoing CABG instead of PCI. The Synergy between Percutaneous Coronary Intervention with Taxus and Cardiac Surgery (SYNTAX) score can be used to semi-quantitate the extent and complexity of disease.

PATIENT SELECTION AND EVALUATION FOR CABG

The decision to proceed with coronary revascularization with CABG starts with a comprehensive patient evaluation. The coronary angiogram will be carefully reviewed to assess for complexity of disease and suitability of distal vessels as targets for revascularization (Figs. 8.5A and B). Anatomic considerations that favor recommendations for CABG include the presence of left main disease (particularly complex and distal left main disease involving the bifurcation), multivessel disease, diffuse disease, bifurcation lesions, chronic total occlusions, and lesions otherwise not amenable to stenting for technical reasons. Each patient's comorbidities are carefully evaluated in

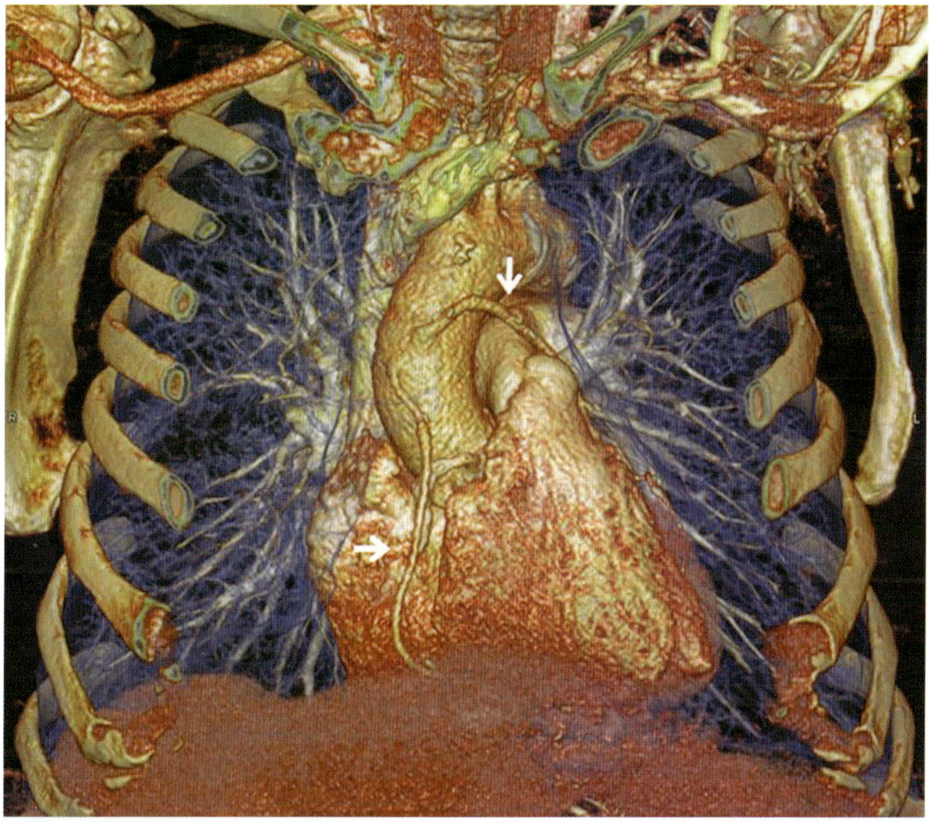

Fig. 8.2A: Chest computed tomography (CT), displayed in a coronal projection, demonstrating saphenous vein bypass grafts (arrows) from the aorta to the posterior descending artery branch (PDA) of the right coronary artery (RCA) and to the obtuse marginal branch of the left circumflex artery.

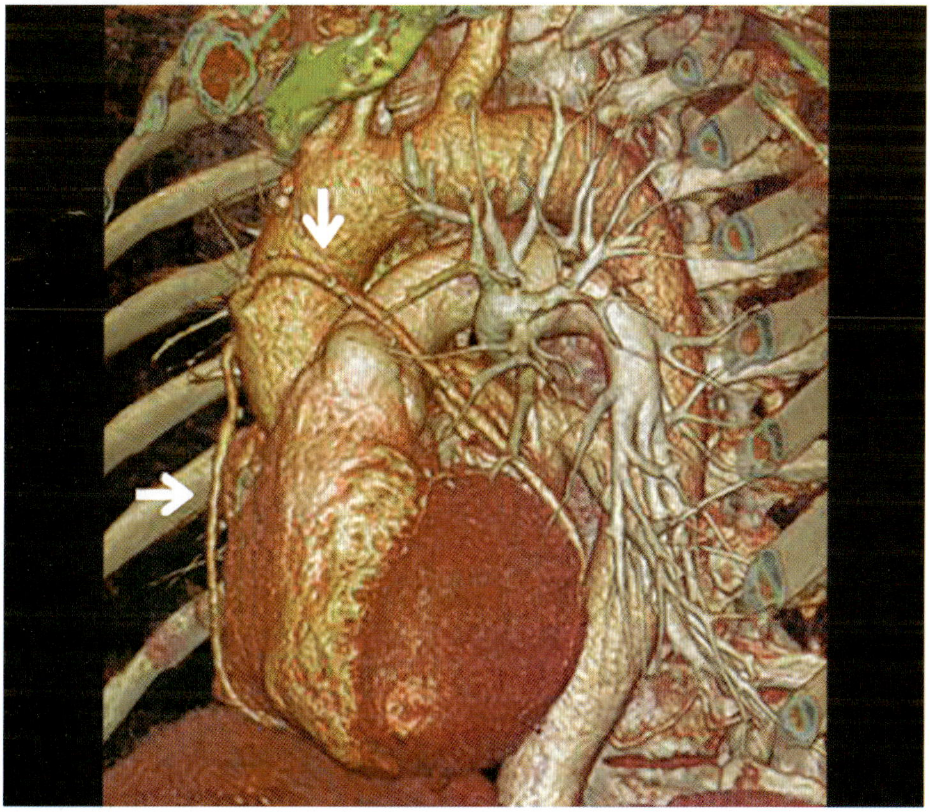

Fig. 8.2B: Chest computed tomography (CT), displayed in an oblique projection, demonstrating saphenous vein bypass grafts (arrows) from the aorta to the posterior descending artery branch (PDA) of the right coronary artery (RCA) and to the obtuse marginal branch of the left circumflex artery.

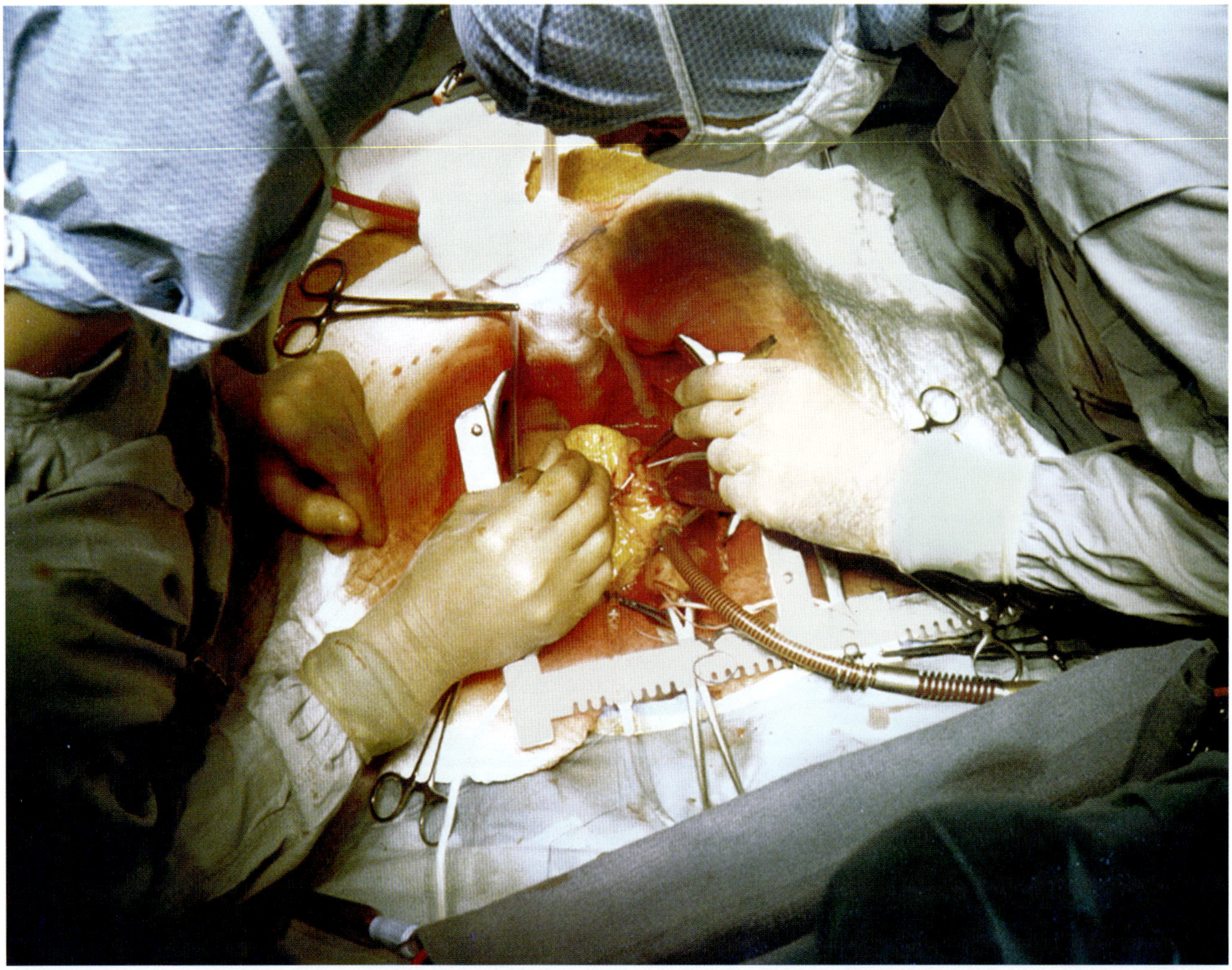

Fig. 8.3: "Birds-eye" view of coronary artery bypass grafting surgery (CABG) procedure. (Image from SeanMack, posted on Wikimedia Commons and en.wikipedia).

the context of perioperative risk profile. Surgical risk can be quantitatively assessed using the STS risk calculator (Table 8.3). Factors that increase risk and may dissuade the surgeon from recommending CABG include poor targets for grafting, cerebrovascular disease (particularly severe carotid stenoses or debilitating stroke), shock, renal failure, immunosuppressants, active malignancy, severe coagulopathy, severe liver disease (Child-Pugh class B or worse), and severely compromised pulmonary status. The presence of diabetes and low LVEF favors recommendation for CABG. Discussion with the patient should include the potential benefits and risks for surgery, expected duration of hospitalization and recovery, and potential alternative treatment options.

CORONARY ARTERY BYPASS PROCEDURES

The technical aspects of CABG have evolved over the last 4 decades. The initial steps in the CABG procedure are induction of general anesthesia with endotracheal intubation and placement of central venous and arterial lines. Next, conduits are harvested to serve as bypass grafts (Figs. 8.6 and 8.7). In most CABG procedures, the left internal mammary artery (LIMA) will be grafted to LAD (Figs. 8.8 to 8.12 and Video 8.1). Use of the LIMA to bypass the LAD is desirable given that this bypass is associated with excellent long-term patency rates and reduced short- and long-term patient mortality. Reversed saphenous vein

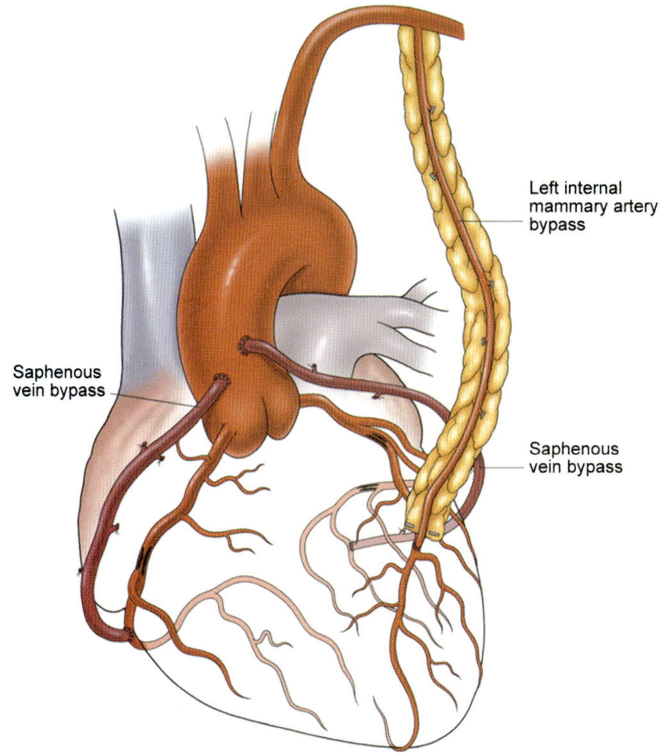

Fig. 8.4A: Schematic illustration of a typical CABG with the left internal mammary artery (LIMA) anastomesed to the left anterior descending artery (LAD) and reverse saphenous vein grafts (SVGs) anastomosed to territories supplied by the left circumflex artery and right coronary artery (RCA), Image courtesy of and by permission of Mayo Foundation for Medical Education and Research. All rights reserved.

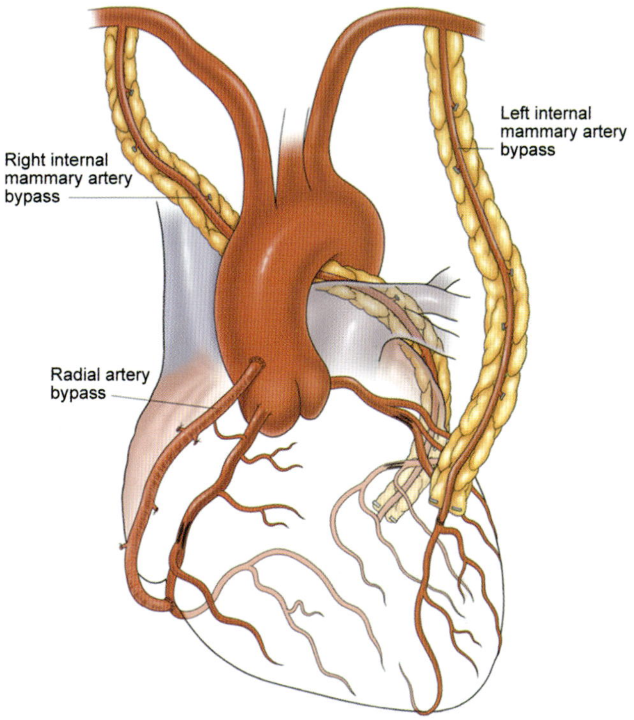

Fig. 8.4B: Schematic illustration of a CABG total arterial revascularization. The left internal mammary artery (LIMA) is anastomosed to the left anterior descending artery (LAD), the right internal mammary artery (RIMA) anastomosed to an obtuse marginal (OM) branch, a free radial artery anastomosed to the right coronary artery (RCA). Image courtesy of and by permission of Mayo Foundation for Medical Education and Research. All rights reserved.

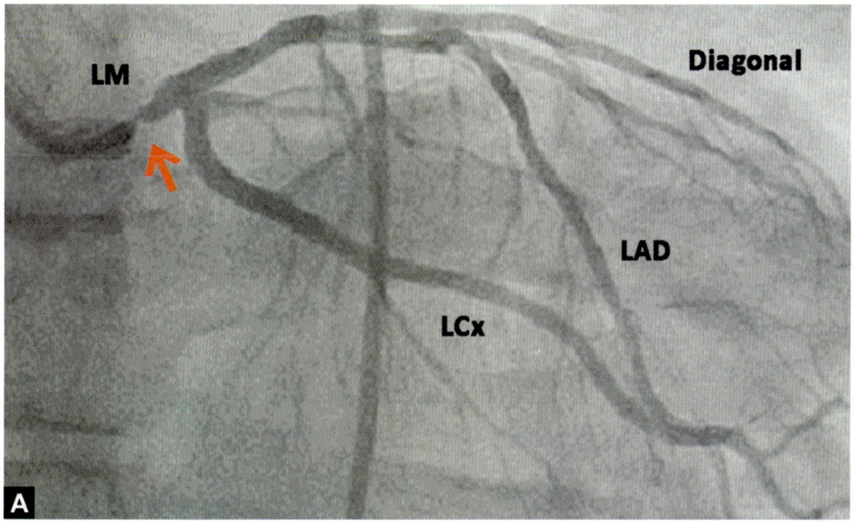

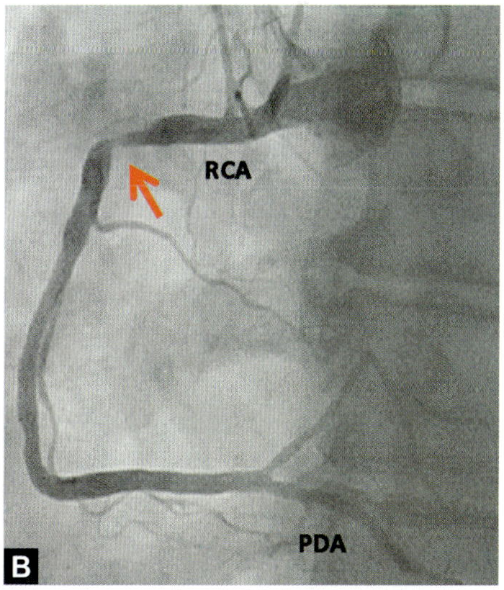

Figs. 8.5A and B: Coronary angiogram in a diabetic patients with acute coronary syndrome. (A) Left coronary artery angiogram showing a tight left main (LM) coronary artery stenosis (arrow). The left circumflex artery (LCx), left anterior descending (LAD) artery, and diagonal branches all appear to be good targets for coronary artery bypass; (B) Angiogram of the right coronary artery (RCA), demonstrating a significant stenosis (arrow) in the proximal segment and a good posterior descending artery (PDA) target for bypass.

Table 8.3: Summary of data input used in the online STS risk calculator for coronary artery bypass surgery.

Procedure • Coronary Artery Bypass (yes/no) • Valve Surgery (yes/no) • VAD implanted or removed(no/implanted/explanted) • Other non-cardiac procedure (yes/no) • Unplanned procedure (yes/no) • Other cardiac procedure (yes/no)
Demographics • Patient age (years) • Gender (male/female) • Black/African American (yes/no) • Asian (yes/no) • Hispanic or Latino (yes/no)
Risk factors • Weight (kg) • Height (cm) • Diabetes (yes/no) • Last Creatinine (mg/dL) • Dialysis (yes/no) • Hypertension (yes/no) • Infectious endocarditis (yes/no) • Chronic lung disease (no/mild/moderate/severe) • Immunosuppresive Rx (yes/no) • Peripheral vascular disease (yes/no) • Cerebovascular disease (yes/no)
Previous CV interventions • Previous CABG (yes/no) • Previous valve (yes/no) • Previous other cardiac – PCI (yes/no)
Preoperative cardiac status • Myocardial infarction (yes/no) • Cardiac presentation (no angina/stable angina/NSTE-ACS/STEMI) • Congestive heart failure (yes/no) • Cardiogenic shock (yes/no) • Rescucitation (yes/no) • Arrhythmia (yes/no)
Preoperative Medications • Inotropes (yes/no)
Hemodynamics and Cath • Number Diseased Vessels (none/one/two/three) • Left Main Disease ≥50% (yes/no) • Ejection Fraction (%) • Aortic Stenosis (yes/no) • Mitral Stenosis (yes/no) • Aortic insufficiency (none/mild/moderate/severe) • Mitral insufficiency (none/mild/moderate/severe) • Tricuspid insufficiency (none/mild/moderate/severe)
Operative • Incidence (first CV surgery/first re-op/second re-op/third re-op/≥Fourth re-op) • Status of the procedure (elective/urgent/emergent/emergent salvage) • IABP (yes/no)

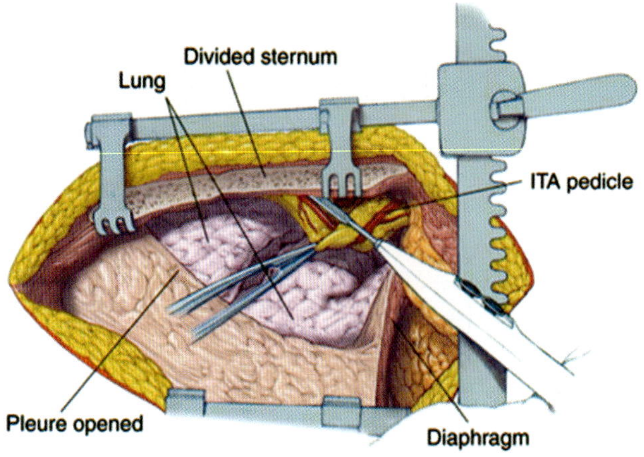

Fig. 8.6: Operative harvest of the left internal mammary artery (LIMA) for use in bypass grafting, Image courtesy of and by permission of Mayo Foundation for Medical Education and Research. All rights reserved.

conduit is the most common choice for additional grafts, to bypass the left circumflex artery (via obtuse marginal grafts), right coronary artery (usually via posterior descending artery and/or posterolateral branch grafts), diagonal branches, and the ramus artery (Figs. 8.13 to 8.16 and Videos 8.2 and 8.3). The choice between endoscopic vein harvesting (EVH) and open harvesting for greater saphenous vein remains somewhat controversial due to reports of possible worsened graft patency rates with EVH, and is the subject on ongoing studies. The right internal mammary artery (RIMA) (Fig. 8.17) or radial artery (Figs. 8.18 and 8.19) may also be used for bypass grafting.

Although the CPB machine (Figs. 8.20A and B) is used in the majority (> 80%) of CABG operations performed today, "off-pump" techniques have also been evolving since the first reports in the 1990s. The CPB involves placing a patient temporarily on a machine to supply circulation and oxygenation, so that cardiac contractions and respiration can be temporarily stopped to facilitate the bypass procedure. The bypass circuit consists of the tubing, a collection chamber, oxygenator, heat exchanger, and the pump (Fig. 8.21). Systemic anticoagulation, usually with heparin 300 units/kg, is administered before inserting the CPB circuit, in order to prevent thrombus formation in the circuit. An aortic cannula is secured into the distal ascending aorta (Fig. 8.22), and a dual stage venous cannula is secured in the right atrium, and advanced down into the inferior vena cava. The venous cannula will collect

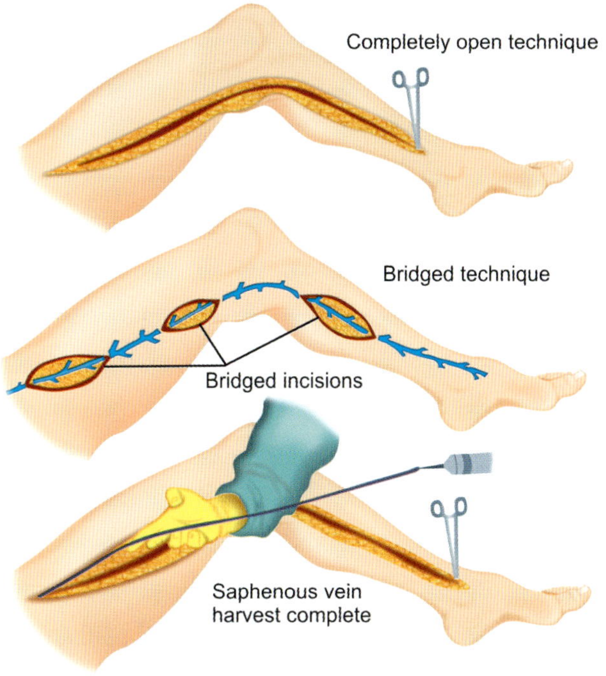

Fig. 8.7A: Open harvesting of the greater saphenous vein. Image courtesy of and by permission of Mayo Foundation for Medical Education and Research. All rights reserved.

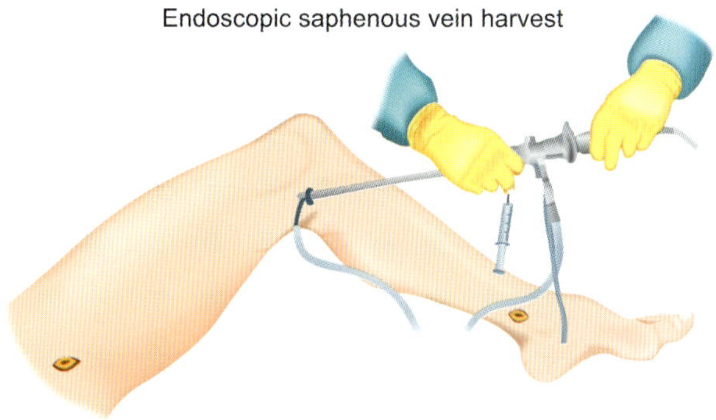

Fig. 8.7B: Endoscopic harvesting of the greater saphenous vein. Image courtesy of and by permission of Mayo Foundation for Medical Education and Research. All rights reserved.

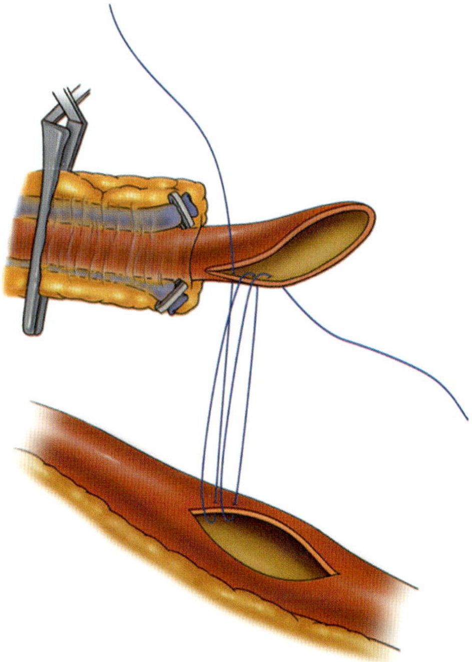

Fig. 8.8: Operative technique of anastomosing the left internal mammary artery (LIMA) to the LAD. Image courtesy of and by permission of Mayo Foundation for Medical Education and Research. All rights reserved.

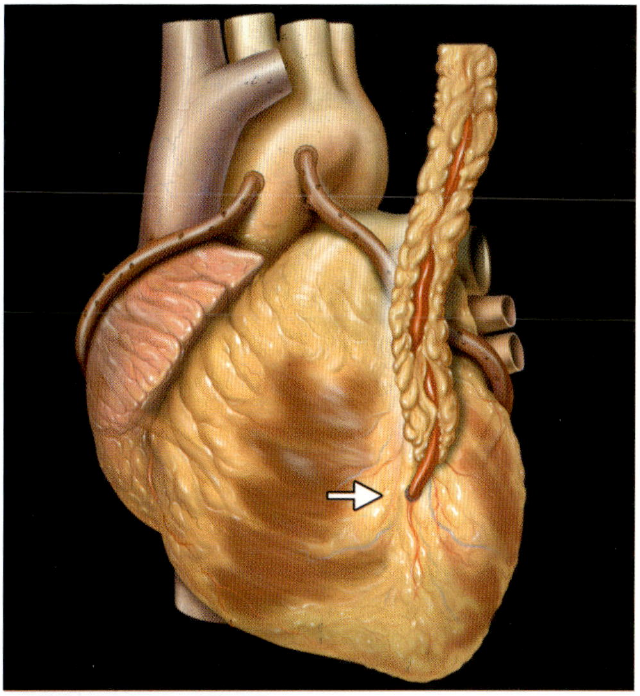

Fig. 8.9: LIMA anastomosis to the LAD (arrow). Two SVGs are also visualized. Image from Patrick J. Lynch and C. Carl Jaffe, MD., posted on Wikimedia Commons.

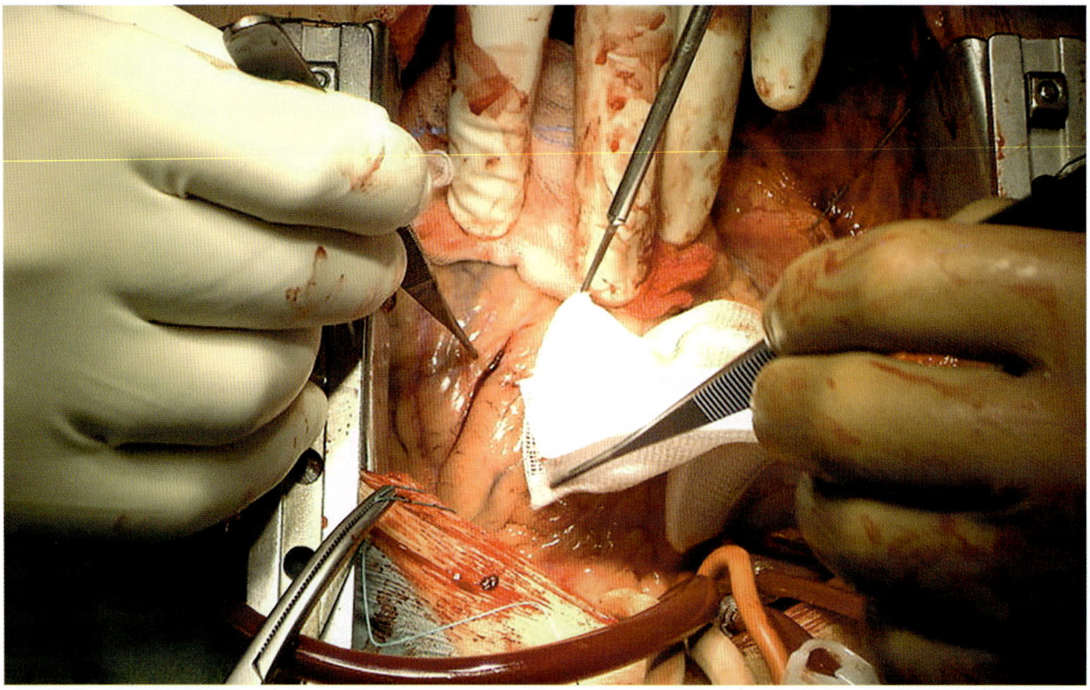

Fig. 8.10: Operative room (OR) image demonstrating dissection of the left anterior descending (LAD) artery from epicardial fat, in preparation for a left internal mammary artery (LIMA) to LAD anastomoses. (From image posted by Dr Arifnajafov, posted on Wikimedia Commons).

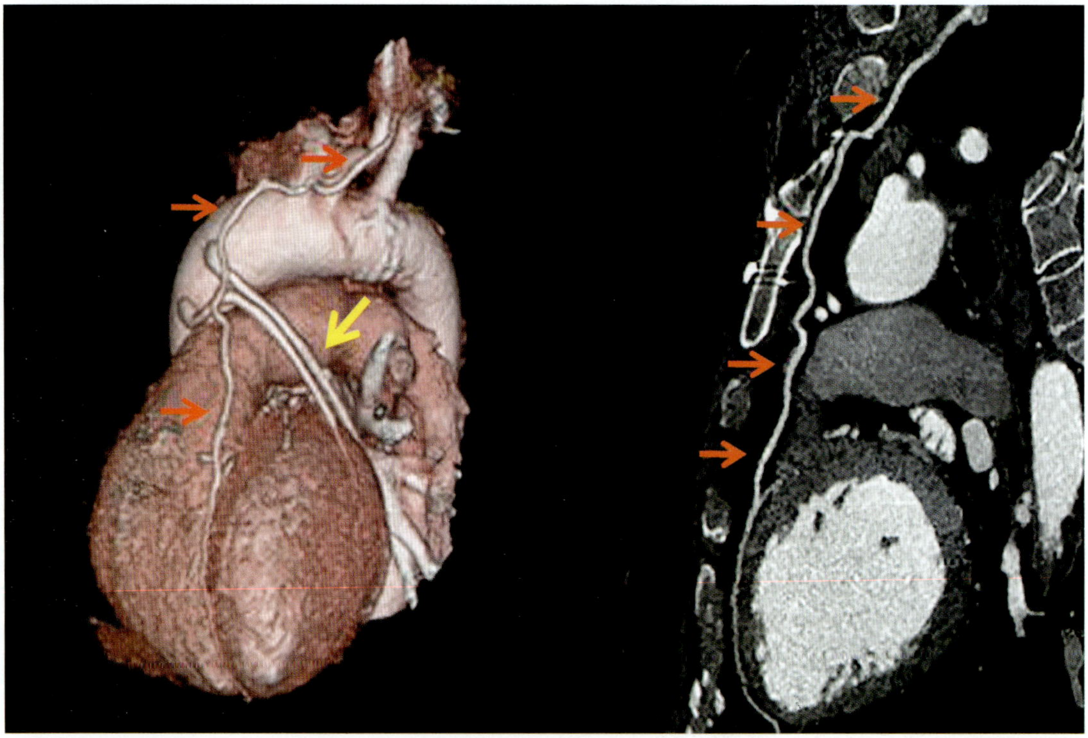

Fig. 8.11: Computed tomography (CT) coronary angiography demonstrating left internal mammary artery (LIMA) (red arrows) to the left anterior descending (LAD). A saphenous vein graft (SVG) to an obtuse marginal (OM) branch (yellow arrow) is also visualized. [Images from Balghith M. (2013). Artery bypass versus PCI using new generation DES. [online] Available from www.intechopen.com/books/artery-bypass/artery-bypass-versus-pci-using-new-generation-des. Accessed February, 2014].

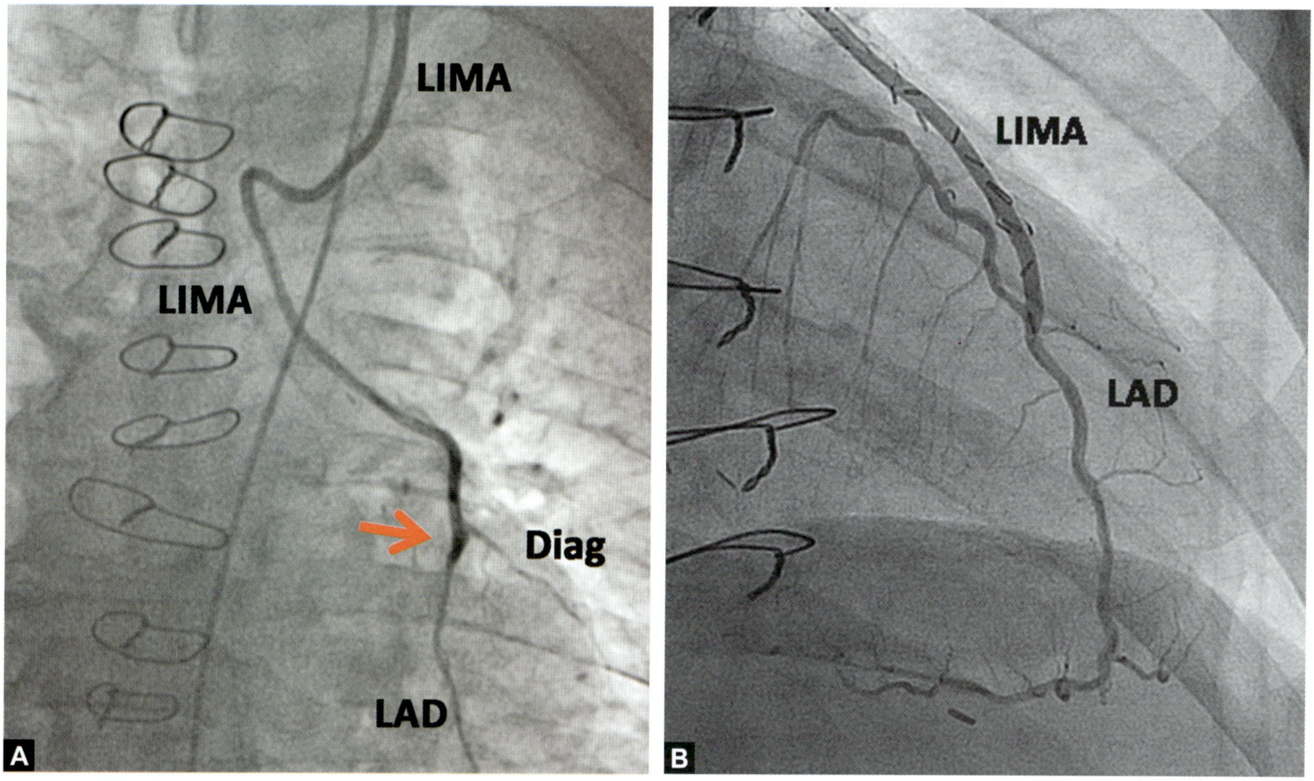

Figs. 8.12A and B: Coronary angiogram of the left internal mammary artery (LIMA) anastomosed to the left anterior descending (LAD). (LIMA: Left internal mammary artery; LAD: Left anterior descending).

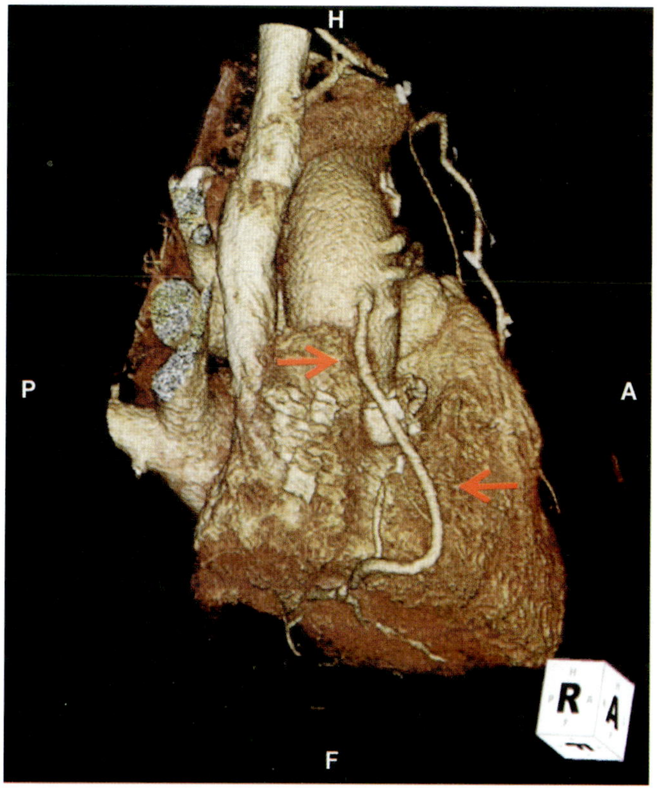

Fig. 8.13: Computed tomography (CT) coronary angiography image of saphenous vein graft (SVG) (arrows) to the right coronary artery (RCA). [Image from Ananthasubramaniam K, Bhatti S, Hakeem A. (2013). Noninvasive modalities for coronary angiography. [online] Available from www.intechopen.com/books/what-should-we-know-about-prevented-diagnostic-and-interventional-therapy-in-coronary-artery-disease/noninvasive-modalities-for-coronary-angiography. (Accessed February, 2014)].

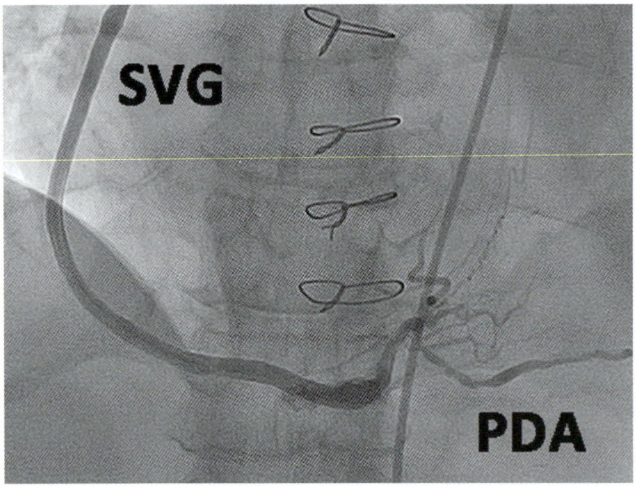

Fig. 8.14: Saphenous vein graft (SVG) anastomosed to the right coronary artery. (PDA: Posterior descending artery).

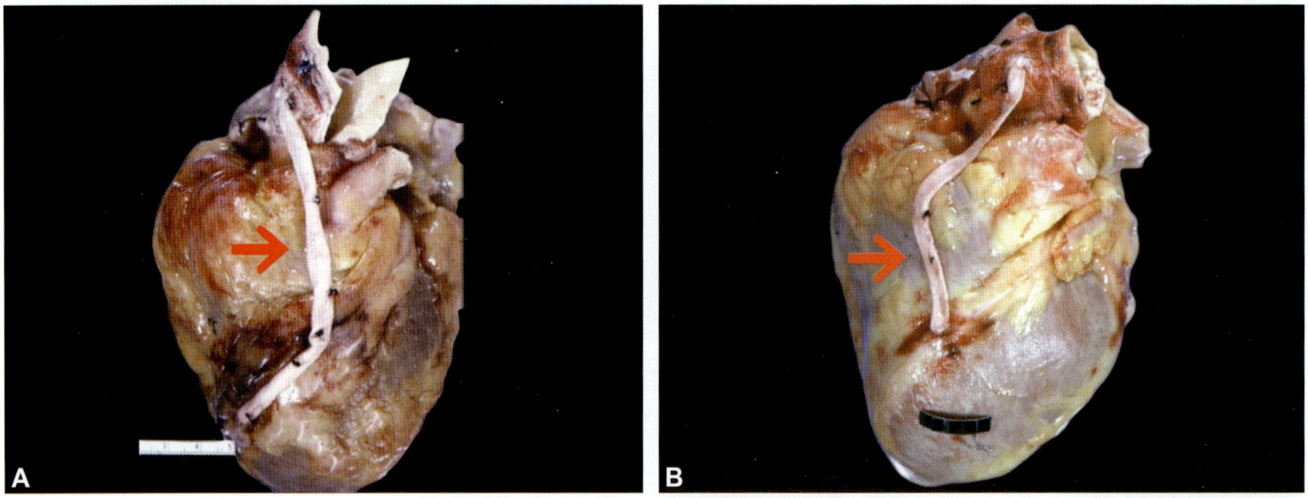

Figs. 8.15A and B: (A) Excised heart specimen showing saphenous vein graft (SVG) to right coronary artery (RCA); (B) SVG to left anterior descending (LAD). [Images from Wikidoc (no author credited)].

venous blood and return it to the pump, where it will then be oxygenated and returned to the arterial circulation via the aortic cannula.

In the "on-pump" technique for CABG, the heart is then arrested by placing a cross-clamp across the ascending aorta, below the aortic cannula, which eliminates blood flow to the coronary arteries. Cardioplegia containing high-dose potassium is then administered to induce cardiac arrest, and can be administered both antegrade, into the aortic root, and retrograde, via the coronary sinus. Once cardioplegia has been administered and the heart is at standstill, the distal coronary anastomoses are then performed. The target site is opened at a location suitable for revascularization, and fine 7-0 or 8-0 polypropylene sutures are generally used to create an end-to-side anastomosis. The technical benefit of using full CPB is that the surgical site will be dry and still. Once the distal anastomoses are completed, the blood is rewarmed, the proximal anastomoses to the aorta are then performed, and the patient is then weaned off CPB.

"Off-pump" CABG, where the heart remains beating throughout the procedure, has the potential benefit of avoiding side effects of the CPB machine. However, in recent clinical trials, including randomized studies, off-pump surgery has not shown significant clinical advantage compared to on-pump. The off-pump procedure is performed by using suction devices to position the heart and to stabilize the target site to allow surgical

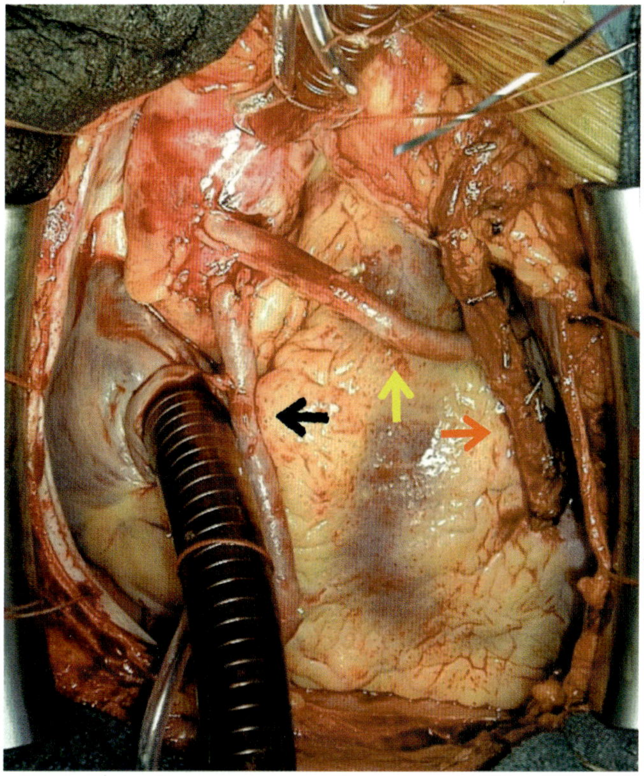

Fig. 8.16: Operative room (OR) image showing left internal mammary artery (LIMA) to left anterior descending (LAD) (red arrow), saphenous vein graft (SVG) to obtuse marginal (OM) (yellow arrow), and SVG to posterior descending artery (PDA) (black arrow). The large venous cannula in the right atrium (RA) is also visualized. [Image from Mandak J. (2013). Peripheral tissue oxygenation during standard and miniaturized cardiopulmonary bypass (direct oxymetric tissue perfusion monitoring study). (online) Available from www.intechopen.com/books/artery-bypass/peripheral-tissue-oxygenation-during-standard-and-miniaturized-cardiopulmonary-bypass-direct-oxymetr. Accessed February, 2014].

manipulation (Figs. 8.23 to 8.25). The coronary target is then temporarily occluded, with the option to place a shunt at the site if needed, and the anastomosis is then completed in a similar fashion as the on-pump technique. There are certain scenarios for which off-pump techniques are important options, such as in patients with severely calcified aorta (porcelain aorta, Fig. 8.26), which is not suitable to the cannulation and clamping required for CPB. In addition, some studies have demonstrated a benefit in outcomes for higher risk patients, such as those with stroke history or renal insufficiency. However, despite the use of these techniques for more than a decade, the technical aspects of off-pump remain more challenging than the on-pump technique, and studies have shown that fewer grafts are performed, resulting in a greater incidence of incomplete revascularization and need for repeat revascularization. The large Randomized On/Off Bypass (ROOBY) trial showed worse short- and midterm outcomes with the off-pump technique. In addition, the CABG Off or On Pump Revascularization Study (CORONARY) and German Off Pump Coronary Artery Bypass Grafting in Elderly Study (GOPCABE) trials did not demonstrate any benefit of off-pump CABG in higher risk patients in the hands of experienced off-pump surgeons when compared to on-pump bypass surgery.

More recent innovations in bypass surgery have included use of robotics and minimally invasive CABG, in which smaller incisions can be used to accomplish off-pump bypass, and hybrid procedures. With hybrid procedures, off-pump techniques are used for the LIMA to LAD anastomosis, and the non-LAD targets are revascularized by stenting. Although these options are now used only in a minority of cases worldwide, further technical developments may increase their use in the future.

COMPLICATIONS OF CABG

Complications of CABG include stroke (1–3%), bleeding (2–4%), mediastinitis (1–2%), arrhythmias (atrial fibrillation 20–40%), myocardial infarction (MI) (1–5%), heart failure, and death (2%). Death is uncommon in patients undergoing elective CABG, but the risk of death is increased in patients undergoing emergency CABG, CABG in the days after an acute MI (particularly a large transmural MI), and patients in cardiogenic shock. Other important factors that increase the risk of death include renal insufficiency, stroke, and peripheral vascular disease.

Immediate graft thrombosis is unusual, accounting for low rates of postoperative MI, because the surgeon will check the grafts meticulously in the operating room. There are several technical methods available to check the graft flow for completeness of revascularization. Most commonly a flow meter is used, which uses Doppler interrogation of the graft directly to confirm adequate flow with minimal obstruction. Another method is to perform fluorescent angiography while the chest is still open, to confirm patent anastomosis and runoff (Figs. 8.27A to C).

Early failure of the LIMA bypass is most commonly related to technical issues in anastomosing the LIMA to the LAD, which is fortunately infrequent (approximately

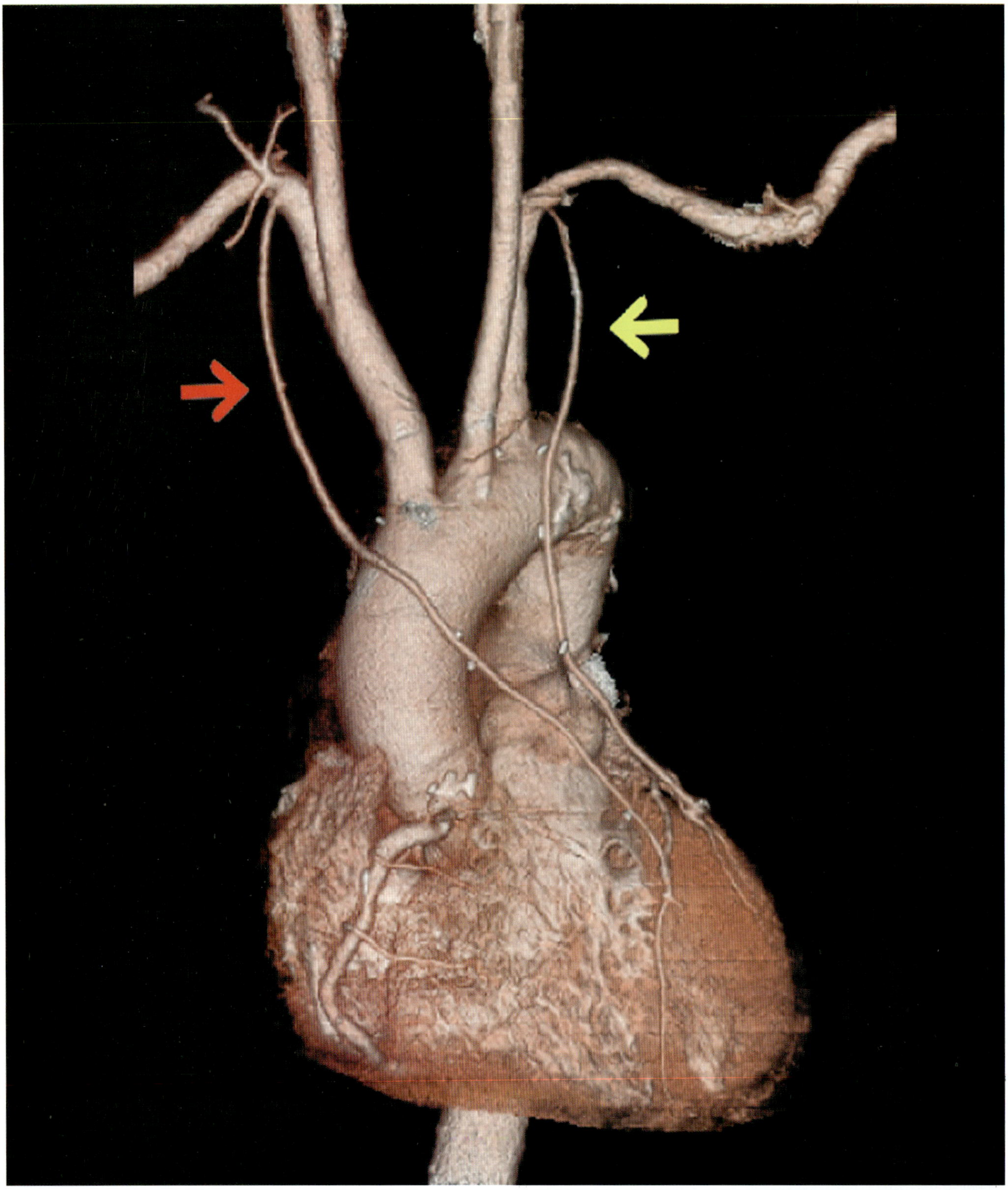

Fig. 8.17: Three-dimensional (3D) volume rendered computed tomography (CT) coronary angiogram showing a right internal mammary artery (RIMA) going to the left anterior descending (LAD) (red arrow). A left internal mammary artery (LIMA) is also present (yellow arrow), anastomosed to a diagonal branch. (Image from Jinzaki M, Yamada M, Kuribayashi S. (2011). Image post-processing and interpretation. [online] Available from www.intechopen.com/books/advances-in-the-diagnosis-of-coronary-atherosclerosis/image-post-processing-and-interpretation. Accessed February, 2014).

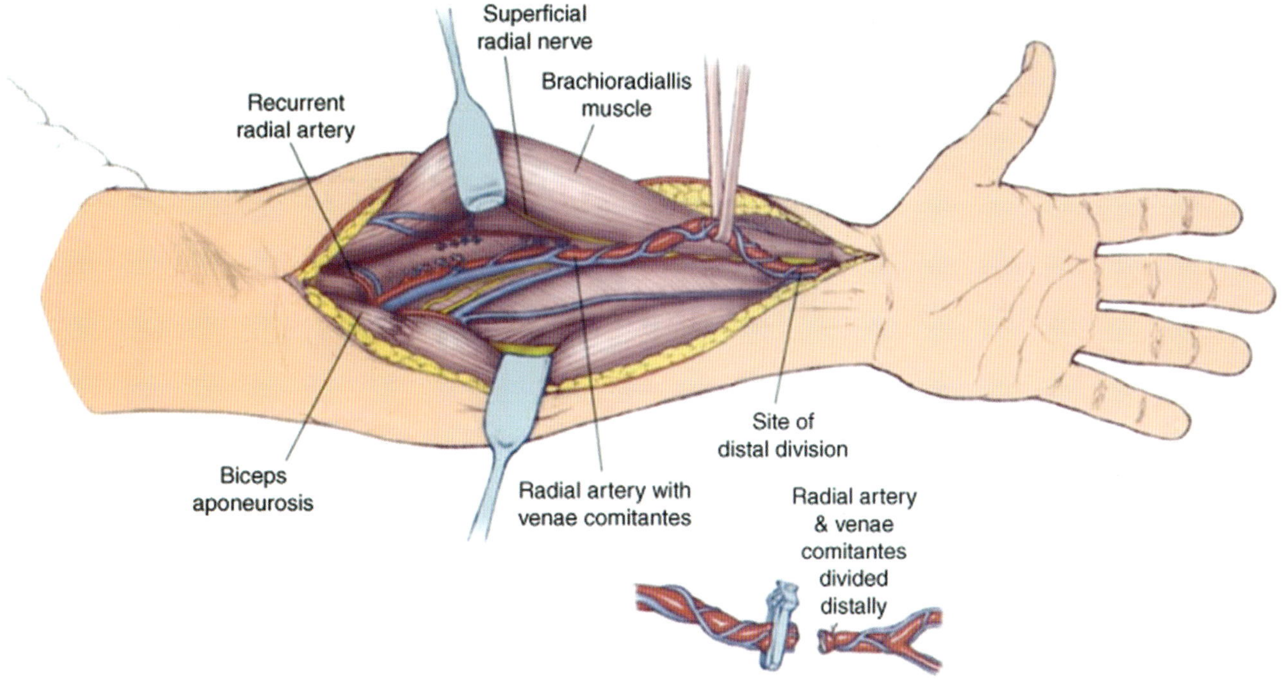

Fig. 8.18: Illustration of operative harvesting of the radial artery for free radial artery bypass grafting. Image courtesy of and by permission of Mayo Foundation for Medical Education and Research. All rights reserved.

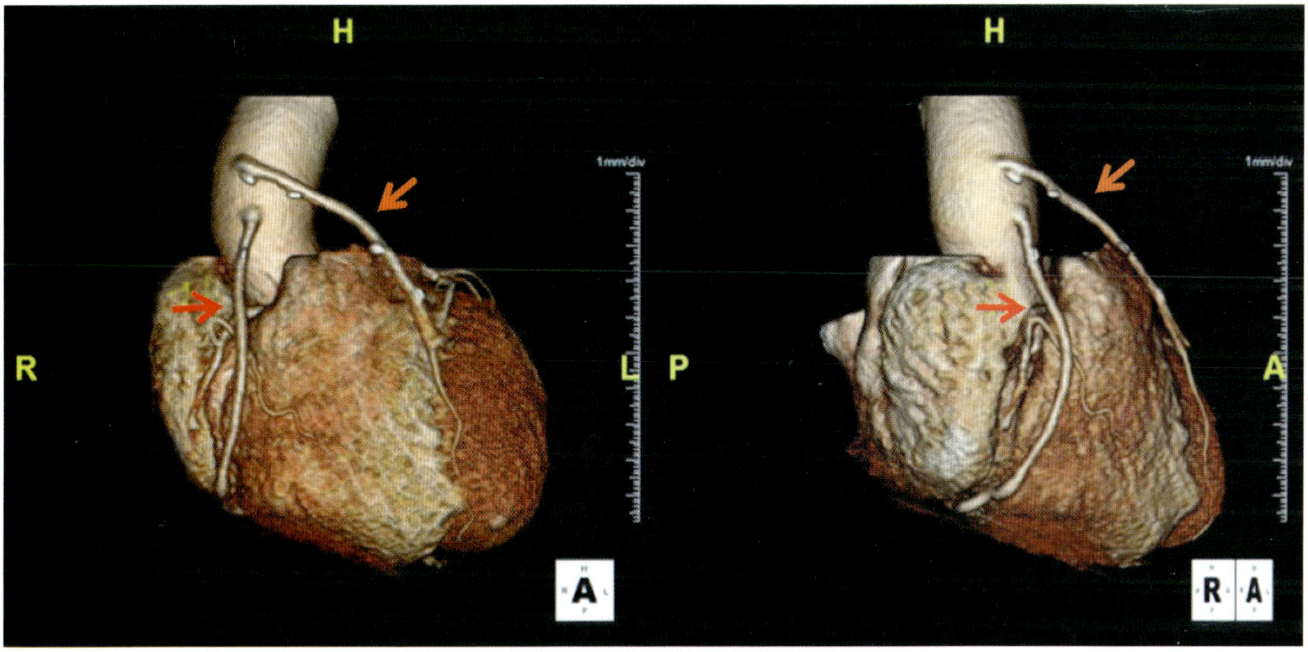

Fig. 8.19: Computed tomography (CT) coronary angiography images showing a free radial artery bypass to the left anterior descending (LAD) (orange arrow). A saphenous vein graft to the posterior descending artery (PDA) (red arrow) is also visualized. [Image from Pelgrim GJ, Oudkerk M, Vliegenthart R. (2013). Computed tomography imaging of the coronary arteries. (online) Available from www.intechopen.com/books/what-should-we-know-about-prevented-diagnostic-and-interventional-therapy-in-coronary-artery-disease/computed-tomography-imaging-of-the-coronary-arteries. Accessed February, 2014].

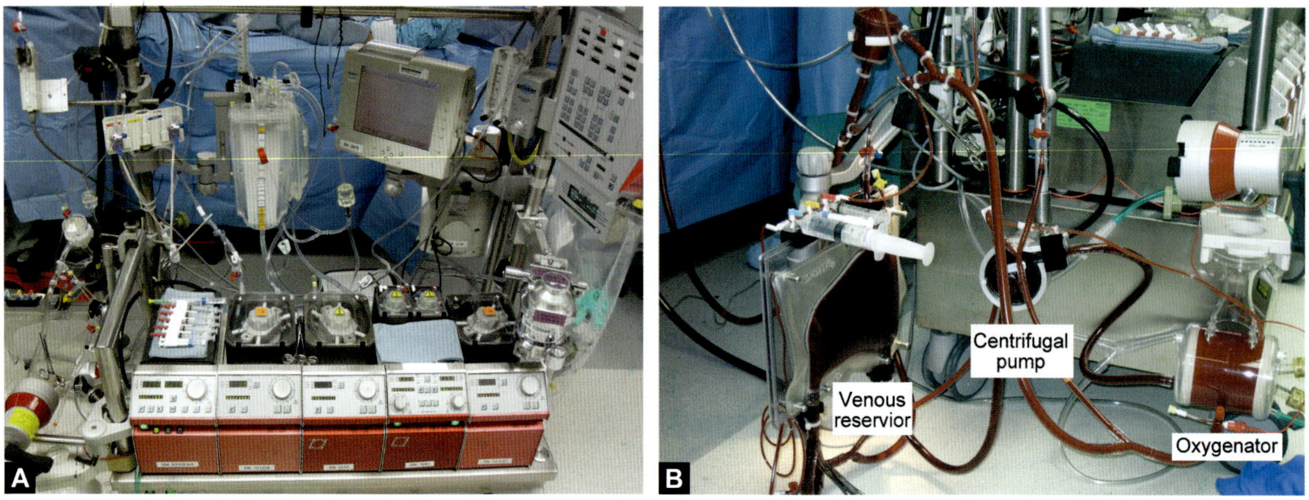

Figs. 8.20A and B: Modern-day cardiopulmonary bypass (CPB) system.

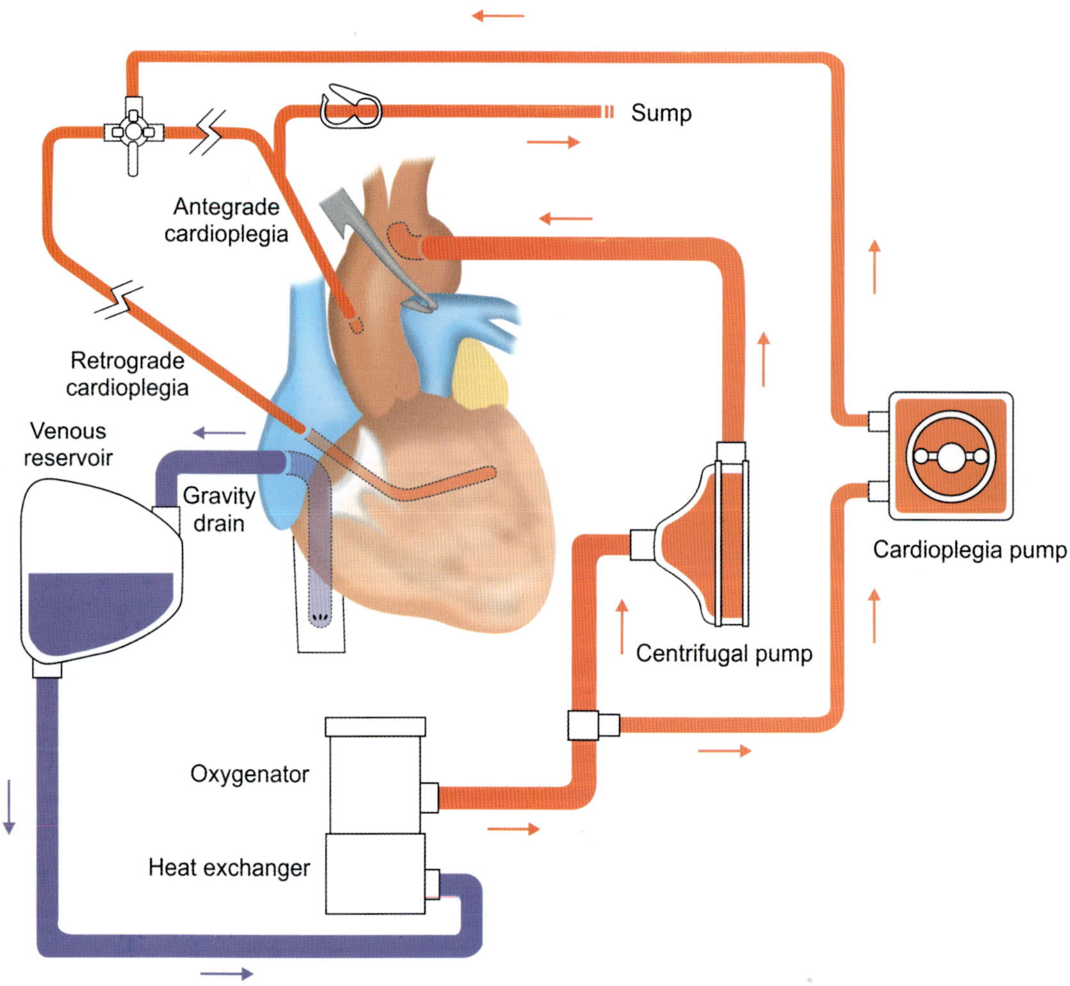

Fig. 8.21: Schematic of the cardiopulmonary bypass (CPB) circuit.

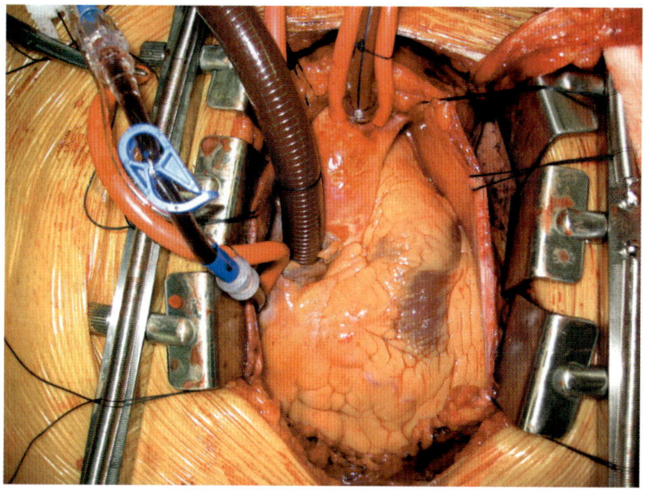

Fig. 8.22A: Cannulation of the ascending aorta and right atrium in a patient on complete cardiopulmonary bypass.

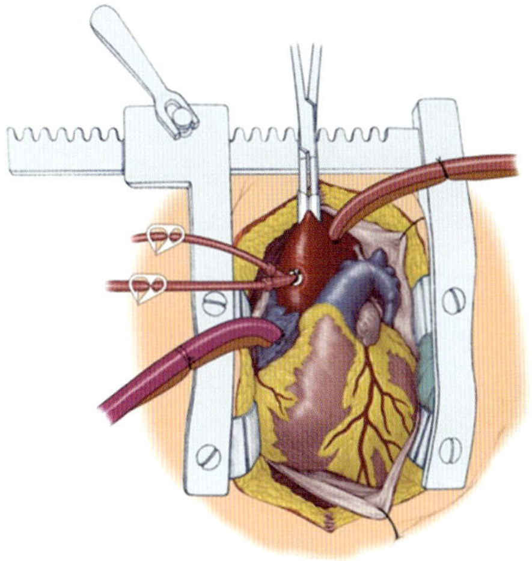

Fig. 8.22B: Illustration of cannulation of the ascending aorta and right atrium for cardiopulmonary bypass. Image courtesy of and by permission of Mayo Foundation for Medical Education and Research. All rights reserved.

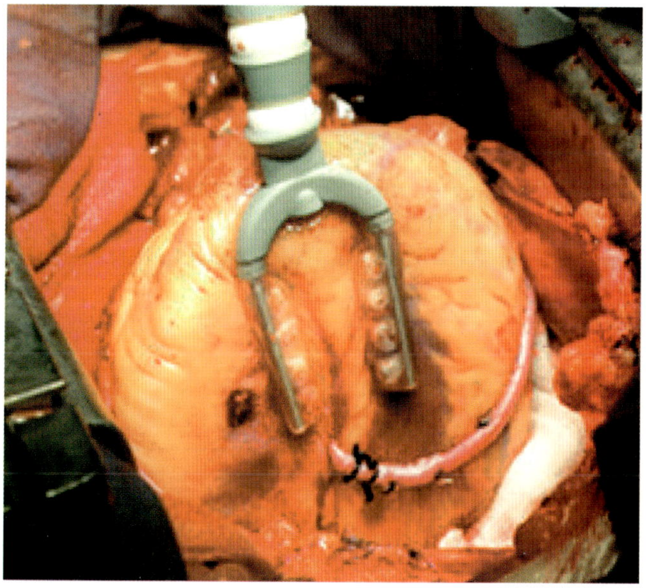

Fig. 8.23: Off-pump, beating heart CABG. Saphenous vein graft distal anastomosis has been performed to the right posterior descending artery with heart stabilizer in place. Image from Gu CX et al. Surgical treatment for diffuse coronary artery disease. In Aronow W (ed). Artery Bypass. Intechweb.org.

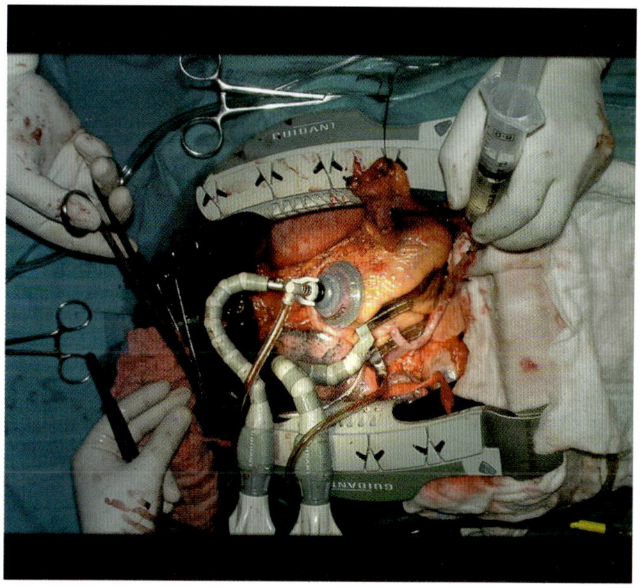

Fig. 8.24: Use of the off-pump suction positioner on the RV free wall in a patient undergoing off-pump CABG. Image from Vettath MP et al. Re-engineering in OPCAB surgery. In Narin C (ed). Special topics in cardiac surgery. Intechweb.org.

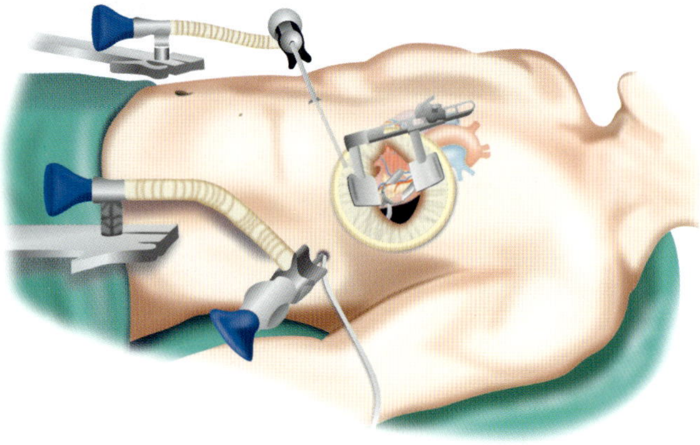

Fig. 8.25A: Illustration of minimally invasive direct coronary artery bypass (Mid-CAB) procedure. Image courtesy of Medtronic, Inc.

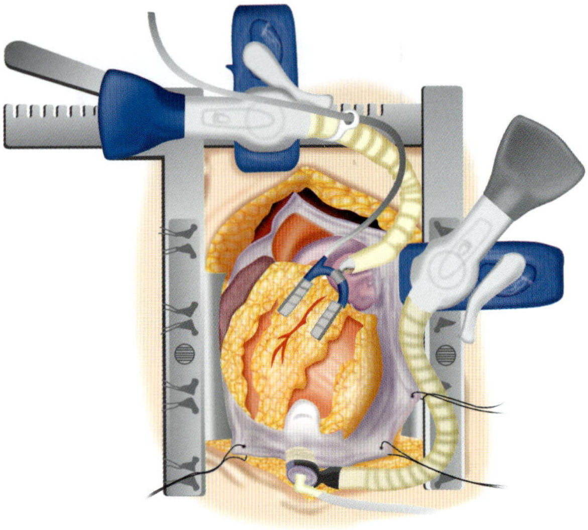

Fig. 8.25B: Stabilizer used in beating heart surgery.

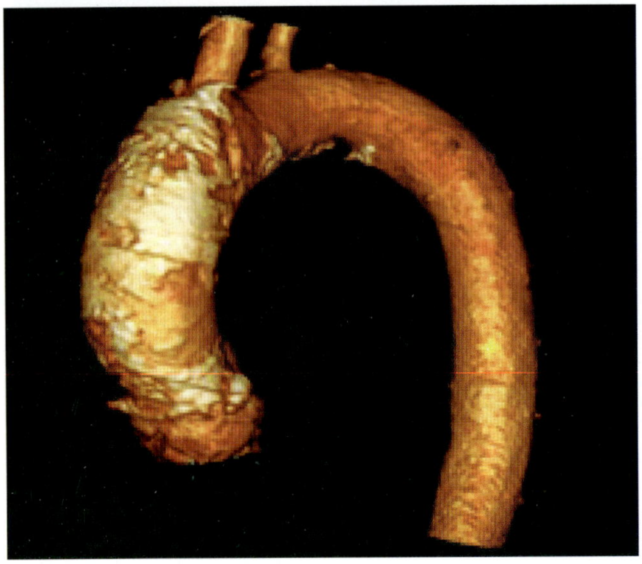

Fig. 8.26: Electrocardiogram (ECG)-gated computed tomography (CT) scan of a patient with a heavily calcified ascending aorta (porcelain aorta). [Image from Akin I et al. Current indications for transcatheter aortic valve implanation. In Chen YF and Luo CY (Ed). Aortic valve. Intechweb.org].

2–10%), and late failure is unusual if the LAD target runoff is good. In contrast, the incidence of saphenous vein graft (SVG) occlusion is higher, at approximately 10–20% after 1 year and approximately 25–50% at 10 years (Figs. 8.28 and 8.29 and Video 8.4). Early occlusion is related to thrombosis, possibly caused by endothelial injury or technical factors, or poor conduit or target quality, whereas longer-term stenosis and occlusion is related to development of intimal hyperplasia, which then provides a foundation for development of atherosclerosis.

A very rare complication of CABG is pseudoaneurysm formation at the site of the proximal anastomosis between a SVG and the ascending aorta (Figs. 8.30A and B).

PATIENT MANAGEMENT AND FOLLOW-UP

Postdischarge, patients are instructed to refrain from activities such as heavy lifting which can compromise sternal healing for 6–8 weeks. Short-term follow-up includes assessment of patient clinical status and inspection of the mediastinal wound and vein graft incision sites. Routine stress testing or bypass imaging by CT angiography or cardiac catheterization in asymptomatic patients is not recommended. Aspirin has been shown to increase the incidence of SVG patency for the first year after bypass surgery, and almost all patients who undergo CABG should be treated with lifelong aspirin therapy. Whether additional treatment with a second antiplatelet agent, such as clopidogrel, has any additional benefit has not been established.

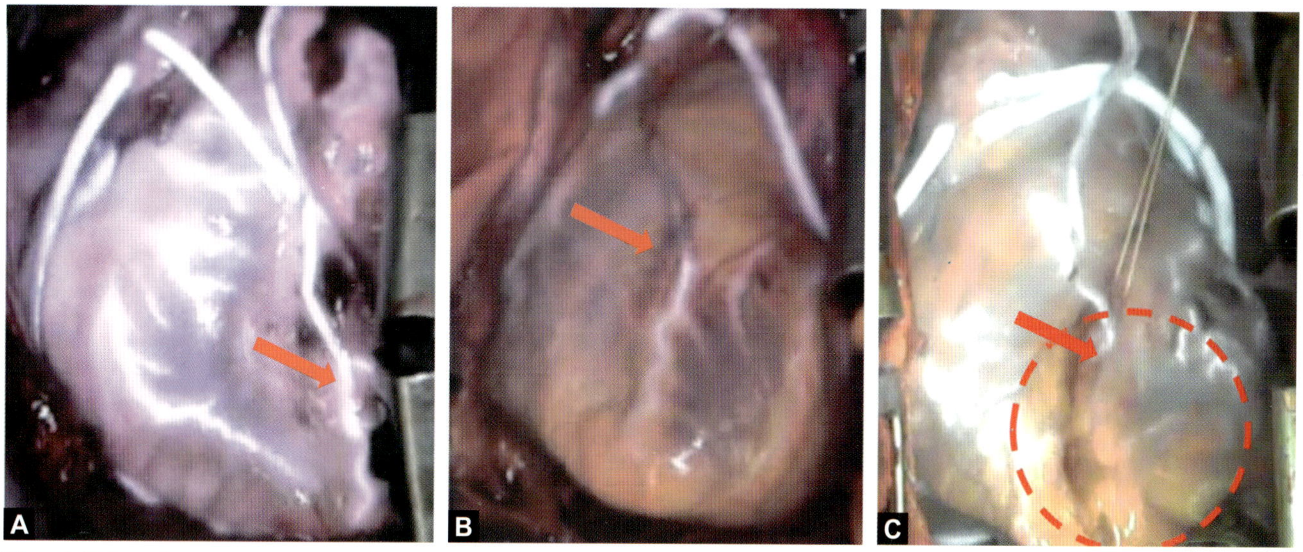

Figs. 8.27A to C: HyperEye Medical System (HEMS) assessment of coronary arterial grafts. Arrows indicate coronary anastomose. (A) Smooth opacification of graft and distal coronary artery; (B) Delayed graft flow; (C) Absence of fluorescence in the left anterior descending (LAD) despite opacification of the left internal mammary artery (LIMA) raft. Dashed circle represents area of compromised blood flow. [Image and figure legend from Yamamoto M et al. Intraoperative Indocyanine Green Imaging Technique in Cardiovascular Surgery. In Aronow W (ed), Artery Bypass. Intechweb.org].

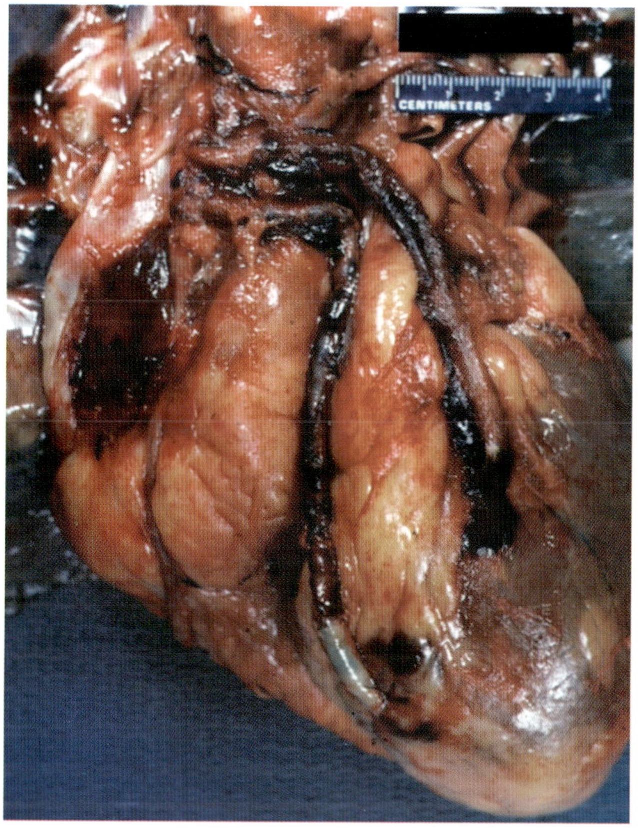

Fig. 8.28: Gross pathology specimen demonstrating completely thrombosed saphenous vein grafts (SVGs). (Image from Cafer Zorkun, posted on Wikidoc).

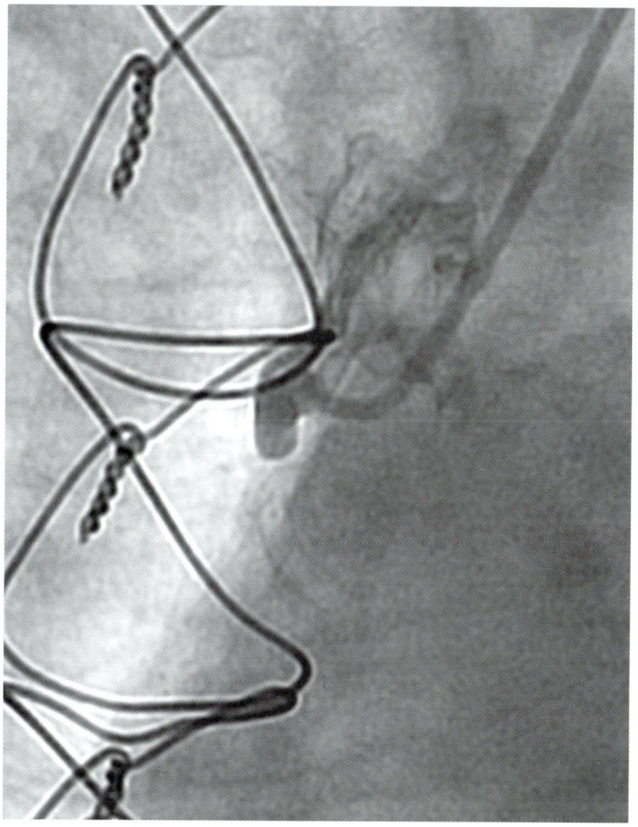

Fig. 8.29: Cineangiogram demonstrating an occluded saphenous vein graft to the right coronary artery. Image courtesy of Glenn N Levine, MD.

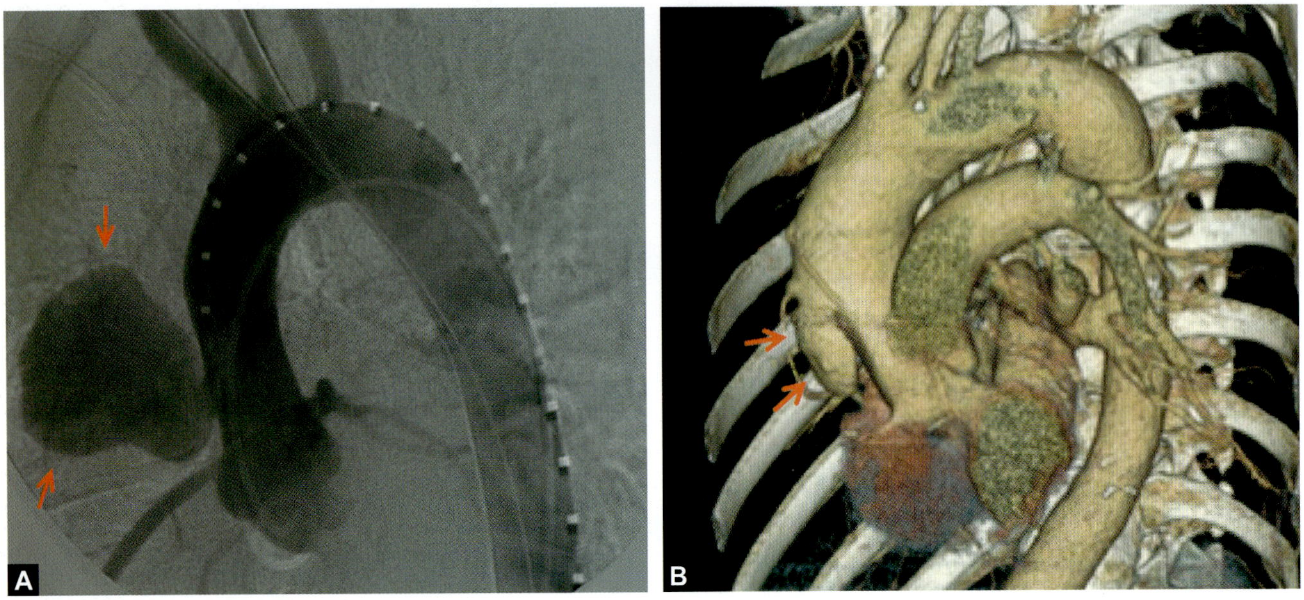

Figs. 8.30A and B: Pseudoaneurysm formation (arrows) in the area of saphenous vein graft (SVG) anastomosis to the ascending thoracic aorta. (A) Digital subtraction angiography. (B) Three-dimensional (3D) volume rendered computed tomography (CT) angiography. [Images from Saadi EK et al. Endovascular treatment of ascending aorta: the last frontier?. In Aronow W (ed), Artery Bypass. Intechweb.org].

VIDEO LEGENDS

Video 8.1: Left internal mammary artery (LIMA) to left anterior descending (LAD).

Video 8.2: Saphenous vein graft (SVG) to obtuse marginal (OM) branch.

Video 8.3: Saphenous vein graft (SVG) to posterior descending artery (PDA).

Video 8.4: Saphenous vein graft (SVG) occluded.

REFERENCES

Favaloro RG. Critical analysis of coronary artery bypass graft surgery: a 30-year journey. J Am Coll Cardiol. 1998;31(4 Suppl B): 1-63B.

Loop FD, Lytle BW, Cosgrove DM, et al. Influence of the internal-mammary-artery graft on 10-year survival and other cardiac events. N Engl J Med. 1986;314 (1):1-6.

Mohr F, Morice MC, Kappetein AP, et al. Coronary artery bypass graft surgery versus percutaneous coronary intervention in patients with three-vessel disease and left main coronary disease: 5 year follow-up of the randomized, clinical SYNTAX trial. Lancet. 2013;381:629-38.

Section 2

Valvular Heart Disease

Chapters

- Normal Valve Anatomy and Function
- Aortic Stenosis
- Aortic Regurgitation
- Mitral Stenosis and Percutaneous Mitral Valvotomy
- Mitral Regurgitation
- Mitral Valve Prolapse
- Right-Sided Valvular Heart Disease
- Endocarditis
- Transcatheter Aortic Valve Replacement
- Valve Surgery and Prosthetic Heart Valves

CHAPTER

9

Normal Valve Anatomy and Function

Alvin S Blaustein, Anita Deswal, Glenn N Levine

INTRODUCTION

The heart valves (Fig. 9.1A) are a marvel of biomechanical engineering. Over the course of a lifetime, a heart valve may open and close a billion times or more. Valve dysfunction, either stenosis or regurgitation, may be a consequence of fetal development, a primary abnormality acquired during adulthood, or as a secondary consequence of secondary processes such as myocardial disease, pulmonary disease, or coronary artery disease.

The two atrioventricular (AV) valves, located between the atria and ventricles are the mitral valve and tricuspid valve. The two semilunar valves, located between the ventricles and pulmonary artery and aorta that exit the heart, are the aortic and pulmonic valves. The mitral, aortic, and tricuspid valves all share the fibrous skeleton, while the pulmonic valve is slightly more basal (Figs. 9.1B to D).

The AV valves are prevented from prolapse or inversion by the chordae tendineae and papillary muscles (collectively referred to as the subvalvular apparatus). Pressure gradients, between the atria and ventricles in the case of the AV valves, and between the ventricles and pulmonary artery/aorta, lead to opening and closing of the valves. Closure of the mitral and tricuspid valves leads to the S1 heart sound; closure of the aortic and pulmonic valves leads to the S2 heart sound (Fig. 9.2).

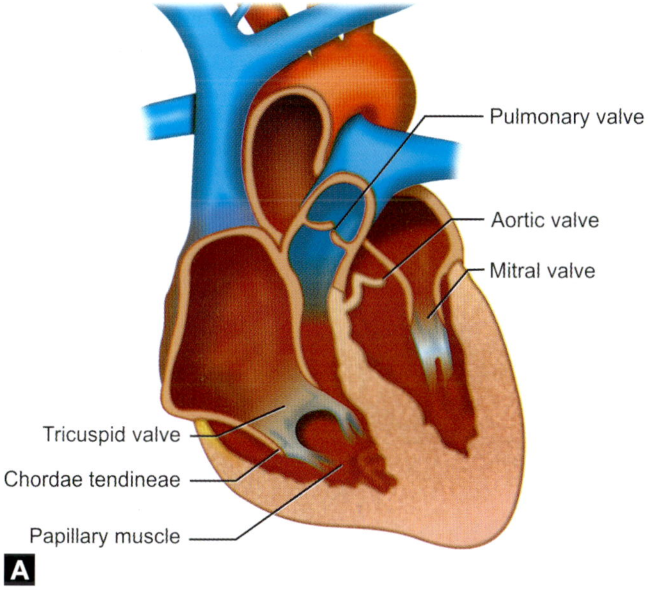

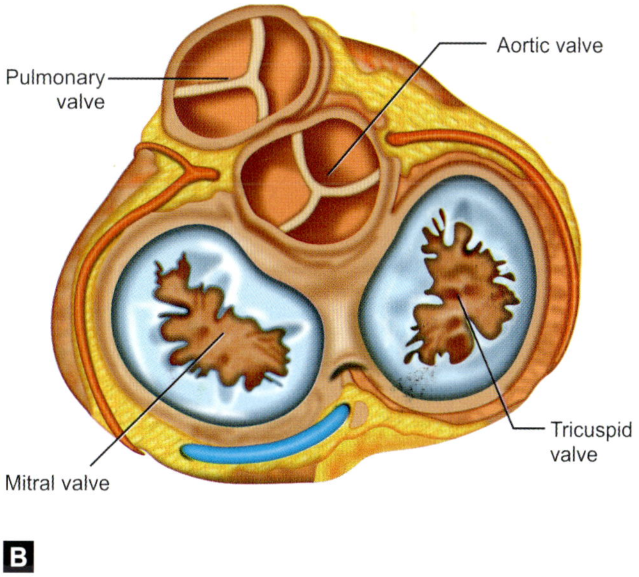

Figs. 9.1A and B: Schematic illustration of the four valves of the heart and their anatomic locations; (B) The four valves of the heart. The aortic, mitral and tricuspid valves are positioned on roughly the same plane on the heart's fibrous skeleton. The pulmonic valve is seated slightly basal to the other valves.

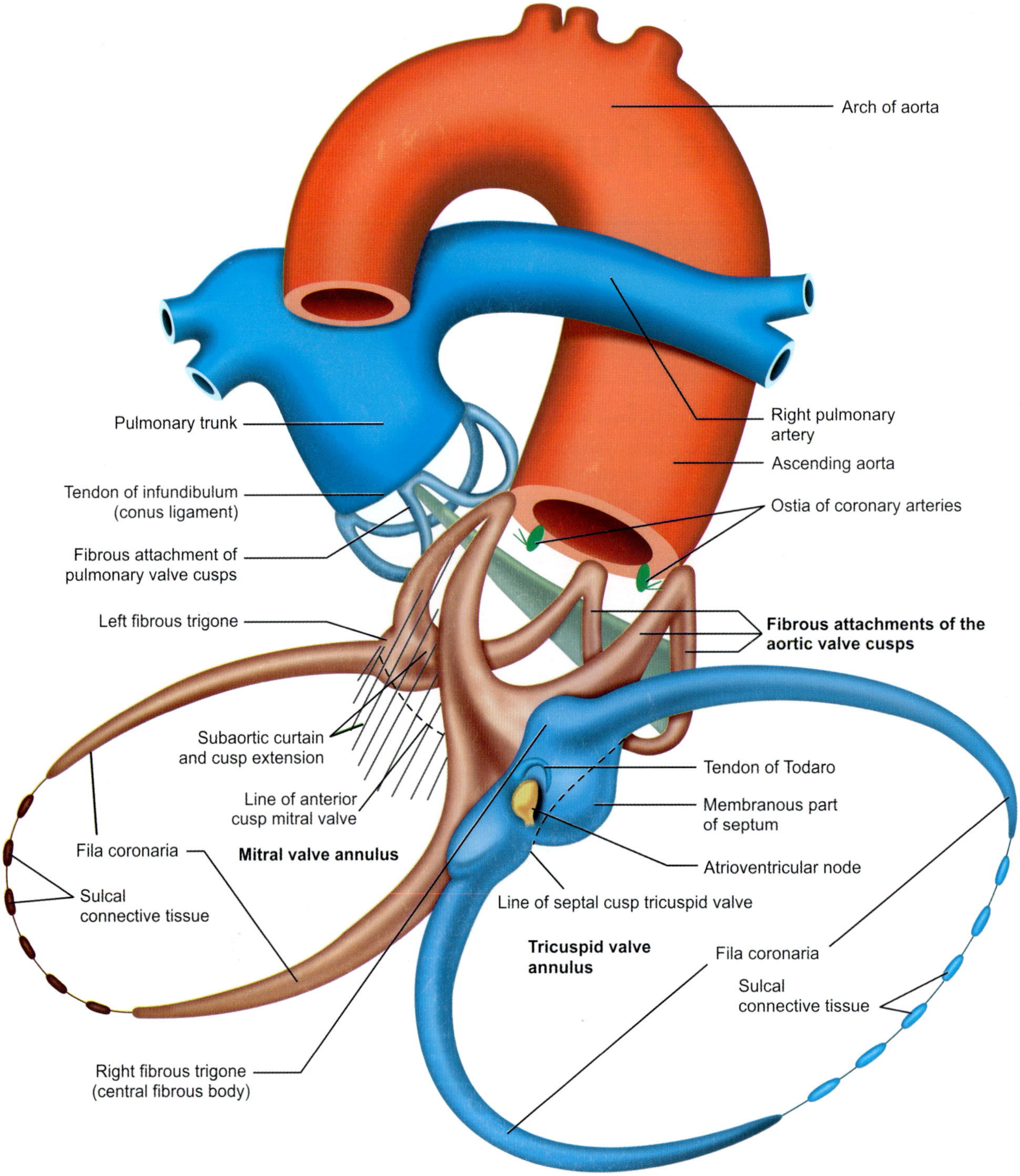

Fig. 9.1C: Schematic illustration of the fibrous skeleton.

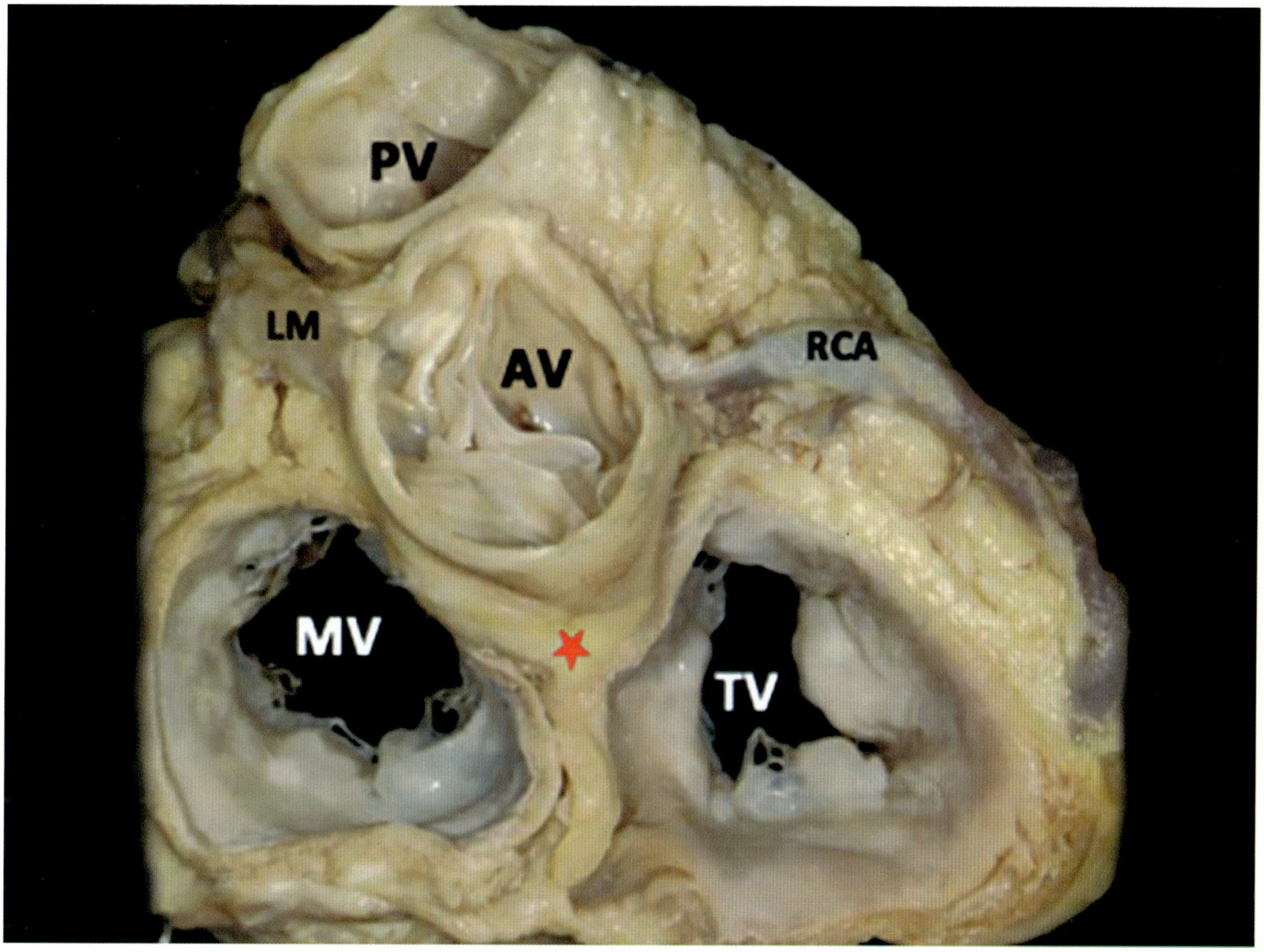

Fig. 9.1D: Gross pathology image of the four cardiac valves in relation to the fibrous skeleton. Viewed from the superior aspect, the base of the heart with most of the atria cutaway shows the aortic valve (AV) wedged between the two atrioventricular valves (MV and TV). Deep to the dissection plane illustrated, the three valves come together at the right fibrous trigone or central fibrous body (red star), while PV is separate from the fibrous skeleton of the heart. [Image and legend text courtesy of Dr Philip C Ursell, Department of Pathology, UCSF. Image from Cheitlin M, Ursell P. Cardiac Anatomy. In Chatterjee K et al. (ed). Cardiology—An Illustrated Textbook. New Delhi, India: Jaypee Brothers Medical Publishers (P) Ltd.]. (MV: Mitral valve; TV: Tricuspid valve; PV: Pulmonary valve; RCA: Right coronary artery; LM: Left main coronary artery).

MITRAL VALVE

The mitral valve is situated between the left atrium and left ventricle and functions to prevent regurgitation of blood back into the left atrium during ventricular systole (Figs. 9.3 and 9.4 and Video 9.1). The mitral valve is a bicuspid valve, and gets its name from its resemblance to a bishop's miter. The two leaflets of the mitral valve are named: (1) the anterior (or anteromedial) leaflet and (2) the posterior (or posterolateral) leaflet. Each leaflet is divided into three scallops, designated from anterolateral to posteromedial location as A1, A2 and A3, and P1, P2 and P3, respectively (Figs. 9.5A and B). Leaflets are inserted into the fibrous cardiac skeleton. The core of the leaflets is largely collagen. Near their origin, there is a layer of atrial musculature, whereas near the leaflet margins there are elastin fibrils that allow the margins to stretch, accommodating changes in pressure and volume. The leaflets are tethered by chordae tendineae to medial and lateral papillary muscles, supported by the ventricular myocardium (Fig. 9.6). The chordae are coiled collagen fibrils surrounded by a thin layer of elastin that function to maintain coaptation, as applied forces vary with load. The collagen components continue into the body of the leaflet,

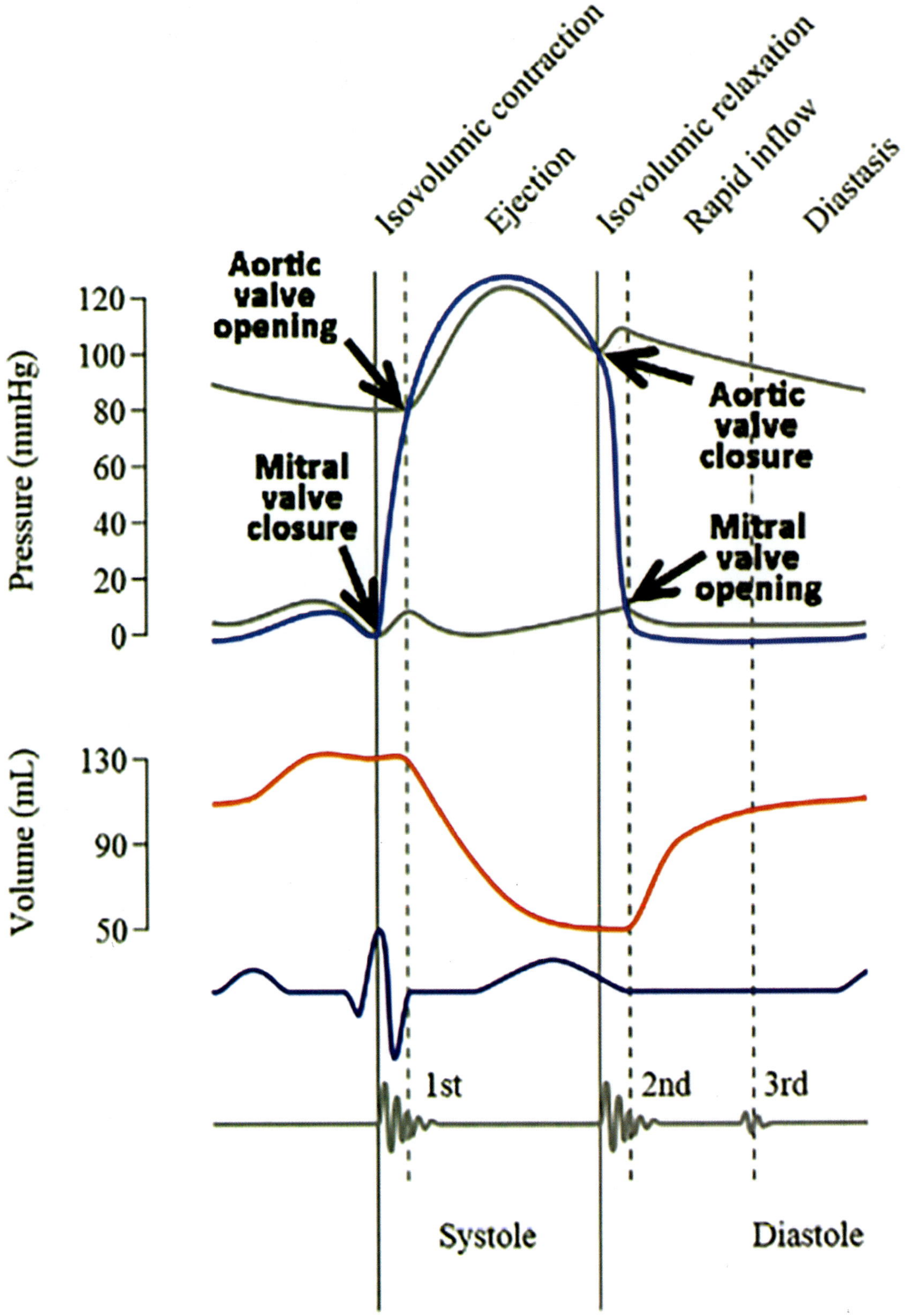

Fig. 9.2: Modified Wiggins diagram, highlighting the timing of and physiology behind the opening and closing of the aortic and mitral valve and S1 and S2. (Image modified from an image created and posted by Daniel Chang, Distny QX, posted on Wikimedia Commons).

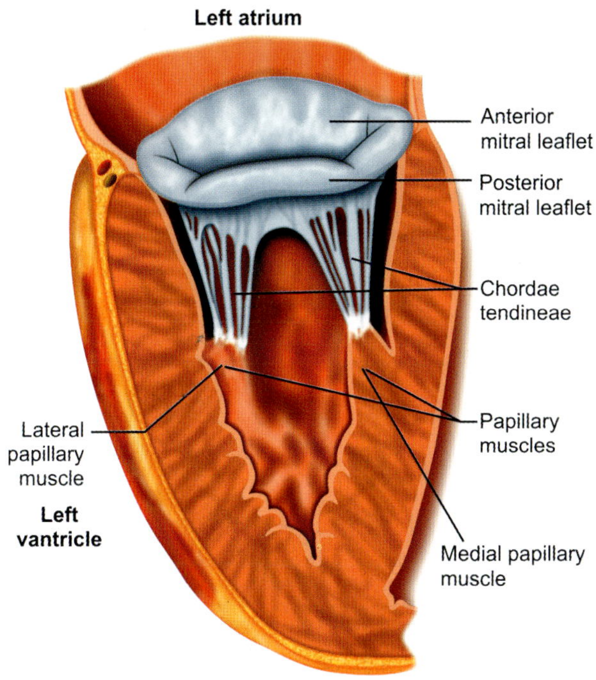

Fig. 9.3: Schematic illustration of the mitral valve.

forming a continuum with leaflet collagen. Chordae from each papillary muscle are connected to both leaflets, distributing forces radially and longitudinally. The anterior leaflet guards approximately 2/3 the area of the mitral valve, and the posterior leaflet occupies about 2/3 of the annular circumference. The mitral and aortic valves are in close proximity, and there is a fibrous continuity between the mitral and aortic valves.

A normal mitral valve orifice is 4–6 cm^2 in area. In a normal heart, approximately 75% of blood that travels across the mitral valve will travel across it in the early diastolic filling phase. This passive blood through is the result of left ventricular relaxation. Blood flow during this time is reflected on Doppler echocardiography as the *E wave*. Left atrial contraction leads to approximately 25% of total blood flow across the mitral valve and is reflected on Doppler echocardiography as the *A wave* (Fig. 9.7).

Numerous primary and secondary disease processes can lead to valve dysfunction. Mitral stenosis is most commonly due to rheumatic heart disease effecting leaflet mobility, and less often in adults, calcification of the annulus and base of the leaflets. Mitral regurgitation may be due to primary processes that affect the valve such as myxomatous degeneration, rheumatic heart disease, or endocarditis. Secondary (functional) mitral regurgitation may result from cardiomyopathies, tethering, mitral annulus dilation, and papillary muscle dysfunction or chordal rupture, as well as numerous other processes.

AORTIC VALVE

The aortic valve (Figs. 9.8 to 9.11 and Videos 9.2 and 9.3) is a semilunar valve that in 99% of persons consists of three leaflets: (1) right cusp, (2) left cusp, and (3) non-coronary cusp. In 1% of patients, the valve is bicuspid. Extremely rarely, the valve is unicuspid or quadricuspid. The aortic valve is situated between the left ventricle and aorta, at the basal ring which forms the base of a configuration known as the coronet. The basal ring is grossly defined by the plane formed by the nadir of the three cusps. The cusps curve up, inserted into the aortic sinuses in which inverted triangles of elastic aortic sinuses interdigitate with more fibrous tissue of the cusps at the surgical annulus. The valve cusps prevent regurgitation of blood from the aorta back into the left ventricle. A small fibrous bulge called the *nodule of Arantius* is present at the center-free edge of each cusp. This structure may help facilitate valve closure and coaptation during ventricular diastole. Commissures between each cusp are composed of collagen fibers attached to the aorta's media and help anchor and support the cusps.

Cusps are composed of collagen and elastic fibers which are arrayed radially along curve of the cusp near its ventricular surface (ventricularis). On the aortic surface (fibrosum) collagen is arrayed circumferentially preventing cusp prolapse. This construct maintains curvature, assuring overlap of the cusp margins and sustaining coaptation during diastole by distributed forces from the column of aortic blood radially as well as longitudinally. The normal aortic valve is approximately 3 cm^2 in area.

Causes of valvular stenosis include degenerative calcified disease (which in reality may be an inflammatory process) and rheumatic disease. Patients with bicuspid aortic valves are predisposed to aortic stenosis and often present in the 5th decade of life. Valvular regurgitation may be the result of degenerative processes, endocarditis, rheumatic heart disease, and dilation of the aortic annulus due to aortic root dilation. Figure 9.12 shows the auscultatory findings with normal aortic valve function, with aortic stenosis, and with aortic regurgitation.

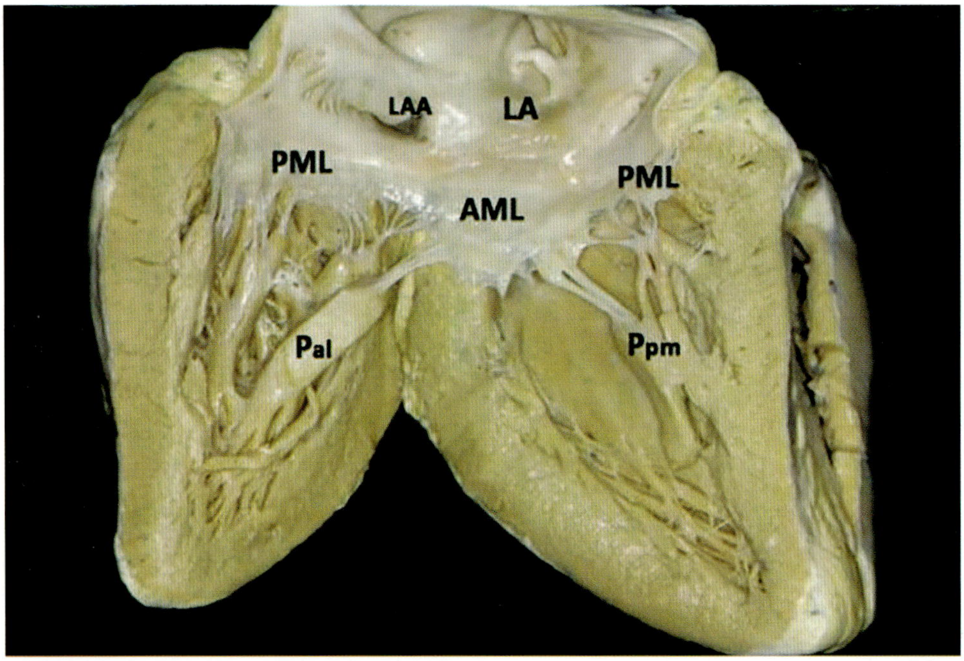

Fig. 9.4A: Pathology specimen showing the mitral valve in relationship to the left ventricle and left atrium. [Image courtesy of Philip C. Ursell, MD, Department of Pathology, UCSF. Image from Cheitlin MD, Ursell PC. Cardiac Anatomy. In Chatterjee K et al. (ed). Cardiology—An Illustrated Textbook]. (AML: Anterior mitral leaflet; LA: Left atrium; LAA: Orifice of the left atrial appendage; Pal: Anterolateral papillary muscle; Ppm: Posteriomedial papillary muscle; PML: Posterior mitral leaflet).

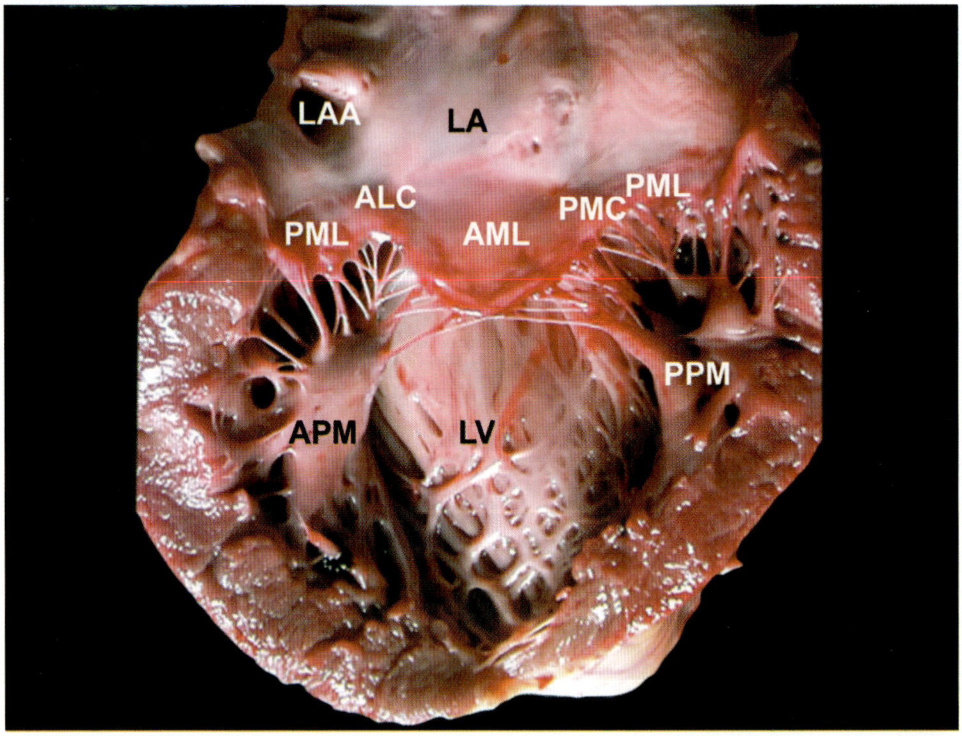

Fig. 9.4B: Gross pathology specimen showing the components of the mitral valve and mitral apparatus. [Image courtesy of Dr Pradeep Vaideeswar, Professor (Additional), Department of Pathology (Cardiovascular & Thoracic Division), Seth GS Medical College, Mumbai, India]. (AML: Anterior mitral leaflet; LA: Left atrium; Ppm: Posteriomedial papillary muscle; PML: Posterior mitral leaflet; ALC: Anterolateral commissures; APM: Anterior papillary muscle; LAA: Left atrial appendage; LV: Left ventricle; PMC: Posteromedial commissures; PPM: Posterior papillary muscle).

TRICUSPID VALVE

The tricuspid valve (Fig. 9.13) is situated between the right atrium and right ventricle, and functions to restrict blood regurgitation into the right atrium during ventricular systole. Functionally, the valve depends on the interaction of annulus, leaflets, chordae and ventricular elements. Unlike the mitral annulus, which is often described as saddle-shaped, the tricuspid valve annulus is asymmetric with a complex shape. The tricuspid valve has three leaflets: (1) anterior, (2) posterior, and (3) septal leaflets. The anterior leaflet is usually the largest of the leaflets. The septal leaflet, the smallest, inserts directly into the interventricular and interatrial septa, and the anterior and posterior trigones. This septal leaflet is always slightly more apical than the visualized mitral leaflet, serving as one means of distinguishing the anatomic right ventricle from the anatomic left ventricle. It has very little mobility so as a result the tricuspid valve is functionally bileaflet. The septal wall chordae connect to the anterior and septal leaflets, and there is usually no formal septal papillary muscle. There are anterior and posterior papillary muscles, each sending chordae to the other leaflets. They are often interconnected by a network of false chordae running to other papillary muscles and to the large trabeculations of the right ventricular apex. The normal tricuspid leaflet has a valve area of 4–6 cm^2.

Numerous congenital heart disease processes affect the tricuspid valve, including tricuspid atresia, tricuspid stenosis, and Ebstein anomaly (discussed in detail in the chapter on Ebstein Anomaly). In adults, the tricuspid valve may become dysfunctional due to endocarditis, which may occur in intravenous drug users or those with indwelling catheters or implantable devices. Secondary valve dysfunction can occur with processes that affect the right ventricle, such as arrhythmogenic rhythm ventricular dysplasia/cardiomyopathy, and pulmonary hypertension, and atrial shunting with resulting volume and pressure overload. Tricuspid regurgitation can also be caused by the presence of a pacemaker or defibrillator lead, which mechanically interferes with tricuspid leaflet coaptation. Tricuspid regurgitation may also occur in patients with repeated right ventricular biopsies, such as those who have undergone cardiac transplantation. Stenosis of the valve most often is due to rheumatic heart disease, but may also occur, along with concomitant tricuspid regurgitation, due to serotonin syndromes (e.g. carcinoid, medication-induced).

PULMONIC VALVE

The pulmonic valve (Fig. 9.14) is situated between the right ventricular outflow tract and the main pulmonary artery. The valve functions to prevent blood regurgitation back

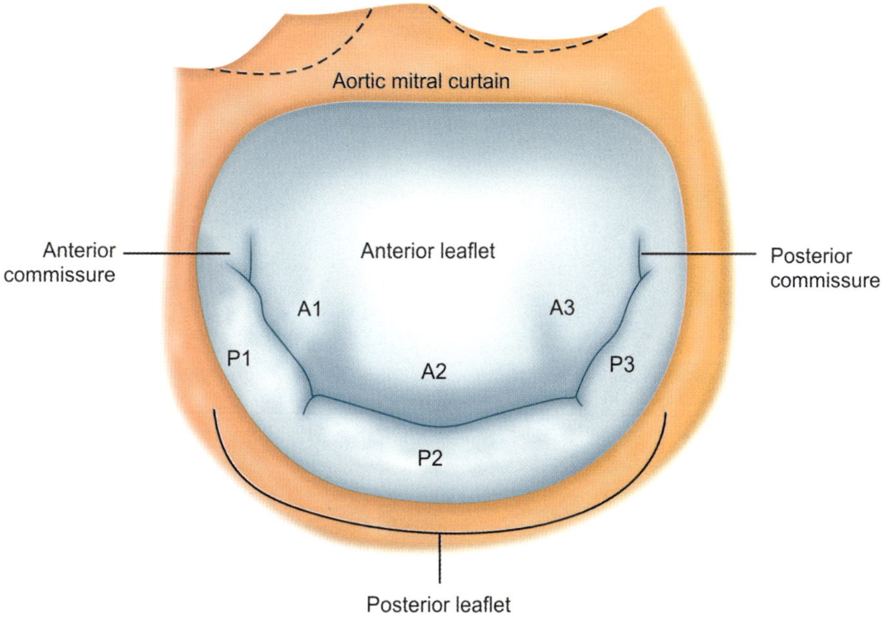

Fig. 9.5A: Schematic illustration of the three scallops of the posterior and anterior mitral leaflets. From anterolateral to posteromedial location, these are denoted as A1, A2, and A3 and P1, P2, and P3.

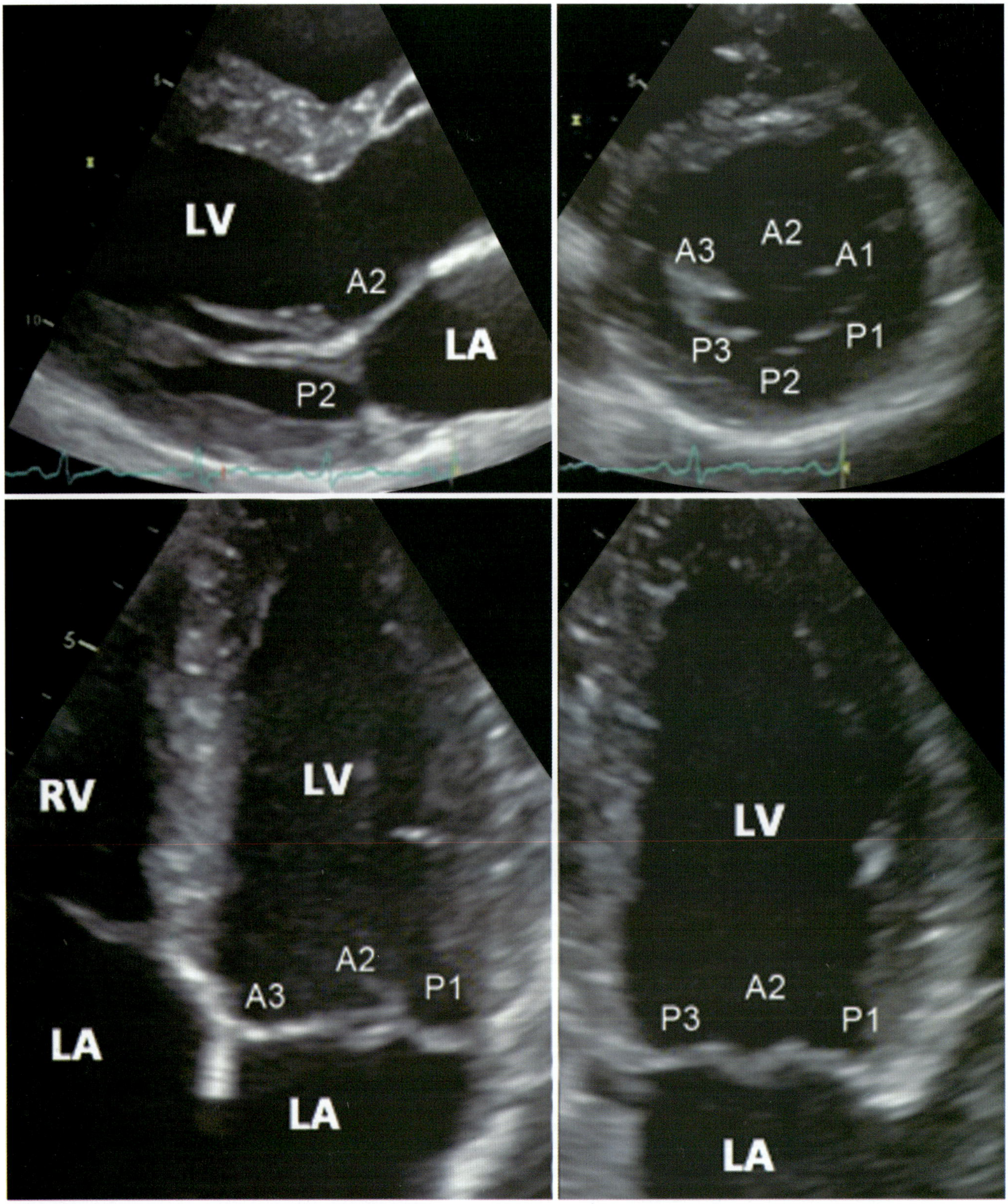

Fig. 9.5B: Echocardiographic images in multiple planes demonstrating the anterior and posterior mitral scallops. [Image from Pierard LA et al. Mitral regurgitation. In Nanda NC (ed). Comprehensive Textbook of Echocardiography. New Delhi, India: Jaypee Brothers Medical Publishers (P) Ltd.].

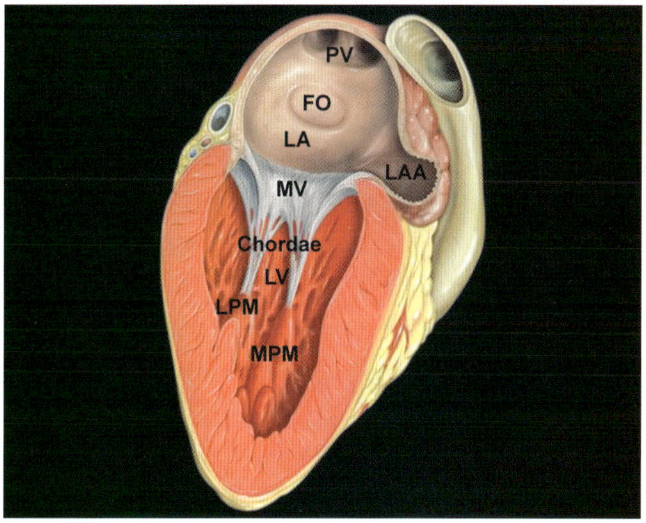

Fig. 9.6: Schematic illustration of the mitral valve and subvalvular apparatus. The mitral valve is attached to the medial papillary muscle (MPM) and lateral papillary muscle (LPM) by chordae. (Image created by Patrick J. Lynch, C. Carl Jaffe, and posted on Wikipedia). (PM: Papillary muscles).

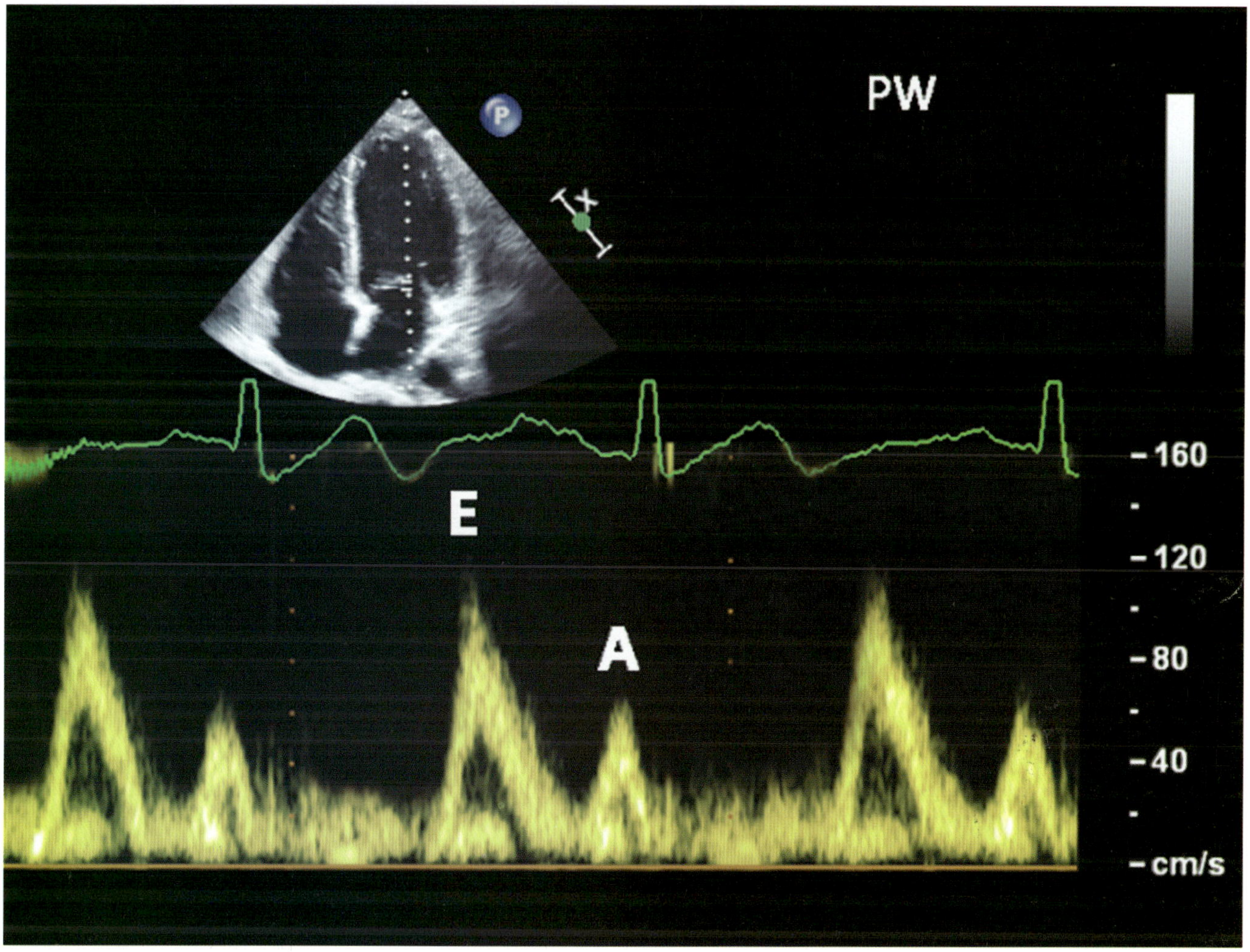

Fig. 9.7: Pulsed wave (PW) spectral Doppler echocardiography image assessing mitral inflow from the left atrium to the left ventricle during ventricular diastole. The E wave represents early diastolic filling, due to opening of the mitral valve and relaxation of the left ventricle. Flow during the A wave is a result of atrial contraction.

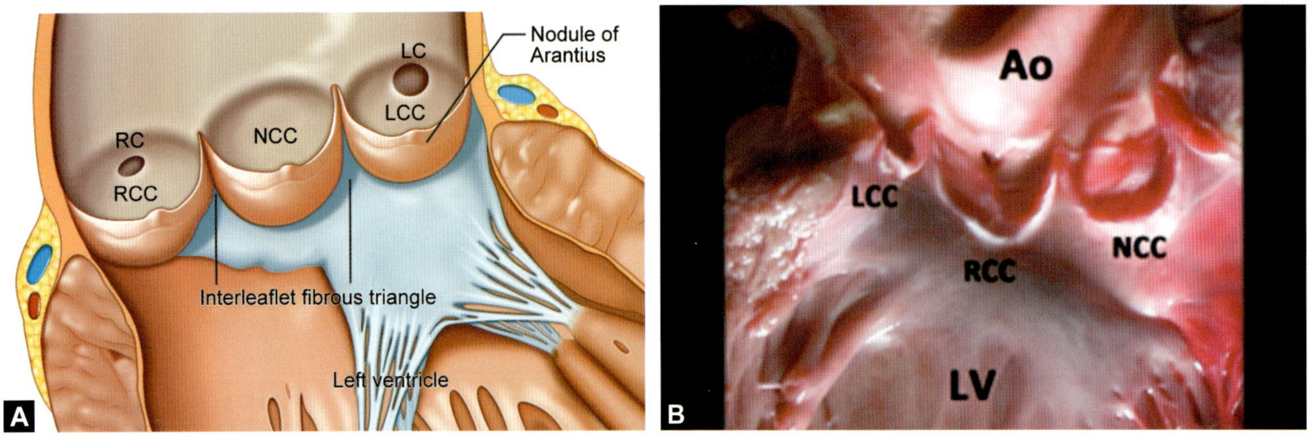

Figs. 9.8A and B: Schematic illustration and gross pathology specimen of the aortic valve. [Image 9.8A from Mishra S, Awashy N. Aortic valve diseases. In Vijayalakshmi IB et al. (ed). Comprehensive approach to congenital heart disease. New Delhi, India: Jaypee Brothers Medical Publishers (P) Ltd. Image 9.8B text courtesy of Dr Pradeep Vaideeswar, Professor (Additional), Department of Pathology (Cardiovascular & Thoracic Division), Seth GS Medical College, Mumbai, India]. (LV: Left coronary artery ostium; LCC: Left coronary cusp; NCC: Non-coronary cusp; RC: Right coronary artery ostium; RCC: Right coronary cusp).

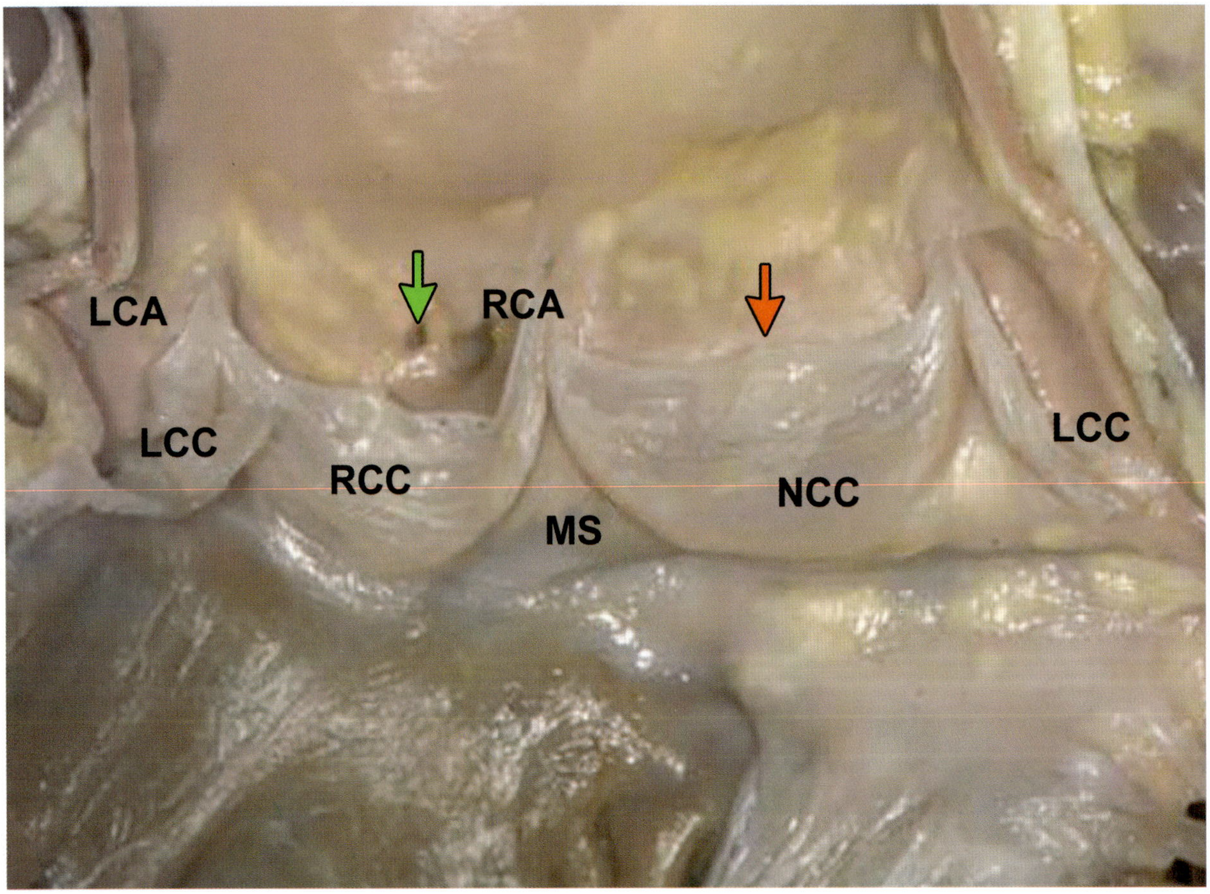

Fig. 9.9A: Anatomy of the aortic valve. The three aortic leaflets are shown, with the left coronary (Lc) leaflet cut in half. Facilitating valve closure, a tiny midline fibrous nodule of the free margin of each semilunar leaflet (red arrow), known as the nodule of Arantius, is present. The left coronary artery (LCA) and right coronary artery (RCA) ostia are visualized arising from the left and right coronary sinuses, respectively. There is also a separate tiny ostium (green arrow) of the conal branch of the RCA, a normal variant. The membranous portion of the interventricular septum (MS) is present between the noncoronary (Nc) and right coronary (Rc) leaflets. [Image and legend text adapted from Cheitlin MD, Ursell PC. Cardiac anatomy. In Chatterjee K et al. (ed). Cardiology—An Illustrated Textbook. New Delhi, India: Jaypee Brothers Medical Publishers (P) Ltd.].

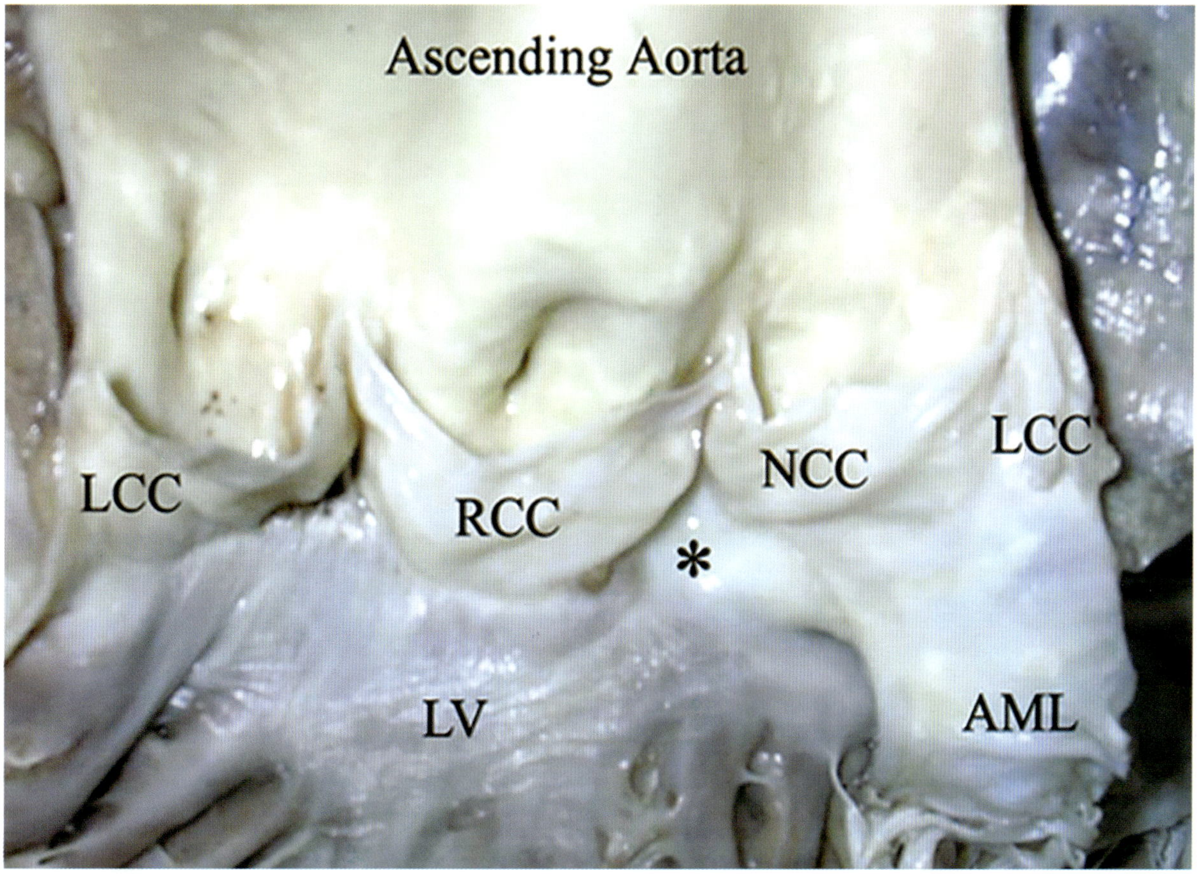

Fig. 9.9B: Anatomy of the normal tricuspid aortic valve. The right coronary cusp (RCC), left coronary cusp (LCC), and non-coronary cusp (NCC) are visualized. There is a fibrous continuity between the adjoining portions of the non-coronary cusp, left coronary cusp, and anterior mitral leaflet (AML). The interventricular septum (asterisk) is also visualized. [Image and legend text adapted from Vaideeswar P. Examination of the heart—a comparative external and internal anatomy. From Vijayalakshmi IB et al. (ed). A Comprehensive Approach to Congenital Heart Disease. New Delhi, India: Jaypee Brothers Medical Publishers (P) Ltd.]. (LV: Left ventricle).

into the right ventricle during ventricular diastole. The pulmonic valve is a semilunar valve and consists of three leaflets: (1) anterior cusp, (2) left cusp, and (3) right cusp.

Pulmonic valve closure at end-systole results in the P2 component of the second heart sound. As pressures are lower in the right-sided vasculature when compared to the left sided vasculature, P2 is usually softer than the A2 sound generated by aortic valve closure.

The most common condition affecting the pulmonic valve encountered in younger persons is congenital pulmonic valve stenosis. Trace or very mild pulmonary regurgitation is present in almost all persons and is a normal finding on echocardiography. More severe, pathological pulmonic regurgitation may develop in patients with severe pulmonary hypertension. Right-sided endocarditis may also lead to pathological pulmonary regurgitation. Rheumatic heard disease and carcinoid tumors may also lead to dysfunction of the pulmonic valve.

VALVE IMAGING AND EVALUATION

Valvular dysfunction may be suggested by auscultation of a cardiac murmur, physical findings suggestive of congestion, cardiovascular symptoms such as dyspnea, angina or presyncope, or abnormal chest X-ray. The workhouse imaging study for the evaluation of valvular dysfunction is transthoracic echocardiography (TTE), including 2D imaging, spectral Doppler imaging, and color Doppler

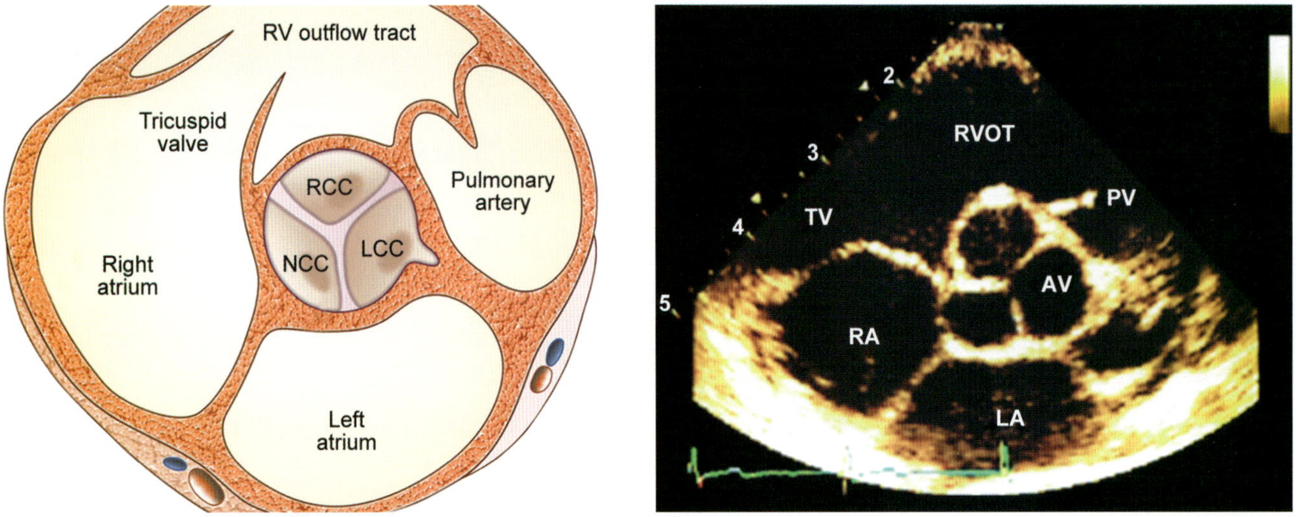

Fig. 9.10A: Anatomy and location of the aortic valve (AV). Schematic (left panel) and parasternal short axis transthoracic echocardiogram (right panel) illustrate the three coronary leaflets and anatomic location of the aortic valve and leaflets with respect to other cardiac structures. [Image from Mishra S, Awashy N. Aortic valve diseases. In Vijayalakshmi IB et al. (ed). Comprehensive Approach to Congenital Heart Disease. New Delhi, India: Jaypee Brothers Medical Publishers (P) Ltd.]. (LCC: Left coronary cusp; NCC: Non-coronary cusp; RCC: Right coronary cusp; LA: Left atrium; PV: Pulmonic valve; RA: Right atrium; RVOT: Right ventricular outflow tract; TV: Tricuspid valve).

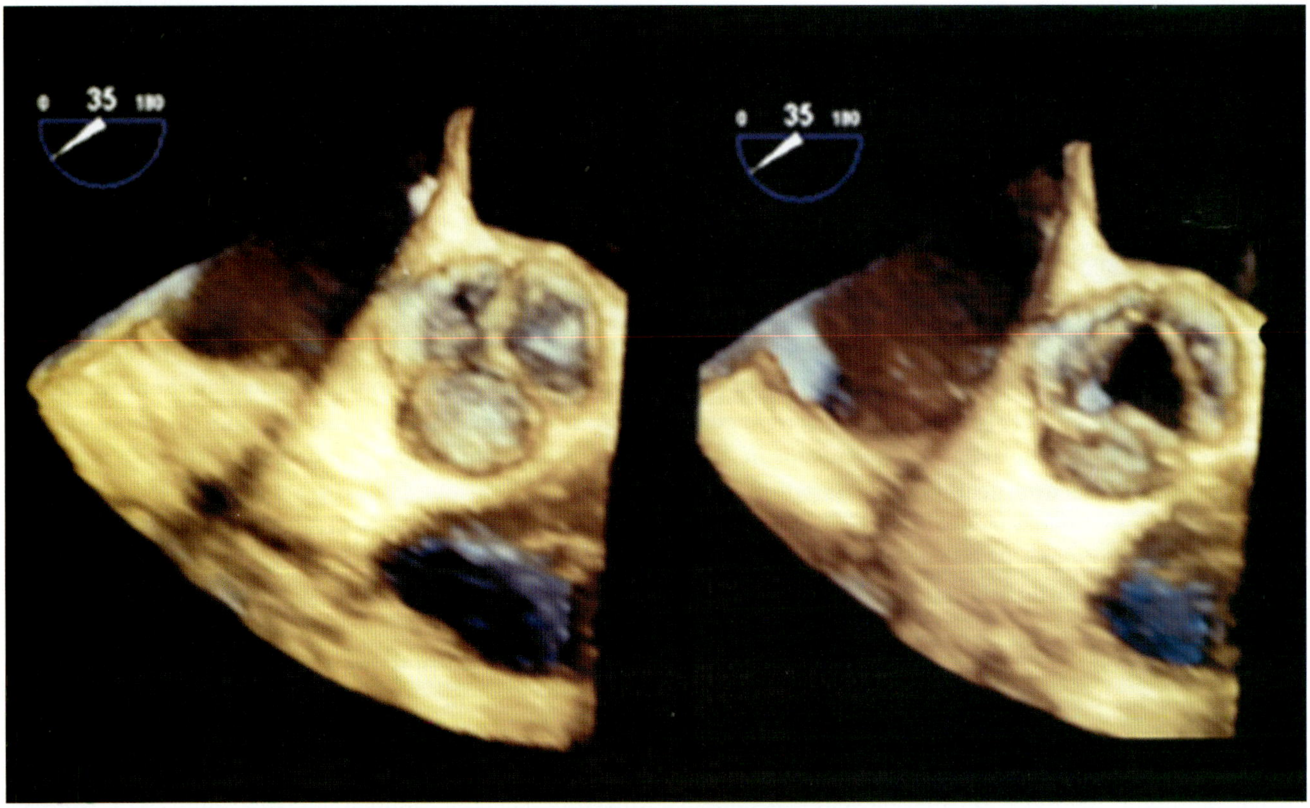

Fig. 9.10B: Normal tricuspid aortic valve visualized by 3D echocardiography during diastole (left panel) and systole (right panel). [Image from Zaragoza-Macias E et al. How to perform a three-dimensional transesophageal echocardiogram. In Nanda NC (ed). Comprehensive Textbook of Echocardiography. New Delhi, India: Jaypee Brothers Medical Publishers (P) Ltd.].

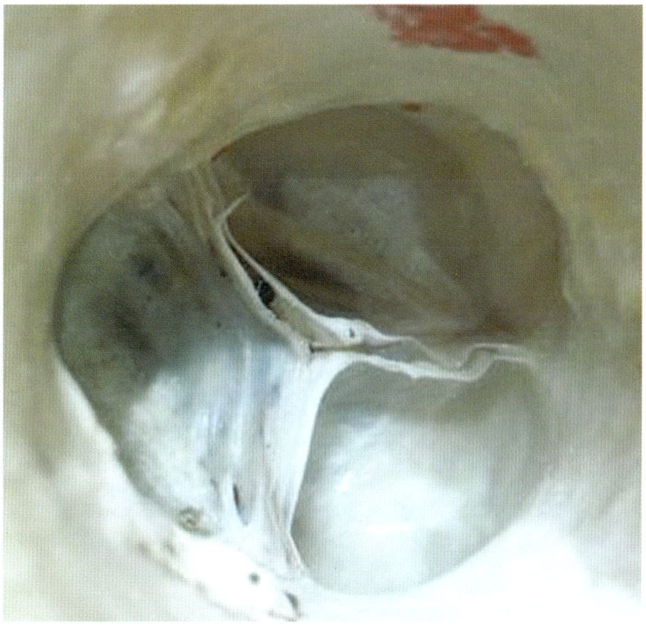

Fig. 9.11: Gross anatomy specimen of a trileaflet aortic valve. (Image created by Anatomist90 and posted on Wikipedia Commons CC).

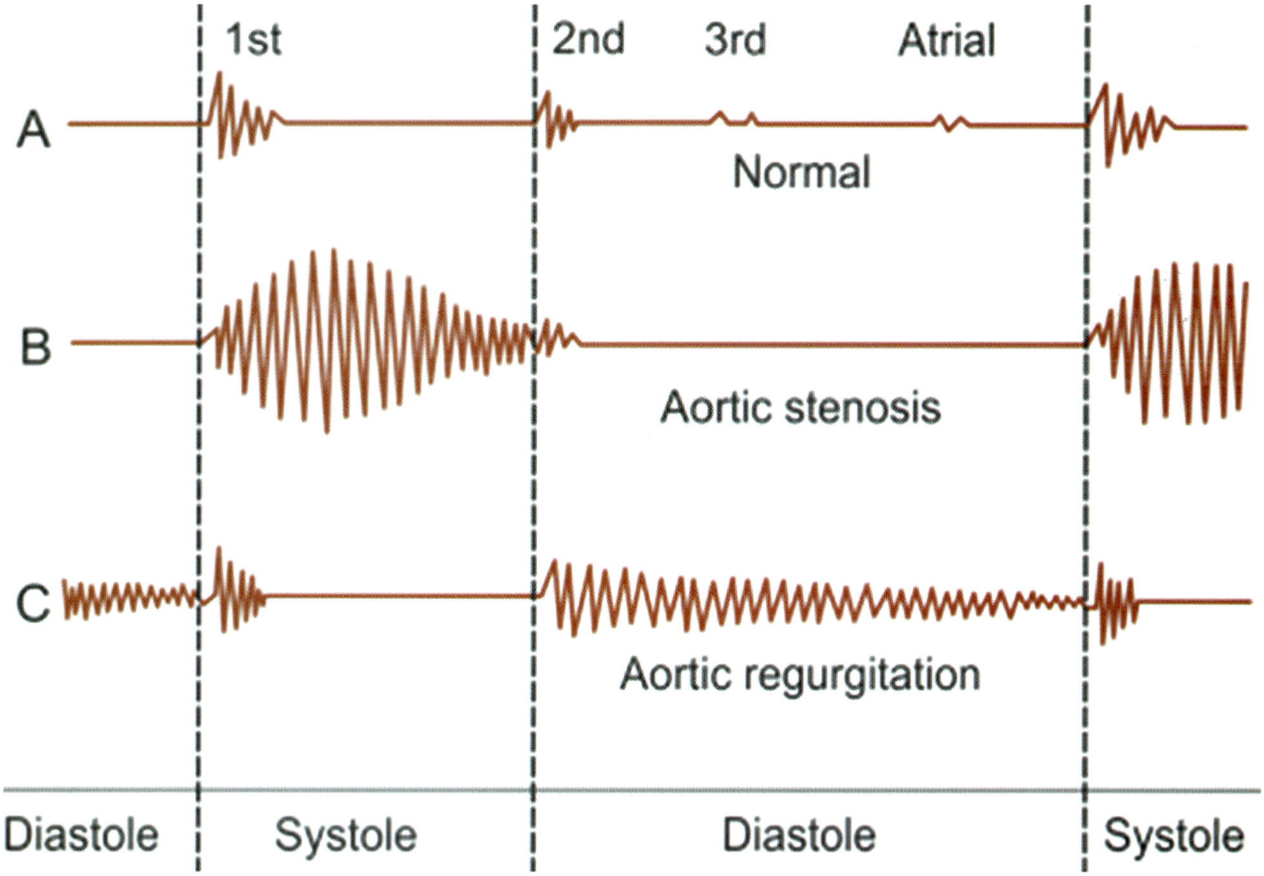

Fig. 9.12: Phonocardiogram of normal heart sounds (A), aortic stenosis (B), and aortic regurgitation (C). [Image from Mishra S, Awashy N. Aortic valve diseases. In Vijayalakshmi IB et al. (ed). Comprehensive Approach to Congenital Heart Disease. New Delhi, India: Jaypee Brothers Medical Publishers (P) Ltd. Image originally from a Creative Commons site (unattributed)].

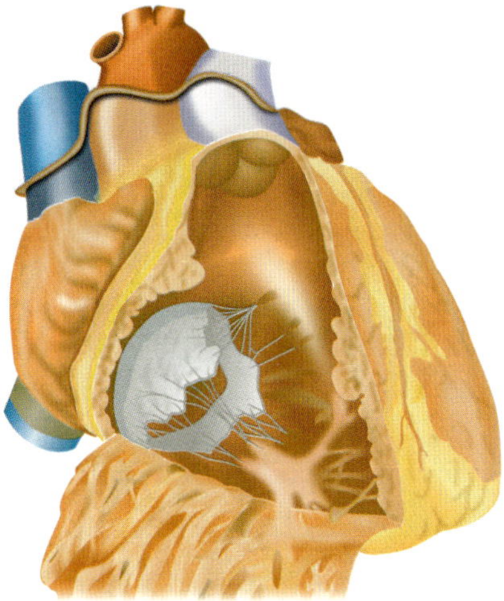

Fig. 9.13: Schematic representation of the tricuspid valve.

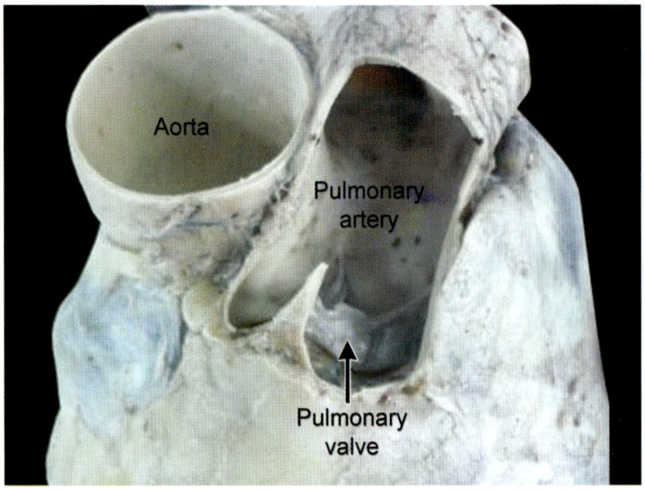

Fig. 9.14: Gross pathology specimen of the pulmonic valve. (Image created by anatomist90 and posted on Wikipedia Commons).

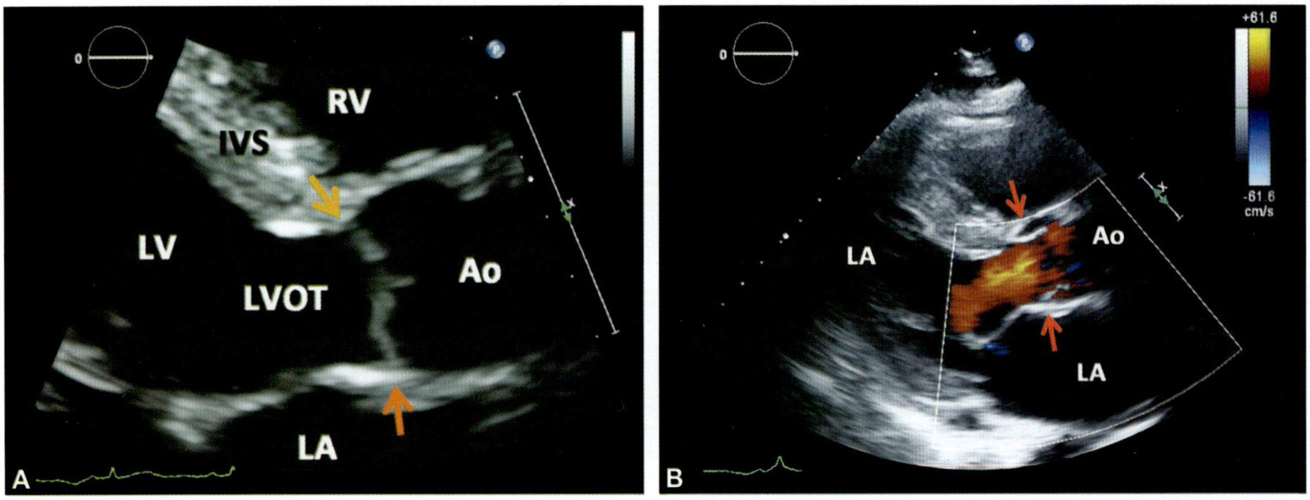

Figs. 9.15A and B: Parasternal long-axis transthoracic echocardiography (TTE) images of the aortic valve. (A) 2D image taken during diastole. The cusp near the interventricular septum (IVS) in this image (orange arrow) is the right coronary cusp; the cusp seen proximate to the left atrium (LA) may be either the left coronary cusp or the non-coronary cusp; (B) Color Doppler image during systole showing normal, laminar flow across a non-stenotic aortic valve (arrows). (Ao: Aorta; LA: Left atrium; LV: Left ventricle; LVOT: Left ventricular outflow tract; RV: Right ventricle).

imaging (Figs. 9.15A and B). 3D imaging is being increasingly utilized for valve assessment, particular of the mitral valve. Transesophageal echocardiography (Figs. 9.16A and B) is used primarily in those in whom the degree or mechanism of valve dysfunction are still in question after TTE, in those in whom reparative valve surgery is being contemplated, in those with complex congenital heart disease, and in those in whom a diagnosis of endocarditis is still in question. Cardiac magnetic resonance (CMR) imaging (Figs. 9.17A and B) is increasingly being used for assessment of valve pathology and physiology. Cardiac CT scanning (Fig. 9.18) may occasionally be used to provide adjunctive information on valve pathology.

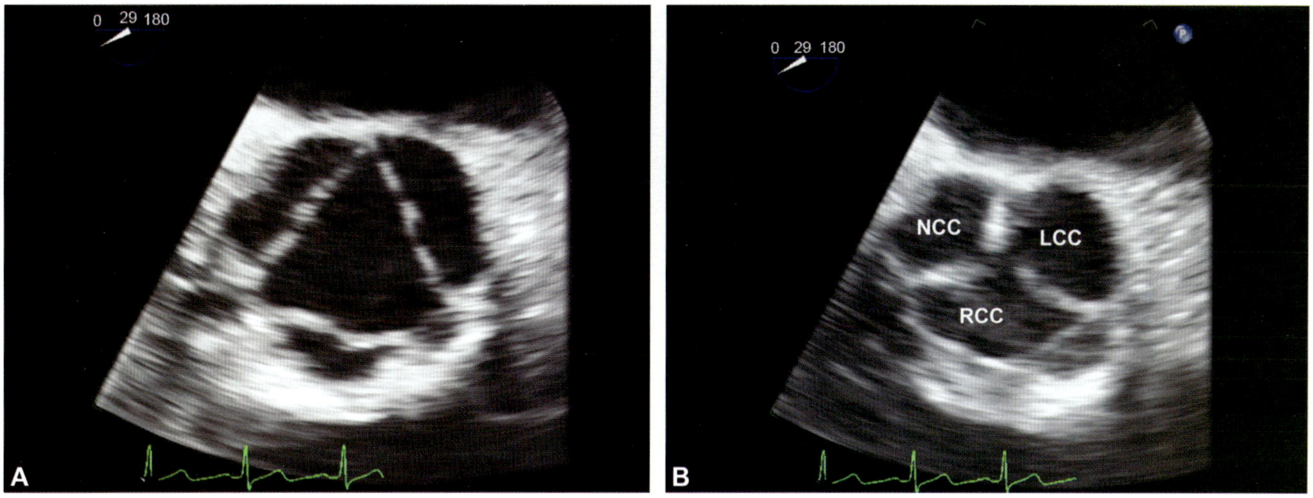

Figs. 9.16A and B: Transesophageal echocardiograms (TEE) of the aortic valve. (A) Image obtained during systole, showing a normal trileaflet aortic valve. (B) Image from same patient obtained during diastole, showing good coaptation of the leaflets. (LCC: Left coronary cusp; NCC: Non-coronary cusp; RCC: Right coronary cusp).

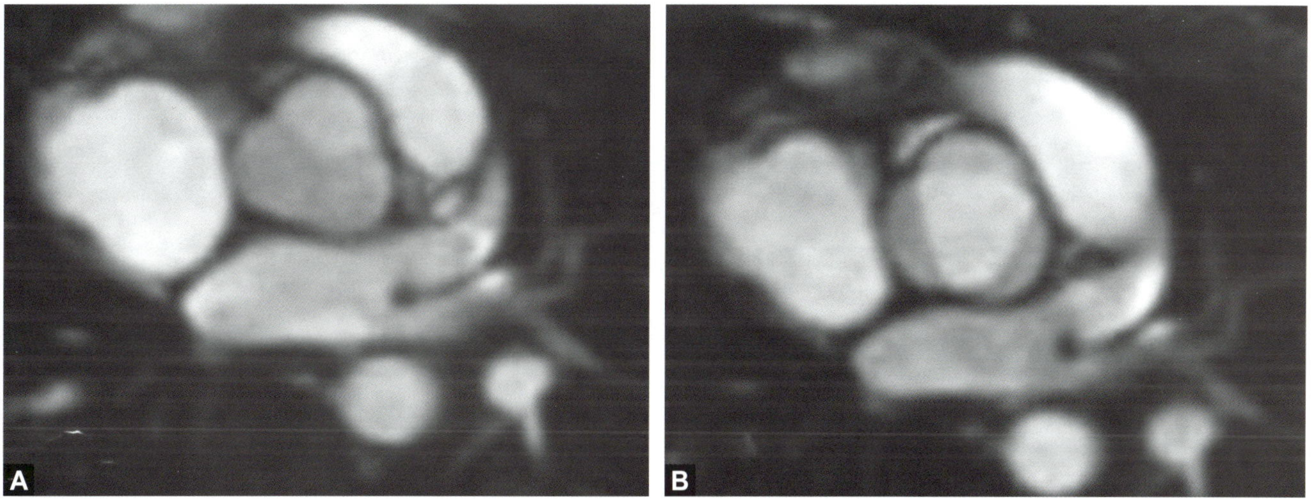

Figs. 9.17A and B: Cardiac magnetic resonance imaging of a normal tricuspid aortic valve in diastole (A) and systole (B). [Image from Tokmaji G et al. Bicuspid aortic valve. In Aikawa E (ed). Calcific Aortic Valve Disease. Intechweb.org. CC].

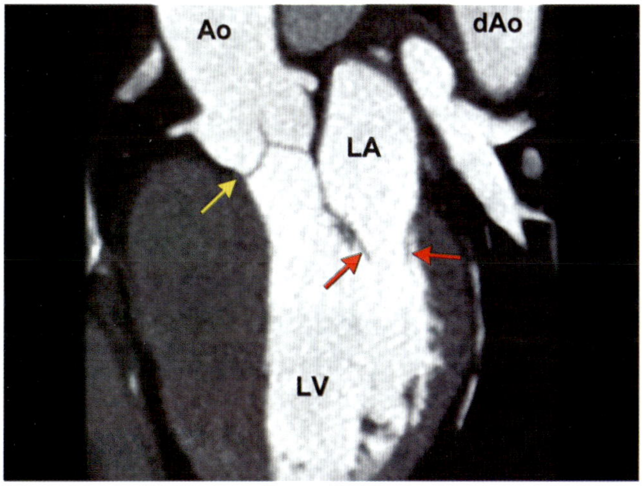

Fig. 9.18: Cardiac CT image during diastole showing the aortic valve leaflets (yellow arrow) and mitral leaflets (red arrows). [Image from Sriharan M et al. Non-invasive coronary angiography. In Baskot B (ed). Coronary Angiography—Advances in Noninvasive Imaging Approach for Evaluation of Coronary Artery Disease. Intechweb.org. CC].

VIDEO LEGENDS

Video 9.1: Apical four chamber TTE showing a mitral valve with good coaptation.

Video 9.2: Parasternal short-axis showing a trileaflet aortic valve (center of image). The tricuspid valve is visible at the 9 O'clock position in the image. The pulmonic valve, which is usually not well visualized, is imaged at the 2 O'clock position.

Video 9.3: Parasternal long-axis TTE showing a normal aortic valve.

CHAPTER

10

Aortic Stenosis

Blase A Carabello

ETIOLOGY OF AORTIC STENOSIS

Once considered a degenerative disease, it is now clear that aortic stenosis (AS) in developed countries is caused by an active inflammatory process that bears many similarities to atherosclerosis. The initial plaque of AS often has a lipid core covered by a fibrous cap similar to the plaque of coronary artery disease (CAD). It is postulated that shear stress created by leaflet inhomogeneity (bicuspid valve is the most extreme case) and hypertension causes endothelial cell activation of tissue growth factor beta (TGF-β), tissue necrosis factor, and other cytokines, amplified by circulating factors included oxidized low-density lipoprotein (LDL). This cascade leads to lymphocyte activation and inflammation, and in turn initiates calcification (Fig. 10.1) and even true bone formation. As calcium nodules build up on the aortic side of the valve, valve opening is impaired and aortic valve orifice area is reduced (Figs. 10.2 to 10.4 and Videos 10.1 to 10.3). Because of similarities between the pathology of aortic stenosis and CAD, statins, which are so effective in treating CAD, have been administered to AS patients in hope of slowing the progression of the coronary disease. While randomized trials of statins have failed, this new understanding of the nature of AS may lead to other pharmacologic targets in the future.

Bicuspid aortic valve (Figs. 10.5 to 10.7 and Video 10.4) is another important cause of AS. Bicuspid aortic valve is extremely common, affecting approximately 1–2% of the population. About one-third of such valves become severely stenotic.

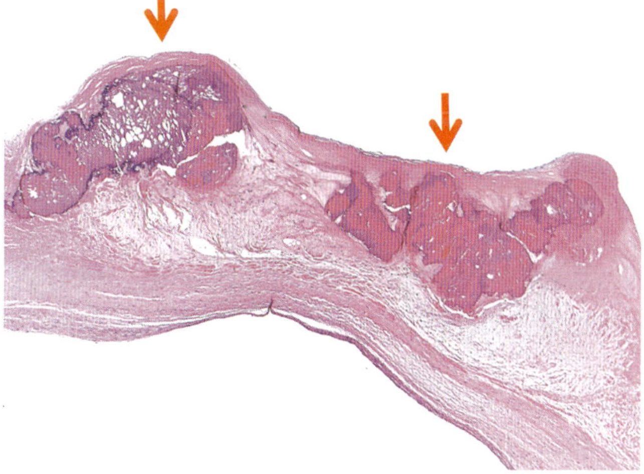

Fig. 10.1: Photomicrograph of a stenotic aortic valve showing the presence of calcifications (arrows) on the aortic side of the valve. [Image and legend text from Ker J, Van Heerden WFP. Cellular and neuronal aspects in aortic stenosis. In: Hirota M (Ed). Aortic Stenosis—Etiology, Pathophysiology and Treatment. InTech; 2011].

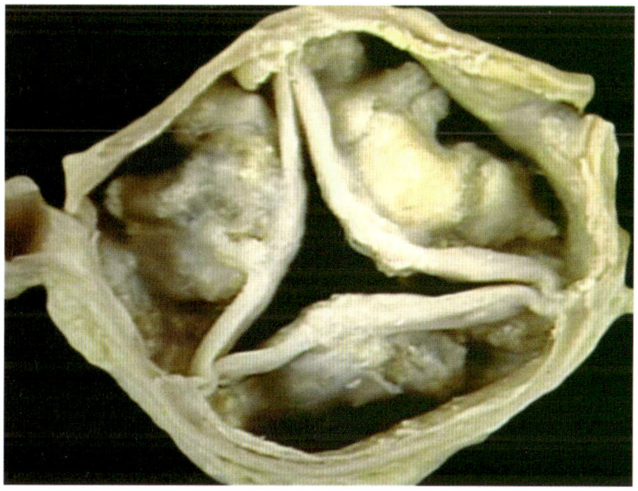

Fig. 10.2: Gross pathology specimen of calcific aortic stenosis. (Image from Armed Forces Institute of Pathology).

In developing countries, rheumatic heart disease (Figs. 10.8A and B) remains an important cause of AS, as well as other valvular diseases discussed in this section of the book.

Other causes of AS include prior chest irradiation and a variety of congenital abnormalities in addition to bicuspid valve such as congenital unicuspid (Figs. 10.9 to 10.11) and quadricuspid valve (Figs. 10.12 and 10.13).

PATHOPHYSIOLOGY OF AORTIC STENOSIS AND ITS RELATIONSHIP TO SYMPTOMS

Compromise of the valve orifice to half of its normal area produces little change in left ventricular hemodynamics. However, further narrowing results in progressively more obstruction in flow, requiring the left ventricle (LV) to

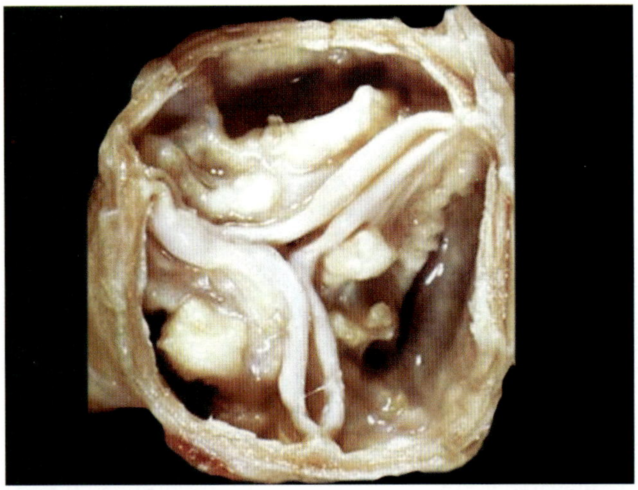

Fig. 10.3: Gross pathology specimen of calcific aortic stenosis. (Image courtesy of Renu Virmani, MD, and Edwards Lifesciences, Inc).

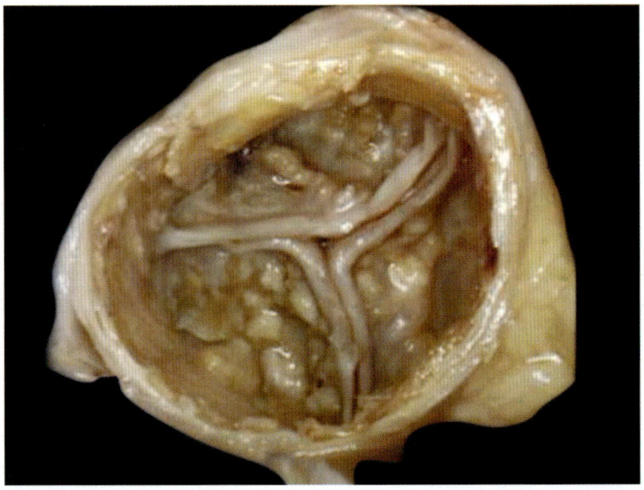

Fig. 10.4: Gross pathology specimen of calcific aortic stenosis. (Image courtesy of Renu Virmani, MD, and Edwards Lifesciences, Inc).

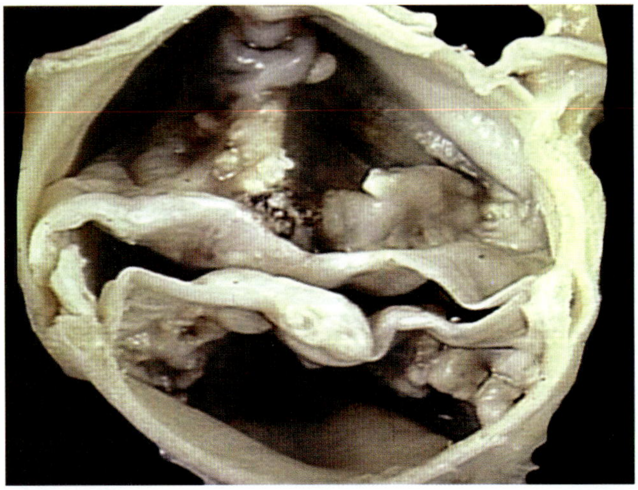

Fig. 10.5A: Gross pathology specimen of a stenotic bicuspid aortic valve. (Image from Armed Forces Institute of Pathology).

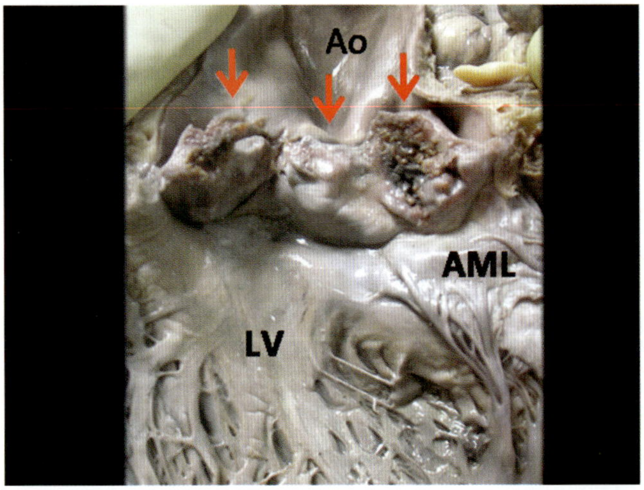

Fig. 10.5B: Gross pathology specimen of a severely calcified and ulcerated bicuspid aortic valve (arrows). [Image courtesy of Dr Pradeep Vaideeswar, Professor (Additional), Department of Pathology (Cardiovascular and Thoracic Division), Seth GS Medical College, Mumbai, India]. (AML: Anterior mitral leaflet; Ao: Aorta; LV: Left ventricle).

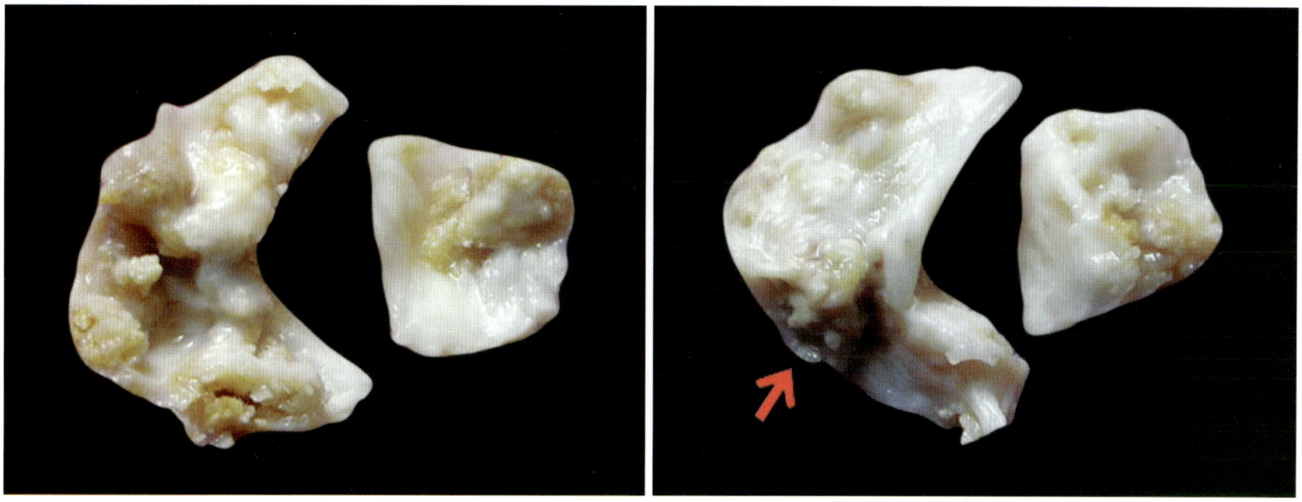

Fig. 10.5C: Surgically excised calcified cusps from a patient with bicuspid aortic stenosis. Left panel shows the flow surfaces; Right panel shows the non-flow surfaces. Note presence of calcified raphae (arrow). [Image and legend text courtesy of Dr Pradeep Vaideeswar, Professor (Additional), Department of Pathology (Cardiovascular and Thoracic Division), Seth GS Medical College, Mumbai, India].

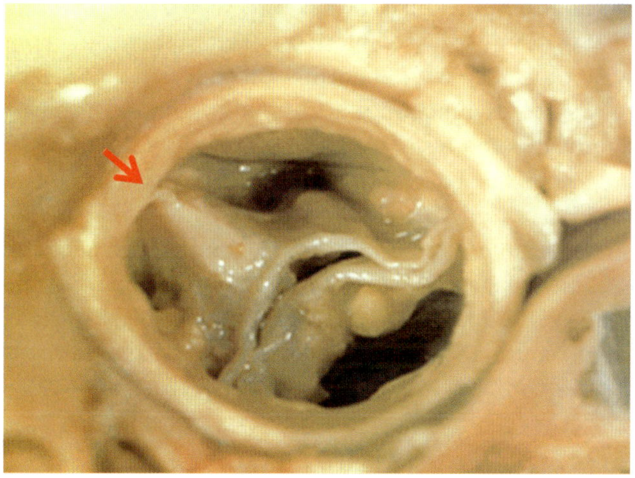

Fig. 10.6: Stenotic bicuspid aortic valve. The raphae (arrow) is clearly visible. [Image from Mishra S, Awasthy N. Aortic valve diseases. In: Vijayalakshmi IB, Rao PS, Chugh R (Eds). A Comprehensive Approach to Congenital Heart Diseases. New Delhi, India: Jaypee Brothers Medical Publishers (P) Ltd. 2013].

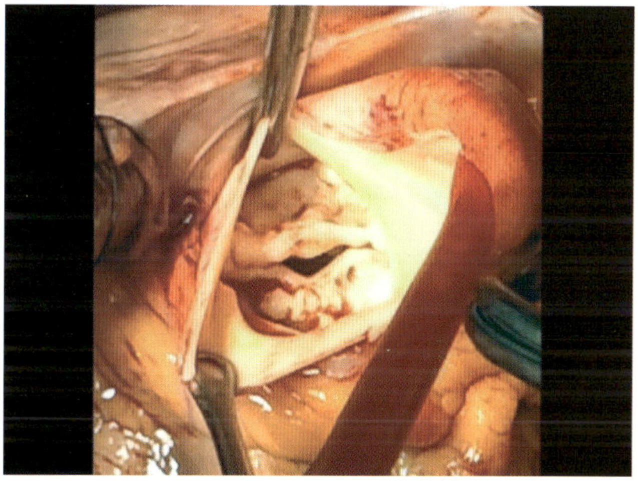

Fig. 10.7: Intraoperative image of a stenotic bicuspid aortic valve. [Image from Akkus MN. A case-control investigation of the relationship between bicuspid aortic valve disease and coronary heart disease. In Chen YF, Luo CY (Ed). Aortic Valve. InTech; 2011].

produce progressively greater pressure to drive blood past the obstructed orifice. When valve area is reduced to one-third its normal area (1/3 of 3 cm^2 = 1.0 cm^2) at a normal cardiac output a gradient of about 25 mm Hg results. When valve area is reduced to 0.75 cm^2 this gradient approximately doubles. Figure 10.14 demonstrates the pressure gradient taken from a patient with severe AS. This gradient (green area) represents the pressure overload imposed upon the LV. This pressure overload is compensated by left ventricular concentric hypertrophy wherein increased muscle mass and increased wall thickness (Figs. 10.15A and B) helps to normalize the load on any given muscle fiber (afterload). Afterload is often approximated as LV wall stress (σ):

$$\sigma = (p \times r)/(2 \times th)$$

Where,

p = LV systolic pressure

r = radius

th = wall thickness

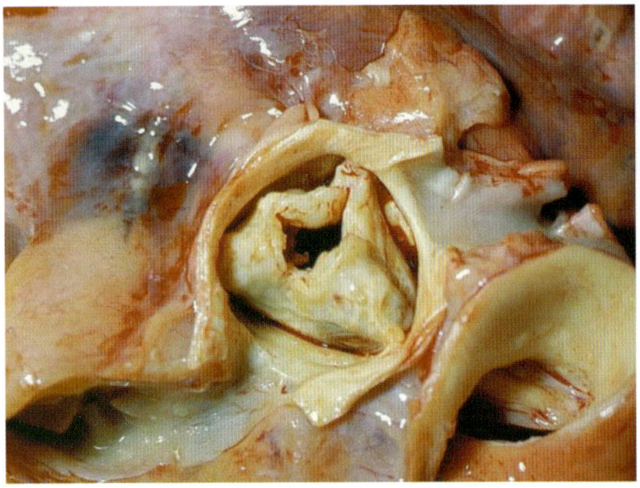

Fig. 10.8A: Gross pathology image of rheumatic aortic stenosis. (Image from Dr Edwin P Ewing Jr and CDC).

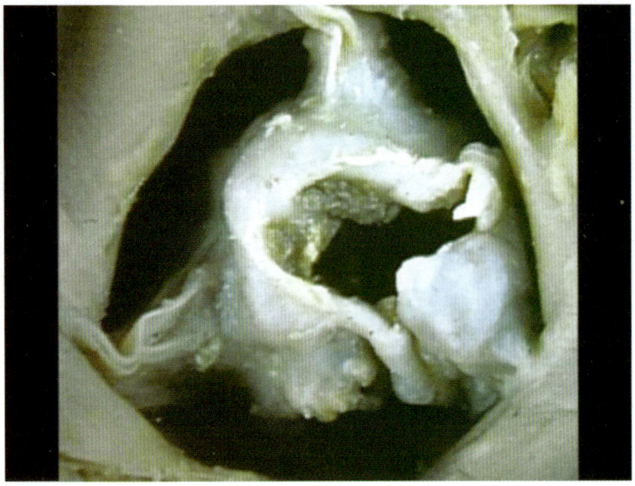

Fig. 10.8B: Rheumatic aortic stenosis. Note the fusion of the commissures. (Image from Armed Forces Institute of Pathology).

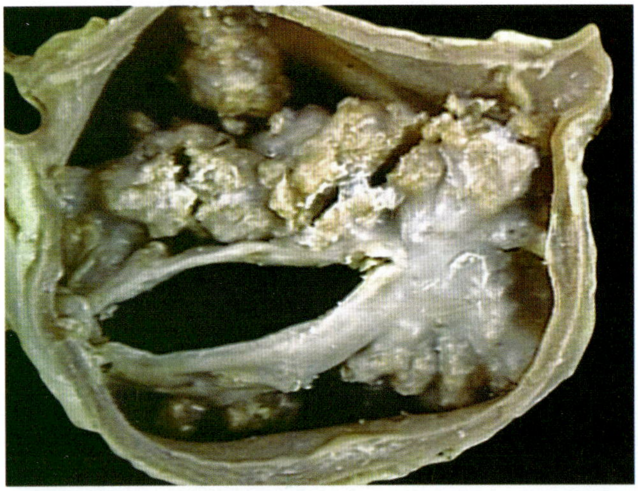

Fig. 10.9: Gross pathology specimen of a unicommissural aortic valve. (Image from Armed Forces Institute of Pathology).

As pressure in the numerator increases from the overload, it is offset by increased LV wall thickness in the denominator. Because LV ejection is inhibited by afterload, maintenance of normal afterload by left ventricular hypertrophy (LVH) helps maintain normal LV ejection and cardiac output. Unfortunately, the compensatory nature of LVH is complicated by pathological properties that in turn are related to the symptoms of the disease.

The onset of symptoms increases the expected mortality of AS from < 1%/year to > 25%/year (Fig. 10.16). The classic symptoms of AS are angina, syncope and dyspnea (and the other symptoms of heart failure). Concentric LVH limits coronary blood flow and thus is partially responsible for producing angina in AS. The thickened LV requires higher than normal diastolic pressure for LV filling (diastolic dysfunction), leading to the symptoms of heart failure. Diastolic dysfunction is further exacerbated by myocardial fibrosis. Fibrosis also interferes with systolic function, which together with abnormal calcium handling, leads to systolic dysfunction and further contributes to heart failure. In some cases, inadequate LVH allows afterload to increase, adding to worsened systolic function. Concentric hypertrophy may also reduce chamber volume, reducing stroke volume, contributing to the symptom of syncope.

The change in etiology of AS from rheumatic fever 50 years ago to that of an atherosclerotic-like disease today has advanced the age of onset by about 15 years. However, the dire consequences of symptom onset remain the same.

PHYSICAL EXAMINATION

The diagnosis of AS is often suspected for the first time when the patient's clinician hears the murmur characteristic of the disease. Importantly, since there is no foolproof technique for diagnosing the severity of the obstruction, physical examination sets the pre-test probability of the accuracy of the ensuing diagnostic tests employed to establish the diagnosis.

Palpation of the apical impulse usually finds it in its normal position but enlarged in size, prolonged, and forceful in character. Palpation of the carotid arteries finds their upstrokes both delayed in timing and diminished in volume (parvus et tardus) (Fig. 10.17). The simultaneous palpation of a powerful apical beat and a weakened carotid upstroke strongly suggests obstruction to outflow, leading the examiner toward the diagnosis of AS before auscultation is even performed.

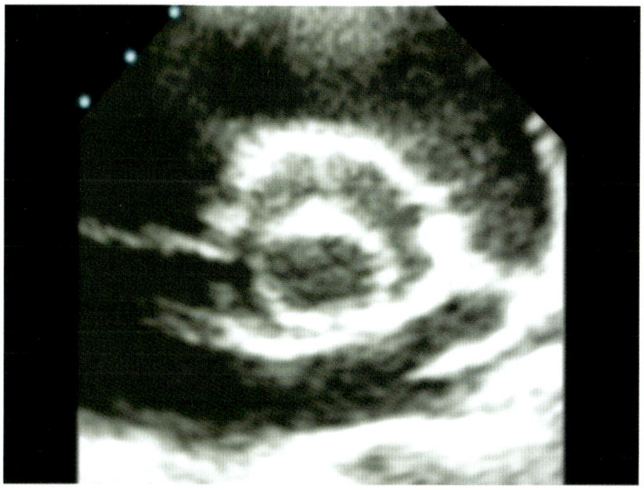

Fig. 10.10A: Enface view on parasternal short axis echocardiography of a unicuspid aortic valve. [Image from Mishra S, Awasthy N. Aortic valve diseases. In: Vijayalakshmi IB, Rao PS, Chugh R (Eds). A Comprehensive Approach to Congenital Heart Diseases. New Delhi, India: Jaypee Brothers Medical Publishers (P) Ltd. 2013].

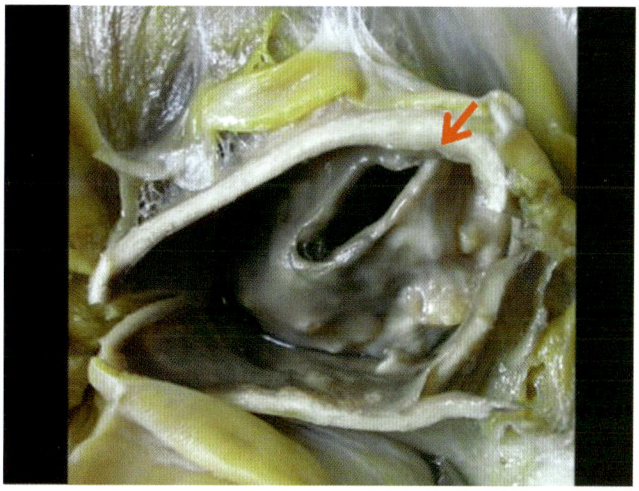

Fig. 10.10B: Unicuspid aortic stenosis with unicommissural (arrow) valve. [Image courtesy of Dr Pradeep Vaideeswar, Professor (Additional), Department of Pathology (Cardiovascular and Thoracic Division), Seth GS Medical College, Mumbai, India].

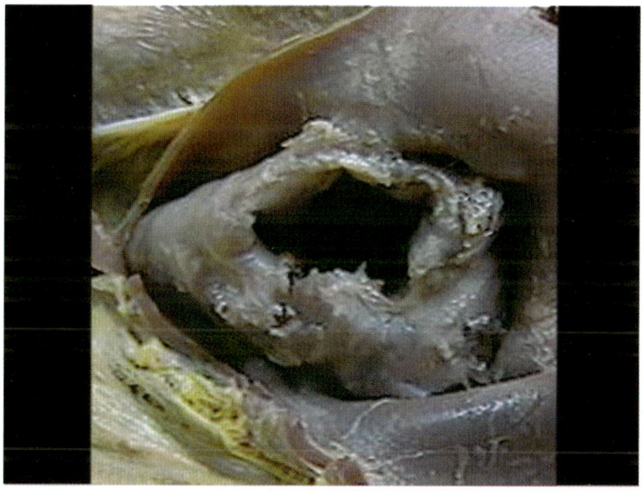

Fig. 10.10C: Gross pathology specimen of a unicuspid acommissural stenotic aortic valve. [Image and legend text courtesy of Dr Pradeep Vaideeswar, Professor (Additional), Department of Pathology (Cardiovascular and Thoracic Division), Seth GS Medical College, Mumbai, India].

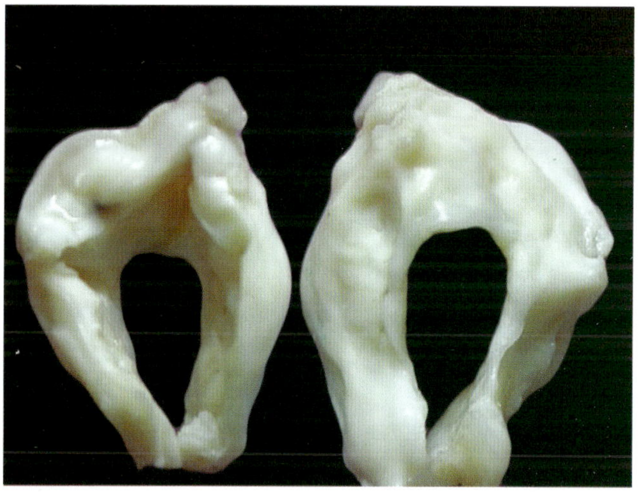

Fig. 10.10D: Surgically excised calcified unicuspid calcified valve showing typical exclamation mark orifice. The flow (left panel) and non-flow (right panel) surfaces are shown. [Image and legend text courtesy of Dr Pradeep Vaideeswar, Professor (Additional), Department of Pathology (Cardiovascular and Thoracic Division), Seth GS Medical College, Mumbai, India].

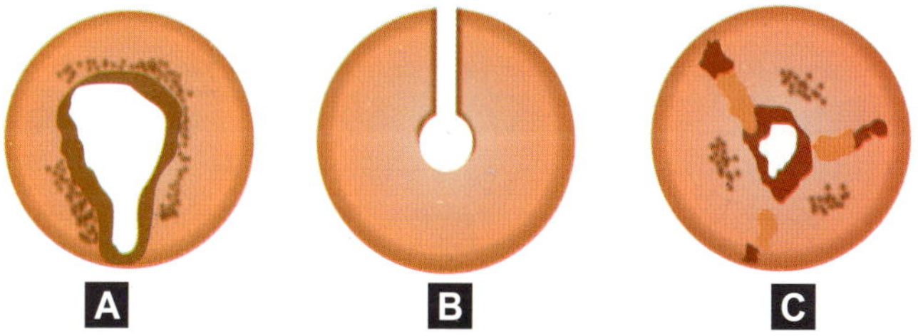

Figs. 10.11A to C: Schematic illustration of unicuspid aortic valves. (A) Unicommisural valve (toilet-seat shape); (B) Unicommissural valve (tear-drop shape); (C) Acommissural valve (only raphae seen, no commissures seen reaching the wall of aorta and centrally stenotic opening). [Image and legend text from Mishra S, Awasthy N. Aortic valve diseases. In: Vijayalakshmi IB, Rao PS, Chugh R (Eds). A Comprehensive Approach to Congenital Heart Diseases. New Delhi, India: Jaypee Brothers Medical Publishers (P) Ltd. 2013].

Although the murmur of AS is often described as crescendo-decrescendo in nature, this quality pertains to relatively mild disease. As AS worsens, the murmur intensity peaks progressively, later in systole, until only a crescendo murmur is heard (Fig. 10.18), usually best in the aortic area, and radiating to the neck. As obstruction worsens, stroke volume often falls, reducing the loudness of the murmur so that there is weak negative correlation between murmur intensity and disease severity. In some cases the murmur is heard well over the aortic area, diminishes over the sternum, and reappearing in intensity over the LV apex, giving the false impression that a second murmur of mitral regurgitation is present (Gallavardin phenomenon).

Other clues to AS severity are the absence of the A2 component of the second heart sound because the aortic valve neither opens nor closes well, and an S4 gallop. There may be paradoxical splitting of the second heart sound due to slow emptying of the LV in advanced disease, but this sign is rarely seen today unless left bundle branch block is also present.

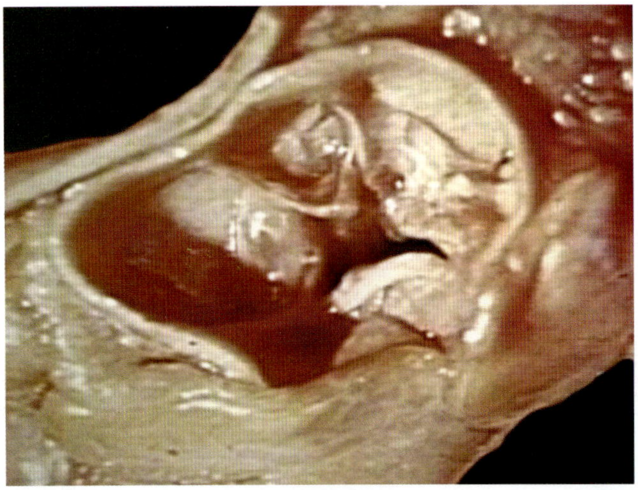

Fig. 10.12: Gross pathology specimen of a quadracuspid aortic valve. (Image from Armed Forces Institute of Pathology).

DIAGNOSIS

The electrocardiogram (ECG) may show signs of LVH (Fig. 10.19) and the chest X-ray may demonstrate a boot-shaped heart consistent with LVH, but the *sine quo non* for diagnosis is the echocardiogram (Figs. 10.20 and 10.21).

Echocardiographic evaluation can assess LV function, the presence of LVH, aortic valve motion (Video 10.1), transvalvular gradient, and aortic valve area (AVA). For blood flow volume to remain constant it must accelerate when it reaches a narrowed orifice. This increase in flow velocity (V) is used to calculate the instantaneous transvalvular pressure gradient (G) where,

$$G = 4V^2$$

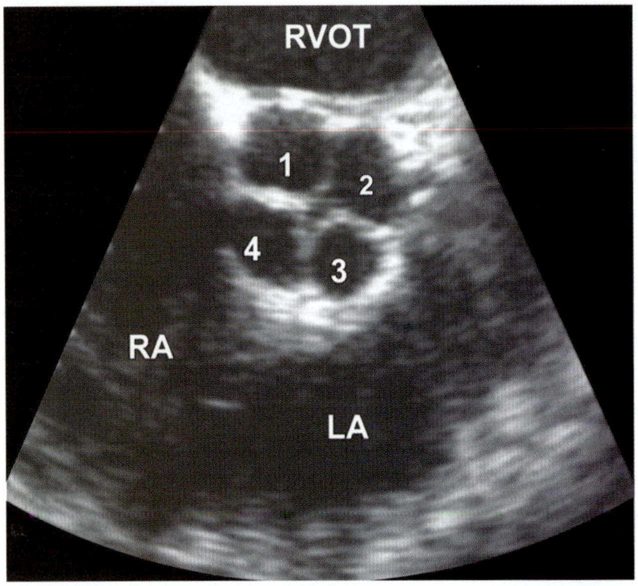

Fig. 10.13A: Parasternal short-axis images of a quadracuspid aortic valve imaged in (A) diastole. (LA: Left atrium; RA: Right atrium; RVOT: Right ventricular outflow tract).

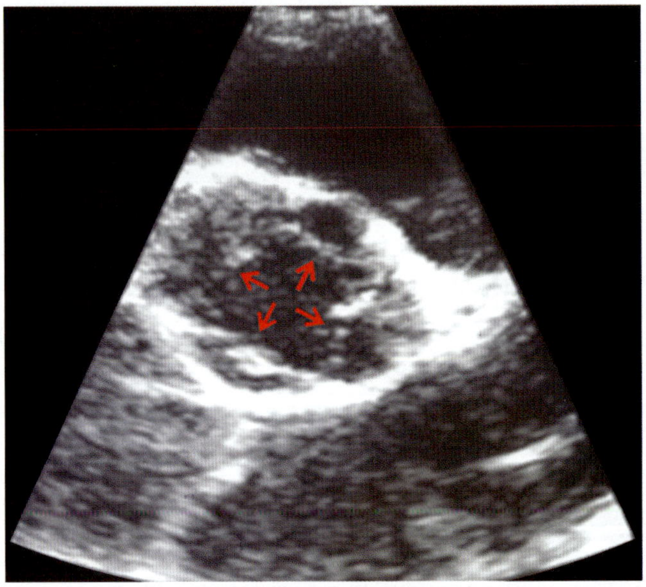

Fig. 10.13B: Systole. [Image adapted from Mishra S, Awasthy N. Aortic valve diseases. In: Vijayalakshmi IB, Rao PS, Chugh R (Eds). A Comprehensive Approach to Congenital Heart Diseases. New Delhi, India: Jaypee Brothers Medical Publishers (P) Ltd. 2013].

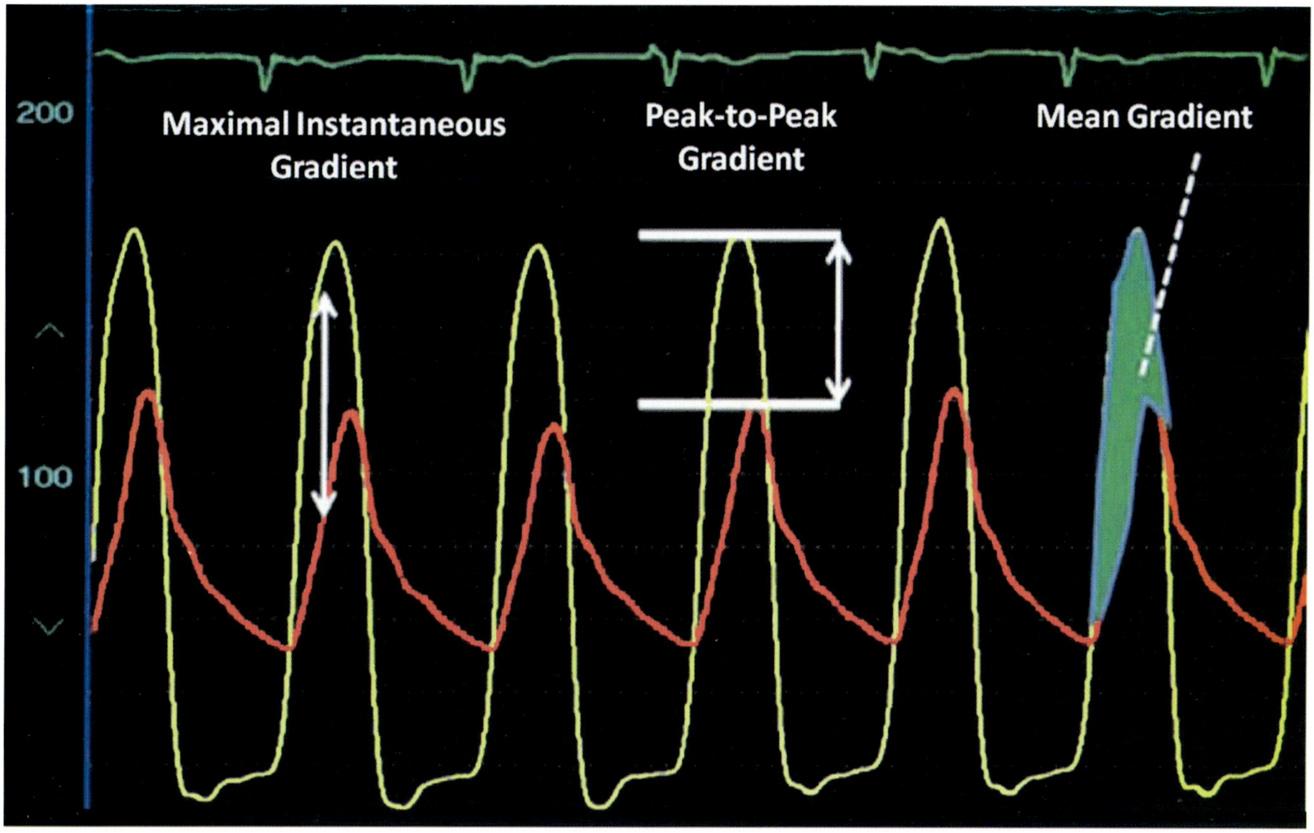

Fig. 10.14: Hemodynamic tracing in aortic stenosis. Maximal instantaneous gradient is the maximum pressure gradient between the aorta (red) and left ventricle (yellow) at a single point in time. Peak-to-peak gradient is the absolute difference between peak aortic systolic pressure and peak left ventricular systolic pressure. Mean gradient is defined by the area between the systolic left ventricular and aortic hemodynamic tracings (green shaded area). [Image and legend text from Singh AK, Boyle A, Yeghiazarians Y. Cardiac hemodynamics and coronary physiology. In: Chatterjee K, Anderson M, Heistad D, Kerber RE (Eds). Cardiology—An Illustrated Textbook. New Delhi, India: Jaypee Brothers Medical Publishers (P) Ltd. 2012].

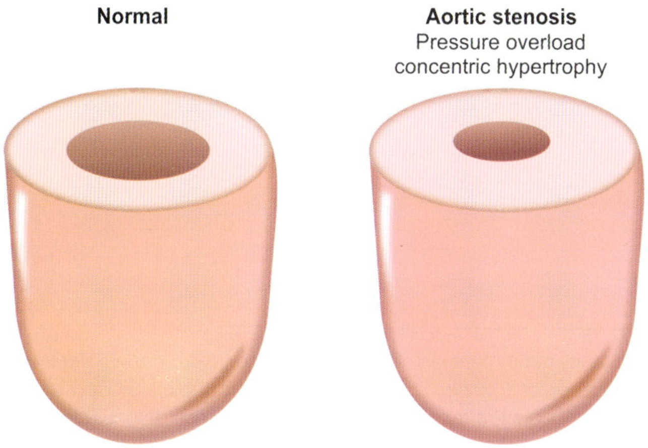

Fig. 10.15A: Schematic illustration of the compensatory concentric left ventricular hypertrophy in severe aortic stenosis. [Image adapted from Ursula P, Wolfgang D. Asymptomatic aortic stenosis—prognosis, risk stratification and follow-up. In: Hirota M (Ed). Aortic Stenosis—Etiology, Pathophysiology and Treatment. InTech; 2011].

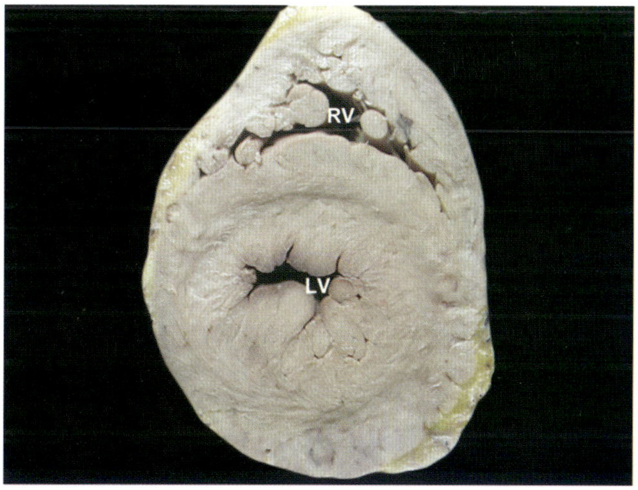

Fig. 10.15B: Severe concentric LVH from a patient with severe aortic stenosis. [Image courtesy of Dr Pradeep Vaideeswar, Professor (Additional), Department of Pathology, (Cardiovascular and Thoracic Division). Seth GS Medical College, Mumbai, India]. (LV: Left ventricle; RV: Right ventricle).

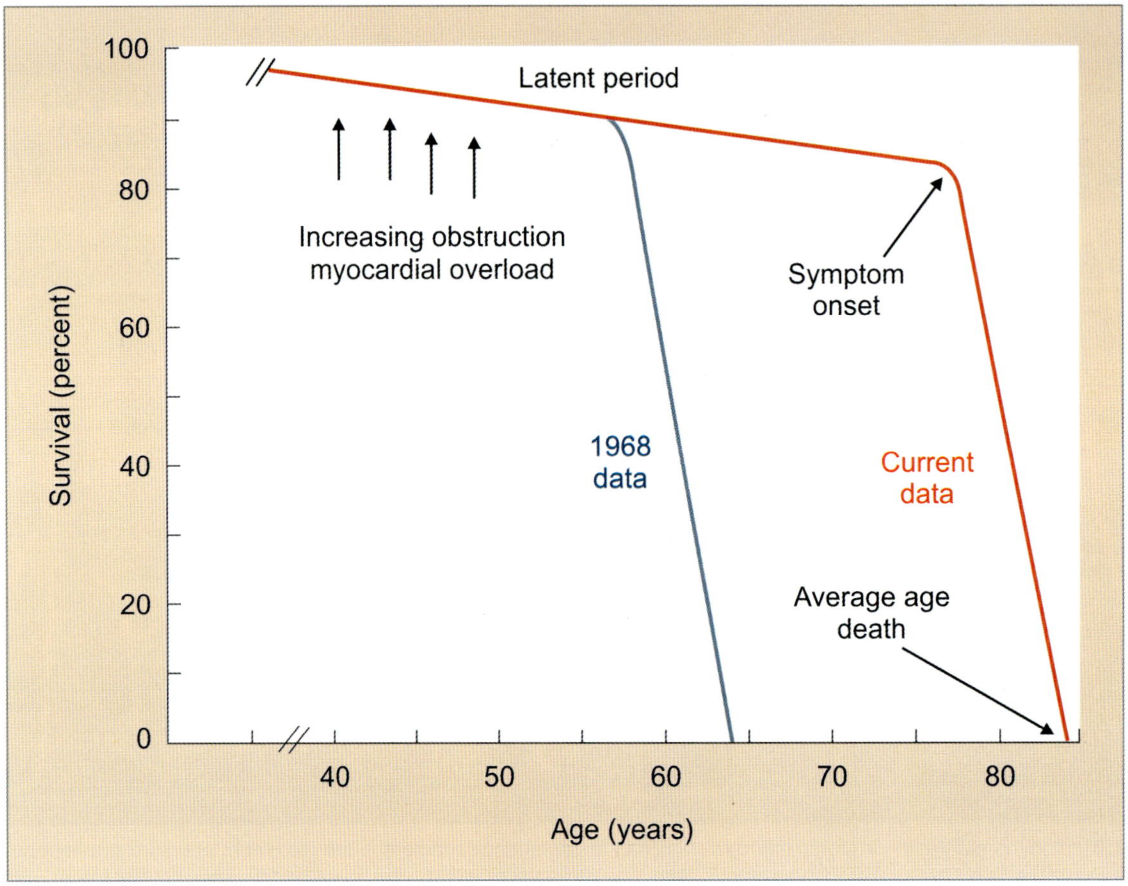

Fig. 10.16: The survival for aortic stenosis patients as of 1968 (light blue line) and for the present day (pink line). The onset of symptoms dramatically alters survival while symptom onset typically occurs later in life. (Image courtesy of Robert Bonow).

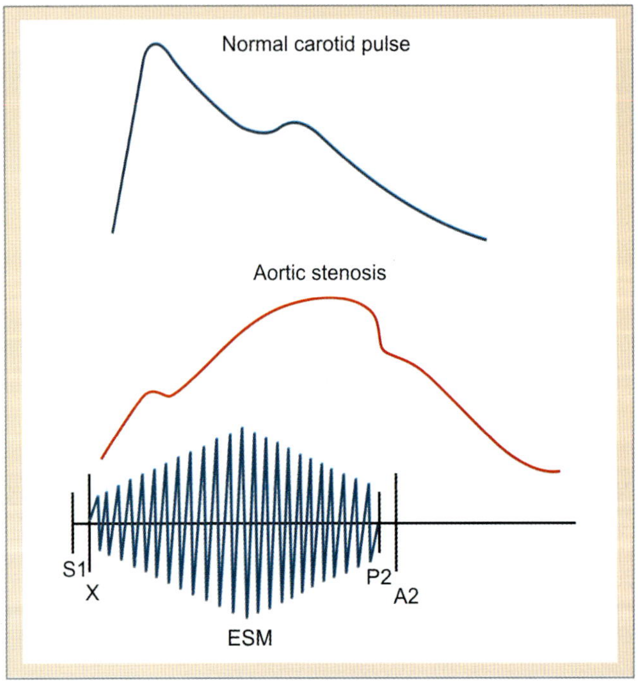

Fig. 10.17: Schematic illustration of the *parvus et tardus* carotid pulse in aortic stenosis. The upper image green tracing depicts a normal carotid pulse. The lower red tracing depicts the low amplitude and delayed pulse in aortic stenosis. Image also displays the corresponding crescendo-decrescendo ejection murmur seen in patients with mild or moderate aortic stensosis. [Image adapted from Chatterjee K. Physical examination. In: Chatterjee K, Anderson M, Heistad D, Kerber RE (Eds). Cardiology—An Illustrated Textbook. New Delhi, India: Jaypee Brothers Medical Publishers (P) Ltd. 2012].

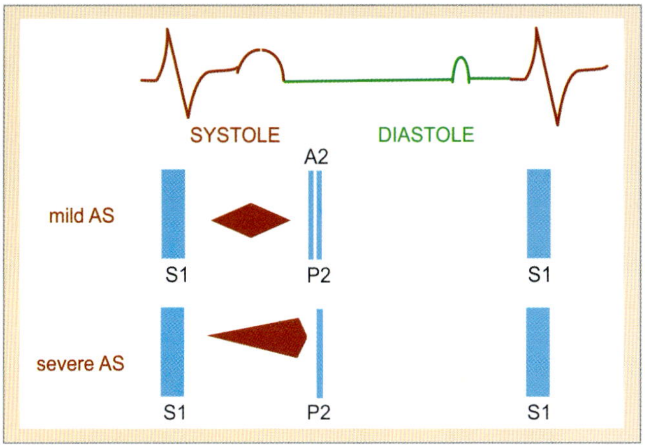

Fig. 10.18: The auscultatory findings for a patient with mild (upper panel) and severe (lower panel) AS are shown. As the disease severity worsens, the systolic ejection murmur peaks progressively later in systole and the A_2 component of the second heart sound is often lost. [Image adapted from Ursula P, Wolfgang D. Asymptomatic aortic stenosis—prognosis, risk stratification and follow-up. In: Hirota M (Ed). Aortic Stenosis—Etiology, Pathophysiology and Treatment. InTech; 2011].

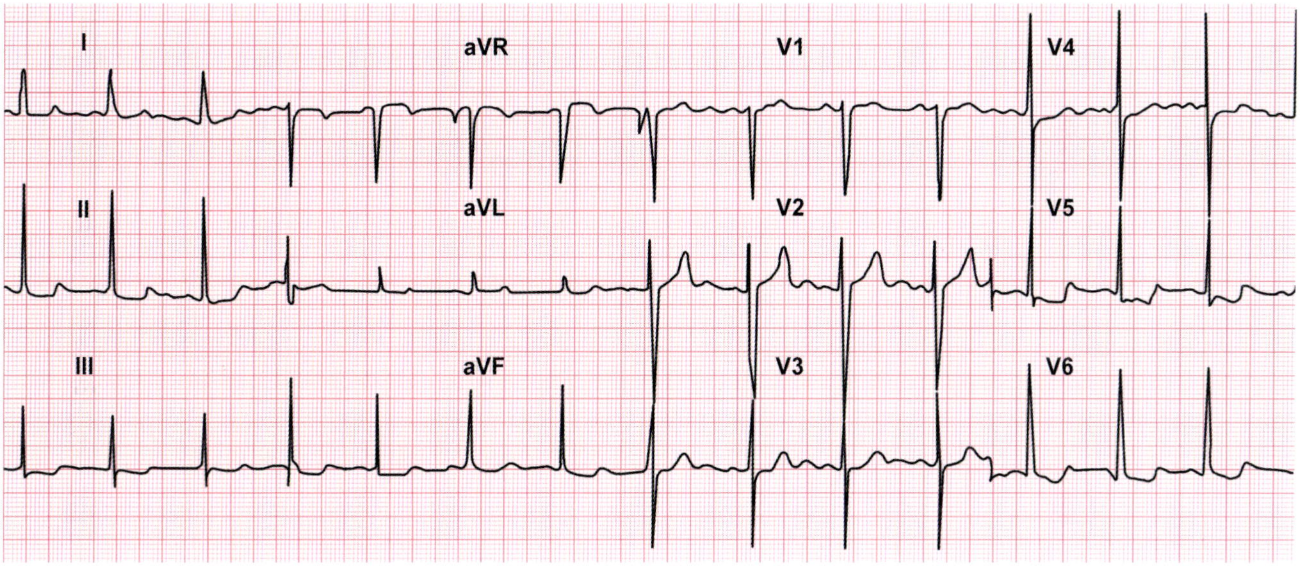

Fig. 10.19: A 12 lead electrocardiogram demonstrating left ventricular hypertrophy with a "strain pattern" in a patient with severe aortic stenosis. [Image from Mishra S, Awasthy N. Aortic valve diseases. In: Vijayalakshmi IB, Rao PS, Chugh R (Eds). A Comprehensive Approach to Congenital Heart Diseases. New Delhi, India: Jaypee Brothers Medical Publishers (P) Ltd. 2013].

It should be noted that the peak velocity determined echocardiographically differs from the peak to peak pressure gradient obtained from invasively-recorded pressure tracings as the pressure peaks obtained invasively do not occur instantaneously or simultaneously.

Because flow must remain constant on either side of the valve, the continuity equation is used to calculate AVA (Fig. 10.22).

If the patient has symptoms of AS, physical signs typical of AS, and the AVA is <1.0 cm^2 (or indexed to body service area 0.6 cm^2/m^2) or the mean transvalvular pressure gradient is above 40 mm Hg or peak jet velocity is > 4.0 m/sec, the AS is generally regarded as being "severe" in nature, and if untreated will have a predictably fatal progression. On the other hand, there are patients with an AVA of 1.0 cm^2 who have no other features consistent with severe AS, and no one single parameter should be used to diagnose life-threatening AS. Rather the whole clinical picture should be analyzed to arrive at a diagnosis.

In about 80% of AS cases the diagnosis of severity is obvious (i.e., the patient with syncope and an 80 mm Hg mean transvalvular pressure gradient and an AVA of 0.6 cm^2). However, in some cases, the degree of severity after echocardiography is still in doubt and other diagnostic modalities must be used to clarify the clinical picture. In most cases of severe AS the valve has become

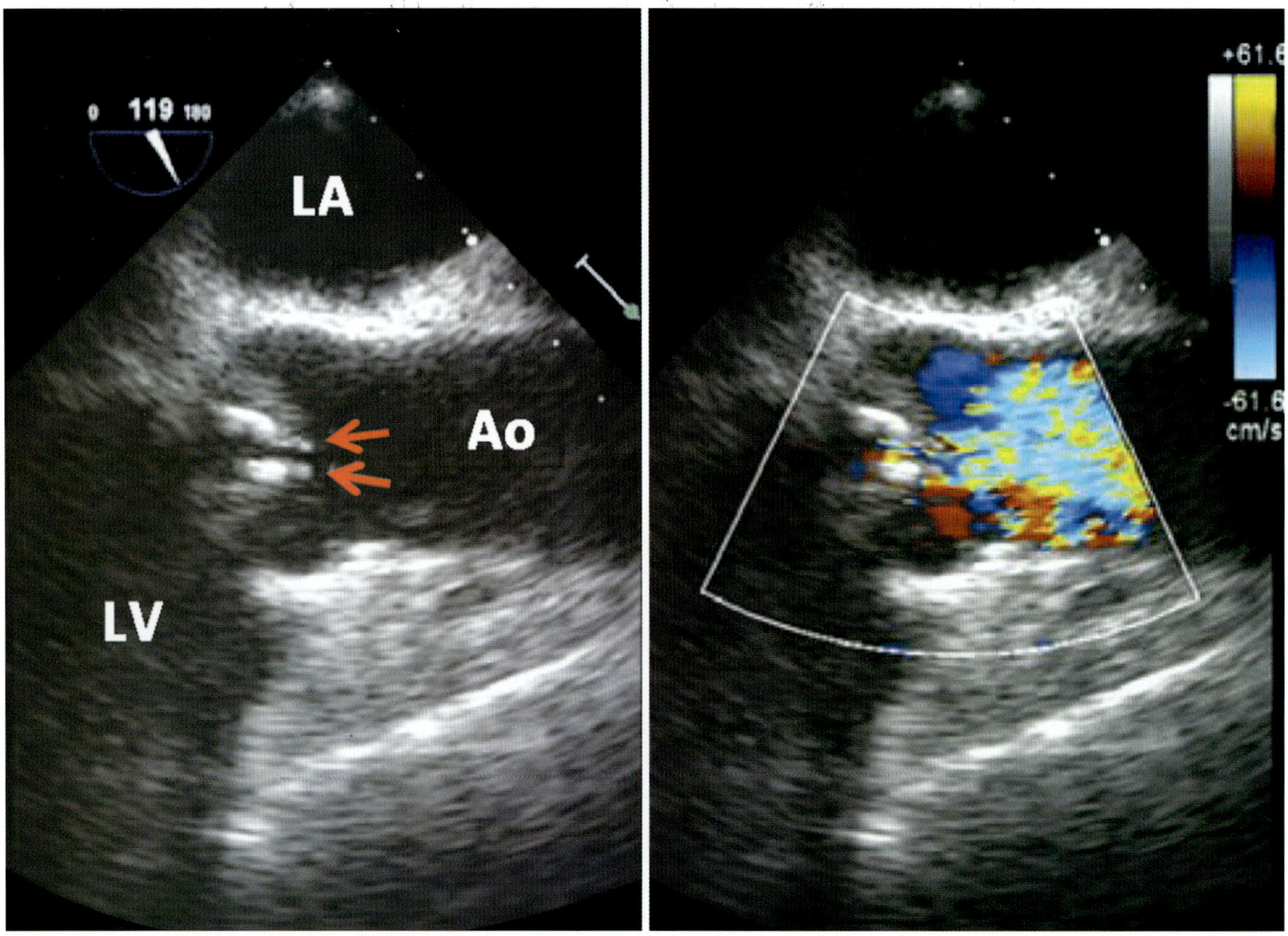

Fig. 10.20: Transesophageal long-axis view image demonstrating severe aortic stenosis. There is severely restricted leaflet mobility (left panel, arrows), resulting in turbulent blood flow (right panel). [Image and legend text from Hashemi SM, Lindower P, Kerber RE. Transesophageal echocardiography. In: Chatterjee K, Anderson M, Heistad D, Kerber RE (Eds). Cardiology—An Illustrated Textbook. New Delhi, India: Jaypee Brothers Medical Publishers (P) Ltd. 2012]. (Ao: Aortic valve; LA: Left atrium; LV: Left ventricle).

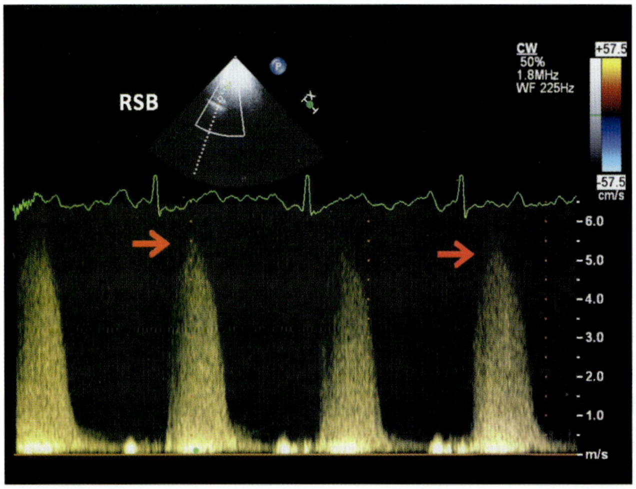

Fig. 10.21: Pedoff Doppler interrogation of the aortic valve from the right sternal border (RSB), revealing a peak jet velocity of greater than 5 m/sec, indicative of severe aortic stenosis. Using the formula $G = 4V^2$, this velocity translates to a peak pressure gradient of 100 mm Hg. (Image courtesy of Glenn N Levine, MD).

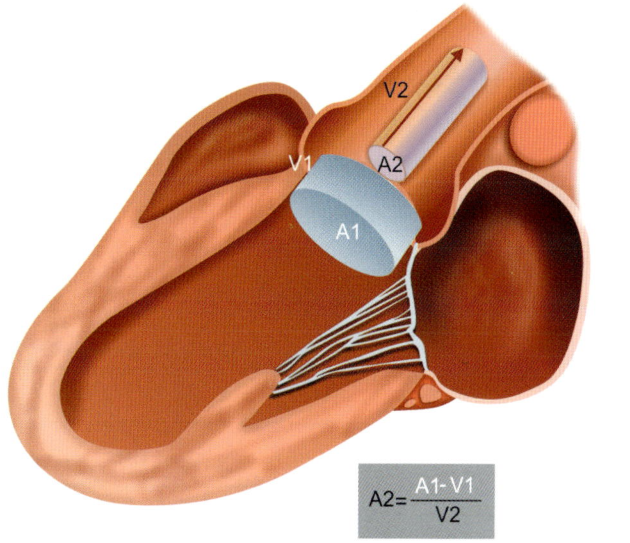

Fig. 10.22: A schematic of the continuity equation is shown. A1 is the area of the aortic outflow tract and A2 is the aortic valve area. As blood enters the valve it must accelerate creating V2. [Image adapted with permission from Baumgartner H et al. Echocardiographic assessment of valve stenosis: EAE/ASE recommendations for clinical practice 2009;22:1-23].

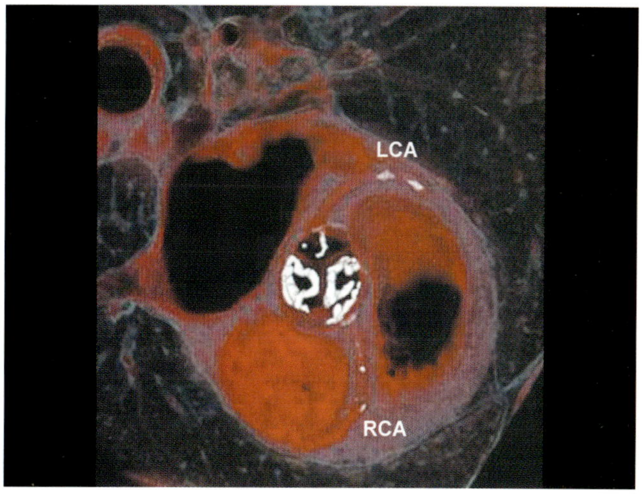

Fig. 10.23: Cardiac CT imaging demonstrating severe aortic valve calcification in a patient with aortic stenosis. [Image adapted from Ursula P, Wolfgang D. Asymptomatic aortic stensosis—prognosis, risk stratification and follow-up. In: Hirota M (Ed). Aortic Stenosis—Etiology, Pathophysiology and Treatment. InTech; 2011]. (LCA: Left coronary artery; RCA: Right coronary artery).

severely calcified and calcification roughly correlates with disease severity. Cardiac CT can be used to ascertain the extent of calcification, wherein the finding of a severely calcified valve supports the diagnosis of severe AS (Fig. 10.23). CT images can also be used in some cases to visualize and directly measure the aortic orifice area, recognizing that this anatomic area must be differentiated from the physiologic area usually used to quantify stenosis severity (Fig. 10.24).

Magnetic resonance imaging is increasingly used in the assessment of cardiac valve pathology and can also be used to establish jet velocity to calculate a valve area (Figs. 10.25A and B).

When diagnosis is still in doubt, direct measurement of the transvalvular gradient (Fig. 10.26) during a carefully performed heart catheterization adds further data to assess AS severity, including gradients and calculated AVA. For an invasive study to be helpful, there must be fastidious attention to catheter placement and transducer calibration. Simultaneous measurement of cardiac output and transvalvular gradient allows calculation of AVA using the Gorlin formula.

Summary tables of the classification of degree of AS are given in Tables 10.1 and 10.2.

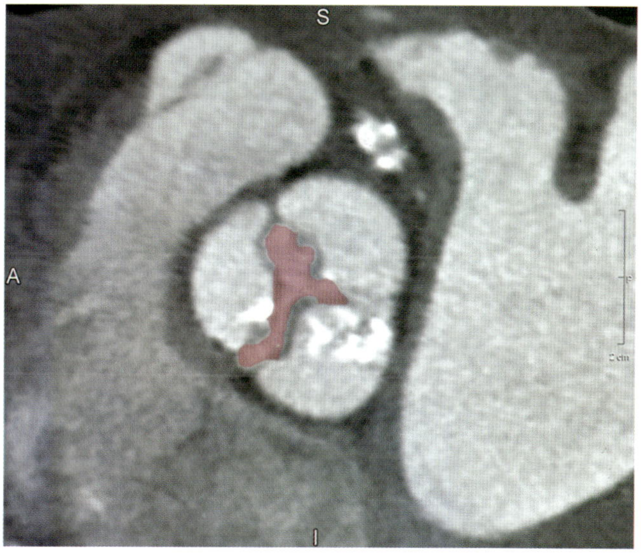

Fig. 10.24: Cardiac CT showing valve calcification. The pink area is the valve opening and can be planimetered to obtain a valve area. (Image courtesy of Glenn N Levine).

MANAGEMENT OF AORTIC STENOSIS

The only effective therapy for AS is aortic valve replacement (AVR). There is no effective medical therapy for the disease. Balloon valvotomy (Figs. 10.27 and 10.28) is a

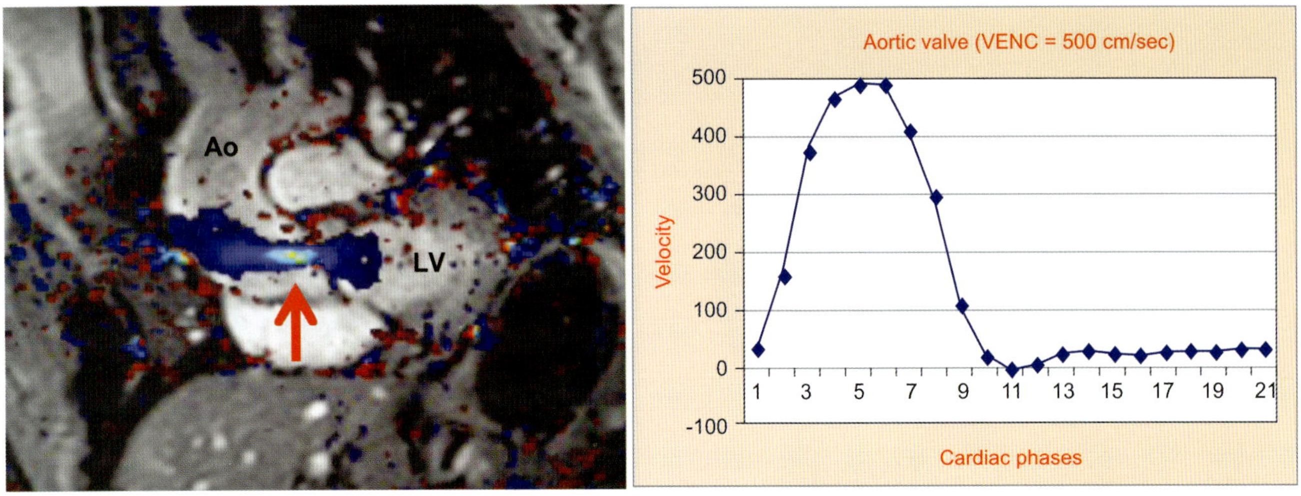

Fig. 10.25A: Example of MRI assessment of flow acceleration across the aortic valve. An area of flow interrogation in the area of the aortic valve is interrogated (arrow). Peak flow velocity can be seen to be almost 5 m/sec, indicating severe aortic stenosis. (Image courtesy of Dr Scott Flamm).

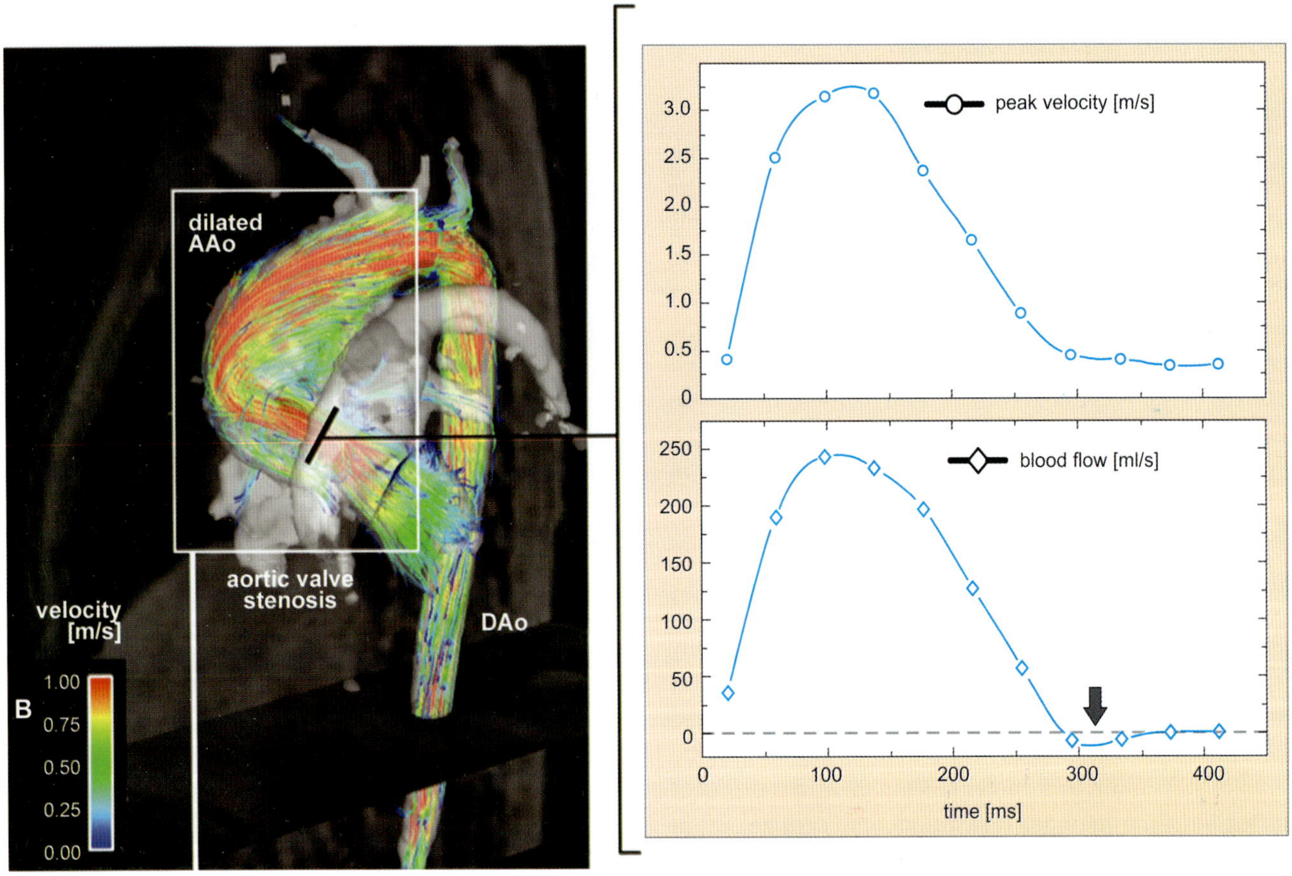

Fig. 10.25B: 3D flow visualization and flow quantification using MRI in a young patient with aortic stenosis and dilation of the ascending aorta. Peak velocity is 3.2 m/sec. (Image from Markl M, Kilner PJ, Ebbers T. Comprehensive 4D velocity mapping of the heart and great vessels by cardiovascular magnetic resonance. J Cardiovasc Magn Reson. 2011;13:7). (Ao: Aorta; LV: Left ventricle).

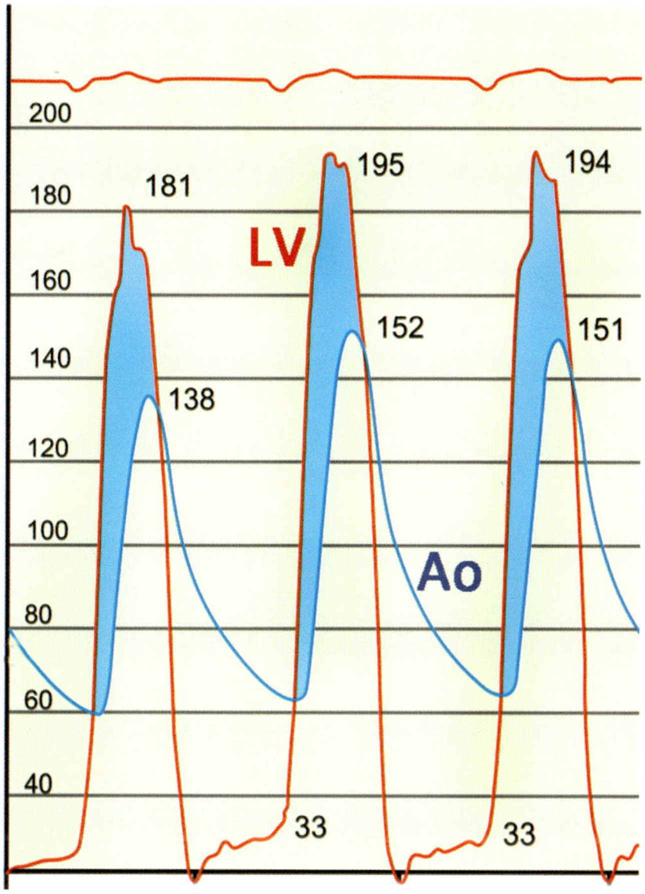

Fig. 10.26: Hemodynamic tracings of left ventricular (red tracing, LV) and aortic (blued tracing, Ao) pressures demonstrating a pressure gradient (shaded blue area) due to the presence of aortic stenosis. [Image adapted from Mishra S, Awasthy N. Aortic valve diseases. In: Vijayalakshmi IB, Rao PS, Chugh R (Eds). A Comprehensive Approach to Congenital Heart Diseases. New Delhi, India: Jaypee Brothers Medical Publishers (P) Ltd. 2013].

palliative therapy that does not extend life but is sometimes used as a bridge to AVR. Valve replacement is usually performed surgically, although transcatheter aortic valve replacement (TAVR) (Figs. 10.29A to C) is a lifesaving therapy in selected patients who are either inoperable or at very high risk for surgery. This therapy will evolve rapidly over the next decade and will likely be used more frequently in the future.

Aortic valve replacement is indicated in symptomatic patients or in those in whom there is reduced ejection fraction (EF) without symptoms. There is also a subset of asymptomatic patients who, although asymptomatic, are at higher than average risk for sudden death. These include those with poor exercise tolerance, those with very severe AS (AVA <0.6 cm^2), those with a rising B-type natriuretic protein (BNP) level, those with severe LVH, and those with heavy valve calcification. In such patients earlier AVR may be pursued in the absence of symptoms.

Tables 10.3 and 10.4 summarize the guideline recommendations for surgical AVR. Guidelines for the performance of TAVR are given in Chapter 17.

Table 10.1: Summary of the European Society of Cardiology (ESC) and European Association for Cardiothoracic Surgery (EACTS) guidelines on the management of valvular heart disease criteria for the diagnosis of severe aortic stenosis. Gradient and jet velocity criteria apply for patients with normal cardiac output/transvalvular flow.

• Valve area < 1.0 cm^2
• Indexed valve area 0.6 cm^2/m^2 body surface area
• Mean gradient > 40 mm Hg
• Maximum jet velocity > 4.0 (m/sec)
• Velocity ratio < 0.25

Low Flow, Low Gradient, Low Ejection Fraction Aortic Stenosis

In patients with reduced EF (< 30%) and low mean transvalvular gradient (< 30 mm Hg) there is invariably severe LV muscle dysfunction and patient prognosis is not favorable. Additionally, at reduced cardiac output, especially when cardiac output is < 5 L/minute, a damaged LV may be unable to open a mildly but not severely stenotic valve to its full orifice area, resulting in calculation of a small AVA, a condition called *pseudoaortic stenosis*. A critical patient management dilemma is to distinguish whether such patients with reduced EF and low transvalvular gradients have true AS or pseudoaortic stenosis. In such cases, administration of a positive inotrope such as dobutamine serves two purposes. Augmentation of cardiac output helps distinguish between true AS, wherein increased output increases gradient and AVA increases only slightly, versus pseudo AS, where increased output increases AVA significantly (to greater than 1.0 cm^2) but gradient increases only slightly. These latter patients probably will not benefit from AVR and have a prognosis similar to other patients treated medically for heart failure. On the other hand, if there is true AS and stroke volume is augmented by at least 20% (inotropic reserve), these patients are likely to benefit from AVR, particularly if their resting mean gradient exceeds 20 mm Hg.

Table 10.2: Summary of the new American College of Cardiology Foundation/American Heart Association guidelines classification of aortic stenosis. (AS: Aortic stenosis; LVEF: Left ventricular ejection fraction; LV: Left ventricle; EF: Ejection fraction; AVA: Aortic valve area).

Stage/Definition	*Valve Anatomy and Hemodynamics*	*Hemodynamic Consequences and Symptoms*
A - At risk of AS	• Bicuspid aortic valve (or other congenital valve anomaly) • Aortic valve sclerosis • Aortic jet velocity < 2 m/s	• No hemodynamic consequences • No symptoms
B - Progressive AS	• Mild-to-moderate leaflet calcification of a bicuspid or trileaflet valve with some reduction in systolic motion or • Rheumatic valve changes with commissural fusion • *Mild AS*: Aortic jet velocity 2.0–2.9 m/s or mean ΔP < 20 mm Hg • *Moderate AS*: Aortic jet velocity 3.0–3.9 m/s or mean ΔP 20–39 mm Hg	• Early LV diastolic dysfunction may be present • Normal LVEF • No symptoms
C1 - Asymptomatic severe AS	• Severe leaflet calcification or congenital stenosis with severely reduced leaflet opening • Aortic jet velocity ≥ 4 m/s or mean ΔP ≥ 40 mm Hg • AVA typically is ≤ 1 cm^2 • Very severe AS is a jet velocity ≥ 5 m/s, or mean ΔP ≥ 60 mm Hg	• LV diastolic dysfunction • Mild LV hypertrophy • Normal LVEF • No symptoms
C2 - Asymptomatic severe AS with LV dysfunction (LVEF < 50%)	• Severe leaflet calcification or congenital stenosis with severely reduced leaflet opening • Aortic jet velocity ≥ 4 m/s or mean ΔP ≥ 40 mm Hg • AVA typically is ≤ 1 cm^2	• LVEF < 50% • No symptoms
D1 - Symptomatic severe high-gradient AS	• Severe leaflet calcification or congenital stenosis with severely reduced leaflet opening • Aortic jet velocity ≥ 4 m/s, or mean ΔP ≥ 40 mm Hg • AVA typically is ≤ 1 cm^2 but may be larger with mixed AS/AR	• LV diastolic dysfunction • LV hypertrophy • Pulmonary hypertension may be present • Exertional dyspnea, angina, syncope or presyncope, or decreased exercise tolerance
D2 - Symptomatic severe low-flow/low-gradient AS with reduced LVEF	• Severe leaflet calcification with severely reduced leaflet motion • AVA ≤ 1 cm^2 with • Resting aortic jet velocity < 4 m/s or mean ΔP < 40 mm Hg • Dobutamine stress echo shows AVA ≤ 1 cm^2 with jet velocity ≥ 4 m/s at any flow rate	• LV diastolic dysfunction • LV hypertrophy • LVEF < 50% • Heart failure, angina, syncope, or presyncope
D3 - Symptomatic severe low-gradient AS with normal LVEF or paradoxical low-flow severe AS	• Severe leaflet calcification with severely reduced leaflet motion • AVA ≤ 1 cm^2 with aortic jet velocity < 4 m/s, or mean ΔP < 40 mm Hg • Stroke volume index < 35 mL/m^2	• Increased LV relative wall thickness • Small LV chamber with low-stroke volume. • Restrictive diastolic filling • LVEF ≥ 50% • Heart failure, angina, syncope, or presyncope

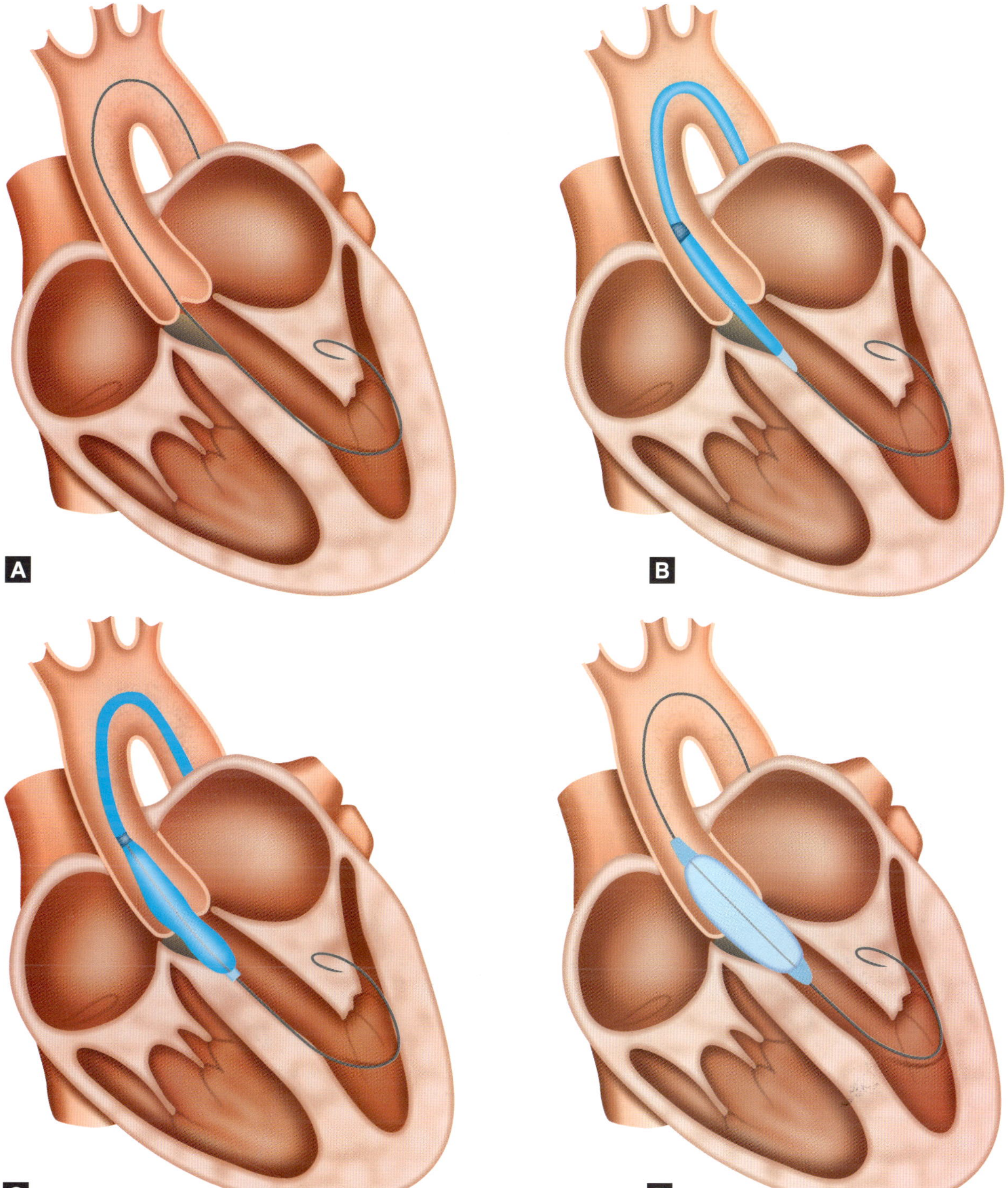

Figs. 10.27A to D: Schematic illustration of the steps in balloon aortic valvuloplasty (BAV). [Image from Gudmundsson H, Horwitz PA. Catheter-based treatment of valvular heart disease. In: Chatterjee K, Anderson M, Heistad D, Kerber RE (Eds). Cardiology—An Illustrated Textbook. New Delhi, India: Jaypee Brothers Medical Publishers (P) Ltd. 2012].

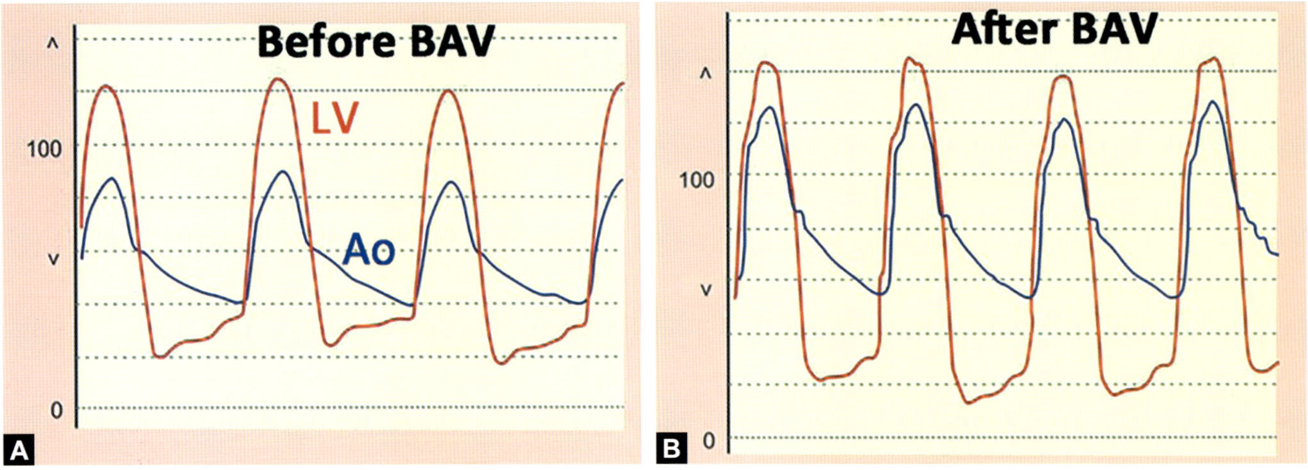

Figs. 10.28A and B: Hemodynamic tracings (A) before and (B) after balloon aortic valvuloplasty (BAV). Simultaneous pressure tracings from the left ventricle (red line, LV) and aorta (blue line, Ao) are shown. [Images from Gudmundsson H, Horwitz PA. Catheter-based treatment of valvular heart disease. In: Chatterjee K, Anderson M, Heistad D, Kerber RE (Eds). Cardiology—An Illustrated Textbook. New Delhi, India: Jaypee Brothers Medical Publishers (P) Ltd. 2012].

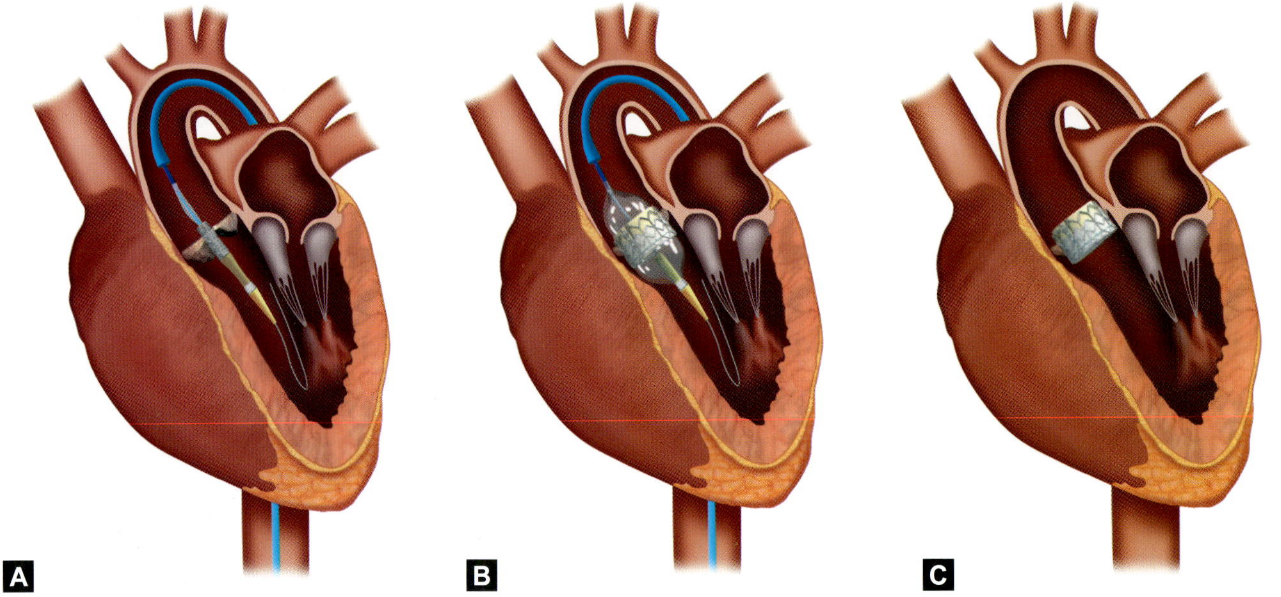

Figs. 10.29A to C: Deployment of the balloon-expandable Edwards Sapien valve via the transfemoral route. (A) Valve is delivered retrograde from the femoral artery and positioned at the level of the aortic annulus; (B) Balloon inflated, deploying the valve; (C) Deployed valve. (Images courtesy of Edwards Lifesciences).

Low Flow, Low Gradient, Normal Ejection Fraction Aortic Stenosis

In some patients, extensive concentric LVH reduces LV chamber volume, which in turn reduces stroke volume, despite the presence of a normal EF. Because it is stroke volume that generates the transvalvular gradient, the gradient in such patients is also low, potentially misleading the clinician into underestimating the severity of the AS. If such patients have features consistent with severe AS, including a typical physical exam, a small AVA and valvular calcification, AVR is indicated.

Table 10.3: Summary of the European Society of Cardiology (ESC) and European Association for Cardiothoracic Surgery (EACTS) guidelines for the performance of surgery for severe aortic stenosis. The level of evidence (LOE) supporting the recommendation is given in parenthesis, where LOE = A denotes a recommendation derived from multiple randomized clinical trials or meta-analyses; LOE = B denotes a recommendation derived from a single randomized clinical trial or large non-randomized studies; and LOE = C denotes a recommendation based on consensus of expert opinion or based on small studies, retrospective studies, or registries. (AS: Aortic stenosis; CABG: Coronary artery bypass surgery; LVEF: Left ventricular ejection fraction; LV: Left ventricle; EF: Ejection fraction; BNP: B-type natriuretic protein; LOE: Level of evidence).

Class I (is recommended; is indicated)
• Symptomatic patients with severe AS (LOE=B)
• Asymptomatic patients with severe AS with systolic LV dysfunction (LVEF ≤ 50%) not due to another cause (LOE = C)
• Asymptomatic patients with severe AS and abnormal exercise test showing symptoms on exercise clearly related to AS (LOE = C)
• Patients with severe AS undergoing CABG, surgery on the ascending aorta, or surgery on another valve (LOE = C)
Class IIa (should be considered)
• Asymptomatic patients with severe AS and abnormal exercise test showing fall in blood pressure below baseline (LOE = C)
• Patients with moderate AS undergoing CABG, surgery of the ascending aorta, or surgery on another valve (LOE = C)
• Symptomatic patients with low flow, low gradient (< 40 mm Hg) AS with normal EF only after careful confirmation of severe AS (LOE = C)
• Symptomatic patients with severe AS, low flow, low gradient with reduced EF, and evidence of flow (contractile) reserve (LOE = C)
• Asymptomatic patients with normal EF and no exercise test abnormalities if the surgical risk is low and there is very severe AS (peak transvalvular velocity > 5.5 m/sec) and/or severe valve calcification and a rate of peak transvalvular velocity progression of ≥ 0.3 m/sec/year (LOE = C)
• High risk patients with severe symptomatic AS who are suitable for TVI, but in whom surgery is favored by a “heart team” based on individual risk profile and anatomic suitability (LOE = B)
Class IIb (may be considered)
• Symptomatic patients with severe AS low flow, low gradient, and LV dysfunction without flow (contractile) reserve (LOE = C)
• Asymptomatic patients with severe AS, normal EF, and no exercise test abnormalities, if surgical risk is low, and one or more of the following are present (LOE = C):
– Markedly elevated BNP levels confirmed by repeated measurement and without other explanation
– Increase of mean pressure gradient with exercise by > 20 mm Hg
– Excessive LV hypertrophy in the absence of hypertension

Table 10.4: Summary of the new American College of Cardiology Foundation/American Heart Association guidelines for the performance of aortic valve replacement in patients with aortic stenosis. (LOE: Level of evidence; LVEF: Left ventricular ejection fraction; AS: Aortic stenosis).

Class I (is recommended; is indicated)
• Severe high-gradient AS with symptoms by history or on exercise testing (LOE = B)
• Asymptomatic patients with severe AS and LVEF< 50% (LOE = B)
• Severe AS when undergoing other cardiac surgery (LOE = B)
Class IIa (is reasonable)
• Asymptomatic patients with very severe AS (aortic jet velocity ≥ 5 m/sec) and low surgical risk (LOE = B)
• Asymptomatic patients with severe AS and decreased exercise tolerance or an exercise fall in BP (LOE = B)
• Symptomatic patients with low-flow/low-gradient severe AS with reduced LVEF with a low-dose dobutamine stress study that shows an aortic jet velocity ≥ 4 m/sec and a valve area ≤ 1.0 cm^2 (LOE = B)
• Symptomatic patients who have low-flow/low-gradient severe AS who are normotensive and have an LVEF ≥ 50% if clinical, hemodynamic, and anatomic data support valve obstruction as the most likely cause of symptoms (LOE = C)
• Patients with moderate AS who are undergoing other cardiac surgery (LOE = C)
Class IIb (may be considered)
• Asymptomatic patients with severe AS and rapid disease progression and low surgical risk (LOE = C)

SUMMARY

Aortic stenosis in developed countries accrues from a process similar to atherosclerosis. Once severe AS causes symptoms, life span is shortened with a death rate of 25% per year. Diagnosis is based upon physical examination and echocardiography in most cases. The only effective therapy for AS is AVR which is usually performed surgically although transcatheter techniques available today offer lifesaving relief to those at high surgical risk.

VIDEO LEGENDS

Videos 10.1 to 10.3: Parasternal long-axis transthoracic echocardiography (TTE) of heavily calcified and stenotic aortic valves. Note the markedly decreased excursion of the aortic valve leaflets during systole. Videos (Video courtesy of Glenn N Levine, MD).

Video 10.4: MRI of a stenotic bicuspid aortic valve. (Video courtesy of Scott D Flamm, MD).

REFERENCES

Carabello BA. Introduction to aortic stenosis. Circ Res. 2013;113(2):179-85.

Carabello BA. George Ohm and the changing character of aortic stenosis: it's not your grandfather's oldsmobile. Circulation 2012;125(19):2295-7.

Carabello BA, Paulus WJ. Aortic stenosis. Lancet. 2009;373(9667):956-66.

Monin JL, Quéré JP, Monchi M, et al. Low-gradient aortic stenosis: operative risk stratification and predictors for long-term outcome: a multicenter study using dobutamine stress hemodynamics. Circulation. 2003;108(3):319-24.

Nishimura RA, Carabello BA, Faxon DP, et al. ACC/AHA 2008 Guideline update on valvular heart disease: focused update on infective endocarditis: a report of the American College of Cardiology/American Heart Association Task Force on Practice Guidelines endorsed by the Society of Cardiovascular Anesthesiologists, Society for Cardiovascular Angiography and Interventions, and Society of Thoracic Surgeons. J Am Coll Cardiol. 2008;52(8):676-85.

Otto CM, Kuusisto J, Reichenback DD, et al. Characterization of the early lesion of "degenerative" valvular aortic stenosis. Histological and immunohistochemical studies. Circulation. 1994;90(2):844-53.

Pellikka PA, Sarano ME, Nishimura RA, et al. Outcome of 622 adults with asymptomatic, hemodynamically significant aortic stenosis during prolonged follow-up. Circulation. 2005;111(24):3290-5.

Ross J Jr, Braunwald E. Aortic stenosis. Circulation. 1968;38(1 Suppl):61-7.

CHAPTER

11

Aortic Regurgitation

Kanu Chatterjee, James D Rossen, Phillip A Horwitz

INTRODUCTION

The normal aortic valve consists of three cusps (leaflets), attached to the aortic annulus and base of the heart and situated in the aortic root (Figs. 11.1 and 11.2). Normal coaptation of the leaflets during diastole prevents aortic regurgitation. Aortic regurgitation results when there is incompetence of the aortic valve. Aortic regurgitation (Figs. 11.3A and B and Videos 11.1 to 11.5) can result from abnormalities of leaflets, the aortic root or the annulus. As the mechanisms and management of acute and chronic aortic regurgitation differ, these two conditions are discussed separately.

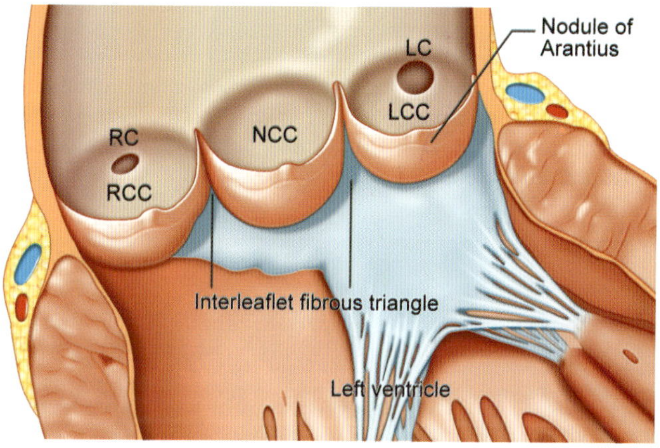

Fig. 11.1: The aortic leaflets and their attachment to the aortic root [Image from Mishra S, Awasthy N. Aortic valve diseases. In: Vijayalakshmi IB et al. (Eds). A Comprehensive Approach to Congenital Heart Diseases. New Delhi, India: Jaypee Brothers Medical Publishers (P) Ltd.].

ACUTE AORTIC REGURGITATION

Infective endocarditis (Fig. 11.4) is the most common cause of acute aortic regurgitation. Infective endocarditis

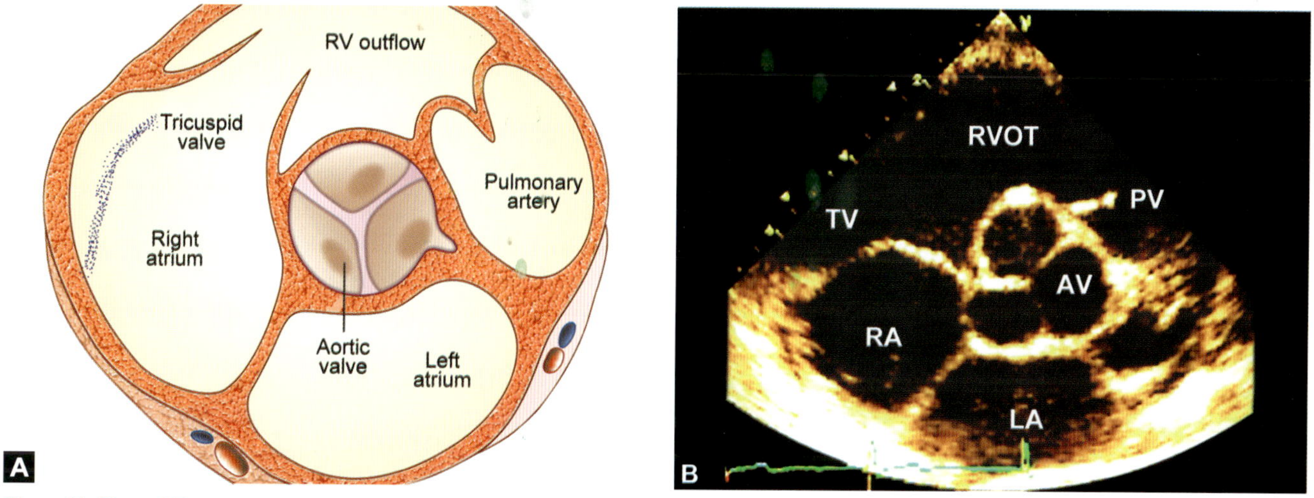

Figs. 11.2A and B: The aortic valve. (A) cartoon showing the base of the heart; (B) The corresponding parasternal short-axis view of the aortic valve. [Images from Mishra S, Awasthy N. Aortic valve diseases. In: Vijayalakshmi IB et al. (Eds). A Comprehensive Approach to Congenital Heart Diseases. New Delhi, India: Jaypee Brothers Medical Publishers (P) Ltd.].

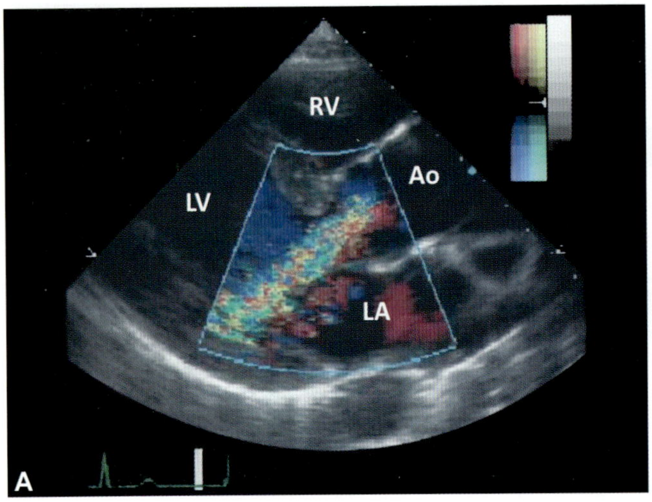

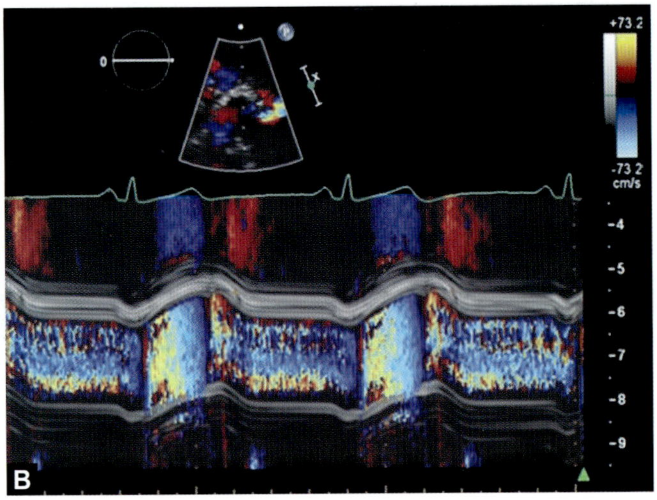

Figs. 11.3A and B: (A) Parasternal long axis echocardiogram demonstrating severe aortic regurgitation; (B) Color Doppler M-mode demonstrating pan-diastolic aortic regurgitation [Haleem K et al. M-mode examination. In: Nanda NC (Ed). Comprehensive Textbook of Echocardiography. New Delhi, India: Jaypee Brothers Medical Publishers (P) Ltd.]. (Ao: Aorta; LA: Left atrium; LV: Left ventricle; RV: Right ventricle).

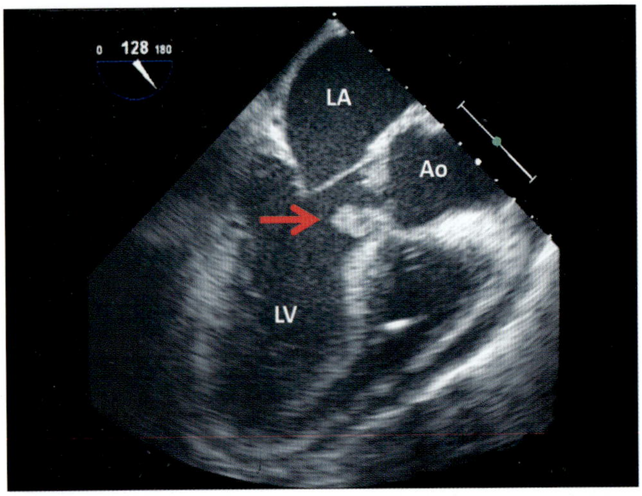

Fig. 11.4: Transesophageal echocardiogram of a patient with bacterial endocarditis showing a large aortic valve vegetation (arrow). (Ao: Aorta; LA: Left atrium; LV: Left ventricle).

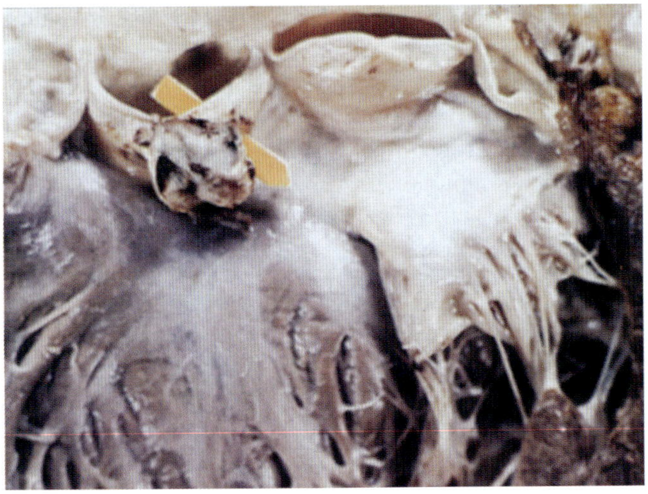

Fig. 11.5: Perforation (arrow) of the aortic cusp from endocarditis.

can result in perforation of the leaflet (Fig. 11.5). Aortic dissection (Figs. 11.6 and 11.7) and trauma are other causes of acute aortic regurgitation. In Type A aortic dissection, aortic regurgitation occurs if there is prolapse of the sinus of Valsalva.

Acute aortic regurgitation results in a sudden increase in volume load to the left ventricle, causing a disproportionate increase in left ventricular diastolic pressure, which may precipitate acute pulmonary edema. Analysis of the pressure volume loop in acute severe aortic regurgitation (Fig. 11.8) demonstrates that there is only a slight increase in left ventricular diastolic volume, but there is a marked increase in left ventricular diastolic pressure, resulting in pulmonary edema. As left ventricular diastolic pressure is markedly increased, the differences between aortic diastolic pressure and left ventricular diastolic pressure (transmural pressure gradient) is decreased, which can lead to impaired subendocardial perfusion and subendocardial ischemia. Subendocardial ischemia may cause myocardial injury and myocyte loss.

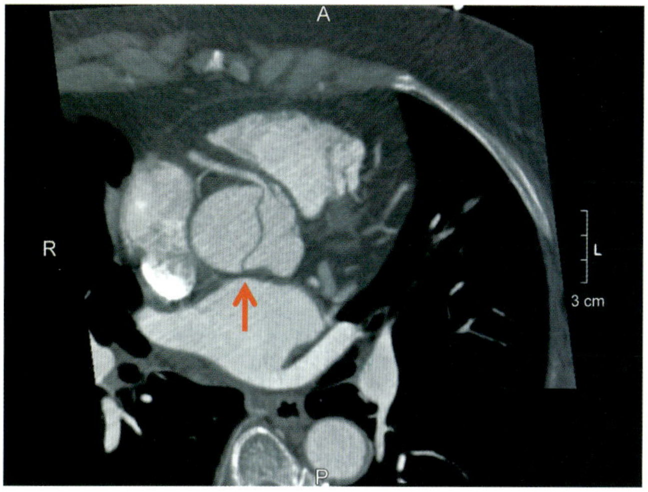

Fig. 11.6: CT scan demonstrating type A aortic dissection. The intimal flap (arrow) extends to and partially compromises the right coronary artery.

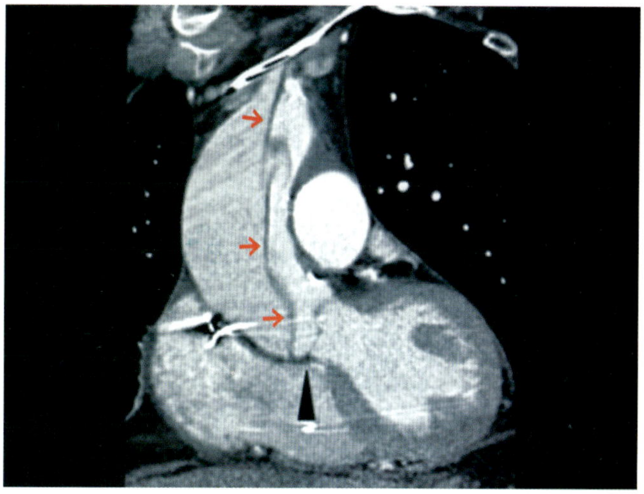

Fig. 11.7: Contrast-enhanced CT examination showing type A dissection. The dissection flap compromises the aortic leaflets and valve. (Image courtesy of Dr Alan C Braverman, Washington University School of Medicine).

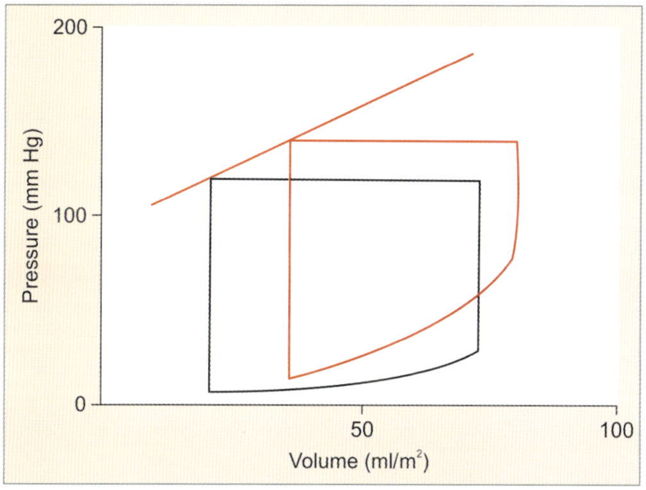

Fig. 11.8: Pressure volume loops in acute severe aortic regurgitation. The diastolic pressure—volume relation shifts upward and to the right with a marked increase in left ventricular diastolic pressure. Stroke volume is reduced. There is no change in contractile function as there was no shift of the isovolumic pressure line.

EVALUATION OF THE PATIENT WITH ACUTE AORTIC REGURGITATION

Physical examination in patients with severe acute aortic regurgitation reveals evidences of low cardiac output. There is tachycardia and the arterial pulse amplitude is decreased. Jugular venous pressure is elevated in those patients who have secondary right ventricular failure due to post-capillary pulmonary arterial hypertension. The intensity of the pulmonic component of the second heart sound (P2) is increased. The character of the left ventricular apical impulse is normal, indicating normal left ventricular ejection fraction. Over the cardiac apex, an atrial filling sound (S4) is present and an early filling sound (S3) is usually absent. The early diastolic murmur over the aortic area and along the left sternal border is usually of short duration, as equalization of aortic diastolic pressure and left ventricular diastolic pressure occurs soon after onset of diastole. The physical findings in patients with acute AR are illustrated in Figure 11.9.

The chest X-ray in patients with severe acute aortic regurgitation will demonstrate pulmonary edema (Fig. 11.10).

Echocardiographic studies are essential to establish the severity and cause of acute aortic regurgitation. In patients with infective endocarditis and aortic valve vegetation, cusp perforation and paravalvular leak can be recognized. Echocardiogram in patients with severe acute aortic regurgitation also reveals a short aortic diastolic pressure half time (Figs. 11.11A and B), a short mitral deceleration time, and premature closure of aortic valve.

During cardiac catheterization, simultaneous measurements of femoral arterial pressure and left ventricular pressure (Fig. 11.12) reveal that femoral arterial systolic pressure is significantly higher than left ventricular systolic pressure (Hill's sign). There is a rapid equalization of

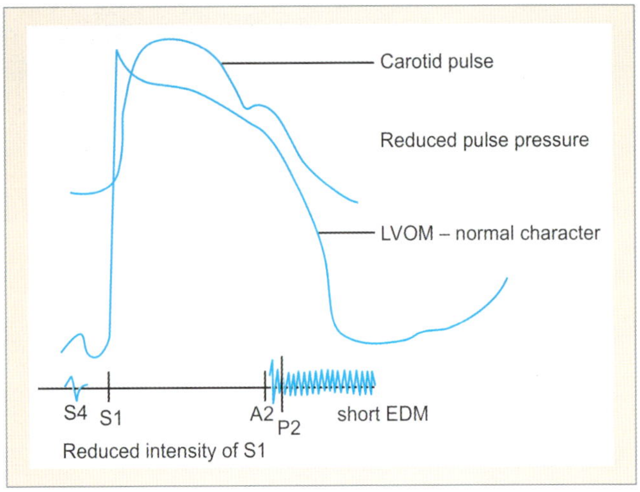

Fig. 11.9: The physical findings of severe acute aortic regurgitation are illustrated. Due to decreased stroke volume, the pulse pressure is decreased. Left ventricular outward movement (LVOM) has a normal character, indicating normal left ventricular ejection fraction. The intensity of the first heart sound (S1) is reduced due to increased left ventricular end-diastolic pressure. A fourth heart sound (S4) is present due to increased end-diastolic pressure. The intensity of the pulmonic component of the second heart sound (P2) is increased compared to the aortic component (A2), indicating pulmonary hypertension. The duration of the early diastolic murmur of aortic regurgitation is short because of rapid equalization of aortic and left ventricular diastolic pressures.

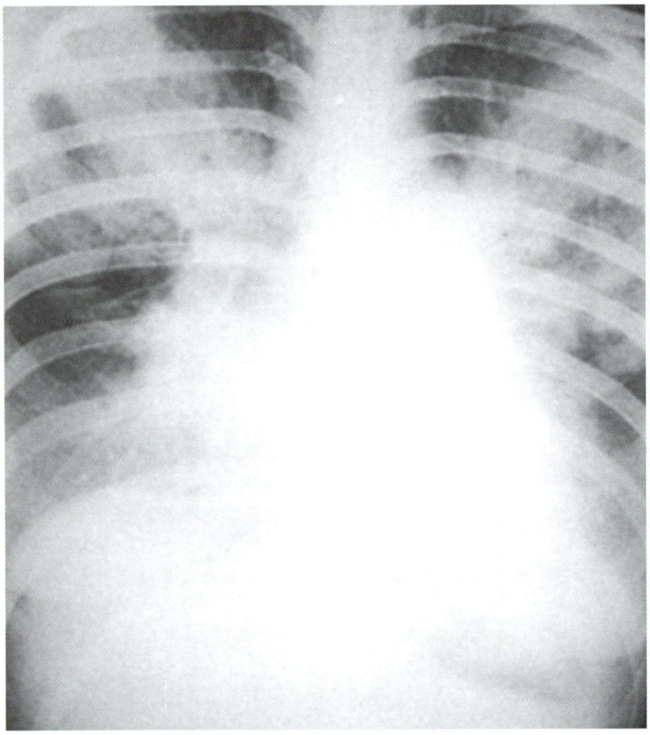

Fig. 11.10: Chest X-ray of a patient with acute severe aortic regurgitation showing florid pulmonary edema with a normal heart size.

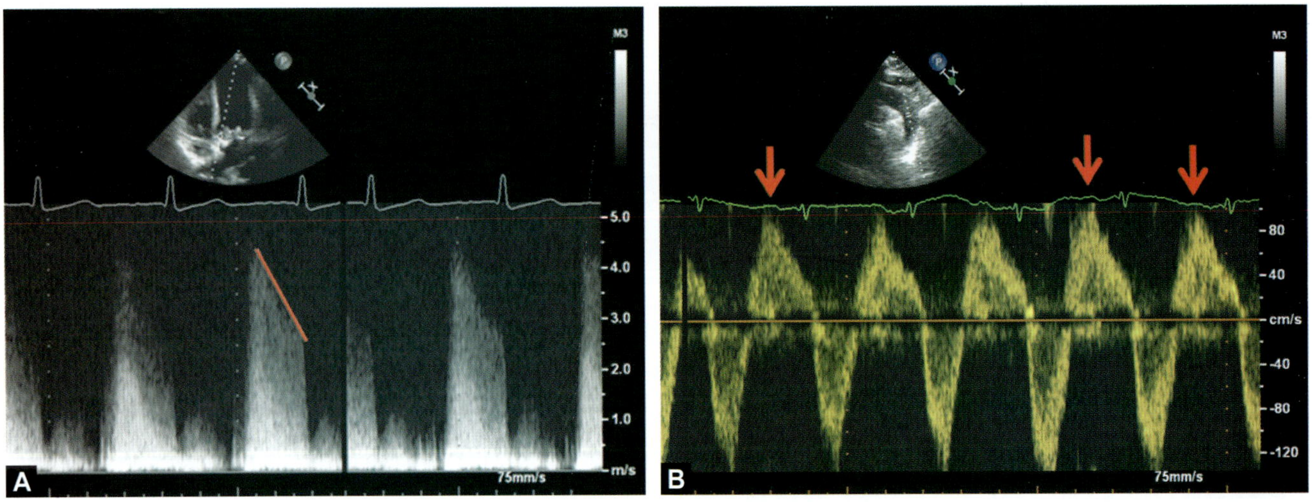

Figs. 11.11A and B: Spectral Doppler examination of a patient with severe aortic regurgitation. (A) Spectral Doppler of the aortic valve in a patient with severe acute aortic regurgitation. The steep deceleration slope (red line) and short pressure half-time reflect rapid equalization of LV and aortic diastolic pressures; (B) Pulsed wave examination of the proximal thoracic descending aorta demonstrating reversal of flow during diastole (arrows).

left ventricular and arterial diastolic pressures. Aortic root contrast angiography can be used to establish the diagnosis of aortic dissection and also to assess the severity of aortic regurgitation.

The prognosis of patients with severe acute aortic regurgitation either due to bacterial endocarditis or type A aortic dissection is poor unless early surgical intervention is undertaken.

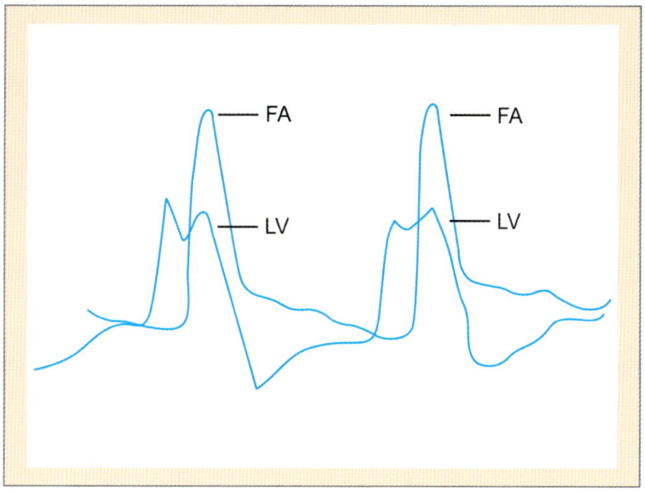

Fig. 11.12: Hemodynamic tracings of a patient with severe aortic regurgitation. During cardiac catheterization, simultaneous measurements of femoral arterial (FA) pressure and left ventricular (LV) pressure reveal that femoral arterial systolic pressure is significantly higher than left ventricular systolic pressure (Hill's sign). There is a rapid equalization of left ventricular and arterial diastolic pressures.

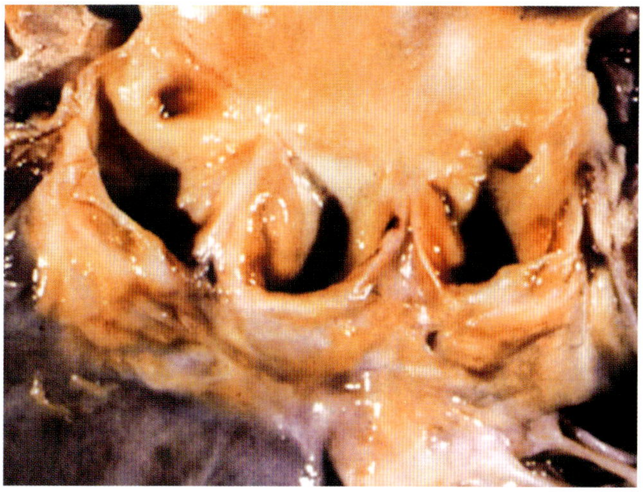

Fig. 11.13: Aortic annular dilatation, a cause of chronic aortic regurgitation.

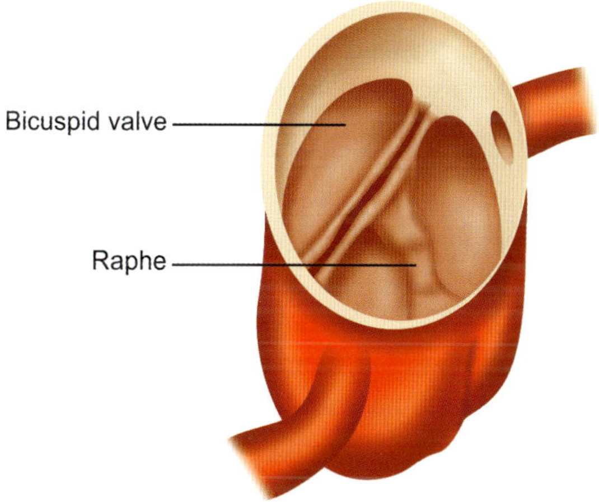

Fig. 11.14: Schematic illustration of a bicuspid aortic valve. [Images from Mishra S, Awasthy N. Aortic valve diseases. In: Vijayalakshmi IB et al. (Eds). A Comprehensive Approach to Congenital Heart Diseases. New Delhi: Jaypee Brothers Medical Publishers (P) Ltd.].

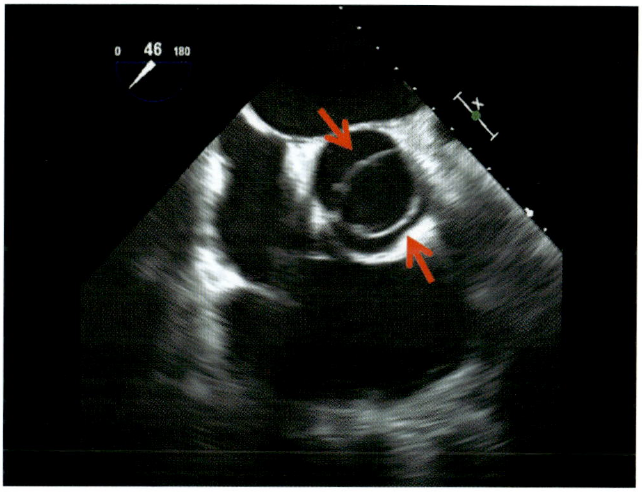

Fig. 11.15: Transesophageal echocardiogram demonstrating bicuspid aortic valve.

CAUSES OF CHRONIC AORTIC REGURGITATION

Chronic aortic regurgitation can result from abnormalities of the aortic valve leaflets, the aortic root, or the annulus. Aortic root or aortic annular dilatation (Fig. 11.13) without the involvement of the aortic valve leaflets usually causes only mild aortic regurgitation. Chronic causes of aortic regurgitation include healed (resolved) endocarditis, rheumatic valvular disease, bicuspid aortic valve (Figs. 11.14 to 11.16), dilation of the aortic root and annulus, and degenerative valvular disease. Rheumatic etiology should be considered in the countries where rheumatic fever is still prevalent. Isolated aortic regurgitation due to rheumatic heart disease is uncommon; rheumatic mitral valve disease is usually also present.

Bicuspid aortic valve is the most common congenital heart disease in the adults. The prevalence of bicuspid aortic valve is about 1–2% in the general population. Infective endocarditis is a complication of bicuspid aortic valve and severe aortic regurgitation may result from valve leaflet perforation. Aortic regurgitation due to valve

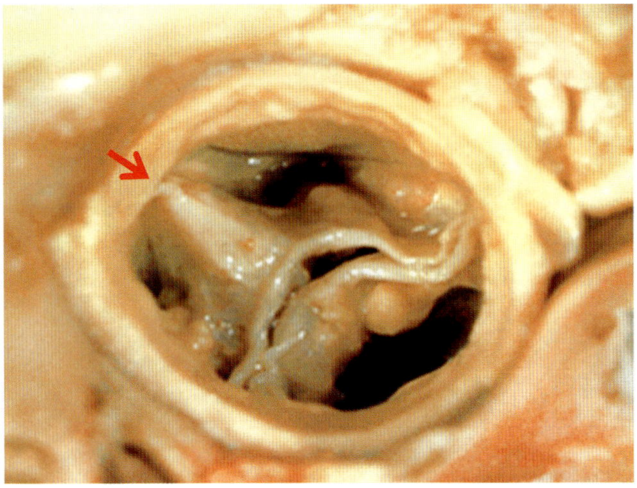

Fig. 11.16: Pathology specimen demonstrating a bicuspid aortic valve. The raphe (arrow) is clearly visible. [Image from Mishra S, Awasthy N. Aortic valve diseases. In: Vijayalakshmi IB et al. (Eds). A Comprehensive Approach to Congenital Heart Diseases. New Delhi: Jaypee Brothers Medical Publishers (P) Ltd.].

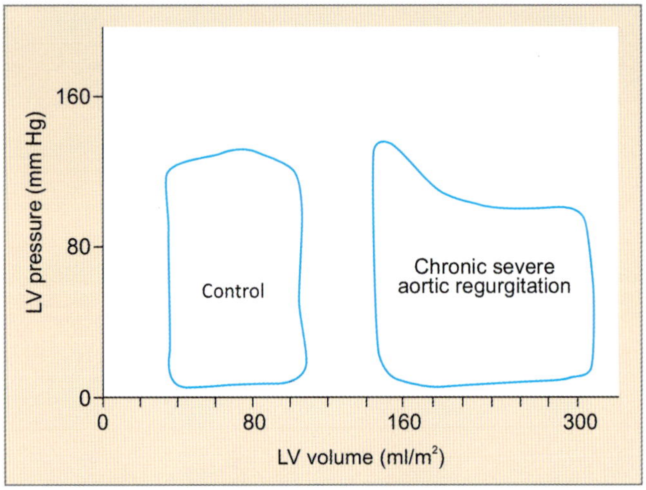

Fig. 11.17: Pressure volume loop of a patient with chronic aortic regurgitation. Left ventricular compliance is increased in chronic aortic regurgitation, resulting in very little increase in left ventricular diastolic pressure despite a marked increase in left ventricular diastolic volume. The area within the pressure volume loop is substantially increased; indicating increased left ventricular stroke work.

deformity alone is usually mild. Very rarely, severe aortic regurgitation can occur due to retraction and fibrosis of the valve leaflets.

Syphilitic aortic root and aortic valve disease is a rare cause of aortic regurgitation in the present era. Ascending aortic aneurysm can occasionally cause significant aortic regurgitation. Ankylosing spondylitis and connective tissue diseases such as lupus erythematosus are uncommon causes of significant aortic regurgitation. Marfan's and Ehlers-Danlos syndromes can cause aortic regurgitation due to aortic root and aortic annular dilatation, and also due to structural abnormalities of the valve leaflets.

Functional aortic regurgitation due to systemic hypertension is almost always mild. Similarly, aortic regurgitation associated with anemia is also mild and there is no hemodynamic compromise.

PHYSIOLOGY OF CHRONIC AORTIC REGURGITATION

In patients with chronic severe aortic regurgitation, there is both volume and pressure overload of the left ventricle. The magnitude of volume overload is related to the severity of aortic regurgitation. The pressure overload results from increased left ventricular wall stress. In patients with chronic severe aortic regurgitation, left ventricular end-diastolic volume is markedly increased, which is associated with increased wall stress. Although the increase in systolic wall stress (left ventricular afterload) decreases stroke volume, the magnitude of increase in stroke volume by Frank-Starling mechanism is greater than the decrease in stroke volume due to increased wall stress. Thus, the net effect is an increase in forward stroke volume. As the increase in forward stroke volume is proportional to increase in end-diastolic volume, left ventricular ejection fraction (stroke volume/end-diastolic volume) is maintained in patients with compensated chronic aortic regurgitation. Left ventricular compliance is increased in chronic aortic regurgitation. As a result there is very little increase in left ventricular diastolic pressure despite a marked increase in left ventricular diastolic volume.

Analysis of the pressure volume loops in patients with chronic severe aortic regurgitation (Fig. 11.17) demonstrates that the diastolic pressure volume curve shifts to the right with little or no upward shift; thus there is very little increase in left ventricular diastolic pressure despite a marked increase in end-diastolic volume. The area within the pressure volume loop is substantially increased; indicating increased left ventricular stroke work. There is no change in contractile function.

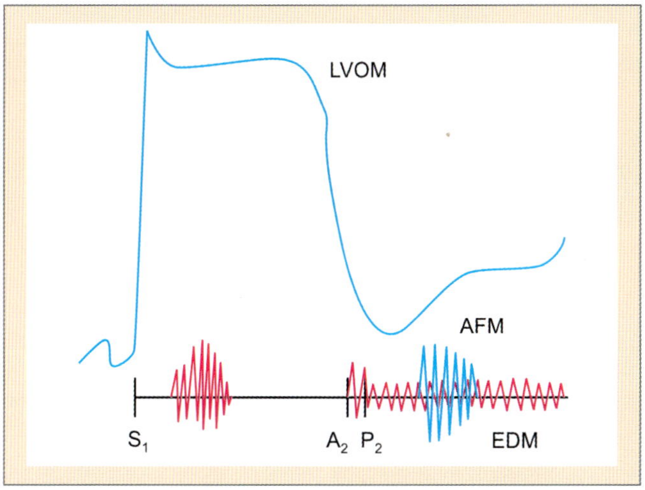

Fig. 11.18: The auscultatory findings of significant chronic aortic regurgitation. The auscultatory findings of significant chronic aortic regurgitation with normal systolic function are characterized by a long early diastolic murmur, an Austin-Flint murmur, and occasionally a presystolic murmur. There is an ejection systolic murmur due to increased stroke volume. The first heart sound (S1) is usually normal, and the second heart sound is often paradoxically split due to a marked increase in forward stroke volume. A third heart sound (S3) can be presented.

EVALUATION OF THE PATIENT WITH CHRONIC AORTIC REGURGITATION

The physical findings of significant chronic aortic regurgitation with normal systolic function are characterized by a long early diastolic murmur, an Austin-Flint murmur, and occasionally a presystolic murmur. There is an ejection systolic murmur due to increased stroke volume. The first heart sound (S1) is usually normal, and the second heart sound is often paradoxically split due to marked increase in forward stroke volume. A third heart sound (S3) can be present. The left ventricular apical impulse (left ventricular outward movement) has a normal character, indicating normal left ventricular ejection fraction. The auscultatory findings of patients with chronic aortic regurgitation are summarized in Figure 11.18.

Systolic blood pressure is often higher than normal due primarily to increased stroke volume. Because of the "peripheral runoff" aortic diastolic pressure is lower and thus the pulse pressure is increased in patients with severe chronic aortic regurgitation.

The electrocardiogram in patients with chronic severe aortic regurgitation is characterized by left ventricular eccentric hypertrophy with repolarization changes. The chest X-ray of those with chronic severe untreated AI will demonstrate cardiomegaly and evidence of left ventricular enlargement (Fig. 11.19).

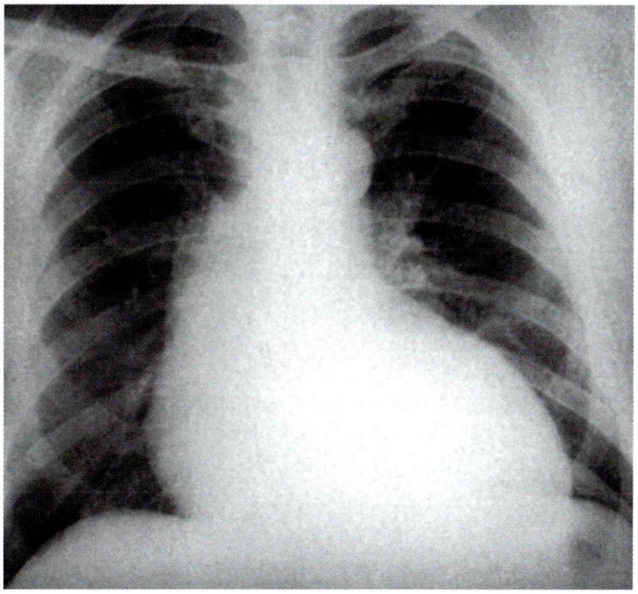

Fig. 11.19: Chest X-ray of a patient with chronic AR demonstrating cardiomegaly with prominent left ventricular enlargement.

Echocardiographic and Doppler-echocardiographic studies should be routinely performed to assess the severity of aortic regurgitation, the degree of left ventricular enlargement, and the left ventricular ejection fraction. In patients with severe or moderately severe aortic regurgitation, echocardiography reveals increased left ventricular size and volume (Fig. 11.20). Color Doppler jet width more than 25% of left ventricular outflow tract (LVOT) dimension and Doppler vena contraction width greater than 0.6 indicate severe aortic regurgitation (Fig. 11.21). Spectral Doppler of the AI jet (Fig. 11.22) may demonstrate less pronounced reduction of the pressure half time than in patients with acute severe AR. Color and spectral Doppler examination in patients with chronic severe AR may also reveal reversal of flow in the descending thoracic aorta (Video 11.2) and abdominal aorta (Fig. 11.23). Echocardiography can also reveal valve pathology such as annular dilatation, healed endocarditis and fibrosis of the valve leaflets. Table 11.1 to 11.3 summarize the American College of Cardiology Foundation (ACCF)/American Heart Association (AHA) and European Society of Cardiology (ESC) classification of the severity of aortic regurgitation in adults, based primarily on echocardiographic findings.

Table 11.1: Summary of the older ACCF/AHA classification of the severity of aortic regurgitation in adults.

	Mild	*Moderate*	*Severe*
Angiography grade	1+	2+	3–4+
Color Doppler central jet width	< 25% LVOT	Greater than mild but no signs of severe AR	> 65% LVOT
Doppler vena contracta width	< 0.3 cm	0.3–0.6 cm	> 0.6 cm
Regurgitant volume (mL/beat)	30 mL	30–59 mL	≥ 60 mL
Regurgitant fraction	< 30%	30–49%	≥ 50%
Regurgitant orifice area	< 0.10 cm^2	0.10–0.29 cm^2	≥ 0.30 cm^2
LV size			Increased

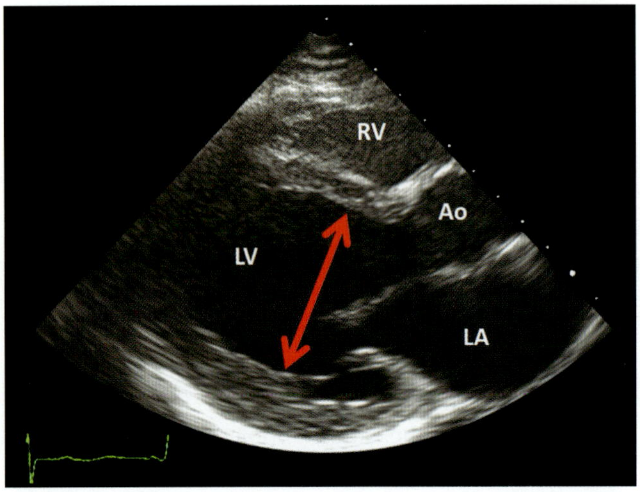

Fig. 11.20: Parasternal long-axis transthoracic echocardiogram of a patient with chronic severe aortic regurgitation showing left ventricular enlargement. The left ventricular end-diastolic diameter (arrow) is notably increased. (Ao: Aortic valve; LA: Left atrium; LV: Left ventricle; RA: Right ventricle).

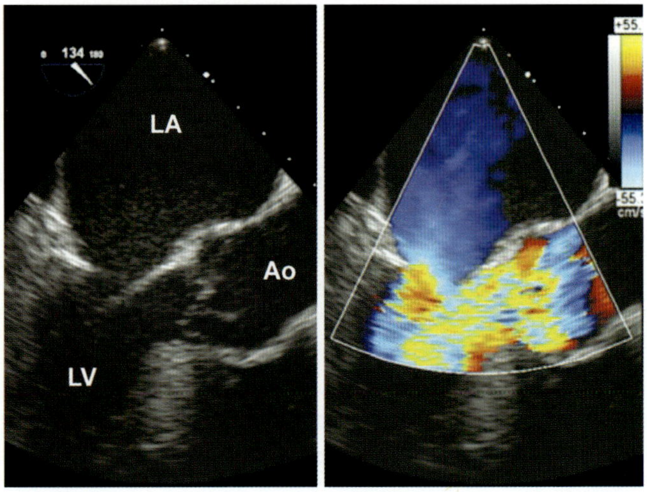

Fig. 11.21: Three-chamber view transesophageal echocardiography showing long-axis of the aortic valve with severe aortic regurgitation. [Image from Hashemi SM et al. Transesophageal echocardiography. In: Chatterjee K et al. (Eds). Cardiology—An Illustrated Textbook. New Delhi, India: Jaypee Brothers Medical Publishers (P) Ltd.]. (Ao: Aorta; LA: Left atrium; LV: Left ventricle).

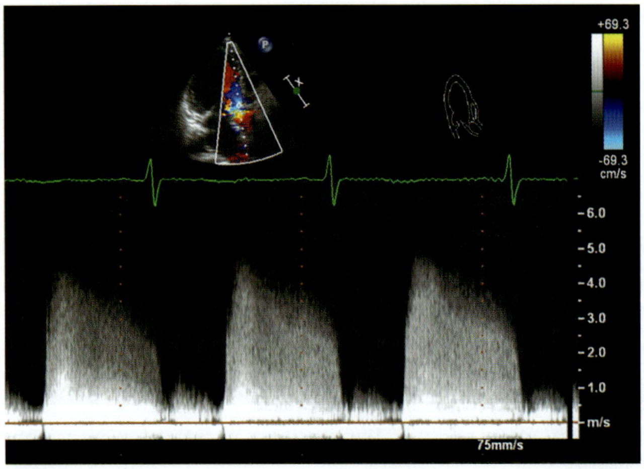

Fig. 11.22: Continuous wave spectral Doppler of the aortic regurgitation jet. Spectral Doppler of the AI jet may demonstrate less pronounced reduction of the pressure half time than in patients with acute severe AR.

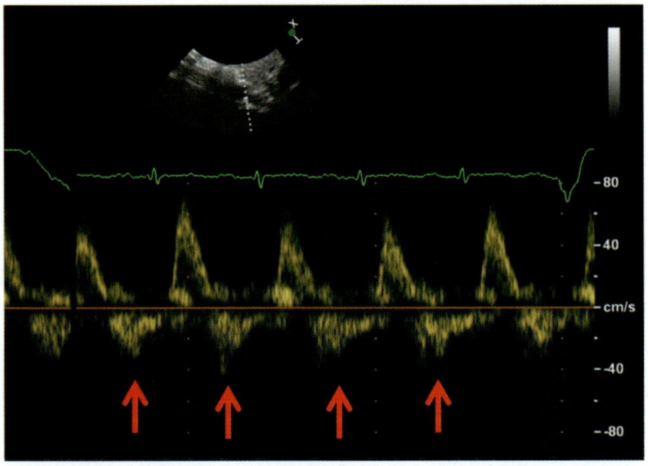

Fig. 11.23: Pulsed wave spectral Doppler demonstrating flow reversal in the abdominal aorta during diastole in a patient with severe aortic regurgitation.

Table 11.2: Summary of the new American College of Cardiology Foundation (ACCF)/American Heart Association (AHA) classification of the stages of chronic aortic regurgitation (AR). (ERO: Effective regurgitant oriface; LVEF: Left ventricular ejection fraction; LVESD: Left ventricular end-systolic diameter; LVOT: Left ventricular outflow tract).

Stage/Definition	*Valve Anatomy*	*Valve Hemodynamics*	*Hemodynamic Consequences and Symptoms*
A—At risk of AR	• Bicuspid aortic valve (or other congenital valve anomaly) • Aortic valve sclerosis • Diseases of the aortic sinuses or ascending aorta	• AR severity none or trace	• No hemodynamic consequences • No symptoms
B—Progressive AR	• Mild-to-moderate calcification of a trileaflet valve • Mild-to-moderate calcification of a bicuspid aortic valve (or other congenital valve anomaly) • Dilated aortic sinuses • Rheumatic valve changes • Valve damage from previous IE	**Mild AR** • Jet width < 25% of LVOT • Vena contracta < 0.3 cm • Regurgitant volume < 30 mL/beat • Regurgitant fraction < 30% • ERO < 0.10 cm^2 • Angiography grade 1+ **Moderate AR** • Jet width 25–64% of LVOT • Vena contracta 0.3–0.6 cm • Regurgitant volume 30–59 mL/beat • Regurgitant fraction 30–49% • ERO 0.10–0.29 cm^2 • Angiography grade 2+	• Normal LV systolic function • Normal LV volume or mild LV dilation • No symptoms
C—Asymptomatic severe AR • *C1*: Normal LVEF (≥ 50%) and mild-to-moderate LV dilation (LVESD ≤ 50 mm) • *C2*: LVEF < 50% or severe LV dilatation (LVESD > 50 mm or indexed LVESD > 25 mm/m^2)	• Calcific aortic valve disease • Bicuspid valve (or other congenital abnormality) • Dilated aortic sinuses or ascending aorta • Rheumatic valve changes • Previous IE with abnormal leaflet closure or perforation	• Jet width ≥ 65% of LVOT • Vena contracta > 0.6 cm • Holodiastolic flow reversal in the proximal abdominal aorta • Regurgitant volume ≥ 60 mL/beat • Regurgitant fraction ≥ 50% • ERO ≥ 0.3 cm^2 • Angiography grade 3+ to 4+ • Evidence of LV dilation	• Normal or depressed LV systolic function • Mild, moderate or severe LV dilatation • No symptoms; exercise testing is reasonable to confirm symptom status
D—Symptomatic severe AR	• Calcific valve disease • Bicuspid valve (or other congenital abnormality) • Dilated aortic sinuses or ascending aorta • Rheumatic valve changes • Previous IE with abnormal leaflet closure or perforation	• Doppler jet width ≥ 65% of LVOT • Vena contracta > 0.6 cm, • Holodiastolic flow reversal in the proximal abdominal aorta • Regurgitant volume ≥ 60 mL/beat • Regurgitant fraction ≥ 50% • ERO ≥ 0.3 cm^2 • Angiography grade 3+ to 4+ • Evidence of LV dilation	• Symptomatic severe AR may occur with normal systolic function (LVEF ≥ 50%), mild-to-moderate LV dysfunction (LVEF 40% to 50%) or severe LV dysfunction (LVEF < 40%); • Moderate-to-severe LV dilation is present. • Exertional dyspnea or angina, or more severe HF symptoms

Cardiac magnetic resonance imaging (CMRI) can also provide accurate assessment of the severity of aortic regurgitation, as well as left ventricular volume and mass (Figs. 11.24A and B).

Cardiac catheterization is performed primarily to assess presence or absence of obstructive coronary artery disease. Determination of hemodynamics, however, can reveal magnitude of elevation of left ventricular end-diastolic

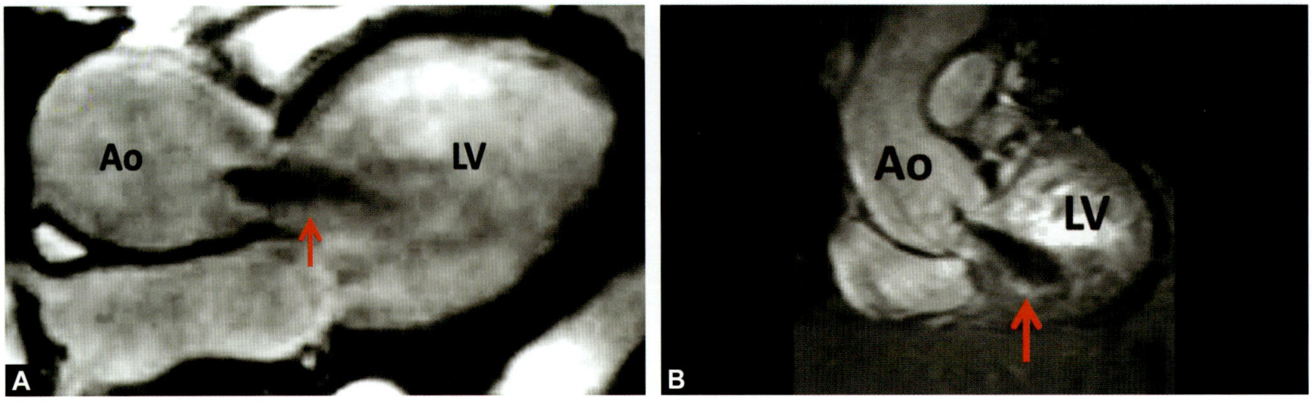

Figs. 11.24A and B: Magnetic resonance imaging demonstrating aortic regurgitation. Dephased blood, corresponding to the AI jet, appears dark (arrows). The Ao is clearly dilated. (LV: Left ventricle; Ao: Ascending aorta).

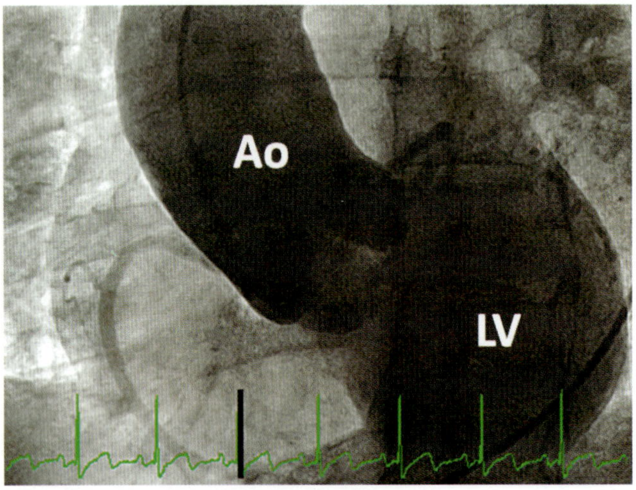

Fig. 11.25: Aortography demonstrates severe aortic regurgitation. The density of contrast in the left ventricle (LV) equals that in the aorta (Ao) within 1 beat, indicating severe AR.

Table 11.3: Summary of the European Society of Cardiology (ESC) and European Association for Cardio-Thoracic Surgery (EACTS) Guidelines echocardiographic criteria for the diagnosis of severe aortic regurgitation.

Qualitative	Abnormal/flail/large valve coaptation defect
	Large central color flow regurgitant jets, variable eccentric jets
	Dense CW signal of regurgitant jet
	Holodiastolic flow reversal in the descending aorta (EDV > 20 cm/sec)
Semiquantitative	Vena contract width > 6 mm
	Pressure half-time < 200 msec
Quantitative	EROA ≥ 30 mm^2
	Regurgitant volume ≥ 60 mL/beat
	Enlarged left ventricle

pressure. Aortic root injection can be used to assess the severity of aortic regurgitation and valve leaflet and aortic root pathology (Fig. 11.25).

MANAGEMENT OF CHRONIC AORTIC REGURGITATION

Medical therapy in patients with AI should be considered only as palliative therapy. In such cases, vasodilators with predominantly arteriolar dilating properties, such as hydralazine, are recommended. Surgical therapy should be considered in all patients with symptomatic chronic aortic regurgitation irrespective of left ventricular ejection fraction. In asymptomatic patients with severe aortic regurgitation, surgical therapy is indicated if left ventricular ejection fraction is less than 50%. Indications for aortic valve replacement or repair are given in Tables 11.4 and 11.5.

Table 11.4: Summary of the new ACCF/AHA recommendations for aortic valve replacement (AVR) in patients with aortic regurgitation. AR = aortic regurgitation; LVEDD = left ventricular end-diastolic diameter; LVESD = left ventricular end-systolic diameter. The level of evidence (LOE) supporting the recommendation is given in parenthesis, where LOE = A denotes a recommendation derived from multiple randomized clinical trials or meta-analyses, LOE = B denotes a recommendation derived from a single randomized clinical trial or non-randomized studies, and LOE = C denotes a recommendation based on consensus of expert opinion, standard of care, or case reports.

Class I (is indicated)
• Symptomatic patients with severe AR regardless of LV systolic function (LOE = B)
• Asymptomatic patients with chronic severe AR and LV systolic dysfunction (LVEF < 50%) (LOE = B)
• Patients with severe AR while undergoing cardiac surgery for other indications (LOE = C)
Class IIa (is reasonable)
• Asymptomatic patients with severe AR with normal LV systolic function (LVEF ≥ 50%) but with severe LV dilation (LVESD > 50 mm) (LOE = B)
• Patients with moderate AR who are undergoing other cardiac surgery (LOE = C)
Class IIb (may be considered)
• Asymptomatic patients with severe AR and normal LV systolic function (LVEF ≥ 50%) but severe LV dilation (LVEDD > 65 mm) if surgical risk is low (LOE = C)

Table 11.5: Summary of the European Society of Cardiology (ESC) and European Association for Cardio-Thoracic Surgery (EACTS) guidelines for surgery in severe aortic regurgitation. The level of evidence (LOE) supporting the recommendation is given in parenthesis, where LOE = A denotes a recommendation derived from multiple randomized clinical trials or meta-analyses, LOE = B denotes a recommendation derived from a single randomized clinical trial or large non-randomized studies, and LOE = C denotes a recommendation based on consensus of expert opinion or based on small studies, retrospective studies, or registries. (AR: Aortic regurgitation; CABG: Coronary artery bypass surgery; LVEF: Left ventricular ejection fraction).

Class I (is recommended and indicated)
• Symptomatic patients with severe AR (LOE = B)
• Asymptomatic patients with severe AR with LVEF ≤ 50% (LOE = B)
• Patients with severe AR undergoing CABG, surgery on the aorta, or surgery on another valve (LOE = C)
Class IIa (should be considered)
• Asymptomatic patients with severe AR with normal LV systolic function (EF > 50%) but with severe LV dilation (LVEDD > 75 mm or LVESD > 55 mm) (LOE = B)

ACKNOWLEDGMENT

We sincerely thank Ms Teresa Ruggle , Ms Melissa Davis, Dr Robert Weiss and Dr Garder Sirgudsson for providing the illustrations. We also sincrely thank Ms Cari Bermel and Ms Linda Berg for their invaluable secretarial help.

VIDEO LEGENDS

Video 11.1: Parasternal long axis echocardiographic image demonstrating severe AI (Video courtesy of Glenn N. Levine, MD).

Video 11.2: Color Doppler imaging in the parasternal long axis view showing mild AI due to a dilated aortic annulus (Video courtesy of Glenn N. Levine, MD).

Videos 11.3A and B: Severe aortic regurgitation due to a flail right aortic leaflet. (A) 2D video and (B) Corresponding color Doppler video (Video courtesy of Glenn N. Levine, MD).

Video 11.4: Five-chamber view showing AI in a patient with heavily calcified aortic leaflets (Video courtesy of Glenn N. Levine, MD).

Video 11.5: MRI demonstrating aortic regurgitation in a patient with a dilated aortic annulus and proximal ascending aorta (Video courtesy of Scott D. Flamm, MD).

REFERENCES

Bonow RO, Carabello BA, Chatterjee K, et al. 2008 focussed update incorporated into the ACC/AHA 2006 guidelines for the management of patients with valvular heart disease: a report of the American College of Cardiology/American Heart Association Task Force on Practice Guidelines (Writing Committee to revise the 1998 guidelines for the management of patients with valvular heart disease). Endorsed by the Society of Cardiovascular Anesthesiologists, Society of Cardiovascular Angiography and Interventions, and Society of Thoracic Surgeons. J Am Coll Cardiol. 2008;(13):e1-142.

Borer JS, Bonow RO. Contemporary approach to mitral and aortic regurgitation. Circulation. 2003;108:2432-8.

Carabello BA. Aortic valve disease. In: Chatterjee K, Anderson M, Heistad D, Kerber R (Eds). Cardiology—An Illustrated Textbook. India: Jaypee Brothers Medical Publishers (P) Ltd. 2012. pp. 985-99.

Carabello BA. Progress in mitral and aoric regurgitation. Prog Cardiovasc Dis. 2001;43:457-75.

Neyou A. Aortic dissection. In: Chatterjee K, Anderson M, Heistad D, Kerber R (Eds). Cardiology—An Illustrated Textbook. India: Jaypee Brothers Medical Publishers (P) Ltd. 2012. pp. 1166-74.

CHAPTER 12

Mitral Stenosis and Percutaneous Mitral Valvotomy

Sivadasanpillai Harikrishnan, Sanjay Ganapathi

INTRODUCTION

The mitral valve (MV) is a bileaflet valve guarding the left atrioventricular orifice which prevents the regurgitation of blood from the left ventricle back into the left atrium during ventricular systole. The valve is named so because of its resemblance to a Bishop's miter. Mitral stenosis (MS) is the narrowing of the MV, leading to the hindrance of blood flow from left atrium to the left ventricle.

Mitral stenosis (Fig. 12.1) can be congenital, but the most common cause of MS is rheumatic heart disease, especially in the developing world. Table 12.1 enumerates some of the common etiologies of MS.

PATHOLOGY OF RHEUMATIC MITRAL STENOSIS

The orifice area of normal MV is about 4–6 cm^2. Chronic rheumatic processes may lead to one or more of the following pathological processes after a variable latent period, often decades after the initial infection (Figs. 12.2 to 12.7):

- Fusion of valve commissures
- Thickening, fibrosis, retraction of edges of valve leaflets
- Calcification of leaflet tissue
- Shortening, thickening and fusion of chordae.

These pathological processes result in a funnel-shaped mitral apparatus, in which the orifice of the MV (primary orifice) is reduced in size. Interchordal fusion obliterates the secondary orifices.

At the histological level, abnormalities in the leaflet include acute and chronic inflammation, neovascularization, and myxoid degeneration (Figs. 12.8A to D).

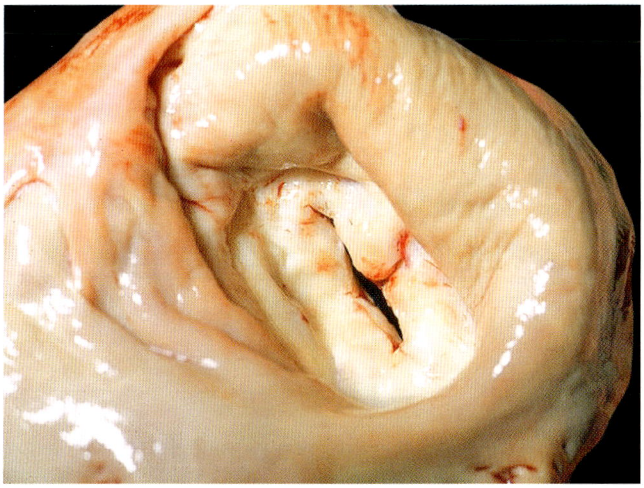

Fig. 12.1: Gross pathology specimen of mitral stenosis (MS). (Image from Dr Ewing EP and the Center for Disease Control).

HEMODYNAMICS OF MITRAL STENOSIS

When the valve area is reduced to less than 2.5 cm^2, blood can flow from left atrium to left ventricle only if

Table 12.1: Etiologies of mitral stenosis (MS).

Rheumatic heart disease (most common)
Congenital mitral stenosis (MS)
Systemic diseases (rare causes): • Rheumatoid arthritis • Systemic lupus erythematosus • Mucopolysaccharidosis • Fabry disease • Whipple disease • Malignant carcinoid syndrome • Methysergide
Mitral inflow obstruction: • Left atrial (LA) myxoma • Valve thrombosis • Large vegetation • Cor-triatriatum

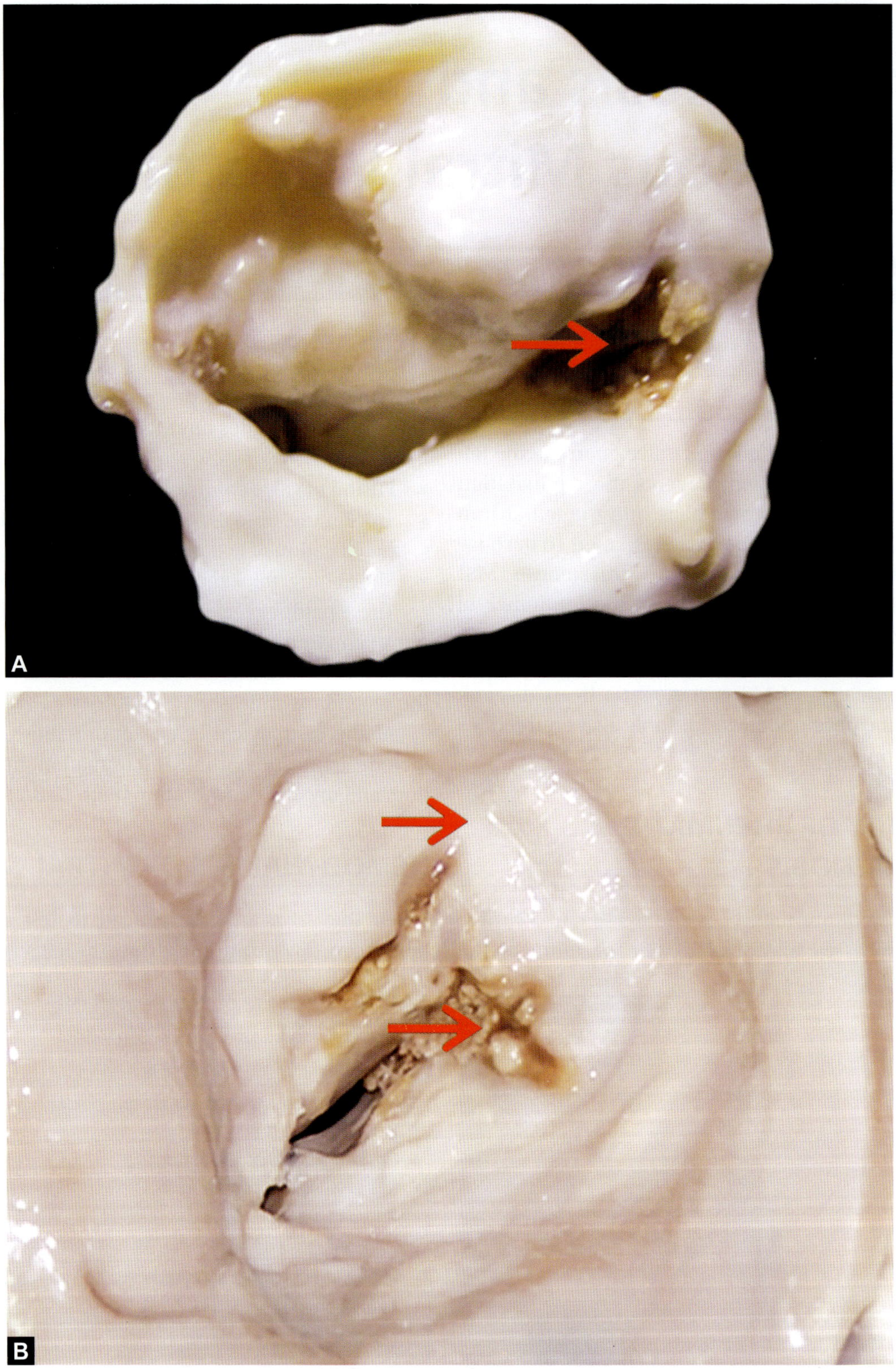

Figs. 12.2A and B: Gross photomicrographs of surgically excised mitral valves (MV). (A) MV specimen showing thickened, opaque and scarred valve leaflets with commissural fusion (arrow). Pearly white calcified nodules are seen focally; (B) Near the valve closure line, there are erosion and microthrombi (arrow). [Image courtesy of Professor Ray R, AIIMS New Delhi, India. Image reproduced from Ray R, Das P. Pathological aspects of rheumatic mitral stenosis. In: Harikrishnan S (Ed). Percutaneous Mitral Valvotomy, 1st edition. New Delhi, India: Jaypee Brothers Medical Publishers (P) Ltd; 2012. pp. 24-33].

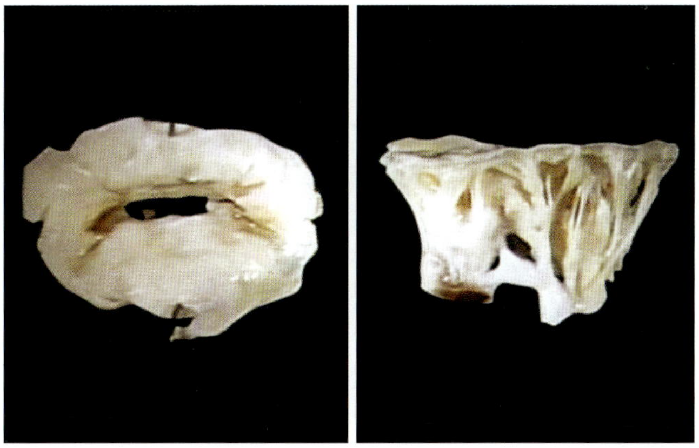

Fig. 12.3A: Rheumatic mitral stenosis (MS). (Image from Armed Forces Institute of Pathology).

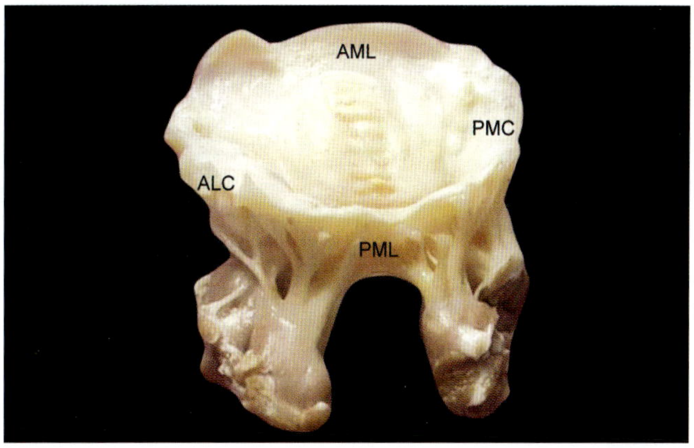

Fig. 12.3B: Surgically excised stenotic mitral valve (MV) with severe subvalvular affliction. The papillary muscles (PM) appear directly attached to the valve leaflets. [Image and legend text courtesy of Dr Vaideeswar P, Professor (Additional), Department of Pathology (Cardiovascular and Thoracic Division), Seth GS Medical College, Mumbai, India]. (AML: Anterior mitral leaflet; PML: Posterior mitral leaflet; ALC: Anterolateral commissure; PMC: Posteromedial commissure).

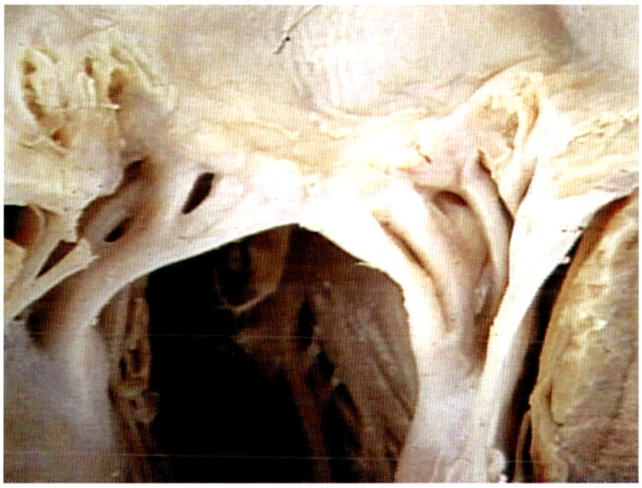

Fig. 12.4: Rheumatic fibrosis of the mitral valve (MV). (Image from Armed Forces Institute of Pathology).

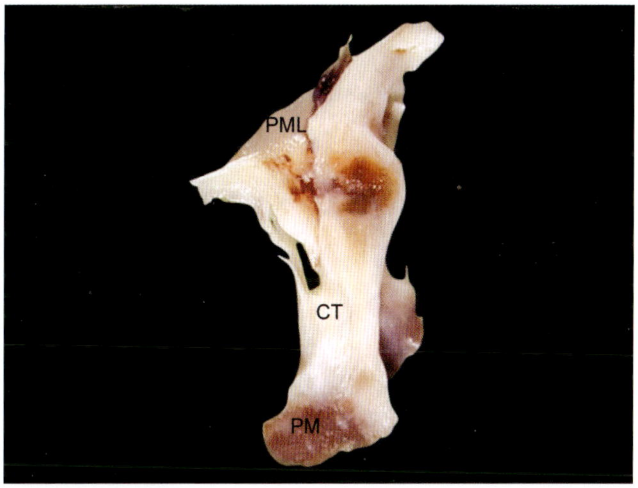

Fig. 12.5: Gross pathology from a patient with rheumatic mitral disease showing fusion and agglutination of the chordae tendineae (CT) with absence of interchordal space, leading to the phenomenon of subvalvular stenosis. [Image and figure legend from Turgeman Y. Subvalvular apparatus in rheumatic mitral stenosis—methods of assessment and therapeutic implications. In: Harikrishnan S (Ed). Percutaneous Mitral Valvotomy, 1st edition. New Delhi, India: Jaypee Brothers Medical Publishers (P) Ltd. 2012. pp 118-28]. (CT: Chordae tendineae; PM: Papillary muscle; PML: Posterior mitral leaflet).

propelled by a pressure gradient. While the left ventricular mean diastolic pressure remains at its normal value of approximately 5 mm Hg, the left atrial mean pressure rises progressively, and can rise to 25 mm Hg or more (Fig. 12.9).

A second major circulatory change is reduction of blood flow across the MV, leading to reduction in cardiac output, the severity of which is augmented by development of atrial fibrillation, increased pulmonary arteriolar resistance and tricuspid regurgitation in advanced disease.

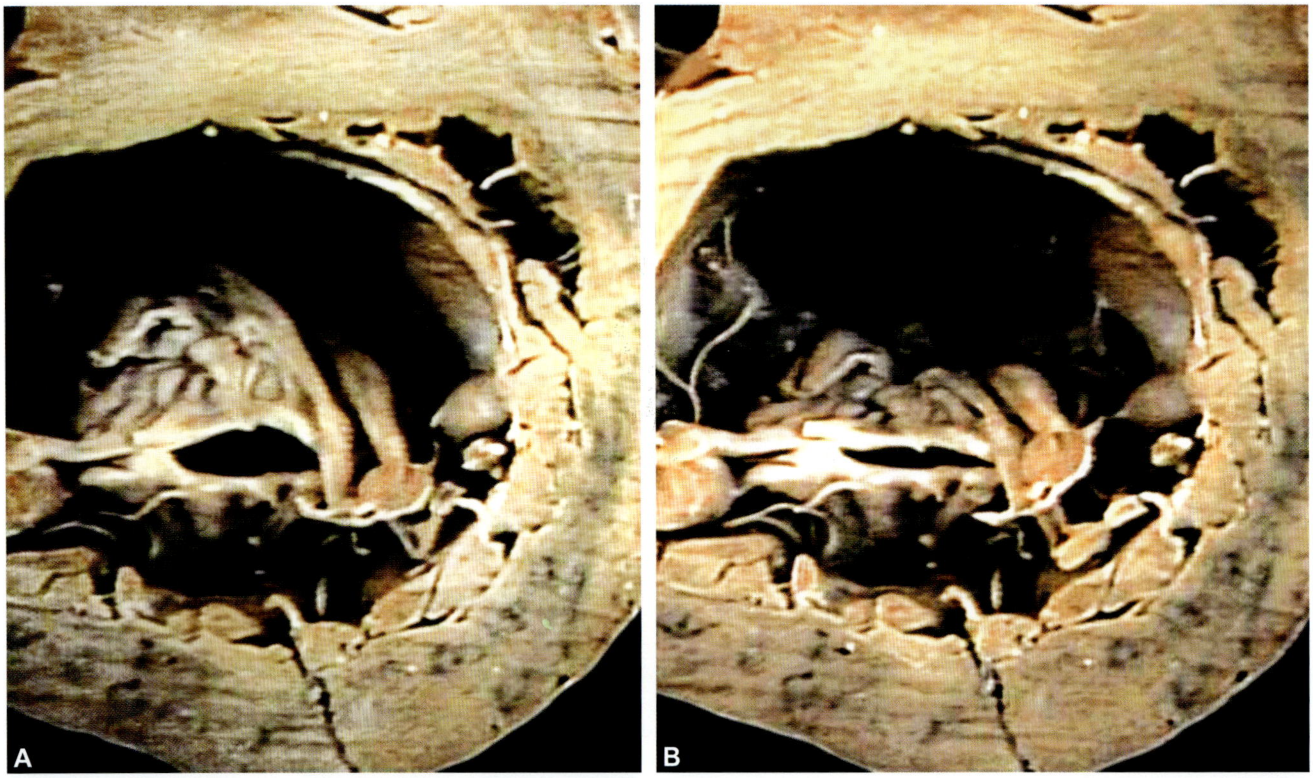

Figs. 12.6A and B: Gross pathology of mitral stenosis (MS). Note the "fish mouth" appearance of the mitral orifice. (Image from Armed Forces Institute of Pathology).

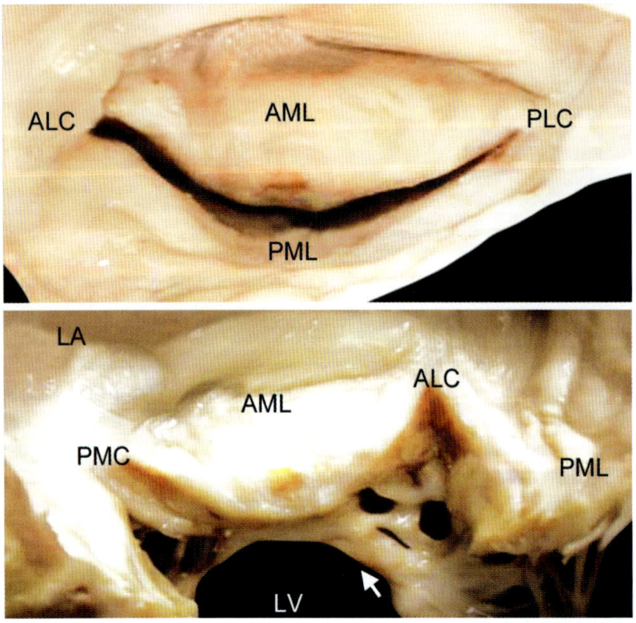

Fig. 12.7: Pathology of mitral stenosis (MS). Upper panel: Mitral valve (MV) viewed from left atrial (LA) aspect showing crescentic appearance of the valve orifice. Lower panel: The opened-out valve highlights the commissural and chordal fusion (arrow) and leaflet thickening in rheumatic MS. [Image adapted and legend text from Sharma S, Dalvi VH. Mitral valve disease. In: Chatterjee K, Anderson M, Heistad D, Kerber RE (Eds). Cardiology: An Illustrated Textbook, 1st edition. New Delhi, India: Jaypee Brothers Medical Publishers (P) Ltd; 2012. pp. 1000-1017]. (AML: Anterior mitral leaflet; PML: Posterior mitral leaflet; ALC: Anterolateral commissure; PMC: Posteromedial commissure; LV: Left ventricle).

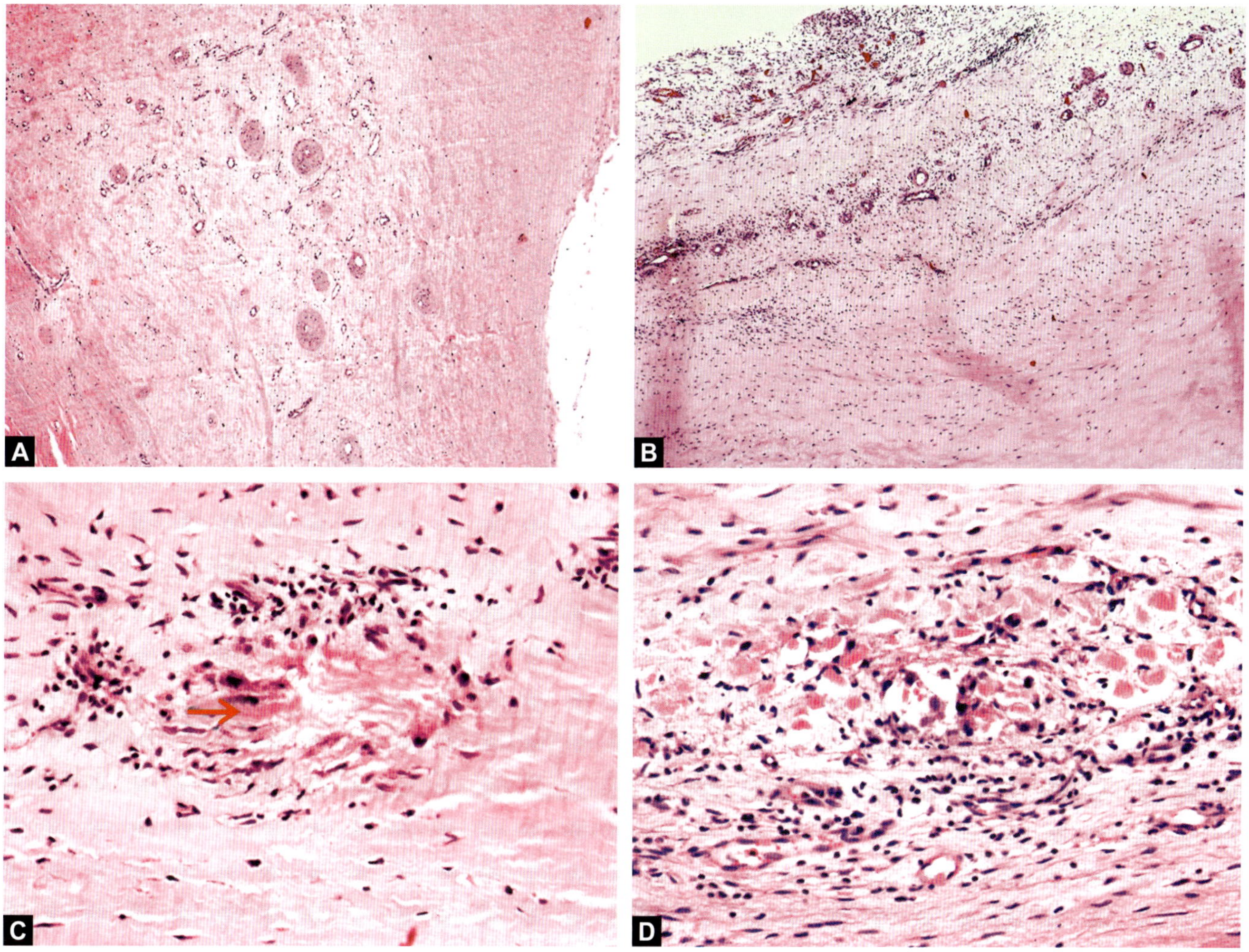

Figs. 12.8A to D: Histopathologic changes in rheumatic mitral leaflets. (A) Myxoid degeneration of the stroma and neovascularization; (B) Prominent neovascularization and subendothelial collection of moderately dense chronic inflammatory cell infiltrate; (C) Aschoff nodule in granulomatous phase, with fibrinoid necrosis in the center of the nodule (arrow), surrounded by lymphocytes, plasma cells and histiocytes with typical caterpillar-like nuclear chromatin; (D) Aschoff nodule in the acute phase with inflammatory cell infiltrate around the lamina fibrosa with fibrinoid necrosis. [Images and figure legends from Ray R, Das P. Pathological aspects of rheumatic mitral stenosis. In: Harikrishnan S (Ed). Percutaneous Mitral Valvotomy, 1st edition. New Delhi, India: Jaypee Brothers Medical Publishers (P) Ltd; 2012. pp. 24-33].

The third hemodynamic sequel of MS is the stagnation of blood in the left atrium, which can lead to thrombus formation and embolic complications.

Longstanding MS will also lead to pulmonary hypertension (PH) (Fig. 12.10). PH results due to passive back-transmission of elevated pulmonary venous pressures and to reactive changes, including pulmonary arterial and arteriolar vasoconstriction, hypertrophy of the muscular layer of the pulmonary arteries, and obliterative changes in the pulmonary vascular bed.

Figure 12.11 illustrates the various hemodynamic evolutions of a patient with chronic MS.

NATURAL HISTORY OF RHEUMATIC MITRAL STENOSIS

In one series, the mean duration from carditis to first symptom of MS was 19 years. In patients with no or minimal symptoms, survival is greater than 80% at 10 years. Ten-year survival of untreated patients presenting

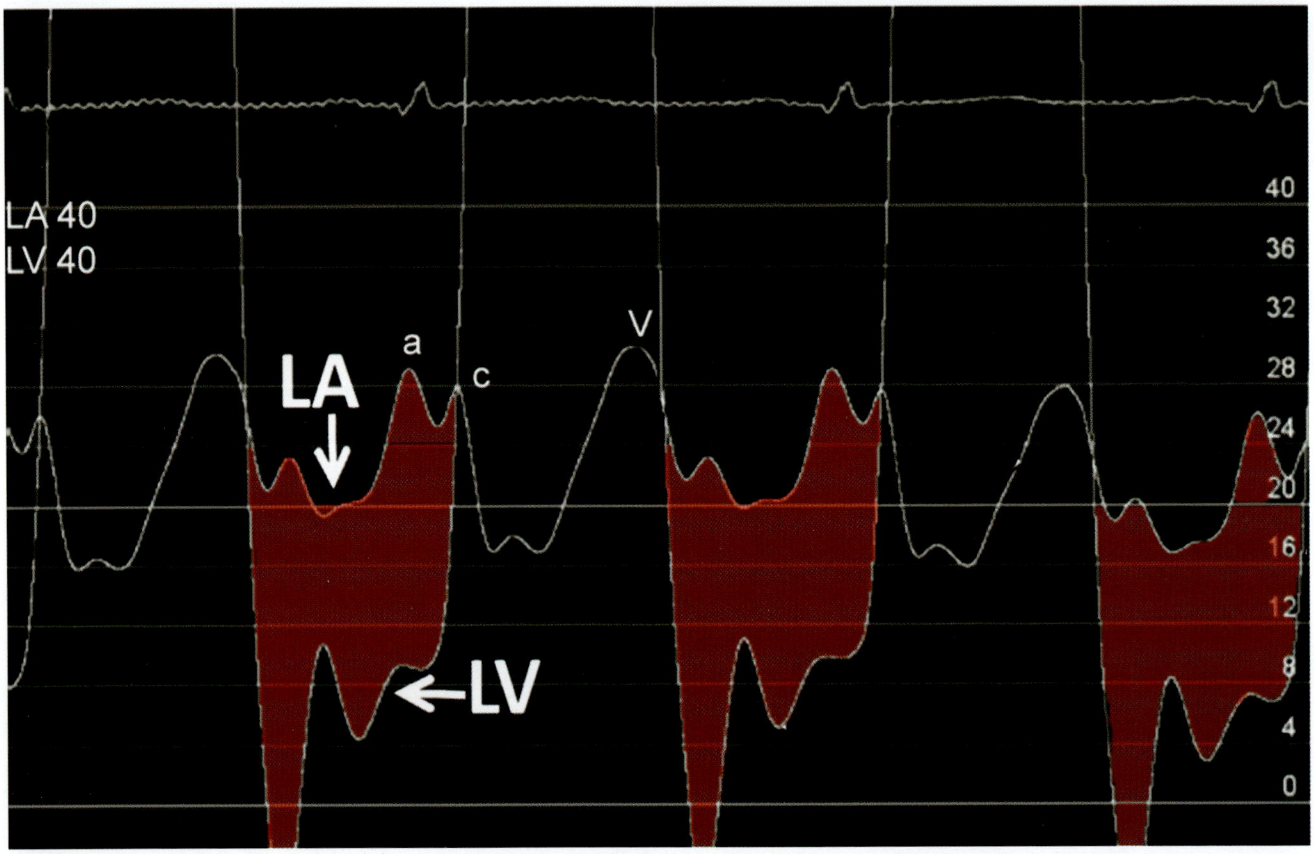

Fig. 12.9: Simultaneous left atrial (LA) and left ventricular (LV) pressure tracings in a patient with hemodynamically significant mitral stenosis (MS). The red-shaded area represents the significant gradient across the mitral leaflet during diastole. [Image from Krishnakumar M, Mahesh SK, Arun SR. Pathophysiology, natural history and hemodynamics of mitral stenosis. In: Harikrishnan S (Ed). Percutaneous Mitral Valvotomy, 1st edition. New Delhi, India: Jaypee Brothers Medical Publishers (P) Ltd; 2012. pp. 34-43]. (LA: Left atrium; LV: Left ventricle).

with MS and significantly limiting symptoms [New York Heart Association (NYHA) class III/IV)] is less than 15%. Mean survival of patients with untreated MS and severe pulmonary artery (PA) hypertension is less than years. Systemic embolization occurs in up to 25% of patients with significant MS.

Juvenile MS refers to MS occurring in patients less than 20 years of age. The term was coined by SB Roy and colleagues to refer to patients of very young age presenting with severe MS, mostly in the developing world where rheumatic fever is rampant. MS at this age is often associated with severe symptoms, high transmitral gradients and high PA pressures.

CLINICAL EVALUATION OF PATIENTS WITH RHEUMATIC MITRAL STENOSIS

The physical examination of patients with MS typically reveals a mid-diastolic murmur, with presystolic augmentation in those in sinus rhythm. This presystolic augmentation of the murmur is lost when the patient develops atrial fibrillation.

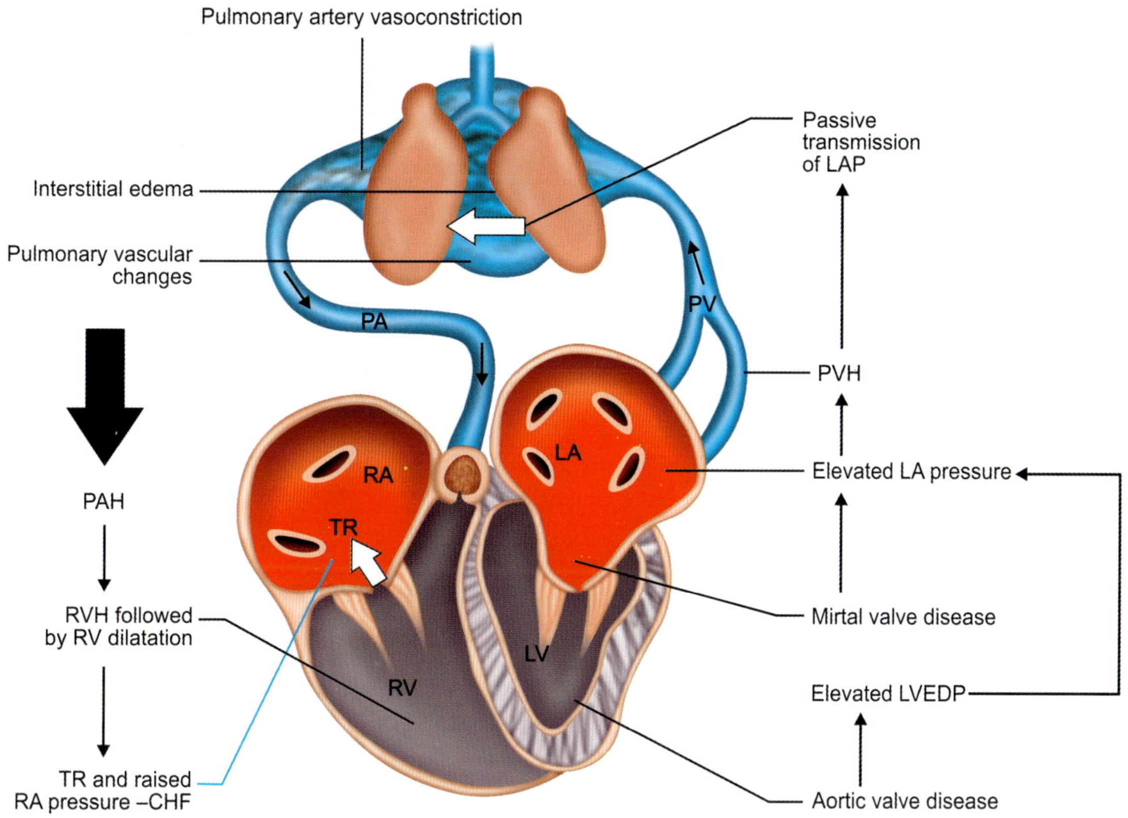

Fig. 12.10: Pathophysiology of pulmonary hypertension (PH) in valvular heart disease. (Image from Harikrishnan S, Kartha CC. Pulmonary hypertension in rheumatic heart disease. PVRI Review. 2009;1(1):13-9). (LV: Left ventricle; LVEDP: Left ventricular end-diastolic pressure; LA: Left atrial; PVH: Pulmonary venous hypertension; LAP: Left atrial pressure; PV: Pulmonary veins; PA: Pulmonary artery; PAH: Pulmonary arterial hypertension; RVH: Right ventricular hypertrophy; RV: Right ventricular; TR: Tricuspid regurgitation; RA: Right atrium; CHF: Congestive heart failure).

Electrocardiogram often demonstrates right axis deviation (RAD), left atrial enlargement (LAE) and evidence of PH (Fig. 12.12). Many patients with chronic, untreated, and MS will develop atrial flutter or fibrillation.

The chest X-ray of patients with chronic MS will demonstrate LAE and pulmonary venous hypertension, and in later stages, features of pulmonary arterial hypertension (Fig. 12.13).

Echocardiography is the mainstay of diagnosis in MS (Figs. 12.14 to 12.19 and Videos 12.1 to 12.3). M mode, two-dimensional echocardiogram, Doppler and color flow imaging are helpful in assessing the severity of MS and for assessing the need and suitability of interventional procedures. Valves without significant mitral regurgitation (MR) and without significant commissural calcium are suitable for balloon mitral valvotomy (BMV), which is the procedure of choice in pliable MS. Table 12.2 lists the current system of classifying the degree of MS, which is based to a significant extent on echocardiographic findings.

Several findings on echocardiography are contraindications to BMV. Already significant MR (*see* Chapter 13) may be worsened by BMV and thus is considered a

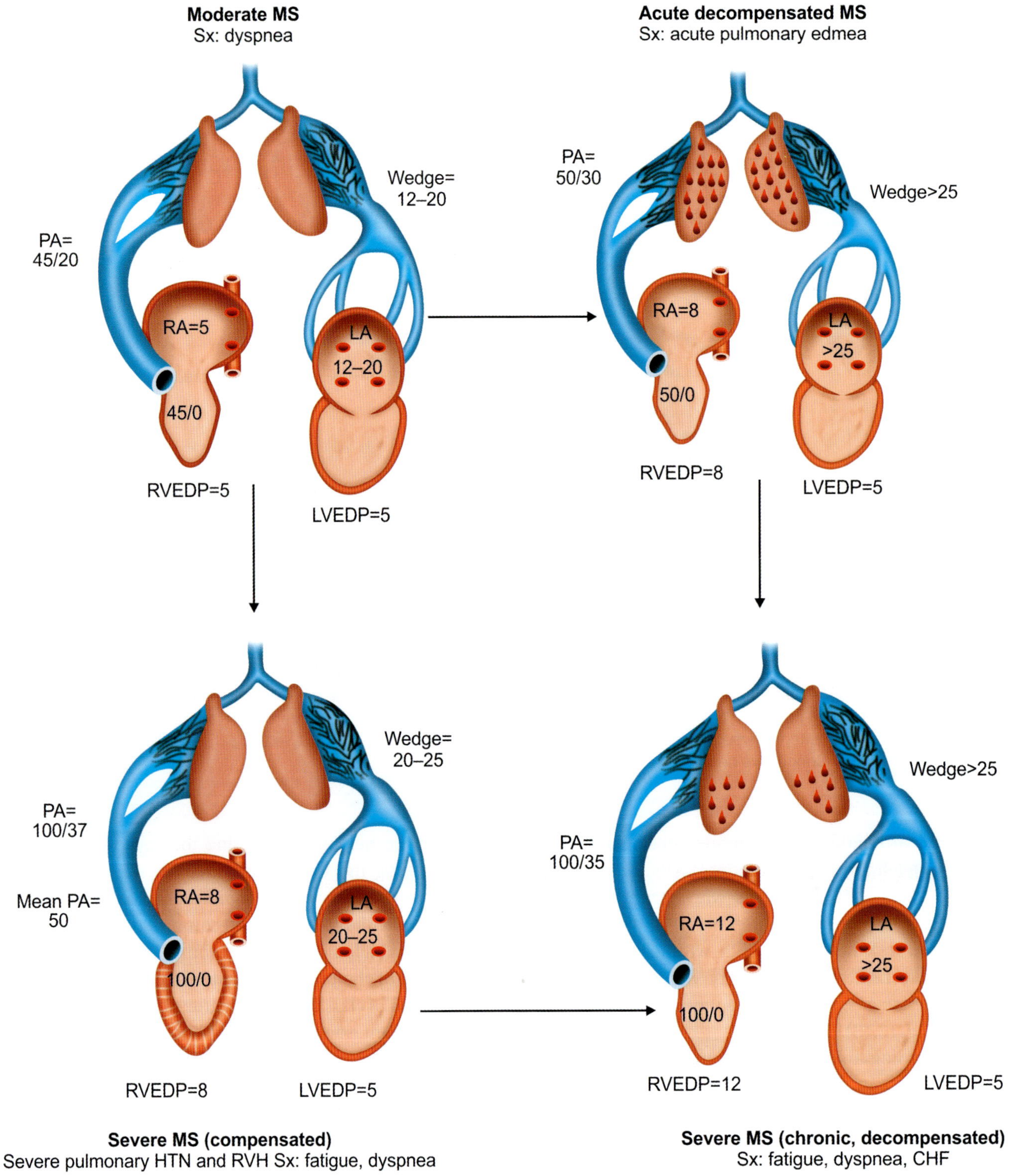

Fig. 12.11: The different hemodynamic stages of mitral stenosis (MS). (Image from Krishnakumar M, Mahesh SK, Arun SR. Pathophysiology, natural history and hemodynamics of mitral stenosis. In: Harikrishnan S (Ed). Percutaneous Mitral Valvotomy, 1st edition. New Delhi, India: Jaypee Brothers Medical Publishers (P) Ltd. 2012. pp. 34-43). (MS: Mitral stenosis; CHF: Congestive heart failure; PH: Pulmonary hypertension; RVH: Right ventricular hypertrophy).

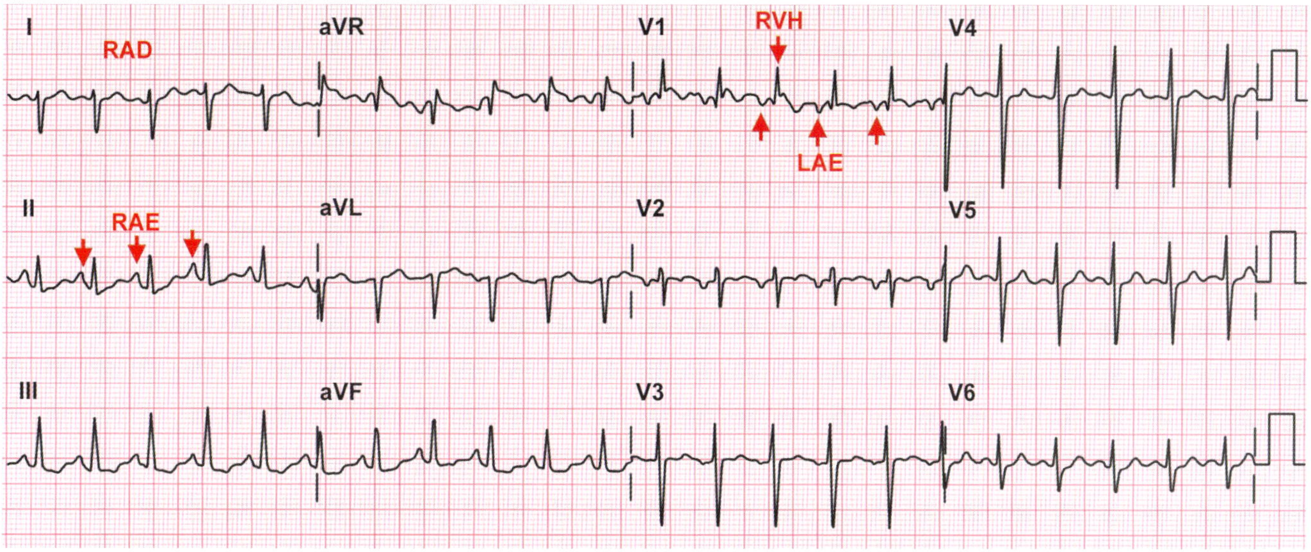

Fig. 12.12: Electrocardiogram (ECG) findings in mitral stenosis (MS). The deep P wave in lead V1 indicates left atrial enlargement (LAE, arrows). The tall R wave in lead V1, deep S wave in V6, and right axis deviation (RAD) [predominantly negative QRS in lead I and upright QRS in lead avF] all suggest right ventricular hypertrophy (RVH). The tall P waves in the inferior leads suggest the presence of right atrial enlargement (RAE, arrows). The findings of LAE, RAE, and RVH, without the presence of left ventricular hypertrophy (LVH) are highly suggestive of the presence of MS. [Image from Wang K. Atlas of Electrocardiography, 1st edition. New Delhi, India: Jaypee Brothers Medical Publishers (P) Ltd. 2013].

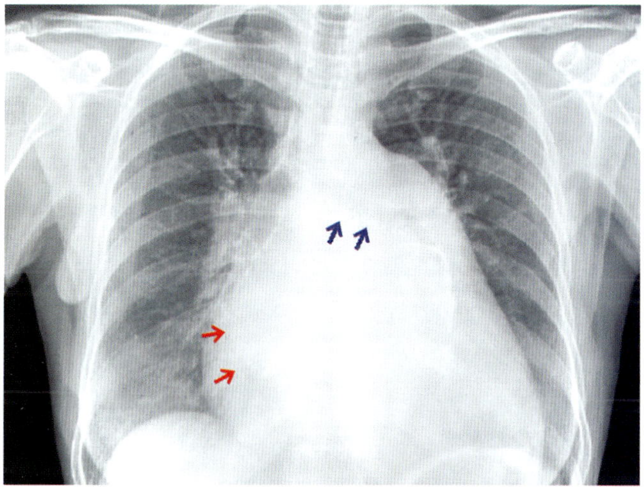

Fig. 12.13: Chest X-ray of a patient with severe mitral stenosis (MS). Left atrial enlargement (LAE) is seen as double shadow (blue arrows). There is an uplifted left main stem bronchus (splaying of the right and left bronchi) (red arrows) suggestive of LAE. Pulmonary arterial hypertension is evident as dilated central pulmonary arteries. Note the calcified wall of left atrium. [Image from Harivadan B, Harikrishnan S. Radiological evaluation in mitral stenosis. In: Harikrishnan S (Ed). Percutaneous Mitral Valvotomy, 1st edition. New Delhi, India: Jaypee Brothers Medical Publishers (P) Ltd; 2012. pp. 69-75].

contraindication. BMV is not performed if thrombus is detected by echocardiography in the left atrium (Fig. 12.19) or left atrial appendage (Fig. 12.20), due to the risk of embolization. In patients who are not significantly symptomatic and who are found to have a small thrombus, echocardiography can be repeated after 8–12 weeks of anticoagulation.

Several scoring systems have been devised to assess the suitability of the MV for percutaneous BMV and are given in Tables 12.3 to 12.5.

If the severity of MS remains in doubt after echocardiography, exercise testing and cardiac catheterization may additionally be performed. Like echocardiography, cardiac catheterization can assess the valve gradient (Fig. 12.21) and calculate the valve area. Ventriculography can provide another means of assessing left ventricular function and the degree of MR present (Fig. 12.22). Grade III or IV MR on ventriculography is considered as a contraindication to BMV.

MANAGEMENT OF MITRAL STENOSIS

Principles of management for patient with rheumatic MS include secondary rheumatic prophylaxis should be instituted as per guidelines. Tachycardia, particularly if during atrial fibrillation, leads to greater gradients and should be controlled with beta blockers (preferred), non-dihydropyridine calcium-channel blockers (verapamil

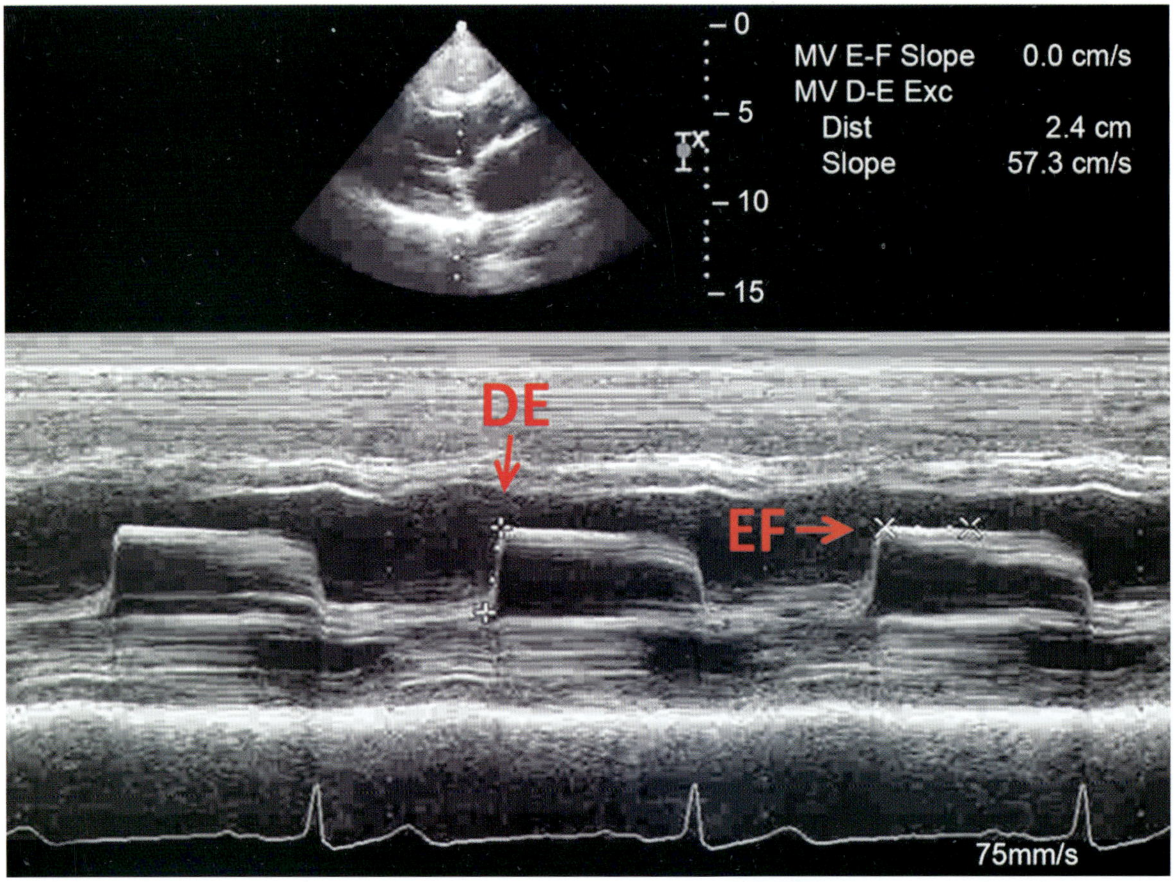

Fig. 12.14: M-mode echocardiogram of mitral valve (MV) in a patient with severe MS. Note the DE amplitude of 24 mm and EF slope of 0 cm/sec. This indicates severe and pliable MS. (Image from Harivadan B, Harikrishnan S. Radiological evaluation in mitral stenosis. In: Harikrishnan S (Ed). Percutaneous Mitral Valvotomy, 1st edition. New Delhi, India: Jaypee Brothers Medical Publishers (P) Ltd; 2012. pp. 69-75).

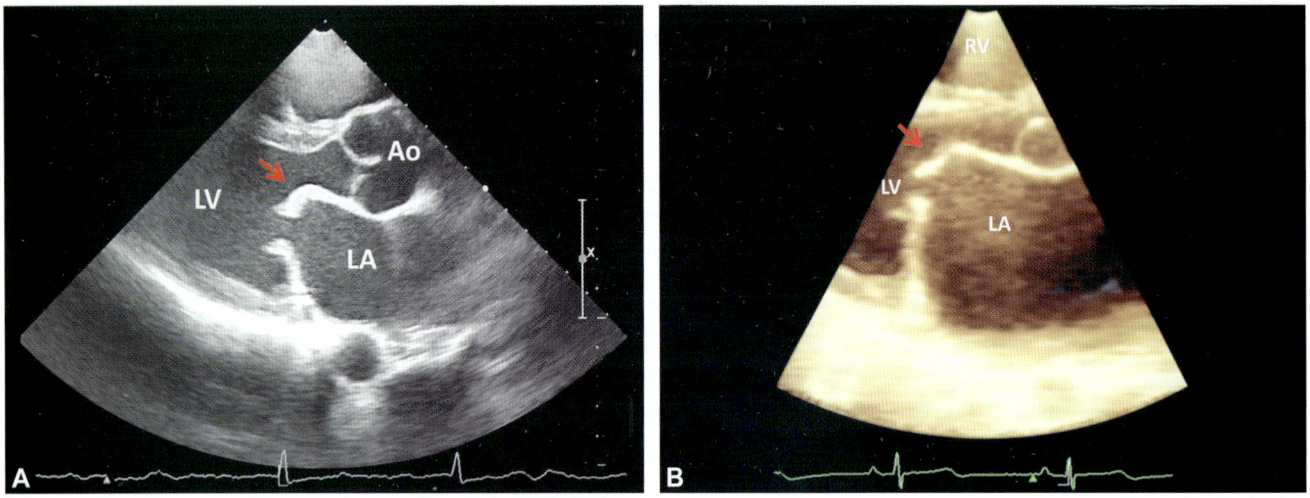

Figs. 12.15A and B: "Hockey stick" finding in mitral stenosis (MS). (A) Two-dimensional (2D) parasternal long axis echocardiogram demonstrating the grossly thickened mitral valve (MV) with the doming anterior mitral leaflet (AML) showing the characteristic "hockey-stick" appearance (arrow); (B) Three-dimensional (3D) echocardiographic image recorded online using a matrix arrow probe demonstrating a dilated left atrium (LA) and thickened and doming MV with "hockey stick" appearance of the AML (arrow). [Images from Harivadan B, Harikrishnan S. Radiological evaluation in mitral stenosis. In: Harikrishnan S (Ed). Percutaneous Mitral Valvotomy, 1st edition. New Delhi, India: Jaypee Brothers Medical Publishers (P) Ltd; 2012. pp. 69-75].

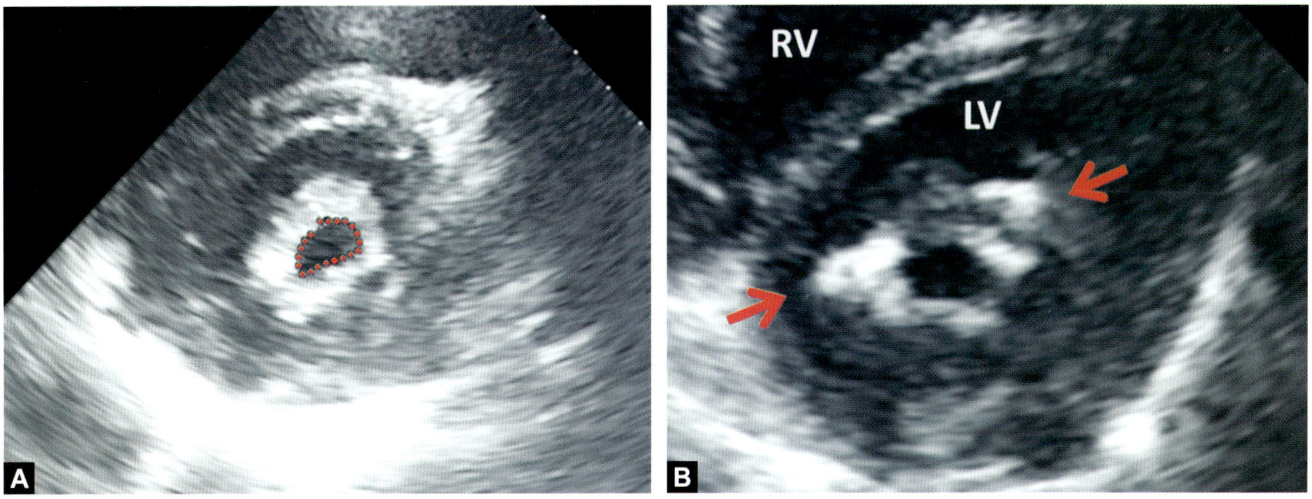

Figs. 12.16A and B: Parasternal short-axis echocardiographic assessment of the mitral valve (MV). (A) Assessment of mitral valve area (MVA) by planimetry. The two-dimensional (2D) MVA obtained is 0.894 cm^2, indicating severe mitral stenosis (MS). Both the commissures are fused. This valve is suitable for balloon mitral valvotomy (BMV); (B) Short axis view at the level of MV showing bilateral commissural calcium in a 60-year-old female with severe MS. This is a contraindication for BMV. [Images from Harivadan B, Harikrishnan S. Radiological evaluation in mitral stenosis. In: Harikrishnan S (Ed). Percutaneous Mitral Valvotomy, 1st edition. New Delhi, India: Jaypee Brothers Medical Publishers (P) Ltd; 2012. pp. 69-75].

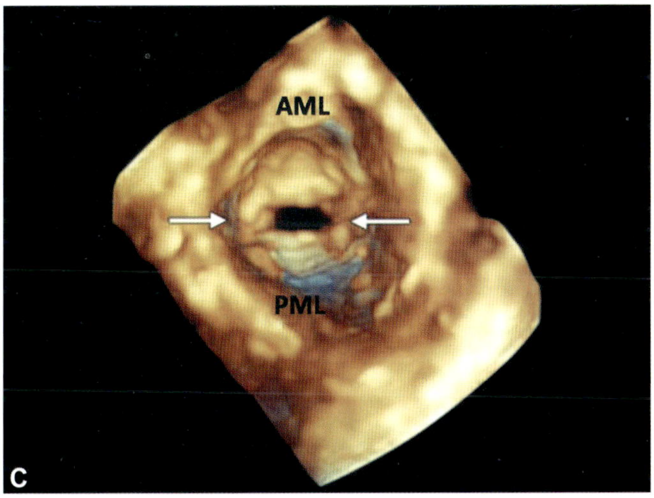

Fig. 12.16C: (C) Three-dimensional (3D) transesophageal echocardiography (TEE) of MS demonstrating fusion of the commissures (arrows). [Image from Saric M, Benenstein R. Three-dimensional echocardiographic guidance of percutaneous procedures. In: Nanda NC (Ed). Comprehensive Textbook of Echocardiography. New Delhi, India: Jaypee Brothers Medical Publishers (P) Ltd; 2013]. (AML: Anterior mitral leaflet; PML: Posterior mitral leaflet).

or diltiazem, or digoxin). Anticoagulation with vitamin K antagonists are indicated in patients with history of atrial fibrillation, and irrespective of the cardiac rhythm in patients with history of embolism, atrial thrombus and possibly in patients with left atrial dimension > 55 mm by echocardiography with or without spontaneous echo contrast. The newer oral anticoagulants may also be considered, although these have not been specifically tested in patients with rheumatic MS.

The prognosis of patients with severe MS and significant symptoms (NYHA class III/IV) is poor without mechanical interventions, and such patients should be

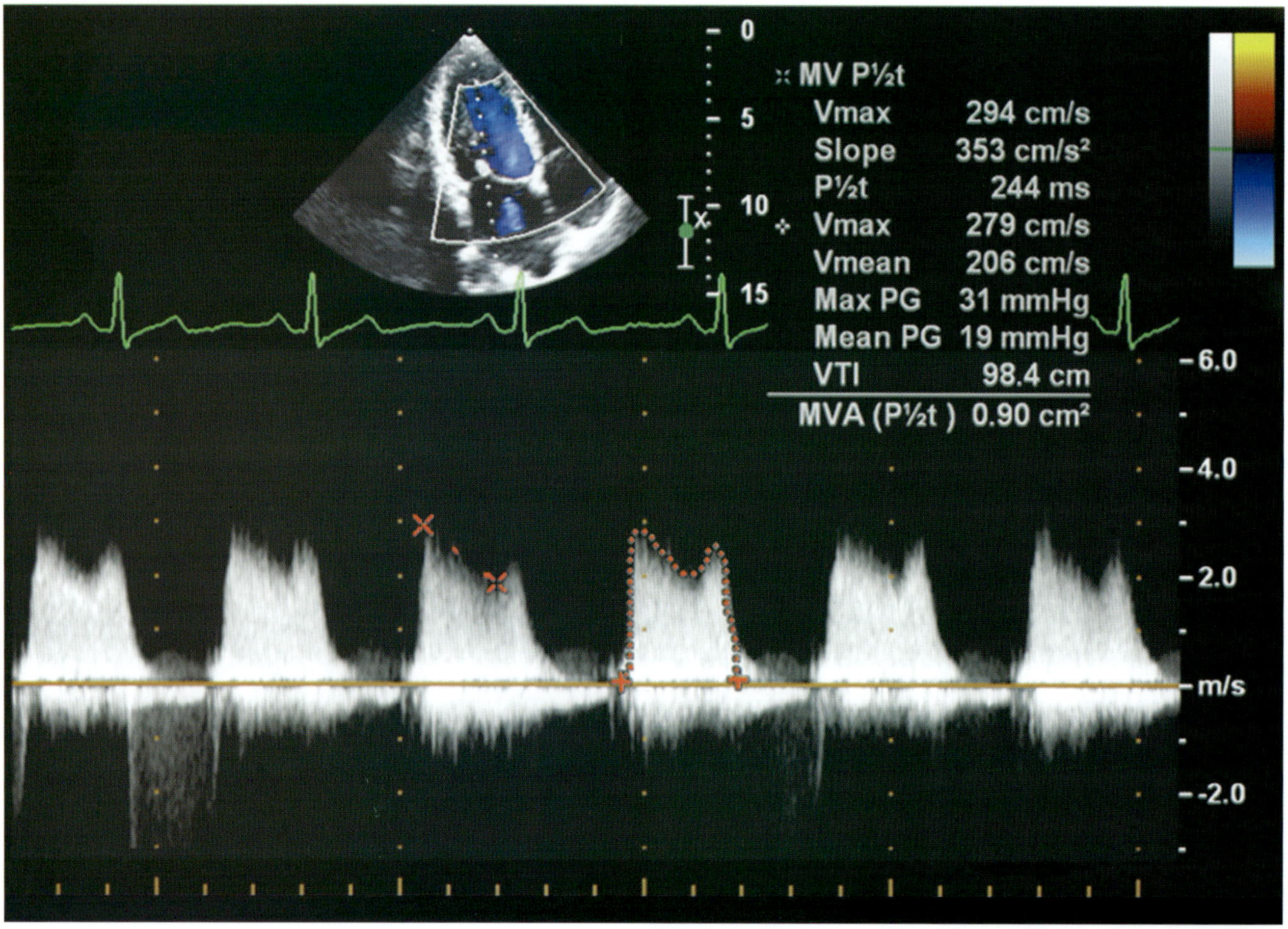

Fig. 12.17: Continuous wave (CW) spectral Doppler of mitral inflow velocities in a patient in sinus rhythm showing a "M" pattern. There is a peak gradient of 31 mm Hg and a mean gradient of 19 mm Hg, indicating severe mitral stenosis (MS). The image also illustrates the calculation of valve area using the Pressure half time method, which by this method is determined to be 0.9 cm². [Image from Hasan-Ali H, Harikrishnan S. Balloon mitral valvotomy—role of echocardiography. In: Harikrishnan S (Ed). Percutaneous Mitral Valvotomy, 1st edition. New Delhi, India: Jaypee Brothers Medical Publishers (P) Ltd; 2012. pp. 75-118].

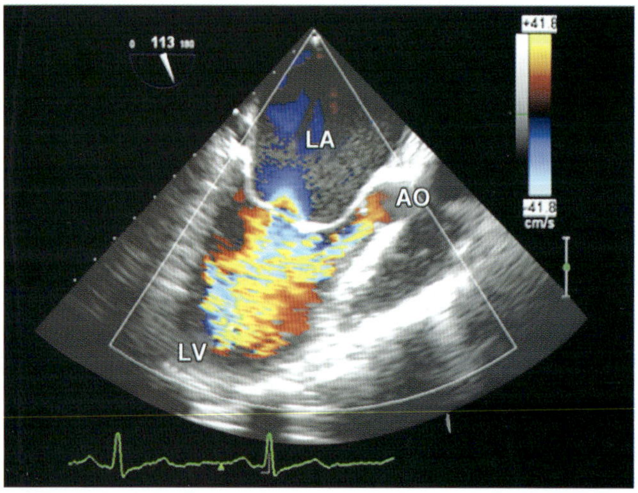

Fig. 12.18: Color Doppler transesophageal echocardiography (TEE) demonstrating severe turbulent blood flow across the mitral valve (MV). Note the doming of the mitral leaflets. Some aortic insufficiency is also visible in this patient with rheumatic valvular disease. (Image from Harivadan B, Harikrishnan S. Radiological evaluation in mitral stenosis. In: Harikrishnan S (Ed). Percutaneous Mitral Valvotomy, 1st edition. New Delhi, India: Jaypee Brothers Medical Publishers (P) Ltd; 2012. pp. 69-75). (Ao: Aorta; LA: Left atrial; LV: Left ventricle).

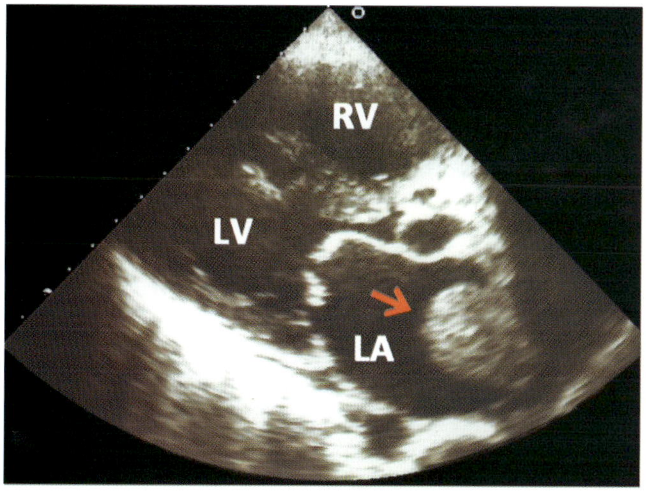

Fig. 12.19: Parasternal long axis transthoracic echocardiography (TTE) demonstrating a large thrombus (arrow) in this patient with mitral stenosis (MS). [Image from Mocumbi AO. Role of echocardiography in research into neglected cardiovascular disease in sub-Saharan Africa. In: Gaze DC (Ed). The Cardiovascular System—Physiology, Diagnostics and Clinical Implications. Intechopen.com].

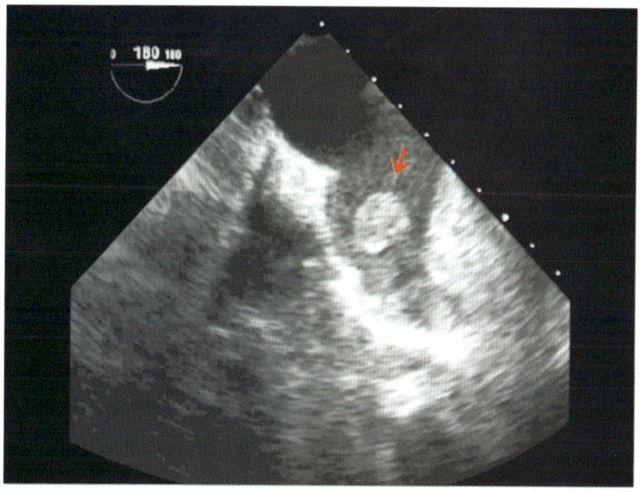

Fig. 12.20: Transesophageal echocardiogram (TEE) showing a mobile left atrial appendage (LAA) thrombus (arrow) in a patient with severe mitral stenosis (MS). [Image from Jacob SP. Left atrial thrombosis in rheumatic mitral stenosis. In: Harikrishnan S (Ed). Percutaneous Mitral Valvotomy, 1st edition. New Delhi, India: Jaypee Brothers Medical Publishers (P) Ltd; 2012. pp. 385-94].

Table 12.2: Summary of the American College of Cardiology Foundation (ACCF)/American Heart Association (AHA) guidelines criteria for the classification of degree of mitral stenosis (MS). (MVA: Mitral valve area; LA: Left atrial; PASP: Pulmonary artery systolic pressure.

Stage/Definition	*Valve Anatomy and Hemodynamics*	*Hemodynamic Consequences and Symptoms*
A - At risk of MS	• Mild valve doming during diastole • Normal transmitral flow velocity	• No hemodynamic consequences • No symptoms
B - Progressive MS	• Rheumatic valve changes with commissural fusion and diastolic doming of the mitral valve leaflets • Increased transmitral flow velocities • MVA >1.5 cm^2 • Diastolic pressure half-time <150 msec	• Mild-to-moderate LA enlargement • Normal pulmonary pressure at rest • No symptoms
C - Asymptomatic severe MS	• Rheumatic valve changes with commissural fusion and diastolic doming of the mitral valve leaflets • MVA ≤ 1.5 cm^2; MVA ≤ 1 cm^2 with very severe MS • Diastolic pressure half-time ≥ 150 msec; diastolic pressure half-time ≥ 220 msec with very severe MS	• Severe LA enlargement • Elevated PASP > 30 mm Hg • No symptoms
D - Symptomatic severe MS	• Rheumatic valve changes with commissural fusion and diastolic doming of the mitral valve leaflets • MVA ≤ 1.5 cm^2; MVA ≤ 1 cm^2 with very severe MS • Diastolic pressure half-time ≥ 150 m/sec; diastolic pressure half-time ≥ 220 msec with very severe MS	• Severe LA enlargement • Elevated PASP >30 mm Hg • Decreased exercise tolerance • Exertional dyspnea

referred for either surgery [closed mitral commissurotomy, open mitral commissurotomy, or mitral valve replacement (MVR)] or BMV.

Indications for intervention in patients with MS are summarized in Tables 12.6 and 12.7. There are some differences between how the American College of Cardiology Foundation/American Heart Association (ACCF/AHA) and the European Society of Cardiology (ESC) guidelines are organized and presented, although both convey the same basic messages:

- Intervention is recommended in symptomatic patients with severe MS (MVA ≤ 1.5 cm^2)

Table 12.3: Summary of the assessment of the mitral valve (MV) as a candidate for balloon mitral valvuloplasty using the Wilkins scoring system.

Grade	*Leaflet Mobility*	*Valvular Thickening*	*Subvalvular Thickening*	*Valvular Calcification*
1	Highly mobile valve with restriction of only the leaflet tips	Leaflet near normal (4–5 mm)	Minimal thickening of chordal structures just below the valve	A single area of increased echo brightness
2	Midportion and base of the leaflet have reduced mobility	Mild leaflet thickening, marked thickening at the margins	Thickening of chordae extending up to one third of chordal length	Scattered areas of brightness confined to leaflet margin
3	Valve leaflets move forward in diastole mainly at the base	Thickening extends through the entire leaflets (5–8 mm)	Thickening extending to the distal third of the chordae	Brightness extending to the midportion of the leaflets
4	No or minimal forward movement of the leaflets in diastole	Marked thickening of all leaflet tissue (> 8–10 mm)	Extensive thickening and shortening of all chordae extending to the papillary muscles (PM)	Extensive brightness through most of the leaflet tissue

Table 12.4: Summary of the Reid scoring system for mitral valve (MV) evaluation prior to percutaneous mitral valvotomy. (H: Height of doming of mitral valve; L: Length of dome of mitral valve; MV: Mitral valve; PWAo: Posterior wall of aorta).

Morphologic Feature	*Definition*	*Grade*	*Score*
Leaflet motion (H/L ratio)	≥ 0.45	Mild	0
	0.26–0.44	Moderate	1
	< 0.25	Severe	2
Leaflet thickness (MV/PWAo ratio)	1.5–2	Mild	0
	2.1–4.9	Moderate	1
	≥ 5.0	Severe	2
Subvalvular disease	Thin faintly visible chordae tendineae (CT)	Absent-mild	0
	Areas of increased density equal to endocardium	Moderate	1
	Areas denser than endocardium with thickened CT	Severe	2
Commissural calcium	Homogenous density of mitral valve orifice	Absent	0
	Increased density of anterior/posterior	One commissure	1
	Increased density of both commissures	Two commissures	2

Table 12.5: Summary of the lung and Cormeir scoring system for assessing mitral valve (MV) suitability for percutaneous mitral valvuloplasty (PMV).

Echocardiographic group	*Mitral valve (MV) anatomy*
Group 1	Pliable non-calcified anterior mitral leaflet (AML) and mild subvalvular disease (thin chordae, ≥ 10 mm long)
Group 2	Pliable non-calcified AML and severe subvalvular disease (thick chordae, < 10 mm long)
Group 3	Calcification of MV of any extent, as assessed by fluoroscopy, whatever the state of subvalvular apparatus

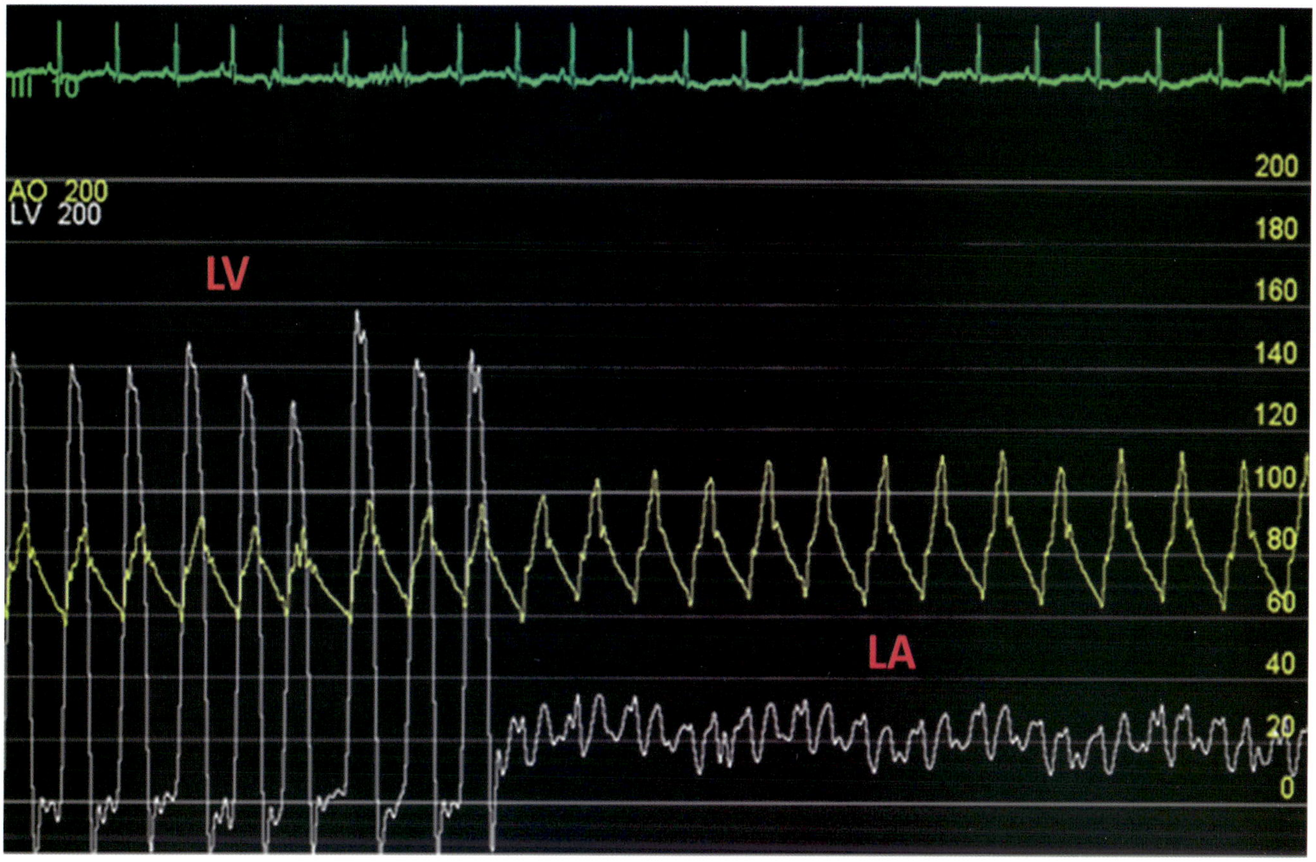

Fig. 12.21: Hemodynamic tracing in the cardiac catheterization laboratory in a patient with combined rheumatic mitral and aortic stenosis. The white tracing shows a pull-back from left ventricle (LV) to left atrium (LA), with simultaneous pressure in the ascending aorta (yellow line). Note the elevated LA pressure. [Image from Harikrishnan S, Choudhary D. PMV performed with other percutaneous interventions. In: Harikrishnan S (Ed). Percutaneous Mitral Valvotomy, 1st edition. New Delhi, India: Jaypee Brothers Medical Publishers (P) Ltd; 2012. pp. 349-57].

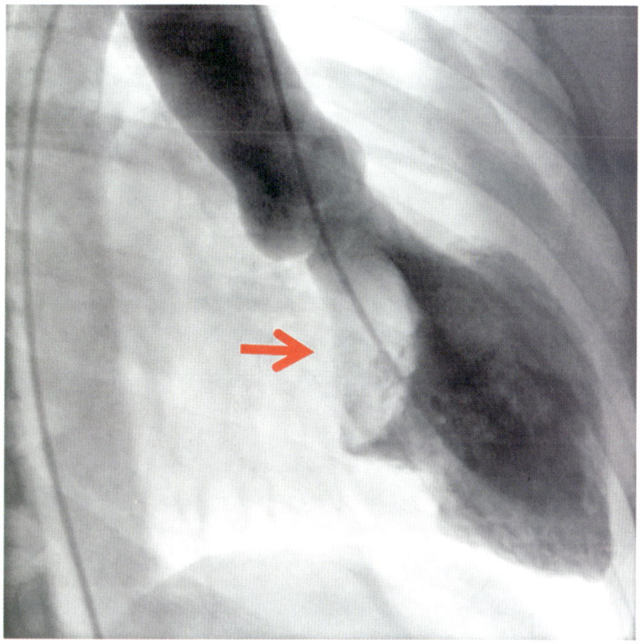

Fig. 12.22: Left ventricular angiogram in a patient with severe mitral stenosis (MS). Still frame in diastole demonstrates the doming mitral valve (MV) (arrow), with bulging of the mitral leaflets into the contrast-filled left ventricle (LV) (egg sign). No mitral regurgitation (MR) is seen. [Image from Harivadan B, Harikrishnan S. Radiological evaluation in mitral stenosis. In: Harikrishnan S (Ed). Percutaneous Mitral Valvotomy, 1st edition. New Delhi, India: Jaypee Brothers Medical Publishers (P) Ltd; 2012. pp. 69-75].

Table 12.6: Summary of the ACCF/AHA guidelines for indications for intervention in patients with mitral stenosis. The level of evidence (LOE) supporting the recommendation is given in parenthesis, where LOE=A denotes a recommendation derived from multiple randomized clinical trials or meta-analyses, LOE=B denotes a recommendation derived from a single randomized clinical trial or non-randomized studies, and LOE=C denotes a recommendation based on consensus of expert opinion, standard of care, or case reports. (MS: Mitral stenosis; MVA: Mitral valve area; NYHA: New York Heart Association; PMBC: Percutaneous mitral balloon commissurotomy).

Class I (is recommended)
• PMBC in symptomatic patients with severe MS (MVA ≤ 1.5 cm^2) and favorable valve morphology in the absence of contraindications (LOE=A)
• MV surgery in severely symptomatic patients with severe MS (MVA ≤ 1.5 cm^2) who are not high risk for surgery and who are not candidates for or failed previous PMBC (LOE=B)
• Concomitant MV surgery in patients with severe MS (MVA ≤ 1.5 cm^2) undergoing other cardiac surgery (LOE=C)
Class II (is reasonable)
• PMBC in asymptomatic patients with very severe MS (MVA ≤ 1.0 cm^2) and favorable valve morphology in the absence of contraindications (LOE=C)
• MV surgery in severely symptomatic patients with severe MS (MVA ≤ 1.5 cm^2) provided there are other operative indications (LOE=C)
Class IIb (may be considered)
• PMBC in symptomatic patients with severe MS (MVA ≤ 1.5 cm^2) and favorable valve morphology who have new onset of atrial fibrillation, in the absence of contraindications (LOE=C)
• PMBC in symptomatic patients with MVA > 1.5 cm^2 if there is evidence of hemodynamically significant MS during exercise (LOE=C)
• PMBC in severely symptomatic patients with severe MS (MVA ≤ 1.5 cm^2) who have suboptimal valve anatomy and are not candidates or are at high risk for surgery (LOE=C)
• Concomitant MV surgery in patients with moderate MS (MVA 1.6-2.0 cm^2) undergoing other cardiac surgery (LOE=C)
• MV surgery and excision of the left atrial appendate in patients with severe MS (MVA ≤ 1.5 cm^2) who have had recurrent embolic events while receiving adequate anticoagulation.

Table 12.7: Summary of the European Society of Cardiology (ESC) and European Association for Cardiothoracic Surgery (EACTS) guideline indications and contraindications for percutaneous mitral commissurotomy in mitral stenosis (MS) with valve area ≤ 1.5 cm^2. The level of evidence (LOE) supporting the recommendation is given in parenthesis, where LOE=A denotes a recommendation derived from multiple randomized clinical trials or meta-analyses, LOE=B denotes a recommendation derived from a single randomized clinical trial or large nonrandomized studies, and LOE=C denotes a recommendation based on consensus of expert opinion or based on small studies, retrospective studies, or registries.

Class I (is recommended; is indicated)
• Symptomatic patients with favorable characteristics (LOE=B)
• Symptomatic patients with contraindication or high risk for surgery (LOE=C)
Class IIa (should be considered)
• As initial treatment in symptomatic patients with unfavorable anatomy but without unfavorable clinical characteristics (LOE=C)
• Asymptomatic patients without unfavorable characteristics and (LOE=C):
– High thromboembolic risk (previous history of embolism, dense spontaneous contrast in the left atrium (LA), recent or paroxysmal atrial fibrillation) and/or
– High risk of hemodynamic decompensation (systolic pulmonary pressure > 50 mm Hg at rest, need for major non-cardiac surgery, desire for pregnancy)
Class III (contraindicated, should not be performed)
• Mitral valve area (MVA) > 1.5 cm^2
• Left atrial (LA) thrombus
• More than mild mitral regurgitation
• Severe or bicommissural calcification
• Absence of commissural fusion
• Severe concomitant aortic valve disease, or severe combined tricuspid stenosis and regurgitation
• Concomitant coronary artery disease requiring bypass surgery

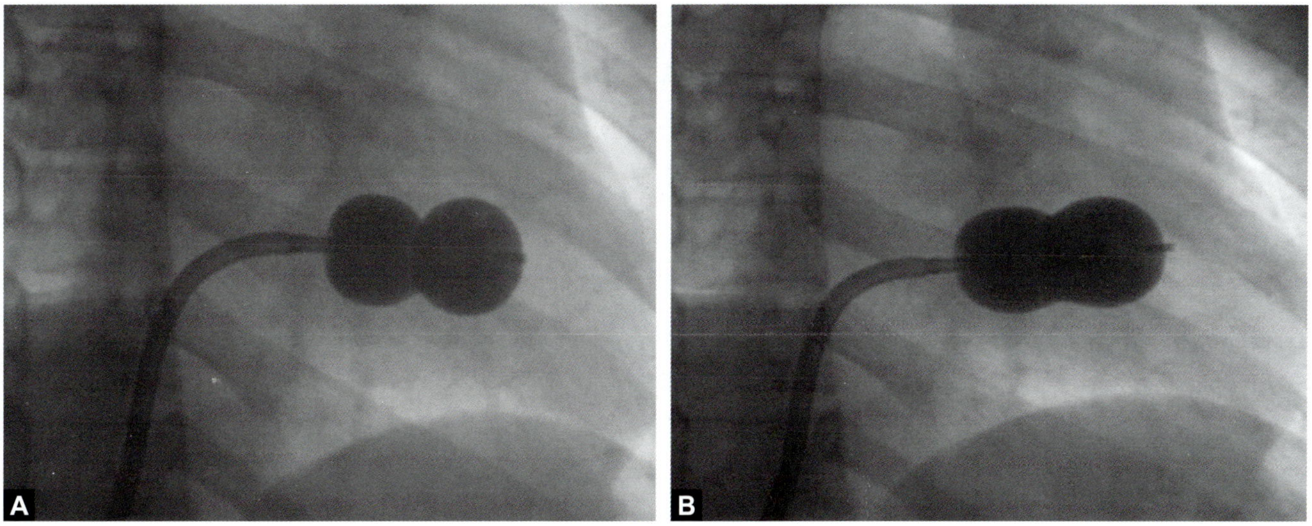

Figs. 12.23A and B: Fluoroscopy image of Accura balloon in partially open position (A) and in fully expanded "give-way" position B. [Image from Harikrishnan S, Sanjay G, Rajesh M. Percutaneous mitral valvotomy (PMV)—procedure. In: Harikrishnan S (Ed). Percutaneous Mitral Valvotomy, 1st edition. New Delhi, India: Jaypee Brothers Medical Publishers (P) Ltd; 2012. pp. 163-72].

- Percutaneous mitral balloon commissurotomy (PMBC) is generally preferred over surgical intervention when there is favorable valve morphology for PMBC and the absence of contraindications

In general, surgical intervention is recommended over percutaneous BMV in patients with: Significant MR (Grade III or IV): For MVR

- Non-pliable valve or bi-commissural calcium: MVR/repair if feasible
- *LA clot*: Open mitral commissurotomy with clot extraction.

Balloon mitral valvotomy is performed by crossing intra-atrial septum and inflating a specially designed balloon-tipped catheter at the level of the stenotic MV. The procedure can be performed using either one balloon (Figs. 12.23A and B) or two side-by-side balloons (Fig. 12.24). A successfully treated MV is demonstrated in Figures 12.25A and B.

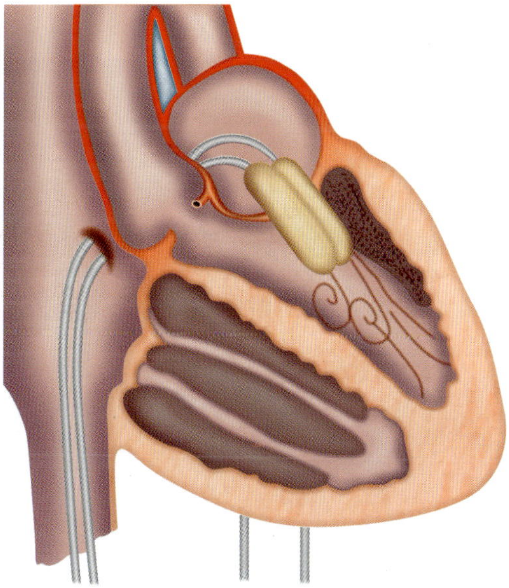

Fig. 12.24: Schematic illustration of the two balloon mitral valvotomy (BMV) technique.

Numerous complications from BMV can result, including MR (Fig. 12.26). Although some degree of MR will usually result from the procedure, a modest degree of MR is acceptable, and may be found to be decreased on follow-up echocardiography (Figs. 12.27A and B). In occasionally cases though, overt tearing of the leaflet can occur (Fig. 12.28). Iatrogenic atrial septal defect (ASD) is an accepted potential consequence of the procedure (Fig. 12.29), but is usually not hemodynamically or clinically significant.

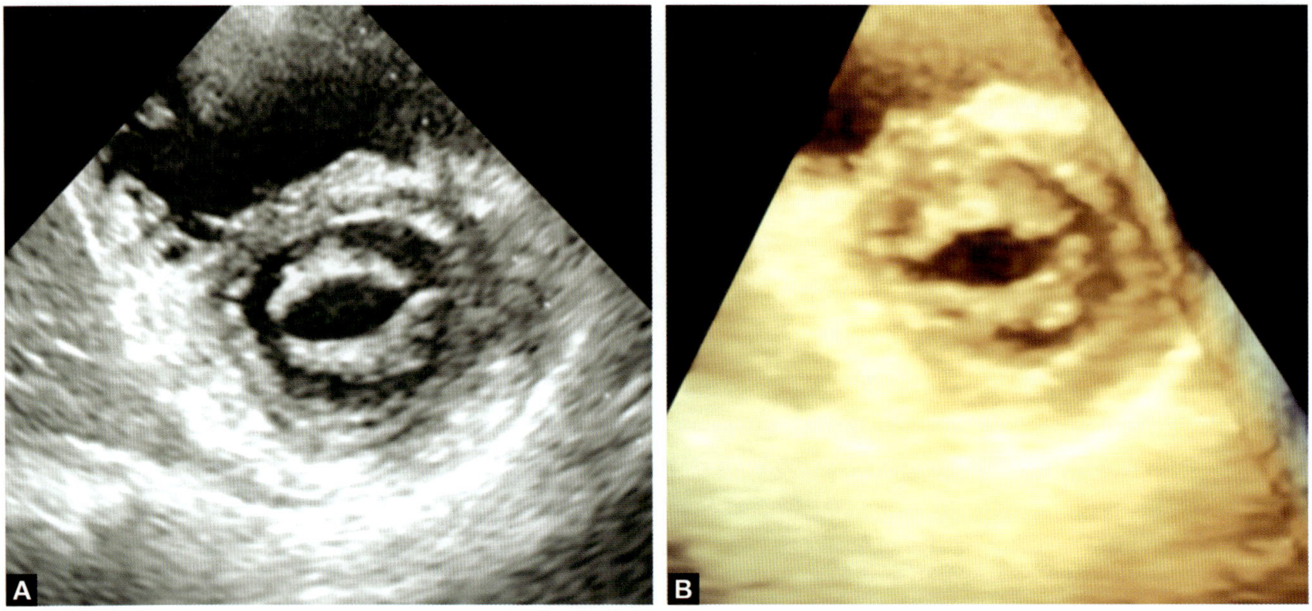

Figs. 12.25A and B: Echocardiograms obtained post-balloon mitral valvotomy (BMV). (A) Two-dimensional (2D) short axis view demonstrating mitral valve (MV) with well-split commissures; (B) The same valve imaged by three-dimensional (3D) matrix array probe. [Images from Harivadan B, Harikrishnan S. Radiological evaluation in mitral stenosis. In: Harikrishnan S (Ed). Percutaneous Mitral Valvotomy, 1st edition. New Delhi, India: Jaypee Brothers Medical Publishers (P) Ltd; 2012. pp. 69-75].

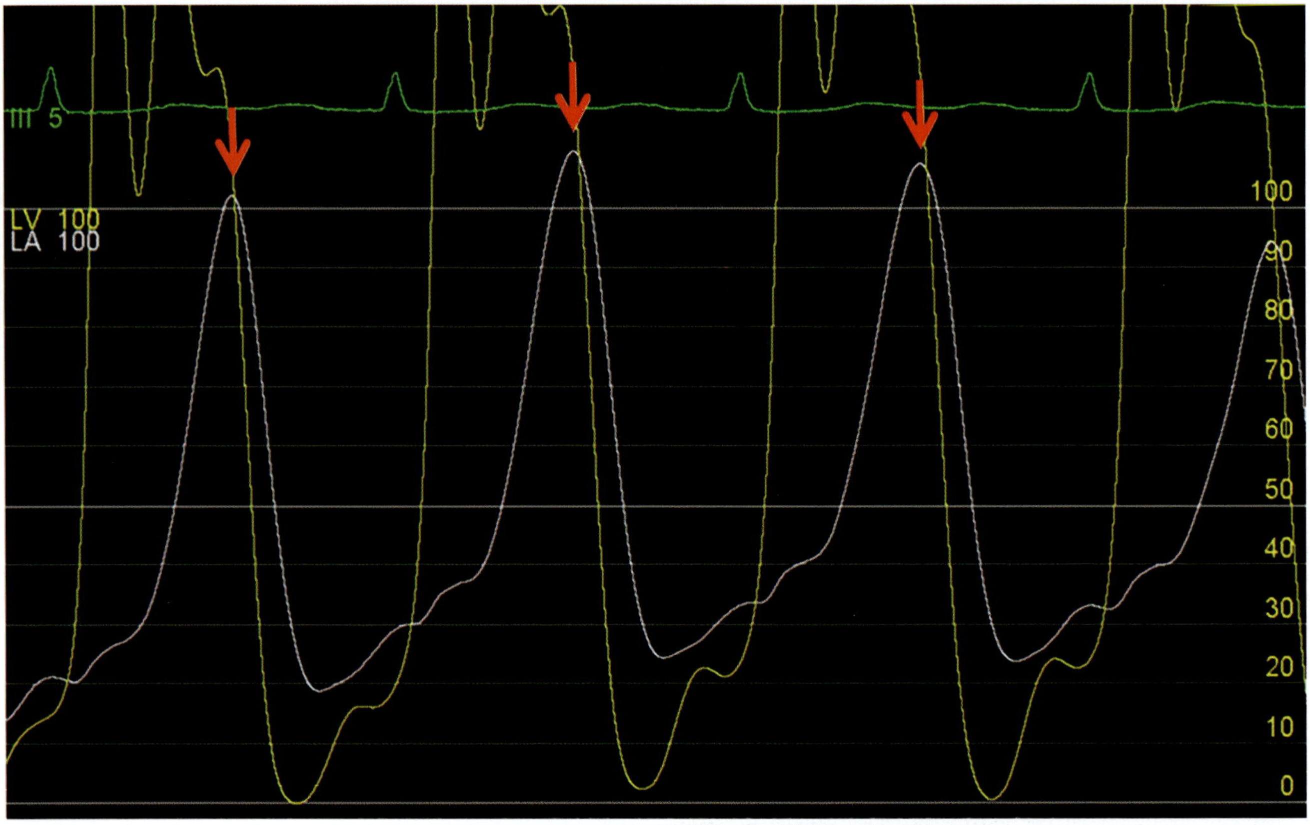

Fig. 12.26: Hemodynamic tracing in a patient who developed severe mitral regurgitation (MR) due to tear of anterior mitral leaflet (AML) following balloon mitral valvotomy (BMV). Note the huge "V" waves (arrows) measuring more than 100 mm Hg.

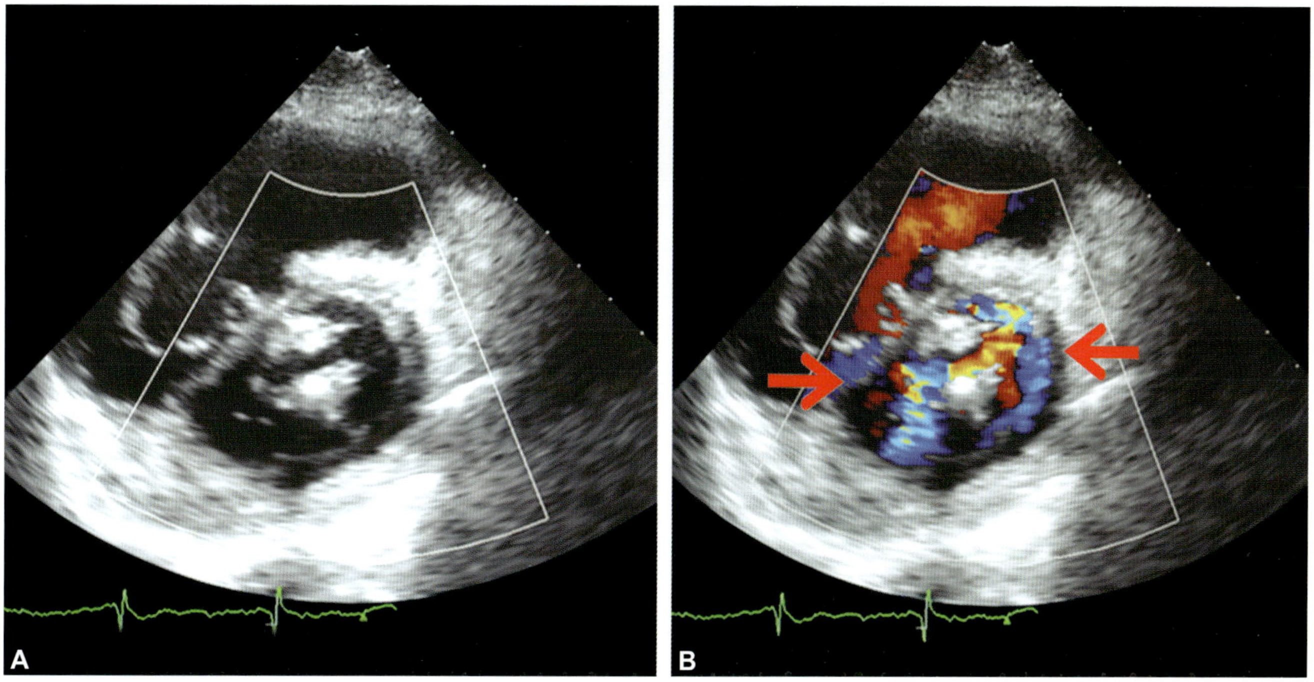

Figs. 12.27A and B: Commissural mitral regurgitation (MR) after balloon mitral valvotomy (BMV). (A) Echocardiographic image in parasternal short axis view showing a very fibrotic mitral valve (MV) following a successful percutaneous mitral balloon valvuloplasty (PMV) with both commissures open; (B) Color Doppler imaging revealing MR through both the commissures (arrows). MR through the commissures is usually benign and will be found to have diminished on follow-up echocardiographic examination. [Image from Harivadan B, Harikrishnan S. Radiological evaluation in mitral stenosis. In: Harikrishnan S (Ed). Percutaneous Mitral Valvotomy, 1st edition. New Delhi, India: Jaypee Brothers Medical Publishers (P) Ltd; 2012. pp. 69-75].

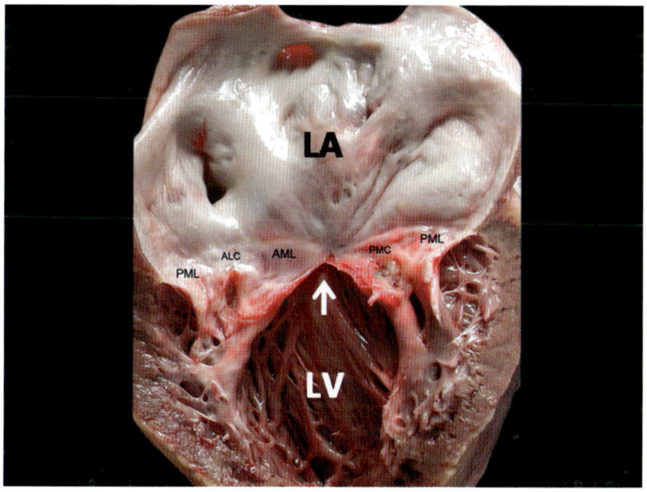

Fig. 12.28: Balloon mitral valvotomy (BMV) in a patient with mitral stenosis (MS) resulting in inadvertent tear (white arrow) of the anterior mitral leaflet (AML) extending from the free margin to its base, leading to torrential mitral regurgitation. [Image and legend text courtesy of Dr Pradeep Vaideeswar, Professor (Additional), Department of Pathology (Cardiovascular and Thoracic Division), Seth GS Medical College, Mumbai, India].

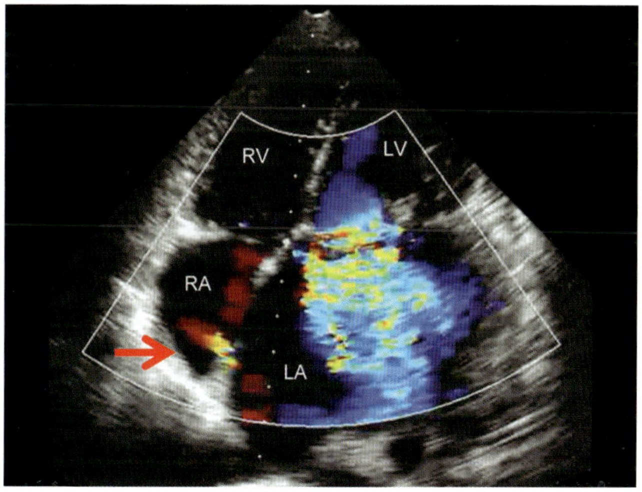

Fig. 12.29: Color Doppler image obtained post-balloon mitral valvotomy (BMV) showing moderate to severe mitral regurgitation (MR) and iatrogenic atrial septal defect (ASD) following transseptal puncture with left to right shunting (arrow). [Image from Harivadan B, Harikrishnan S. Radiological evaluation in mitral stenosis. In: Harikrishnan S (Ed). Percutaneous Mitral Valvotomy, 1st edition. New Delhi, India: Jaypee Brothers Medical Publishers (P) Ltd; 2012. pp. 69-75].

VIDEO LEGENDS

Video 12.1: Parasternal long axis transthoracic echocardiography (TTE) showing mitral stenosis (MS) in a patient with rheumatic heart disease. The anterior mitral leaflet (AML) forms a "hockey stick" as it tries to open during ventricular diastole. Note also aortic stenosis is present in this patient. (Video courtesy of Levine GN, MD).

Video 12.2: Parasternal short axis transthoracic echocardiography (TTE) of a patient with mitral stenosis (MS). A "fish mouth" appearance of the stenotic mitral valve (MV) is present.

Video 12.3: Transesophageal echocardiography (TEE) of a patient showing mitral stenosis (MS).

CHAPTER

Mitral Regurgitation

13

Alvin S Blaustein, Glenn N Levine

INTRODUCTION

The mitral valve consists of an anterior leaflet, a posterior leaflet, and an annulus to which the leaflets are attached (Figs. 13.1 and 13.2). Each leaflet is divided into three scallops, designated from anterolateral to posteromedial location as A1, A2 and A3, and P1, P2, and P3, respectively (Figs. 13.3 and 13.4). The leaflets are tethered by chordae tendineae to medial and lateral papillary muscles, supported by the ventricular myocardium.

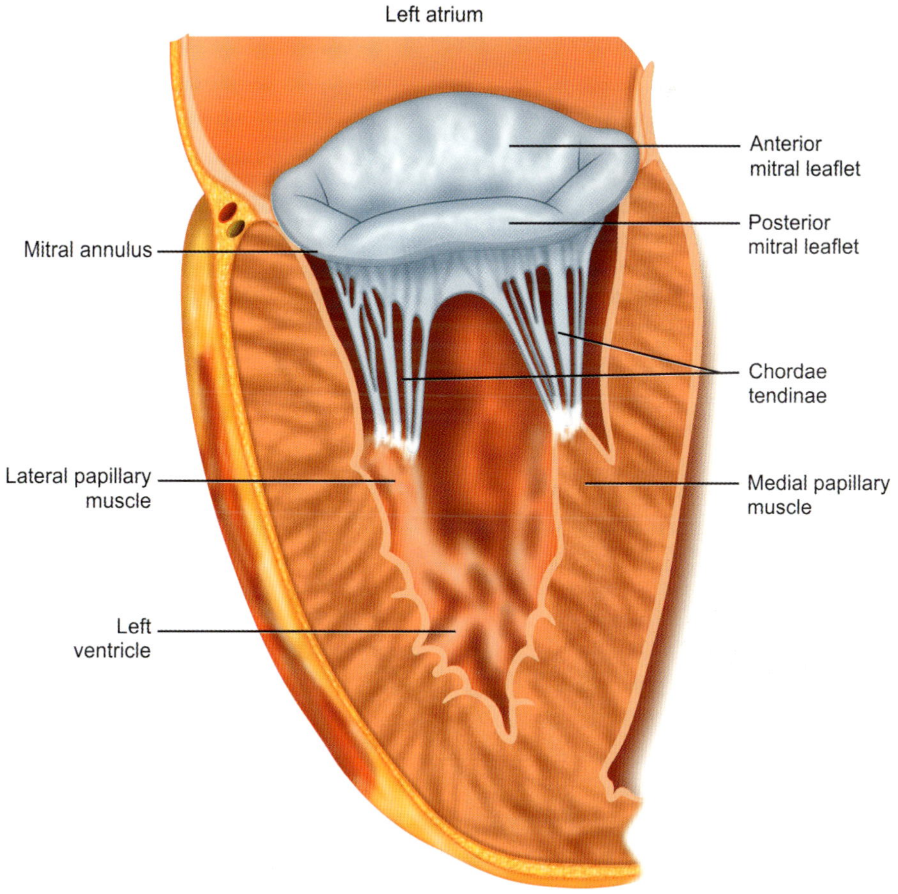

Fig. 13.1: Anatomy of the mitral valve and apparatus. The mitral valve consists of anterior and posterior leaflets. The mitral apparatus consist of medial and lateral papillary muscles, connected to the mitral leaflets by the chordae tendineae and supported by the ventricular myocardium.

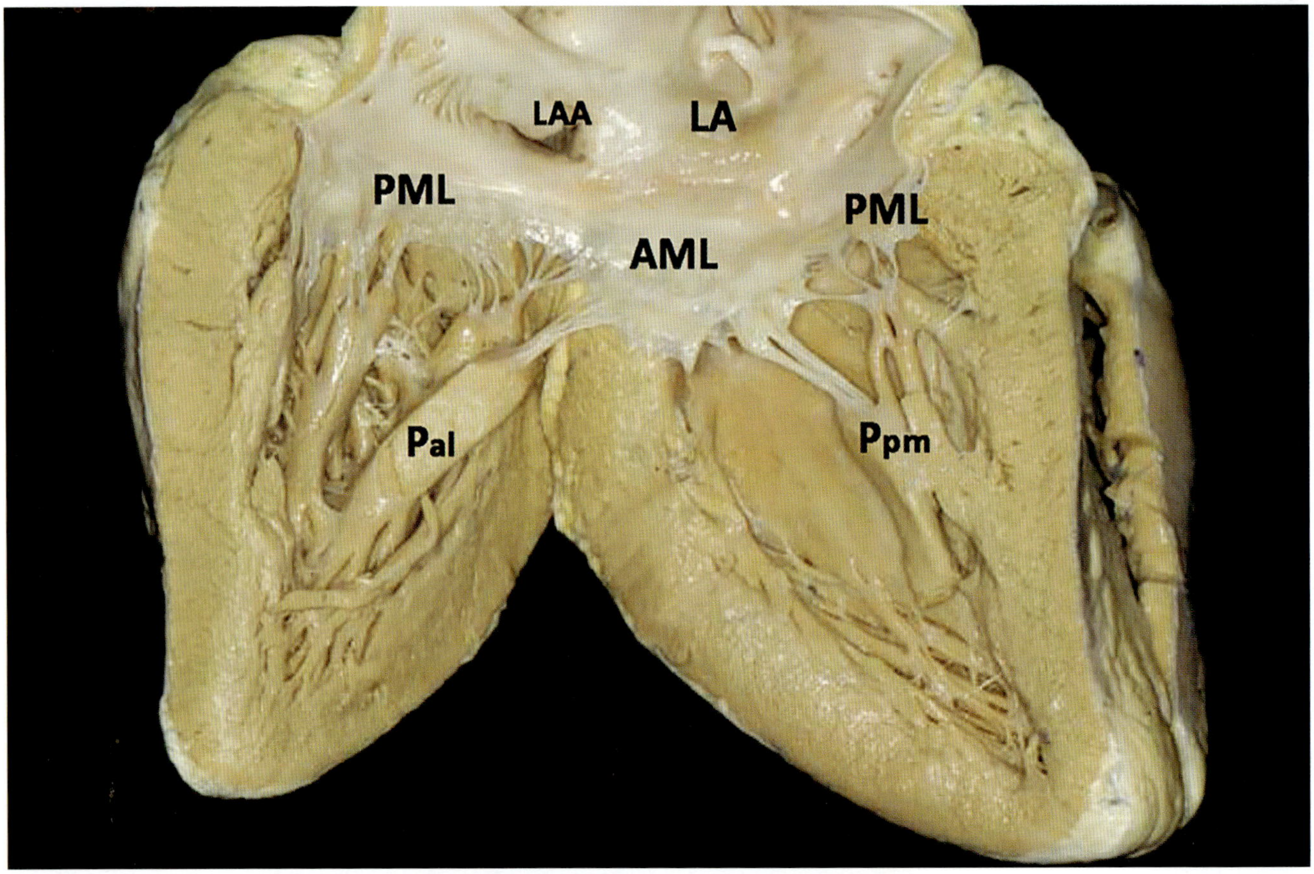

Fig. 13.2A: Pathology specimen showing the mitral valve in relationship to the left ventricle and left atrium. [Image from Cheitlin MD, Ursell PC. Cardiac anatomy. In: Chatterjee K, Anderson M, Heistad D, Kerber RE (Eds). Cardiology: An Illustrated Textbook. New Delhi, India: Jaypee Brothers Medical Publishers (P) Ltd; 2013; image courtesy of Philip C Ursell, MD, Department of Pathology, UCSF].

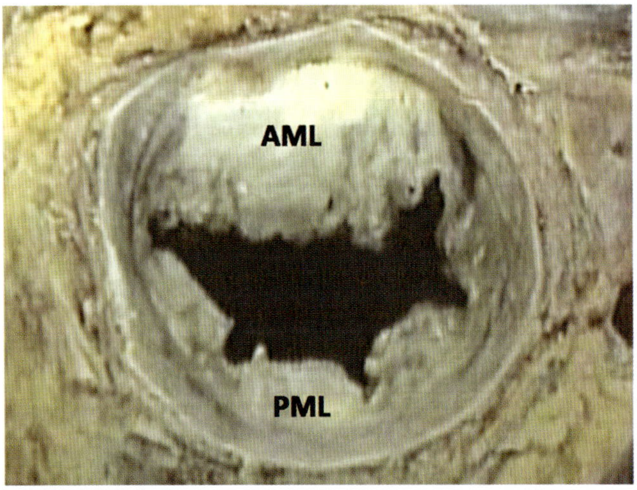

Fig. 13.2B: Gross pathology image of the mitral valve. (AML: Anterior mitral leaflet; PML: Posterior mitral leaflet).

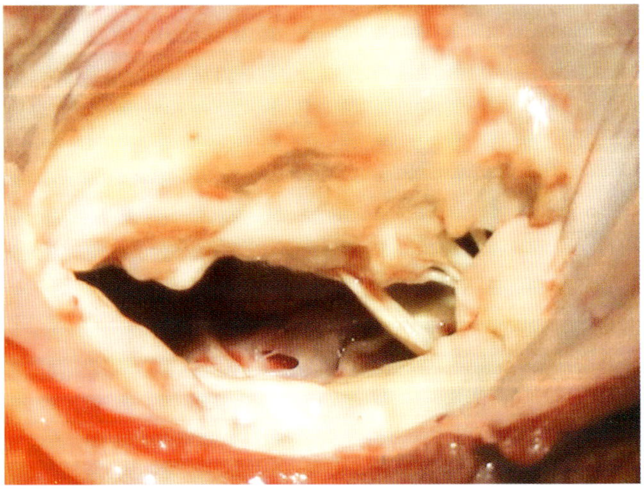

Fig. 13.2C: Operative image of the mitral valve. [Image from Boldyrev SY, Barbukhatty KO, Rossokha OA, et al. Mitral valve subvalvular apparatus repair with artificial neochords application. In: Nazari S (Ed). Front Lines of Thoracic Surgery. InTech; 2012]. (AML: Anterior mitral leaflet; LA: Left atrium; LAA: Orifice of the left atrial appendage; Pal: Anterolateral papillary muscle; Ppm: Posteromedial papillary muscle; PML: Posterior mitral leaflet).

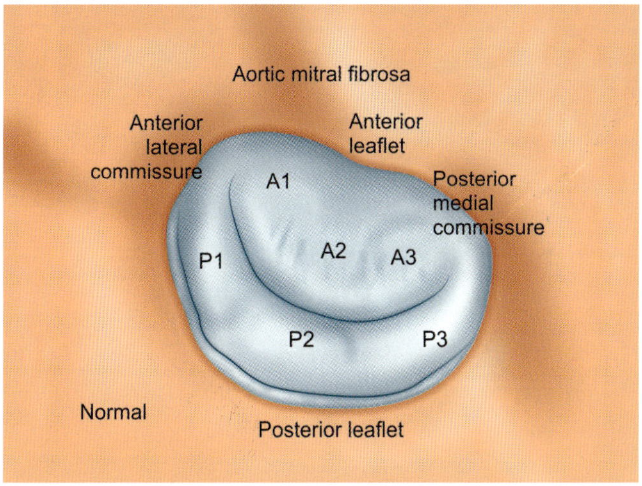

Fig. 13.3: Scallops of the mitral valve. The anterior and posterior mitral leaflets each consist of three scallops. From anterolateral to posteromedial location, these are denoted as A1, A2, and A3 and P1, P2, and P3.

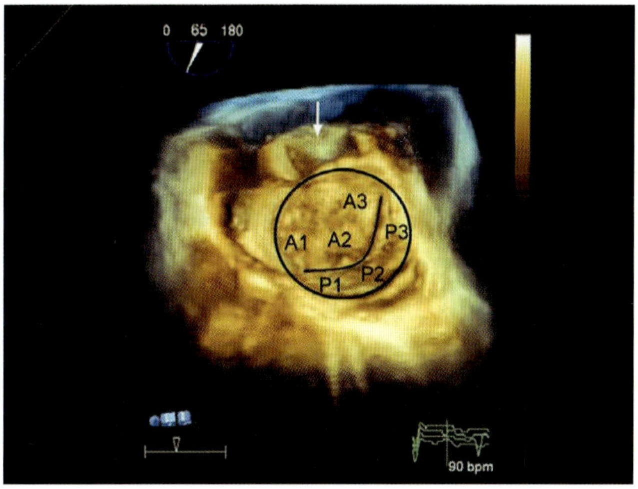

Fig. 13.4: Real time 3D echocardiography of the mitral valve, demonstrating the three anterior and three posterior scallops. The image is oriented such that the valve is viewed from the left atrium, oriented to surgeon's view, with the aortic valve (white arrow) at 12 O'clock position and the left atrial appendage (black arrowhead) at 9 O'clock position. [Image from Burri MV, Kerber RE. Real time three-dimensional echocardiography. In: Chatterjee K, Anderson M, Heistad D, Kerber RE (Eds). Cardiology: An Illustrated Textbook. New Delhi, India: Jaypee Brothers Medical Publishers (P) Ltd; 2013].

The mitral valve functions to prevent regurgitation of blood during systole from the left ventricle into the left atrium (LA). The mitral valve and support apparatus also play a key role in preserving the geometry of the left ventricle.

Mitral regurgitation (MR) is the second most common valvular disease. The causes of MR can be divided up between primary (organic) and secondary (functional) causes (Table 13.1). Primary (organic) causes involve damage to or dysfunction of the valve leaflets. Causes include myxomatous degeneration (Figs. 13.5 to 13.7), infective endocarditis (Figs. 13.8 and 13.9), mitral valve prolapse (MVP) syndrome (Figs. 13.10A to C), rheumatic heart disease (Figs. 13.11 to 13.13) and collagen vascular disease. Secondary causes include mitral annulus dilation due to left ventricular (LV) dilation (which prevents the leaflets from coapting), papillary muscle dysfunction, tethering (Figs. 13.14 and 13.15) or rupture (such as with ischemia or infarction), and rupture of the chordae, leading to a flail mitral leaflet (Fig. 13.16). Several of the primary and secondary causes of MR are shown schematically in Figures 13.17A to D and illustrated in Videos 13.1 to 13.9.

Table 13.1: Primary and secondary causes of mitral regurgitation.

Primary (organic) causes	*Secondary (functional) causes*
Myxomatous degeneration	Papillary muscle ischemia
Mitral valve prolapse	Papillary muscle tethering
Endocarditis	Papillary muscle or chordal rupture
Rheumatic heart disease	Mitral annulus dilation
Collagen vascular disease	

EVALUATION OF MITRAL REGURGITATION

Prior to the wide adoption of echocardiography, left ventriculography (Fig. 13.18A) was the primary modality utilized to assess the degree of MR. Grading was based on the degree of opacification of the left ventricle, with 1+ MR being mild, 2+ MR being moderate, and 3–4+ MR being considered severe and a potential indication for surgery. A large V wave (Fig. 13.18B) seen during right heart catheterization was a supportive finding that the MR was more severe, although a large V wave is a somewhat non-specific finding. Although, as discussed below, echocardiography has generally supplanted cardiac catheterization in the diagnosis of MR, cardiac catheterization may still be of value in patients in whom there is a discrepancy between echocardiographic and clinical findings regarding the degree of MR.

In current practice, echocardiography is the primary modality for assessing not only the degree of MR but also the cause of the MR. 2D echocardiography, 3D echocardiography, transesophageal echocardiography (TEE), color Doppler, spectral Doppler (Fig. 13.19), and even M-mode

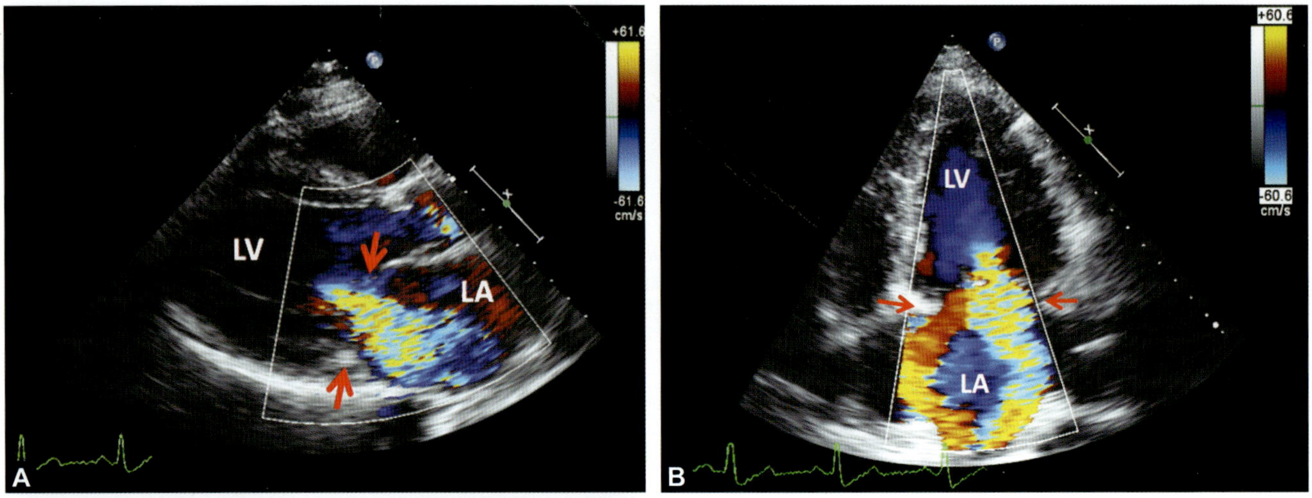

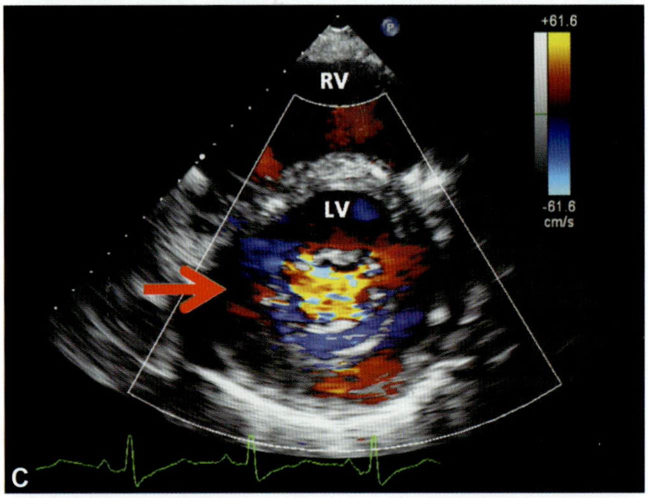

Figs. 13.5A to C: Mitral regurgitation (MR) due to myxomatous degeneration. (A) Parasternal long axis echocardiogram demonstrating severe MR due to myxomatous degeneration. Turbulent blood flow from the left ventricle into the left atrium appears on color Doppler examination as the blue-yellow mosaic color. The red arrows indicate the mitral annulus plane; (B) Apical 4 chamber echocardiogram demonstrating severe MR due to myxomatous degeneration. Turbulent blood flow from the left ventricle into the left atrium appears on color Doppler examination as the blue-yellow mosaic color. The red arrows indicate the mitral annulus plane; (C) Parasternal short axis echocardiogram demonstrating the same severe MR. (LA: Left atrium; LV: Left ventricle; RV: Right ventricle).

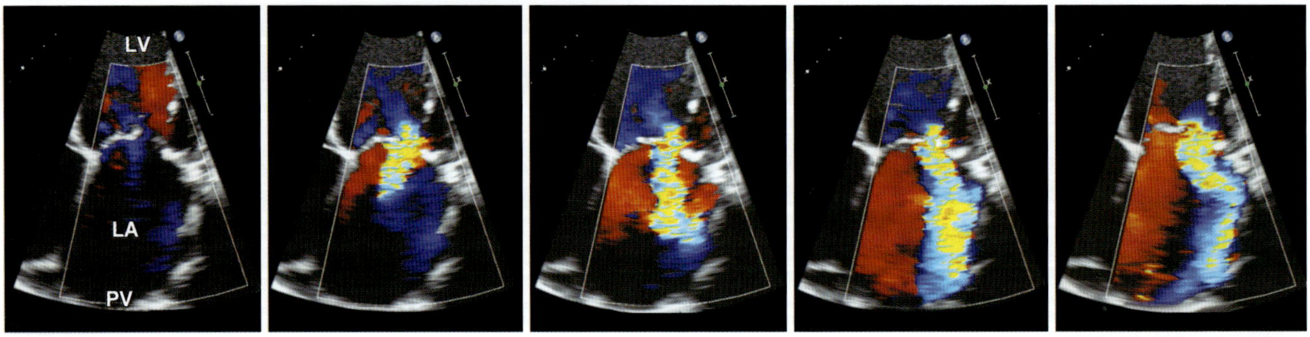

Fig. 13.5D: Multiple time-elapse frames from a color Doppler transesophageal echocardiogram demonstrating the path across the mitral valves and through the left atrium (LA) to the pulmonary vein (PV) of severe mitral regurgitation. (LV: Left ventricle).

color Doppler (Fig. 13.20), can all be employed to assess the severity and cause of MR. In general, findings suggestive of only mild MR include a small central jet (<4 cm^2) filling $<20\%$ of the left atrial area, Doppler vena contracta (jet width at maximum convergence in orifice) width <0.3 cm, regurgitant volume <30 mL, regurgitant fraction $>30\%$, and a calculated effective regurgitant orifice area ≤ 0.20 cm^2. Corresponding measurements for severe MR

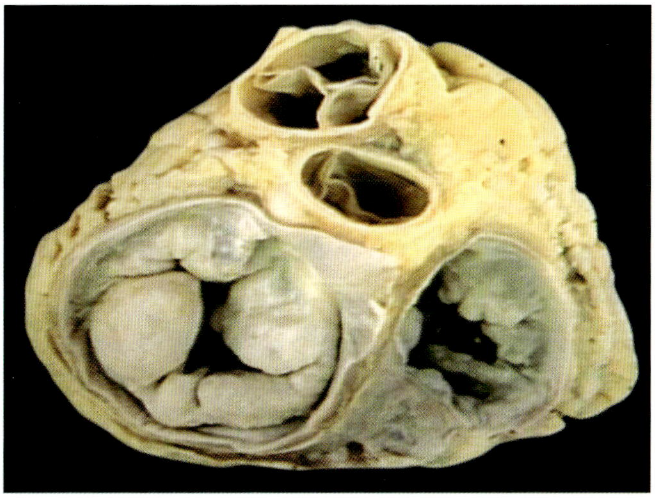

Fig. 13.6: Gross pathology specimen demonstrating myxomatous degeneration of the mitral valve. (Image from Armed Forces Institute of Pathology).

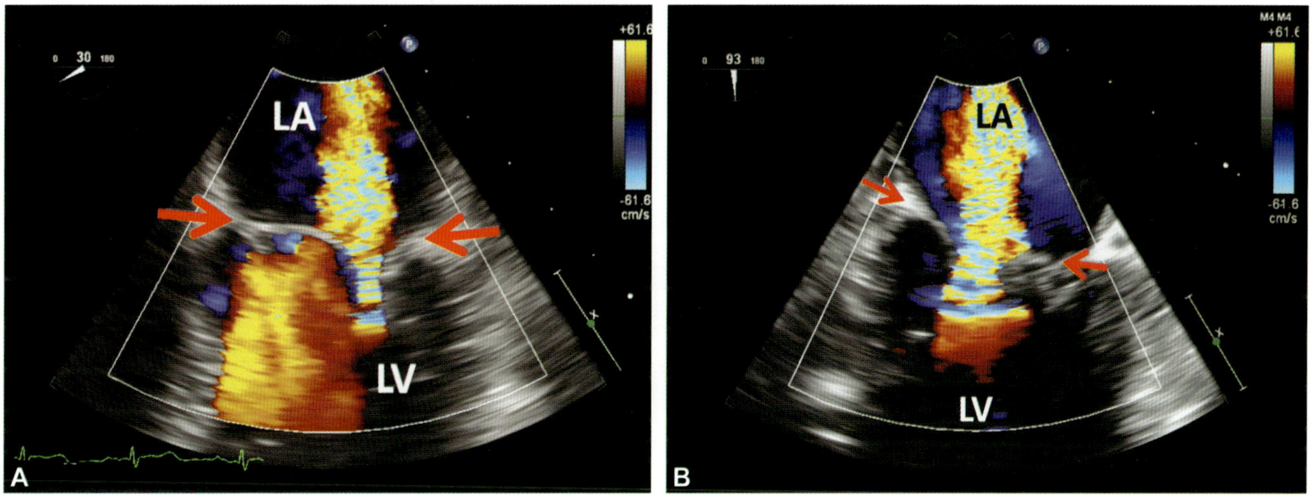

Figs. 13.7A and B: Transesophageal echocardiogram demonstrating mitral regurgitation (MR) due to fibrodegenerative disease. The thickened leaflets have restricted motion and fail to coapt. The red arrows indicate the mitral annulus plane. (LA: Left atrium; LV: Left ventricle).

are jet width > 0.7 cm, regurgitant volume > 60 mL, regurgitant fraction > 50% and effective regurgitant orifice area >0.4 cm^2. Other features of severe MR include a wall-impinging MR jet hugging the LA wall, any swirling of the MR jet in the LA, and reversal of systolic flow in the pulmonary veins (Fig. 13.21). Criteria for the grading of MR are summarized in Tables 13.2 and 13.3.

In patients with acute severe MR, transthoracic echocardiography may underestimate the degree of MR by inadequate imaging of the color flow jet extinguished by rapid rise in LA pressure. In a patient with acute severe heart failure, the finding of a hyperdynamic left ventricle should raise suspicion for acute severe MR.

In recent years, cardiac magnetic resonance imaging (MRI) has become a recognized imaging modality to assess and quantify MR (Fig. 13.22).

MANAGEMENT OF PATIENTS WITH MITRAL REGURGITATION

There is currently no well-accepted medical therapy for asymptomatic patients with chronic MR. No agents, including vasodilators such as angiotensin converting enzyme (ACE) inhibitors, have been shown to improve prognosis in asymptomatic patients with preserved LV systolic function.

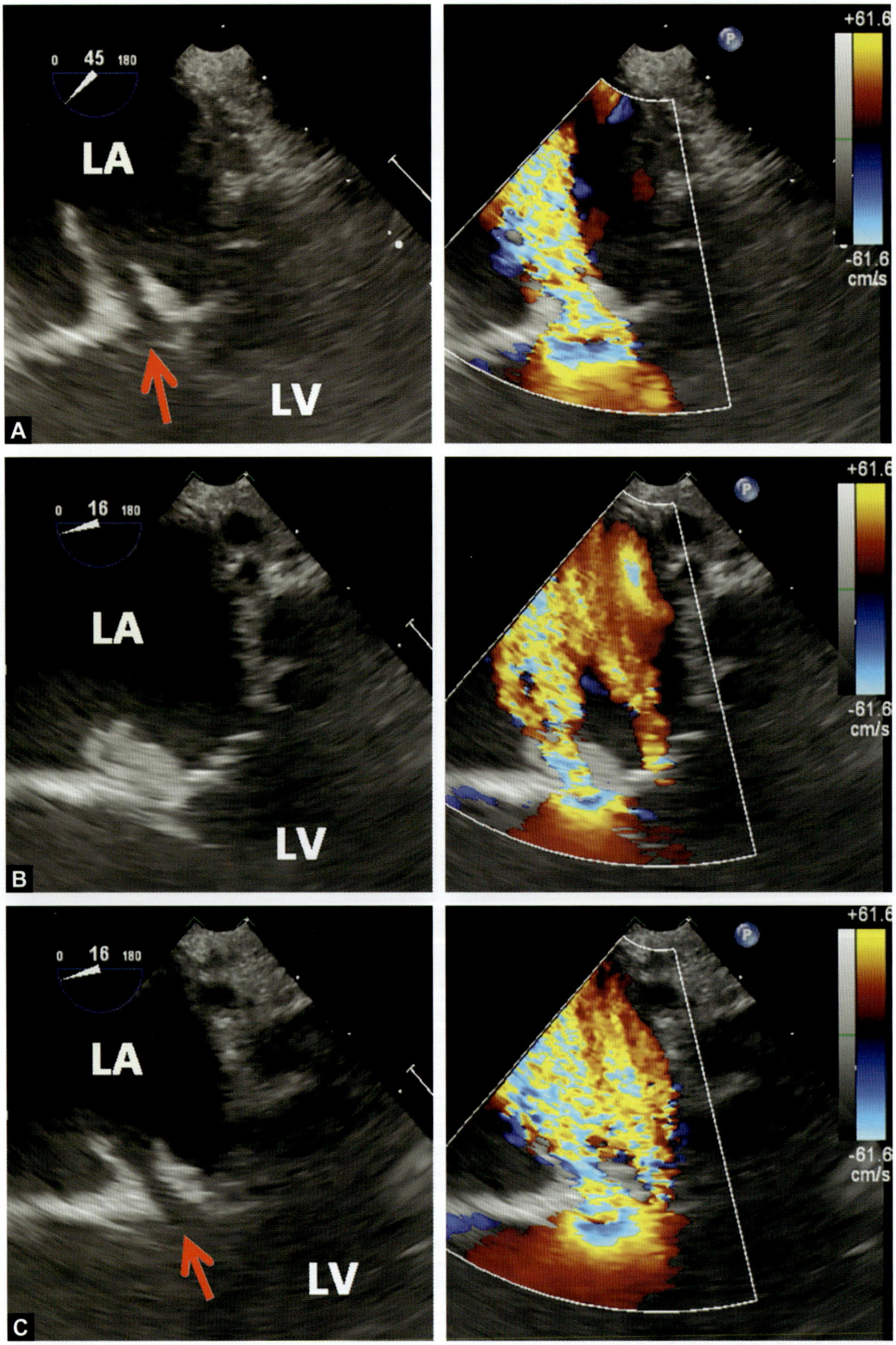

Figs. 13.8A to C: 2D and color Doppler transesophageal echocardiography (TEE) images demonstrating severe mitral regurgitation (MR) due to endocarditis. Images demonstrate that endocarditis of the anterior mitral leaflet has lead to multiple areas of leaflet perforation and resulting MR. The most obvious areas of leaflet perforation are labeled with a red arrow, but other areas of perforation are clearly present based on the multiple color Doppler jets. (LA: Left atrium; LV: Left ventricle).

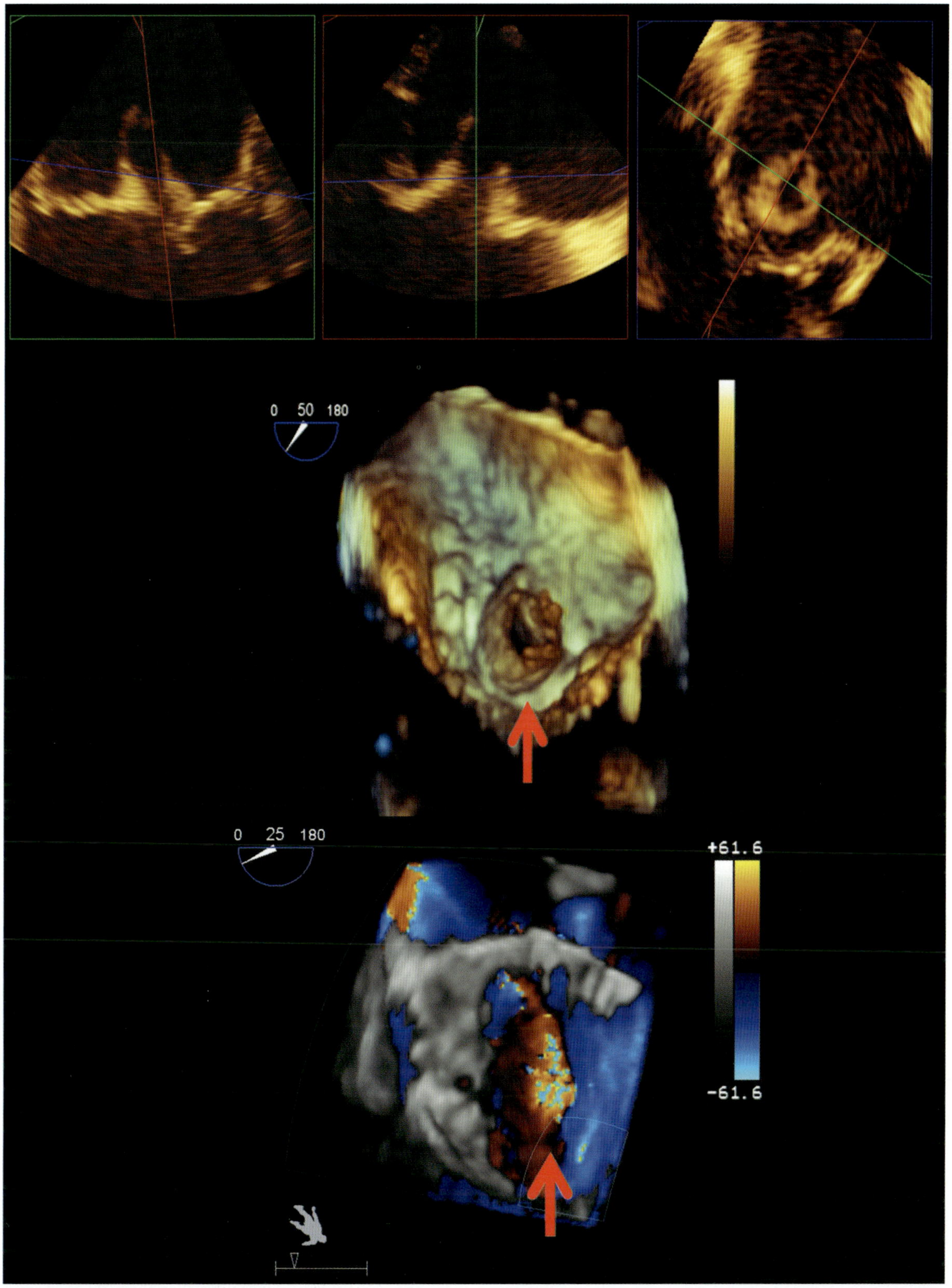

Fig. 13.9: Echocardiograms demonstrated mitral regurgitation due to leaflet perforation as a result of endocarditis. Upper panel images show the 2D images generated from the 3D image acquisition. Middle panel image is the 3D image, demonstrating the leaflet perforation (arrow). Bottom panel image is the 3D color Doppler image demonstrating the regurgitant jet through the perforation (arrow).

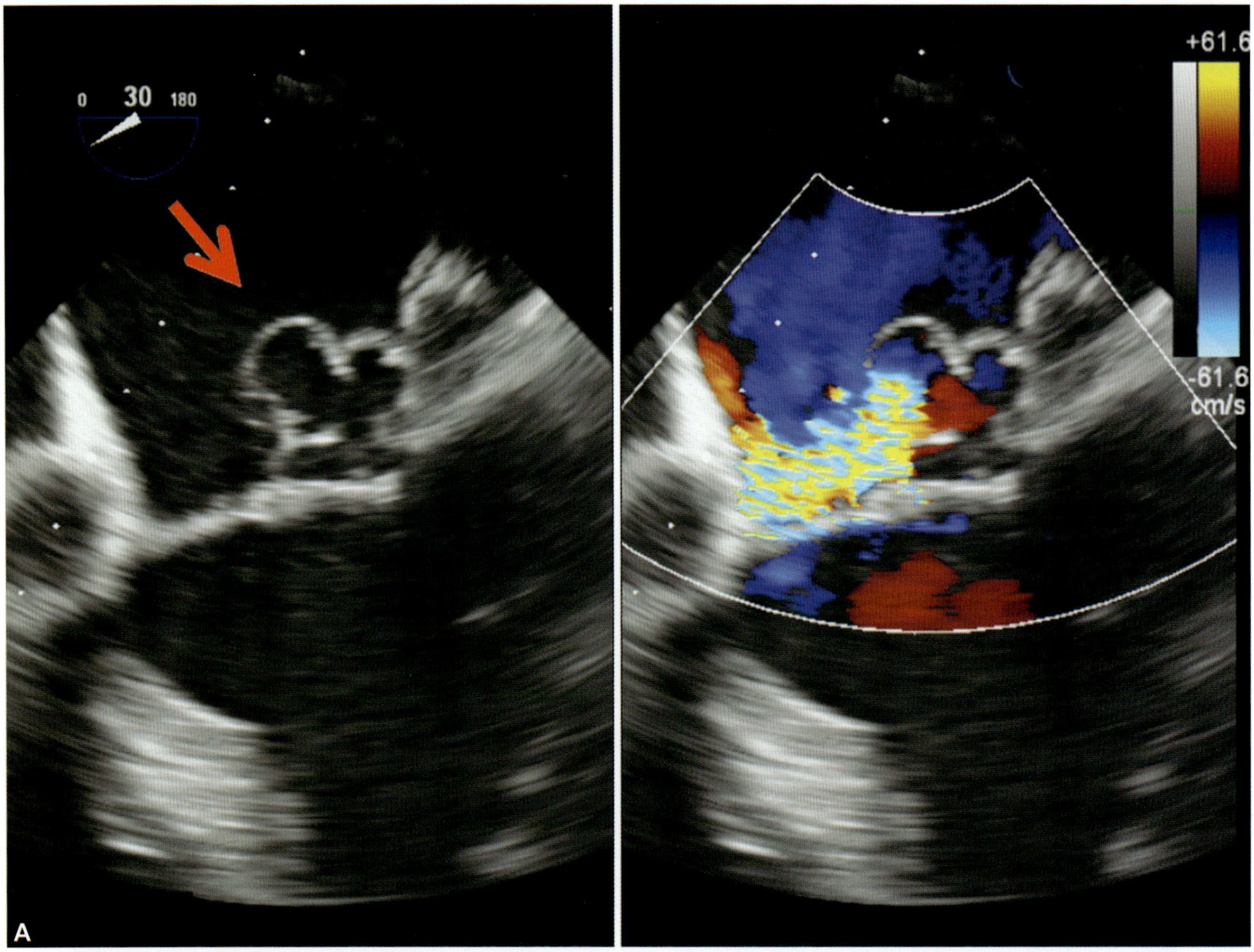

Fig. 13.10A: Transesophageal echocardiography (TEE) images showing marked posterior mitral leaflet prolapse and resulting eccentric mitral regurgitation (MR). (A) 2D Doppler TEE demonstrating the marked mitral valve prolapse (red arrow) and corresponding eccentric MR.

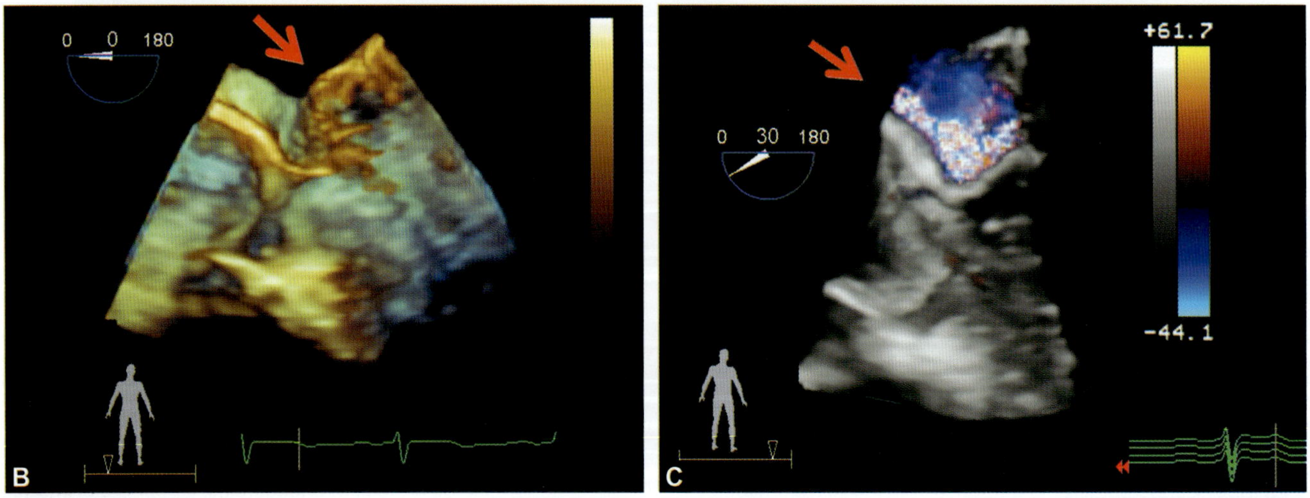

Figs. 13.10B and C: (B) 3D TEE showing the posterior leaflet prolapse (red arrow); (C) Corresponding 3D color TEE showing the resulting eccentric MR (red arrow).

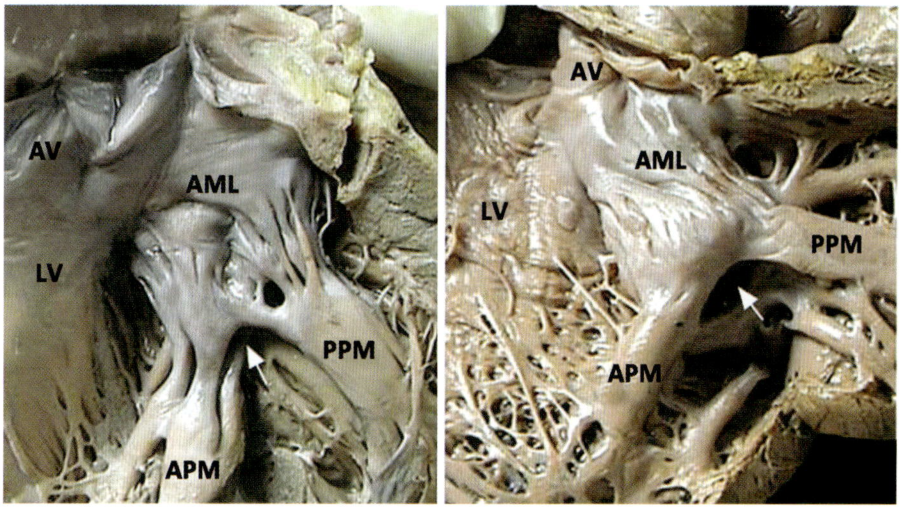

Fig. 13.11A: Chordal shortening and interchordal fusion of the mitral apparatus in a patient with rheumatic heart disease. [Image from Vaideeswar P. Pathology of chronic rheumatic heart disease. In: Vijayalakshmi IB (Ed). Acute Rheumatic Fever and Chronic Rheumatic Heart Disease. New Delhi, India: Jaypee Brothers Medical Publishers (P) Ltd; 2011. pp. 87-101]. (AML: Anterior mitral leaflet; APM: Anterior papillary muscle; AV: Aortic valve; LV: Left ventricle; PPM: Posterior papillary muscle).

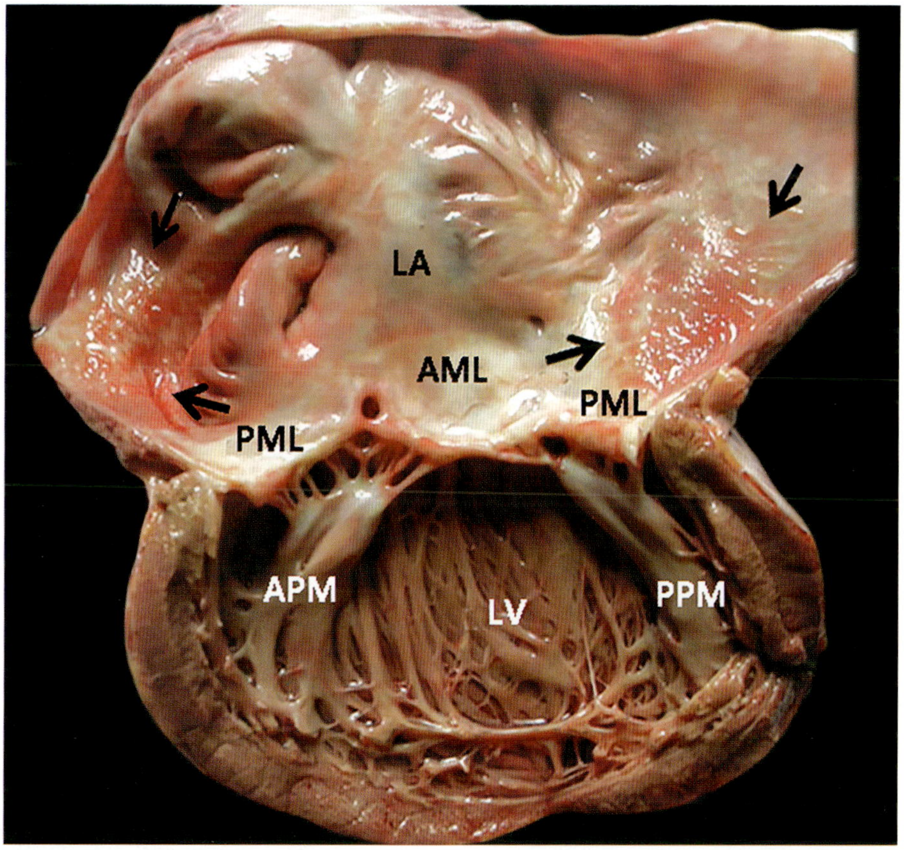

Fig. 13.11B: Opened out left ventricular inflow tract shows extremely large left atrial cavity with jet lesion of mitral regurgitation appearing as endocardial rugosity (arrows). The commissures are mildly fused with leaflet thickening and rolling. Note that despite chordal involvement, the interchordal spaces are still preserved. [Image and legend text courtesy of Dr Pradeep Vaideeswar, Professor (Additional), Department of Pathology (Cardiovascular & Thoracic Division), Seth GS Medical College, Mumbai, India]. (AML: Anterior mitral leaflet; APM: Anterior papillary muscle; LV: Left ventricle; PPM: Posterior papillary muscle; LA: Left atrium; PML: Posterior mitral leaflet).

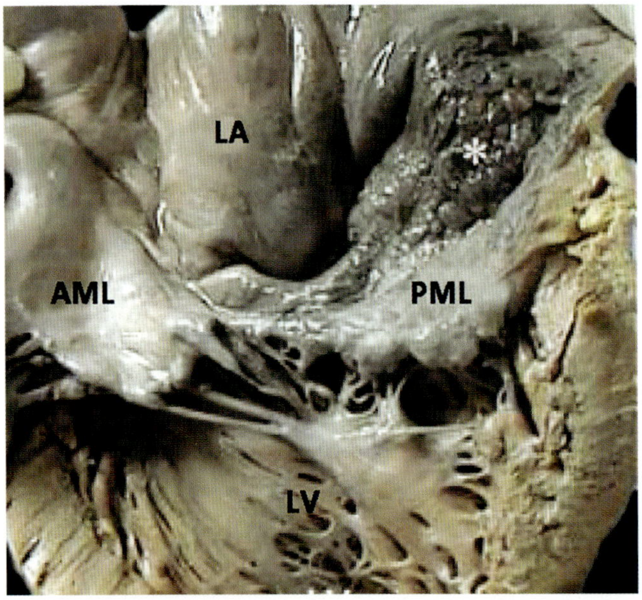

Fig. 13.12: Thickening and retraction of the anterior mitral leaflet (AML) and posterior mitral leaflet (PML) in a patient with mitral regurgitation as a result of rheumatic heart disease. [Image from Vaideeswar P. Pathology of chronic rheumatic heart disease. In: Vijayalakshmi IB (Ed). Acute Rheumatic Fever and Chronic Rheumatic Heart Disease. New Delhi, India: Jaypee Brothers Medical Publishers (P) Ltd; 2011. pp. 87-101]. (AML: Anterior mitral leaflet; LA: Left atrium; LV: Left ventricle; PML: Posterior mitral leaflet).

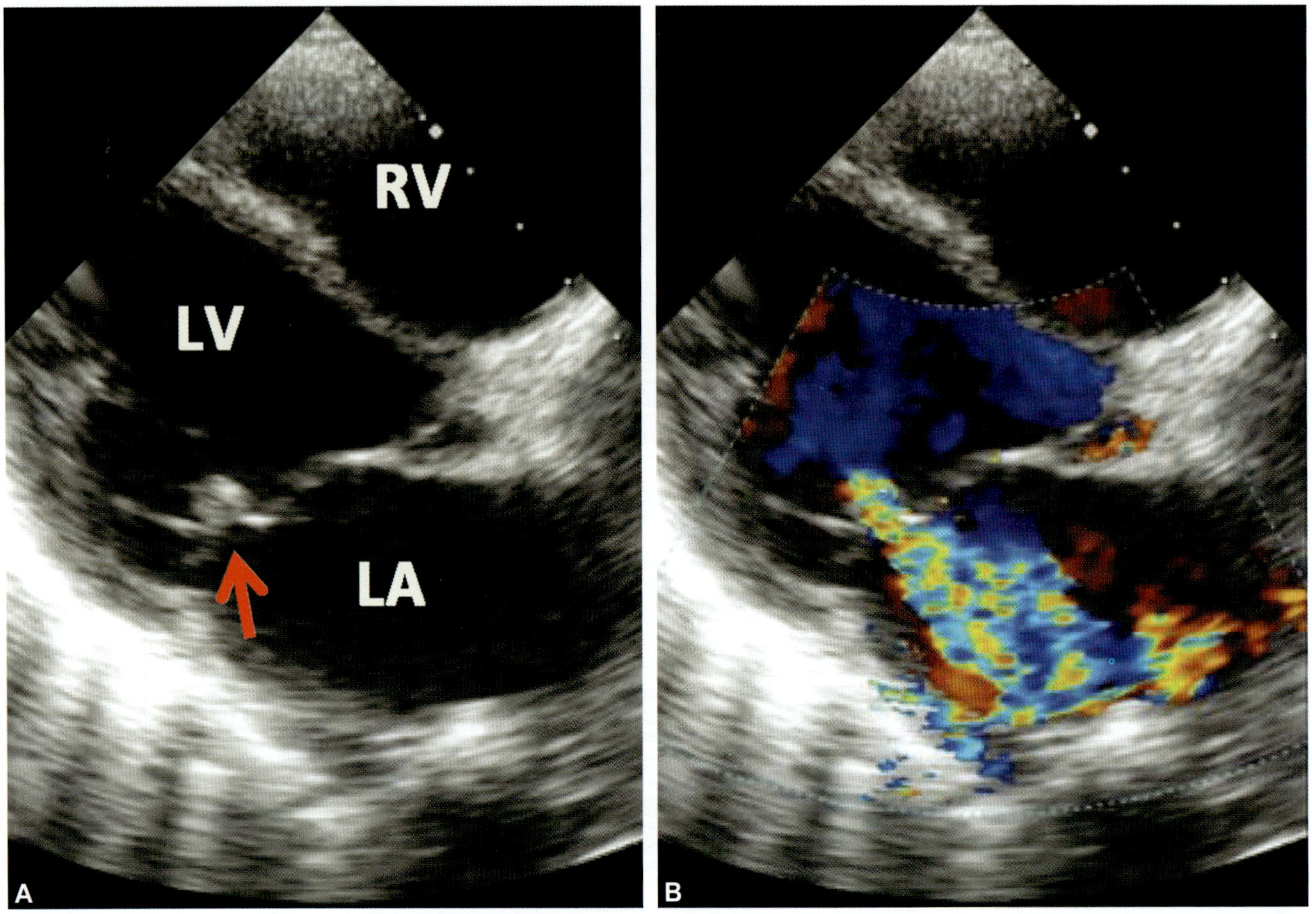

Figs. 13.13A and B: Parasternal long axis echocardiogram demonstrating mitral regurgitation in a patient with rheumatic mitral valve disease. On the left panel, the red arrow points to the area of fused clordae and scarred leaflets. [Image from Vijayalakshmi IB, Narasimhan C. Role of echocardiography in rheumatic heart disease. In: Vijayalakshmi IB (Ed). Acute Rheumatic Fever and Chronic Rheumatic Heart Disease. New Delhi, India: Jaypee Brothers Medical Publishers (P) Ltd; 2011. pp. 87-101].

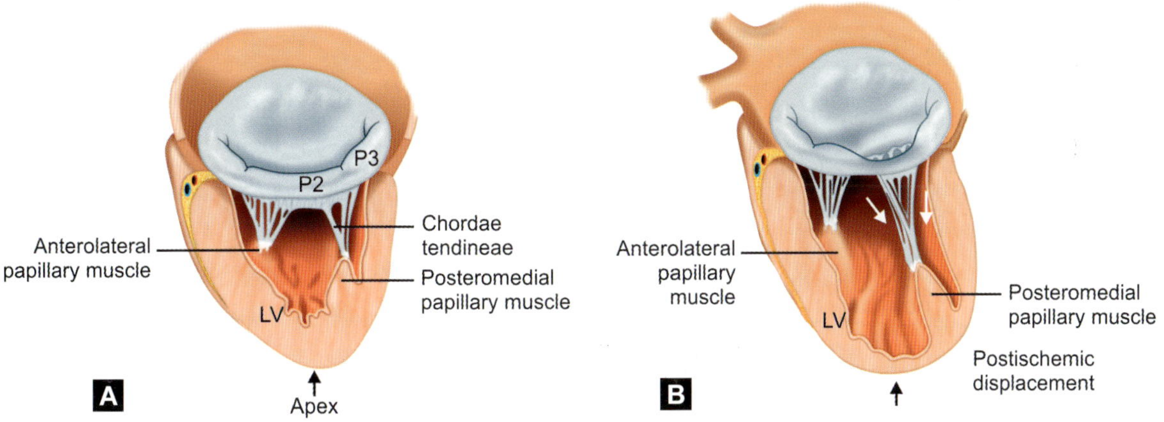

Figs. 13.14A and B: Tethering of the posterior mitral leaflet which will result in mitral regurgitation. Tethering may occur in patients with dilated left ventricle, prior myocardial infarction, or other conditions that affect the left ventricle.

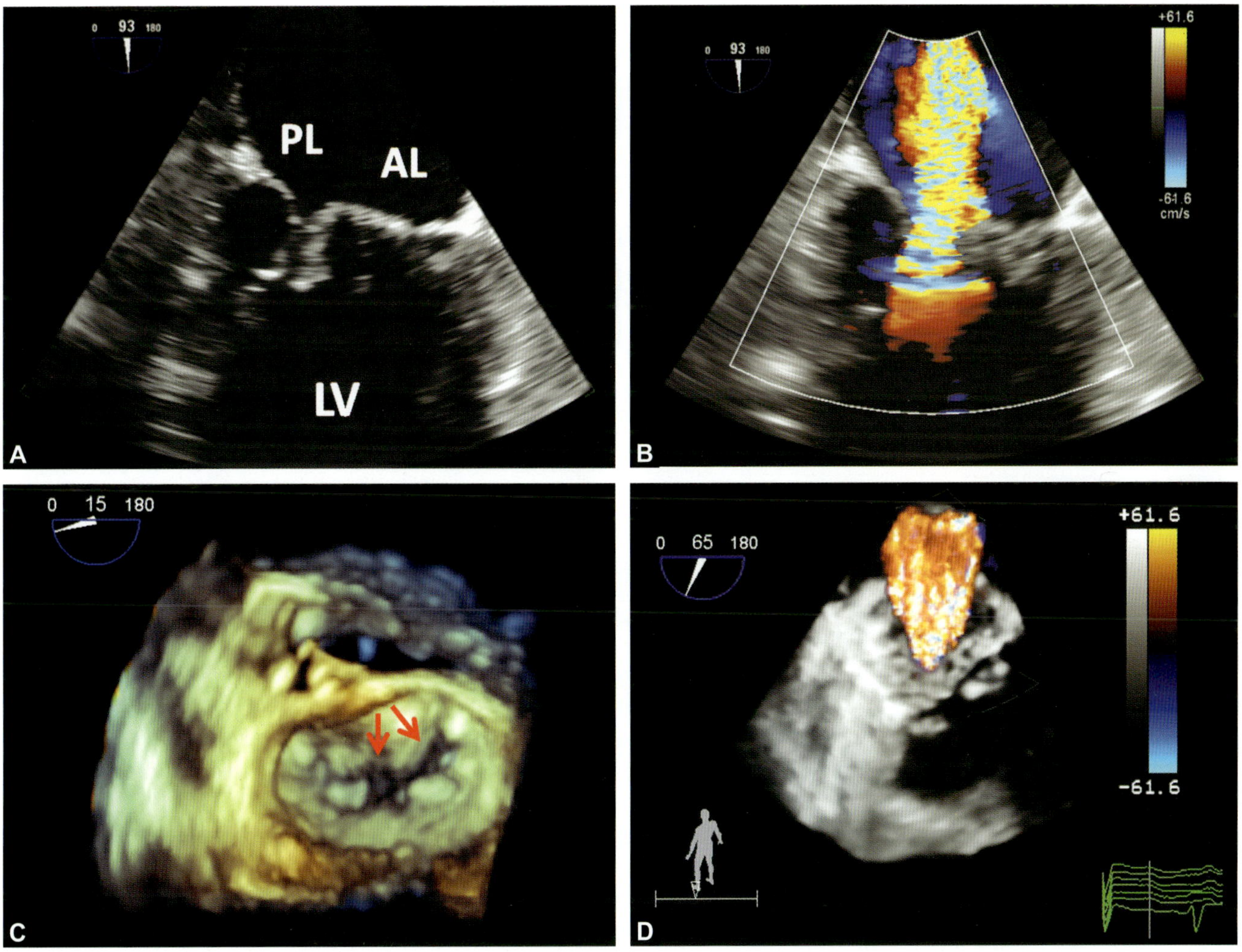

Figs. 13.15A to D: Tethering of the mitral leaflets, resulting in mitral regurgitation. (A) 2D Transesophageal echocardiogram (TEE) demonstrating tethering of the mitral leaflets and incomplete coaptation; B) Corresponding 2D color Doppler TEE showing mitral regurgitation at the area of malcoaptation; (C) Corresponding 3D TEE showing tethering of the mitral leaflet leading to incomplete coaptation; (D) Corresponding 3D color Doppler TEE showing the resulting mitral regurgitation. (AL: Anterior mitral leaflet; LV: Left ventricle; PL: Posterior mitral leaflet).

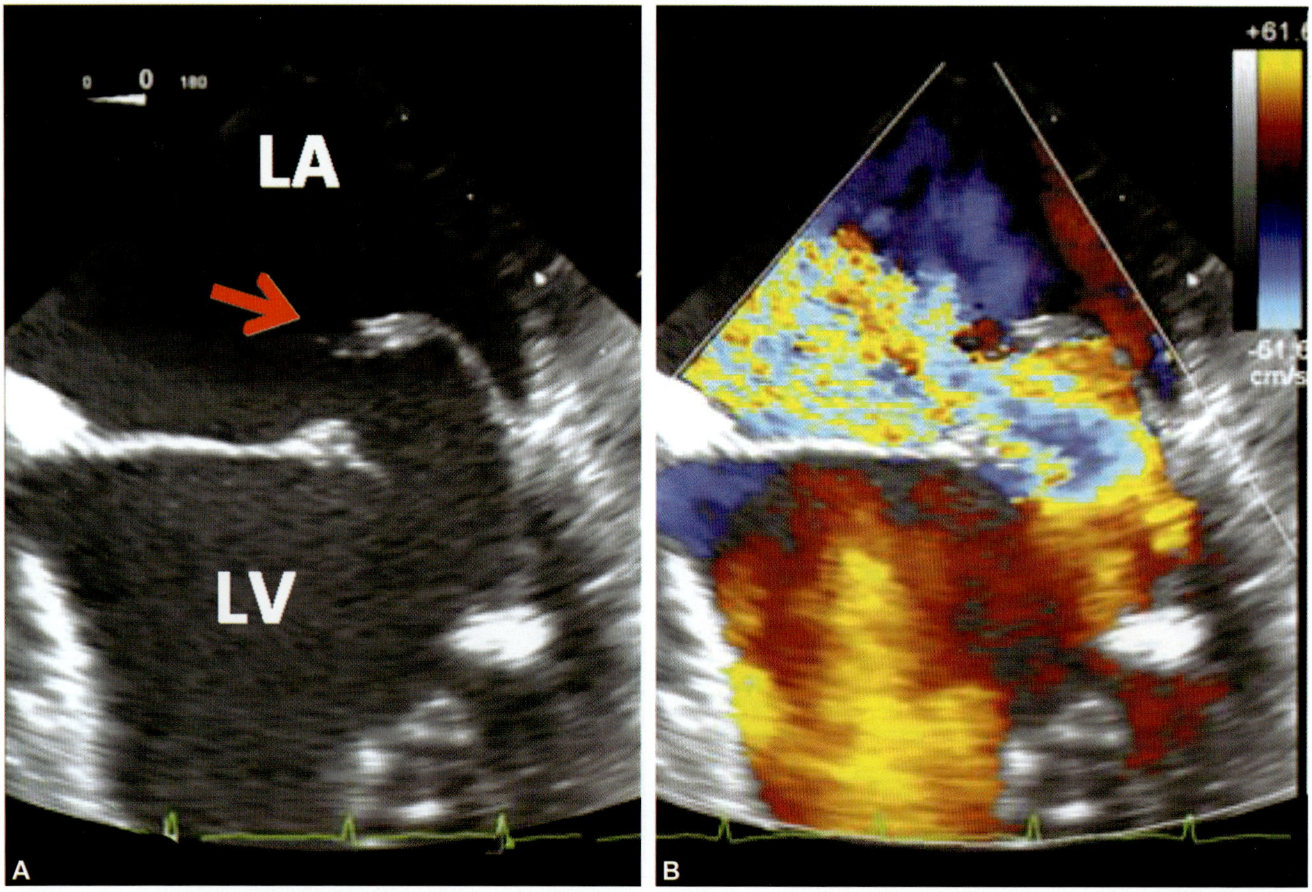

Figs. 13.16A and B: Transesophageal echocardiogram showing flail posterior mitral leaflet (arrow) as a result of chordae rupture, leading to eccentric mitral regurgitation.

In patients for whom there is an indication for mitral valve surgery, mitral valve repair is preferred to mitral valve replacement whenever possible. When mitral valve replacement is required, preservation of the mitral apparatus (chordal preservation) is recommended when possible to preserve LV geometry and LV function. Preservation of the chordae has been associated with improved postoperative LV function and lower long-term morbidity.

Recommendations regarding mitral valve surgery are summarized in Tables 13.4 and 13.5. In general American College of Cardiology Foundation (ACCF)/American Heart Association (AHA) and European Society of Cardiology (ESC) guidelines for mitral valve surgery are relatively similar. Both organizations given separate recommendations for patients with primary mitral regurgitation and for those with secondary mitral regurgitation. Both organizations recommend (Class I) mitral valve surgery for symptomatic patients with chronic severe primary MR and left ventricular ejection fraction (LVEF) > 30%. Both organizations also recommend (Class I) mitral valve surgery for asymptomatic patients with chronic severe primary MR and LV dysfunction. For severe secondary MR, both organizations are less enthusiastically address mitral valve surgery, using class IIa and IIb recommendations (is reasonable, may be considered). Mitral valve surgery should not be undertaken for patients with only mild to moderate MR. Mitral valve surgery should not be undertaken for patients with only mild to moderate MR.

In certain symptomatic patients with mitral regurgitation who have an indication for intervention but are poor candidates for surgical repair, the percutaneously deployed MitraClip (Figs. 13.23 to 13.25) may be an option. Transcatheter mitral valve repair for severely symptomatic patients with chronic severe primary MR who have a reasonable life expectancy but a prohibitive risk is given a class IIb recommendation (may be considered) in the ACCF/AHA guidelines.

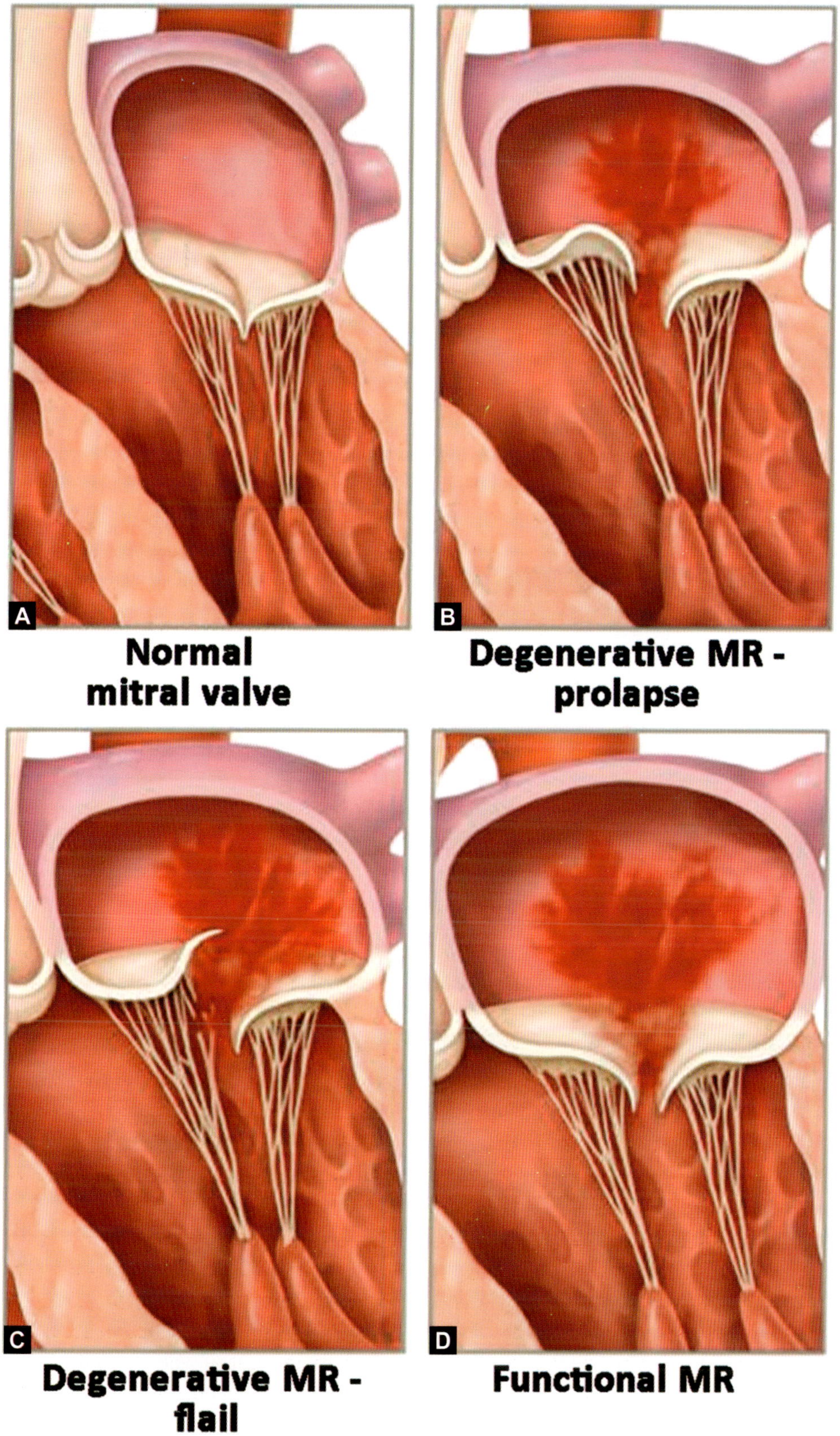

Figs. 13.17A to D: Schematic illustration of a normal mitral valve and of primary and secondary causes of mitral regurgitation. [Image courtesy of and copyright (2013) by Abbott Vascular].

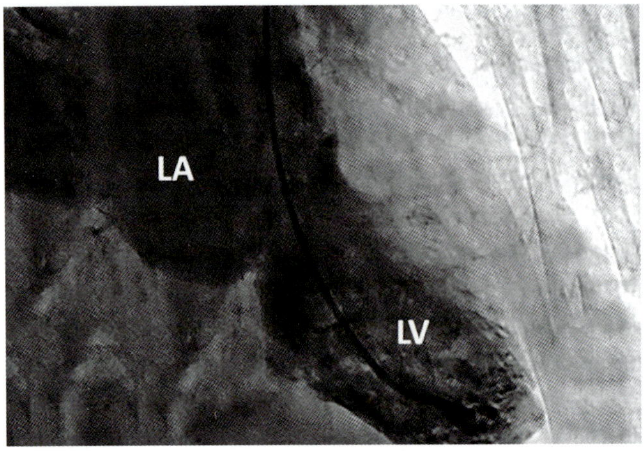

Fig. 13.18A: Left ventriculogram demonstrating severe mitral regurgitation (MR). Radio-opaque iodinated contrast is seen refluxing from the left ventricle (LV) into the left atrium (LA). The density of contrast in the LA is equal to the density of contrast in the LV, indicating 3+ to 4+ MR.

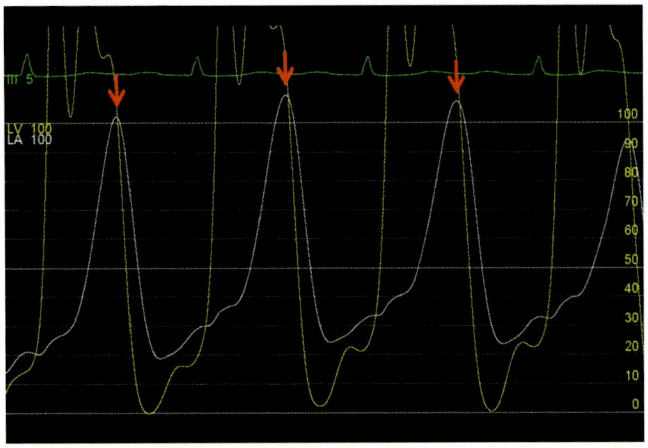

Fig. 13.18B: Pulmonary artery (Swan-Ganz) catheter tracing of the pulmonary capillary wedge pressure (PCWP), showing a large V wave as a result of severe mitral regurgitation. A large V wave (red arrows) is present, beginning after the QRS complex, due to severe mitral regurgitation. [Image from Daniel R, Thajudeen A, Harikrishnan S. Mitral regurgitation following percutaneous mitral valvotomy. In: Harikrishnan S (Ed). Percutaneous Mitral Valvotomy. New Delhi, India: Jaypee Brothers Medical Publishers (P) Ltd; 2012. p. 406].

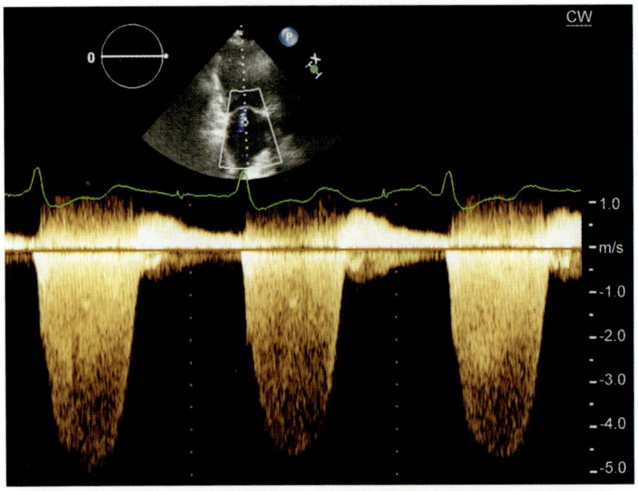

Fig. 13.19: Spectral Doppler performed in the apical 2 chamber echocardiographic view demonstrating mitral regurgitation.

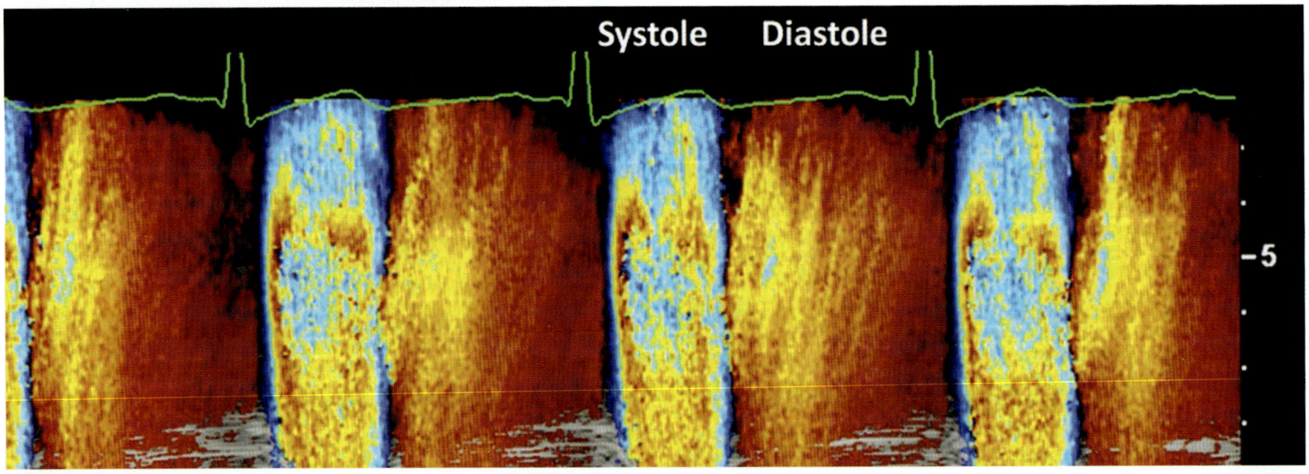

Fig. 13.20: M-Mode color Doppler demonstrating mitral regurgitation (MR). The MR jets are seen to occur during systole, immediately after the QRS complexes. (Image courtesy of the British Society of Echocardiography).

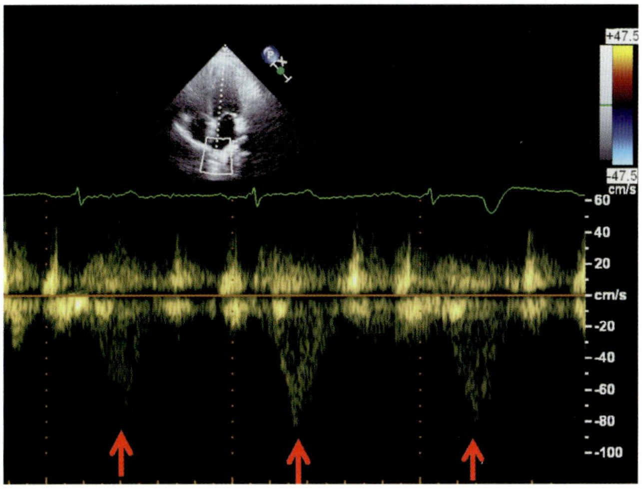

Fig. 13.21: Pulsed wave spectral Doppler echocardiography demonstrating reversal of flow (red arrows) in the pulmonary vein in a patient with severe mitral regurgitation.

Table 13.2A: Summary of echocardiograph grading of mitral regurgitation, based on criteria in the 2008 American College of Cardiology Foundation (ACCF)/American Heart Association (AHA) valvular heart disease guidelines. This "traditional" grading system has been supplanted in the newer ACCF/AHA valvular guidelines by "stages" of mitral regurgitation, but is still supplied to the reader as many will be familiar with this system and may continue to use it. (LA: Left atrium; LV: Left ventricle; MR: Mitral regurgitation).

	Mild	*Moderate*	*Severe*
Color Doppler jet area	Small central jet (< 4 cm^2 or < 20% LA area)	Signs of MR greater than mild present but no criteria for severe MR	Vena contracta width > 0.7 cm with large central MR jet (area> 40% LA area), any wall-impinging jet, or any swirling in LA
Doppler vena contracta width	< 0.3 cm	0.3–0.69 cm	≥ 0.7 cm
Regurgitant volume	< 30 mL	30–59 mL	≥ 60 mL
Regurgitant fraction	< 30%	30–49%	≥ 50%
Regurgitant orifice area	< 0.20 cm^2	0.2–0.39 cm^2	≥ 0.40 cm^2
Chamber size			Enlarged LA or LV

Table 13.2B: Summary of the new ACCF/AHA valvular guidelines classification of the stages of primary mitral regurgitation. (LVEF: Left ventricular ejection fraction; LVESD: LV end-systolic diameter; LA: Left atrium; MR: Mitral regurgitation; ERO: Effective regurgitant orifice).

Grade/Definition	*Valve Anatomy and Hemodynamics*	*Hemodynamic Consequences and Symptoms*
A - At risk of MR	• Mild mitral valve prolapse with normal coaptation • Mild valve thickening and leaflet restriction • No MR jet or small central jet area < 20% LA on Doppler • Small vena contracta < 0.3 cm	• No hemodynamic consequences • No symptoms
B - Progressive MR	• Severe mitral valve prolapse with normal coaptation • Rheumatic valve changes with leaflet restriction and loss of central coaptation • Prior IE • Central jet MR 20%–40% LA or late systolic eccentric jet MR • Vena contracta < 0.7 cm • Regurgitant volume < 60 cc • Regurgitant fraction < 50% • ERO < 0.40 cm^2 • Angiographic grade 1–2+	• Mild LA enlargement • No LV enlargement • Normal pulmonary pressure • No symptoms

Contd...

Contd...

Grade/Definition	Valve Anatomy and Hemodynamics	Hemodynamic Consequences and Symptoms
C - Asymptomatic severe MR	• Severe mitral valve prolapse with loss of coaptation or flail leaflet • Rheumatic valve changes with leaflet restriction and loss of central coaptation • Prior IE • Thickening of leaflets with radiation heart disease • Central jet MR > 40% LA or holosystolic eccentric jet MR • Vena contracta ≥ 0.7 cm • Regurgitant volume ≥ 60 cc • Regurgitant fraction ≥ 50% • ERO ≥ 0.40 cm^2 • Angiographic grade 3–4+	• Moderate or severe LA enlargement • LV enlargement • Pulmonary hypertension may be present at rest or with exercise • C1: LVEF > 60% and LVESD < 40 mm • C2: LVEF ≤ 60% and LVESD ≥ 40 mm • No symptoms
D -Symptomatic severe MR	• Severe mitral valve prolapse with loss of coaptation or flail leaflet • Rheumatic valve changes with leaflet restriction and loss of central coaptation • Prior IE • Thickening of leaflets with radiation heart disease • Central jet MR > 40% LA or holosystolic eccentric jet MR • Vena contracta ≥ 0.7 cm • Regurgitant volume ≥ 60 cc • Regurgitant fraction ≥ 50% • ERO ≥ 0.40 cm^2 • Angiographic grade 3–4+	• Moderate or severe LA enlargement • LV enlargement • Pulmonary hypertension present • Decreased exercise tolerance • Exertional dyspnea

Table 13.2C: Summary of the new ACCF/AHA valvular guidelines classification of the stages of secondary mitral regurgitation. (LA: Left atrium; LV: Left ventricle; MR: Mitral regurgitation; HF: Heart failure; ERO: Effective regurgitant orifice).

Grade/Definition	Valve Anatomy and Hemodynamics	Associated Cardiac Findings and Symptoms
A - At risk of MR	• Normal valve leaflets, chords, and annulus in a patient with coronary disease or a cardiomyopathy • No MR jet or small central jet area < 20% LA on Doppler • Small vena contracta < 0.30 cm	• Normal or mildly dilated LV size with fixed or inducible regional wall motion abnormalities • Primary myocardial disease with LV dilation and systolic dysfunction • Symptoms due to coronary ischemia or HF may be present that respond to revascularization and appropriate medical therapy
B - Progressive MR	• Regional wall motion abnormalities with mild tethering of mitral leaflet • Annular dilation with mild loss of central coaptation of the mitral leaflets • ERO < 0.20 cm^2 • Regurgitant volume < 30 cc • Regurgitant fraction < 50%	• Regional wall motion abnormalities with reduced LV systolic function • LV dilation and systolic dysfunction due to primary myocardial disease • Symptoms due to coronary ischemia or HF may be present that respond to revascularization and appropriate medical therapy
C - Asymptomatic severe MR	• Regional wall motion abnormalities and/or LV dilation with severe tethering of mitral leaflet • Annular dilation with severe loss of central coaptation of the mitral leaflets • ERO ≥ 0.20 cm^2 • Regurgitant volume ≥ 30 cc • Regurgitant fraction ≥ 50%	• Regional wall motion abnormalities with reduced LV systolic function • LV dilation and systolic dysfunction due to primary myocardial disease • Symptoms due to coronary ischemia or HF may be present that respond to revascularization and appropriate medical therapy
D - Symptomatic severe MR	• Regional wall motion abnormalities and/or LV dilation with severe tethering of mitral leaflet • Annular dilation with severe loss of central coaptation of the mitral leaflets • ERO ≥ 0.20 cm^2 • Regurgitant volume ≥ 30 cc • Regurgitant fraction ≥ 50%	• Regional wall motion abnormalities with reduced LV systolic function • LV dilation and systolic dysfunction due to primary myocardial disease. • HF symptoms that persist, even after revascularization performed • Decreased exercise tolerance

Table 13.3: Summary of the European Society of Cardiology (ESC) and European Association for Cardio-Thoracic Surgery (EACTS) guidelines echocardiographic criteria for the diagnosis of severe mitral regurgitation (MR). (CW: Continuous wave; EROA: Effective regurgitant orifice area; MR: Mitral regurgitation; TVI: Time-velocity integral).

Qualitative	Flail leaflet, ruptured papillary muscle, large coaptation defect
	Very large central color flow regurgitant jet or eccentric jet adhering, swirling, and reaching the posterior wall of the left atrium
	Dense/triangular CW signal of regurgitant jet
	Large flow convergence zone at Nyquist limit of 50–60 cm/sec
Semiquantitative	Vena contracta width ≥ 7 mm (> 8 for biplane)
	Systolic pulmonary vein flow reversal
	E-wave dominant ≥ 1 m/sec
	TVI mitral/TVI aortic > 1.4
Quantitative	EROA ≥ 40 mm^2 for primary MR; ≥ 20 mm^2 for secondary MR
	Regurgitant volume ≥ 60 mL/beat for primary MR; ≥ 30 mL/beat for secondary MR
	Enlarged left ventricle and left atrium for primary MR

Table 13.4A: Summary of the ACCF/AHA valvular heart disease guidelines recommendation for mitral valve intervention in patients with chronic *primary* MR. The level of evidence (LOE) supporting the recommendation is given in parenthesis, where LOE = A denotes a recommendation derived from multiple randomized clinical trials or meta-analyses, LOE = B denotes a recommendation derived from a single randomized clinical trial or non-randomized studies, and LOE = C denotes a recommendation based on consensus of expert opinion, standard of care, or case reports. (LVEF: Left ventricular ejection fraction; LVESD: LV end-systolic diameter; MR: Mitral regurgitation).

Class I (is recommended; is indicated)
• MV surgery for symptomatic patients with chronic severe primary MR and LVEF > 30% (LOE = B)
• MV surgery for asymptomatic patients with chronic severe primary MR and LV dysfunction (LVEF 30–60% and/or LVESD ≥ 40 mm (LOE = B)
• Concomitant MV repair or replacement in patients with chronic severe primary MR undergoing cardiac surgery for other indications
• MV repair in preference to MV replacement when surgical treatment is indicated for patients with chronic severe primary MR limited to the posterior leaflet (LOE = B)
• MV repair in preference to MV replacement when surgical treatment is indicated for patients with chronic severe primary MR involving the anterior leaflet or both leaflets when a successful and durable repair can be accomplished (LOE = B)
Class IIa (is reasonable)
• MV repair in asymptomatic patients with chronic severe primary MR with preserved LV function (LVEF > 60^ and LVESD < 40 mm) in whom the likelihood of a successful and durable repair without residual MR is > 95% with an expected mortality < 1% when performed at a Heart Valve Center of Excellence (LOE = B)
• MV for asymptomatic patients with chronic severe non-rheumatic primary MR and preserved LV function in whom there is a high likelihood of a successful and durable repair with (1) new onset of atrial fibrillation or (2) resting pulmonary hypertension (PA arterial pressure > 50 mm Hg) (LOE = B)
• Concomitant MV repair in patients with chronic moderate primary MR undergoing cardiac surgery for other indications (LOE = C)
Class IIb (may be considered)
• MV surgery in patients with rheumatic mitral valve disease when surgical treatment is indicated if a durable and successful repair is likely or if the reliability of long-term anticoagulation management is questionable (LOE = B)
• Transcatheter MV repair for severely symptomatic patients with chronic severe primary MR who have a reasonable life expectancy, but a prohibitive surgical risk because of severe comorbidities (LOE = B)
Class III (should not be performed)
• MV replacement for the treatment of isolated severe primary MR limited to less than one half of the posterior leaflet unless MV repair has been attempted and was unsuccessful (LOE = B)

Table 13.4B: Summary of the ACCF/AHA valvular heart disease guidelines recommendation for mitral valve intervention in patients with chronic *secondary* MR. The level of evidence (LOE) supporting the recommendation is given in parenthesis, where LOE = A denotes a recommendation derived from multiple randomized clinical trials or meta-analyses, LOE = B denotes a recommendation derived from a single randomized clinical trial or non-randomized studies, and LOE = C denotes a recommendation based on consensus of expert opinion, standard of care, or case reports. (AVR: Aortic valve replacement; CABG: Coronary artery bypass grafting; MR: Mitral regurgitation).

Class IIa (is reasonable)
• MV surgery for patients with chronic severe secondary MR who are undergoing CABG or AVR (LOE = C)
Class IIb (may be considered)
• MV surgery for severely symptomatic patients with chronic severe secondary MR (LOE = B)
• MV repair for patients with chronic moderate secondary MR who are undergoing other cardiac surgery (LOE = C)

Table 13.5A: Summary of the European Society of Cardiology (ESC) and European Association for Cardio-Thoracic Surgery (EACTS) guidelines for surgery in severe primary mitral regurgitation (MR). The level of evidence (LOE) supporting the recommendation is given in parenthesis, where LOE = A denotes a recommendation derived from multiple randomized clinical trials or meta-analyses, LOE = B denotes a recommendation derived from a single randomized clinical trial or large non-randomized studies, and LOE = C denotes a recommendation based on consensus of expert opinion or based on small studies, retrospective studies, or registries. (LV: Left ventricle; LVEF: Left ventricular ejection fraction; LVESD: Left ventricular end-systolic diameter).

Class I (is recommended; is indicated)
• Symptomatic patients with severe primary MR with LVEF > 30% and LVESD < 55 mm (LOE = B)
• Asymptomatic patients with severe primary MR LV dysfunction (LVESD ≥ 45 mm and/or LVEF ≤ 60% (LOE = C)
Class IIa (should be considered)
• Asymptomatic patients with severe primary MR with preserved LV function and new onset of atrial fibrillation or pulmonary hypertension (LOE = C)
• Asymptomatic patients with severe primary MR with preserved LV function, high likelihood of durable repair, low surgical risk, flail leaflet and LVESD ≥ 40 mm (LOE = C)
• Patients with severe primary MR and severe LV dysfunction (LVEF < 30% and/or LVESD > 55 mm) refractory to medical therapy with high likelihood of durable repair and low comorbidity (LOE = C)
Class IIb (may be considered)
• Patients with severe primary MR with severe LV dysfunction (LVEF < 30% and/or LVESD > 55 mm) refractory to medical therapy with low likelihood of durable repair and low comorbidity (LOE = C)
• Asymptomatic patients with severe primary MR with preserved LV function, high likelihood of durable repair, low surgical risk and either severe left atrial dilatation or pulmonary hypertension on exercise (LOE = C)

Table 13.5B: Summary of the European Society of Cardiology (ESC) and European Association for Cardio-Thoracic Surgery (EACTS) guidelines for surgery in secondary mitral regurgitation (MR). The level of evidence (LOE) supporting the recommendation is given in parenthesis, where LOE = A denotes a recommendation derived from multiple randomized clinical trials or meta-analyses, LOE = B denotes a recommendation derived from a single randomized clinical trial or large non-randomized studies, and LOE = C denotes a recommendation based on consensus of expert opinion or based on small studies, retrospective studies, or registries. (CABG: Coronary artery bypass grafting; LVEF: Left ventricular ejection fraction; LVESD: Left ventricular end-systolic diameter).

Class I (is recommended; is indicated)
• Patients with severe secondary MR undergoing CABG and LVEF > 30% (LOE = C)
Class IIa (should be considered)
• Patients with moderate secondary MR undergoing CABG (LOE = C)
• Symptomatic patients with severe secondary MR, LVEF < 30%, option for revascularization, and evidence of viability (LOE = C)
Class IIb (may be considered)
• Patients with severe secondary LVEF > 30% who remain symptomatic despite optimal medical management and have low comorbidity, when revascularization is not indicated (LOE = C)

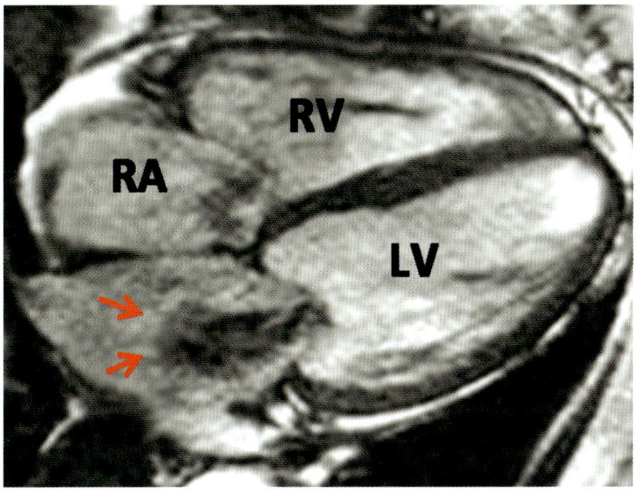

Fig. 13.22: Magnetic resonance imaging (MRI) demonstrating mitral regurgitation (arrows). (Image from PLoSOne). (LV: Left ventricle; RV: Right ventricle; RA: Right atrium).

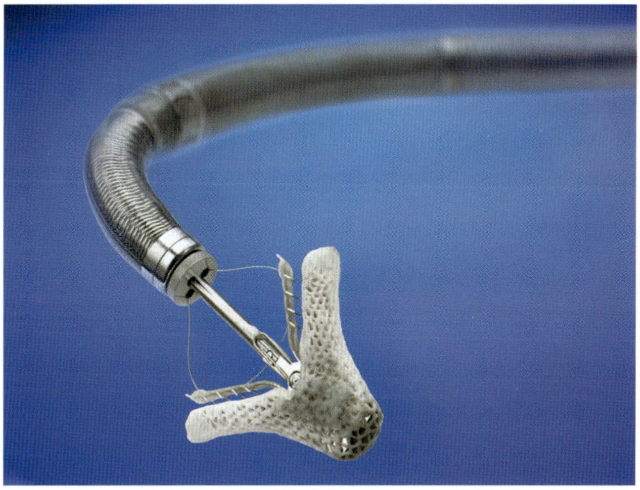

Fig. 13.23: Close-up image of the MitraClip. [Image courtesy of and copyright (2013) by Abbott Vascular].

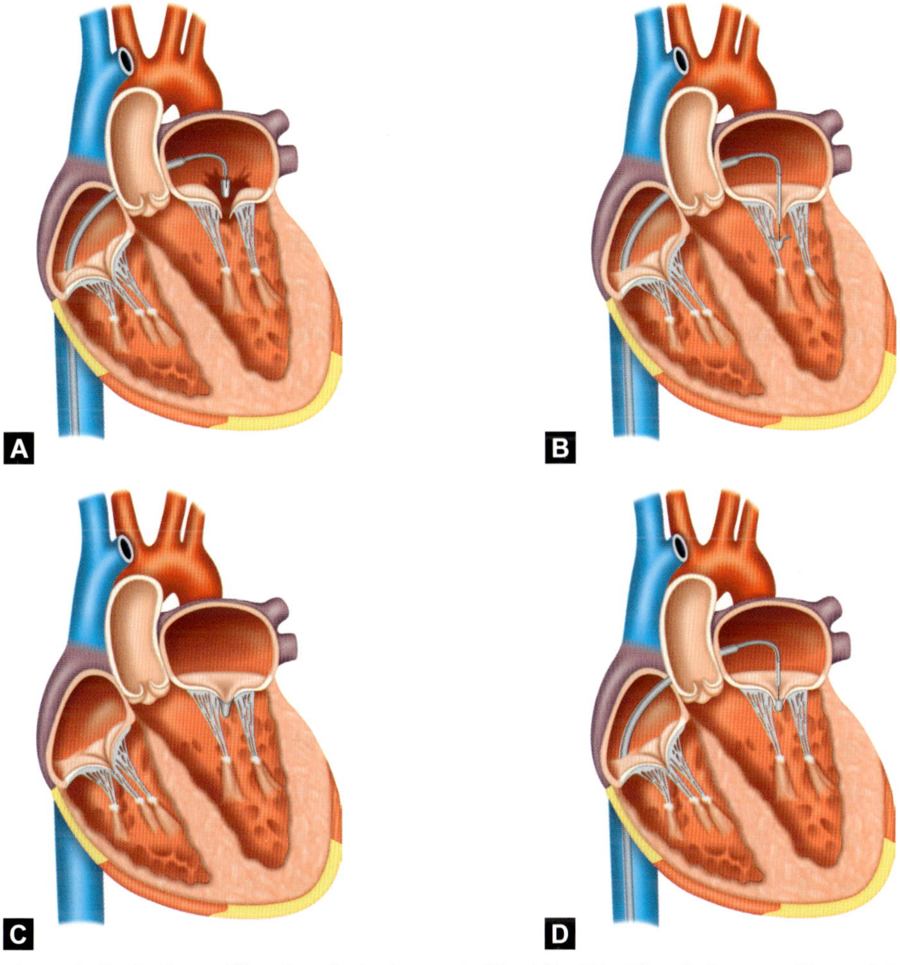

Figs. 13.24A to D: Schematic illustrations of the steps in deployment of the MitraClip. The clip is passed through the interatrial septum, across the mitral valve, and positioned below the mitral leaflets. The clip is then opened. Guided by transesophageal echocardiography, the leaflet margins are then captured in the clip. The degree of mitral regurgitation is then evaluated and if acceptable the cable is disengaged, leaving in place the clip, teathering the leaflets. [Images courtesy of and copyright (2013) by Abbott Vascular].

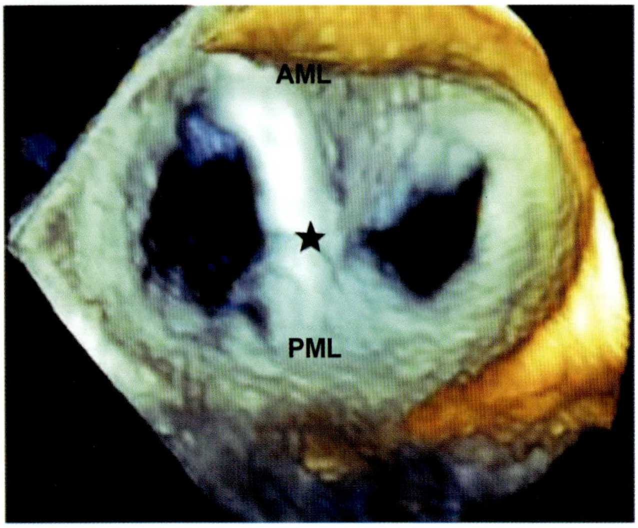

Fig. 13.25: 3D transesophageal echocardiography (TEE) of a mitral valve treated with the MitraClip (star). Note that there are now two mitral orifices. [Image from Saric M, Benenstein R. Three-dimensional echocardiographic guidance of percutaneous procedures. In: Nanda NC (Ed). Comprehensive Textbook of Echocardiography. New Delhi, India: Jaypee Brothers Medical Publishers (P) Ltd; 2014]. (AML: Anterior mitral leaflet; PML: Posterior mitral leaflet).

VIDEO LEGENDS

Video 13.1: Parasternal long axis transthoracic echocardiography (TTE) showing mild mitral regurgitation (MR) in a patient with myxomatous mitral leaflets.

Videos 13.2A and B: Transesophageal echocardiography (TEE) study showing (A) endocarditis of mitral valve and (B) resulting mitral regurgitation.

Video 13.3: Transesophageal echocardiography (TEE) showing endocarditis of the mitral valve and resulting regurgitation.

Video 13.4: Apical 4 chamber transthoracic echocardiography (TTE) showing severe, somewhat eccentric, mitral regurgitation (MR). Tethering of the posterior mitral leaflet is contributing to the MR.

Videos 13.5A and B: Transesophageal echocardiography (TEE) study showing (A) a restricted posterior mitral leaflet with (B) resulting mitral regurgitation.

Video 13.6: Mitral regurgitation due to mitral valve prolapse

Video 13.7: Transesophageal echocardiography (TEE) showing mitral regurgitation due to a flail mitral leaflet.

Video 13.8: Transesophageal echocardiography (TEE) showing a flail A1 scallop with resulting mitral regurgitation (MR).

Video 13.9: Functional mitral regurgitation (MR) in a patient with dilated cardiomyopathy and a dilated mitral annulus.

REFERENCES

Adams DH, Rosenhek R, Falk V. Degenerative mitral valve regurgitation: best practice revolution. Eur Heart J. 2010;31 (16):1958-66.

Bonow RO, Carabello BA, Chatterjee K, et al. 2008 focused update incorporated into the ACC/AHA 2006 guidelines for the management of patients with valvular heart disease: a report of the American College of Cardiology/American Heart Association Task Force on Practice Guidelines (Writing Committee to revise the 1998 guidelines for the management of patients with valvular heart disease). Endorsed by the Society of Cardiovascular Anesthesiologists, Society for Cardiovascular Angiography and Interventions, and Society of Thoracic Surgeons. J Am Coll Cardiol. 2008;52(13):e1-142.

Chikwe J, Adams DH. State of the art: degenerative mitral valve disease. Heart Lung Circ. 2009;18(5):319-29.

De Bonis M, Maisano F, La Canna G, et al. Treatment and management of mitral regurgitation. Nat Rev Cardiol. 2011; 9(3):133-46.

Joint Task Force on the Management of Valvular Heart Disease of the European Society of Cardiology (ESC); European Association for Cardio-Thoracic Surgery (EACTS), Vahanian A, et al. Guidelines on the management of valvular heart disease (version 2012). Eur Heart J. 2012;33(19):2451-96.

Piérard LA, Carabello BA. Ischaemic mitral regurgitation: pathophysiology, outcomes and the conundrum of treatment. Eur Heart J. 2010;31(24):2996-3005.

CHAPTER

14

Mitral Valve Prolapse

Pravin V Patil, Mohammad A Kashem, T Sloane Guy

INTRODUCTION

Mitral valve prolapse (MVP) (Figs. 14.1 to 14.3 and Videos 14.1 to 14.3) was first recognized in the 1960s by Reid and further validated by Barlow and colleagues. MVP is an abnormal bulge of mitral valve leaflets into the left atrium during ventricular systole. The overwhelming majority of patients with MVP remain asymptomatic throughout their lives; however, complications such as significant mitral regurgitation (MR) are known to occur and require surveillance. The spectrum of MVP ranges from a small left ventricle with relative lengthening of chordae to severely redundant leaflets that exhibit myxomatous degeneration and deformity. The result of severe mitral prolapse is severe MR (Fig. 14.4), and increased risk for stroke, arrhythmia and endocarditis.

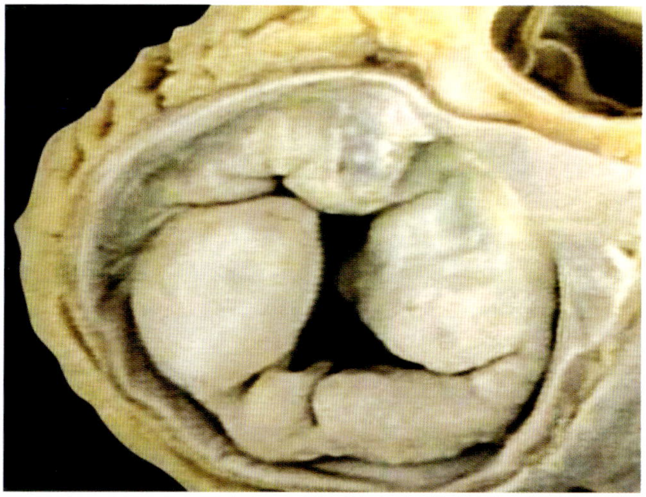

Fig. 14.1: Enface gross pathology example of mitral valve prolapse. There is myxomatous degeneration of the mitral leaflets and abnormal bulging of leaflets across the mitral annulus. (Image from Armed Forces Institute of Pathology).

PATHOPHYSIOLOGY

Mitral valve prolapse can be the result of a number of processes. These range from myxomatous diseases like fibroelastic deficiency or Barlow's disease (Table 14.1) to papillary muscle diseases, acute rheumatic disease, or connective tissue disorders like Marfan syndrome.

Fibroelastic deficiency is a degenerative myxomatous disease more commonly seen in elderly patients. The inciting event which may lead to symptoms is often rupture of a single chord, resulting in leaflet dysfunction. For this reason, patients typically have a shorter history of valvular regurgitation. Aside from the ruptured chord and prolapsing leaflet, valve morphology, including the mitral annulus size and leaflet sizes, is often quite normal (Fig. 14.5).

Barlow's disease was first described in the 1960s. It is classically described as excess leaflet tissue with large billowing and thick leaflets. In contrast to fibroelastic deficiency, these patients typically have an enlarged mitral annulus. In conjunction with the leaflets, the chordae tendinae are usually thickened. As the chordae elongate, prolapse of multiple scallops occurs. In contrast to fibroelastic deficiency, Barlow's disease is generally seen in younger patients. The spectrum of mitral valve disease that can result in MVP is illustrated in Figure 14.6.

CLINICAL PRESENTATION

The classic finding on physical examination for MVP is a midsystolic click followed by a late systolic murmur (Fig. 14.7). The click occurs when the chordae tendineae are snapped taut by a prolapsing leaflet in mid-systole. Prolapse results in MR and a late systolic murmur. Any maneuver to decrease left ventricular (LV) size (nitrates, Valsalva, etc.) will result in an earlier click and earlier occurrence of MR; the MR will usually be louder.

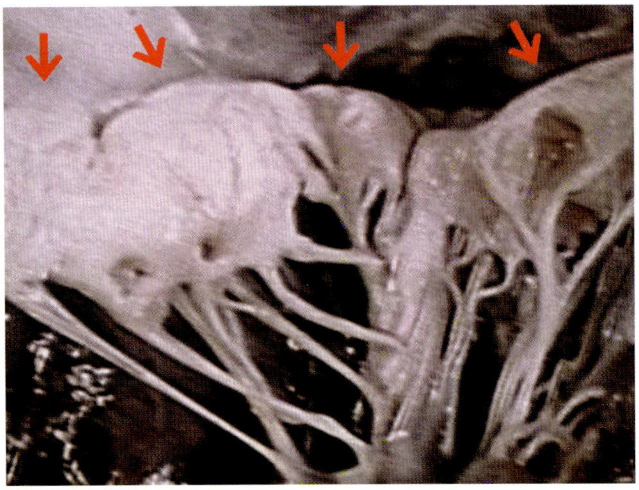

Fig. 14.2A: Gross pathology example of degenerated mitral valve leaflets in mitral valve prolapse. (From Armed Forces Institute of Pathology).

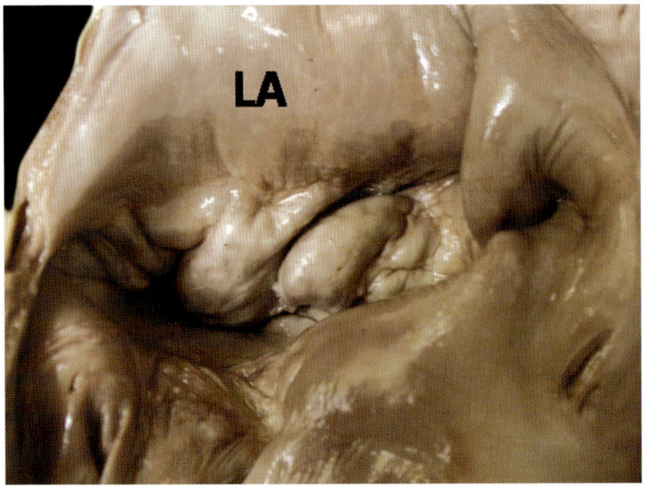

Fig. 14.2B: Opened out left atrium LA showing prolapse of the posterior mitral leaflet PML into the cavity. [Image and legend text courtesy of Dr Pradeep Vaideeswar, Professor (Additional), Department of Pathology (Cardiovascular & Thoracic Division), Seth GS Medical College, Mumbai, India].

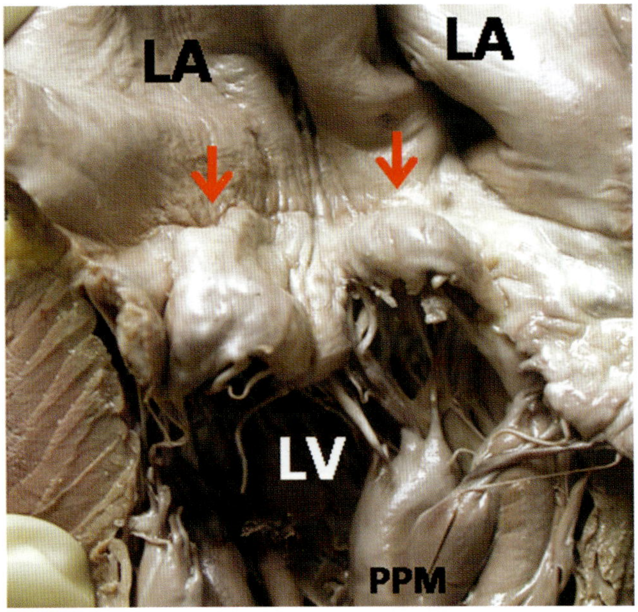

Fig. 14.2C: Marked myxomatous changes of the posterior mitral leaflet with billowing and prolapse. [Image and legend text courtesy of Dr. Pradeep Vaideeswar, Professor (Additional), Department of Pathology (Cardiovascular & Thoracic Division), Seth GS Medical College, Mumbai, India]. (LA: Left atrium; LV: Left ventricle; PPM: Posterior papillary muscle).

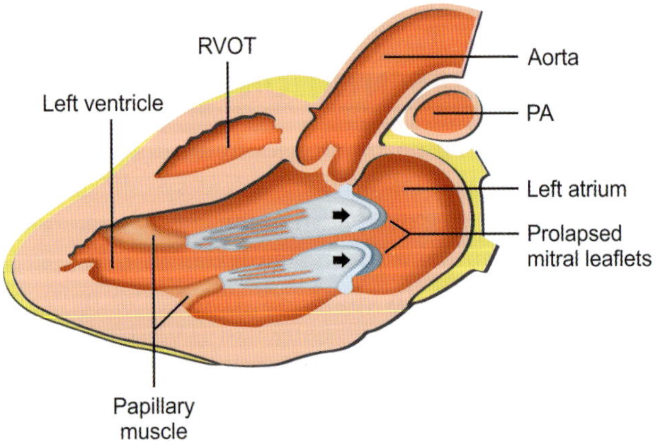

Fig. 14.3: Schematic illustration of mitral valve prolapse. The heart is shown as imaged in the parasternal long transthoracic echocardiography window. The mitral leaflets can be seen prolapsing across the mitral valve annulus into the left atrium. Diagnostic criteria for the diagnosis of mitral valve prolapse is prolapse of the leaflet >2 mm across a virtual line of the mitral annulus into the left atrium.

Table 14.1: Comparison of the two types of myxomatous degeneration: Barlow's disease and fibroelastic deficiency.

	Barlow's Disease	***Fibroelastic Deficiency***
Pathology	Myxoid infiltration	Impaired production of connective tissue
Typical age	Young (<60 years)	Older (60+ years)
Duration of known mitral disease	Several years to decades	Months
Long history of murmur	Usually	No
Familial history	Sometimes	No
Marfanoid features	Sometimes	No
Auscultation	Midsystolic click and late systolic murmur	Holosystolic murmur
Echocardiography	Bulky, billowing leaflets, multi-segmental prolapse	Thin leaflets, prolapse of single segment, ruptured chord(s)
Surgical lesions	Excess tissue, thickened and tall leaflets, chordal thickening or thinning, chordal elongation or rupture, atrialization of leaflets, fusion, fibrosis or calcification of chords, papillary muscle calcification, annular calcification	Thin leaflets, thickening and excess tissue (if present) limited to prolapsing segment, ruptured chordae
Mitral valve repair	More complex	Less complex

Source: Table adapted from Anyanwu, et al. Semin Thorac Cardiovasc Surg 2007.

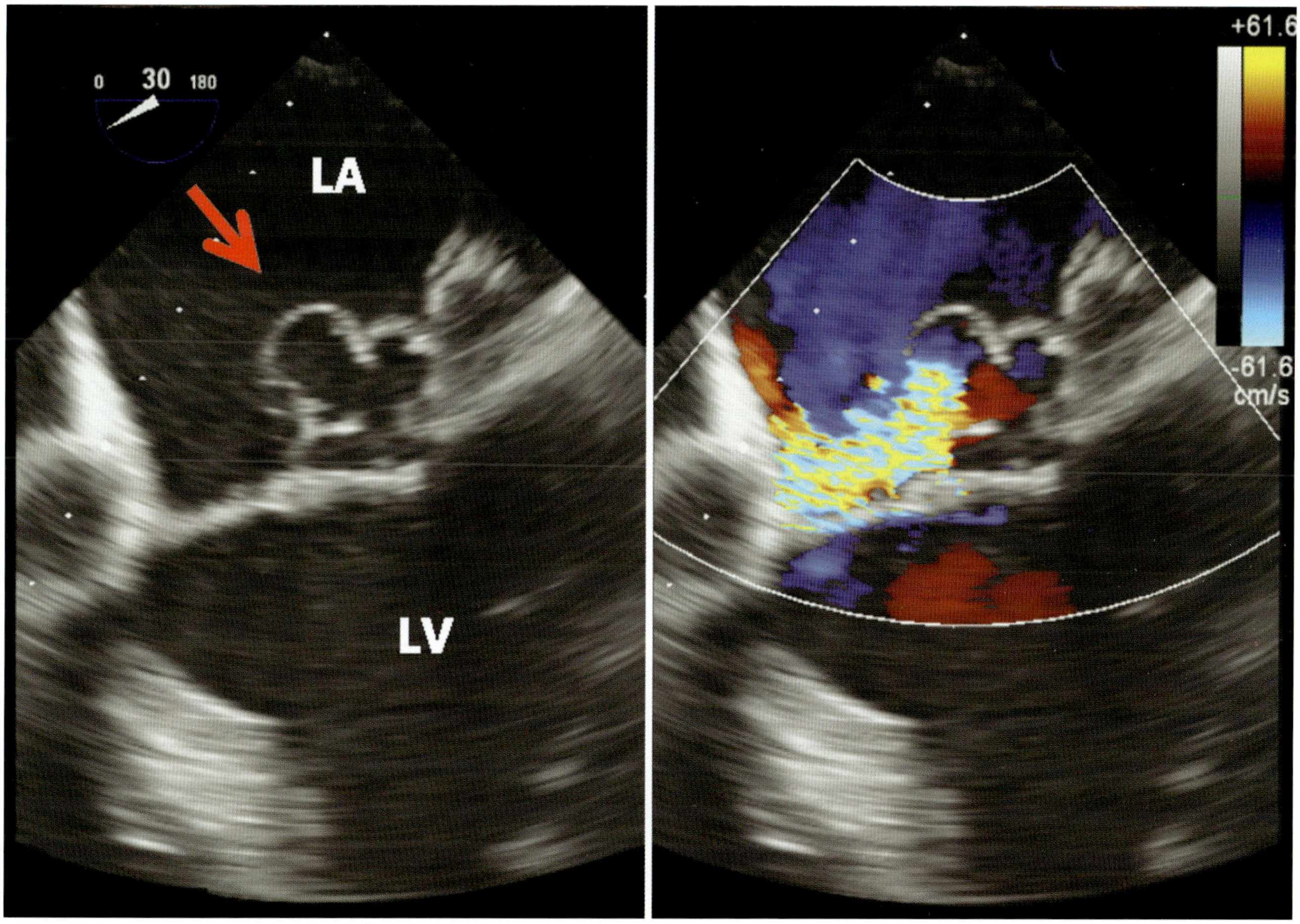

Fig. 14.4: Transesophageal echocardiography 2d (left panel) and color Doppler (right panel) images showing marked mitral valve prolapse (arrow) resulting in eccentric mitral regurgitation. (Image courtesy of Glenn N Levine, MD and Vinnie Blaustein, MD).

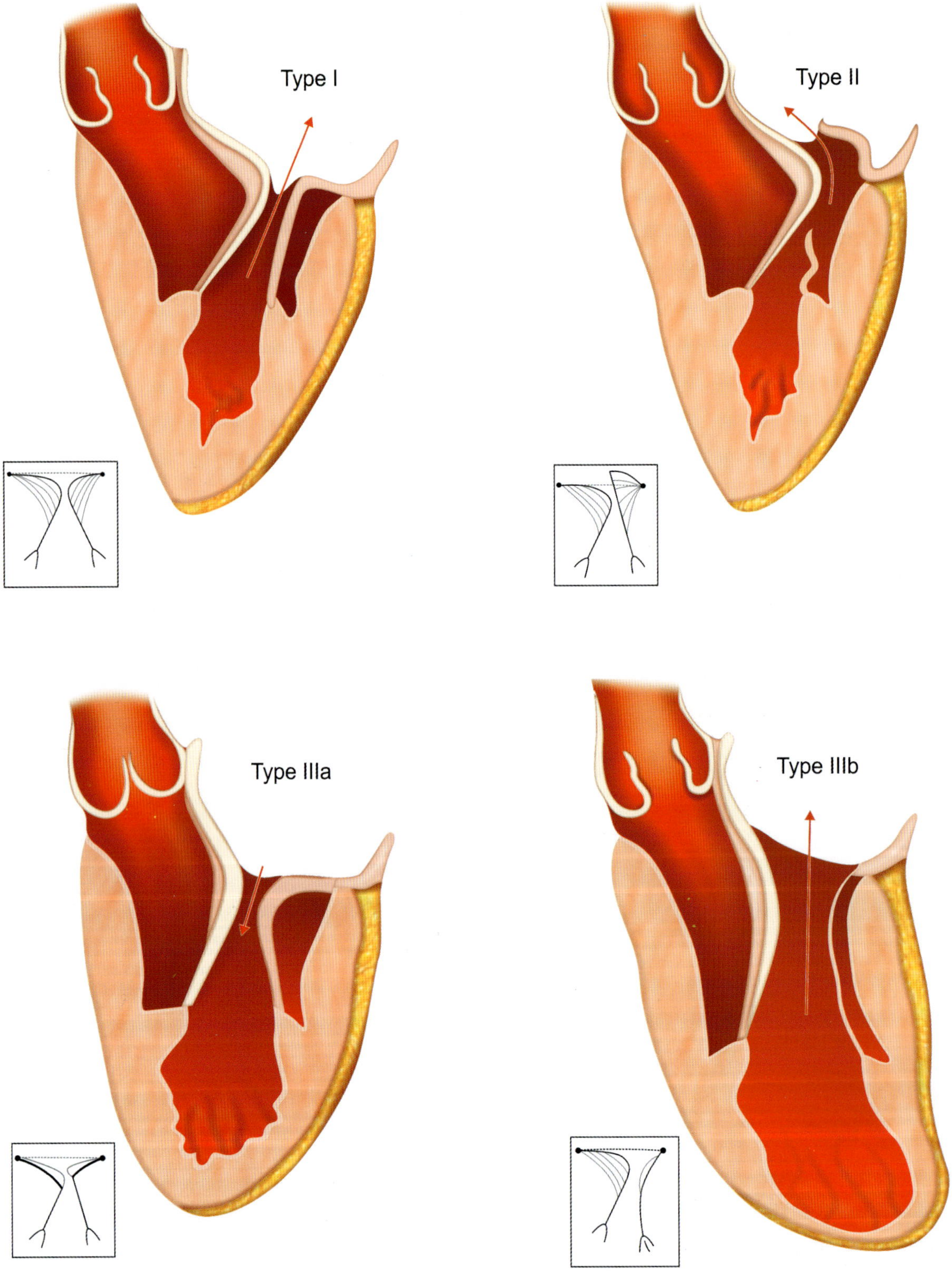

Fig. 14.5: Carpentier functional classifications of mitral valve disease. In order to facilitate multidisciplinary communication this classification delineates etiology, lesions and subsequent valve dysfunction. Mitral valve prolapse has been classically described as type II. (Image adapted from Carpentier 2010).

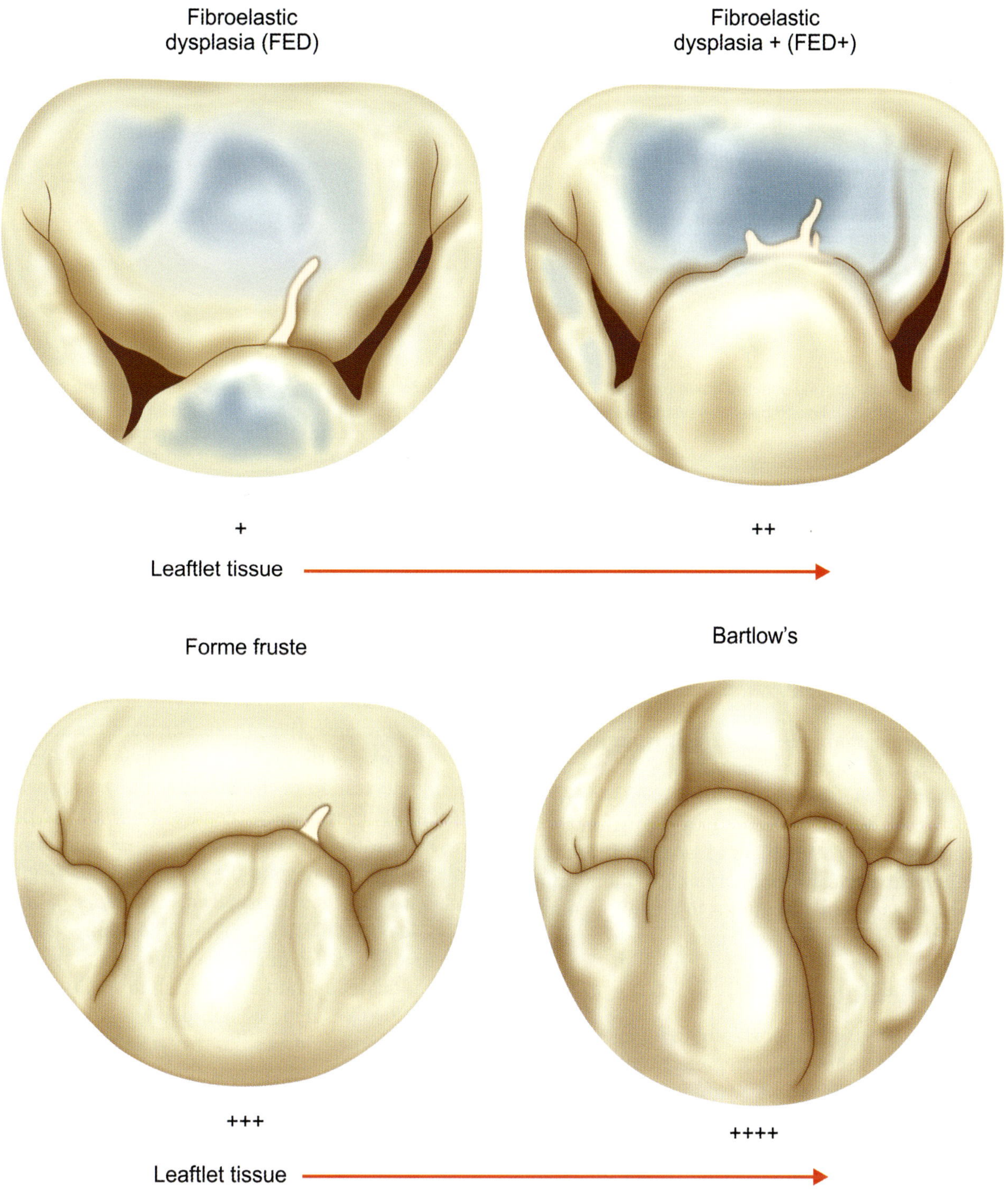

Fig. 14.6: Spectrum of degenerative mitral valve disease. In isolated fibroelastic dysplasia (FED) there is deficiency of collagen and a ruptured thin chordae. In long-standing prolapse, myxomatous changes occur with leaflet thickening (FED+). Forme fruste has excessive tissue, myxomatous changes in one or more leaflets, but does not involve a large valve size. In Barlow's the hallmarks are large valve size, with diffuse myxomatous changes and excess leaflet tissue, with thickened, elongated and often ruptured chordae. [Image and legend text from Sharma S and Dalvi BV. Mitral valve disease. In: Chatterjee K, et al (ed). Cardiology—an illustrated textbook. New Delhi, India: Jaypee Brothers Medical Publishers (P) Ltd.].

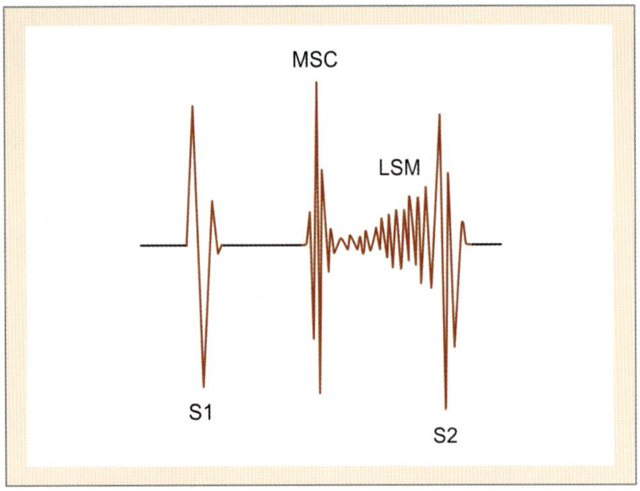

Fig. 14.7: Phonocardiography in mitral valve prolapse. There is a mid-systolic click (MSC) followed by a late-systolic murmur (LSM).

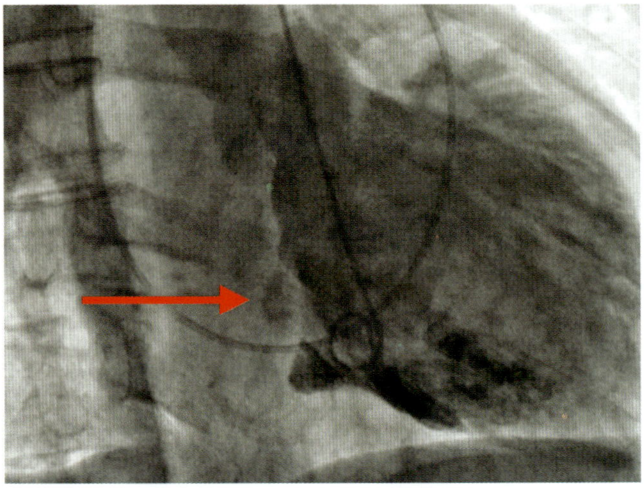

Fig. 14.8: Left ventriculography performed in the right anterior oblique projection with a straight pigtail catheter (end-systole) demonstrating prolapse of a posteromedial scallop (arrow). A discrete area of contrast is visualized beyond the mitral valve plane due to the prolapsing mitral valve scallop.

In some cases of MVP, however, none of these physical exam findings will be present, and the diagnosis will only be made after an imaging study.

DIAGNOSTIC TESTING

ECG

The electrocardiogram (ECG) in MVP is typically normal in patients who are asymptomatic. Although a wide variety of arrhythmias have been seen in patient with MVP, including atrial, ventricular and bradyarrhythmias, the mechanism by which MVP might cause such arrhythmias remains unclear. Typically, ambulatory ECG monitoring is performed in symptomatic patients to identify significant arrhythmias.

Left Ventriculography

Angiocardiograms (ventriculography) were initially felt to be the diagnostic test of choice in patients with suspected MVP (Fig. 14.8 and Video 14.4). Although there was good diagnostic consistency for the presence of mitral valve prolapse, interobserver agreement on prolapsing leaflet morphology was varied. This has led to echocardiography supplanting ventriculography as a diagnostic technique.

Echocardiography

Echocardiography is the most readily available and useful tool available for the diagnosis of mitral valve prolapse. The primary goal of an echocardiogram is to define chamber sizes and ventricular function. The mitral valve structure and function can be accurately assessed with 2-dimensional, M-mode, color flow and spectral Doppler imaging.

M-mode transthoracic echocardiography has excellent temporal resolution and allows visualization and timing of leaflet prolapse (Fig. 14.9). The parasternal long-axis view is particularly useful, as it allows visualization of the middle scallop of the anterior and posterior leaflets (A2 and P2, Carpentier). Diagnostic criteria for prolapse have been established in this view as visualization leaflet prolapse > 2 mm beyond the mitral annulus (Fig. 14.10). In classic MVP, there is usually also evidence of increased mitral leaflet thickness. Echocardiography allows one to assess the leaflet thickness, evaluate for redundancy, annular dilatation and chordal abnormalities. Additionally, the assessment of subsequent MR severity and intracardiac hemodynamics by echocardiography can be accomplished using color flow and spectral Doppler techniques.

Transesophageal echocardiography affords improved spatial resolution, limited artifacts and excellent views of the mitral valve. In addition to transthoracic echocardiography, it allows for scallop-by-scallop evaluation and detailed visualization of the chordal structures. Transesophageal echocardiography is considered the gold standard for dynamic evaluation of mitral valve disease (Figs. 14.11 and 14.12, Videos 14.5 and 14.6).

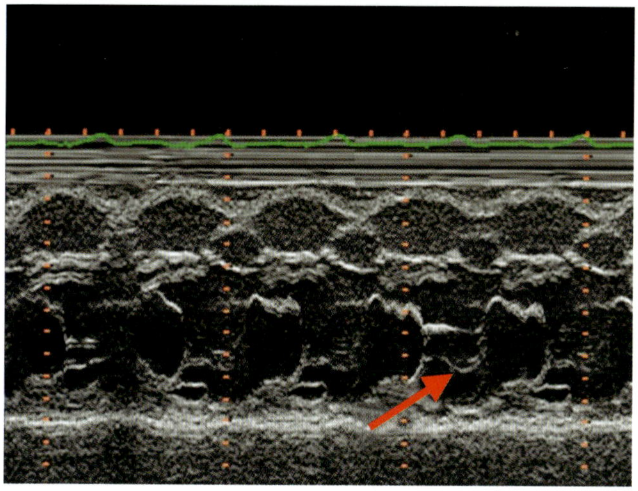

Fig. 14.9: M-mode echocardiography at the level of the mitral valve demonstrating late systolic posterior leaflet prolapse (arrow).

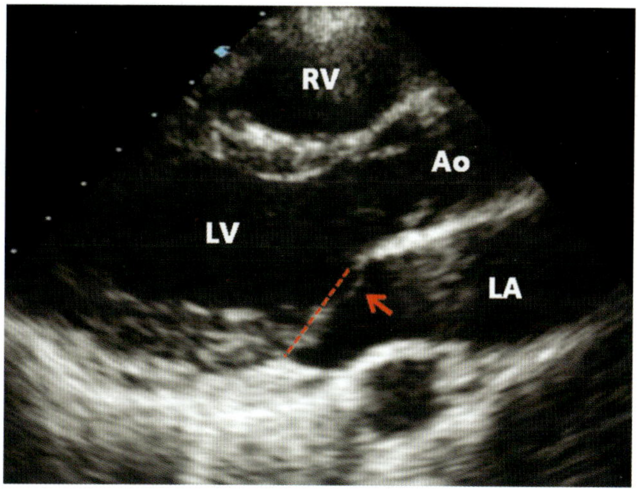

Fig. 14.10: 2-Dimensional transthoracic echocardiography in the parasternal long-axis view showing end-systolic protrusion of the anterior leaflet (arrow) by > 2 mm beyond the mitral annulus (dashed line) consistent with mitral valve prolapse. (Ao: Aorta; LA: Left atrium; LV: Left ventricle; RV: Right ventricle).

Real-time three-dimensional echocardiography has been particularly useful in conjunction with transesophageal echocardiography. It allows the physician to obtain a "surgical" view of the mitral valve from behind the left atrium. These images can be manipulated in a multiplanar reformat to allow interrogation of cardiac structures (Figs. 14.13 to 14.17, Videos 14.7 to 14.10). Color flow Doppler data can also be obtained in 3D and be superimposed onto conventional 3D datasets.

Cardiac Computed Tomography

Cardiac computed tomography (CT) is a novel adjunctive method to assess cardiac morphology and the coronary arteries for preoperative planning prior to mitral valve repair. Cardiac CT is particularly useful in the evaluation of the cardiac structures associated with mitral annulus, as well as the entire mitral valve apparatus from myocardium to leaflet (Figs. 14.18A to C).

Cardiac Magnetic Resonance

Cardiovascular magnetic resonance (CMR) imaging is the gold standard for the quantification of LV function and measuring cardiac volumes. Magnetic resonance offers the benefit of avoiding ionizing radiation exposure and a relatively non-toxic contrast agent. CMR allows for non-invasive cardiac imaging with good spatial resolution and excellent temporal resolution.

Criterion established for transthoracic echocardiography (i.e. leaflet excursion of > 2 mm into the LA in the long-axis view) has been validated in CMR. This criterion has been proven in CMR to be highly sensitive and specific for mitral valve prolapse. CMR also allows for assessment of delayed gadolinium hyperenhancement (DHE). DHE has been utilized to identify areas of scar or fibrosis within the LV myocardium. It has also been used in patient with mitral valve prolapse, where DHE has been identified in the papillary muscles and/or leaflets (Figs. 14.19A and B). These areas of potential scar in the papillary muscle have been implicated as a source of arrhythmia in these patients.

MANAGEMENT

The majority of patients with mitral valve are asymptomatic, and therefore therapy is often unnecessary. This is particularly true if there is no evidence of adverse remodeling, such as cavity dilatation and/or systolic dysfunction seen in the presence of any MR. These low-risk patients should be reassured, as they have a benign prognosis.

Patients who experience palpitations and symptoms of autonomic dysfunction often find that beta-blockers are effective in relieving their symptoms. They usually benefit from cessation of stimulants, such as caffeine, nicotine and/or alcohol. Ambulatory ECG can help to identify significant arrhythmia.

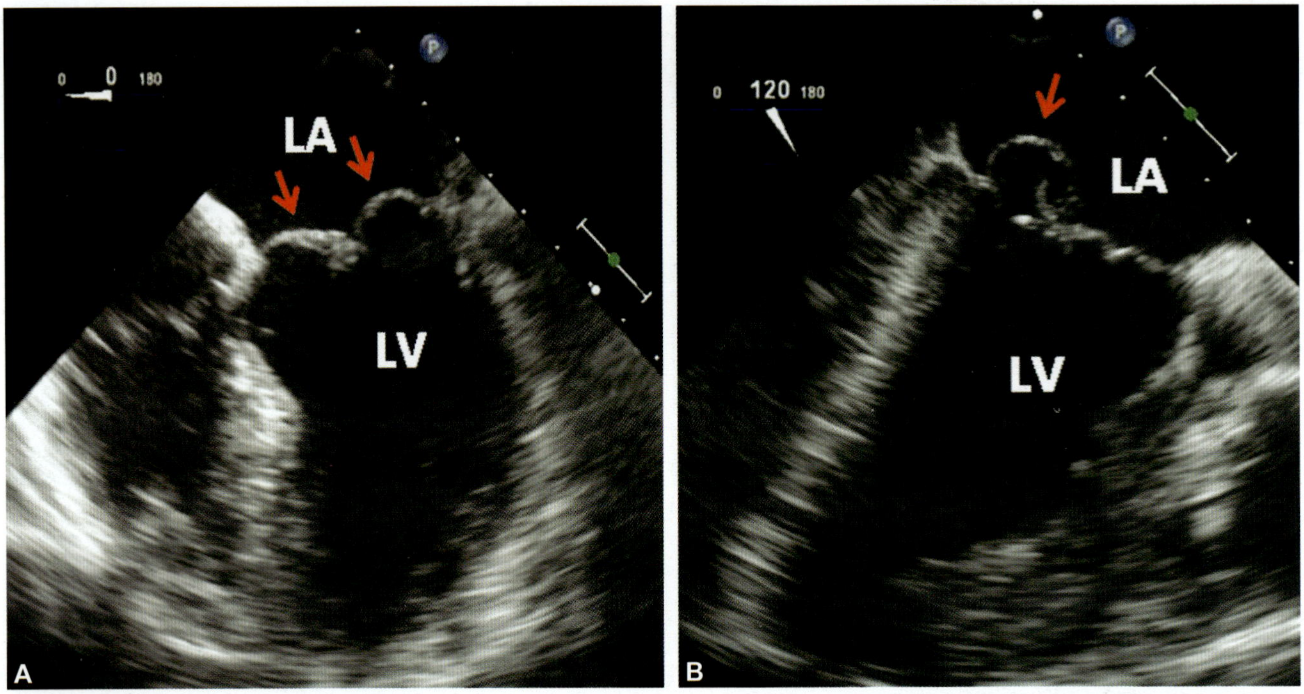

Figs. 14.11A and B: 2-Dimensional transesophageal echocardiography (TEE) of mitral valve prolapse. (A) Barlow's disease with thickened leaflets and bileaflet prolapse (arrows); (B) Fibroelastic deficiency with thin leaflets and focal scallop prolapse (arrow). (LA: Left atrium; LV: Left ventricle).

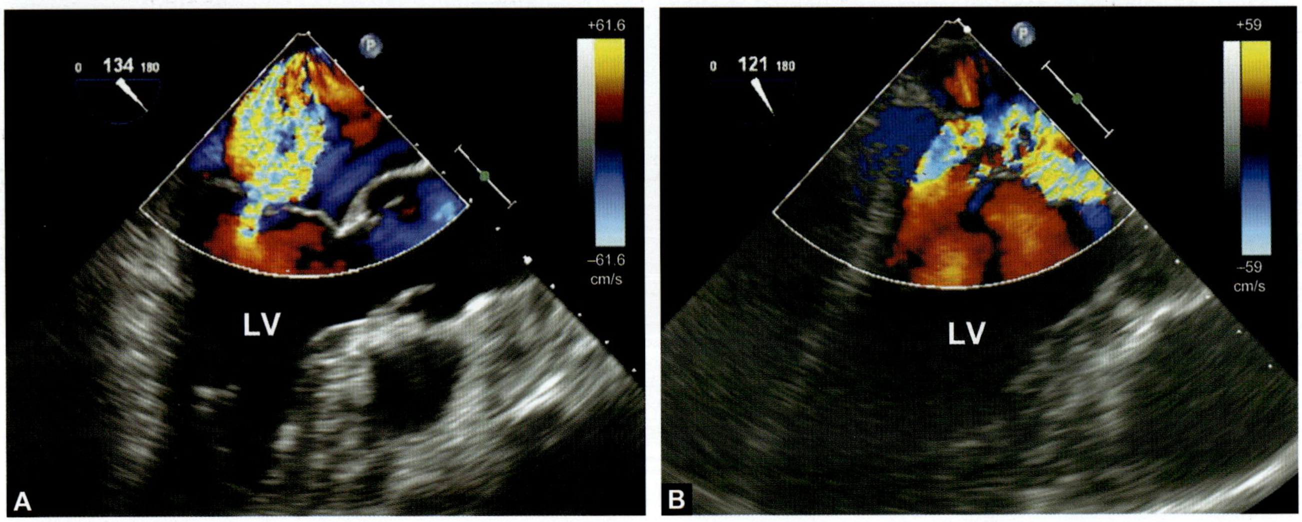

Figs. 14.12A and B: 2-Dimensional transesophageal echocardiography (TEE) with color flow Doppler of two cases of mitral valve prolapse. (A) Barlow's disease with bileaflet prolapse and severe central mitral regurgitation; (B) Fibroelastic deficiency with focal scallop prolapse and highly eccentric severe mitral regurgitation. (LV: Left ventricle).

Those patients with significant/severe MR should be followed closely. Their management should be per established guidelines, as discussed in the chapter on MR. This includes close clinical follow-up and early referral for mitral valve repair before adverse remodeling (LV dilatation and systolic dysfunction) occurs. Even asymptomatic patients who have significant MR, LV dilatation and/or pulmonary hypertension should be considered for surgical referral if local repair versus replacement rates are high.

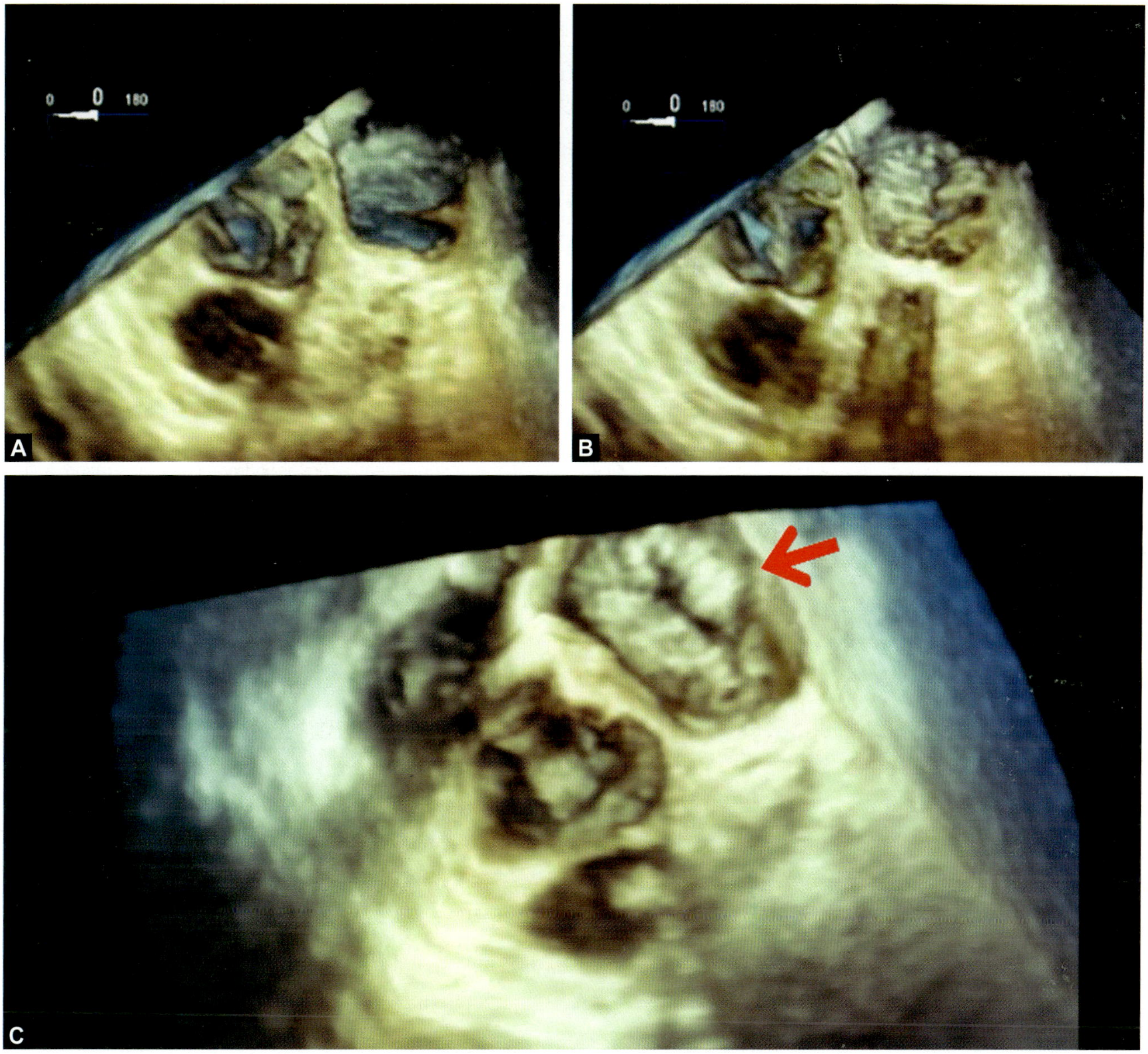

Figs. 14.13A to C: Real-time full volume (wide-angle) 3-dimensional transesophageal echocardiography of MVP. (A) Diastole with the mitral leaflets widely open; (B) End-systole with bileaflet mitral prolapse; (C) Zoomed and repositioned 3D data set to highlight the bileaflet prolapse (arrow) in end-systole.

SURGICAL TREATMENT

Sternotomy

There are several different surgical techniques. Median sternotomy is the most commonly used surgical approach in mitral valve surgery. It provides excellent access to all cardiac structures, allowing central cannulation. It remains the surgical approach of choice in patients undergoing complex mitral valve, multi-valve, combined mitral and coronary artery bypass grafting, and reoperative surgery. Standard cardiopulmonary bypass (CPB) is instituted in such intervention. An schematic illustration of the steps in mitral valve repair is given in Figures 14.20A to D.

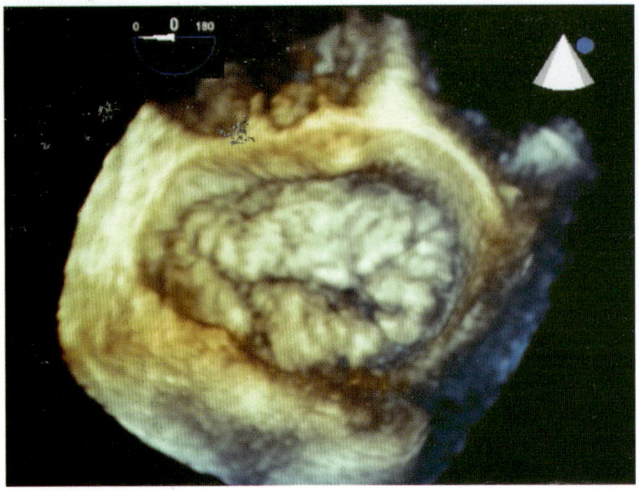

Fig. 14.14: Real-time 3D zoom/live 3D (narrow-angle) 3-dimensional transesophageal echocardiography demonstrating bileaflet prolapse.

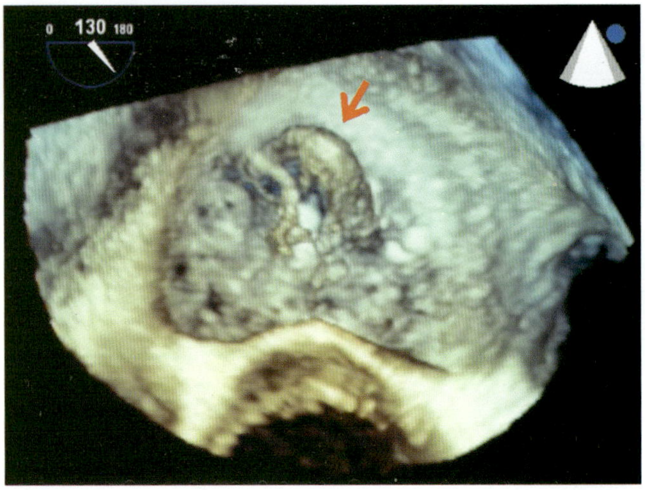

Fig. 14.15: Real-time 3D zoom/live 3D (narrow-angle) 3-dimensional transesophageal echocardiography demonstrating a flail P2 leaflet (arrow) with a ruptured chordae, typical of fibroelastic deficiency.

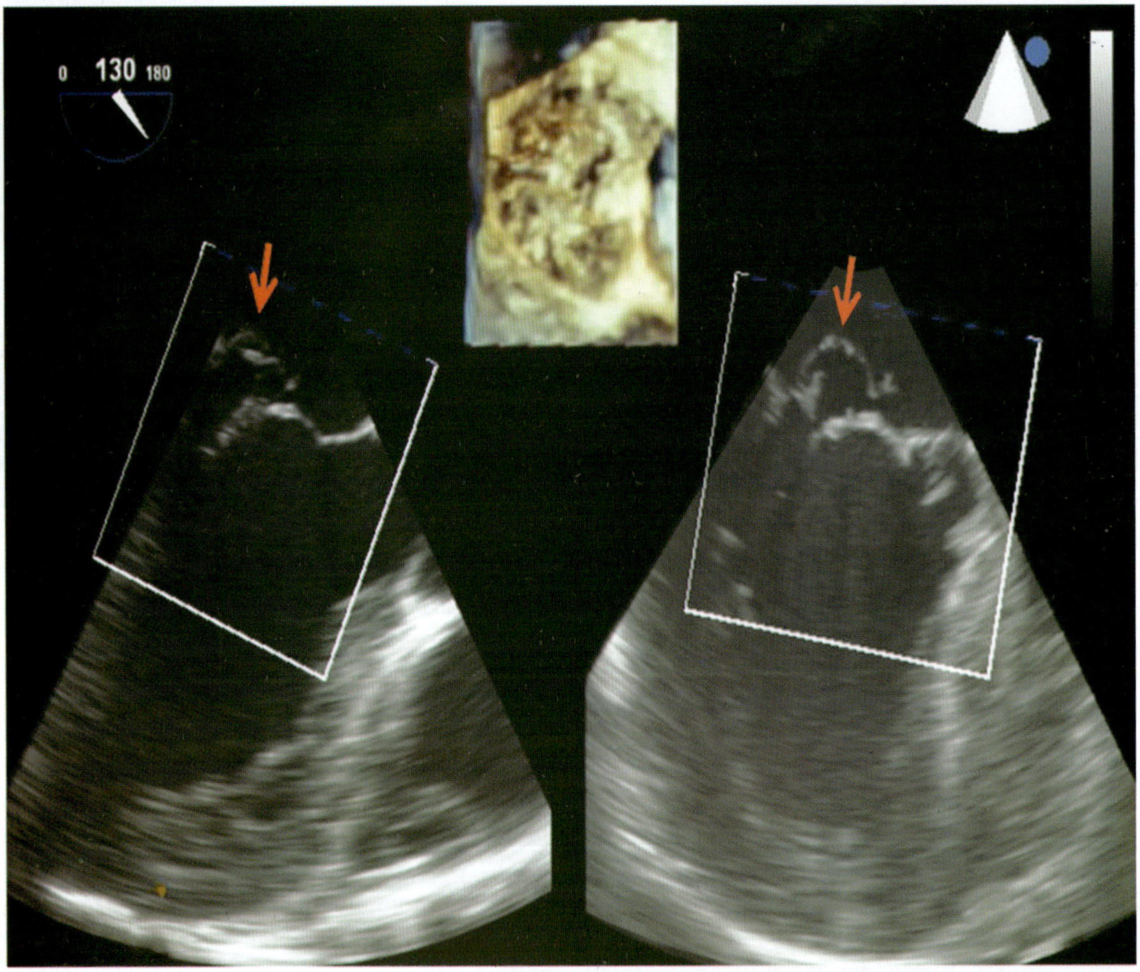

Fig. 14.16: Real-time full volume (wide-angle) 3-dimensional transesophageal echocardiography utilizing a simultaneous display of a multiplanar reformat in orthogonal planes and a 3D volume rendering of the region of interest (flail P2 scallop, arrows).

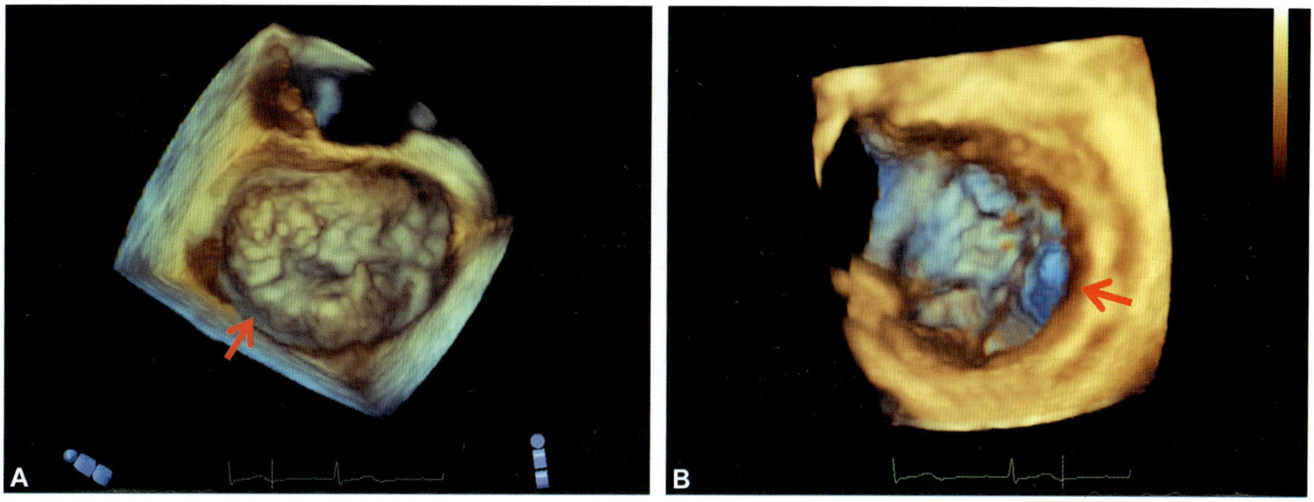

Figs. 14.17A and B: Real-time 3D zoom/live 3D (narrow-angle) 3-Dimensional transesophageal echocardiography demonstrating multi-scallop prolapse A1, P1 and P2 (arrows) shown in (A) left atrial view and (B) left ventricular view.

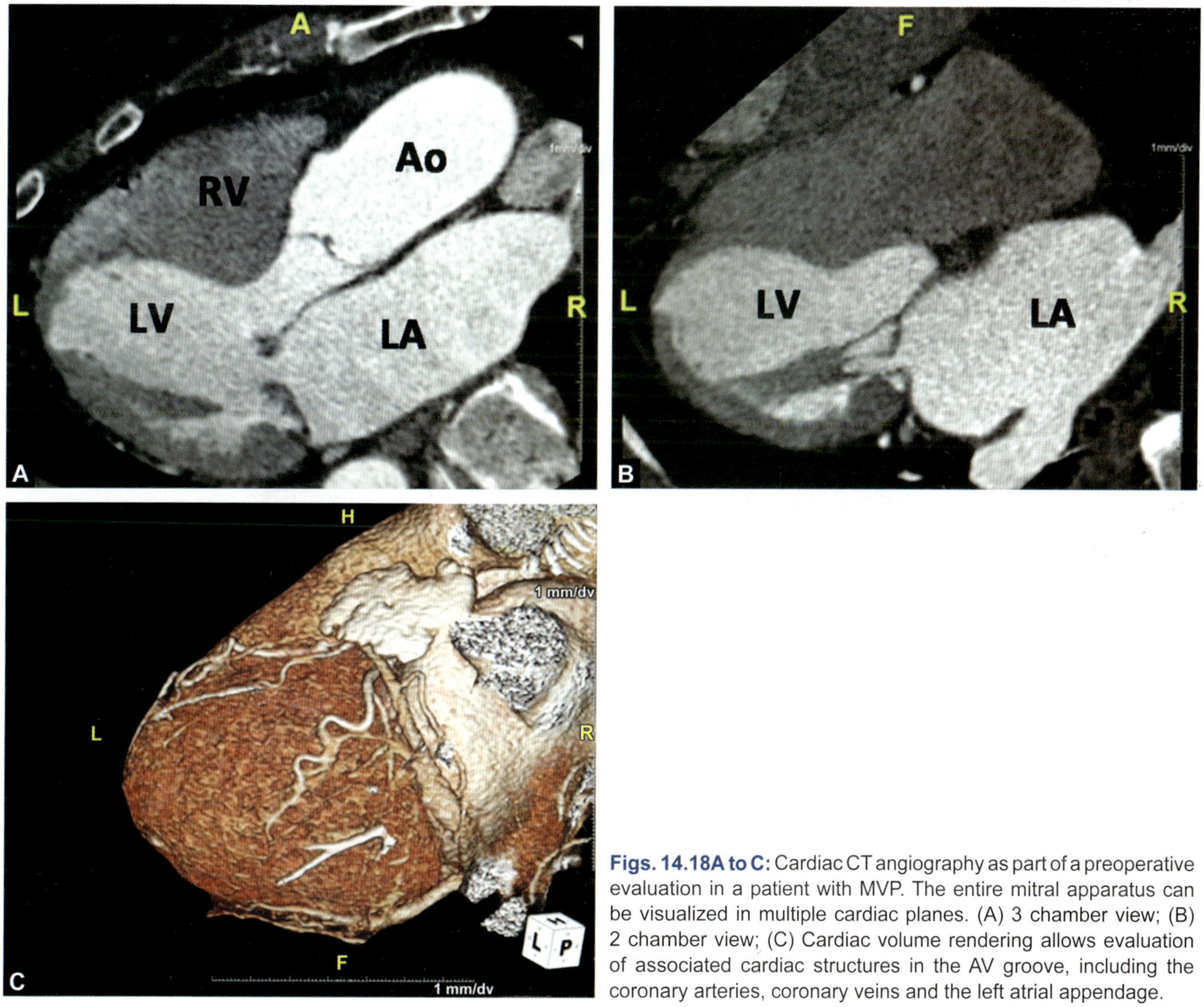

Figs. 14.18A to C: Cardiac CT angiography as part of a preoperative evaluation in a patient with MVP. The entire mitral apparatus can be visualized in multiple cardiac planes. (A) 3 chamber view; (B) 2 chamber view; (C) Cardiac volume rendering allows evaluation of associated cardiac structures in the AV groove, including the coronary arteries, coronary veins and the left atrial appendage.

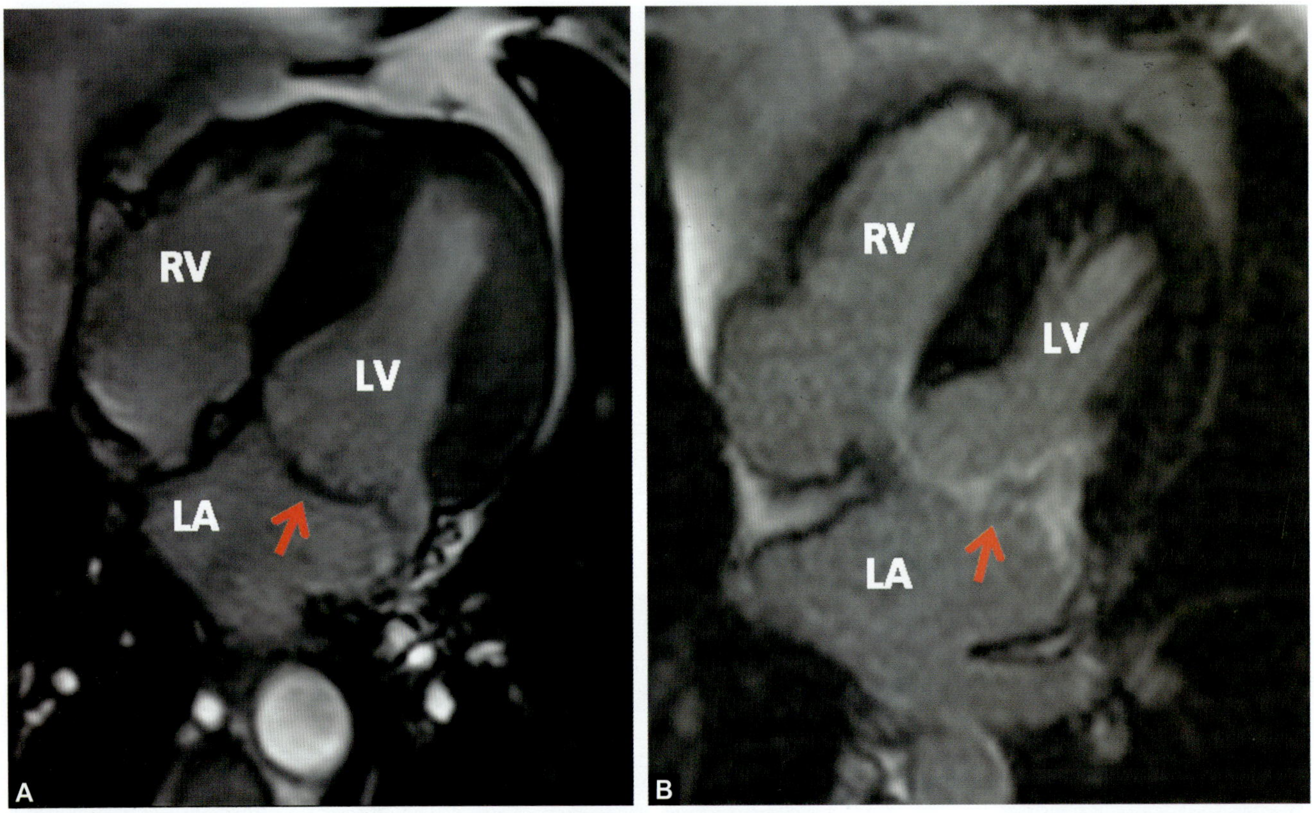

Figs. 14.19A and B: Cardiac MRI with and without contrast in a patient with MVP. (A) Steady-state free precession (SSFP) cine sequence in the 4-chamber plane demonstrating bileaflet mitral valve prolapse (arrow); (B) Delayed gadolinium hyperenhancement (arrow) of both mitral leaflets consistent with myxomatous degeneration.

Right Anterolateral Approach

Right anterolateral thoracotomy approach is typically performed in the fourth intercostal space and useful in patients with prior coronary artery bypass grafting, patent internal thoracic grafts, and in patients with prior aortic valve replacement. This technique avoids extensive mediastinal dissection and is useful in those with mediastinal adhesions. This technique is contraindicated in patients with previous right-sided chest surgery, severe chronic obstructive pulmonary disease (COPD), and significant aortic regurgitation.

Minimally Invasive Mitral Valve Surgery

These are many new surgical techniques that are currently used, including: limited incision with direct visualization; video assisted, video directed and robot assisted; and totally endoscopic robotic surgery. The first three options involve partial hemisternotomy, right mini-thoracotomy or additional incisions. Totally endoscopic mitral valve surgery can be a good option in certain patients (Figs. 14.21 to 14.23).

Totally Endoscopic Robotic Mitral Valve Repair

In our center, totally endoscopic robotic mitral valve repair is performed (Video 14.11) with five small incisions (ranging from 7–20 mm in size) and we avoid spreading of the ribs if only repair is planned. The da Vinci Robotic System™ allows all members of the cardiac team to visualize the surgical field. Cardioplegia and heart-lung bypass is established using a catheter based approach. In our experience with over 100 robotic mitral valve surgeries, 90% of patients underwent mitral repair without any operative deaths.

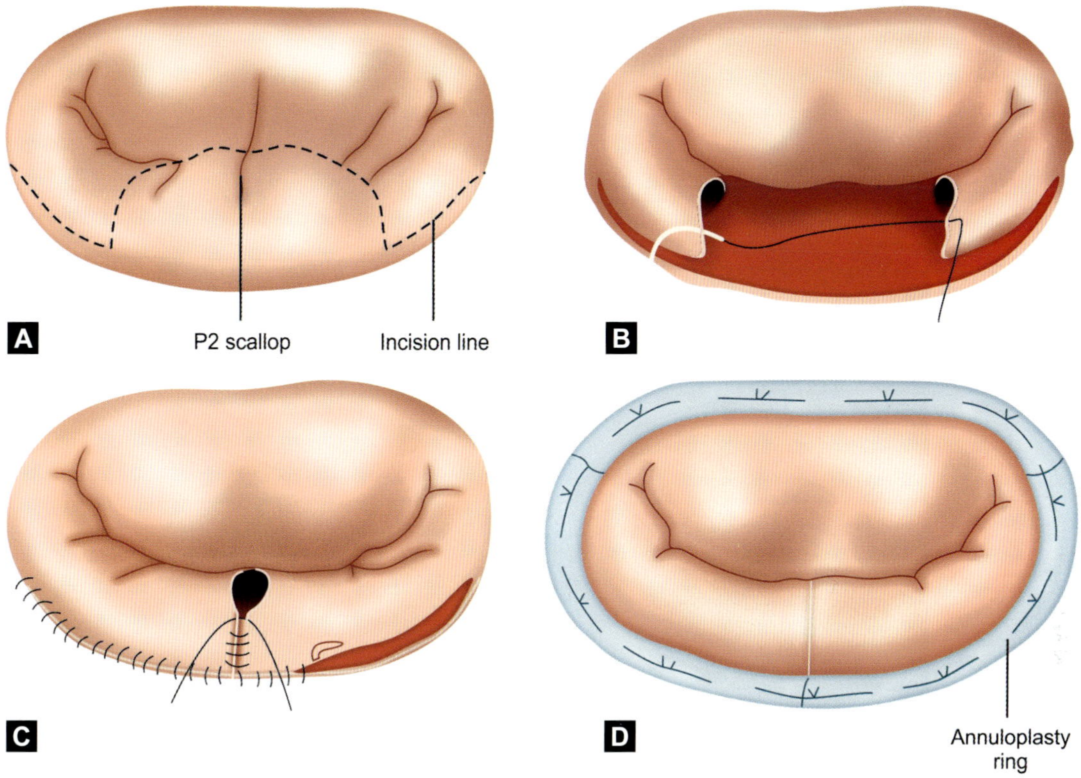

Figs. 14.20A to D: Steps for surgery for mitral valve prolapse. (A) Surgeon's view, from the atrium of a valve with a flail P2 scallop. Dashed line shows the planned incision of ruptured and elongated chordae; (B) View after resection of the diseased portion; (C) Re-apposition of the leaflet edges; (D) Reconstructed valve with an annuloplasty ring. [Image and legend text from Sharma S and Dalvi BV. Mitral valve disease. In Chatterjee K, et al. (ed). Cardiology—an illustrated textbook. New Delhi, India: Jaypee Brothers Medical Publishers (P) Ltd.].

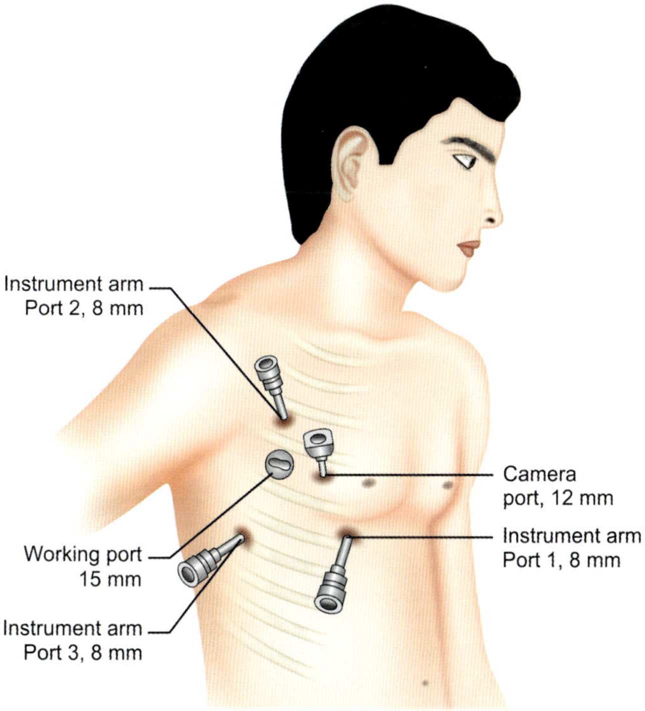

Fig. 14.21: Schematic demonstrating typical locations of port access during totally endoscopic robotic mitral valve repair.

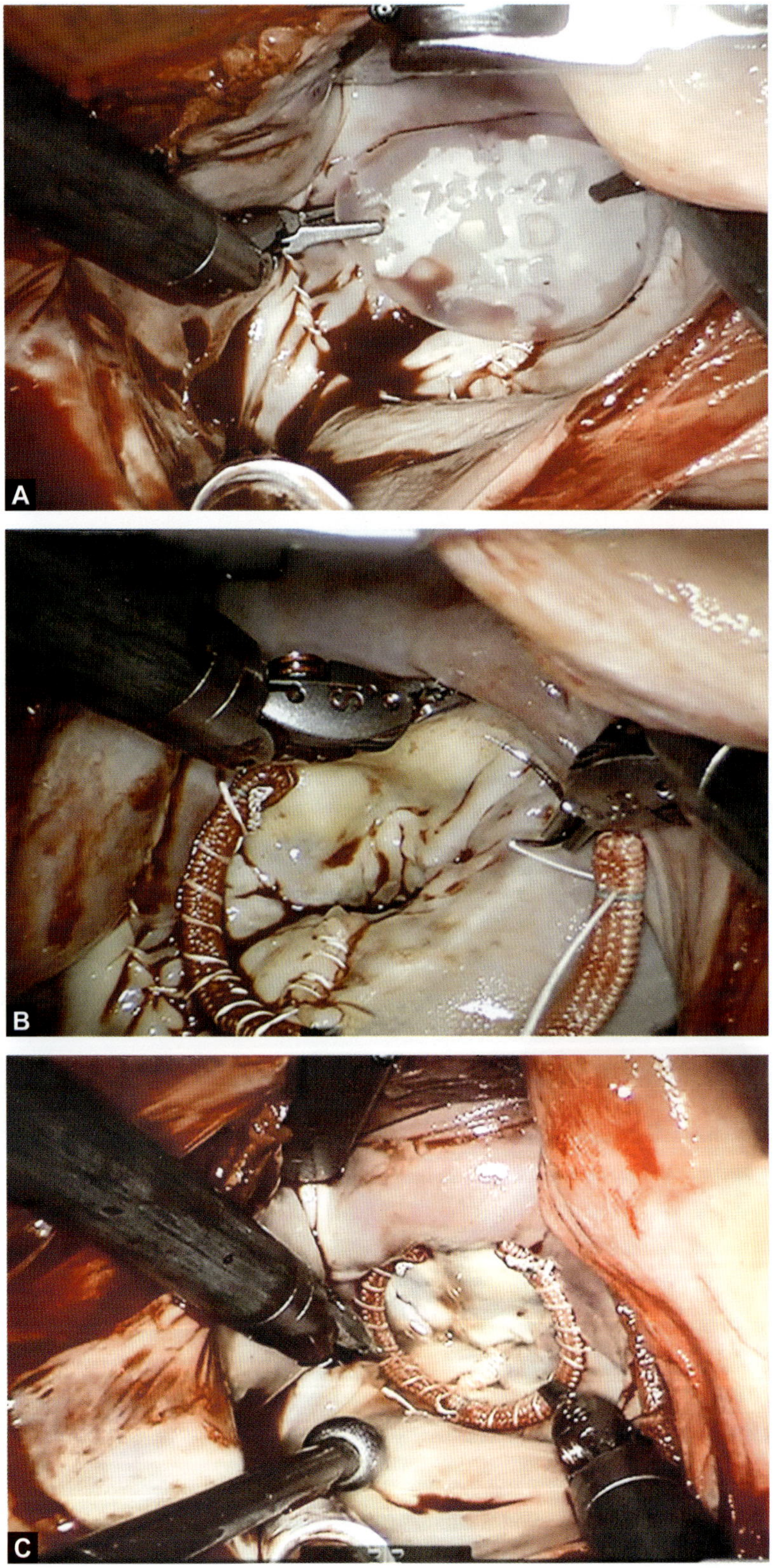

Figs. 14.22A to C: Totally endoscopic robotic repair of the mitral valve. (A) Following resection of the prolapsing P2 leaflet, the mitral valve has been sutured and ring sizing is performed; (B) Suturing of the annuloplasty ring prosthesis with the robotic arms; (C) Final repair result with the annuloplasty ring in place and the posterior leaflet repair evident.

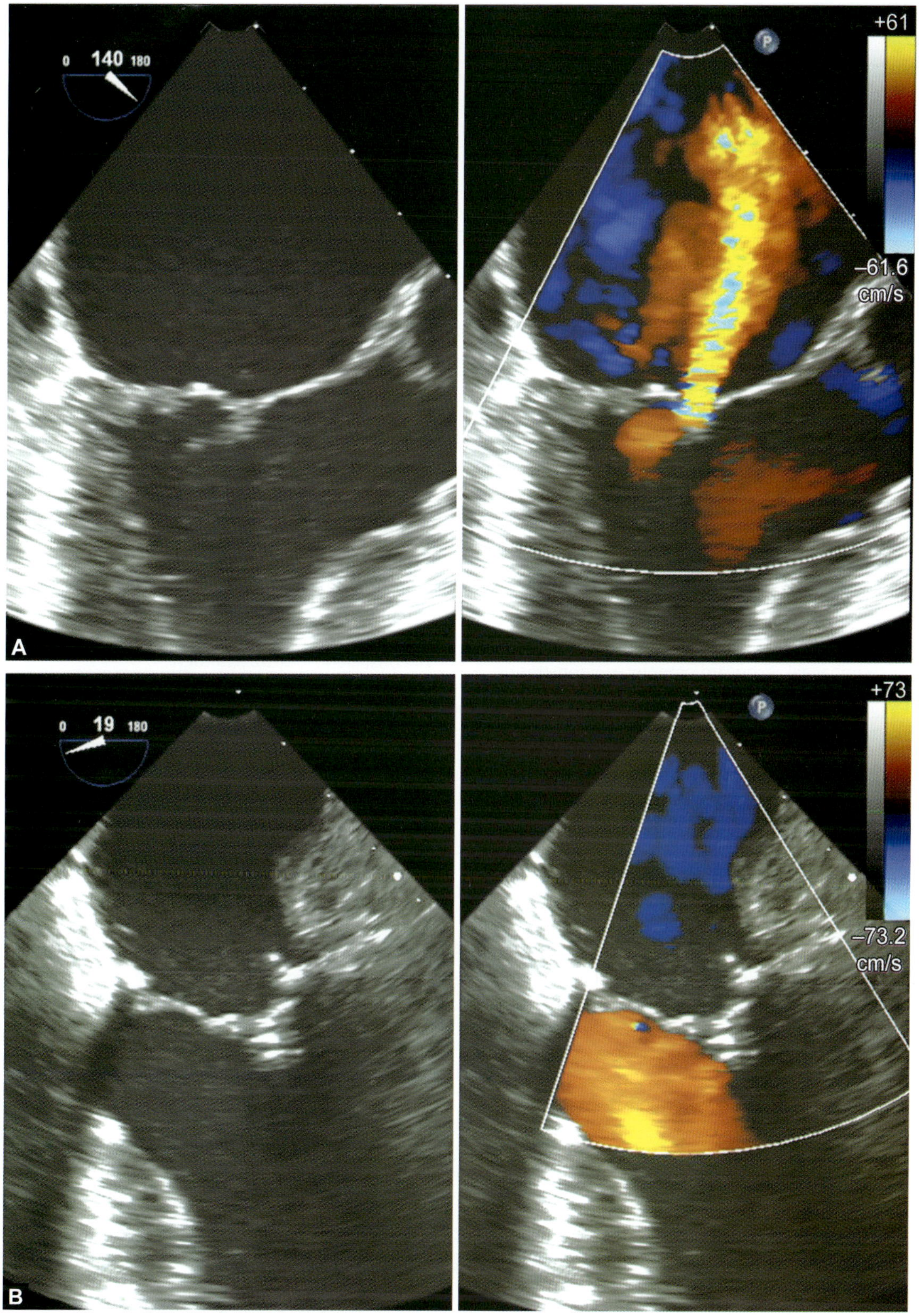

Figs. 14.23A and B: Intraoperative transesophageal echocardiography without and with color flow Doppler in a patient with MVP and mitral regurgitation. (A) Preoperative evaluation demonstrating significant mitral regurgitation related to posterior leaflet prolapse; (B) Postoperative evaluation demonstrating a new annuloplasty ring and no evidence of mitral regurgitation.

VIDEO LEGENDS

Video 14.1: Parasternal long-axis TTE showing mitral valve prolapse. During systole both the anterior and posterior mitral leaflets are seen prolapsing into the left atrium. Video courtesy of Glenn N. Levine, MD.

(TTE: Transthoracic echocardiogram).

Video 14.2: Zoomed parasternal long-axis TTE demonstrating mitral valve prolapse (MVP).

(TTE: Transthoracic echocardiogram).

Video 14.3: TEE showing mitral regurgitation in a patient with mitral valve prolapse.

(TEE: Transesophageal echocardiography).

Video 14.4: Left ventriculography performed in the right anterior oblique projection with a straight pigtail catheter (end-systole) demonstrating prolapse of a posteromedial scallop (arrow).

Video 14.5: 2-Dimensional transesophageal echocardiography (TEE) of mitral valve prolapse demonstrating Barlow's disease with thickened leaflets and bileaflet prolapse

Video 14.6: 2-Dimensional transesophageal echocardiography (TEE) of mitral valve prolapse. Fibroelastic deficiency with thin leaflets and focal scallop prolapse (arrow).

Video 14.7: Real-time full volume (wide-angle) 3-dimensional transesophageal echocardiography of MVP

Video 14.8: Real-time 3D zoom/live 3D (narrow-angle) 3-dimensional transesophageal echocardiography demonstrating a flail P2 leaflet with a ruptured chordae, typical of fibroelastic deficiency.

Video 14.9: Real-time full volume (wide-angle) 3-dimensional transesophageal echocardiography utilizing a simultaneous display of a multiplanar reformat in orthogonal planes and a 3D volume rendering of the region of interest (flail P2 scallop)

Video 14.10: Real-time 3D zoom/live 3D (narrow-angle) 3-dimensional transesophageal echocardiography demonstrating multi-scallop prolapse A1, P1 and P2 shown in from a left atrial view.

Video 14.11: Intraoperative video. Totally endoscopic robotic repair of the mitral valve. Following resection of the prolapsing P2 leaflet, the mitral valve has been sutured. Suturing of the annuloplasty ring prosthesis with the robotic arms is underway.

REFERENCES

Anyanwu AC, Adams DH. Etiologic Classification of Degenerative Mitral Valve Disease: Barlow's Disease and Fibroelastic Deficiency. Semin Thorac Cardiovasc Surg. 2007;19:90-6.

Barlow JB, Pocock WA. The significance of late systolic murmurs and mid-late systolic clicks. Md State Med J. 1963;12:76-7.

Bonow RO, onow RO, Carabello BA, et al. ACC/AHA 2006 guidelines for the management of patients with valvular heart disease. A report of the American College of Cardiology/ American Heart Association Task Force on Practice Guidelines (Writing Committee to Revise the 1998 Guidelines for the Management of Patients with Valvular Heart Disease). Circulation. 2006;114(5):e84-e231.

Carpentier A, Chauvaud S, Fabiani JN, et al. Reconstructive surgery of mitral valve incompetence: ten-year appraisal. J Thorac Cardiovasc Surg. 1980;79(3):338-48.

Carpentier A. Cardiac valve surgery—the "French correction". J Thorac Cardiovasc Surg. 1983;86(3):323-37.

Carpentier A, Adams DA, Filsoufi F. Textbook of Carpentier's Reconstructive Valve Surgery: From Valve Analysis to Valve Reconstruction. 2010, Saunders.

Filsoufi F, Chikwe J, Adams DH. Sabiston Textbook of Surgery 18th edition Philadelphia: Saunders 2008:Chapter 78.

Guy TS, Hill AC. Mitral Valve Prolapse. Annu Rev Med. 2012; 63:277-92.

Han Y, Peters DC, Salton CJ, et al. J Am Coll Card Imag. 2008; 1(3):294-303.

Kennett JD, Rust PF, Martin RH, et al. Observer Variation in the Angiocardiographic Diagnosis of Mitral Valve Prolapse. Chest. 1981;79:2.

Nifong LW, Chitwood WR, Pappas PS, et al. Robotic Mitral Valve Surgery: A United States Multicenter Trial. J Thorac Cardiovasc Surg. 2005;129(6):1395-404.

CHAPTER

Right-Sided Valvular Heart Disease

15

Ivan Anderson, Jason H Rogers

TRICUSPID REGURGITATION

Tricuspid Valve Anatomy

The tricuspid valve apparatus has three leaflets: (1) anterior; (2) posterior; and (3) septal. The leaflets are tethered by chordae tendineae, which are attached to papillary muscles contiguous with the right ventricular myocardium. While there are discrete anterior and posterior papillary muscles, the septal insertion of the chordae is directly on to the septal wall. The valve annulus is surrounded by the coronary sinus posteriorly, the atrioventricular node medially, and the right coronary artery, which courses in the atrioventricular groove anteriorly and posteriorly (Figs. 15.1 and 15.2). All of these structures become important considerations during tricuspid valve repair or replacement.

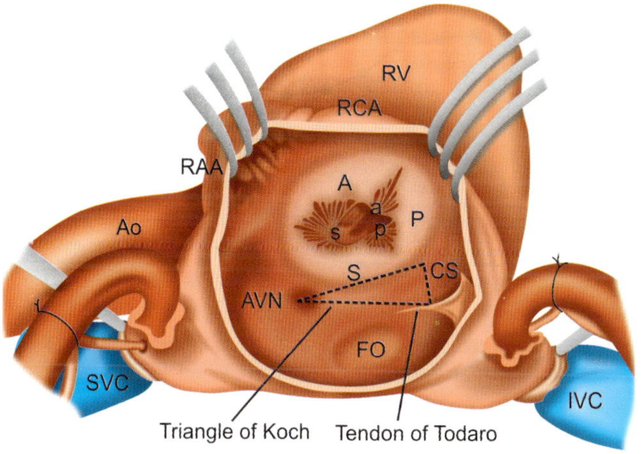

Fig. 15.1A: The tricuspid valve apparatus, surgical view. Note the three leaflets: anterior (A), posterior (P), and septal (S). There are three discrete papillary muscles: anterior (a), posterior (p), and septal (s). Directly adjacent to the septal leaflet is the triangle of Koch defined at its apex by the atrioventricular node (AVN), anteriorly by the septal leaflet, posteriorly by the coronary sinus (CS), and septally by the tendon of Todaro. (IVC: Inferior vena cava; SVC: Superior vena cava; FO: Fossa ovalis; Ao: Aorta; RAA: Right atrial appendage; RV: Right ventricle; RCA: Right coronary artery).

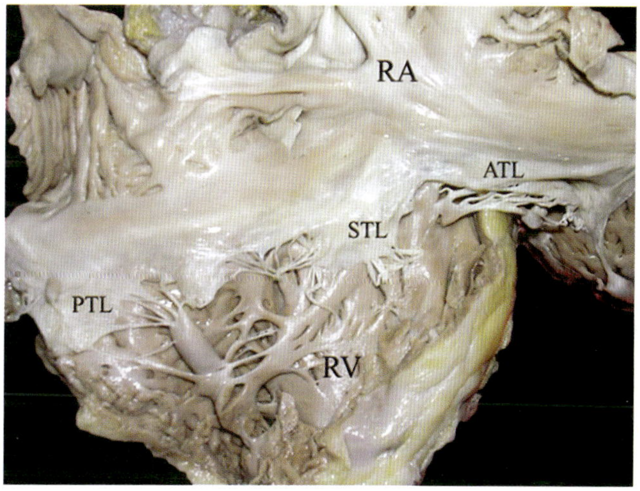

Fig. 15.1B: Anatomy of the tricuspid valve (TV). The TV has three leaflets: anterior (ATL), septal (STL) and posterior (PTL) and hence three commissures: anteroseptal, posteroseptal and anteroposterior. The leaflets are anchored to the RV endocardium via the chordae tendineae to the papillary muscles. The anterior group is constant, while the posterior is usually developed and the medial is occasionally developed [Image and legend text from Vaideeswar P. Examination of the heart—a comparative external and internal anatomy. In: Vijayalakshmi IB et al. (Ed). A Comprehensive Approach to Congenital Heart Disease. New Delhi, India: Jaypee Brothers Medical Publishers (P) Ltd]. (RA: Right atrium).

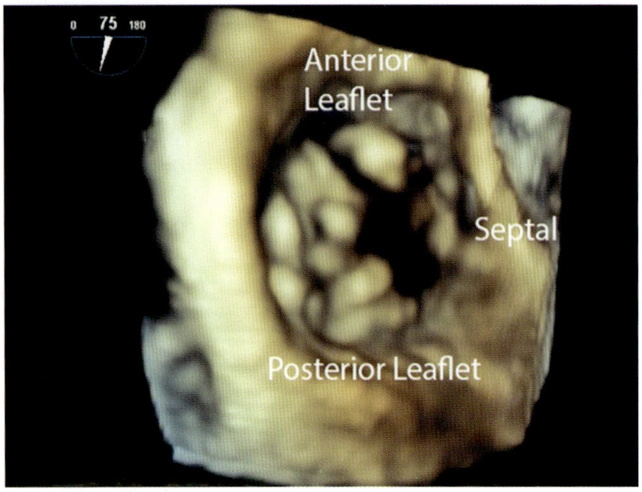

Fig. 15.2: The tricuspid valve as seen on transesophageal echocardiogram looking from right ventricle.

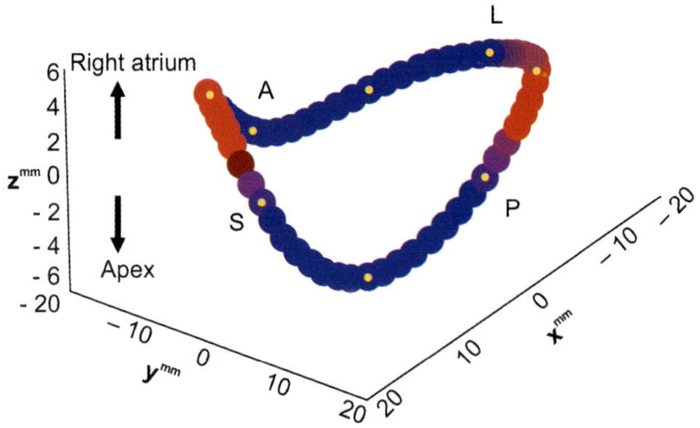

Fig. 15.3: Schematic demonstrating saddle shape of the tricuspid annulus. In the normal tricuspid valve annulus, the areas in red are closer to the atrium. Points in blue are closer to the right ventricle and apex of the heart. (Reproduced from Fukuda S et al. Three-dimensional geometry of the tricuspid annulus in healthy subjects and in patients with functional tricuspid regurgitation: a real-time, 3-dimensional echocardiographic study. Circulation. 2006;114:I492-8, with permission).

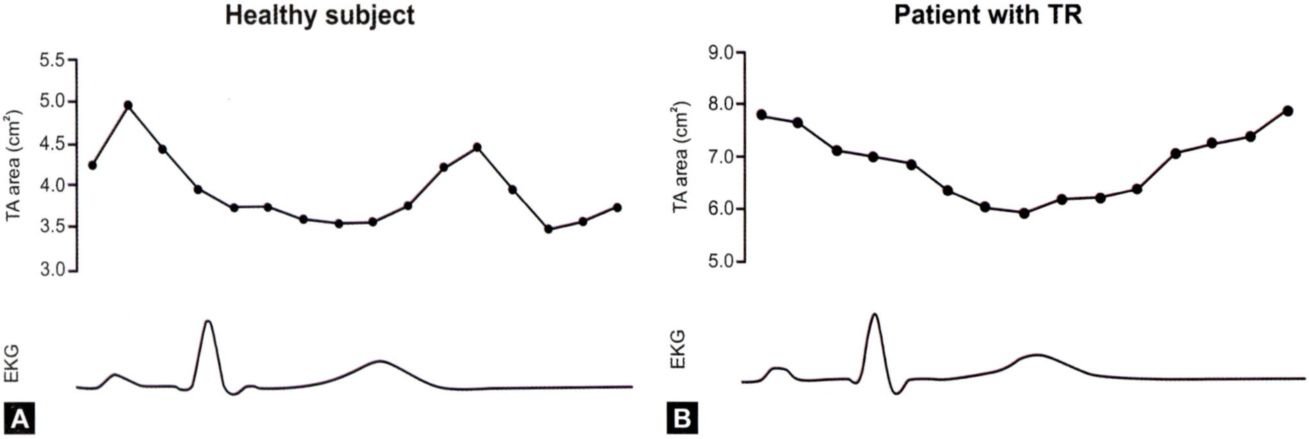

Figs. 15.4A and B: Tricuspid annulus (TA) excursion in a healthy subject (A) and in a patient with functional tricuspid regurgitation (TR). Notice that the healthy tricuspid annulus has the ability to dilate in early and late diastole. Reproduced from Circulation. 2006;114:1492-8 with permission from the Editor.

The tricuspid valve annulus is saddle shaped (Fig. 15.3). A healthy tricuspid annulus is dynamic through the cardiac cycle. As the annulus dilates, it becomes more planar and its motion becomes less dynamic throughout the cardiac cycle (Figs. 15.4A and B). There is a strong association between tricuspid annulus motion and right ventricular systolic function. In fact, tricuspid annular plane systolic excursion (TAPSE) as assessed with transthoracic echocardiography is a useful single measurement for the estimation of right ventricular systolic function (Fig. 15.5), although cardiac MRI provides much more refined measurement of right ventricular ejection fraction (Figs. 15.6A to F). As the tricuspid valve and right ventricle fail together, volume overload and dilation of the right ventricle are often seen on echocardiogram (Figs. 15.7A and B).

Causes of Tricuspid Regurgitation

Regurgitation (Figs. 15.7A and B & 15.8, videos 15.1 to 15.3) is by far more common as a cause of tricuspid valve pathology than stenosis. Functional regurgitation is the most common cause of tricuspid regurgitation (TR). Functional TR is typically the consequence of chronic pressure (Fig. 15.7A) and/or volume overload associated with

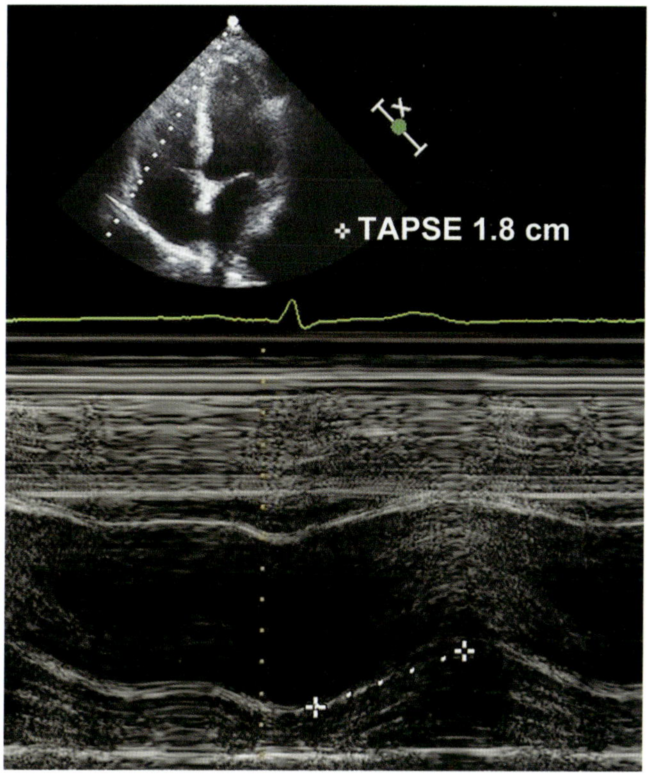

Fig. 15.5: Tricuspid annular plane systolic excursion (TAPSE). A pulse wave Doppler signal is placed on the plane of the tricuspid annulus, and M mode measurements are used to quantify the motion of the tricuspid annulus through the cardiac cycle.

congestive pulmonary venous hypertension from left heart failure. As the right ventricle dilates, the tricuspid annulus enlarges mostly in the anteroposterior dimension. This is because the septal annulus is contiguous with the interventricular septum and is relatively fixed in position.

Although the most common cause of functional TR is left-sided heart failure, a broader differential for primary and secondary TR exists and should be considered (Table 15.1). Pacer/defibrillator wire-associated TR is increasingly being recognized as an important cause of TR (Fig. 15.9). Endocarditis can cause leaflet destruction (Figs. 15.10A and B). Alternatively, myxomatous degeneration of the tricuspid valve can be seen (Fig. 15.11). A variety of other rarer causes of TR can include congenital defects, such as congenitally corrected transposition of the great vessels (Fig. 15.12).

Clinical Presentation and Diagnosis

A patient presenting with moderate to severe tricuspid valve regurgitation would typically present with signs of right-sided heart failure including lower extremity edema and elevated jugular venous pressure. Estimation of right heart pressure by measurement of jugular venous pulsation in centimeter of H_2O above the right atrium is frequently compromised in severe TR. This is because large V waves result from transmission of the higher right ventricular pressure being regurgitated through the incompetent tricuspid valve. Figure 15.13 demonstrates a hemodynamic tracing in a patient with CV fusion resulting in giant V waves.

A variety of echocardiographic and Doppler parameters have been established and codified in guidelines to classify the severity of TR (Table 15.2). As TR becomes severe, the jet density becomes more dense and early peaking (Fig. 15.14). The large regurgitant jet reaches the hepatic veins, leading to systolic flow reversal in the hepatic veins (Fig. 15.15). The vena contracta (Fig. 15.16) and proximal isovelocity surface area may be useful similar to as with mitral regurgitation to estimate TR severity. Valve morphology and right-sided chamber and inferior vena cava (IVC) size are also used in assessing severity of TR.

Valve Repair and Replacement

Surgical repair or replacement of the tricuspid valve (Figs. 15.17A to D) is generally not performed for asymptomatic severe TR alone. Rather, it is appropriately performed concomitantly at the time of other valvular heart surgery, or in cases of right ventricular failure (Tables 15.3 and 15.4). When repair or replacement of the tricuspid valve is necessary, a variety of surgical techniques are available. In general, rigid ring annuloplasty is preferred and gives the most durable result. In patients who require replacement, a bioprosthesis is usually preferred. Figures 15.18A to F show percutaneous valve-in-valve therapy, which can be used for the treatment of a failed bioprosthesis.

Pulmonic Regurgitation

The pulmonary valve is a semilunar valve (Figs. 15.19A and B), and is the most difficult valve to image by echocardiography due to poor echocardiographic windows in adults. The anterior location of the pulmonic valve also limits effectiveness of transesophageal echocardiography in capturing high-resolution imaging. Rarely, the pulmonary valve can be visualized in the parasternal short-axis view (Fig. 15.20).

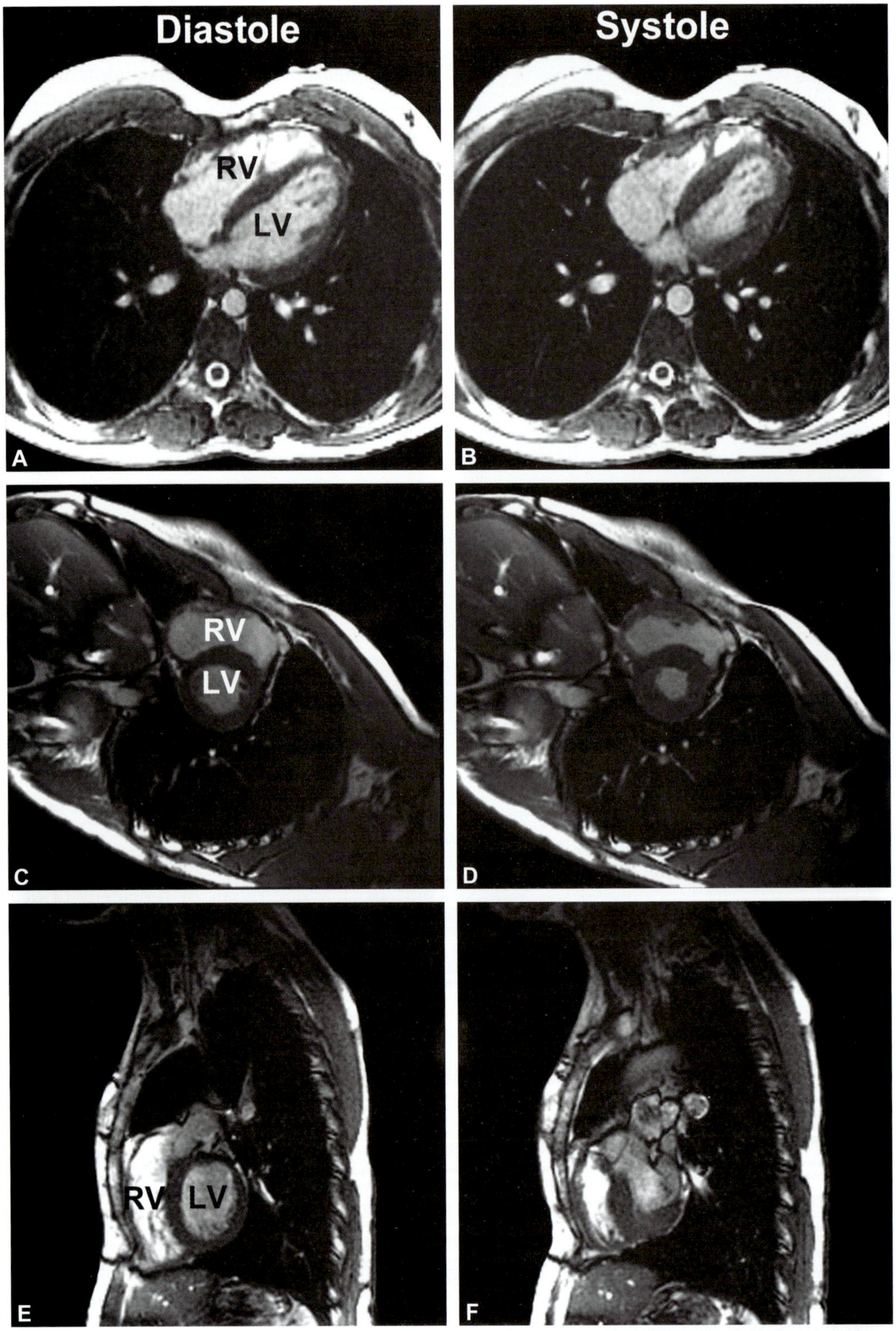

Figs. 15.6A to F: Cardiac MRI demonstrating views of the right ventricle used in calculation of the right ventricular ejection fraction. (A) Sagittal section through the right ventricle in a 4-chamber view with the right ventricle in diastole; (B) Sagittal section from (A) in systole; (C) Sagittal section through the right ventricle in a short-axis view in diastole; (D) The short-axis view from (C) in systole; (E) Coronal section of the right ventricle in diastole; (F) Coronal section of the right ventricle in systole. The ability of MRI to capture the complex structure of the right ventricle makes it the preferred imaging modality to assess right ventricular systolic function.

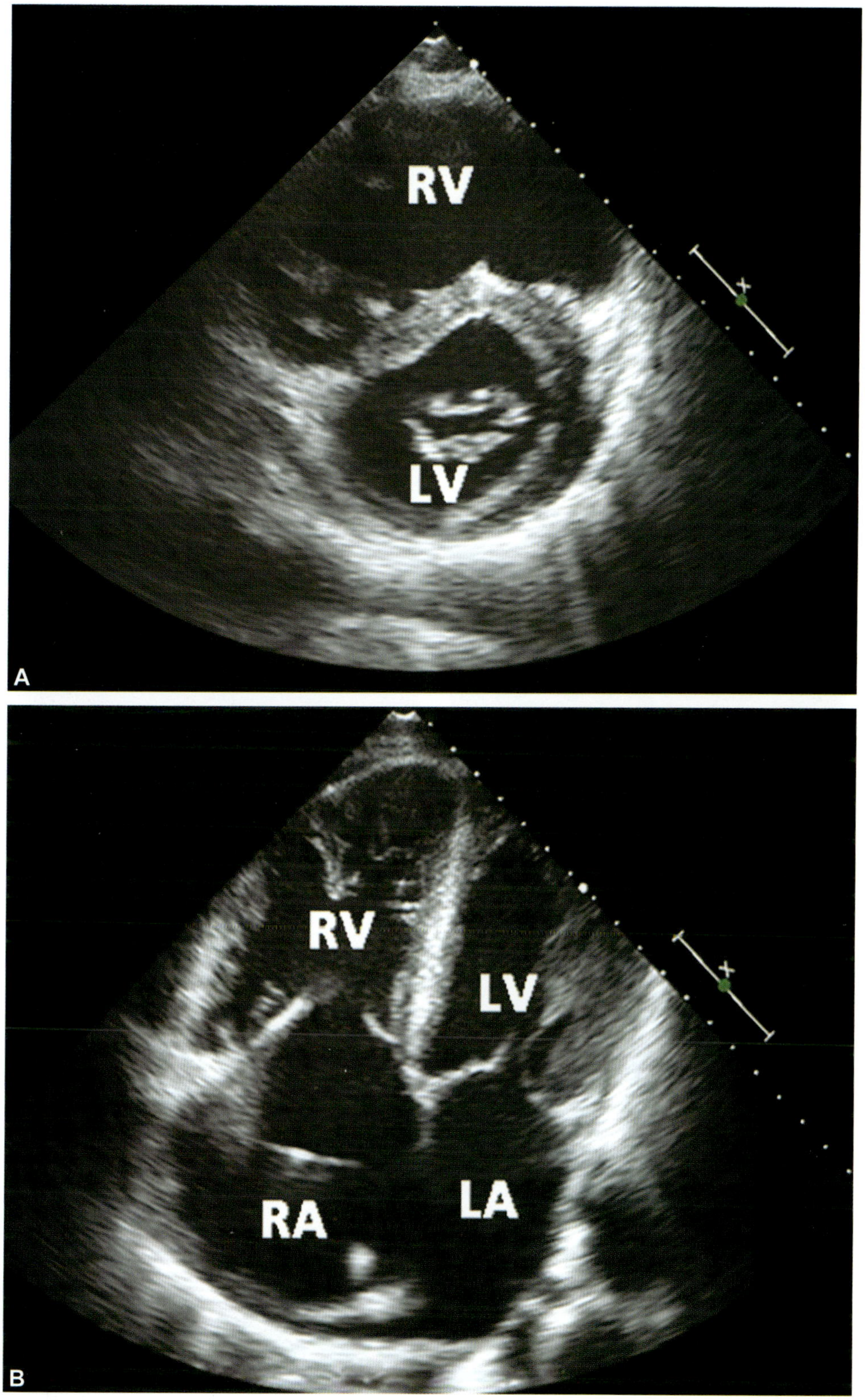

Figs. 15.7A and B: Right ventricular volume overload with resultant right ventricular dilation and tricuspid regurgitation. (A) Note the large right ventricular size in comparison with the left ventricle. The right ventricle itself is hypertrophied, and volume overload during diastole results in a D-shaped interventricular septum; (B) Right ventricle is markedly enlarged and the dilated tricuspid valve annulus has poor leaflet coaptation.

Table 15.1: Etiologies of tricuspid regurgitation.

Primary Causes (25%)	*Secondary Causes (75%)*
• Rheumatic • Myxomatous • Ebstein's anomaly • Endomyocardial fibrosis • Endocarditis • Carcinoid disease • Traumatic (blunt chest injury) • Iatrogenic (pacemaker/defibrillator)	• Left heart disease (left ventricular dysfunction or valve disease) • Any cause of pulmonary hypertension (idiopathic, pulmonary thrombo-embolism, left to right shunt) • Any cause of right ventricular dysfunction (myocardial disease, RV ischemia/infarction, chronic volume overload, e.g. from dialysis)

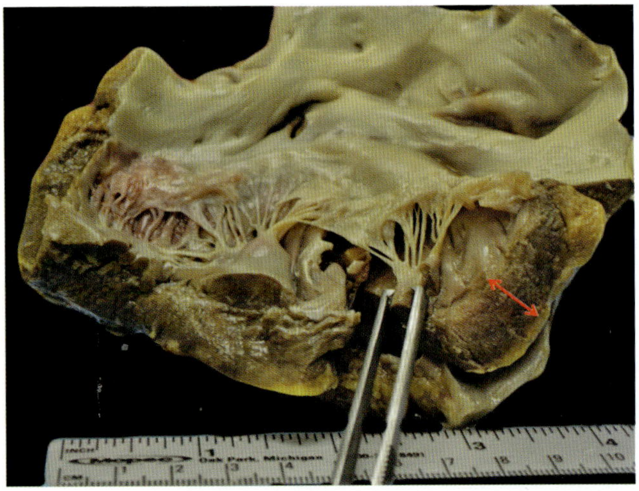

Fig. 15.8: A tricuspid valve situated within a hypertrophied right ventricle. In this patient, pulmonary hypertension led to right ventricular hypertrophy. Here the right ventricular wall thickness is around 11 mm in diameter. The normal right ventricular wall thickness is 5 mm or less.

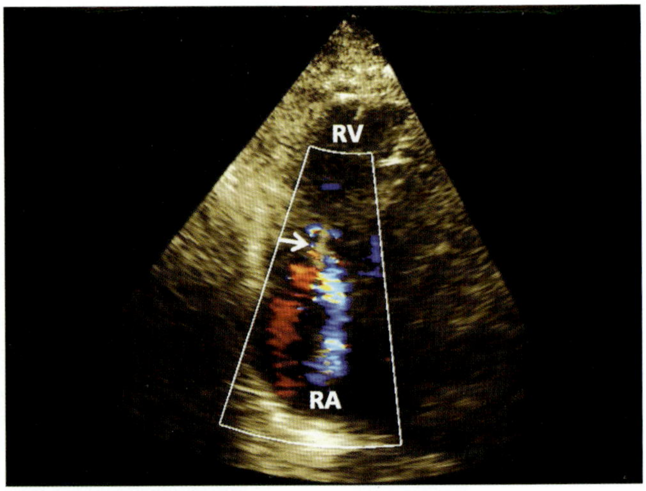

Fig. 15.9: Tricuspid regurgitation associated with a pacer wire. The echodensity central to the tricuspid valve is a pacer wire with a regurgitant jet seen on either side of it.

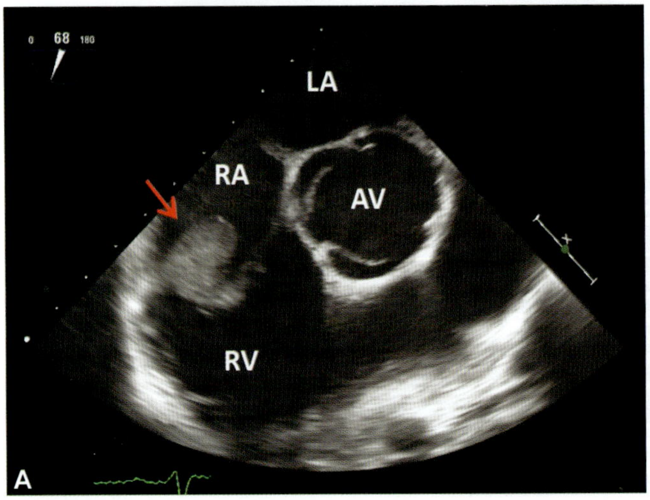

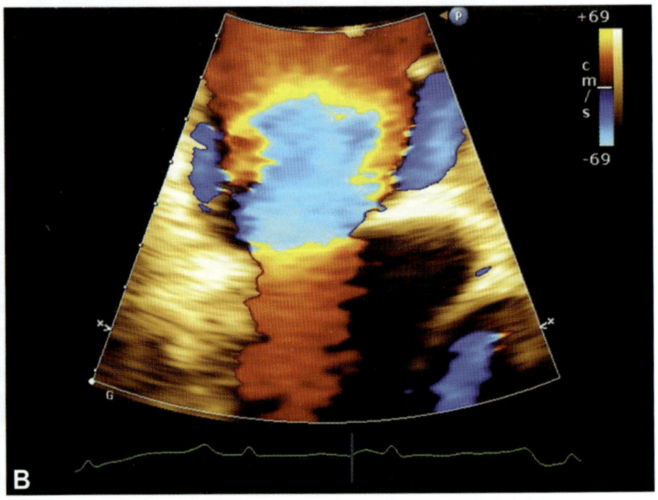

Figs. 15.10A and B: Transesophageal short-axis image showing tricuspid valve endocarditis (arrow) (Image courtesy of Glenn N Levine, MD); (B) Tricuspid regurgitation related to endocarditis. Note near total leaflet destruction. Notice the large, nonstandard isosurface velocity [Proximal isovelocity surface area (PISA) radius, the hemispherical Doppler signal projecting into the right atrium from the tricuspid valve].

Table 15.2: Parameters used in grading tricuspid regurgitation. Adapted from the American Society of Echocardiography Guidelines.

	Mild	*Moderate*	*Severe*
Valve leaflets	Normal	+/– Normal	Flail, poor coaptation, otherwise abnormal
IVC/RA/RV size	Normal	+/– Dilated	Dilated
Jet area (cm²)	< 5	5–10	> 10
Vena contracta width (cm)	Undefined	< 0.7	> 0.7
PISA radius (cm)	≤ 0.5	0.6–0.9	> 0.9
Jet density/contour	Soft and parabolic	Dense with variable contour	Dense with early peaking triangular contour
Hepatic vein flow	Systolic dominant	Systolic blunting	Systolic reversal

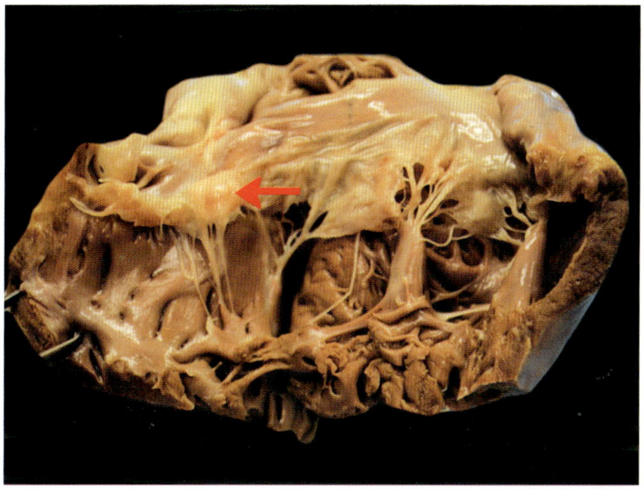

Fig. 15.11: Myxomatous degeneration of the septal leaflet (arrow) of the tricuspid valve. This is more commonly incidentally found post-mortem as it was in this patient.

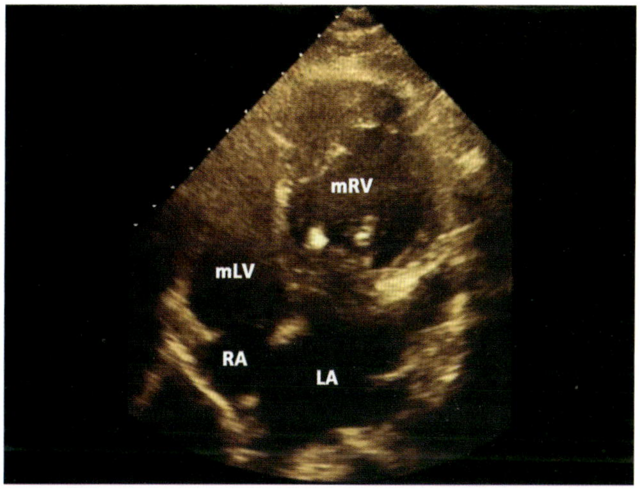

Fig. 15.12: Congenitally corrected levo-transposition of great vessels. In this case, a failing tricuspid valve manages the pressure load of the sub-systemic ventricle (right side of image, morphologic right ventricle mRV). A tipoff to this pathology is the relative position of the valve annuli. Typically, the tricuspid valve annulus is more apically displaced (as it is here within the morphologic RV/systemic ventricle). mLV, morphologic left ventricle which is the sub-pulmonic ventricle. Figure 15.7 provides a traditional 4-chamber view in a patient with preserved atrioventricular concordance to compare.

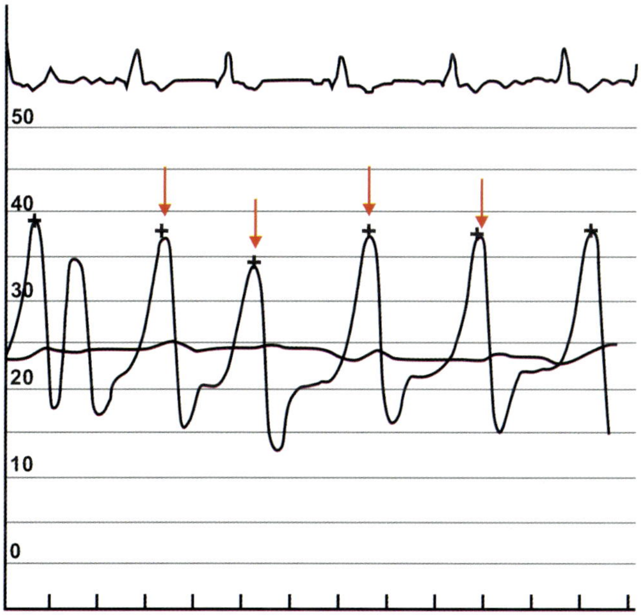

Fig. 15.13: Right atrial CV wave fusion waves seen with severe tricuspid regurgitation.

Similar to TR, minor pulmonic regurgitation (PR) is present in a large percentage of the healthy population. Pathologic PR is rare, and typically the consequence of pulmonary hypertension causing dilation of the pulmonary artery, right ventricular outflow tract (RVOT) and hence the pulmonic valve. Moderate to severe PR may be observed in the setting of prior congenital heart surgery. This is most common after surgical repair (Figs. 15.21A and B).

Given that the pulmonic valve is so difficult to image, establishing the severity of regurgitation by valve morphology is difficult and often not possible. Grading of severity relies heavily on Doppler parameters. Figures 15.21A and B demonstrate severe pulmonic insufficiency

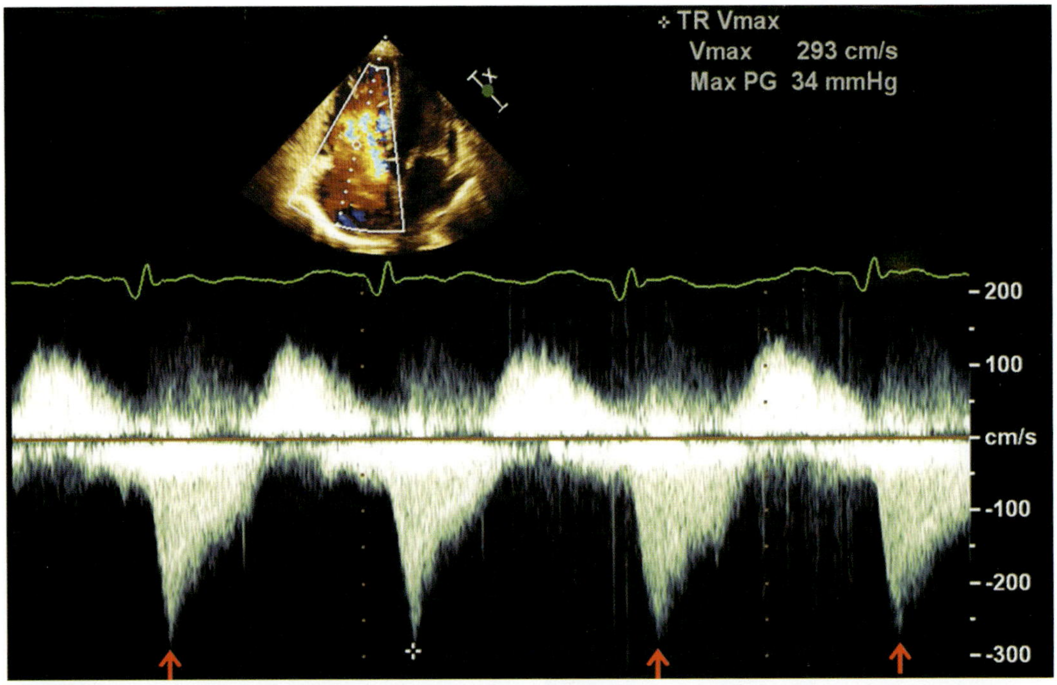

Fig. 15.14: Jet density as a measure of the severity of tricuspid regurgitation. This jet is very dense and early peaking.

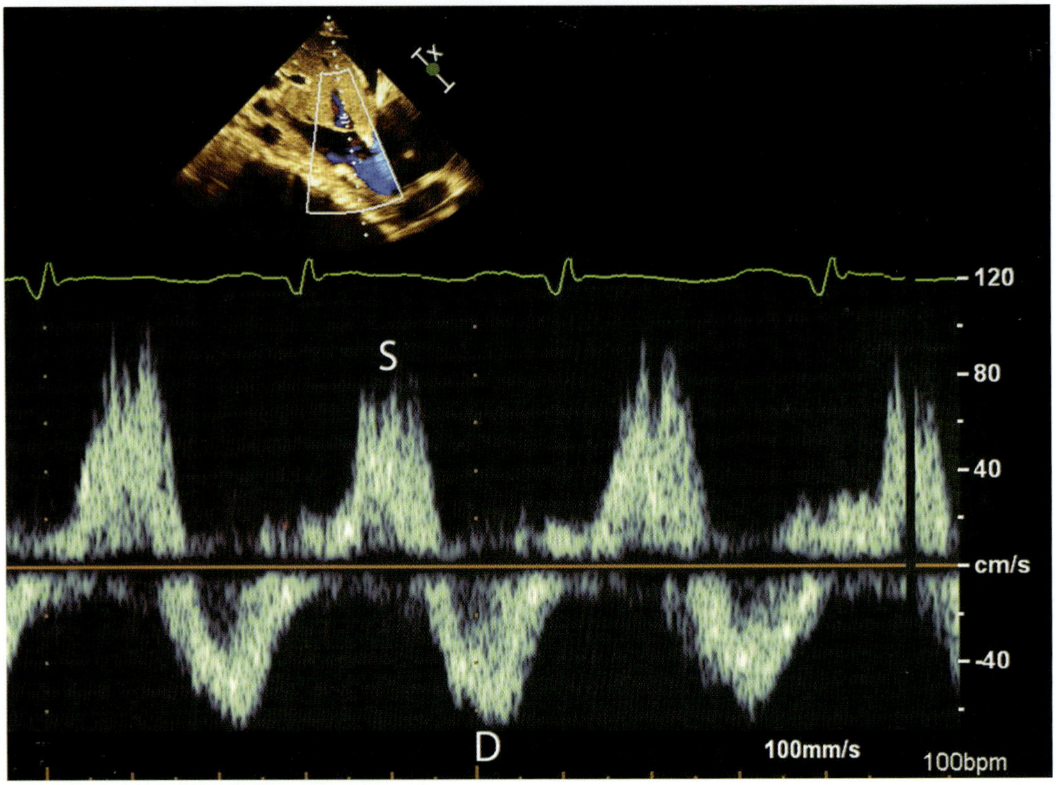

Fig. 15.15: Hepatic vein flow is a measure of the severity of tricuspid regurgitation. Notice that with severe regurgitation, there is systolic (S) blood flow reversal of hepatic vein flow. Normal hepatic vein flow is into the right atrium in both systole (S) and diastole (D) i.e. the S and D waves normally are in the same direction with negative velocities as imaged from this vantage point.

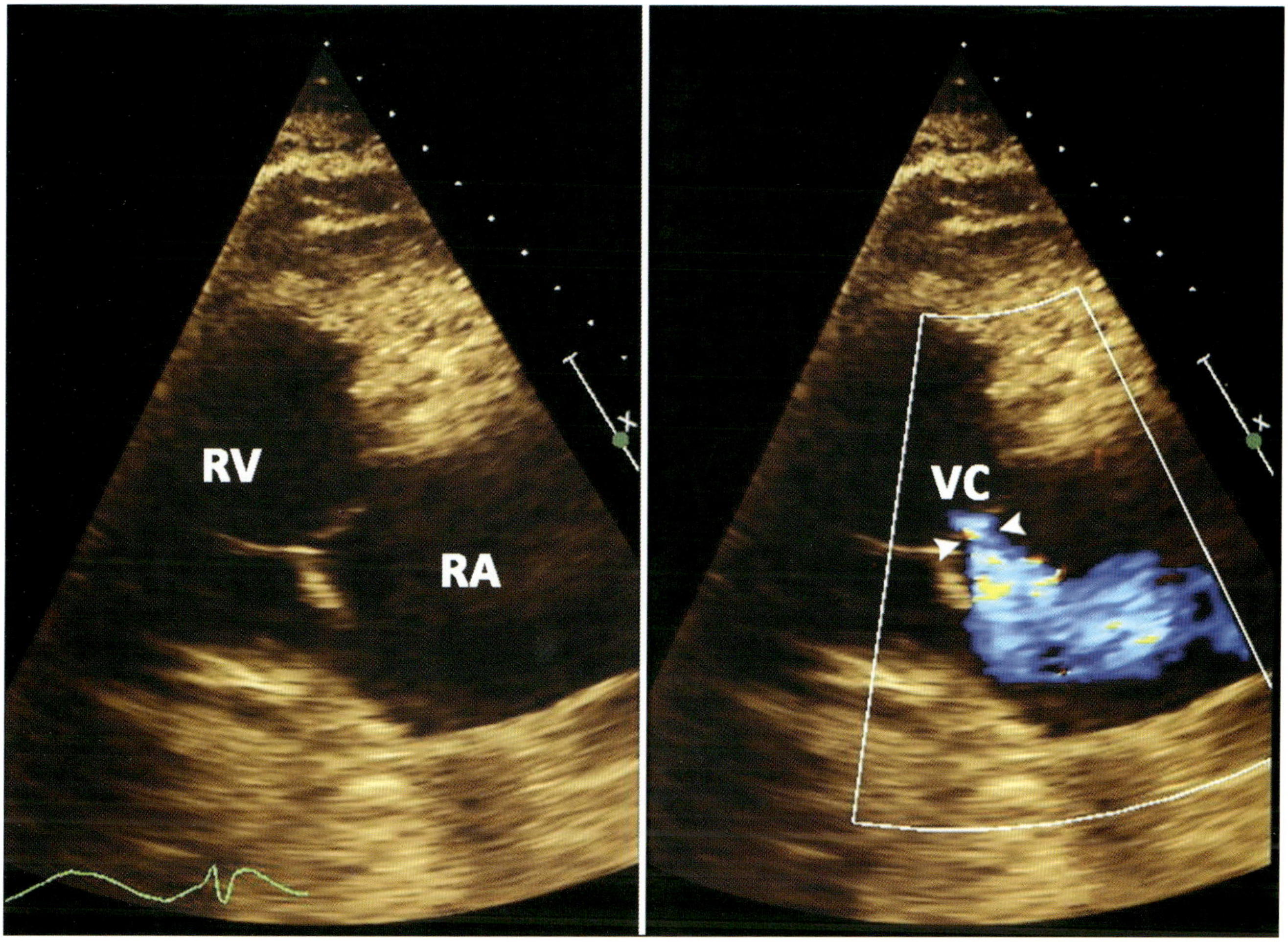

Fig. 15.16: The convergence point (between the arrowheads), labeled VC for vena contracta, is one parameter used in establishing severity of tricuspid regurgitation.

Table 15.3: Summary of the European Society of Cardiology/the European Association for Cardiothoracic Surgery (ESC/EACTS) guidelines for surgery in patients with tricuspid valve disease. The level of evidence (LOE) supporting the recommendation is given in parenthesis, where LOE = A denotes a recommendation derived from multiple randomized clinical trials or meta-analyses, LOE = B denotes a recommendation derived from a single randomized clinical trial or large non-randomized studies, and LOE = C denotes a recommendation based on consensus of expert opinion or based on small studies, retrospective studies, or registries.

Class I (is recommended and indicated)
• Surgery is indicated in patients with severe TS undergoing left-sided valve surgery (LOC = C) • Surgery is indicated in symptomatic patients with severe primary isolated TR without severe right ventricular dysfunction (LOE = C) • Surgery is indicated in symptomatic patients with severe TS (LOE = C)
Class IIa (should be considered)
• Surgery should be considered in patients with moderate primary TR undergoing left-sided valve surgery (LOE = C) • Surgery should be considered in patients with mild or moderate secondary TR with dilated annulus (> 40 mm or > 21 mm/m^2) undergoing left-sided valve surgery (LOE = C) • After left-sided valve surgery, surgery should be considered in patients with severe TR who are symptomatic or have progressive right ventricular dilation/dysfunction, severe right or left ventricular dysfunction, and severe pulmonary vascular disease (LOE = C)

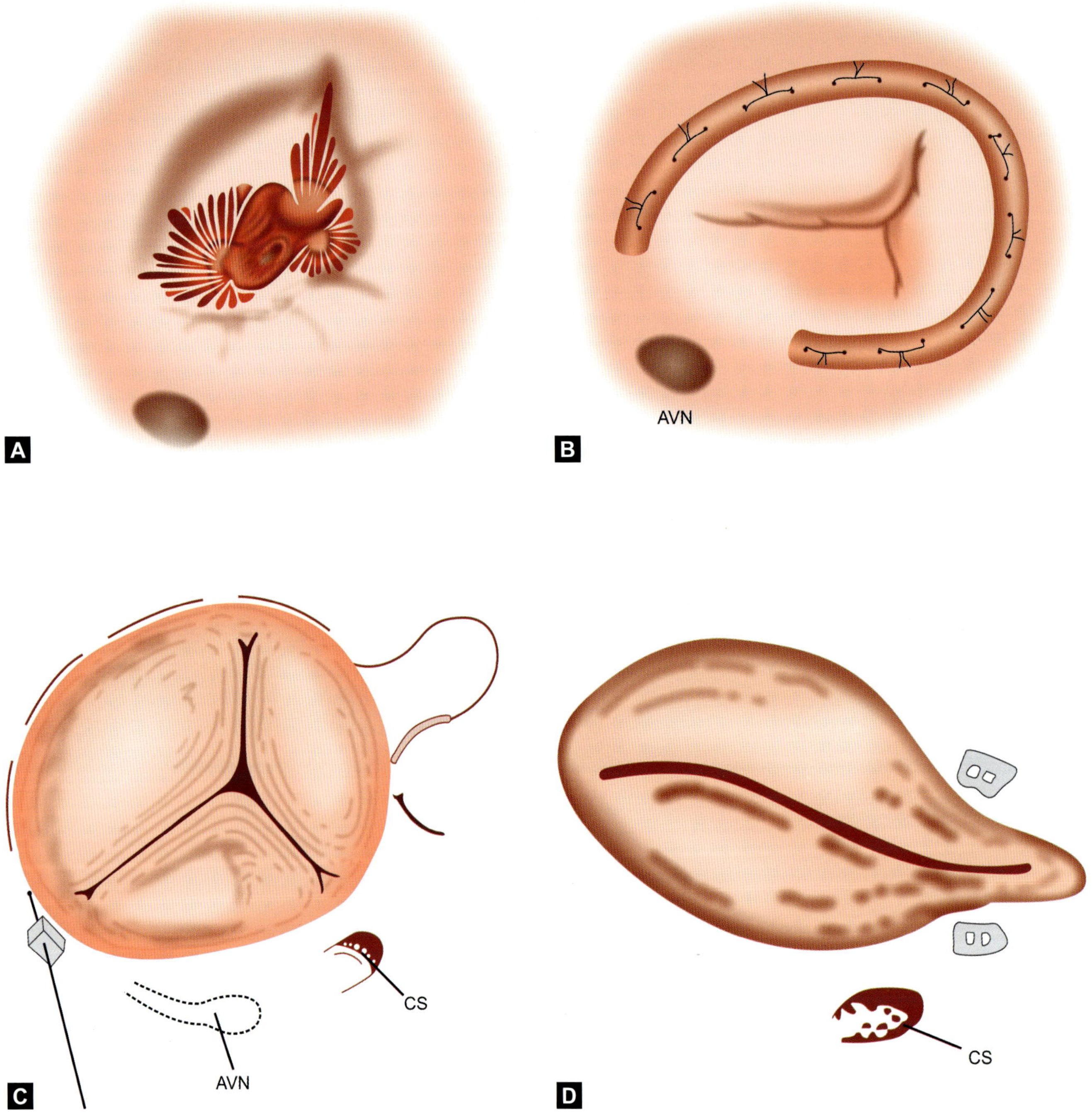

Figs. 15.17A to D: Surgical techniques for tricuspid valve repair: (A) functional TR with annular dilation, (B) rigid tricuspid annuloplasty ring, (C) suture (DeVega) annuloplasty, (D) bicuspidalization. (Adapted from Rogers JH, Bolling SF. The tricuspid valve: current perspective and evolving management of tricuspid regurgitation. Circulation. 2009;119:2718-25, with permission).

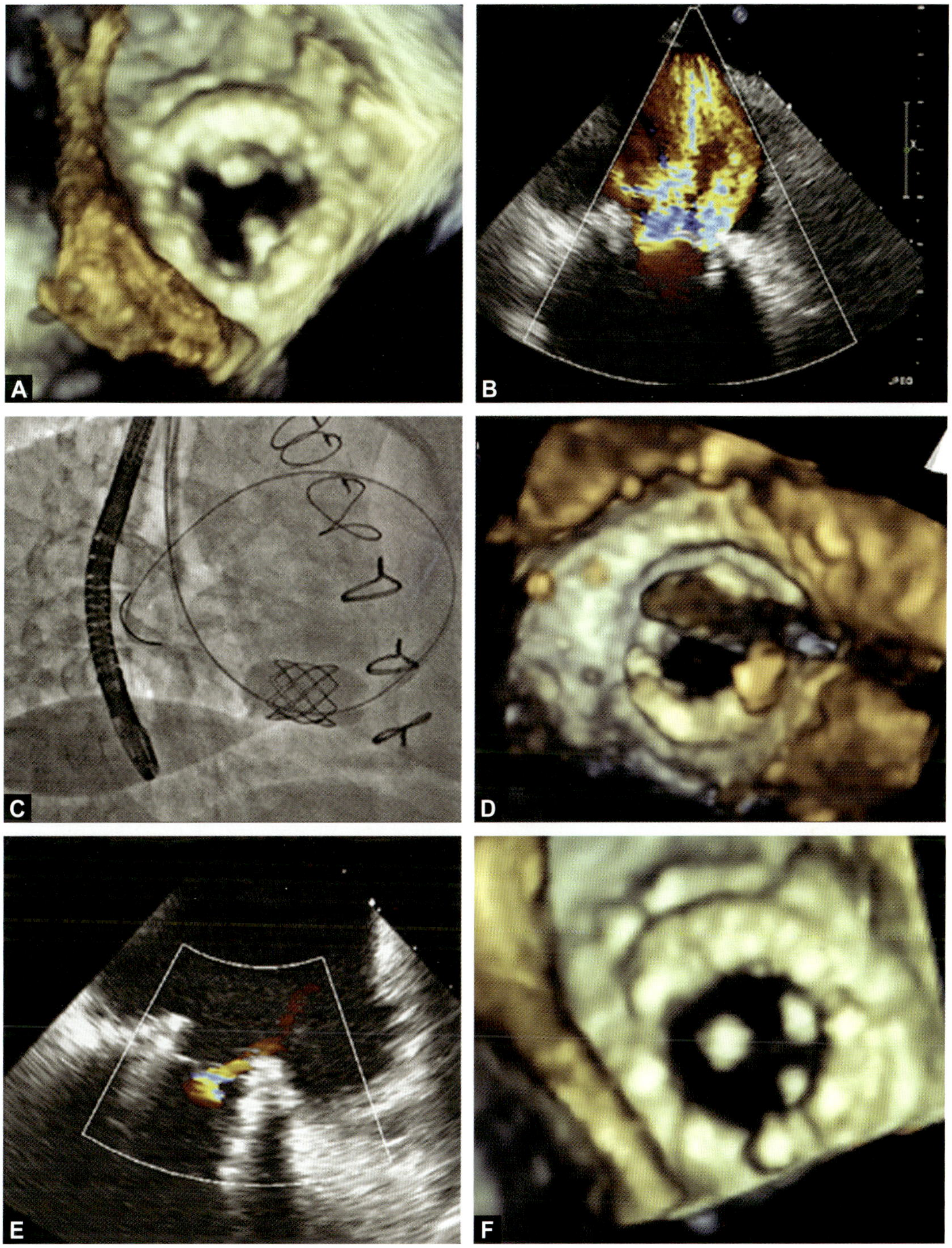

Figs. 15.18A to F: Transcatheter valve-in-valve therapy for a failed bioprosthesis. Shown above is a Melody valve, designed to be implanted in a failed bioprosthesis. In this case a failed bioprosthetic tricuspid valve is replaced. (A) A failed bioprosthetic tricuspid valve on a three-dimensional transesophageal echocardiogram (3-D TEE); (B) Severe tricuspid regurgitation of a previously implanted bioprosthesis is seen (the chamber closer to the echo probe is the right atrium); (C) The valve is deployed over a balloon in the tricuspid position. Venous access if through the right internal jugular vein. A wire is seen seated in the pulmonary artery, as is a transesophageal echo probe in this right anterior oblique view on fluoroscopy; (D) The melody valve is seen inside the failed bioprosthesis on 3-D TEE prior to deployment; (E) Post-procedure tricuspid regurgitation through the new valve is markedly reduced when compared with (B) above; (F) A post-procedure 3-D TEE shows the stent struts of the Melody valve (Reproduced from the editors). (Reprinted from Cullen MW et al. Transvenous, antegrade melody valve-in-valve implantation for bioprosthetic mitral and tricuspid valve dysfunction: a case series in children and adults. JACC. Cardiovascular Interventions. 2013;6:598-605, with permission).

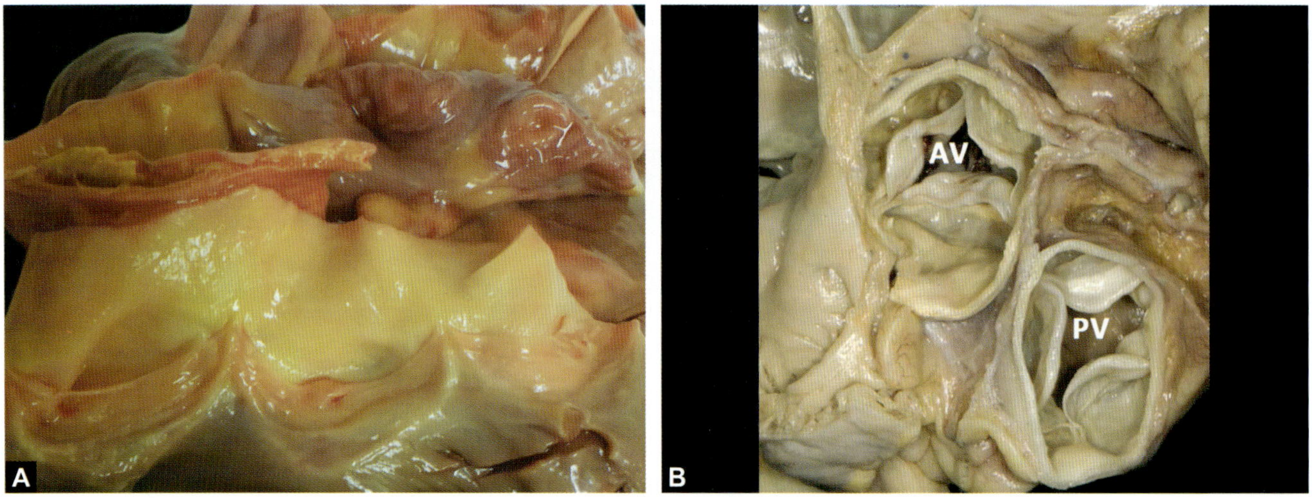

Figs. 15.19A and B: (A) Autopsy specimen of a normal pulmonic valve. There are three leaflets: right, left, and anterior. Note the normal fibrous node seen at the midpoint of each leaflet; (B) Gross pathology specimen of the semilunar valves. [Image courtesy of Dr. Philip C. Ursell, Department of Pathology, UCSF. Image from Cheitlin M, Ursell P. Cardiac anatomy. In: Chatterjee K et al. (Ed). Cardiology—An Illustrated Textbook. New Delhi, India: Jaypee Brothers Medical Publishers (P) Ltd.]. (AV: Aortic valve; PV: Pulmonic valve).

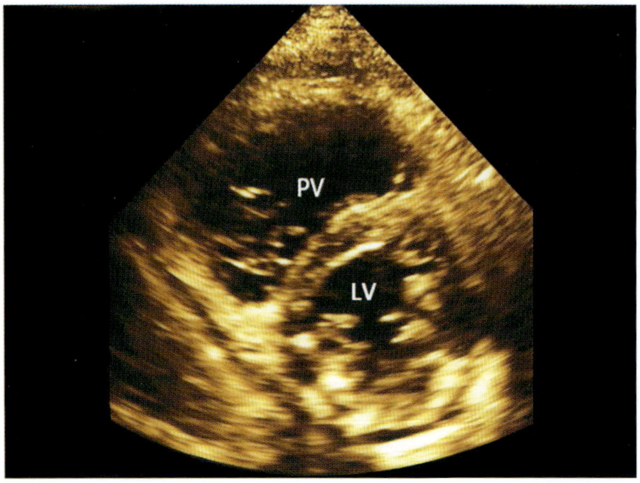

Fig. 15.20: Parasternal short-axis view demonstrates the trileaflet, semilunar pulmonic valve (PV) rarely visualized in this view.

that occurred years after surgical repair. Figure 15.22 demonstrates a Doppler recording of the valve seen in Figures 15.21A and B. An example of the hemodynamics of severe PR is shown in Figure 15.23. Guidelines suggest that it is reasonable to replace the pulmonic valve in the setting of severe regurgitation and ≥NYHA II symptoms.

TRICUSPID STENOSIS

Tricuspid stenosis (TS) is the least common valve pathology of the heart. A variety of causes of TS exist. The differential diagnosis for TS has significant overlap with secondary causes of TR and includes carcinoid syndrome, pacemaker-induced adhesions, lupus valvulitis, rare congenital malformations (Fig. 15.24), and obstructive tumors. Assessment of the severity of TS is akin to that for mitral stenosis (MS). Measurements should be taken at heart rates less than 100 bpm, ideally at 70–80 bpm. Unlike MS, planimetry of the tricuspid valve is rarely feasible, and the estimated valve area is more accurately assessed by pressure half-time ($T_{1/2}$) using a constant of 190 as opposed to 220 for MS. ACCF/AHA valvular heart disease guidelines include stages C and D (severe TS) findings of a pressure half-time of ≥190 msec and a valve area of ≤1.0 cm^2. Figures 15.25 and 15.26 demonstrate a case of TS related to a large mass of endocarditis with valve area calculated by velocity time integral. Guidelines for treatment of TS are given in Table 15.3.

PULMONIC STENOSIS

The vast majority (95%) of cases of pulmonic stenosis (PS) are congenital. A classic dome-shaped conical valve is the most common morphology seen with congenital PS, and is the result of fusion of the commissures. Other described malformations include dysplastic thickened leaflets, and congenital bicuspid pulmonic valves (Fig. 15.27). Rheumatic PS has also been described. Subvalvular or infundibular PS has been described, especially in the setting of ASD (Figs. 15.28A to D).

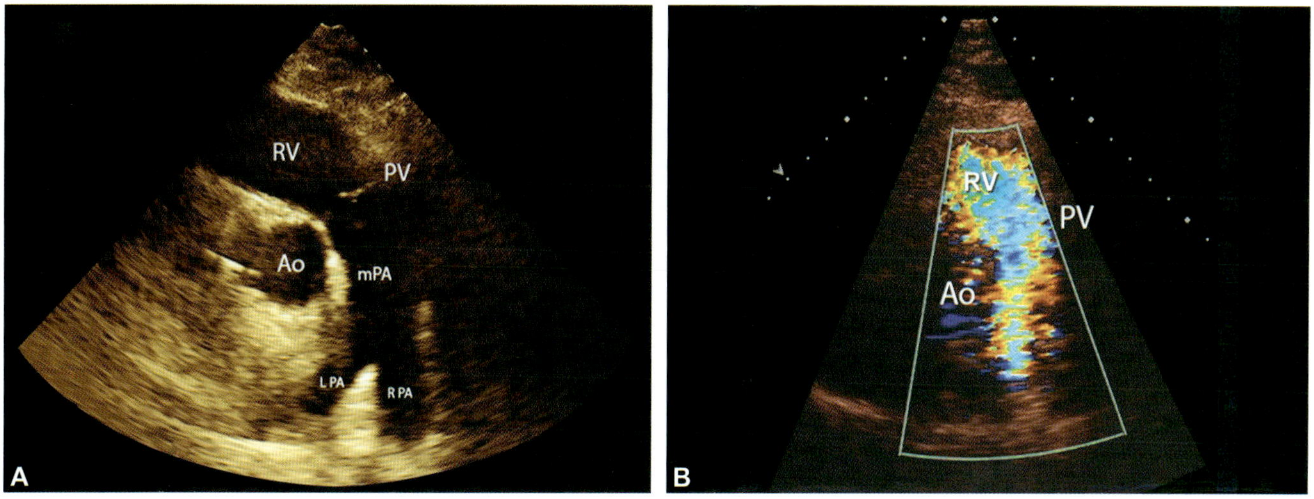

Figs. 15.21A and B: Pulmonic insufficiency from failed homograft. The figure shows normal anatomy seen on a parasternal short-axis view; (B) A failed pulmonic valve homograft (PV) is seen in the same view (parasternal short axis). There is turbulence seen related to pulmonary stenosis as well as pulmonary regurgitation with color flowing back into the right ventricle through the pulmonic valve. (Ao: Aortic valve; LPA: Left pulmonary artery; mPA: Main pulmonary artery; PV: Pulmonic valve; RPA: Right pulmonary artery; Ao: Aortic valve; PV: Pulmonic valve; RV: Right Ventricle)

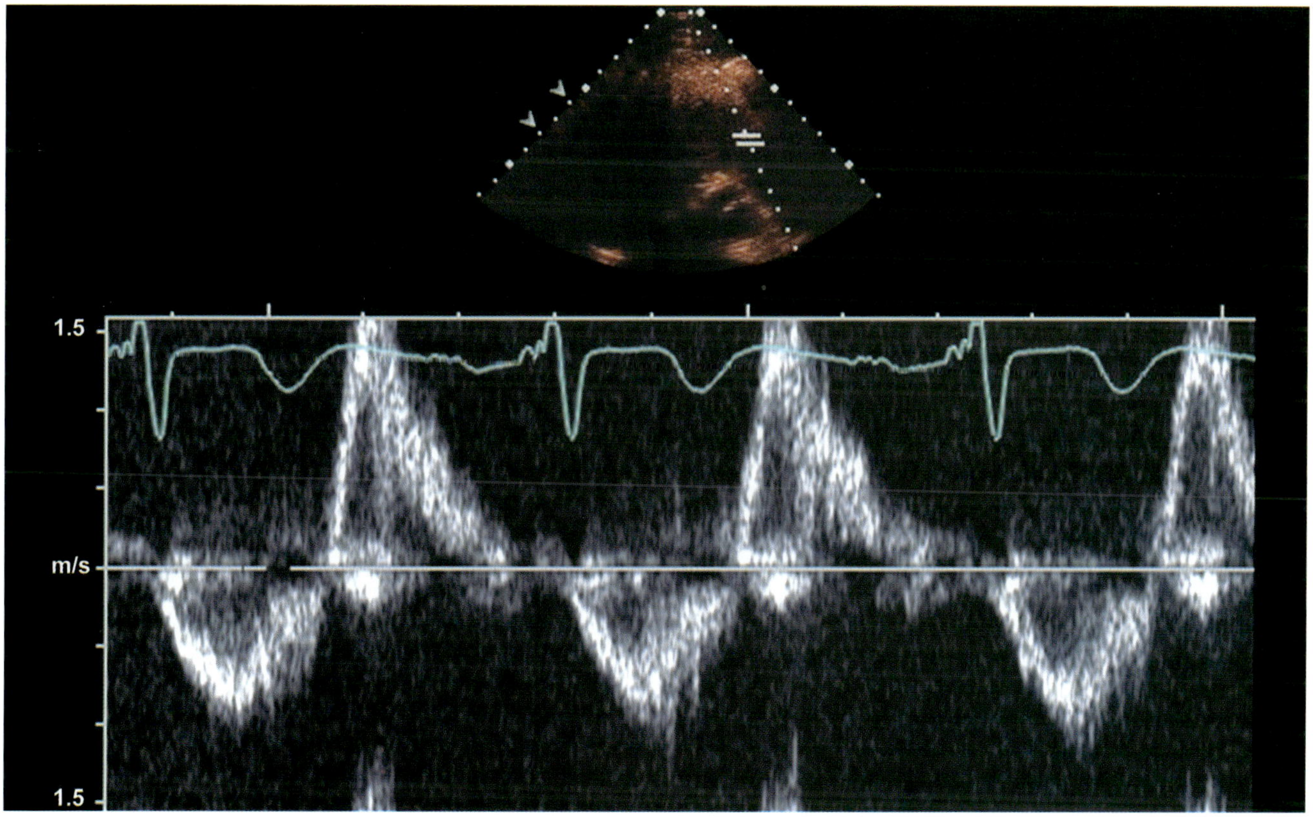

Fig. 15.22: Pulsed wave Doppler across the pulmonic valve seen above in Figure 15.21 shows the sine wave pattern associated with concomitant stenosis and regurgitation.

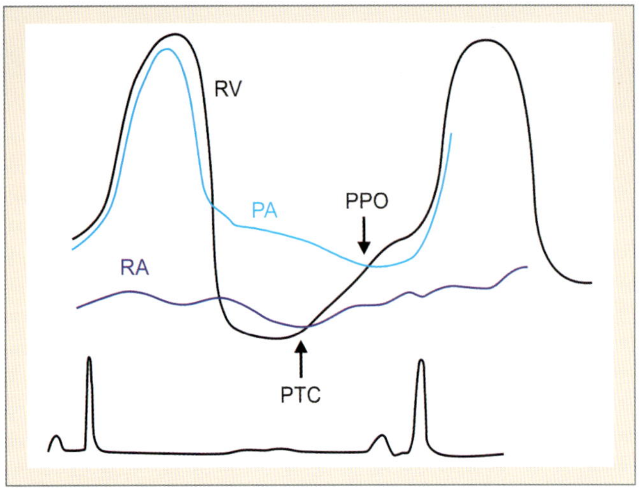

Fig. 15.23: Right heart hemodynamics in severe pulmonary regurgitation. Premature tricuspid valve closure (PTC) occurs in mid-diastole, when right ventricular diastolic pressure (RV; black line) exceeds right atrial pressure (RA; purple line). Premature pulmonic valve opening (PPO) occurs when right ventricular end-diastolic pressure rises above pulmonary artery (PA) diastolic pressure. [Image and legend text from Moorthy A, Kallarakkal JT. Pulmonary valve disease. In: Vijayalakshmi IB et al. (Ed). A Comprehensive Approach to Congenital Heart Disease. New Delhi, India: Jaypee Brothers Medical Publishers (P) Ltd.].

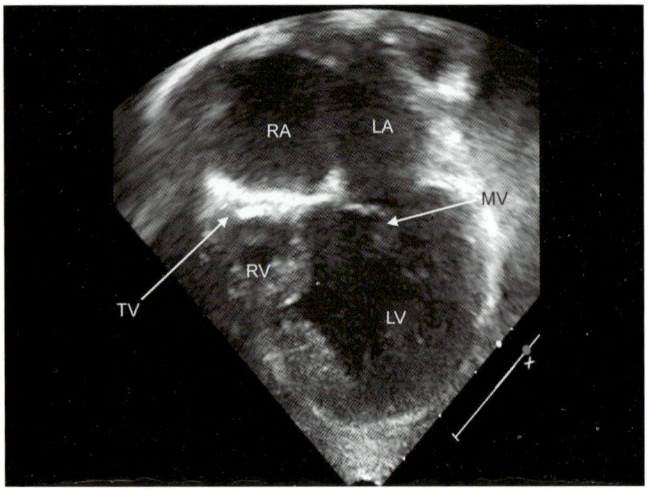

Fig. 15.24: Apical 4-chamber transthoracic echocardiogram (TTE) showing tricuspid atresia, an extreme form of tricuspid stenosis. There is a dense echodensity at the site of where the tricuspid valve should be [Image from Rao PS. Tricuspid atresia. In: Vijayalakshmi IB et al. (Ed). A Comprehensive Approach to Congenital Heart Disease. New Delhi, India: Jaypee Brothers Medical Publishers (P) Ltd.].

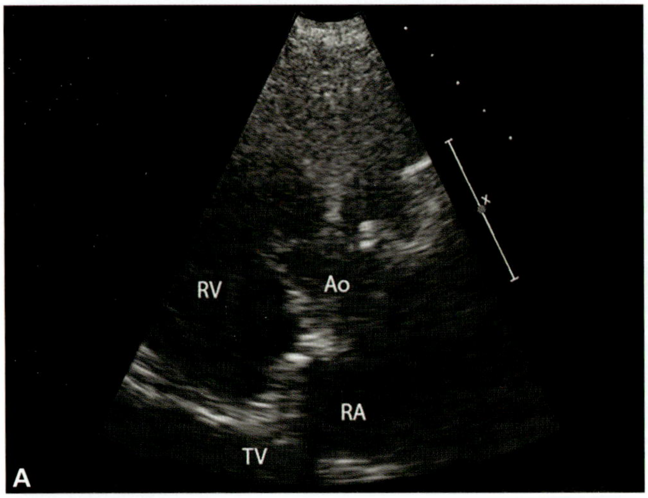

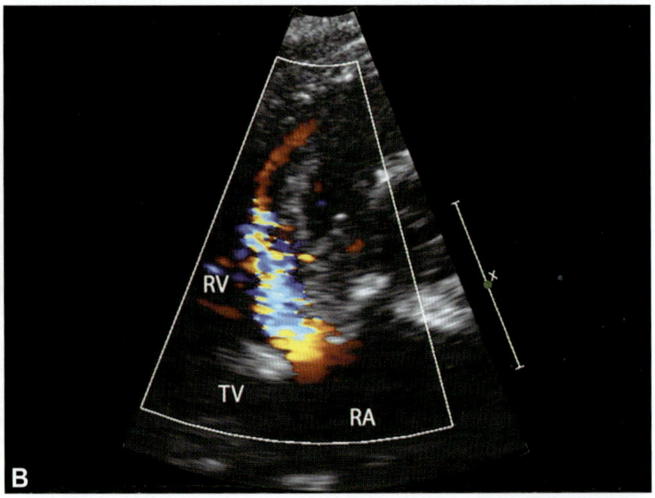

Figs. 15.25A and B: Predominant tricuspid stenosis with mild regurgitation resulting from recurrent endocarditis in a patient with a previous tricuspid valve replacement. Figure A shows the tricuspid valve in the parasternal short axis on a transthoracic echocardiogram. Figure B shows the same view with Doppler color added.

Table 15.4: ACCF/AHA guidelines for tricuspid valve repair or replacement in patients with tricuspid valve disease. The level of evidence (LOE) supporting the recommendation is given in parenthesis, where LOE = A denotes a recommendation derived from multiple randomized clinical trials or meta-analyses, LOE = B denotes a recommendation derived from a single randomized clinical trial or non-randomized studies, and LOE = C denotes a recommendation based on consensus of expert opinion, standard of care, or case reports. MS = mitral stenosis; MVA = mitral valve area; NYHA = New York Heart Association; PMBC = percutaneous mitral balloon commissurotomy.

Class I (is recommended; is indicated)
• Tricuspid valve surgery for patients with severe TR undergoing left-sided valve surgery (LOE = C)
Class IIa (can be beneficial)
• Tricuspid valve repair for patients with mild, moderate, or greater functional TR at the time of left-sided valve surgery with either (1) tricuspid annular dilation or (2) prior evidence of right-sided heart failure LOE = B)
• Tricuspid valve surgery for patients with symptoms due to severe primary TR that are unresponsive to medical therapy (LOE = C)
Class IIb (may be considered)
• Tricuspid valve repair for patients with moderate functional TR and pulmonary artery hypertension at the time of left-sided valve surgery (LOE = C)
• Tricuspid valve surgery for asymptomatic or minimally symptomatic patients with severe primary TR and progressive degrees of moderate or greater RV dilation and/or systolic dysfunction (LOE = C)
• Reoperation for isolated tricuspid valve repair or replacement for persistent symptoms due to severe TR (stage D) in patients who have undergone previous left-sided valve surgery and who do not have severe pulmonary hypertension or significant RV systolic dysfunction (LOE = C)

Table 15.5: ACCF/AHA criteria for severe (stage C and D) pulmonic stenosis.

Valve Anatomy	*Valve Hemodynamics and Hemodynamic Consequences*	*Symptoms*
• Thickened, distorted, calcified leaflets with systolic doming and/or reduced excursion • Other anatomic abnormalities such as narrowed RVOT	• Vmax >4 m/s • Peak instantaneous gradient >64 mm Hg • RVH • Possible RV, RA enlargement • Poststenotic enlargement of main PA	• None or variable symptoms, depending on the severity of obstruction

Auscultatory findings characteristic of PS include a crescendo-decrescendo murmur, and, depending on PS severity, may include an ejection click, and/or widely split second heart sound (Fig. 15.29). With severe PS, the ECG shows right ventricular hypertrophy and right axis deviation (Fig. 15.30). Spectral Doppler echocardiography demonstrates a significant transvalvular gradient (Fig. 15.31). ACCF/AHA valvular guidelines list hemodynamic findings in severe pulmonic stenosis stages (stages C and D) as a peak velocity of >4 m/sec and a peak instantaneous gradient >64 mm Hg (Table 15.5). Associated hemodynamic consequences with severe PS include right ventricular hypertrophy, possible right ventricular and right atrial enlargement, and poststenotic enlargement of the main pulmonary artery.

Guidelines support balloon valvulotomy (Figs. 15.32A to C) for PS in symptomatic patients. For pulmonic valves with stenosis and leaflet destruction or where balloon valvuloplasty is not otherwise an option (e.g. with moderate to severe concomitant pulmonic insufficiency) pulmonary valve replacement is an option. Figures 15.33A and B demonstrates a three-dimensional transesophageal echocardiogram of a pulmonic bioprosthesis.

ASSESSMENT OF RIGHT VENTRICULAR FUNCTION IN PATIENTS WITH RIGHT-SIDED VALVE DISEASE

All right-sided valvular heart disease must be taken in the overall context of right ventricular function. As discussed above, TAPSE (Fig. 15.34) can be used to assess right ventricular systolic function on echocardiography. TAPSE of < 16 mm is considered to be a sign of right ventricular dysfunction. A limitation of TAPSE is that it measures the right ventricle in only one dimension. The shape of the right ventricle (similar to a bellows) is complicated and lends poorly to mathematical modeling of systolic function, especially when assessed in only one or two views. Doppler tissue imaging (DTI) is also used to assess right ventricular systolic function. Right ventricular systolic velocity (Fig. 15.35) measured during DTI of < 10 cm/sec is considered to be abnormal. Right ventricular systolic function is best approximated with cardiac CT or MRI (Figs. 15.36 and 15.37).

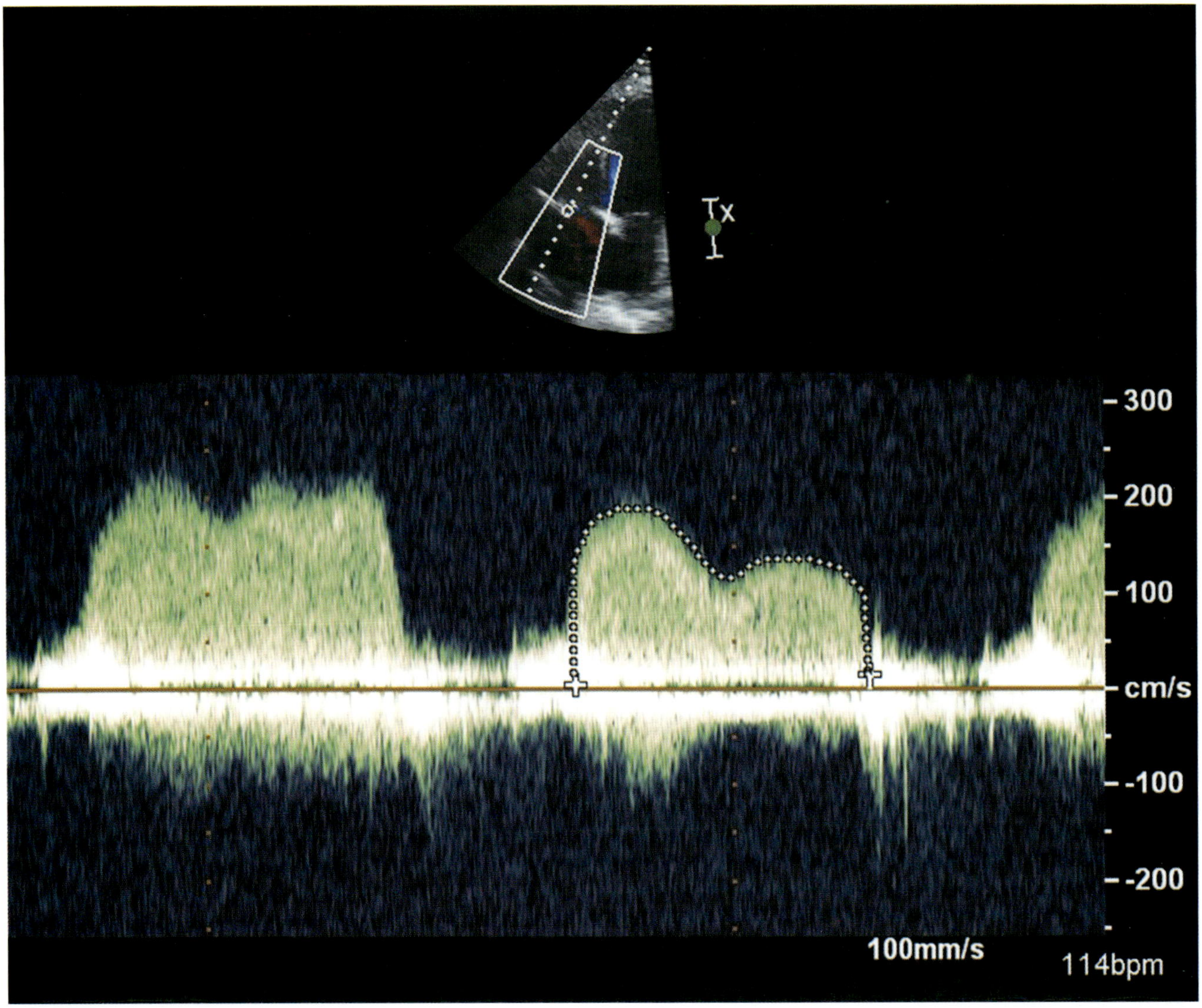

Fig. 15.26: Velocity time integral (VTI) is one means used to establish a gradient in tricuspid stenosis similarly to mitral stenosis. The mean gradient across this stenotic tricuspid valve is 9 mm Hg.

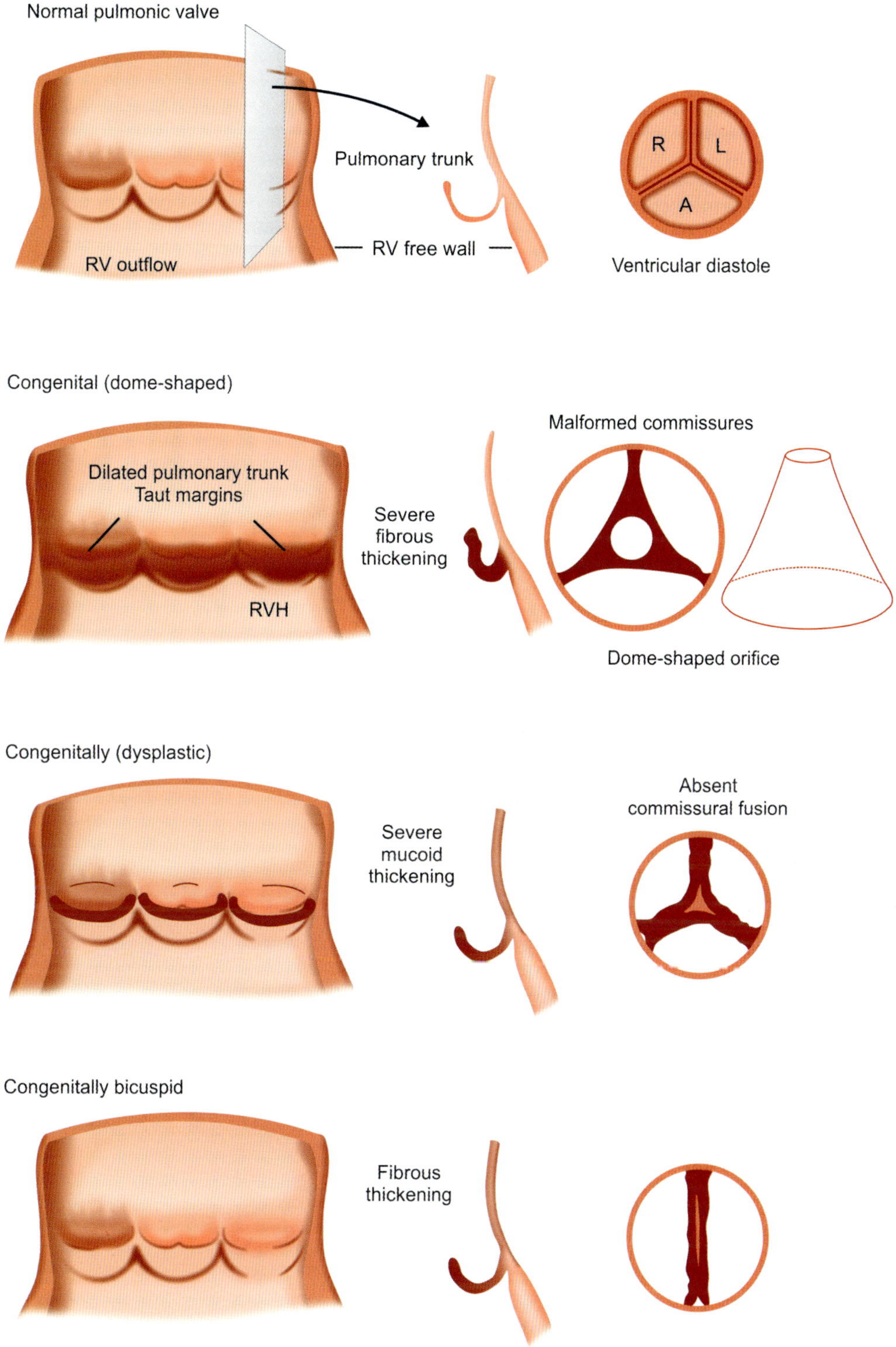

Fig. 15.27: Anatomy of the normal pulmonary valve and various congenital causes of pulmonic stenosis (Adapted from Waller BF et al. Pathology of pulmonic valve stenosis and pure regurgitation. Clinical Cardiology. 1995;18:45-50, with permission).

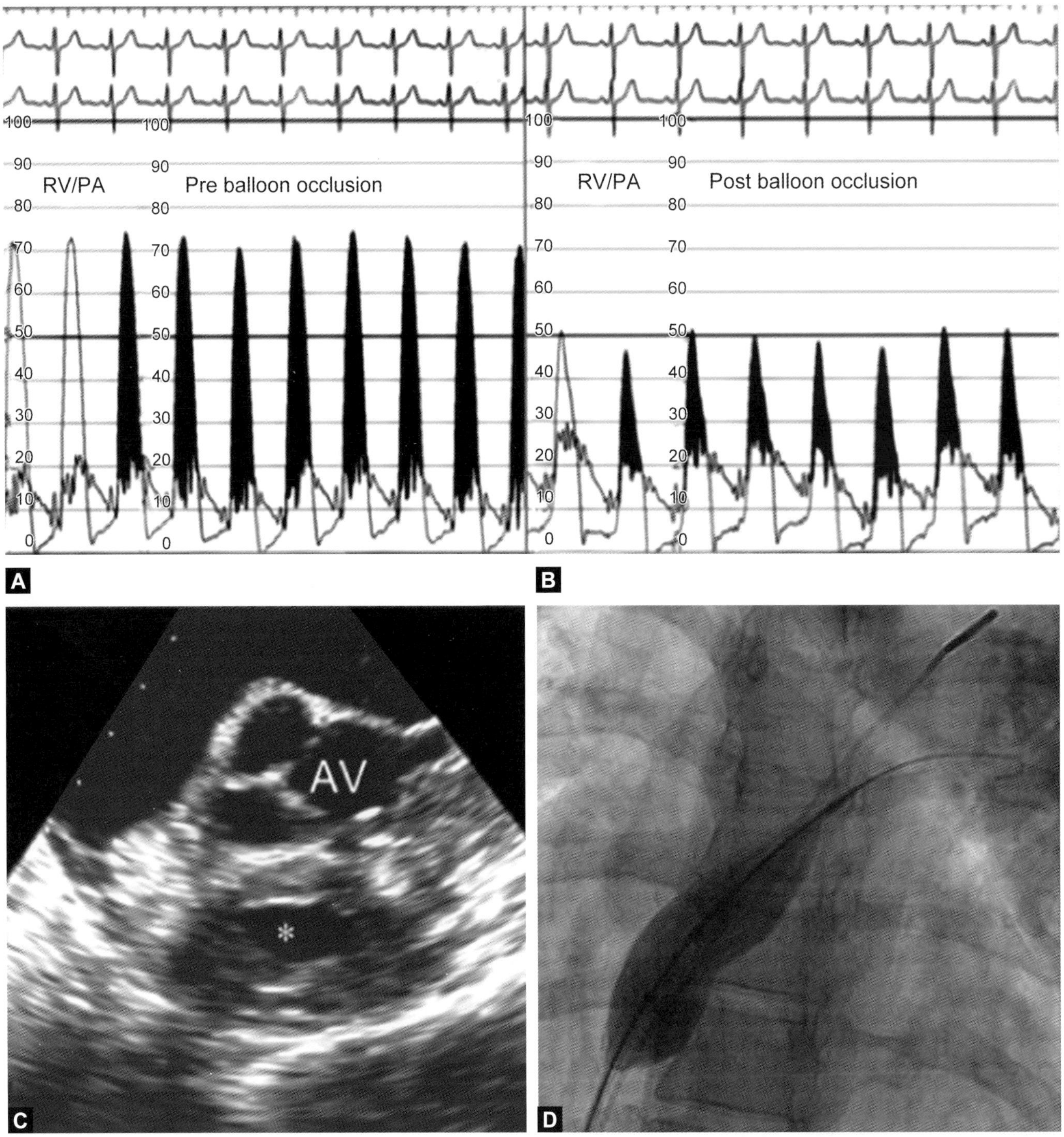

Figs. 15.28A to D: Pulmonic stenosis assessment with simultaneous right ventricular (RV) and pulmonary artery (PA) pressures before (A) and after (B) temporary balloon occlusion of a moderate-sized atrial septal defect (D). Note that the transpulmonic gradient decreases significantly with balloon occlusion as a result of decreased left-to-right shunting through the ASD. (C) Patient has mild muscular narrowing of the right ventricular outflow tract (asterisk) which is not clinically significant. (Adapted from Javed U, Levisman J, Rogers JH. A tale of two balloons: assessment of hemodynamics with atrial septal defect temporary balloon occlusion. The Journal of Invasive Cardiology. 2012;24:248-9, with permission).

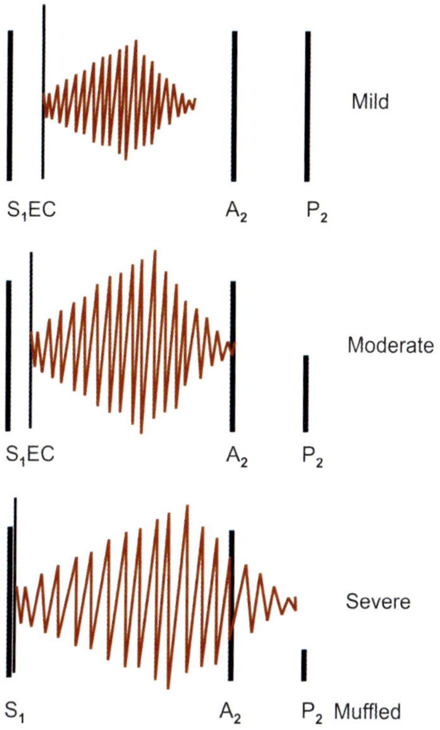

Fig. 15.29: Schematic illustration of auscultatory findings in valvular pulmonic stenosis. In mild stenosis, the ejection click (EC) is clearly separated from the first heart sound (S1). The murmur starts with the click, peaks in early systole, and ends before the aortic component of the second heart sound (A2). The pulmonary component of the second heart sound (P2) is normal or decreased in intensity. In moderate pulmonic stenosis, the click is closer to the first heart sound, the ejection murmur peaks later in the systole and the murmur reaches A2 and the second heart sound is widely split with soft pulmonary component. In severe valvar obstruction, the click is either absent or occurs so close to S1 that it cannot be heard separately, and the murmur peaks late in systole and extends beyond the A2. The second heart sound is widely split with an extremely soft or inaudible P2. [Image and legend text from Moorthy A, Kallarakkal JT. Pulmonary valve disease. In: Vijayalakshmi IB et al. (Ed). A Comprehensive Approach to Congenital Heart Disease. New Delhi, India: Jaypee Brothers Medical Publishers (P) Ltd.].

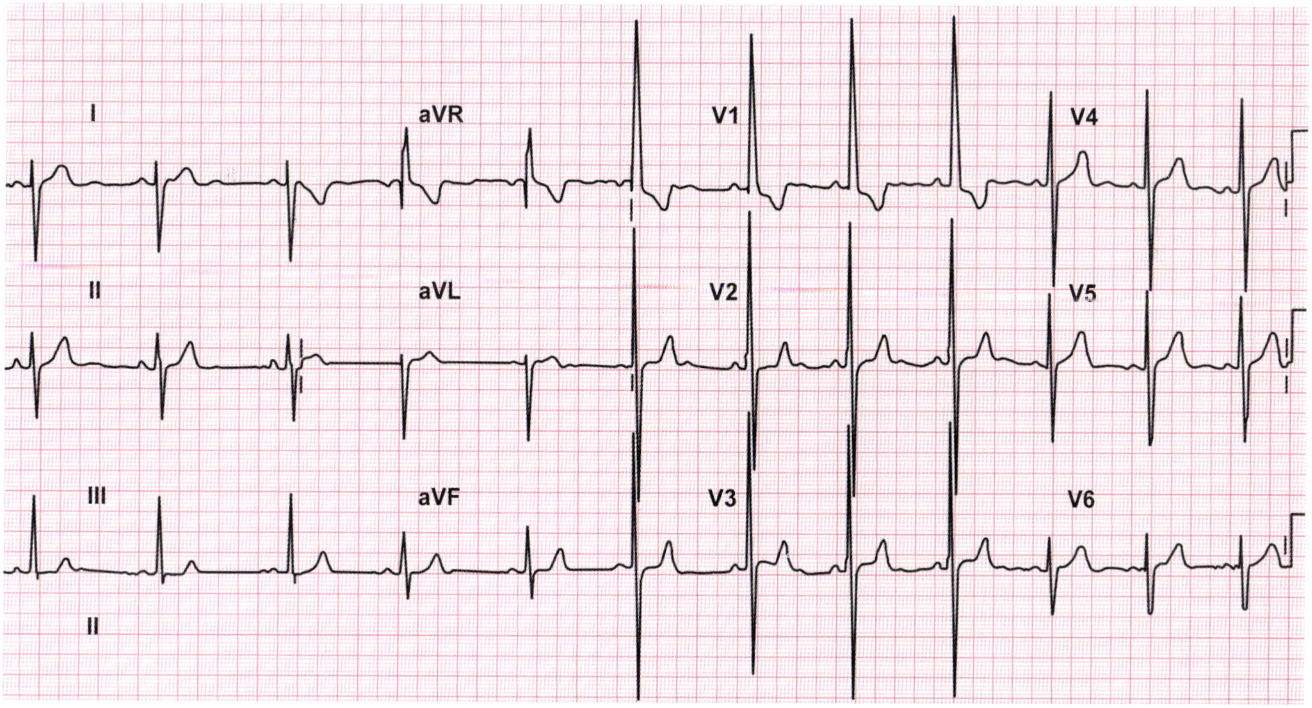

Fig. 15.30: 12 lead ECG from a patient with severe pulmonic valve stenosis. The ECG shows right axis deviation and marked right ventricular hypertrophy with RV strain pattern in lead V1. [Image from Moorthy A, Kallarakkal JT. Pulmonary valve disease. In: Vijayalakshmi IB et al. (Ed). A Comprehensive Approach to Congenital Heart Disease. New Delhi, Inida: Jaypee Brothers Medical Publishers (P) Ltd.].

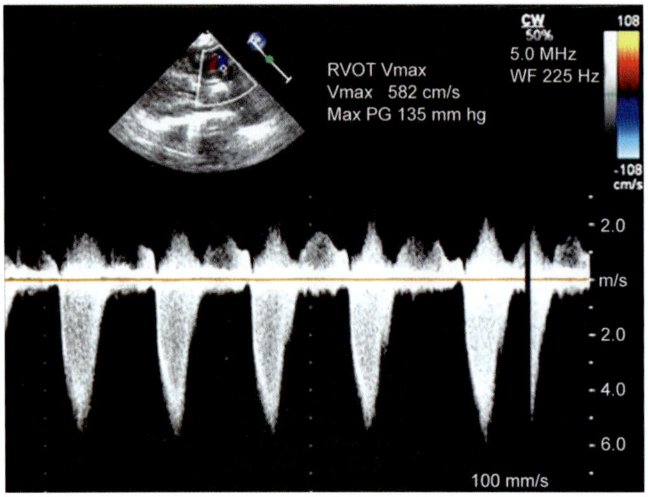

Fig. 15.31: Continuous wave (CW) Doppler across the pulmonic valve demonstrating severe pulmonic valve stenosis, with a peak velocity of 5.8 m/sec and a peak gradient of 135 mm Hg. [Image from Moorthy A, Kallarakkal JT. Pulmonary valve disease. In: Vijayalakshmi IB et al. (Ed). A Comprehensive Approach to Congenital Heart Disease. New Delhi, India: Jaypee Brothers Medical Publishers (P) Ltd.].

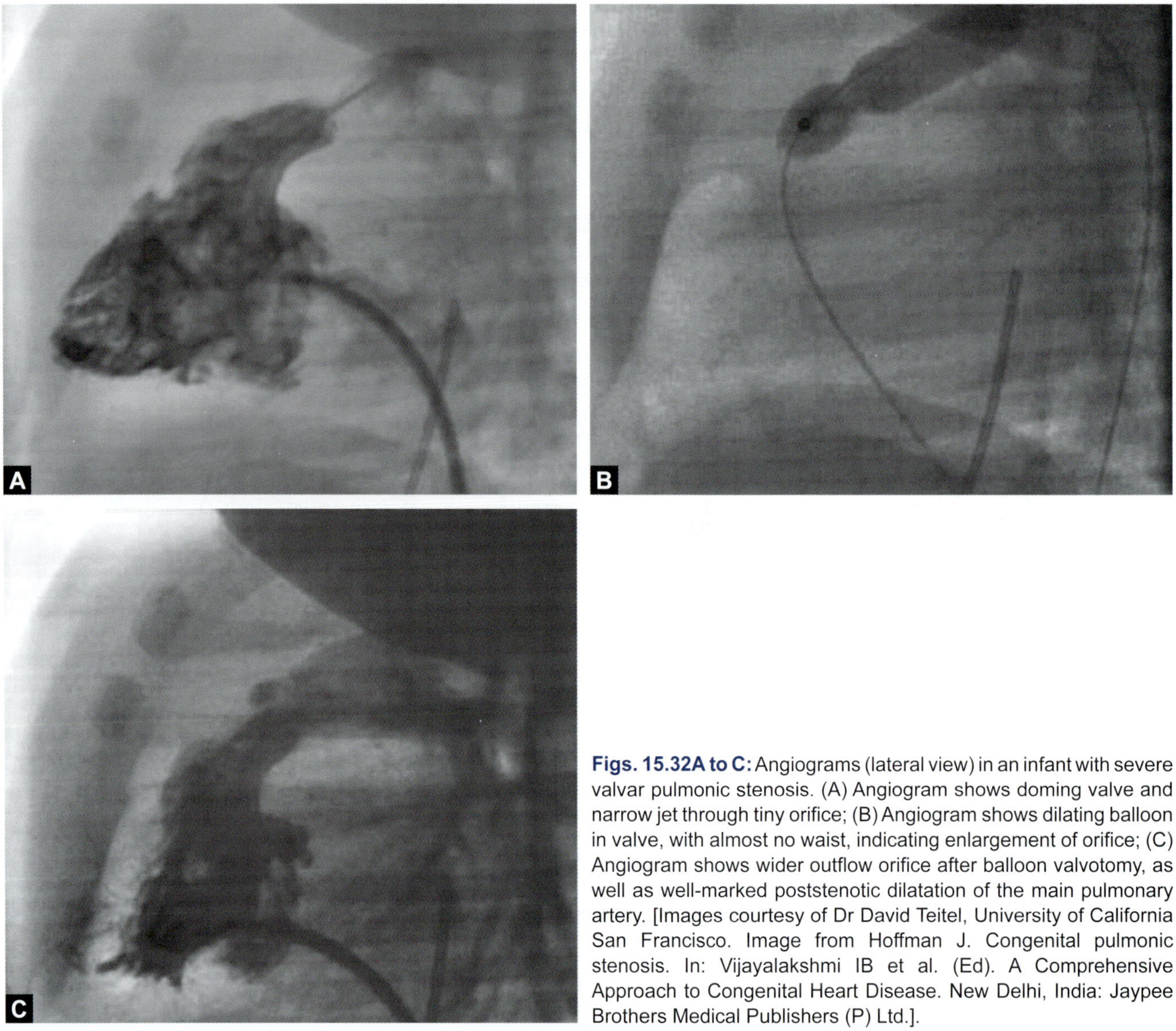

Figs. 15.32A to C: Angiograms (lateral view) in an infant with severe valvar pulmonic stenosis. (A) Angiogram shows doming valve and narrow jet through tiny orifice; (B) Angiogram shows dilating balloon in valve, with almost no waist, indicating enlargement of orifice; (C) Angiogram shows wider outflow orifice after balloon valvotomy, as well as well-marked poststenotic dilatation of the main pulmonary artery. [Images courtesy of Dr David Teitel, University of California San Francisco. Image from Hoffman J. Congenital pulmonic stenosis. In: Vijayalakshmi IB et al. (Ed). A Comprehensive Approach to Congenital Heart Disease. New Delhi, India: Jaypee Brothers Medical Publishers (P) Ltd.].

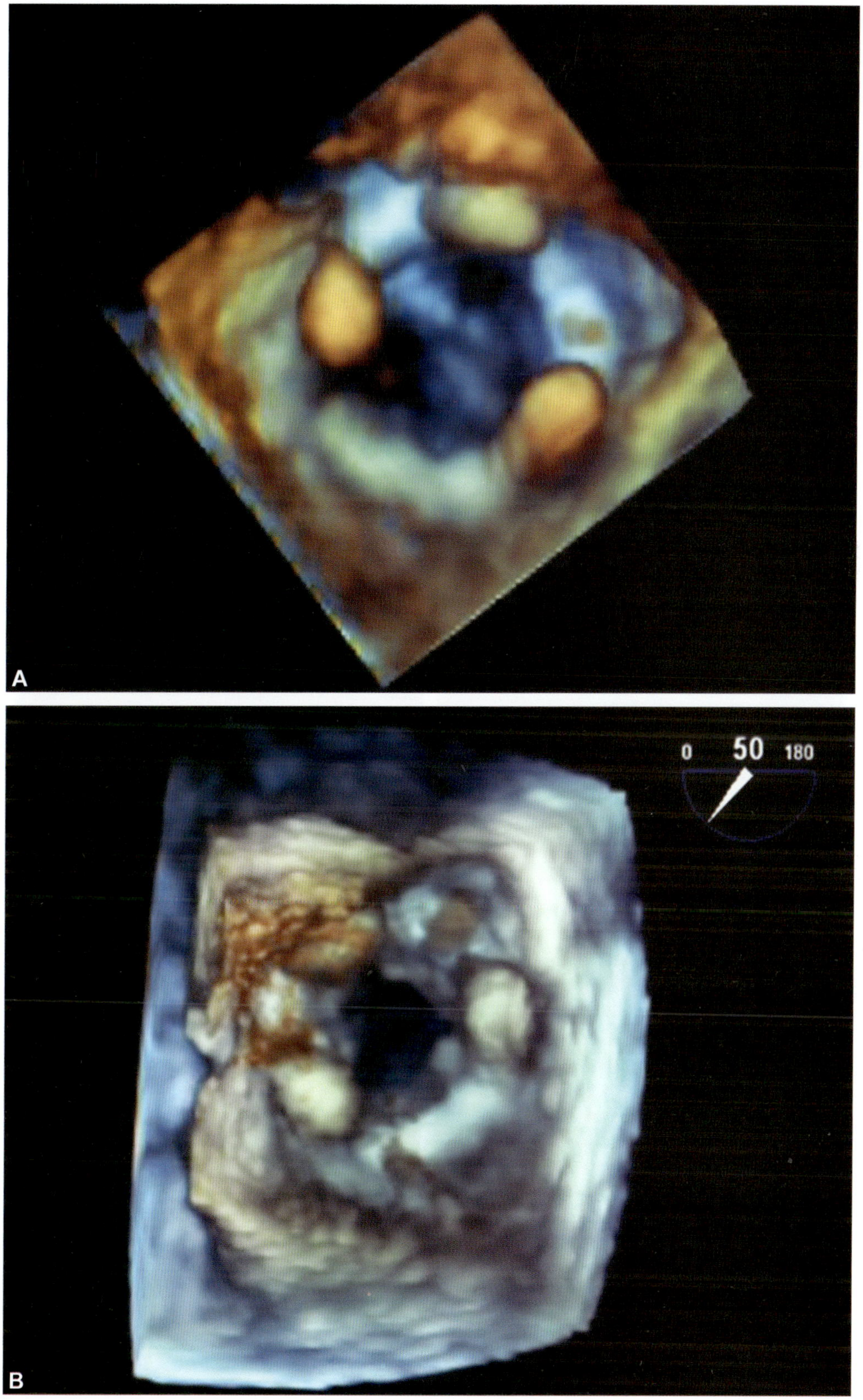

Figs. 15.33A and B: Three-dimensional transesophageal echocardiographic images of a surgically replaced bioprosthetic pulmonary valve. (A) The valve in the closed position; (B) The valve in the open position.

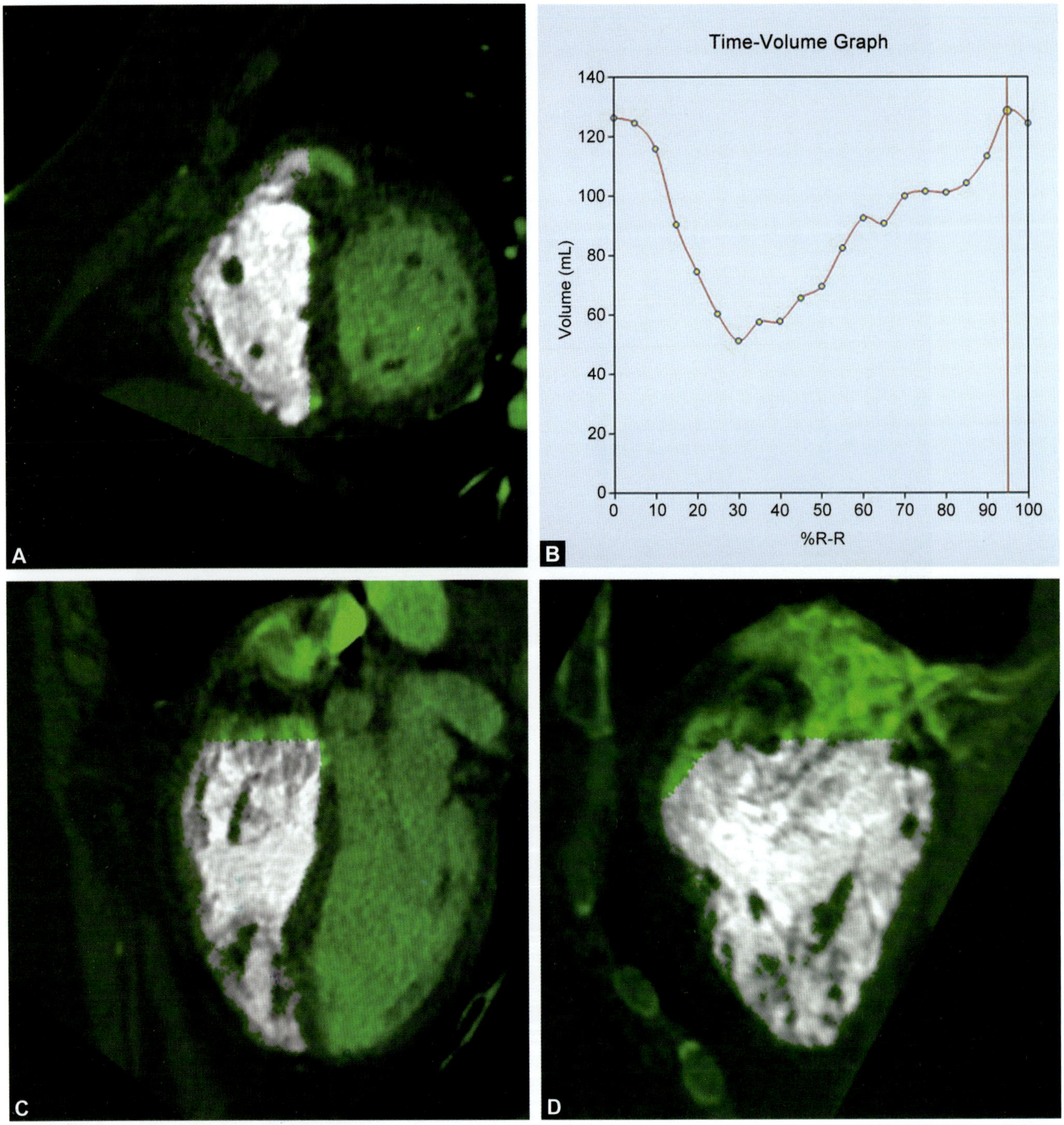

Figs. 15.34A to D: Cardiac CT scan demonstrating various projections of the right ventricle used to calculate the right ventricular volume in diastole. Figure A shows a short-axis view of the right ventricle. Figures C and D demonstrate long-axis views of the right ventricle in orthogonal projections. In Figures A, C and D, chambers other than the right ventricle are deselected as shown by green highlighting. Integration of the remaining volume yields a volume.

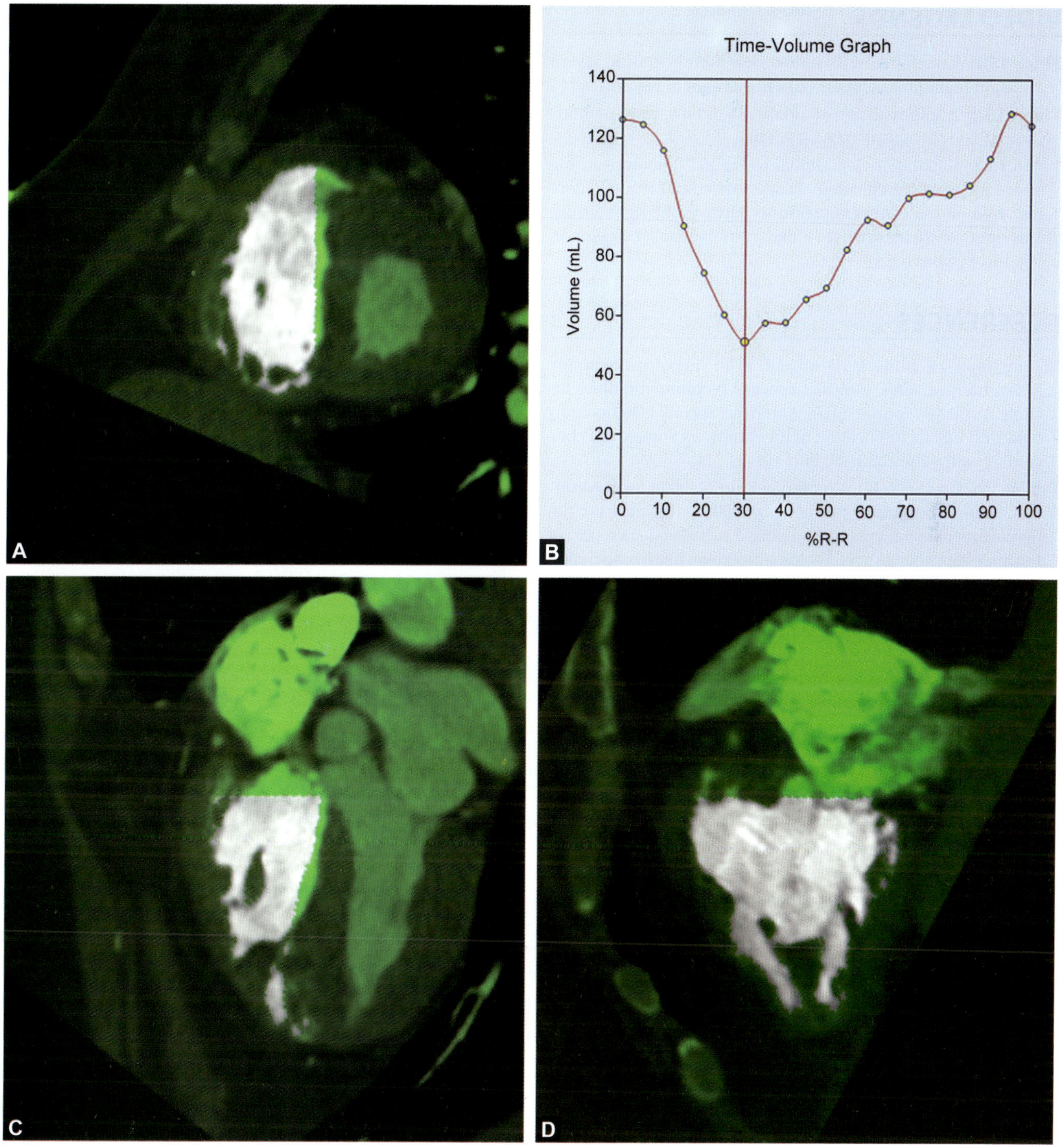

Figs. 15.35A to D: The right ventricle with volume measured in systole by cardiac CT. Figures A, C and D demonstrate orthogonal views of the RV with volume measured and shown in Figure B. Compare these images to those in Figure 15.28.

VIDEO LEGENDS

Video 15.1: Non-standard RV inflow view demonstrating severe tricuspid regurgitation in the patient pictured in Fig. 15.7.

Video 15.2: Additional non-standard RV inflow view demonstrating severe tricuspid regurgitation.

Video 15.3: 4-chamber view similar to Fig 15.7B demonstrating severe tricuspid regurgitation. In severe tricuspid regurgitation, the rapid normalization of pressures between the right atrium and right ventricle results in a dense, triangular jet as seen in Fig. 15.14 (red arrows).

REFERENCES

Baumgartner H, Hung J, Bermejo J, et al. Echocardiographic assessment of valve stenosis: eae/ase recommendations for clinical practice. Journal of the American Society of Echocardiography : official publication of the American Society of Echocardiography. 2009;22:1-23; quiz 101-2.

Bonow RO, Carabello BA, Chatterjee K, et al. 2008 focused update incorporated into the acc/aha 2006 guidelines for the management of patients with valvular heart disease: a report of the american college of cardiology/american heart association task force on practice guidelines (writing committee to revise the 1998 guidelines for the management of patients with valvular heart disease). Endorsed by the society of cardiovascular anesthesiologists, society for cardiovascular angiography and interventions, and society of thoracic surgeons. Journal of the American College of Cardiology. 2008;52:e1-142.

Choong CY, Abascal VM, Weyman J, et al. Prevalence of valvular regurgitation by Doppler echocardiography in patients with structurally normal hearts by two-dimensional echocardiography. American heart journal. 1989;117:636-42.

Cullen MW, Cabalka AK, Alli OO, et al. Transvenous, antegrade melody valve-in-valve implantation for bioprosthetic mitral and tricuspid valve dysfunction: a case series in children and adults. JACC. Cardiovascular Interventions. 2013;6:598-605.

Fukuda S, Saracino G, Matsumura Y, et al. Three-dimensional geometry of the tricuspid annulus in healthy subjects and in patients with functional tricuspid regurgitation: a real-time, 3-dimensional echocardiographic study. Circulation. 2006;114:I492-8.

Javed U, Levisman J, Rogers JH. A tale of two balloons: assessment of hemodynamics with atrial septal defect temporary balloon occlusion. The Journal of Invasive Cardiology. 2012;24:248-9.

Klein AL, Burstow DJ, Tajik AJ, et al. Age-related prevalence of valvular regurgitation in normal subjects: a comprehensive color flow examination of 118 volunteers. Journal of the American Society of Echocardiography: official publication of the American Society of Echocardiography. 1990;3:54-63.

Lavie CJ, Hebert K, Cassidy M. Prevalence and severity of Doppler-detected valvular regurgitation and estimation of right-sided cardiac pressures in patients with normal two-dimensional echocardiograms. Chest. 1993;103:226-31.

Rogers JH, Bolling SF. The tricuspid valve: current perspective and evolving management of tricuspid regurgitation. Circulation. 2009;119:2718-25.

Singh JP, Evans JC, Levy D, et al. Prevalence and clinical determinants of mitral, tricuspid, and aortic regurgitation (the framingham heart study). The American Journal of Cardiology. 1999;83:897-902.

Takao S, Miyatake K, Izumi S, et al. Clinical implications of pulmonary regurgitation in healthy individuals: detection by cross sectional pulsed Doppler echocardiography. British Heart Journal. 1988;59:542-50.

Waller BF, Howard J, Fess S. Pathology of pulmonic valve stenosis and pure regurgitation. Clinical Cardiology. 1995;18:45-50.

Zoghbi WA, Enriquez-Sarano M, Foster E, et al. Recommendations for evaluation of the severity of native valvular regurgitation with two-dimensional and Doppler echocardiography. Journal of the American Society of Echocardiography: official publication of the American Society of Echocardiography. 2003;16:777-802.

CHAPTER

16

Endocarditis

Tina Shah

INTRODUCTION

Endocarditis is an inflammation of the inner layer of the heart; i.e. the endocardium. Although, most commonly it involves the heart valves (Figs. 16.1 to 16.4 and Videos 16.1 to 16.7), it can also involve the mural endocardium, septal defects and surfaces of intracardiac devices (Fig. 16.5). Depending on the etiology, it is further classified as infective endocarditis (IE) or non-infective endocarditis, depending on whether a microorganism is

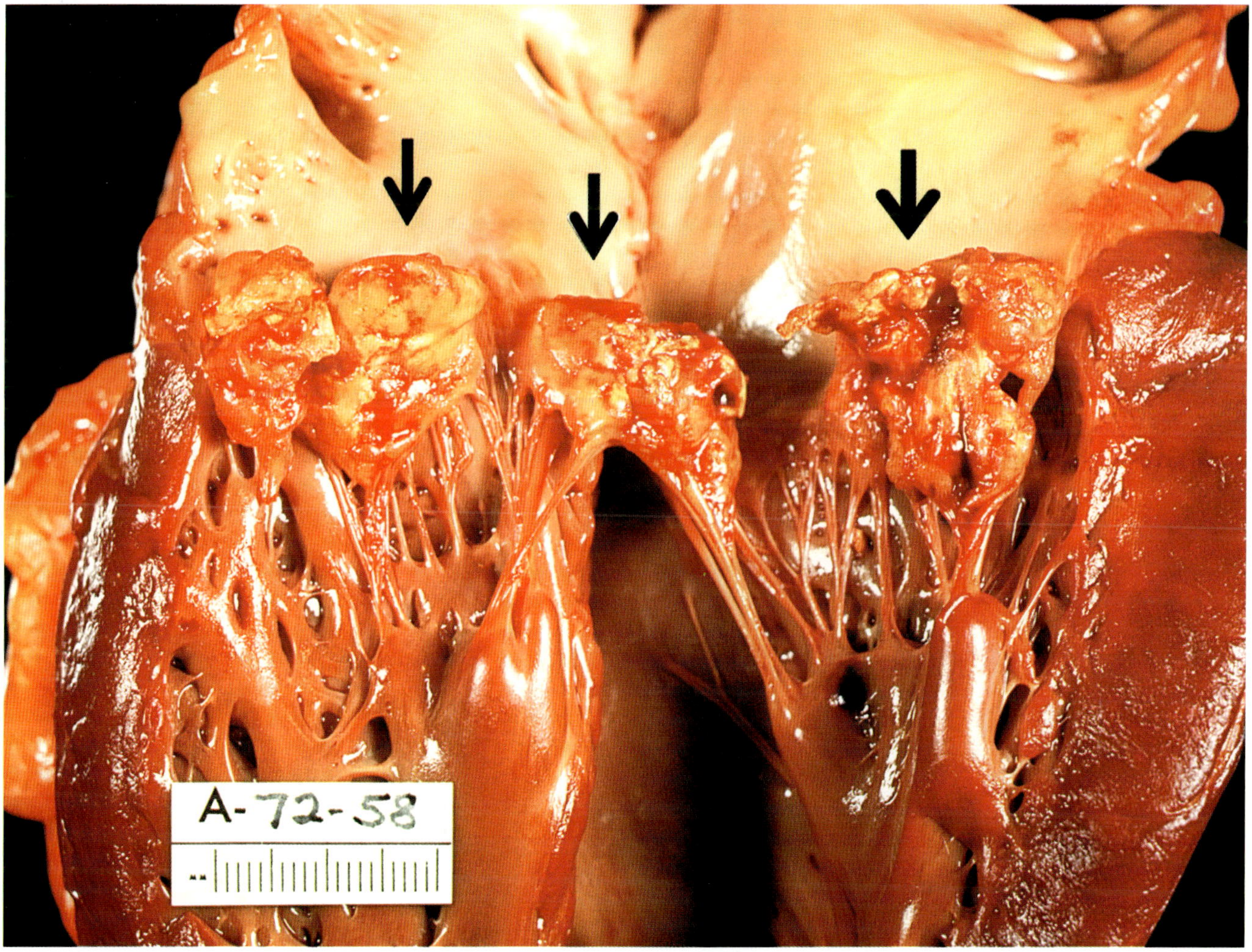

Fig. 16.1A: Vegetations on the mitral valve (arrows) in a patient with infective endocarditis. [Image courtesy of Dr Edwin P Ewing Jr. and the Centers for Disease Control and Prevention (CDC)].

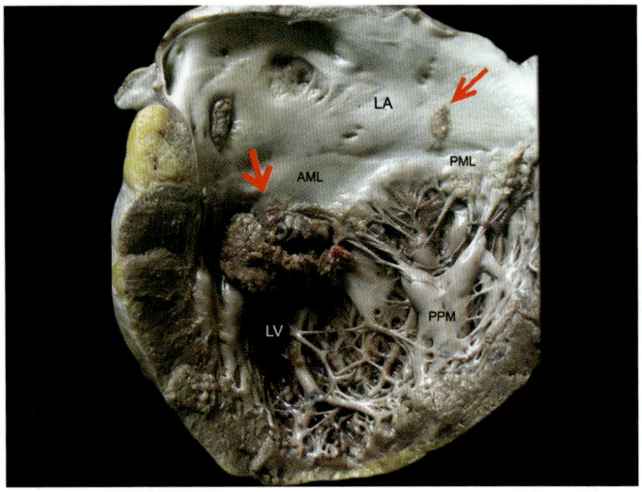

Fig. 16.1B: Bulky friable red-brown infective vegetation completely obscures the free margin of anterior mitral leaflet, its chords and apices of anterior papillary muscle (thick arrow). Flat vegetations are also seen over posterior leaflet and posterior wall of left atrium LA (thin arrow). [Image courtesy of Pradeep Vaideeswar, Department of Pathology (Cardiovascular & Thoracic Division), Seth GS Medical College, Mumbai, India]. (AML: Anterior mitral leaflet; LA: Left atrium; LV: Left ventricle; PPM: Posteromedial papillary muscle; PML: Posterior mitral leaflet).

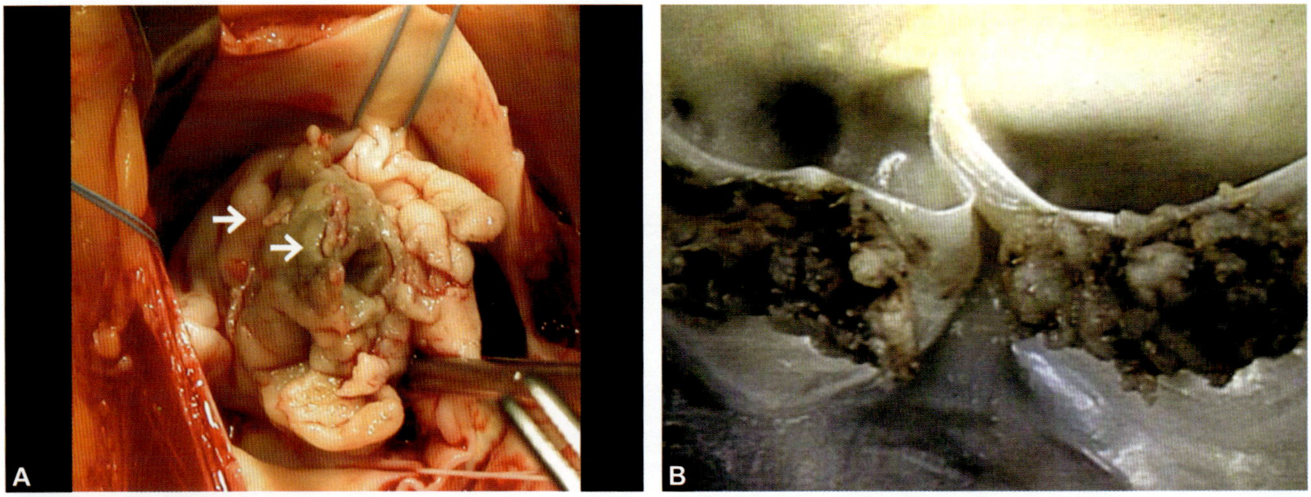

Figs. 16.2A and B: (A) Surgical view of vegetations (arrows) on the aortic valve; (B) Pathologic specimen demonstrating aortic valve endocarditis. [Image 16.2A from Velicki L, et al. Aortic valve endocarditis. In: Chen YF, Luo CY (eds). Aortic Valve. Intechweb.org. Image 16.2B from Armed Forces Institute of Pathology].

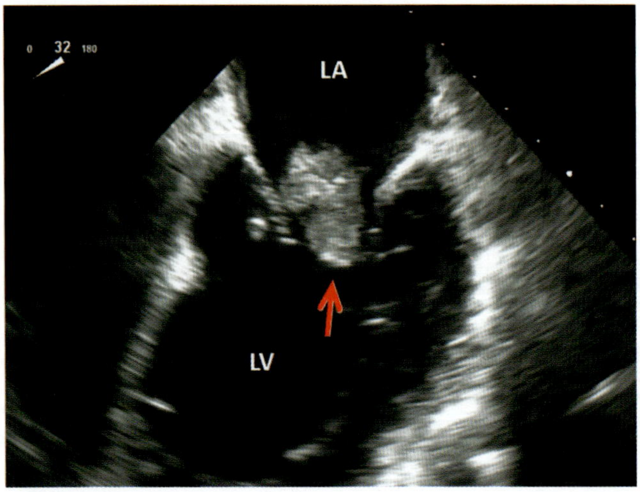

Fig. 16.3: Transesphogeal echocardiogram demonstrating a large vegetation (arrow) on the mitral valve in a patient with infective endocarditis.

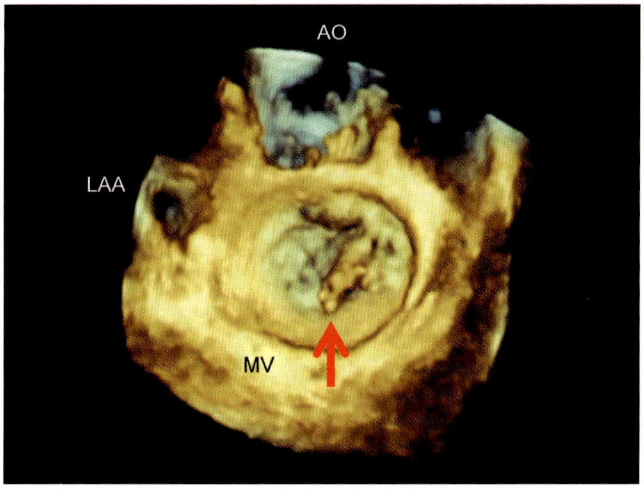

Fig. 16.4: 3D TEE demonstrating a large vegetation (arrow) on the A3 segment of the anterior mitral leaflet. [Image from Lopez J. Echocardiography in infective endocarditis. In: Nanda NC (ed). Comprehensive textbook of echocardiography. New Delhi, India: Jaypee Brothers Medical Publishers (P) Ltd.]. (TEE: Transesophageal echocardiogram; LAA: Orifice of the left atrial appendage; MV: Mitral valve; AO: Aorta).

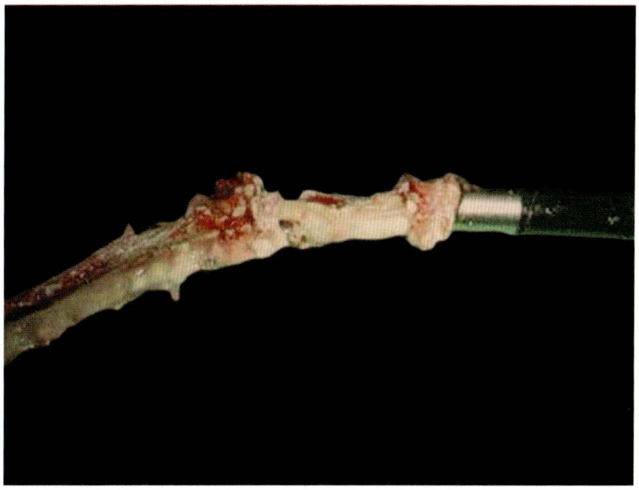

Fig. 16.5: Endocarditis on an explanted right atrial pacer lead. (Image courtesy of Dr Irakli Giorgberidze).

the source of the inflammation. Most of the discussion that follows describes IE as it is much more common compared to non-infective endocarditis. The prototypic lesion of IE is the vegetation, which is a mass of platelets, fibrin, microcolonies of microorganisms, and scant inflammatory cells.

The variability in clinical presentation of IE requires a diagnostic strategy that is both sensitive for disease detection and specific for its exclusion across all forms of the disease. In 1994, Durack and colleagues from Duke University Medical Center proposed a diagnostic schema termed *"the Duke criteria"*. A diagnosis of IE is based on the presence of either major or minor clinical criteria. Major criteria in the Modified Duke strategy included IE documented by data obtained at the time of open heart surgery or autopsy (pathologically definite) or by well-defined microbiological criteria (high-grade bacteremia or fungemia) plus echocardiographic data (clinically definite) (Tables 16.1 and 16.2).

RISK FACTORS OF INFECTIVE ENDOCARDITIS

A number of factors predispose to the development of IE, including intravenous (injection) drug use, prosthetic heart valves or other intracardiac devices, structural heart disease (congenital, rheumatic or degenerative), prior history of IE, hemodialysis and HIV infection.

Table 16.1: Diagnosis of infective endocarditis (IE) according to the modified Duke criteria.

DEFINITIVE IE
Pathological criteria
• Microorganisms demonstrated by culture or histological examination of a vegetation, a vegetation that has embolized, or an intracardiac abscess specimen;
or
• Pathological lesions; vegetation or intracardiac abscess confirmed by histological examination showing active endocarditis
Clinical criteria
• 2 major criteria
or
• 1 major criterion and 3 minor criteria
or
• 5 minor criteria
POSSIBLE IE
• 1 major criterion and 1 minor criterion
or
• 3 minor criteria
REJECTED IE
• Firm alternative diagnosis explaining evidence of IE
or
• Resolution of IE syndrome with antibiotic therapy for </equal to 4 days
or
• No pathological evidence of IE at surgery or autopsy, with antibiotic therapy for </equal to 4 days
or
• Does not meet criteria for possible IE as above

Table 16.2: Definition of terms used in the modified Duke criteria for the diagnosis of infective endocarditis (IE).

MAJOR CRITERIA
Blood culture positive for IE
• Typical microorganisms consistent with IE from 2 separate blood cultures: *Viridans streptococci*, *Streptococcus bovis*, *HACEK* group, *Staphylococcus aureus*; or community-acquired *enterococci* in the absence of a primary focus;
or
• Microorganisms consistent with IE from persistently positive blood cultures defined as follows: At least 2 positive cultures of blood samples drawn 12 hours apart; or all of 3 or a majority of 4 separate cultures of blood (with first and last sample drawn at least 1 hours apart);
or
• Single positive blood culture for *Coxiella burnetii* or anti–phase 1 IgG antibody titer >1:800
Evidence of endocardial involvement
• Echocardiogram positive for IE (TEE recommended for patients with prosthetic valves, rated at least "possible IE" by clinical criteria, or complicated IE (paravalvular abscess); TTE as first test in other patients) defined as follows:
• Oscillating intracardiac mass on valve or supporting structures, in the path of regurgitant jets, or on implanted material in the absence of an alternative anatomic explanation;
or
• Abscess; or new partial dehiscence of prosthetic valve; new valvular regurgitation (worsening or changing or pre-existing murmur not sufficient)
MINOR CRITERIA
• Predisposition, predisposing heart condition, or intravenous drug use
• Fever, temperature ≥ 38°C
• Vascular phenomena, major arterial emboli, septic pulmonary infarcts, mycotic aneurysm, intracranial hemorrhage, conjunctival hemorrhages, and Janeway's lesions
• Immunologic phenomena: glomerulonephritis, Osler's nodes, Roth's spots, and rheumatoid factor
• Microbiological evidence: positive blood culture but does not meet a major criterion as noted above or serological evidence of active infection with organism consistent with IE
• Some Echocardiographic minor criteria were previously defined but they have been eliminated from the Modified Duke's criteria.

PATHOGENESIS OF INFECTIVE ENDOCARDITIS

The endothelial lining of the heart and its valves is normally resistant to infection with bacteria and fungi. Although a few highly virulent organisms such as *Staphylococcus aureus* are capable of infecting normal human heart valves, the initial step in the formation of a vegetation is injury to the endocardium, followed by focal adherence of platelets and fibrin (Figs. 16.6 and 16.7). The primary event is bacterial adherence to damaged valves. The organisms that have the greatest ability to adhere to damaged tissues are usually responsible for IE. The second step involves persistence and growth of bacteria within the cardiac lesions usually associated with local extension and tissue damage. During this phase, the bacteria must be able to survive and avoid host defense. Dissemination of septic emboli to distant organs then takes place.

A variety of microorganisms Can cause IE. *Staphylococci* and *streptococci* account for the majority of cases. Organisms associated with endocarditis are listed in Table 16.3.

DIAGNOSIS OF INFECTIVE ENDOCARDITIS

The diagnosis of IE is usually based upon a combination of factors, including a careful history and physical examination, blood cultures, selected laboratory results, an electrocardiogram (ECG), a chest radiograph, and an echocardiogram. In evaluating a patient with suspected endocarditis, a detailed history should be obtained about prior structural cardiac disease, prosthetic valves or intracardiac devices. The history should also include questioning on whether subjective or documented fever has occurred, general malaise or other symptoms have been present, and any intravenous drug use.

The physical exam includes not only a thorough cardiac exam to evaluate for murmurs, but also examination of the entire body to look for stigmata of IE. Associated peripheral cutaneous or mucocutaneous lesions of IE include purpura (Fig. 16.8), splinter hemorrhages (Fig. 16.9), Janeway lesions (Figs. 16.10 and 16.11), Osler's nodes (Figs. 16.12 and 16.13), and Roth spots (Fig. 16.14).

- Three sets of blood cultures are usually obtained in patients being evaluated for possible endocarditis. In patients with culture-negative endocarditis, additional measures may have to be taken. Blood cultures should be obtained prior to initiation of antibiotic therapy.
- Standard blood tests include white blood cell (WBC) count and erythrocyte sedimentation rate (ESR). White blood cell count and ESR are elevated in patients with endocarditis. Elevated level of C-reactive protein may also be seen. A normochromic normocytic anemia is seen in patients with subacute endocarditis.

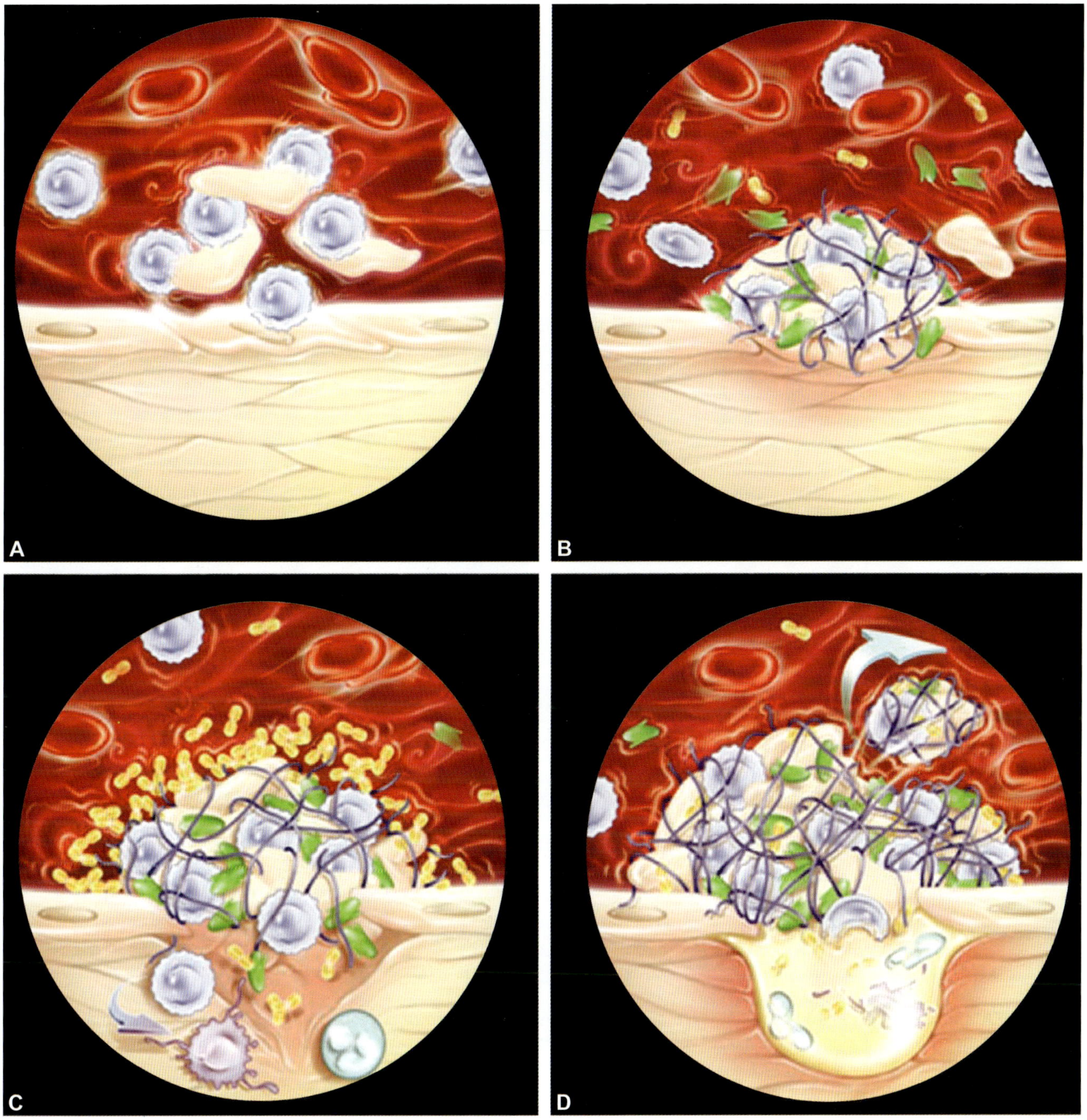

Figs. 16.6A to D: The natural history of IE may be decomposed in successive steps. (A) Cell apoptosis that may be promoted by blood turbulence in the vicinity of valve lesion; (B) Procoagulant activity that results in fibrin and platelet deposition; (C) Bacterial colonization and chemoattraction of neutrophils increasing vegetation size; (D) Tissue remodeling and neoangiogenesis leading to the functional destruction of the valve. [Image and text legend from Benoit M, et al. The Transcriptional Programme of Human Heart Valves Reveals the Natural History of Infective Endocarditis. PLoS ONE 5(1): e8939].

A baseline ECG should be obtained in all patients. The presence or development of heart block (Fig. 16.15) can suggest the presence or development of abscess formation from aortic valve endocarditis, which is now extending in the area of the AV node. Rare embolization of part of the vegetation into the coronary artery likely results in acute ischemia or infarction, which will manifest on follow-up ECGs.

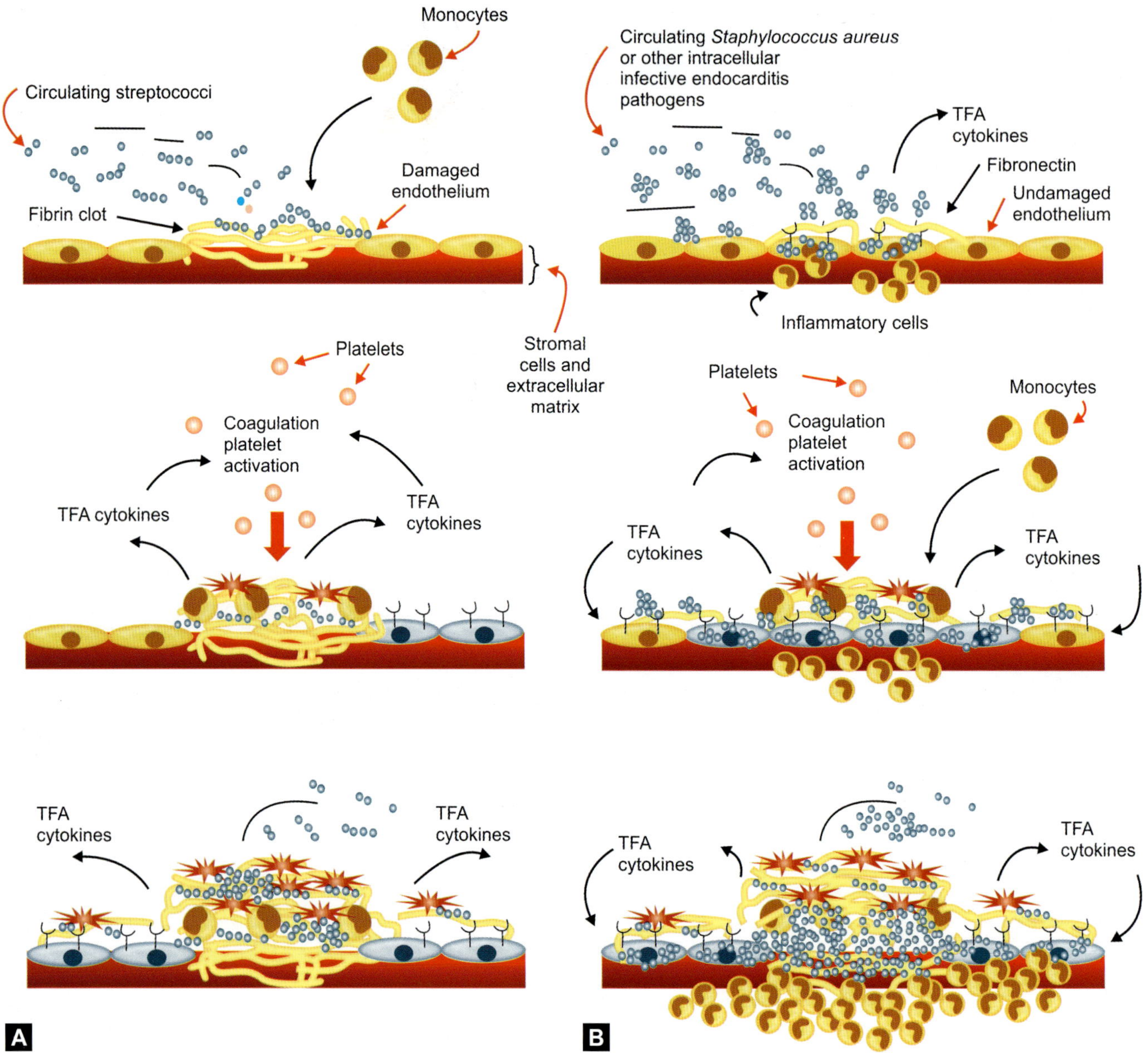

Figs. 16.7A and B: Early steps in bacterial valve colonization. (A) *Colonization of damaged epithelium*: exposed stromal cells and extracellular matrix proteins trigger deposition of fibrin-platelet clots to which *Streptococci* bind (upper panel); fibrin-adherent *Streptococci* attract monocytes and induce them to produce tissue-factor activity (TFA) and cytokines (middle panel); these mediators activate coagulation cascade, attract and activate blood platelets, and induce cytokine, integrin, and TFA production from neighboring endothelial cells (lower panel), encouraging vegetation growth; (B) *Colonization of inflamed valve tissues*: in response to local inflammation, endothelial cells express integrins that bind plasma fibronectin, which microorganisms adhere to via wall-attached fibronectin-binding proteins, resulting in endothelial internalization of bacteria (upper panel); in response to invasion, endothelial cells produce TFA and cytokines, triggering blood clotting and extension of inflammation, and promoting formation of the vegetation (middle panel); internalised bacteria eventually lyse endothelial cells (green cells) by secreting membrane-active proteins—e.g. hemolysins (lower panel). [Reproduced with permission from Philippe Moreillon, Yok-Ai Que. Infective endocarditis. The Lancet. 2004;363(9403):139-49].

Chest X-ray may reveal pulmonary edema in patients with mitral or aortic valve endocarditis who have developed significant valvular regurgitation due to valve perforation or extensive damage. In patients with right-sided endocarditis of the pulmonary or tricuspid valve, chest X-ray may reveal the typical "cannon shot" pattern of infiltrates from multiple septic emboli to the lungs (Fig. 16.16).

Echocardiography in patients with a low clinical probability of endocarditis is usually unrevealing and of low yield. However, in those with moderate or high suspicion of endocarditis, performance of echocardiography is mandatory. An echocardiogram should be performed in all patients with a moderate or high suspicion of endocarditis. Transthoracic echocardiography (TTE) is a good initial test to evaluate for the presence of endocarditis (Figs. 16.17 to 16.20). TTE has a low sensitivity and high specificity. Hence, the absence of vegetation does not preclude the diagnosis and, TEE is usually warranted if clinical suspicion of endocarditis is high. Transesophageal echocardiography (TEE) has a higher spatial resolution than TTE and hence has better sensitivity for the diagnosis of vegetations (Figs. 16.21 to 16.23). TEE is especially

Table 16.3: Organisms associated with endocarditis.

• *Staphylococcus aureus*
• *Viridans* group *streptococci*
• *Enterococci*
• *Coagulase-negative staphylococci*
• *Streptococcus bovis*
• Other *streptococci*
• Non-HACEK Gram-negative bacteria
• *Fungi*
• HACEK- Organisms in this category include a number of fastidious gram-negative bacilli: *Haemophilus aphrophilus; Actinobacillus actinomycetemcomitans; Cardiobacterium hominis; Eikenella corrodens*; and *Kingella kingae*.

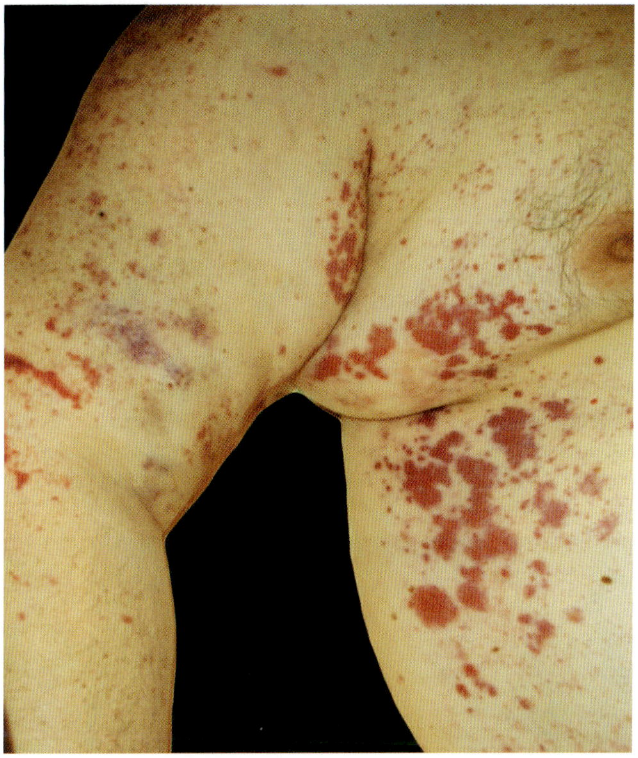

Fig. 16.8: Vascular purpura in a patient with infective endocarditis. [Image from Amandine S. Importance of dermatology in infective endocarditis. In: Gaze D (ed). The cardiovascular system—physiology, diagnosis and clinical implication. Intechopen.com].

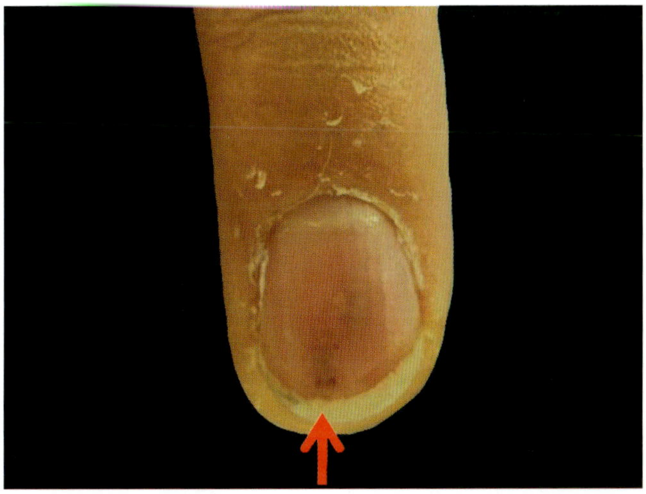

Fig. 16.9A: (A) Splinter hemorrhage (arrow) in a patient with infective endocarditis. [Reproduced with permission from Park MY, Jeon HK, Shim BJ, et al. Complete Atrioventricular Block due to Infective Endocarditis of Bicuspid Aortic Valve. J Cardiovasc Ultrasound. 2011;19(3):140-3].

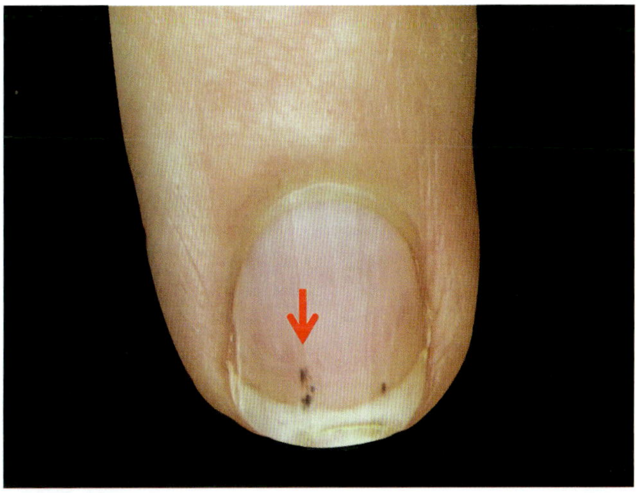

Fig. 16.9B: Splinter hemorrhage (arrow) in a patient with infective endocarditis. (Image posted by Splarkla on Wikimedia Commons).

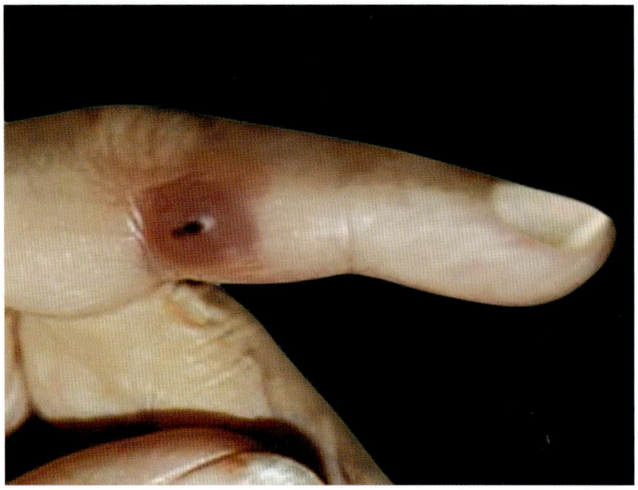

Fig. 16.10: Janeway lesion (usually seen in *staphylococcal endocarditis; painless, septic emboli*). [Image from Bhalerao JC. Bacterial endocarditis. In: Bhalerao JC (ed). Essentials of clinical cardiology. New Delhi, Inida: Jaypee Brothers Medical Publishers (P) Ltd.].

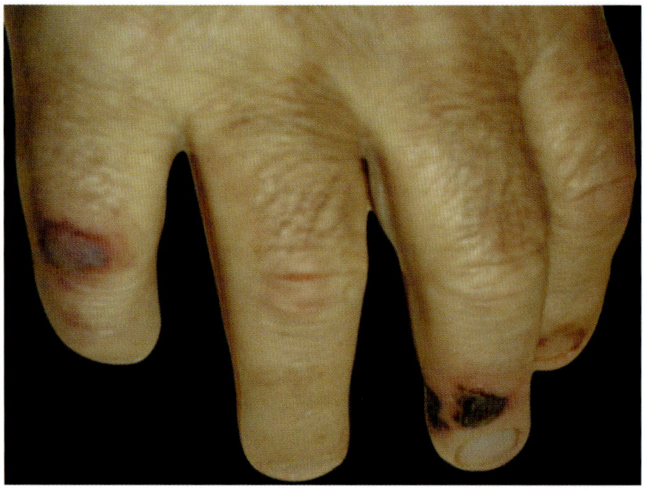

Fig. 16.11: Janeway lesions in a patient with IE. [Image from Amandine S. Importance of dermatology in infective endocarditis. In: Gaze D (ed). The cardiovascular system—physiology, diagnosis and clinical implication. Intechopen.com].

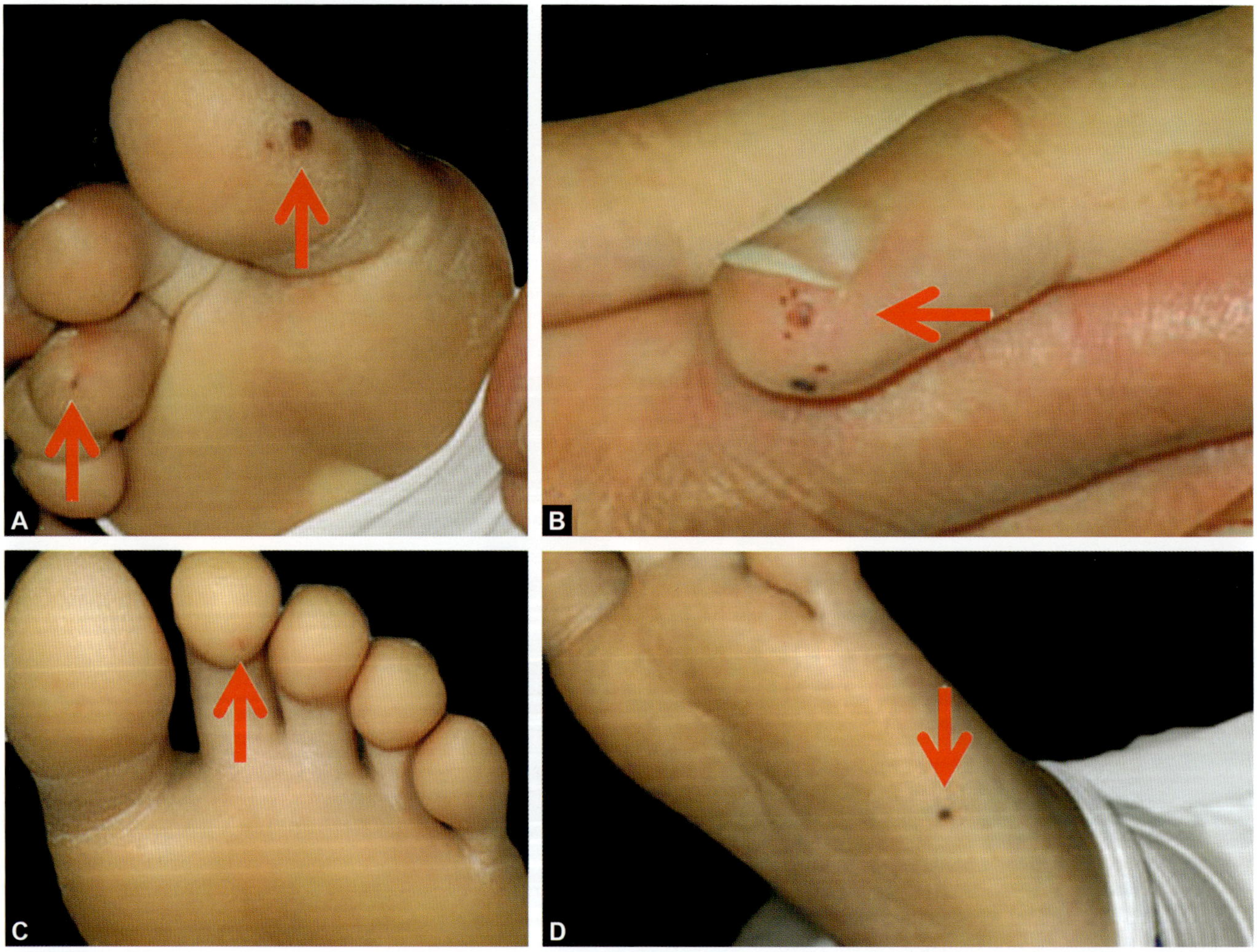

Figs. 16.12A to D: Examples of Osler's nodes painful, immune complex microvasculitis. [Image from Bhalerao JC. Bacterial endocarditis. In: Bhalerao JC (ed). Essentials of Clinical Cardiology, New Delhi, India: Jaypee Brothers Medical Publishers (P) Ltd.].

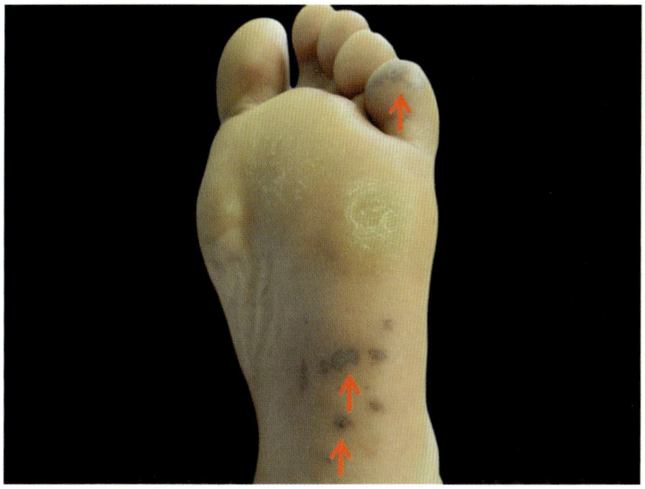

Fig. 16.13: Osler's nodes (arrows). [Image reproduced with permission from Park MY, Jeon HK, Shim BJ, et al. Complete Atrioventricular Block due to Infective Endocarditis of Bicuspid Aortic Valve. J Cardiovasc Ultrasound. 2011;19(3):140-3].

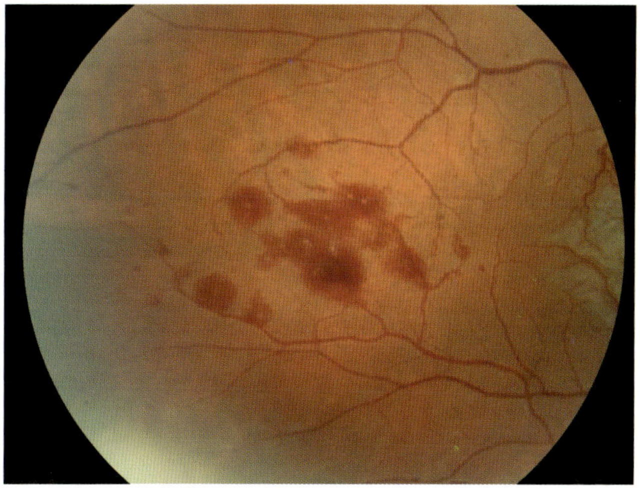

Fig. 16.14: Roth spots. [Image from Sahin O. Ocular complications of endocarditis. In: Breijo-Marquez FR (ed). Endocarditis. Intechweb.org].

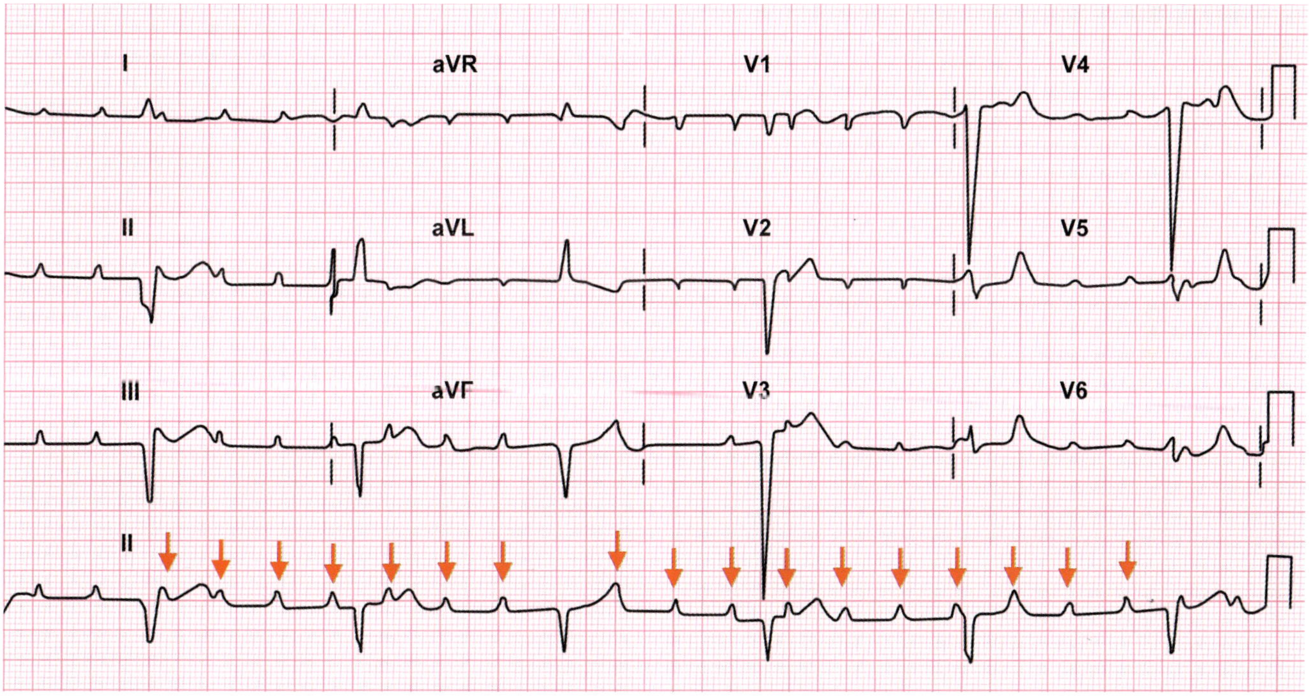

Fig. 16.15: ECG showing sinus tachycardia with complete heart block and junctional escape in a patient with aortic valve endocarditis and abscess formation compromising the AV node. [Image adapted from Abhilash SP. Congenital heart blocks and bradyarrhythmias. In: Vijayalakshmi IB (ed). A Comprehensive Approach to Congenital Heart Diseases. New Delhi, India: Jaypee Brothers Medical Publishers (P) Ltd.].

helpful in the setting of prosthetic valve endocarditis (Fig. 16.24) and in diagnosing aortic valve abscesses.

ECG-gated cardiac CT imaging may in select cases provide incremental benefit in the pre-operative assessment of patients with IE. CT scans are also helpful in assessing the presence and extent of septic pulmonary emboli in patients with right-sided endocarditis.

Magnetic resonance imaging (MRI) has a relatively modest resolution and will often not detect small or medium sized vegetations, although larger vegetations

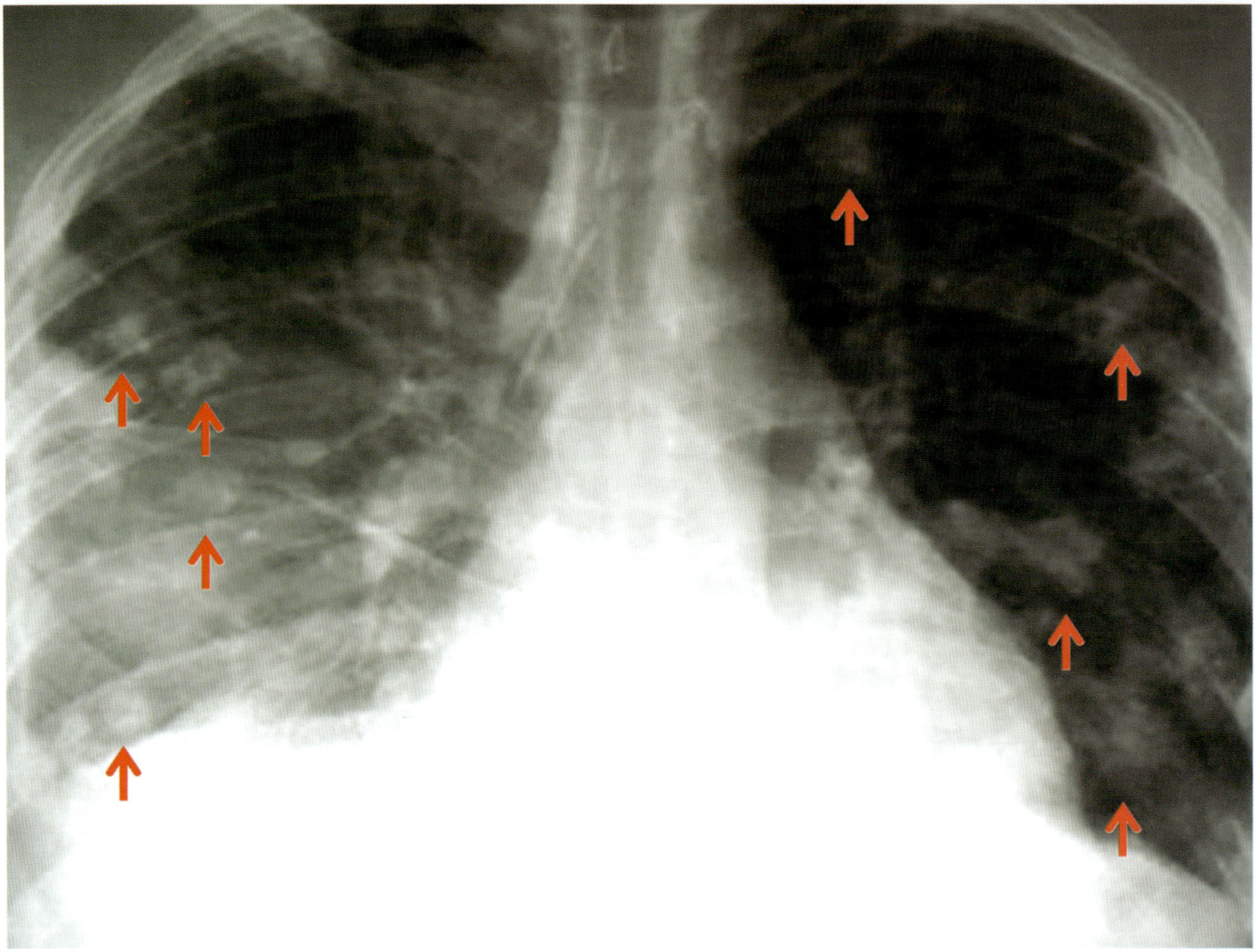

Fig. 16.16: Chest X-ray showing multiple "cannon shot" lesions due to septic emboli in a patient with tricuspid valve infective endocarditis. [Image from Prados C. Radiology in infective endocarditis. In: Breijo-Marquez FR (ed). Endocarditis. Intechweb.org].

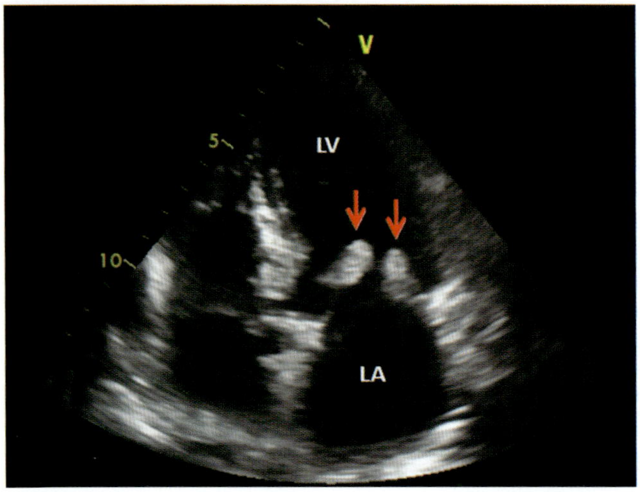

Fig. 16.17: TTE showing vegetations (arrows) on both leaflets of the mitral valve. (TTE: Transthoracic echocardiography).

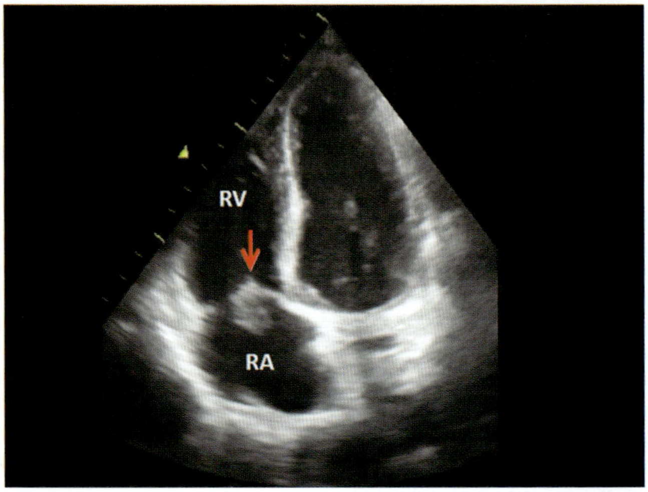

Fig. 16.18: TTE showing large vegetation (arrow) on the tricuspid valve. (TTE: Transthoracic echocardiography).

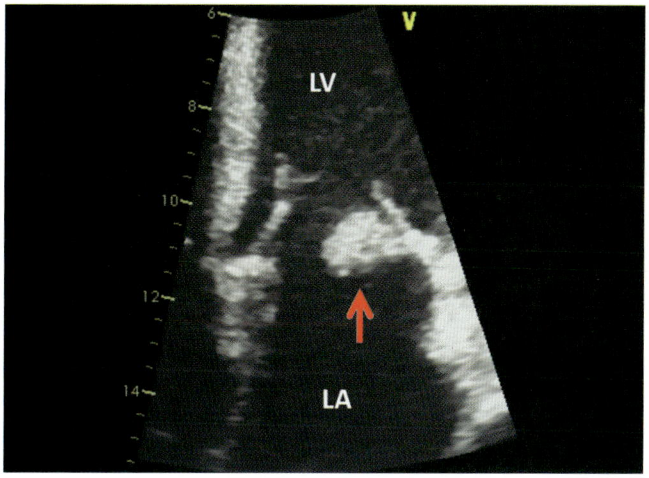

Fig. 16.19: Zoomed TTE image of a vegetation (arrow) on the mitral valve. (TTE: Transthoracic echocardiography).

may be seen on some MRI examinations. MRI is a useful tool in assessing for valve perforation, mycotic aneurysm formation, and other complications of endocarditis.

NON-INFECTIVE ENDOCARDITIS

Several conditions are associated with the formation of valve vegetations not due to infectious etiologies (Fig. 16.25). As opposed to IE, the vegetation in non-bacterial thrombotic endocarditis (NBTE) are small, sterile. The vegetations consist of degenerating platelets interwoven with strands of fibrin. NBTE usually occurs during a hypercoagulable state such as system wide bacterial infection and cancers, particularly mucinous adenocarcinoma. Another form of sterile endocarditis, is termed Libman-Sacks endocarditis; this form occurs more often in patients with lupus

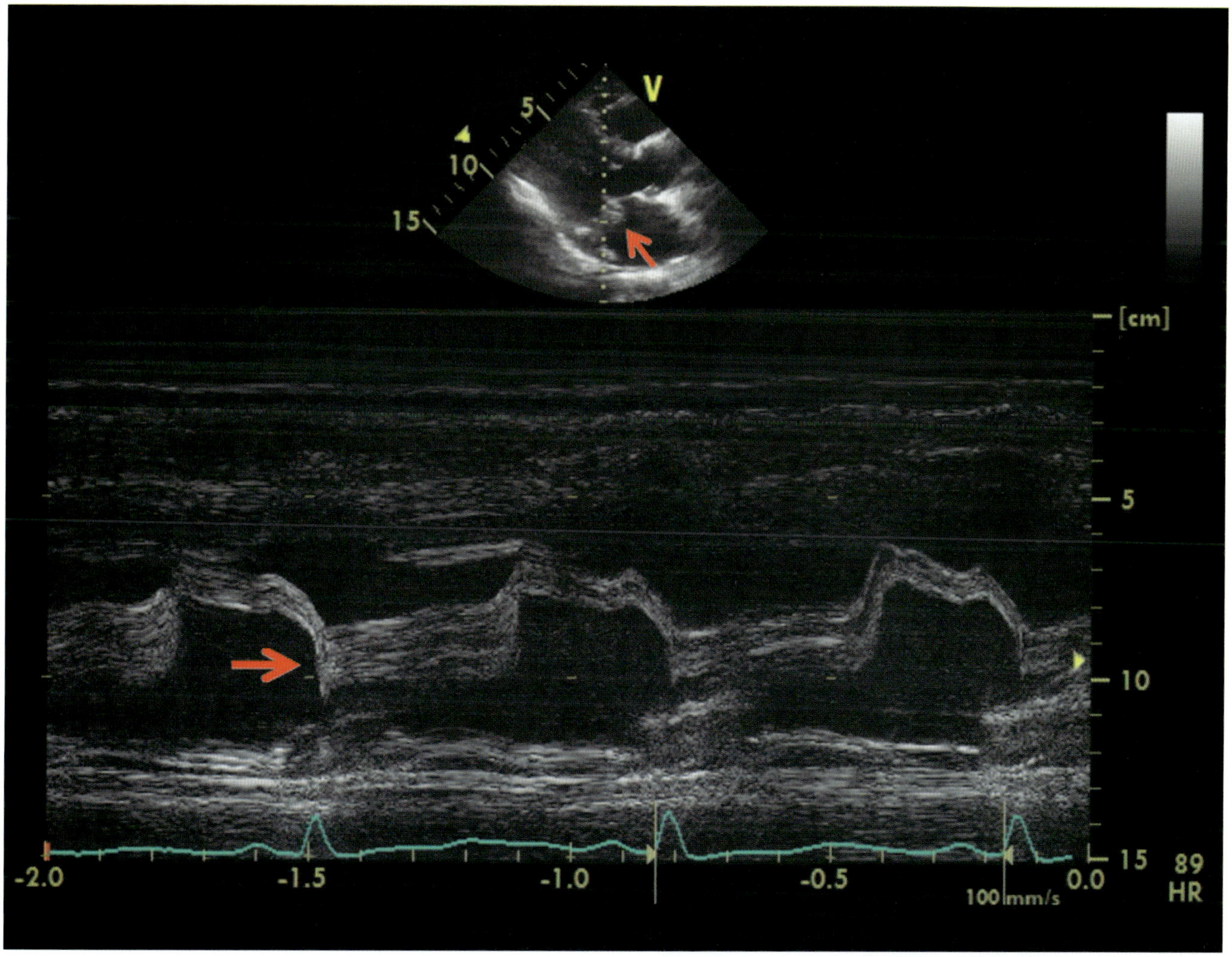

Fig. 16.20: M-mode TTE of a patient with mitral valve endocarditis (arrows). (TTE: Transthoracic echocardiography).

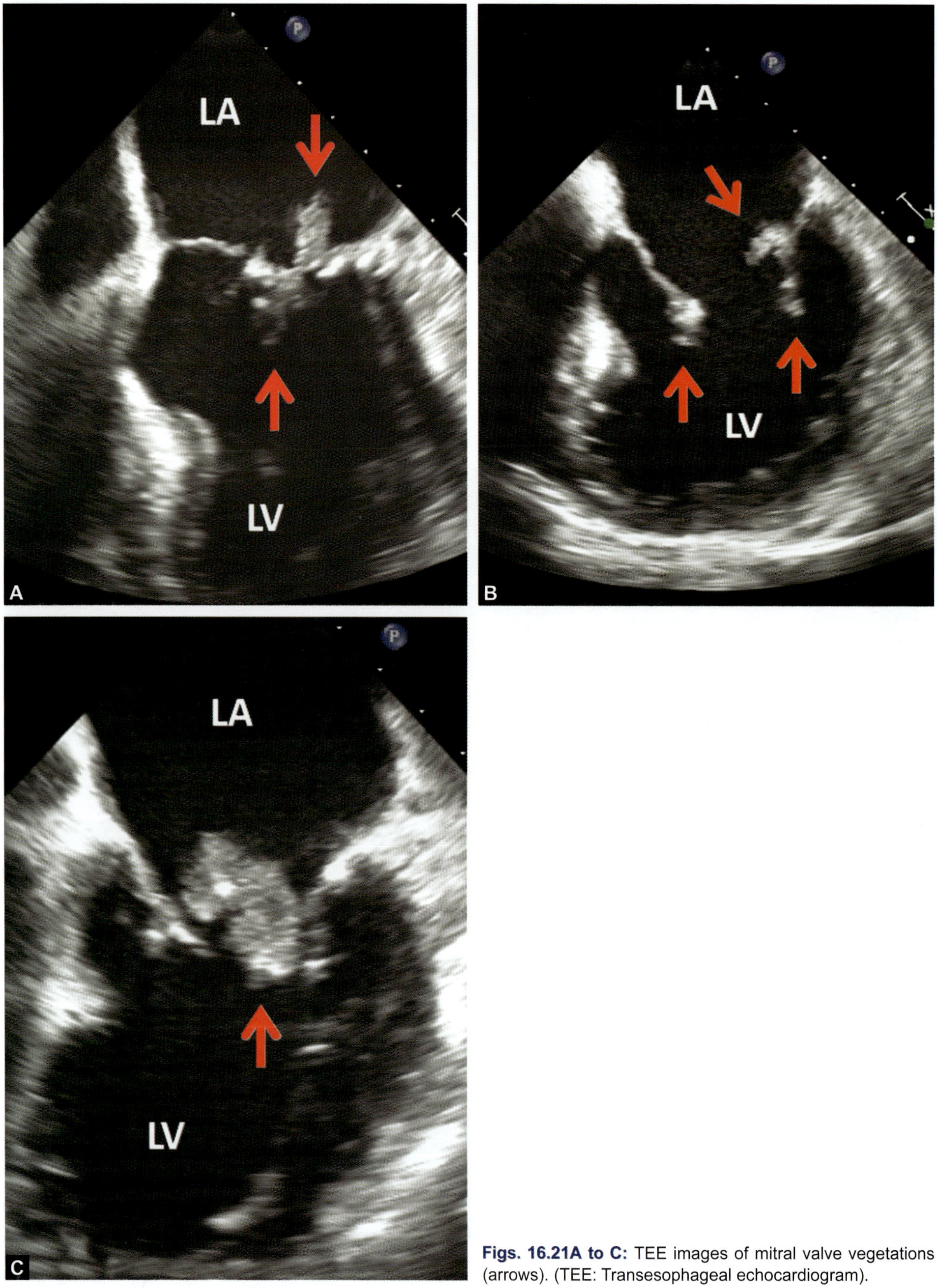

Figs. 16.21A to C: TEE images of mitral valve vegetations (arrows). (TEE: Transesophageal echocardiogram).

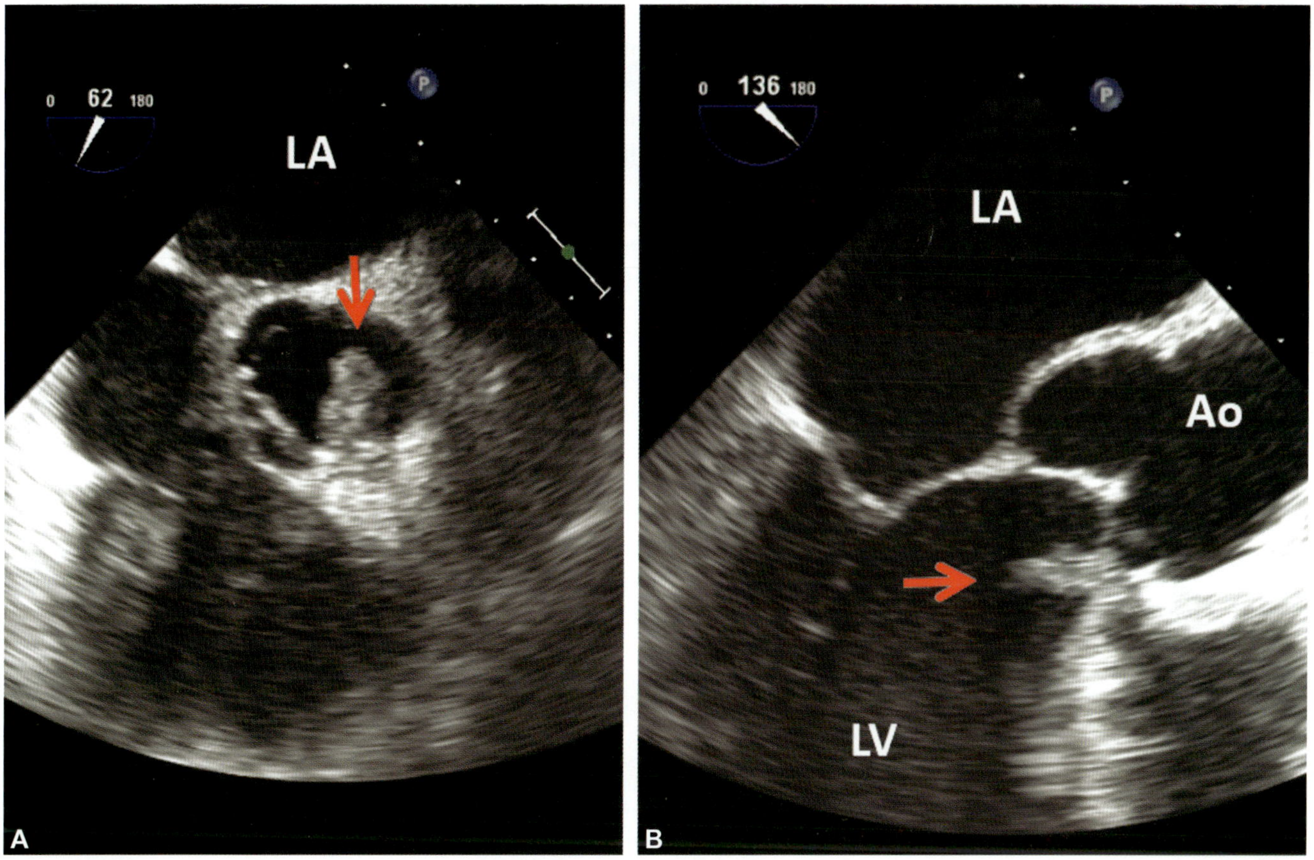

Figs. 16.22A and B: TEE of a large aortic valve vegetation. (A) Short-axis view; (B) Long-axis view. (TEE: Transesophageal echocardiogram).

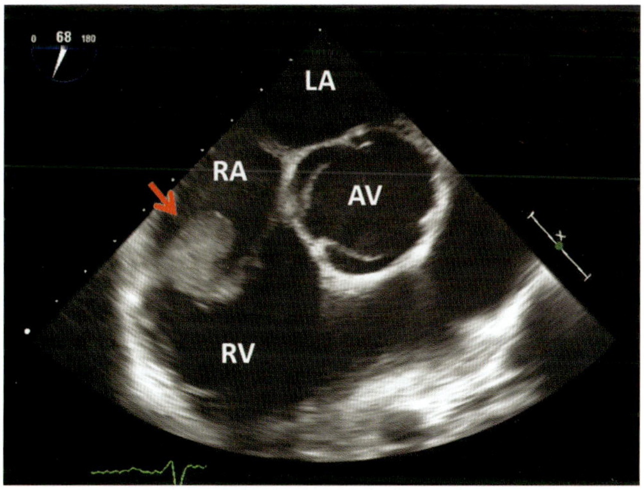

Fig. 16.23: Short-axis TEE image demonstrating a large vegetation on the tricuspid valve. (TEE: Transesophageal echocardiogram).

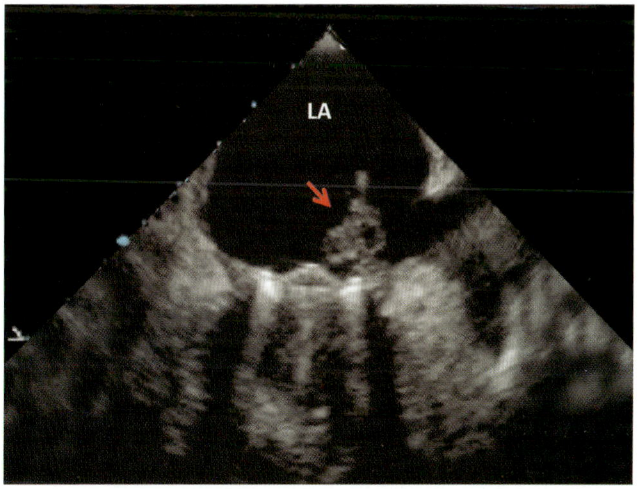

Fig. 16.24: TEE demonstrating infective endocarditis (arrow) in a patient with a mechanical prosthetic mitral valve. (TEE: Transesophageal echocardiogram).

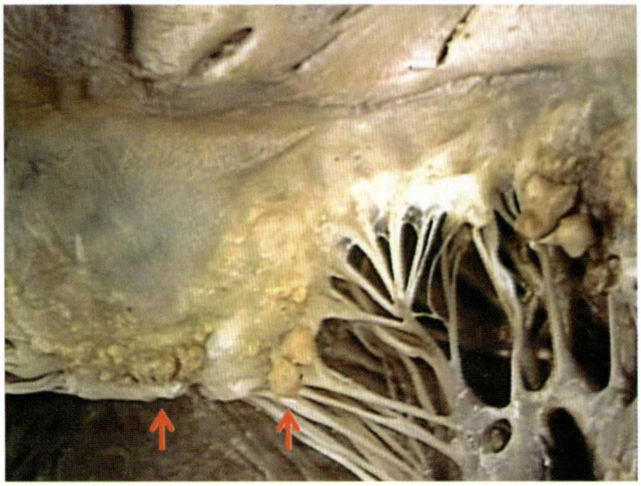

Fig. 16.25: Pathology specimen from a patient with mitral valve Libman-Sacks endocarditis. Libman-Sacks endocarditis can be observed in patients with systemic lupus erythematosus and is a form of non-bacterial endocarditis. [Image from Armed Forces Institute of Pathology (public domain)].

erythematosus and is thought to be due to the deposition of immune complexes. It is often difficult based on echocardiography alone to distinguish between infectious and non-infectious causes of vegetations detected on echocardiographic examination.

COMPLICATIONS OF INFECTIVE ENDOCARDITIS

Numerous life-threatening complications can arise in patients with IE. Such complications include valvular degeneration or perforation (Figs. 16.26 to 16.29 and Video 16.8), leading to regurgitation and pulmonary edema, abscess formation (Fig. 16.30), pseudoaneurysm (Fig. 16.31), and septic emboli (Figs. 16.32 and 16.33) and mycotic aneurysms (Figs. 16.34 and 16.35). The development of any of these complications is often an indication for surgery, as discussed below.

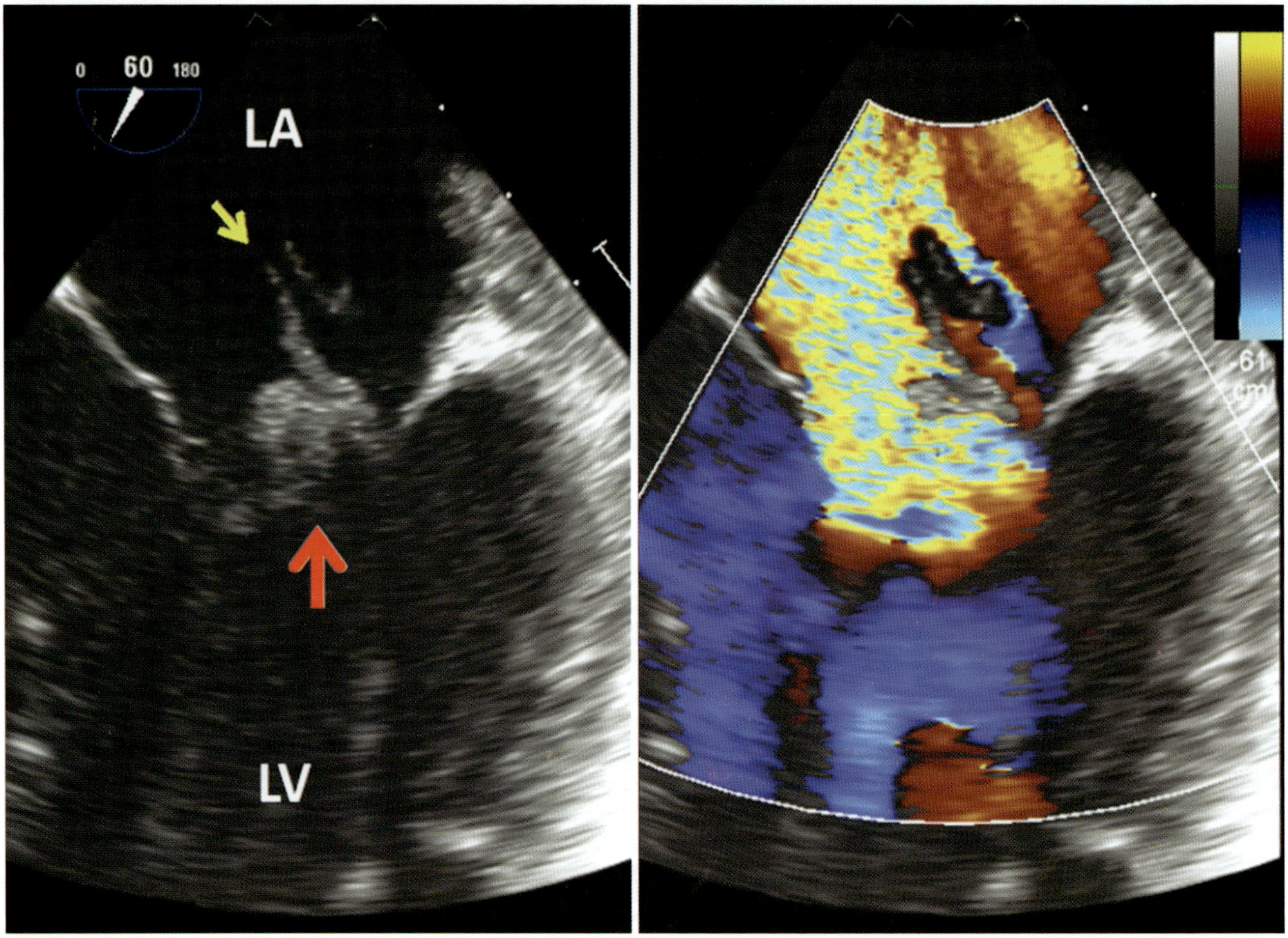

Fig. 16.26: Mitral valve endocarditis (red arrow, left panel) complicated by the development of severe mitral regurgitation (right panel). Note the filamentous vegetations seen on the atrial side of the leaflet (yellow arrow, left panel).

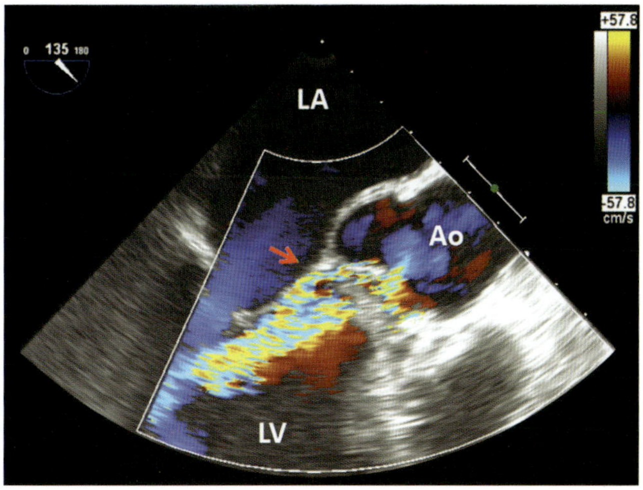

Fig. 16.27: TEE demonstrating perforation of the aortic valve and resulting aortic regurgitation in a patient with aortic valve endocarditis. (TEE: Transesophageal echocardiogram).

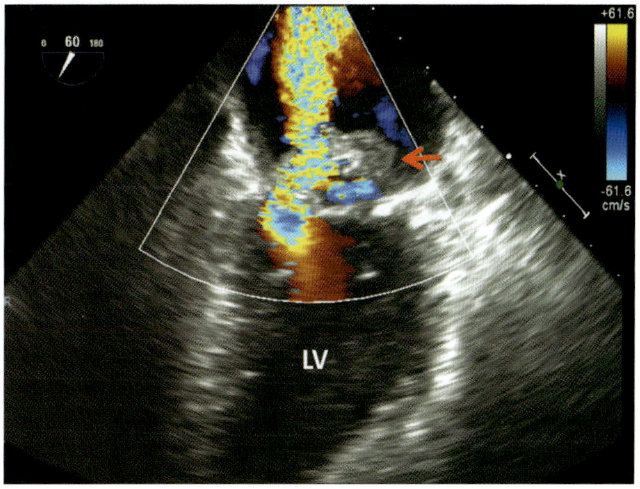

Fig. 16.28: Mitral valve endocarditis (arrow), leading to destruction of the valve and mitral regurgitation.

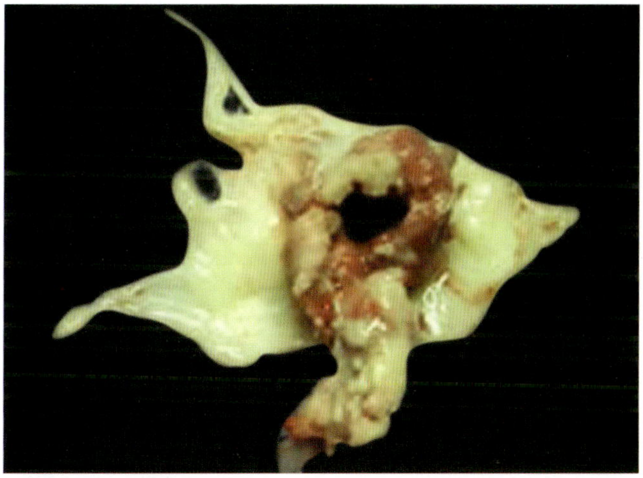

Fig. 16.29: Gross pathology specimen demonstrating mitral valve endocarditis with resultant leaflet perforation. (From Al-Attar N and the European Society of Cardiology. Image from Al-Attar N. Infective endocarditis. Vol 7; number 15. Dec 31, 2008. http://www.escardio.org/communities/councils/ccp/e-journal/volume7/Pages/infective-endocarditis.aspx. Image is copyright of the E-journal of the European Society of Cardiology).

TREATMENT OF INFECTIVE ENDOCARDITIS

Medical treatment consists primarily of antibiotic therapy dictated by the organism isolated on cultures and the organism sensitivity. In most cases of endocarditis, treatment is for 4–6 weeks depending on the organism.

Decisions regarding surgical intervention in patients with IE should be individualized, with input from both the cardiologist and the cardiovascular surgeon. Numerous criteria exist for indications for surgical intervention, and are summarized in Table 16.4.

ENDOCARDITIS PROPHYLAXIS

The American Heart Association (AHA) guidelines for antibiotic prophylaxis were dramatically revised in 2007. Other major national and international organizations have similarly signficantly revised their recommendations regarding endocarditis prophylaxis over the last decade. These revisions are based on the fact that most cases of bacteremia occur during normal daily activities (e.g. tooth brushing, flossing) and that dental or surgical procedures likely account for a very small proportion of the time that a person may be transiently bacteremic. In addition, no study has ever shown that antibiotic prophylaxis actually decreases the risk of developing endocarditis. Current AHA guidelines recommend antibiotic prophylaxis in the setting of dental procedures that involve manipulation of gingival tissue or the periapical region of teeth or perforation of the oral mucosa in "high risk patients" Among the groups of patients who are considered to be "high risk" include those with prosthetic cardiac valve or prosthetic material used for cardiac valve repair; prior history of IE, unrepaired cyanotic congenital heart disease (CHD), including palliative shunts and conduits; completely repaired congenital heart defect with prosthetic material or device, whether placed by surgery

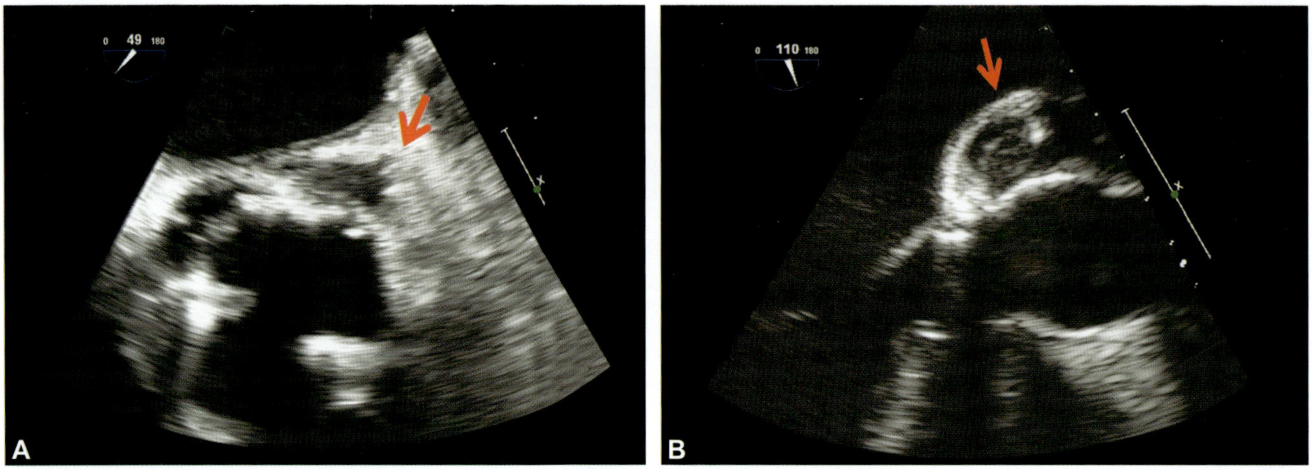

Figs. 16.30A and B: TEE (A) short-axis and (B) long-axis images showing abscess formation (arrows) in a patient with aortic valve endocarditis. (TEE: Transesophageal echocardiogram).

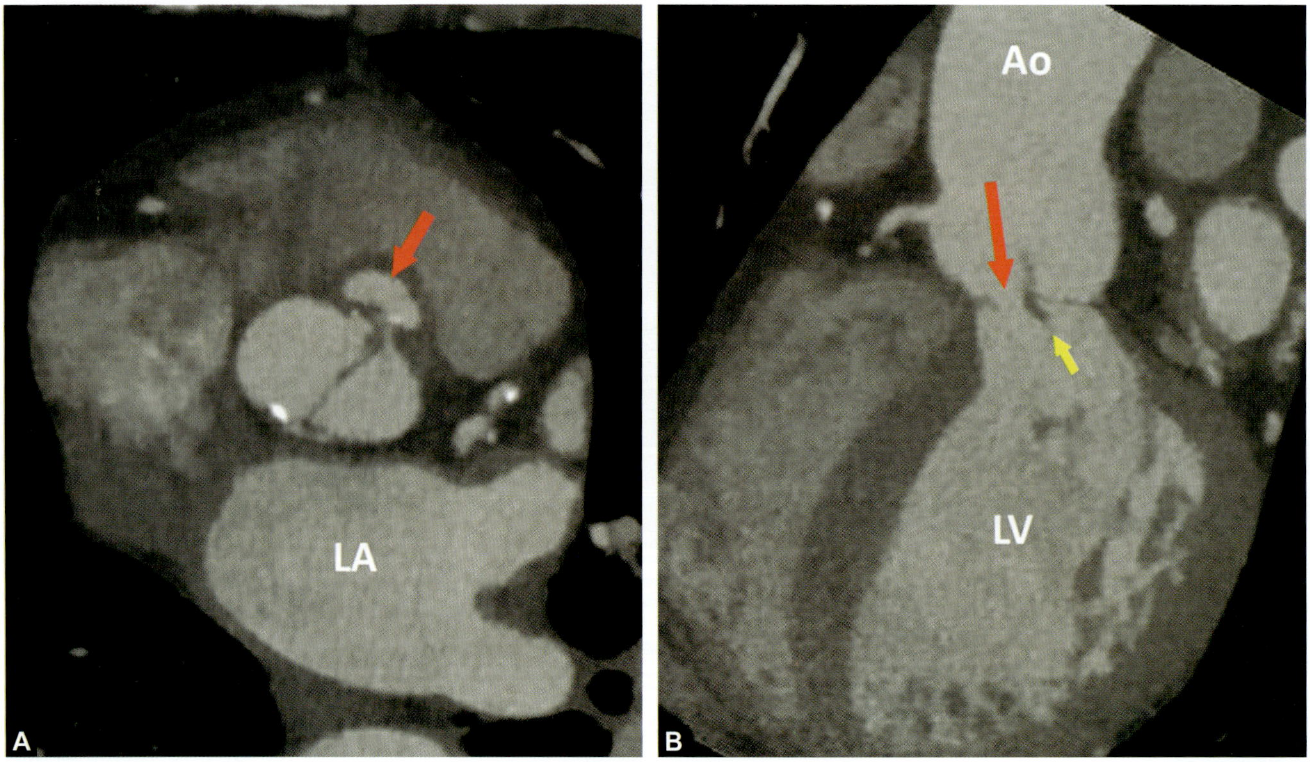

Figs. 16.31A and B: Preoperative CT-scan in a patient with bicuspid aortic valve and aortic valve endocarditis. (A) Bicuspid aortic valve with an infectious pseudoaneurysm red (arrow) arising from the left coronary cusp, anterior to the aorta. (B) Fenestration of the right coronary cusp with a large regurgitant orifice (red arrow) and prolapse of some cusp fibers into the LVOT (yellow arrow). (Images courtesy of Dr Suhny Abbara, University of Texas Southwestern Medical Center).

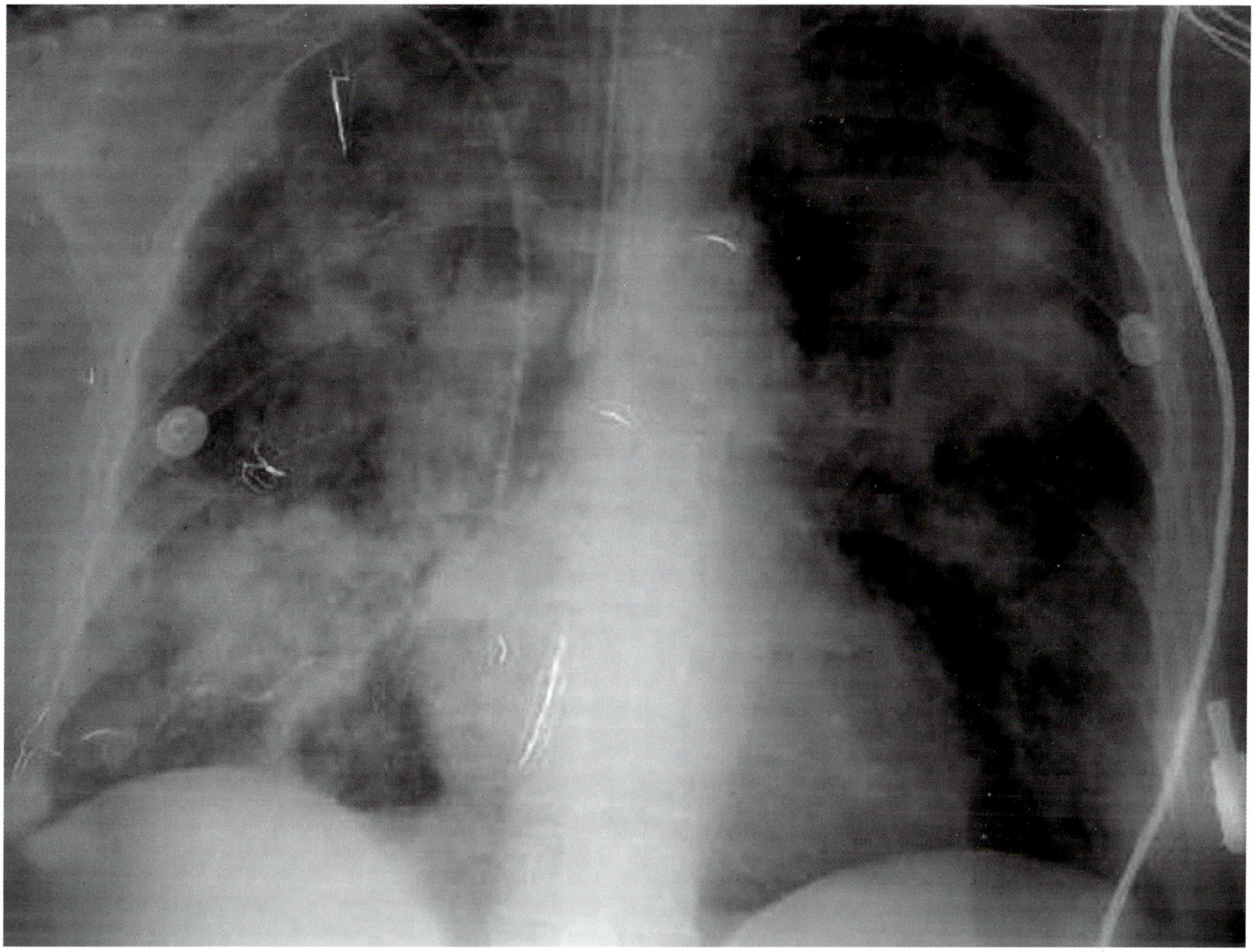

Fig. 16.32: Chest X-ray showing innumerable septal emboli in a patient with tricuspid valve endocarditis. [Image courtesy of Dr Felipe G, Rendón-Elías, Servicio de Cirugía Cardiovascular y Torácica, Hospital Universitario "Dr José Eleuterio González". Image from Rendon-Elias FG. Surgical management of infective endocarditis: 10 years experience. Medicina Universitaria 2012;14(57):196-204].

Table 16.4: Indications for surgical intervention in patients with endocarditis.

• Acute aortic insufficiency or mitral regurgitation leading to congestive heart failure.
• Cardiac abscess formation/perivalvular extension
• Persistence of infection despite adequate antibiotic treatment
• Increase in vegetation size despite appropriate antibiotic therapy
• Recurrent peripheral emboli
• Cerebral emboli
• Infection due to microorganisms with a poor response to antibiotic treatment (e.g. fungi)
• Prosthetic valve endocarditis, particularly if hemodynamic compromise exists
• Prosthetic valve dehiscence
• "Mitral kissing infection" – when cardiac echo demonstrates a large vegetation on the aortic valve that "kisses" the anterior mitral leaflet
• Some also consider large (> 10 mm) mobile vegetations an indication for surgery

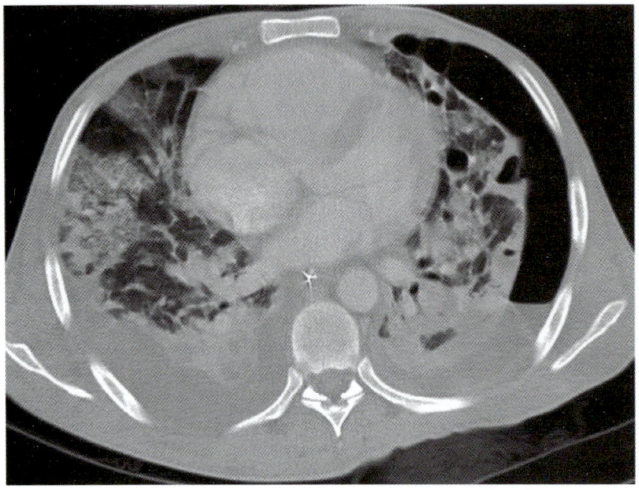

Fig. 16.33: Computed tomography scan demonstrating florid embolic lung abscesses with cavitation, bronchopleural fistula and pyopneumothorax in a patient with septic emboli from pulmonary valve endocarditis due to *Staphylococcus aureus*; [Image and legend text from Kang N, Smith W. Surgical Management of Infective Endocarditis. In: Kerrigan SW (ed). Recent Advances in Infective Endocarditis, Intechweb.org].

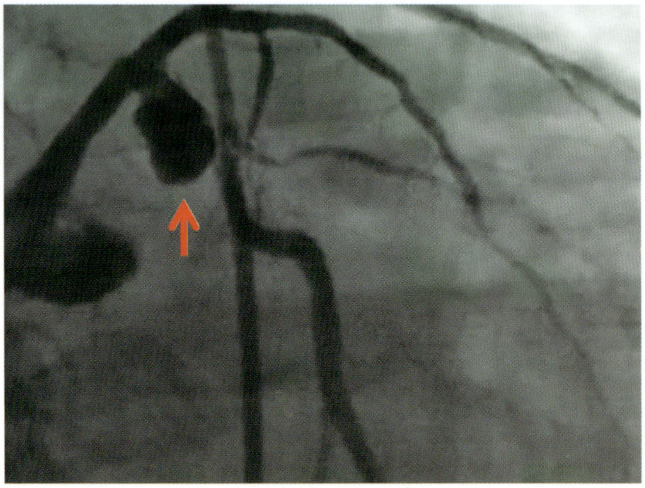

Fig. 16.34: Large mycotic aneurysm (arrow) in the distal left main coronary artery in a patient with endocarditis.

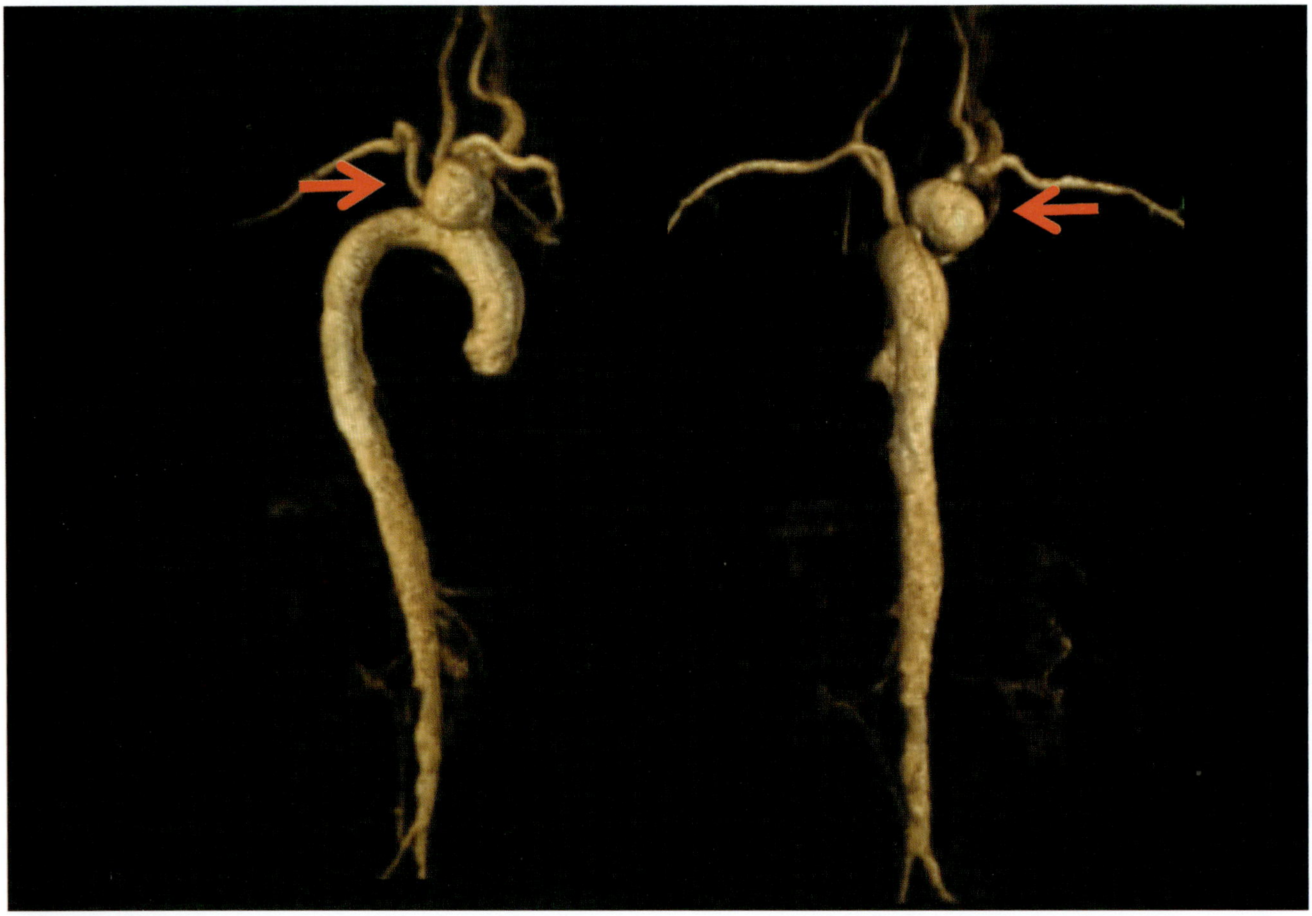

Fig. 16.35: MRA showing mycotic aneurysm (arrows) of the innominate artery. (MRA: Magnetic resonance angiography).

or by catheter intervention, during the first 6 months after the procedure; repaired CHD with residual defects at the site or adjacent to the site of a prosthetic patch or prosthetic device (which inhibit endothelialization); and cardiac transplantation recipients who develop cardiac valvulopathy.

VIDEO LEGENDS

Video 1: Parasternal long axis TTE showing small vegetations on the aortic valve. Video courtesy of Glenn N. Levine, MD.

Video 2: Transesophageal echocardiography (TEE) videoclip showing complex vegetation on the posterior mitral leaflet. Video courtesy of Alvin Blaustein, MD.

Video 3: Transesophageal echocardiography (TEE) videoclip showing complex vegetation on the mitral valve in a patient with endocarditis. Video courtesy of Alvin Blaustein, MD.

Video 4: TEE videoclip of large, highly mobile vegetation on a prosthetic mitral valve.

Video 5: TEE showing a mobile vegetation on a prosthetic mitral valve in a patient with endocarditis. Video courtesy of Alvin Blaustein, MD.

Video 6: TEE showing a complex and highly mobile vegetation on a prosthetic mitral valve in a patient with endocarditis. Video courtesy of Alvin Blaustein, MD.

Video 7: Large, complex vegetation on a prosthetic mitral valve in a patient with blood-culture documented endocarditis.

Video 8: Color Doppler TEE showing mitral regurgitation as a result of mitral valve endocarditis and valve destruction. Video courtesy of Alvin Blaustein, MD.

REFERENCES

Baddour LM, Wilson WR, Bayer AS, et al. Infective endocarditis: diagnosis, antimicrobial therapy, and management of complications: a statement for healthcare professionals from the Committee on Rheumatic Fever, Endocarditis, and Kawasaki Disease, Council on Cardiovascular Disease in the Young, and the Councils on Clinical Cardiology, Stroke, and Cardiovascular Surgery and Anesthesia, American Heart Association: endorsed by the Infectious Diseases Society of America. Circulation. 2005;111:e394-e434.

Durack DT, Lukes AS, Bright DK. New criteria for diagnosis of infective endocarditis: utilization of specific echocardiographic findings. Duke Endocarditis Service. Am J Med. 1994; 96(3):200-9.

Karchmer AW. Infective endocarditis. In: Zipes DP, Libby P, Bonow R, Braunwald E (eds). Braunwald's Heart Disease: A Textbook of Cardiovascular Medicine, 7th edition. Philadelphia: WB Saunders Co; 2005:1633-58.

Karchmer AW. Infective endocarditis. In: Kasper DL, Braunwald E, Hauser S, Longo D, Jameson JL, Fauci As. Harrison's Principles of Internal Medicine, 16th ed. New York: McGraw-Hill; 2005:731-40.

Wilson W, Taubert KA, Gewitz M, et al. Prevention of infective endocarditis: guidelines from the American Heart Association: a guideline from the American Heart Association Rheumatic Fever, Endocarditis, and Kawasaki Disease Committee, Council on Cardiovascular Disease in the Young, and the Council on Clinical Cardiology, Council on Cardiovascular Surgery and Anesthesia, and the Quality of Care and Outcomes Research Interdisciplinary Working Group. Circulation. 2007;116(15):1736-54.

CHAPTER

Transcatheter Aortic Valve Replacement

17

Michael J Mack, Ambarish Gopal

INTRODUCTION

Transcatheter aortic valve replacement (TAVR), alternately called transcatheter aortic valve implantation (TAVI), has now become the standard of care for the extremely high-risk or the "inoperable" patients with symptomatic severe aortic stenosis, and is also an alternative to surgery for many high-risk but "operable" patients. The two most commonly used valves are the Edwards Sapien balloon-expandable valve (Fig. 17.1A) and the self-expanding Medtronic CoreValve (Figs. 17.1B to D). While in the United States only several valves are being used or are approved, many more are in various states of development, have been CE approved for use in Europe, and are used worldwide (Figs. 17.2A to F).

Two routes of delivery for TAVR are commonly employed for the balloon expandable Edwards Sapien platform valve, the transfemoral route (Fig. 17.3A, Videos 1 and 2) and the transapical route (Fig. 17.3B, Video 3), although direct aortic delivery (Fig. 17.4) is also used in some patients. Delivery of the CoreValve can be performed via transfemoral, trans-subclavian and transaortic routes (Fig. 17.5). These delivery routes can be used with other transcatheter valves as well.

Formal guidelines for TAVI (Table 17.1) have been made by the European Society of Cardiology (ESC) and the European Association for Cardio-Thoracic Surgery (EACTS). Current treatment recommendations have also been summarized in a US expert consensus document (Table 17.2). Recommendations regarding TAVR and now also included in the new American College of Cardiology Foundation (ACCF)/American Heart Association (AHA) guidelines on valvular heart disease (Table 17.3).

PATIENT AND PROCEDURAL CONSIDERATIONS FOR TAVR

Evaluation of a patient for TAVR involves a multidisciplinary team (the "Heart Team") approach, which may include the patient's primary cardiologist, a cardiac surgeon, an interventional cardiologist, an echocardiographer, an imaging specialist (cardiac CT or CMR), a heart failure and valve disease specialist, the cardiac anesthesiologist, a nurse practitioner, and cardiac rehabilitation specialists. The goals of this multidisciplinary team are to assess the patient's suitability for open chest, surgical aortic valve replacement (SAVR), and TAVR. Although the risk of open chest, SAVR in terms of morbidity and mortality can be estimated using the Society of Thoracic Surgeons (STS) score, even some patients with a relatively low STS score may not be candidates for SAVR due to conditions such

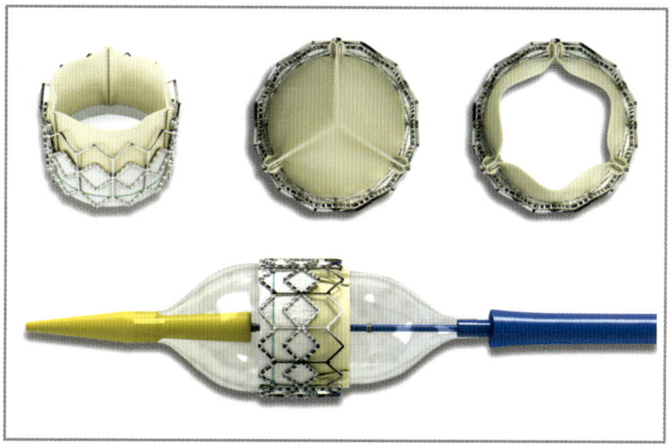

Fig. 17.1A: The balloon-expandable Edwards Sapien valve along with the delivery system. (Image courtesy of Edwards Lifesciences).

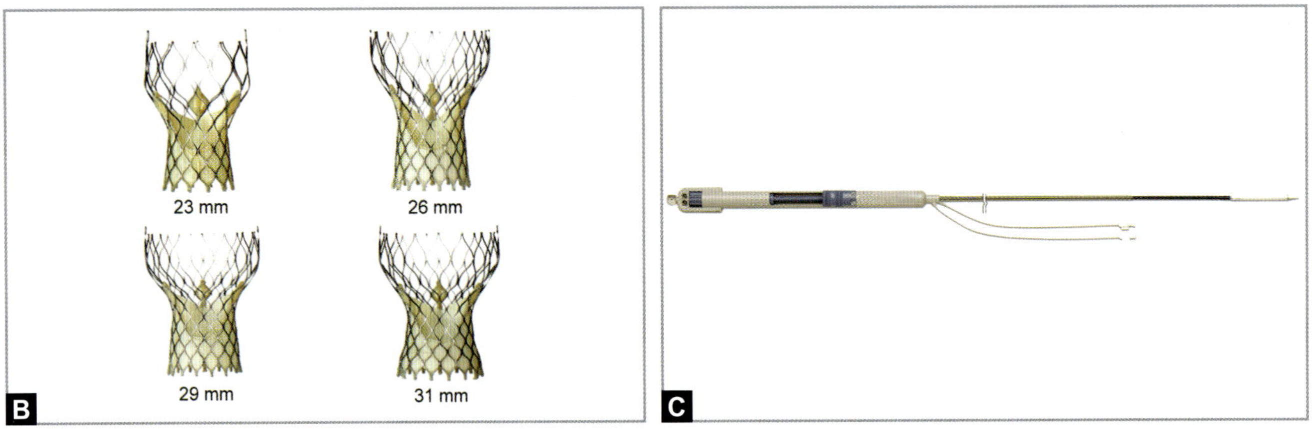

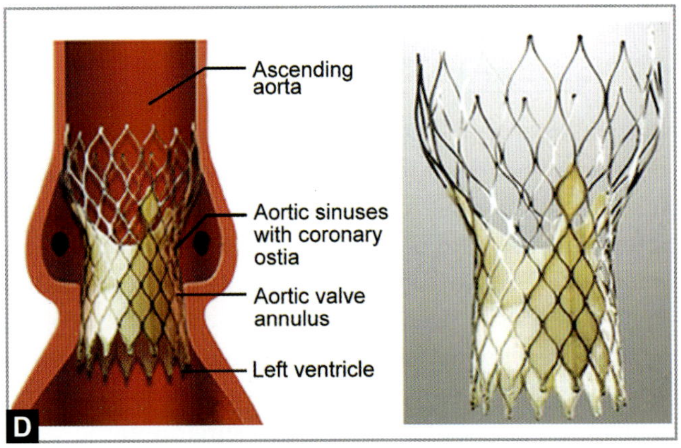

Figs. 17.1B to D: The Medtronic CoreValve. (B) CoreValve pictured in different sizes; (C) CoreValve delivery system; (D) Schematic of the CoreValve 2 deployed in the aortic root. (Images courtesy of Medtronic, Inc).

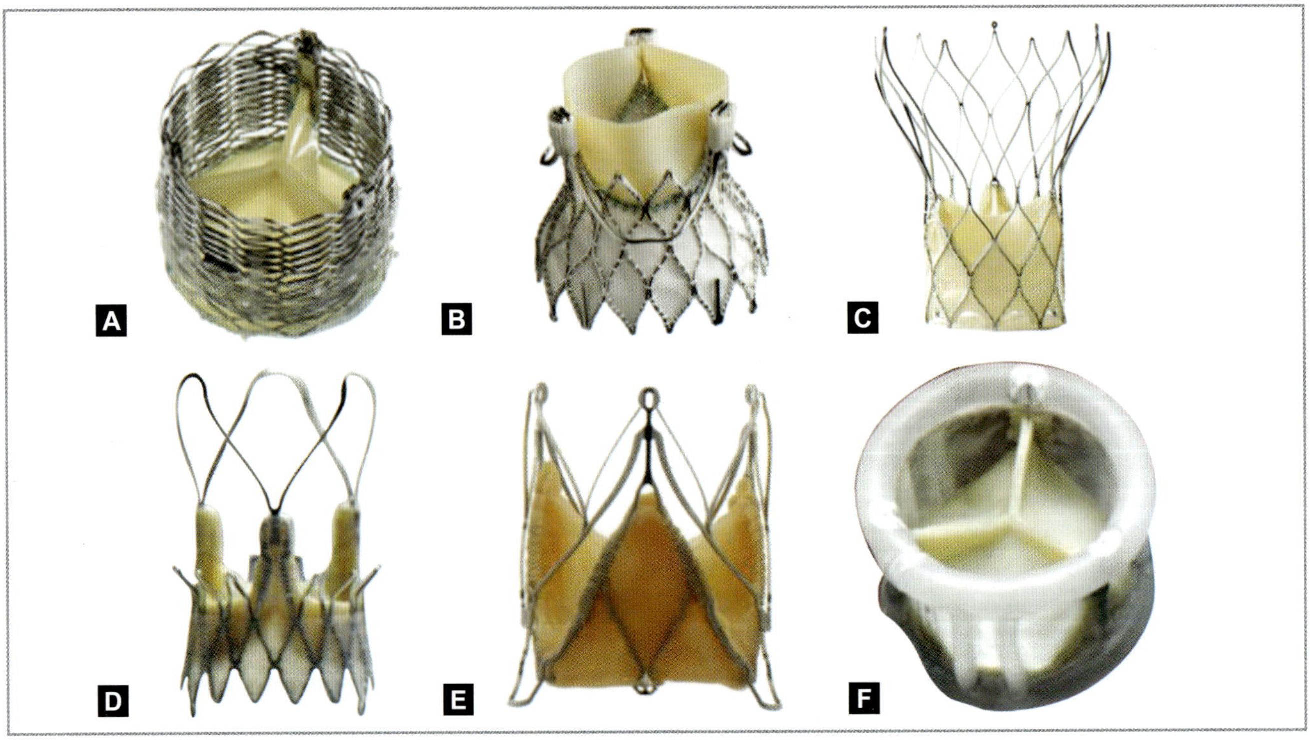

Figs. 17.2A to F: Examples of other transcatheter heart valves in development or available in parts of the world. (A) Sadra Lotus (Boston Scientific, Inc.); (B) Medtronic Engager; (C) St. Jude Portico 23; (D) Symetis Acurate; (E) JenaValve TA; (F) Direct Flow Valve. (Direct Flow Medical, Inc).

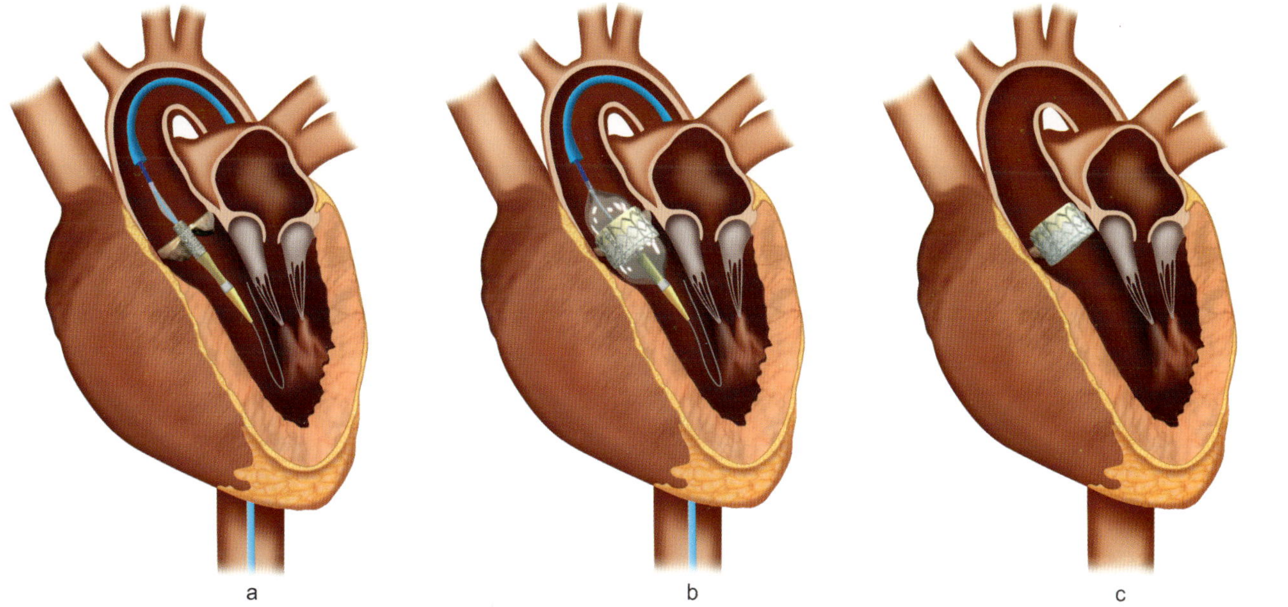

Fig. 17.3A: Deployment of the balloon-expandable Edwards Sapien valve via the transfemoral route. (a) Valve is delivered retrograde from the femoral artery and positioned at the level of the aortic annulus. (b) Balloon inflated, deploying the valve. (c) Deployed valve. (Images courtesy of Edwards Lifesciences).

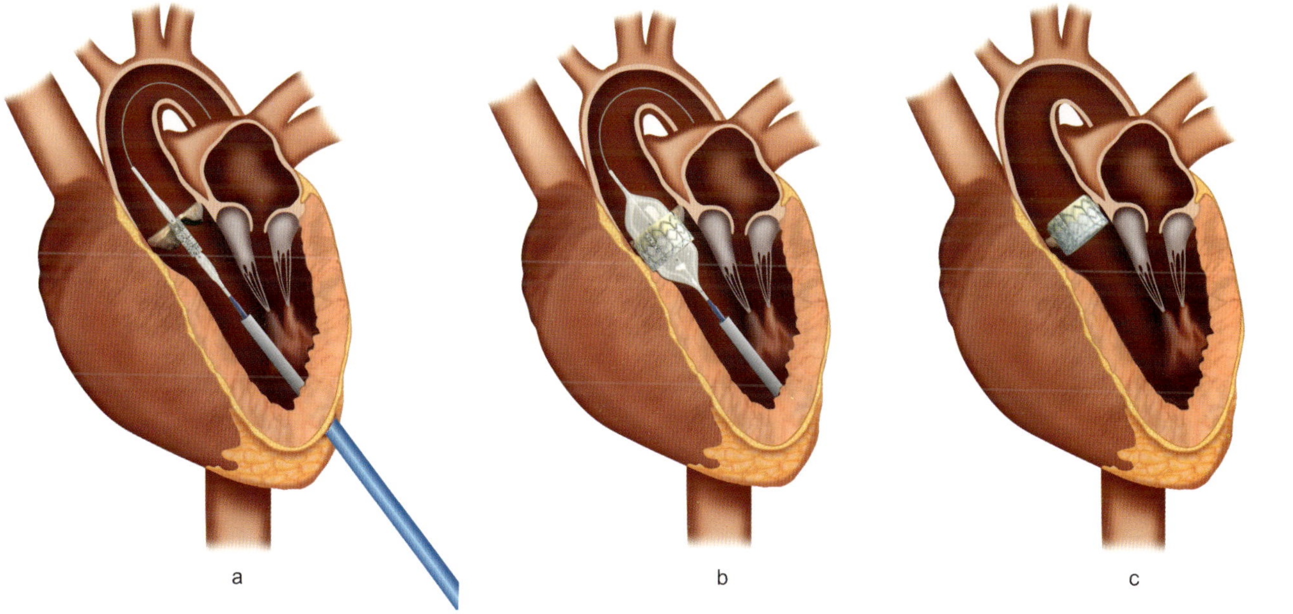

Fig. 17.3B: Deployment of the balloon-expandable Edwards Sapien valve via the transapical route. (a) Valve delivered antegrade to the aortic annulus via a small incision in the left ventricular apex. (b) Balloon inflated, deploying the valve. (c) Deployed valve. (Images courtesy of Edwards Lifesciences).

as heavily calcified (porcelain) aorta (Figs. 17.6A and B), chest wall deformity, oxygen-dependent lung disease, or frailty, and may thus be considered for TAVR.

An accurate sizing of the aortic valve annulus is critical in achieving a successful result. Annulus assessment is performed both to assess the most appropriate size valve and to assess if the annulus is too large or two small for TAVR. However, the aortic root and attachment of the aortic leaflets to the root is complex, and not well suited to simple axial two-dimensional (2D) assessment. Further,

Table 17.1: Summary of the European Society of Cardiology (ESC) and European Association for Cardio-Thoracic Surgery (EACTS) guidelines for transcatheter aortic valve implantation (TAVI). The level of evidence (LOE) supporting the recommendation is given in parenthesis, where LOE = A denotes a recommendation derived from multiple randomized clinical trials or meta-analyses; LOE = B denotes a recommendation derived from a single randomized clinical trial or large non-randomized studies; and LOE = C denotes a recommendation based on consensus of expert opinion or based on small studies, retrospective studies, or registries.

Class I (is recommended; is indicated)
• TAVI should only be undertaken with a multidisciplinary "heart team" (LOE = C)
• TAVI should only be performed in hospitals with on-site cardiac surgery capability (LOE = C)
• TAVI in patients with severe aortic stenosis (AS) who are not suitable for AVR, as assessed by a "heart team", and who are likely gain improvement in their quality of life and to have a life expectancy of >1 year after consideration of their comorbidities (LOE = B)
Class IIa (should be considered)
• TAVI in high-risk patients with severe symptomatic AS who may still be suitable for surgery, but in whom TAVI is favored by a "heart team" based on individual risk profile and anatomic suitability (LOE = B)

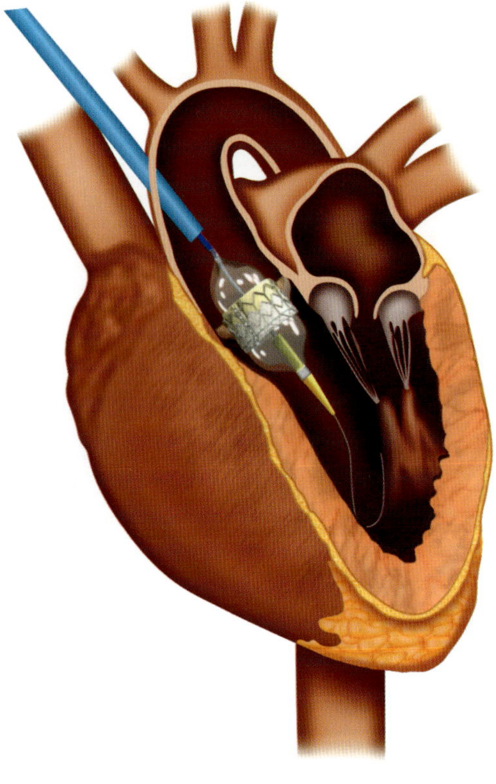

Fig. 17.4: Schematic illustration of the transaortic delivery of the Edwards Sapien valve. (Image courtesy of Edwards Lifesciences).

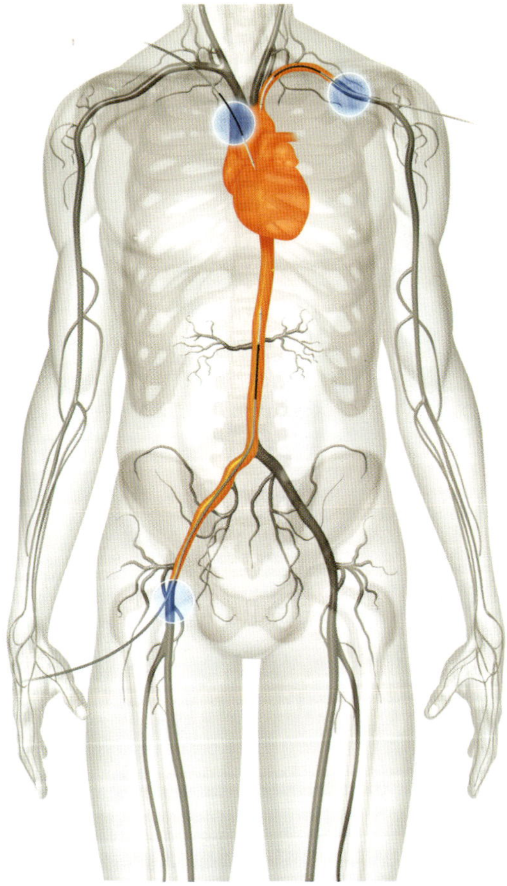

Fig. 17.5: Available delivery options (transfemoral, trans-subclavian and transaortic) for the Medtronic CoreValve. (Images courtesy of Medtronic, Inc).

Table 17.2: Summary of the American College of Cardiology Foundation (ACCF)/American Association of Thoracic Surgeons (AATS)/Society for Cardiovascular Angiography and Intervention (SCAI) and the Society of Thoracic Surgeons (STS) expert consensus document of transcatheter aortic valve replacement (TAVR) recommendations for TAVR in patients with aortic stenosis.

Class I (is recommended; is indicated)
• TAVR in patients with severe, symptomatic, calcified stenosis of a trileaflet aortic valve who have aortic and vascular anatomy suitable for TAVR and have a predicted survival > 12 months, and who have a prohibitive surgical risk as defined by an estimated 50% or greater risk of mortality or irreversible morbidity at 30 days or other factors such as frailty, prior radiation therapy, porcelain aorta, and severe hepatic or pulmonary disease
Class IIa (is reasonable)
• TAVR as an alternative to surgical AVR in patients at high surgical risk (PARTNER trial criteria: STS ≥ 8%)

Table 17.3: Summary of the recommendations regarding TAVR in the new American College of Cardiology Foundation (ACCF)/American Heart Association (AHA) guidelines on valvular heart disease.

Class I (is recommended)
• Surgical AVR (not TAVR) in low to intermediate surgical risk patients (LOE = A)
• Heart Valve Team collaboration in deciding between TAVR or high-risk surgical AVR (LOE = C)
• TAVR for patients who meet an indication for AVR for AS who have prohibitive surgical risk and a predicted post-TAVR survival > 12 months (LOE = B)
Class IIa (is reasonable)
• TAVR as an alternative to surgical AVR for AS in patients who meet an indication for AVR and who have high surgical risk (LOE = B)
Class IIb (may be considered)
• Percutaneous aortic balloon dilation as a bridge to surgical or transcatheter AVR in severely symptomatic patients with severe AS (LOE = C)
Class III (no benefit)
• Performance of TAVR in patients in whom the existing comorbidities would preclude the expected benefit from correction of AS (LOE = B)

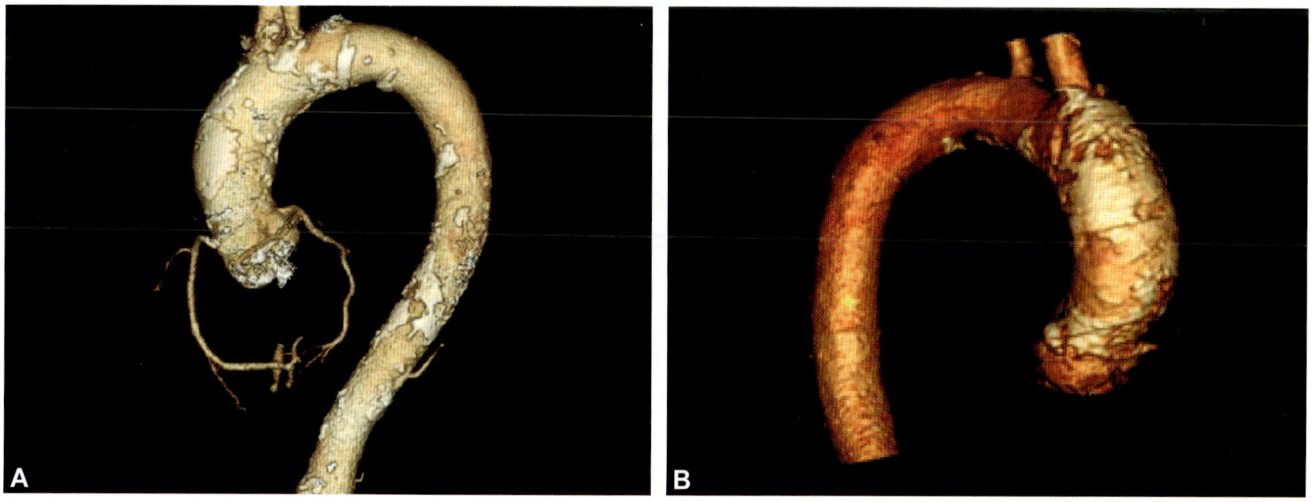

Figs. 17.6A and B: CT imaging demonstrating a heavily calcified (porcelain) aorta, making the patient high-risk for open surgical aortic valve replacement (as well as transaortic transcatheter heart valve delivery). The patient in Figure 17.6B had previously been treated with radiation therapy, a likely cause of the porcelain aorta. [Figure 17.6A courtesy of Edwards Lifesciences; Figure 17.6B from Akin I, Kische S, Schneider H, et al. Current indications for transcatheter aortic valve implantation. In: Chen YF, Luo CY (Eds). Aortic Valve. InTech, 2011].

the aortic valve annulus is not a perfectly circular entity. It is an elliptical structure with variable degree of eccentricity that is formed by a virtual ring that connects the three hinge points or anchor points of the three cusps of the aortic valve leaflets. These considerations are illustrated in Figures 17.7A to C.

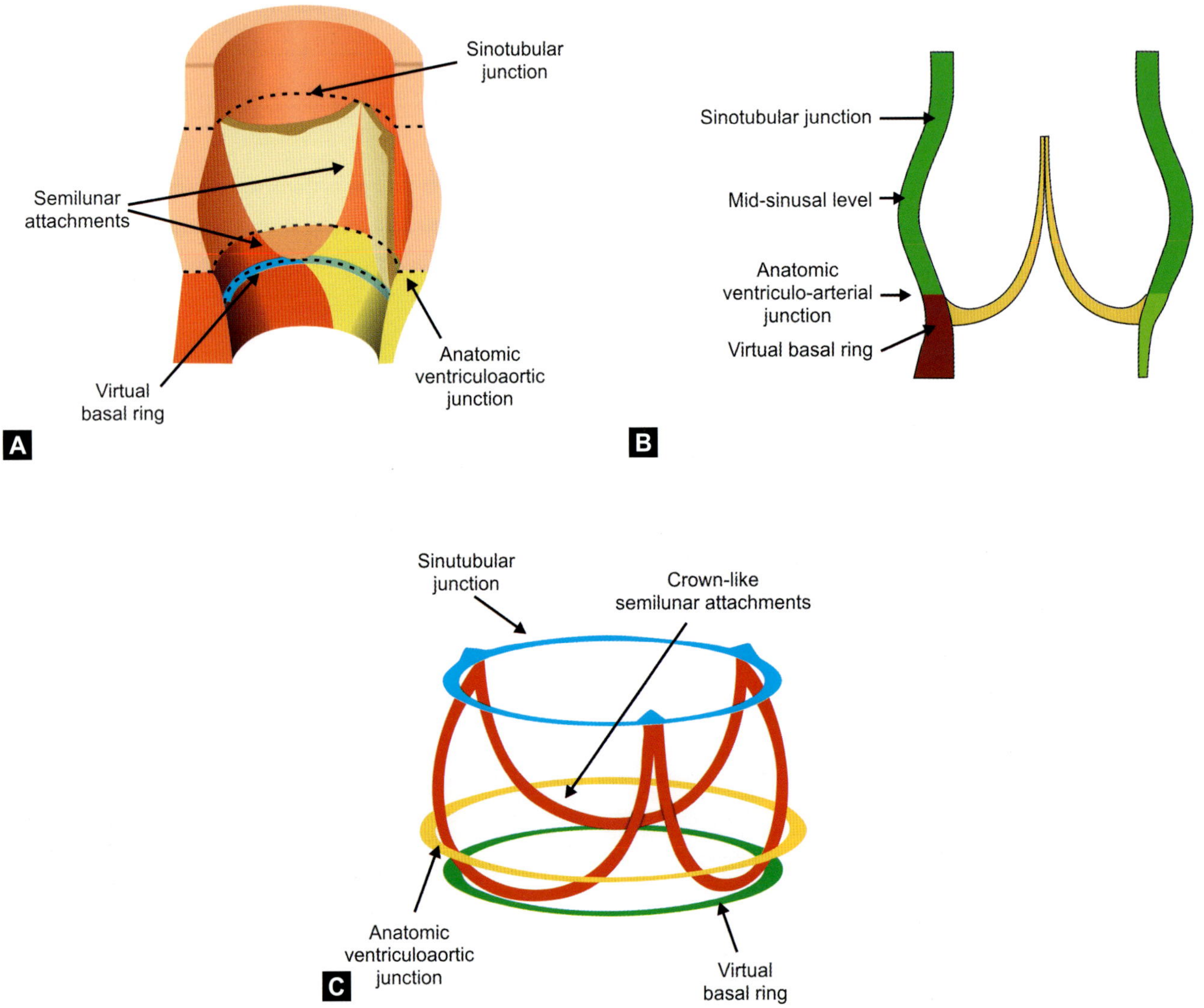

Figs. 17.7A to C: (A) This illustration shows a bisected aortic root, and illustrates how the semilunar attachment of the valvular leaflets incorporates aortic wall in the intersinusal triangles, and ventricular tissues at the base of each of the coronary aortic sinuses; (B) This illustration shows how measurement of the basal ring provides information relating only to the entrance of the aortic root. To provide full details, measurements should be taken also of the diameter of the sinotubular junction, and at mid-sinusal level. None of these measurements take account of the diameter at the anatomic ventriculoaortic junction; (C) This figure shows an idealized aortic root. The attachments of the valvular leaflets, shown in red, extend through the entire length of the root, from the sinotubular junction, in blue, to the virtual basal ring, shown in green, and produced by joining together the basal attachments of the leaflets. The crown-like attachments of the leaflets cross the anatomic ventriculoaortic junction, shown in yellow. Image courtesy of Dr Robert Anderson, Institute of Genetic Medicine, Newcastle University, United Kingdom and Gemma Price. [Figures and legend text from Anderson RH. The surgical anatomy of the aortic root. Multimed Man Cardiothorac Surg. 2007;2007(102):mmcts.2006.002527].

Although 2D echocardiography (Fig. 17.8) has been used to assess the aortic root and valve annulus, this strategy in itself is not favored. In contrast, a three-dimensional (3D) imaging technique, such as gated cardiac computed tomography (Figs. 17.9A and B) or a cardiac MRI (CMR), provides the ability to align the three anchor points of the aortic annulus virtual ring and to more accurately size the annulus. Three-dimensional transesophageal electrocardiography (TEE) is also used to measure the aortic annulus (Fig. 17.10). Accurate major and minor axes, maximum annulus area, and annulus perimeter measures are ideally obtained during systole (between 5% and 30% of the R-R interval during ECG-gated image acquisition).

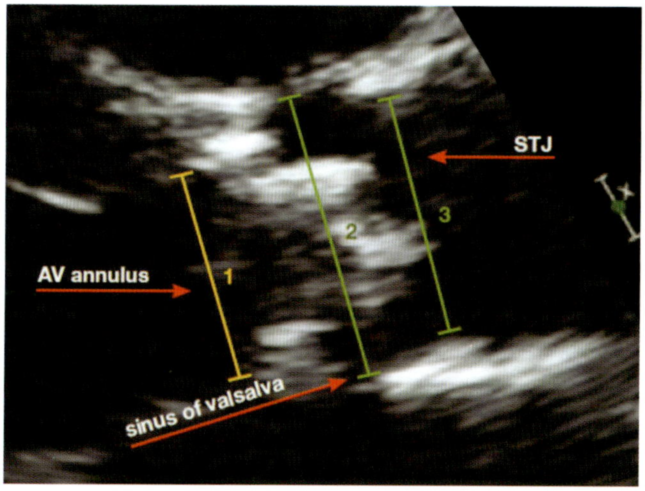

Fig. 17.8: Two-dimensional (2D) transesophageal electrocardiography images of the aortic root and annulus. Because of the complex nature of the aortic root and annulus, and the elliptical geometry of the annulus, valve sizing based solely on 2D measurements are not favored. (Image courtesy of Edwards Lifesciences). (AV: Aortic valve; STJ: Sinatubular junction).

An undersized transcatheter heart valve (THV) can result in paravalvular regurgitation (Fig. 17.11), which in some cases may be severe. An oversized THV can potentially result in annulus rupture. Based on an accurate sizing with a 3D modality, an optimal acceptable annulus area-based oversizing of about 10–15% with the THV is desirable (this can range from 1% to 20%). In some practices, when the area-based oversizing exceeds 20%, the concept of controlled oversizing with an intentional THV balloon "underfill" is recommended. This is a consideration in the small elderly female patient or in a patient with high-risk patterns of calcification, in order to avoid rupturing the annulus.

Cardiac CT provides details regarding the burden and the patterns of calcification of the aortic valve annulus and neighboring structures (Figs. 17.12A to D). Cardiac CT imaging allows for identification of patients at increased risk for annulus rupture and paravalvular leak, even if there is accurate annulus sizing, as well as the assessment of the distance of the coronary ostia from the aortic annulus (Figs. 17.13A and B).

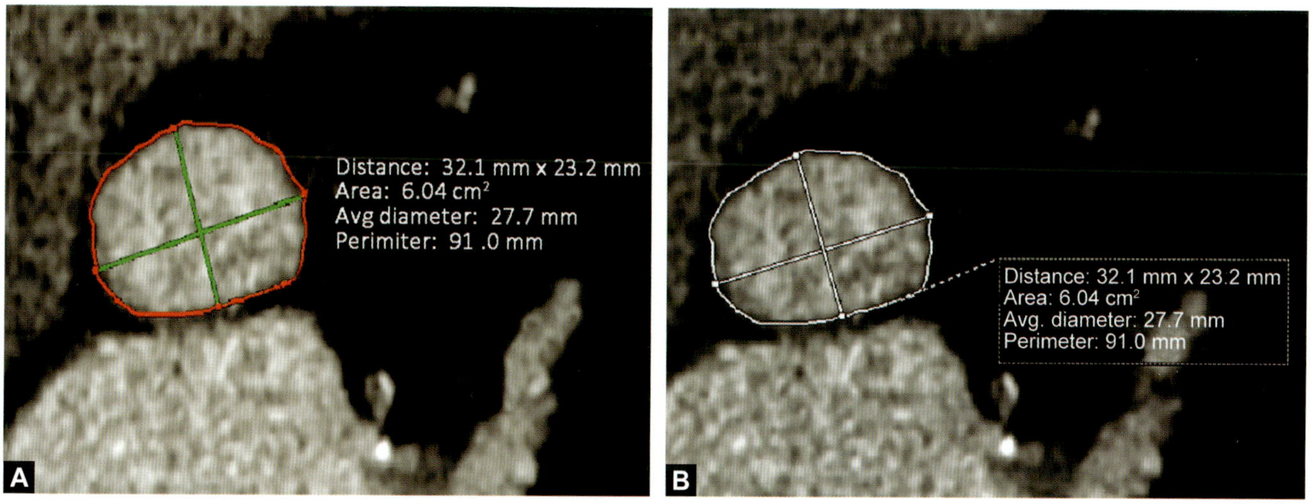

Figs. 17.9A and B: CT multiplanar reformatted images used to measure the aortic annulus. Measurements include major and minor axis dimensions, cross-sectional area, and circumference.

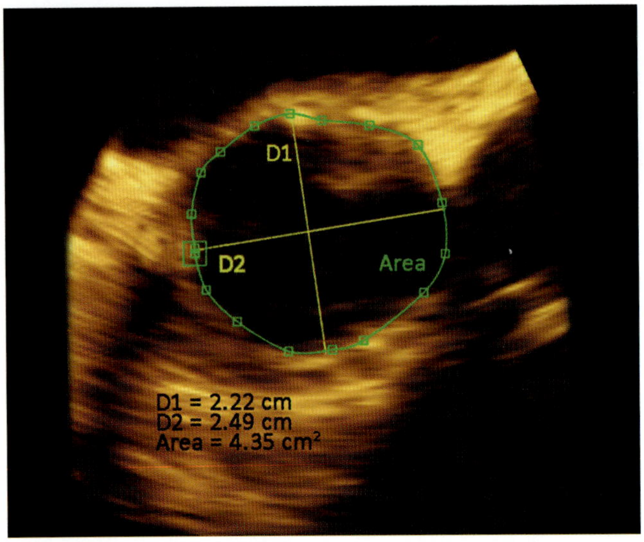

Fig. 17.10: 3D transesophageal echocardiography assessment of the aortic annulus dimensions.

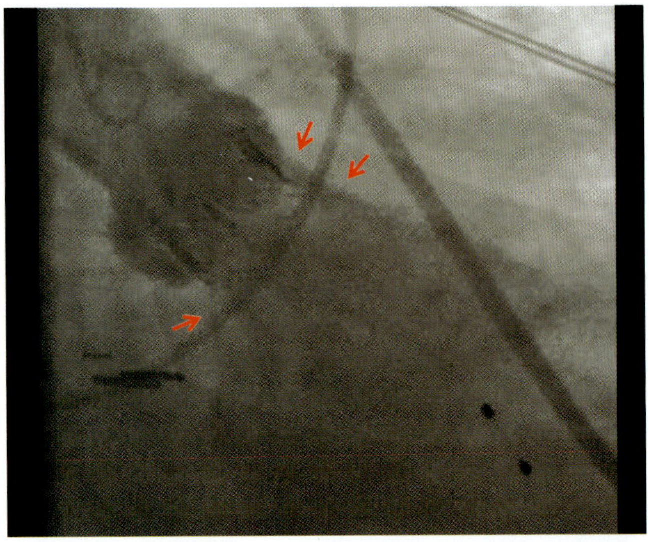

Fig. 17.11: Aortography after valve deployment of an undersized transcatheter heart valve demonstrates significant perivalvular leak (arrows).

During the TAVR procedure, fluoroscopy and aortography are used to optimally position the image intensifier to visualize all three cusps in a single plane (Figs. 17.14A to C). For many if not most procedures, pre-procedural CT imaging and analysis is used to pre-select optimal image intensifier position (Fig. 17.15). Fluoroscopic-guided deployment of the THV is shown in Figures 17.16A to C. Intraoperative CT imaging to guide angulation and THV deployment has also been used (Figs. 17.17A to C), although this is not routinely done in most TAVR procedures.

ROUTE OF DELIVERY CONSIDERATIONS IN TAVR

Once an appropriate THV size has been determined, the next step in TAVR planning is to select an appropriate approach for THV delivery. The different access routes with their advantages and disadvantages are listed in Table 17.4. In most patients, CT angiography is performed not only to assess the aortic annulus, but also to assess and plan vascular access (Figs. 17.18 and 17.19).

The presence of moderate to severe calcification in the iliofemoral arteries (Figs. 17.20A to E) predicts a three-fold increase in vascular complications (29% vs 9%). Sheath-to-femoral artery ratio (SFAR) of >1.05 is predictive of a four-fold increased risk of vascular complication (23% vs 5%). If moderate to severe calcification is noted in the iliofemoral arteries, a SFAR cutoff of >1.00 is recommended. Considerations for transfemoral access route delivery are listed in Table 17.5.

In patients in whom a transfemoral approach is not feasible, several options are available, depending somewhat on the THV used. In some patients, uses of a conduit anastomosed to the proximal iliac artery may allow peripheral THV delivery in a patient with relatively healthy proximal iliac arteries but diseased more distal iliac and/or femoral arteries. Conduit anastomosis to the left iliac artery is favored for anatomical reasons.

In some patients, a subclavian or direct aortic approach can be utilized. CT imaging is used to assess suitability for THV delivery (Figs. 17.21 to 17.23). Heavy calcification of the ascending aorta (Figs. 17.24A and B) may be an issue when considering a direct aortic approach. The transapical approach allows antegrade delivery of the THV in patients in whom retrograde delivery is not feasible or is high-risk. Transapical TAVR requires a small left thoracotomy incision (Fig. 17.25) and direct instrumentation of the left ventricular apex, but does not require cardiopulmonary bypass.

COMPLICATIONS

As with most surgical and transcatheter procedures, TAVR is associated with risk of complication. Stroke may occur due to atheroembolic or other mechanisms. The incidence of stroke ranges from approximately 1–7%. Annulus rupture is a catastrophic complication and is associated

Table 17.4: Considerations for transfemoral access route delivery. After assessing the minimal luminal diameter of a transfemoral route and with true outer diameter (OD) of the chosen delivery sheath, one can calculate the sheath-to-femoral access ratio (SFAR). SFAR of > 1.05 is predictive of a 4-fold increased risk of vascular complication (23% vs 5%). The presence of moderate to severe calcification in the iliofemoral arteries predicts a 3-fold increase in vascular complications (29% vs 9%). If moderate to severe calcification is noted in the iliofemoral arteries, an SFAR cutoff of > 1.00 is recommended. The actual luminal distance of the ilio-femoral access from the iliac bifurcation to the common femoral artery divided by the distance between the two points "as the crow flies" is used to calculate the iliofemoral tortuosity index. An ilio-femoral tortuosity index of > 1.5 and/or the most acute angle determined in the iliofemoral access route of </= 120 degrees are more likely to make the transfemoral access more challenging and not a recommended route particularly in the presence of moderate-severe calcification.

Minimum luminal diameter	xx mm			
True OD of the sheath selected	xx mm			
SFAR (calculated for patient)	X:Y			
Burden of TF calcification	None to Mild		Moderate to Severe	
Required SFAR cutoff (Ca^{++} modified)	< 1.10	< 1.05		< 1.00
Iliofemoral tortuosity Index	≤ 1.25	1.25 to ≤ 1.5	1.5 to ≤ 1.6	> 1.6
Iliofemoral angle (degrees)	160 to 180	121 to 159	90 to 120	< 90
Grade	0	1	3	4

Table 17.5: Considerations for transfemoral access route delivery.

Access route	***Advantages***	***Disadvantages***	***Comments***
Transfemoral	• Least invasive • Access can be closed with a percutaneous "preclosure" technique without the need for a cut down	• Requires an iliofemoral access route that can safely accommodate the delivery system • Vascular complications have substantially come down with better pre-procedural screening	• Most commonly used
Transapical	• Practically all patients are candidates for this • The straight delivery line to the aortic valve, short distance and a more rigid delivery system (valve-on-a-stick rather than valve-on-a-catheter) all help with accurate valve positioning and deployment	• Need for invasive surgical thoracotomy particularly in elderly, debilitated patients and those with significant lung disease • Early bleeding complications due to apical tissue fragility have come down due to better apical purse string suturing techniques • Apical access and closure devices allow possibility of a percutaneous trocar-based transapical approach to provide a safe less invasive method	• Currently, the second most common access route • Recommend periprocedural trans-esophageal echocardiography (TEE) to verify the initial guidewire has not accidentally gone through a mitral chordal structure before going through the aortic valve (TEE will show either a new mitral regurgitation or worsening of pre-existing mitral regurgitation). Fortunately, this is not a common issue
Transaortic	• Includes direct passage at a brief distance from the aortic valve apparatus via a purse string suture in the ascending aorta	• A surgical incision is still required, either an upper partial sternotomy or small right anterior thoracotomy (these are regarded as less invasive than the surgical incision required for the transapical approach)	• Also referred to as direct aortic • Though there were concerns that ascending aorta calcification would preclude this approach, recent data demonstrates that almost all patients are candidates for this approach as the most important requisite is the presence of a "calcification free zone" for the cannulation in the distal portion of the ascending aorta
Subclavian/ Axillary	• Has been used when transfemoral access is not possible	• Use of the left subclavian artery in patients with a previous patent left internal mammary graft has the possible risk of occlusion • Thought not frequent, the subclavian artery can be relatively small in caliber, and can have the risk of dissection or disruption owing to the relative lack of a muscular component of the arterial wall	• Losing favor given the availability of a direct aortic approach • Both left and right subclavian arteries may be used. The left subclavian artery is used more commonly due to a favorable angle of delivery relative to the aortic valve

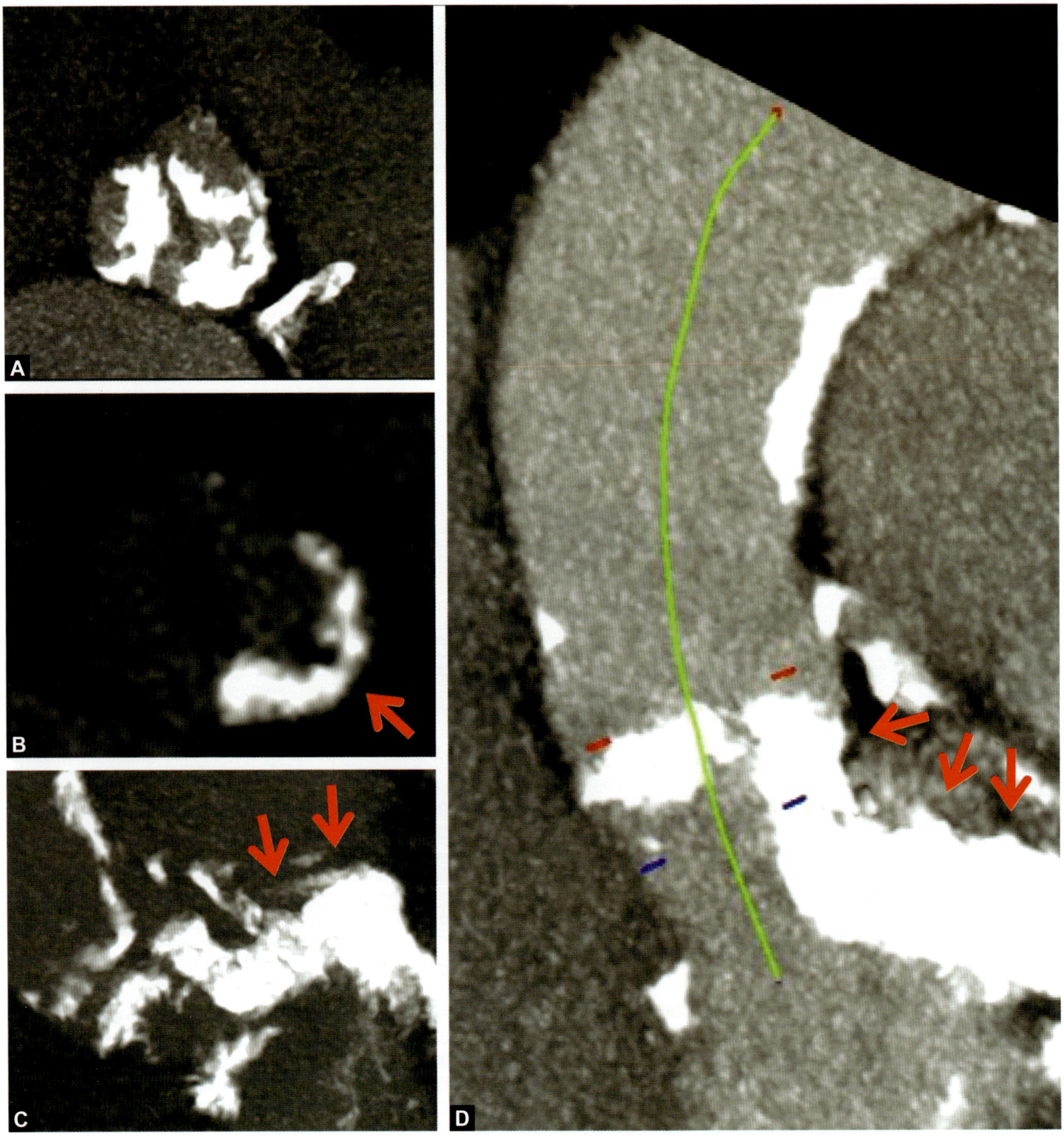

Figs. 17.12A to D: CT images used in the assessment of patient suitability for transcatheter aortic valve replacement (TAVR). (A) Maximum intensity projection (MIP) cross-section of the aortic valve showing severe calcification (grade 3) of the aortic valve leaflets; (B) Sub-millimeter multiplanar reformatted image showing crescentic calcification (arrow) in the left cusp zone, a finding associated with higher risk of procedural complication; (C) Curved multiplanar reformat maximum intensity projection image demonstrating heavy calcification of the aortic valve apparatus and its neighboring structures (arrows). This finding is a high-risk predictor for annular rupture with TAVR; (D) Straightened curved multiplanar reformatted view showing the same findings of extensive calcification (arrows) as in Figure C.

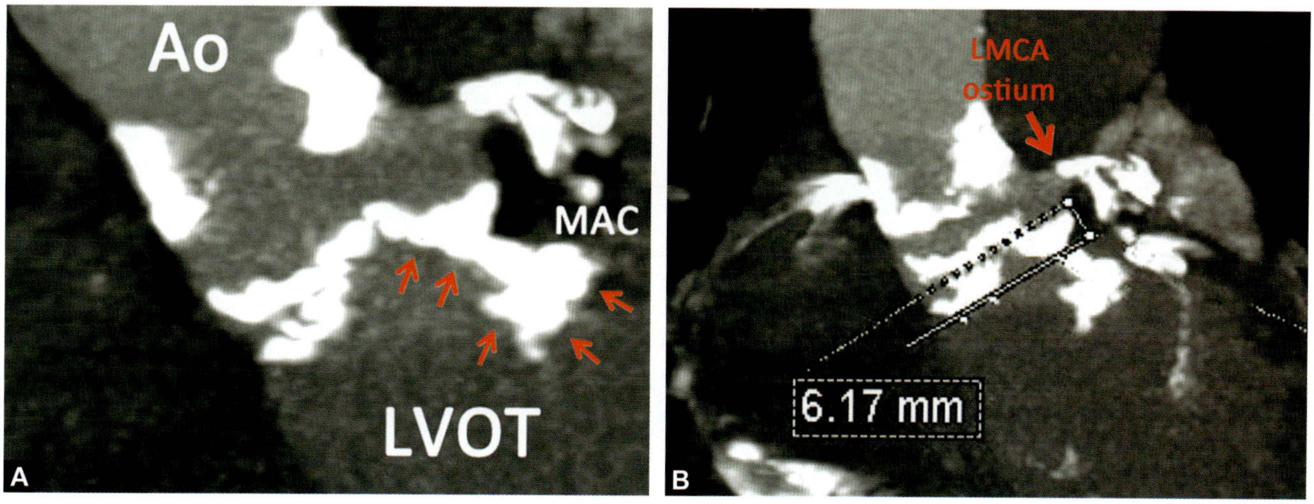

Figs. 17.13A and B: CT images used in the assessment of patient suitability for transcatheter aortic valve replacement (TAVR). (A) Significant calcification of the left coronary cusp sector extending into the left ventricular outflow tract (LVOT) in continuity with mitral annular calcification (MAC), a finding associated with increased risk of annulus rupture; (B) CT imaging demonstrates the low origin of the left main ostium with respect to the annulus, a high-risk finding associated with increased risk of left main coronary artery (arrow) compromise during TAVR deployment. This finding makes the patient not suitable for TAVR.

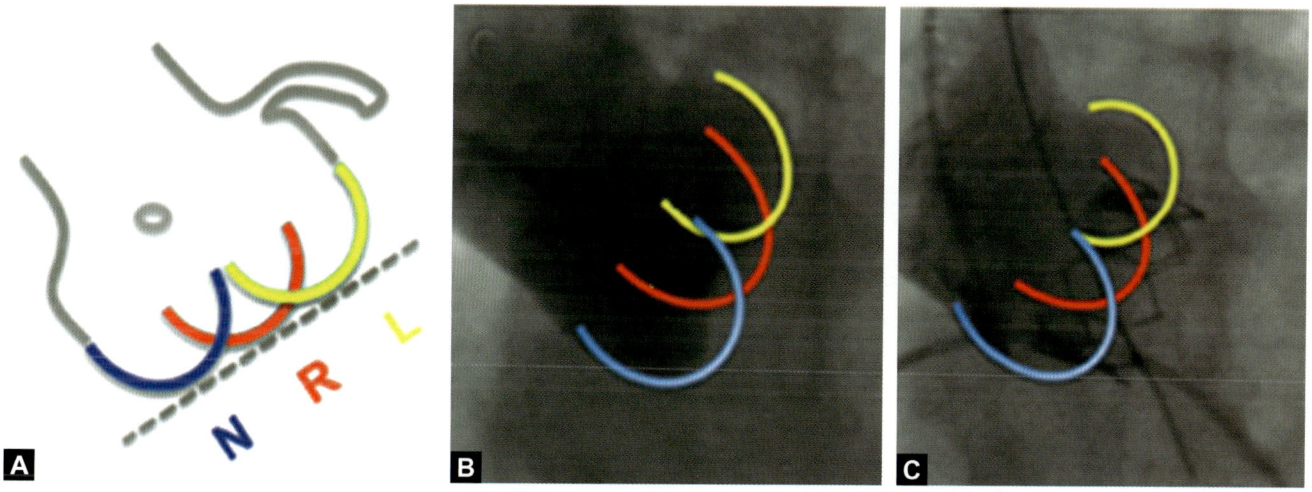

Figs. 17.14A to C: Optimal alignment of all three cusps forming the virtual aortic annulus in one plane, allowing more precise deployment of the transcatheter heart valve at the level of the virtual annulus. (Images courtesy of Edwards Lifesciences).

with a high incidence of death. Annulus rupture is likely related to significant oversizing of the TAVR balloon and THV, although other mechanisms may also contribute to annulus rupture. The atrioventricular (AV) node is located in direct proximity of the AV, and TAVR may lead to heart block and the need for permanent pacemaker implantation. The risk of heart block is greater with the CoreValve than with the Edwards Sapien valve. Vascular complications include arterial dissection, avulsion or perforation, and access site bleeding. Vascular complications are understandably less frequent with the apical approach than with a transarterial approach. Obstruction of the coronary ostia by the valve is a rare complication of the procedure but one that needs to be considered in pre-procedure planning. The distance between the leaflet origin/annulus and coronary ostia origin (particularly the left main coronary artery) are routinely measured pre-procedure. As with any iodine-based contrast procedure, TAVR is associated with a modest risk of acute kidney injury.

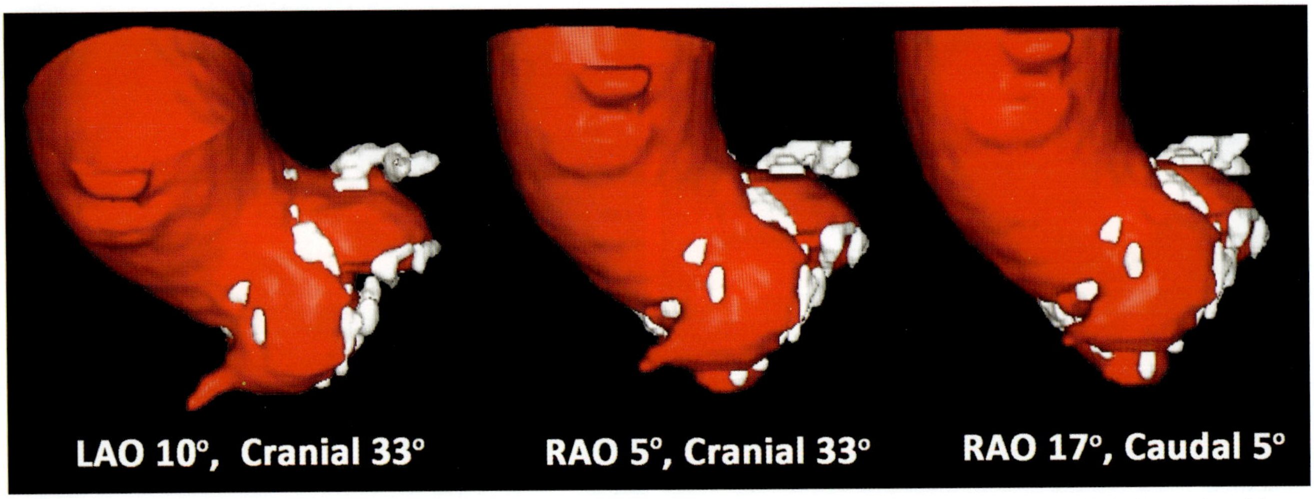

Fig. 17.15: Use of pre-procedural CT imaging and analysis to pre-select optimal image intensifier position. (LAO: Left anterior oblique; RAO: Right anterior oblique).

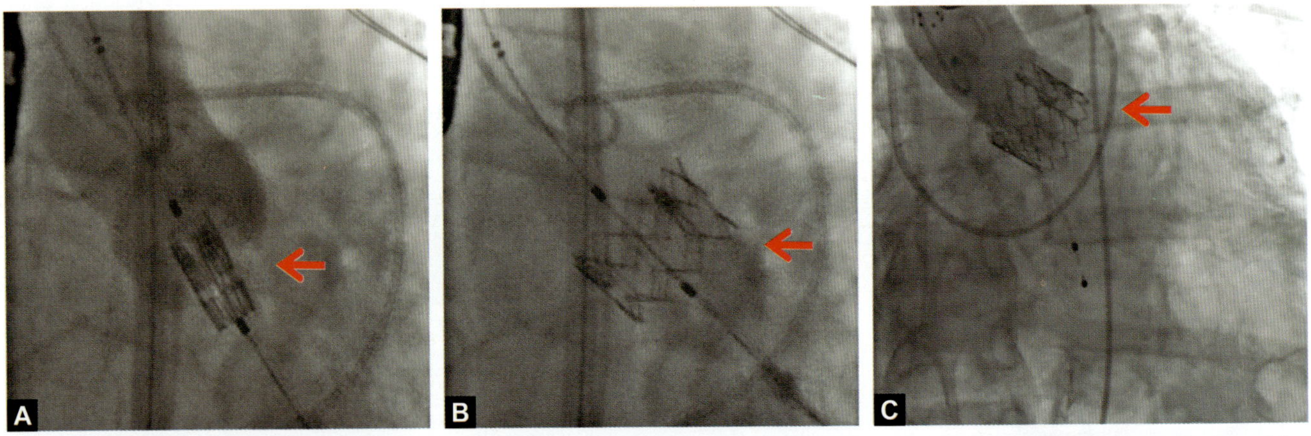

Figs. 17.16A to C: Fluoroscopic images of transcatheter heart valve (THV) deployment. (A) Image shows optimal positioning of the unexpanded THV (arrow); (B) Fully deployed valve (arrow); (C) Aortography demonstrating no paravalvular lead or valvular insufficiency.

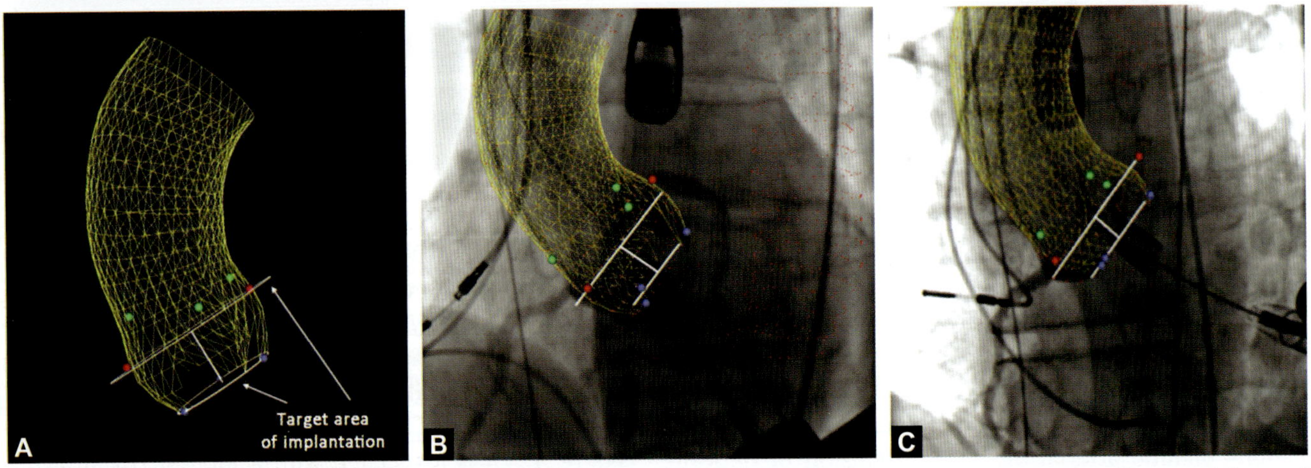

Figs. 17.17A to C: Intraoperative CT imaging and 3D modeling of the aortic root used to guide image intensifier angulation and transcatheter heart valve positioning and deployment. Red dots represent the coronary ostia, green dots the commissures, and blue dots the lowest points of the leaflet cusps. White lines represent the estimated target area of the valve implantation. (Images from Karar ME, Holzhey D, John M, et al. Image-guided transcatheter aortic valve implantation assistance system. In: Chen YF, Luo CY (Eds). Aortic Valve. InTech, 2011).

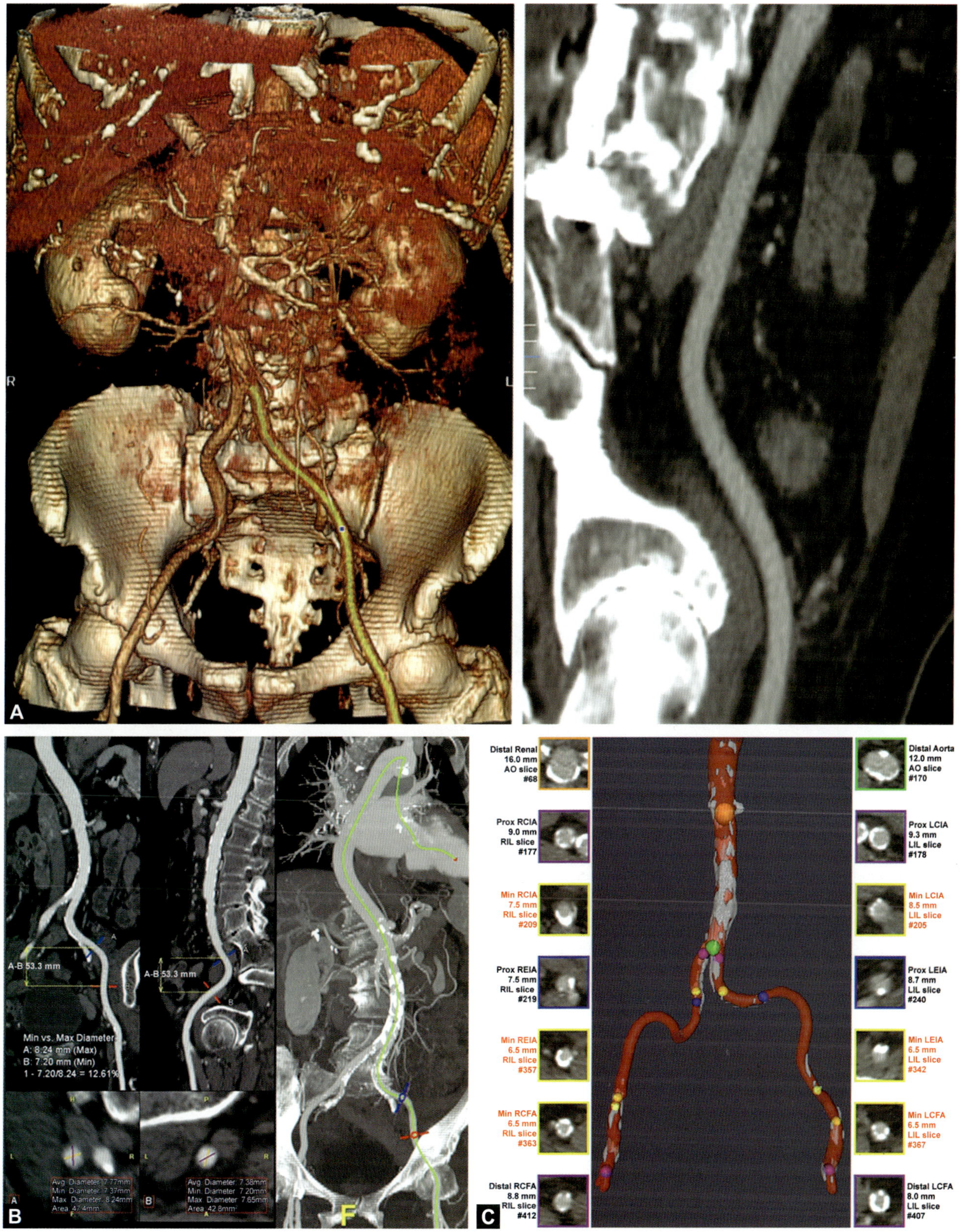

Figs. 17.18A to C: Examples of CT angiography of the peripheral arteries performed to evaluate access options for delivery of the transcatheter heart valve. Minimal lumen diameters (MLDs) are measured in the common iliac, external iliac, and common femoral arteries. The arteries are also assessed for tortuosity and degree of calcification.

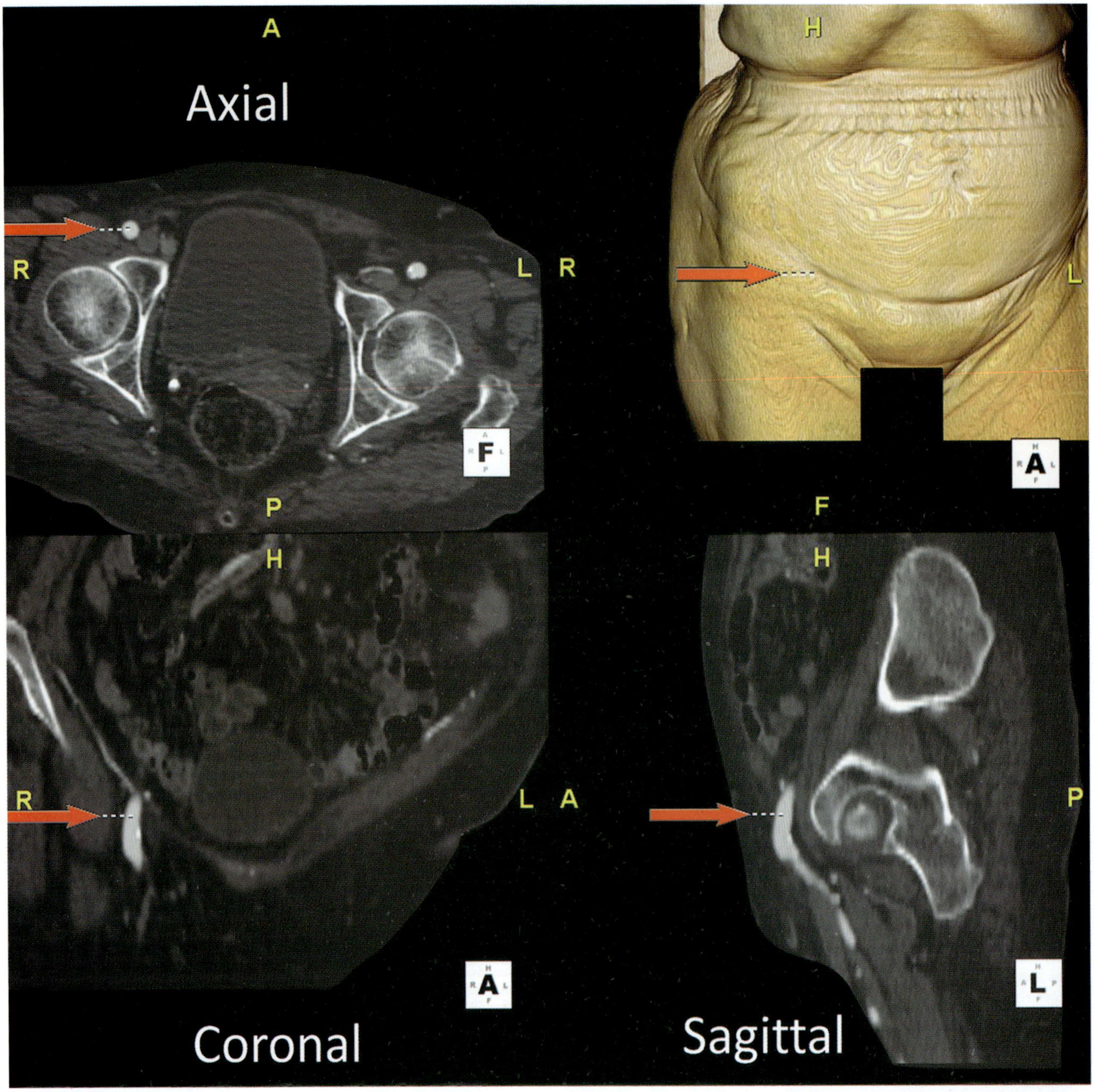

Fig. 17.19: Use of CT imaging to assess relationship of target arterial access area in the femoral artery in relationship to surface anatomy. Axial, coronary and sagittal 2D images, as well as a full body 3D reconstruction, are shown. This approach may be particularly useful in obese and elderly patients in which the inguinal crease may shift in relationship to the underlying femoral artery.

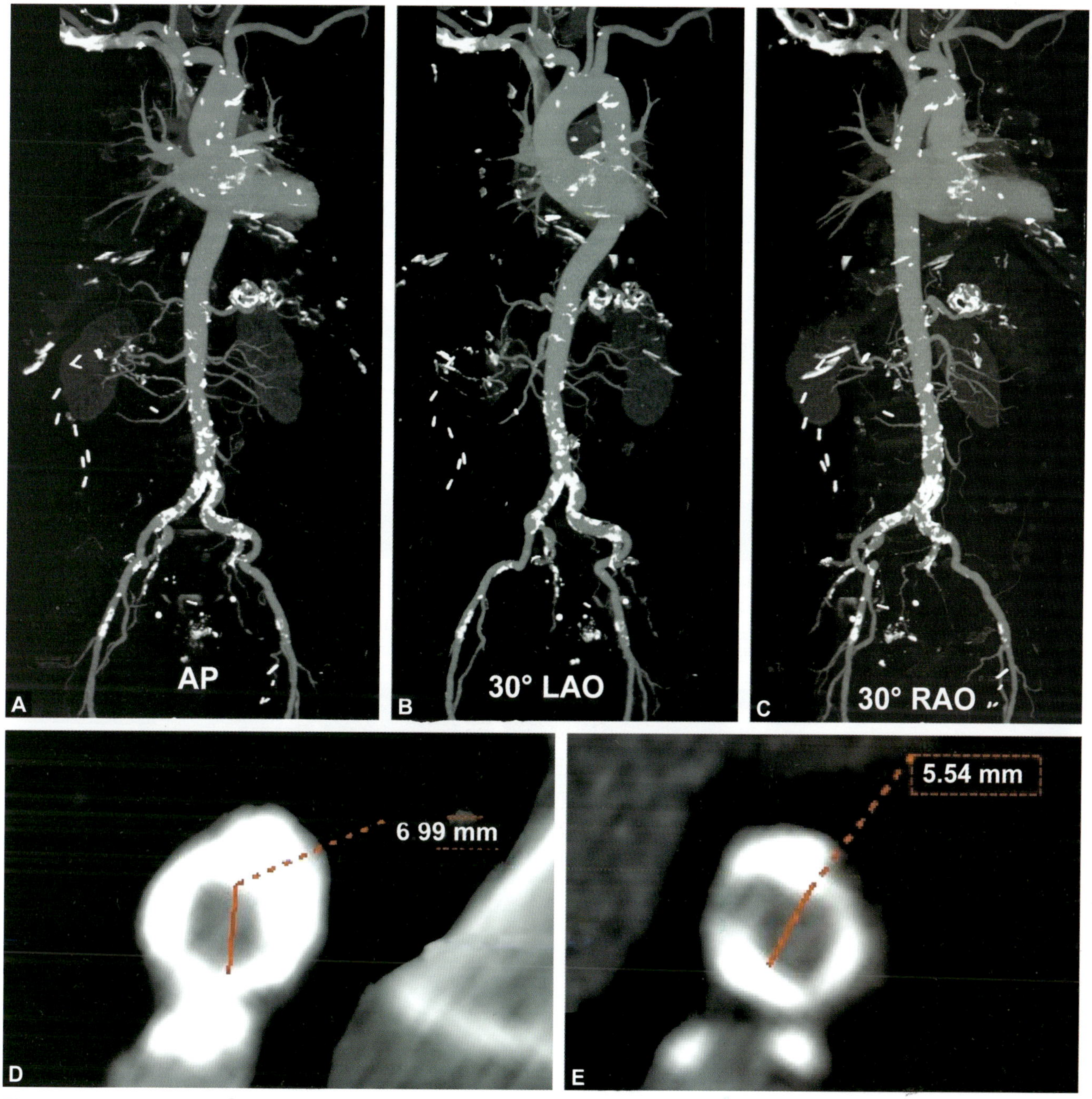

Figs. 17.20A to E: CT assessment of iliofemoral access for transcatheter aortic valve replacement. CT maximum intensity projection (MIP) images in (A) the anteroposterior view with (B) 30° left anterior oblique (LAO) angulation and with (C) 30° right anterior oblique (RAO) angulation. Severe aortoiliac bifurcation disease is present, a marker for increased risk of vascular complication and inability to delivery of the transcatheter heart valve (THV) via a transfemoral approach. True cross-sectional images of the (D) right and (E) left iliac arteries demonstrating (D) circumferential and (E) near circumferential calcification. Circumferential and "horseshoe" patterns of calcification are predictors of increased risk of vascular complications. Note also that the small lumen diameters, along with the calcification, would preclude delivery of most THV devices. The heavy ostial and proximal iliac disease would also preclude use of an iliac artery conduit for device delivery.

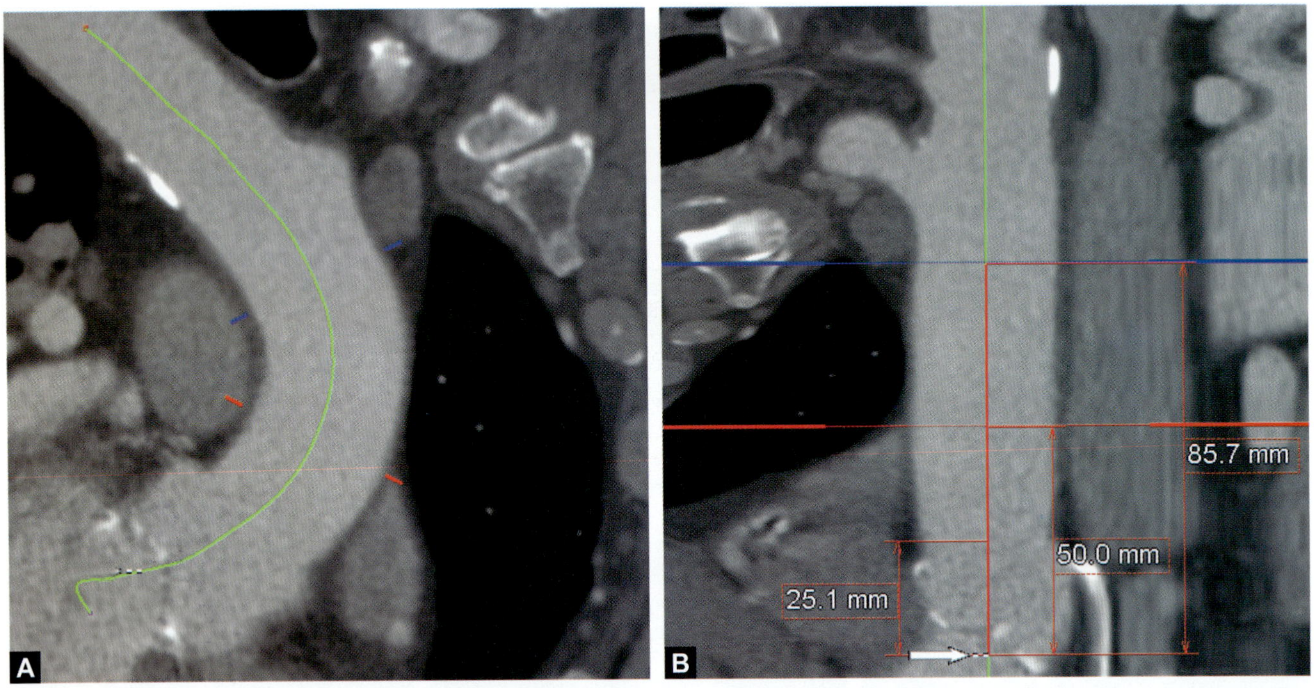

Figs. 17.21A and B: CT multiplanar reformatted reconstructions of the aortic root and ascending aorta. Area between the red and blue lines is referred to the transaortic zone (TAo). The red line represents the area in the ascending aorta 50 mm above the aortic annulus. The blue line is placed proximal to the origin of the brachiocephalic artery. Imaging of this area is used to assess for the suitability of transaortic access when transfemoral access is not possible. Importantly, no calcification is identified in this area.

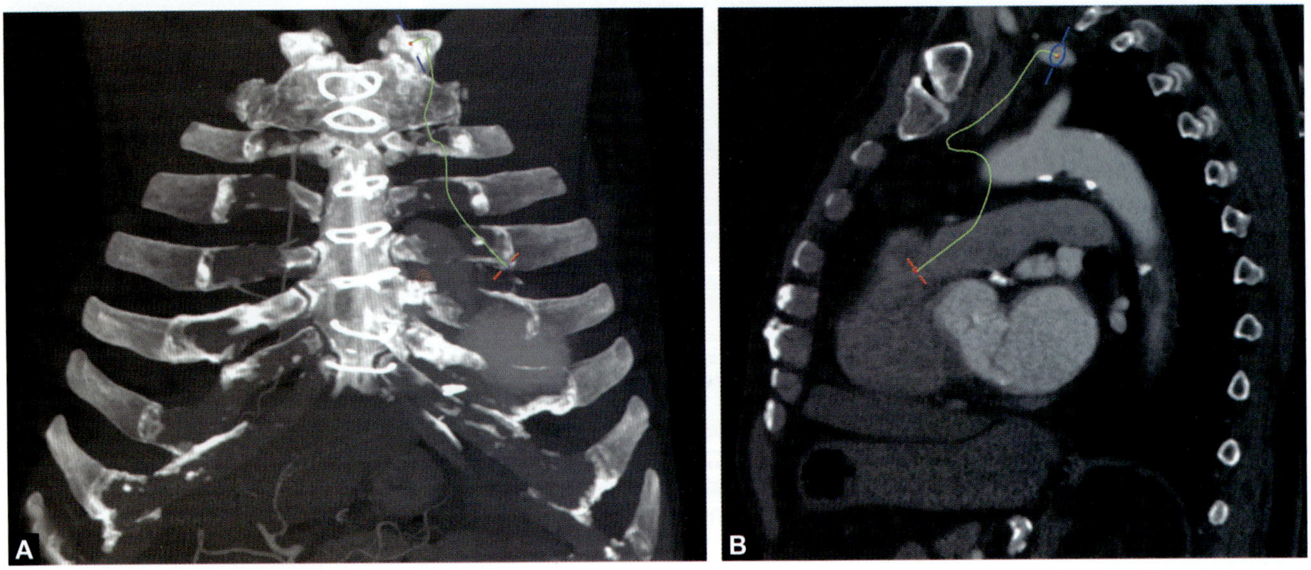

Figs. 17.22A and B: CT imaging of the LIMA in assessing approach options for transcatheter heart valve delivery. (A) Coronal and (B) sagittal images of the chest demonstrate the course of the LIMA, which has been used for LAD artery bypass. CT is used to assess the position of the LIMA in relationship to the sternum and whether it is adherent to the sternum, as well as its overall course. A LIMA adherent to the sternum makes the patient a higher risk for repeat open chest surgical AVR.

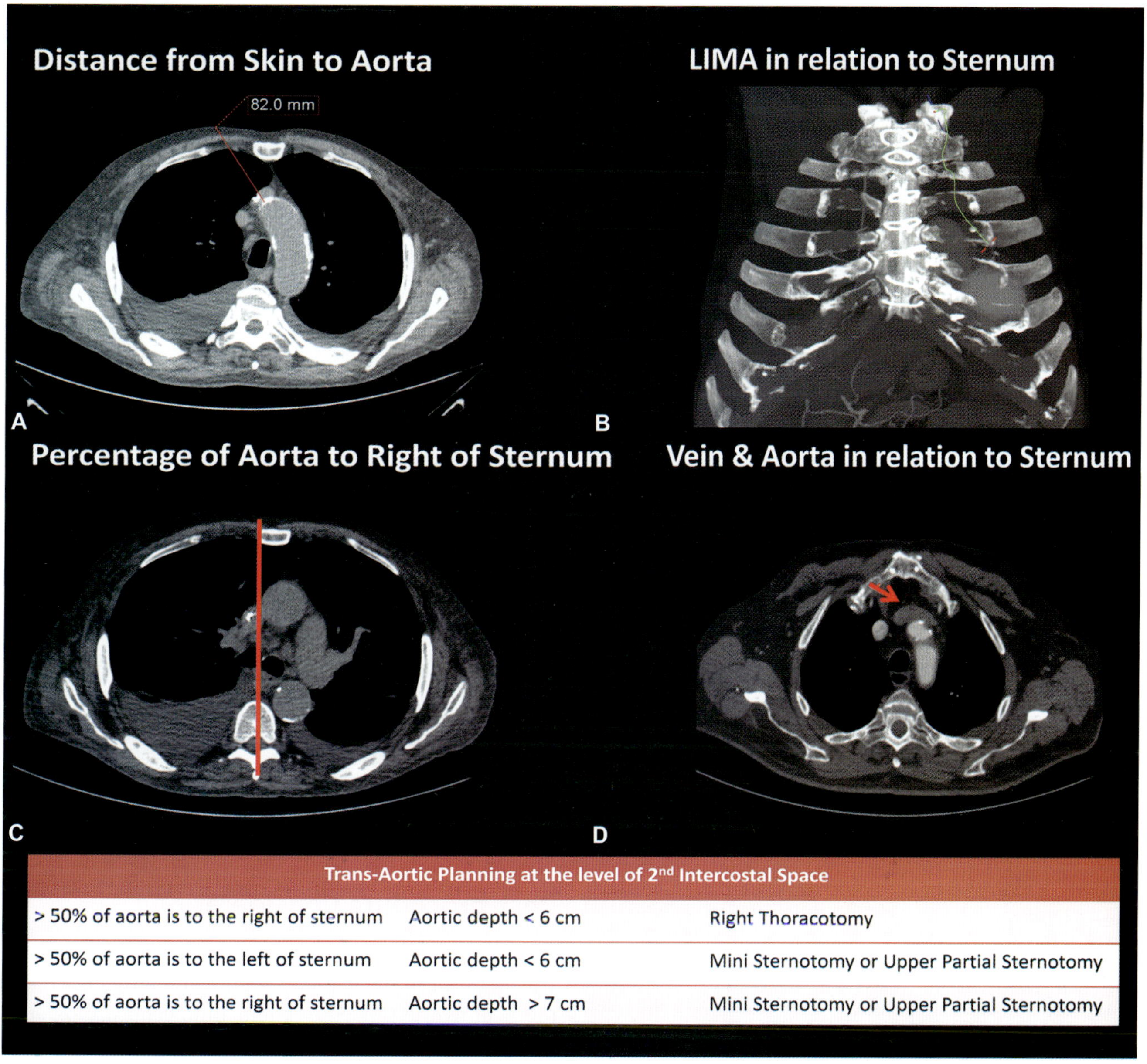

Trans-Aortic Planning at the level of 2nd Intercostal Space		
> 50% of aorta is to the right of sternum	Aortic depth < 6 cm	Right Thoracotomy
> 50% of aorta is to the left of sternum	Aortic depth < 6 cm	Mini Sternotomy or Upper Partial Sternotomy
> 50% of aorta is to the right of sternum	Aortic depth > 7 cm	Mini Sternotomy or Upper Partial Sternotomy

Figs. 17.23A to D: Considerations in the planning of transaortic route delivery transcatheter aortic valve replacement. Considerations include (A) distance from the skin to the aorta, (B) course of the LIMA (green line) and RIMA, and (C and D) position of the aorta in relationship to the sternum as well as the position of other vessels such as the innominate vein (arrow).

Paravalvular aortic insufficiency (AI) is a not uncommon finding (Figs. 17.26A to C). Proper selection of device size, as well as thorough assessment of the annulus, may decrease the risk of paravalvular AI. Paravalvular leak may occasionally be treated with implantation of a second THV (Figs. 17.27A to F). The presence of significant paravalvular post-procedure is associated with a clear increased risk of mortality.

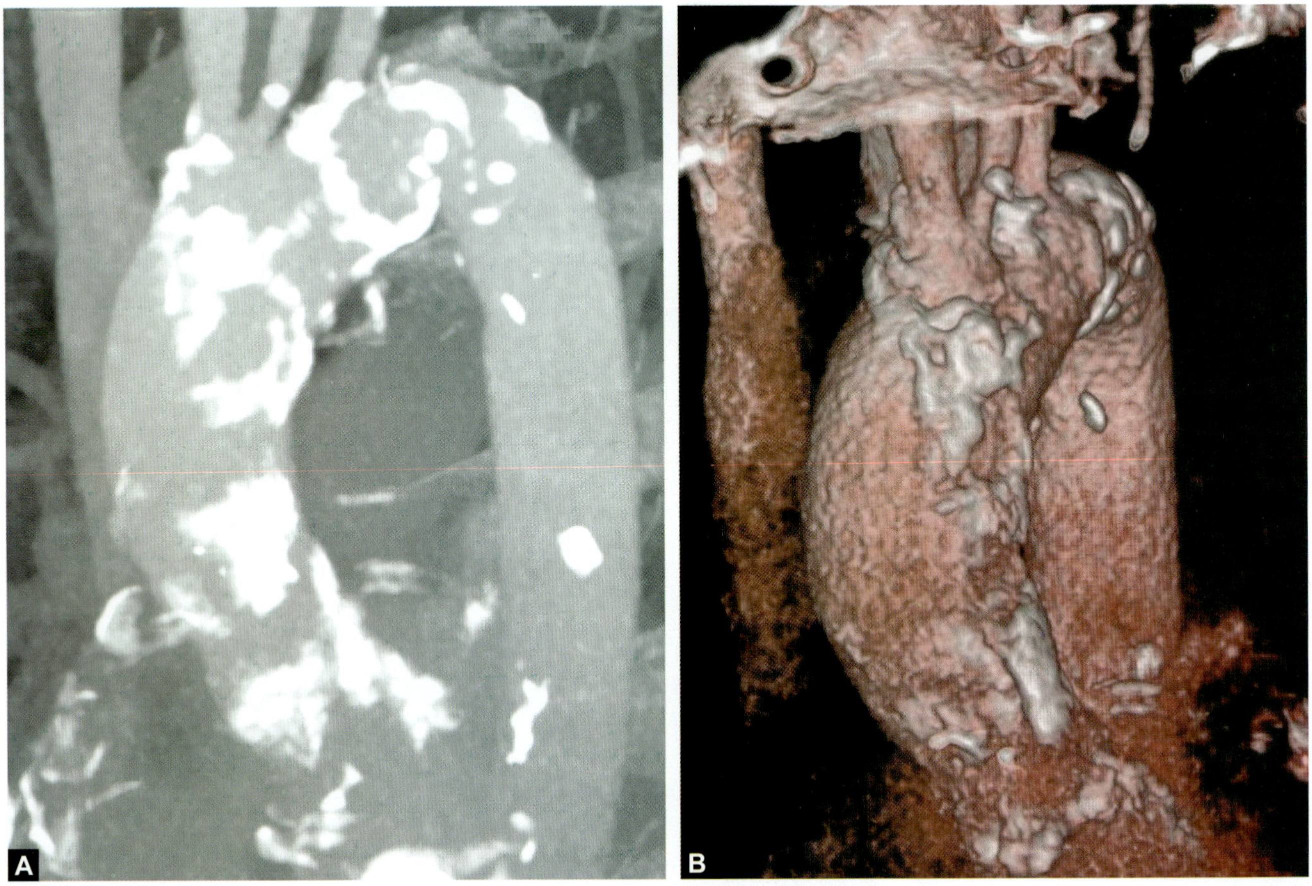

Figs. 17.24A and B: (A) CT maximum intensity projection (MIP) and (B) volume rendered 3D image demonstrating significant calcification in the ascending aorta. The presence of such calcification makes the patient a poor candidate for transaortic delivery of a transcatheter heart valve.

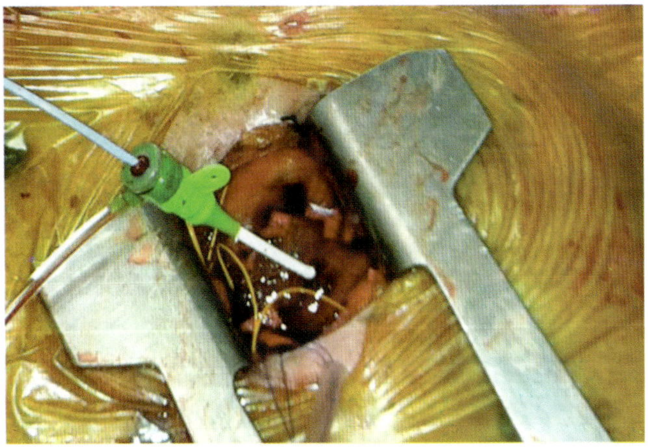

Fig. 17.25: Hybrid OR room picture of a small incision used during apical delivery of the transcatheter heart valve. [From Leal O, Bustamante J, Cánovas S, et al. New therapeutic approaches to conventional surgery for aortic stenosis in high-risk patients. In: Aikawa E (Ed). Calcific Aortic Valve Disease. InTech, 2013].

Post-procedure Considerations

Immediate procedural success or complication is usually assessed in the catheterization laboratory, operating room, or hybrid procedure room. Both echocardiography (often TEE) and aortic angiography may be utilized to assess for paravalvular aortic regurgitation. Transthoracic echocardiography is usually performed before patient discharge to assess for prosthetic valve function, paravalvular aortic regurgitation, and improvement in left ventricular function (if left ventricle systolic function was depressed pre-procedure).

Patients are usually treated with weeks to several months of antiplatelet therapy. In some patients, monotherapy with aspirin is prescribed, while in others dual antiplatelet therapy with aspirin and clopidogrel may be utilized.

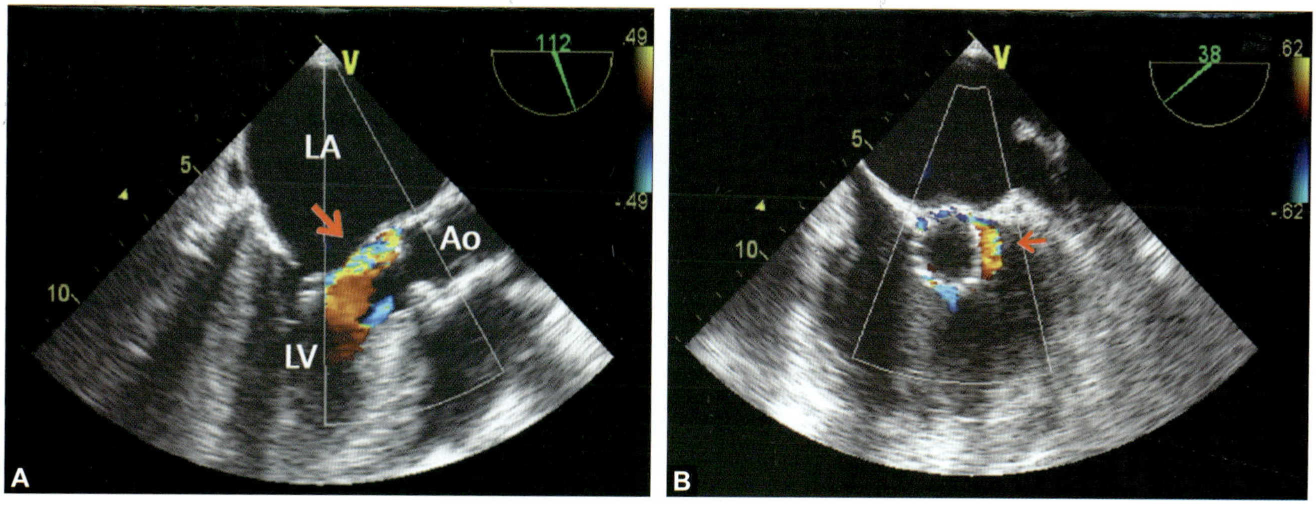

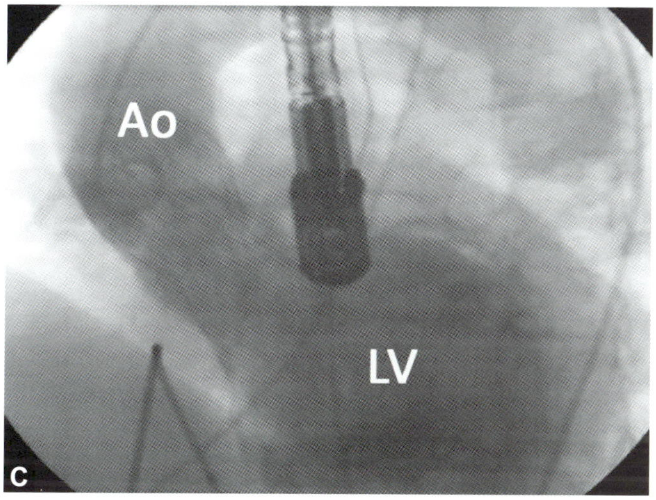

Figs. 17.26A to C: Paravalvular leak. (A) TEE intraoperative long-axis and (B) short-axis images immediately after transcatheter heart valve deployment, demonstrating significant paravalvular aortic regurgitation (arrows). (C) Aortograph also had demonstrated significant regurgitation. [Images from Calé R, Neves J, Teles R, et al. Surgical bailout therapy after implantation of a Medtronic CoreValve bioprosthesis. Case Reports in Cardiology. Volume 2012 (2012), Article ID 387103. Available from http://www.hindawi.com/crim/cardiology/2012/387103/].

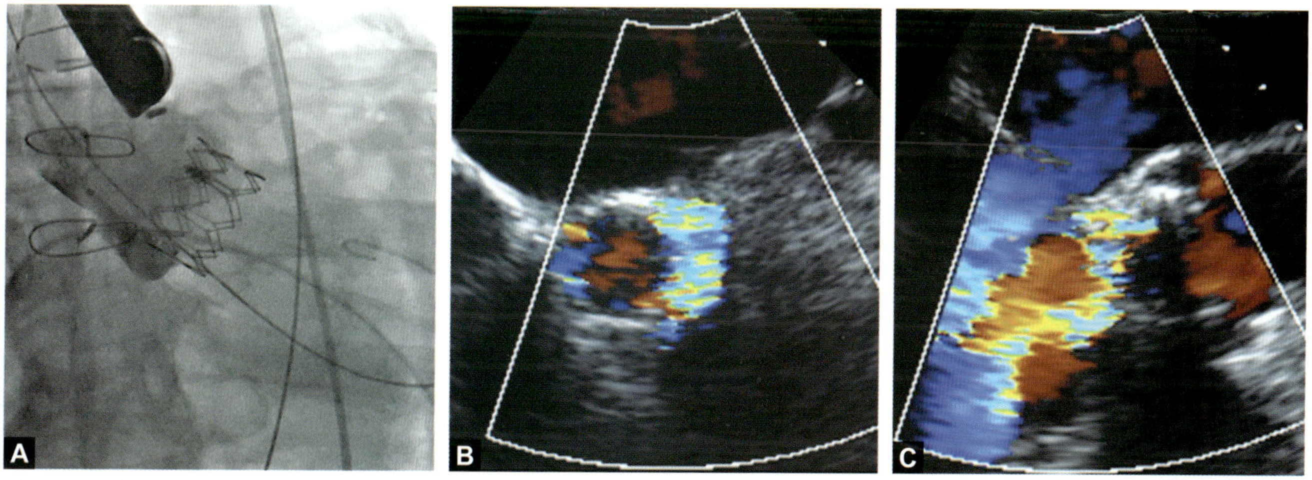

Figs. 17.27A to C: Perivalvular aortic regurgitation treated by implantation of a second transcatheter heart valve. Low implantation of (A) a Edwards Sapien XT valve results in severe paravalvular aortic regurgitation seen on intraoperative TEE in (B) the short-axis and (C) long-axis. Implantation of a second valve, implanted in a higher position.

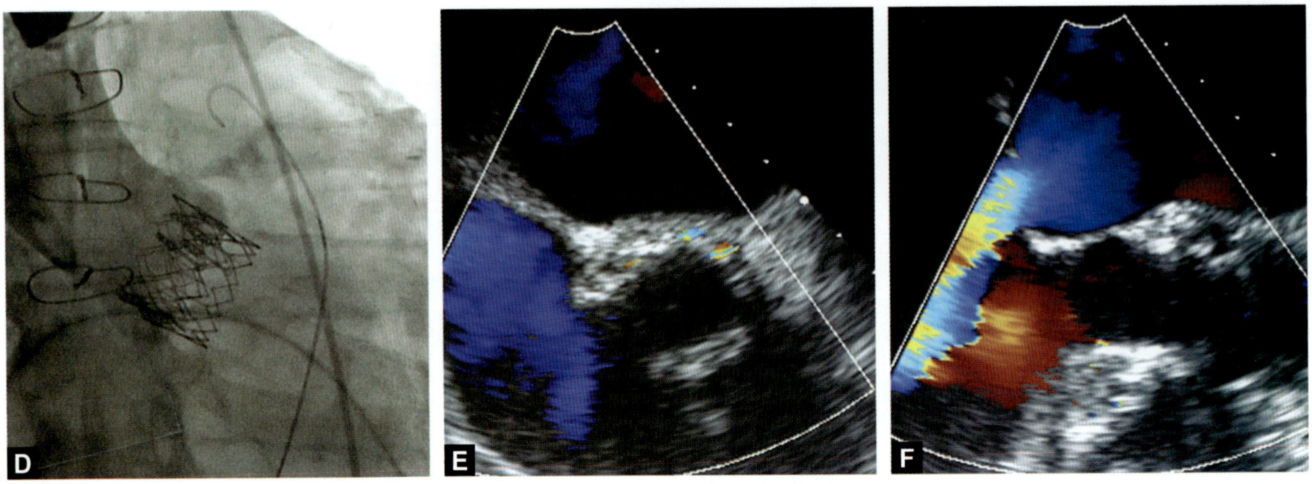

Figs. 17.27D to F: (D) extending the annular seal, and (E and F) resulting in a marked decrease in paravalvular leak. (Images with permission courtesy of Toggweiler S, Webb JG. Challenges in transcatheter aortic valve implantation. Swiss Med Wkly. 2012;142:w13735).

VIDEO LEGENDS

Video 17.1: Animation of transfemoral transcatheter aortic valve replacement with the Edwards Sapian valve. (Video courtesy of Edwards Lifesciences).

Video 17.2: Fluoroscopy of deployment of a Edwards Sapien valve. (Video courtesy of Edwards Lifesciences).

Video 17.3: Animation of apical transcatheter aortic valve replacement with the Edwards Sapian valve. (Video courtesy of Edwards Lifesciences).

REFERENCES

Achenbach S, Delgado V, Hausleiter J, et al. SCCT expert consensus document on computed tomography imaging before transcatheter aortic valve implantation (TAVI)/ transcatheter aortic valve replacement (TAVR). J Cardiovasc Comput Tomogr. 2012;6(6):366-80.

Bapat VN, Attia RQ, Thomas M. Distribution of calcium in the ascending aorta in patients undergoing transcatheter aortic valve implantation and its relevance to the transaortic approach. JACC Cardiovasc Interv. 2012;5(5):470-6.

Blanke P, Russe M, Leipsic J, et al. Conformational pulsatile changes of the aortic annulus: impact on prosthesis sizing by computed tomography for transcatheter aortic valve replacement. JACC Cardiovasc Interv. 2012;5(9):984-94.

Holmes DR Jr, Mack MJ. Transcatheter valve therapy a professional society overview from the american college of cardiology foundation and the society of thoracic surgeons. J Am Coll Cardiol. 2011;58(4):445-55.

Holmes DR Jr, Rich JB, Zoghbi WA, et al. The heart team of cardiovascular care. J Am Coll Cardiol. 2013;61(9):903-7.

Mack MJ. Access for transcatheter aortic valve replacement: which is the preferred route? JACC Cardiovasc Interv. 2012;5(5):487-8.

Mack MJ. Transcatheter aortic valve implantation: changing patient populations and novel indications. Heart. 2012;98 Suppl 4:iv73-9.

The Joint Task Force on the Management of Valvular Heart Disease of the European Society of Cardiology (ESC); European Association for Cardio-Thoracic Surgery (EACTS), Vahanian A, et al. Guidelines on the management of valvular heart disease (version 2012). Eur Heart J. 2012;33(19): 2451-96.

Walther T, Simon P, Dewey T, et al. Transapical minimally invasive aortic valve implantation: multicenter experience. Circulation. 2007;116(11 Suppl):I240-5.

CHAPTER

Valve Surgery and Prosthetic Heart Valves

18

Sebastian A Iturra, Arul D Furtado, Vinod H Thourani

SURGICAL APPROACH

Traditionally, aortic valve replacement (AVR) is done with a full sternotomy (Figs. 18.1 to 18.3). This allows having an adequate exposure of the major vessels, atriums, ventricles and valves and facilitates cannulation. The principles of minimally invasive surgery utilizing small sternal incisions are to maintain the same rate of surgical success, without increasing the operative risk. One can also obtain safe access to the aortic valve with partial sternotomy, right thoracotomy or by the use of transcatheter techniques. Alternative access to the mitral valve can be obtained by a right thoracotomy or a robotic assisted approach through the right chest. Potential benefits include improved smaller incisions, cosmesis, less deep and superficial wound infection and less sternal dehiscence. Patients are mobilized more quickly which aids recovery, which is especially important in elderly patients. However, availability of minimally invasive surgery is generally limited to experienced centers, and no data shows clear benefit in elderly patients with such procedures.

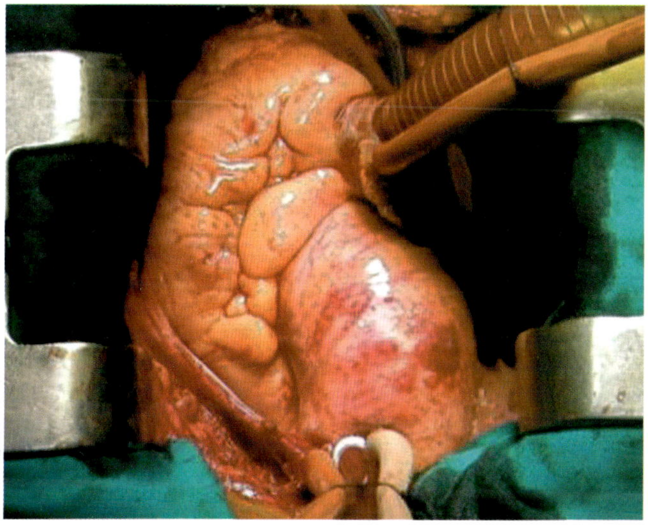

Fig. 18.1: Upper hemisternotomy approach to the aortic valve and central aortic and right atrial cannulation in preparation for cardiopulmonary bypass.

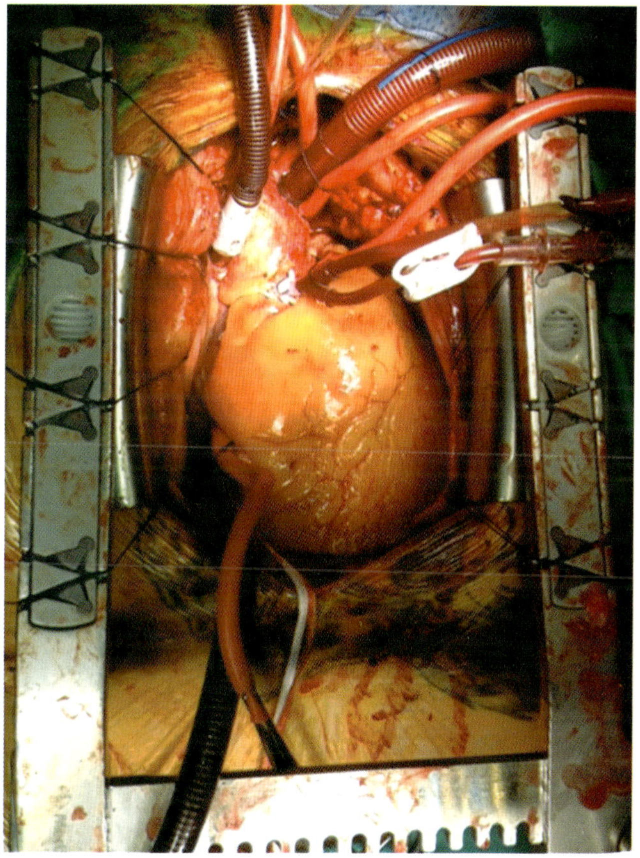

Fig. 18.2: Median sternotomy and exposure of the heart. Cannulation of the ascending aorta and right atrium is performed in preparation for using cardiopulmonary bypass, and cannulation of the coronary sinus for administration of cardioplegic solution. [Image from Sanz-Ayan MP et al. Neurological complications in aortic valve surgery and rehabilitation treatment used. In: Motomura N (Ed). Aortic Valve Surgery. Intechweb.org. CC].

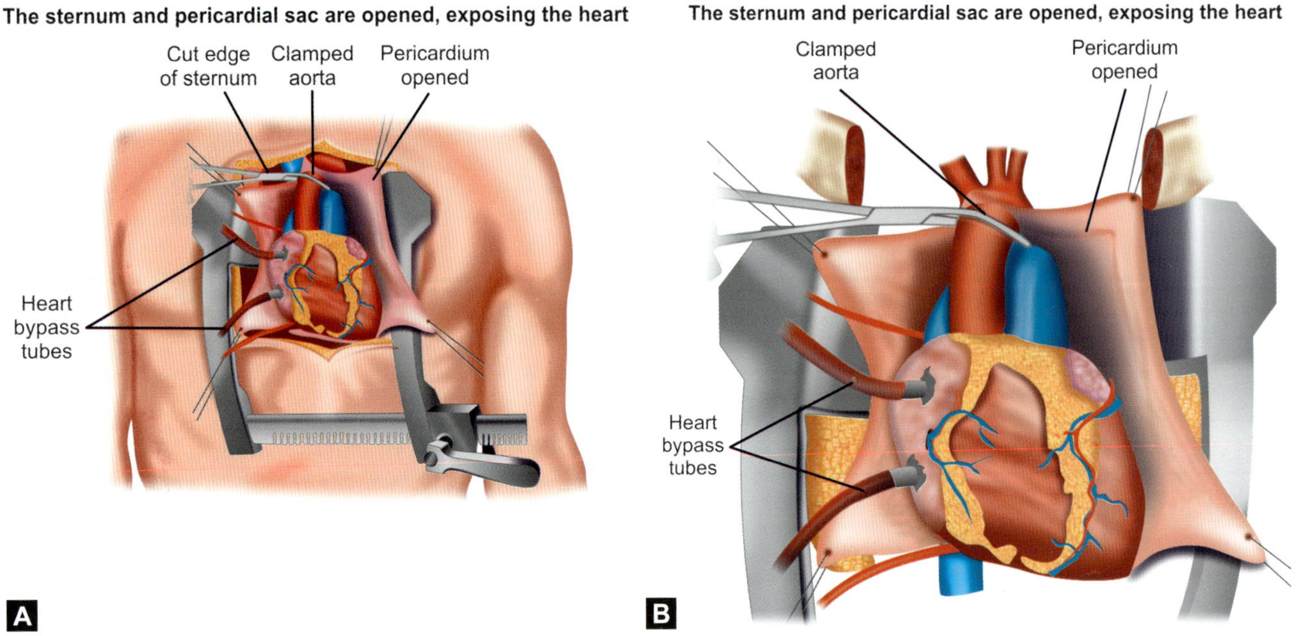

Figs. 18.3A and B: Schematic illustration of median sternotomy and heart cannulation.

AORTIC VALVE SURGERY

Aortic valve stenosis (Fig. 18.4) is the most common valve pathology requiring surgical intervention. The Aortic valve replacement (AVR) is performed with full anticoagulation under cardiopulmonary bypass with direct cannulation of the ascending aorta for arterial inflow and a right atrial cannula for venous drainage. The ascending aorta is clamped after the patient is on cardiopulmonary support. After successful cardiac protection and arrest, aortotomy and excision of the diseased valve is performed. Following adequate exposure of the aortic annulus, placement of multiples sutures to secure the sewing ring of the prosthesis is performed (Figs. 18.5A to D). After the implantation is done, the aortotomy is closed, the patient weaned from cardio-pulmonary bypass anticoagulation is reversed followed by decannulation.

Aortic valve surgery is also performed in appropriately selected patients with severe aortic insufficiency. While valve replacement is performed in most cases, in select cases and at highly experienced centers, aortic valve repair may instead be performed.

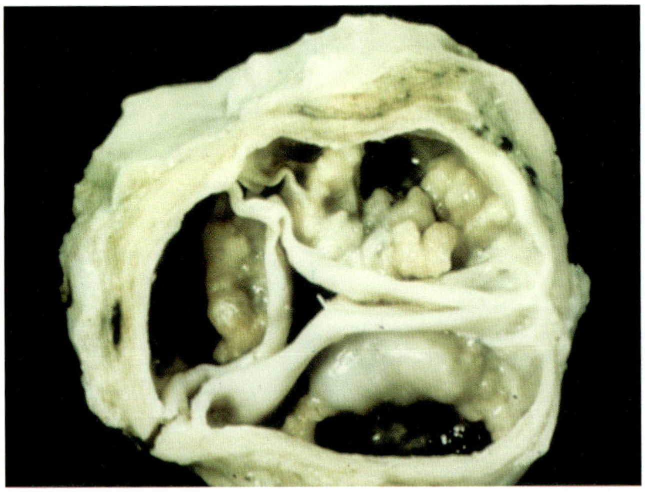

Fig. 18.4: Gross pathology image of a stenotic aortic valve.

MITRAL VALVE SURGERY

Mitral valve repair (Figs. 18.6A to D), often with placement of a mitral ring (Fig. 18.6E) or annuloplasty band (Fig. 18.6F), is preferred over mitral valve replacement (Figs. 18.7A and B) whenever feasible. During mitral valve surgery, after connecting the patient to cardiopulmonary bypass and arresting the heart, access to the mitral valve is achieved routinely by a direct left atriotomy or through the right atrium and inter-atrial septum. Whenever possible, the posterior mitral leaflet and the anterior subvalvular apparatus are preserved so as to maintain the left ventricular geometry and function. Placement of multiples sutures to secure the sewing ring of the prosthesis is performed in a similar fashion as with an aortic prosthesis.

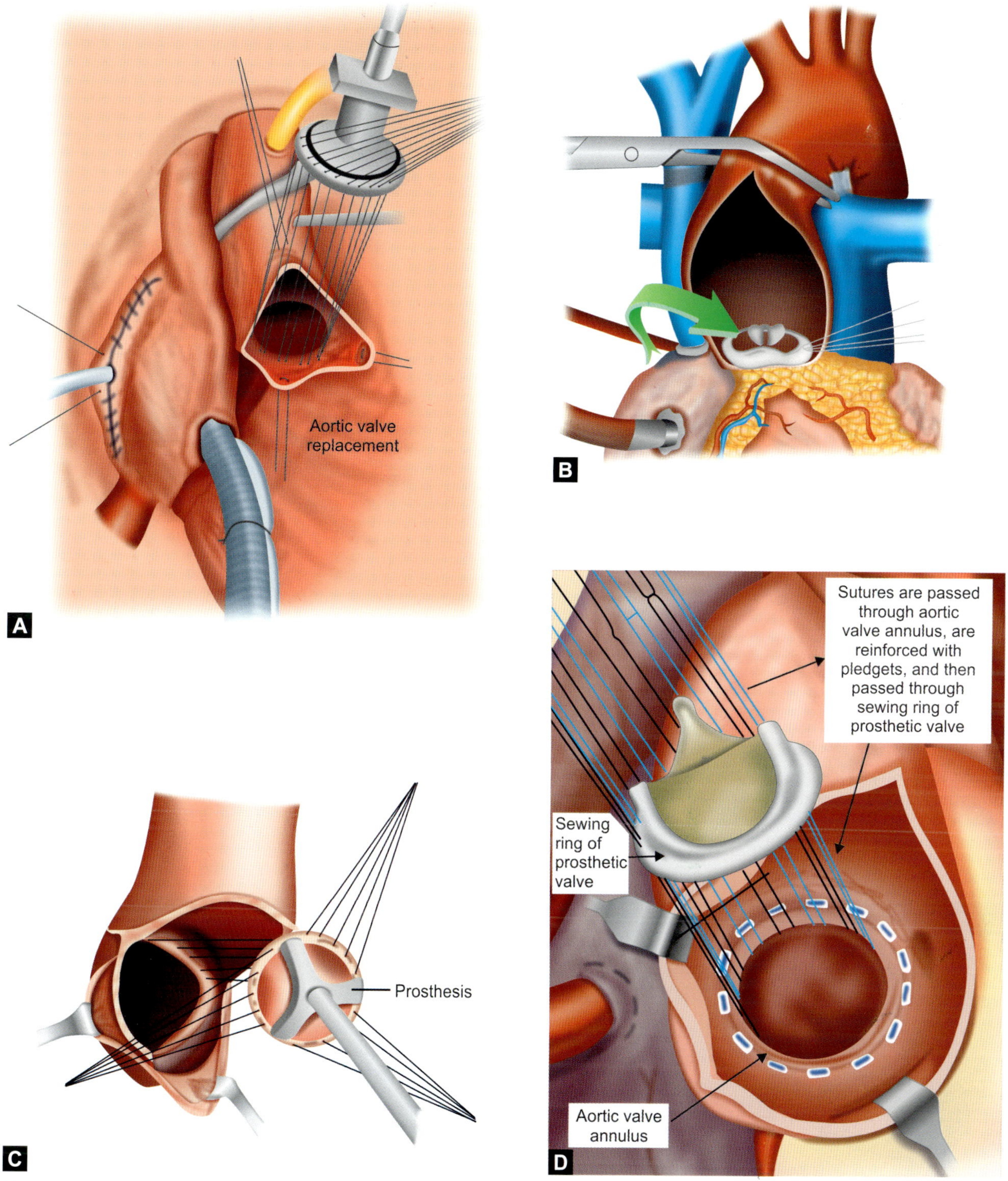

Figs. 18.5A to D: Schematic illustration of implantation of a prosthetic aortic valve.

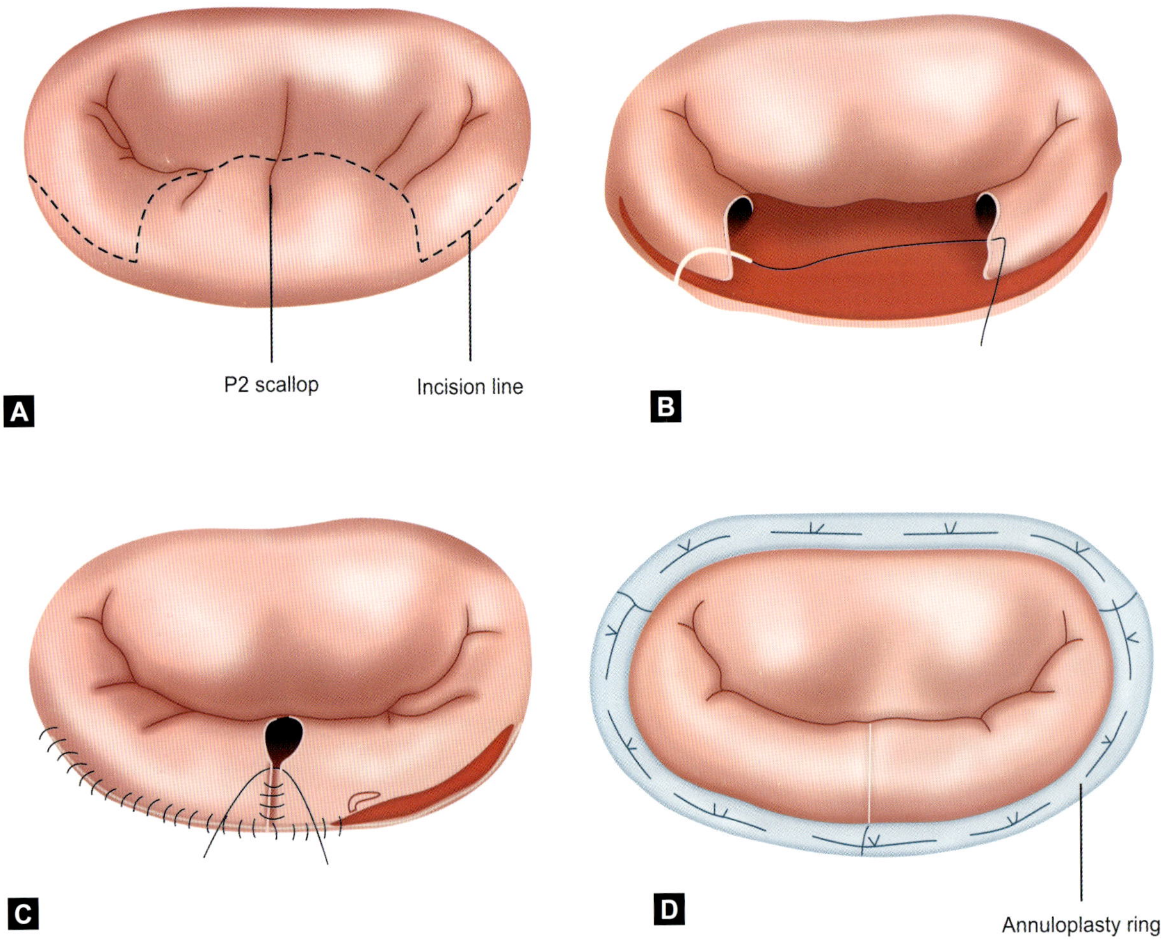

Figs. 18.6A to D: Steps for surgery for mitral valve repair. (A) Surgeon's view, from the atrium of a valve with a flail P2 scallop. Dashed line shows the planned excision of ruptured and elongated chordae; (B) View after resection of the diseased portion; (C) Re-apposition of the leaflet edges; (D) Reconstructed valve with an annuloplasty ring. [Image and legend text from Sharma S, Dalvi BV. Mitral valve disease. In: Chatterjee K et al. (Ed). Cardiology—An Illustrated Textbook. New Delhi, India; Jaypee Brothers Medical Publishers (P) Ltd].

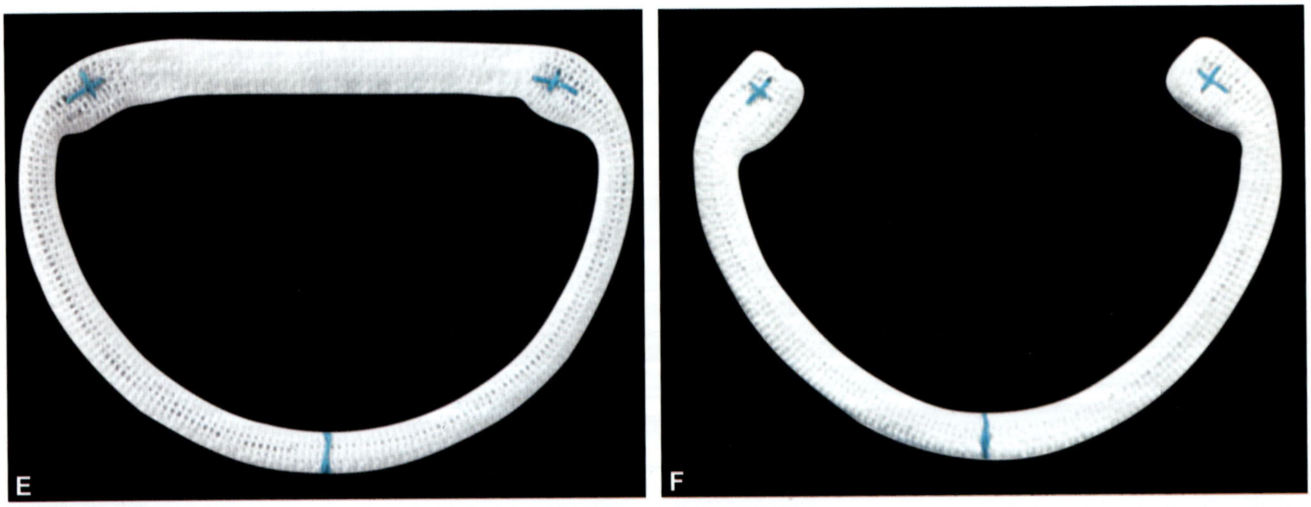

Figs. 18.6E and F: Examples of a mitral ring (E) and annuloplasty band (F) frequently used in patients undergoing mitral valve repair.

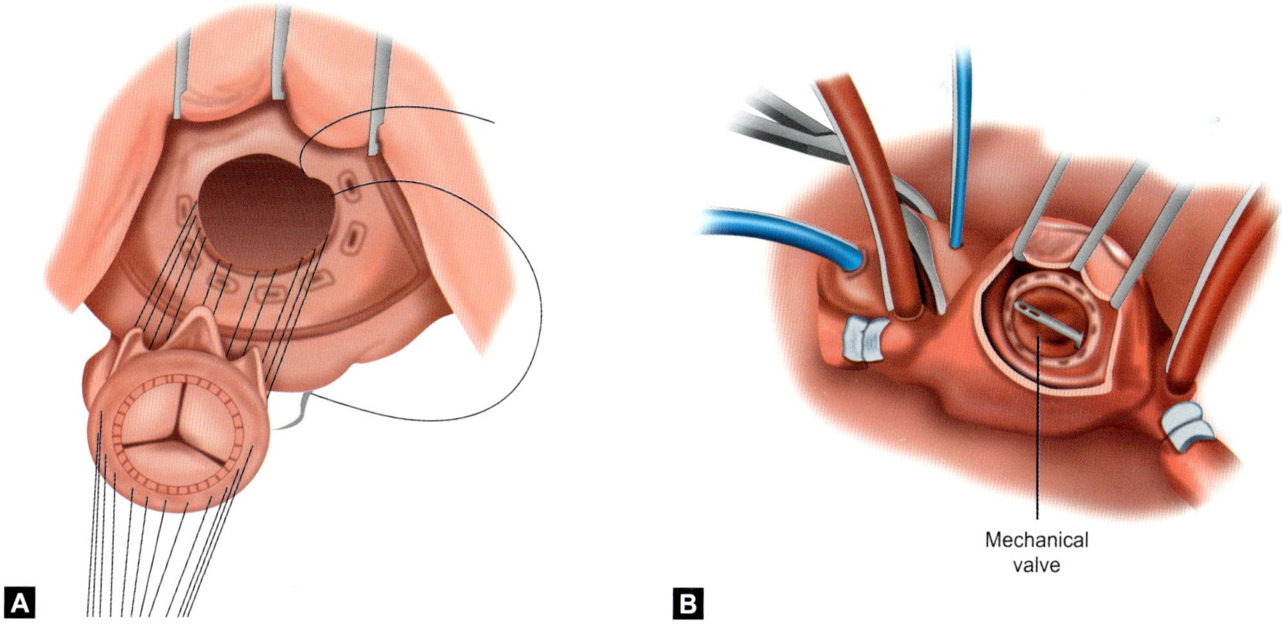

Figs. 18.7A and B: Schematic illustration of implantation of a prosthetic mitral valve.

BIOPROSTHETIC AORTIC VALVES

The first bioprosthetic valves were native homografts or xenografts that were decellularized to reduce immune rejection. The Achilles' heel of bioprosthetic valves is structural valve deterioration which limits long-term success. To mitigate this, pretreatment with glutaraldehyde stabilizes collagen linkage and reduces matrix fiber calcification (Figs. 18.8 and 18.9). The rate of structural valve deterioration is inversely proportional to age, with low rates in the elderly population because of lower metabolic activity and less extracellular calcium. Importantly, new fixation techniques are continuing to develop.

In recent years, evolution in stent design has led to better valve hemodynamics. Finite element analysis and computational fluid dynamics have yielded models which simulate the stress distribution on valve leaflets. Applying this information, new designs have lessened the concentration of stress on the leaflets. Four commonly used stented valves for AVR include: (1) the Carpentier-Edwards Magna-Ease (Fig. 18.10) which is composed of bovine pericardial leaflets, metal alloy wire-form, low profile commissural posts, a thin stent base, and a contoured and compliant sewing ring; (2) the Medtronic Mosaic valve (Fig. 18.11) which is treated with alpha-amino oleic acid to reduce calcification and is made of porcine valve leaflets with preserved leaflet structure and retained leaflet collagen crimp; (3) the St Jude Trifecta valve (Fig. 18.12); and (4) the Sorin Mitroflow valve (Fig. 18.13) made of bovine pericardium wrapped around the outside of a stent with a soft silicone sewing ring as the base; its design is meant to accommodate small, narrow aortic roots. Numerous other valves are commonly used in Europe, Asia, and worldwide, with constant revision and improvement of valve design.

Taking these design innovations further, stentless valves remove the apparatus of a rigid stent, strut and sewing ring in an attempt to reduce the transvalvular gradient. Because loss of native root geometry causes turbulence and leaflet stress, improved valve hemodynamics can be achieved by recreating physiologic leaflet motion. In theory, maintaining the conformity of the native coronary sinuses facilitates smooth closure of the valve and avoids buildup of stress in leaflet. Examples of stentless valves for AVR are the Medtronic 3f valve (Fig. 18.14) and the Medtronic Freestyle valve (Fig. 18.15). The 3f valve has felt tabs that must be tacked to the sinotubular junction in order to preserve sinus form and function. Equine pericardium is used for the leaflets because of low phospholipid content. The Freestyle valve is a porcine root that has 2-alpha-amino oleic acid tissue treatment, root pressure fixation, leaflets fixed at zero pressure, and minimal polyester covering. It can be implanted in a complete subcoronary fashion where the valve is placed in the native valve annulus

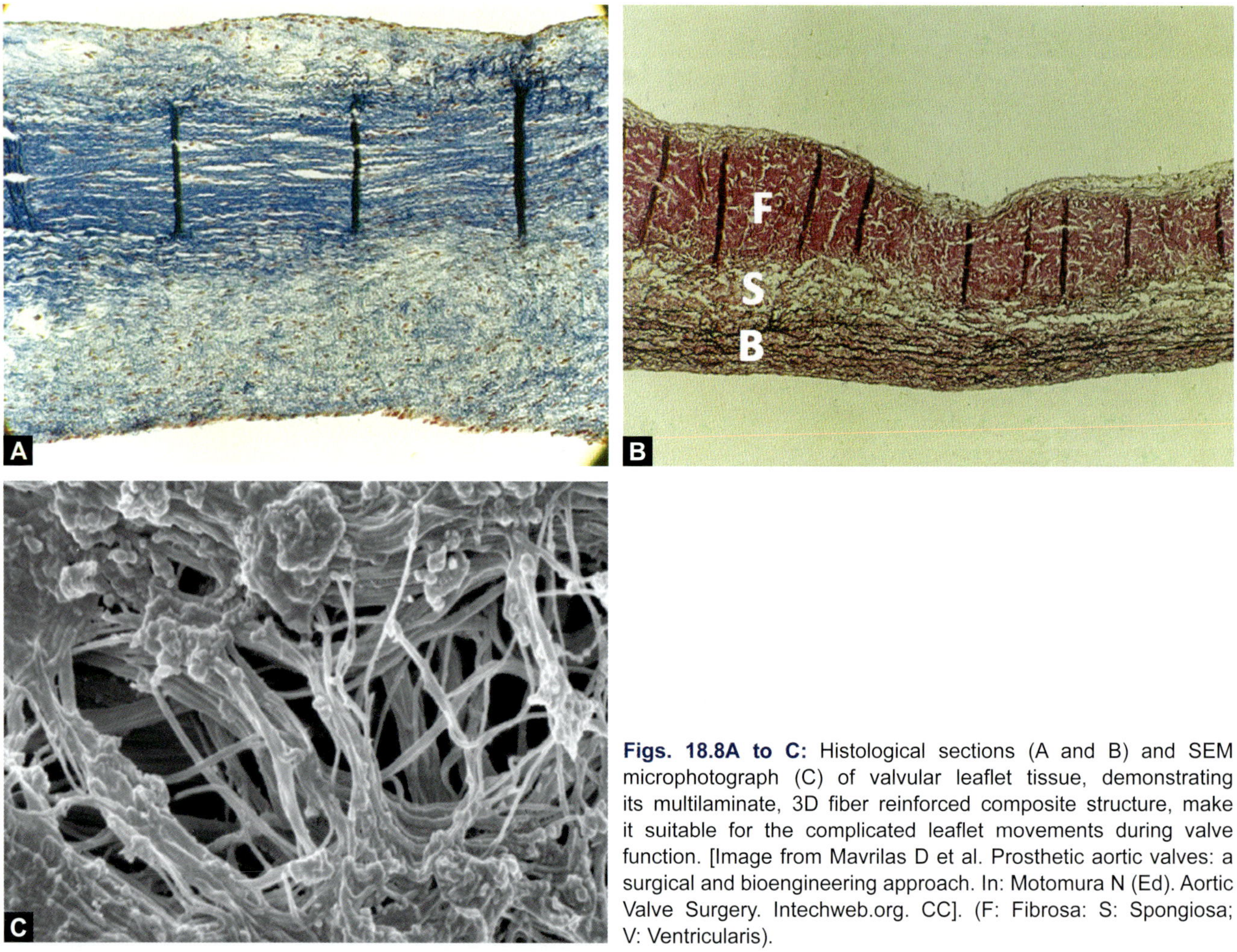

Figs. 18.8A to C: Histological sections (A and B) and SEM microphotograph (C) of valvular leaflet tissue, demonstrating its multilaminate, 3D fiber reinforced composite structure, make it suitable for the complicated leaflet movements during valve function. [Image from Mavrilas D et al. Prosthetic aortic valves: a surgical and bioengineering approach. In: Motomura N (Ed). Aortic Valve Surgery. Intechweb.org. CC]. (F: Fibrosa: S: Spongiosa; V: Ventricularis).

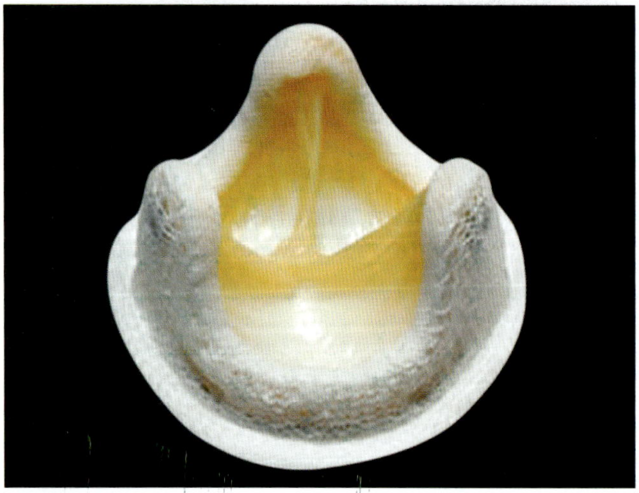

Fig. 18.9: Example of a modern bioprosthetic valve.

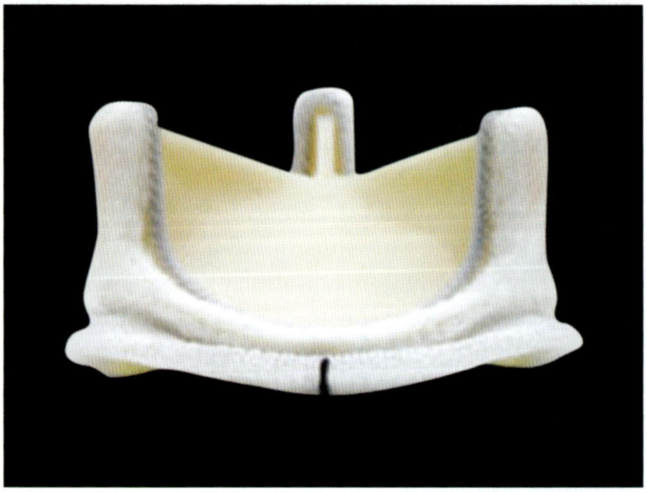

Fig. 18.10: The Carpentier-Edwards Magna-Ease bioprosthetic valve composed of bovine pericardial leaflets, metal alloy wire-form, low profile commissural posts, a thin stent base, and a contoured and compliant sewing ring.

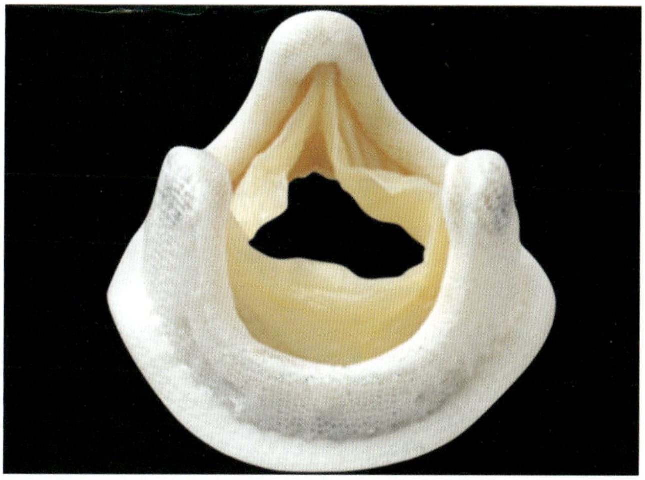

Fig. 18.11: The Medtronic Mosaic bioprosthetic valve, which is treated with alpha-amino oleic acid to reduce calcification and is made of porcine valve leaflets with preserved leaflet structure and retained leaflet collagen crimp.

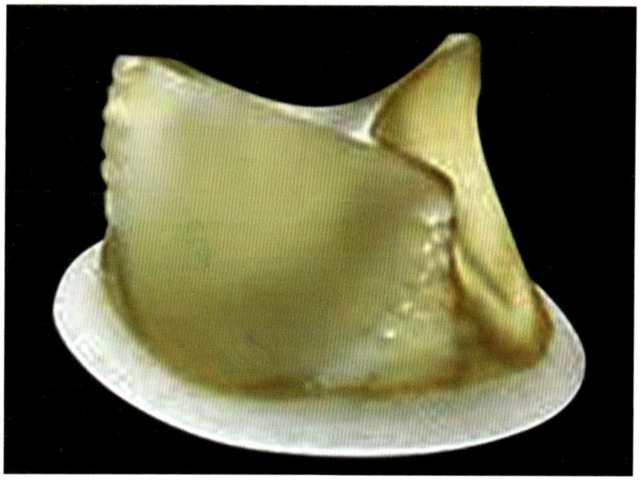

Fig. 18.12: The St Jude Trifecta bioprosthetic valve.

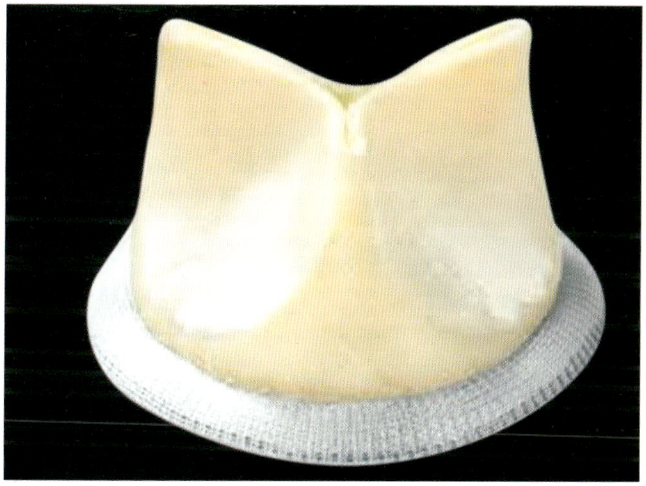

Fig. 18.13: The Sorin Mitroflow bioprosthetic valve, made of bovine pericardium wrapped around the outside of a stent with a soft silicone sewing ring as the base; its design is meant to accommodate small, narrow aortic roots.

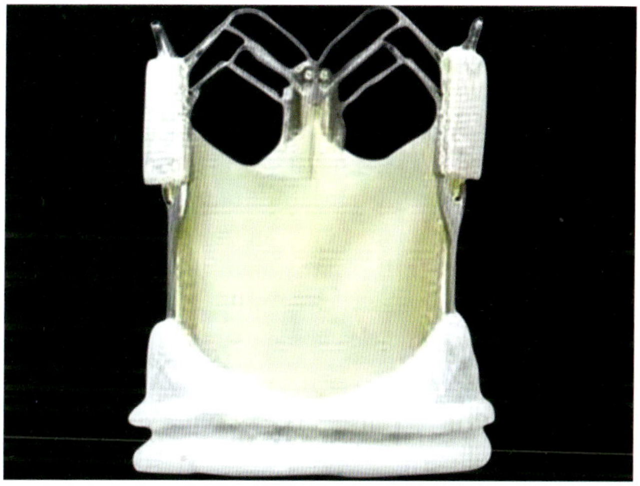

Fig. 18.14: The Medtronic 3f stentless bioprosthetic valve.

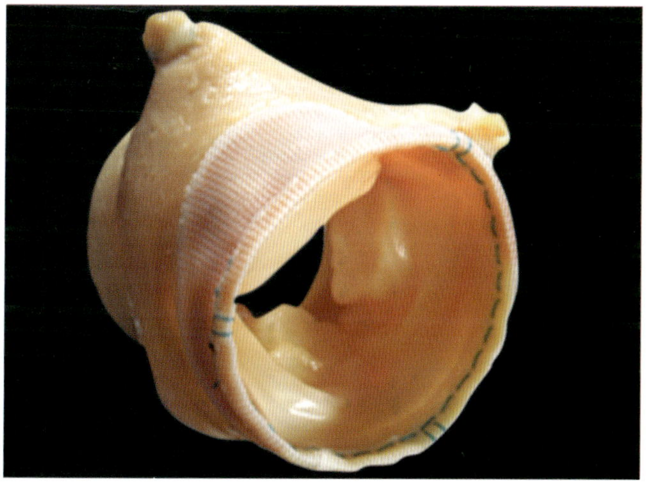

Fig. 18.15: The Medtronic Freestyle stentless bioprosthetic valve.

and is supported by the aortic root. The valve can also be implanted as a full root where the patient's entire native aortic root and aortic valve are replaced with the Freestyle anastomosed to the ascending aorta. One meta-analysis concluded that stentless valves did not have improved LV mass regression or postoperative mean gradients, but did display improved hemodynamics in terms of peak gradients. No long-term benefit or survival advantage from improved hemodynamics has been proven in randomized controlled trials with stentless valves.

The Sorin Solo valve (Fig. 18.16) was introduced in Europe in 2004 and is implanted using a proven single-suture line technique. This stentless valve design utilizes two pericardial sheets constructed to maximize leaflet opening and closing and the supra-annular position potentially reduces the risk of mismatch between the annulus of the patient and the size of the valve.

The newest aortic valve bioprosthesis include the sutureless aortic valves that incorporate the use of transcatheter technology with stentless valve hemodynamics. This may potentially reduce ischemic time by eliminating the need to place sutures in the aortic annulus and sewing ring. Such valves include the Perceval S sutureless valve (Figs. 18.17A and B), the Edwards Intuity sutureless valve (Figs. 18.18A and B), and the Medtronic/ATS 3f Enable sutureless valve (Fig. 18.19). In comparison to transcatheter aortic valves, sutureless valves have the advantage of resection of the stenotic leaflets and direct visualization of implantation.

Examples of delivery of modern bioprosthetic valves are shown in Figures 18.20 and 18.21.

MECHANICAL AORTIC VALVES

Mechanical heart valves have also improved significantly in parallel to bioprosthetic valves. Improvements in design aided by simulation of fluid mechanics have lowered transvalvular gradients and enhanced durability. Older ball-cage designs (Fig. 18.22) have been replaced by bileaflet designs with superior hemodynamics. However, life-long anticoagulation with a vitamin K antagonist (VKA) such as warfarin is needed to prevent thrombus formation in hinge recesses. Commonly used mechanical

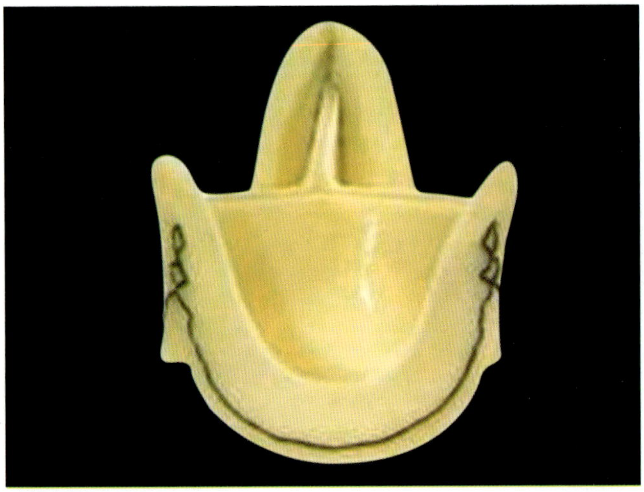

Fig. 18.16: The Sorin Solo valve, which is implanted using a proven single-suture line technique. This stentless valve design utilizes two pericardial sheets constructed to maximize leaflet opening and closing and the supra-annular position potentially reduces the risk of mismatch between the annulus of the patient and the size of the valve.

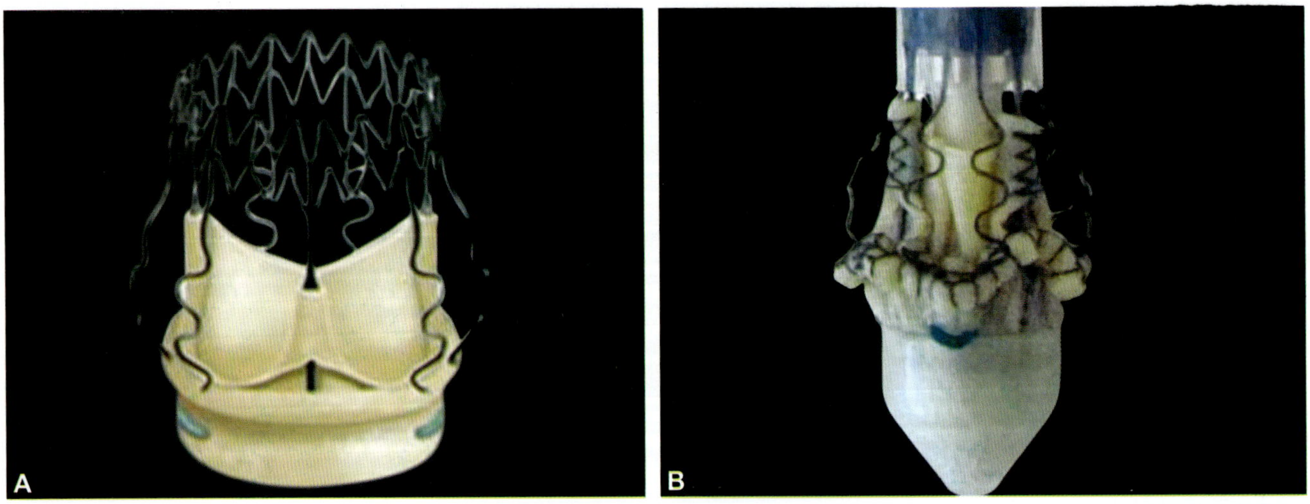

Figs. 18.17A and B: The Perceval S sutureless bioprosthetic valve.

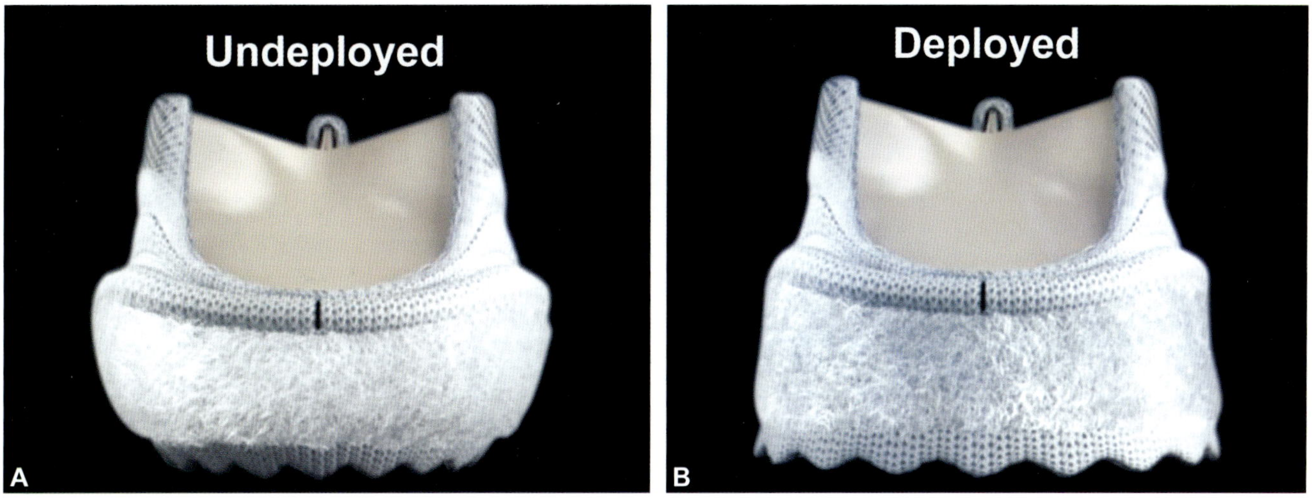

Figs. 18.18A and B: The Edwards Intuity sutureless bioprosthetic valve.

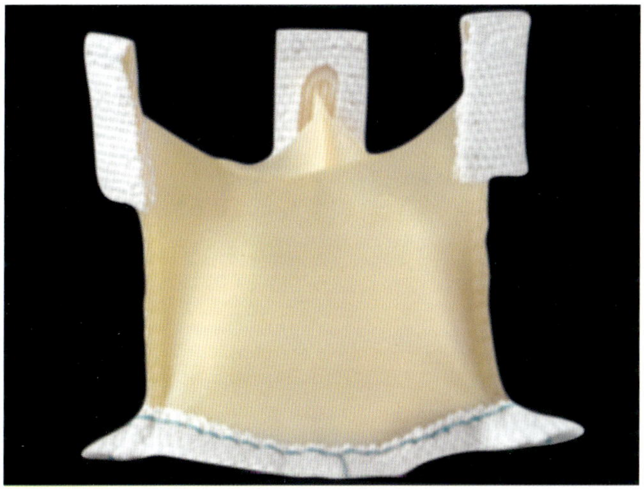

Fig. 18.19: The Medtronic/ATS 3f Enable sutureless bioprosthetic valve.

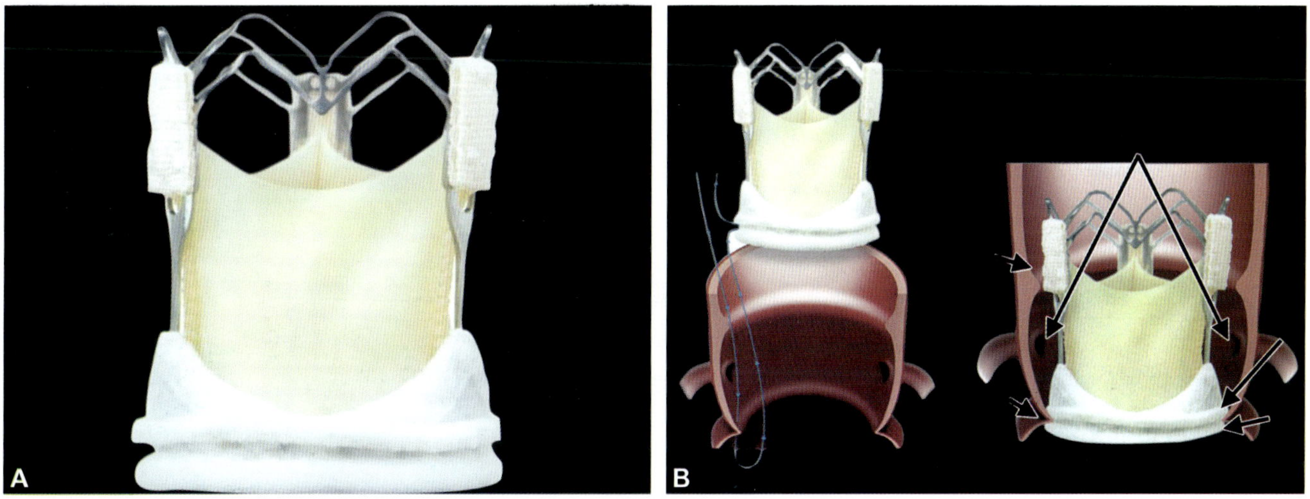

Figs. 18.20A and B: The Medtronic Enable valve (A) and schematic of valve insertion in the aortic position (B).

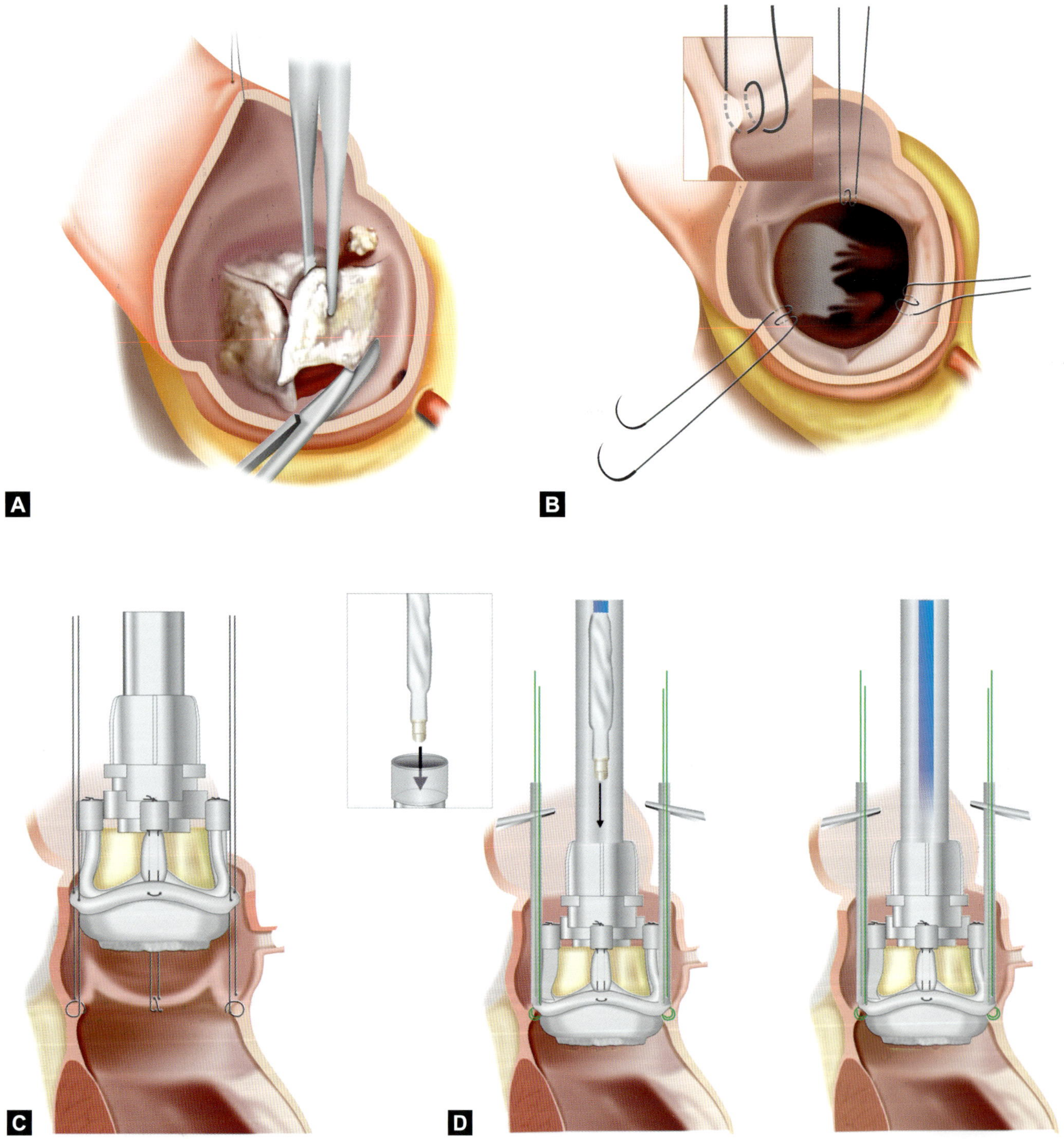

Figs. 18.21A to D: Implantation of the Edwards Aortic Quick Connect Bioprosthetic valve.

valves include the St Jude Regent valve (Fig. 18.23), the On-X aortic valve (Fig. 18.24), the Medtronic Open Pivot valve (Fig. 18.25), and the Sorin Tophat valve (Fig. 18.26).

BIOPROSTHETIC VERSUS MECHANICAL VALVE DECISIONS

Tissue prostheses carry a low risk of thromboembolic events (between 0.5% and 1% risk per year without anticoagulation), but with a higher change of valvular degeneration, requiring the potential need of a new surgical intervention. The decision between using mechanical versus tissue prosthesis is based on the specific patient characteristics. The decision is influenced by the valve-related risk of thromboembolism (especially with the mechanical prosthesis) and valvular structural degeneration of the tissue valves. Generally accepted indications for a mechanical valve are the use of chronic anticoagulation and young age of the patient. A randomized trial showed no difference in valve-related complications or survival at 15–20 years of follow-up among patients receiving a mechanical versus a bioprosthetic valve, but greater structural valve deterioration within the later group in patients <65 years of age. Newer technology with transcatheter valve replacement with valve-in-valve procedure on previous replacements is shifting

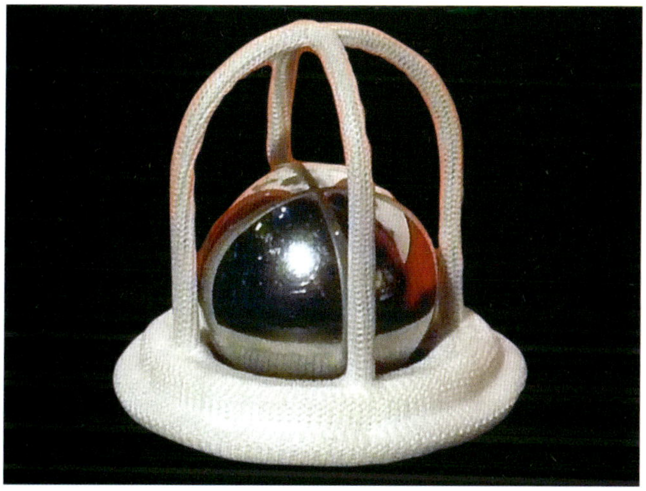

Fig. 18.22: The Starr-Edwards ball-cage design mechanical heart valve. While used decades ago, this valve design is no longer used in modern practice.

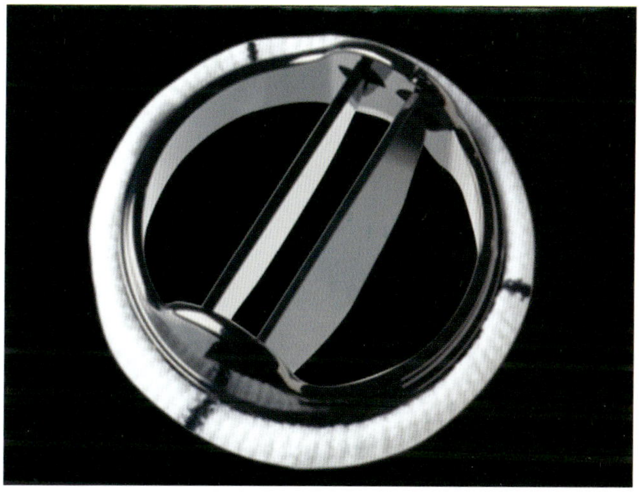

Fig. 18.23: The St Jude Regent bileaflet mechanical heart valve.

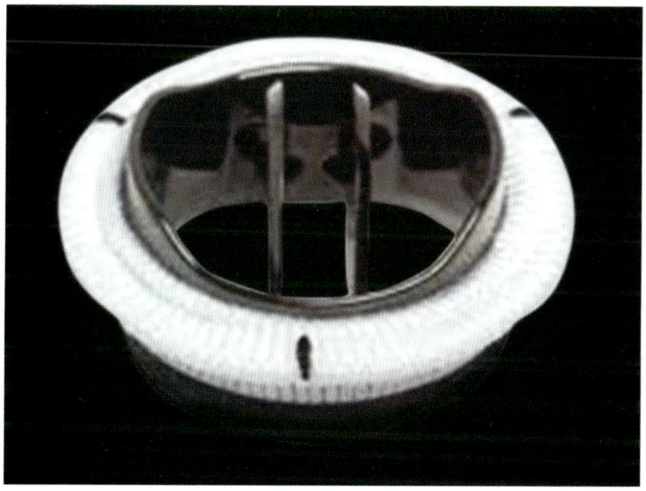

Fig. 18.24: The On-X bileaflet mechanical heart valve.

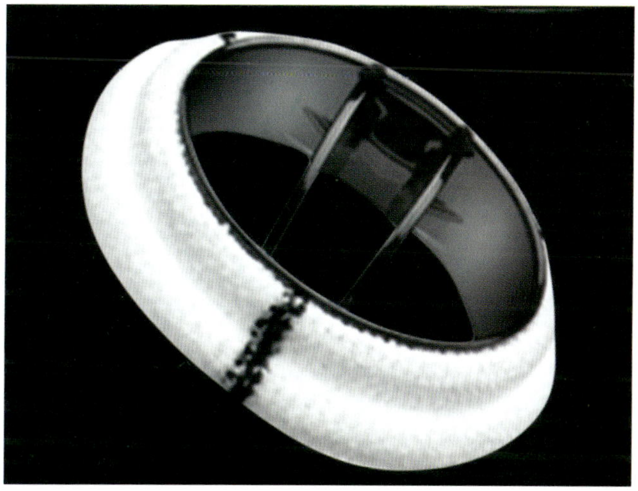

Fig. 18.25: The Medtronic Open Pivot bileaflet mechanical heart valve.

the trend to increase the use of bioprostheses in even younger population without the need of a future repeat sternotomy. Tables 18.1A, B and 18.2 summarize European and American guideline recommendations with regard to the choice of bioprosthetic or mechanical heart valve implantation.

POSTOPERATIVE MANAGEMENT

The initial goals in postoperative cardiac recovery are to obtain normothermia, adequate oxygenation and ventilation, control of bleeding, restoration of intravascular volume, optimization of blood pressure and cardiac output to maintain organ perfusion and metabolic stabilization. This initial management in the postoperative care after routine cardiac surgery has shifted toward a more efficient use of limited postoperative care facilities, early extubation and rapid discharge in the majority of the patients.

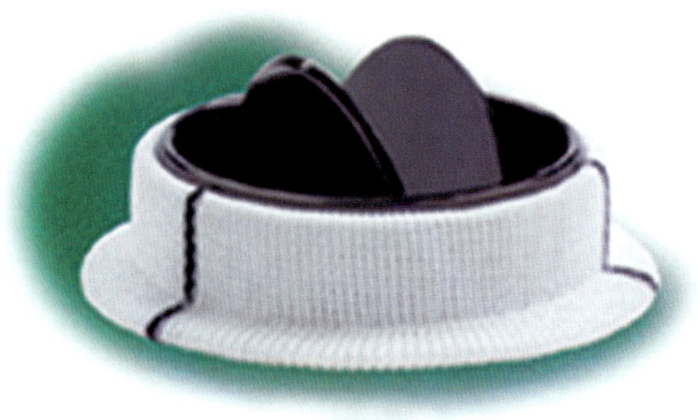

Fig. 18.26: The Sorin Tophat bileaflet mechanical heart valve.

SURGICAL COMPLICATIONS

Complications can be encountered during the surgical procedure or immediately postoperatively. These include: stroke, myocardial infarction, bleeding, cardiogenic shock, respiratory failure, acute kidney decompensation, conduction abnormalities requiring a pacemaker, liver failure, or gastrointestinal and vascular ischemia. Remote valve-related complications include anticoagulation-related hemorrhage, thromboembolism, valve thrombosis (Figs. 18.27 and 18.28), prosthetic valve endocarditis (Fig. 18.29), annulus abscess (Figs. 18.30A and B), valve dehiscence and paravalvular leak (Figs. 18.31 to 18.34, Videos 18.1 and 18.2), structural valve deterioration, patient-prosthesis mismatch, arrhythmia, and cardiac failure.

CLINICAL FOLLOW-UP

Clinical follow-up is recommended approximately 6–12 weeks after surgery, and includes clinical assessment, CBC (to screen for hemolysis or bleeding), ECG, and

Table 18.1A: Summary of the European Society of Cardiology (ESC) and European Association for Cardio-Thoracic Surgery (EACTS) guidelines for choice of aortic/mitral prosthesis, in regards to factors favoring choice of a mechanical prosthesis over a bioprosthesis. The level of evidence (LOE) supporting the recommendation is given in parenthesis, where LOE = A denotes a recommendation derived from multiple randomized clinical trials or meta-analyses, LOE = B denotes a recommendation derived from a single randomized clinical trial or large nonrandomized studies, and LOE = C denotes a recommendation based on consensus of expert opinion or based on small studies, retrospective studies, or registries.

Class I (is recommended and indicated)
• Mechanical prosthesis recommended according to the desire of the informed patient and if there are no contraindications for long-term anticoagulation (LOE = C) • Mechanical prosthesis recommended in patients at risk of accelerated structural valve deterioration (LOE = C) • Mechanical prosthesis recommended in patients already on anticoagulation as a result of having a mechanical prosthesis in another valve position (LOE = C)
Class IIa (should be considered)
• Mechanical prosthesis should be considered in patients aged < 60 years for prostheses in the aortic position and < 65 years for prostheses in the mitral position (LOE = C) • Mechanical prosthesis should be considered in patients with a reasonable life expectancy, for whom future redo valve surgery would be at high risk (LOE = C)
Class IIb (may be considered)
• Mechanical prosthesis may be considered in patients already on long-term anticoagulation due to high risk of thromboembolism (LOE = C)

Table 18.1B: Summary of the European Society of Cardiology (ESC) and European Association for Cardio-Thoracic Surgery (EACTS) guidelines for choice of aortic/mitral prosthesis, in regards to factors favoring choice of a bioprosthesis over a mechanical prosthesis. The level of evidence (LOE) supporting the recommendation is given in parenthesis, where LOE = A denotes a recommendation derived from multiple randomized clinical trials or meta-analyses, LOE = B denotes a recommendation derived from a single randomized clinical trial or large nonrandomized studies, and LOE = C denotes a recommendation based on consensus of expert opinion or based on small studies, retrospective studies, or registries.

Class I (is recommended and indicated)
• Bioprosthesis recommended according to the desire of the informed patient (LOE = C)
• Bioprosthesis recommended when good quality anticoagulation is unlikely or contraindicated because of high bleeding risk (LOE = C)
• Bioprosthesis recommended for reoperation for mechanical valve thrombosis despite good long-term anticoagulant control (LOE = C)
Class IIa (should be considered)
• Bioprosthesis should be considered in patients for whom future redo valve surgery would be at low risk (LOE = C)
• Bioprosthesis should be considered in young women contemplating pregnancy (LOE = C)
• Bioprosthesis should be considered in patients aged > 65 years for prosthesis in aortic position or > 70 years in mitral position, or those with life expectancy lower than the presumed durability of the bioprosthesis (LOE = C)

Table 18.2: Summary of the American College of Cardiology Foundation (ACCF)/American Heart Association (AHA) recommendations for choice of prosthetic heart valve. The level of evidence (LOE) supporting the recommendation is given in parenthesis, where LOE = A denotes a recommendation derived from multiple randomized clinical trials or meta-analyses, LOE = B denotes a recommendation derived from a single randomized clinical trial or nonrandomized studies, and LOE = C denotes a recommendation based on consensus of expert opinion, standard of care, or case reports.

Class I (is recommended; is indicated)
• Bioprosthesis in patients of any age for whom anticoagulation therapy is contraindicated, cannot be managed appropriately, or is not desired (LOE=C)
Class IIa (is reasonable)
• Mechanical valve for AVR or MVR in patients < 60 years of age who do not have a contraindication to anticoagulation (LOE = B)
• Bioprosthetic valve in patients > 70 years of age (LOE = B)
• Either a bioprosthetic or mechanical valve in patients between 60 and 70 years of age (LOE = B)
Class IIb (may be considered)
• Replacement of the aortic valve by a pulmonary autograft (the Ross procedure), when performed by an experienced surgeon, in young patients when anticoagulation is contraindicated or undesirable (LOE = C)

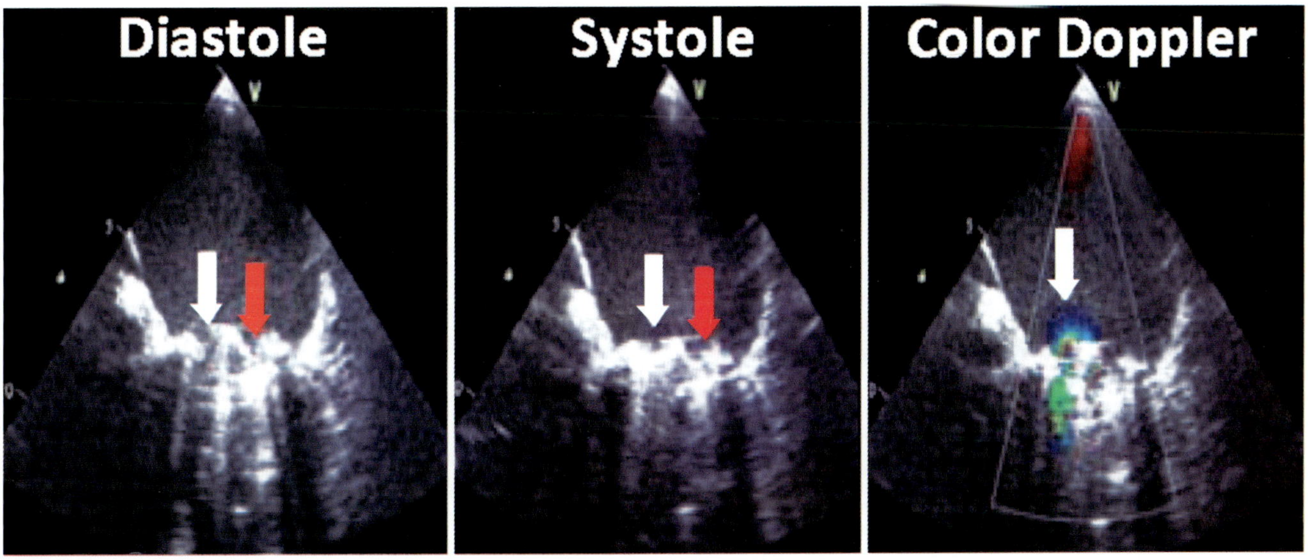

Fig. 18.27: Transesophageal echocardiography showing reduced mobility of the prosthetic valve with functional stenosis. The white and red arrows point to the mobile and immobile leaflets, respectively. Right panel shows color Doppler during diastole. [Image from Wilke A et al. Thrombosis of a prosthetic mitral valve after withdrawal of phenprocoumon therapy. Cardiol Res. 2011;2(6):298-300. CC].

transthoracic echocardiography (TTE). All patients who undergo valve replacement surgery should be followed by a cardiologist. Clinical assessment is generally recommended yearly. TTE is recommended if any new symptoms occur after valve surgery or if complications are suspected. Yearly echocardiography examination is recommended beginning five years after placement of a bioprosthetic valve. Transprosthetic gradients are better interpreted in comparison to baseline values (early postoperative TTE), rather than with theoretical values for a given prosthesis.

Transesophageal echocardiography (TEE) should be conserved if TTE is of poor quality, and should be performed in cases of suspected prosthetic valve dysfunction or endocarditis.

Cinefluoroscopy or cardiac CT can be utilized to provide additional information in cases of suspected valve thrombus or pannus.

ANTITHROMBOTIC THERAPY

Aspirin is now favored over VKA for the first 3 months in patients with bioprosthetic aortic valves. Oral anticoagulation with a VKA is recommended for the first 3 months in patients treated with bioprosthetic mitral valves, and in all patients treated with mechanical valves. The addition of low-dose aspirin should be considered in patients with mechanical valves, particularly those with concomitant coronary artery disease and in those at low

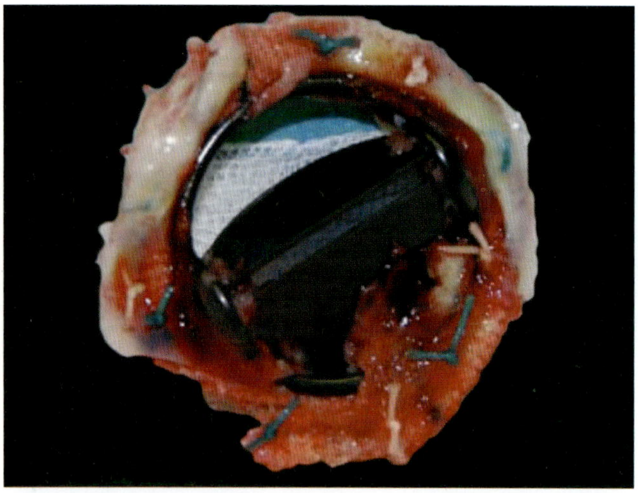

Fig. 18.28: Excised thrombosed valve shown in Figure 18.27. [Image from Wilke A et al. Thrombosis of a prosthetic mitral valve after withdrawal of phenprocoumon therapy. Cardiol Res. 2011;2(6):298-300. CC].

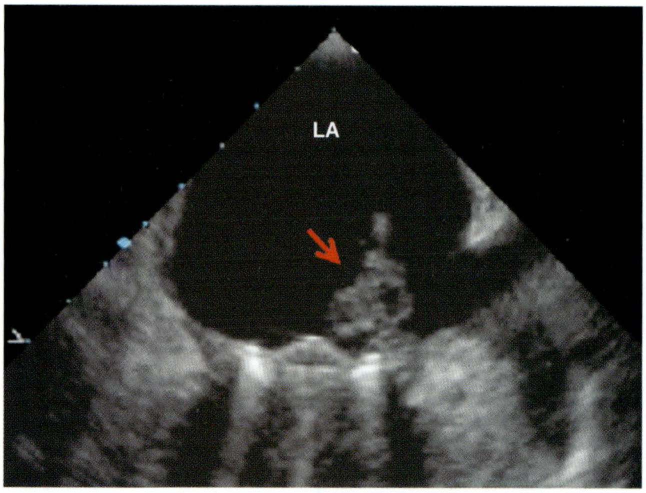

Fig. 18.29: TEE demonstrating infective endocarditis (arrow) in a patient with a mechanical prosthetic mitral valve. (Image courtesy of Glenn N Levine, MD).

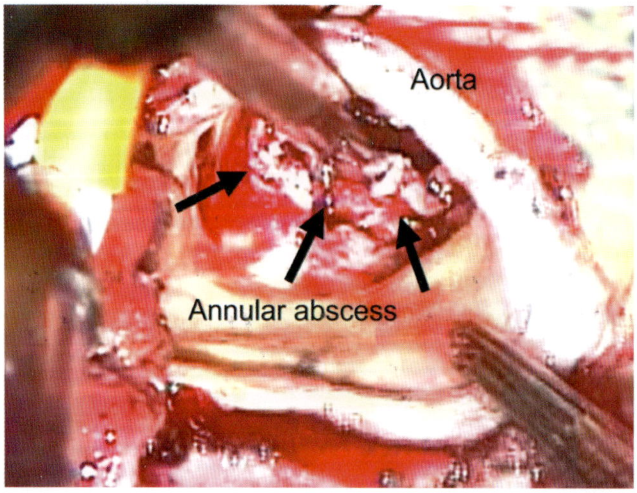

Fig. 18.30A: Annulus abscess. Operative findings demonstrating an abscess on the aortic annulus and partial valvular dehiscence in a patient with prosthetic aortic valve. (Image from Nonaka M et al. Case of prosthetic valve endocarditis with osteomyelitis associated with disregarded skin infection. Research Journal of Infectious Diseases 2013. DOI: http://dx.doi.org/10.7243/2052-5958-1-4. CC).

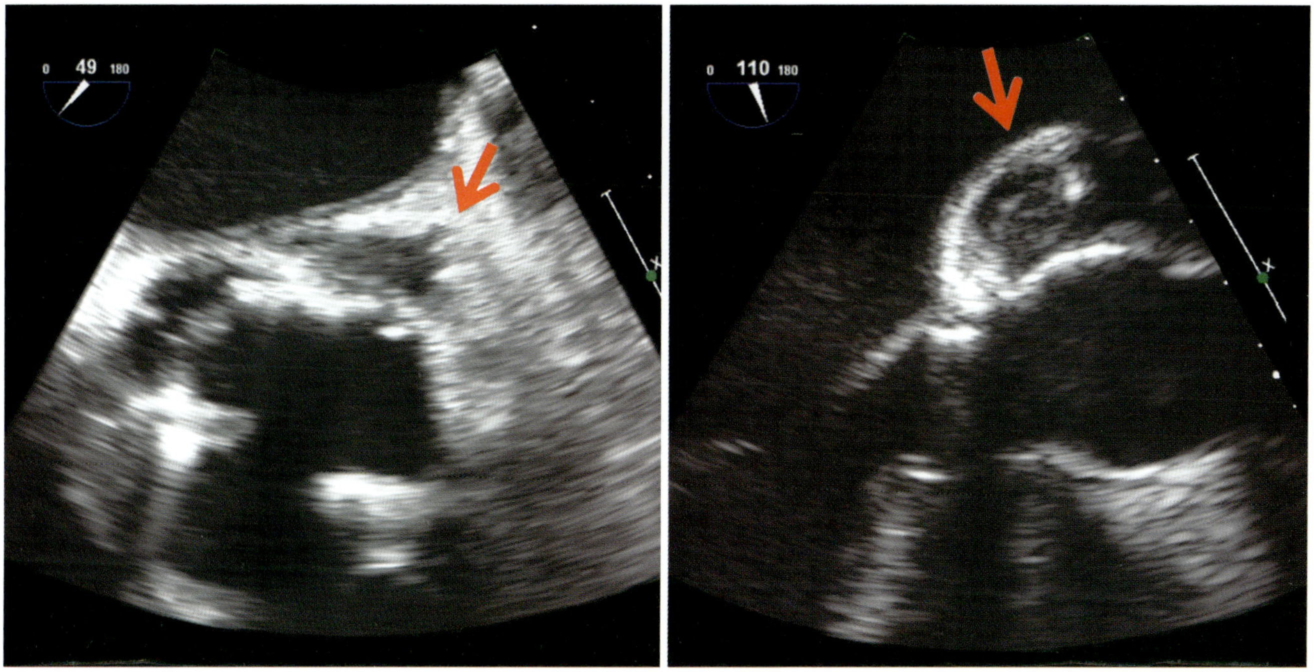

Fig. 18.30B: TEE short-axis (left panel) and long-axis (right panel) images showing abscess formation (arrow) in a patient with aortic valve endocarditis. (Image courtesy of Glenn N Levine, MD).

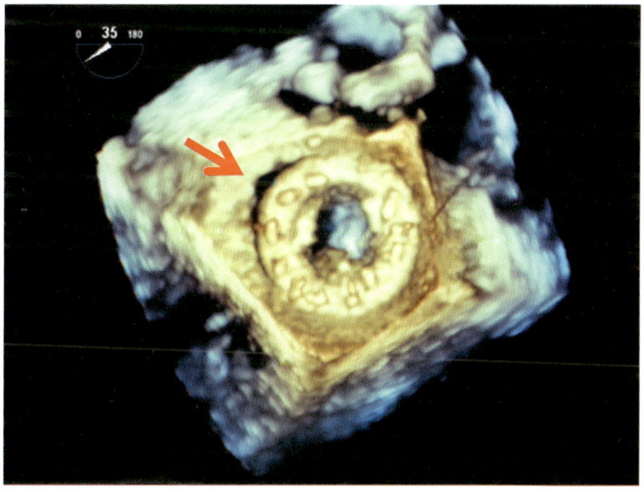

Fig. 18.31: Prosthetic mitral valve paravalvular defect (arrow). [Image from Zaragoza-Macias E et al. How to Perform a Three-Dimensional Transesophageal Echocardiogram. In: Nanda NC. Comprehensive Textbook of Echocardiography. New Delhi, India: Jaypee Brothers Medical Publishers (P) Ltd].

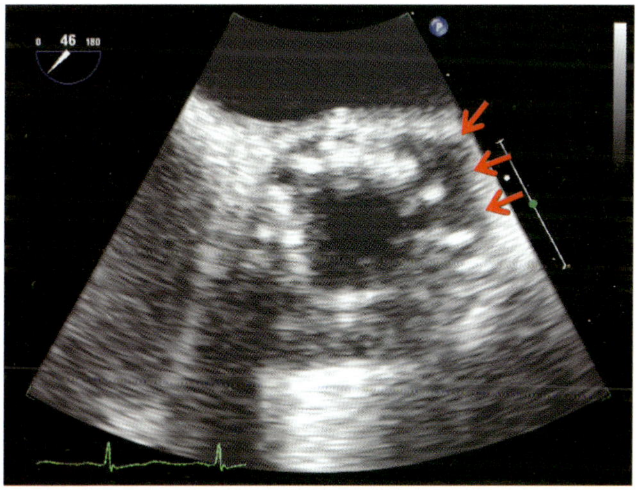

Fig. 18.32: TEE showing dehiscence (arrows) of a prosthetic aortic valve. (Image courtesy of Glenn N Levine, MD).

risk of bleeding complications. As of this writing, the newer oral anticoagulants (direct factor IIa or Xa inhibitors) have not been recommended as substitutes for VKA therapy. Recommendations regarding antithrombotic therapy in patients treated with prosthetic heart valves are summarized in Tables 18.3 to 18.5.

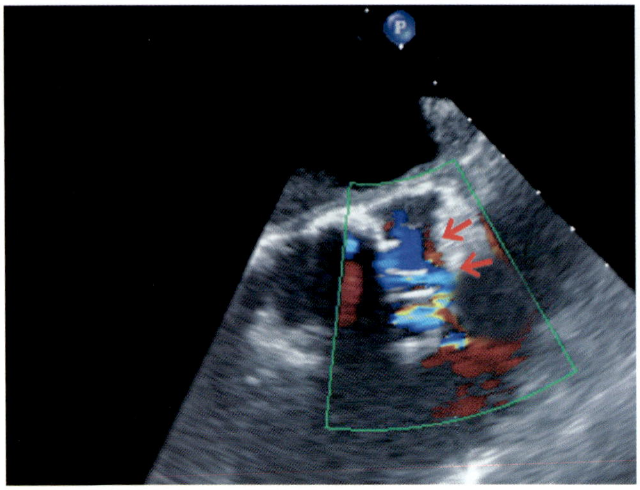

Fig. 18.33: TEE showing dehiscence of a prosthetic aortic valve with perivalvular leak (arrows). Videos 18.1 and 18.2 show the 2D and color Dopper video loops corresponding to this still frame image. (Image courtesy of Glenn N Levine, MD).

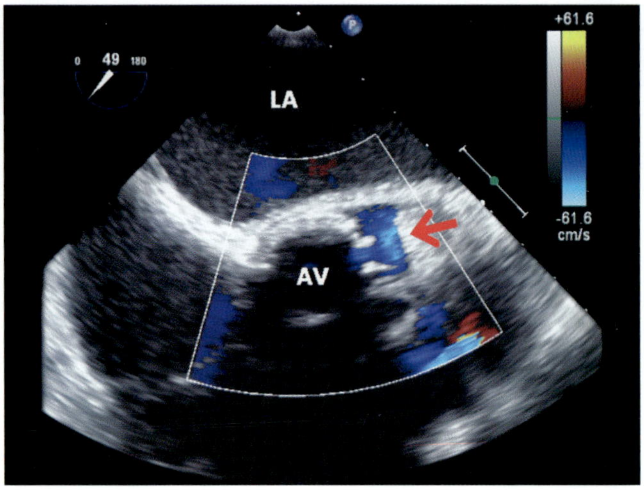

Fig. 18.34: TEE showing dehiscence and resultant paravalvular leak (arrow) in a patient with a prosthetic aortic valve. (Image courtesy of Glenn N Levine, MD).

Table 18.3: Summary of the European Society of Cardiology (ESC) and European Association for Cardio-Thoracic Surgery (EACTS) guidelines antithrombotic therapy after valvular surgery. The level of evidence (LOE) supporting the recommendation is given in parenthesis, where LOE = A denotes a recommendation derived from multiple randomized clinical trials or meta-analyses, LOE = B denotes a recommendation derived from a single randomized clinical trial or large nonrandomized studies, and LOE = C denotes a recommendation based on consensus of expert opinion or based on small studies, retrospective studies, or registries.

Class I (is recommended and indicated)
• Lifelong for all patients with a mechanical prosthesis (LOE = B)
• Lifelong for patients with bioprostheses who have other indications for anticoagulation (LOE = C)
Class IIa (should be considered)
• Addition of low-dose aspirin in patients with a mechanical prosthesis and concomitant atherosclerotic disease (LOE = C)
• Addition of low-dose aspirin in patients with a mechanical prosthesis after thromboembolism despite adequate INR (LOE = C)
• Oral anticoagulation for the first 3 months after implantation of a mitral- or tricuspid bioprosthesis (LOE = C)
• Oral anticoagulation for the first 3 months after mitral valve repair
• Low-dose aspirin for the first 3 months after implantation of an aortic bioprosthesis (LOE = C)
Class IIb (may be considered)
• Oral anticoagulation for the first 3 months after implantation of an aortic bioprosthesis (LOE = C)

Table 18.4: Summary of the American College of Chest Physicians (ACCP) 9th edition recommendations for antithrombotic and thrombolytic therapy after valve surgery. Recommendations assume patient is in sinus rhythm.

Valve/Position	*Recommendation*	*Grade*
Bioprosthetic heart valves—first 3 months after implantation		
Bioprosthetic aortic valve	Aspirin (50–100 mg/day) for first 3 months	2C
Transcatheter aortic bioprosthetic valve	Aspirin (50–100 mg/day) and clopidogrel (75 mg/day) for first 3 months	2C
Bioprosthetic mitral valve	VKA therapy (target INR 2.5; range 2.0–3.0) for first 3 months	2C
Bioprosthetic heart valves—3 months and beyond after implantation		
Bioprosthetic valve after 3 months postoperative	Aspirin therapy	2C
Mechanical heart valve		
Mechanical heart valves	VKA therapy in preference to no VKA therapy	1B
Mechanical aortic valves	VKA therapy with target INR 2.5; range 2.0–3.0 in preference to lower targets	2C

Contd...

Contd...

Valve/Position	*Recommendation*	*Grade*
Mechanical aortic valves	VKA therapy with target INR 2.5; range 2.0–3.0 in preference to higher targets	1B
Mechanical mitral valve	VKA therapy with target INR 3.0; range 2.5–3.5	2C
Mechanical aortic and mitral valves	VKA therapy with target INR 3.0; range 2.5–3.5	2C
Mechanical aortic or mitral valves; patient at low risk of bleeding	Addition of low dose aspirin (50–100 mg/day) to VKA therapy	1B
Valve repair		
Aortic valve repair	Aspirin (50–100 mg/day)	2C
Mitral valve repair with a prosthetic band/ring	Antiplatelet therapy for the first 3 months	2C
Prosthetic valve thrombosis (PVT)		
Right-sided PVT	Fibrinolytic therapy (if no contraindications) over surgical intervention	2C
Left-sided PVT and large thrombus area (≤ 0.8 cm^2)	Early surgery suggested over fibrinolytic therapy; fibrinolytic therapy suggested if contraindication to surgery	2C
Left-sided PVT and small thrombus area (> 0.8 cm^2)	Fibrinolytic therapy in preference to surgery	2C
Left-sided PVT and very small, non obstructive, thrombus	IV unfractionated heparin and serial Doppler echocardiography	2C

Table 18.5: Summary of the European Society of Cardiology (ESC) guidelines for target INR in patients with mechanical heart valves.

Prosthesis thrombogenicity	***Patient-related risk factors***	
	No risk factors	***≥ 1 risk factor*** *(mitral or tricuspid valve replacement, previous thrombo-embolism, atrial fibrillation, mitral stenosis, LVEF < 35%)*
Low (Carbomedics, Medronic Hall, St Jude Medical bileaflet valves)	2.5	3.0
Medium (other bileaflet valves)	3.0	3.5
High (tilting-disk valves)	3.5	4.0

VIDEO LEGENDS

Video 18.1: TEE video of a prosthetic aortic valve showing valve dehiscence, visible most prominently from 1 o'clock to 3 o'clock. The sutures are visualized.

Video 18.2: Color Doppler TEE video corresponding to Video 18.1, showing that the valve dehiscence has led to significant paravalvular leak.

REFERENCES

Franco KL, Thourani VH. Cardiothoracic Surgery Review, 1st edition. Philadelphia: Lippincott Williams & Wilkins; 2012.

Hammermiester K, Sethi GK, Henderson WG, et al. Outcomes 15 years after valve replacement with a mechanical versus a bioprosthetic valve: final report of the veterans affairs randomized trial. J Am Coll Cardiol. 2000;36:1152-8.

Payne DM, Koka HP, Karanicolas PJ, et al. Hemodynamic performance of stentless versus stented vlaves: a systematic review and meta-analysis. J Card Surg. 2008;23(5):556-64.

Schelbert EB, Vaughan-Sarrazin MS, Welke KF, et al. Valve type and long-term outcomes after aortic valve replacement in older patients. Heart. 2008;94:1181-8.

Vahanian A, Alfieri O, Andreotti F, et al. Guidelines on the management of valvular heart disease (version 2012). The Joint Task Force on the Management of Valvular Heart Disease of the European Society of Cardiology (ESC) and the European Association for Cardio-Thoracic Surgery (EACTS). European Heart Journal. 2012;33:2451-96.

Webb JG, Wood DA, Ye J, et al. Transcatheter valve-in-valve implantation for failed bioprosthetic heart valves. Circulation. 2012;121:1848-57.

Whitlock RP, Sun JC, Fremes S, et al. Antithrombotic and thrombolytic therapy for valvular disease. Antithrombotic Therapy and Prevention of Thrombosis, 9th edition. American College of Chest Physicians Evidence-Based Clinical Practice Guidelines. Chest. 2012;141(2)(Suppl):e576S-e600S.

Section 3

Heart Failure and Cardiomyopathy

Chapters

CHAPTER

Normal Cardiac Anatomy and Function

19

Jin T Kim, Pradeep Vaideeswar, Glenn N Levine

INTRODUCTION

The heart is contained in the mediastinal cavity (Figs. 19.1A and B). In all but a very few patients, the heart consists of left and right atria and ventricles (Figs. 19.2 to 19.5). Imaging of the heart and heart chambers in current practice to assess chamber size and ventricular function is performed via echocardiography, cardiac computed tomography (CT) and cardiac magnetic resonance imaging (MRI). Nuclear cardiology imaging and ventriculography can also be used to assess left and right ventricular size and function.

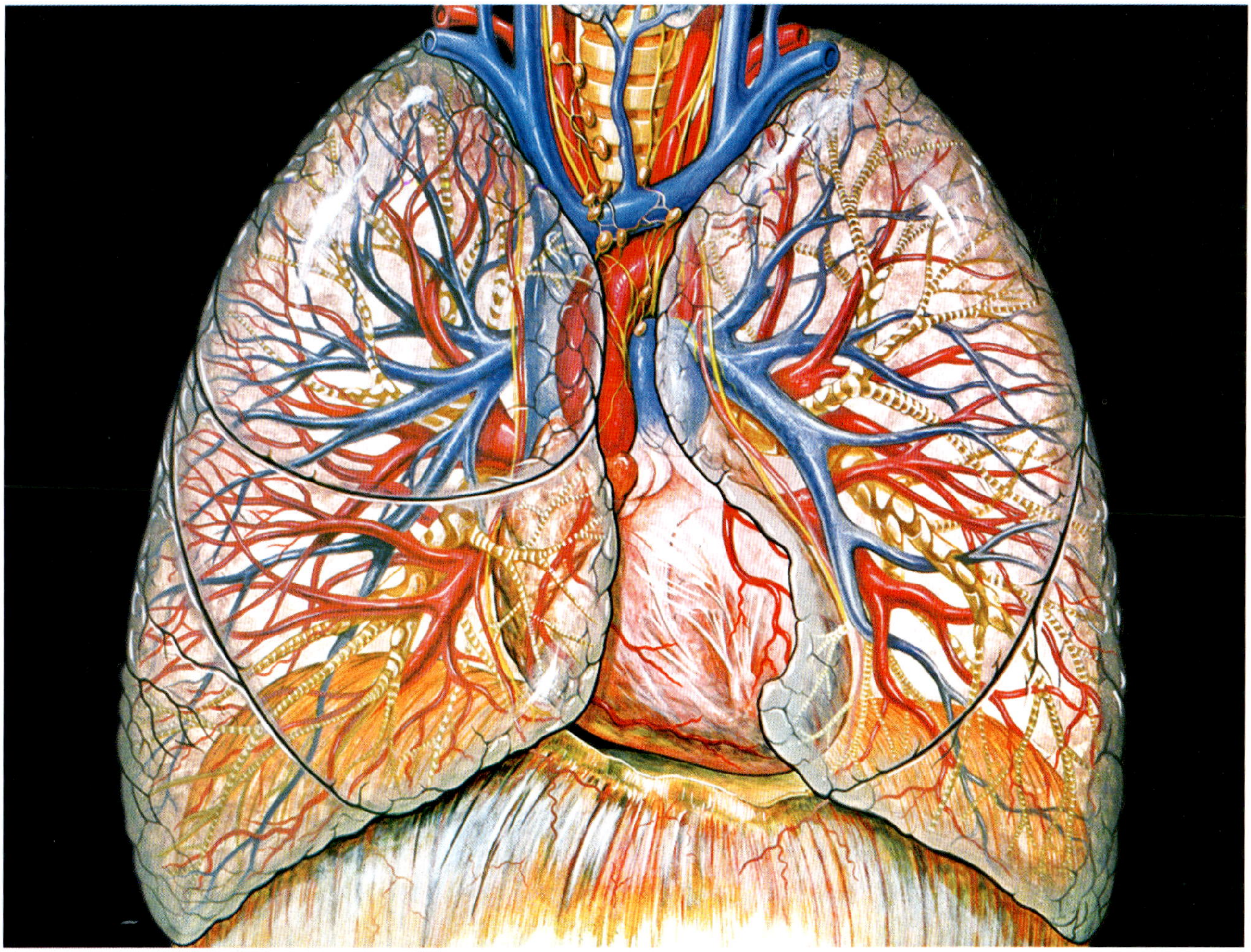

Fig. 19.1A: Anatomic location of the heart in the mediastinum. (Image created by Patrick J Lynch and C Carl Jaffe, MD, and posted on Wikipedia).

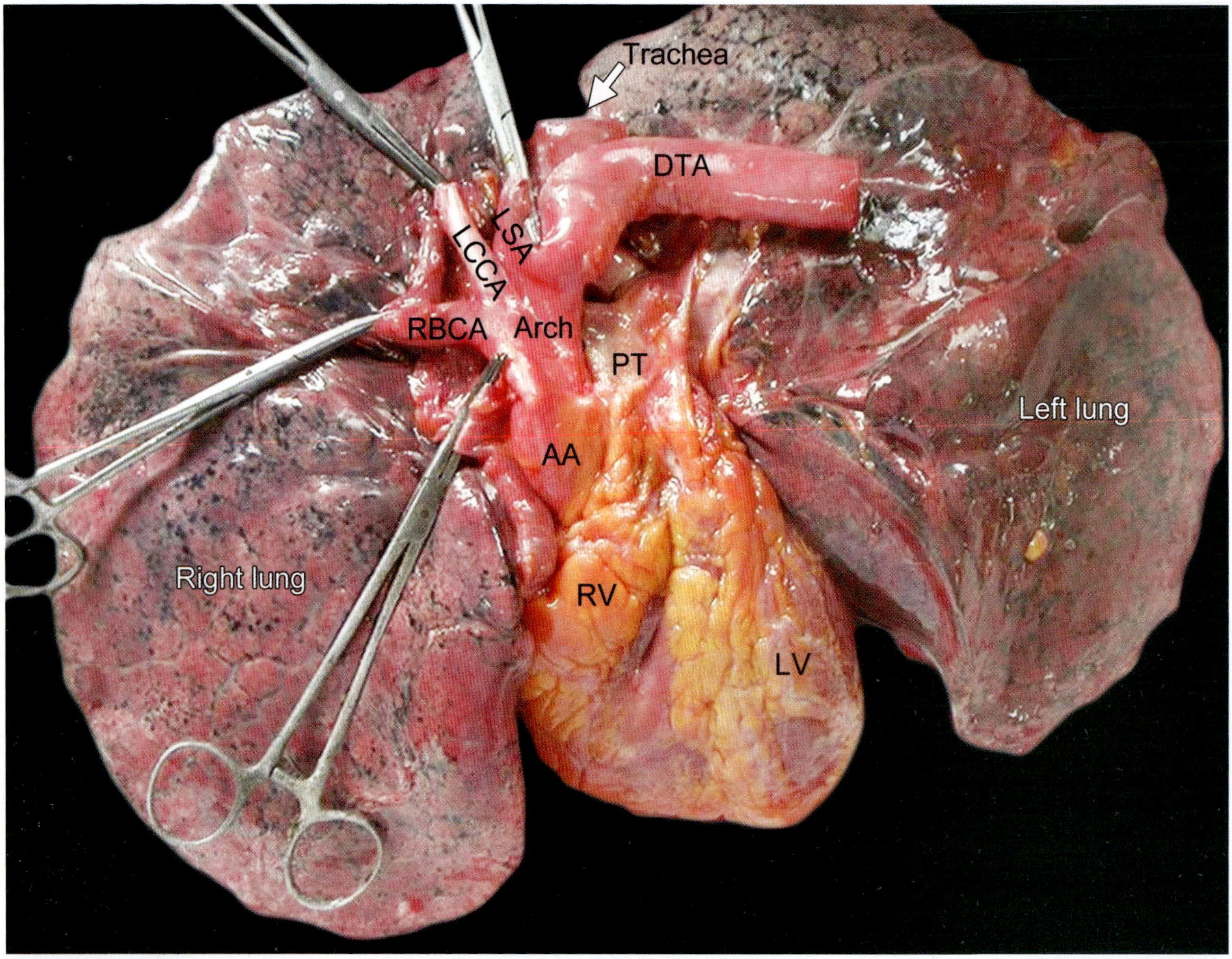

Fig. 19.1B: Gross pathology of the heart, aorta and branches, and the lungs. [Courtesy of Pradeep Vaideeswar, Professor (Additional), Department of Pathology, Cardiovascular & Thoracic Division, Seth Gordhandas Sunderdas Medical College, Mumbai, India]. (AA: Ascending aorta; DTA: Descending thoracic aorta; LCCA: Left common carotid artery; LSA: Left subclavian artery; PT: Pulmonary trunk; RBCA: Right brachiocephalic artery; RV: Right ventricle; LV: Left ventricle).

THE CARDIAC CHAMBERS

The left atrium (LA) (Fig. 19.6) usually receives oxygenated blood returning from the lungs by two sets of right and left pulmonary veins, although there is some variation in this (Fig. 19.7). Oxygenated blood returning from the lungs passes through the LA and mitral valve in to the left ventricle (LV) by both passive and active processes. The LA is actually a structure of complex and varying geometry. That said, an approximation of LA size can be made using standard echocardiographic techniques. LA size is generally slightly greater in men than women. Assessment of LA size should be adjusted based on a patient's body surface area (BSA). The right atrium (RA) serves as a conduit between returning deoxygenated blood from the superior and inferior vena cava and the right ventricle (RV) (Fig. 19.8). There is less data on assessment of right atrial (RA) size. RA area of >18 cm^2, measured on an apical four chamber transthoracic echocardiogram, is considered to be abnormal.

The left and right atria each have an appendage (Fig. 19.9). The left atria appendage contains pectinate muscles and is often the source of thrombus formation (Fig. 19.10) in patients who have suffered cardioembolic stroke.

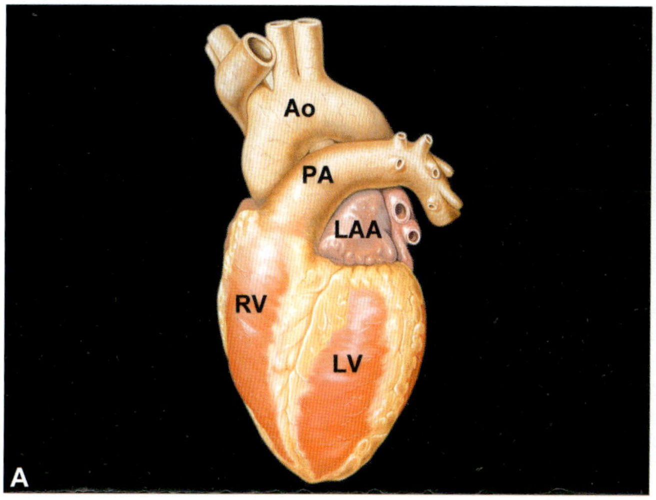

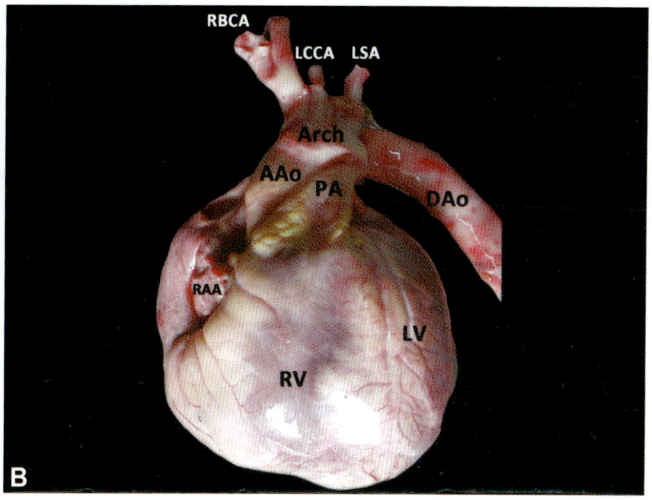

Figs. 19.2A and B: External anatomy of the heart and great vessels. (A) Schematic left oblique view of the normal external anatomy of the heart; (B) Gross pathology specimen. [Figure 19.2A created by Patrick J Lynch and C Carl Jaffe, MD, and posted on Wikipedia. Figure 19.2B courtesy of Pradeep Vaideeswar, Professor (Additional), Department of Pathology, Cardiovascular & Thoracic Division, Seth Gordhandas Sunderdas Medical College, Mumbai, India]. (AAo: Ascending aorta; Ao: Aorta; DAo: Descending aorta; LAA: Left atrial appendage; LCCA: Left common carotid artery; LSA: Left subclavian artery; LV: Left ventricle; PA: Pulmonary artery; RAA: Right atrial appendage; RBCA: Right brachiocephalic artery; RV: Right ventricle).

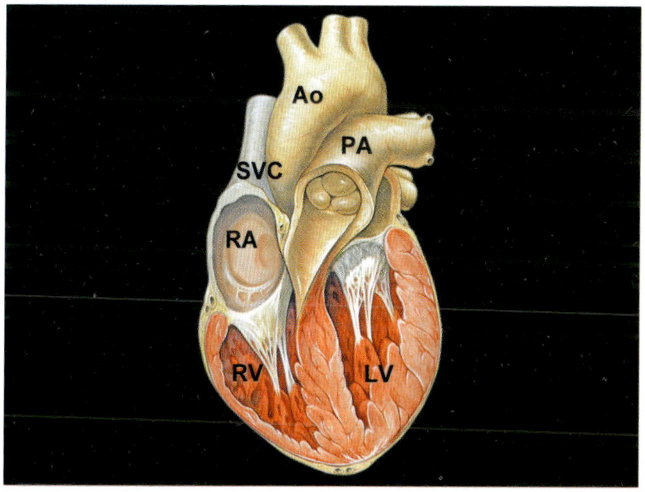

Fig. 19.3: Left oblique view of the normal internal anatomy of the heart. [Image created by Patrick J Lynch and C Carl Jaffe, MD, and posted on Wikipedia]. (Ao: Aorta; LV: Left ventricle; PA: Pulmonary artery; RA: Right atrium; RV: Right ventricle; SVC: Superior vena cava).

Right heart pressures and left heart diastolic filling pressure can usually be assessed through noninvasive means, primary echocardiography. When necessary, right heart pressures and indirect assessment of left atrial pressure can be measured by right heart catheterization (Figs. 19.11A to D).

The RV is the most anterior cardiac chamber and is delimited by the tricuspid valve annulus and the pulmonary valve. The RV is highly trabeculated and has several prominent muscular bands. Trabeculations in the RV are coarser than those in the LV (Fig. 19.12). One of these bands, the moderator band, is frequently prominent on echocardiography examination. The RV may be divided into two or three parts. In the two-part schema, the RV is divided into the inflow portion and the outflow portion. In the three-part schema, it is divided into an inlet part, an apical trabecular part, and an outlet (or infundibular) part. In reality though, the RV has a complex geometric shape, which makes assessment of right ventricular function challenging. RV mass is approximately one-sixth that of left ventricular mass, with a much thinner free wall when compared to the free walls of the LV (Fig. 19.13). This roughly corresponds to the finding that the RV pumps against approximately one-fifth to one-sixth the resistance of the LV. Right ventricular function is usually assessed qualitatively or semiquantitatively. Several objective parameters have been established to more quantitatively assess RV systolic function as normal or abnormal and are summarized in Table 19.1.

The LV (Fig. 19.14) is shorter and more conical than the RV, with a wall thickness 3-6 times that of the RV.

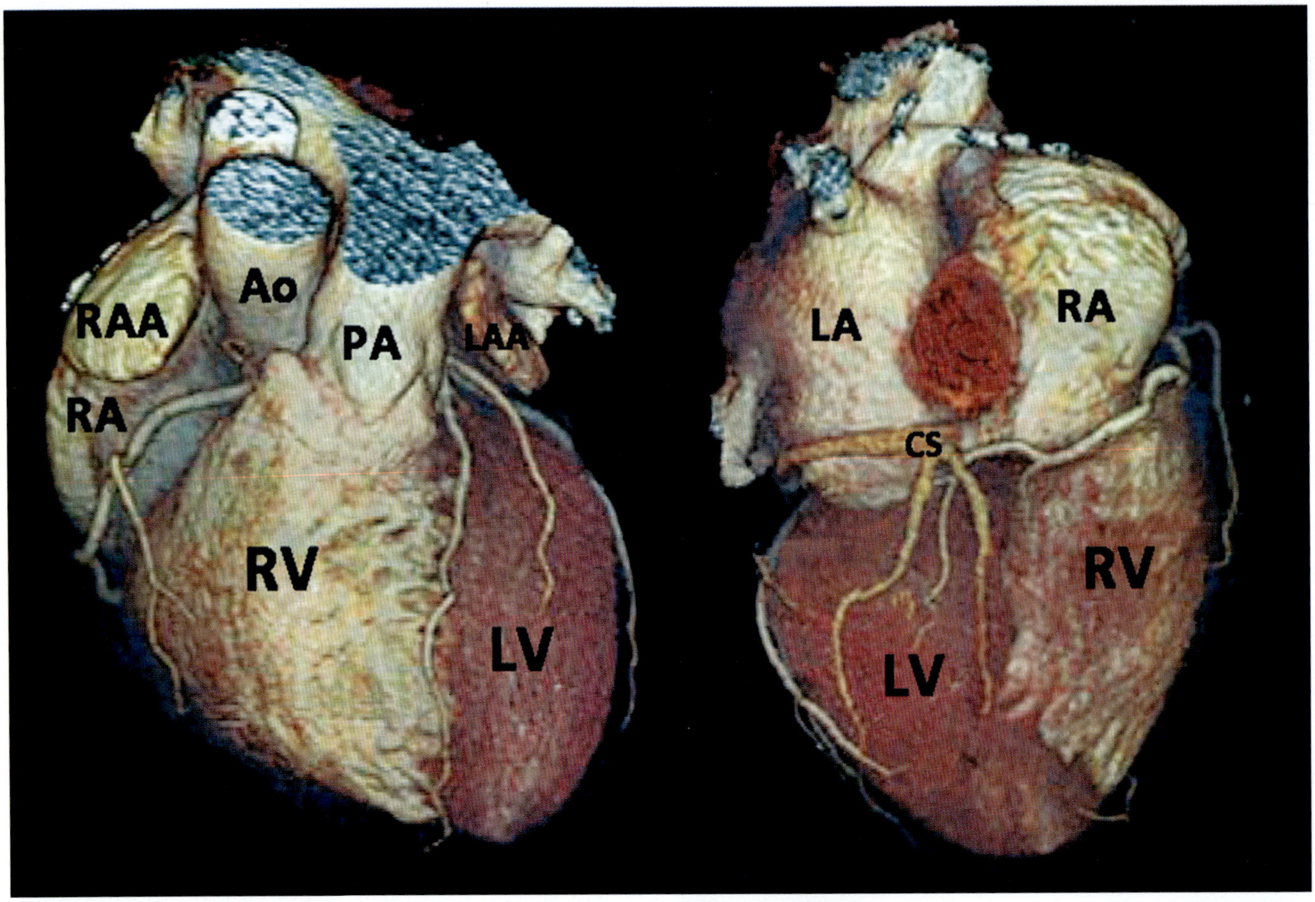

Fig. 19.4: Volume-rendered CT scan of the heart. Anterior view is displayed on the left panel; posterior view on the right panel. [Image adapted from Okere IC, Sigurdsson G. Cardiac computed tomography. In: Chatterjee K, Anderson M, Heistad D, Kerber RE (Eds). Cardiology: An Illustrated Textbook. New Delhi, India: Jaypee Brothers Medical Publishers (P) Ltd; 2012]. (Ao: Aorta; CS: Coronary sinus; LA: Left atrium; LAA: Left atrial appendage; LV: Left ventricle; PA: Pulmonary artery; RA: Right atrium; RAA: Right atrial appendage; RV: Right ventricle).

Normal LV diastolic diameters are modestly higher in men than women (4.2–5.9 cm versus 3.9–5.3 cm, respectively). Normal LV diastolic volumes are similarly modestly higher in men than women (67–155 mL versus 56–104 mL, respectively). Normal LV wall thickness, according to the American Society of Echocardiography (ASE), is 0.6-1.0 cm in men and 0.6-0.9 cm in women. Typical left ventricular output is 5 liters/minute. This may increase to up to 25 liters/minute in nonathletes and up to 45 liters/minute for Olympic level athletes. Different sources and organizations have developed modestly different criteria for that classification of LV ejection fraction (LVEF). Table 19.2 presents criteria from the ASE.

Blood supply to the LV is via the three coronary arteries. Although there is some overlap and variation, in general, the left anterior descending (LAD) artery supplies the anterior wall and superior septum, the left circumflex artery supplies the anterolateral and inferolateral walls, and the right coronary artery (RCA) supplies the inferior wall and inferior septum (Fig. 19.15).

ASSESSMENT OF CARDIAC FUNCTION

Assessment of left ventricular function in the past was commonly performed during cardiac catheterization (Figs. 19.16A and B). Although both right anterior oblique (RAO) and left anterior oblique (LAO) imaging is performed to assess all walls, in the majority of patients only RAO imaging was performed for practical reasons. During ventriculography, ejection fraction is most commonly visually estimated, although quantification of ejection fraction can be performed.

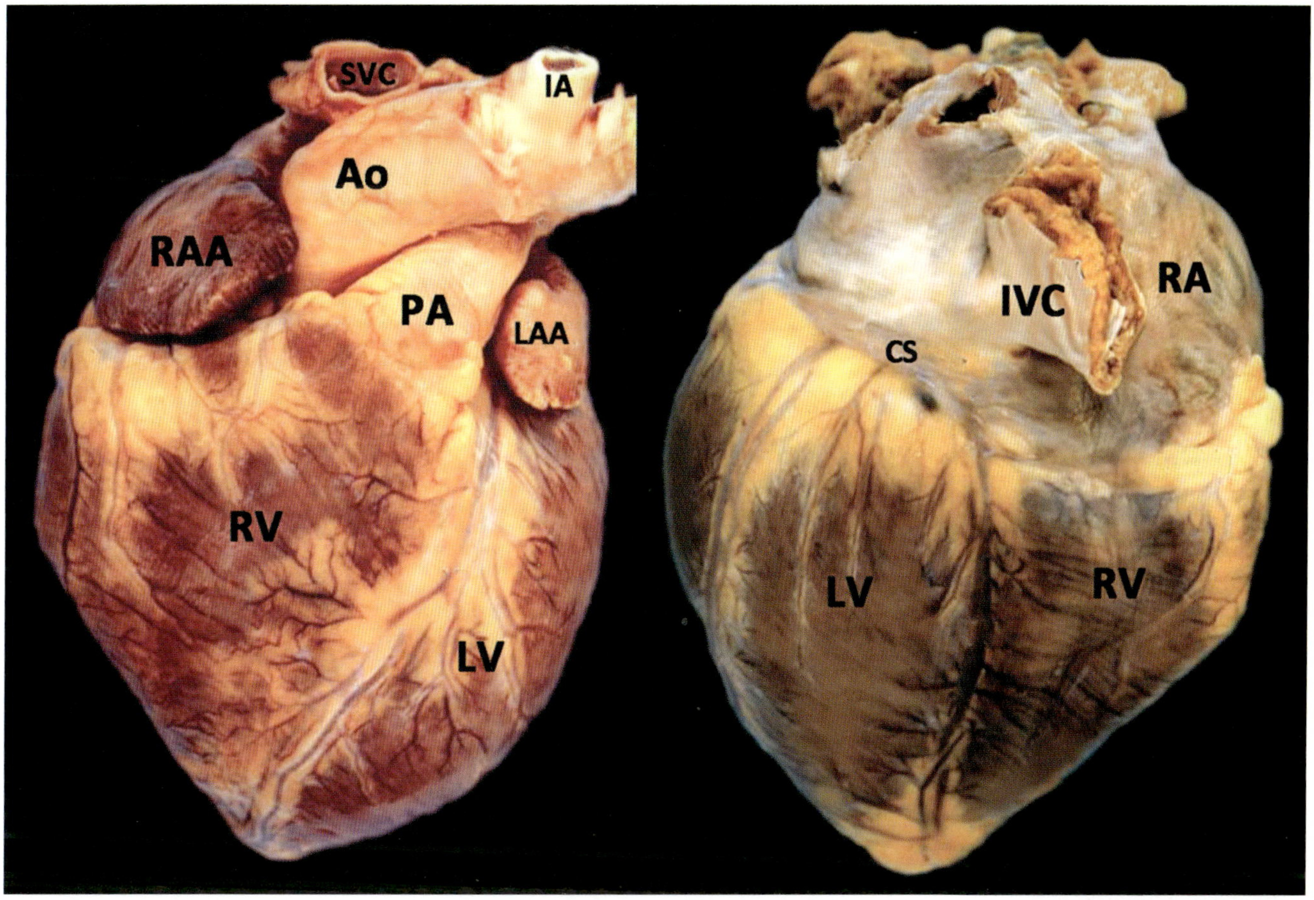

Fig. 19.5: Epicardial anatomy of the heart. Left panel displays an anterior view; right panel displays the inferior surface of the heart. (Images courtesy of Philip C Ursell, Department of Pathology, UCSF. [Image from Cheitlin MD, Ursell PC. Cardiac anatomy. In: Chatterjee K, Anderson M, Heistad D, Kerber RE (Eds). Cardiology: An Illustrated Textbook. New Delhi, India: Jaypee Brothers Medical Publishers (P) Ltd; 2012]. (Ao: Aorta; CS: Coronary sinus; IA: Innominate artery; IVC: Inferior vena cava; LV: Left ventricle; PA: Pulmonary artery; RA: Right atrium; RAA: Right atrial appendage; RV: Right ventricle; SVC: Superior vena cava).

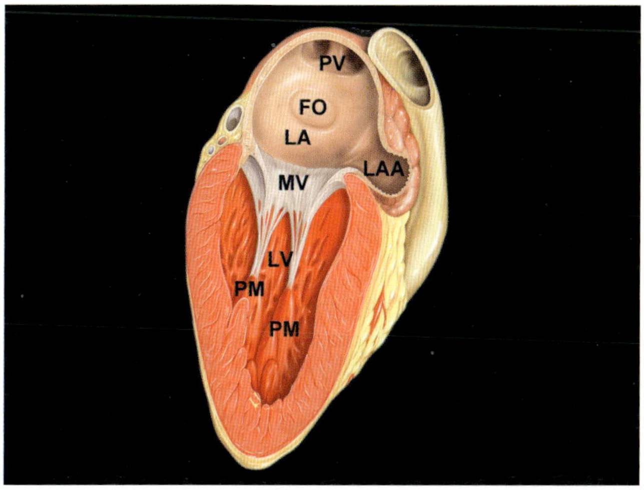

Fig. 19.6: Schematic illustration of the smooth-walled left atrium and the more muscular left atrial appendage with pectinate muscles. Two pulmonary veins are visualized returning oxygenated blood to the left atrium. The fossa ovalis is the site where patent foramen ovale or secundum atrial septal defect occurs. Regurgitation of blood from the left ventricle back into the left atrium is prevented by the presence of the mitral valve (left ventricle). (Image created by Patrick J Lynch and C Carl Jaffe, MD, and posted on Wikipedia). (ASD: Atrial septal defect; FO: Fossa ovalis; LA: Left atrium; LAA: Left atrial appendage; LV: Left ventricle; PM: Papillary muscles; PFO: Patent foramen ovale; PV: Pulmonary veins).

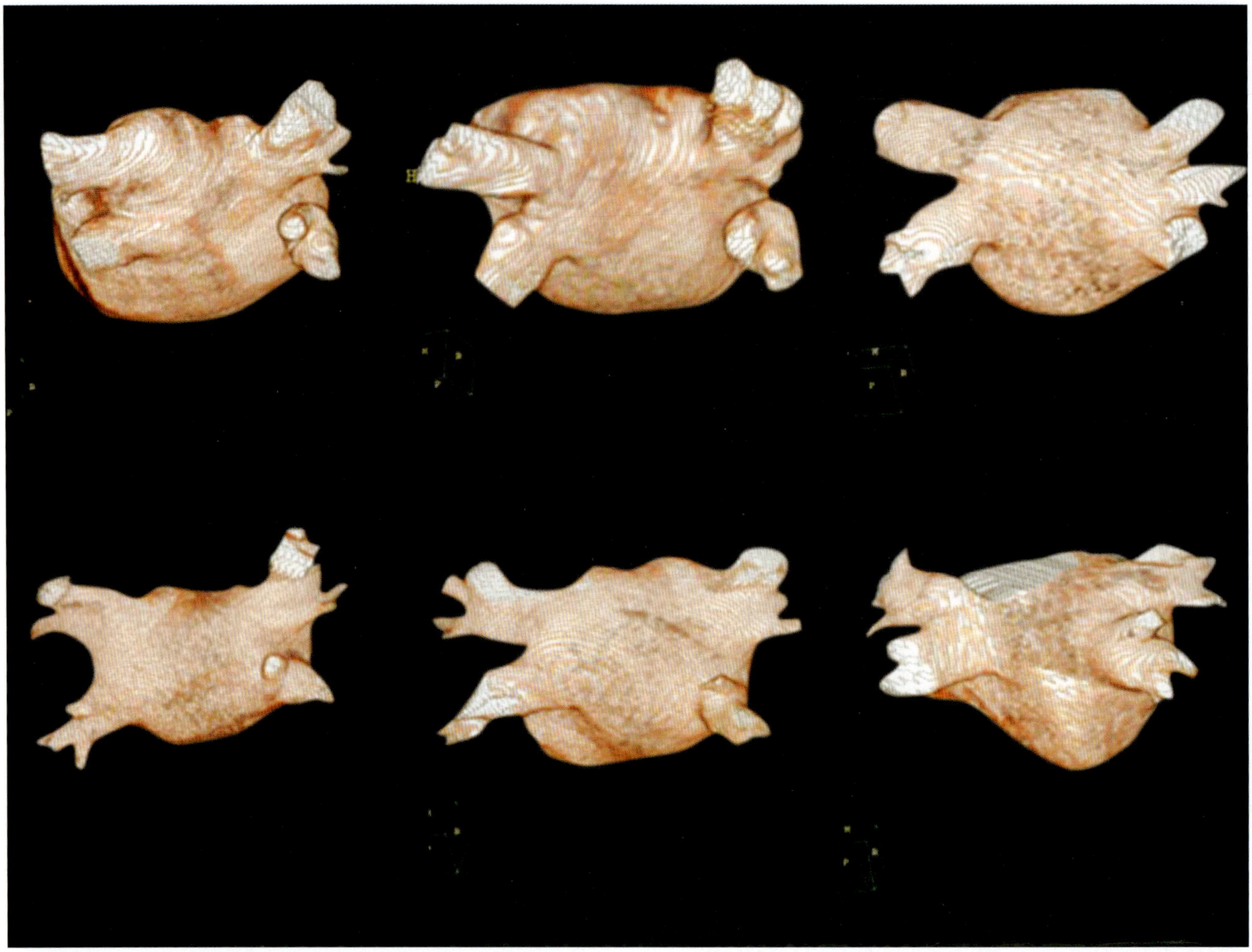

Fig. 19.7: Variation in pulmonary vein drainage into the left atrium. [Image from Okere IC, Sigurdsson G. Cardiac computed tomography. In: Chatterjee K, Anderson M, Heistad D, Kerber RE (Eds). Cardiology: An Illustrated Textbook. New Delhi, India: Jaypee Brothers Medical Publishers (P) Ltd; 2012].

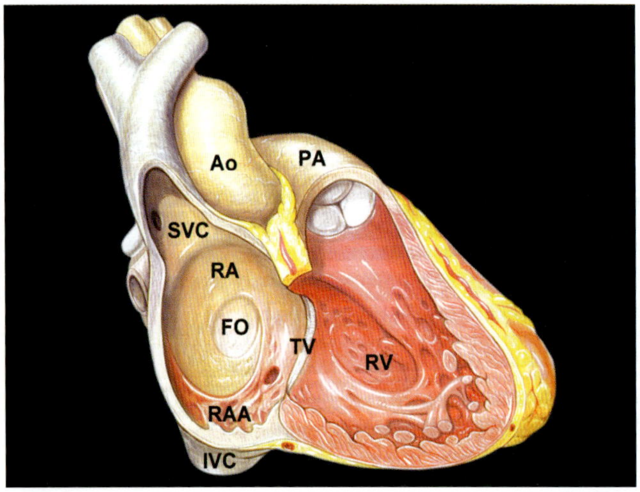

Fig. 19.8: Schematic illustration of the right atrium and surrounding structures. Deoxygenated blood returns to the right atrium via the superior vena cava and inferior vena cava. Deoxygenated blood flows through the tricuspid valve (cut away in this illustration) into the right ventricle (RV), and is subsequently pumped to the lungs through the pulmonary artery (PA). These relationships will be different in patients with transposition of the great arteries (TGA), discussed later in the book. [Image created by Patrick J Lynch, C Carl Jaffe, MD, and posted on Wikipedia]. (Ao: Aorta; FO: Fossa ovalis; RAA: Right atrial appendage IVC: Inferior vena cava; RA: Right atrium; RV: Right ventricle; SVC: Superior vena cava; TV: Tricuspid valve).

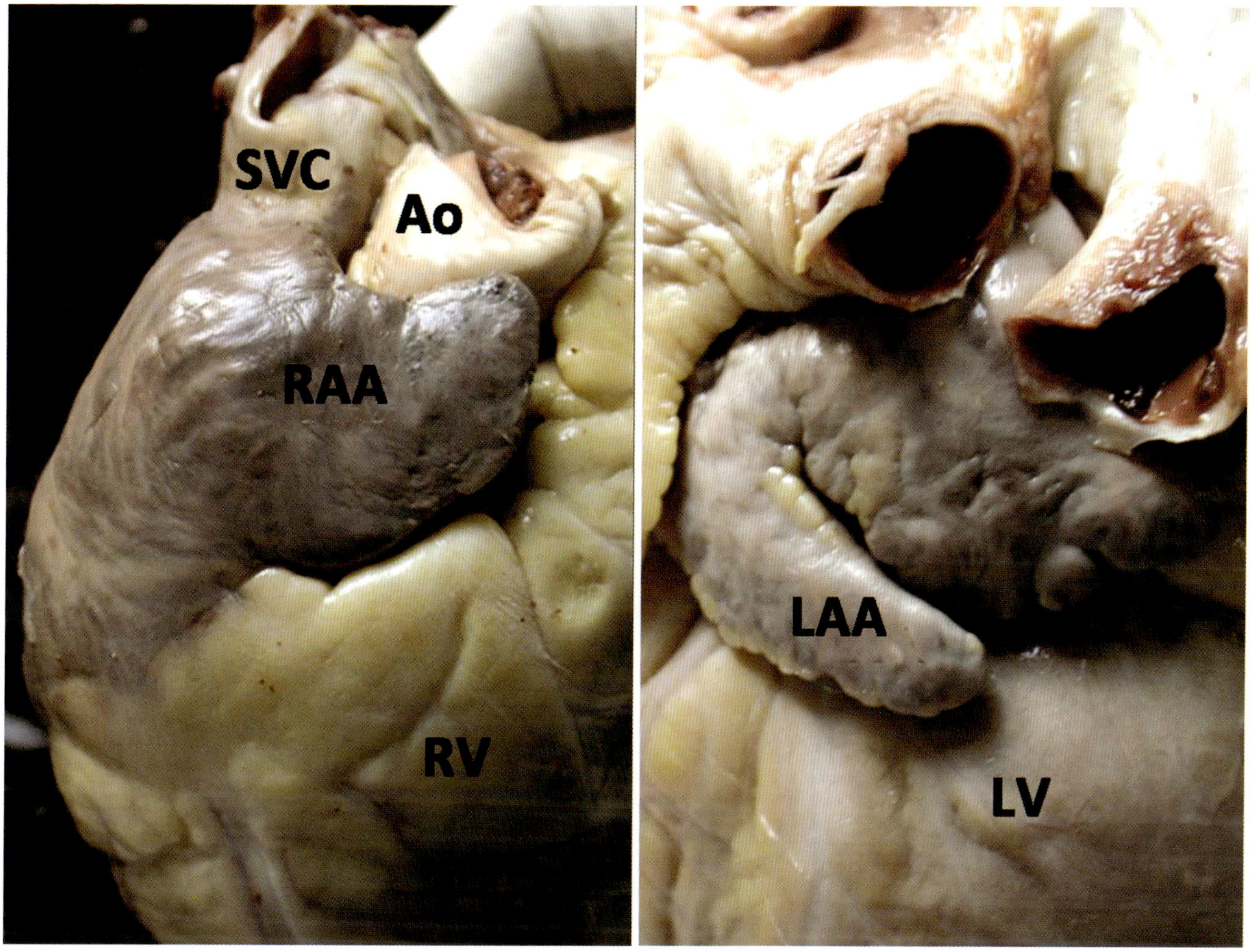

Fig. 19.9: The right atrial appendage and left atrial appendage (LAA), and adjacent structures. [Image from Vaideeswar P. Examination of the heart—a comparative external and internal anatomy. In: Vijayalakshmi IB, Rao PS, Chugh R (Eds). A Comprehensive Approach to Congenital Heart Disease. New Delhi, India: Jaypee Brothers Medical Publishers (P) Ltd; 2013]. (Ao: Aorta; LV: Left ventricle; RAA: Right atrial appendage; RV: Right ventricle; SVC: Superior vena cava).

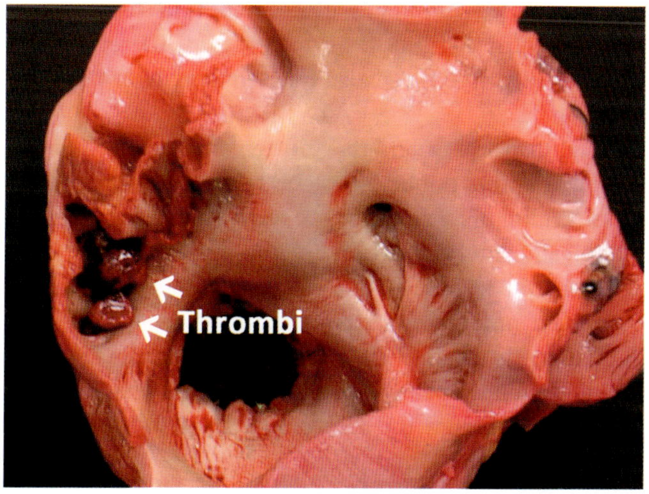

Fig. 19.10: Pathological specimen demonstrating thrombi (arrows) that have formed in the left atrial appendage. [Image from Feng D, Klarich K, Oh JK. Intracardiac thrombosis, embolism, and anticoagulation therapy in patients with cardiac amyloidosis—inspiration from a case observation. In: Guvenc IA (Ed). Amyloidosis—An Insight to Disease of Systems and Novel Therapies. Shanghai: InTech; 2011].

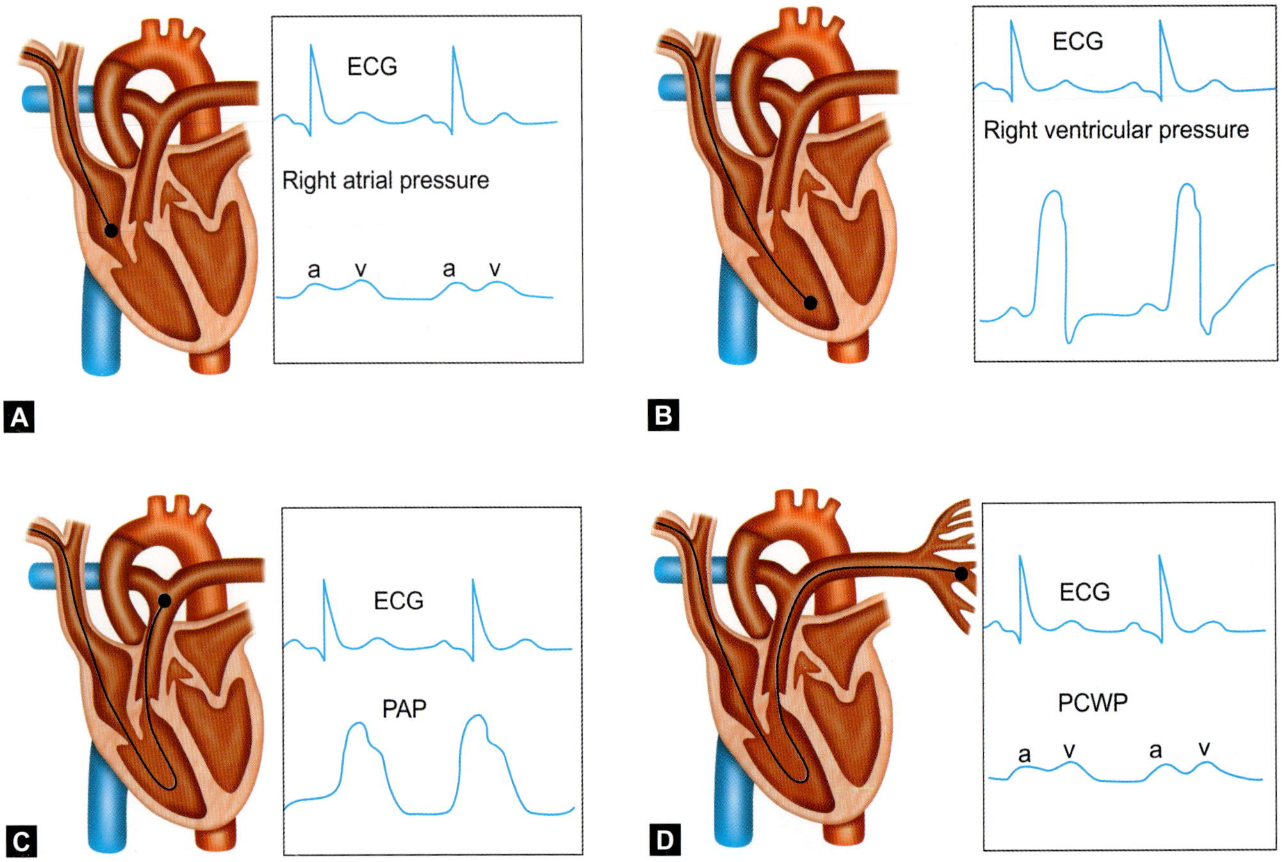

Figs. 19.11A to D: Normal tracings during a right heart catheterization. (A) Right atrial pressure, with "a" and "v" waves; (B) Right ventricular pressure. A rapid upstroke in systole is followed by an end-systolic dip. After a rapid filling phase, there is diastasis and then the atrial filling phase; (C) Pulmonary artery pressure waveform characterized by a rapid upstroke at the beginning of the ejection phase and then the dicrotic notch and downstroke; (D) Pulmonary capillary wedge pressure (PCWP) waveform, similar to that of the right atrial pressure waveform. [Image and legend text from Gupta D, Karrowni W, Chatterjee K. Swan-Ganz catheters: Clinical Applications. In: Chatterjee K, Anderson M, Heistad D, Kerber RE (Eds). Cardiology: An Illustrated Textbook. New Delhi, India: Jaypee Brothers Medical Publishers (P) Ltd; 2012]. (PAP: Pulmonary artery pressure; PCWP: Pulmonary artery wedge pressure).

In current practice, the "workhorse" of left ventricular functional assessment is 2D transthoracic echocardiography. M-mode imaging (Fig. 19.17) was used in earlier times to assess LV systolic function, and though M-mode assessment of the ventricle is still performed, assessment of LV systolic function is based on 2D imaging. For experienced echocardiographers, visual assessment of LV systolic ejection fraction on 2D echocardiography has a test-to-test reliability of approximately ±5%. Interobserver reliability for visual differentiation between normal, hypokinetic, and akinetic segments is reasonable for classification of normal and akinetic segments but poor for hypokinetic segments. In current practice, quantitative assessment of LV ejection fraction is performed using two- and four-chamber apical echocardiographic views using Simpson's method of LVEF assessment (Fig. 19.18). More advanced 2D (Figs. 19.19A1 to A3) and 3D techniques (Figs. 19.19B1 to B3) can also be used to assess LV systolic function.

Slightly varying criteria and terminology have been used in different publications and textbooks regarding the classification of LV systolic function based on echocardiographically derived ejection fraction with regards to what is considered hyperdynamic, normal, "low normal", mildly depressed, moderately depressed, and severely depressed. The currently established terminology and criteria of the ASE and the European Society of Echocardiography (ESE) are similar, though the ESE organization does not give a specific criteria for hyperdynamic. The classification system of the ASE is summarized in Table 19.1.

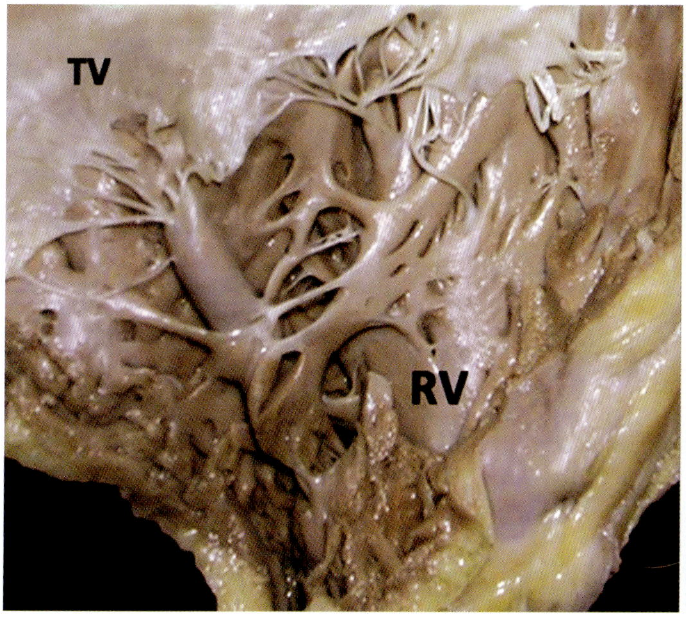

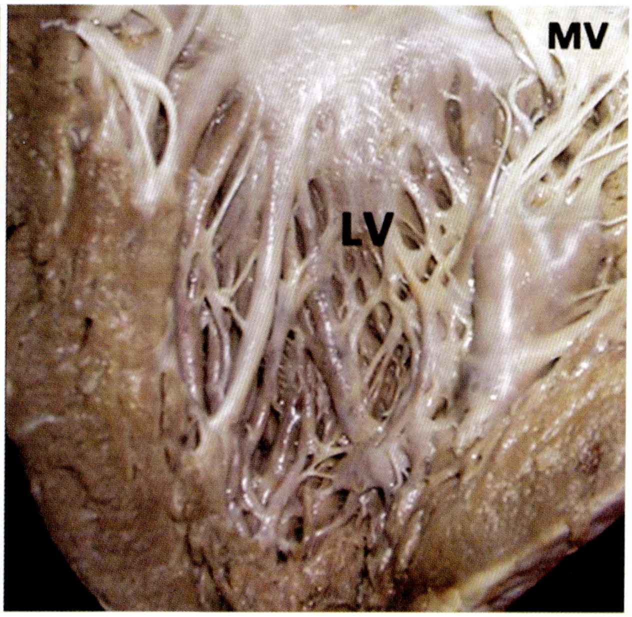

Fig. 19.12: Comparison of the right ventricle and left ventricle. The right ventricle is coarsely trabeculated with a thin compact portion that measures 0.5–0.7 cm. The trabeculation extends even into the outflow tract. The LV is finely trabeculated with a thick compact portion measuring approximately 1 cm. The septal surface is smooth and covered by the thicker endocardium. [Image and legend text adapted from Vaideeswar P. Examination of the heart–a comparative external and internal anatomy. In: Vijayalakshmi IB, Rao PS, Chugh R (Eds). A Comprehensive Approach to Congenital Heart Disease. New Delhi, India: Jaypee Brothers Medical Publishers (P) Ltd; 2013].

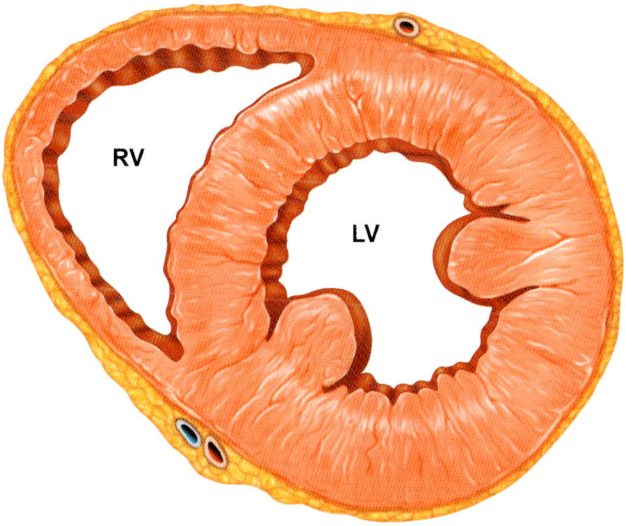

Fig. 19.13: Cross section of the heart at the midventricular level. The mass of the right ventricle (RV) is much less than that of the left ventricle (LV). Note the relative thickness of the RV free wall compared to that of the LV free wall. (Image created by Patrick J Lynch and C Carl Jaffe and posted on Wikimedia Commons).

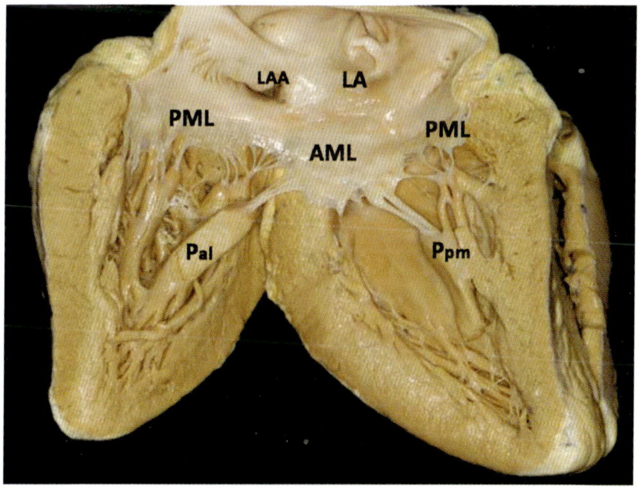

Fig. 19.14: Pathology specimen of the left ventricle, also showing the mitral valve and left atrium. [Image courtesy of Philip C Ursell, Department of Pathology, University of California, San Francisco, CA. Image from Cheitlin MD, Ursell PC. Cardiac anatomy. In: Chatterjee K, Anderson M, Heistad D, Kerber RE (Eds). Cardiology: An Illustrated Textbook. New Delhi, India: Jaypee Brothers Medical Publishers (P) Ltd; 2012]. (AML: Anterior mitral leaflet; LA: Left atrium; LAA: Orifice of the left atrial appendage; Pal: Anterolateral papillary muscle; Ppm: Posteromedial papillary muscle; PML: Posterior mitral leaflet).

Table 19.1: Classification of left ventricular ejection fraction based on criteria developed by the American Society of Cardiology (ASE). Classification by the European Society of Echocardiography (ESE) is similar, though that organization does not give a specific criteria for hyperdynamic.

Ejection Fraction	*Classification of Left Ventricular Function*
> 70%	Hyperdynamic
55–70%	Normal
45–54%	Mildly depressed
30–44%	Moderately depressed
< 30%	Severely depressed

Table 19.2: Summary of the classification of left ventricular (LV) function based on echocardiography measurement of the continuous wave spectral Doppler mitral regurgitation signal. LV dP/dT = 32,000 mm Hg/[$T_{3m/s} - T_{1m/s}$], where ΔT is in ms.

Classification	*LV dp/dT*
Normal	> 1200 mm Hg/s
Mildly depressed	1000–1200 mm Hg/s
Moderately depressed	800–999 mm Hg/s
Severely depressed	< 800 mm Hg/s

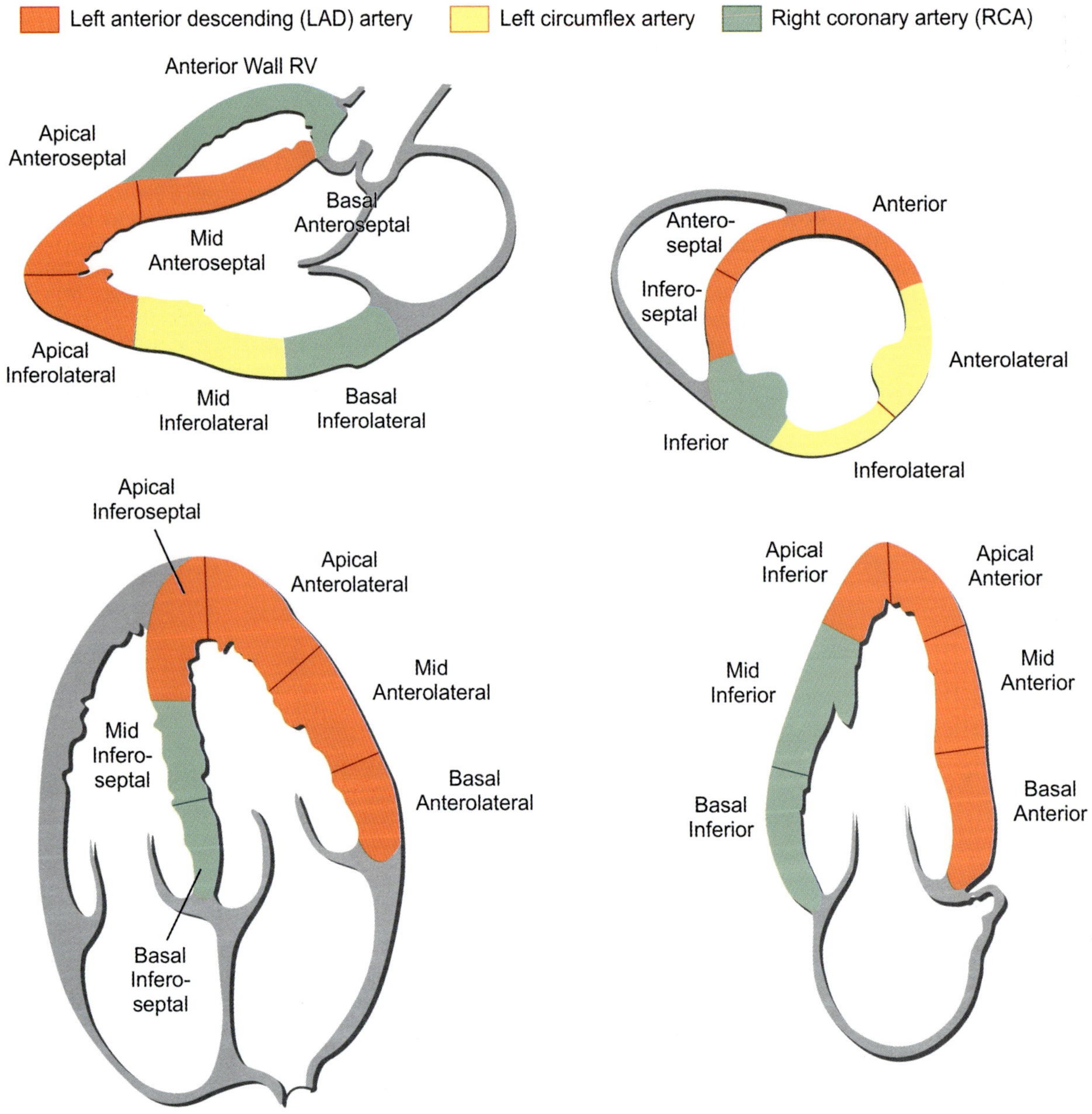

Fig. 19.15: Schematic illustration of the blood supply to the left ventricle.

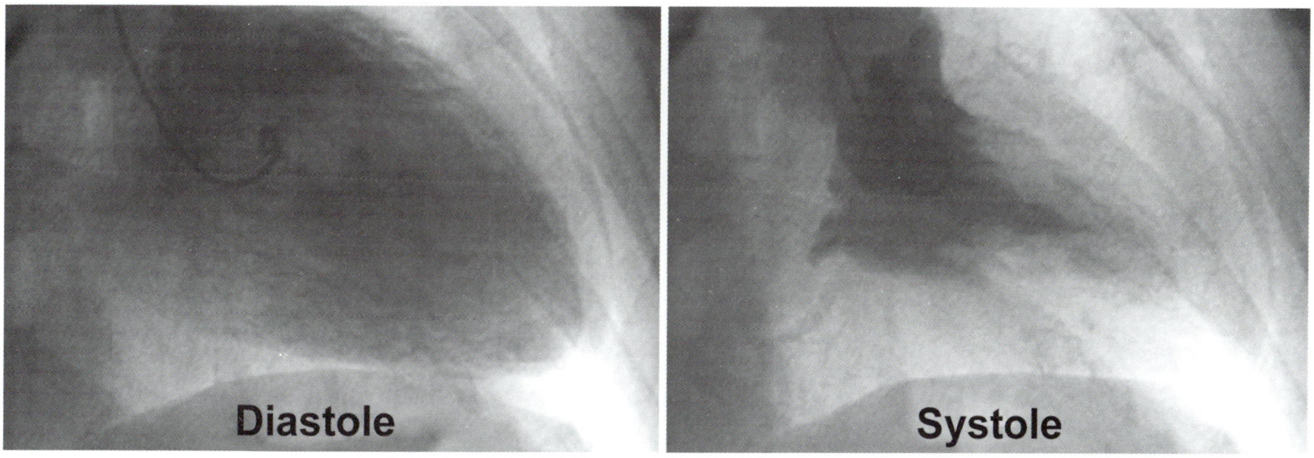

Fig. 19.16A: Right anterior oblique (RAO) projection ventriculogram in diastole (left panel) and systole (right panel) demonstrating normal left ventricular ejection fraction. [Image modified from Kawano H. Torsades de pointes in Takotsubo cardiomyopathy with QT prolongation. In: Veselka J (Ed). Cardiomyopathies–From Basic Research to Clinical Management. Shanghai: InTech; 2012].

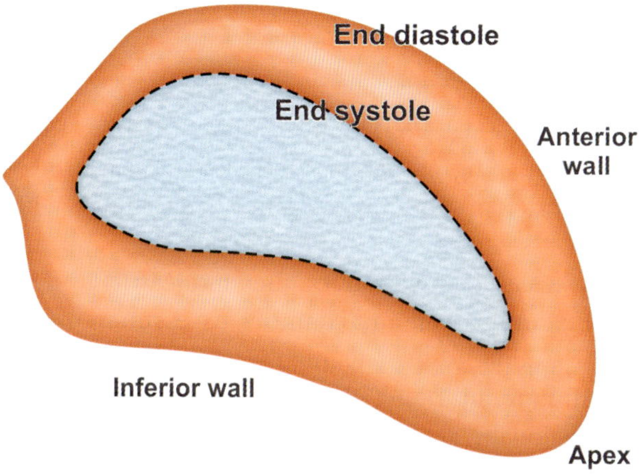

Fig. 19.16B: Schematic illustration of contrast ventriculography to determine left ventricular ejection fraction based on left ventricular tracing at end-systole and end-diastole. Illustration shows the ventriculogram as obtained in the right anterior oblique (RAO) projection. [Image and legend text adapted from Chatterjee K, Karrowni W, Parmley W. Ventricular function—assessment and clinical application. In: Chatterjee K, Anderson M, Heistad D, Kerber RE (Eds). Cardiology: An Illustrated Textbook. New Delhi, India: Jaypee Brothers Medical Publishers (P) Ltd; 2012].

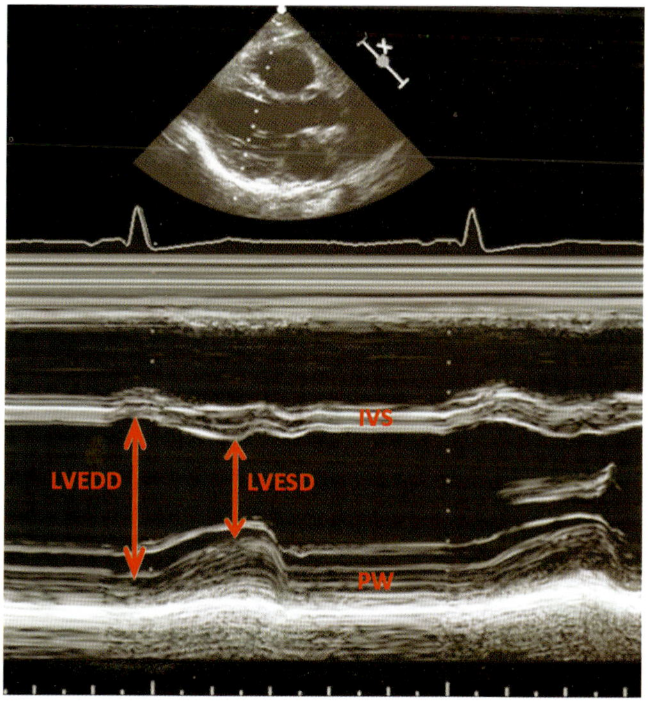

Fig. 19.17: M-mode transthoracic echocardiogram. Left ventricular function was assessed by comparing left ventricular end-diastolic diameter and left ventricular end-systolic diameter. [Image adapted from Vanderberg BF, Kerber RE. Transthoracic echocardiography. In: Chatterjee K, Anderson M, Heistad D, Kerber RE (Eds). Cardiology: An Illustrated Textbook. New Delhi, India: Jaypee Brothers Medical Publishers (P) Ltd; 2012]. (IVS: Interventricular septum; LVEDD: Left ventricular end-diastolic diameter; LVESD: Left ventricular end-systolic diameter; PW: Posterior wall).

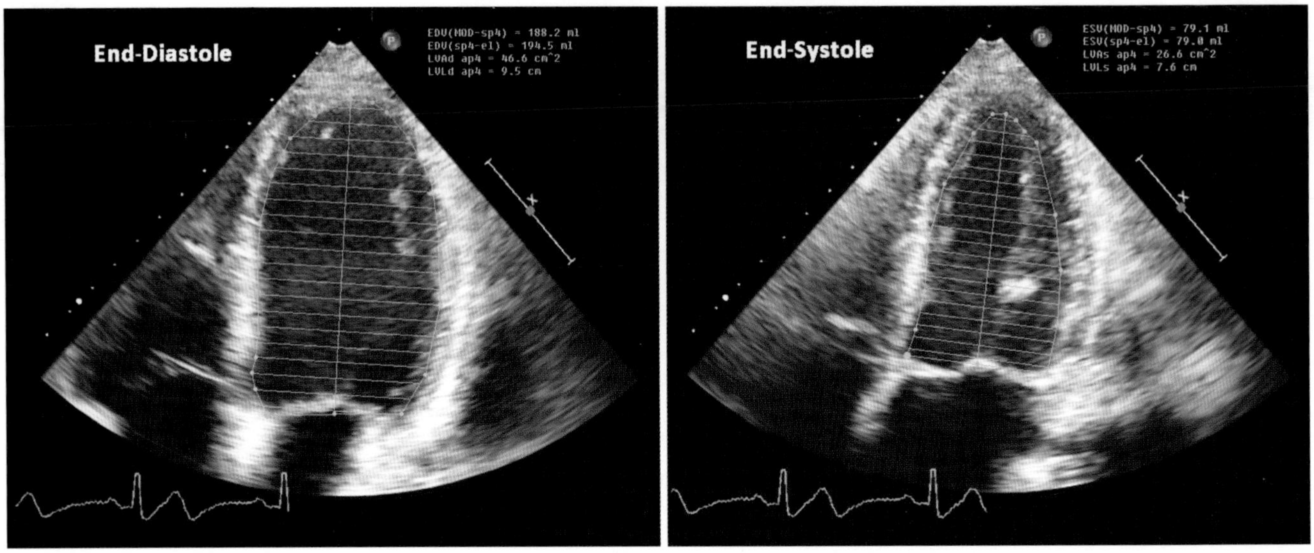

Fig. 19.18: Two-dimensional echocardiographic assessment of LV ejection fraction using Simpson's method. Apical four-chamber images of the left ventricle are shown at end-diastole (left panel) and end-systole (right panel).

Importantly, ejection fraction should not be equated with left ventricular myocardial contractility or function, as numerous factors can influence calculated ejection fraction. With routine 2D echocardiographic examination, ventricular wall thickening is carefully scrutinized, with wall thickening during systole of <50% of end-diastolic values considered to be abnormal. Left ventricular dP/dT is not used in daily clinical practice, but can also be used as an assessment of left ventricular contractility, though this assessment is somewhat preload and afterload dependent. dP/dT can be assessed during left heart catheterization, and can be approximated noninvasively using standard 2D echo assessment in patients with an adequate continuous wave spectral Doppler mitral regurgitation signals. Criteria that have been established to classify left ventricular systolic function based on echocardiographically derived dP/dT are summarized in Table 19.2.

Nuclear cardiology (Fig. 19.20) can also be used to assess LV function. Although ejection fraction is reported as part of a routine nuclear stress test, dedicated multigated acquisition scan (MUGA) for the assessment of LV systolic function and wall motion is considered to be more accurate.

Cardiac CT (Fig. 19.21) and cardiac MRI (Fig. 19.22) are newer imaging modalities that also can be used to assess ventricular function. As these modalities allow direct 3D assessment of chamber morphology and usually allow clear delineation of the endocardial border between chamber wall and chamber, assessment of ventricular function is usually highly accurate. Advanced MRI technique, including 4D velocity (three-dimensional, three-directionally encoded, time resolved velocity acquisition), can also be used to more generally assess blood flow in the cardiac chambers and in the great vessels (Figs. 19.23 to 19.26).

Left ventricular function can be described using pressure-volume loop diagrams (Fig. 19.27). With systolic dysfunction, the loop is shifted downward and to the right. Pressure generated is lower for any given preload. With diastolic dysfunction (heart failure with preserved ejection fraction), the pressure-volume loop is shifted upward and to the left. Left ventricular diastolic pressure is higher for any given preload. Effects on the relationship between stroke volume and ventricular filling pressure in normal and depressed LV and RV systolic function are shown in Figure 19.28.

Right ventricular size and function are somewhat more challenging given complex right ventricular geometry. Echocardiographic assessment of right ventricular function includes 2D assessment (particularly of the RV free wall), tissue Doppler imaging/velocity (TDI or TVI) assessment of systolic motion of the tricuspid annulus (Fig. 19.29), and M-mode assessment of tricuspid annular plane systolic excursion (TAPSE) (Fig. 19.30). According to criteria established by the ASE, a pulsed Doppler peak velocity at the annulus of < 10 cm/s and a TAPSE of < 1.6 cm/s are considered to be abnormal. Criteria established by the ASE in the assessment of right ventricular systolic function are summarized in Table 19.3. Given their ability to better visualize and more fully assess the RV in three dimensions, cardiac CT (Figs. 19.31A to D) and MRI are increasingly being utilized to assess right ventricular function. Newer techniques and methodologies are being used to quantify RV ejection fraction during nuclear-imaging as well.

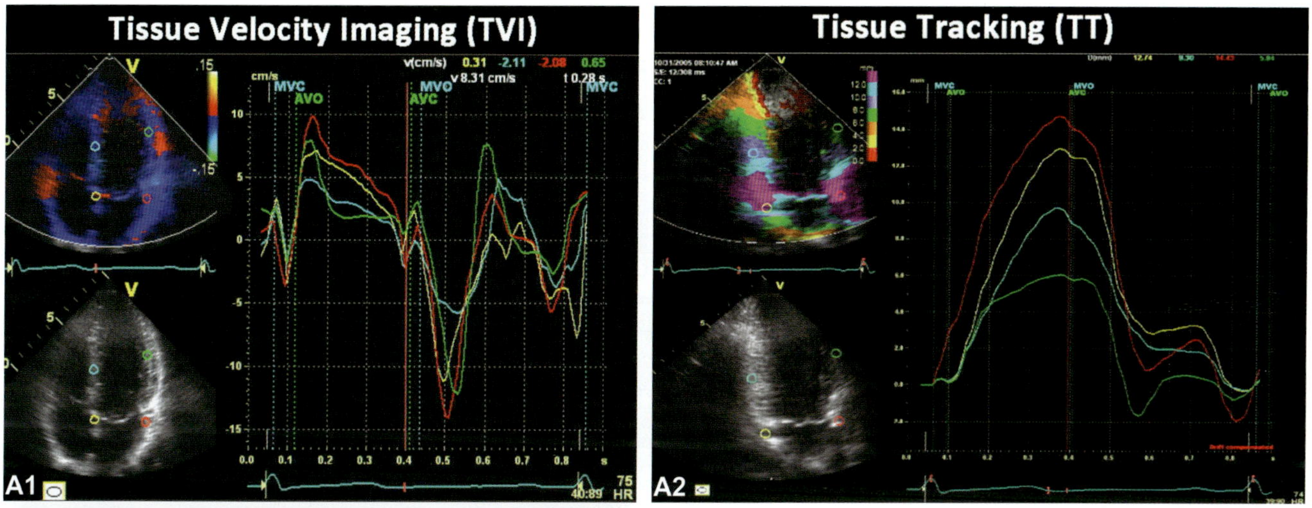

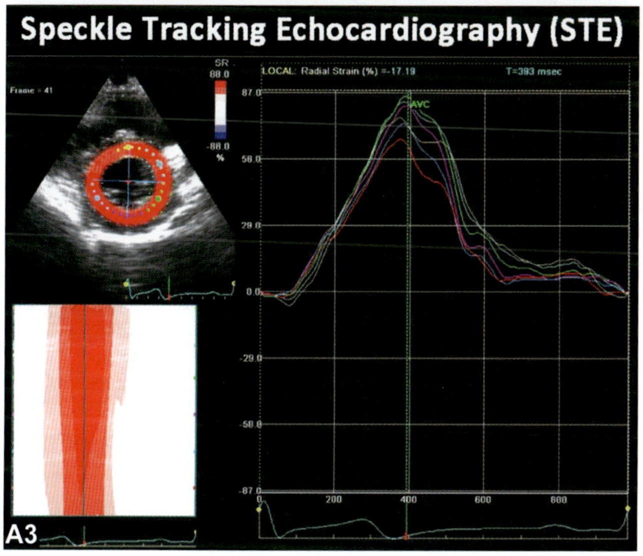

Figs. 19.19A1 to A3: Advanced 2D transthoracic echocardiography techniques to assess left ventricular systolic function and synergy. (A1) Tissue velocity imaging (TVI), also called tissue Doppler imaging (TDI), of a normal heart. The systolic velocity curves of each wall segment overlap and reach peak systolic velocity at the same time; (A2) Tissue tracking (TT) of a normal heart. Displacement over time is plotted. All wall segments reach peak displacement at the same time; (A3) Speckle tracking echocardiography (STE), with radial strain over time plotted. The strain curves in this heart with normal left ventricular function and synchrony all overlap and peak at the same time. [Images from Burns KV, Gage RM, Bank AJ, et al. Right ventricular pacing and mechanical dyssynchrony. In: Oraii S (Ed). Electrophysiology–From Plants to Heart. Shanghai: InTech; 2012].

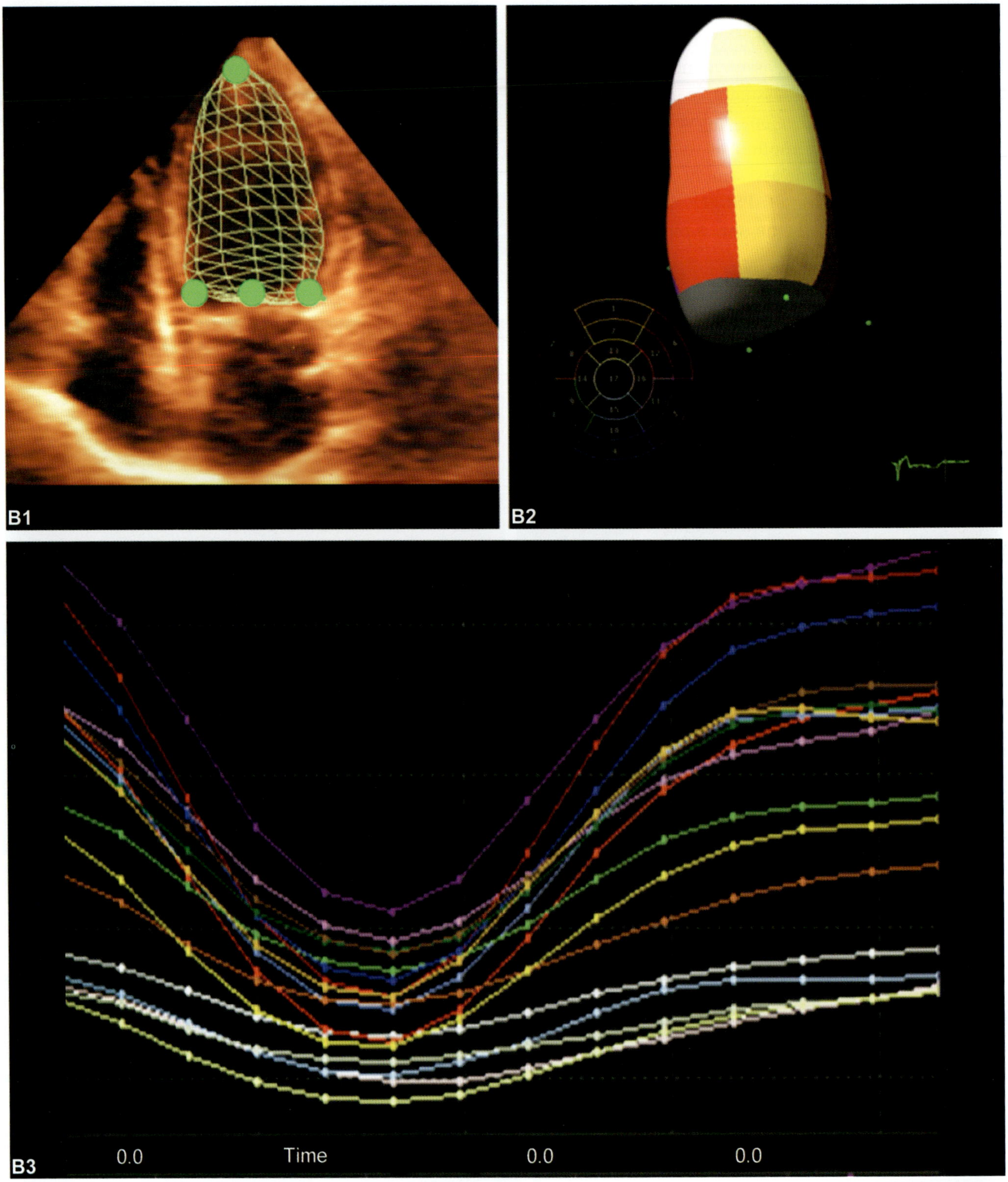

Figs. 19.19B1 to B3: Three-dimensional (3D) assessment of ventricular function. (B1) A 3D data set of the heart is acquired. Image shown is apical four chambers; not shown is apical two chambers; (B2) A segmented model of the heart is constructed; (B3) Graphical display of the volume change over time for each heart segment is shown. There is normal and synchronous contraction of all segments. [Image adapted from Jamil G, Abbas A, Shehab A, et al. Echocardiography findings in common primary and secondary cardiomyopathies. In: Milei J, Ambrosia G (Eds). Cardiomyopathies. Shanghai: InTech; 2013].

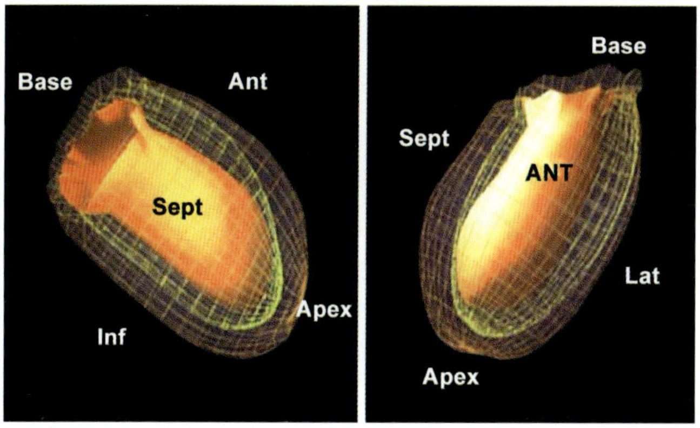

Fig. 19.20: Nuclear cardiology assessment of left ventricular wall motion and systolic function. Image shows the epicardial (orange mesh) and endocardial contours at end diastole (yellow mesh) and end systolic (solid orange region). [Image courtesy of Dr Eli Botvinick, UCSF. Image reproduced from Mahenthiran J. Cardiac stress testing. In: Levine GN (Ed). Color Atlas of Clinical Cardiology. New Delhi, Inida: Jaypee Brothers Medical Publishers (P) Ltd; 2004].

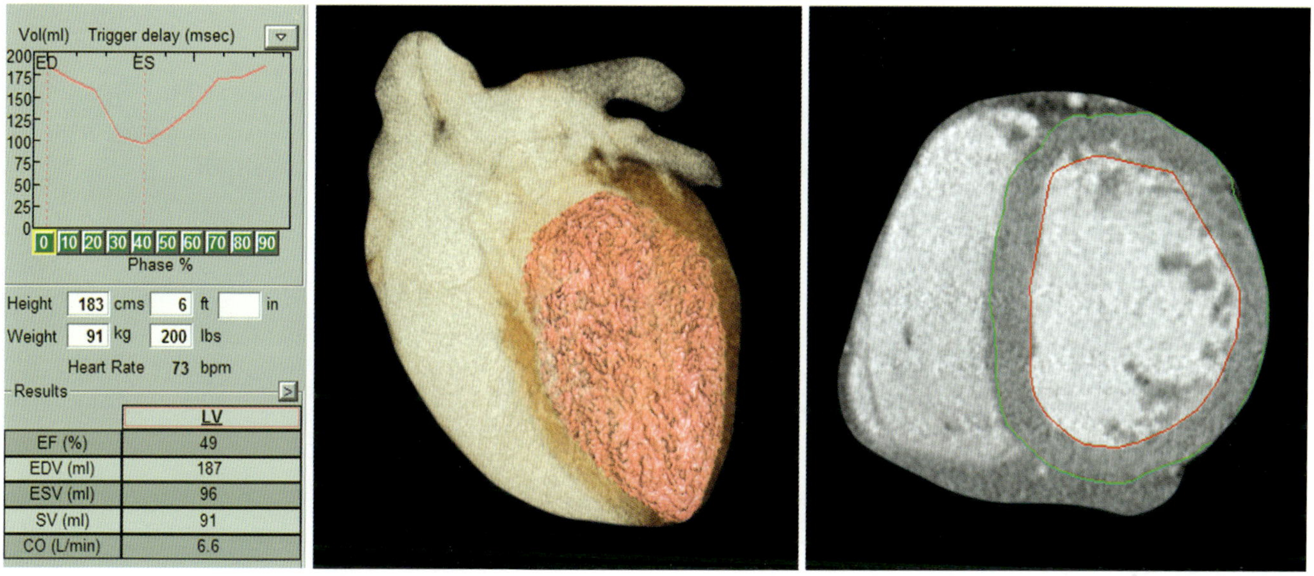

Fig. 19.21: Cardiac CT assessment of left ventricular systolic function. Retrospective gating is used to acquire and analyze ventricular function. Images are usually analyzed at every 10% of the cardiac phase, and maximum and minimum ventricular volumes used to calculate ejection fraction.

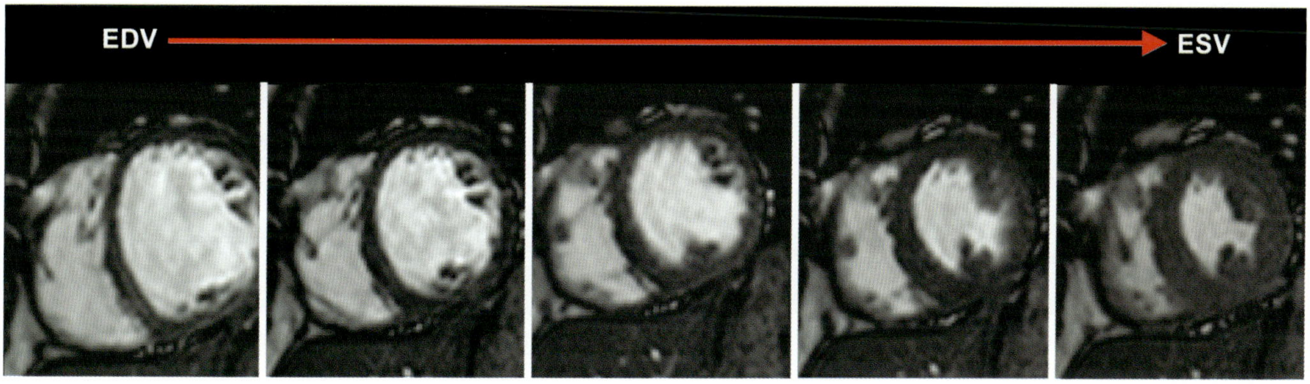

Fig. 19.22: Short-axis midventricular images at different phases of the cardiac cycle. MRI can be used to accurately assess LV ejection fraction and stroke volume, by comparing end-diastolic volume (EDV) to end-systolic volume (ESV). Usually, 8–10 short-axis slices from base to apex are used to quantify left ventricular function in this manner. [Image adapted from Marlon AGM, Galjee MA, Jan van E, et al. The use of contrast-enhanced cardiovascular magnetic resonance imaging in cardiomyopathies. In: Veselka J (Ed). Cardiomyopathies–From Basic Research to Clinical Management. Shanghai: InTech; 2011].

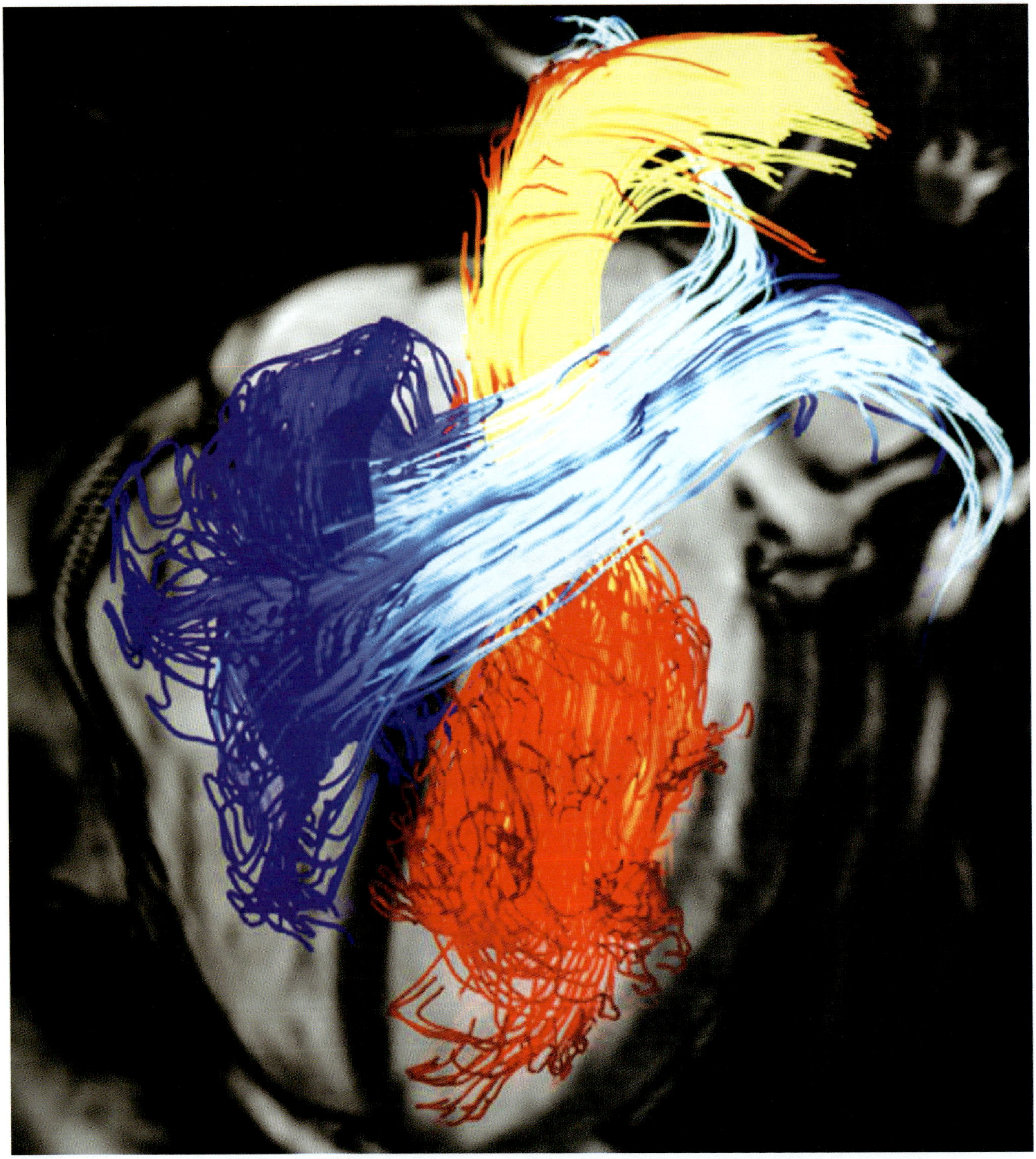

Fig. 19.23: Path line visualization of cardiac blood flow in the heart and great vessels. [Image from Markl M, Kilner PJ, Ebbers T. Comprehensive 4D velocity mapping of the heart and great vessels by cardiovascular magnetic resonance. J Cardiovasc Mag Reson. 2011;13:7].

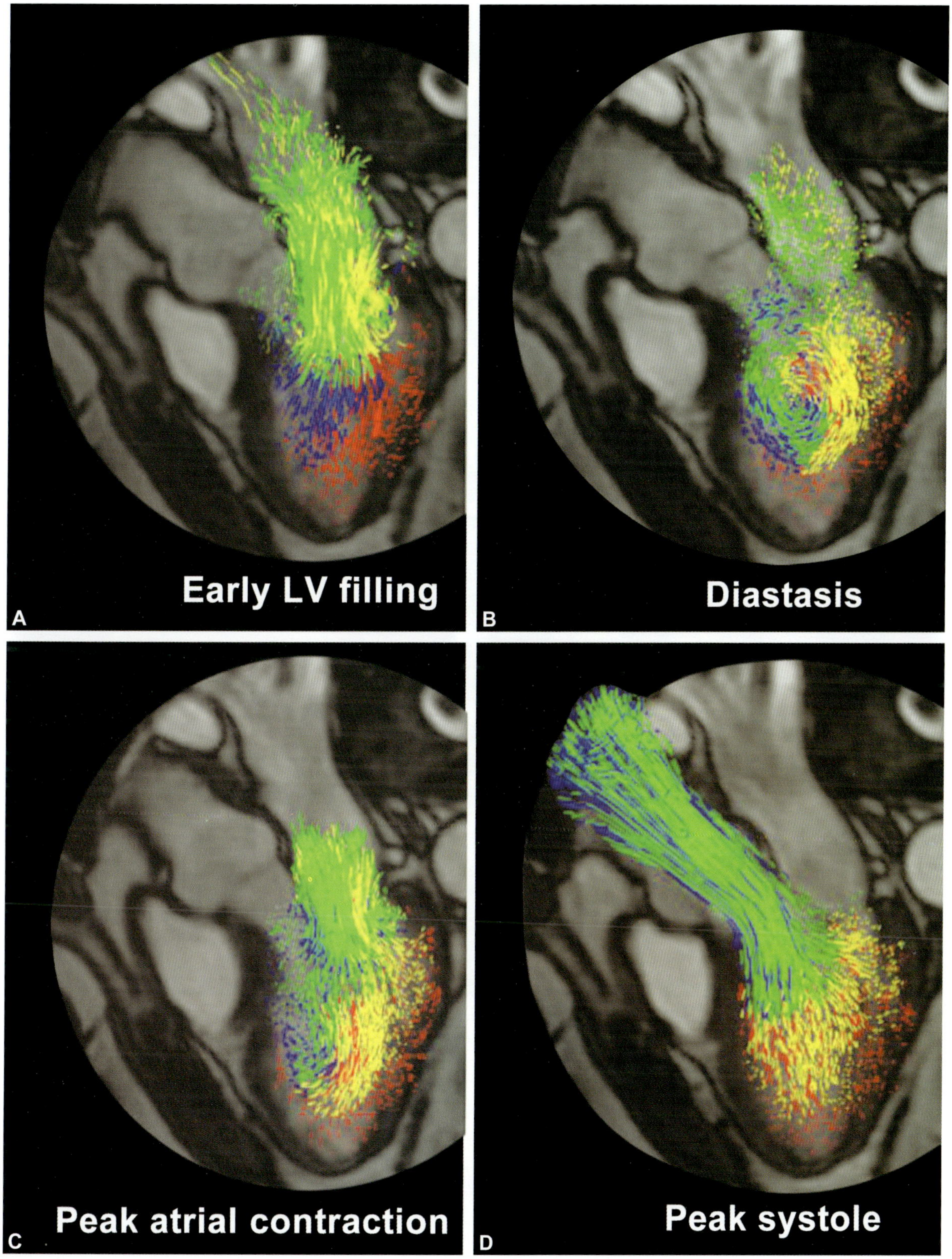

Figs. 19.24A to D: Path line visualization of blood flow through the left ventricle during one cardiac cycle. (Image from Markl M, Kilner PJ, Ebbers T. Comprehensive 4D velocity mapping of the heart and great vessels by cardiovascular magnetic resonance. J Cardiovasc Mag Reson. 2011;13:7).

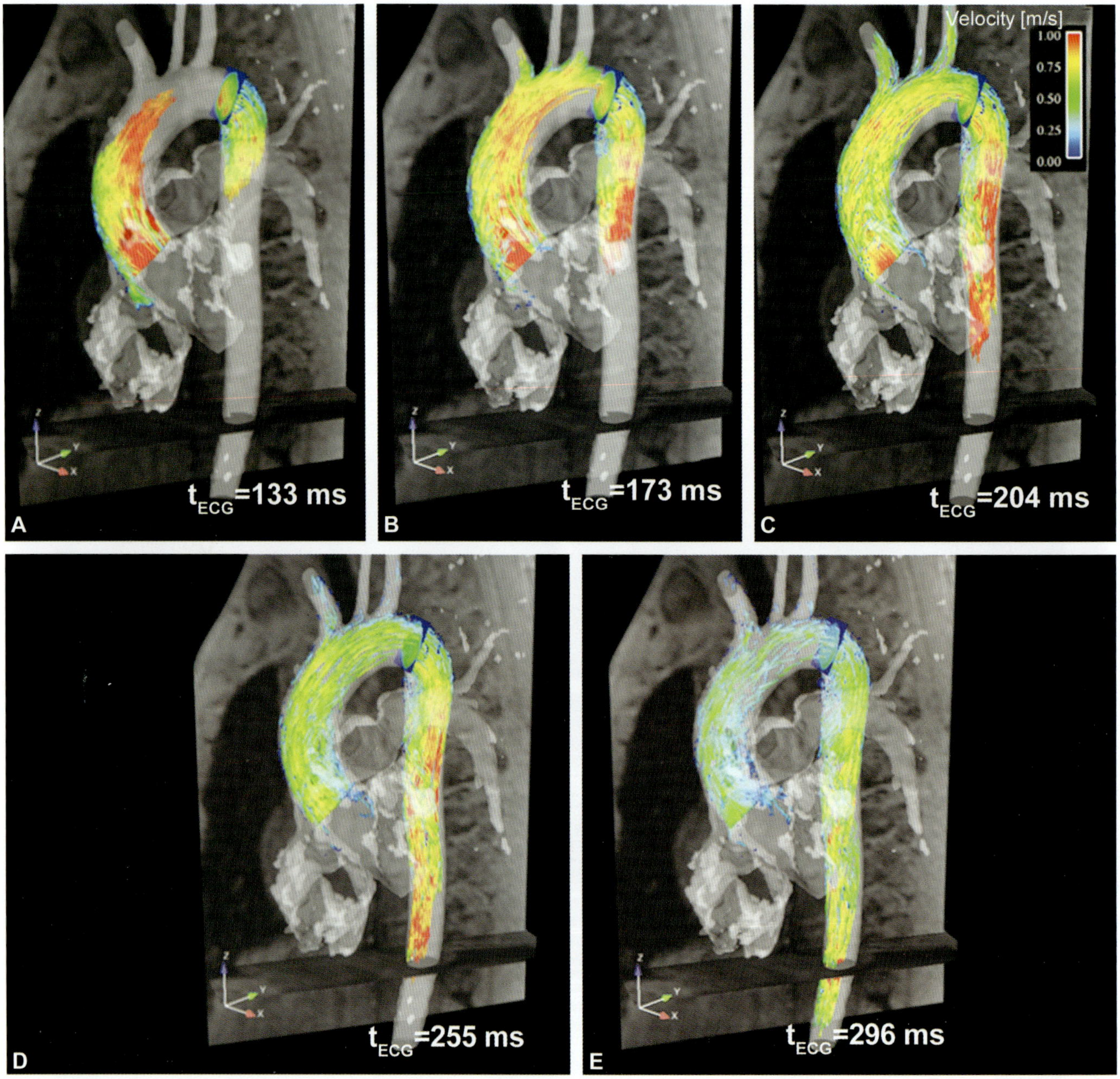

Figs. 19.25A to E: Three-dimensional path lines demonstrating flow velocities in the aorta at different time points in systole. (Image from Markl M, Kilner PJ, Ebbers T. Comprehensive 4D velocity mapping of the heart and great vessels by cardiovascular magnetic resonance. J Cardiovasc Mag Reson. 2011;13:7).

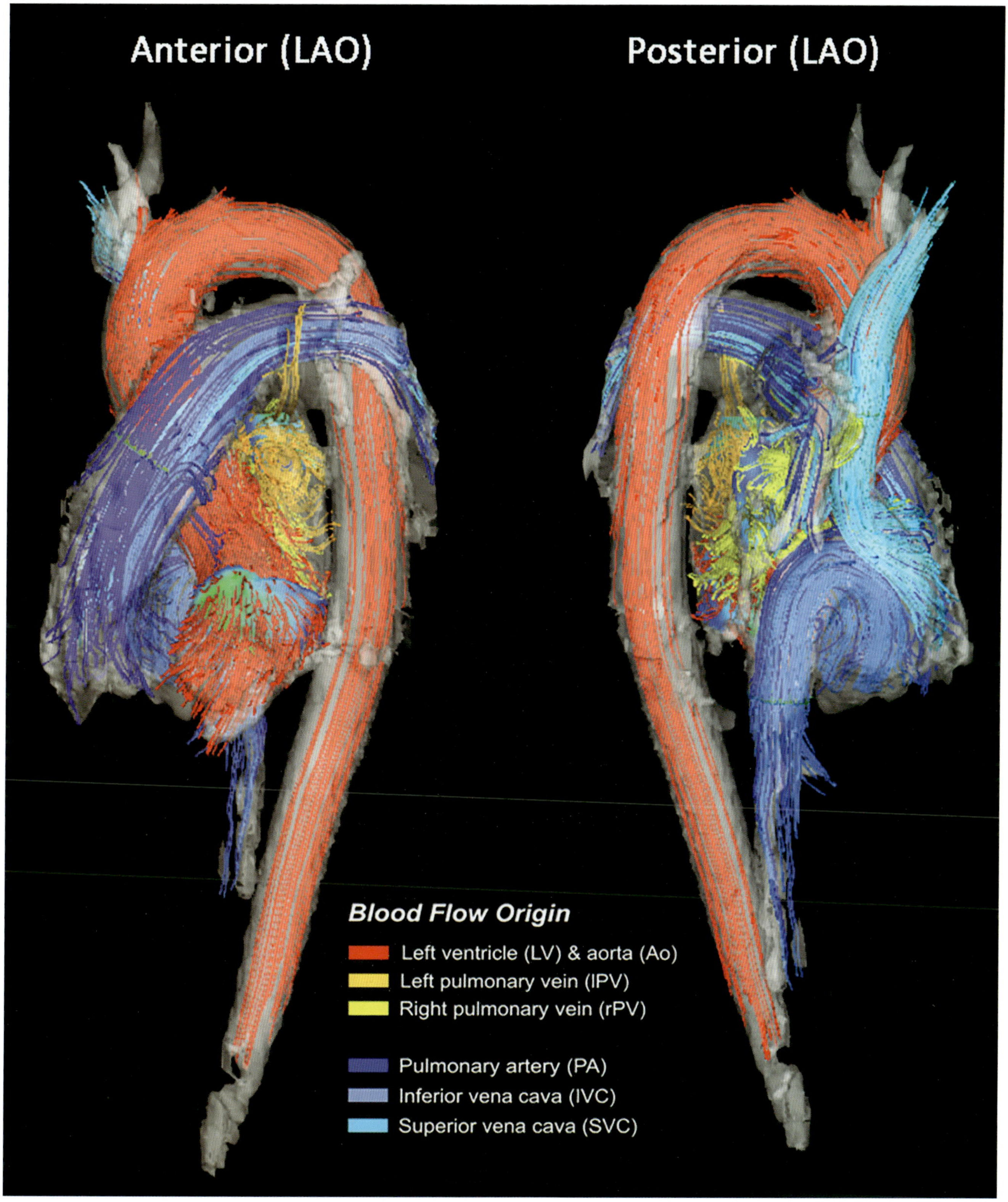

Fig. 19.26: Flow visualization of the heart and large vessels using streamlines in a patient with normal systolic heart function. (Image from Markl M, Kilner PJ, Ebbers T. Comprehensive 4D velocity mapping of the heart and great vessels by cardiovascular magnetic resonance. J Cardiovasc Mag Reson. 2011;13:7).

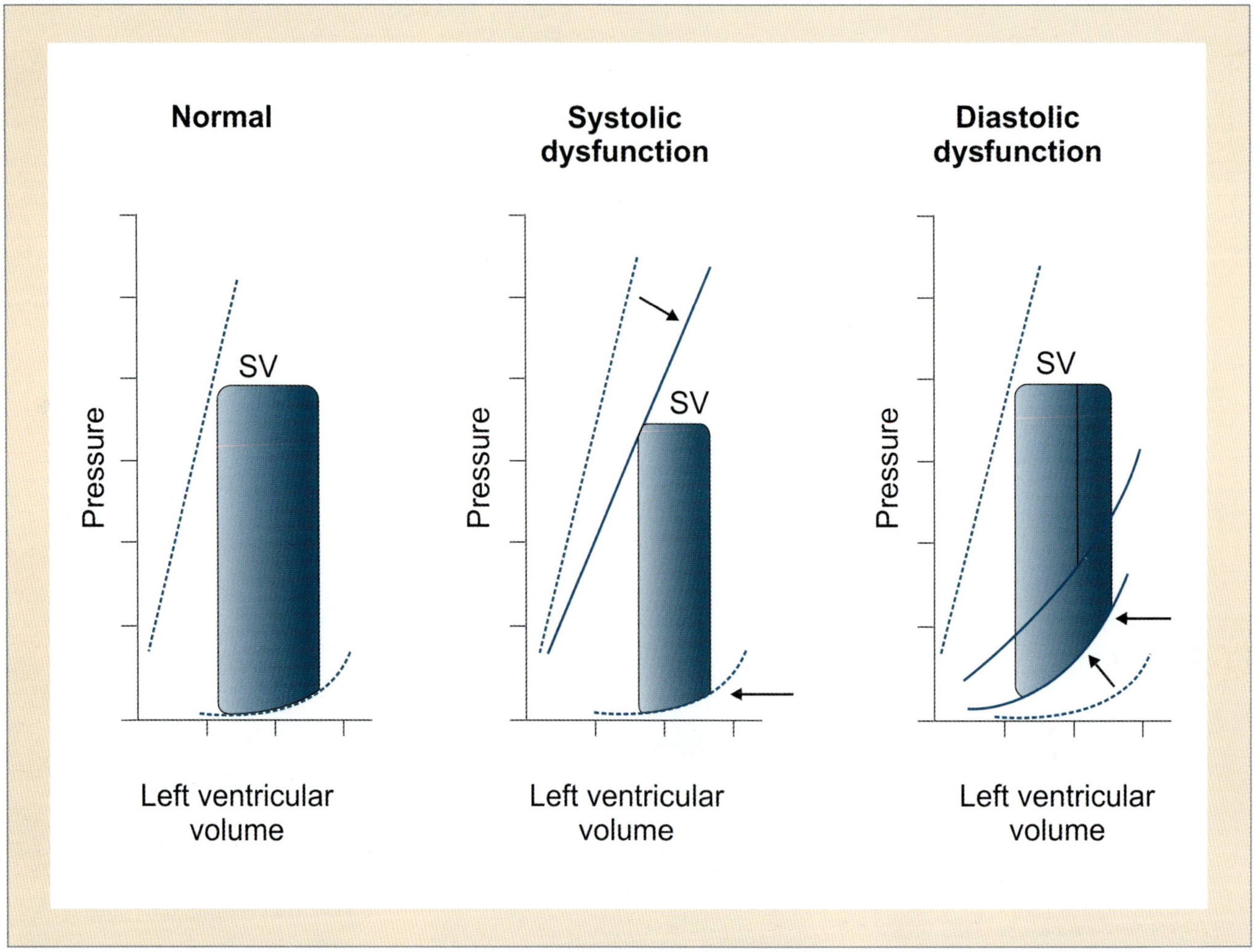

Fig. 19.27: Left ventricular pressure-volume loops with normal left ventricular dysfunction and with systolic and diastolic dysfunction. Left panel shows a normal pressure-volume loop. Middle panel shows the pressure-volume loop with left ventricular systolic dysfunction, in which the loop shifts downward and to the right. Right panel shows the pressure-volume loop with left ventricular diastolic dysfunction (heart failure with preserved ejection fraction), in which the loop shifts upward and to the left. [Image and legend text adapted from Chatterjee K, Karrowni W, Parmley W. Ventricular function—assessment and clinical application. In: Chatterjee K, Anderson M, Heistad D, Kerber RE (Eds). Cardiology: An Illustrated Textbook. New Delhi, India: Jaypee Brothers Medical Publishers (P) Ltd; 2012].

Table 19.3: Summary of criteria for the quantitative assessment of right ventricular (RV) systolic function as either normal or abnormal, based on criteria established by the American Society of Echocardiography.

Parameter	***Abnormal (impaired)***
• RV systolic tissue Doppler	< 10 cm/s
• RV TAPSE (Tricuspid Annular Plane Systolic Excursion)	< 1.6 cm
• RV fractional area change	< 35%
• RV Pulsed Doppler MPI (myocardial performance index)	> 0.40

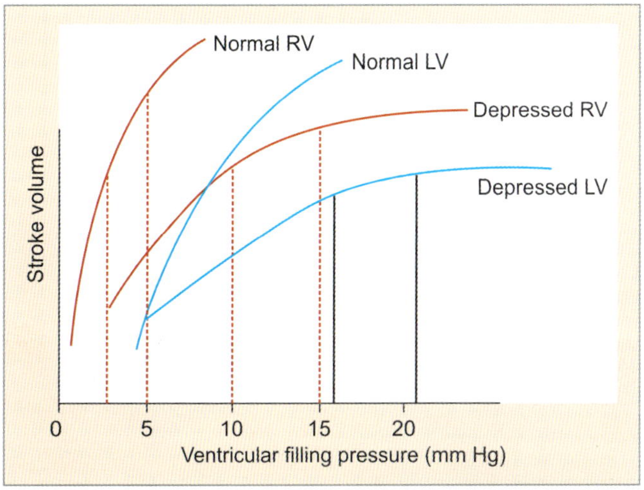

Fig. 19.28: Ventricular function curves showing the relationship between stroke volume and ventricular filling pressure with left ventricular and right ventricular normal systolic function and with depressed systolic function. [Image from Chatterjee K, Karrowni W, Parmley W. Ventricular function—assessment and clinical application. In: Chatterjee K, Anderson M, Heistad D, Kerber RE (Eds). Cardiology: An Illustrated Textbook. New Delhi, India: Jaypee Brothers Medical Publishers (P) Ltd; 2012].

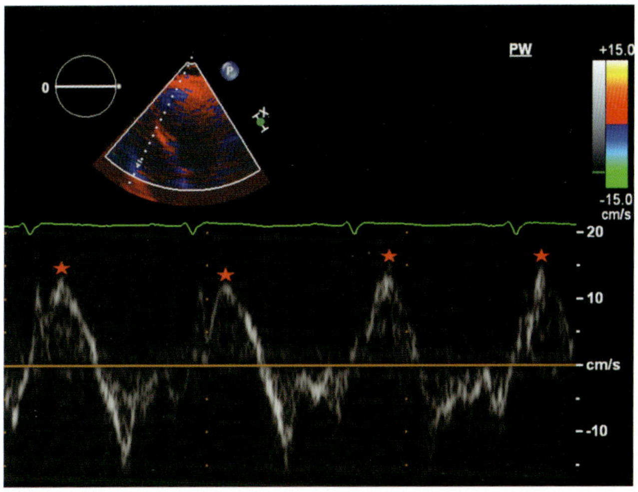

Fig. 19.29: An example of tissue Doppler imaging to assess systolic motion of the tricuspid annulus as part of the evaluation of right ventricular systolic dysfunction. A measured peak systolic velocity of < 10 cm/s is considered to be abnormal.

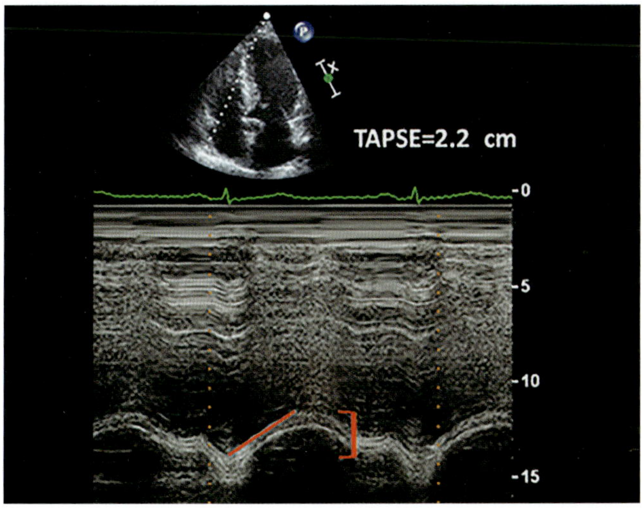

Fig. 19.30: An example of M-mode assessment of tricuspid annular plane systolic excursion (TAPSE) as part of the evaluation of right ventricular systolic dysfunction. A TAPSE of < 1.6 cm is considered abnormal.

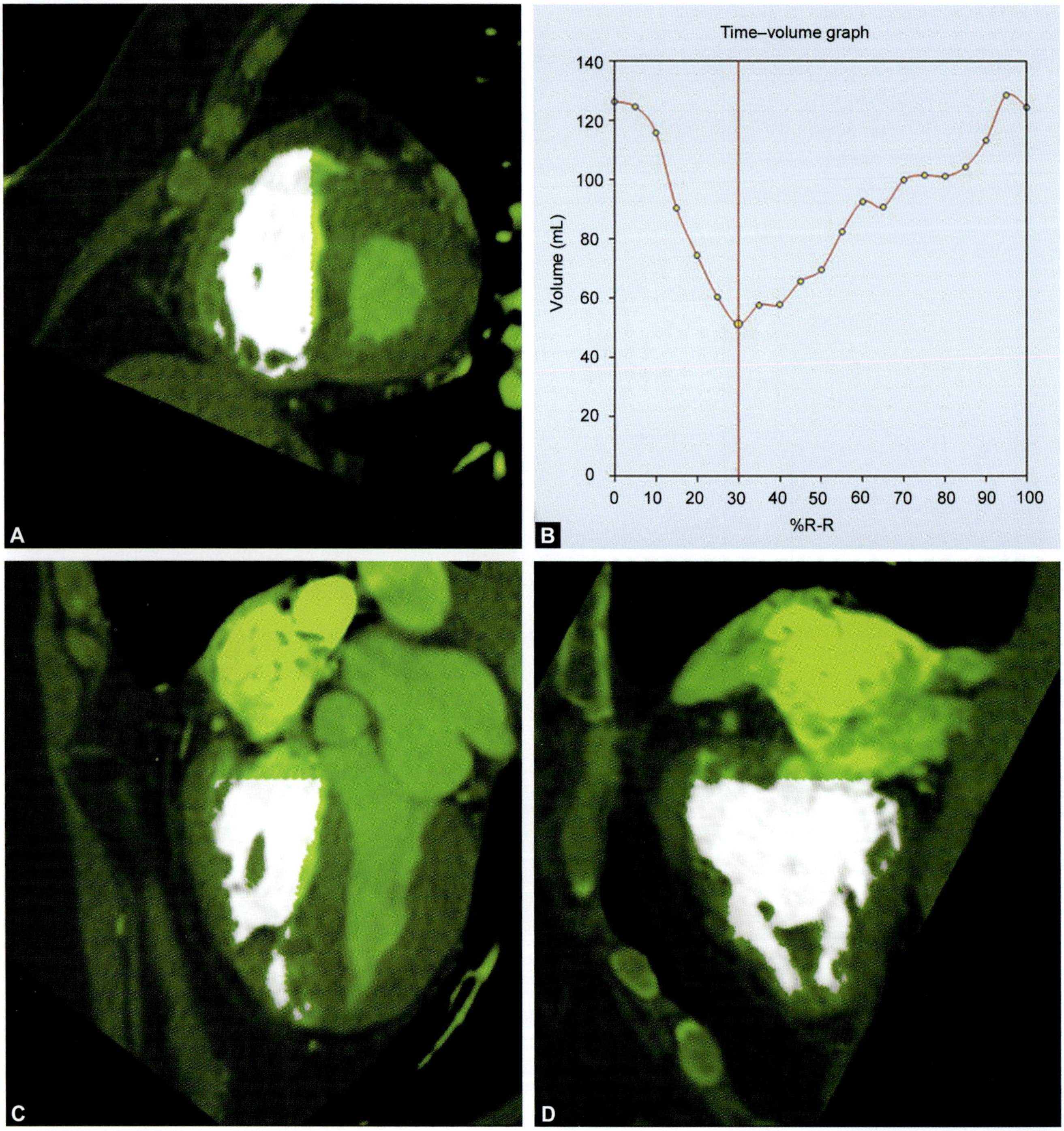

Figs. 19.31A to D: An example of assessment of right ventricular volume in three dimensions by contrast-enhanced CT examination during ECG-gated image acquisition, which is used in the assessment of right ventricular volume and systolic function. (Image courtesy of Sanjiv J Shah, MD).

REFERENCES

Blondheim DS, Beeri R, Feinberg MS, et al. Reliability of visual assessment of global and segmental left ventricular function: a multicenter study by the Israeli Echocardiography Research Group. J Am Soc Echocardiogr. 2010;23(3):258-64.

Rudski LG, Lai WW, Afilalo J, et al. Guidelines for the echocardiographic assessment of the right heart in adults: a report from the American Society of Echocardiography. J Am Soc Echocardiogr. 2010;23:685-713.

Lang RM, Bierig M, Devereux RB, et al. Recommendations for chamber quantification. Eur J Echocardiogr. 2006;7:79-108.

CHAPTER 20

Systolic Heart Failure and Dilated Cardiomyopathy

Allison M Pritchett, Ravi S Hira, Biykem Bozkurt

DEFINITION AND ETIOLOGY

Heart failure (HF) is a progressive, clinical syndrome due to a structural or functional impairment that results in the inability of the heart to adequately fill with or eject blood to meet the body's demands. The terms "HF" and "cardiomyopathy" are not synonymous. The former implies the association of symptoms such as fatigue, dyspnea on exertion, orthopnea, and peripheral edema with an underlying cardiac structural disorder or cardiomyopathy (Figs. 20.1A and B). The ejection fraction (EF), a measure of left ventricular (LV) systolic function, has been utilized to classify cardiomyopathies into those with HF with preserved ejection fraction (HFpEF) (generally EF > 50%) and those with HF with reduced ejection fraction (HFrEF) (EF ≤ 40%). HFpEF is typified by increased myocardial stiffness, often due to ischemia, fibrosis, or myocardial hypertrophy. HFrEF is characterized by LV dilatation and reduced systolic function, and may also exhibit increased myocardial stiffness. These hemodynamic alterations are depicted graphically in Figure 20.2. This chapter will focus on HFrEF or systolic HF. Of the patients with HF, approximately 50% have systolic HF.

The development and progression of HF has been divided into stages (Table 20.1). The spectrum includes those with risk factors for the development of HF (stage A), those with asymptomatic structural heart disease (stage B), those with symptomatic HF (stage C), and those with refractory HF (stage D). Hypertension and coronary artery disease (CAD) are among the most common causes of HF. In fact, hypertension is the most modifiable risk factor for HF. Aggressive hypertension management may reduce the risk of HF by ~50%. Other etiologies of HF include exposure to toxins, endocrine and infectious etiologies, and pregnancy and other systemic diseases (Table 20.2). The incidence of HF increases with age, and is highest in blacks compared to other racial groups. HF is associated with ~50% mortality within 5 years of diagnosis.

PHYSIOLOGY OF HEART FAILURE

The development and subsequent progression of a dilated cardiomyopathy is due to the complex interaction of multiple mechanisms. To begin, LV dilatation increases LV wall stress as dictated by the Law of Laplace:

$$\text{wall stress} = \frac{\text{pressure} \times \text{radius}}{2 \times \text{wall thickness}}$$

This increased wall stress increases the myocardial oxygen requirement and triggers the development of eccentric hypertrophy. The reduced cardiac output induces activation of the adrenergic and renin-angiotensin-aldosterone (RAS) systems, which act to cause compensatory vasoconstriction, reabsorption of sodium and free water, increased heart rate, stimulation of myocardial hypertrophy and fibrosis.

CLINICAL EVALUATION OF HEART FAILURE

Evaluation of patients with HF requires a careful history, including a detailed family history, to elucidate possible contributory risk factors or etiologies of the underlying cardiomyopathy, as well as defining the patient's current symptoms. The New York Heart Association (NYHA) functional classification (Table 20.3) is useful when assessing the severity of HF symptoms.

The physical examination requires a detailed cardiovascular examination as well as assessment for features of systemic diseases which may cause a cardiomyopathy. It is also important to evaluate the patient's volume status by

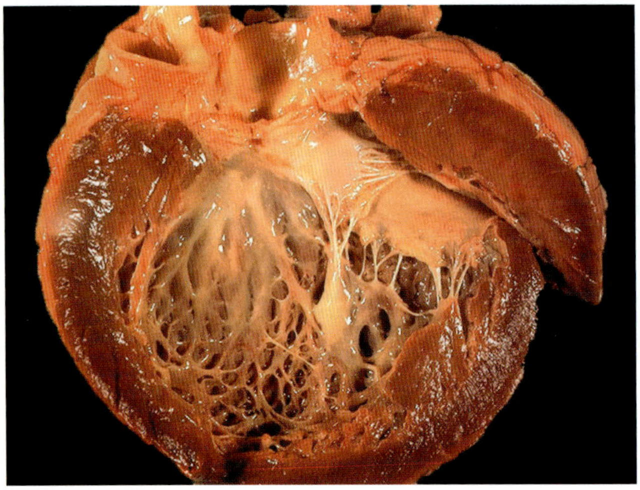

Fig. 20.1A: Gross cardiac specimen of dilated cardiomyopathy. The left ventricle is dilated taking on a more spherical shape. (Image from Dr Edwin P Ewing and the Center for Disease Control).

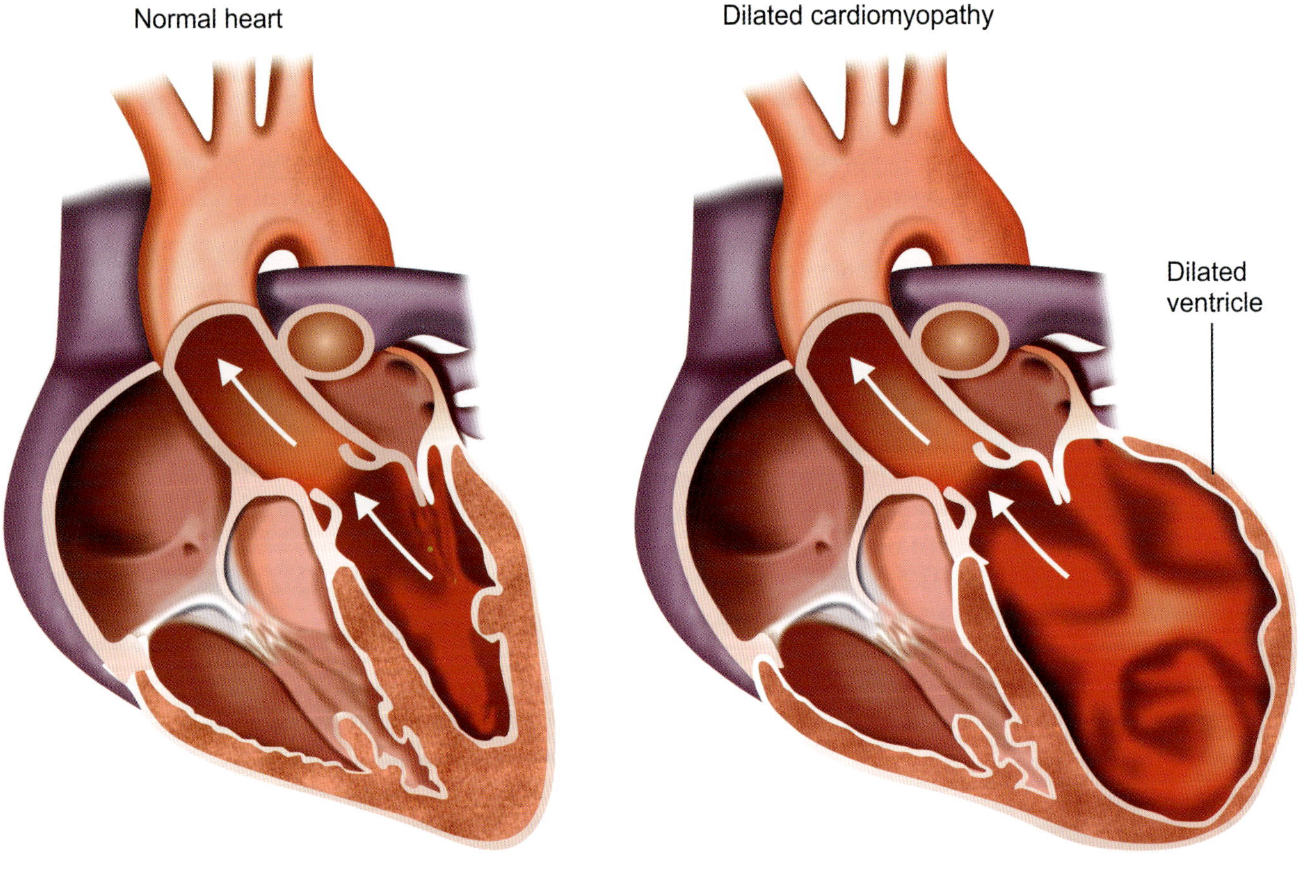

Fig. 20.1B: Diagrammatic depiction of dilated cardiomyopathy. The dilated left ventricle takes on a more spherical shape. [Image from Sofijanova A, Jordanova O. Pediatric cardiomyopathies. In: Milei J, Ambrosia G (Eds). Cardiomyopathies. InTech. 2013].

Table 20.1: The stages of heart failure (HF).

Stage	Definition
A	Those at risk for development of structural heart disease
B	Structural heart disease without signs or symptoms of heart failure (HF)
C	Structural heart disease with prior or current symptoms of HF
D	Refractory HF despite optimal medical therapy

Table 20.2: Causes of cardiomyopathy.

Cause	Specific Examples
Hypertension	• Primary hypertension • Secondary hypertension
Coronary artery disease (CAD)	• Myocardial infarction (MI) • Hibernating myocardium
Endocrine	• Diabetes • Obesity • Hyper- and hypothyroid • Acromegaly
Rheumatologic	• Lupus • Scleroderma
Infectious	• Human immunodeficiency virus • Lyme disease • Chagas' disease • Other viruses
Infiltrative	• Hemochromatosis • Amyloidosis • Sarcoidosis
Genetic/familial	• Muscular dystrophies • Familial • Storage diseases
Valvular pathology	• Aortic valve stenosis or insufficiency • Mitral regurgitation
Arrhythmia-related disease	• Atrial fibrillation • Tachycardia mediated • Frequent ventricular ectopy
Congenital heart disease	• Atrial septal defect (nonrestrictive) • Ventricular septal defect (nonrestrictive) • Cyanotic congenital heart disease
Toxin	• Chemotherapy (anthracyclines, trastuzumab, cyclophosphamide) • Radiation • Alcohol, cocaine, ephedra
Others	• Pregnancy • Noncompaction • Sleep disturbed breathing • Beri beri • High output states • Stress-induced (Takotsubo)

Table 20.3: New York Heart Association (NYHA) classification of heart failure (HF) symptoms.

Class	Definition
I	No symptoms or limitation with normal activity (walking, climbing stairs, etc.)
II	Mild symptoms with normal activity
III	Symptoms with less than normal activity (showering, dressing), comfortable at rest
IV	Symptomatic at rest

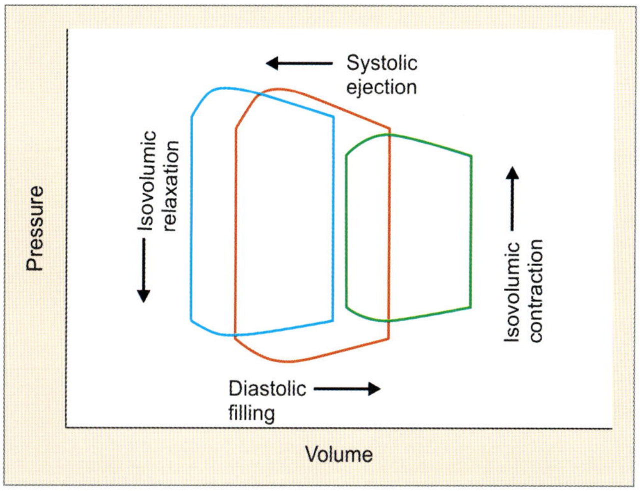

Fig. 20.2: Schematic diagram of left ventricular (LV) pressure volume loop. The cardiac cycle of the normal left ventricle is demonstrated by the red pressure volume loop. For a dilated cardiomyopathy (green line), the end-diastolic and end-systolic volumes are larger with a lower end-systolic pressure for a given LV volume (decreased inotropy). For a stiff ventricle (blue line), typified in heart failure with preserved ejection fraction (HFpEF), the end-diastolic pressure is increased often with smaller end-diastolic volume, yet follows the normal ejection curve.

documenting weight, estimating jugular venous pressure (JVP) (Figs. 20.3A to C), and assessment for ascites or peripheral edema (Figs. 20.4A and B). Given the chronicity of HF and need for frequent follow-up, especially during titration of the medical regimen, it is important to reassess NYHA class and volume status on each subsequent visit.

Recommended diagnostic tests (Table 20.4) include basic laboratory studies, electrocardiogram, posterior-anterior (PA) and lateral chest radiographs (Fig. 20.5), and an echocardiogram. It may be appropriate to screen for systemic diseases such as hemochromatosis, human immunodeficiency virus, amyloid, or pheochromocytoma in selected patients if there is a clinical suspicion. A brain natriuretic peptide (BNP) level may be useful to determine if HF is the cause of dyspnea. This hormone is released in

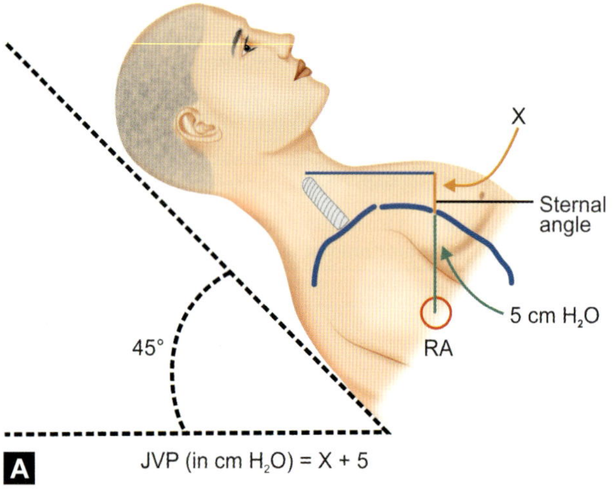

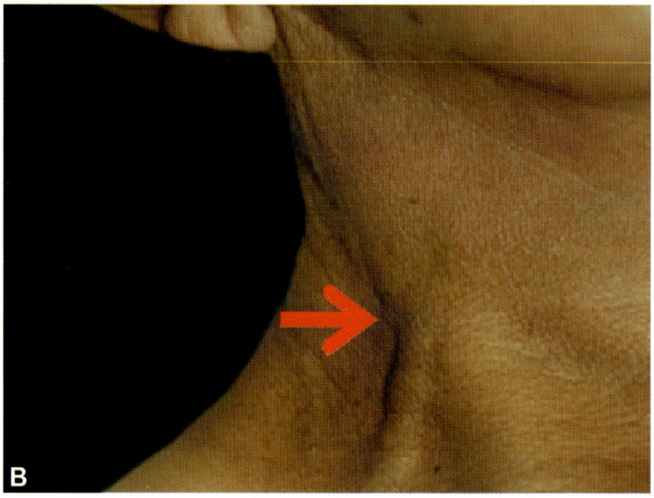

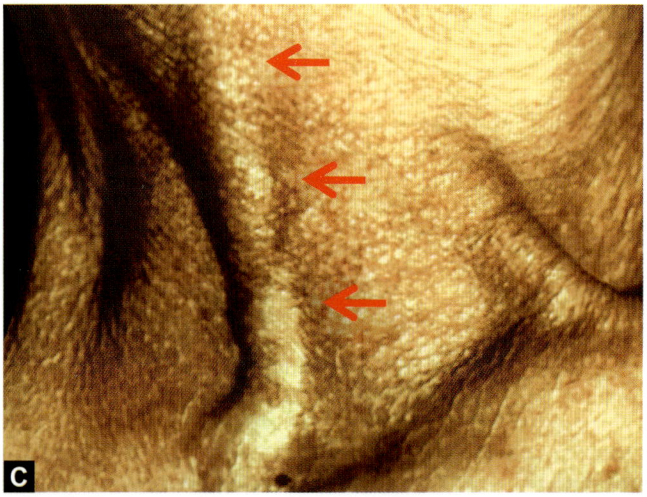

Figs. 20.3A to C: Jugular venous pressure (JVP). (A) With the patient positioned at 45°, estimate the number of centimeters the venous column extends above the sternal angle. Add 5 cm for the depth of the right atrium below the sternal angle. This estimates the right atrial pressure with a normal value < 8 cm H_2O. Giant V waves can be seen in the presence of severe tricuspid regurgitation; (B) In the example shown, the venous column is approximately 5 cm above the sternal angle, so a JVP of 10 cm H_2O is reported; (C) More profound jugular venous distention is shown. [Figure 20.3B courtesy of Harris Health System. Figure 20.3C from Chatterjee K. Physical examination. In: Chatterjee K, Anderson M, Heistad D, Kerber RE (Eds). Cardiology: An Illustrated Textbook, 1st edition. New Delhi, India: Jaypee Brothers Medical Publishers (P) Ltd; 2012. pp. 151-73].

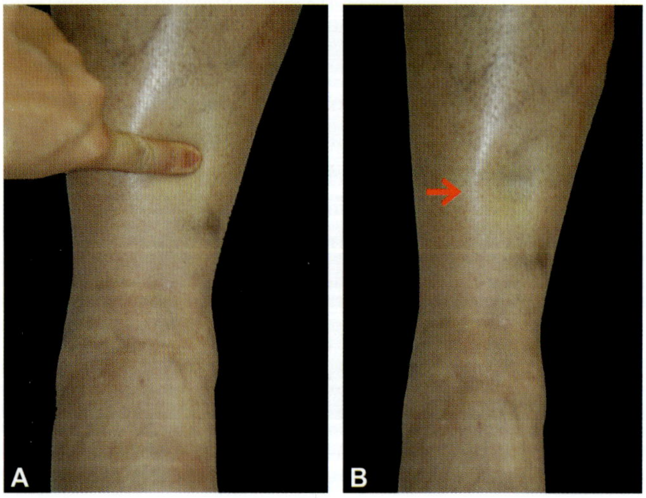

Figs. 20.4A and B: Peripheral edema. Pressure is applied to the pretibial area (A) and results in a marked depression or pitting of the skin (B). Edema is graded on a scale of 1-4 based on depth of pit and time for it to rebound. This is an example of 4+ pitting edema. (Image courtesy of Harris Health System).

Table 20.4: Laboratory and radiographic examinations to evaluate the etiology of heart failure (HF).

Laboratory:
• Complete blood count
• Electrolytes
• BUN/Creatinine
• Liver function tests
• Glucose
• Lipid panel
• TSH
• Urinalysis
• BNP or NT-BNP
Electrocardiogram
Chest radiograph
Transthoracic echocardiogram
Others—in selected patients, consideration of:
• Coronary angiography
• MRI
• CT
• Nuclear imaging
• Holter monitoring
• Exercise testing

(BUN: Blood urea nitrogen; TSH: Thyroid-stimulating hormone; BNP: Brain natriuretic peptide; NT-BNP: N-terminal prohormone of brain natriuretic peptide; MRI: Magnetic resonance imaging; CT: Computed tomography).

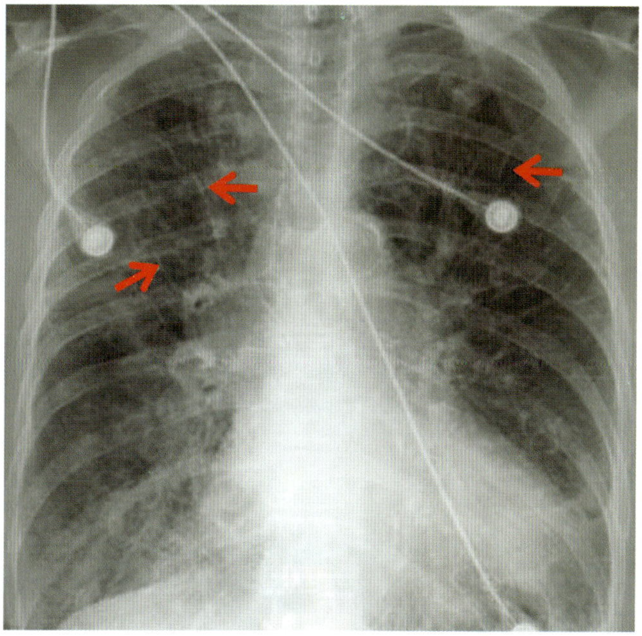

Fig. 20.5: Chest radiograph demonstrating features of heart failure (HF). This posterior-anterior (PA) image demonstrates an enlarged cardiac silhouette, increased pulmonary vascular markings as well as Kerley lines. Kerley lines represent edema within the intralobular septae of the lung parenchyma. [Image from Thompson BH, van Beek EJ. Plain film imaging of adult cardiovascular disease. In: Chatterjee K, Anderson M, Heistad D, Kerber RE (Eds). Cardiology: An Illustrated Textbook, 1st edition. New Delhi, India: Jaypee Brothers Medical Publishers (P) Ltd.; 2012. pp. 174-88].

response to ventricular stretch and counteracts some of the effects of sympathetic and RAS activation described above by augmenting sodium and water excretion and inducing vasorelaxation.

Echocardiography

Performance of a transthoracic echocardiogram is one of the most common imaging examinations to define cardiac structural and functional abnormalities in patients with signs and symptoms of HF. This modality is safe, able to be performed at bedside, does not require exposure to contrast or radiation, and can be repeated serially to evaluate changes with medication optimization or alteration in symptoms. The primary findings in those with systolic HF are dilatation of the left ventricle with decreased global systolic function (Videos 20.1 and 20.2). Right ventricular (RV) involvement may also be seen. The LV can be measured by an end-diastolic dimension from the parasternal long-axis view (Fig. 20.6) or by volumetric analysis with a modified Simpson's technique, where the endocardium of the left ventricle is traced at end-diastole in the apical four- and two-chamber images (Fig. 20.7). The normal values for LV dimension are 3.9–5.3 cm for women and 4.2–5.9 cm for men. Normal LV volume is 56–104 mL and 67–155 mL for women and men, respectively. In general, as the LV dilates it takes on a more spherical, rather than elliptical shape. With this LV remodeling, the papillary muscles are displaced, creating tenting or apical displacement of the mitral valve (MV) leaflet coaptation point. The MV annulus also dilates. Both mechanisms contribute to the development of functional mitral regurgitation (Figs. 20.8A and B).

The EF is the most commonly utilized measure of systolic function. While often this is performed semiquantitatively by an experienced observer, the EF can be quantified using the following formula:

$$EF\,(\%) = \frac{\text{end diastolic volume} - \text{end systolic volume}}{\text{end systolic volume}} \times 100$$

The LV volumes are traced at end-diastole and end-systole according to the method demonstrated in Figure 20.7.

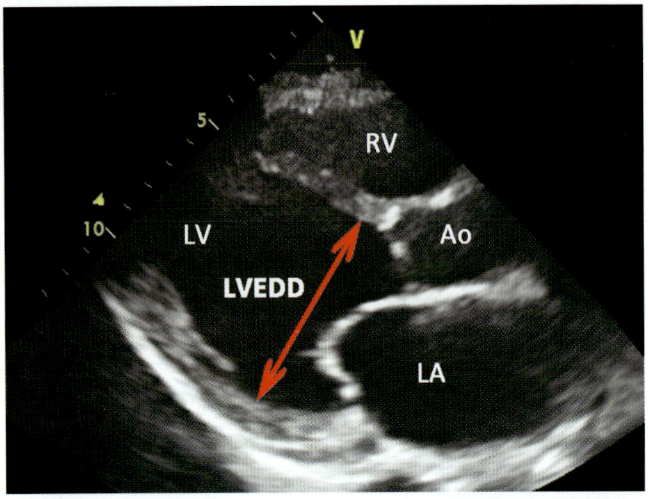

Fig. 20.6: Left ventricular (LV) dilatation by transthoracic echocardiography. In this parasternal long-axis image, the LV dimension is measured at the level of the mitral leaflet tips. The LV is severely dilated in this example with a dimension of 7 cm. (Image courtesy of Harris Health System). (LV: Left ventricle; RV: Right ventricle; Ao: Aorta; LVEDD: Left-ventricular end-diastolic dimension; LA: Left atrium).

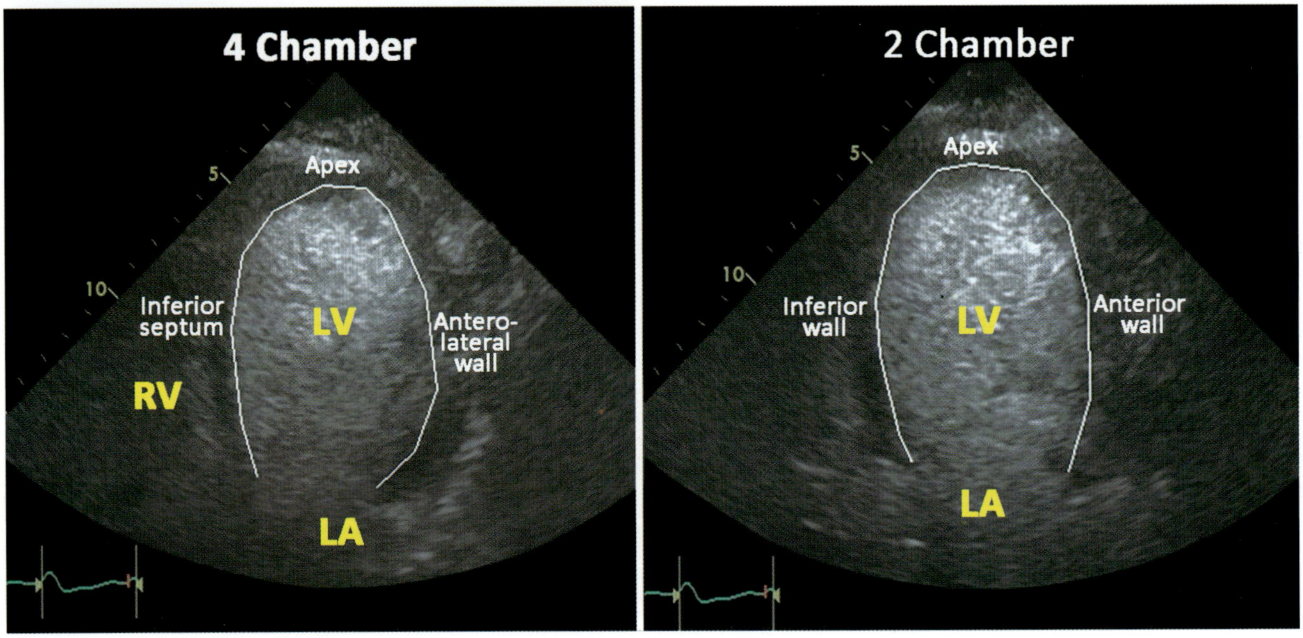

Fig. 20.7: Left ventricular (LV) volume is obtained by tracing the endocardium of two orthogonal apical views (four-chamber- and two-chamber views) of the left ventricle at end-diastole. The volume is calculated by summing the volume of stacked elliptical disks (modified Simpson's rule). In this example, perfluorocarbon contrast was utilized to enhance the endocardial borders. It is important that the images are not foreshortened. This LV is severely dilated with the volume exceeding 200 mL. (Image courtesy of Harris Health System).

In addition to a reduced EF, the majority of patients with systolic HF also exhibit concomitant abnormalities of diastolic function. While the echocardiographic features of diastolic dysfunction will be covered in greater detail in the chapter on diastolic HF, an example of restrictive LV filling is shown in Figures 20.9A and B. Echocardiographic features associated with a worsened prognosis include severe LV dilatation, a shortened mitral inflow E wave deceleration time, and the severity of mitral regurgitation. Other echocardiographic findings of a severe cardiomyopathy are failure to sustain aortic valve opening throughout systole (Fig. 20.10), reduced excursion of the mitral leaflets due to low cardiac output, beat-to-beat variation in the LV outflow tract Doppler signals suggesting pulsus alternans, atrial and RV enlargement, and the apical mural thrombus (Figs. 20.11A and B).

Cardiovascular Magnetic Resonance

Cardiovascular magnetic resonance (CMR) provides excellent three-dimensional visualization of cardiac structure and function, yet is expensive, less readily available than

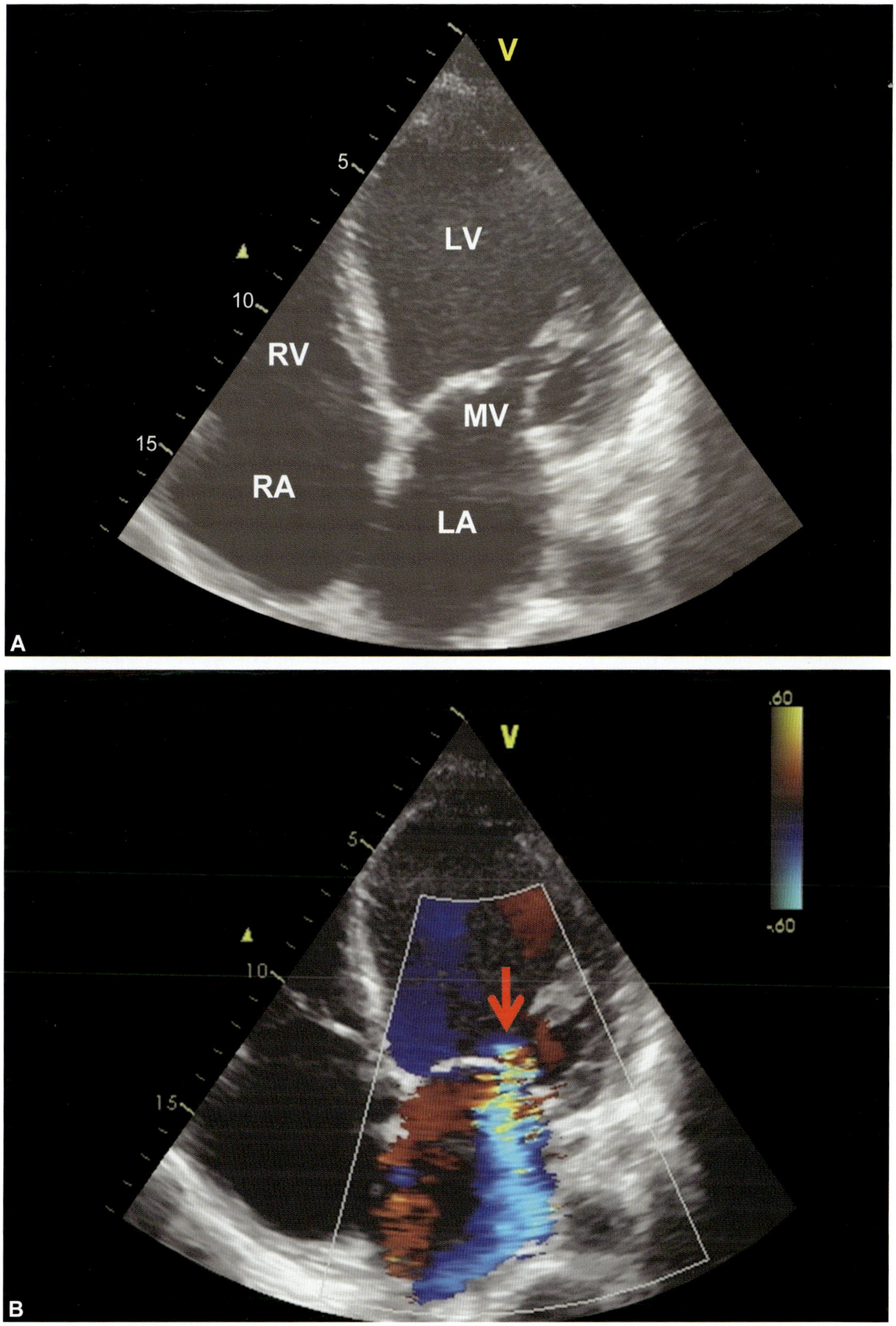

Figs. 20.8A and B: Severely dilated left ventricle with displacement of the papillary muscle and resultant functional mitral regurgitation. (A) Left ventricular (LV) dilatation causes mitral annular dilatation as well as displacement of the papillary muscles and tenting of the mitral valve (MV) leaflets. (B) This results in malcoaptation of the MV leaflets and resultant severe mitral regurgitation (arrow). (Image courtesy of Harris Health System). (LA: Left atrium; RA: Right atrium; RV: Right ventricle; LV: Left ventricle; MV: Mitral valve).

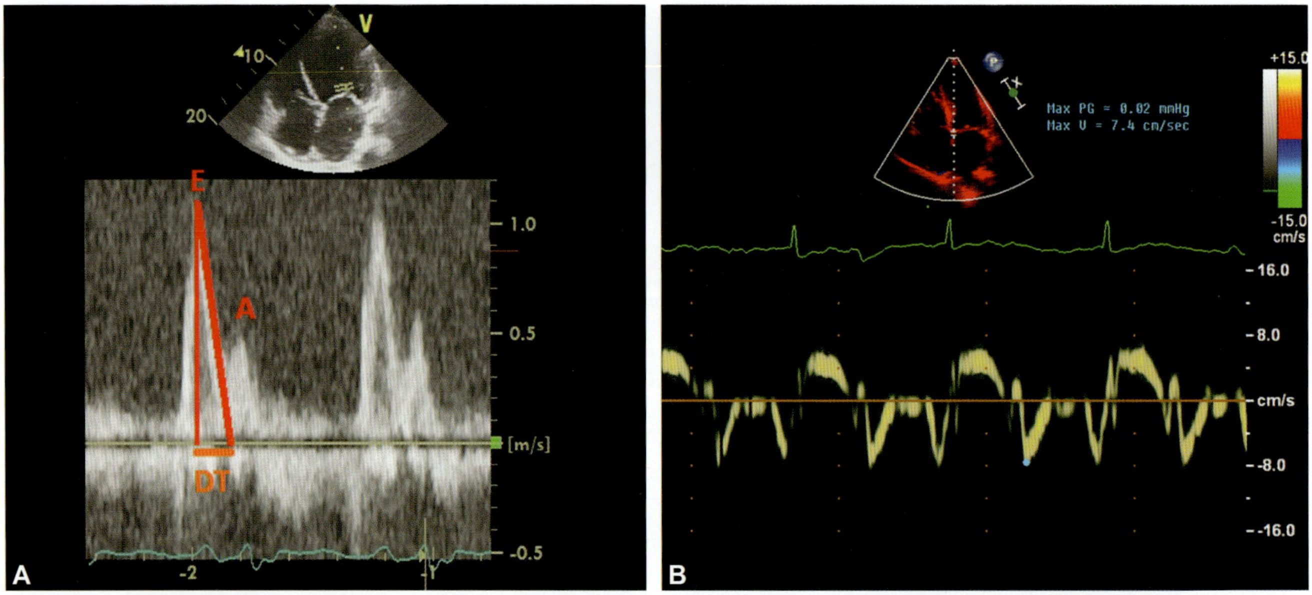

Figs. 20.9A and B: Restrictive left ventricular (LV) filling. (A) Mitral inflow pulsed wave Doppler signal obtained at the leaflet tips in the apical four-chamber view. In severe systolic heart failure (HF), the reduced cardiac output, as well as fibrosis and increased stiffness of the LV myocardium contribute to increased left atrial (LA) pressure. The increased LA pressure results in a large E velocity with blood rushing into the LV only to be met by a stiff, noncompliant myocardium. The rapid equalization of the LV and LA pressures is manifested as a shortened deceleration time (< 160 msec). The left atrium at this stage is often severely dilated with reduced systolic function. As well, the increased LV end-diastolic pressure limits atrial forward flow and augments flow reversal back into the pulmonary veins. Both mechanisms contribute to a diminutive A wave. This pattern is consistent with restrictive LV filling which is a marker of poor prognosis; (B) Tissue Doppler signals performed at the septal and lateral mitral valve (MV) annulus demonstrate reduced e' velocities. An E/e' ratio > 15 correlates with an increase in LV filling pressure. (Images courtesy of Harris Health System).

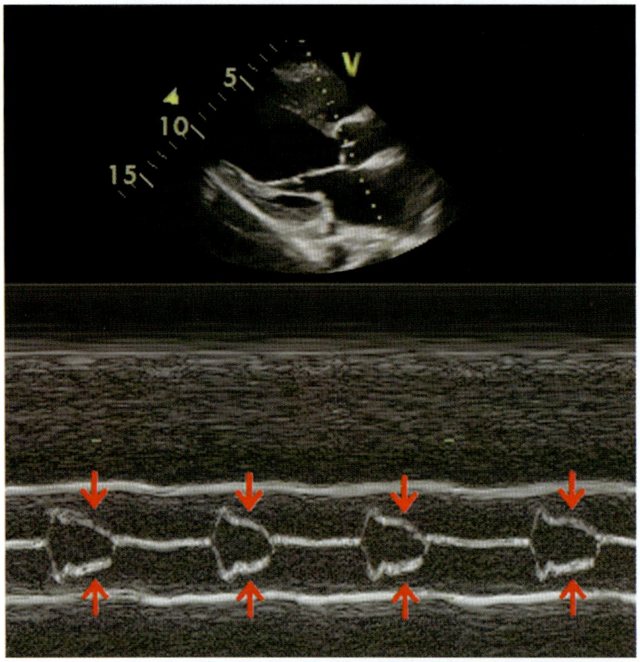

Fig. 20.10: M-mode image through the aortic valve and aortic root. This demonstrates a gradual closure of the aortic valve in late systole and is a sign of severely depressed myocardial systolic function. (Image courtesy of Harris Health System).

echocardiography, and is relatively contraindicated in patients with pacemakers or most implantable cardioverter defibrillators. CMR allows accurate quantification of ventricular volumes and systolic function. Use of late gadolinium enhancement allows characterization of the myocardial tissue to better determine the etiology of an underlying cardiomyopathy. Gadolinium contrast accumulates extracellularly. In areas of infarction, gadolinium typically localizes to the subendocardium and may extend transmurally in a coronary distribution (Fig. 20.12). In dilated cardiomyopathy, gadolinium enhancement may occur in the mid-wall in a noncoronary distribution (Figs. 20.13A and B). This pattern correlates with myocardial fibrosis and predicts an adverse outcome. CMR is also useful in patients with suspected infiltrative diseases that may result in LV systolic dysfunction, such as amyloidosis and sarcoidosis, and can be used to assess for cardiac involvement in patients with hemochromatosis.

Endomyocardial Biopsy

While endomyocardial biopsy should not be performed routinely in HF patients, it may be considered in the

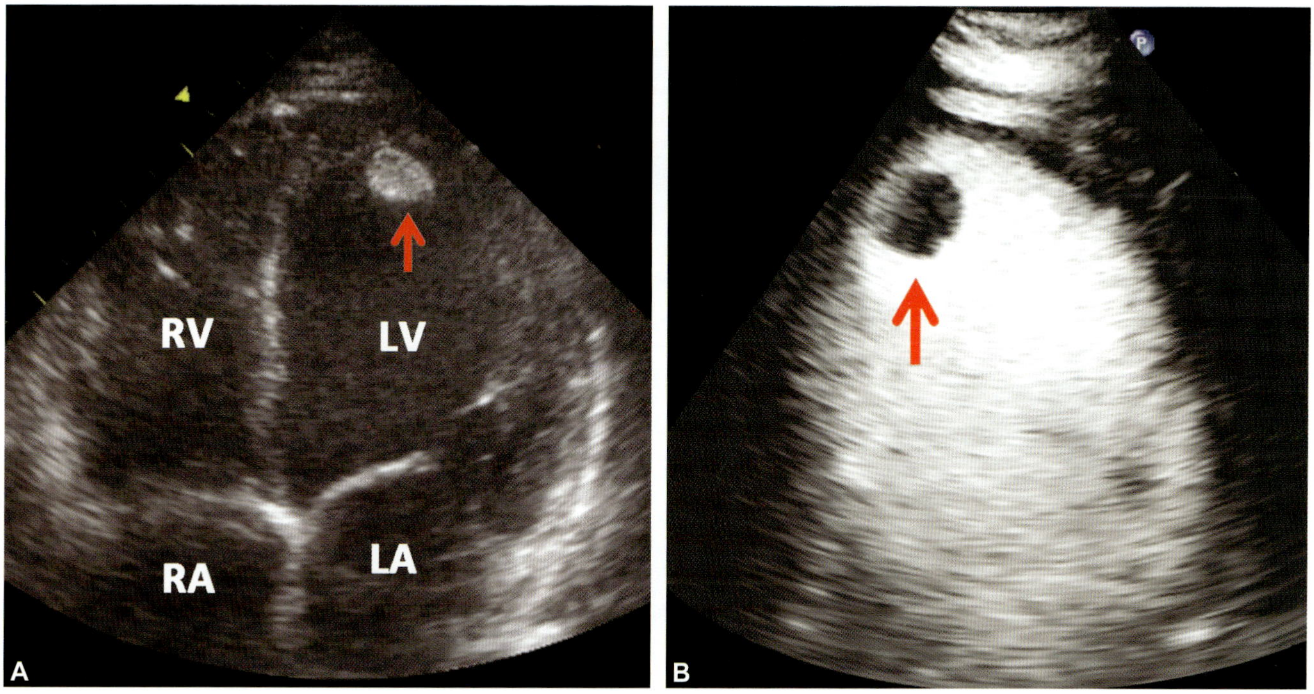

Figs. 20.11A and B: Left ventricular (LV) apical thrombus (red arrow). Apical four-chamber view without (A) and with perfluorocarbon contrast (B) demonstrating a circular mass in the LV apex consistent with thrombus. Perfluorocarbon contrast is often helpful to better delineate the apical cavity to assess for the presence of thrombus. The use of an echo-contrast agent should be considered, especially if the apex is akinetic, to assess for the presence of apical thrombus. (Images courtesy of Glenn N Levine, MD).

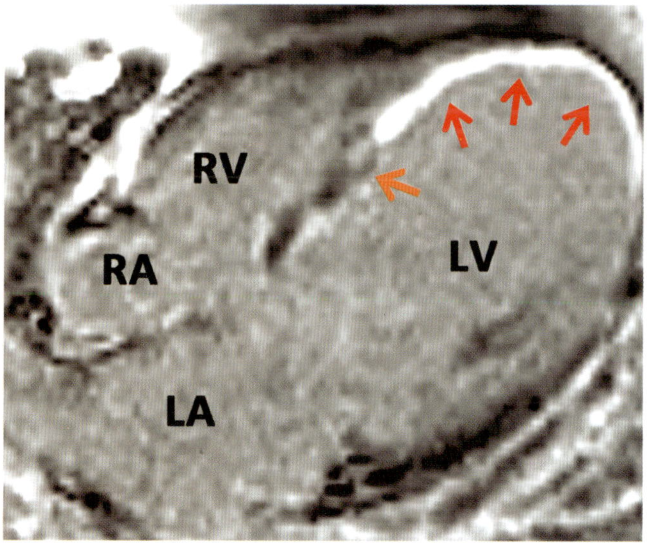

Fig. 20.12: Cardiovascular magnetic resonance image (MRI) of ischemic cardiomyopathy. Image acquired 10 minutes following administration of gadolinium contrast demonstrates a transmural infarction (red arrows) in the septum and apex, as well as microvascular obstruction in the basal septum (orange arrow). [Image from Weiss RM. Cardiovascular magnetic resonance. In: Chatterjee K, Anderson M, Heistad D, Kerber RE (Eds). Cardiology: An Illustrated Textbook, 1st edition. New Delhi, India: Jaypee Brothers Medical Publishers (P) Ltd.; 2012. pp. 431-49].

following situations: acute onset (< 2 weeks duration) of severe HF with hemodynamic compromise; HF of 2 weeks to 3 months duration with dilated left ventricle and associated ventricular arrhythmias; HF with second- or third-degree heart block; or HF with failure to respond to standard therapy. These situations would lead to consideration of diagnoses such as lymphocytic myocarditis, giant cell myocarditis, or necrotizing eosinophilic myocarditis (Figs. 20.14A to C).

Medical Therapy

Table 20.5 lists the most common medications and their associated indications for patients with symptomatic (stage 3) HF, based on the recent 2013 American College of Cardiology Foundation (ACCF)/American Heart Association (AHA) guideline for the management of HF. In general, patients should be on an angiotensin-converting-enzyme (ACE) inhibitor and one of the HF-specific beta-blockers, unless contraindicated, to reduce mortality and HF hospitalizations. ACE inhibitors can cause hyperkalemia, angioedema, and are teratogenic. Potassium and renal function should be measured within 1–2 weeks of initiation and periodically thereafter. An

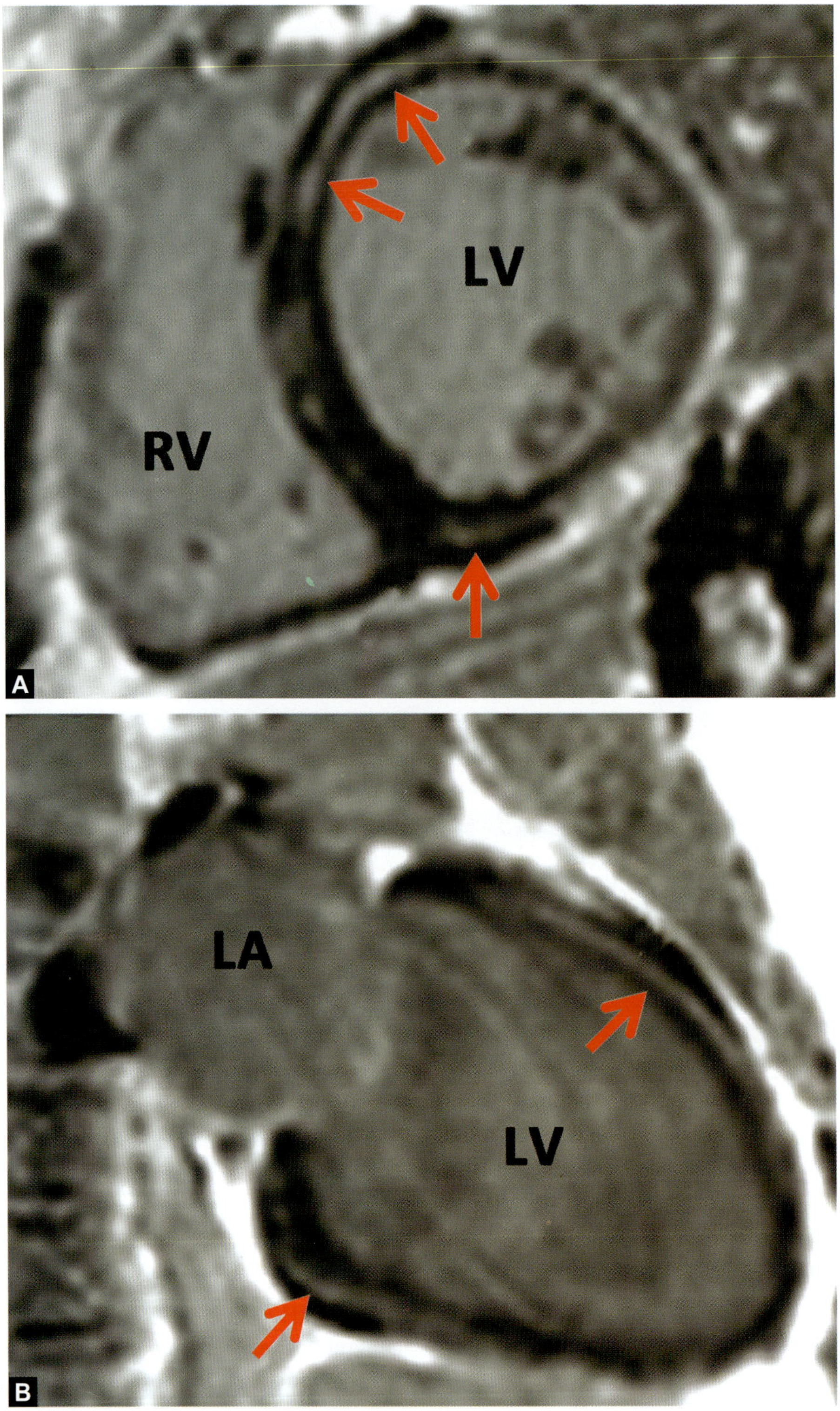

Figs. 20.13A and B: Cardiovascular magnetic resonance image (MRI) of dilated cardiomyopathy. Short-axis (A) and two-chamber—long-axis (B) images acquired 10 minutes following administration of gadolinium contrast demonstrate mid-myocardial late gadolinium enhancement (LGE) in the anterior and inferior left ventricular (LV) walls (arrows). LGE is evidence for myocardial fibrosis, is associated with an increased risk of death or hospitalization, and may predict a lower likelihood to respond to therapy. [Images from Weiss RM. Cardiovascular magnetic resonance. In: Chatterjee K, Anderson M, Heistad D, Kerber RE (Eds). Cardiology: An Illustrated Textbook, 1st edition. New Delhi, India: Jaypee Brothers Medical Publishers (P) Ltd; 2012. pp. 431-49].

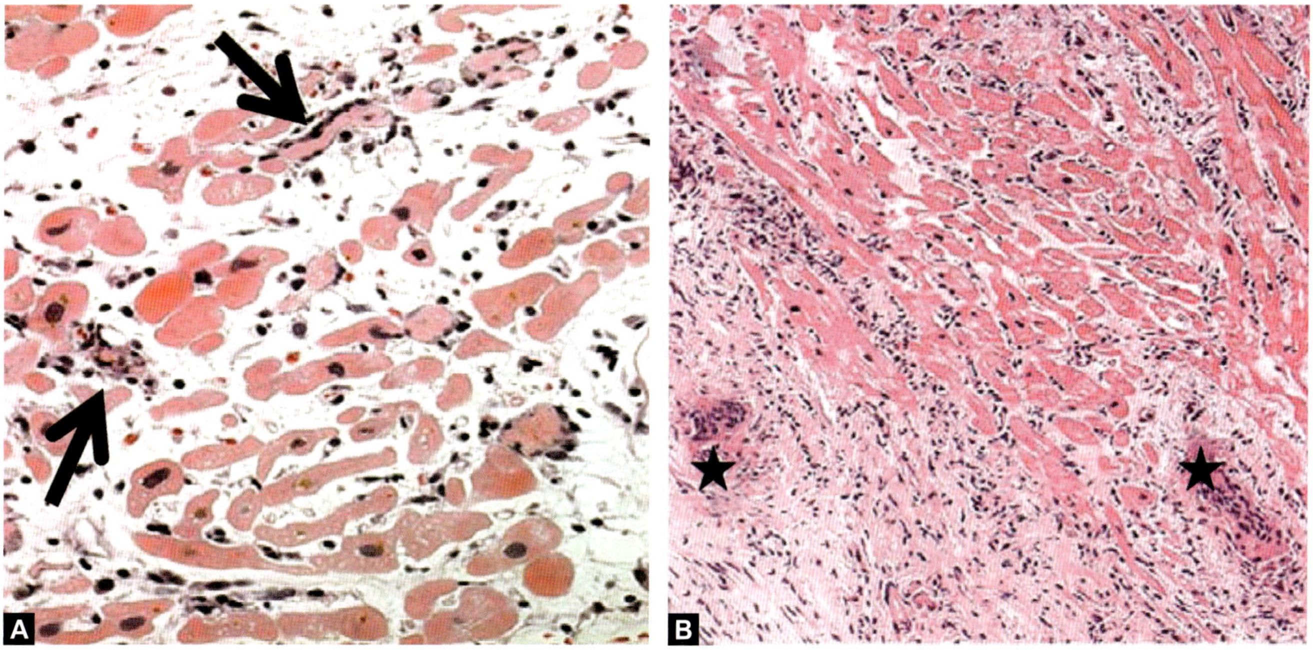

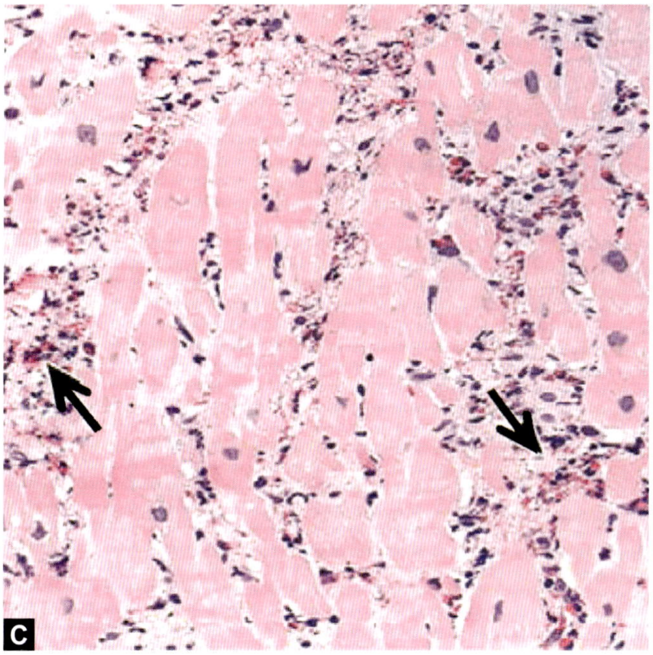

Figs. 20.14A to C: (A) Endomyocardial biopsy specimens demonstrating myocarditis: Lymphocytic myocarditis, typified by mononuclear cells within the interstitium surrounding damaged or dying myocytes (arrows); (B) Giant cell myocarditis biopsy specimen demonstrating extensive mononuclear cell infiltration, myocyte necrosis, and giant cells (stars); (C) Hypersensitivity myocarditis. Numerous interstitial eosinophils are seen with necrotizing eosinophilic myocarditis. [Figures 20.14A to C courtesy of Ursell PC, MD, Department of Pathology, UCSF. Images from Rao VU, de Marco T. Cardiac biopsy. In: Chatterjee K, Anderson M, Heistad D, Kerber RE (Eds). Cardiology: An Illustrated Textbook, 1st edition. New Delhi, India: Jaypee Brothers Medical Publishers (P) Ltd; 2012. pp. 485-502].

Table 20.5: Select class I and class III indications and contraindications, respectively, for medical therapy in stage C systolic heart failure (HF) with reduced ejection fraction (HFrEF) according to 2013 American College of Cardiology Foundation (ACCF)/American Heart Association (AHA) guideline for the management of HF. (HF: Heart failure; NYHA, New York Heart Association; EF: Ejection fraction; CrCl: Creatinine clearance; K^+: Potassium; MI: Myocardial infarction).

Medication	*Class of Recommendation*
Angiotensin-converting enzyme (ACE) inhibitors or angiotensin-receptor blockers (ARBs)	Class I: For all patients with current or prior HF symptoms, unless contraindicated, to reduce morbidity and mortality. ARBs may be utilized in those who are intolerant of ACE inhibitors.
Beta-blockers	Class I: 1 of 3 beta-blockers proven to reduce mortality (bisoprolol, carvedilol, or sustained-release metoprolol succinate) should be utilized in all patients with current or prior HF symptoms, unless contraindicated, to reduce morbidity and mortality
Loop diuretic	Class I: For all NYHA II-IV patients with volume overload
Hydralazine/nitrate	Class I: For persistently symptomatic NYHA III-IV African American patients already receiving optimal therapy with ACE inhibitors and beta-blockers
Aldosterone antagonist	Class I: • For NYHA II-IV patients with EF ≤ 35% with CrCl > 30 mL/min/1.73 m^2 and K^+ < 5.0 mEq/dL • In patients post-acute MI, with EF ≤ 40% who develop symptoms of HF or have diabetes, unless contraindicated
Aldosterone antagonist	Class III: • Combined use of an ACE inhibitor, ARB, and aldosterone antagonist is potentially harmful • There is significant potential harm if aldosterone antagonists are used inappropriately due to risk of hyperkalemia and renal insufficiency

angiotensin-receptor blocker (ARB) may be considered if an ACE-inhibitor induced cough develops. Both ACE inhibitors and beta-blockers should be initiated at low doses and titrated upward gradually as tolerated.

Loop diuretics are utilized to control symptoms of volume overload. Both aldosterone antagonists and the hydralazine/nitrate combination are utilized if patients remain symptomatic despite optimal ACE inhibitor and beta-blocker therapy. Potassium levels and renal function must be monitored closely with use of aldosterone antagonists. The hydralazine/nitrate combination is of particular benefit to African American patients. Digoxin can be beneficial in patients with HFrEF to crease hospitalizations for HF (class IIa recommendation). Guideline-directed medical therapy (GDMT) can potentially improve LV systolic function. A repeat echocardiogram should be performed approximately 3–6 months after the patient has been treated with GDMT to reassess LV systolic function, especially prior to consideration of an implantable cardiac-defibrillator.

CORONARY REVASCULARIZATION

Decisions regarding revascularization to improve survival in patients with systolic HF are complex. Most data on the benefits of revascularization in patients with LV systolic function are from noncontemporary studies, and compared coronary artery bypass surgery (CABG) to contemporaneous therapy. A more recent study of CABG versus medical therapy in patients with LVEF < 35% produced mixed results, with a similar primary endpoint with CABG or medical therapy, but better secondary endpoint outcomes with CABG. CABG is considered to be reasonable (class IIa indication by guidelines) to improve survival in patients with mild-to-moderate LV systolic function (EF 35–50%) and significant multivessel CAD or proximal left anterior descending (LAD) stenosis when viable myocardium is present in the intended region(s) of revascularization. Furthermore, in patients with ischemic heart disease and severe LV systolic function (EF < 35%), CABG may be considered to improve survival (class IIb), even whether or not viable myocardium is present in the areas to undergo revascularization. Percutaneous coronary intervention (PCI) has not been demonstrated in any study to improve survival in patients with LV systolic dysfunction.

DEVICE THERAPY

Patients with systolic HF are at risk of ventricular arrhythmias and sudden cardiac death. Almost all patients with systolic HF who have sustained ventricular tachycardia, ventricular fibrillation, unexplained syncope, or cardiac arrest, and who otherwise have a reasonable life expectancy of at least 1 year will be treated with implanted cardioverter-defibrillator (ICD) for secondary prevention. For primary prevention of sudden cardiac death, ICD is recommended in: (1) selected patients LVEF ≤ 35% and NYHA class II or III symptoms on chronic GDMT and who have reasonable expectation of meaningful survival for more than 1 year; and (2) in selected patients at least 40 days post-MI with LVEF ≤ 30% and NYHA class I symptoms while receiving GDMT.

Approximately one-third of patients with systolic HF will have a significantly prolonged QRS interval. This finding in itself is associated with worse outcome. In patients with widened QRS intervals, which are usually associated with ventricular dyssynchrony, cardiac resynchronization therapy (CRT), also referred to as "biventricular pacing", can improve ventricular function, decrease secondary mitral regurgitation, reverse ventricular remodeling, and improve LVEF. Implantation of a biventricular pacer is recommended in patients with LVEF ≤ 35%, NYHA class II, III, or ambulatory IV symptoms on GDMT, and sinus rhythm with a left bundle-branch block and QRS duration of ≥ 150 msec. This subgroup of patients has been shown to derive the greatest benefit from CRT. CRT can also be considered in other subgroups of patients with depressed LVEF and prolonged QRS duration.

SPECIFIC CARDIOMYOPATHIES

While there are multiple causes of dilated cardiomyopathy, unique features of several are highlighted in Figures 20.15 to 20.20 and Videos 20.3 to 20.5. These may have specific diagnostic and treatment strategies. Etiologies such as amyloidosis, sarcoidosis, and hemochromatosis typically initially present as restrictive/infiltrative cardiomyopathies, but may eventually progress to systolic dysfunction or a dilated cardiomyopathy.

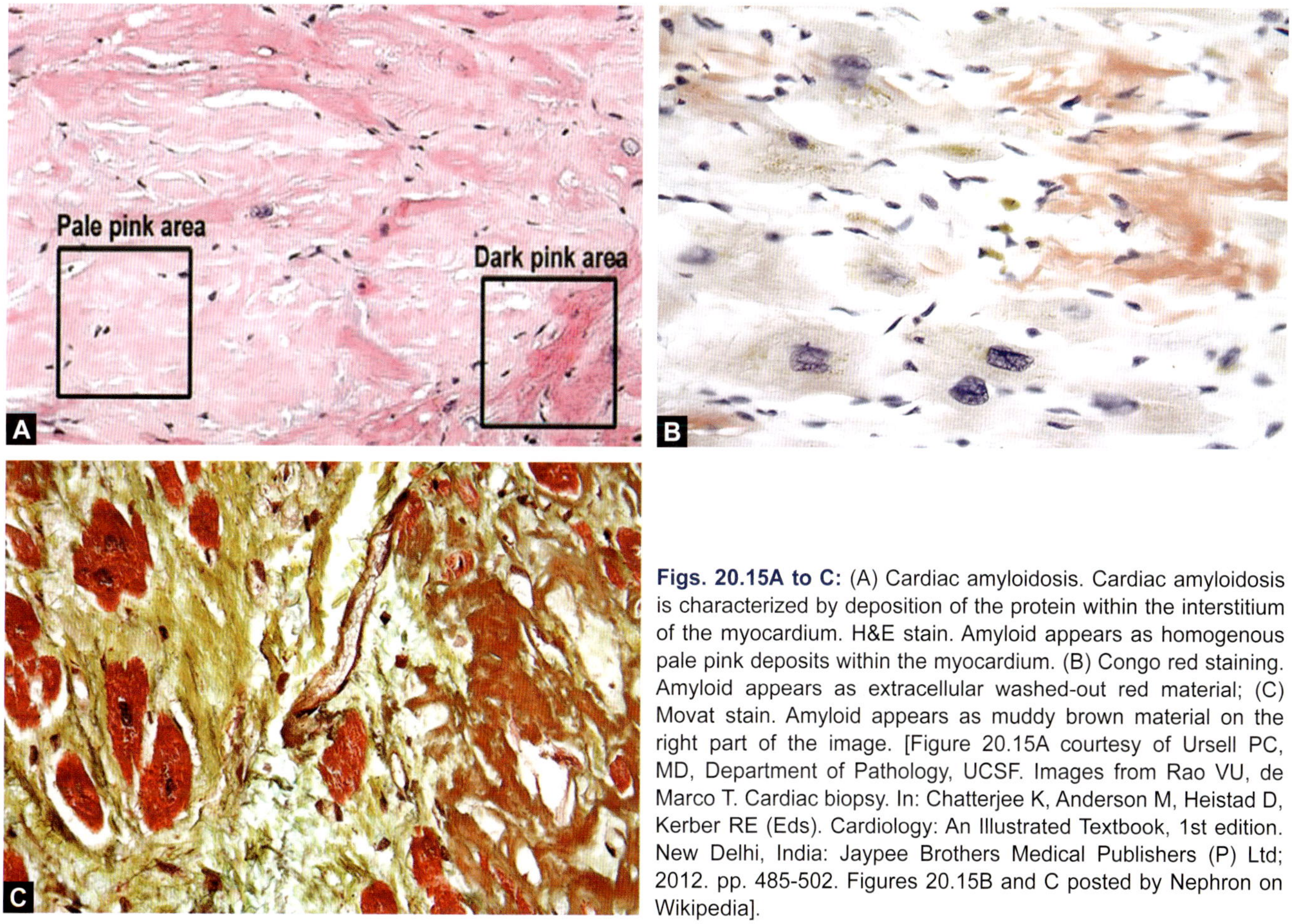

Figs. 20.15A to C: (A) Cardiac amyloidosis. Cardiac amyloidosis is characterized by deposition of the protein within the interstitium of the myocardium. H&E stain. Amyloid appears as homogenous pale pink deposits within the myocardium. (B) Congo red staining. Amyloid appears as extracellular washed-out red material; (C) Movat stain. Amyloid appears as muddy brown material on the right part of the image. [Figure 20.15A courtesy of Ursell PC, MD, Department of Pathology, UCSF. Images from Rao VU, de Marco T. Cardiac biopsy. In: Chatterjee K, Anderson M, Heistad D, Kerber RE (Eds). Cardiology: An Illustrated Textbook, 1st edition. New Delhi, India: Jaypee Brothers Medical Publishers (P) Ltd; 2012. pp. 485-502. Figures 20.15B and C posted by Nephron on Wikipedia].

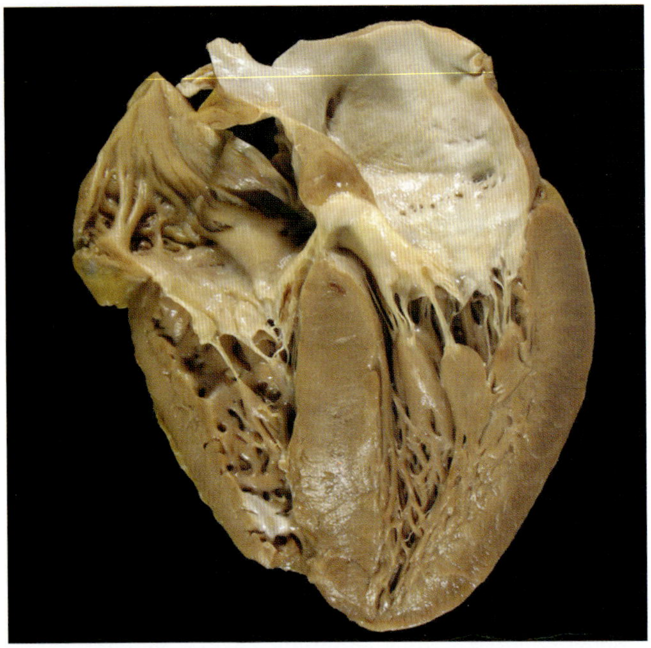

Fig. 20.15D: Gross pathology of cardiac amyloidosis. (Image courtesy of Padera R, MD, PhD, Department of Pathology, Brigham and Women's Hospital).

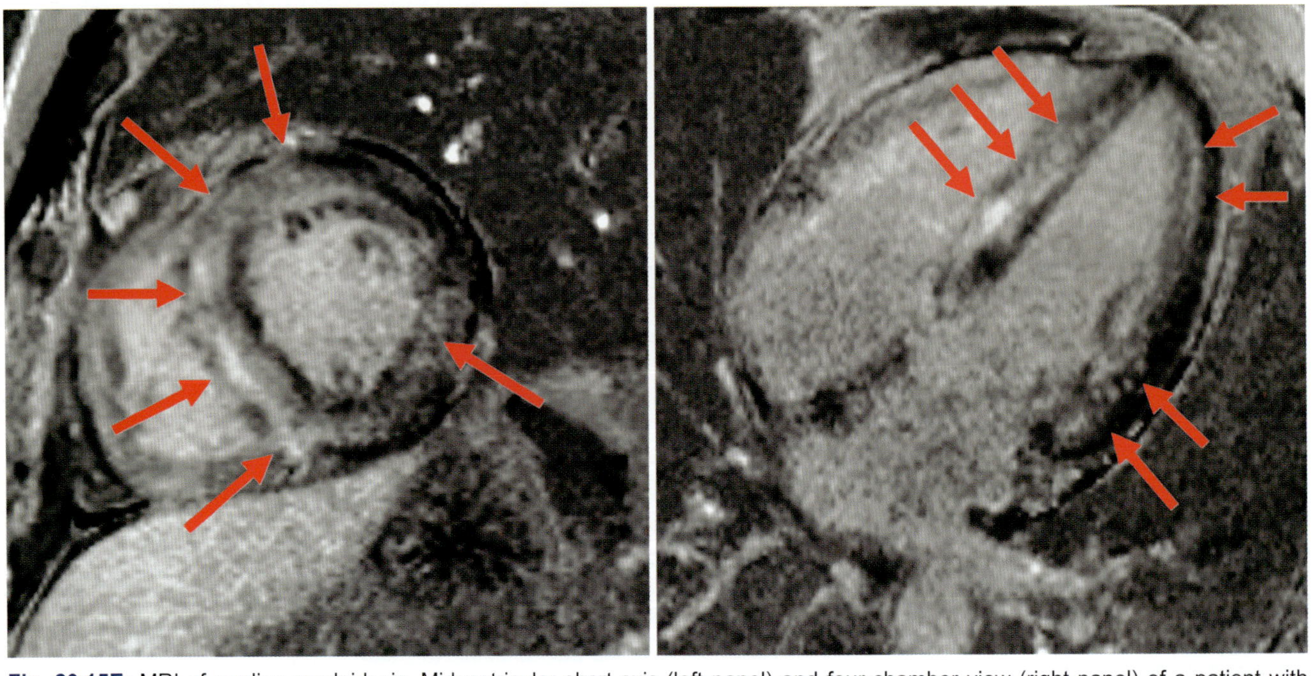

Fig. 20.15E: MRI of cardiac amyloidosis. Midventricular short-axis (left panel) and four-chamber view (right panel) of a patient with amyloid cardiomyopathy. Red arrows point to uniform deposition of amyloid in the myocardium. This commonly results in low voltage on the electrocardiogram. [Image adapted from Liu D, Hu K, Niemann M, et al. Impact of regional left ventricular function on outcome for patients with AL amyloidosis. PLoS ONE. 2013;8(3):e56923].

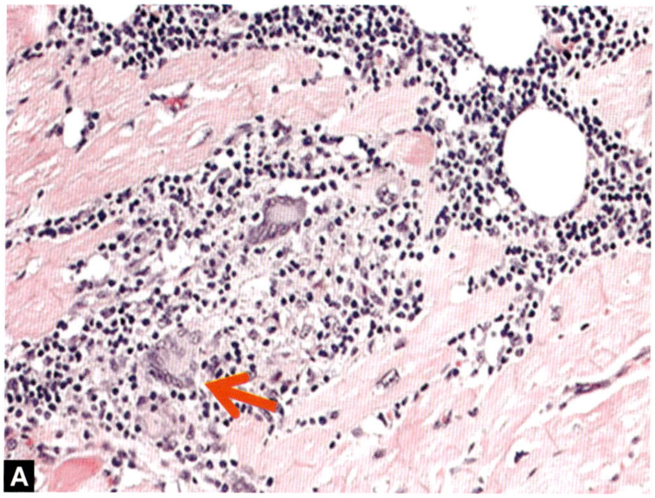

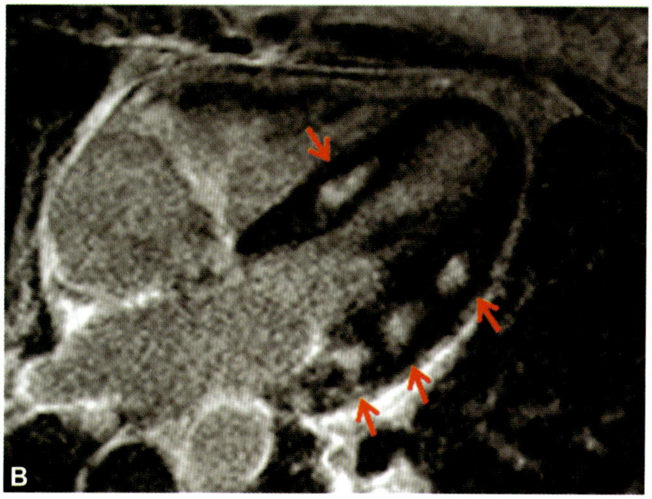

Figs. 20.16A and B: Cardiac sarcoidosis. (A) Biopsy specimen demonstrating myocardial granulomas characterized by clusters of mononuclear cells and giant cells (arrow); (B) Cardiac magnetic resonance imaging (MRI) of a patient with cardiac sarcoidosis showing patchy infiltration (red arrows) of the myocardium. [Figure 20.16A courtesy of Ursell PC, MD, Department of Pathology, UCSF. Images from Rao VU, de Marco T. Cardiac biopsy. In: Chatterjee K, Anderson M, Heistad D, Kerber RE (Eds). Cardiology: An Illustrated Textbook, 1st edition. New Delhi, India: Jaypee Brothers Medical Publishers (P) Ltd; 2012. pp. 485-502. Figure 20.16B courtesy of Levine GN, MD].

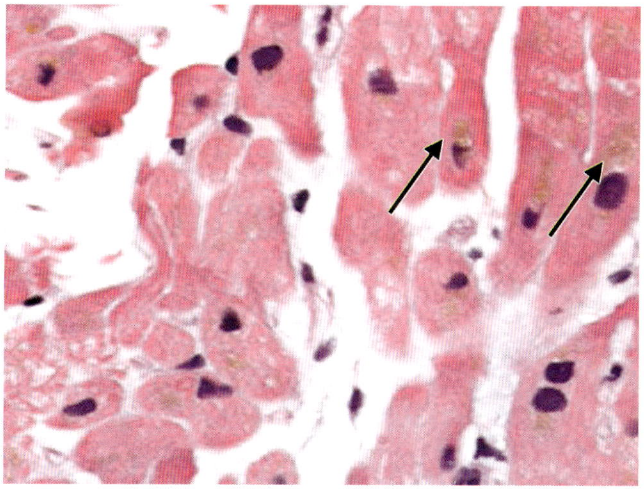

Fig. 20.17A: Hemochromatosis. Biopsy specimen demonstrating pigmented granules within myocytes consistent with iron deposition (arrows).

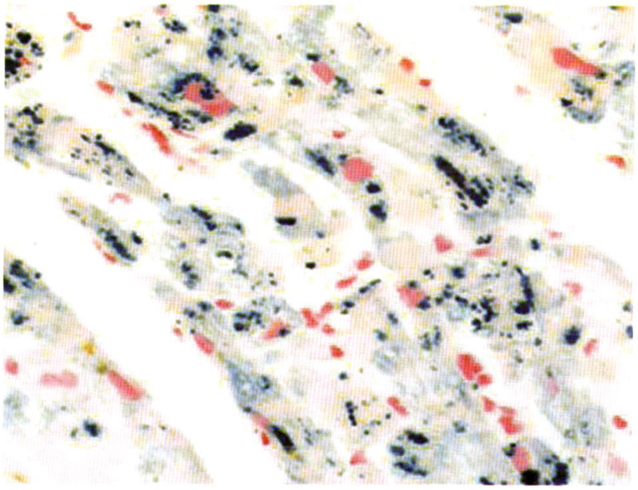

Fig. 20.17B: Hemochromatosis. Special stain shows abundant bluish pigment consistent with iron deposition in the myofibers. [Images courtesy of Ursell PC, MD, Department of Pathology, UCSF. Images from Rao VU, de Marco T. Cardiac biopsy. In: Chatterjee K, Anderson M, Heistad D, Kerber RE (Eds). Cardiology: An Illustrated Textbook, 1st edition. New Delhi, India: Jaypee Brothers Medical Publishers (P) Ltd; 2012. pp. 485-502].

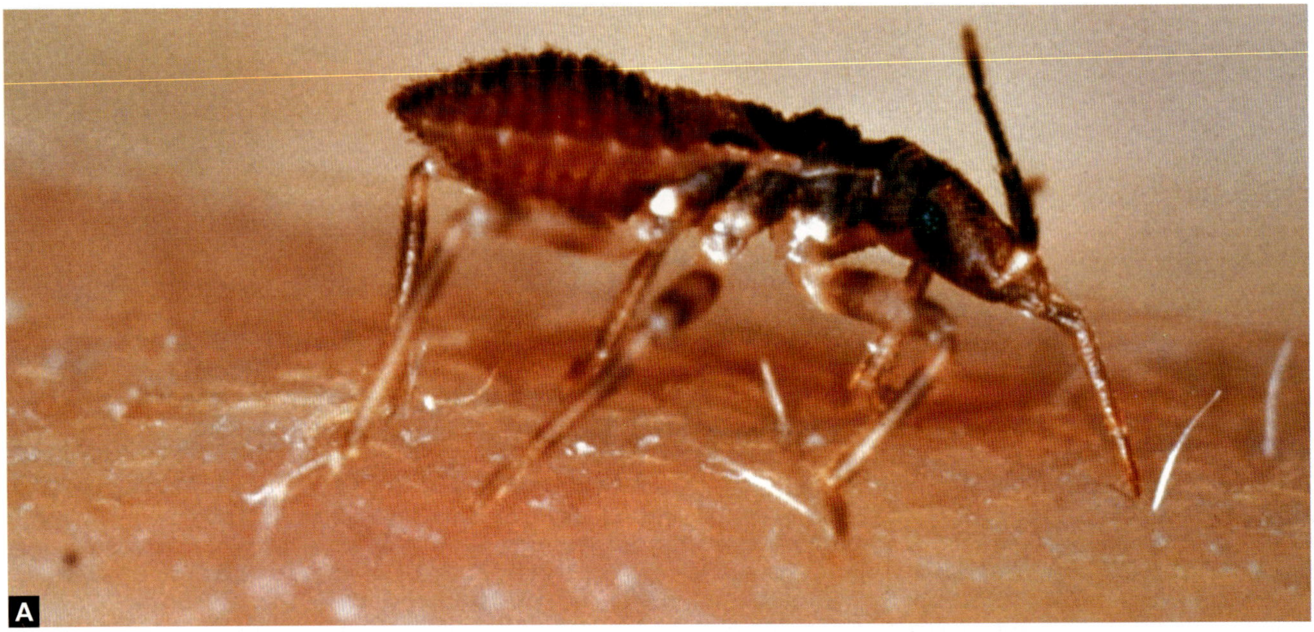

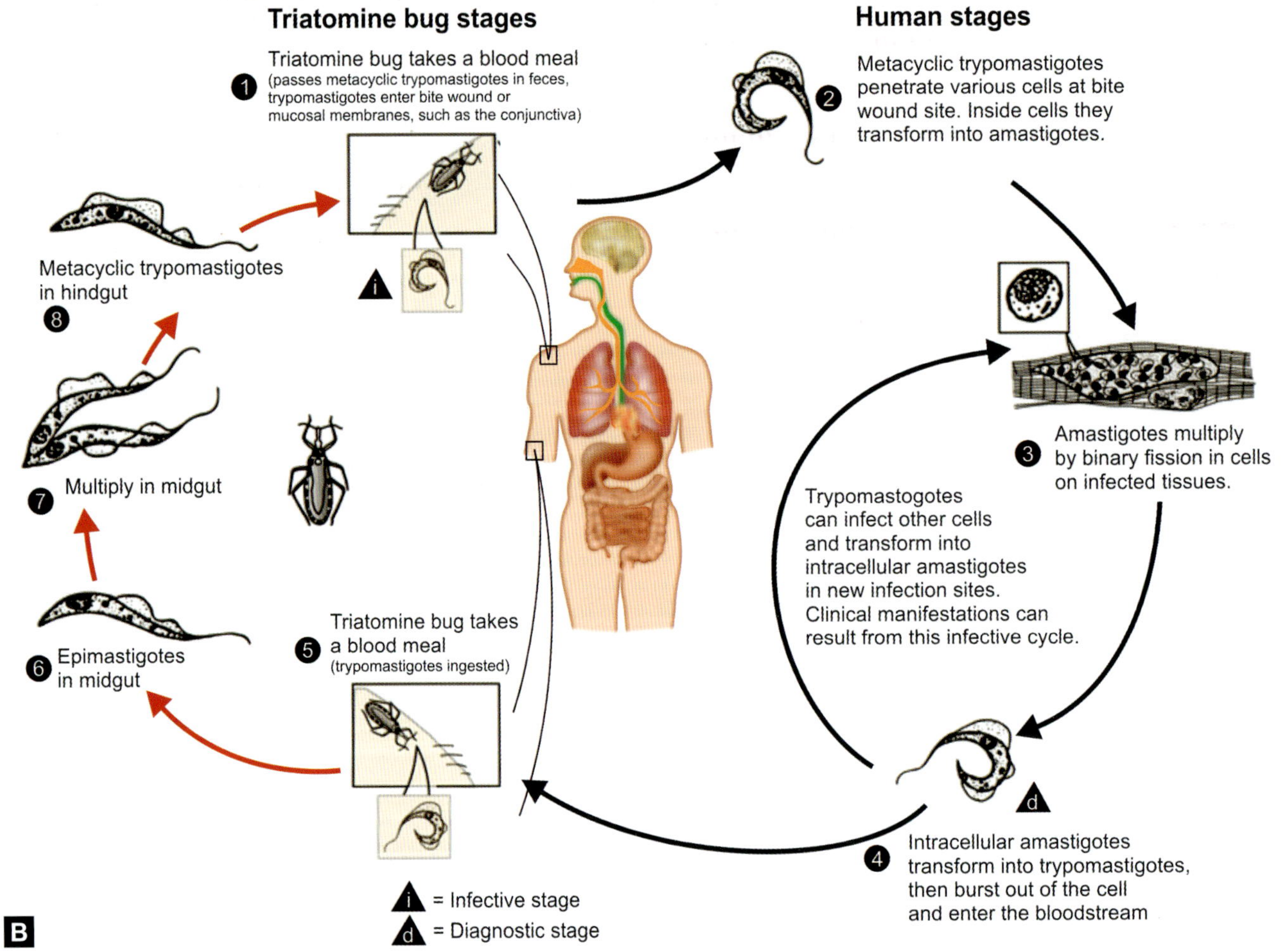

Figs. 20.18A and B: Chagas disease. (A) The vector for Chagas disease is *Triatoma infestans* of the family *Reduviidae*. It is also known as the "Kissing Bug", "Assassin Bug", or "Cone-Nose Bug". Chagas disease is caused by the parasitic protozoan *Trypanosoma cruzi*; (B) The lifecycle of T. Cruzi involves a trypomastigote form in the vector and an amastigote form in the human.

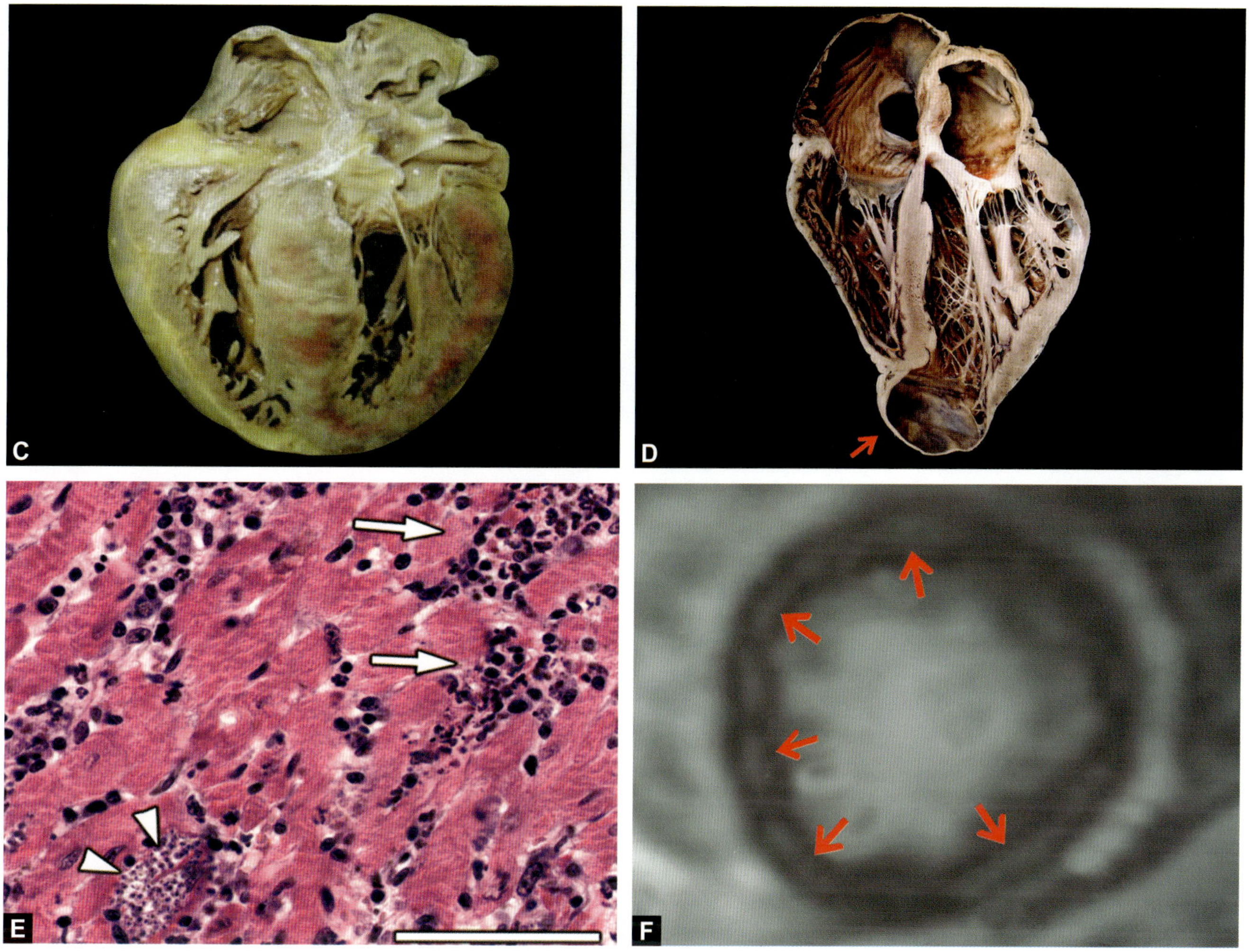

Figs. 20.18C to F: Pathological and histological findings and MRI in Chagas Disease: (C) Chagas disease gross specimen with pale and red areas corresponding to focuses of inflammation, necrosis, and hemorrhage; (D) Gross pathology specimen showing dilation of all four chambers and a large apical aneurysm (arrow); (E) Biopsy specimen with foci of mycocytolytic necrosis and degeneration are seen with an intense inflammatory infiltrate around ruptured pseudocysts of parasite (short white arrows). Intact intramyocyte parasite nest without inflammatory response (long white arrows); (F) Cardiac magnetic resonance imaging (MRI) of patient with Chagas disease with late gadolinium enhancement showing areas of mid-myocardial fibrosis. [Figure 20.18A from Center for Disease Control and Wikimedia Commons. Figures 20.18B and F from Kraft DC, Kerber RE. Chagas disease. In: Chatterjee K, Anderson M, Heistad D, Kerber RE (Eds). Cardiology: An Illustrated Textbook, 1st edition. New Delhi, India: Jaypee Brothers Medical Publishers (P) Ltd; 2012. pp. 1513-9. Figure 20.18C from Gonzales CI, Mantilla JC. Chagas heart disease. In: Veselka J (Ed) Cardiomyopathies—From Basic Research to Clinical Management. InTech. 2012. Figures 20.18D and E from Rossi MA, Tanowitz HB, Malvestio LM, et al. Coronary microvascular disease in chronic Chagas cardiomyopathy including an overview on history, pathology, and other proposed pathogenic mechanisms. PLoS Negl Trop Dis. 2010;4(8):e674].

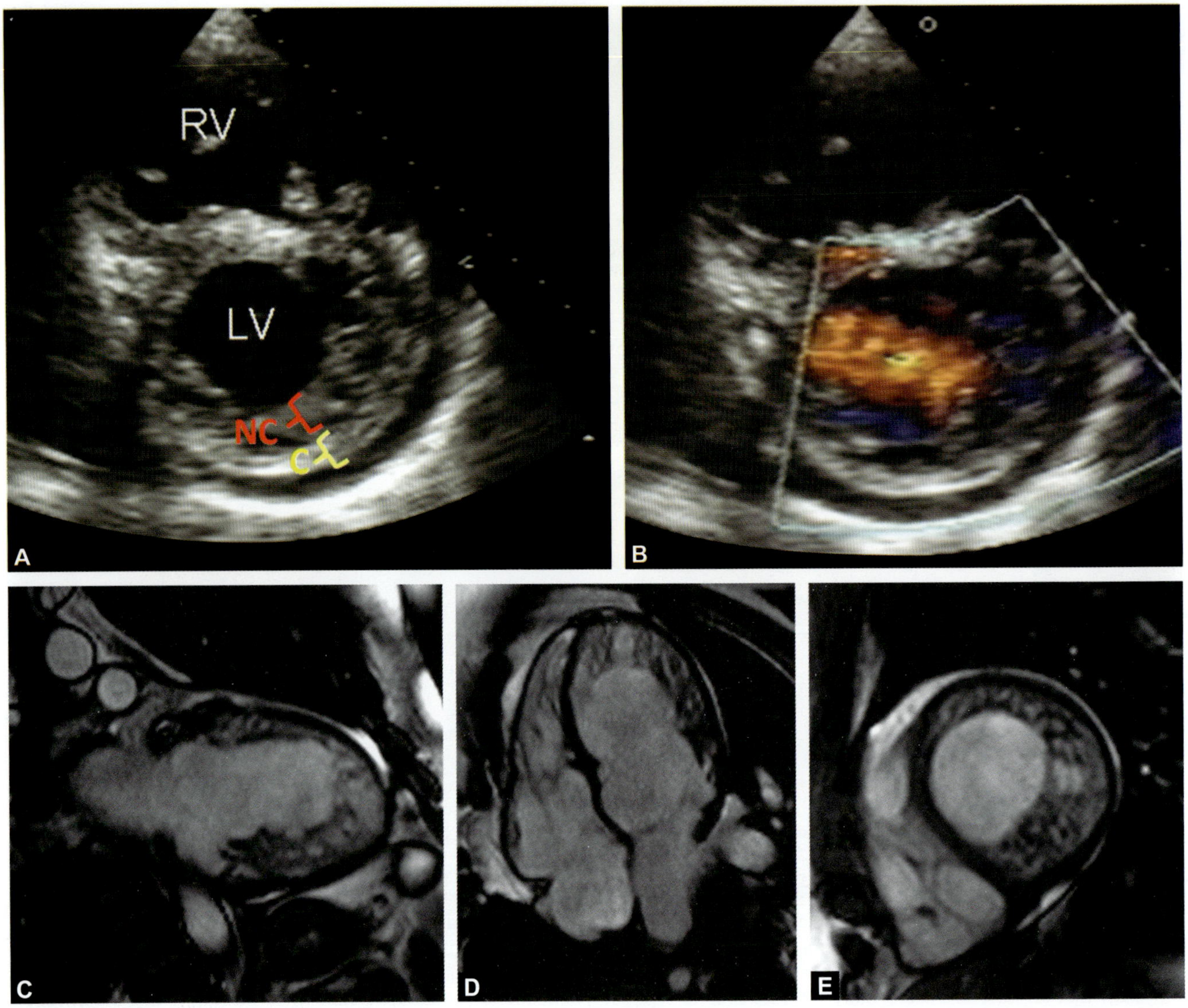

Figs. 20.19A to E: Noncompacted (NC) cardiomyopathy. NC cardiomyopathy is a congenital cardiomyopathy of defective endomyocardial morphogenesis resulting in failure of trabecular compaction of the developing myocardium. (A and B) Echocardiographic images—midventricular short-axis view. In the inferior and inferolateral walls, a portion of myocardium appears trabeculated and is NC compared to the compacted portion of the myocardium [C]; (C to E) Cardiac magnetic resonance imaging (MRI) with long-axis, four-chamber- and midventricular short-axis views in a patient with noncompaction. A portion of the left ventricular (LV) myocardium appears trabeculated [similar to the right ventricular (RV)] and is noncompacted compared to the compacted portion of the myocardium. Videos 20.3 to 20.5 show the MRI findings in noncompaction.

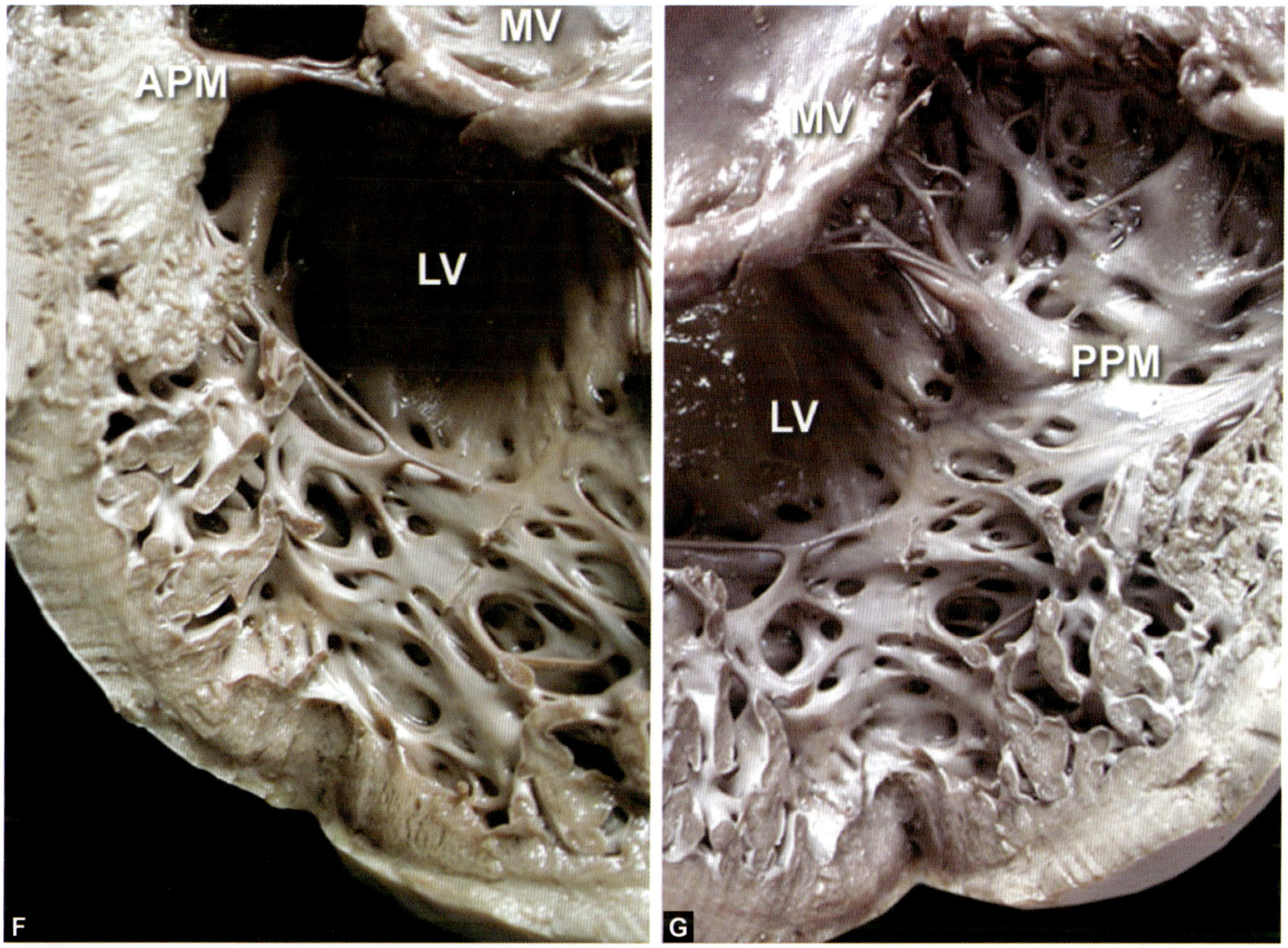

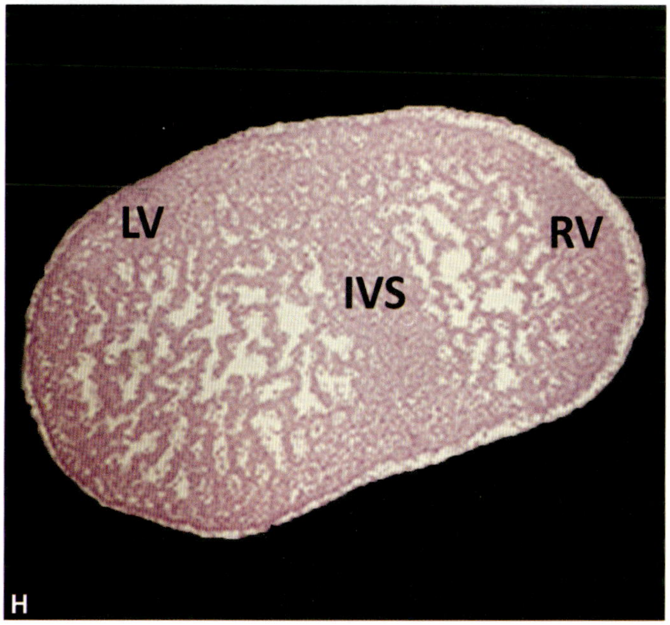

Figs. 20.19F to H: Pathology findings in non-compaction. (F and G) Gross pathology specimens of noncompaction; (H) Micrograph of a transverse section of the heart at the level of both ventricles showing noncompaction and extensively developed trabeculae that fill the ventricular lumen. [Figures 20.19A, B and H from Espinola-Zaveleta N, Soto ME, Castellanos LM, et al. Non-compacted cardiomyopathy: clinical-echocardiography study. Cardiovascular ultrasound. 2006;4:35. Figures 20.19C to E adapted from Strohm O, Shehab A, Qureshi A. Role of advanced cardiac magnetic resonance imaging in atypical cardiomyopathies such as Stress-Induced cardiomyopathies and left-ventricular non-compaction cardiomyopathy. In: Veselka J (Ed). Cardiomyopathies—From Basic Research to Clinical Management. InTech. 2012. Figures 20.19F and G courtesy of Dr Pradeep Vaideeswar, Professor (Additional), Department of Pathology (Cardiovascular and Thoracic Division), Seth SG Medical College, Mumbai, India. Image from Vijayalakshmi IB. Non-compaction of the ventricles. In: Vijayalakshmi IB, Rao PS, Chugh R (Eds). A Comprehensive Approach to Congenital Heart Diseases, 1st edition. New Delhi, India: Jaypee Brothers Medical Publishers (P) Ltd.; 2013. pp. 697-711]. (NC: Noncompacted; LV: Left ventricle; RV: Right ventricle; MV: Mitral valve; APM: Anterior papillary muscle; PPM: Posterior papillary muscle; IVS: Interventricular septum).

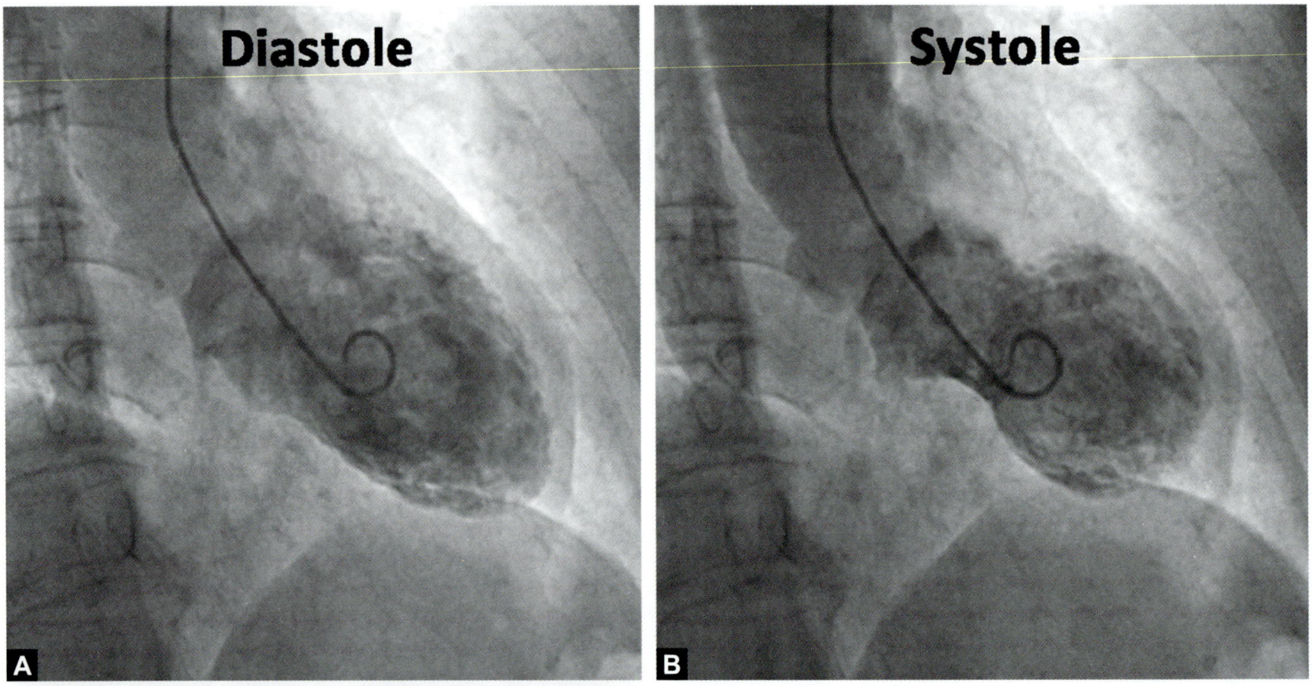

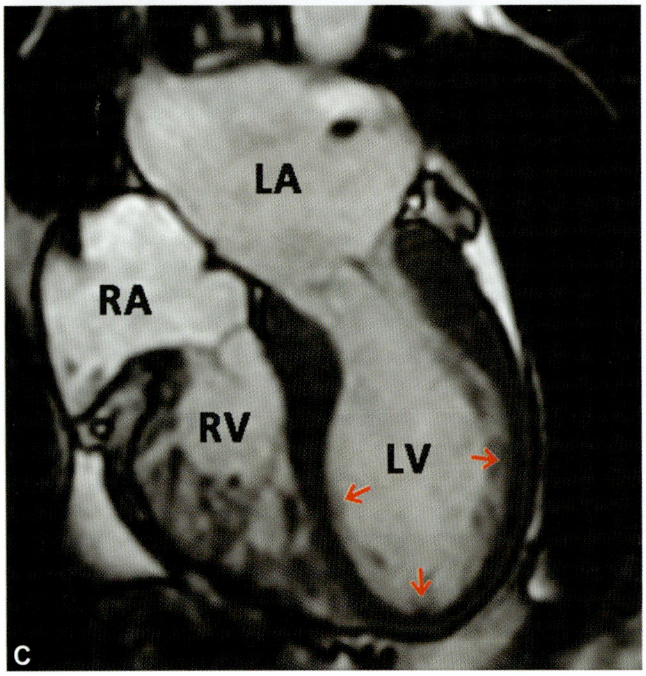

Figs. 20.20A to C: Takotsubo cardiomyopathy (stress-induced cardiomyopathy). Takotsubo cardiomyopathy is a type of nonischemic cardiomyopathy which occurs suddenly, can be triggered by severe emotional stress, and is usually reversible. It is characterized by transient apical ballooning as shown. (A) Left ventricular (LV) angiogram at end diastole; and (B) at end systole. At end systole, the mid and apical walls are hypo- to akinetic while the base contracts normally. This gives the appearance of a Japanese fishing device called "Takotsubo" which is used to catch an octopus. (C) Cardiac magnetic resonance imaging (MRI) of a patient with Takotsubo cardiomyopathy. Mid and apical akinesis to dyskinesias (arrows) with normal basal contraction is seen. [Figures 20.20A and B from Lee JW, Lim HK, Kim JY, et al. Stress-induced cardiomyopathy: clinical observation. In: Veselka J (Ed). Cardiomyopathies—From Basic Research to Clinical Management. InTech. 2012. Figure 20.20C from Olimulder MA, Galjee MA, Es JV, et al. The use of contrast-enhanced cardiovascular magnetic resonance imaging in cardiomyopathies. In: Veselka J (Ed). Cardiomyopathies—From Basic Research to Clinical Management. InTech. 2012].

VIDEO LEGENDS

Videos 20.1 to 20.3: Representative magnetic resonance imaging (MRI) video clips of left ventricular (LV) noncompaction. (Videos courtesy of Flamm SD, MD).

Video 20.4: Example of noncompaction demonstrated on four chamber magnetic resonance imaging (MRI).

Video 20.5: Example of noncompaction demonstrated on short-axis magnetic resonance imaging (MRI).

REFERENCES

Cooper LT, Baughman KL, Feldman AM, et al. The role of endomyocardial biopsy in the management of cardiovascular disease: A Scientific Statement from the American Heart Association, the American College of Cardiology, and the European Society of Cardiology. J Am Coll Cardiol. 2007; 50(19):1914-31.

Go AS, Mozaffarian D, Roger VL, et al. Heart disease and stroke statistics—2013 Update: a report from the American Heart Association. Circulation. 2013;127(1):e6-245.

Kubanek M, Sramko M, Maluskova J, et al. Novel Predictors of Left Ventricular Reverse Remodeling in Individuals With Recent-Onset Dilated Cardiomyopathy. J Am Coll Cardiol. 2013;61(1):54-63.

Lang RM, Bierig M, Devereux RB, et al. Recommendations for chamber quantification: a report from the American Society of Echocardiography's Guidelines and Standards Committee and the Chamber Quantification Writing Group, developed in conjunction with the European Association of Echocardiography, a branch of the European Society of Cardiology. J Am Soc Echocardiogr. 2005;18(12):1440-63.

Pinamonti B, Zecchin M, Di Lenarda A, et al. Persistence of restrictive left ventricular filling pattern in dilated cardiomyopathy: an ominous prognostic sign. J Am Coll Cardiol. 1997;29(3):604-12.

Quarta G, Sado DM, Moon JC. Cardiomyopathies: focus on cardiovascular magnetic resonance. Br J Radiol. 2011;84 (Spec No 3):S296-305.

Rao VU, De Marco T. Cardiac Biopsy. In Cardiology—an illustrated Textbook. Chatterjee R et al. New Delhi, India: Jaypee Brothers Medical Publishers (P) Ltd.

Yancy CW, Jessup M, Bozkurt B, et al. 2013 ACCF/AHA Guideline for the Management of Heart Failure: a report of the American College of Cardiology Foundation/American Heart Association Task Force on Practice Guidelines. J Am Coll Cardiol. 2013;62(16):e147-239.

CHAPTER 21

Heart Failure with Preserved Ejection Fraction

A Afşin Oktay, Sanjiv J Shah

INTRODUCTION

Heart failure with preserved ejection fraction (HFpEF) is a common clinical syndrome that is increasing in frequency (Fig. 21.1). Patients with HFpEF (huff-puff) are predominantly elderly, more likely female than male, and have a high prevalence of comorbidities, such as hypertension, obesity, diabetes mellitus, chronic kidney disease, coronary artery disease (CAD), anemia, and atrial fibrillation. HFpEF is a leading cause of morbidity and mortality. Patients with HFpEF have impaired quality of life similar to end-stage renal disease, and they require frequent hospitalizations. Five-year survival after heart failure (HF) hospitalization is only 35–40% in patients with HFpEF.

Although HFpEF has been variably termed "diastolic dysfunction" and "diastolic heart failure", diastolic dysfunction is a pathophysiologic condition (rather than a clinical syndrome) due to impaired myocardial relaxation and/or decreased ventricular compliance. Diastolic dysfunction is often present in patients with HFpEF; however, it is now well-known that left ventricular (LV) longitudinal systolic dysfunction occurs in HFpEF, and there are

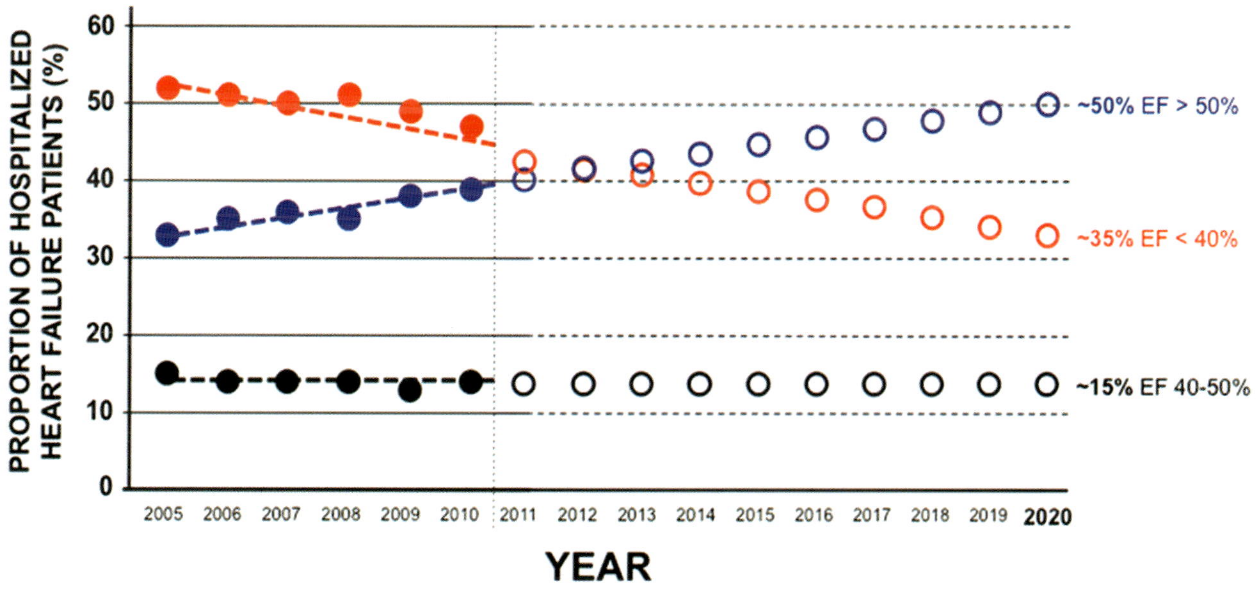

Fig. 21.1: The changing landscape of heart failure (HF): the projected trajectory of heart failure with preserved ejection fraction (HFpEF) in hospitalized HF patients. Based on results from Get with the Guidelines® Heart Failure (GWTG-HF) Study (Steinberg BA, Zhao X, Heidenreich PA, et al. Trends in patients hospitalized with heart failure and preserved left ventricular ejection fraction: prevalence, therapies, and outcomes. Circulation. 2012;126(1):65-75; N=110,621), using actual data on the proportion of hospitalized patients with three types of HF [HFpEF (EF > 50%); HFrEF (EF < 40%); and HF borderline-EF (EF 40–50%)] at each time point between 2005 and 2010. The trajectories for 2011–2020 were estimated for HFpEF and heart failure with reduced ejection fraction (HFrEF) using linear regression analyses, while HF borderline-EF was held at a constant 14% proportion of hospitalized HF patients. The regression equation for the projected HFpEF trajectory = −0.86 (Year) + 1771 (P = 0.015 for the trend of decreasing HFrEF over time); the equation for the projected HFrEF trajectory = 1.086 (Year) − 2144 (P = 0.008 for the trend of increasing HFpEF over time). [Image reproduced from Oktay AA, Rich JD, Shah SJ. The emerging epidemic of heart failure with preserved ejection fraction. Curr Heart Fail Rep. 2013;10(4):401-10, with permission].

several pathophysiologic mechanisms underlying HFpEF. It is therefore important to understand the difference between the terms "diastolic dysfunction", "diastolic heart failure", and "heart failure with preserved ejection fraction" (Fig. 21.2).

PATHOGENESIS AND PHENOTYPES OF HFpEF

The pathogenesis of HFpEF is multifactorial (Flow chart 21.1), and clinical presentations can vary considerably. What is consistent in patients with HFpEF is the presence of exercise intolerance. Environmental triggers, poor diet, comorbidities, and genetic susceptibility all unite to create a susceptibility to the HFpEF syndrome. However, patients can present as: (1) exercise intolerance alone (i.e. exercise-induced diastolic dysfunction); (2) volume overload; or (3) significant pulmonary hypertension and right HF (Flow chart 21.2). The clinical course, risk profile, and B-type natriuretic peptide (BNP) elevation varies by type of HFpEF clinical presentation.

From a clinical perspective, there are several distinct HFpEF phenotypes (Table 21.1). Understanding these HFpEF phenotypes can improve detection of the HFpEF syndrome and can guide treatment decisions. Examples of the specific types of HFpEF include right HF-predominant HFpEF with significant pulmonary hypertension (Fig. 21.3); hypertrophic cardiomyopathy-like HFpEF, which mimics genetic forms of hypertrophic cardiomyopathy; valvular-type HFpEF, the presence of multiple moderate valvular lesions in an elderly patient (Fig. 21.4, Videos 21.1 to 21.3); high-output HFpEF (Fig. 21.5); and rare causes of HFpEF (zebras) such as constrictive pericarditis (Figs. 21.6 and 21.7, Videos 21.4 to 21.6) and restrictive cardiomyopathies (Figs. 21.8 and 21.9, Videos 21.7 to 21.10).

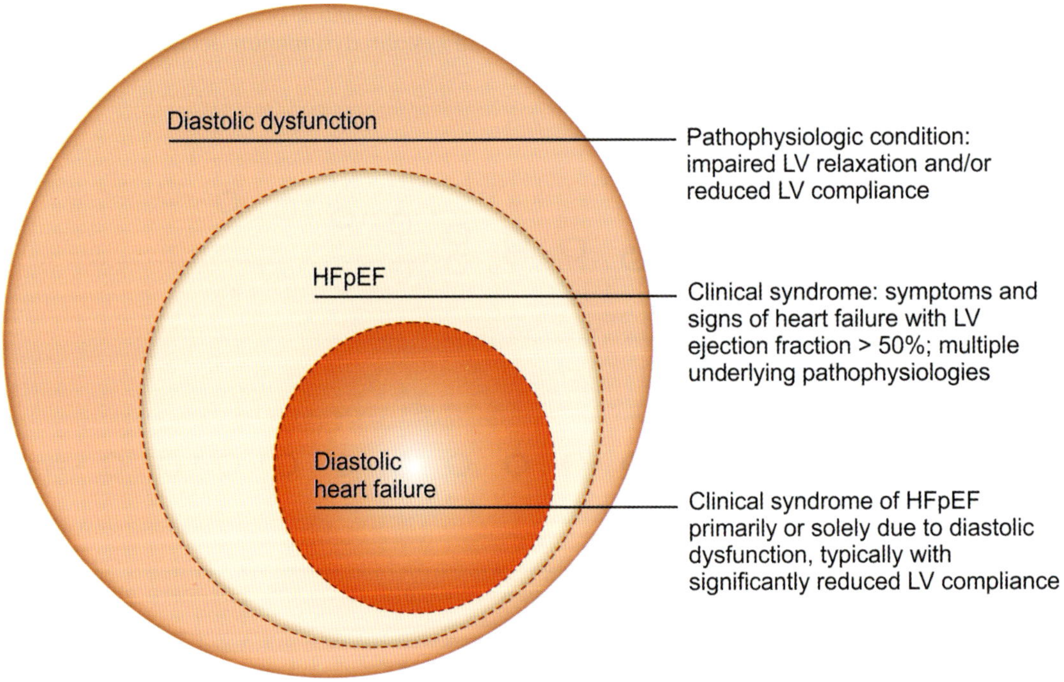

Fig. 21.2: Nomenclature of heart failure with preserved ejection fraction (HFpEF). Diastolic dysfunction is a pathophysiologic condition that is common in the general population and not necessarily associated with symptoms. HFpEF is present in the subset of patients with diastolic dysfunction who have evidence of signs and symptoms of heart failure and who also have a left ventricular (LV) ejection fraction > 50%. Of the large number of patients with HFpEF, some will have "pure" diastolic heart failure in which the pathophysiology of their HFpEF syndrome is primarily or solely due to diastolic dysfunction (typically with significantly reduced LV compliance). Although pathophysiologic studies of HFpEF have focused on this smaller subset of diastolic heart failure, most patients with HFpEF will have a more complex, multifactorial pathophysiology underlying their heart failure symptoms.

Flow chart 21.1: Pathophysiologic heterogeneity in heart failure with preserved ejection fraction (HFpEF). Although previously thought to be due to diastolic dysfunction alone, it is now clear that multiple pathophysiologic abnormalities are present mostly in HFpEF patients.

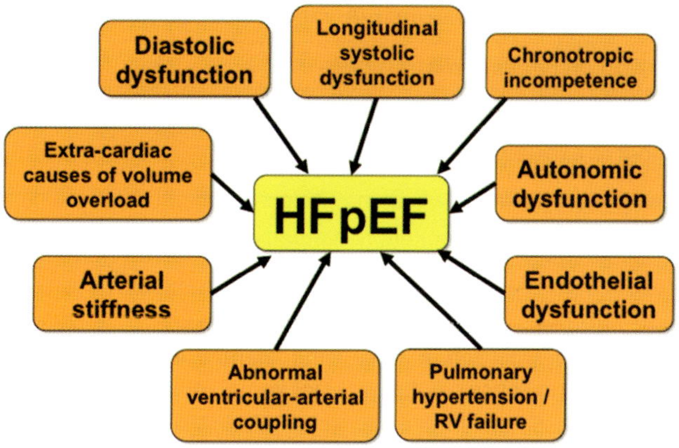

Flow chart 21.2: Theoretical schema of heart failure with preserved ejection fraction (HFpEF) patient types with sample patient risk profiles. Image modified with permission from Shah SJ. J Am Coll Cardiol 2013;62(15):1339-42.

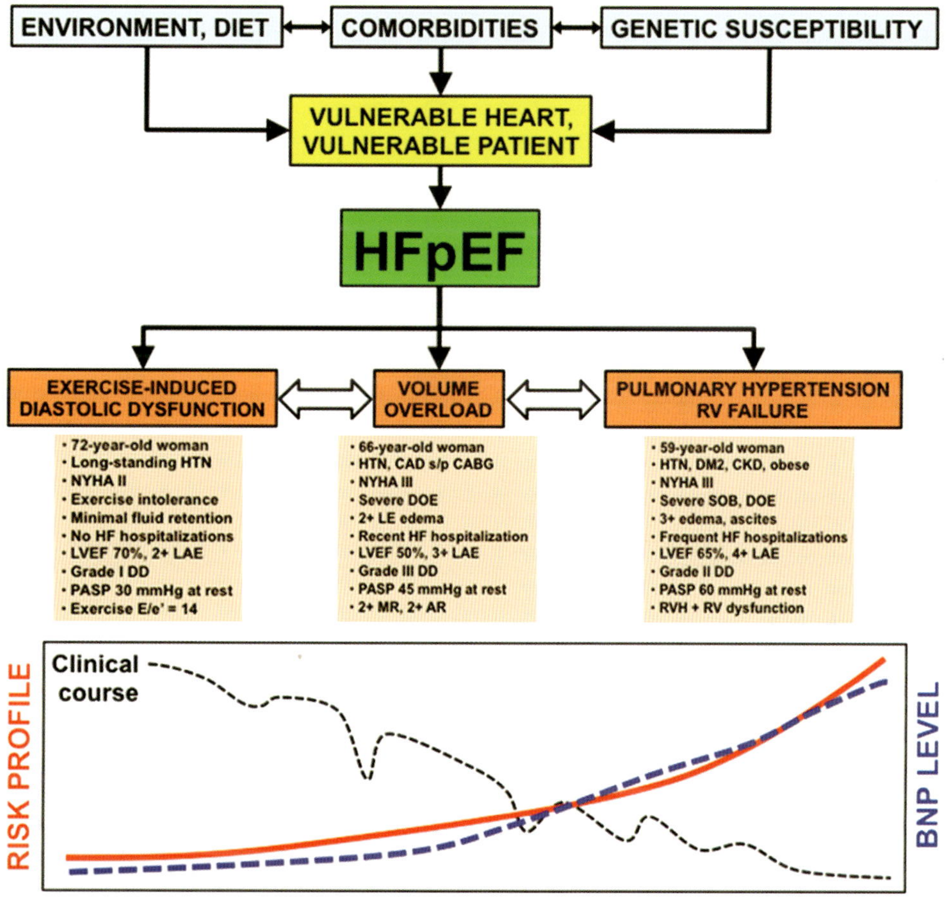

(HTN: Hypertension; NYHA: New York Heart Association functional class; HF: Heart failure; LVEF: Left ventricular ejection fraction; LAE: Left atrial enlargement; DD: Diastolic dysfunction; PASP: Pulmonary artery systolic pressure; E/e': Ratio of early mitral inflow to early mitral annular diastolic tissue velocity; CAD s/p CABG: Coronary artery disease status-post coronary artery bypass grafting; DOE: Dyspnea on exertion; MR: Mitral regurgitation; AR: Aortic regurgitation; DM2: Type 2 diabetes mellitus; CKD: Chronic kidney disease; SOB: Shortness of breath; RVH: Right ventricular hypertrophy; RV: Right ventricular; BNP: B-type natriuretic peptide).

Table 21.1: Phenotypic classification of heart failure with preserved ejection fraction. (HFpEF: heart failure with preserved ejection fraction; PAH: pulmonary arterial hypertension; PDE5: phosphodiesterase-5; PA: pulmonary artery; LV: left ventricular; AV: arterio-venous; MRI: magnetic resonance imaging; HF: heart failure; E/A: ratio of peak early to late diastolic filling velocity).

HFpEF phenotype	*Diagnosis and management strategies*
Garden-variety HFpEF	• Besides treatment of hypertension and fluid overload, management of comorbidities will be essential • Remember to exclude other causes of HFpEF
Coronary artery disease-HFpEF	• Consider revascularization which may help symptoms • Aggressive medical management of coronary artery disease is essential
Right heart failure-predominant HFpEF	• Differentiate from PAH using history/risk factors, echocardiography, and invasive hemodynamic testing • On echocardiography, increased left atrial size, interatrial septum bowing from left to right, grade 2 or worse diastolic dysfunction, and elevated lateral E/e' ratio all favor HFpEF over PAH (i.e. intrinsic pulmonary vascular disease); note that right ventricular size and systolic dysfunction, and interventricular septal flattening do not differentiate pulmonary hypertension due to HFpEF versus PAH • Treatment strategies include diuresis, ultrafiltration, digoxin, midodrine (to support systemic blood pressure in cases of systemic hypotension due to poor forward stroke volume due to right heart failure), and PDE5 inhibition if superimposed PAH is present (i.e. if PA diastolic pressure—pulmonary capillary wedge pressure > 5 mm Hg)
Atrial fibrillation-predominant HFpEF	• Typically have normal or easily controlled blood pressure with atrial fibrillation driving their clinical symptoms • Typically require rate/rhythm control more than antihypertensive therapy • Trial of cardioversion or ablation, especially if very symptomatic with loss of atrial contraction • Anticoagulation unless contraindicated
Hypertrophic cardiomyopathy-like HFpEF	• Echocardiography indistinguishable from genetic forms of hypertrophic cardiomyopathy but these patients present later in life and often have a history of long-standing hypertension • Verapamil, diltiazem, long-acting metoprolol; cautious use of diuretics and vasodilators (use only if absolutely necessary)
Multivalvular HFpEF	• Severe valvular disease (stenotic or regurgitant) is typically an exclusion criteria for the diagnosis of HFpEF • Some patients, particularly the elderly will have multiple moderate valvular lesions, which combine with evidence of diastolic dysfunction and LV hypertrophy to produce the HF syndrome • Medical treatment of underlying valve disease if possible • Surgical treatment of valvular disease if indicated
High output HFpEF	• Look for 4-chamber enlargement, increased LV outflow tract velocity-time integral (> 22 cm at a heart rate of > 60 bpm), and/or high cardiac output at the time of right heart catheterization • Determine underlying cause of high output state (i.e. anemia, liver disease, AV fistula, hyperthyroidism, etc.) • Treat underlying cause of high output state • Diuretics/ultrafiltration typically necessary
Rare causes of HFpEF (zebras)	• Clues to the presence of a restrictive cardiomyopathy as a cause of HFpEF include systemic hypotension, severe diastolic dysfunction at a young age (< 60 years old), low QRS voltage on electrocardiography with increased LV wall thickness on echocardiography, decreased longitudinal systolic tissue velocities (s' < 5 cm/s) • Clues to the presence of constrictive pericarditis include a prominent diastolic interventricular septal bounce which is exaggerated on inspiration (can be seen on echocardiography or cardiac MRI), respiratory variation in the mitral inflow Doppler tracings, significant diastolic dysfunction (increased E/A ratio and short deceleration time) in the setting of preserved or normal e' tissue velocities, and discordance on simultaneous right and left heart catheterization • Cardiac MRI can be very useful in the work-up on these patients • Determine the underlying etiology and treat the underlying cause

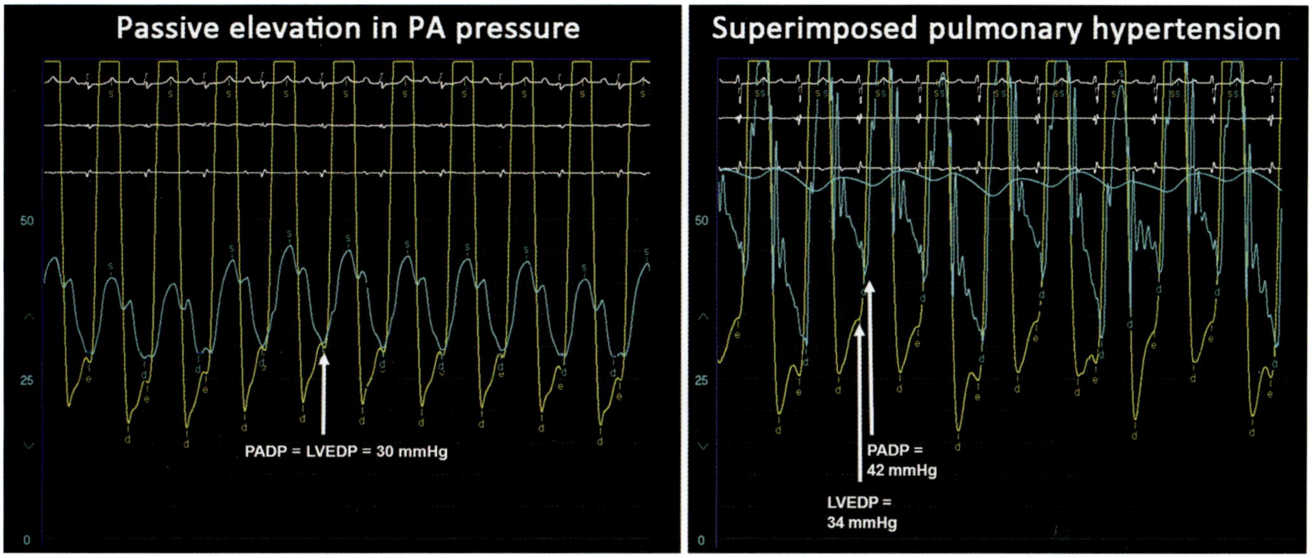

Fig. 21.3: Invasive hemodynamic profiles of pulmonary hypertension in the setting of heart failure and preserved ejection fraction. The majority of patients with heart failure with preserved ejection fraction (HFpEF) have pulmonary hypertension due to passive elevation in pulmonary artery pressures from increased left ventricular filling pressure. In these cases, as in the example shown in the left panel, pulmonary artery diastolic pressure (PADP, blue tracing) is equal to left ventricular end-diastolic pressure (LVEDP, yellow tracing), and both are elevated. The panel on the right demonstrates a patient with HFpEF and superimposed pulmonary arterial hypertension, which occurs but is a less common clinical scenario. In this patient, PADP exceeds the LVEDP by 8 mm Hg (normal PADP-LVEDP gradient < 5 mm Hg).

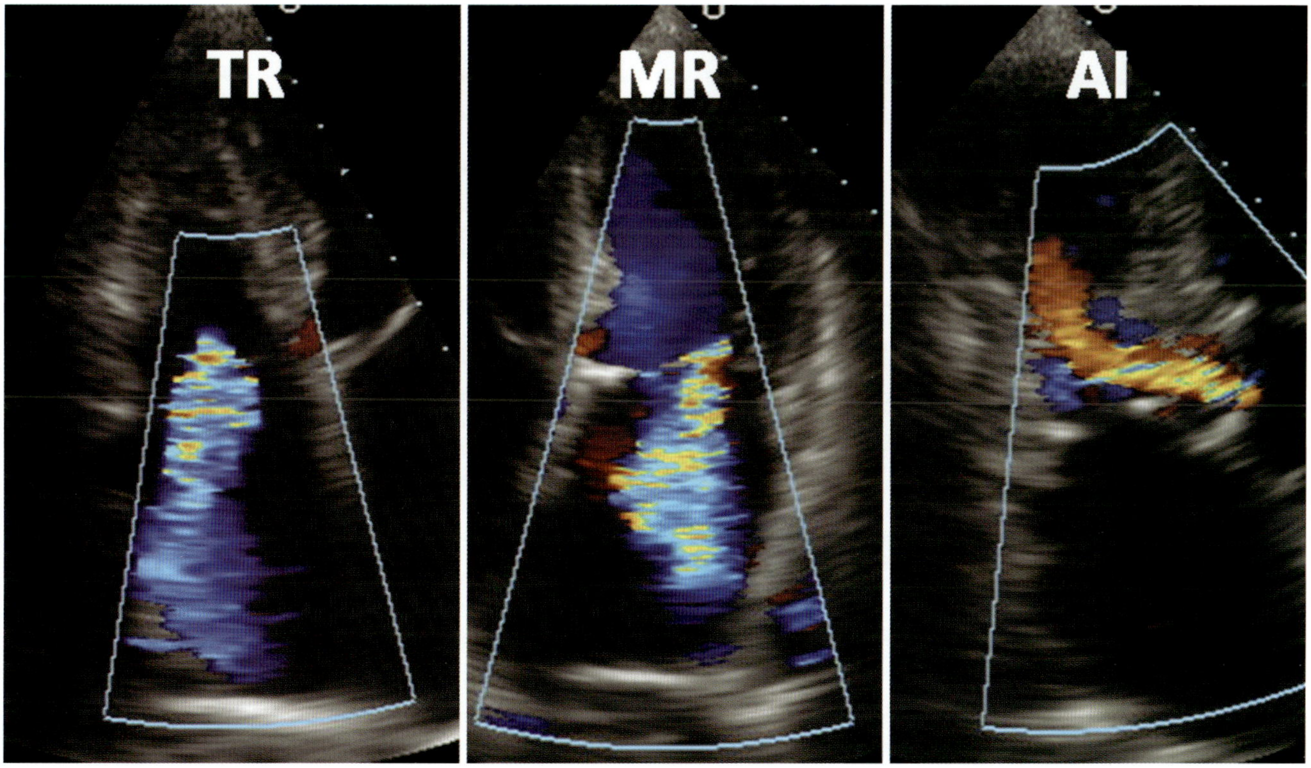

Fig. 21.4: Multivalvular heart failure with preserved ejection fraction (HFpEF). Some elderly patients with HFpEF have evidence of multiple valvular lesions. Although none of these valvular abnormalities (stenosis or regurgitation) are severe, in combination they can result in increased left ventricular (LV) filling pressure, and ultimately, the HFpEF syndrome. In the example shown, the left panel shows moderate tricuspid regurgitation, the middle panel shows moderate mitral regurgitation, and the right panel shows moderate aortic regurgitation. Besides these abnormalities, the patient also had concentric LV hypertrophy with basal septal hypertrophy, diastolic dysfunction, and significant left atrial enlargement, all of which are consistent with the HFpEF syndrome.

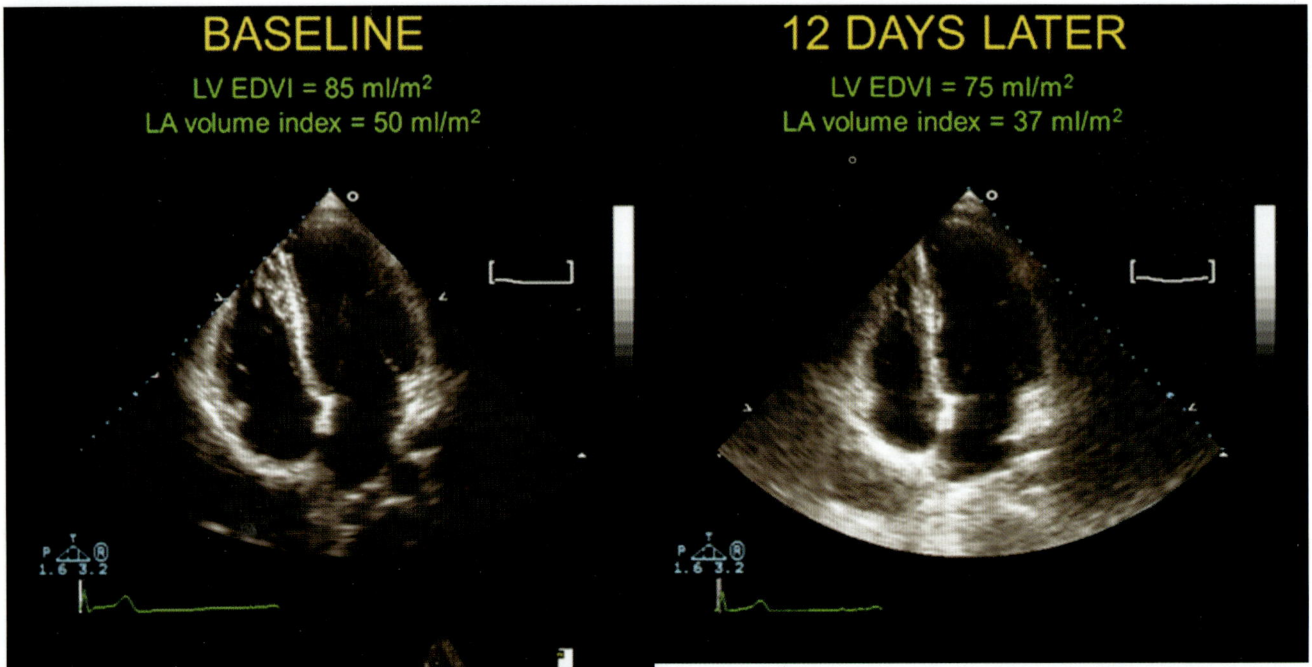

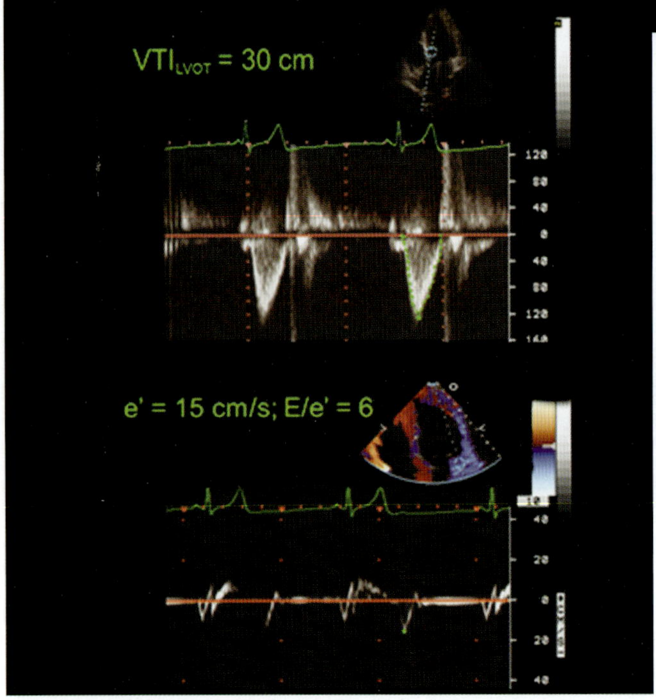

Fig. 21.5: High-output heart failure with preserved ejection fraction (HFpEF). Some patients with signs and symptoms of HFpEF have cardiac chamber enlargement, which is a clue to the presence of high-output heart failure. The example shown is of a young woman who was fasting while training for a marathon who developed shortness of breath, ankle edema, and an elevated B-type natriuretic peptide. Images in the left side of the figure show moderate left ventricular (LV) enlargement, severe left atrial enlargement, increased LV outflow tract velocity time integral, and normal diastolic function with preserved e' velocities, taken together as suggesting high-output heart failure. In this case, based on the history, thiamine (Vitamin B1) level was checked and found to be severely decreased. Thiamine supplementation resulted in rapid improvement of LV chamber sizes and symptoms. After only 12 days on thiamine supplementation, cardiac chamber sizes had decreased (right side of diagram) and the patient's symptoms had resolved.

DIAGNOSIS OF HFpEF

The diagnosis of HFpEF requires the simultaneous presence of signs and symptoms of HF, evidence of preserved LV ejection fraction [(EF) > 50%], and evidence of increased LV filling pressures at rest or with exertion.

There is no significant difference between clinical presentations of patients with HFpEF and heart failure with reduced ejection fraction (HFrEF). Exertional dyspnea, impaired exercise tolerance, paroxysmal dyspnea, and orthopnea are the most common symptoms in both conditions. Each may have similar signs of HF, such

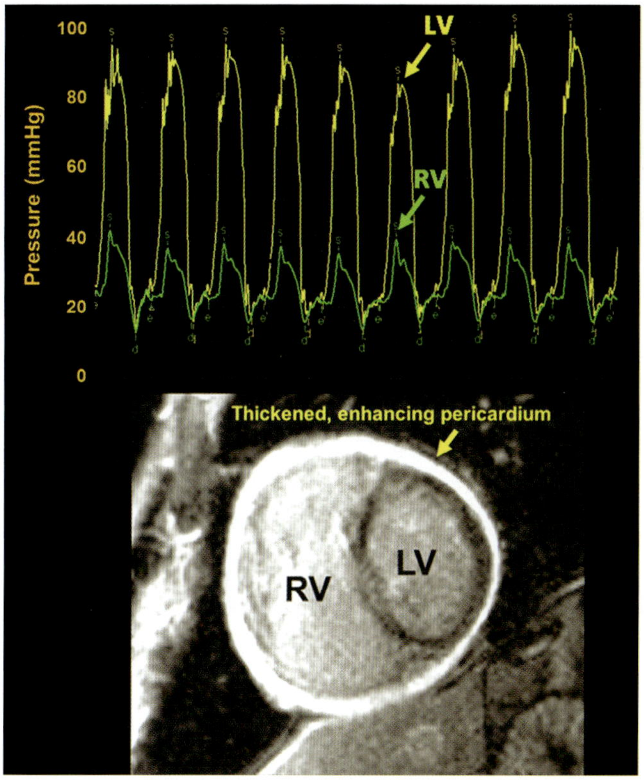

Fig. 21.6: Constrictive pericarditis presenting as heart failure with preserved ejection fraction. Top panel shows pressure tracing of the left ventricle (LV, yellow tracing) and the right ventricle (RV, green tracing). Diastolic pressure is elevated in both chambers. There is ventricular discordance, in which LV systolic pressure is increased when RV systolic pressure decreases, and vice versa. Lower panel shows magnetic resonance imaging (MRI) study with late gadolinium enhancement of a thickened pericardium.

as rales, edema, jugular venous distension, S3, S4, and hepatomegaly. Chest radiography findings, which include cardiomegaly, pulmonary vascular congestion, interstitial edema, and pulmonary edema are also common to both types of HF.

B-type natriuretic peptide is thought to have high negative predictive value in the diagnosis of HF as a cause of dyspnea. However, BNP is less helpful in the evaluation of patients with HFpEF compared to those with HFrEF. A normal BNP or N-terminal pro-BNP level does not exclude the diagnosis of HFpEF, especially in the outpatient setting. Overall, BNP levels tend to be lower in patients with HFpEF compared to those with HFrEF because diastolic wall stress (= LV diastolic pressure x chamber radius/wall thickness), thought to be the stimulus for BNP secretion from the myocardium, is lower in HFpEF compared to HFrEF. In addition, obesity is very common in HFpEF, and obesity has been associated with decreased BNP levels due to decreased BNP production and increased BNP clearance. Despite the lower BNP values in HFpEF, elevated BNP is still a potent predictor of adverse events in these patients.

Echocardiography is the cornerstone of the evaluation of patients with HFpEF due to its widespread availability and ability to provide comprehensive information about cardiac structure, systolic function, diastolic function, wall motion, valvular abnormalities, and hemodynamics (Fig. 21.10). These is no clear consensus for the EF cutoff for the definition of HFpEF; however, a "normal" or "preserved" EF is usually defined as EF>50% with LV end-diastolic volume index<97 mL/m^2 (i.e. absence of severe LV enlargement).

Invasive hemodynamic testing remains the gold standard for diagnosing elevated LV filling pressures. However, routine use of cardiac catheterization for the diagnosis of HFpEF is not common due to the invasive nature of the procedure. Thus, elevated LV filling pressures and diastolic dysfunction are most often diagnosed by echocardiography using spectral Doppler and tissue Doppler techniques (Figs. 21.11 and 21.12). Diagnosis of HFpEF may be challenging in patients with early stages of the HFpEF syndrome since echocardiography may show only mild diastolic dysfunction and normal or intermediate LV filling pressures. In patients with unexplained dyspnea or exercise intolerance, in whom HFpEF may be a possibility, exercise echocardiography (Figs. 21.13A and B) and cardiopulmonary exercise testing can be used to evaluate the patient. If the cause of dyspnea is still equivocal, exercise cardiac catheterization can be useful for the further evaluation of possible HFpEF (Fig. 21.14).

Although it is not as commonly performed as echocardiography, cardiac magnetic resonance imaging (MRI; Figs. 21.15A to D) can be very helpful in quantitating cardiac function, mass, and chamber sizes, and in elucidating the underlying cause of HFpEF, especially in cases where subendocardial microvascular ischemia, diffuse myocardial fibrosis, infiltrative cardiomyopathies, or constrictive pericarditis are diagnostic considerations. Advanced 4D MRI techniques are being used to assess diastolic blood flow over time (Fig. 21.16).

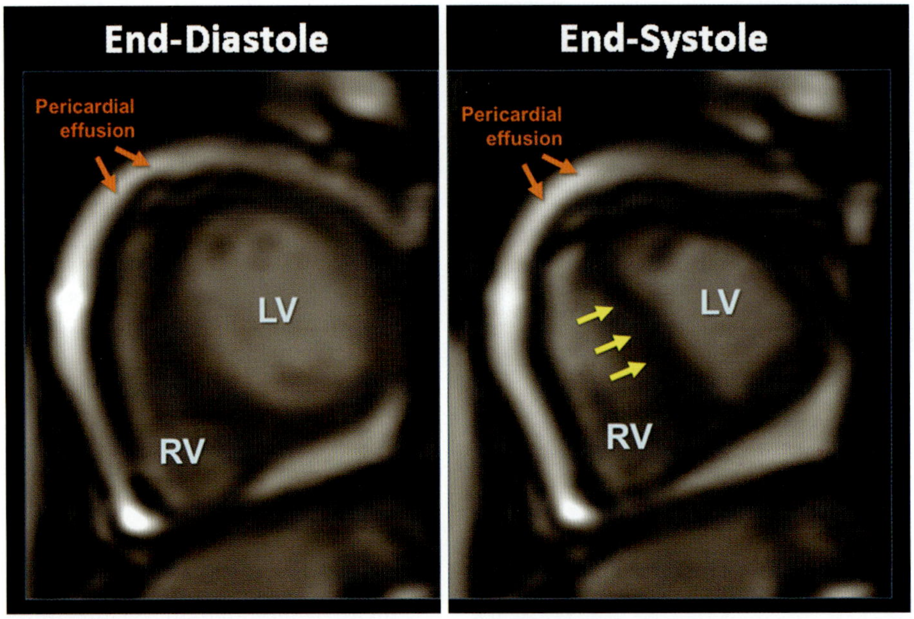

Fig. 21.7: Pericardial effusion and constriction causing heart failure with preserved ejection fraction (HFpEF) in a patient with systemic sclerosis. The example shown is from a patient with systemic sclerosis and signs and symptoms of HFpEF. There is a small-to-moderate sized pericardial effusion, which is resulting in decreased cardiac chamber compliance and ventricular interdependence. The diagram demonstrates dynamic interventricular septal flattening with inversion of the septum into the left ventricle (LV) during peak inspiration.

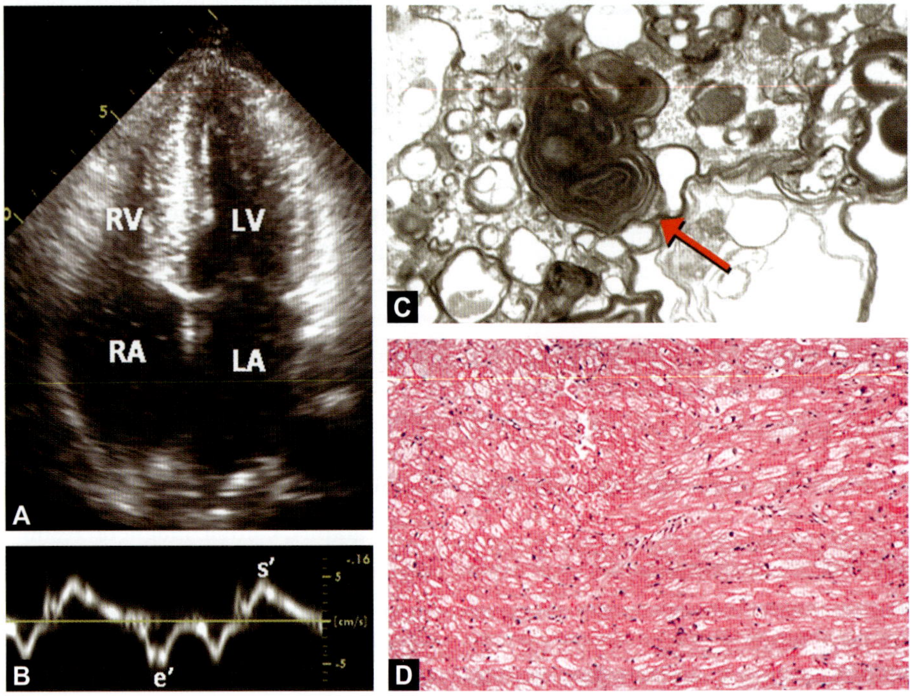

Figs. 21.8A to D: Restrictive cardiomyopathy. An elderly woman with long-standing rheumatoid arthritis and no other traditional cardiac risk factors developed progressive, severe heart failure (HF) symptoms due to hydroxychloroquine toxicity and resultant restrictive cardiomyopathy. (A) Echocardiogram showing small, thickened left ventricle (LV) and right ventricle (RV) with biatrial enlargement consistent with restrictive cardiomyopathy; (B) Tissue Doppler tracings demonstrate severe reduced (< 5 cm/sec) systolic (s') and early diastolic (e') tissue velocities, consistent with cardiomyopathy; (C) Electron microscopy of an endomyocardial biopsy specimen demonstrating myelin bodies (arrow); (D) Hematoxylin and eosin staining of the biopsy showing intense vacuolization (central clearing) of myocytes. These findings were pathognomonic of chronic hydroxychloroquine toxicity. Discontinuation of the drug resulted in improvement of HF symptoms.

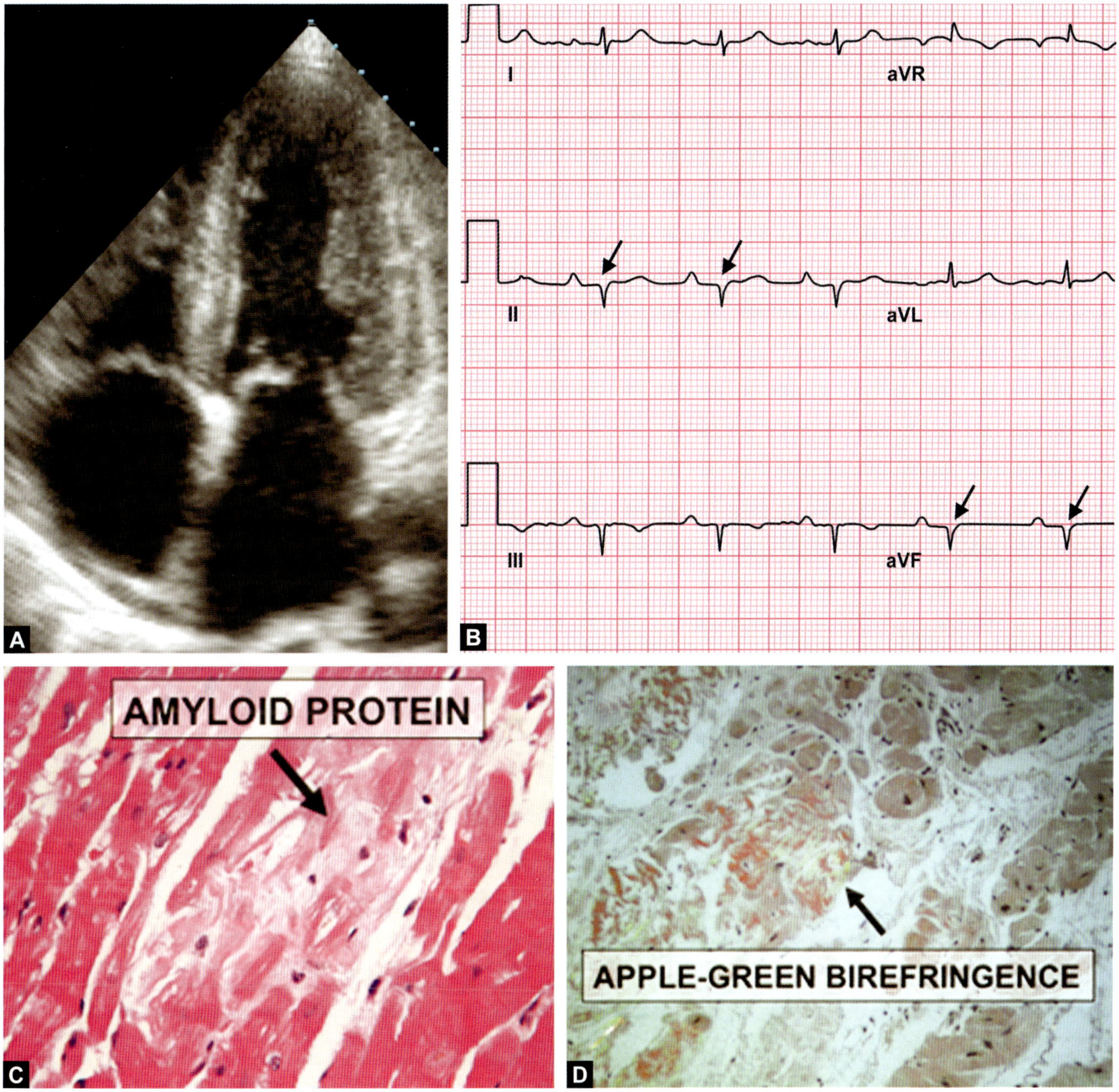

Figs. 21.9A to D: Restrictive cardiomyopathy due to transthyretin (TTR) cardiac amyloidosis. (A) Abnormal myocardial texture and thickened left ventricle (LV) and right ventricle (RV) with biatrial enlargement raise the possibility of infiltrative cardiomyopathy; (B) Electrocardiogram demonstrating low voltage QRS and pseudoinfarct pattern (arrows); (C) Histology of the endomyocardial biopsy specimen demonstrating the waxy-appearing amyloid deposits in the myocytes as well as (D) apple-green birefringence on polarized microscopy with Congo red staining. These findings are consistent with cardiac amyloidosis. Fiber typing revealed that TTR was the infiltrating protein, and the patient was found to have the V122I mutation in the *TTR* gene.

TREATMENT OF HFpEF

Treatment of HFpEF remains challenging due to lack of evidence-based therapeutic options for HFpEF. As described above, patients with HFpEF should be categorized into clinical phenotypes to target specific therapies towards specific types of HFpEF. Patients with HFpEF will

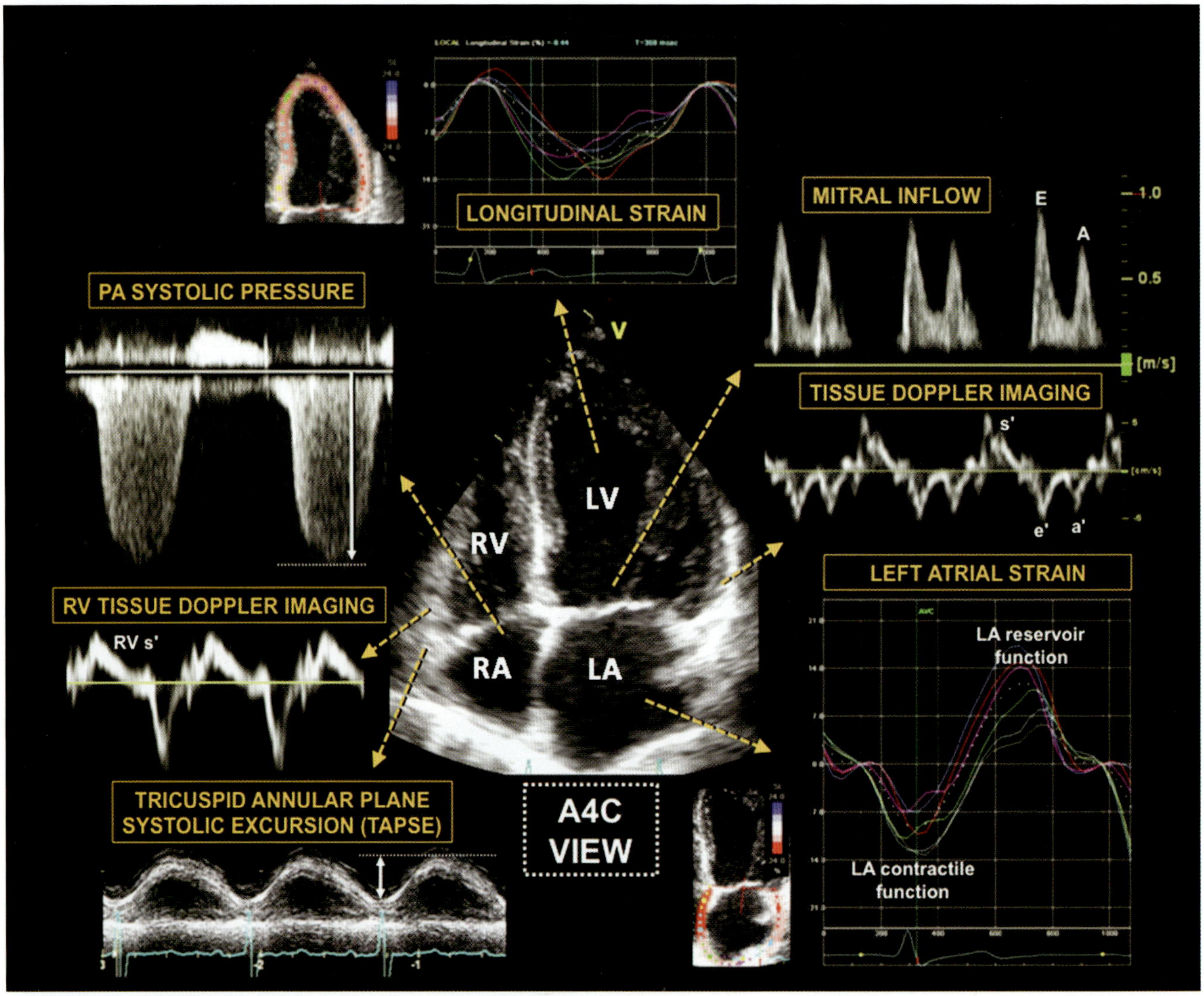

Fig. 21.10: Comprehensive echocardiographic phenotypic analysis of heart failure with preserved ejection fraction. Comprehensive echocardiography, including two dimensional, spectral Doppler, tissue Doppler, and speckle tracking, allows for detailed phenotypic analysis of cardiac structure, function, and mechanics in patients with heart failure with preserved ejection fraction. The figure shows examples of information that can be obtained from the apical 4-chamber view. Clockwise from the top: speckle-tracking echocardiography for assessment of LV regional and global longitudinal strain (early diastolic strain rate can also be obtained in this view). Mitral inflow and tissue Doppler imaging of the septal and lateral mitral annulus provide information on LV diastolic function grade and estimated LV filling pressure (E/e' ratio), along with assessment of longitudinal systolic (s') and atrial (a') function. Speckle-tracking analysis of LA function provides peak LA contractile function (peak negative longitudinal LA strain) and LA reservoir function (peak positive longitudinal LA strain). Tricuspid annular plane systolic excursion (TAPSE) and basal RV free wall peak longitudinal tissue Doppler velocity (RV s') provide information on longitudinal RV function, as does speckle tracking echocardiography of the RV (not shown). Finally, analysis of the tricuspid regurgitant jet Doppler profile, when added to the estimated RA pressure, provides an estimate of the PA systolic pressure. Additional data available from the apical 4-chamber view include assessment of LV volumes and ejection fraction, LA volume, and RV size and global systolic function (e.g. RV fractional area change). (Image reproduced from Butler J, et al. JACC Heart Fail. 2014 Apr;2(2):97-112 with permission). (LV: Left ventricular; LA: Left atrial; PA: Pulmonary artery; RV: Right ventricular; RA: Right atrial; A4C: Apical 4-chamber).

generally benefit from diuresis, blood pressure control, HF education (i.e. dietary sodium restriction, fluid restriction, daily weights), diagnosis and treatment of comorbidities, management of polypharmacy and medication interactions, routine follow-up, and close interaction with primary care and other providers for management of comorbidities. Figure 21.17 summarizes the key steps in diagnosing and treating HFpEF.

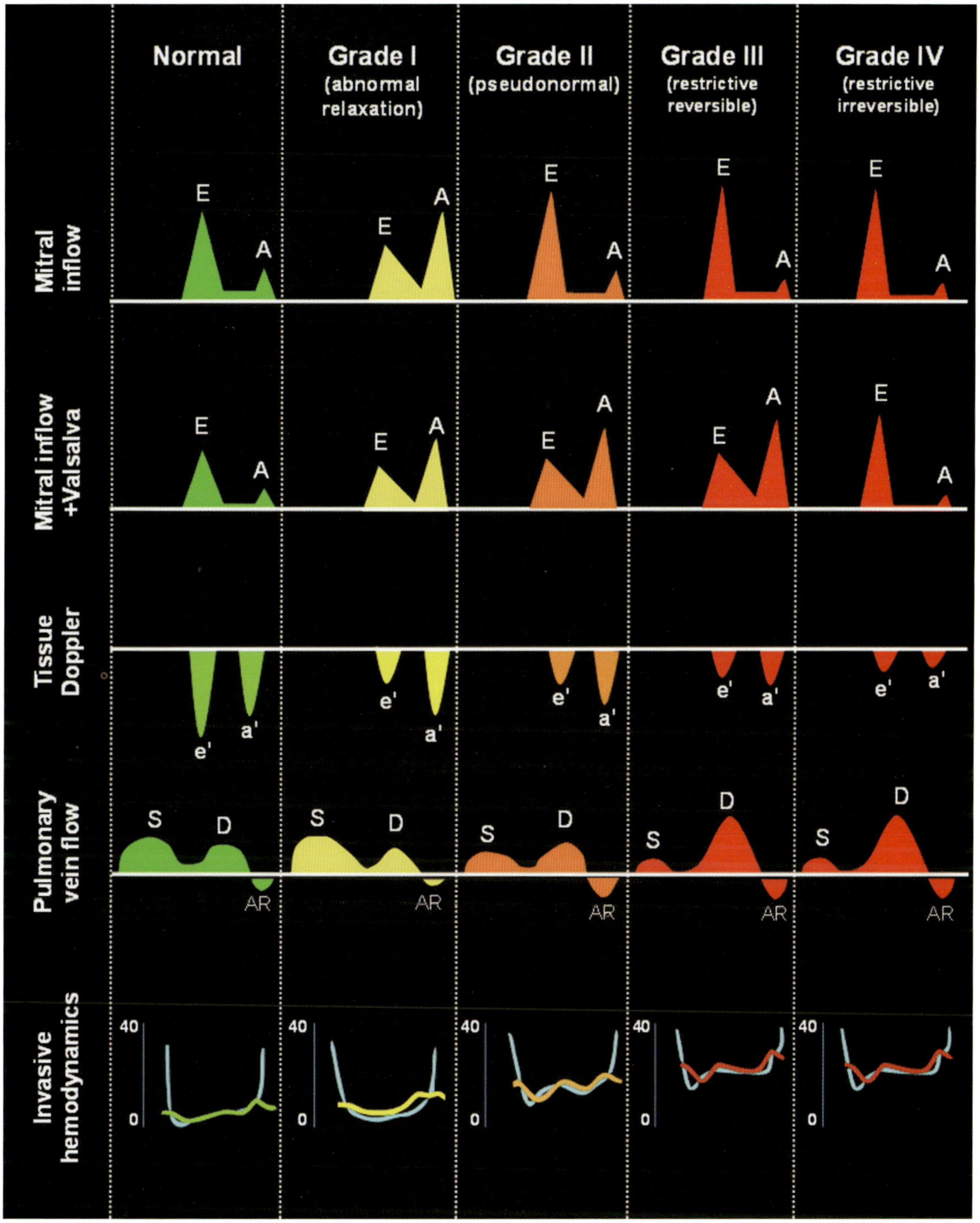

Fig. 21.11: Diagnosis and grading of diastolic dysfunction by spectral and tissue Doppler echocardiography, and the corresponding invasive hemodynamic findings. [Composite image created by Dr Sanjiv J Shah, based on (1) image from Mishra RK, Schiller NB. The left ventricle. In: Chatterjee K, Anderson M, Heistad D, Kerber RE (Eds). Cardiology: An Illustrated Textbook. New Delhi, India: Jaypee Brothers Medical Publishers (P) Ltd; 2013, (2) image created by Glenn N Levine, MD, and (3) image from Galderisi M. Diastolic dysfunction and diastolic heart failure: diagnostic, prognostic and therapeutic aspects. Cardiovasc Ultrasound. 2005;3:9]. (A: Transmitral flow during atrial systole; A_m: Mitral annular motion during atrial systole; E: Early diastolic transmitral flow; E_m: Early diastolic motion of the mitral annulus).

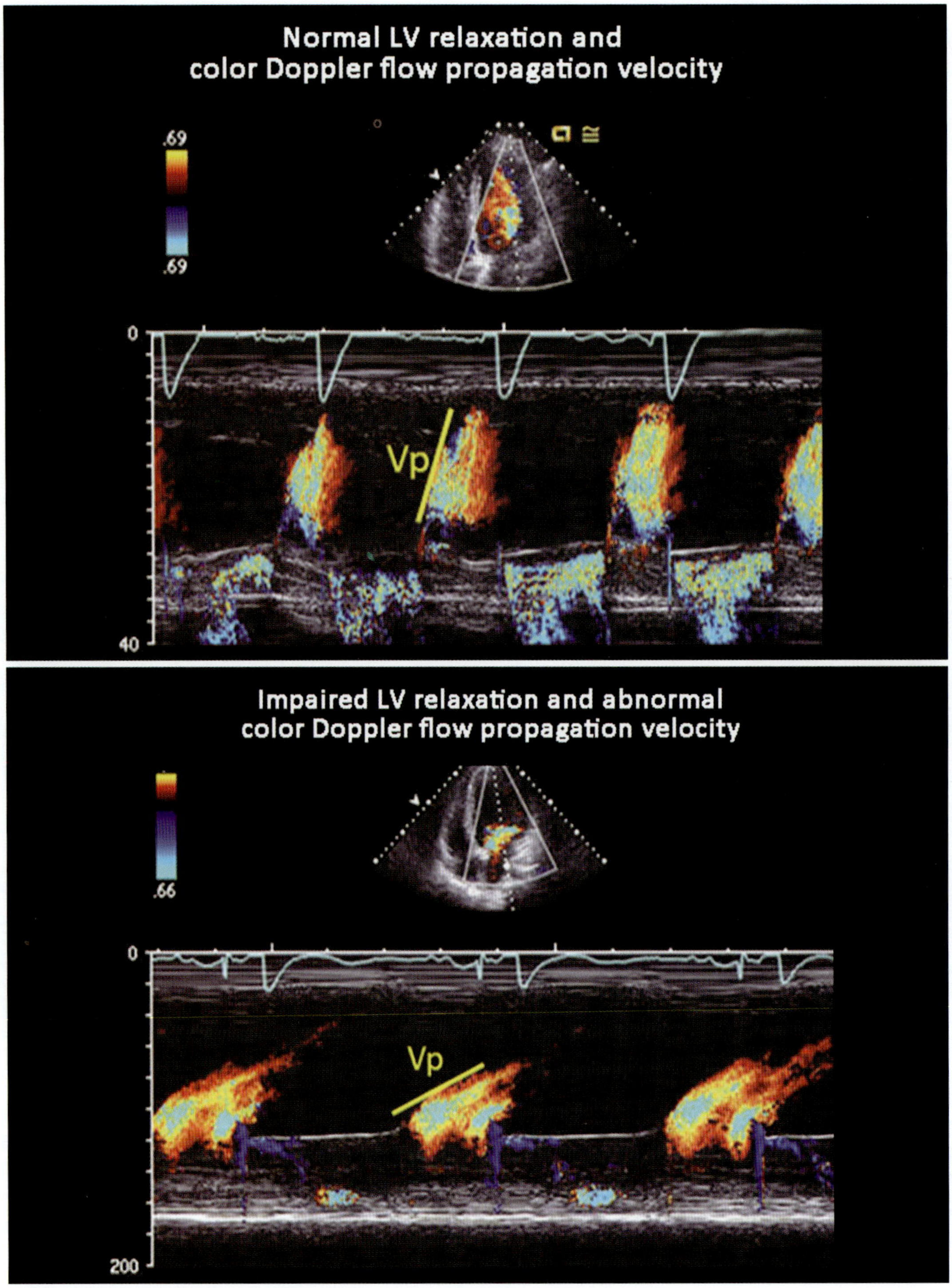

Fig. 21.12: Color Doppler flow propagation velocity (Vp) in the assessment of left ventricular (LV) diastolic function. The more rapid the LV relaxation, the faster blood travels from the mitral annular level to the LV apex, and the more vertical the color Doppler mitral inflow M-mode and the more rapid the Vp slope appears. Color Doppler flow propagation velocity in a patient with normal left ventricular relaxation is shown in the (top panel). In contrast, when there is impaired LV relaxation, it takes longer for blood to go from the mitral annulus to the LV apex, resulting in a "flatter" Vp slope (bottom panel). [Image and legend text adapted from Dokainish H. How to assess diastolic function. In: Nanda NC (Ed). Comprehensive Textbook of Echocardiography. New Delhi, India: Jaypee Brothers Medical Publishers (P) Ltd; 2014].

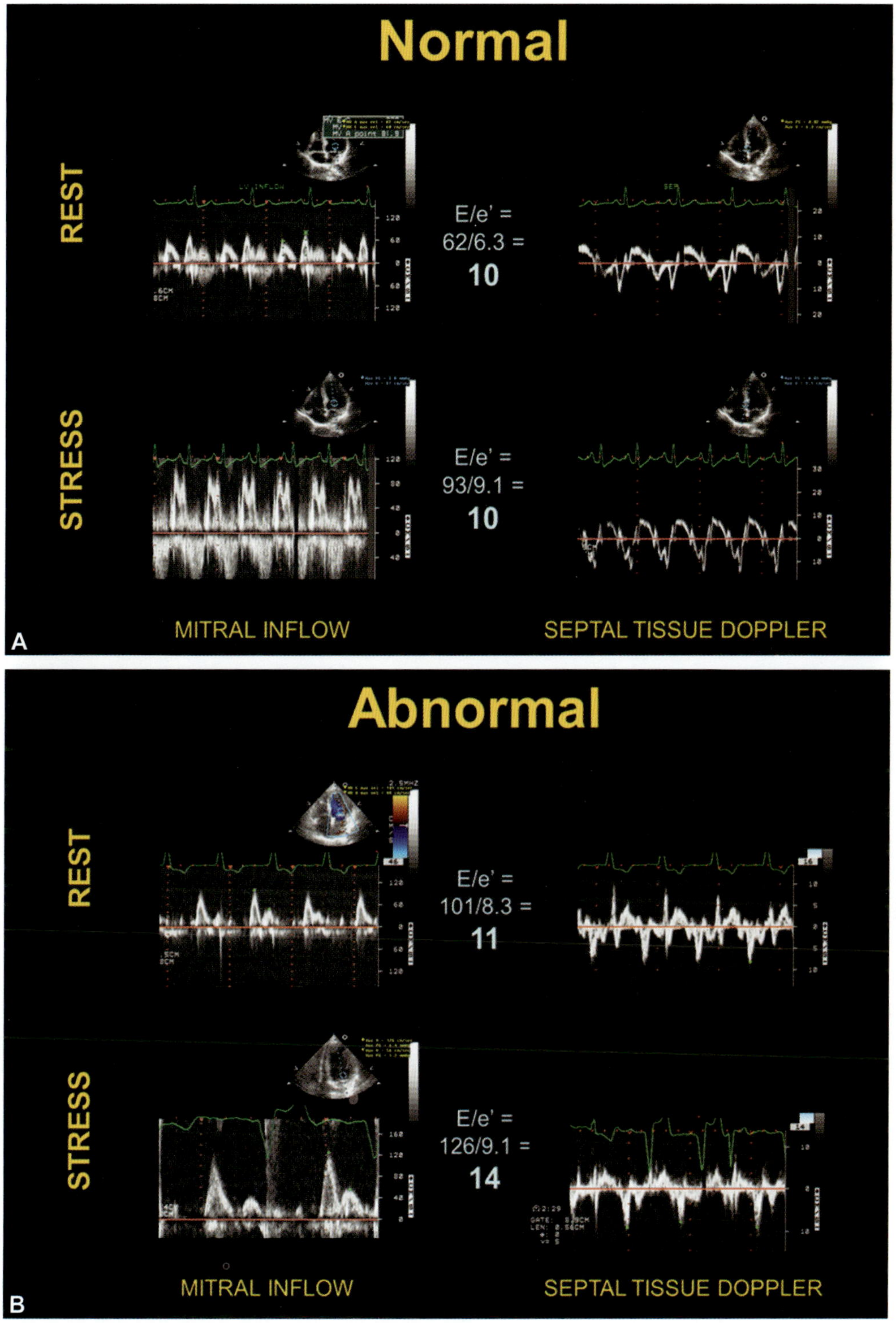

Figs. 21.13A and B: Diastolic stress echocardiography for the diagnosis of exercise-induced elevation in left ventricular filling pressure. (A) Normal mitral inflow and tissue Doppler response to exercise (E/e' ratio=10 at both rest and stress). The bottom panel demonstrates an indeterminate left ventricular filling pressure at rest (septal E/e'=11). In this patient, the grade of diastolic dysfunction, and its clinical significance, are equivocal; (B) Abnormal response to exercise. The E/e' ratio increases to 14 at peak stress, consistent with evidence of exercise-induced increase in left ventricular filling pressure (septal E/e' >13 is the cut-off shown to be associated with a rise in left ventricular filling pressures at peak stress, consistent with clinically significant diastolic dysfunction).

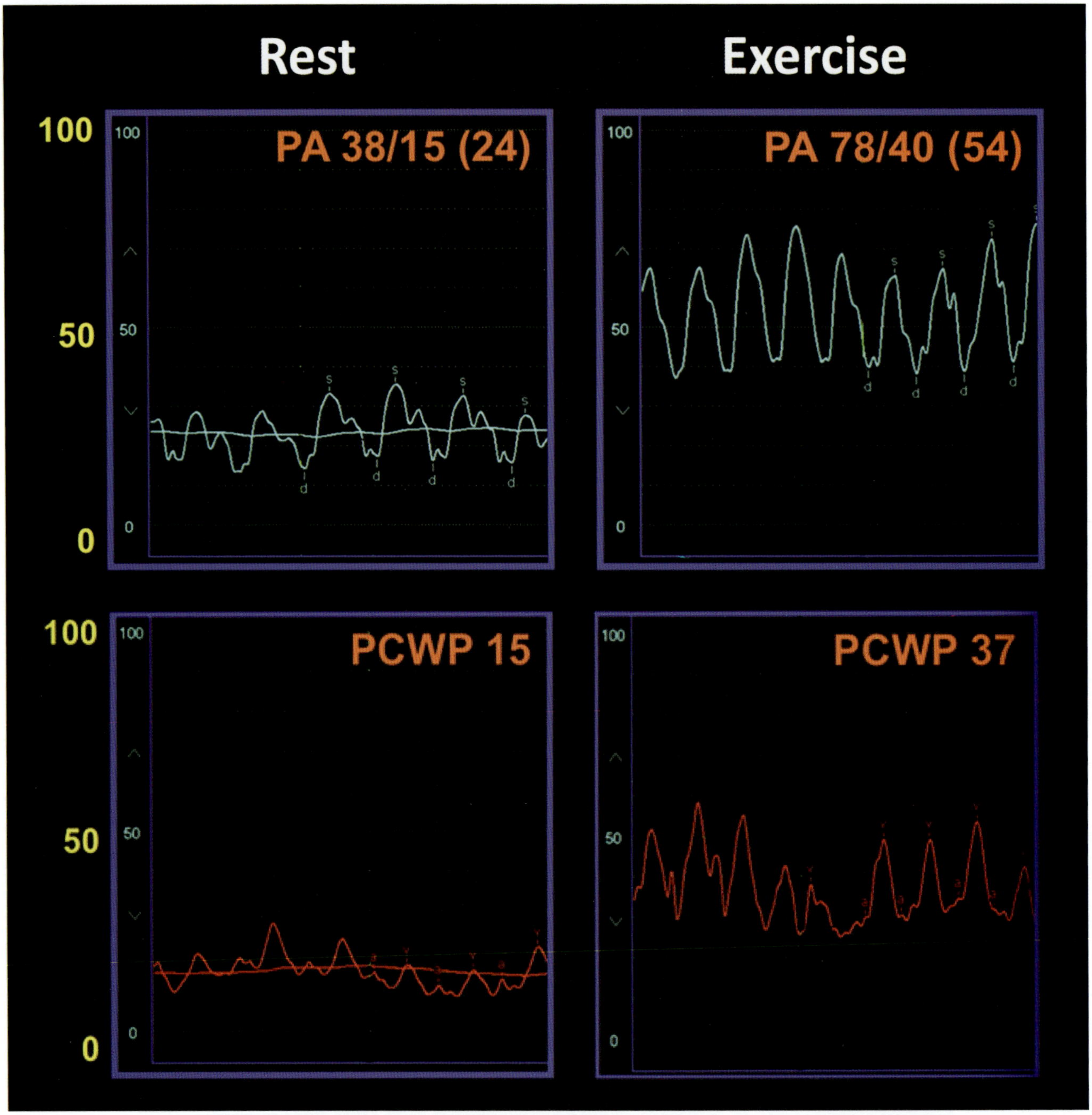

Fig. 21.14: Exercise hemodynamic testing for the diagnosis of exercise-induced elevation in left ventricular filling pressure. The top panels show pulmonary artery pressure and the bottom panels show the pulmonary capillary wedge pressure. In both the top and bottom panels, the Y-axis is pressure in mm Hg. The patient shown here has severe exercise-induced diastolic dysfunction and pulmonary venous hypertension. The rise in both pulmonary artery pressure and pulmonary capillary wedge pressure with minimal exercise (1-minute of supine, 25-watt bicycle exercise) is dramatic. Note the prominent V waves in the peak exercise pulmonary capillary wedge pressure tracing, which suggests a very stiff and non-compliant left ventricle. A resting right heart catheterization would have only revealed borderline mean pulmonary artery pressure and pulmonary capillary wedge pressure, and would have missed the severity of the diastolic dysfunction which was so prominent that the patient experienced exertional hemoptysis. (PA: Pulmonary artery; PCWP: Pulmonary capillary wedge pressure).

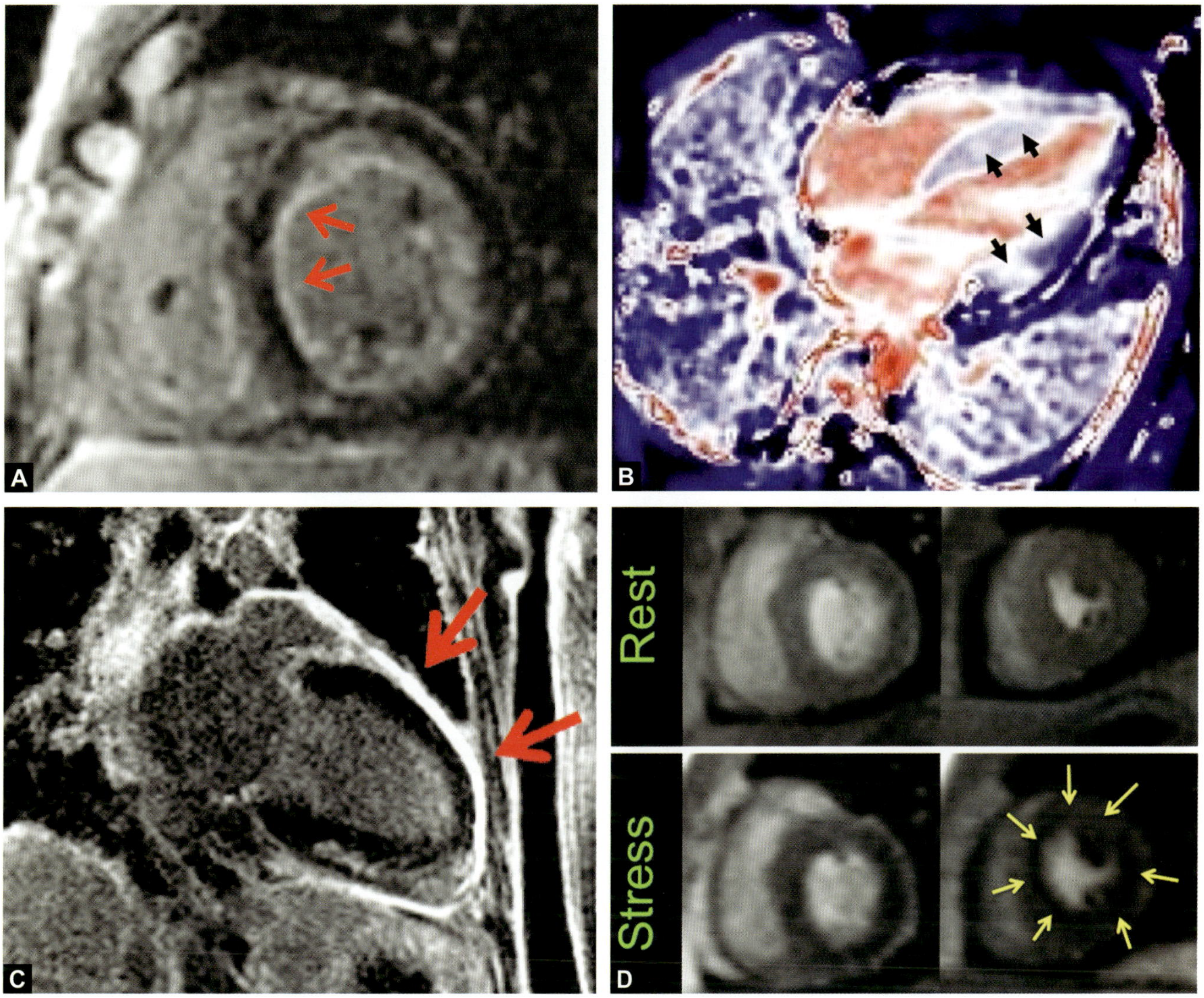

Figs. 21.15A to D: Cardiac magnetic resonance imaging for the diagnosis of myocardial and pericardial abnormalities in heart failure with preserved ejection fraction (HFpEF). (A) An example of subendocardial late gadolinium enhancement in a patient with cardiac amyloidosis (arrows); (B) T1 mapping in a patient with HFpEF showing diffuse myocardial fibrosis (small black arrows), with an extracellular volume fraction of 34%; (C) Pericardial thickening and enhancement in a patient with constrictive pericarditis (arrows); (D) Microvascular ischemia in a patient with HFpEF as denoted by the dark subendocardium at peak stress (arrows).

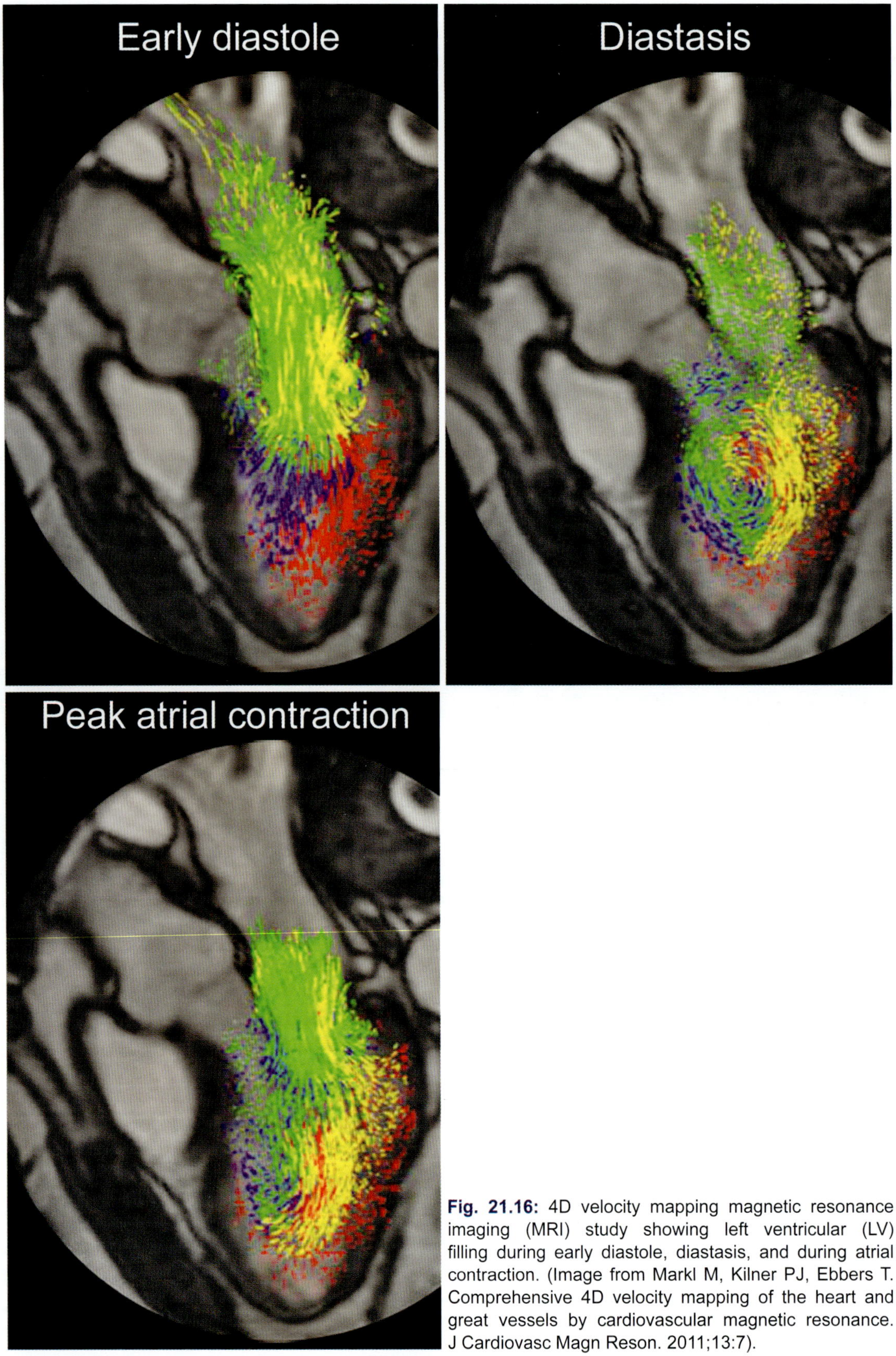

Fig. 21.16: 4D velocity mapping magnetic resonance imaging (MRI) study showing left ventricular (LV) filling during early diastole, diastasis, and during atrial contraction. (Image from Markl M, Kilner PJ, Ebbers T. Comprehensive 4D velocity mapping of the heart and great vessels by cardiovascular magnetic resonance. J Cardiovasc Magn Reson. 2011;13:7).

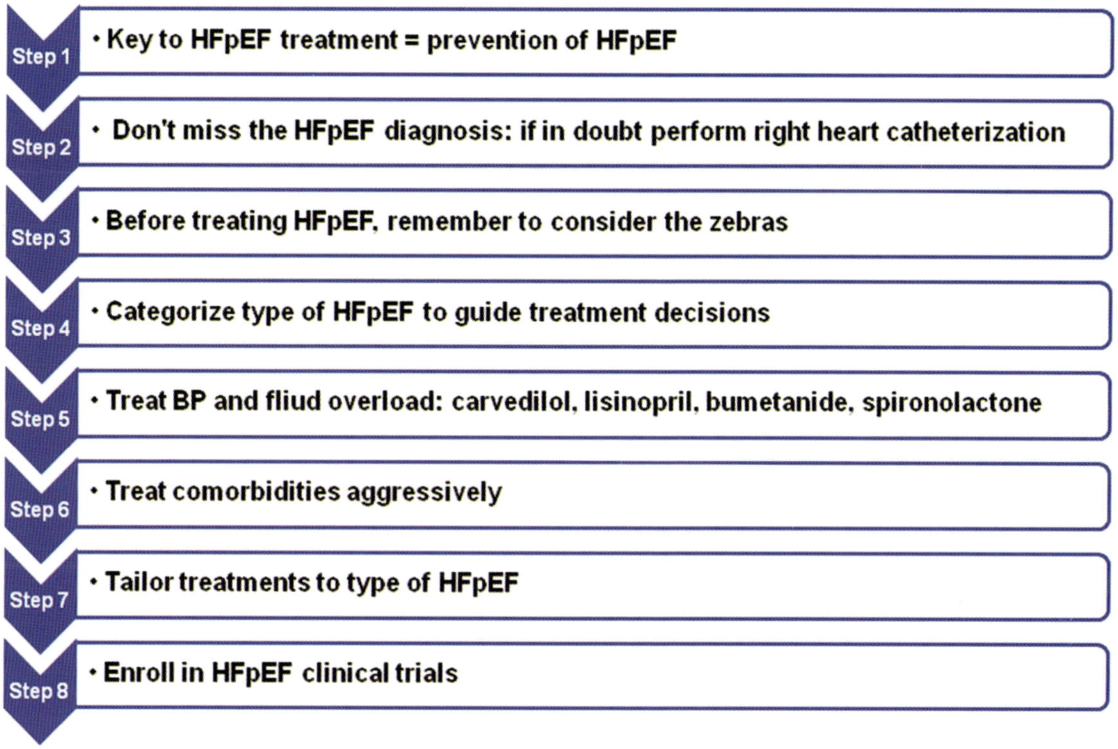

Fig. 21.17: Heart failure with preserved ejection fraction (HFpEF) diagnostic and treatment algorithm. These eight key steps demonstrate a practical approach to the patient with HFpEF. Prevention of HFpEF is critical, because once the syndrome develops, it is challenging to treat. Studies have shown that treatment of blood pressure, for example, can result in decreased incident HFpEF. The diagnosis of HFpEF should not be missed; in equivocal cases, right heart catheterization is useful for making the diagnosis. Even though the majority of HFpEF cases are "garden variety" and due to comorbidities such as hypertension, obesity, diabetes mellitus, coronary artery disease, and chronic kidney disease, among others, it is important not to miss the "zebras". Always consider the rare causes of HFpEF during the diagnostic evaluation so as not to miss these potential treatable etiologies. Categorization of HFpEF type (Table 21.1) can help guide treatment. Almost all patients will benefit from treatment of hypertension and fluid overload. The combination of carvedilol, an angiotensin converting enzyme (ACE)-inhibitor such as lisinopril, a loop diuretic (preferably bumetanide or torsemide, because they are more reliably bioavailable compared to furosemide), and spironolactone typically will result in adequate control of blood pressure and fluid overload. Treatment of comorbidities is essential, especially because proven treatment options for HFpEF are scarce. Once general treatment is administered, tailored treatment based on type of HFpEF can result in improved symptoms. Finally, enrolment in HFpEF clinical trials or referral to a center that is performing HFpEF clinical trials, if possible, is important to further clinical research for these patients, especially since there are few proven therapies for HFpEF.

VIDEO LEGENDS

Video 21.1: Apical 4-chamber transthoracic echocardiography (TTE) showing moderate tricuspid regurgitation.

Video 21.2: Apical 4-chamber transthoracic echocardiography (TTE) showing moderate mitral regurgitation.

Video 21.3: 3-chamber transthoracic echocardiography (TTE) showing moderate aortic insufficiency.

Video 21.4: Short-axis transthoracic echocardiography (TTE) showing prominent "septal bounce" in constrictive pericarditis.

Video 21.5: Apical 4-chamber transthoracic echocardiography (TTE) showing prominent "septal bounce" in constrictive pericarditis.

Video 21.6: MRI of a patient with systemic sclerosis with pericardial effusion and constriction causing heart failure with preserved ejection fraction. The video shows a small-to-moderate sized pericardial effusion, which is resulting in decreased cardiac chamber compliance and ventricular interdependence. There is interventricular septal flattening with inversion of the septum into the left ventricle (LV) during peak inspiration.

Video 21.7: Apical 4-chamber transthoracic echocardiography (TTE) showing small, thickened left ventricle (LV) and right ventricle (RV) with biatrial enlargement in a patient with restrictive cardiomyopathy.

Videos 21.8 to 21.10: Parasternal long-axis (Fig. 21.8), short-axis (Fig. 21.9) and apical 4-chamber (Fig. 21.10) transthoracic echocardiography (TTE) images of a patient with infiltrative cardiomyopathy. The findings of abnormal myocardial texture and thickened left ventricle (LV) and right ventricle (RV) with biatrial enlargement raise the possibility of infiltrative cardiomyopathy from amyloidosis.

REFERENCES

Borlaug BA, Paulus WJ. Heart failure with preserved ejection fraction: pathophysiology, diagnosis, and treatment. Eur Heart J. 2011;32(6):670-9.

Leong DP, De Pasquale CG, Selvanayagam JB. Heart failure with normal ejection fraction: the complementary roles of echocardiography and CMR imaging. JACC Cardiovasc Imaging. 2010;3(4):409-20.

Nagueh SF, Appleton CP, Gillebert TC, et al. Recommendations for the evaluation of left ventricular diastolic function by echocardiography. J Am Soc Echocardiogr. 2009;22(2):107-33.

Oktay AA, Rich JD, Shah SJ. The emerging epidemic of heart failure with preserved ejection fraction. Curr Heart Fail Rep. 2013;10(4):401-10.

Oktay AA, Shah SJ. Diagnosis and Management of Heart Failure with Preserved Ejection Fraction: 10 Key Lessons. Curr Cardiol Rev. 2013 (in press).

Paulus WJ, Tschöpe C, Sanderson JE, et al. How to diagnose diastolic heart failure: a consensus statement on the diagnosis of heart failure with normal left ventricular ejection fraction by the Heart Failure and Echocardiography Associations of the European Society of Cardiology. Eur Heart J. 2007;28(20):2539-50.

CHAPTER

22

Hypertrophic Cardiomyopathy

Christian Prinz, Lothar Faber

INTRODUCTION

The hallmark of hypertrophic cardiomyopathy (HCM) is excessive thickening of the left ventricular (LV) myocardium (Figs. 22.1 to 22.6 and Videos 22.1 to 22.7) without identifiable causes such as arterial hypertension or valve disease. Occasionally, the right ventricle is also involved (Figs. 22.7 and 22.8). The prevalence of this genetically determined cardiomyopathy is estimated to be one case per 500–1,000 in the overall population. The pattern of inheritance is autosomal dominant with incomplete penetrance. Several hundreds of mutations in more than 27 genes have been found to be associated with the HCM phenotype, leading to changes in proteins of the contractile apparatus or those involved in myocardial energy handling (Fig. 22.9).

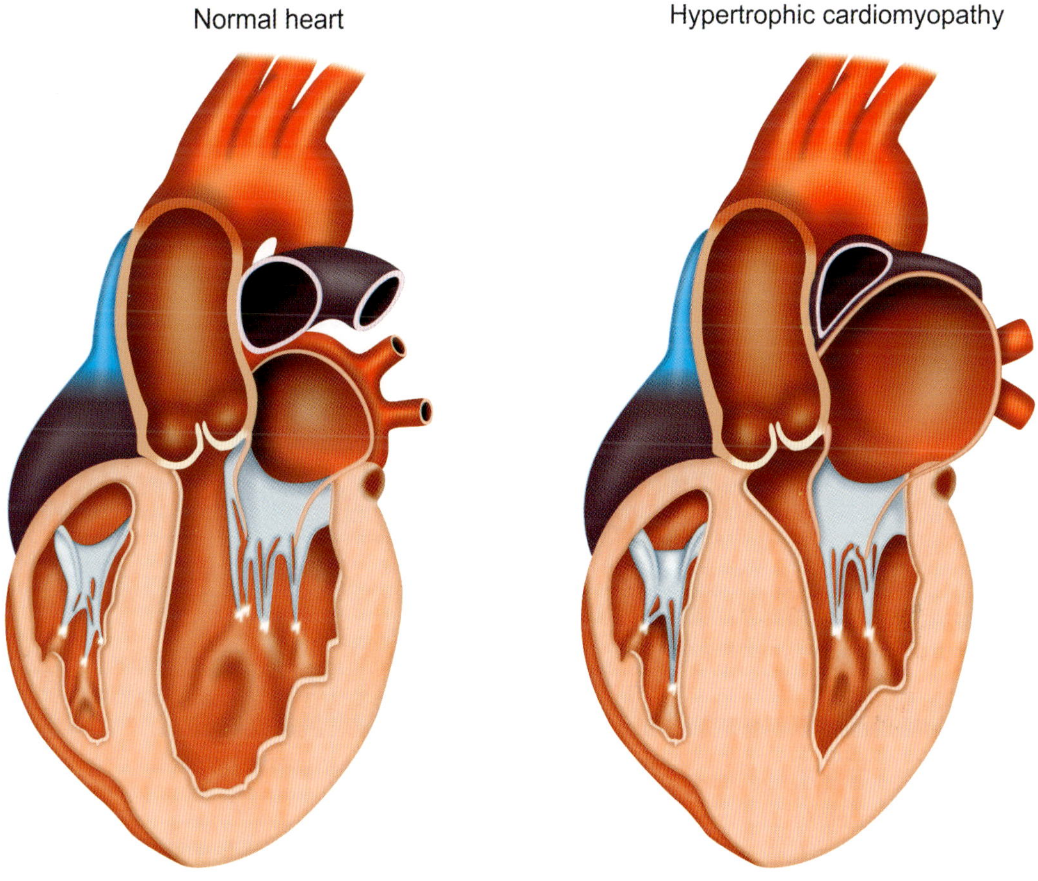

Fig. 22.1: Illustration of a normal heart (left image) and a heart with hypertrophic cardiomyopathy (right image). Note the markedly thickened interventricular septum in the patient with hypertrophic cardiomyopathy. [Image from Sofijanova A, Jordanova O. Pediatric cardiomyopathies. In: Milei J, Ambrosio G (Eds). Cardiomyopathies. Intechweb.org].

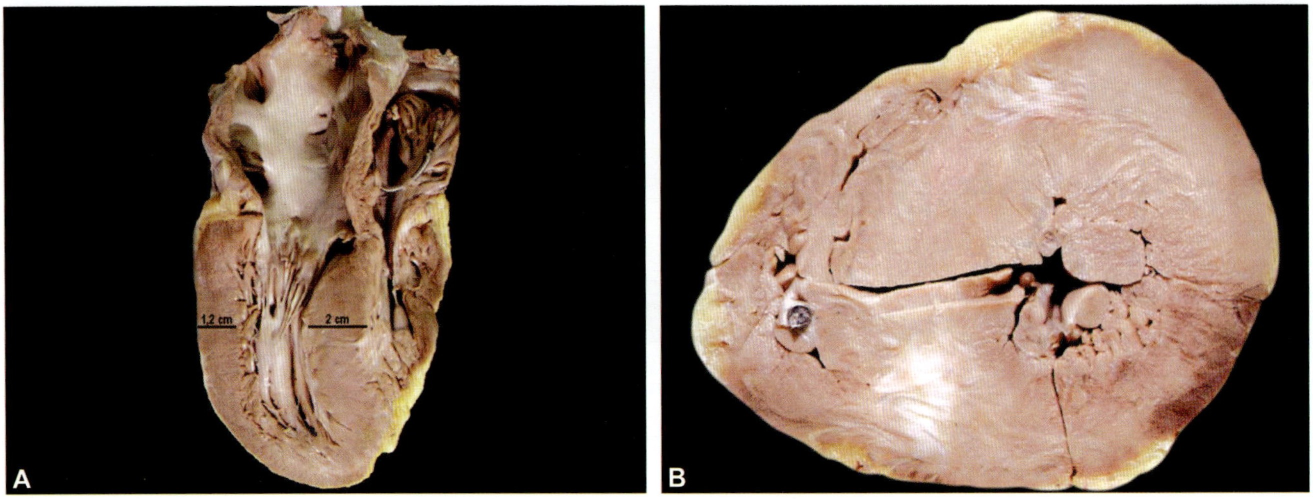

Figs. 22.2A and B: Pathological specimens from a young woman who died from HCM. Note the areas of fibrosis present in the ventricle. (Images from Harada P et al. Case 01/2008—A young female patient with the familial form of hypertrophic cardiomyopathy, who evolved with syncope, complex ventricular arrhythmia, and cardiogenic shock. Arquivos Brasileiros de Cardiologia. 2008:90. CC).

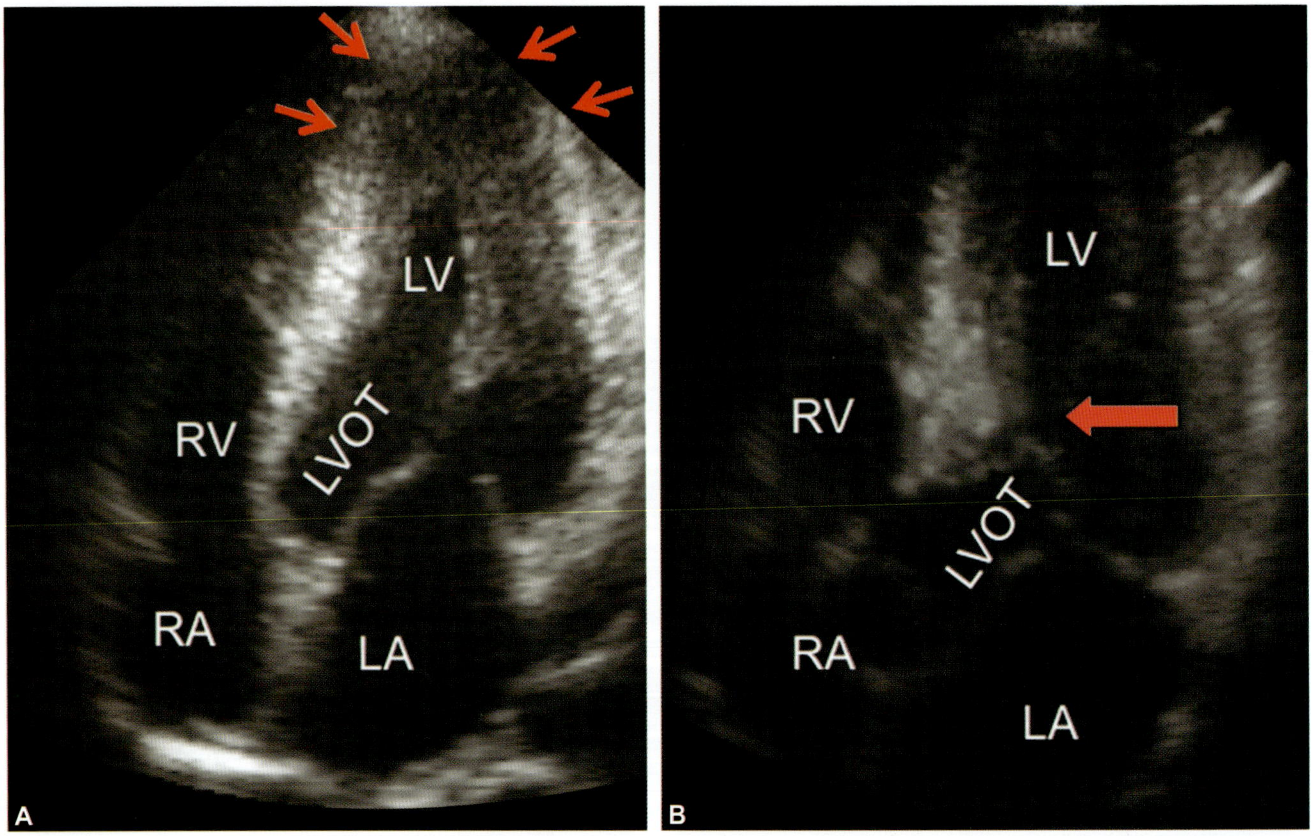

Figs. 22.3A and B: Echocardiography demonstrating 2D echo findings in (A) hypertrophic non-obstructive cardiomyopathy, with hypertrophy primarily in the left ventricular apex (arrows) and (B) hypertrophic obstructive cardiomyopathy with more diffuse wall thickening and a protruding subaortic septum making systolic contact with the mitral valve (arrow). (IVS: Interventricular septum; LA: Left atrium; LV: Left ventricle; LVOT: Left ventricular outflow tract; RA: Right atrium; RV: Right ventricle).

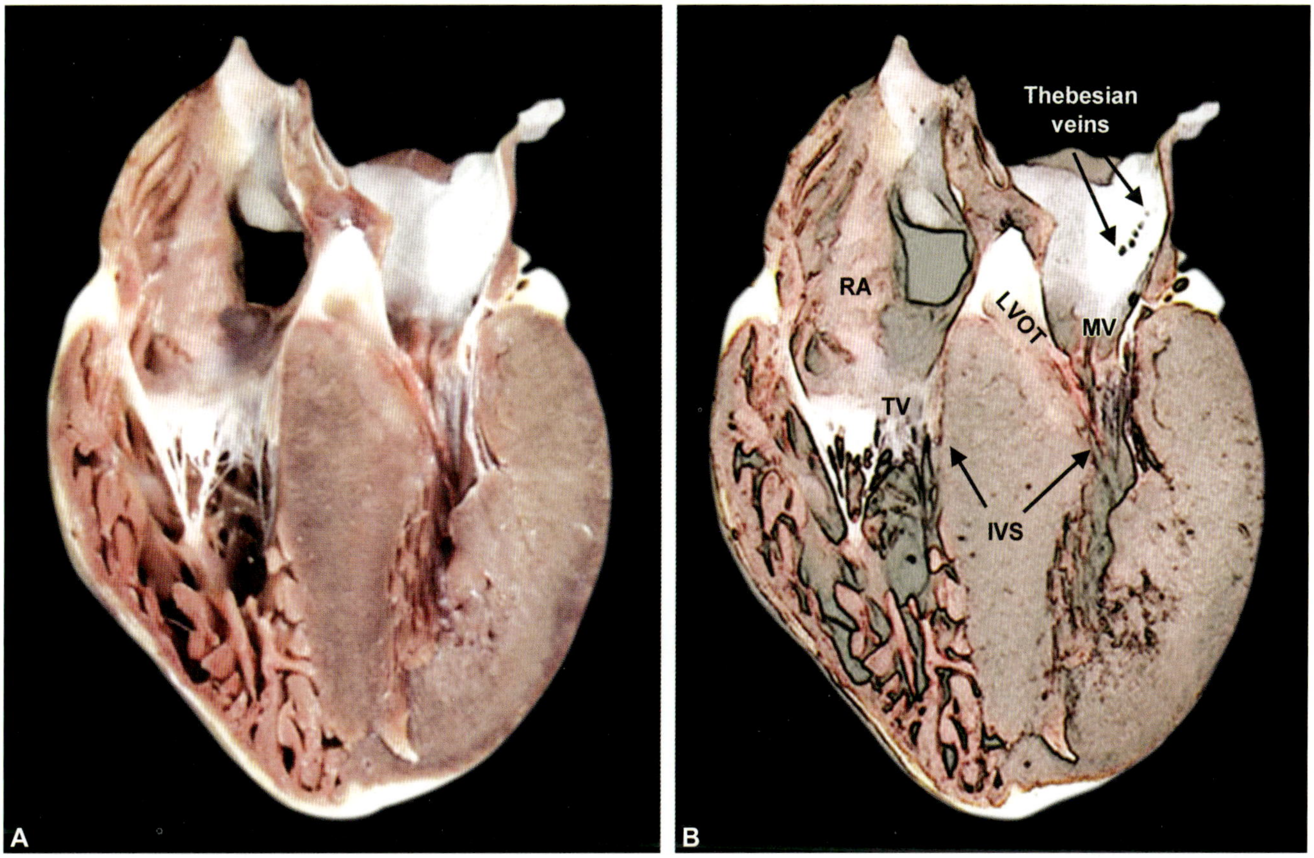

Figs. 22.4A and B: Pathological specimen and accompanying illustration of hypertrophic cardiomyopathy. (Image courtesy of E Rene Rodriguez, Carmela D. Tan. www.e-heart.org).

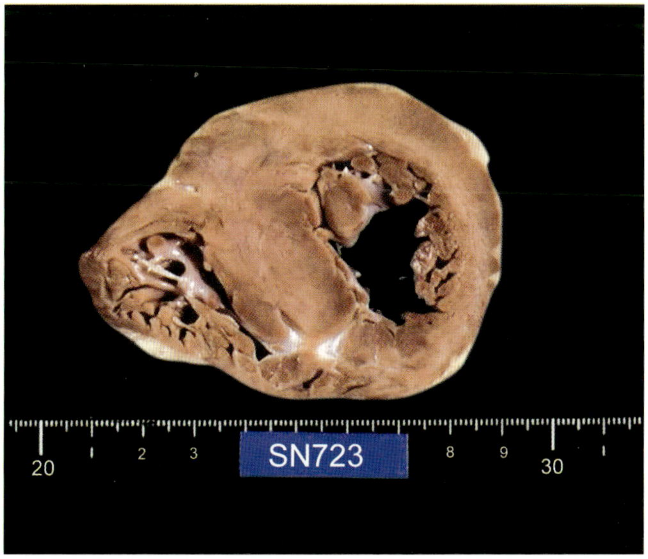

Fig. 22.5: Pathological specimen from a patient with HCM. (Image courtesy of Dr Akio Hasegawa).

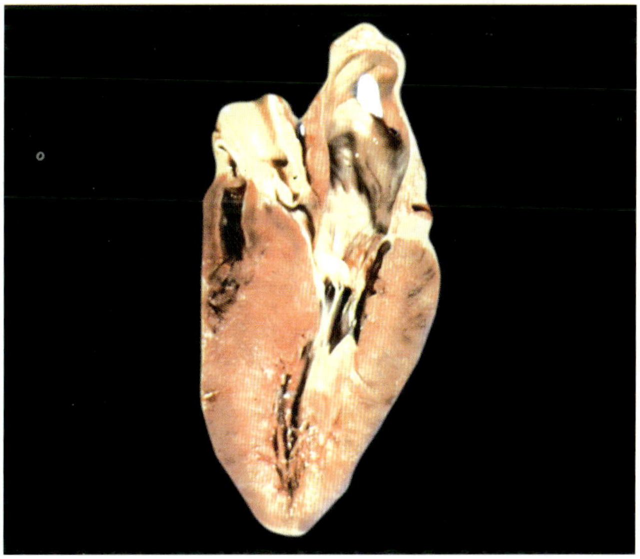

Fig. 22.6: Pathological specimen from a patient with HCM.

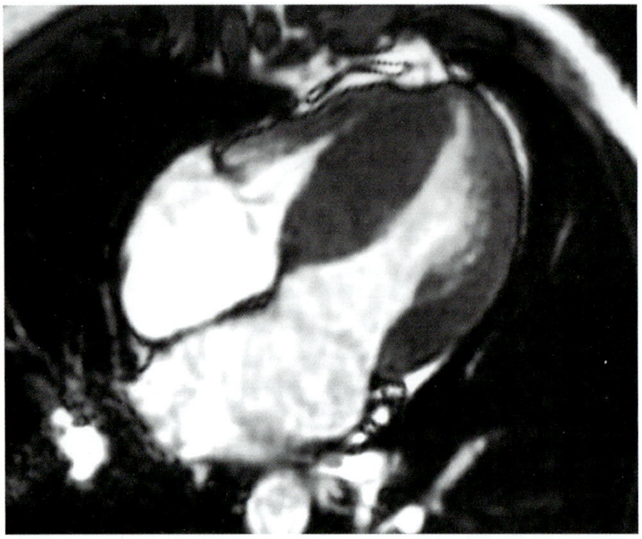

Fig. 22.7: MRI showing hypertrophy in both the left and right ventricles. (Image adapted from Veselka J. Management of hypertrophic obstructive cardiomyopathy with a focus on alcohol septal ablation. Cardiomyopathies—from Basic Research to Clinical Management. Intechweb.org. CC). (IVS: Interventricular septum; LA: Left atrium; LV: Left ventricle; LVOT: Left ventricular outflow tract; RV: Right ventricle).

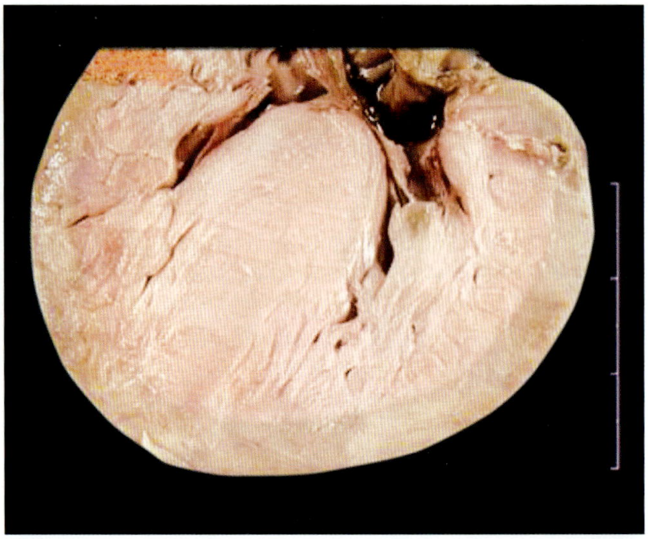

Fig. 22.8: Pathological specimen demonstrating massive biventricular hypertrophy. (Image from Seo HS et al. A case of congenital hypertrophic cardiomyopathy. Korean Circulation Journal. 2013: 43. CC).

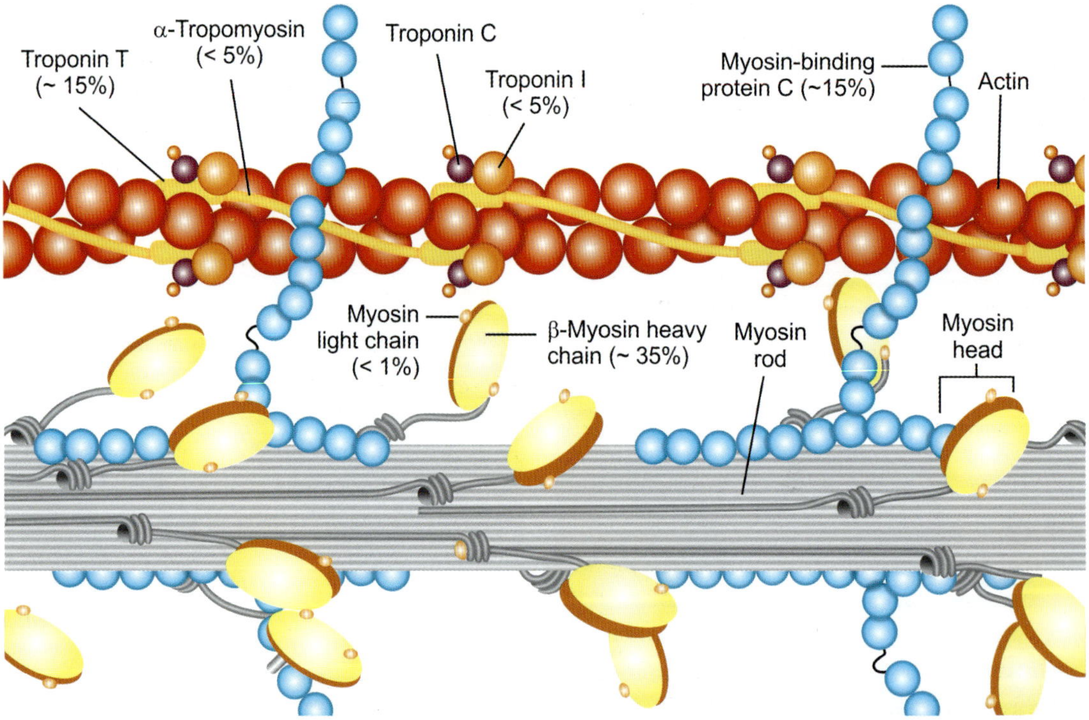

Fig. 22.9: Diagrammatic representation of the molecular structure of the sarcomere showing the thick (myosin) and thin (actin) filaments and the location of the proteins–β myosin heavy chain, myosin light chains, myosin binding protein-C, α-tropomyosin, troponin T and troponin I—that are mutated in HCM. (Redwood CS et al. Properties of mutant contractile proteins that cause hypertrophic cardiomyopathy. Image reproduced from Spirito P, Seidman CE, McKenna WJ, et al. The management of hypertrophic cardiomyopathy. New Engl J Med. 1997;336:775-85, with permission).

The extent and localization of wall thickening in HCM is highly variable. Oftentimes the interventricular septum is specifically involved, leading to the former denomination of asymmetric septal hypertrophy (ASH). The morphological findings may range from isolated thickening of individual myocardial segments that deviate from the normal LV wall thickness (< 12 mm) by only a few millimeters to diffuse and massive hypertrophy (Figs. 22.10A and B) with a wall thickness of up to 60 mm.

Two phenotypes of HCM may be distinguished. The more common obstructive type [hypertrophic obstructive cardiomyopathy (HOCM)] is characterized by a pressure gradient and increased outflow velocities within the LV cavity at rest or with provocation. The less common non-obstructive phenotype (HNCM) shows normal outflow characteristics.

CLINICALLY IMPORTANT PATHOPHYSIOLOGICAL PRINCIPLES

Most patients with HCM present with ECG changes suggesting LV hypertrophy and strain (Figs. 22.11 and 22.12). However, a normal ECG does not necessarily exclude the disease. The combination of thickened walls on imaging and a reduced voltage on ECG should always raise the suspicion of an infiltrative cardiomyopathy (e.g. cardiac amyloidosis).

Left ventricular ejection fraction (LVEF) usually remains normal in patients with HCM. However, due to myocardial hypertrophy and fibrosis, almost all patients present with some degree of diastolic dysfunction, often already present at the time of diagnosis. An indirect but rather reliable sign of diastolic LV dysfunction in HCM is more or less pronounced left atrial enlargement. Furthermore, a delayed EF slope of the anterior mitral leaflet tracing and a reduced early diastolic component of aortic root movement, both on M-mode, a reduced and prolonged early filling phase (E wave) of transmitral flow on flow pulsed-wave flow Doppler, and a reduced velocity of early diastolic mitral annulus motion on tissue Doppler echocardiography (e') all suggest diastolic ventricular dysfunction (Fig. 22.13).

The absence versus the presence of echocardiographic markers of diastolic LV dysfunction may also be used in the differential diagnosis of HCM versus the "athlete's heart" (Fig. 22.14). Moderate wall thickening less than 16 mm has been described in elite athletes engaged in isometric training, at times raising the question whether mild HCM or athlete's heart is present in a given patient.

IMAGING AND HEMODYNAMICS

Due to broad availability and the fact that it does not expose the patient to any radiation, echocardiography is the perfect "workhorse" for diagnosis and follow-up of HCM patients. Careful echocardiography should be performed using standard and "off-axis" views to detect the maximum expression of wall thickening. Comprehensive imaging of the right ventricle should be performed to assess for the rather rare occasion of right ventricular involvement. A maximum wall thickness of more than 30 mm is an established risk marker for sudden cardiac death (SCD). In particular, attention must be paid to the presence of LV outflow tract obstruction causing SAM (Fig. 22.15 and Videos 22.8 to 22.10) and mitral regurgitation. Outflow obstruction can be found in roughly 2/3 of HCM cases. In half of these, obstruction is present during resting conditions. If located in the LV outflow tract, the typical M-mode tracings of the SAM phenomenon can be seen (Figs. 22.16A and B).

Continuous wave (CW) Doppler echocardiography can be used to further quantify outflow tract velocity and to calculate pressure gradients (Figs. 22.17 and 22.18).

The severity of mitral regurgitation can by assessed by Doppler echocardiography. The typical pattern of the obstruction-associated mitral regurgitation is that of a regurgitant jet directed to the posterolateral left atrial wall (Fig. 22.19). If the diagnosis of HCM is in doubt based on echocardiography, additional imaging with cardiac magnetic resonance tomography should be performed (Figs. 22.20A and B).

Less common in patients with HCM is an obstructive gradient in the mid-cavity region (Figs. 22.21 to 22.24) or even in the LV apex (Figs. 22.25 to 22.28). In these cases, other structures, like papillary muscles, or just the thickened myocardial walls themselves, contribute to outflow obstruction and contribute to the systolic outflow gradient. The absence of SAM in the presence of high outflow velocities is characteristic for this type of outflow obstruction.

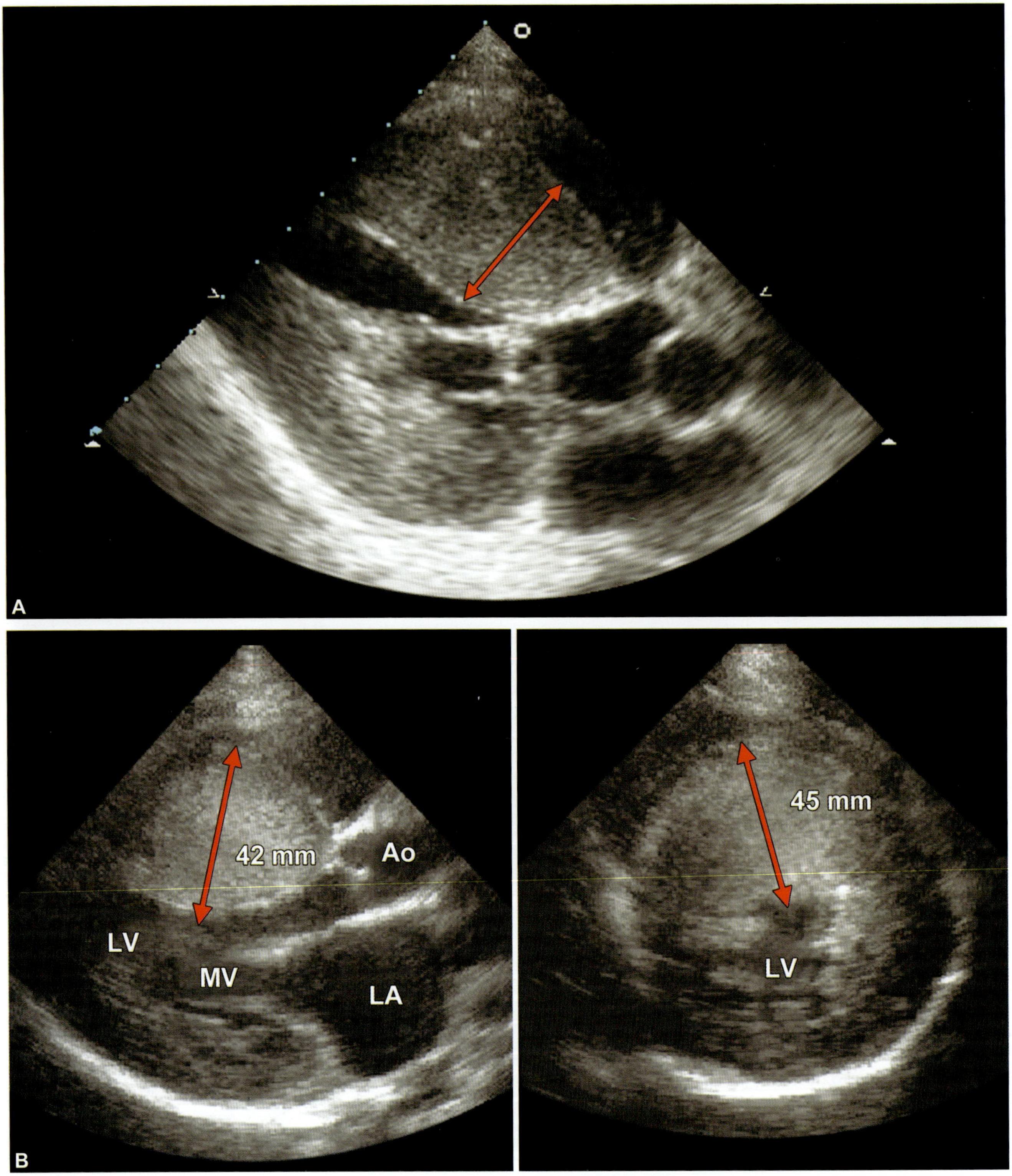

Figs. 22.10A and B: Marked left ventricular hypertrophy demonstrated by echocardiography. (A) Parasternal long-axis 2D transthoracic echocardiogram demonstrating marked left ventricular hypertrophy; (B) Parasternal long-axis and short-axis images of massive hypertrophy of the septum. [Image 22.10A from Veselka J. Management of hypertrophic obstructive cardiomyopathy with a focus on alcohol septal ablation. In: Veselka J (Ed). Cardiomyopathies—from Basic Research to Clinical Management. Intechweb.org]. (Ao: Aorta; IVS: Interventricular septum; LA: Left atrium; LV: Left ventricle; RV: Right ventricle).

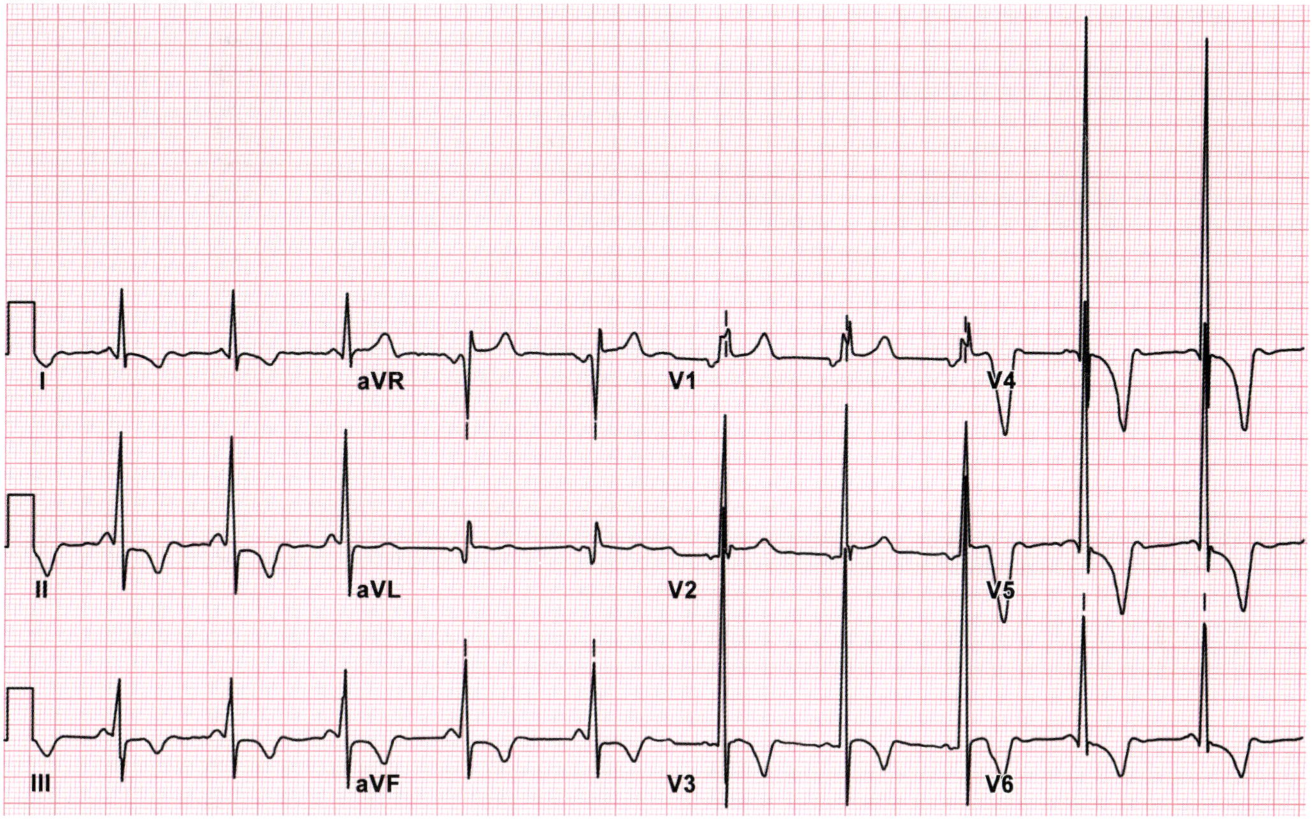

Fig. 22.11: 12 lead ECG demonstrating profound left ventricular hypertrophy (LVH) and a strain pattern.

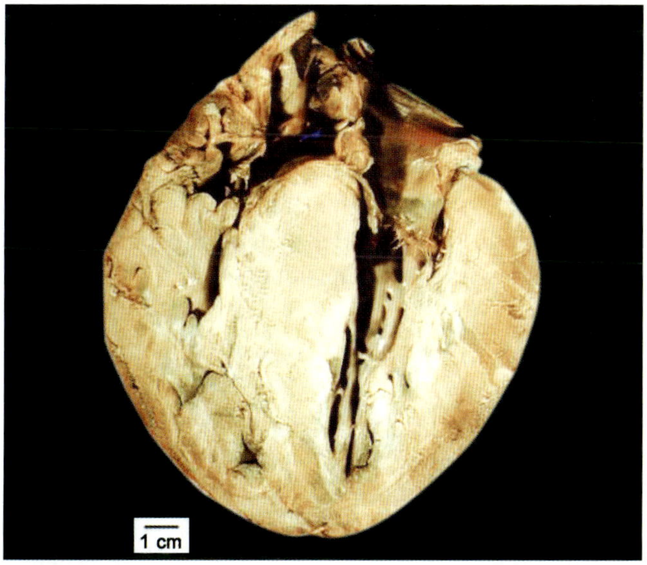

Fig. 22.12: Pathology specimen of a 9-year-old boy who died suddenly during normal activities. There is marked hypertrophy of the septum as well as hypertrophy of the free walls of both ventricles. (Image and text adapted from Alday LE, Moreyra E. Hypertrophic cardiomyopathy in infants and children. In: Veselka J (Ed). Cardiomyopathies—from Basic Research to Clinical Management. Intechweb.org. CC).

Since 50% of HOCM patients show obstruction only with provocation, some maneuver to unmask latent obstruction is mandatory during echocardiographic examination, such as Valsalva maneuver (Fig. 22.29), bicycle or isometric stress, or a pharmacological intervention (e.g. inhalation of amyl nitrite).

INVASIVE DIAGNOSTIC TESTING

Diagnostic angiography may be performed to exclude or verify coexistent coronary artery disease, to evaluate the vascular supply to the septum prior to planned septal ablation, and to assess if myocardial bridging is present. Suspicion of myocardial storage disease (e.g. amyloidosis) "masquerading" as HCM should prompt myocardial biopsy. Invasive hemodynamics usually confirm the noninvasive results regarding diastolic LV properties (e.g. elevation of LV end diastolic pressure) and serve to assess the presence and magnitude of outflow obstruction. During invasive hemodynamic assessment, a postextrasystolic potentiation of the outflow gradient (Brockenbrough-Braunwald-Morrow sign, Fig. 22.30) or another provocative maneuver should be performed.

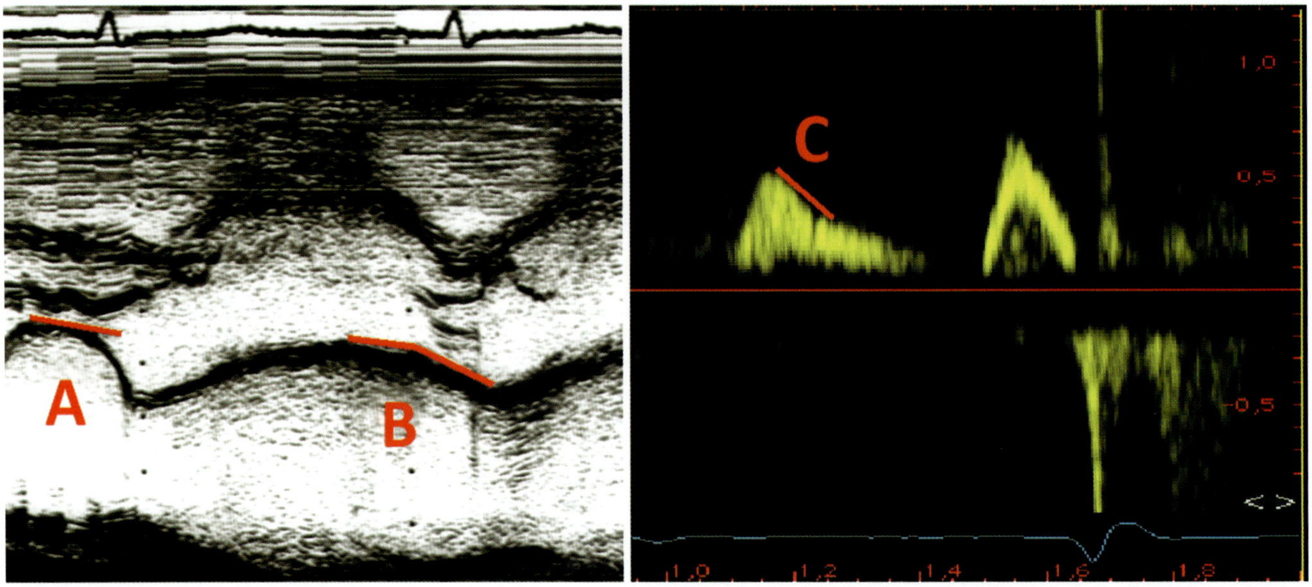

Fig. 22.13: Echocardiographic findings reflecting diastolic dysfunction in HCM: delayed EF-slope of the anterior mitral leaflet excursion (A), reduced early diastolic component of aortic root movement (B), reduced early filling velocity and prolonged early filling phase of transmitral flow (C), all common in hypertrophic cardiomyopathy.

In principle, any variation in afterload (e.g. systemic blood pressure), preload (e.g. hydration status, venous return), or contractility (e.g. endogenous sympathetic drive, pharmacologic interventions) may have profound effects on the outflow gradient. This may explain marked day-to-day variability of pressure gradient severity. Changes associated with therapeutic interventions therefore should be judged with caution, and should exceed 50% in magnitude before being judged as beneficial or therapeutic.

HYPERTROPHY AND MYOCARDIAL FIBROSIS

On pathologic and microscopic examination the thickened myocardium of HCM patients exhibits additional abnormalities. In contrast to normal myocardium showing a side-by-side organization of the myocytes, in HCM the cellular elements are disorganized in swirling and branching patterns called "myocardial disarray" (Figs. 22.31 and 22.32). Furthermore, excess fibrosis is commonly seen, consisting in varying degrees of both replacement fibrosis (scarring) and interstitial fibrosis, distinctly different from fibrosis seen in coronary artery disease or dilated cardiomyopathy. Fibrosis is usually most severe in the areas of greatest myocardial thickening. Myocardial disarry, fibrosis and wall thickenening are contributors to diastolic LV dysfunction. In addition, the presence of fibrosis has been linked to a worse outcome in HCM patients, both with respect to arrhythmic events and to heart failure symptoms.

In vivo detection of myocardial fibrosis has become possible by using cardiac magnetic resonance imaging (MRI) with Gadolinium late enhancement (LGE) (Figs. 22.33 and 22.34), and probably also by cardiac computed tomography (CT). Both techniques rely on different contrast kinetics and a greater volume of distribution in the extracellular matrix as compared to vital myocardium, and make the fibrotic lesions appear brighter.

CLINICAL OBSERVATIONS AND SYMPTOMS

The clinical course of HCM is extremely heterogeneous, and often dissociated from the phenotype. Patients with a marked phenotype may be completely asymptomatic or even be capable of performing competitive sports, while those with a barely recognizable disease may suffer from a severely restricted exercise tolerance. Symptoms may include dyspnea or angina pectoris during physical or

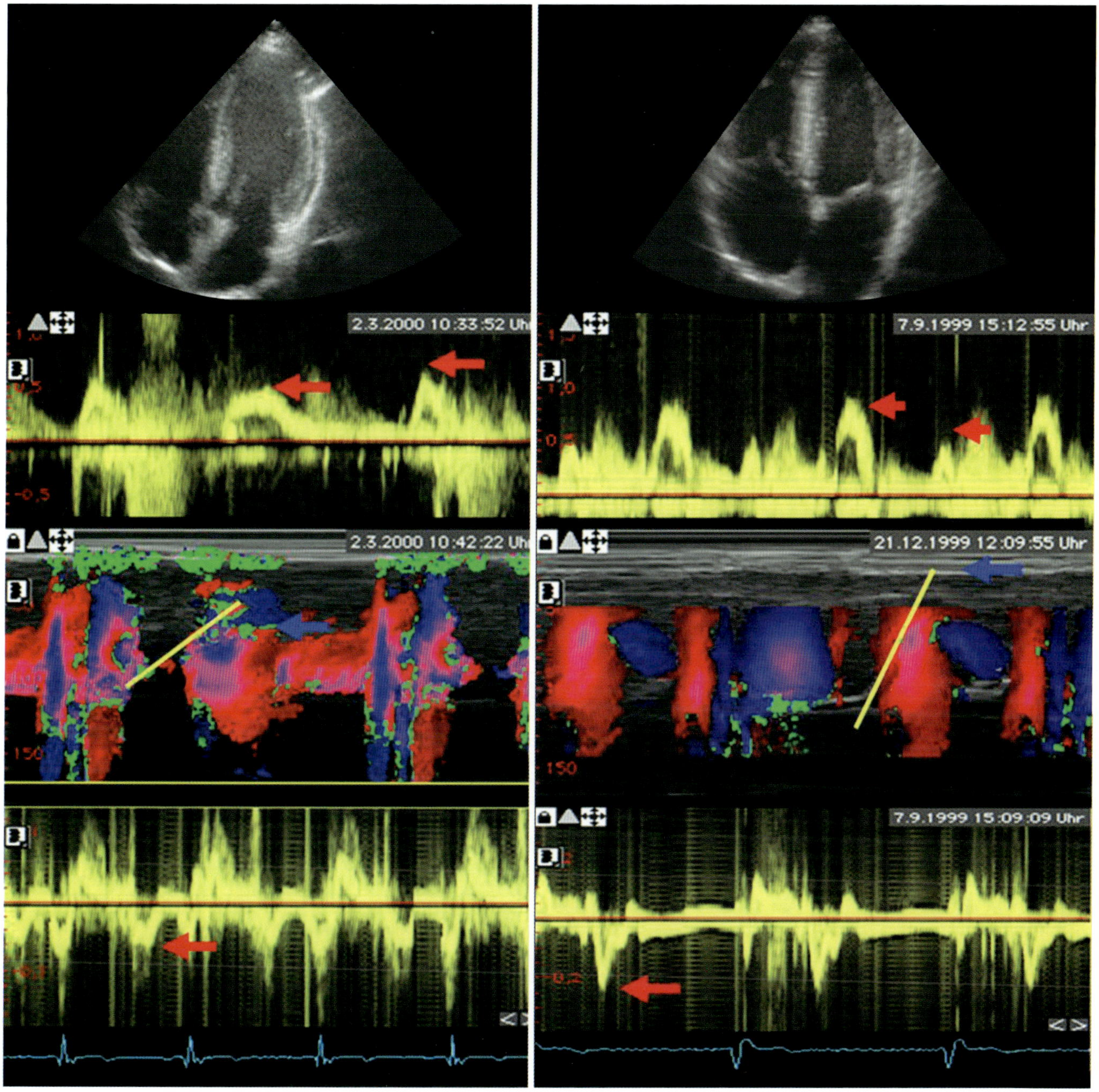

Fig. 22.14: Echocardiographic findings that distinguish HCM (left panel) from athlete's heart (right panel). Both 2D images demonstrate mild left ventricular hypertrophy. However, the HCM heart has an abnormal transmitral flow pattern with a reduced E wave velocity (2nd row of images), a reduced transmitral flow propagation velocity on color m-mode (3rd row of images), and reduced early diastolic mitral annulus velocities on tissue Doppler imaging (4th row of images). These findings of impaired left ventricular relaxation in the heart displayed on the left panel suggest that HCM is present in that heart while the more normal findings on the heart on the right suggest this is athlete's heart.

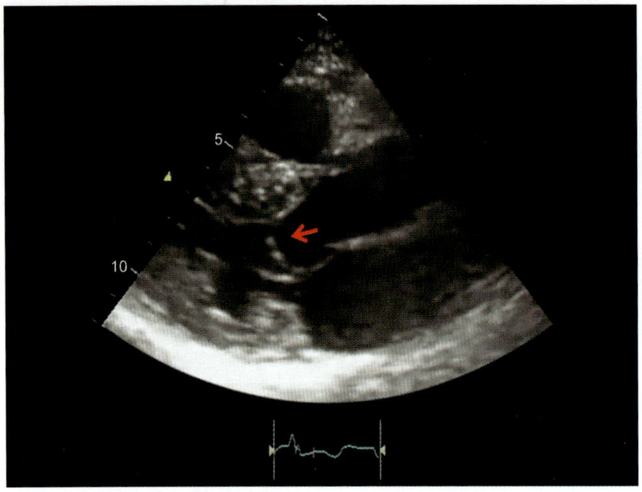

Fig. 22.15: Systolic anterior motion (SAM) of the anterior mitral leaflet (arrow) during systole in a patient with HCM. (Image from Echolab of the Academic Medical Center, the Netherlands, Posted on Echopedia.org. CC). (Ao: Aorta; IVS: Interventricular septum; LA: Left atrium; LV: Left ventricle; LVOT: left ventricular outflow tract; RV, right ventricle).

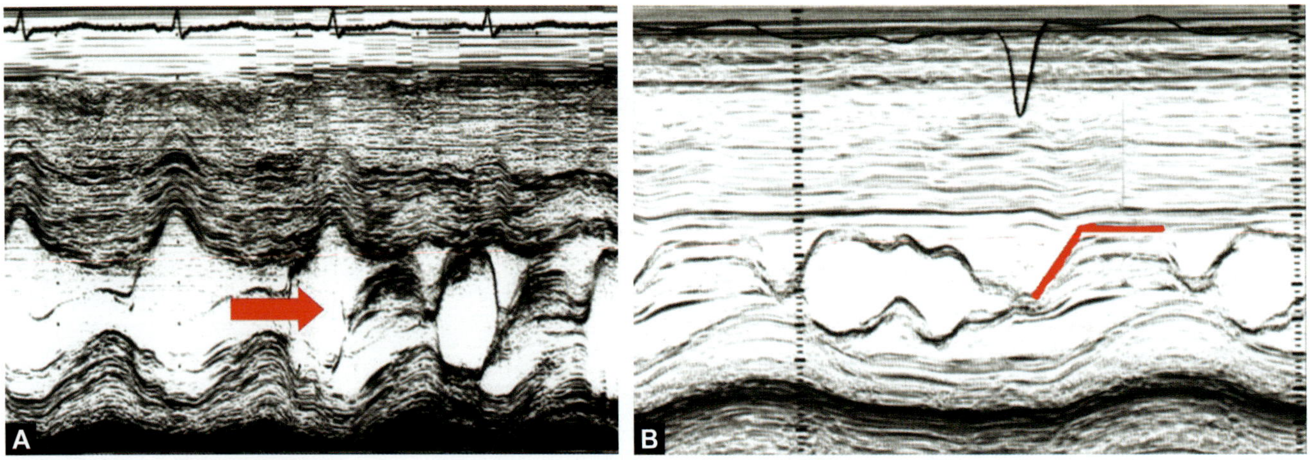

Figs. 22.16A and B: Examples of SAM demonstrated on M-mode echocardiography. In early systole high blood flow velocities within the narrow left ventricular outflow create Venturi forces drawing the mitral valve leaflets toward the interventricular septum. In later phases of systole the mitral leaflets are further dragged toward the septum by the blood flow until making contact (drag effect). This phenomenon is called systolic anterior motion (SAM phenomenon) of the mitral valve (arrow in Figures 22.16A, red line in 22.16B). SAM-related obstruction is the predominant type of outflow obstruction in HCM. [Figure 22.16B from Losi MA et al. Echocardiography in patients with hypertrophic cardiomyopathy: usefulness of old and new techniques in the diagnosis and pathophysiological assessment. Cardiovascular Ultrasound 2010. CC. Figure 22.16B from Haleem K et al. M-mode examination. In: Nanda NC (Ed). Comprehensive Textbook of Echocardiography. New Delhi: Jaypee Brothers Medical Publishers (P) Ltd].

mental stress, dizziness, palpitations, and occasionally syncope. The overall disease-related mortality risk has been reported as 1% per year in unselected patients.

In some patients, SCD is the initial manifestation of the disease. Occult HCM is one of the more common causes of SCD in athletes. Identification of patients with HCM at high risk of SCD has gained considerable clinical attention, and routine management should therefore include repeated risk stratification throughout lifetime.

THERAPEUTIC ALGORITHMS

It is beyond the scope of this article to cover every aspect of therapy in this complex condition. Furthermore, large randomized clinical trials are missing, thus most recommendations are based on observational studies or case series.

A diagnosis of HCM usually disqualifies the patient from competitive sports as well as from engaging in

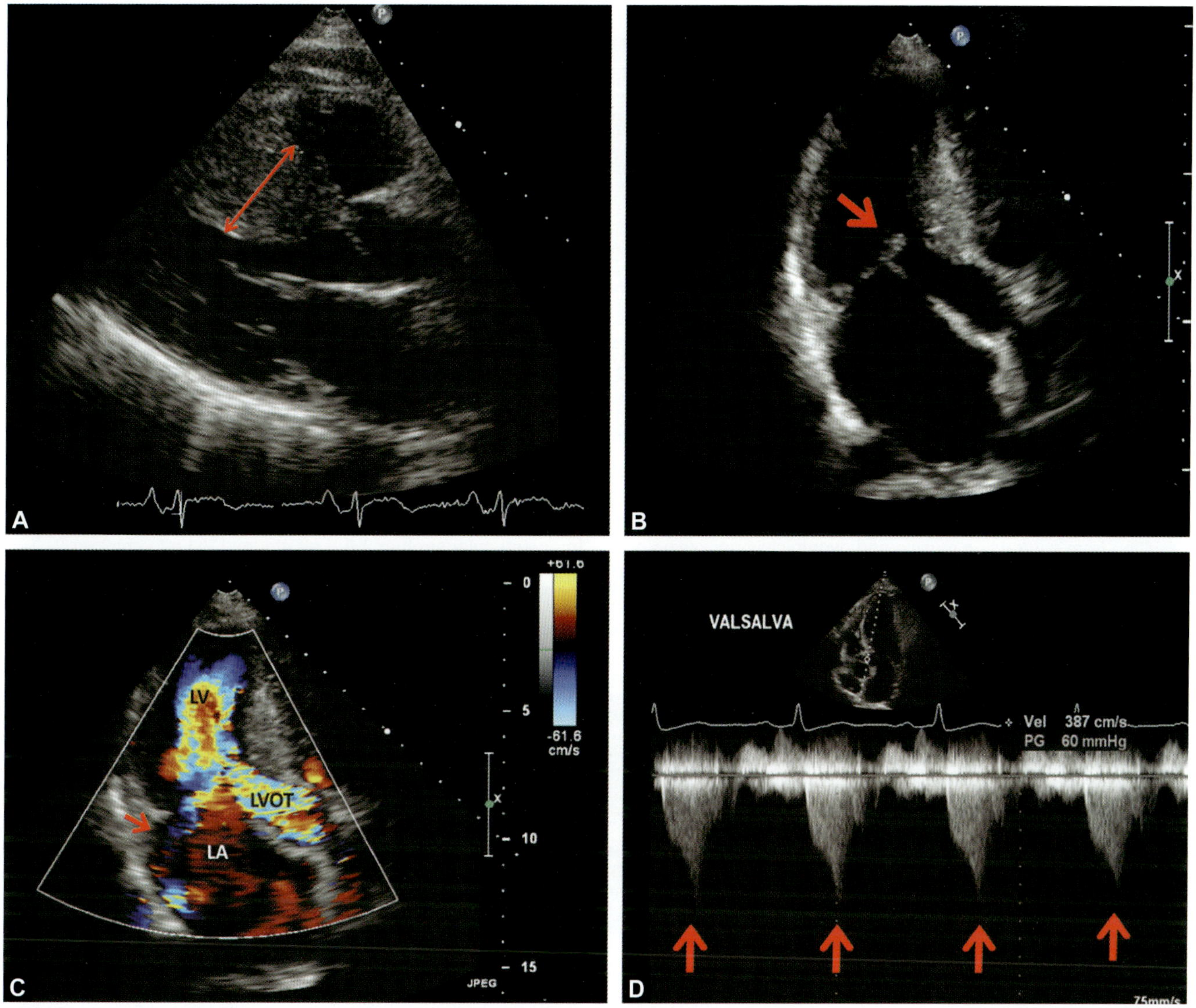

Figs. 22.17A to D: Asymmetric septal hypertrophy (ASH) with SAM and LVOT flow obstruction. (A) Marked asymmetric septal hypertrophy is present; (B) Systolic anterior motion of the anterior mitral valve (arrow) is evident during systole; (C) Color Doppler demonstrates turbulent blood flow through the left ventricular outflow tract (LVOT). As a result of SAM there is also eccentric posterolaterally-directed mitral regurgitation (arrow); (D) Continuous wave spectral Doppler performed during Valsalva maneuver demonstrates a significant gradient across the LVOT. Note the "dagger shaped" pattern (arrows) typical of dynamic flow obstruction. [Images from Jamil G et al. Echocardiography findings in common primary and secondary cardiomyopathies. In: Milei J, Ambrosio G (Eds). Cardiomyopathies. Intechweb.org. CC]. (IVS: Interventricular septum; LA: Left atrium; LV: Left ventricle; LVOT: Left ventricular outflow tract; RV: Right ventricle).

isometric exercise. Physical endurance activity may be performed in the aerobic range. Ingestion of alcohol may lead to aggravation of outflow obstruction due to afterload reduction.

RISK STRATIFICATION

Treatment of high-risk HCM patients with an implantable cardioverter-defibrillator (ICD) has been proven to decrease the risk of SCD. A survived cardiac arrest or a sustained ventricular tachycardia is a clear indication for ICD implantation. The identification of HCM patients for primary SCD prophylaxis remains a challenge. Five major risk factors have been identified with low individually predictive value. However, combining these risk factors increase their significance: patients with more than or equal to 2 risk factors are considered to have an annual SCD rate of approximately 4–5%.

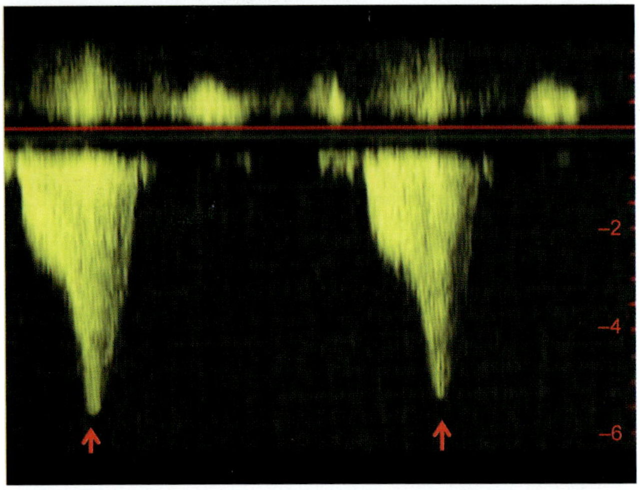

Fig. 22.18: The typical continuous wave (CW) Doppler findings of left ventricular outflow obstruction in HOCM. Note the typical saber-shaped Doppler signal (arrows) indicating dynamic obstruction resulting from contracting muscle and dynamically narrowing outflow, as opposed to the more symmetrical signal of fixed valvular stenosis. The peak pressure gradient equals 4 x (peak velocity).

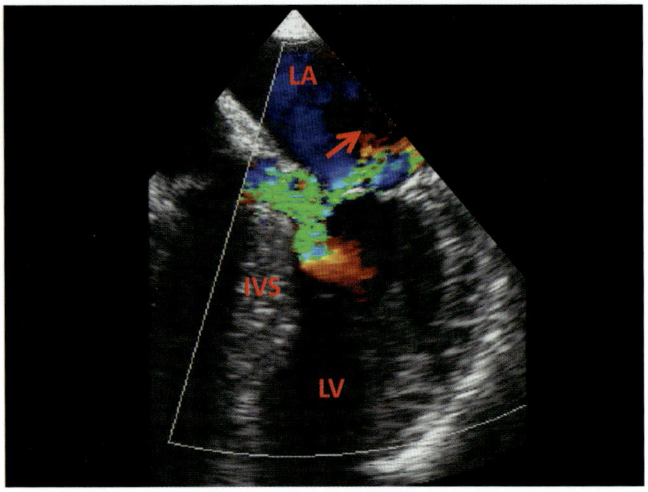

Fig. 22.19: Transesophageal echocardiography view (0 degrees) of the typical pattern of mitral regurgitation seen in HCM with SAM, with a jet orientation toward the posterolateral LA wall. (IVS: Interventricular septum; LA: Left atrium; LV: Left ventricle).

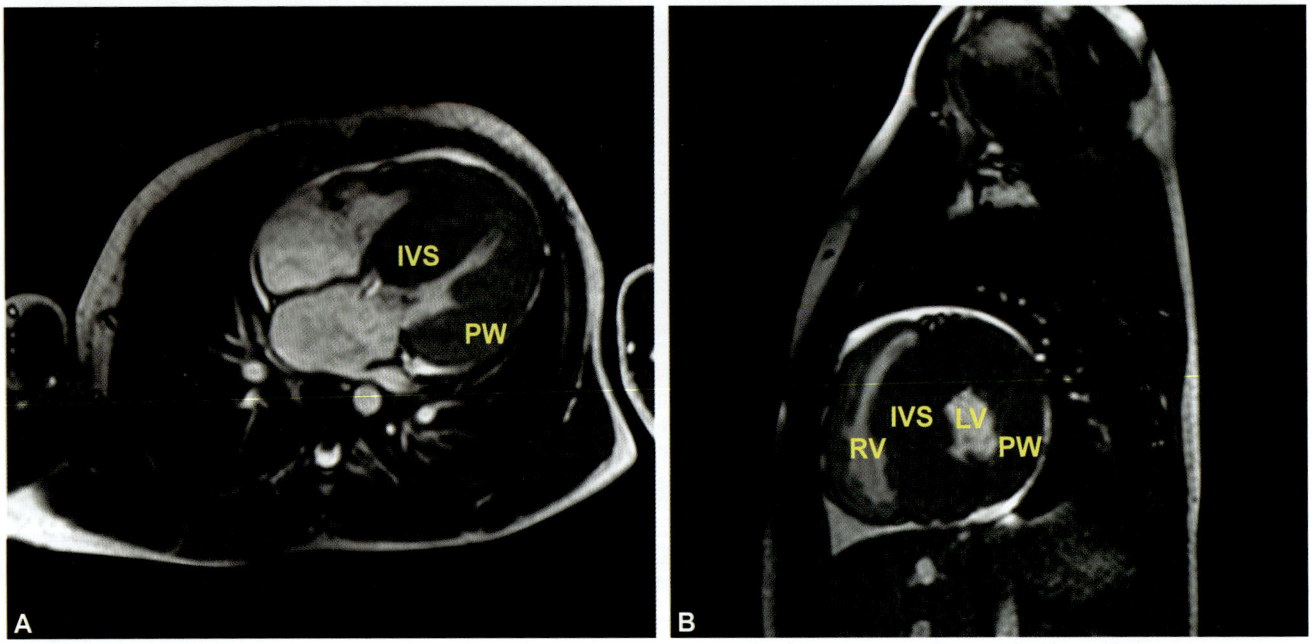

Figs. 22.20A and B: Long-axis (A) and short-axis; (B) cardiac magnetic resonance images of young children with severe hypertrophic cardiomyopathy. (Images courtesy of Dr. Ricardo Pignatelli. Texas Children's Hospital. Images originally published in Alday LE, Moreyra. Hypertrophic cardiomyopathy in infants and children. In: Veselka J. Cardiomyopathies—from Basic Research to Clinical Management. Intechweb.org. CC). (IVS: Interventricular septum; LV: Left ventricle; PW: Posterior wall; RV: Right ventricle).

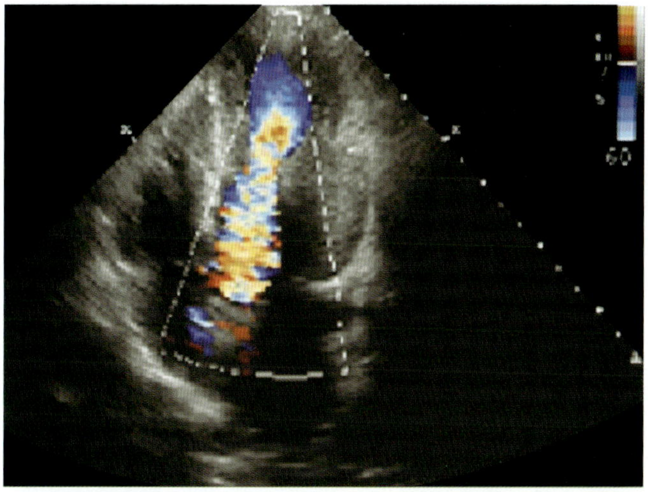

Fig. 22.21A: 2D color Doppler echocardiography demonstrating flow acceleration and turbulent blood flow due to dynamic mid-ventricular obstruction in a patient with HCM. (Image from Vatan MB et al. An unusual type of localized hypertrophic cardiomyopathy with Wolf Parkinson White syndrome presenting with pulmonary edema. Cardiol Res. 2012;3: 133-6. CC).

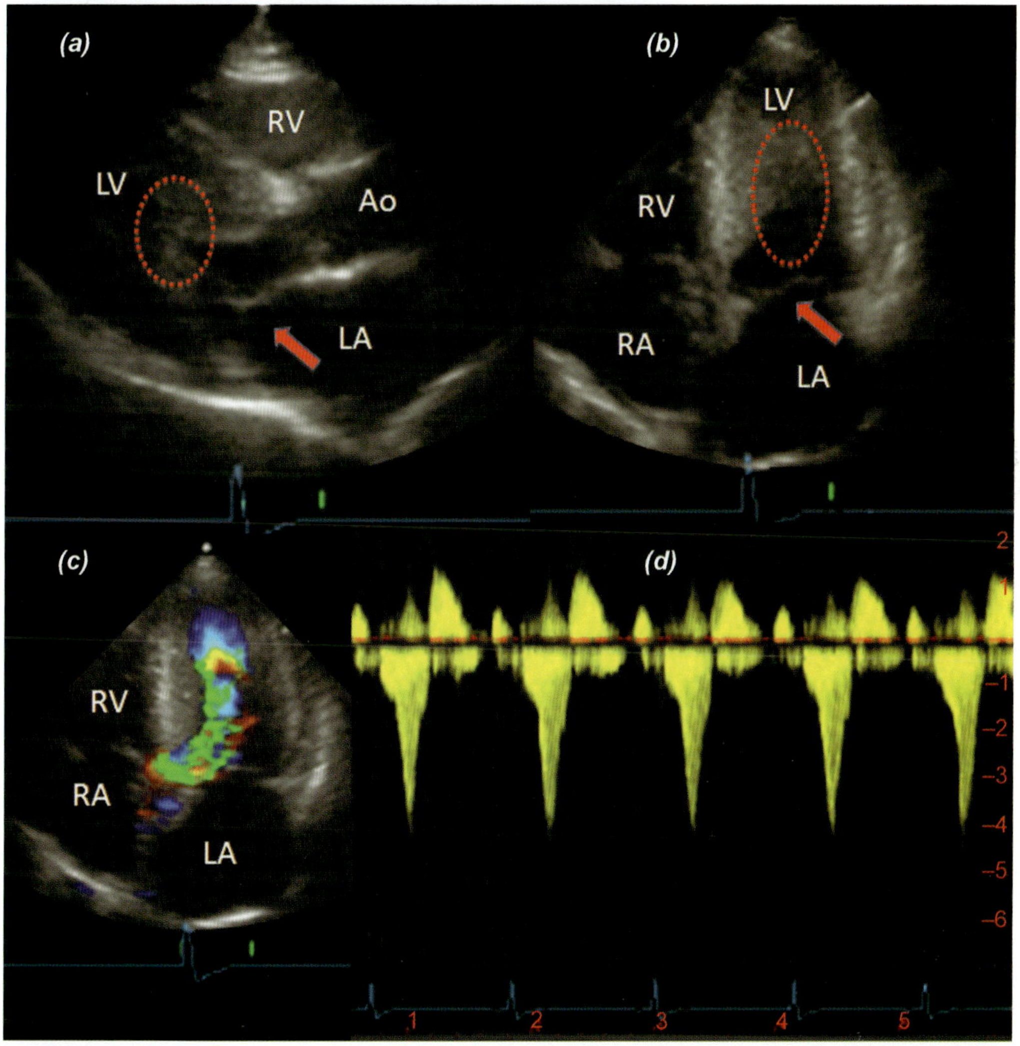

Fig. 22.21B: Transthoracic echo findings in a patient with pure mid-cavity obstruction. The long-axis (a) and the apical 4-chamber views (b) show approximation of the thickened septum and the hypertrophied papillary muscles (dotted area). Flow acceleration as demonstrated by color flow mapping (c) occurs at that level. A gradient of 80 mm Hg is measured by continuous wave (CW) Doppler (d). (Ao: Aorta; LA: Left atrium; LV: Left ventricle; RA: Right atrium; RV: Right ventricle).

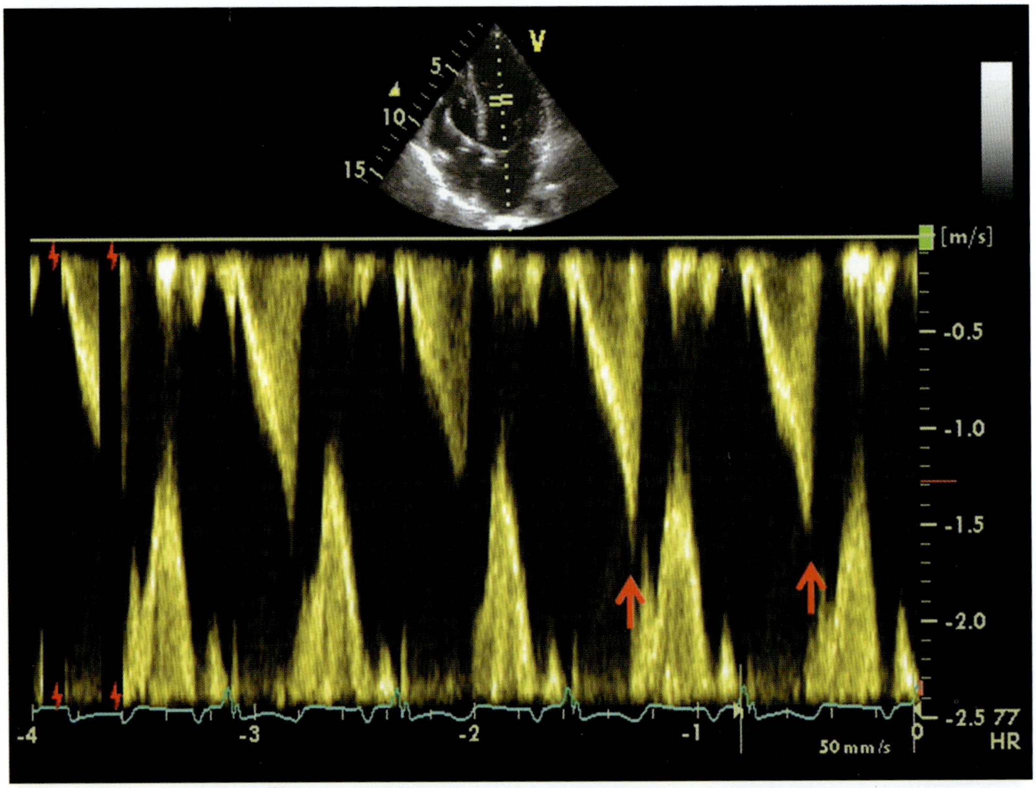

Fig. 22.22: Pulsed wave (PW) spectral echocardiography demonstrating a modest mid-cavitary gradient in a patient with HCM. (Image courtesy of the AMC Echolab, AMC, the Netherlands, posted on Echopedia.org. CC). (Ao: Aorta; LA: Left atrium; LV: Left ventricle; LVOT: Left ventricular outflow tract; RV: Right ventricle).

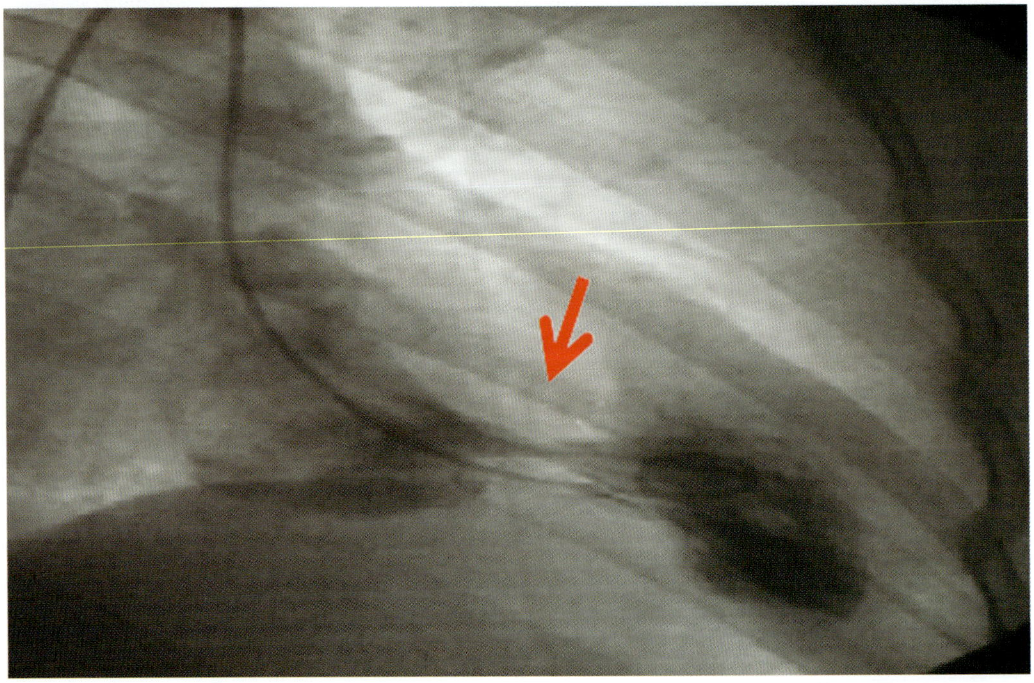

Fig. 22.23: Mid-cavitary dynamic obstruction (arrow) demonstrated by left ventriculogram. (Image from Vatan MB et al. An unusual type of localized hypertrophic cardiomyopathy with Wolf Parkinson White syndrome presenting with pulmonary edema. Cardiol Res. 2012;3:133-6. CC).

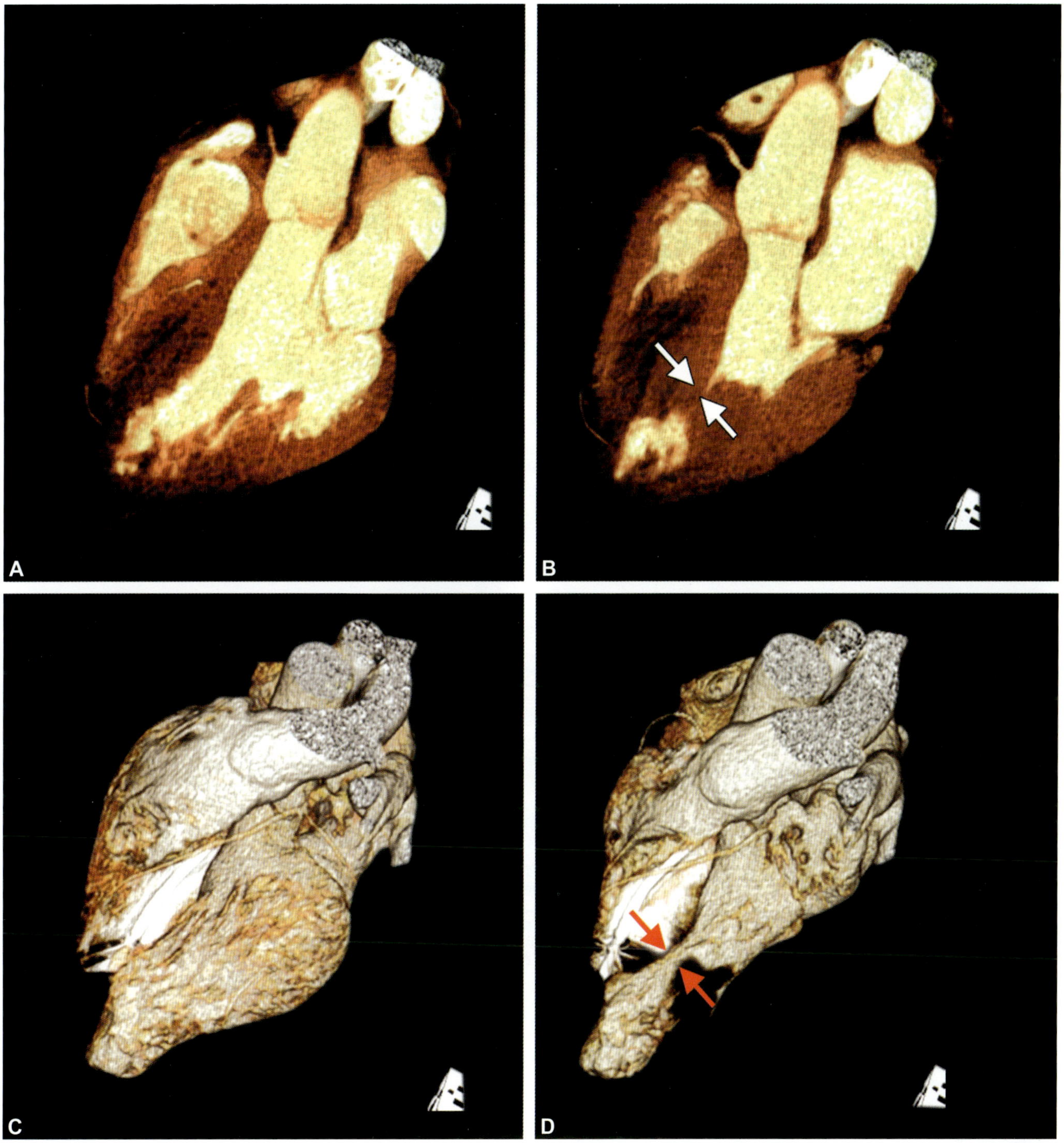

Figs. 22.24A to D: Cardiac CT demonstrating dynamic mid ventricular obstruction (arrow). Figures A and C are during diastole, while Figures B and D during systole. (Image courtesy Hui-Nam Pak, MD, PhD, FHRS).

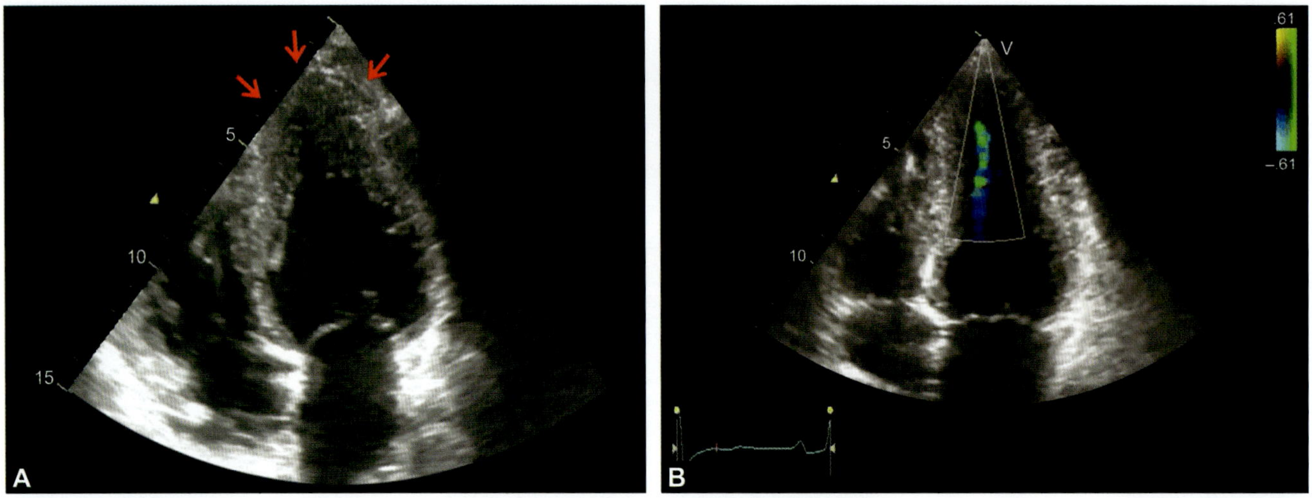

Figs. 22.25A and B: Apical 4-chamber echocardiographic 2D (A) and color Doppler (B) images demonstrating apical HCM (arrows) with dynamic flow obstruction and flow acceleration in the LV apex. (Images courtesy of the AMC Echolab, AMC, the Netherlands, posted on Echopedia.org. CC). (LA: Left atrium; LV: Left ventricle; RA: Right atrium; RV: Right ventricle).

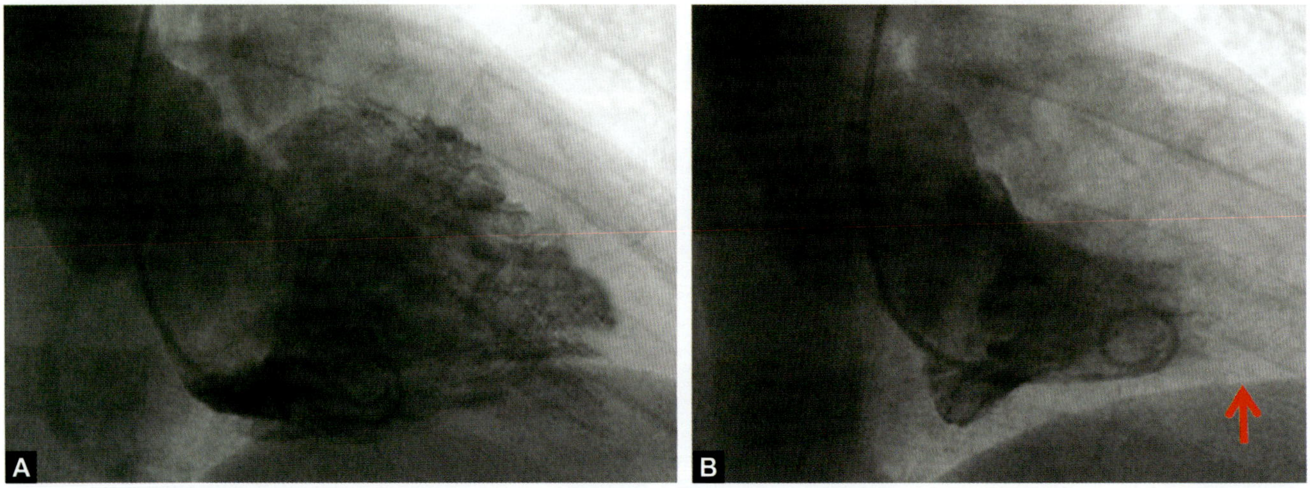

Figs. 22.26A and B: Left ventriculogram of a patient with apical HCM. Figure A is during diastole and Figure B is during systole. Note obliteration of the LV cavity at the apex during systole (arrow). (Image from Lakshmanadoss U et al. All that glitters is not gold: apical hypertrophic cardiomyopathy mimicking acute coronary syndrome. Cardiol Res. 2012;3:137-9. CC).

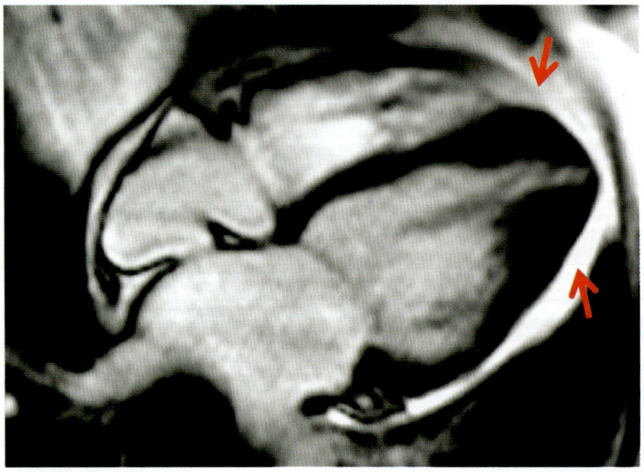

Fig. 22.27: Four-chamber MRI image at end-diastole in a patient initially presenting as acute coronary syndrome with de-novo angina and T wave inversions in the inferolateral ECG leads, Coronary artery disease was invasively ruled out. Standard 2D echocardiography showed normal wall thickness. Cardiac MRI, however, demonstrated wall thickening exclusively in the apical region of the left ventricle (arrows), an area often less well visualized by echocardiography. (LA: Left atrium; LV: Left ventricle; RA: Right atrium; RV: Right ventricle).

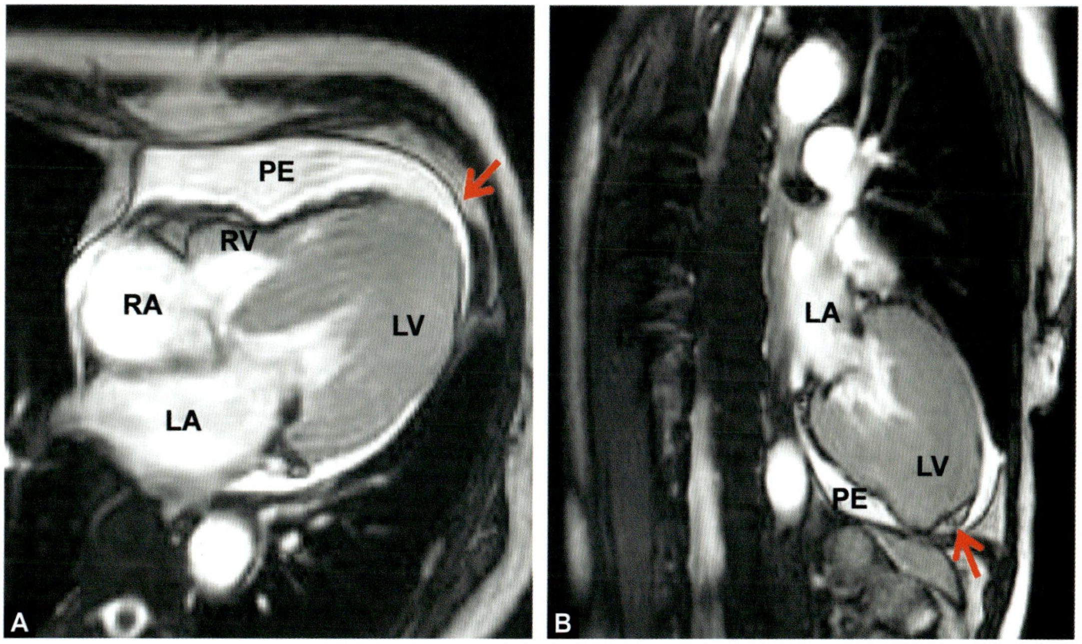

Figs. 22.28A and B: Four-chamber (A) and two-chamber (B) views on MRI using steady state free precession sequence imaging demonstrating predominantly apical hypertrophy (arrows) and "spade-like" configuration of the LV cavity consistent with the apical variant of HCM. (Image and legend from Bishu K et al. Apical variant of hypertrophic cardiomyopathy and systemic scleroderma—a hint for autoimmune mechanism? J Clin Exp Cardiolog. 2012;3:7. CC). (LA: Left atrium; LV: Left ventricle; PE: Pericardial effusion; RA: Right atrium; RV: Right ventricle).

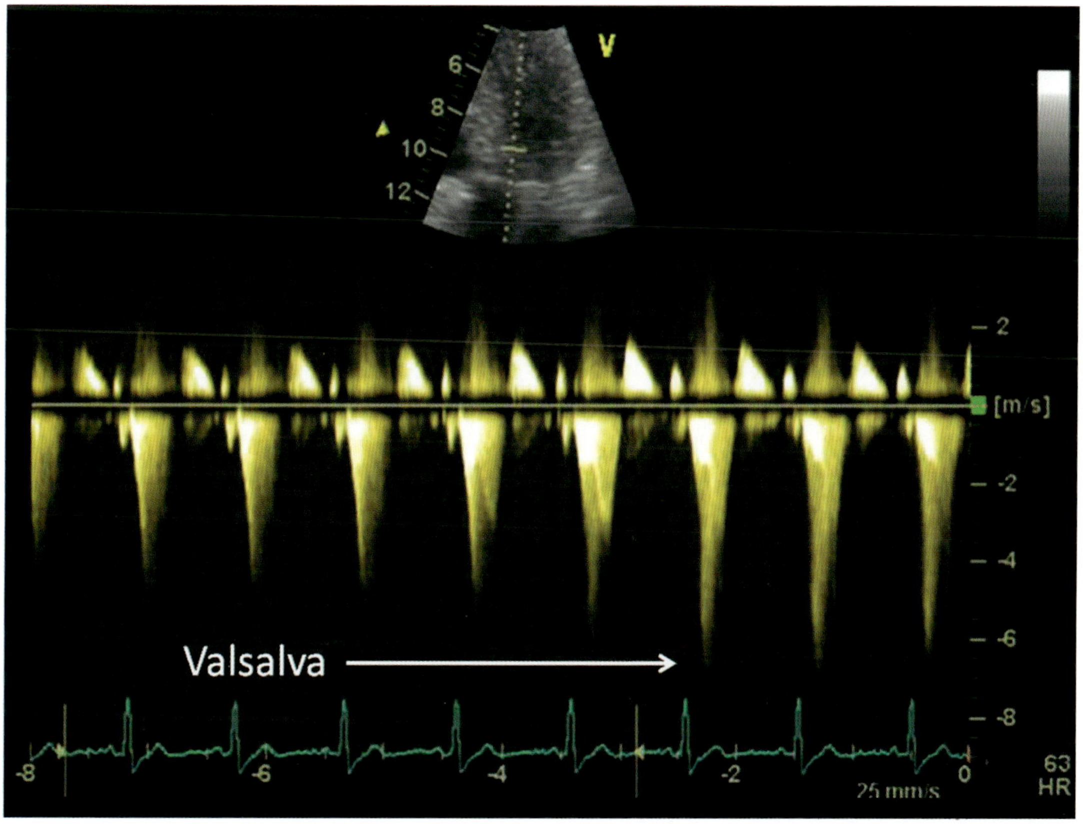

Fig. 22.29: Continuous wave (CW) spectral Doppler demonstrating a notable increase in flow velocity (and thus pressure gradient) with Valsalva maneuver.

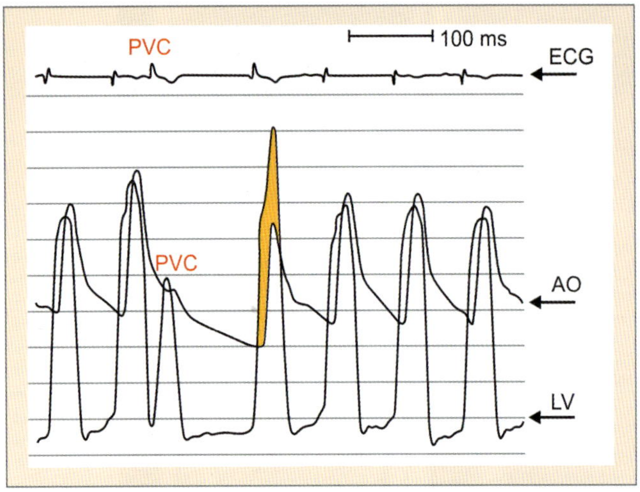

Fig. 22.30: Simultaneous pressure tracing from the LV and the aorta demonstrating the Brockenbrough-Braunwald-Morrow sign. A marked increase of the intra-cavity gradient following a premature ventricular contraction (PVC) is observed as a result of increased myocardial contractility. The post-PVC beat shows a reduction of pulse pressure due to the increased left ventricular outflow tract obstruction. [Image from Wikimedia (no author listed). CC]. (LV: Left ventricle; Ao: Aorta).

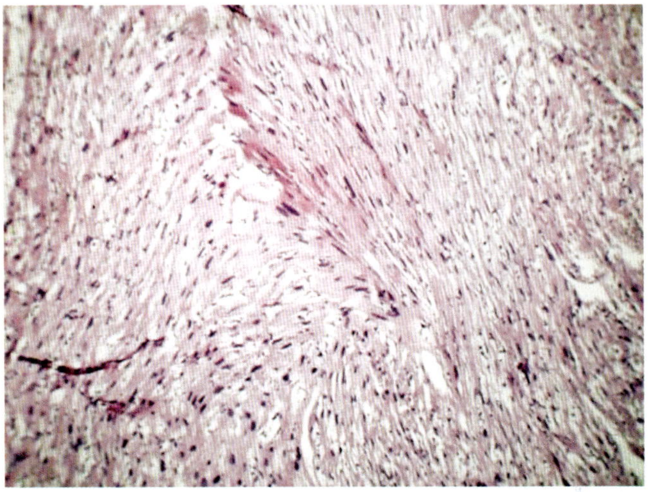

Fig. 22.31: Microscopic view of the myocardium with the typical disarray of hypertrophic cardiomyopathy in an infant who died in congestive heart failure. Myofibers have lost the usual parallel disposition and describe whorls around areas of fibrosis. The disarray is present in the myofibers, among myocytes and in the myofibrils within the myocytes. (Image and legend from Alday LE, Moreyra E. Hypertrophic cardiomyopathy in infants and children. Cardiomyopathies—from Basic Research to Clinical Management. Intechweb.org. CC).

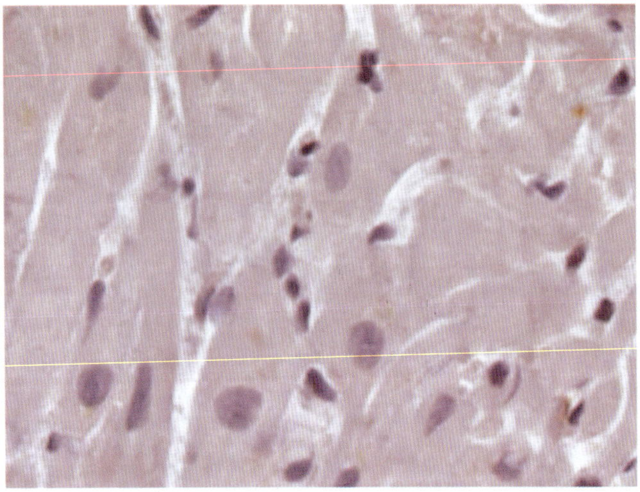

Fig. 22.32: Hematoxylin and eosin staining of ventricular myocardial interstitial fibrosis. The figure also demonstrates myocardial fiber disarray and replacement fibrosis—the microscopic hallmarks of hypertrophic cardiomyopathy.

Additional risk factors that may support ICD implantation are listed in Table 22.1. One of these is the finding of marked fibrosis on Gadolinium-enhanced cardiac MRI. Patients without any of the listed risk markers are considered to have a good prognosis not substantially different from the general population. On the other hand, patients with an apical aneurysm and those who convert into a dilated phenotype with systolic dysfunction very probably in a risk class of its own, warranting close observation with a rather low threshold for ICD implantation.

ASYMPTOMATIC PATIENTS

No evidence-based recommendations can be made for asymptomatic HCM patients due to an absence of data. Based on pathophysiological considerations, beta receptor antagonists and anti-fibrotic interventions may be contemplated.

SYMPTOMATIC HYPERTROPHIC NON-OBSTRUCTIVE CARDIOMYOPATHY PATIENTS

Beta blockers or verapamil-type calcium antagonists may be used for rate control in presence of diastolic dysfunction. A spontaneous or therapy-induced change of phenotype from the non-obstructive to the obstructive variant may occasionally happen, warranting clinical and echocardiographic monitoring. In general, medical therapy for hypertrophic non-obstructive cardiomyopathy follows the recommendations issued for heart failure with preserved ejection fraction (HFpEF), including the management of atrial fibrillation.

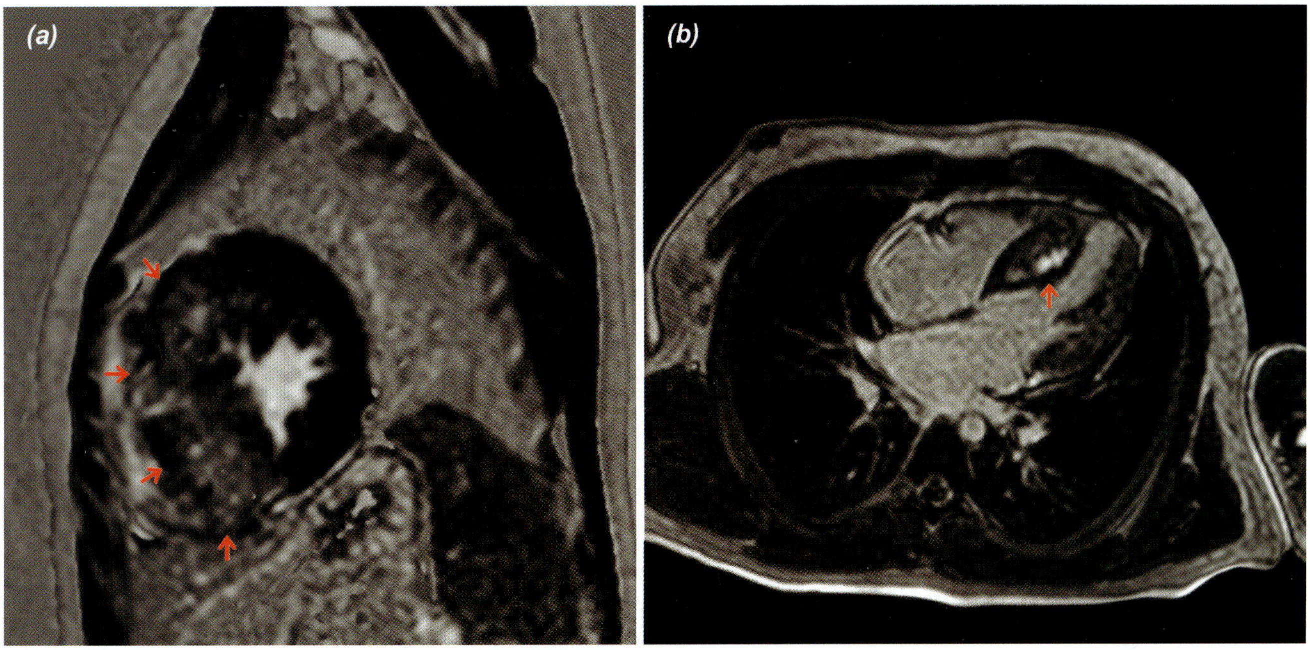

Fig. 22.33A: Cardiac MRI with delayed gadolinium enhancement in two patients with HCM demonstrating diffuse fibrosis (Figure a, arrows) and localized fibrosis in the interventricular septum (Figure b, arrow). [Images courtesy of Dr. Ricardo Pignatelli. Texas Children's Hospital. Images originally published in Alday LE, Moreyra. Hypertrophic cardiomyopathy in infants and children. In: Veselka J (Ed). Cardiomyopathies—from Basic Research to Clinical Management. Intechweb.org. CC]. (LA: Left atrium; LV: Left ventricle; RA: Right atrium; RV: Left ventricle).

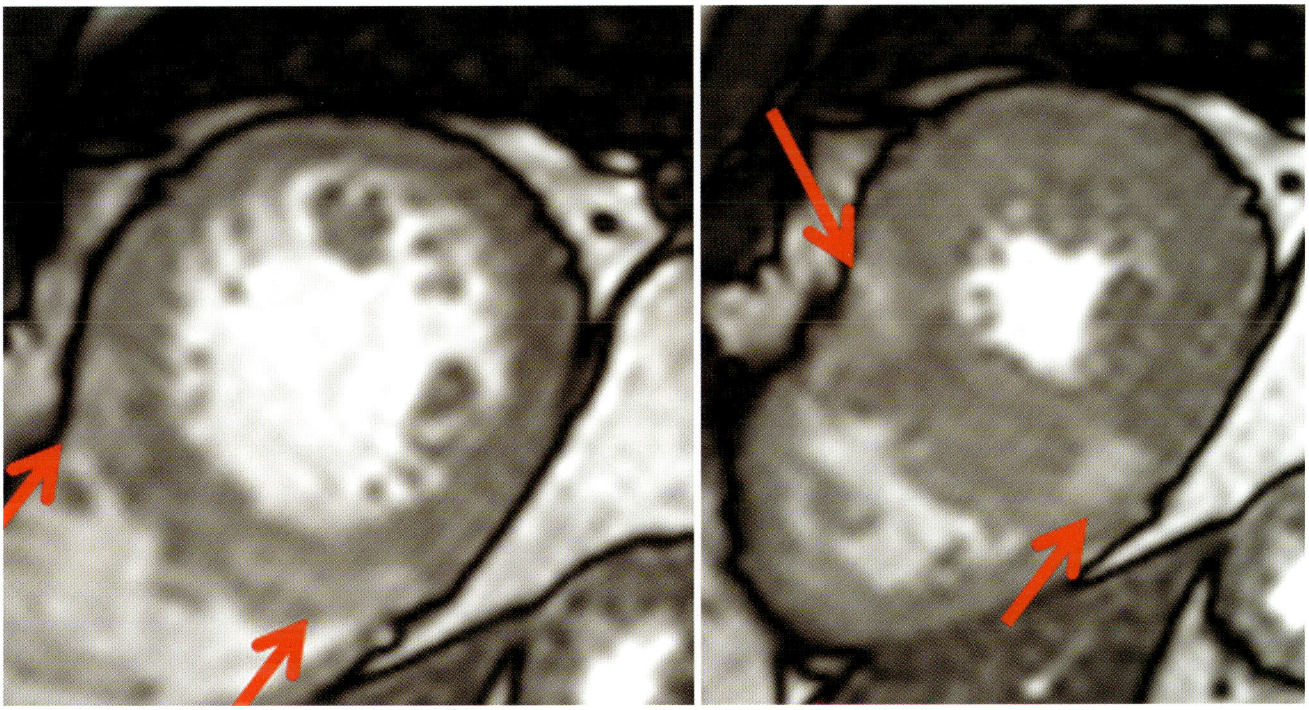

Fig. 22.33B: Gadolinium-enhanced magnetic resonance imaging (LGE-CMR) study of a 69-year-old female with HCM demonstrating areas of myocardial fibrosis (arrows) in the left ventricle.

Table 22.1: Factors which identify patients with HCM at high risk for ventricular arrhythmia and for prophylactic implantation of an ICD.

Risk factor	*Definition*
First degree risk factors	
Positive family history of SCD	SCD < 45 years
Recurrent syncope	≥ 2 incidents
Marked LVH	≥ 30 mm at any site in the LV
Abnormal blood pressure response during exercise	Increase < 20 mm Hg or fall > 20 mm Hg in blood pressure
Non-sustained VT in Holter ECG	≥ 3 consecutive QRS complexes with HR ≥ 120 bpm
Second degree risk factors	
Atrial fibrillation or atrial flutter	
LA dilatation	> 45 mm (M-Mode echo)
High LVOT gradient at rest	> 80 mm Hg (CW-Doppler)
Evidence of myocardial ischemia during exercise	
Early manifestation of HCM	< 30 years of age
Myocardial bridging near the LAD	
Marked fibrosis in cardiac MRI	Fibrosis ≥ 2 segments in 17 segment model of the LV

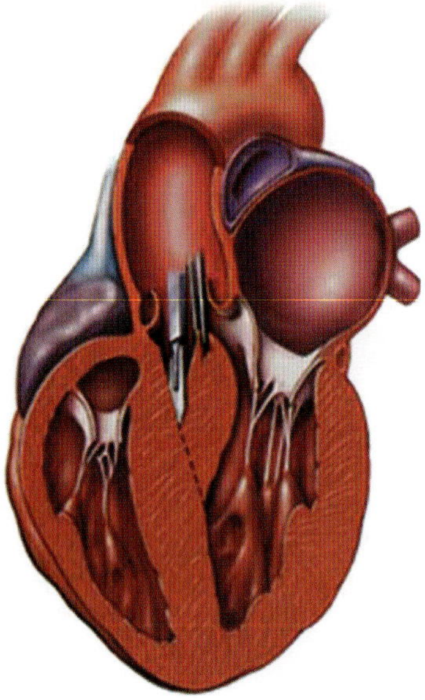

Fig. 22.34: Myomyectomy for asymmetric septal hypertrophy. (Image courtesy of and with permission by Mayo Foundation for Medical Education and Research. All rights reserved. Mayo Clinic retains copyright of this image).

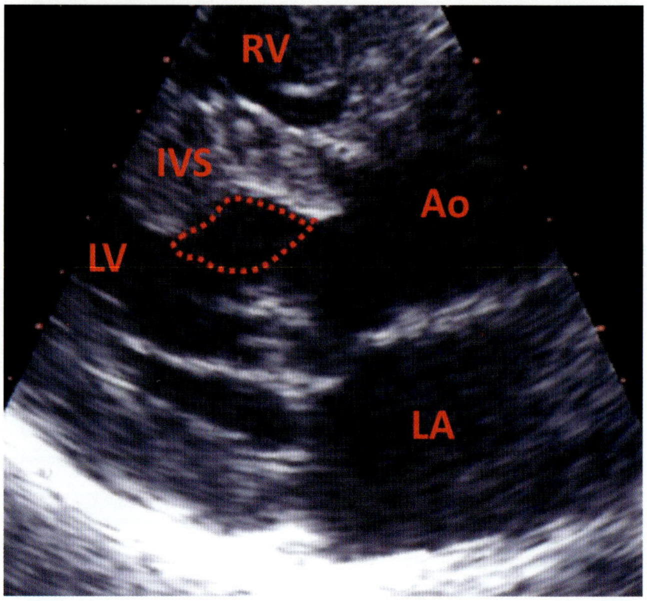

Fig. 22.35: Echocardiographic parasternal long-axis view in a hypertrophic obstructive cardiomyopathy patient years after a septal myectomy procedure. Note the thinned subaortic region where myocardial resection was performed (dotted circle). (Ao: Aorta; IVS: Interventricular septum; LA: Left atrium; LV: Left ventricle; RV: Right ventricle).

SYMPTOMATIC HYPERTROPHIC OBSTRUCTIVE CARDIOMYOPATHY (HOCM) PATIENTS

Positive inotropic agents or those reducing preload or afterload (such as digitalis preparations, nitrates, ACE inhibitors, or nifedipine-type calcium antagonists) should be avoided in HOCM due to possible aggravation of the outflow gradient. Beta blockers or verapamil-type calcium antagonists may be used to improve diastolic LV filling and to reduce the outflow gradient. In cases of coexisting arterial hypertension, diuretics and/or central alpha receptor blockers can be used.

For patients who do not sufficiently respond to pharmacotherapy, septal myectomy (Morrow procedure), developed in the late 1950s, has been the standard of

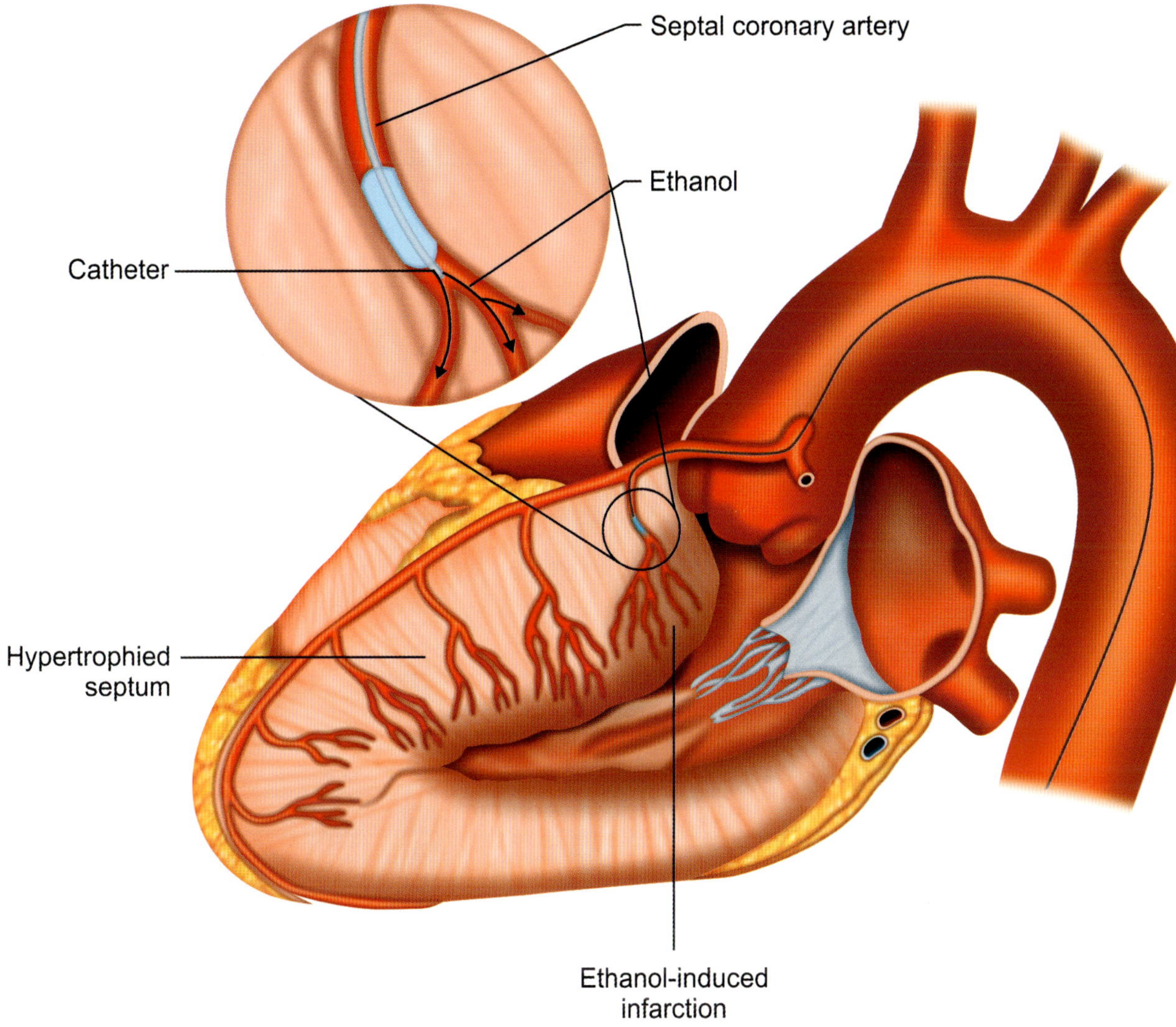

Fig. 22.36: Illustration of the alcohol septal ablation procedure.

therapy over the last several decades. The principle of this procedure is removal of part of the obstructing basal septum during open-heart surgery using cardiopulmonary bypass (Figs. 22.35 and 22.36). Mortality rates of 0–2% have been reported in experienced centers. Whether the clinical and hemodynamic improvement that is usually seen is accompanied by a prognostic improvement is uncertain.

Percutaneous septal ablation therapy (known as PTSMA, TASH, ASA, or ESA) was developed in the 1990s, and aims at reproducing via a catheter-based procedure the morphologic and hemodynamic results of septal myectomy (Figs. 22.36 and 22.37, Flow chart 22.1). Success and complication rates are largely comparable to those reported for myectomy. However, since access to the hypertrophied muscle is linked to availability of an appropriate septal perforator artery, the results are somewhat less predictable, and in a small percentage of patients the procedure is not feasible.

Atrio-right ventricular sequential pacemaker stimulation with a short AV delay may also be used to reduce the outflow gradient in HOCM. This method, delaying contraction of the thickened basal myocardium was somewhat euphorically embraced in the early 1990s. However, results of pacing are far less pronounced as compared to septal myectomy or ablation, so that only niche indications remain. Flow chart 22.1 summarizes a treatment algorithm for HCM patients with drug-refractory symptoms.

Flow chart 22.1: Treatment algorithm for HCM patients with drug-refractory symptoms. (HOCM: Hypertrophic obstructive cardiomyopathy; HNCM: Hypertrophic non-obstructive cardiomyopathy).

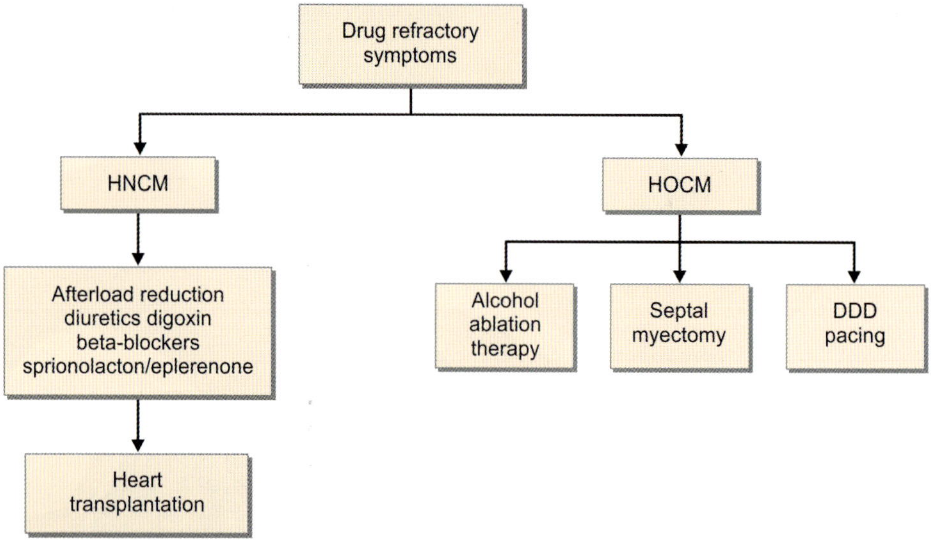

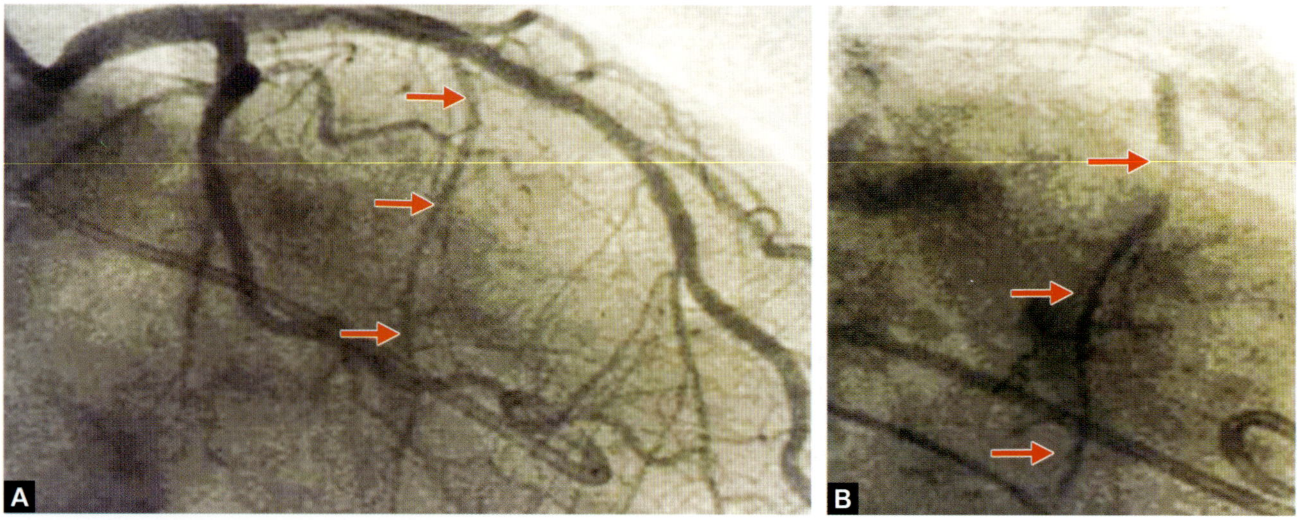

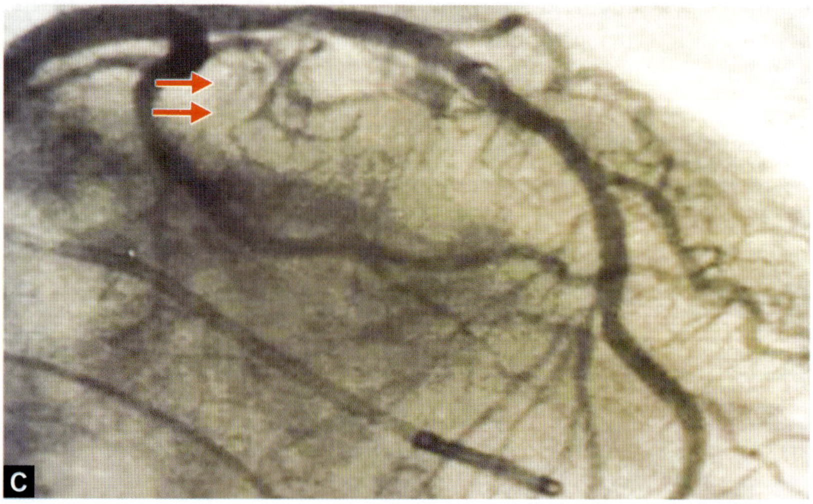

Figs. 22.37A to C: Cine images demonstrating the septal alcohol ablation procedure of a septal perforator artery. The target vessel is identified (Figure A, arrows). After balloon inflation in the proximal part of the target vessel, contrast dye is injected to verify the distal vessel bed (Figure B, arrows). Angiogram also verified that there is complete occlusion of the vessel lumen, preventing any retrograde flow in to the LAD artery. After alcohol injection in to the target septal artery, angiography (Figure C) shows the stump of the septal perforator with complete occlusion of the septal perforator more distally.

VIDEO LEGENDS

Video 22.1: Parasternal long-axis TTE showing septal hypertrophy in a patient with HCM. (Video courtesy of Glenn N. Levine, MD).

Video 22.2: Apical 4-chamber TTE of a patient with marked septal hypertrophy and HCM.

Video 22.3: Parasternal long axis transthoracic echocardiography video clip of a patient with HCM showing thickening of the interventricular septum.

Video 22.4: MRI displayed in the 4-chamber view showing apical hypertrophic cardiomyopathy. (Video courtesy of Scott D. Flamm, MD).

Video 22.5: MRI displayed in the 2-chamber view showing apical hypertrophic cardiomyopathy. (Video courtesy of Scott D. Flamm, MD).

Video 22.6: Apical 4-chamber TTE from a patient with apical HCM. (Video courtesy of Glenn N. Levine, MD).

Video 22.7: Apical 2-chamber TTE from a patient with apical HCM. (Video courtesy of Glenn N. Levine, MD).

Videos 22.8A and B: Apical 4-chamber TTE images of a patient with septal hypertrophy and HCM. (A) 2D video shows systolic anterior motion (SAM) of the anterior mitral leaflet during systole. (B) Corresponding color Doppler video clip shows the resulting mitral regurgitation.

Videos 22.9A and B: Parasternal long-axis TTE images showing modest SAM and resulting mitral regurgitation in a patient with HCM and dynamic outflow obstruction. Note also the turbulent blood flow in the left ventricular outflow tract.

Video 22.10: Three-chamber TTE in a patient with HCM demonstrating SAM and resulting severe eccentric MR during Valsalva maneuver. (Video courtesy of Glenn N. Levine, MD).

REFERENCES

Gersh BJ, Maron BJ, Bonow RO, et al. 2011 ACCF/AHA Guideline for the Diagnosis and Treatment of Hypertrophic Cardiomyopathy. Executive summary: a report of the American College of Cardiology Foundation/American Heart Association Task Force on Practice Guidelines. Circulation. 2011;124:2761-96.

Maron BJ, McKenna WJ, Danielson GK, et al. American College of Cardiology/European Society of Cardiology Clinical Expert Consensus Document on Hypertrophic Cardiomyopathy: a report of the American College of Cardiology Foundation Task Force on Clinical Expert Consensus Documents and the European Society of Cardiology Committee for Practice Guidelines. Eur Heart J. 2003;24:1965-91.

Prinz C, Farr M, Hering D, et al. The diagnosis and treatment of hypertrophic cardiomyopathy. Dtsch Arztebl Int. 2011;108:209-15.

Prinz C, Farr M, Laser KT, et al. Determining the role of fibrosis in hypertrophic cardiomyopathy. Expert Rev Cardiovasc Ther. 2013;11:495-504.

CHAPTER

Infiltrative Heart Disease and Restrictive Cardiomyopathy 23

Salil Ginde, Steven D Zangwill

INTRODUCTION

Restrictive cardiomyopathy (RCM) is a disease of the myocardium characterized by abnormal diastolic function with normal or near normal systolic function. It is associated with a variety of pathologic conditions that cause decreased ventricular compliance, resulting in impaired ventricular filling and reduced diastolic volume of either or both ventricles. Compared to dilated and hypertrophic cardiomyopathy, it is the least common cardiomyopathy in Western countries and accounts for approximately 5% of all cases of primary heart muscle disease.

ETIOLOGY

Restrictive cardiomyopathy can be classified as myocardial (infiltrative or noninfiltrative) or endomyocardial based on the underlying pathology (Table 23.1).

Infiltrative Cardiomyopathies

Infiltrative diseases of the myocardium are a common cause of RCM. Extensive deposition of material between the myocardial fibers or within the myocytes, often in the setting of an underlying systemic condition, results in firm, noncompliant, and often thickened ventricular myocardium.

Amyloidosis (Figs. 23.1A to D) is a disease characterized by the deposition of unique proteins, consisting of twisted beta-pleated sheet fibrils, into various organs. Cardiac infiltration (Fig. 23.2) is most often seen with primary amyloidosis, in which the amyloid protein is composed of portions of immunoglobulin light chain produced by a monoclonal population of plasma cells, as seen with multiple myeloma. RCM is less commonly seen with familial amyloidosis, senile amyloidosis, or secondary amyloidosis, which is associated with protein deposition in patients with a chronic inflammatory disease such as rheumatoid arthritis or tuberculosis. Heart failure occurs in up to one-third of patients with primary amyloidosis and is the most common cause of death. Diagnosis is confirmed by examination of endomyocardial biopsy tissue with special staining, which demonstrates the amyloid deposits within the myocardium.

Sarcoidosis is a granulomatous disorder associated with the deposition of noncaseating sarcoid granulomas into multiple organ systems including the lungs, reticuloendothelial system, skin, and heart (Figs. 23.3 and 23.4).

Table 23.1: Classification of restrictive cardiomyopathy based on underlying pathology.

Myocardial-Infiltrative	*Myocardial-Noninfiltrative*	*Endomyocardial*
• Infiltrative	• Idiopathic restrictive cardiomyopathy	• Endomyocardial fibrosis
• Amyloidosis	• Familial restrictive cardiomyopathy	• Hypereosinophilic syndrome
• Sarcoidosis	• Hypertrophic cardiomyopathy	• Radiation
• Hemochromatosis	• Scleroderma	• Metastatic cancers
• Glycogen storage disease	• Diabetic cardiomyopathy	• Medication toxicity
• Gaucher disease		
• Hurler-Scheie disease		
• Fabry disease		
• Fatty infiltration		

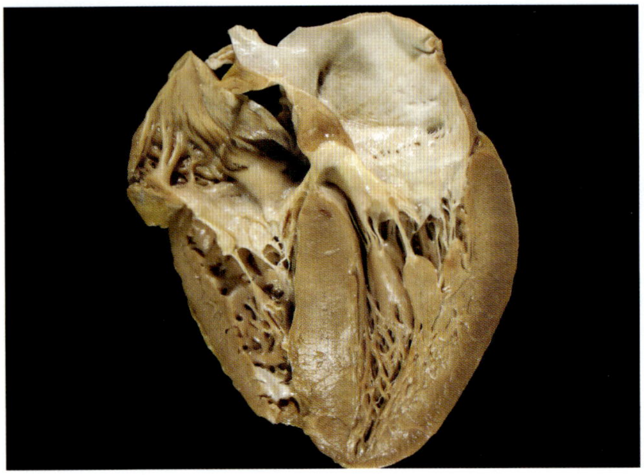

Fig. 23.1A: Gross pathology of cardiac amyloidosis. (Image courtesy of Robert Padera, MD, PhD, Department of Pathology, Brigham and Women's Hospital).

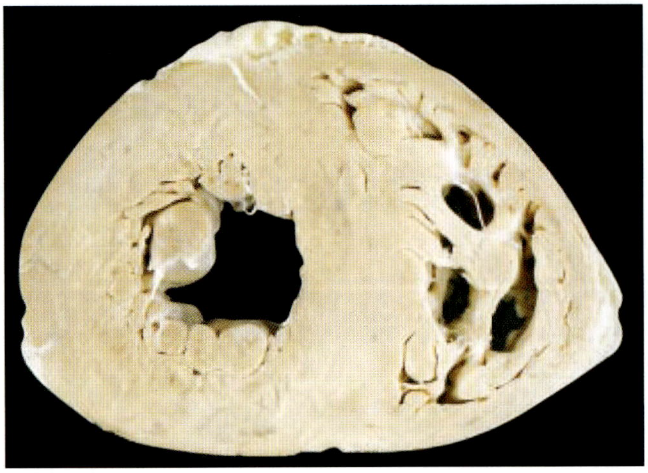

Fig. 23.1B: Gross pathology section from a patient with cardiac amyloidosis and restrictive cardiomyopathy. The ventricular walls are thickened. The heart has a rubbery appearance and is brown with a grayish tone. [Image from Clinicopathologic Session: case 1/00—The patient is a 65-year-old woman with heart failure and proteinuria. Arq Bras Cardiol. 2000;74(2). Available from http://www.scielo.br/pdf/abc/v74n2/2197.pdf].

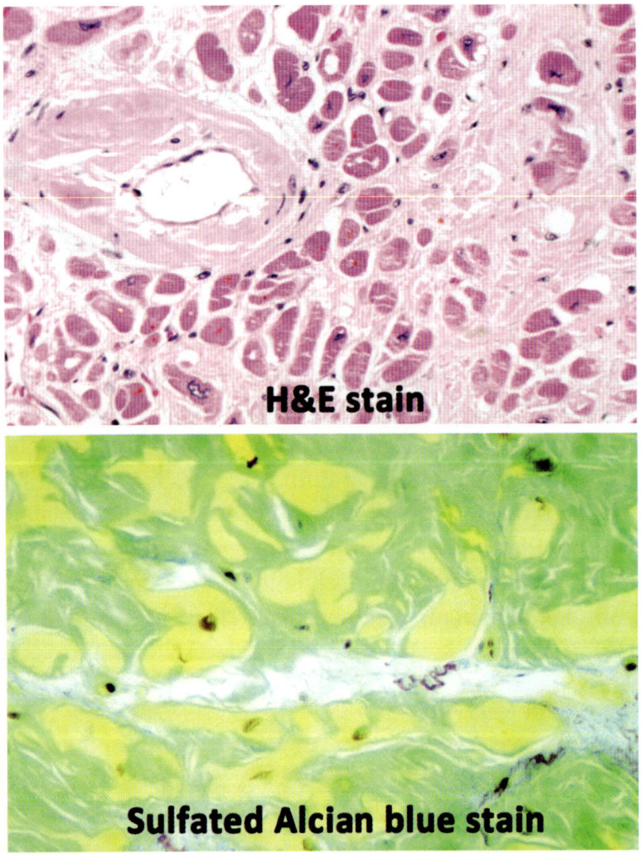

Fig. 23.1C: Endomyocardial biopsy in a patient with cardiac amyloidosis. Upper panel: H&E stain demonstrates an amorphous light pink extracellular material separating the more deeply stained myocytes. Lower panel: Sulfated Alcian blue stain shows the amyloid staining turquoise and the myocytes yellow. [Image from Falk RH. Diagnosis and management of the cardiac amyloidoses. Circulation. 2005;112(13):2047-60, with permission].

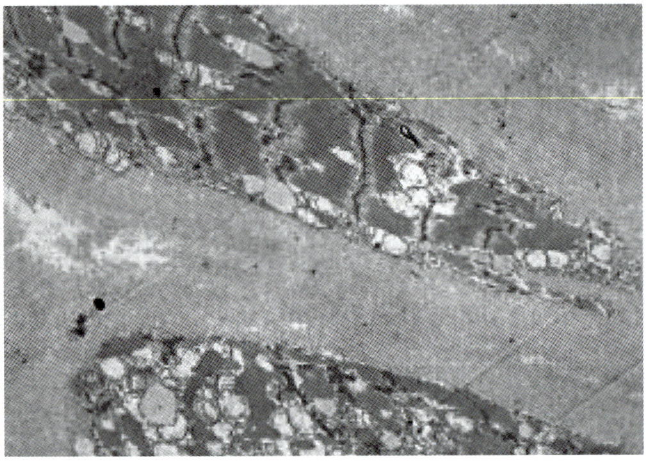

Fig. 23.1D: Electron microscopy of the heart in Figure 23.1A. The interstitium is markedly enlarged due to the presence of the characteristic fibrils of amyloid. [Image from Clinicopathologic Session: case 1/00—The patient is a 65-year-old woman with heart failure and proteinuria. Arq Bras Cardiol. 2000;74(2). Available from http://www.scielo.br/pdf/abc/v74n2/2197.pdf].

Cardiac involvement is found in 20–30% of cases at autopsy, although only about 5% develop clinical manifestations, such as RCM with congestive heart failure, heart block, ventricular arrhythmias, and sudden death.

Hemochromatosis is a systemic disorder characterized by increased deposition of iron in tissue. Cardiac involvement with both intracellular and extracellular iron deposition is common (Fig. 23.5), both with primary (idiopathic)

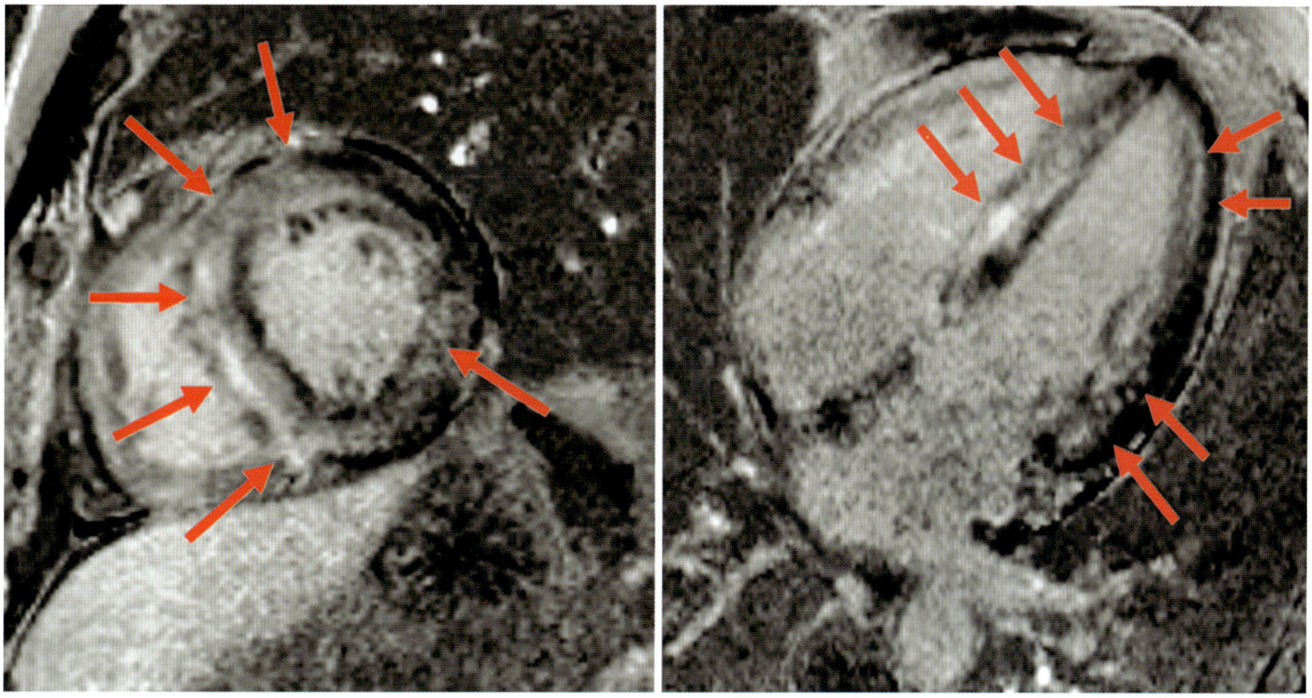

Fig. 23.2: Late gadolinium enhancement images demonstrating diffuse cardiac involvement in a patient with amyloidosis. [Image from Liu D, et al. Impact of regional left ventricular function on outcome for patients with AL amyloidosis. PLoS One. 2013;8(3): e56923].

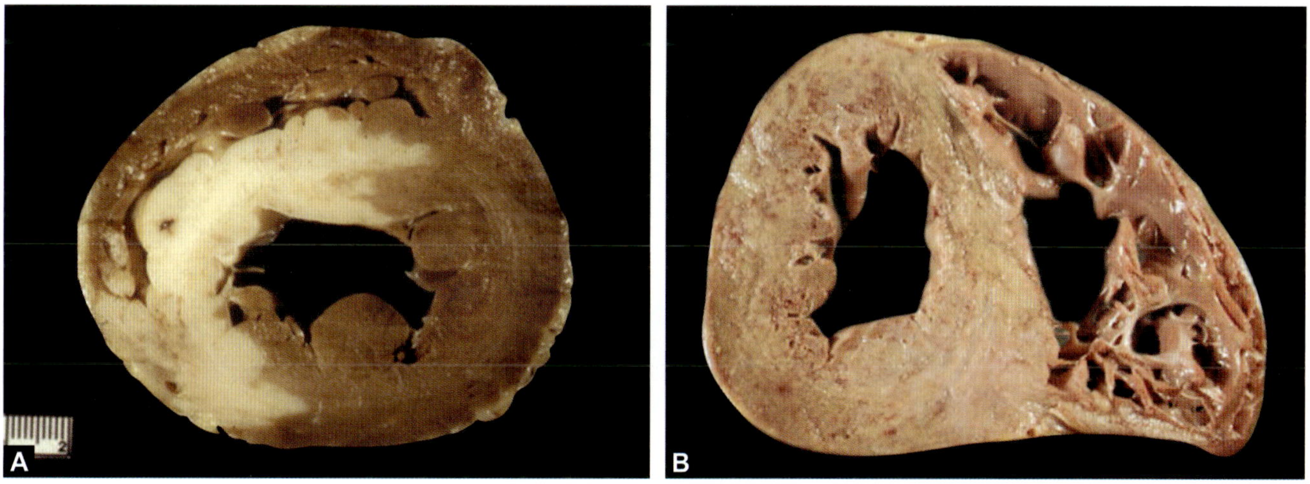

Figs. 23.3A and B: Autopsy cardiac specimens of patients with sarcoidosis with myocardial involvement displayed in the short-axis. (A) The typical pattern of sarcoid involvement with well-demarcated areas involving the ventricular septum and anterior left ventricle with some extension into the anterior right ventricle; (B) Low magnification.

and secondary (i.e. excess blood transfusions or oral iron intake) forms. Both restrictive and dilated cardiomyopathies are associated with hemochromatosis. New magnetic resonance imaging (MRI) techniques have recently been employed for direct assessments of the severity of myocardial iron deposition (Figs. 23.6A to C).

Several forms of metabolic storage disease created by inborn errors of metabolism can result in the accumulation of abnormal metabolites within the cardiac myocytes, producing a restrictive cardiac physiology. Disorders in the metabolism of glycogen (Fig. 23.7) (Pompe disease, Cori disease), lipid (Fabry disease, Gaucher disease), and mucopolysaccharide (Hurler-Scheie, Sanfilippo) have all been associated with myocardial deposition and RCM. Their clinical course is often dictated by the involvement of multiple other organ systems.

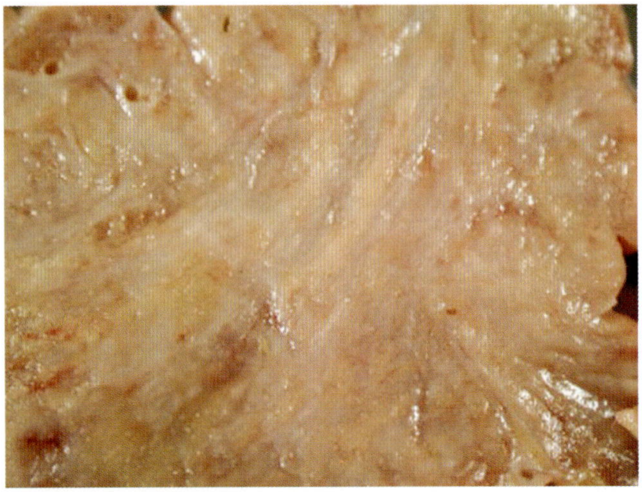

Fig. 23.3C: High magnification views showing a diffuse scarring secondary to the granulomatous disease. [Image reprinted from Tavora F, Cresswell N, Li L, et al. Comparison of necropsy findings in patients with sarcoidosis dying suddenly from cardiac sarcoidosis versus dying suddenly from other causes. Am J Cardiol. 2009;104(4):571-7, with permission from Elsevier].

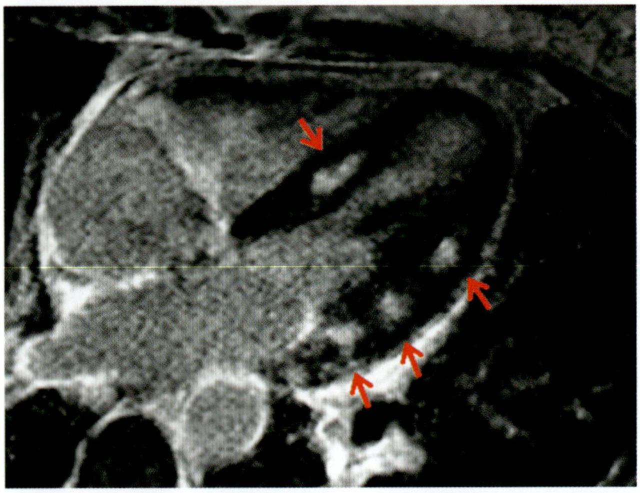

Fig. 23.4: Patchy, mid-myocardial, late gadolinium enhancement, in a patient with sarcoidosis. This finding is highly suggestive of cardiac involvement of sarcoidosis.

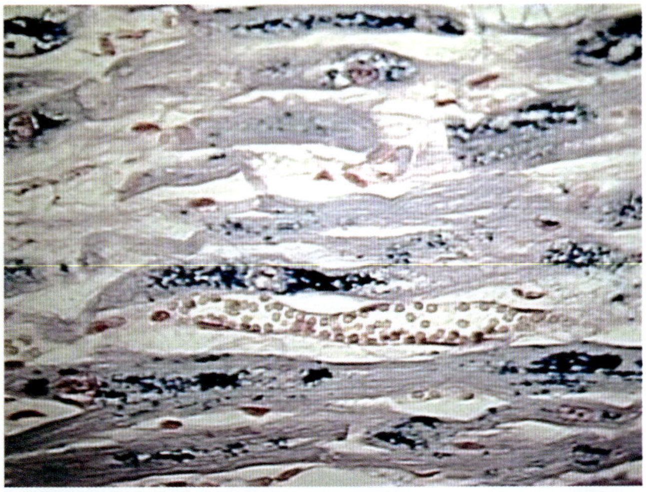

Fig. 23.5: Histological examination of the myocardium in a patient with hemachromatosis. There is diffuse iron deposition in the myocardium. (Image from Armed Forces Institute of Pathology).

Noninfiltrative Diseases

Many cases of RCM are idiopathic. Inherited forms of RCM have been reported, especially in association with atrioventricular block and skeletal myopathy. Hypertrophic cardiomyopathy is a distinct pathologic entity but can have a restrictive physiology similar to RCM.

Endomyocardial Disease

Endomyocardial diseases result in endocardial thickening and/or scarring, which then impairs the diastolic function of the ventricle. Endomyocardial fibrosis is a common form of RCM found in tropical and subtropical regions (Fig. 23.8A), and is characterized by intense endocardial fibrotic thickening of the apex and subvalvular inflow regions of one or both ventricles. Löffler endocarditis (Fig. 23.8B), or hypereosinophilic syndrome, is pathologically and clinically similar to endomyocardial fibrosis, but is differentiated by its occurrence in more temperate climates and its association with marked persistent hypereosinophilia. The etiology of endomyocardial fibrosis and Löffler endocarditis are unknown. Endocardial fibroelastosis is a disorder of infants and young children characterized by thickening of the endocardium due to hyperplasia of the supporting connective tissue and elastic fibers (Figs. 23.9A and B). Finally, radiation therapy and certain medications can result in endomyocardial disease and the development of RCM.

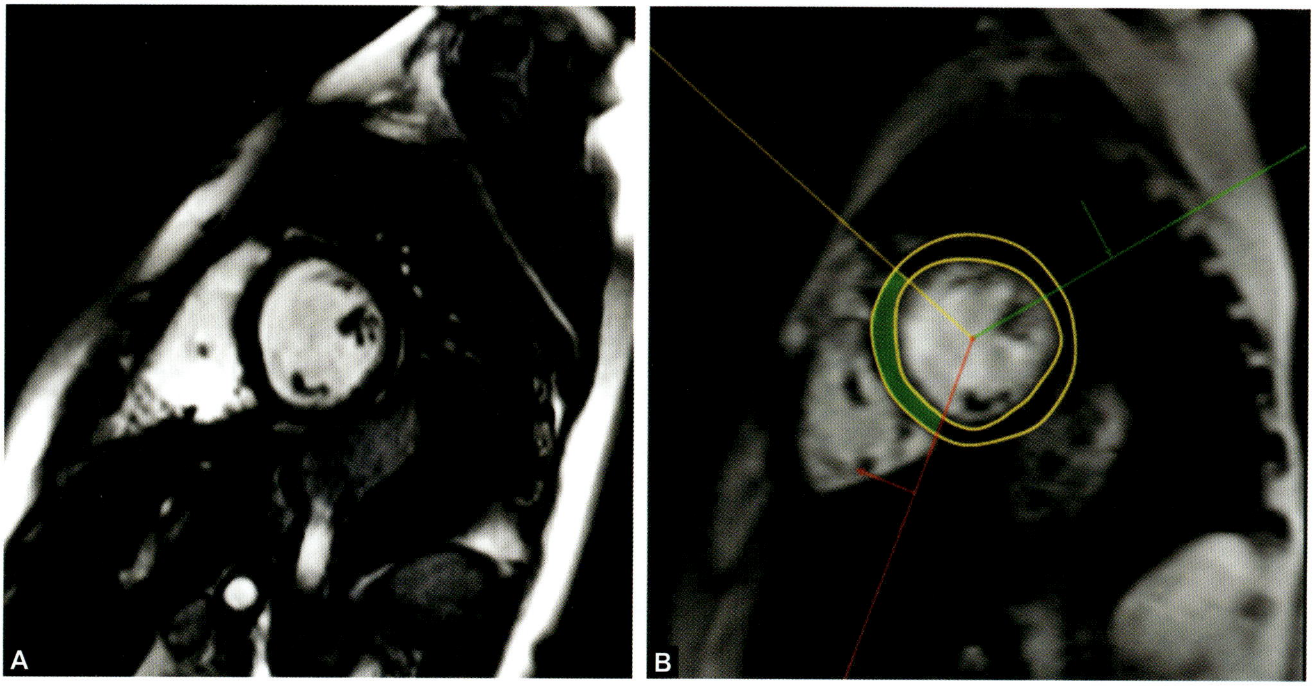

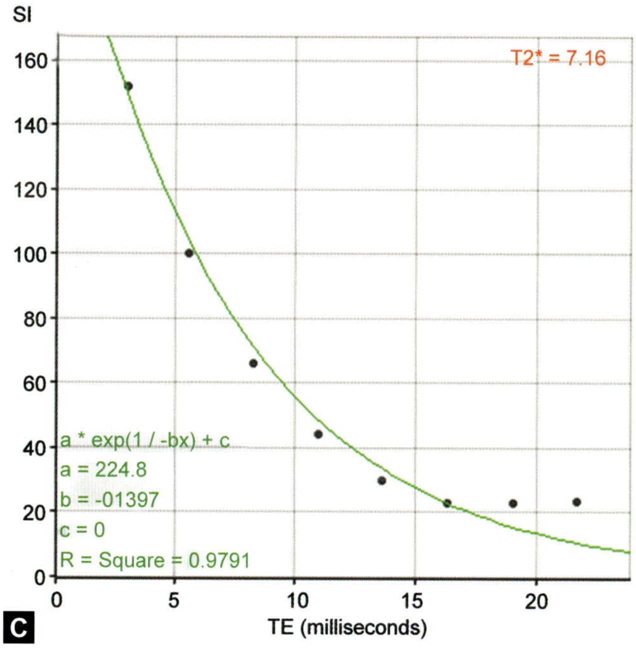

Figs. 23.6A to C: Cardiac magnetic resonance imaging of a patient with Diamond Blackfan anemia and chronic blood transfusions. A short-axis image of the left ventricle (A) with T2* relaxation analysis demonstrates markedly reduced signal intensity of the myocardium and calculated T2* value (B and C) of 7.16 (normal > 20), consistent with severe iron infiltration of the myocardium.

PATHOPHYSIOLOGY

Diastole is defined as the period of the cardiac cycle between closure of the semilunar valves (aortic and pulmonary valves) to closure of the atrioventricular valves (mitral and tricuspid valves), during which time ventricular filling occurs. RCM is characterized by disruption of diastolic function and ventricular filling due to a variety of myopathic processes that affect one or both of two functional properties of the ventricle during diastole: (1) relaxation of the ventricle with active uncoupling of the muscle after systolic contraction, and (2) compliance or stiffness of the ventricle.

These diastolic abnormalities occur in a progressive manner, with delayed active relaxation seen early in the disease process followed by decreased ventricular compliance seen as a later finding. The classic description of RCM is one of severely decreased ventricular compliance

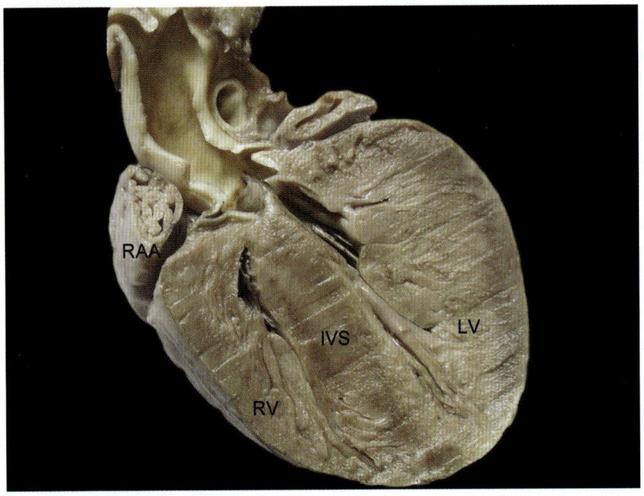

Fig. 23.7: Gross pathology specimen from a patient with glycogen storage disease and restrictive cardiomyopathy. [Image courtesy of Dr Pradeep Vaideeswar, Department of Pathology (Cardiovascular & Thoracic Division), Seth GS Medical College, Mumbai, India]. (Ao: Aorta; LV: Left ventricle; RV: Right ventricle, IVS: Intact ventricular septum; RAA: Right atrial appendage).

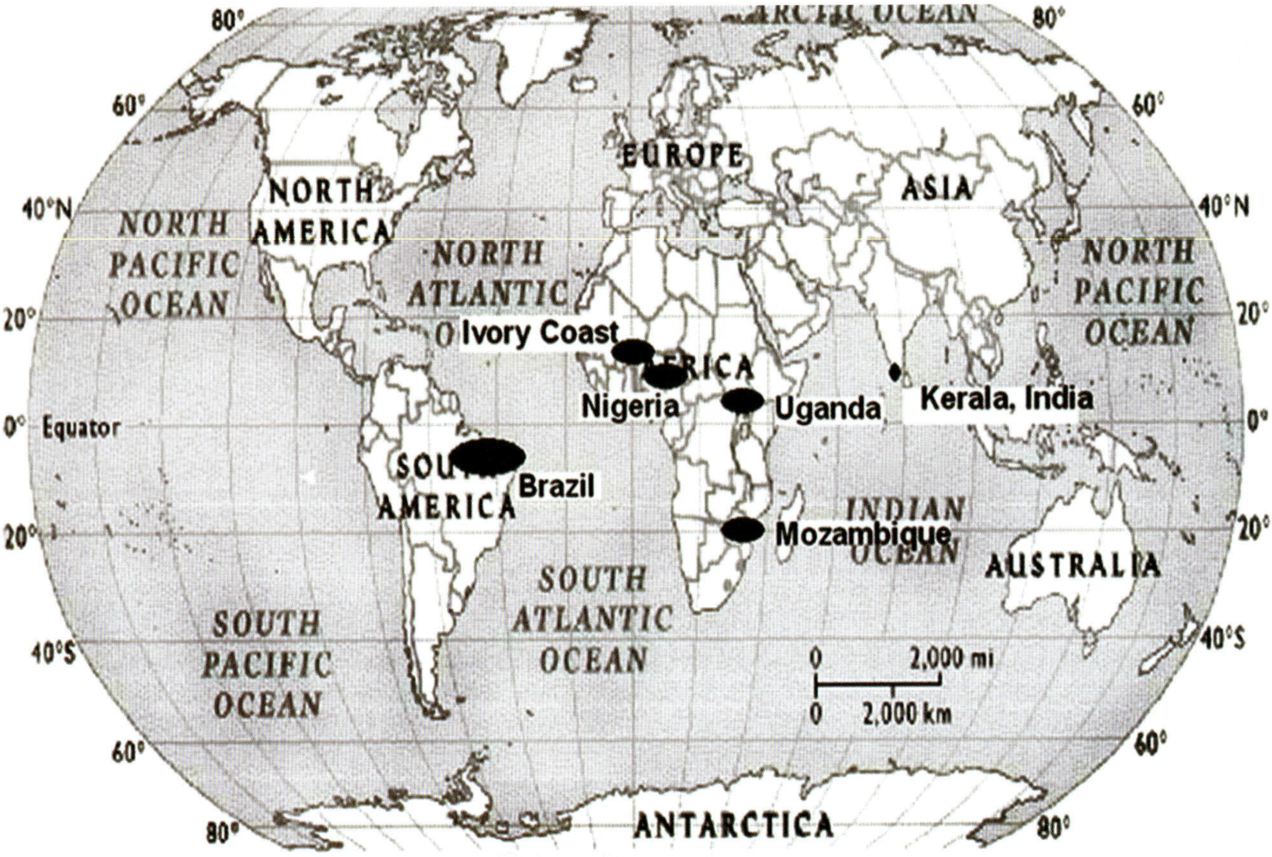

Fig. 23.8A: Map of the world showing the geographic distribution of places which have reported endemic cases of endomyocardial fibrosis. [Image and legend text from Vijayaraghavan G, Sivasankaran S. Restrictive and obliterative cardiomyopathies. In: Chatterjee K, Anderson M, Heistad D, Kerber RE (Eds). Cardiology—An Illustrated Textbook. New Delhi, India: Jaypee Brothers Medical Publishers (P) Ltd. 2012].

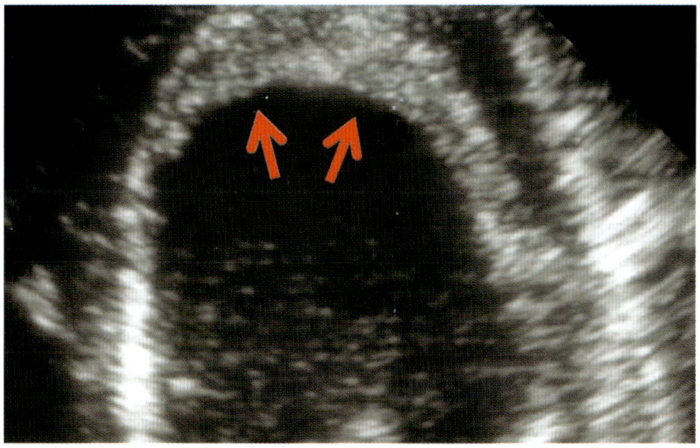

Fig. 23.8B: Zoomed transthoracic image of the left ventricle, showing fibrothrombotic oblieration of the apex (arrows). [Image and legend text from Vijayaraghavan G, Sivasankaran S. Restrictive and obliterative cardiomyopathies. In: Chatterjee K, Anderson M, Heistad D, Kerber RE (Eds). Cardiology—An Illustrated Textbook. New Delhi, India: Jaypee Brothers Medical Publishers (P) Ltd. 2012].

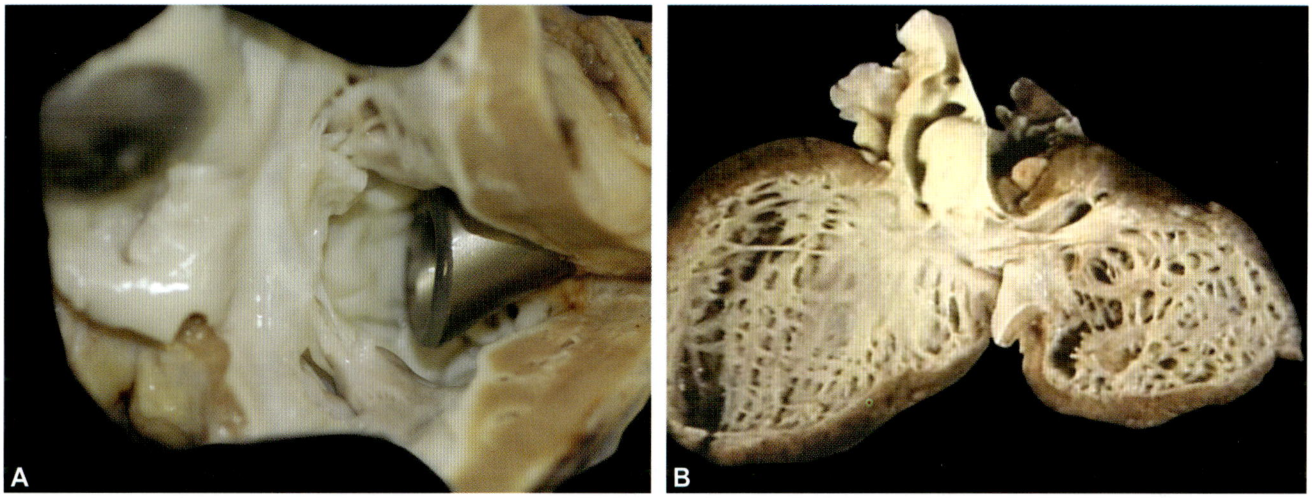

Figs. 23.9A and B: Left ventricular cavity from an explanted heart of a patient with restrictive cardiomyopathy secondary to endocardial fibroelastosis demonstrates a diffuse yellow-white endocardial surface membrane due to deposition of fibrous elastic tissues. Also noted is the left atrial side of an atrial septal defect closure device, as well as the two cannuli of a left ventricular assist device within the left ventricular apex and the ascending aorta. (B) Gross pathology specimen of endocardial fibroelastosis. (Image from Armed Forces Institute of Pathology).

such that ventricular pressure declines rapidly at the onset of diastole, and then rapidly rises in response to a small change in ventricular volume. Ventricular pressure then plateaus with cessation of ventricular filling in early diastole. This dip and plateau is often termed the "square root sign" based on the characteristic ventricular pressure tracing (Figs. 23.10A and B). Although systolic function is preserved, cardiac output is reduced due to impaired ventricular filling. Systolic dysfunction may develop with advanced cases of RCM. Elevation of atrial and ventricular diastolic pressure results in pulmonary and/or systemic venous congestion.

The hemodynamic abnormalities in RCM are similar to those of constrictive pericarditis, which is due to chronic inflammation and subsequent fibrosis of the pericardium. RCM and constrictive pericarditis can be differentiated based on various physical exam, hemodynamic, and diagnostic findings (Table 23.2).

CLINICAL PRESENTATION

Exercise intolerance is a frequent symptom of RCM. It results from the inability to augment cardiac output with tachycardia, due to impaired ventricular filling. Pulmonary

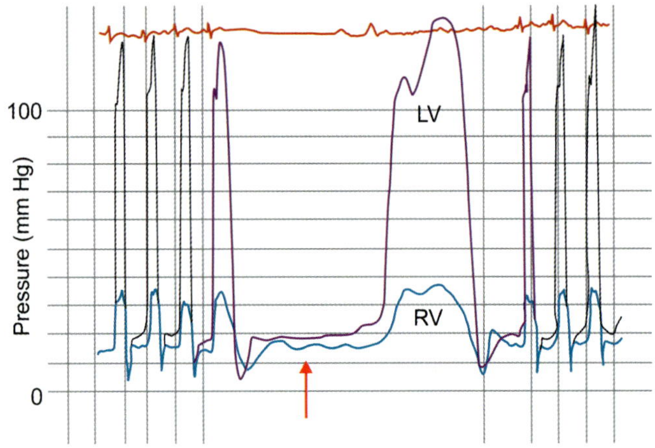

Fig. 23.10A: Simultaneous recordings of left ventricular (LV) and right ventricular (RV) pressures in a patient with restrictive cardiomyopathy illustrating the "square-root sign" with an early diastolic dip and plateau. [Image with permission from Benotti JR, Grossman W, Cohn PF. Clinical profile of restrictive cardiomyopathy. Circulation. 1980;61(6):1206-12].

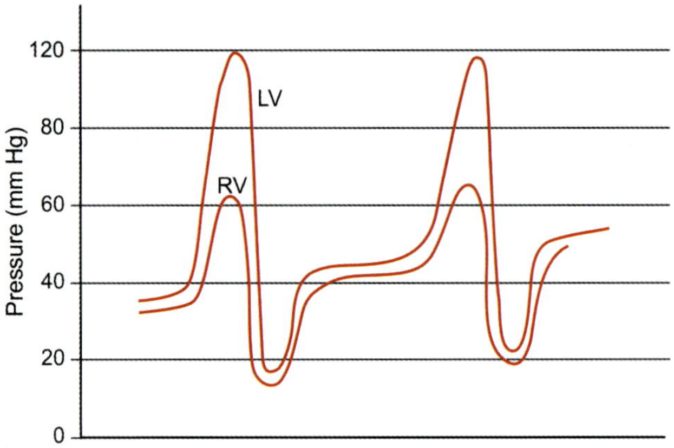

Fig. 23.10B: Schematic diagram showing hemodynamic features of restrictive cardiomyopathy. Left ventricular end-diastolic pressure is higher than the right ventricular end-diastolic pressure. Right ventricular systolic pressure is approximately 60 mm Hg suggesting pulmonary hypertension. Note the dip-and-plateau or square-root contour of the ventricular diastolic pressures (deep and rapid early decline in ventricular pressure at the onset of diastole, with a rapid rise to a plateau in early diastole). [Image and legend text from Karrowni W, Chatterjee K. Radiation-induced heart disease. In: Chatterjee K, Anderson M, Heistad D, Kerber RE (Eds). Cardiology—An Illustrated Textbook. New Delhi, India: Jaypee Brothers Medical Publishers (P) Ltd. 2012].

Table 23.2: Comparison of the clinical and hemodynamic findings of restrictive and constrictive cardiomyopathy. (LVH: Left ventricular hypertrophy; RVH: Right ventricular hypertrophy; RA: Right atrium; RVEDP: Right ventricular end-diastolic pressure; PCWP: Pulmonary capillary wedge pressure; LVEDP: Left ventricular end-diastolic pressure).

	Restrictive Cardiomyopathy	***Constrictive Cardiomyopathy***
Physical examination		
Pulsus paradoxus	Not present	May be present
Pericardial knock	Not present	May be present
Regurgitant murmurs	Common	Uncommon
Electrocardiogram		
Biatrial enlargement	Nearly always present	May be present
LVH/RVH	Common	Rare
Echocardiogram		
Pericardial thickening	Absent	May be present
Atrial size	Marked atrial dilatation	Usually normal
Ventricular wall thickness	Normal to mildly increased	Normal
Septal bounce	Absent	Present
Cardiac catheterization		
Filling pressures: Right-sided (RA/RVEDP) vs left-sided (PCWP/LVEDP)	Left usually 5 mm Hg > right	Equal right-sided and left-sided pressures (RA=PCWP, RVEDP=LVEDP)
Filling pressures > 25 mm Hg	Common	Rare
Pulmonary artery pressure	Usually elevated > 60 mm Hg	Usually < 50 mm Hg
Myocardial biopsy		
Myocardial biopsy	Abnormal	Usually normal

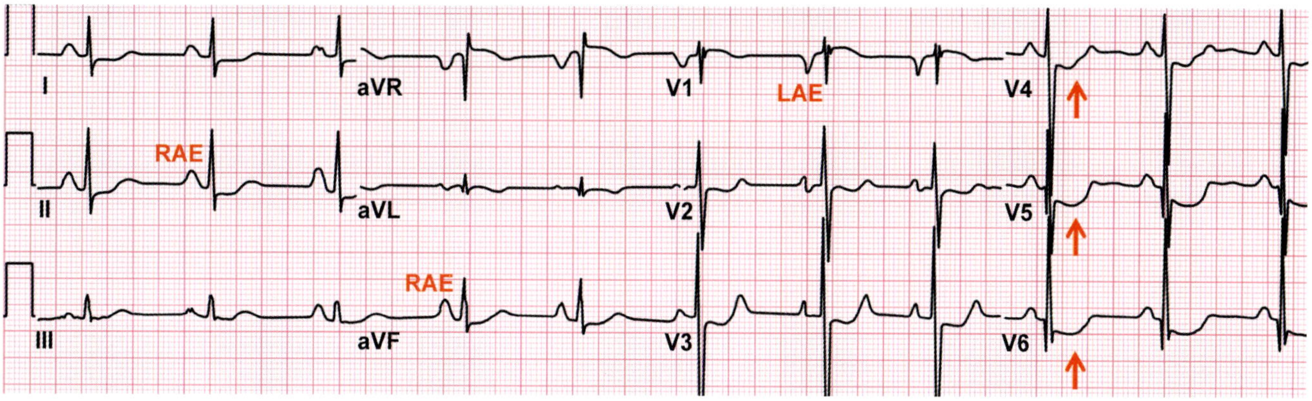

Fig. 23.11: Electrocardiogram in patient with restrictive cardiomyopathy demonstrates biatrial enlargement and ST-segment depression (arrows) in lateral precordial leads.

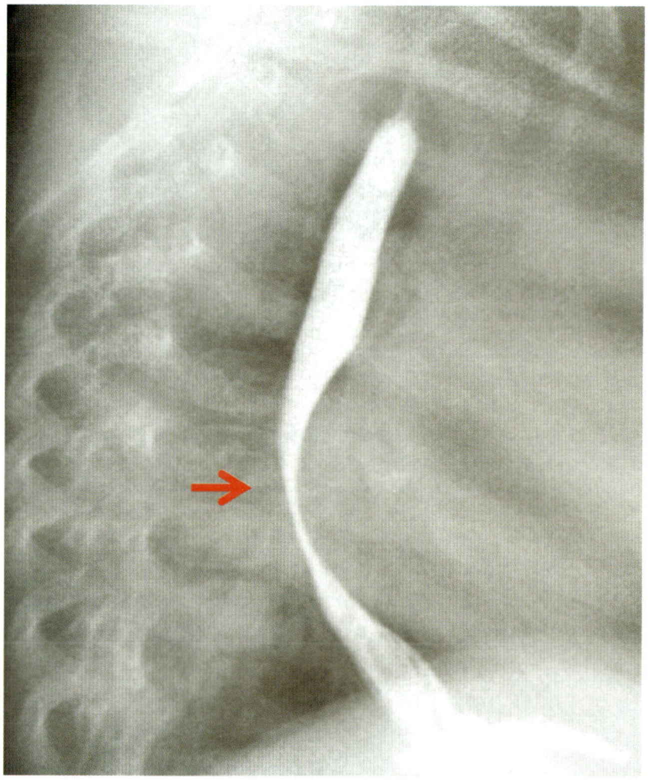

Fig. 23.12: Chest radiograph performed during a barium esophagram on a patient with restrictive cardiomyopathy and dysphagia demonstrates extrinsic compression of the distal esophagus from a dilated left atrium.

venous congestion manifests as dyspnea on exertion, orthopnea, and weakness. Systemic venous congestion may result in peripheral edema, hepatomegaly, and ascites. Syncope and sudden death may occur secondary to ischemia, dysrhythmias, or thromboembolism.

Physical examination of the patient with RCM may demonstrate jugular venous distention and a gallop rhythm with an S3, S4, or both. Kussmaul sign and pulsus paradoxus are more commonly seen with constrictive pericarditis and are typically not present with RCM. Peripheral edema, hepatomegaly, and ascites are present in advanced cases of RCM.

DIAGNOSTIC STUDIES

Electrocardiogram

The electrocardiogram is often abnormal with frequent biatrial enlargement and nonspecific ST-T wave abnormalities (Fig. 23.11). Diffusely diminished voltage is the classic finding with cardiac amyloidosis.

Noninvasive Cardiac Imaging

Chest radiograph is often abnormal, and demonstrates cardiomegaly and left atrial dilation (Fig. 23.12). Echocardiography can be diagnostic for RCM. The classic finding is markedly dilated atria out of proportion to any valvular regurgitation with preserved ventricular systolic function (Fig. 23.13). A granular sparkling texture of the myocardium may be seen with cardiac amyloidosis and Fabry disease. Atrial thrombi may be apparent (Fig. 23.14). Doppler interrogation of atrioventricular valve and venous inflows, as well as regional tissue Doppler assessment of mitral, septal and tricuspid annular velocities, reveal restrictive ventricular filling and increased ventricular end-diastolic pressure, consistent with diastolic dysfunction. In severe cases, the mitral inflow pattern demonstrates a rapid deceleration of the early filling (E) wave, signifying a rapid rise in ventricular pressure during early diastole (Fig. 23.15). Late diastolic filling is diminished

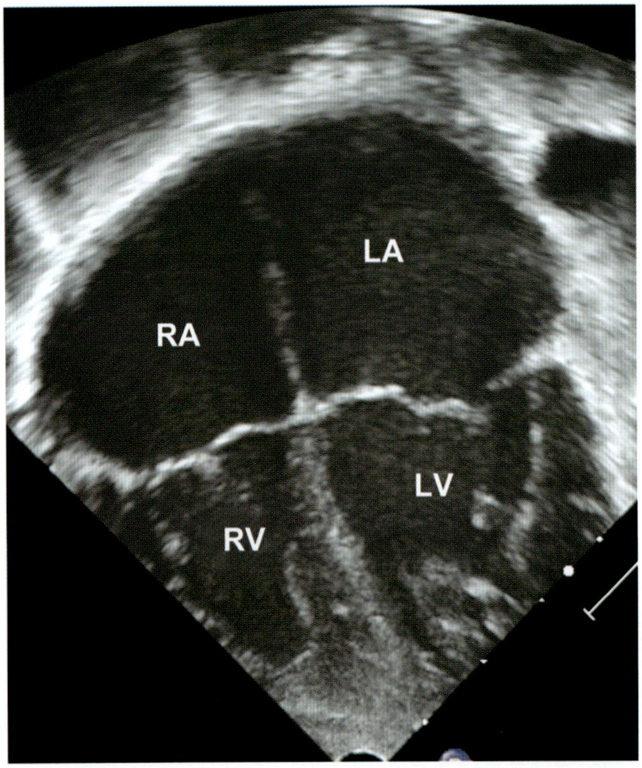

Fig. 23.13: Transthoracic echocardiogram performed in the apical four-chamber view of a patient with familial restrictive cardiomyopathy demonstrates marked biatrial dilatation with preserved ventricular size and geometry. (LA: Left atrium; LV: Left ventricle; RA: Right atrium; RV: Right ventricle).

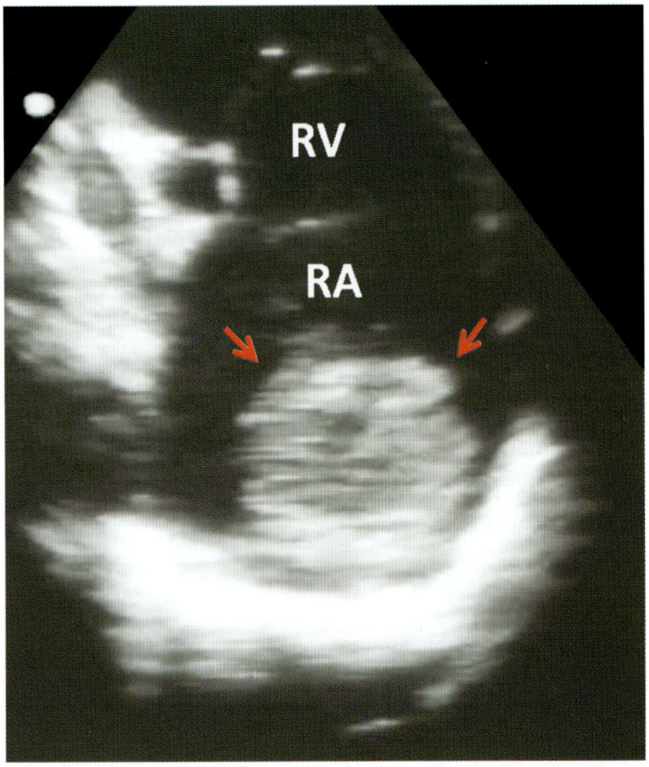

Fig. 23.14: Transthoracic echocardiogram from a patient with right ventricular endomyocardial fibrosis demonstrated a massively dilated right atrium (RA) and a large RA thrombus (arrows). [Image from Vijayaraghavan G, Sivasankaran S. Restrictive and obliterative cardiomyopathies. In: Chatterjee K, Anderson M, Heistad D, Kerber RE (Eds). Cardiology—An Illustrated Textbook. New Delhi, India: Jaypee Brothers Medical Publishers (P) Ltd. 2012]. (RV: Right ventricle).

due to increased ventricular diastolic pressure, and manifests during the mitral inflow Doppler as a low velocity signal during atrial contraction (A-wave) and reversal of flow with atrial contraction (AR) in the pulmonary venous Doppler (Fig. 23.16).

Cardiac MRI has shown increasing utility and versatility in the evaluation of RCM. Particularly useful is the MRI-derived measurements of pericardial thickness, which can assist in the differentiation of RCM with constrictive pericarditis.

Cardiac Catheterization

Invasive hemodynamic assessment can be an important tool in the evaluation of RCM (Fig. 23.17), especially in differentiating RCM from constrictive pericarditis (Table 23.2). Endomyocardial biopsy of patients with idiopathic RCM often demonstrate varying degrees of myocyte hypertrophy and interstitial fibrosis. In certain infiltrative cardiomyopathies, biopsy may reveal the specific etiology of the RCM, although the diagnostic yield can be variable (Figs. 23.18A to F).

MANAGEMENT

Cardiac medications are used for symptomatic treatment of venous congestion and decreased cardiac output. Symptomatic patients often require a combination of diuretics, beta adrenergic blocking agents, and afterload-reducing

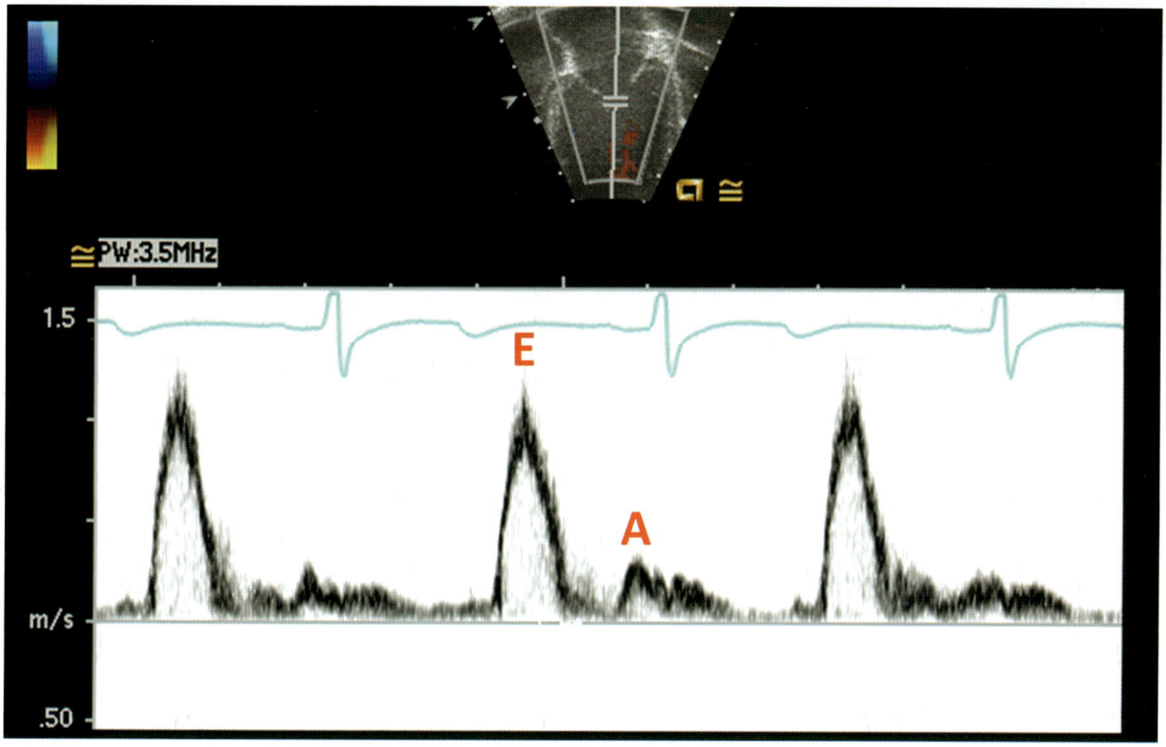

Fig. 23.15: Mitral inflow Doppler tracing in a patient with restrictive cardiomyopathy demonstrating severe diastolic disease. Reduced ventricular compliance and increased atrial diastolic pressures results in rapid deceleration of the early mitral inflow E wave. During late diastole, atrial contraction occurs against a stiff ventricle, resulting is a low velocity mitral inflow A wave.

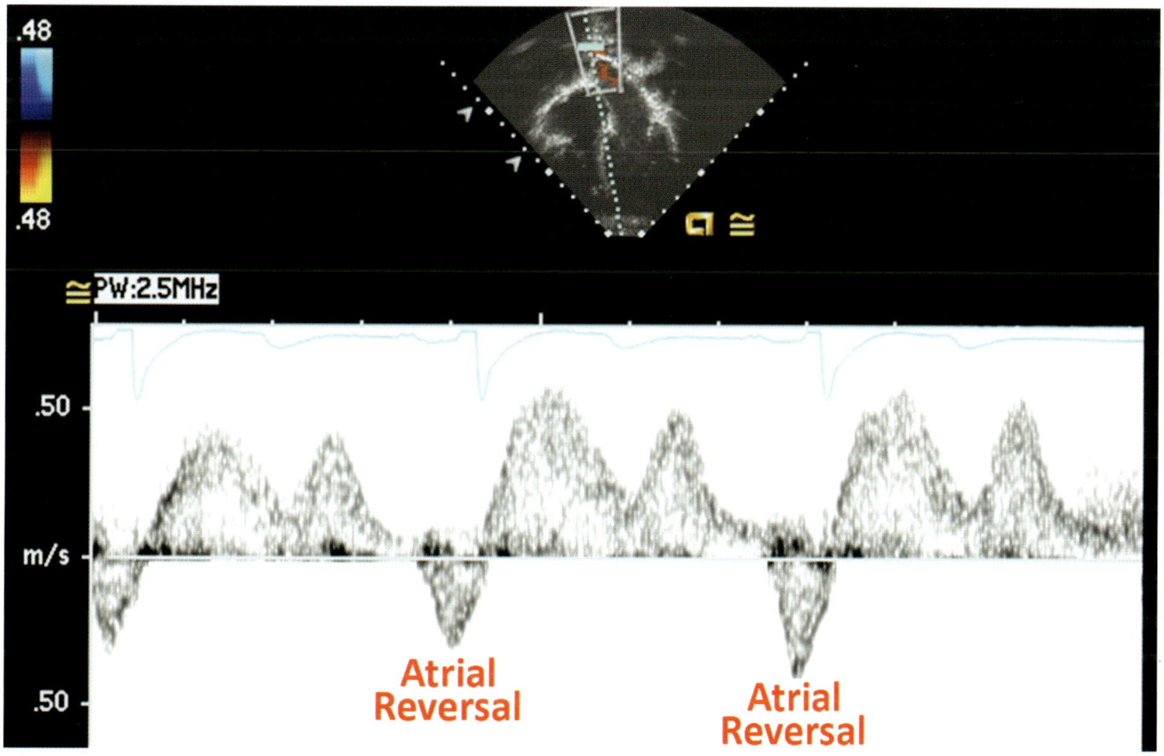

Fig. 23.16: Pulmonary venous inflow Doppler in a patient with restrictive cardiomyopathy and abnormal ventricular compliance. Atrial reversal of flow is seen with atrial contraction, consistent with marked increase in end-diastolic left ventricular pressure.

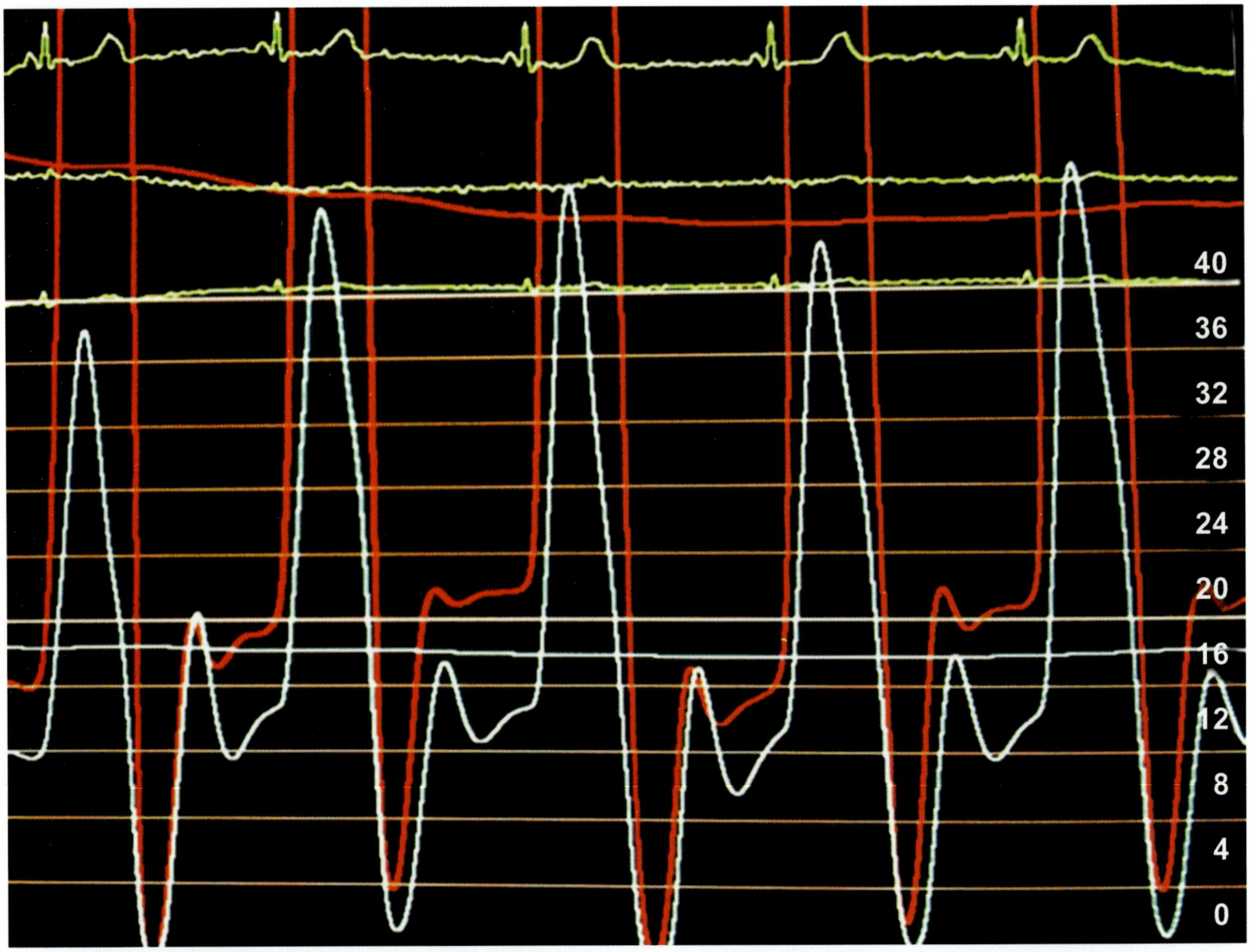

Fig. 23.17: The "dip and plateau" or "square-root sign" observed during cardiac catheterization in patients with restrictive cardiomyopathy. Note that both the left ventricular diastolic pressure (red tracing) and right ventricular diastolic pressure (light blue tracing) are elevated. [Image from Duggal B, Raghani N. Restrictive cardiomyopathy. In: Vijayalakshmi IB, Rao PS, Chugh R (Eds). A Comprehensive Approach to Congenital Heart Diseases. New Delhi, India: Jaypee Brothers Medical Publishers (P) Ltd. 2013].

agents, although data on their long-term benefits for treatment of diastolic dysfunction is lacking. Given the risk of sudden death in children with RCM along with a reported mortality approaching 50% 2 years after diagnosis, early consideration for cardiac transplantation may be warranted. Specific therapies for certain infiltrative cardiomyopathies may be beneficial in slowing the disease process, such as enzyme replacement therapy for metabolic storage diseases or iron chelating agents for hemochromatosis.

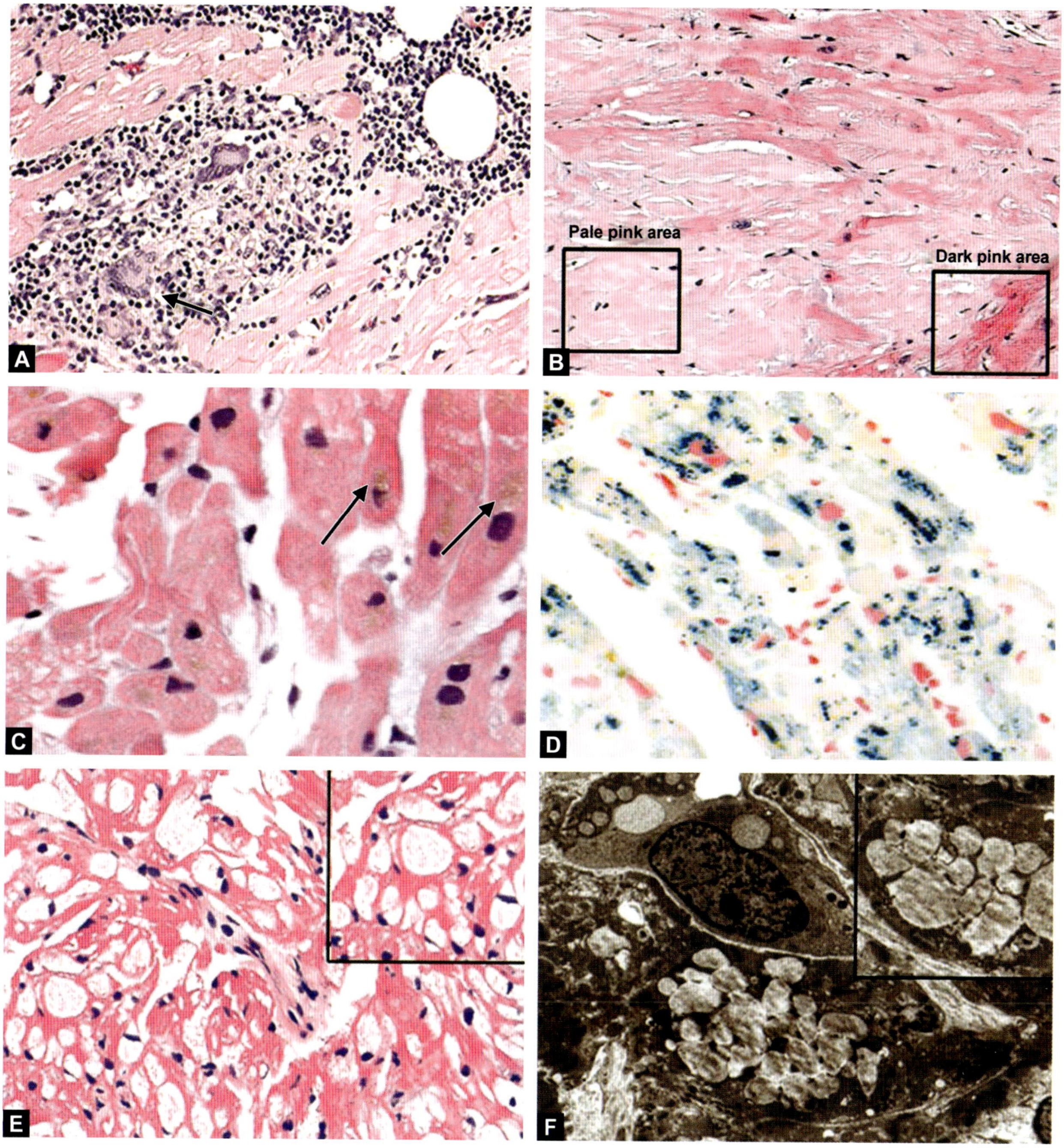

Figs. 23.18A to F: Endomyocardial biopsy specimens from patients with restrictive cardiomyopathy. (A) Cardiac sarcoidosis. In the central portion of the field, there are two myocardial granulomas characterized by clusters of mononuclear cells and giant cells (arrow) (H&E stain, 400x magnification). (B) Cardiac amyloidosis. In this field there are abundant homogenous pale pink deposits of typical amyloid. The remaining viable myofibers (dark pink) are variably hypertrophied or atrophied (H&E stain, 400x magnification); (C and D) Hemochromatosis. Multiple pigmented granules (Figure 23.18C, arrows) are seen within myocytes consistent with iron (H&E stain, 400x magnification). A special stain (Figure 23.18D) discloses abundant bright blue iron in virtually every myofiber (Perl stain, 200x magnification). (E and F) Pompe's disease. At high magnification (Figure 23.18E), light microscopy discloses large empty appearing vacuoles (inset) in virtually every myofiber. A special stain for glycogen (not shown) was markedly positive (H&E stain, 400x magnification). Electron microscopy (Figure 23.18F) shows that the vacuoles are membrane bound aggregates of glycogen (inset) (Uranyl acetate and lead citrate, 5,000x magnification). [Images courtesy of Philip C Ursell, MD, Department of Pathology, UCSF. From Rao VU, de Marco T. Cardiac biopsy. In: Chatterjee K, Anderson M, Heistad D, Kerber RE (Eds). Cardiology—An Illustrated Textbook. New Delhi, India: Jaypee Brothers Medical Publishers (P) Ltd. 2012].

REFERENCES

Hare JM. The dilated, restrictive, and infiltrative cardiomyopathies. In: Bonow RO, Mann DL, Zipes DP, Libby P (Eds). Braunwald's Heart Disease: A Textbook of Cardiovascular Medicine, 9th edition. Philadelphia: Elsevier Health Sciences; 2011.

Levine RA. Echocardiographic assessment of the cardiomyopathies. In: Weyman AE (Ed). Principles and Practice of Echocardiography, 2nd edition. Philadelphia: Lippincott Williams & Wilkins; 1994.

Kushwawa SS, Fallon JT, Fuster V. Restrictive cardiomyopathy. N Engl J Med. 1997;336(4):267-76.

Richardson P, McKenna W, Bristow M, et al. Report of the 1995 World Health Organization/International Society and Federation of Cardiology Task Force on the Definition and Classification of cardiomyopathies. Circulation. 1996;93(5):841-2.

Zangwill S, Hamilton R. Restrictive cardiomyopathy. Pacing Clin Electrophysiol. 2009;32 Suppl 2:S41-43.

CHAPTER

Arrhythmogenic Right Ventricular Cardiomyopathy

24

Darra T Murphy, Rekha Raju, Marc W Deyell

INTRODUCTION

Arrhythmogenic right ventricular cardiomyopathy (ARVC), previously referred to by some as arrhythmogenic right ventricular dysplasia (ARVD) or as ARVC/D, is a rare but increasingly recognized cause of sudden adult death, particularly between the second and the fourth decades. It is a genetic cardiomyopathy leading to progressive fibrofatty replacement of the myocardium (Figs. 24.1A to F) and most commonly manifesting with monomorphic ventricular tachycardia (VT). First described in 1982 as partially or totally absent right ventricular musculature that is replaced by fatty and fibrous tissue, it is estimated that more than 50% of cases have a family history. It is more common in men than in women, has incomplete penetrance, and has variable clinical expression. Sudden death can occur in all stages, including early in the disease well before any symptoms are apparent, and particularly in the second decade of life.

The prevalence of ARVC in the general population is unknown, however, is estimated to be somewhere between 1 in 2,000 and 1 in 5,000. This may though be an

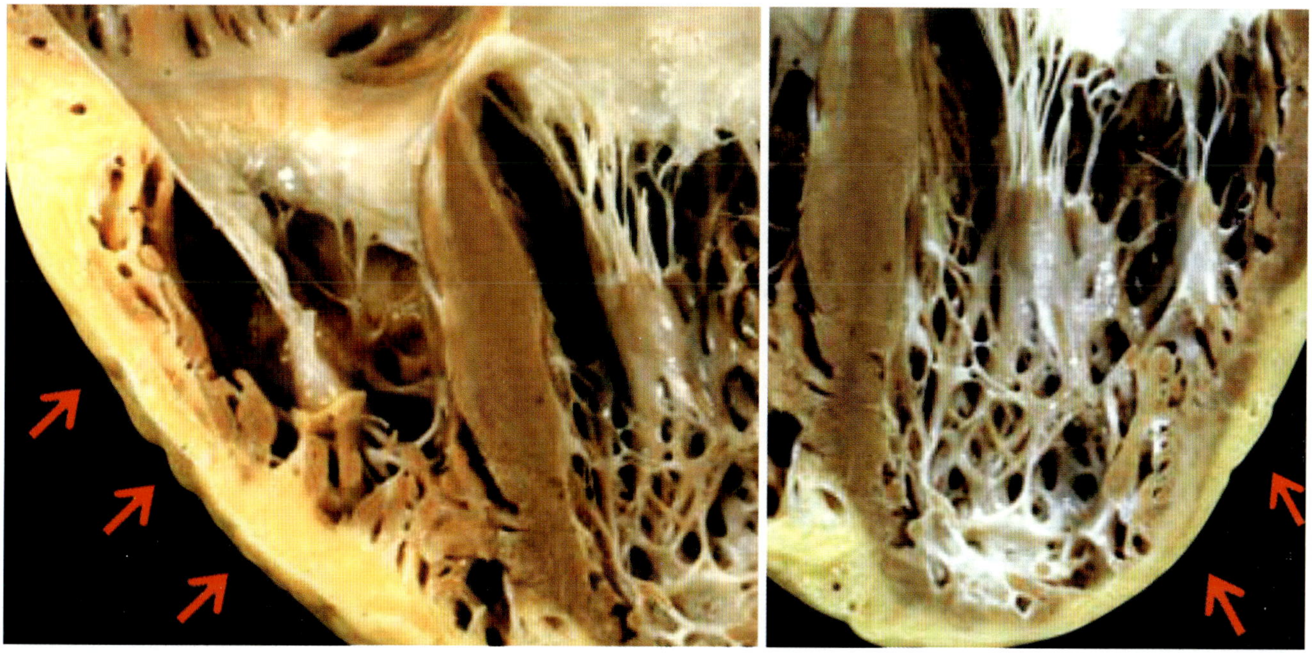

Fig. 24.1A: Gross pathology specimen of arrhythmogenic right ventricular cardiomyopathy/dysplasia. There is fatty infiltration (arrows) of both the RV (left panel) and the LV (right panel). (Image from Thiene G, Corrado D, Basso C. Arrhythmogenic right ventricular cardiomyopathy/dysplasia. Orphanet J Rare Dis. 2007;2:45).

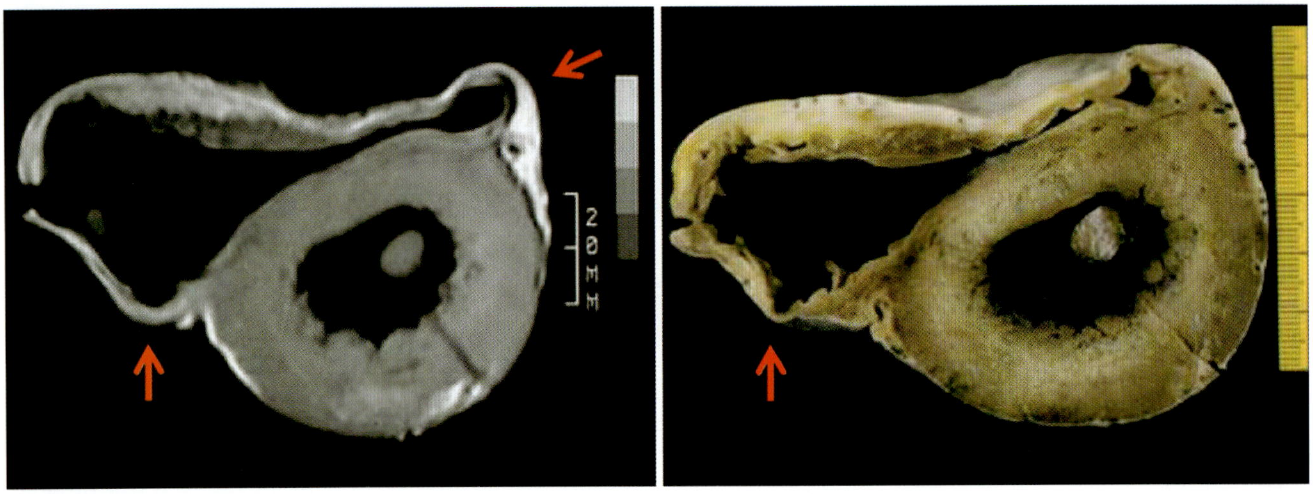

Fig. 24.1B: In vitro MRI and corresponding cross-section of the heart show right ventricle dilatation with anterior and posterior aneurysms (arrows). (Image from Thiene G, Corrado D, Basso C. Arrhythmogenic right ventricular cardiomyopathy/dysplasia. Orphanet J Rare Dis. 2007;2:45).

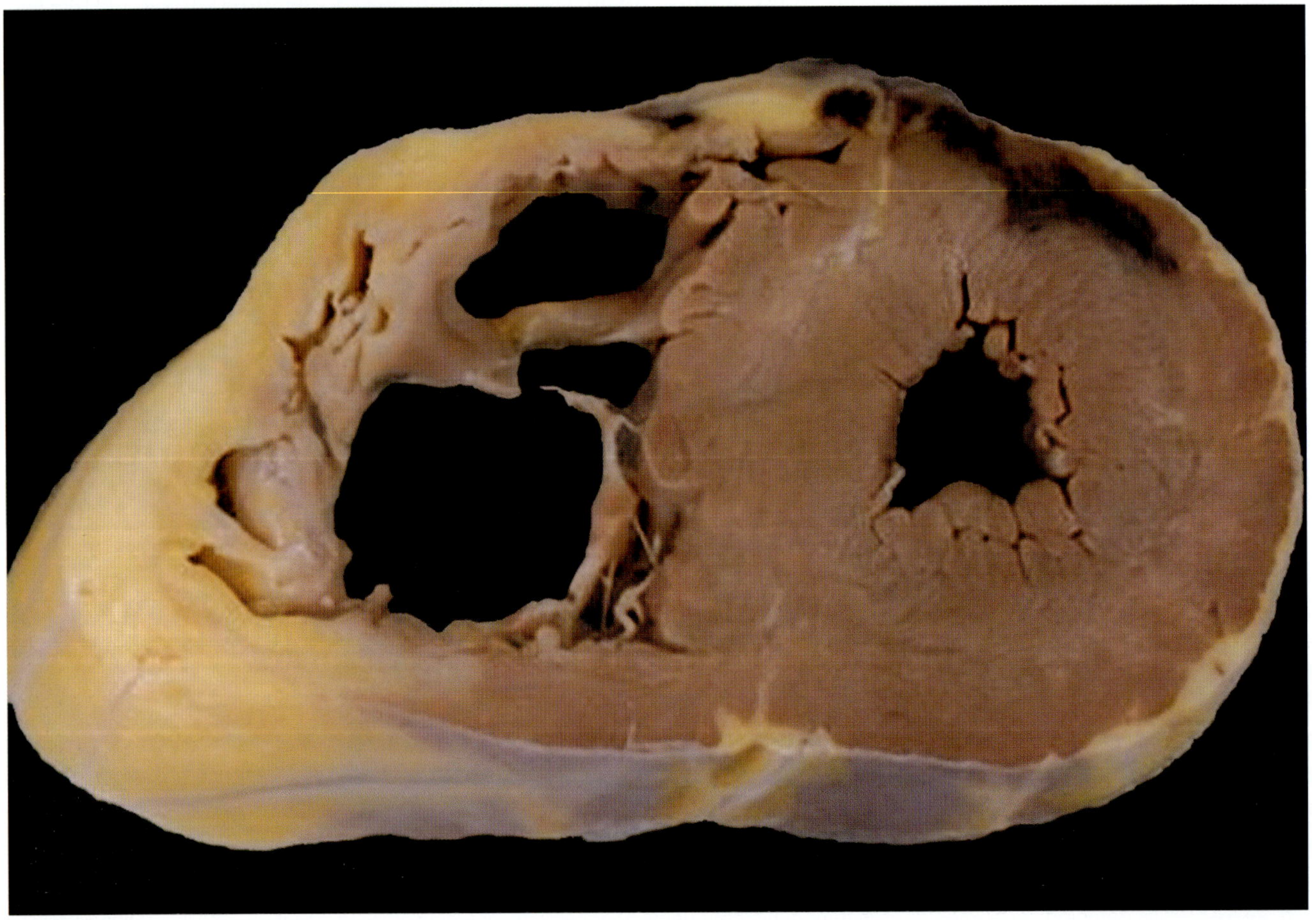

Fig. 24.1C: Gross pathology image demonstrating extensive fatty infiltration of the right ventricle. (Image courtesy of Dr John Partridge).

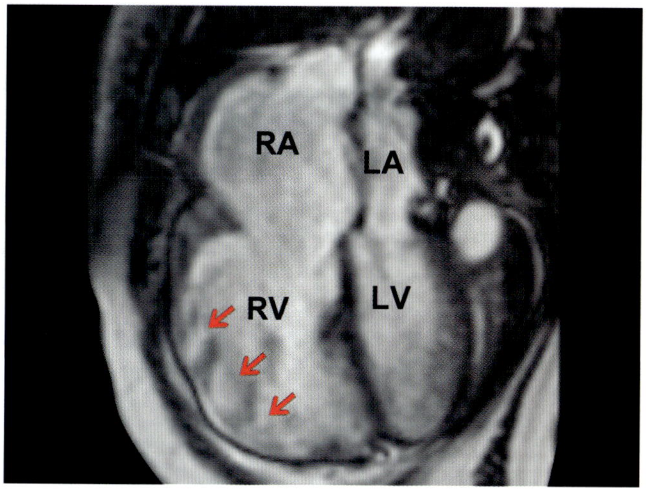

Fig. 24.1D: MRI imaged oriented in the four chamber orientation showing a markedly enlarged right ventricle (RV). Note the thin, dilated and aneurismal right ventricular free wall (arrows). (LA: Left atrium; LV: Left ventricle; RA: Right atrium).

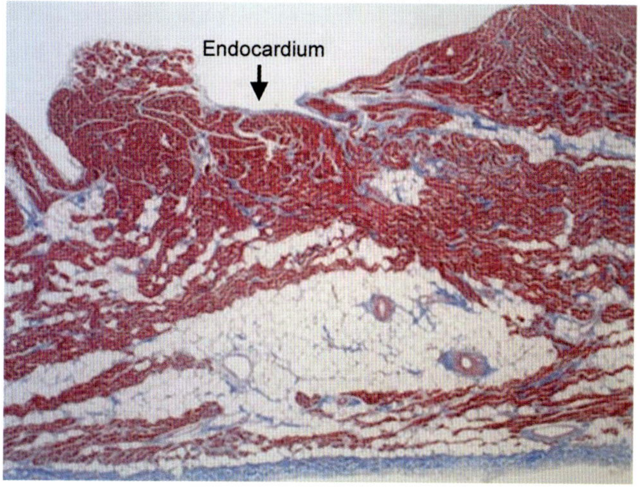

Fig. 24.1E: Histology of right ventricular wall of a patient with ARVC who died suddenly. AZAN stain with cardiac myocytes (red), collagen (blue) and adipocytes (white). Shown is the typical pattern of ARVC with strands of fibrosis reaching all the way to the endocardium (particularly just to the right of the arrow). Bundles of cardiac myocytes are embedded in between the fibrotic strands, particularly in the subendocardial layers. These interconnecting bundles of myocytes give rise to activation delay and re-entrant circuits, the typical electrophysiological substrate for ventricular arrhythmias in ARVD/C. (Image from Hauer RN, Marcus FI, Cox MG. Arrhythmogenic Right Ventricular Dysplasia/Cardiomyopathy. In: Chatterjee K, Anderson M, Heistad D, Kerber RE (Eds). Cardiology—An Illustrated Textbook. New Delhi, India: Jaypee Brothers Medical Publishers (P) Ltd; 2012).

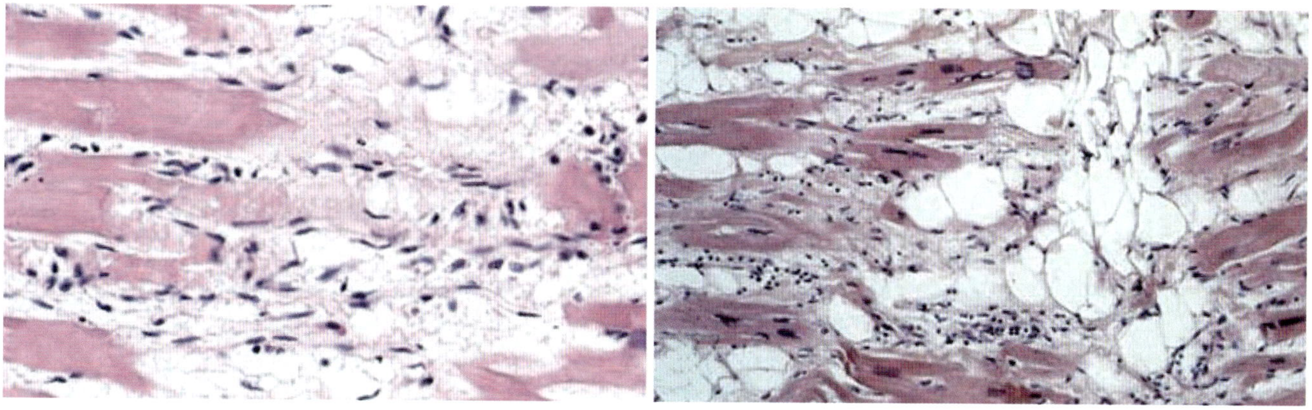

Fig. 24.1F: The typical histologic features of ARVC. Ongoing myocyte death (left panel) with early fibrosis and adipocytes infiltration (right panel). (Image legend text from Thiene G, Corrado D, Basso C. Arrhythmogenic right ventricular cardiomyopathy/dysplasia. Orphanet J Rare Dis. 2007;2:45).

underestimation of its prevalence due to (1) misdiagnosis and (2) under diagnosis, as in one study up to 20% of sudden death occurring in people under 35 years of age have shown evidence of ARVC on postmortem in one study. Many of these persons who died of sudden death were previously asymptomatic.

Although predilection sites in the right ventricle (RV) for structural abnormalities include an area formed by the RV outflow tract, the apex, and the sub tricuspid region, this so-called triangle of dysplasia has recently been called into question.

GENETICS AND PATHOPHYSIOLOGY OF ARVC

A better understanding of the disease in recent years has led it to be grouped as part of the desmosomal diseases (Fig. 24.2), due largely to defective cell adhesion proteins, as well as involving other genes unrelated to the cell adhesion complex. The heart and the epidermis are most commonly affected organs. It is hypothesized that fibrofatty replacement follows myocardial cell-to-cell uncoupling; disruption of the myocardial architecture often leads to arrhythmias, which are occasionally fatal. It is not currently well-known exactly how these desmosomal protein genes affect the individual patient. At least three hypotheses have been proposed, a detailed explanation of which are beyond the scope of this chapter however can be found in more detail elsewhere in the literature.

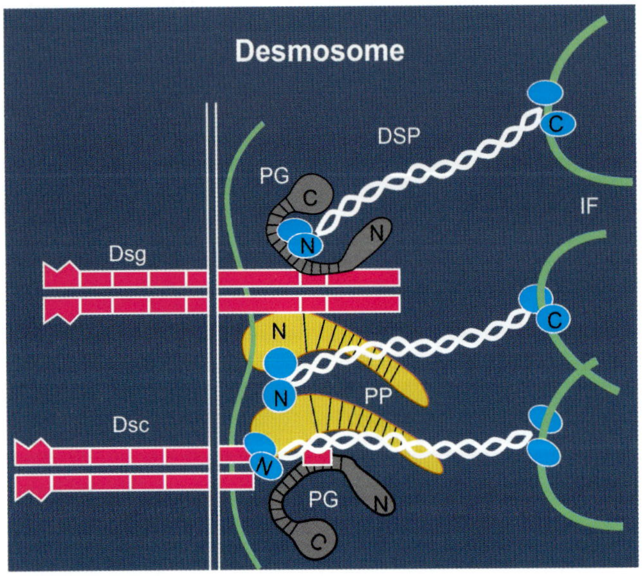

Fig. 24.2: Scheme of the molecular structure of the desmosome, site of defective proteins in ARVC/D. (Image from Thiene G, Corrado D, Basso C. Arrhythmogenic right ventricular cardiomyopathy/dysplasia. Orphanet J Rare Dis. 2007;2:45).

In the classical form of ARVC, the disease is inherited as an autosomal dominant trait. The right ventricle is most commonly affected. However, it is now recognized that there can be biventricular involvement (Figs. 24.3A to C) or even primarily involvement of the left ventricle. Isolated left ventricular involvement is often associated with desmoplakin gene mutations.

Disease progression is common. Four different disease phases have been described for the classical form of ARVC, which primarily affects the right ventricle. These include: (1) a concealed phase (asymptomatic patients with possibly only minor ventricular arrhythmias and subtle structural changes); (2) an overt phase (symptoms due to VT or with more obvious structural abnormalities); (3) RV failure (with relatively preserved LV function); and (4) a biventricular phase (with significant overt LV involvement). Each of these phases has implications for treatment and/or prognostic implications, including risk stratification, surveillance of arrhythmia and surveillance of RV function.

DIAGNOSIS OF ARVC

Diagnosis of ARVC can be very difficult and often only confirmed at surgery or autopsy. Although ventricular fibrillation and sudden death may be the first manifestations of ARVC, symptomatic patients typically present with sustained VT originating from the right ventricle. The criteria for diagnosis of ARVC were initially published in 1994, formulated by a Task Force and published as consensus guidelines using a set of clinically applicable criteria. These guidelines were revised and modified in 2010 and are summarized in Table 24.1. Clinical criteria for the diagnosis of ARVC include global and regional ventricular functional and structural alterations, tissue characterization, depolarization and repolarization abnormalities on ECG, ventricular arrhythmias with a left bundle branch block morphology (Fig. 24.4) and family history. The diagnostic criteria are divided into major and minor criteria, and in order to satisfy the criteria for ARVC diagnosis either two major, one major plus two minor, or four minor criteria are required. Only one criterion can be considered for diagnosis from each group even when multiple criteria from that group are present.

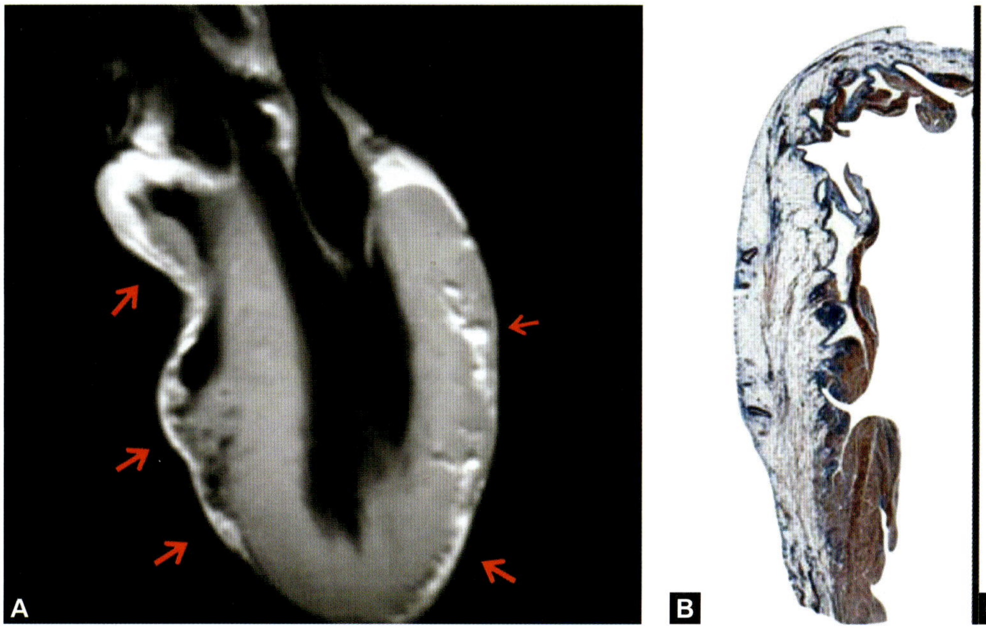

Figs. 24.3A to C: MRI and corresponding histology in ARVC. (A) In vitro MRI demonstrating biventricular involvement. Imaging sequence results in bright signal in areas of fatty infiltrate (arrows); (B) Histological examination demonstrates transmural fibrofatty replacement in the RV free wall and (C) focal subepicardial involvement of the disease in the LV free wall. (Image from Thiene G, Corrado D, Basso C. Arrhythmogenic right ventricular cardiomyopathy/dysplasia. Orphanet J Rare Dis. 2007;2:45).

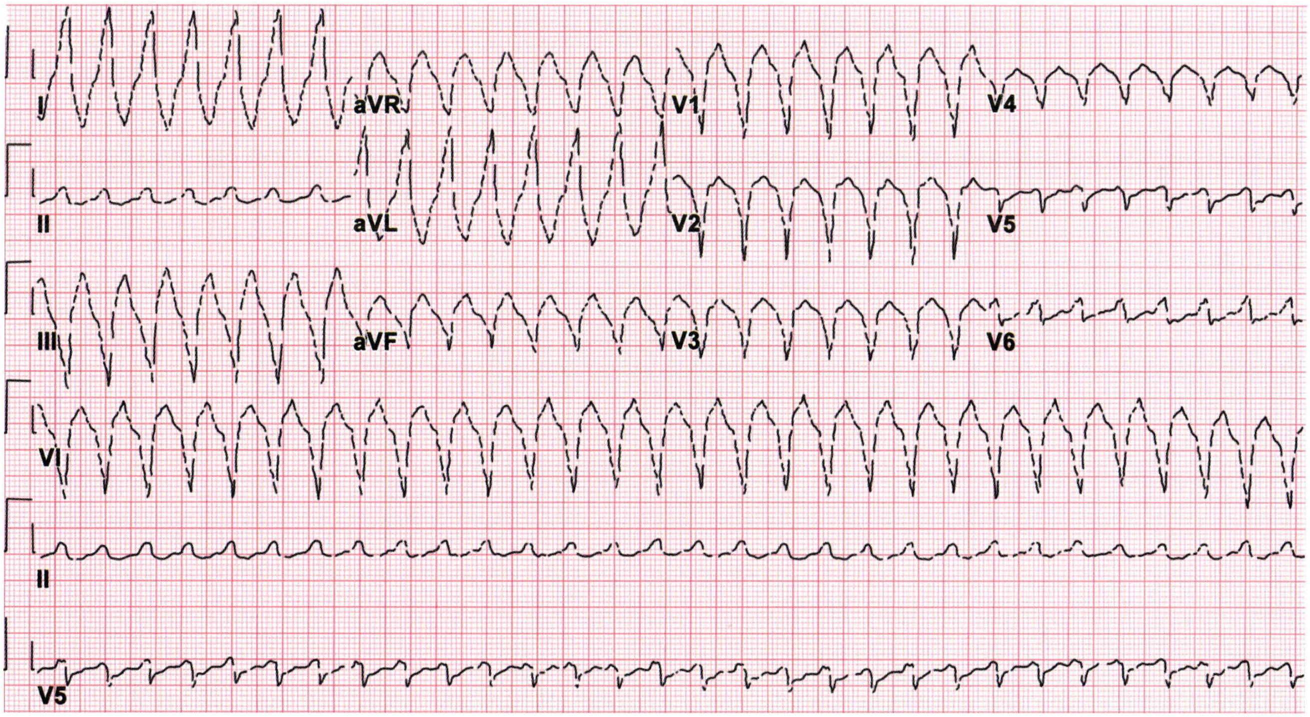

Fig. 24.4: 12 lead ECG demonstrating monomorphic ventricular tachycardia with a left bundle branch block (LBBB) configuration, left superior axis and late precordial transition (V6) indicating origin from the RV free wall. These findings are consistent with ARVC-mediated VT.

Table 24.1: Summary of major and minor diagnostic criteria for the diagnosis of ARVC. (RV: Right ventricle; RVOT: Right ventricular outflow tract; PLAX: Parasternal long axis; BSA: Body surface area; PSAX: Parasternal short axis; FAC: Fractional area change; MRI: Magnetic resonance imaging; RVEDV: Right ventricular end diastolic volume; RVEF: Right ventricular ejection fraction; ECG: Electrocardiogram; LAS: Low amplitude signal; RMS: Root mean square; VT: Ventricular tachycardia; ARVD/C: Arrhythmogenic right ventricular dysplasia/cardiomyopathy).

	Major Criteria	*Minor Criteria*
I. Global and/or regional dysfunction and structural alterations		
• 2D Echocardiography	Regional RV akinesia, dyskinesia or aneurysm and one of: • Parasternal long axis view RVOT ≥ 32 mm or ≥ 19 mm/m² • Parasternal short axis view RVOT ≥ 36 mm or ≥ 21 mm/m² • Fractional area change ≤ 33%	Regional RV akinesia or dyskinesia and one of: • Parasternal long axis view RVOT ≥ 29–31 mm or 16–18 mm/m² • Parasternal short axis view RVOT 32–35 mm or 18–20 mm/m² • Fractional area change ≤ 40%
• MRI	Regional RV akinesia or dyskinesia or dyssynchronous RV contraction and one of: • RV end diastolic volume ≥ 110 ml/m² (male) or ≥ 100 ml/m² (female) • RV ejection fraction ≤ 40%	Regional RV akinesia or dyskinesia or dyssynchronous RV contraction and one of: • RV end diastolic volume ≥ 100 ml/m² (male) or ≥ 90 ml/m² (female) • RV ejection fraction ≤ 45%
• RV Cineangiography	• Regional RV akinesia, dyskinesia or aneurysm	
II. Tissue Characterization of wall	• Residual myocytes < 60% by morphometric analysis, (or < 50%) if estimated), with fibrous replacement of the RV free wall myocardium in at least 1 sample, with or without fatty tissue replacement	• Residual myocytes 60–75% by morphometric analysis, (or 50–65% if estimated), with fibrous replacement of the RV free wall myocardium in at least 1 sample, with or without fatty tissue replacement
III. Repolarization Abnormalities	• Negative T waves in at least leads V1-3	• Negative T waves only in leads V1 and V2 or in V4-6 • In case of complete right bundle branch block: negative T waves in leads V1-4
IV. Depolarization/Conduction abnormalities	• Epsilon wave in one of leads V1-3	• Late potential by signal averaged ECG in at least one of three parameters in the absence of a QRS duration of ≥ 114 msec on the standard ECG • Filtered QRS duration ≥114 msec • Duration of terminal QRS < 40 microVolt (LAS) of ≥ 38 msecs • RMS voltage of terminal 40 msecs ≤ 20 microVolts • Terminal activation duration ≥55 msec
V. Arrhythmias	• (Non-)sustained VT of left bundle branch block morphology with superior axis	• (Non-)sustained VT of left bundle branch block morphology with inferior axis or unknown axis • > 500 ventricular extrasystoles/24 hours by Holter
VI. Family history	• ARVD/c confirmed in a first-degree relative who meets current task force criteria • ARVD/C confirmed pathologically at autopsy or surgery in a first-degree relative • Identification of a pathogenic mutation associated with ARVD/C	• History of ARVC/D in a first-degree relative in whom it is not possible or practical to determine if the family member meets current task force criteria • Premature sudden death (< 35 years) due to suspected ARVD/C in a first-degree relative

Source: Marcus FI, McKenna WJ, Sherrill D, et al. Diagnosis of arrhythmogenic right ventricular cardiomyopathy/dysplasia: proposed modification of the task force criteria. Circulation. 2010;121(13):1533-41.

Electrocardiogram Abnormalities

Electrocardiogram abnormalities are important elements of the diagnostic criteria for ARVC. ECG criteria include both depolarization and repolarization abnormalities, which are believed to be due to electrical uncoupling of the diseased myocardium. Diagnostic abnormalities on the ECG must be from an ECG obtained while in sinus rhythm and with the patient off any antiarrhythmic drugs.

Electrocardiogram abnormalities may develop before any histological evidence of myocyte loss or clinical evidence of disease. Activation delay in the right ventricle is one of the characteristic features of ARVC. This predominantly manifests as epsilon waves and prolonged terminal activation delay, which is defined as the longest value measured from the nadir of the S wave to the end of all depolarization deflections (Figs. 24.5A and B). Although only seen in a minority of patients, epsilon waves (Figs. 24.5C and D) are low amplitude potentials seen in

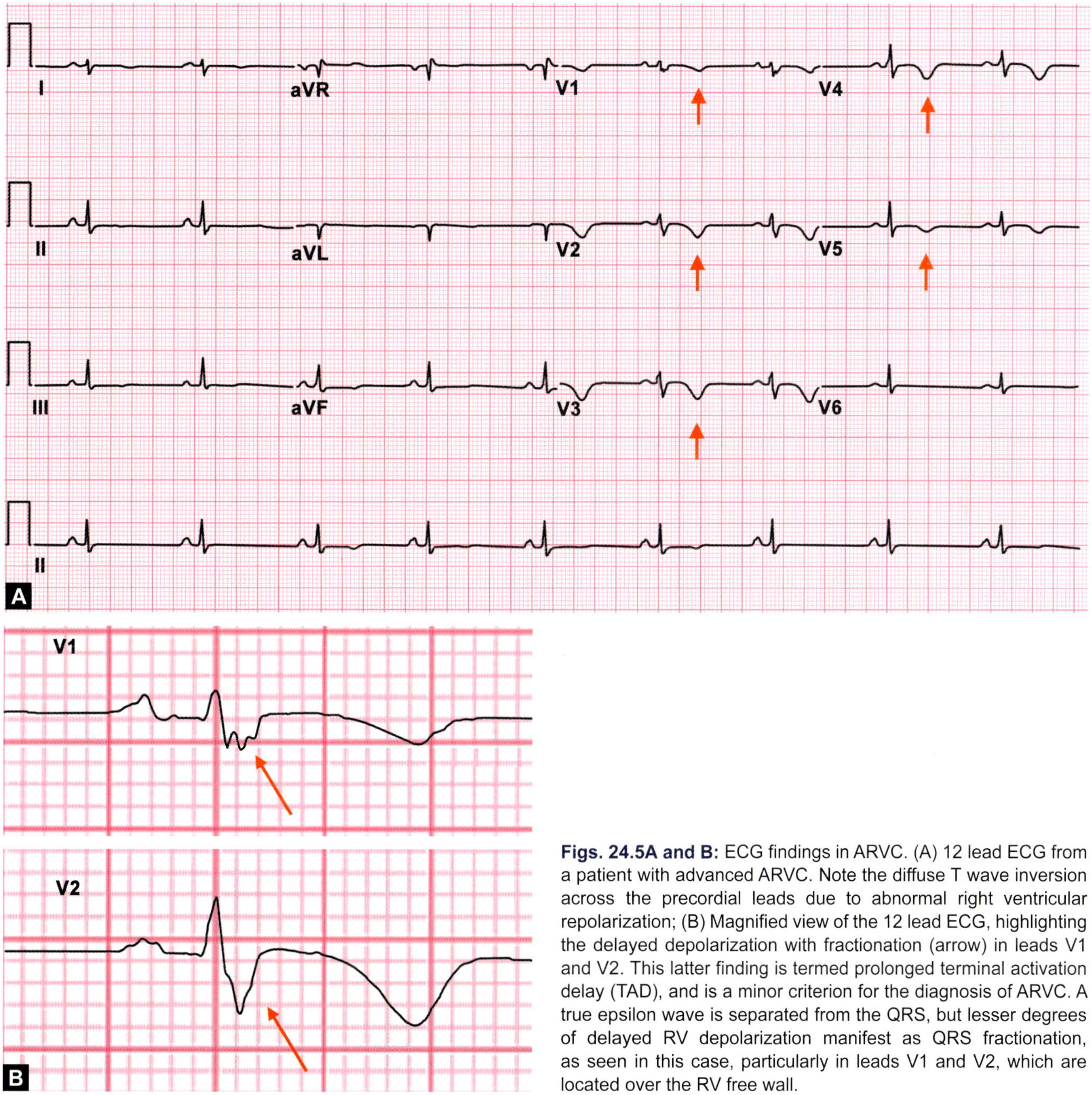

Figs. 24.5A and B: ECG findings in ARVC. (A) 12 lead ECG from a patient with advanced ARVC. Note the diffuse T wave inversion across the precordial leads due to abnormal right ventricular repolarization; (B) Magnified view of the 12 lead ECG, highlighting the delayed depolarization with fractionation (arrow) in leads V1 and V2. This latter finding is termed prolonged terminal activation delay (TAD), and is a minor criterion for the diagnosis of ARVC. A true epsilon wave is separated from the QRS, but lesser degrees of delayed RV depolarization manifest as QRS fractionation, as seen in this case, particularly in leads V1 and V2, which are located over the RV free wall.

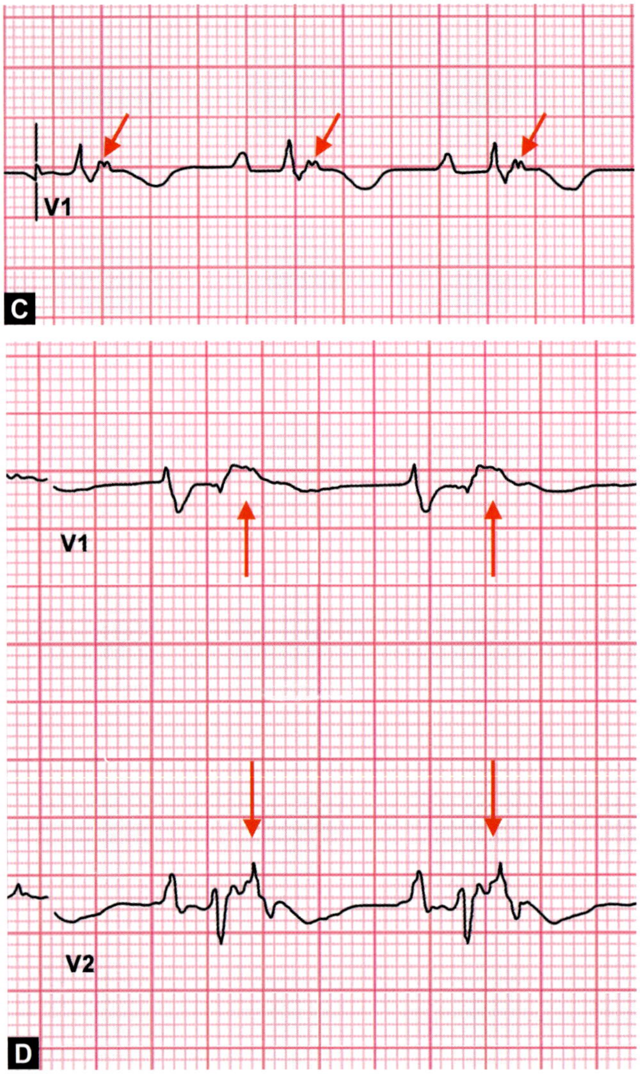

Figs. 24.5C and D: Epsilon waves (arrows) in a patient with ARVC. Epsilon waves are low amplitude potentials seen in leads V1–V3, occurring after and distant from the QRS complex. Epsilon waves are believed to be the result of abnormal repolarization of the affected part of the right ventricle in patients with ARVC. Although true Epsilon waves are only seen in a minority of patients with ARVC, they are highly specific for the disease. Figure 24.5C courtesy of Dr Jayachandran Tejus and Dr Ed Burns, posted on www.lifeinthefastlane.com.

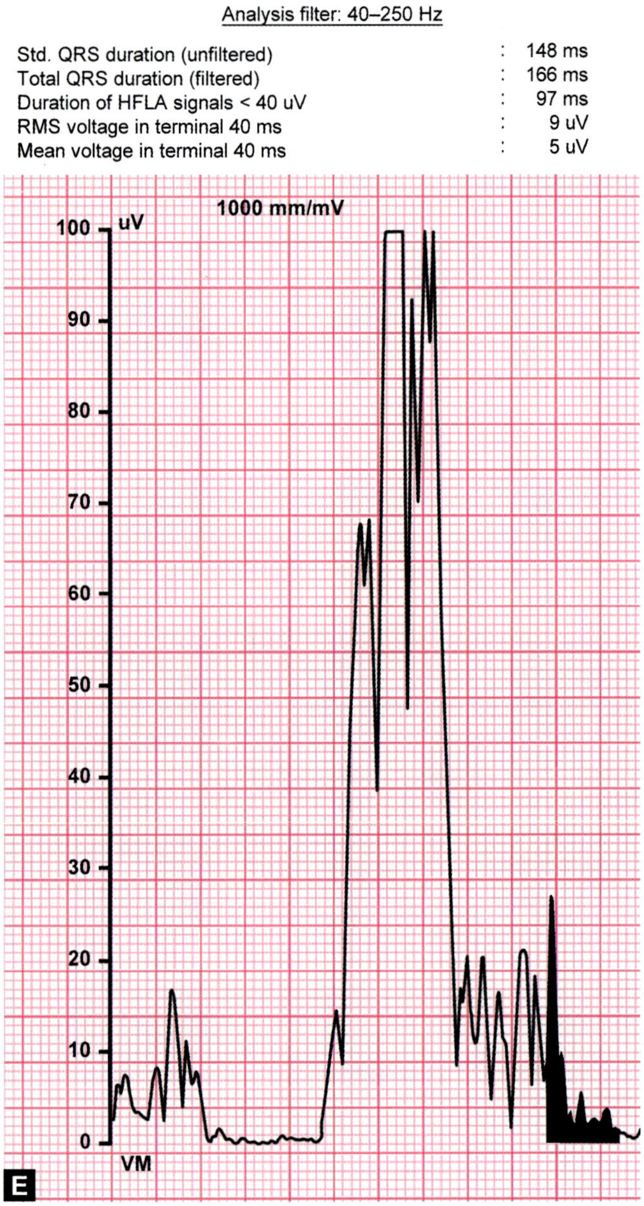

Fig. 24.5E: A highly abnormal signal averaged ECG from a patient with ARVC. The study meets all three ARVC criteria: a filtered total QRS duration of > 114 ms, a low amplitude signal (HFLA) of > 38 ms or a root mean squared (RMS) voltage in the terminal 40 ms < 20 μV. Only one of three criteria is required to be considered abnormal and constitutes a minor revised task force criterion.

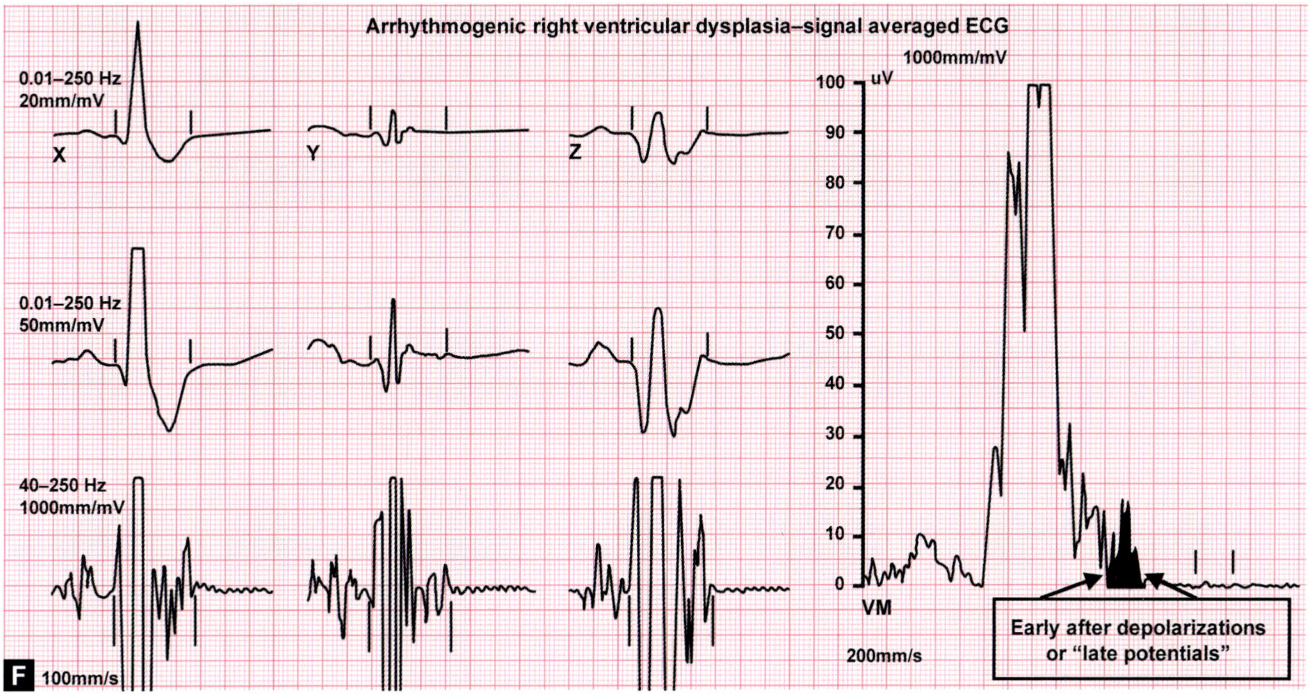

Fig. 24.5F: Example of a signal-averaged ECG (SAECG) in a patient with ARVC. (Image courtesy of Dr Steven Lome. Image from www.learntheheart.com).

the precordial leads (V1–V3) after and separate from the QRS complex, and are highly specific for the diagnosis. TAD (also seen in the precordial leads) is considered prolonged if greater than or equal to 55 ms, and only applicable in the absence of complete right bundle branch block. TAD was added as a minor criterion in the recent modification of ARVC diagnostic criteria, and appears to be equally as sensitive as the presence of late potentials on signal averaged ECG, and much more sensitive than epsilon waves in the diagnosis of ARVC. Disease severity is correlated with all the depolarization criteria.

A positive correlation exists between late potentials and the extent of right ventricular fibrosis and reduction in RV systolic function, as well as with the presence of significant morphological abnormalities seen on imaging studies. Signal-averaged ECG (SAECG) (Figs. 24.5E and F) allows for better quantification of repolarization abnormalities and can help to identify more subtle cases of ARVC.

Imaging Studies in Suspected ARVC

Assessment for global and/or regional dysfunction and structural alterations is most commonly performed using 2D echocardiography (Fig. 24.6) and cardiac MR imaging (Figs. 24.7A to F and Video 24.1). Other imaging modalities, such as cardiac CT (Figs. 24.8A to C) and cineangiography, may occasionally also be utilized in the evaluation of patients with suspected ARVC. Cardiac MR examinations typically focus on the evaluation of right ventricular size, right ventricular ejection fraction and wall motion abnormalities (including dyskinesia and aneurysm formation). While not strictly a part of the diagnostic criteria, the findings of fatty infiltration of the RV or late gadolinium enhancement on delayed MR sequences (suggestive of myocardial fibrosis) are additional helpful information derived from this imaging study. When abnormalities are seen on MRI, the main differential diagnoses for such abnormalities include myocarditis and sarcoidosis.

Endomyocardial Biopsy

Although endomyocardial biopsy (Figs. 24.9 and 24.10) is useful in the assessment of patients with suspected ARVC, the procedure does have some limitations. Although sampling from the interventricular septum, the usual site of endomyocardial biopsy sampling, is relatively safe, in

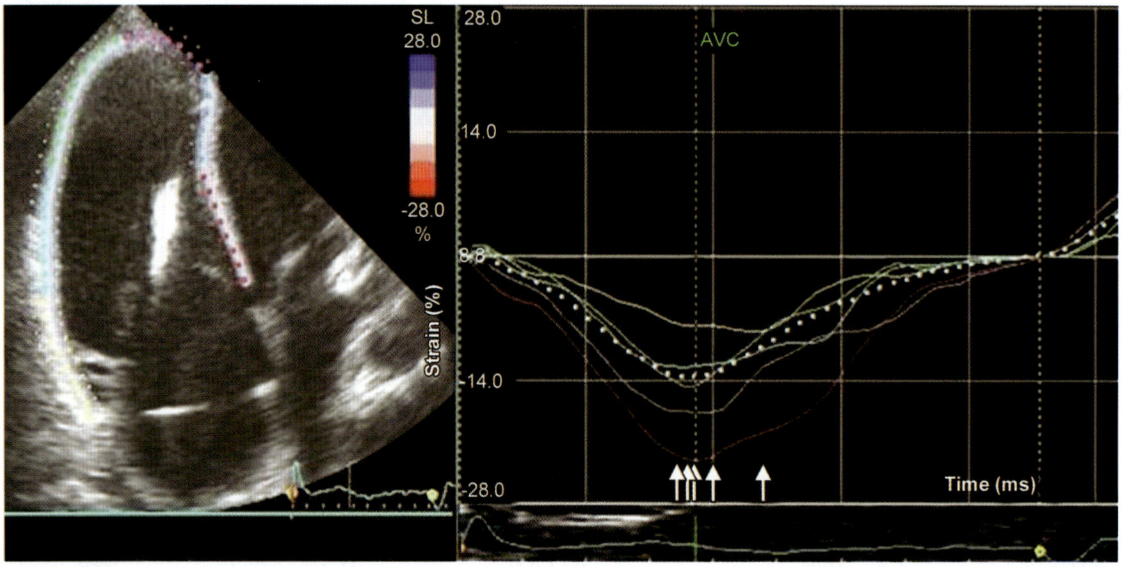

Fig. 24.6: Strain curves from a dilated right ventricle from an apical four-chamber view in a patient with ARVC. Vertical arrows indicate the timing of maximum myocardial shortening in each right ventricular segment and are consistent with pronounced right ventricular mechanical dispersion. (Image from Haugaa KH, Amlie JP, Edvardsen T. Prediction of ventricular arrhythmias in patients at risk of sudden cardiac death. In: Harris JJ (Ed). Cardiac Defibrillation—Prediction, Prevention and Management of Cardiovascular Arrhythmic Events. InTech, 2011).

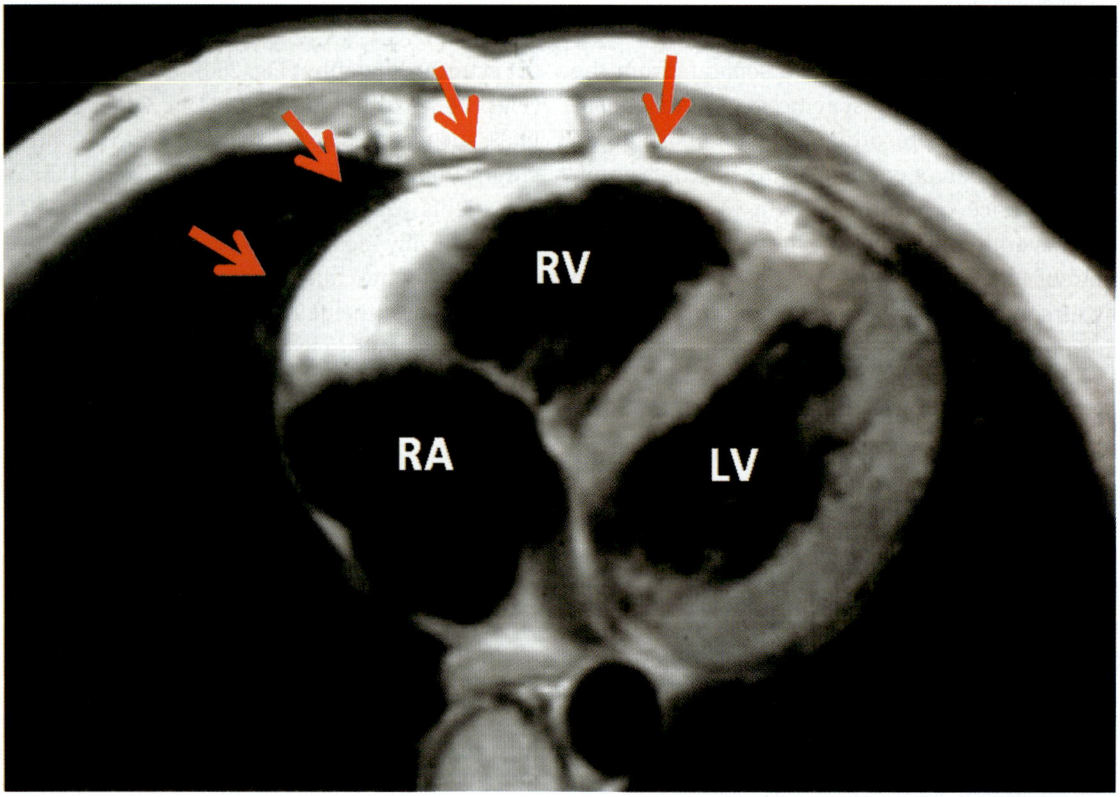

Fig. 24.7A: MRI in a patient with ARVC/D. Spin echo T1 sequence demonstrates transmural bright signal in the RV free wall due to massive myocardial atrophy with fatty replacement. (Image from Thiene G, Corrado D, Basso C. Arrhythmogenic right ventricular cardiomyopathy/dysplasia. Orphanet J Rare Dis. 2007;2:45). (LV: Left ventricle; RA: Right atrium; RV: Right ventricle).

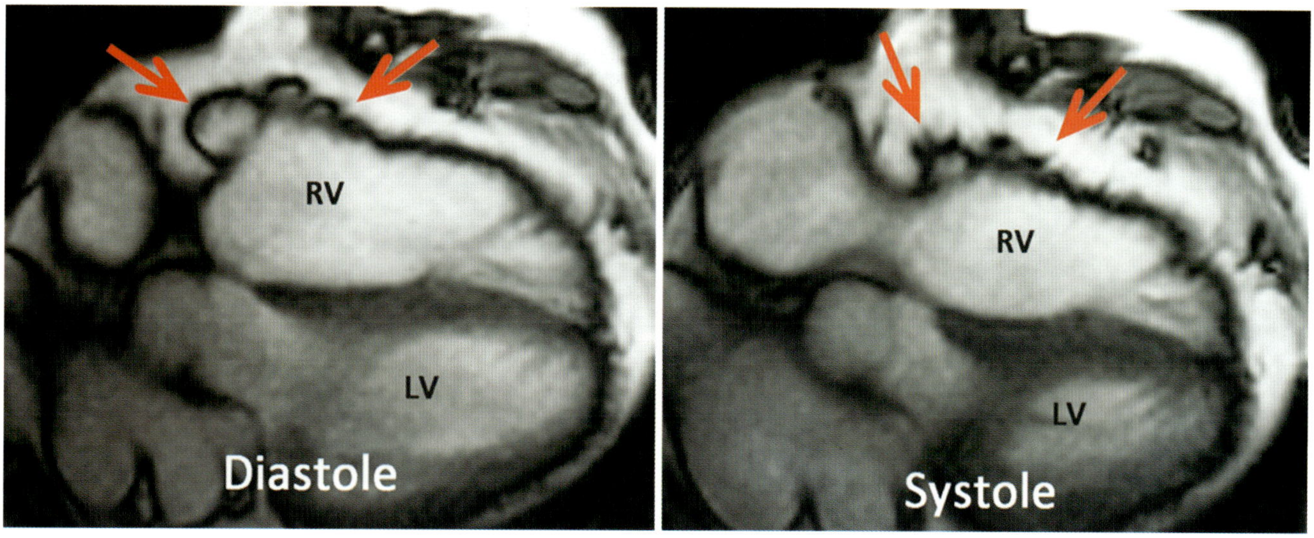

Fig. 24.7B: Images from a cardiac four-chamber MR cine gradient echo sequence in diastole (left panel) and systole (right panel) showing focal aneurysm formation with dyskinesia causing crenation or a "crinkling" effect on the right ventricular free wall (arrows). (LV: Left ventricle; RV: Right ventricle).

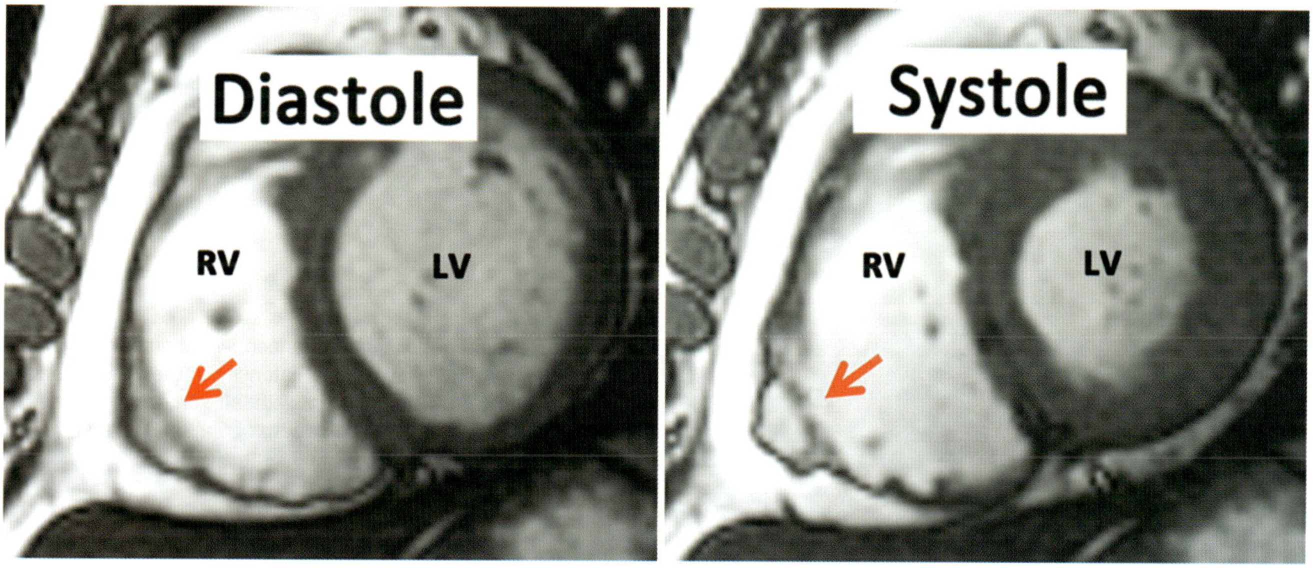

Fig. 24.7C: Images from a cardiac short-axis MR cine gradient echo sequence in diastole (left panel) and systole (right panel) show focal aneurysmal out pouching of the right ventricular myocardium (arrows) in a poorly functioning ventricle. (LV: Left ventricle; RV: Right ventricle).

ARVC the septum is usually spared, and therefore endomyocardial biopsy of the septum may lead to false negative biopsy results due to sampling error. Additionally, the pathology of ARVC can be patchy, and does not always affect the subendocardial layers in the early stages of the disease. Given the endomyocardial biopsies are by design usually not transmural, this also adds to the risk of false negative biopsy results. Voltage mapping or prior imaging often directs optimal biopsy location. However, tissue sampling from the affected, often-thin RV, free wall is associated with a small but non-zero risk of free wall perforation.

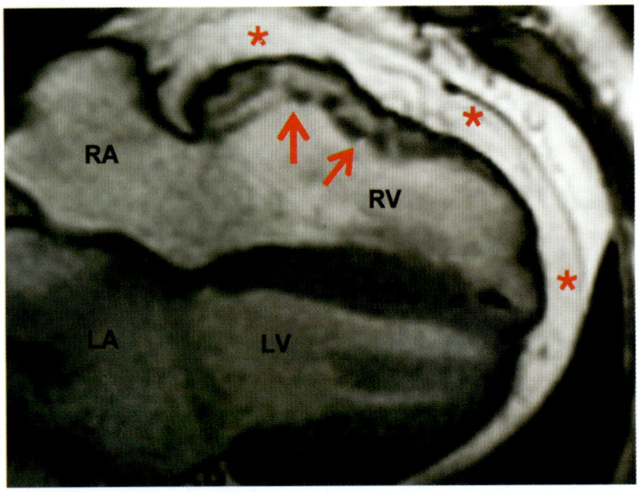

Fig. 24.7D: Four-chamber MR image showing increased signal intensity representing fat (arrows) replacing the right ventricular myocardium. Note this is intrinsic to the myocardium and separate from the epicardial fat (asterisks). (LA: Left atrium; LV: Left ventricle; RA: Right atrium; RV: Right ventricle).

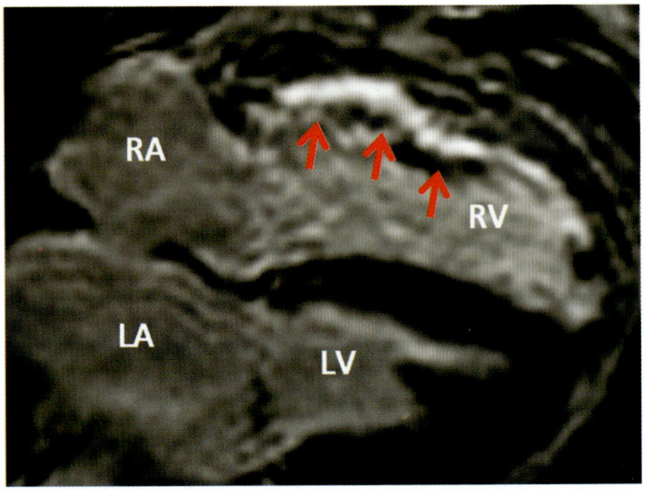

Fig. 24.7E: Delayed post gadolinium four-chamber MR image showing abnormal increased signal intensity in the right ventricular myocardium consistent with scar. (LA: Left atrium; LV: Left ventricle; RA: Right atrium; RV: Right ventricle).

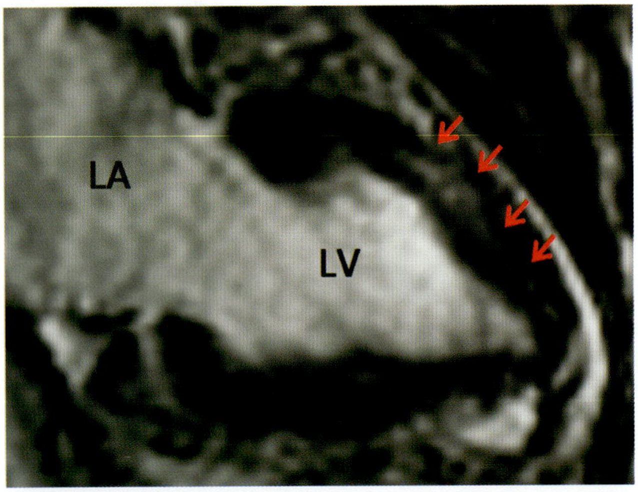

Fig. 24.7F: Delayed gadolinium enhanced two-chamber MR image showing abnormal increased signal intensity in the left ventricular mid-myocardium (arrows) consistent with left ventricular disease in a patient with ARVC with a mixed pattern of right and left ventricular involvement. (LA: Left atrium; LV: Left ventricle).

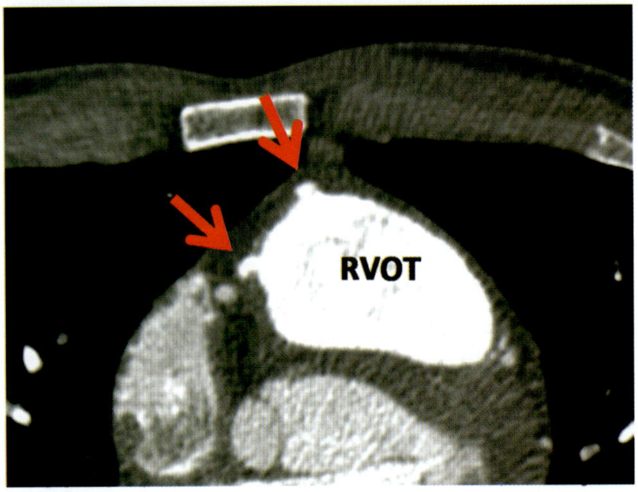

Fig. 24.8A: Contrast CT from a patient with biopsy-proven ARVC showing focal aneurysms (arrows) in the right ventricular outflow tract (RVOT).

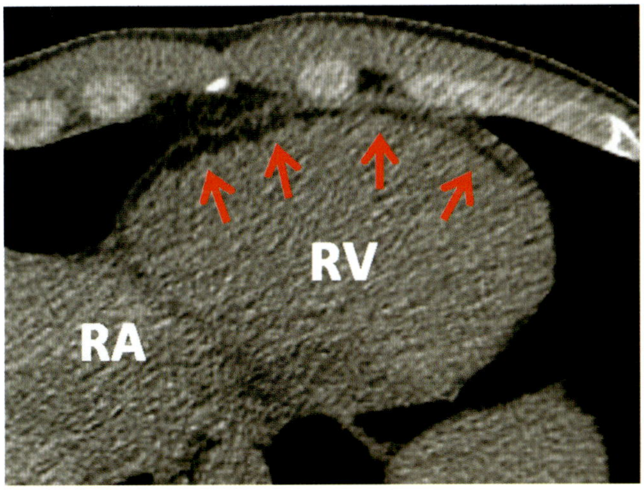

Fig. 24.8B: Noncontrast transverse axial CT image demonstrating subendocardial fat (arrows) in the RV free wall. (RA: Right atrium; RV: Right ventricle).

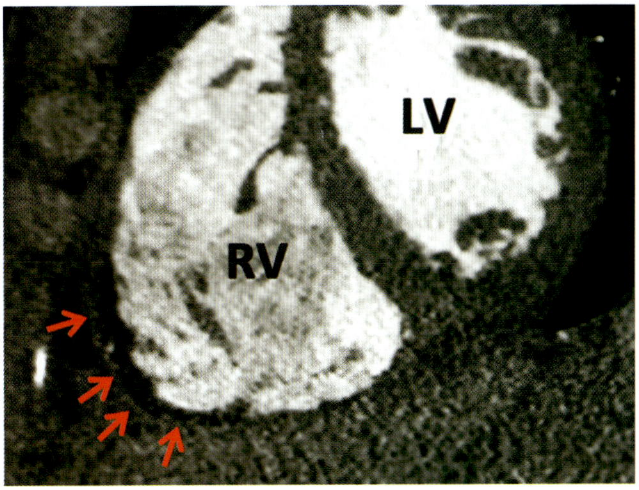

Fig. 24.8C: Contrast-enhanced ECG-gated CT reconstructed in the cardiac short-axis view of the patient in Figure 24.8B demonstrating a dilated right ventricle with hypodensity along the subendocardial right ventricular free wall (arrows), consistent with fibrofatty infiltration and suspected ARVC. (LV: Left ventricle; RV: Right ventricle).

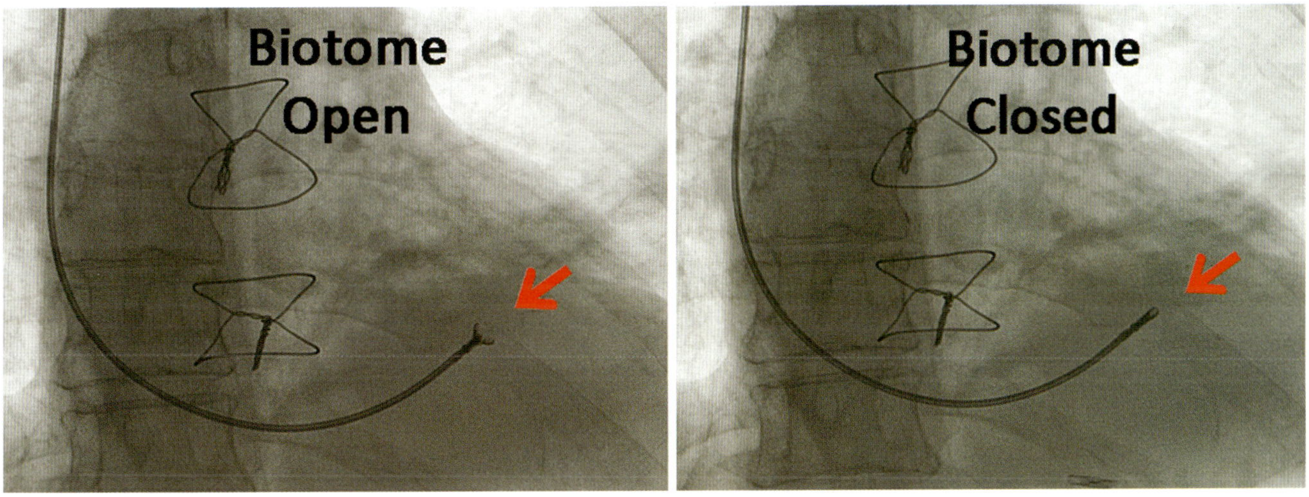

Fig. 24.9: Fluoroscopic images of a right ventricular endomyocardial biopsy showing the biopsy forceps (biotome) both open and closed. (Image courtesy of Dr M Toma).

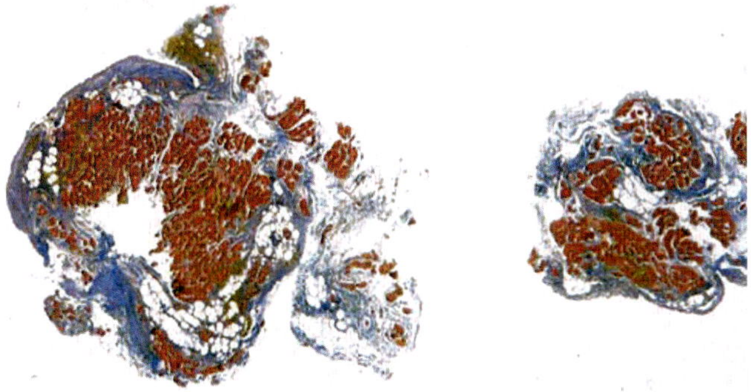

Fig. 24.10: Endomyocardial biopsy specimens from the right ventricle free wall in a patient with ARVC demonstrating fibrofatty replacement of the normal myocardium. (Image from Thiene G, Corrado D, Basso C. Arrhythmogenic right ventricular cardiomyopathy/dysplasia. Orphanet J Rare Dis. 2007;2:45).

PROGNOSIS AND MANAGEMENT OF ARVC PATIENTS

Major risk factors for adverse prognosis include young age, family history of sudden adult death, predominant left ventricular involvement, ventricular tachycardia, syncope, and prior cardiac arrest. Patients who present with VT have a favorable outcome when treated medically and therefore pharmacologic treatment is the first line of therapy. Other treatment options include catheter ablation in those patients with VT refractory to drug treatment (Figs. 24.11A and B) or placement of an implantable cardioverter defibrillator (ICD).

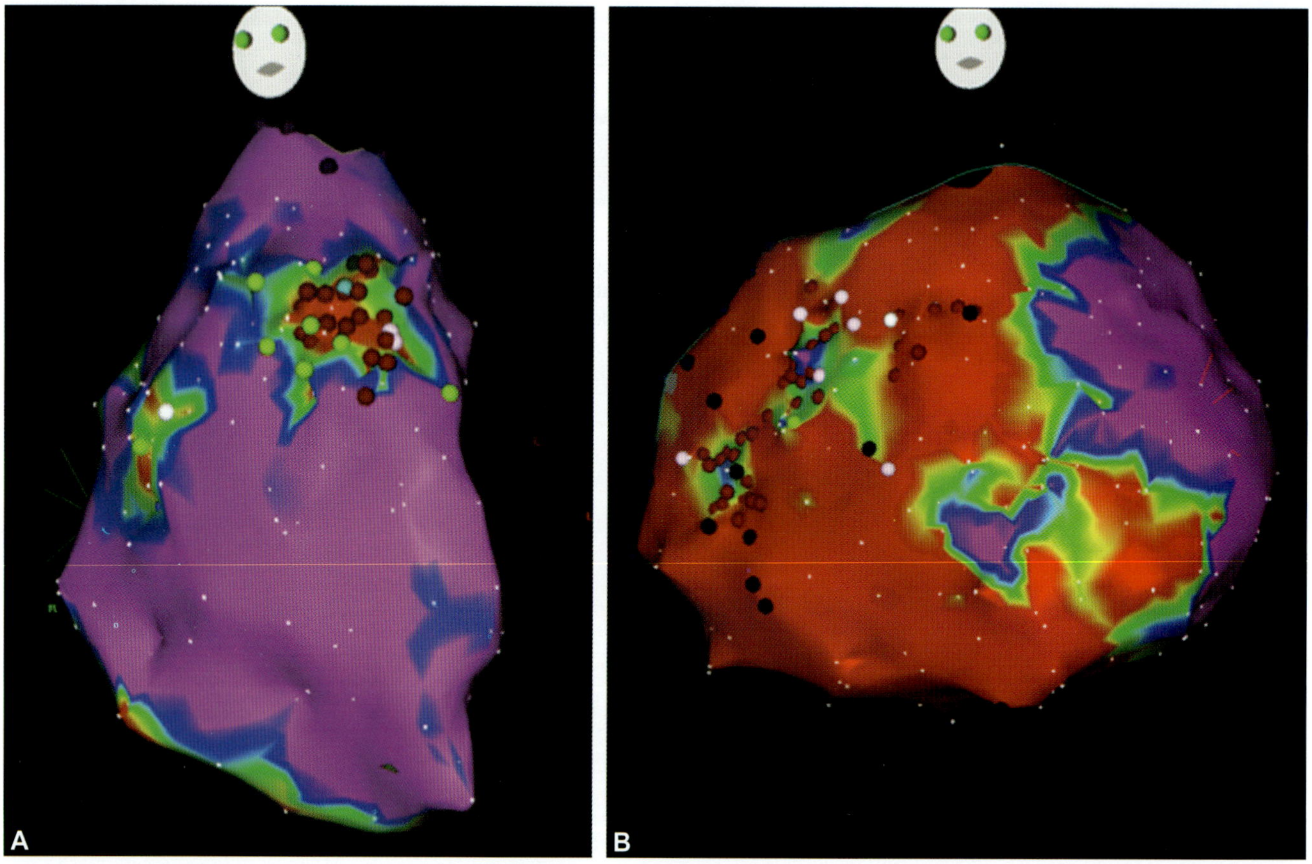

Figs. 24.11A and B: Electroanatomic voltage maps showing right ventricle (RV) abnormalities. RV (A) endocardial and (B) epicardial voltage maps (left anterior oblique projections) from an ablation procedure in a young patient with advanced ARVC and refractory VT. Red, low voltage, purple equals normal voltage. Dark blue and black dots are areas of abnormal electrical signals (fractionation/late potentials). Red dots correspond to ablation lesions while the remaining colors correspond to pacing sites.

VIDEO LEGEND

Video 24.1: MRI of a patient with arrhythmogenic right ventricular dysplasia demonstrating a dilated right ventricle with markedly depressed systolic function. (Video courtesy of Scott D Flamm, MD).

REFERENCES

Basso C, Corrado D, Thiene G. Cardiovascular causes of sudden death in young individuals including athletes. Cardiol Rev. 1999;7(3):127-35.

Basso C, Thiene G, Corrado D, et al. Arrhythmogenic right ventricular cardiomyopathy. Dysplasia, dystrophy, or myocarditis? Circulation. 1996;94(5):983-91.

Ellison KE, Friedman PL, Ganz LI, et al. Entrainment mapping and radiofrequency catheter ablation of ventricular tachycardia in right ventricular dysplasia. J Am Coll Cardiol. 1998;32(3):724-8.

Fontaine G, Umemura J, Di Donna P, et al. Duration of QRS complexes in arrhythmogenic right ventricular dysplasia. A new non-invasive diagnostic marker. Ann Cardiol Angeiol (Paris). 1993;42(8):399-405.

Gemayel C, Pelliccia A, Thompson PD. Arrhythmogenic right ventricular cardiomyopathy. J Am Coll Cardiol. 2001;38(7):1773-81.

Marcus FI, Fontaine GH, Guiraudon G, et al. Right ventricular dysplasia: a report of 24 adult cases. Circulation. 1982;65(2):384-98.

Marcus FI, McKenna WJ, Sherrill D, et al. Diagnosis of arrhythmogenic right ventricular cardiomyopathy/dysplasia: proposed modification of the task force criteria. Circulation. 2010;121(13):1533-41.

McKenna WJ, Thiene G, Nava A, et al. Diagnosis of arrhythmogenic right ventricular dysplasia/cardiomyopathy. Task Force of the Working Group Myocardial and Pericardial Disease of the European Society of Cardiology and of the Scientific Council on Cardiomyopathies of the International Society and Federation of Cardiology. Br Heart J. 1994;71(3):215-8.

Nasir K, Rutberg J, Tandri H, et al. Utility of SAECG in arrhythmogenic right ventricle dysplasia. Ann Noninvasive Electrocardiol. 2003;8(2):112-20.

Oselladore L, Nava A, Buja G, et al. Signal-averaged electrocardiography in familial form of arrhythmogenic right ventricular cardiomyopathy. Am J Cardiol. 1995;75(15):1038-41.

Peters S, Trümmel M. Diagnosis of arrhythmogenic right ventricular dysplasia-cardiomyopathy: value of standard ECG revisited. Ann Noninvasive Electrocardiol. 2003;8(3):238-45.

Pinamonti B, Sinagra G, Salvi A, et al. Left ventricular involvement in right ventricular dysplasia. Am Heart J. 1992;123(3):711-24.

Richardson P, McKenna W, Bristow M, et al. Report of the 1995 World Health Organization/International Society and Federation of Cardiology Task Force on the Definition and Classification of cardiomyopathies. Circulation. 1996;93(5):841-2.

Te Riele AS, James CA, Philips B, et al. Mutation-positive arrhythmogenic right ventricular dysplasia/cardiomyopathy: the triangle of dysplasia displaced. J Cardiovasc Electrophysiol. 2013;24(12):1311-20.

Thiene G, Nava A, Corrado D, et al. Right ventricular cardiomyopathy and sudden death in young people. N Engl J Med. 1988;318(3):129-33.

Turrini P, Angelini A, Thiene G, et al. Late potentials and ventricular arrhythmias in arrhythmogenic right ventricular cardiomyopathy. Am J Cardiol. 1999;83(8):1214-9.

CHAPTER

Left Ventricular Assist Devices

25

Kory J Lavine, Susan M Joseph

INTRODUCTION, TECHNOLOGY, AND OUTCOMES

Left ventricular assist devices (LVADs) are surgically implanted heart pumps that provide support to the left ventricle (LV) to provide adequate blood flow and reduce congestion in patients with advanced systolic heart failure (HF). Hemodynamics acutely improve following LVAD implantation by both a reduction in left ventricular filling pressure ("decongesting" the heart) and by increased cardiac output (Figs. 25.1A and B).

Over the last several decades there has been an evolution of LVAD technology and design (Figs. 25.2 to 25.4). Currently implantable LVADs are approved for (1) "bridge to transplant" and for (2) "destination therapy" (DT) in individuals with advanced HF who are not candidates for a cardiac transplant (in other words, permanent implantation without plans for subsequent transplantation). Implantable durable LVADs include the HeartMate II LVAD (Figs. 25.5 and 25.6) and the HeartWare HVAD (Figs. 25.7A to D).

Randomized trials have demonstrated improved quality of life and survival in patients with refractory severe HF receiving LVADs when compared with medical therapy alone. However, there is still considerable morbidity and mortality with LVAD therapy, particularly in destination therapy LVAD patients, who tend to be older than bridge to transplant patients. The 1- and 2-year survival rates for participants in the HeartMate II DT trial were 68% and 58%, respectively, although more recent registry data show 1-year survival rates exceeding 70%. Careful preoperative assessment of multiple parameters, including hepatic and renal function, coagulopathic measures, lung function, nutritional status, social support network, and capability of adhering to treatment, is performed to enhance patient selection and outcomes. It is anticipated that with improved patient selection, perioperative morbidity and mortality can be further reduced.

The Interagency Registry for Mechanical Assisted Circulatory Support (INTERMACS) has devised a classification for degree of illness prior to LVAD implantation (Table 25.1). At times, a patient with decompensated HF, volume overload, and/or end-organ dysfunction might best be served with preoperative optimization prior to LVAD surgery. Percutaneous ventricular assist devices (Figs. 25.8 and 25.9) or extracorporeal membrane oxygenation (ECMO; Fig. 25.10) may be used to improve patient hemodynamics and clinical status prior to surgical implantation of an LVAD. Table 25.2 summarizes the different types of percutaneous devices. There is no consensus or guideline statement to help clinicians decide how best to acutely support patients with critical cardiogenic shock. The decision is largely individualized, based on patient characteristics and relative risks.

Echocardiography is used to assess device position and function during implantation and during follow-up (Figs. 25.11 to 25.15).

COMPLICATIONS

Though LVADs improve quality and quantity of life, this comes at a considerable cost in the form of frequent hospitalizations for LVAD-related complications. By 6 months post-implant, 60% of patients have experienced at least one hospitalization. Major complications include infection, bleeding, device malfunction, stroke, and death. Managing LVAD complications requires evaluation at a center experienced and equipped to handle these problems, and typically requires multidisciplinary management strategies.

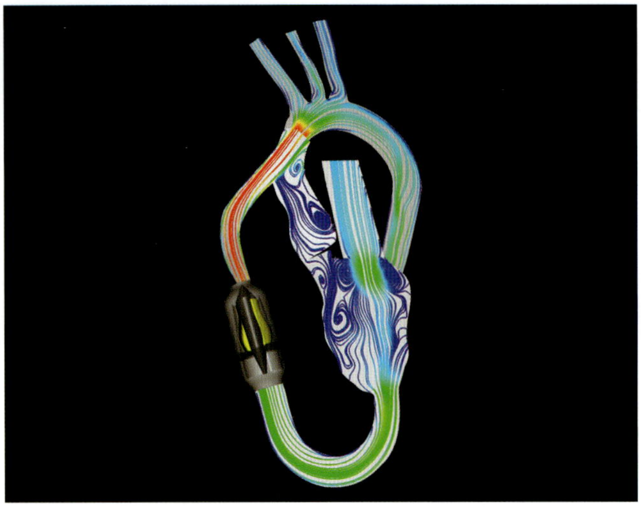

Fig. 25.1A: Simulation of a wave pump human ventricular assist device hemodynamic flow. (Image created by Herbert Oerte and posted on Wikimedia Commons).

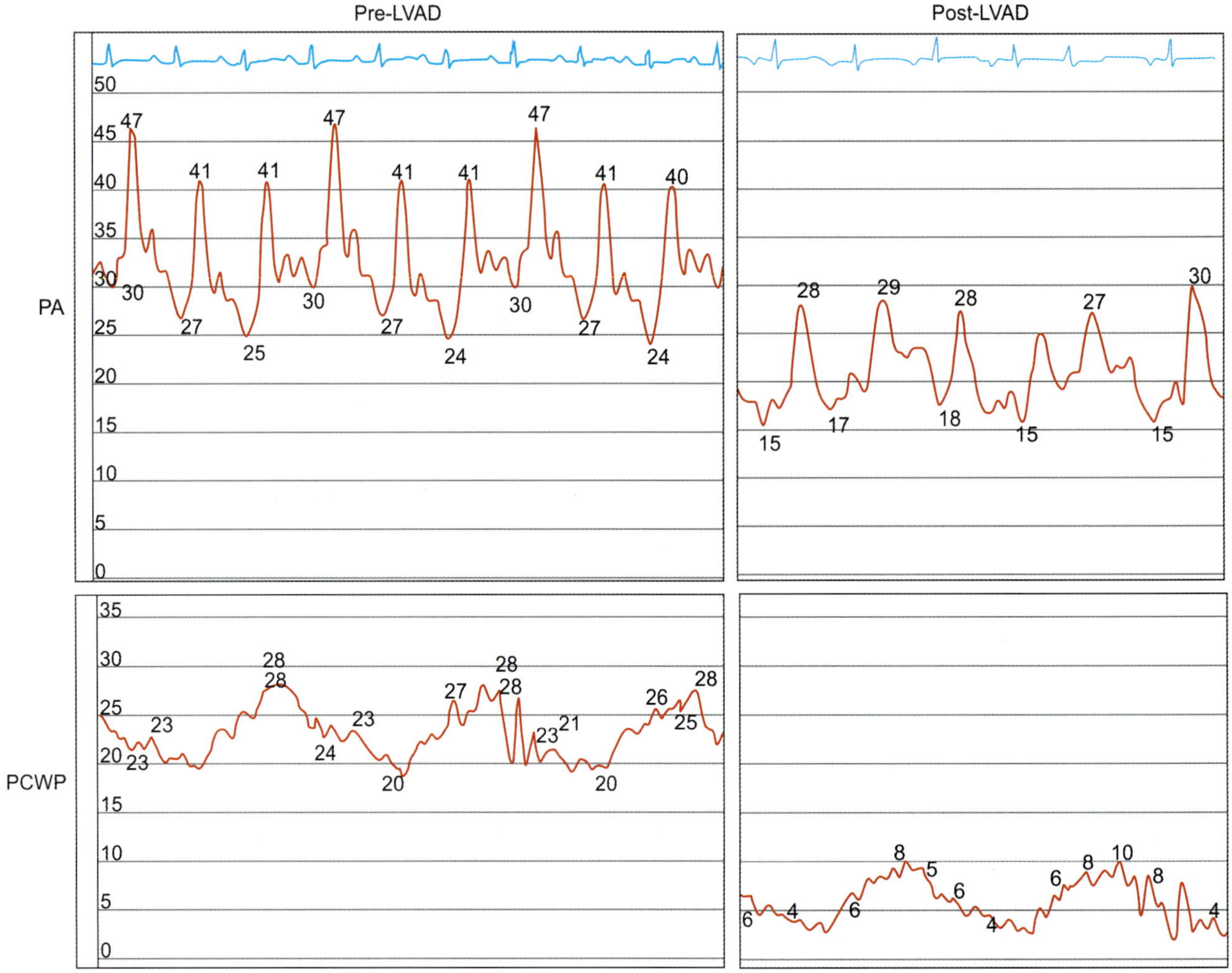

Fig. 25.1B: Hemodynamic changes following left ventricular assist device (LVAD) implantation. Right heart catheterization measurements before (left panels) and after (right panels) LVAD implantation demonstrating evidence of left ventricular unloading with reductions in pulmonary artery (PA) and pulmonary capillary wedge pressure (PCWP).

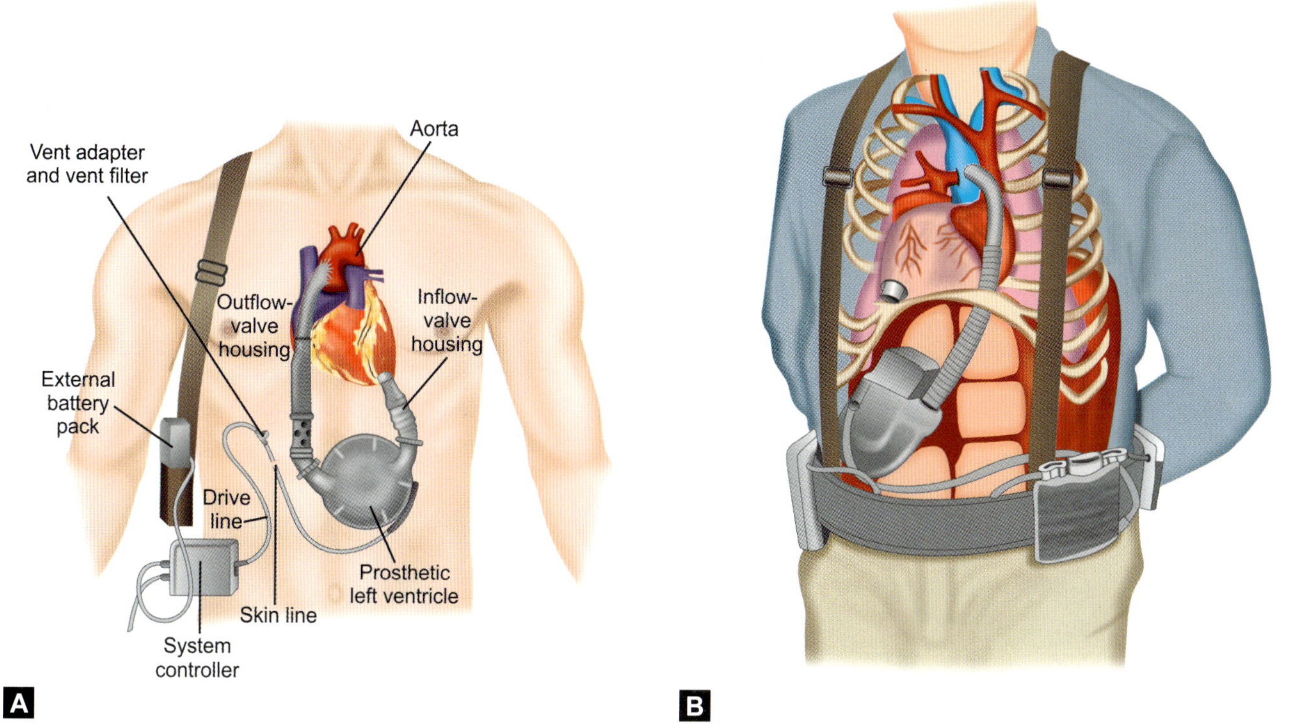

Figs. 25.2A and B: Schematic illustrations of a first-generation left ventricular assist device (LVAD). (Images from Samuels LE. The implantable left ventricular assist device: a bridge to a destination. J Clin Exp Cardiolog. 2013;4:267).

Bleeding Complications

Overall bleeding complications occur at a rate of 1.1 per patient-year on LVAD support, and the most common types of bleeding are gastrointestinal (GI) hemorrhage and epistaxis. Published data suggest that GI bleeding occurs in about 20–30% of LVAD patients. While some GI bleeding is due to gastritis or hemorrhoids, patients with continuous flow LVADs are subject to GI bleeding related to the formation of superficial arteriovenous malformations in the intestinal mucosa. Additionally, these patients develop an acquired von-Willebrand syndrome due to lysis of von-Willebrand factor multimers, resulting in an impairment of primary hemostasis. LVAD patients presenting with significant GI bleeding generally have anticoagulation held or reversed, and often undergo extensive evaluation to determine the source of bleeding. This may include upper GI endoscopy, colonoscopy, capsule endoscopy or, in the case of brisk bleeding, tagged red blood cell nuclear scan or angiography. Hospitalizations are often protracted as anticoagulation is resumed and the patient is observed for any recurrence of bleeding. In patients who have had more than one bleeding episode, anticoagulation is generally reduced, with a lower dose of aspirin and/or lower target international normalized ratio (INR).

Right Ventricular Failure

Right ventricular failure (RVF) is another common challenge on LVAD support because the device supports only the LV (Figs. 25.16A to C). This complication may eventually occur in up to 25% of LVAD-supported patients. Symptoms of RVF include abdominal fullness, anorexia, and peripheral edema. In the perioperative period, right-ventricular assist device implantation may be required, prolonging the hospital course. For those with symptomatic congestion, diuretics are the mainstay of therapy. In patients with concomitant pulmonary hypertension, oral pulmonary vasodilators, such as sildenafil, may have a role in unloading the right ventricle (RV) and reducing central venous pressures. If symptoms are refractory to oral therapies, intravenous inotropes may be required. Pump speed may need to be adjusted to balance RV and LV

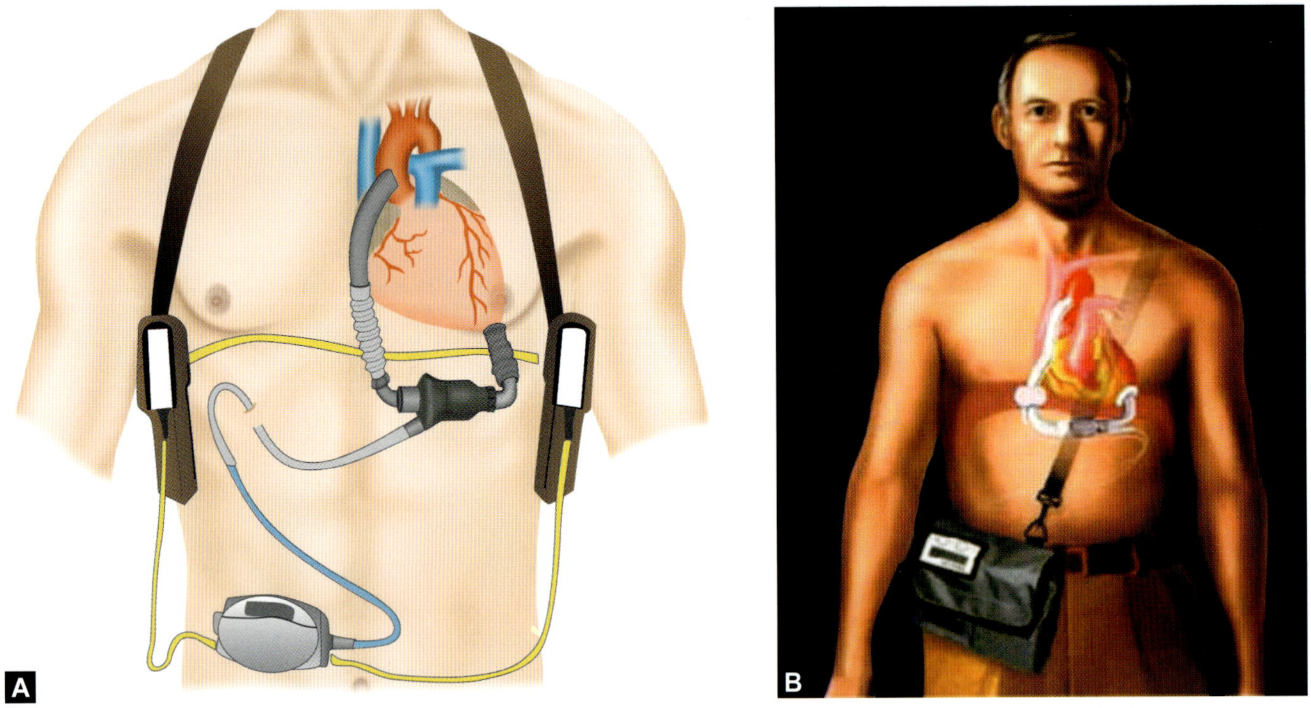

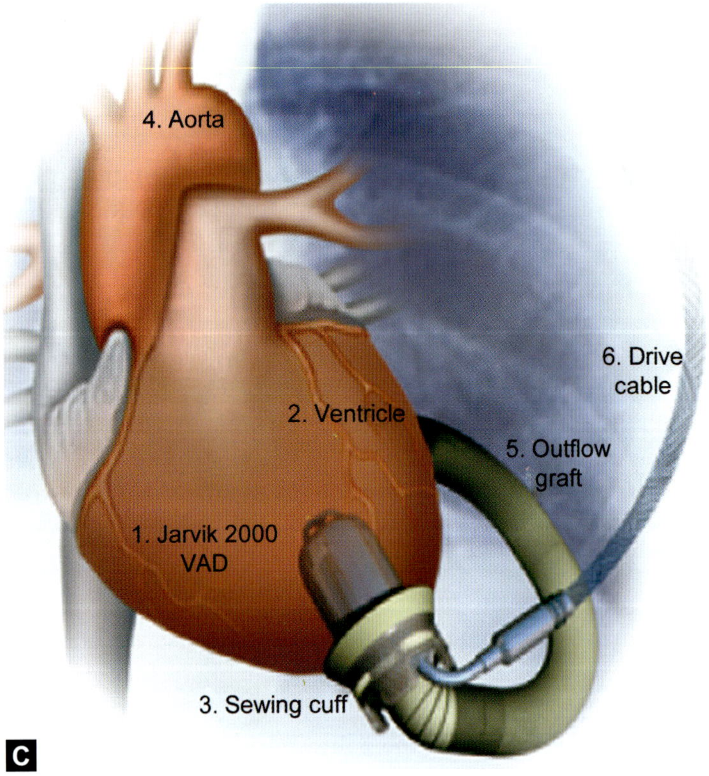

Figs. 25.3A to C: Schematic illustrations of a second-generation left ventricular assist device (LVAD). (Images from Samuels LE. The implantable left ventricular assist device: a bridge to a destination. J Clin Exp Cardiolog. 2013;4:267).

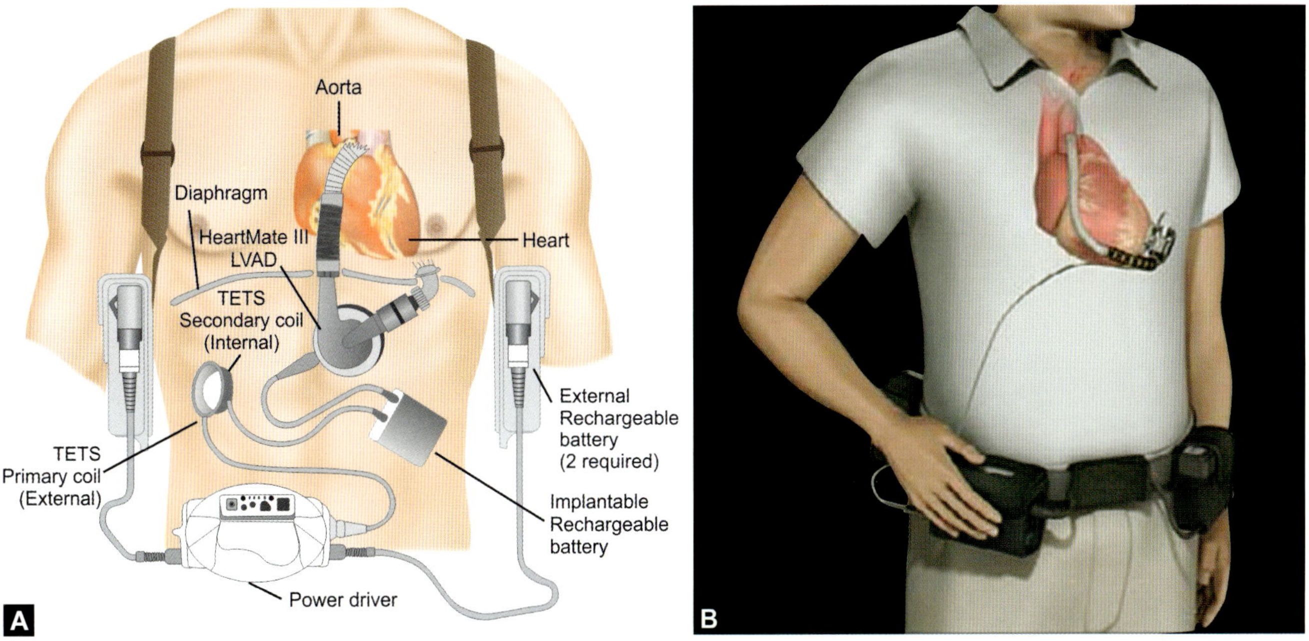

Figs. 25.4A and B: Schematic illustrations of a third-generation left ventricular assist device (LVAD). (Images from Samuels LE. The implantable left ventricular assist device: a bridge to a destination. J Clin Exp Cardiolog. 2013;4:267).

demand. Patients ineligible for heart transplant may benefit symptomatically from continuous intravenous inotropic support. In some cases, palliative care consultation should be considered.

Device Malfunction

Device malfunction occurs at a rate of 0.2 malfunctions per patient-year of support with continuous flow devices and at 2 years approximately 10% of continuous flow pumps fail, leading to pump exchange or death. Clinically, pump dysfunction is usually discovered after the emergence of HF symptoms and/or intravascular hemolysis, which is caused by shearing of red blood cells as they traverse a region of pump thrombosis (Fig. 25.17). Thrombolytic agents have been used in cases of thrombosis with limited success because the clot is often dense and organized by the time a patient presents with symptoms. Pump replacement surgery may be performed, with moderate morbidity and a 1-year survival rate post-exchange of 70%. Alternatively, a patient can be transplanted urgently if a donor is available. Otherwise, patients unwilling to undergo further surgery can elect for inotropic therapy and supportive care. These patients may require blood transfusions to maintain acceptable hemoglobin concentrations. Severe hemolysis may induce arterial vasospasm through a mechanism of nitric oxide depletion resulting in visceral pain.

Neurologic Events

Neurologic events are the most feared complication of LVAD support and occur at rate of 0.2 events per patient-year of support, and at a cumulative rate of 17–20% at 2 years. Strokes may be ischemic, from device-related emboli, or hemorrhagic, resulting from anticoagulation (Fig. 25.18). The severity of neurologic injury varies greatly. The overall prognosis after stroke in LVAD is not well-described and conventional post-stroke consultative services (speech, occupational, and physical therapy) are appropriate. Anticoagulation therapy may be interrupted and a decision to resume therapy must weigh concerns of neurologic bleeding with risk of thrombotic or embolic events.

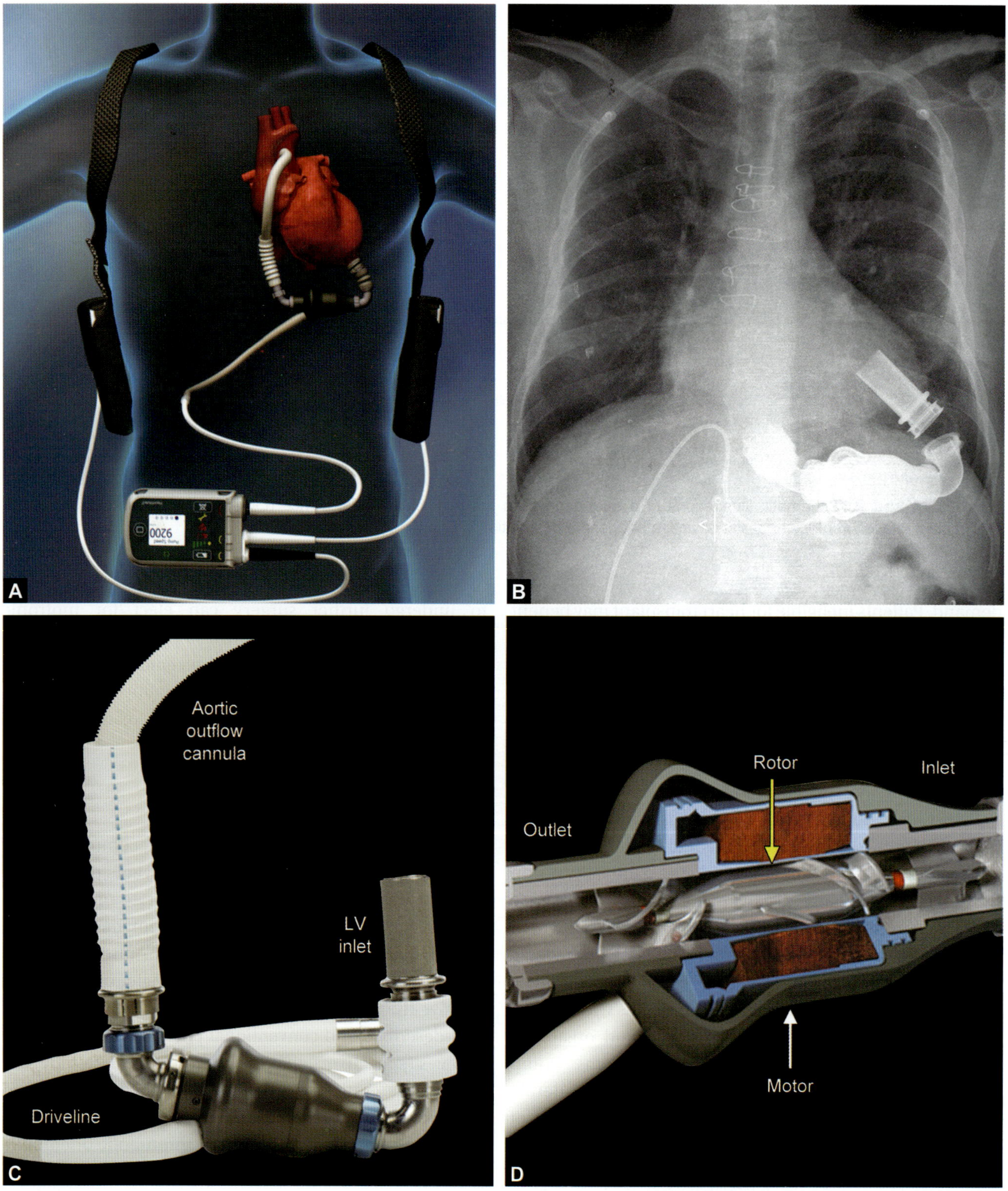

Figs. 25.5A to D: Thoratec HeartMate II left ventricular assist device (LVAD). Schematic (A) and (B) chest radiograph showing the components of the HeartMate II LVAD system. The inlet cannula is placed in the apex of the left ventricle and outflow cannula is inserted in the ascending aorta. The pump is placed in a pocket created above the diaphragm. The driveline is exteriorized through the abdominal wall and connects to a compact portable controller and battery unit. Photograph (C) and schematic (D) of the HeartMate II continuous flow axial pump and rotor.

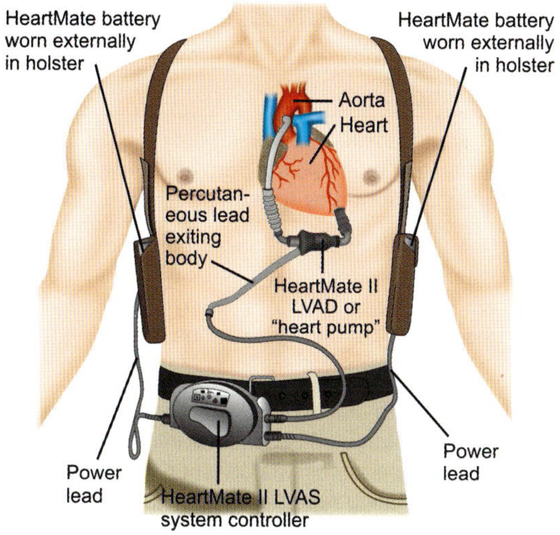

Fig. 25.6: Schematic illustration of the components of the HeartMate II left ventricular assist device (LVAD).

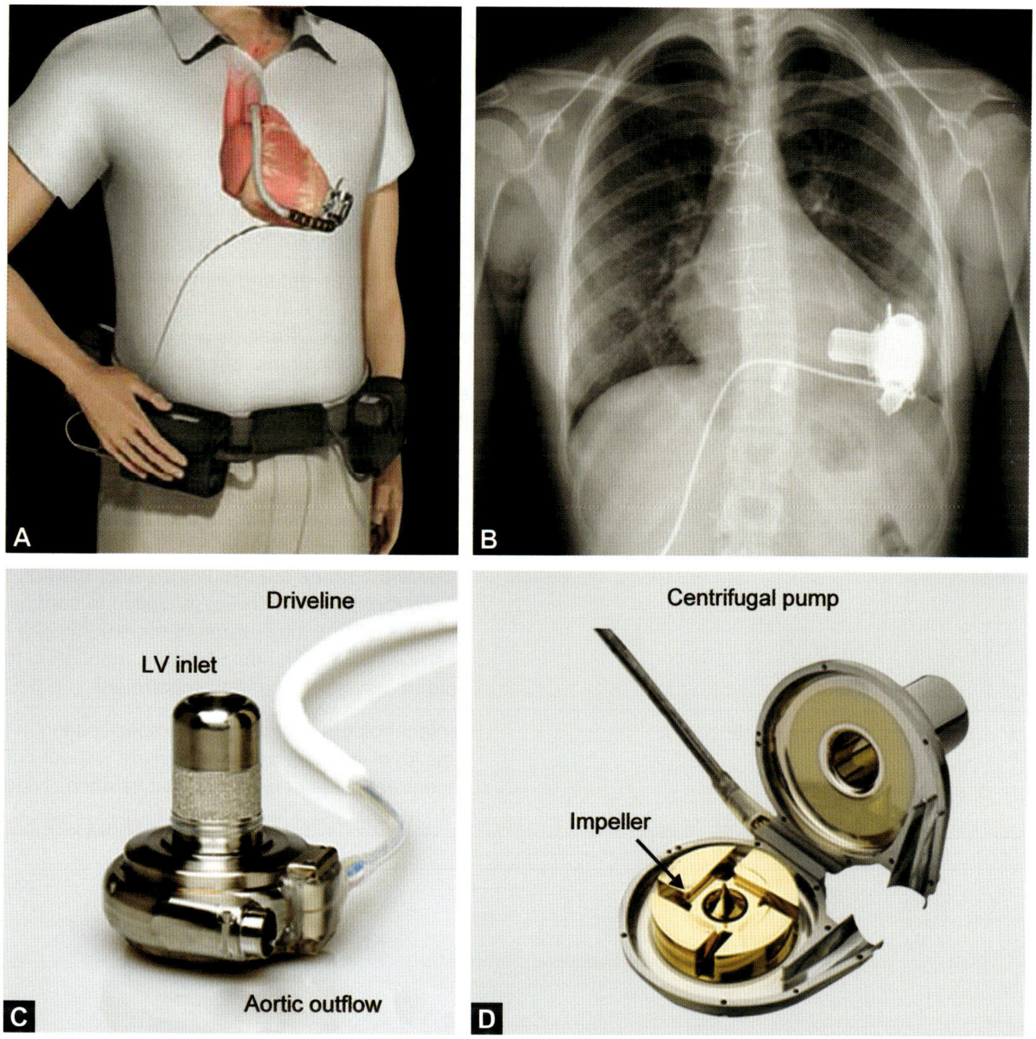

Figs. 25.7A to D: HeartWare HVAD. (A) Schematic illustration and (B) chest radiograph of the intrapericardial HeartWare HVAD system. The inlet cannula is placed in the apex of the left ventricle and outflow cannula is inserted in the ascending aorta; (C and D) The pump is located within the pericardial space between the left ventricle apex and chest wall. The driveline is exteriorized through the abdominal wall and connects to a compact portable controller and battery unit.

Table 25.1: Interagency Registry for Mechanical Assisted Circulatory Support (INTERMACS) patient profiles. (NYHA: New York Heart Association).

Profiles	*Definition*	*Description*
INTERMACS 1	Critical cardiogenic shock (Crash and burn)	Patient with life-threatening hypotension despite rapidly escalating inotropic support, critical organ hypoperfusion, often confirmed by worsening acidosis and lactate levels.
INTERMACS 2	Progressive decline (Sliding fast on inotropes)	Patient with declining function despite intravenous inotropic support, that may manifest by worsening renal function, nutritional depletion, or inability to restore volume balance. Also describes declining status in patients unable to tolerate inotropic therapy.
INTERMACS 3	Stable but inotrope dependent (dependent stability)	Patient with stable blood pressure, organ function, nutrition, and symptoms on continuous intravenous inotropic support (or a temporary circulatory support device or both), but demonstrating repeated failure to wean from support because of recurrent symptomatic hypotension or renal dysfunction.
INTERMACS 4	Resting symptoms on oral therapy at home	Patient can be stabilized close to normal volume status but experiences daily symptoms of congestion at rest or during activities of daily living. Doses of diuretics generally fluctuate at very high levels. More intensive management and surveillance strategies should be considered, which may in some cases reveal poor compliance that would compromise outcomes with any therapy. Some patients may shuttle between 4 and 5.
INTERMACS 5	Exertion intolerant	Comfortable at rest and with activities of daily living but unable to engage in any other activity, living predominantly within the house. Patients are comfortable at rest without congestive symptoms, but may have underlying refractory elevated volume status, often with renal dysfunction. If underlying nutritional status and organ function are marginal, patient may be more at risk than INTERMACS 4, and require definitive intervention.
INTERMACS 6	Exertion limited	Patient without evidence of fluid overload is comfortable at rest, and with activities of daily living and minor activities outside the home but has fatigue after the first few minutes of any meaningful activity. Attribution to cardiac limitation requires careful measurement of peak oxygen consumption, in some cases with hemodynamic monitoring to confirm severity of cardiac impairment.
INTERMACS 7	Advanced NYHA class III	A placeholder for more precise specification in future. This level includes patients who are without current or recent episodes of unstable fluid balance, living comfortably with meaningful activity limited to mild physical exertion.

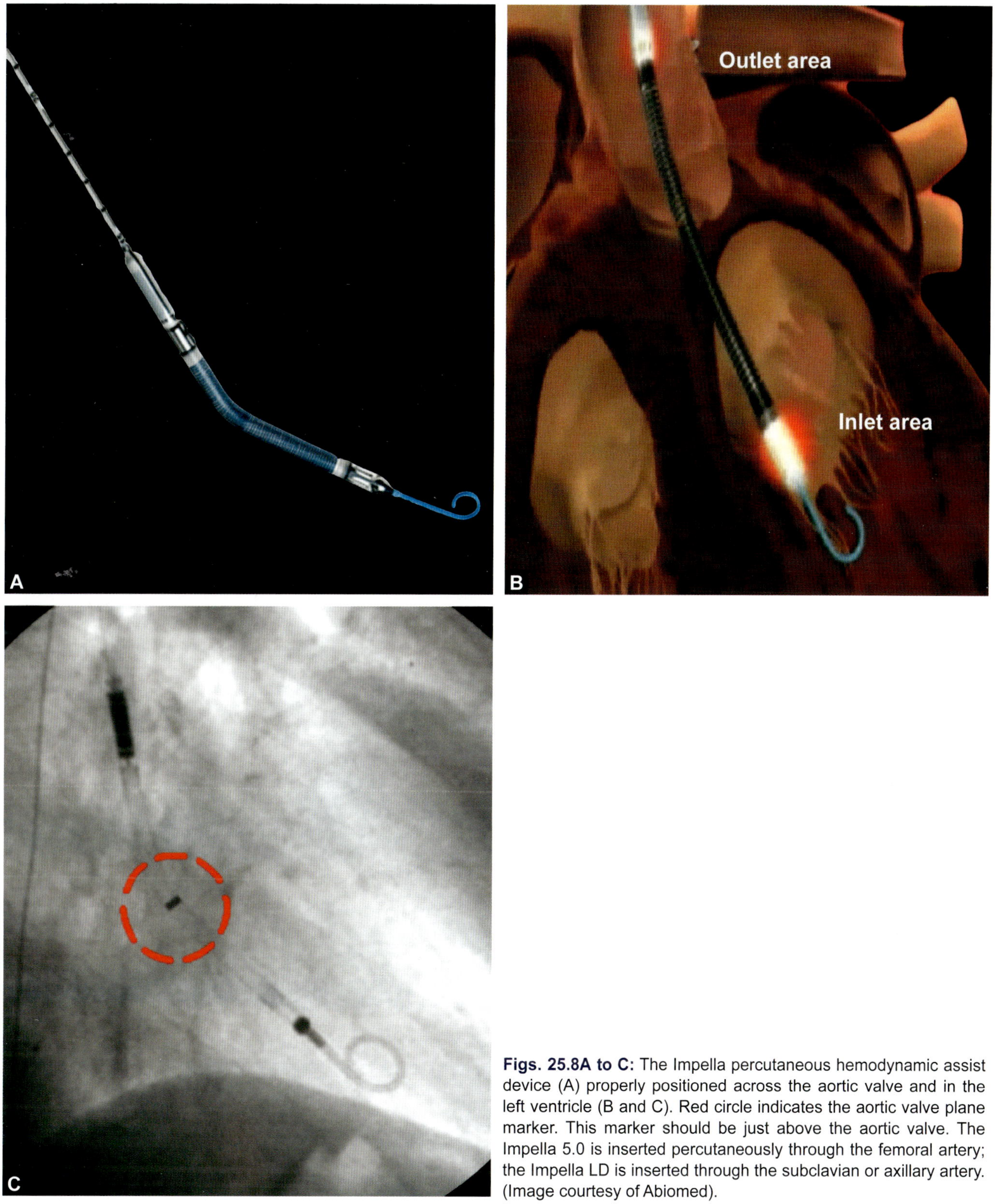

Figs. 25.8A to C: The Impella percutaneous hemodynamic assist device (A) properly positioned across the aortic valve and in the left ventricle (B and C). Red circle indicates the aortic valve plane marker. This marker should be just above the aortic valve. The Impella 5.0 is inserted percutaneously through the femoral artery; the Impella LD is inserted through the subclavian or axillary artery. (Image courtesy of Abiomed).

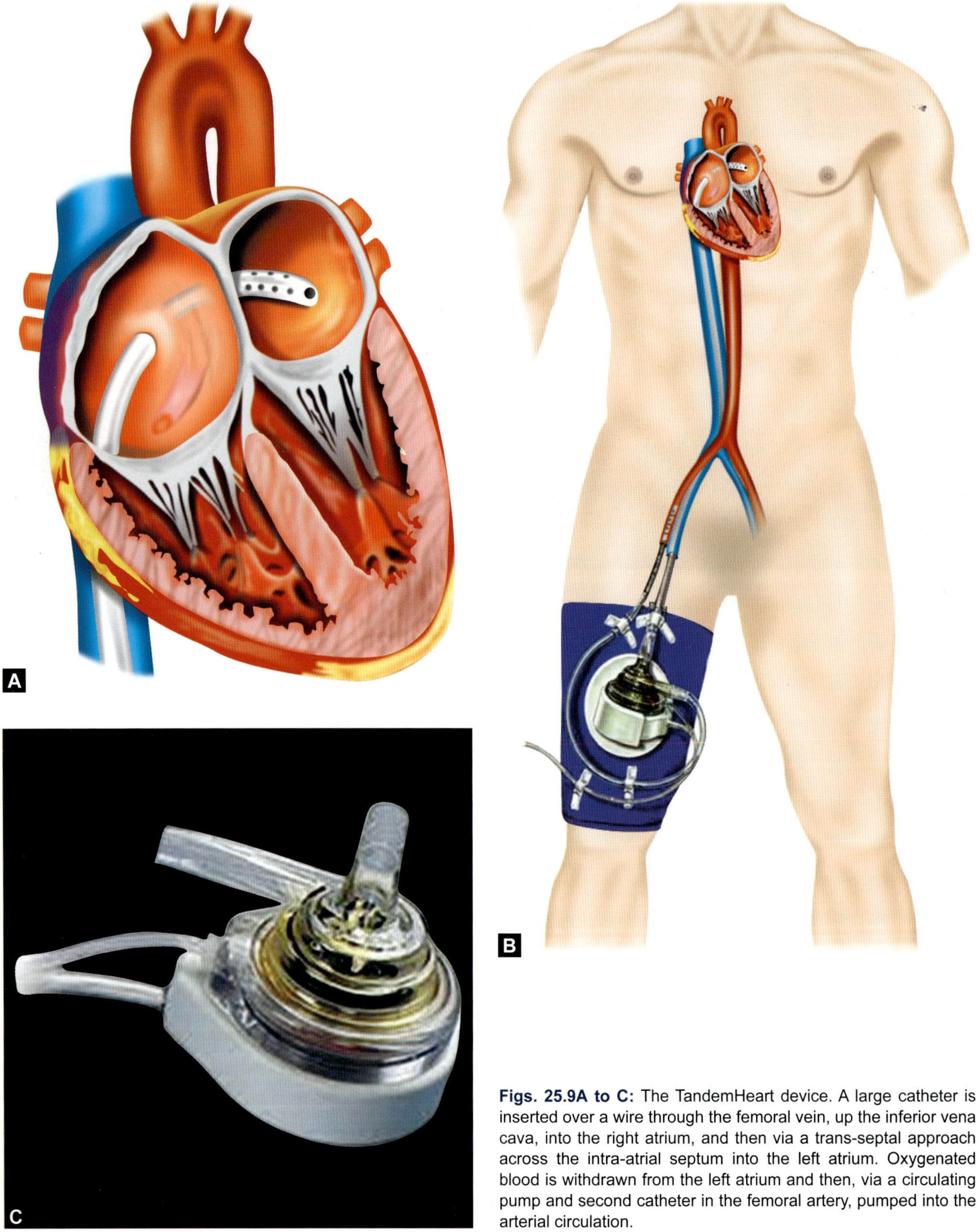

Figs. 25.9A to C: The TandemHeart device. A large catheter is inserted over a wire through the femoral vein, up the inferior vena cava, into the right atrium, and then via a trans-septal approach across the intra-atrial septum into the left atrium. Oxygenated blood is withdrawn from the left atrium and then, via a circulating pump and second catheter in the femoral artery, pumped into the arterial circulation.

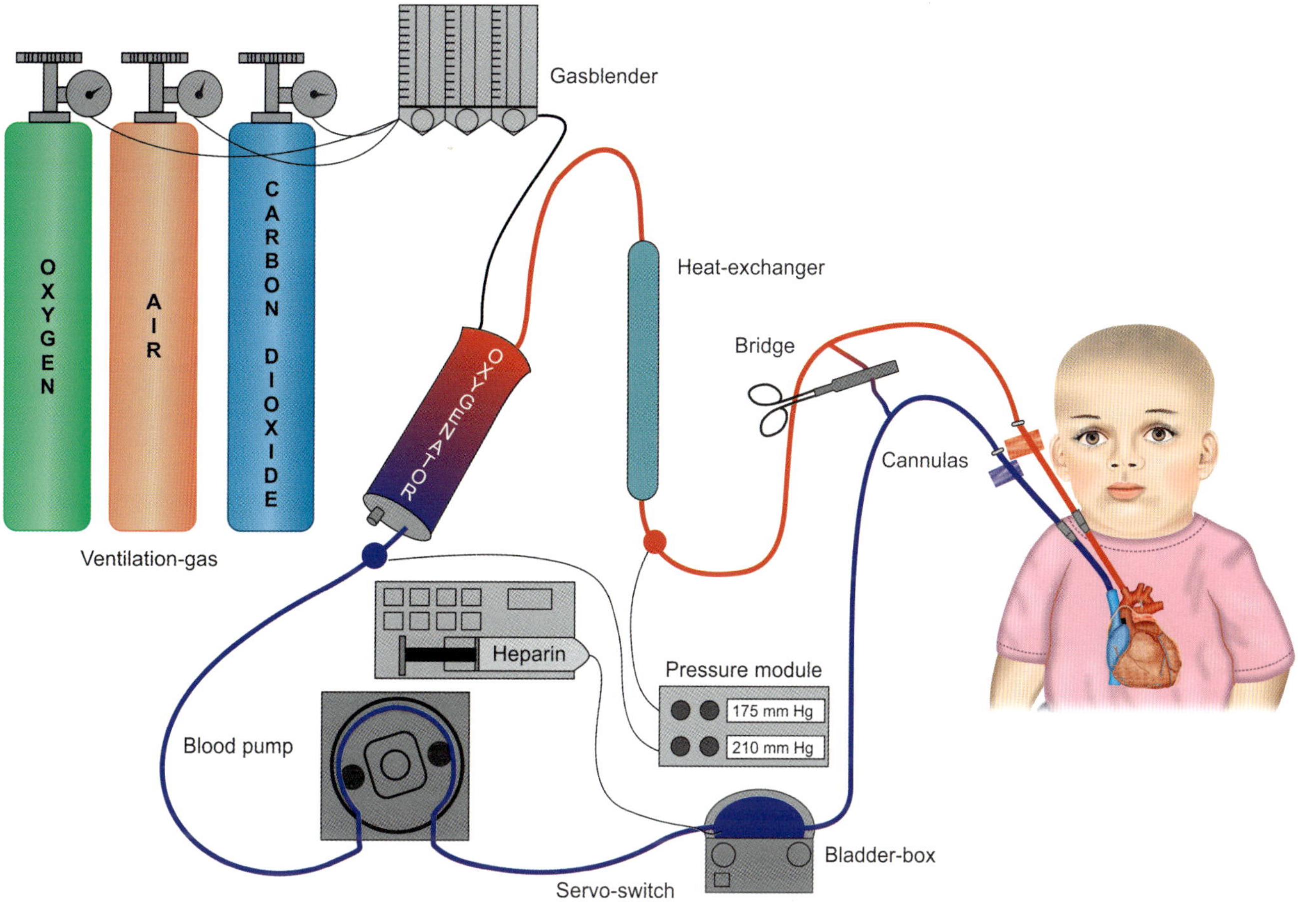

Fig. 25.10: Schematic illustration of extracorporeal membrane oxygenation (ECMO). (Image created by Jurgen Schaub and posted on Wikimedia Commons).

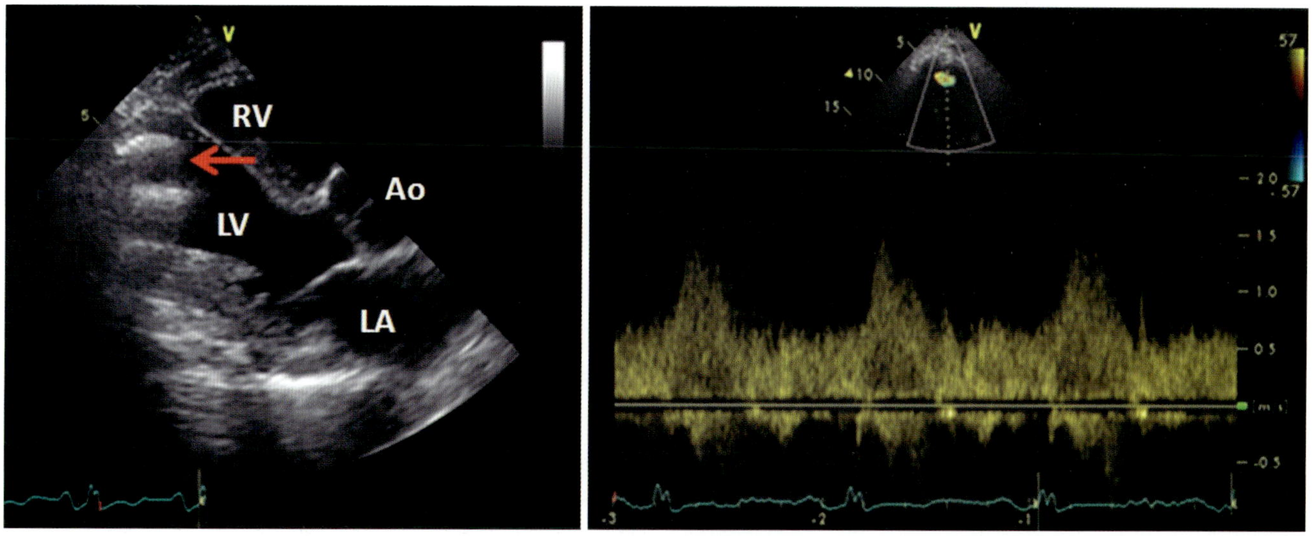

Fig. 25.11: Echocardiographic assessment of left ventricular assist device (LVAD) inflow. Left panel shows 2D parasternal long-axis image, demonstrating position of the inflow cannula (arrow) in the left ventricle. Right panel shows continuous flow Doppler examination demonstrating normal inflow velocities with continuous diastolic and peak systolic components. The aortic valve remains closed throughout the cardiac cycle.

Table 25.2: Comparison of percutaneous devices. (IABP: Intra-aortic balloon pump; ECMO: Extracorporeal membrane oxygenation; LA: Left atrium; AI: Aortic insufficiency; LV: Left ventricle; RV: Right ventricle).

	IABP	*TandemHeart*	*Impella 2.5*	*Impella CP*	*Impella 5.0*	*ECMO*
Pump mechanism	Pneumatic	Centrifugal	Axial flow	Axial flow	Axial flow	Centrifugal
Insertion technique	Femoral artery into descending aorta	Femoral vein into LA via trans-septal puncture and separate femoral artery cannula	Femoral artery retrograde across the aortic valve	Femoral artery retrograde across the aortic valve	Femoral artery retrograde across the aortic valve	Inflow cannula in right atrium via femoral vein, outflow cannula into descending aorta via femoral artery
Cannula size	7–9 Fr	21 Fr inflow, 15–17 Fr outflow cannulas	13 Fr	14 Fr	22 Fr	18–31 Fr inflow, 15–22 Fr outflow
Degree of support (L/min)	0.5	3–4	2.5	3.7	5.0	> 4.5
Time of implantation	10 min	30–60 min	15–25 min	15–25 min	30–75 min	15–45 min
Hemolysis	0	+	+++	+++	++	+
Limb ischemia	+	+++	++	++	++	+++
Bleeding risk	+	+++	++	++	++	++++
Complexity of management	+	++++	++	++	++	+++
Contraindications	Moderate-severe AI	Peripheral arterial disease	Peripheral arterial disease, LV thrombus, ventricular septal defect, severe aortic stenosis, RV failure	Peripheral arterial disease, LV thrombus, ventricular septal defect, severe aortic stenosis, RV failure	Peripheral arterial disease, LV thrombus, ventricular septal defect, severe aortic stenosis, RV failure	Peripheral arterial disease

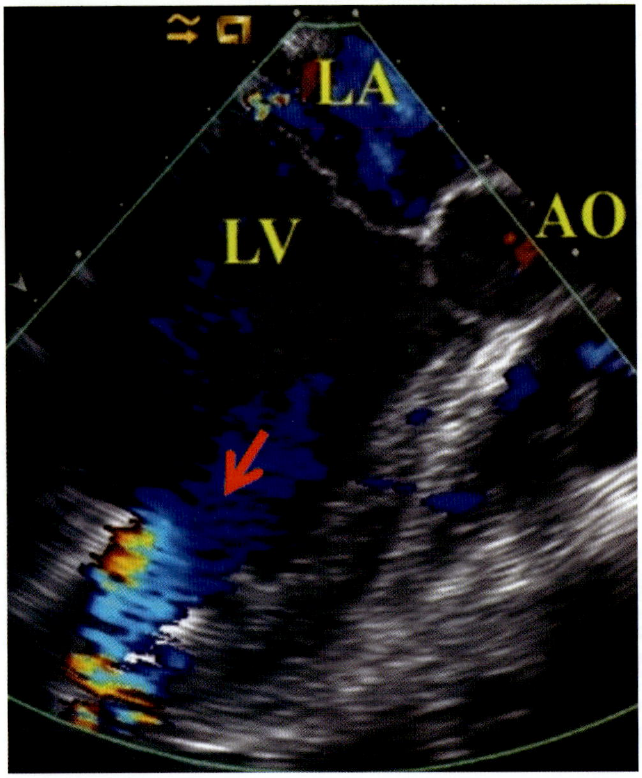

Fig. 25.12: Intraoperative color Doppler transesophageal echocardiography at 115° showing blood flow into the left ventricular assist device (LVAD) conduit at the apex of the left ventricle (LV). [Image from Helmy SM, Albinali A, Hajar R. Echocardiography in left ventricular assist device. Heart Views. 2010;11(2):74-6]. (Ao: Aorta; LA: Left atrium).

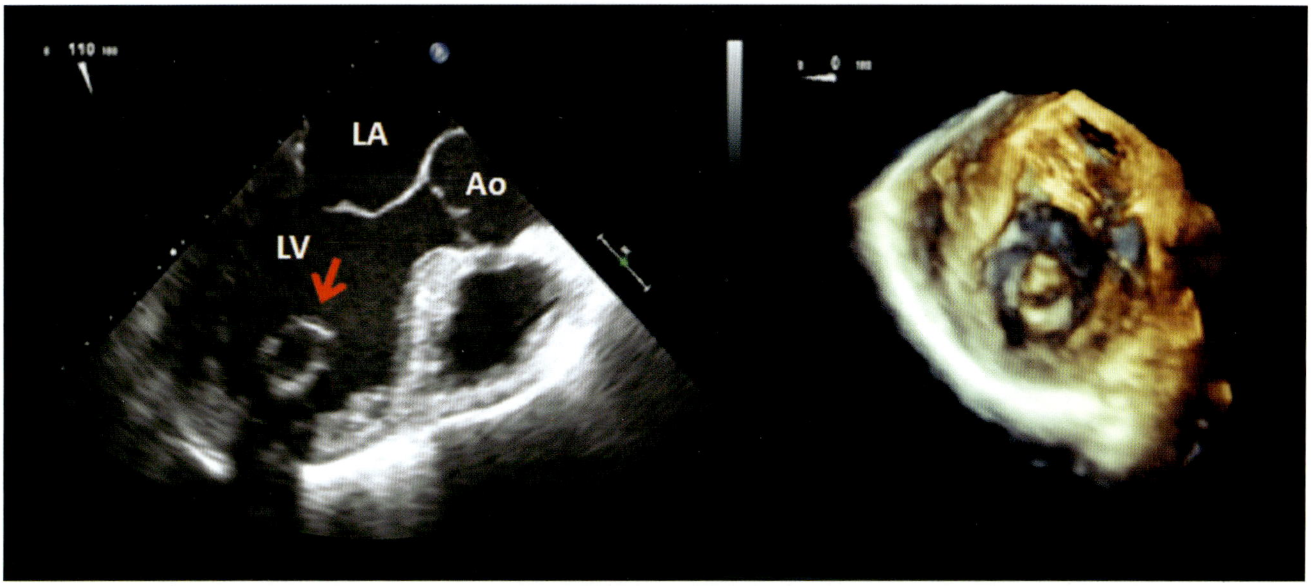

Fig. 25.13: Transesophageal echocardiography (TTE) 2D and 3D images of the left ventricular assist device (LVAD) inflow cannula in the left ventricle (LV). [Image from Platts D. Echocardiographic evaluation of ventricular assist devices. In: Shuhaiber JH (Ed). Ventricular Assist Devices. InTech; 2011]. (Ao: Aorta; LA: Left atrium).

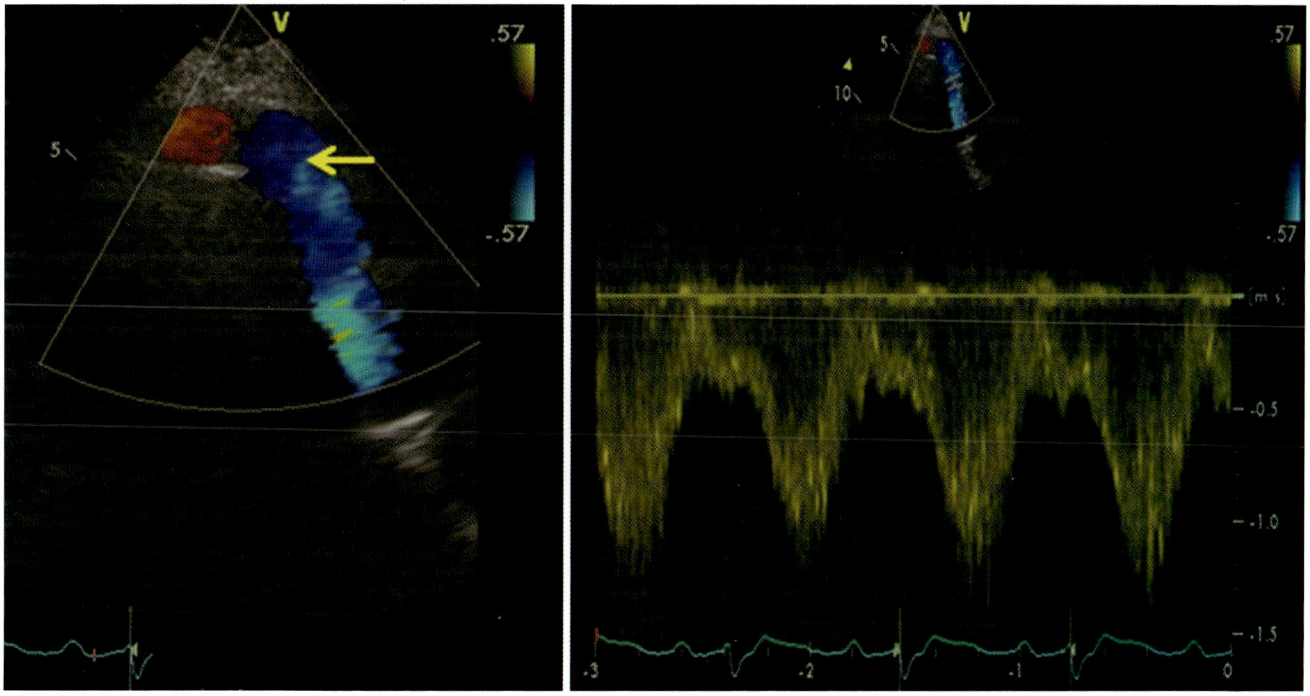

Fig. 25.14: Echocardiographic assessment of left ventricular assist device (LVAD) outflow. Left panel shows color Doppler imaging of the outflow cannula. Right panel shows continuous wave interrogation demonstrating normal outflow diastolic and systolic velocities.

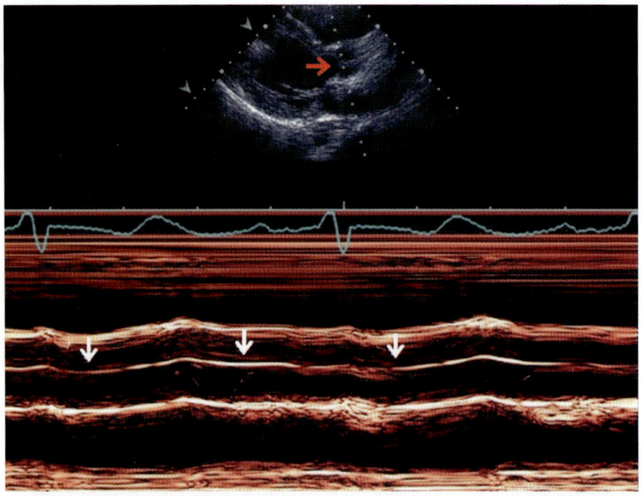

Fig. 25.15: M-Mode of the aortic valve (arrows) in a patient with left ventricular assist device (LVAD). The aortic valve remains closed throughout the cardiac cycle. [Image from Helmy SM, Albinali A, Hajar R. Echocardiography in left ventricular assist device. Heart Views. 2010;11 (2):74-6].

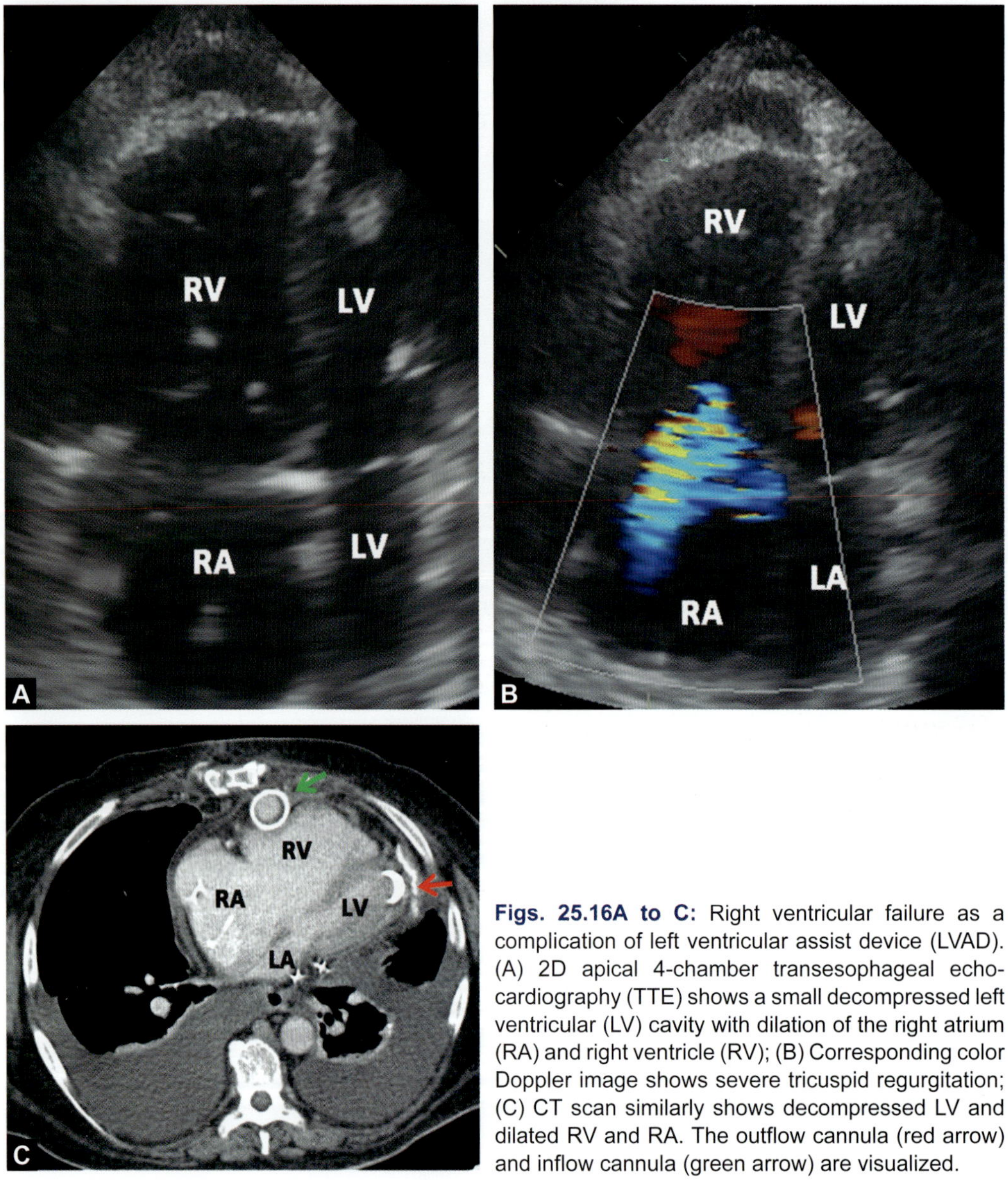

Figs. 25.16A to C: Right ventricular failure as a complication of left ventricular assist device (LVAD). (A) 2D apical 4-chamber transesophageal echocardiography (TTE) shows a small decompressed left ventricular (LV) cavity with dilation of the right atrium (RA) and right ventricle (RV); (B) Corresponding color Doppler image shows severe tricuspid regurgitation; (C) CT scan similarly shows decompressed LV and dilated RV and RA. The outflow cannula (red arrow) and inflow cannula (green arrow) are visualized.

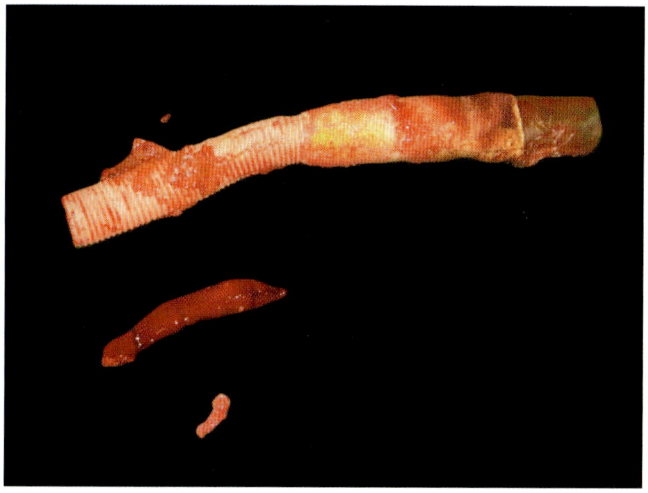

Fig. 25.17: Explanted left ventricular assist device (LVAD) with thrombus. [Image from Platts D. Echocardiographic evaluation of ventricular assist devices. In: Shuhaiber JH (Ed). Ventricular Assist Devices. InTech; 2011].

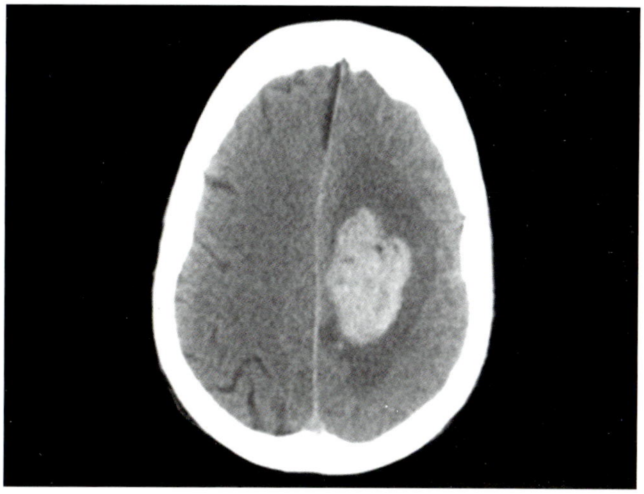

Fig. 25.18: Intracerebral hemorrhage in a patient with left ventricular assist device (LVAD) on anticoagulant therapy.

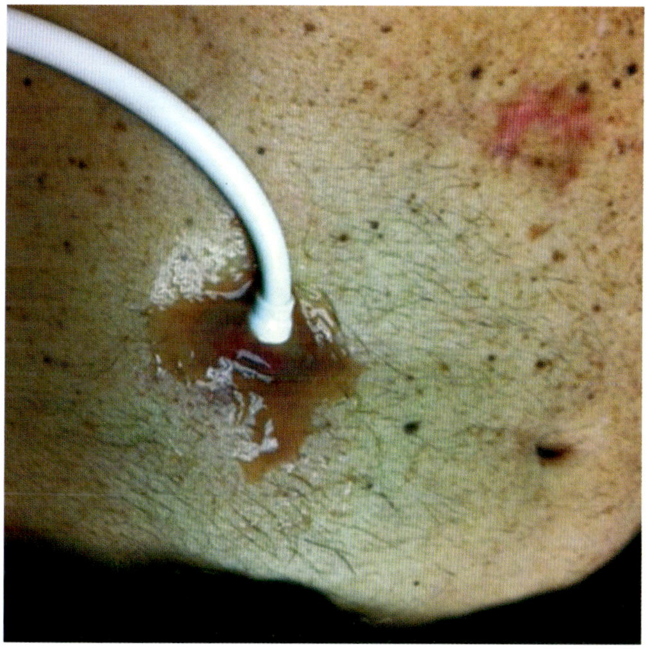

Fig. 25.19: Photograph of a driveline infection with surrounding erythema, induration, and purulent drainage.

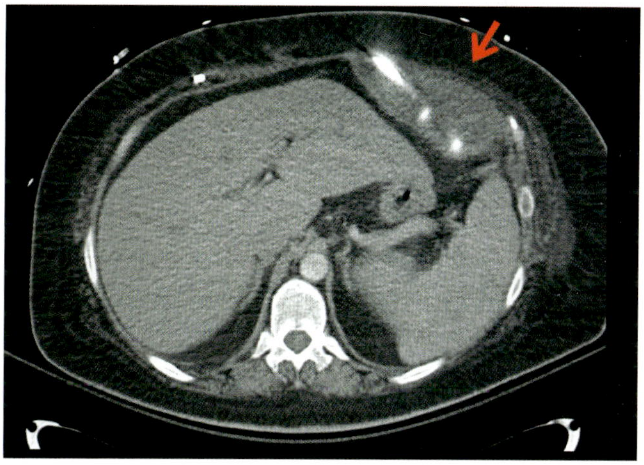

Fig. 25.20: CT imaging demonstrating a fluid collection and abscess (arrow) involving the left ventricular assist device (LVAD) pump pocket.

Infection

Infectious complications occur frequently in continuous-flow LVADs, at a rate of about one infectious complication per patient-year of support. The most frequent complication is infection of the LVAD driveline (Figs. 25.19 and 25.20), which may range in presentation from increased drainage from the exit site at the skin to frank sepsis and deep tissue infection. Extensive infection of the driveline may require surgical debridement with repositioning in healthier tissue. Infection of the pump itself may require revision of the pump pocket.

CHAPTER

26

Cardiac Transplantation

Ajay V Srivastava, Ahmad Y Sheikh, Kiran K Khush

INTRODUCTION

Cardiac transplantation (Fig. 26.1) is an established and proven therapy for patients with end-stage heart failure who continue to decline despite available medical and device therapies. The first successful heart transplant was performed by Christian Barnard (Fig. 26.2) in South Africa in 1967 employing the surgical techniques developed by Norman Shumway (Figs. 26.3A and B) and Richard Lower. Shumway subsequently performed the first heart transplant in the United States at Stanford Hospital, California, in 1968.

Early survival rates were poor, but with the advent of immunosuppressive medications in the 1980s and improved post-transplant management in the ensuing years (Fig. 26.4), heart transplant survival rates improved dramatically. The current 1-year survival rate is approximately 90% and 5-year survival exceeds 70%.

The International Society of Heart and Lung Transplantation (ISHLT) publishes a detailed annual report on the state of heart transplantation. About 5,000 heart transplants are performed annually around the world; about 50–60% are performed in the United States while the remainder are performed primarily in Europe (Fig. 26.5).

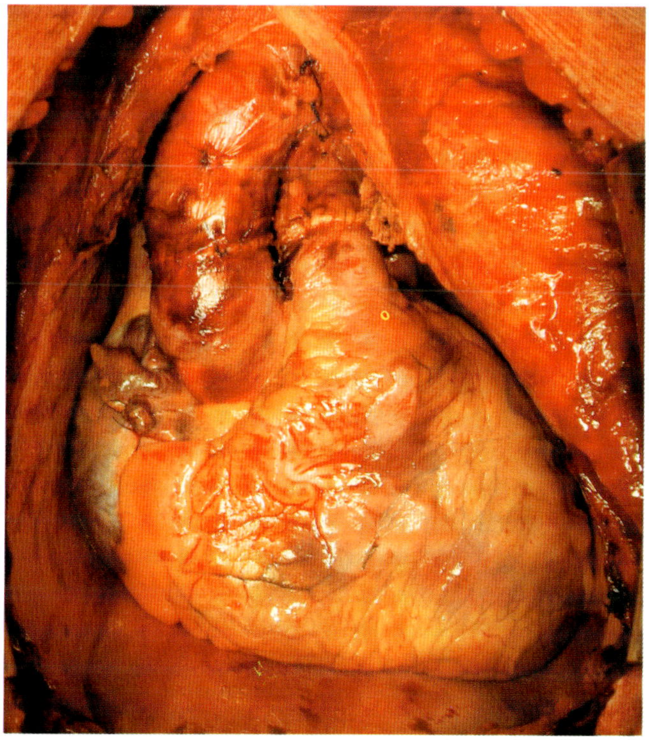

Fig. 26.1: Intraoperative image of a transplanted heart. (Image from Vasily I Kaleda, Wikimedia Commons).

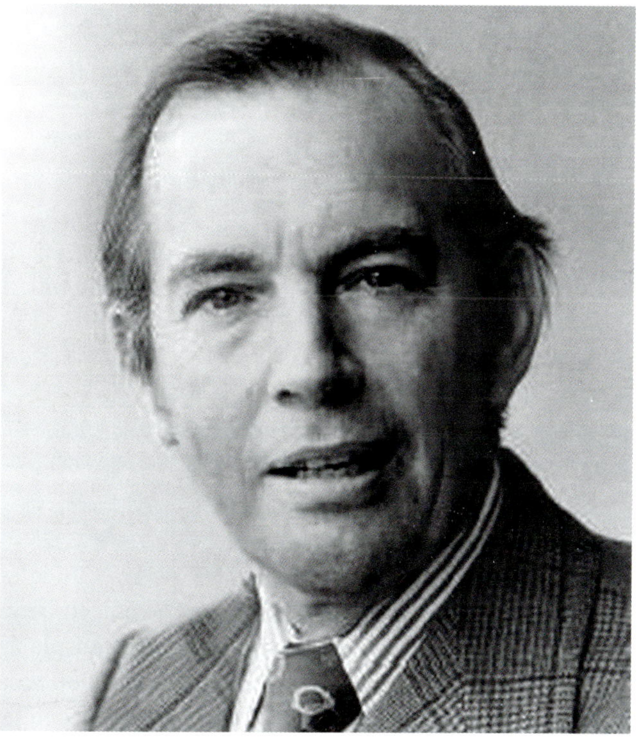

Fig. 26.2: Christian Bernard, who performed the first heart transplant in South Africa in 1967. The recipient lived for 18 days. (Image from HLWIKI International).

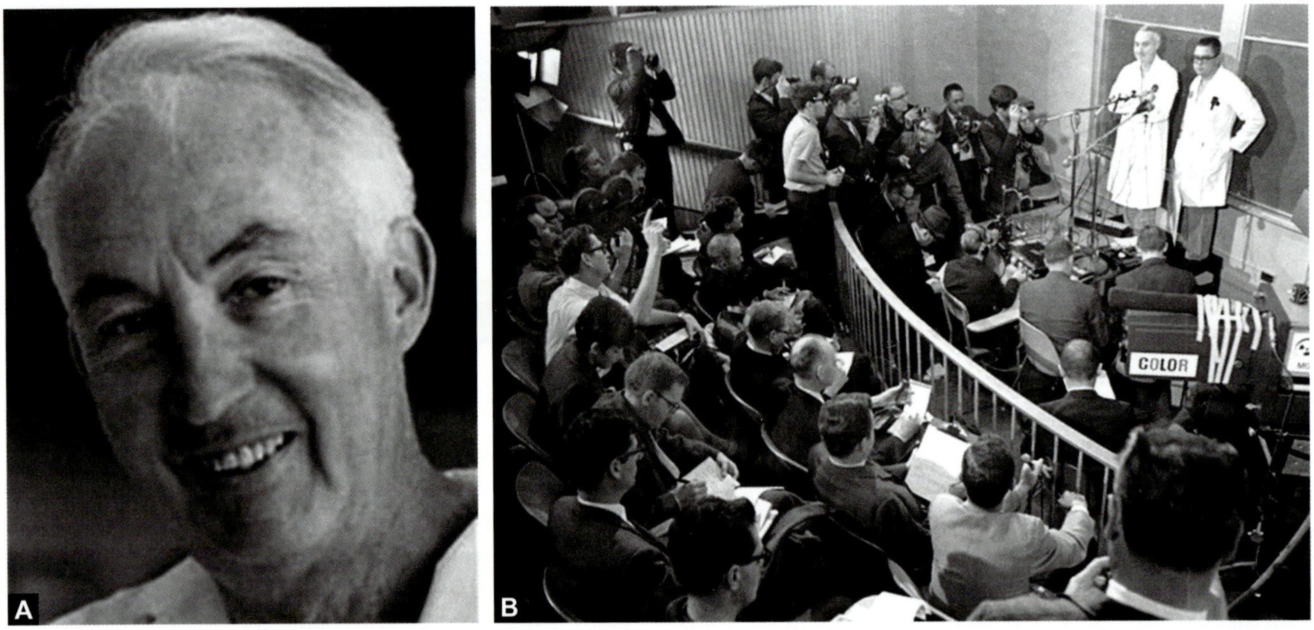

Figs. 26.3A and B: (A) Norman Shumway, who pioneered the field of heart transplantation and performed the first human transplant in the United States in 1968; (B) Reporters from all over the world gathered to hear from Norman Shumway (left) and Donald Harrison after the first successful United States heart transplant was performed. Some journalists also tried to climb the walls of Stanford Hospital to peek into the intensive care unit. (Image from Stanford University Medical Center, United States).

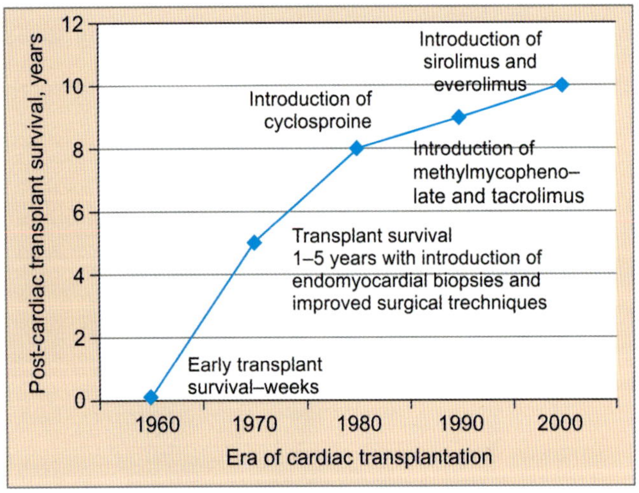

Fig. 26.4: Post-cardiac transplant survival over time. Note how advances in surgical techniques, surveillance for rejection, and particularly immunosuppression have dramatically improved survival.

While the number of patients living with advanced heart failure continues to grow, the number of heart transplants performed has plateaued over time, primarily due to a shortage of donor hearts. Hence, eligible patients must undergo a comprehensive multi-disciplinary evaluation prior to listing for cardiac transplantation. The ACC/AHA recommendations guide providers by listing indications and contraindications for cardiac transplantation (Table 26.1).

SURGICAL TECHNIQUES FOR ORTHOTOPIC HEART TRANSPLANTATION

In the present era, there are two main surgical techniques for orthotopic heart transplantation. The original biatrial technique was first described by Shumway in 1960, in which the donor and recipient right and left atria are anastomosed (Fig. 26.6), resulting in biatrial enlargement, which is easily appreciated on echocardiography (Fig. 26.7). Recipients transplanted by the biatrial technique often demonstrate dual "P" waves on their electrocardiogram (ECG), due to sinoatrial node impulses arising from both atria (Figs. 26.8A and B).

The most common technique used currently is the bicaval approach, whereby the donor right atrium is anastomosed directly to the recipient's inferior and superior vena cava (Fig. 26.9). The posterior wall of the native left atrium is left behind, and anastomosed to the donor left atrium. The bicaval technique has been associated with a reduced need for postoperative pacemaker placement and reduced length of stay post-transplantation.

Table 26.1: Indications and contraindications for cardiac transplantation. (VO_2: Oxygen consumption per unit time; NYHA: New York Heart Association; AIDS: Acquired immunodeficiency syndrome).

Acceptable Indications
• Refractory cardiogenic shock • Intravenous inotropic support required to maintain adequate end-organ perfusion and inability to wean off inotropes • Maximal VO_2 less than 10 mL/kg/minute with achievement of anaerobic metabolism • Severe symptomatic coronary artery disease not amenable to coronary artery bypass surgery or percutaneous coronary intervention • Recurrent ventricular arrhythmias
Probable Indications
• Maximal VO_2 less than 14 mL/kg/minute and major limitation of the patient's activities • Recurrent unstable ischemia not amenable to percutaneous or surgical interventions • Volatility of fluid balance and renal function despite compliance with diet and medications
Inadequate Indications
• Low left ventricular ejection fraction < 20% • Maximal VO_2 greater than 15 mL/kg/minute (and greater than 55% predicted) and absence of other indications • History of NYHA class III or IV heart failure • Prior history of ventricular arrhythmias
Absolute Contraindications
• Systemic non-cardiac illness with a life expectancy less than 2 years • Known current malignancy or recent malignancy within 5 years with a high-risk of recurrence • Untreated systemic infection rendering immunosuppression unsafe • AIDS with opportunistic infections • Significant pulmonary disease despite optimal medical therapy and not expected to improve with cardiac transplantation • Fixed pulmonary hypertension evidenced by pulmonary vascular resistance greater than 5 Wood Units or mean transpulmonary gradient greater than or equal to 16 mm Hg

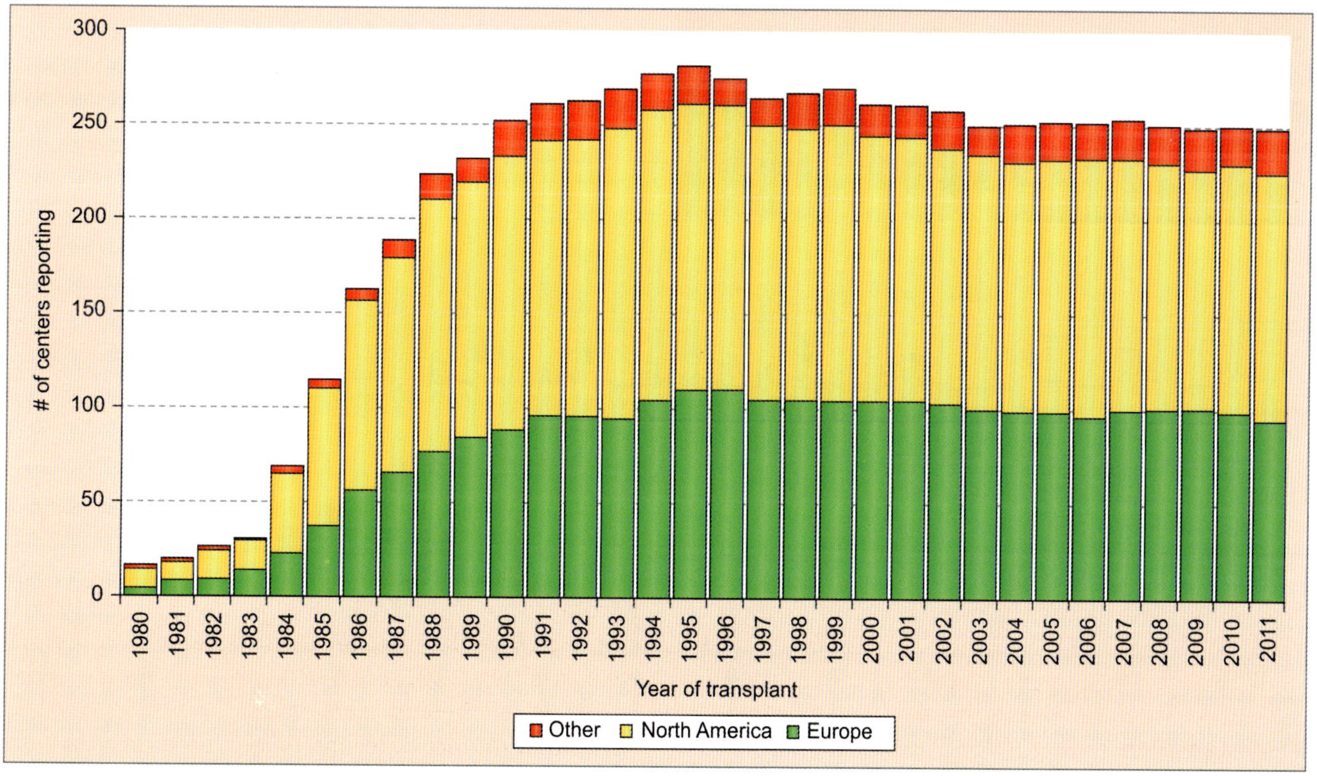

Fig. 26.5: The number of heart transplants by year and location. (Reproduced from the International Society of Heart and Lung Transplantation Heart Transplant Registry).

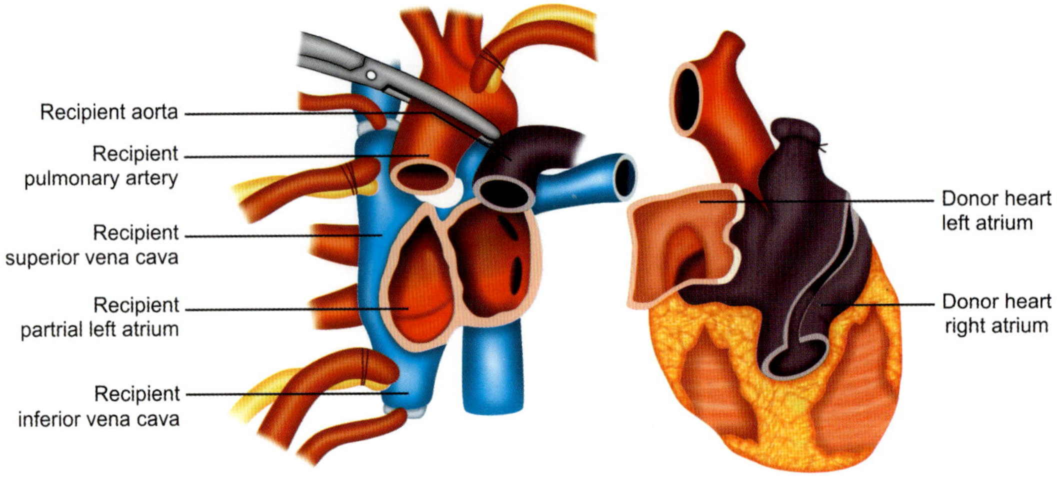

Fig. 26.6: Schematic illustration of biatrial heart transplantation.

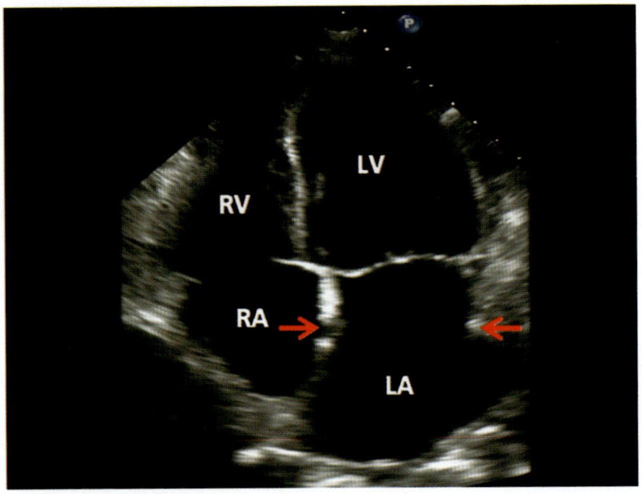

Fig. 26.7: Apical four-chamber view by transthoracic echocardiography illustrating an enlarged left atrium in a heart transplant recipient transplanted by the biatrial technique. Arrows point to the anastomosis site between the donor and recipient left atria. (LA: Left atrium; LV: Left ventricle; RA: Right atrium; RV: Right ventricle).

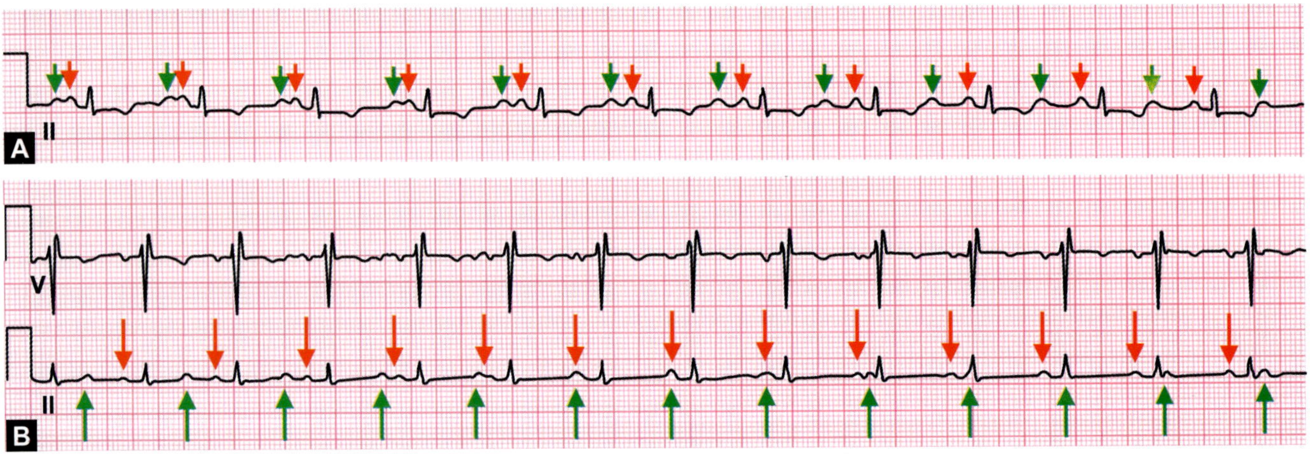

Figs. 26.8A and B: Electrocardiograms in biatrial heart transplant recipients demonstrating two distinct P waves arising from the donor and recipient atria.

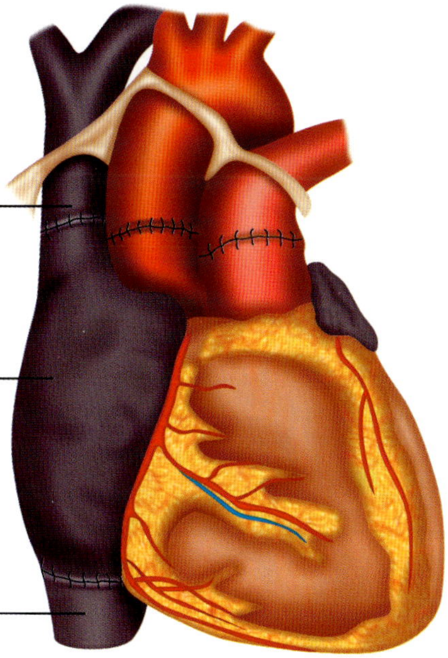

Fig. 26.9: Schematic illustration of the bicaval surgical approach to cardiac transplantation.

Table 26.2: Routinely used immunosuppressive medications after cardiac transplantation.

Immunosuppressive Agent	*Comment*
Corticosteroids	Usually weaned off or to low doses within 6–12 months post-transplant
Mycophenolate mofetil	Routinely used as part of post-transplant immunosuppressive regimens along with corticosteroids and calcineurin inhibitors or proliferation signal inhibitors
Calcineurin inhibitors • Tacrolimus • Cyclosporine	Tacrolimus is the preferred calcineurin inhibitor due to more effective prevention of acute rejection
Proliferation signal inhibitors • Sirolimus • Everolimus	Have been shown to reduce the development and progression of cardiac allograft vasculopathy
Polyclonal antibody • Anti-thymocyte globulin	Primarily used in induction therapy
Basiliximab	Used in induction therapy
Rituximab	Used in the treatment of antibody-mediated rejection
Intravenous immunoglobulin	Used in the treatment of antibody-mediated rejection or in treatment of allosensitized patients prior to transplantation

HETEROTOPIC HEART TRANSPLANTATION

In a heterotopic heart transplant (Figs. 26.10A to C), the patient's heart is not removed. Instead, a donor heart is additionally implanted in the chest, in essence in parallel with the native recipient heart. Heterotopic heart transplantation may be performed in cases where the recipient heart may recover over time or if the donor heart may not be strong enough to function and main adequate circulation only by itself. Heterotopic heart transplantation may be chosen in patients with severe pulmonary hypertension. In the early era of heart transplantation, heterotopic heart transplantation allowed for the continuing functioning of the recipient's native heart to support the patient in case of life-threatening acute rejection. With the evolution of cyclosporine use and other anti-rejection medications, this rationale for the performance of heterotopic heart transplantation has waned.

The heterotopic heart transplant procedure entails leaving the recipient's heart in place and connecting the donor's heart in parallel with the native heart. The donor aorta is anastomosed into the native ascending aorta. A graft (or one of the donor blood vessels) connects the donor's pulmonary artery to the main pulmonary artery of the recipient. The donor's superior vena cava is anastomosed to the recipient's right atrium. The donor and recipient's left atria are anastomosed together.

MANAGEMENT OF POST-TRANSPLANT PATIENTS

As illustrated in Figure 26.4, post-transplant outcomes were poor in the early years of heart transplantation, primarily due to the lack of effective immunosuppressive therapies. Survival improved dramatically in the early 1980s with the development of cyclosporine—a potent immune suppressive medication. Survival rates improved further with the introduction of tacrolimus and mycophenolate mofetil in the 1990s. Currently used post-transplant immunosuppressive medications include corticosteroids, calcineurin inhibitors, mycophenolate mofetil, and proliferation signal inhibitors (Table 26.2).

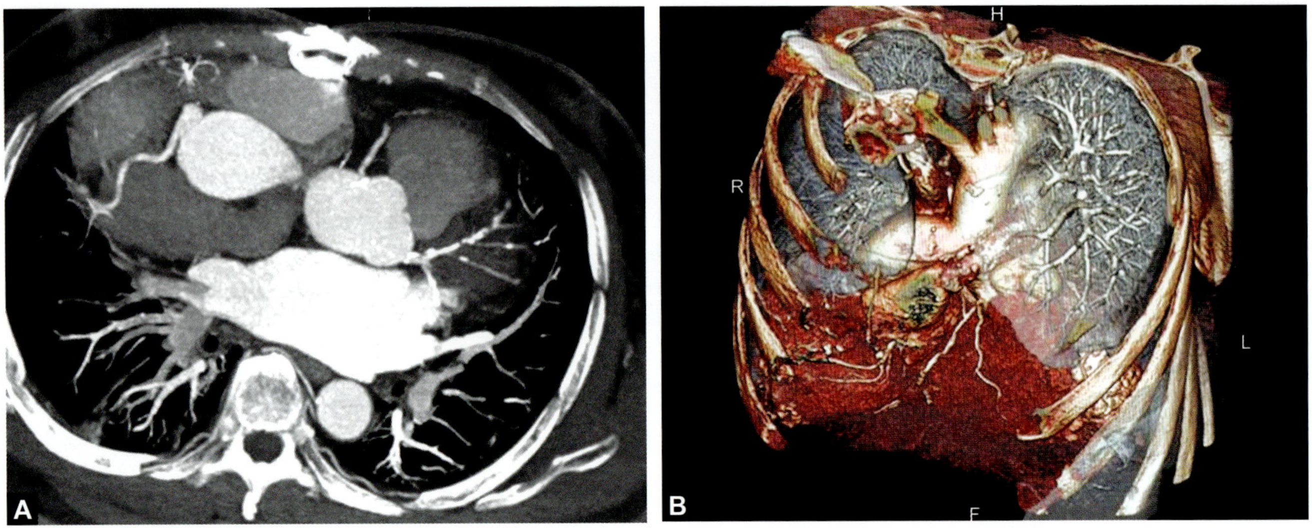

Figs. 26.10A and B: CT images of a heterotopic heart transplant. (Images courtesy of Dr Shu-Hsun Chu, Cardiovascular Center, Far Eastern Memorial Hospital, Taipei, Taiwan).

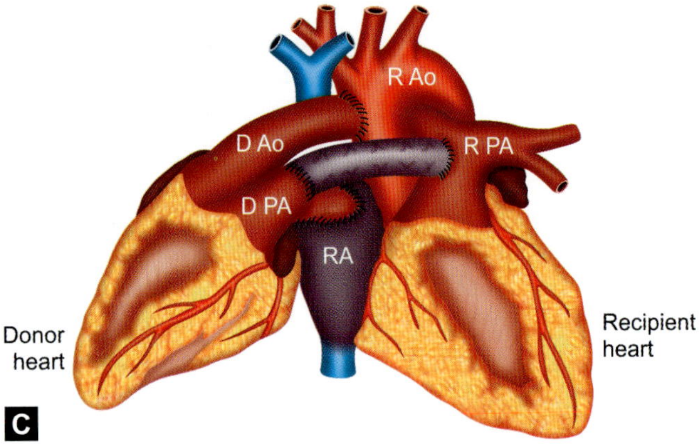

Fig. 26.10C: Schematic illustration of a heterotopic heart transplantation. The recipient's heart is left in place and the donor's heart is connected in parallel with the native heart. The donor aorta is anastomosed into the native ascending aorta. A graft (or one of the donor blood vessels) connects the donor's pulmonary artery to the main pulmonary artery of the recipient. The donor's superior vena cava is anastomosed to the recipient's right atrium. The donor and recipient's left atria are anastomosed together.

Despite being on immunosuppressive medications, the transplanted heart is at risk for immune-mediated graft injury, which can occur as a result of cellular- or antibody-mediated mechanisms. Hence, graft surveillance is routinely performed as part of post-transplant management. The gold standard for diagnosing acute rejection is the endomyocardial biopsy. Normal transplanted myocardium with no evidence of rejection is shown in Figure 26.11A. A common finding known as "Quilty lesion" is said to be present when histology specimens demonstrate a focal endocardial mononuclear lymphocytic infiltrate (Fig. 26.11B). This finding is distinct from acute cellular rejection but can be confused with acute rejection if the infiltrate extends to the myocardium. In acute cellular rejection, T-lymphocytes mediate the inflammatory response. Examination of a sample of myocardial tissue obtained via endomyocardial biopsy facilitates the diagnosis of acute cellular rejection (Fig. 26.12), and also permits grading of its severity (Table 26.3). Antibody-mediated rejection (AMR), also known as humoral rejection, occurs when the recipient generates antibodies against donor human leukocyte antigens (HLA) (Fig. 26.13).

Endomyocardial biopsies (Figs. 26.14A and B) are performed frequently during the first year after heart transplantation and less frequently thereafter, due to diminishing risk of acute rejection and potential trauma to the tricuspid valve during the biopsy procedures (Figs. 26.15A and B). At the present time, pulse corticosteroids form the mainstay of treatment for acute rejection.

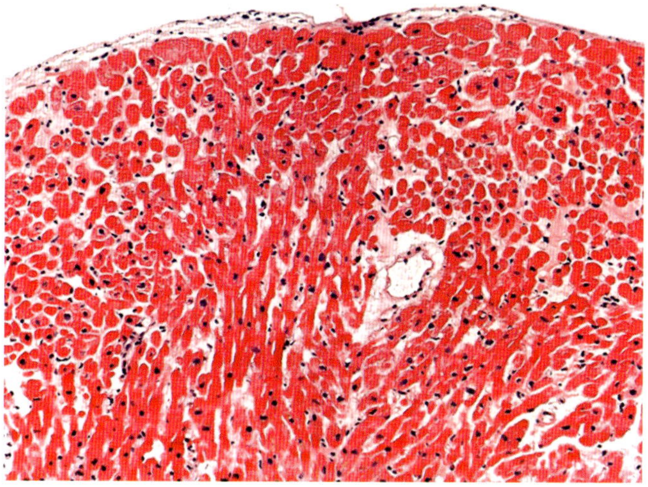

Fig. 26.11A: Histology specimen from an endomyocardial biopsy demonstrating normal myocardium with no evidence of rejection.

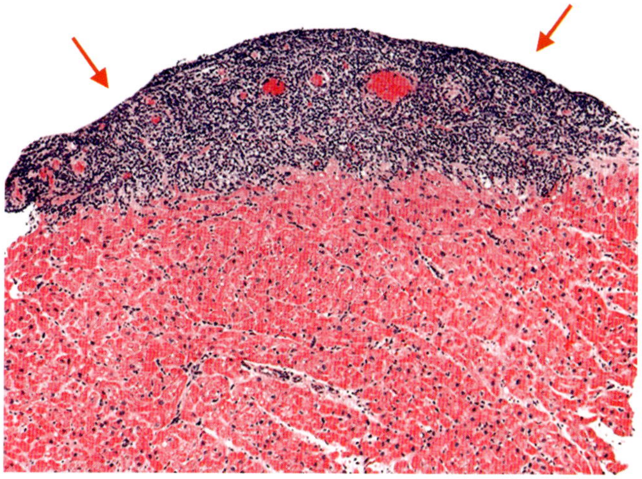

Fig. 26.11B: Histology specimen from an endomyocardial biopsy demonstrating a "Quilty lesion" which is a focal endocardial mononuclear lymphocytic infiltrate but can be confused with cellular rejection.

Table 26.3: International Society of Heart and Lung Transplantation grading system for acute cellular rejection.

Grade/Degree of rejection	*Findings*
Grade 0	No rejection
Grade 1 R—mild	Interstitial and/or perivascular infiltrate with up to one focus of myocyte damage
Grade 2 R—moderate	Two or more foci of infiltrate with associated myocyte damage
Grade 3 R—severe	Diffuse infiltrate with multifocal myocyte damage, with or without edema, hemorrhage, or vasculitis

Echocardiography serves as a very useful adjunct to myocardial tissue examination and is the mainstay for evaluating the transplanted heart's function noninvasively. An acute decrease in left ventricular systolic function and/or an increase in left ventricular end-diastolic volume (Figs. 26.16A and B) should raise concern and an immediate evaluation for etiologies of heart transplant dysfunction should be pursued.

In patients who survive the first few years after heart transplantation, coronary artery disease in the transplanted heart is an important cause of mortality. Compared to the general population, the pathology of coronary disease in transplant recipients is unique, and is characterized by diffuse intimal hyperplasia along the lumen of the donor coronary arteries. This process leads to luminal narrowing and distal tapering of the coronary arteries, rather than the focal stenoses due to atherosclerotic plaque that are seen in the general population (Figs. 26.17A and B). This phenomenon is referred to as cardiac allograft vasculopathy (CAV). In patients with CAV, the coronary arteries may appear normal on two-dimensional coronary angiography and thus the use of intravascular ultrasound (IVUS) imaging may be required to confirm the presence of diffuse coronary artery intimal thickening (Figs. 26.18A and B). Transplant recipients are not only at risk for developing CAV, but can also develop focal epicardial coronary artery stenoses just as in the general population. Hence, serial screening for flow-limiting CAD is often performed annually, either by Dobutamine stress echocardiography or by myocardial perfusion imaging with vasodilator stress (Fig. 26.19).

Other significant causes of morbidity and mortality in heart transplant recipients include primary graft failure, malignancy, cytomegalovirus infection, and renal failure (Table 26.4).

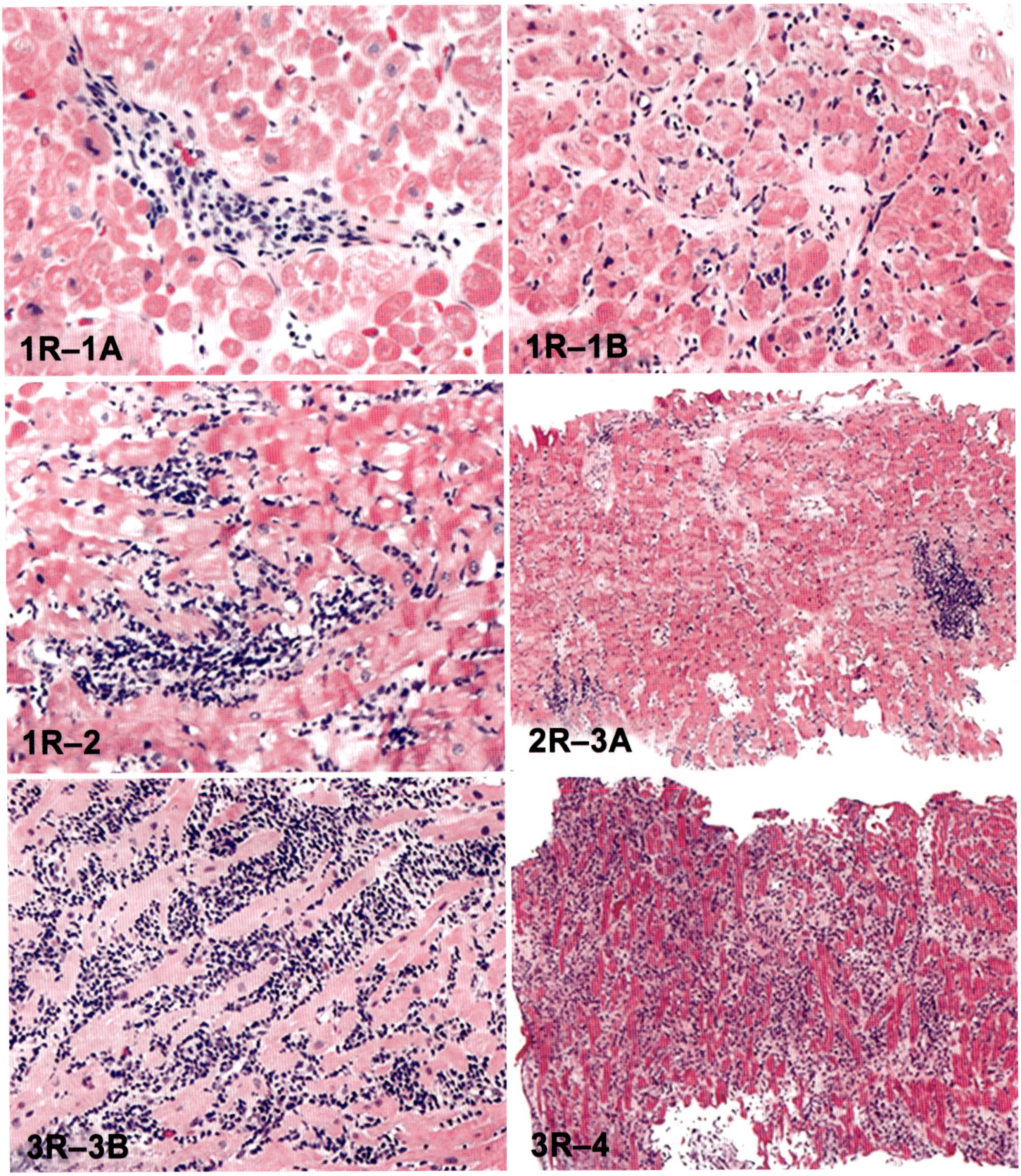

Fig. 26.12: Histology specimens of transplanted myocardium illustrating the various grades of acute cellular rejection per the 2004 ISHLT Standardized Cardiac Biopsy Grading: Grade 1R implies *mild rejection* "Interstitial and/or perivascular infiltrate with up to 1 focus of myocyte damage—Includes grades 1R-1A, 1R-1B and 1R-2 from the 1990 grading scheme. Grade 2R implies *moderate rejection* "Two or more foci of infiltrate with associated myocyte damage"—Includes grade 3A from the 1990 grading scheme. Grade 3R implies severe rejection "Diffuses infiltrate with multifocal myocyte damage ± edema, ± hemorrhage ± vasculitis—Includes grades 3B and 4 from the 1990 grading scheme.

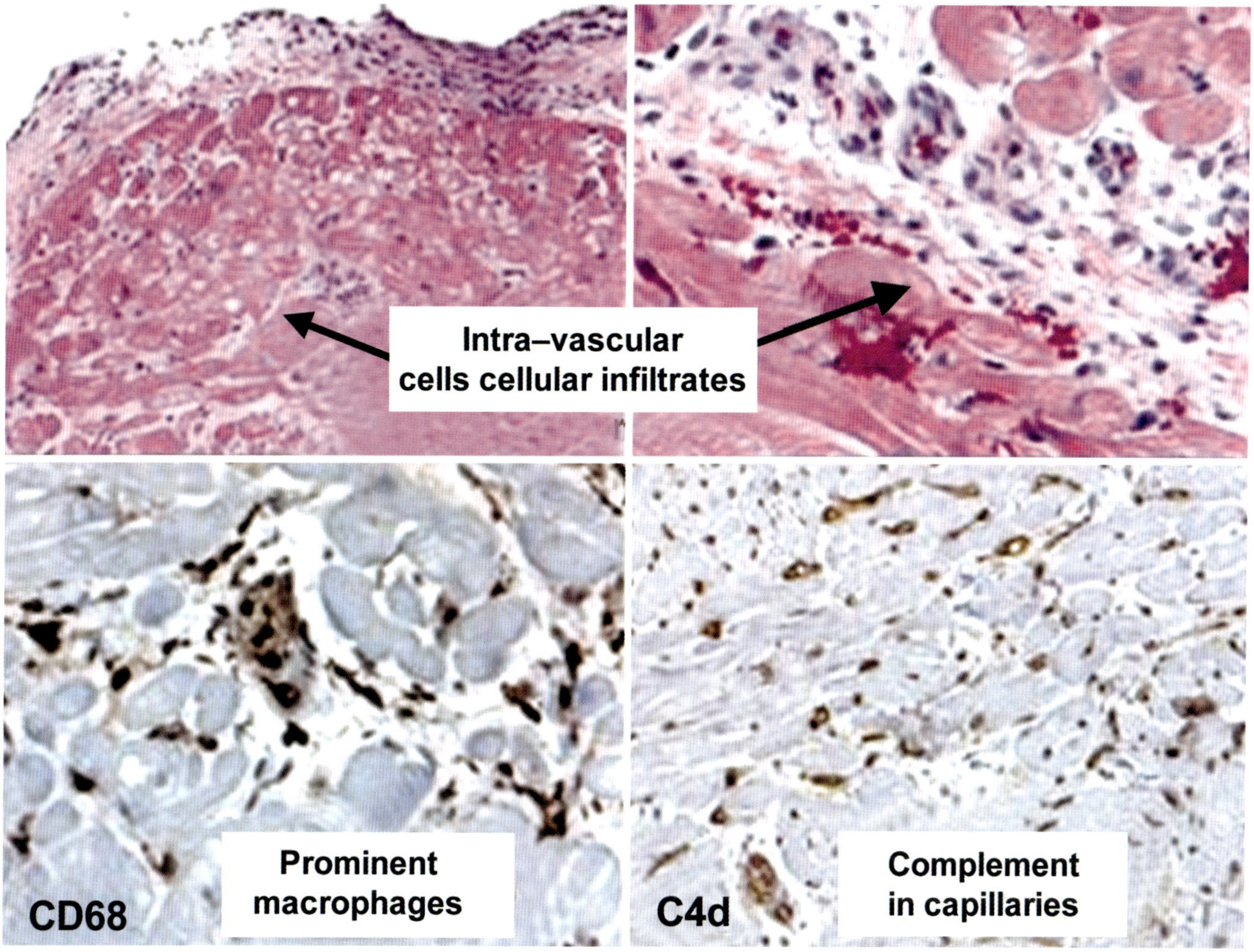

Fig. 26.13: Antibody-mediated (humoral) rejection. Figures in top row are histology specimens of transplanted myocardium stained with hematoxylin and eosin, showing cellular infiltrates within vessels along with endothelial swelling. Figures in bottom row are immunoperoxidase stains of transplanted myocardium that are strongly positive for CD68 and C4d which confirm the intravascular cells to be macrophages thereby allowing a diagnosis of antibody mediated rejection to be made.

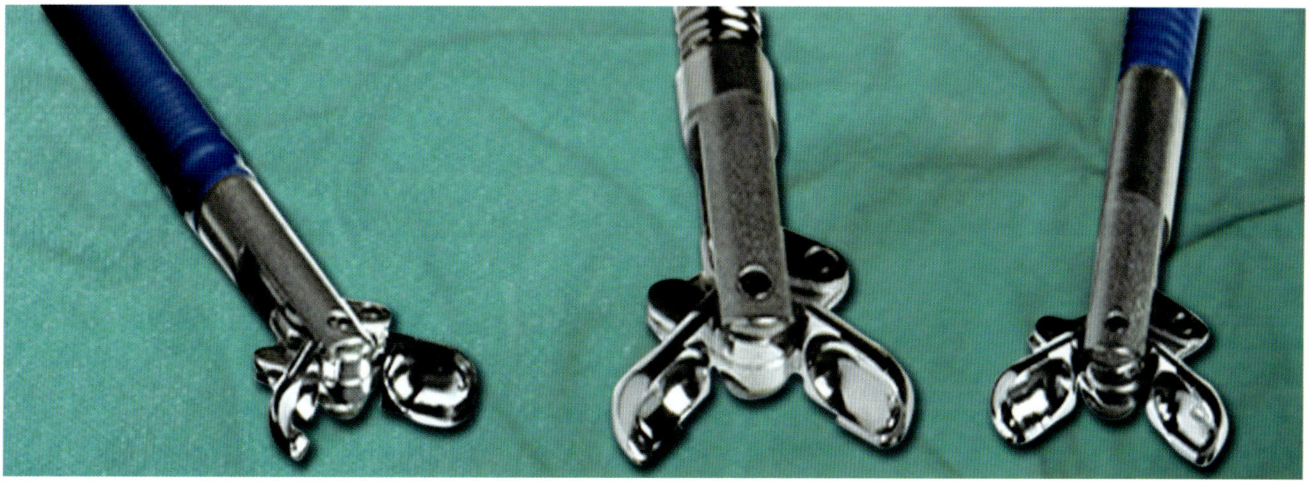

Fig. 26.14A: Images of bioptome tips used in endomyocardial biopsy.

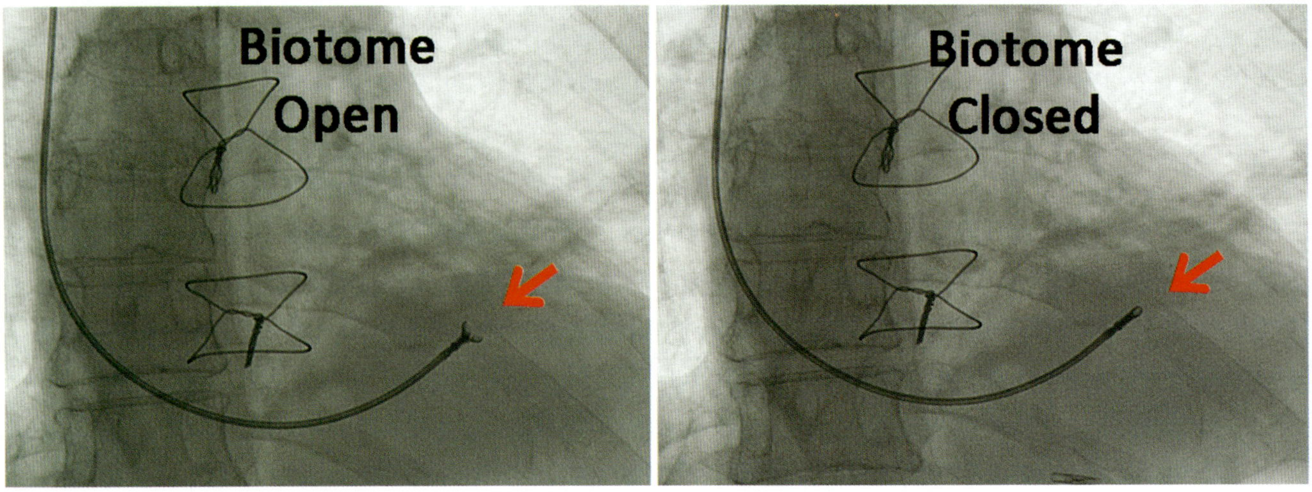

Fig. 26.14B: Fluoroscopic images of a right ventricular endomyocardial biopsy showing the biopsy forceps (bioptome) both open and closed. (Image courtesy of Dr M Toma, Dr Darra T Murphy, and Dr Marc W Deyell).

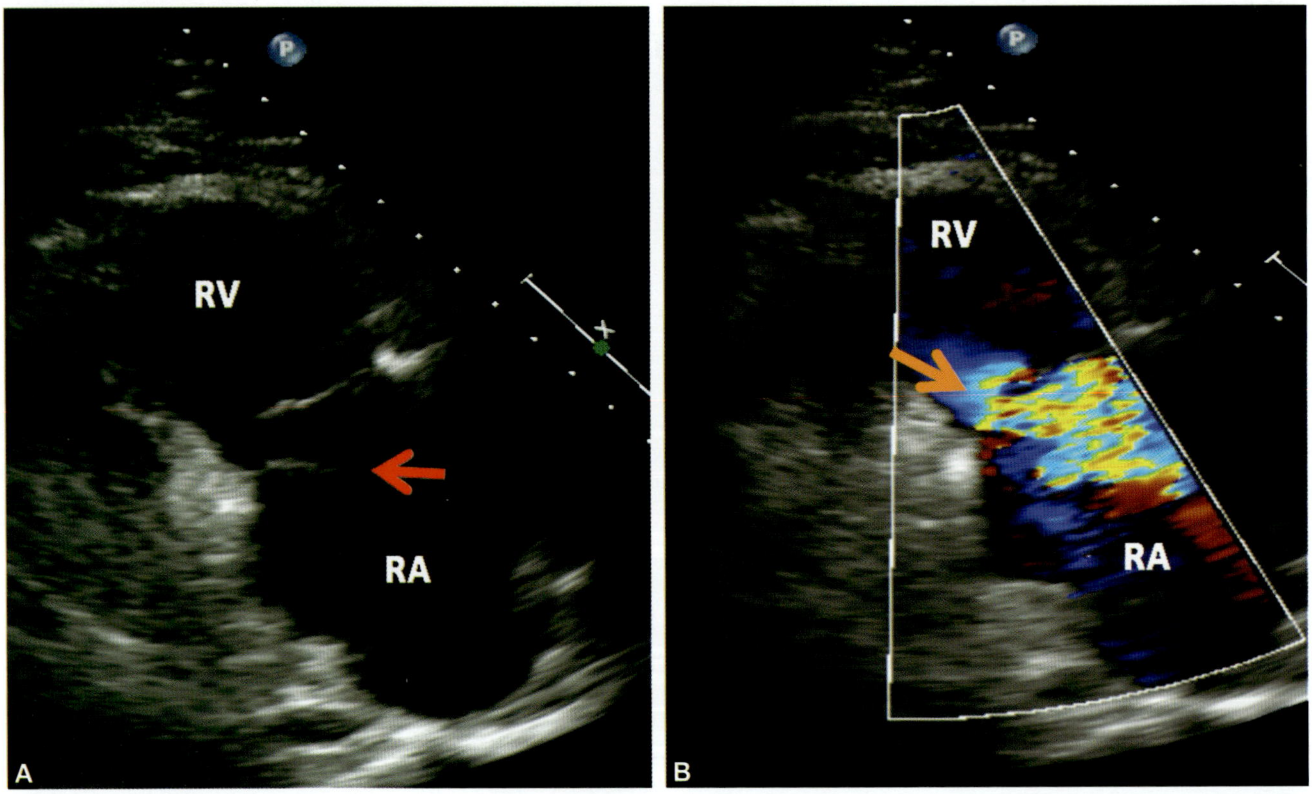

Figs. 26.15A and B: Damage to the tricuspid valve after endomyocardial biopsy. (A) Two-chamber transthoracic echocardiography view of the right atrium (RA) and right ventricle (RV) showing a damaged and flail tricuspid valve leaflet (red arrow) secondary to an endomyocardial biopsy procedure; (B) Corresponding color Doppler image demonstrating severe tricuspid regurgitation (yellow arrow) as a result of the damaged and flail tricuspid leaflet.

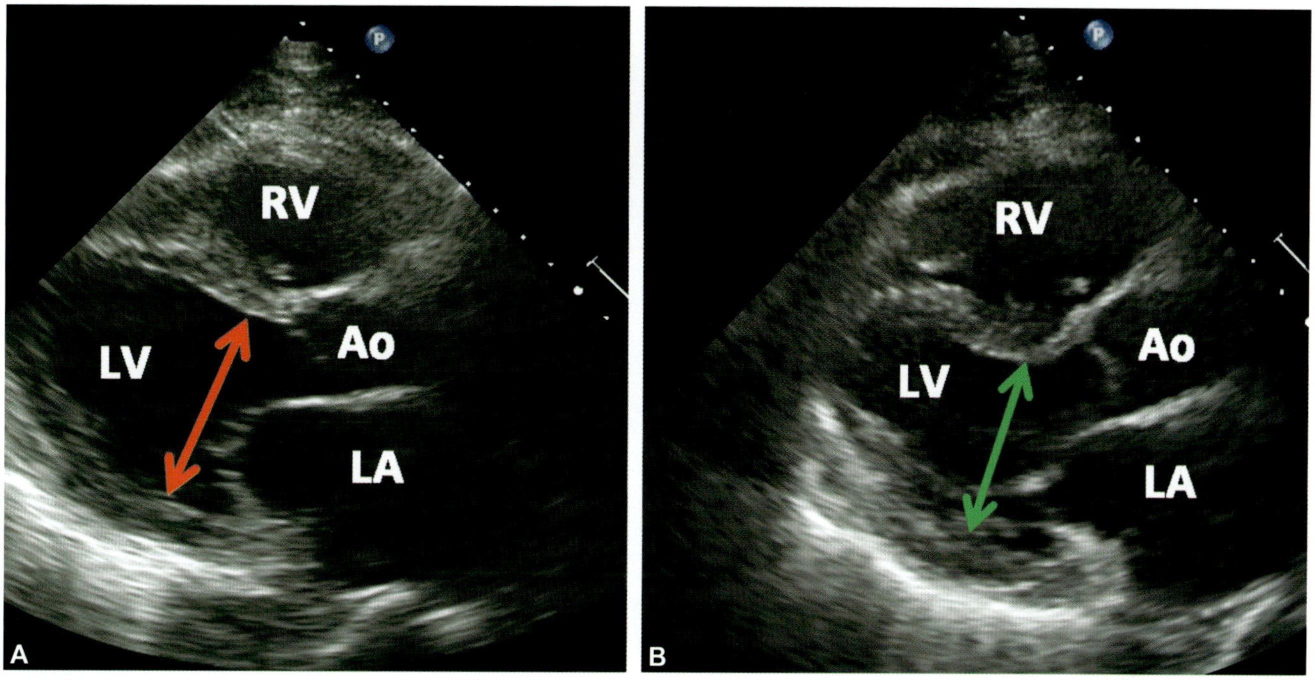

Figs. 26.16A and B: Echocardiography assessment of the post-transplant heart. (A) Parasternal long-axis view of the left ventricle showing an increase in left ventricular end-diastolic dimensions with severe acute rejection; (B) Same patient after treatment for acute rejection. A favorable response to treatment is evidenced by a decrease in left ventricular end-diastolic dimensions.

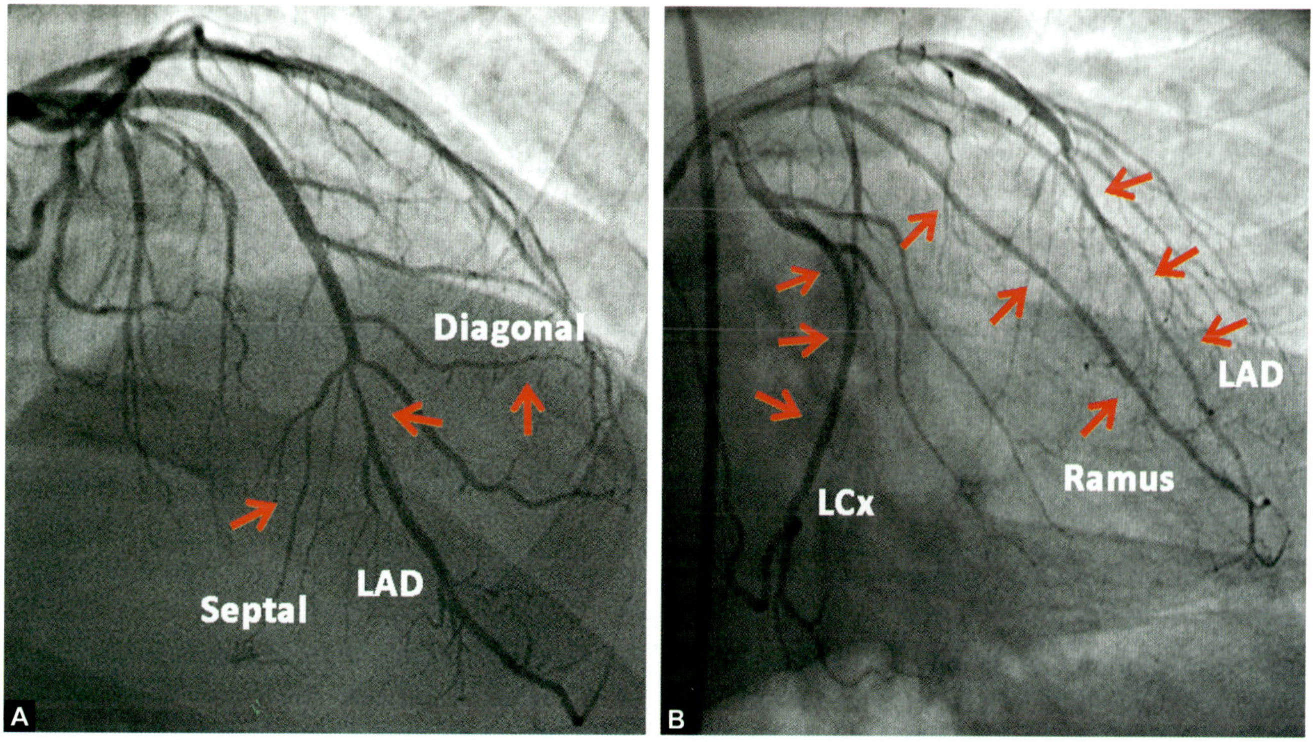

Figs. 26.17A and B: Coronary angiograms demonstrating cardiac allograft vasculopathy. (A) Angiogram demonstrates reduced caliber of the left anterior descending coronary artery and its branches, with distal pruning; (B) Coronary angiogram in a heart transplant recipient with significant cardiac allograft vasculopathy, demonstrating severe narrowing of the entire left coronary arterial system.

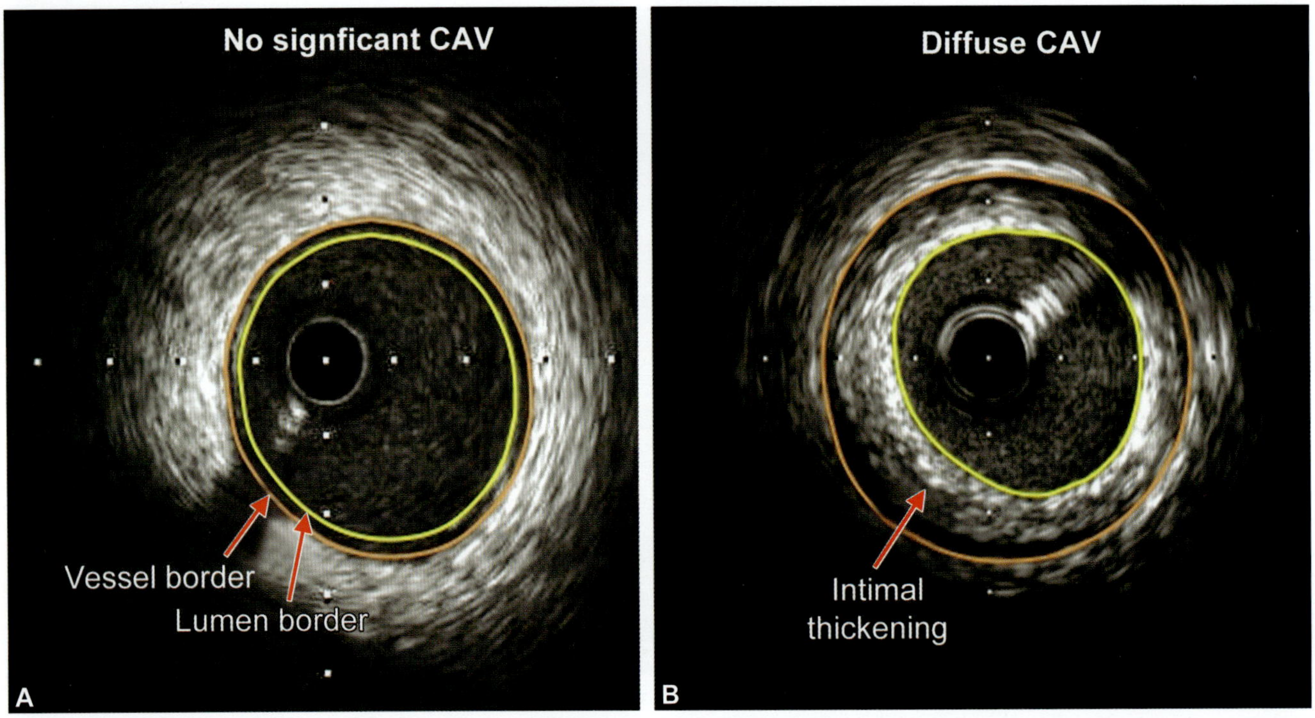

Figs. 26.18A and B: Intravascular ultrasound (IVUS) of post-transplant coronary arteries. (A) IVUS shows no significant cardiac allograft vasculopathy (CAV) and minimal intimal thickening; (B) IVUS demonstrates diffuse CAV with significant intimal thickening.

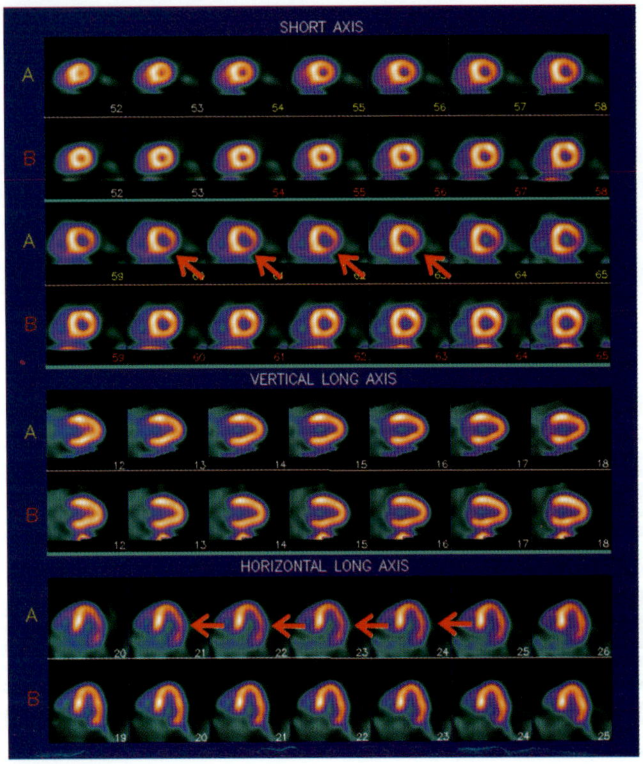

Fig. 26.19: Presence in a post-transplant patient of inferolateral and lateral myocardial perfusion defects (arrows) on ^{82}rubidium positron emission tomography (PET) scan with pharmacologic vasodilator stress testing. Rows with yellow letter "A" are images acquired during stress; rows with red letter "B" are images acquired during rest.

Table 26.4: Adult heart transplant recipients: cause of death (1994–2011). Data from the International Society of Heart and Lung Transplantation.

Cause of Death	*0–30 Days (N = 4,092)*	*31 Days–1 Years (N = 3,801)*	*>1–3 Years (N = 2,846)*	*>10–15 Years (N = 4,221)*	*>15 Years (N = 1,937)*
Cardiac allograft vasculopathy	71 (1.7%)	161 (4.2%)	373 (13.1%)	619 (14.7%)	248 (12.8%)
Acute rejection	222 (5.4%)	394 (10.4%)	296 (10.4%)	42 (1.0%)	13 (0.7%)
Lymphoma	3 (0.1%)	59 (1.6%)	81 (2.8%)	163 (3.9%)	66 (3.4%)
Malignancy, other	1 (0.0%)	91 (2.4%)	326 (11.5%)	847 (20.1%)	345 (17.8%)
Cytomegalovirus (CMV)	3 (0.1%)	42 (1.1%)	14 (0.5%)	2 (0.0%)	0
Infection, non-CMV	548 (13.4%)	1,155 (30.4%)	354 (12.4%)	432 (10.2%)	226 (11.7%)
Graft failure	1,522 (37.2%)	631 (16.6%)	688 (24.2%)	670 (15.9%)	305 (15.7%)
Technical	307 (7.5%)	53 (1.4%)	21 (0.7%)	59 (1.4%)	27 (1.4%)
Other	199 (4.9%)	305 (8.0%)	253 (8.9%)	311 (7.4%)	167 (8.6%)
Multiple organ failure	716 (17.5%)	533 (14.0%)	164 (5.8%)	345 (8.2%)	175 (9.0%)
Renal failure	31 (0.8%)	39 (1.0%)	45 (1.6%)	359 (8.5%)	175 (9.0%)
Pulmonary	142 (3.5%)	158 (4.2%)	123 (4.3%)	173 (4.1%)	88 (4.5%)
Cerebrovascular	327 (8.0%)	180 (4.7%)	108 (3.8%)	199 (4.7%)	102 (5.3%)

REFERENCES

Hunt SA, Haddad F. The changing face of heart transplantation. J Am Coll Cardiol. 2008;52(8):587-98.

Hunt SA, Abraham WT, Chin MH, et al. 2009 Focused Update incorporated into the ACC/AHA 2005 guidelines for the diagnosis and management of heart failure in adults: a report of the American College of Cardiology Foundation/American Heart Association task force on practice guidelines: developed in collaboration with the International Society for Heart and Lung Transplantation. Circulation. 2009;119(14):e391.

Lund LH, Edwards LB, Kucheryavaya AY, et al. The Registry of the International Society for Heart and Lung Transplantation: thirtieth adult lung and heart-lung transplant report—2013. J Heart Lung Transplant. 2013;32(10):951-64.

Mancini D, Lietz K. Selection of cardiac transplantation candidates in 2010. Circulation. 2010; 22:174.

Weiss ES, Nwakanma LU, Russell SB, et al. Outcomes in bicaval versus biatrial techniques in heart transplantation: an analysis of the UNOS database. J Heart Lung Transplant. 2008;27(2): 178-83.

Section 4

Arrhythmias

Chapters

CHAPTER

27

Normal Cardiac Depolarization and Impulse Conduction

Irakli Giorgberidze, Hamid Afshar, Glenn N Levine

The electrical system of the heart (Fig. 27.1) consists of a highly evolved and specialized series of myocardial cells which function to orchestrate synchronized electrical stimulation and subsequent contraction of the atria and ventricles more than one billion times over the course of a person's lifetime.

CARDIAC ACTION POTENTIALS AND ACTION OF ANTIARRHYTHMIC DRUGS

Myocyte depolarization and repolarization is mediated by a complex interaction of ion movement through specialized transmembrane ion channels. In the specialized pacemaker cells of the heart (e.g. SA node), a slow rise in membrane potential occurs due to increased inward current of sodium, as well as calcium, and a slow decrease in potassium outward current. Once a threshold (≅ –40 mV) is reached, the depolarization impulse is initiated (Figs. 27.2 and 27.3). The action potential of non-pacemaker cells is, in contrast to that of pacemaker cells, characterized by a flat (horizontal) phase 4. Electrical activation of these cells leads to a rapid influx on sodium ions (Figs. 27.4 and 27.5). This Na^+ inward current causes rapid depolarization of the cell membrane and constitutes phase 0 of the action potential. Sodium inward current quickly ceases once membrane potential is reversed (i.e. depolarized). This is followed by a brief rapid repolarization (phase 1) as a result of activation of transient outward K^+ current (I_{to}).

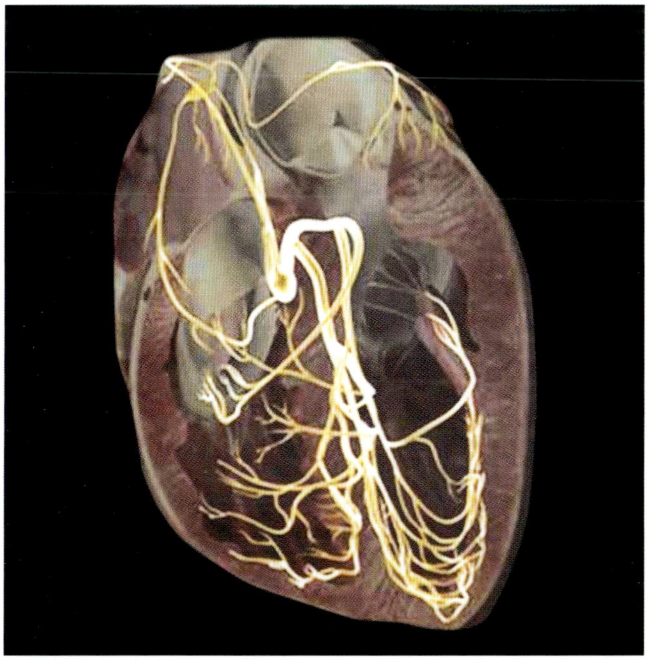

Fig. 27.1: Ghosted image of the cardiac conduction system (Image from circuitsurfers.com; image creator not listed. CC).

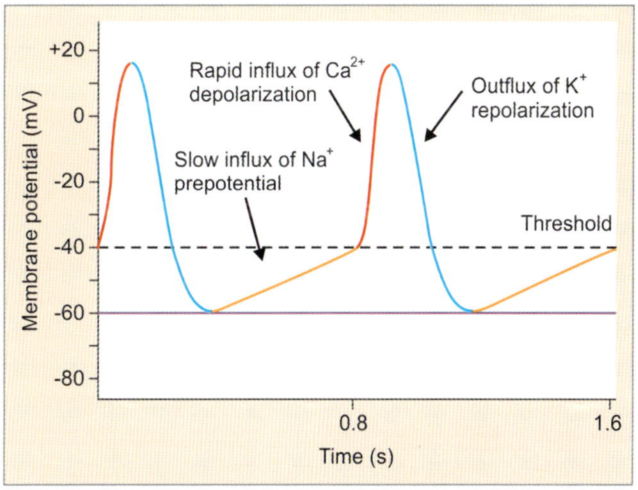

Fig. 27.2: Action potential of a cardiac pacemaker cell. The prepotential is due to a slow influx of sodium ions until the threshold is reached followed by a rapid depolarization and repolarization. The prepotential accounts for the membrane reaching threshold and initiates the spontaneous depolarization and contraction of the cell. Note the lack of a resting potential (Image from OpenStax College. Cardiac Muscle and Electrical Activity. Connexions. 19 June 2013 http://cnx.org/content/m46664/1.3/. CC).

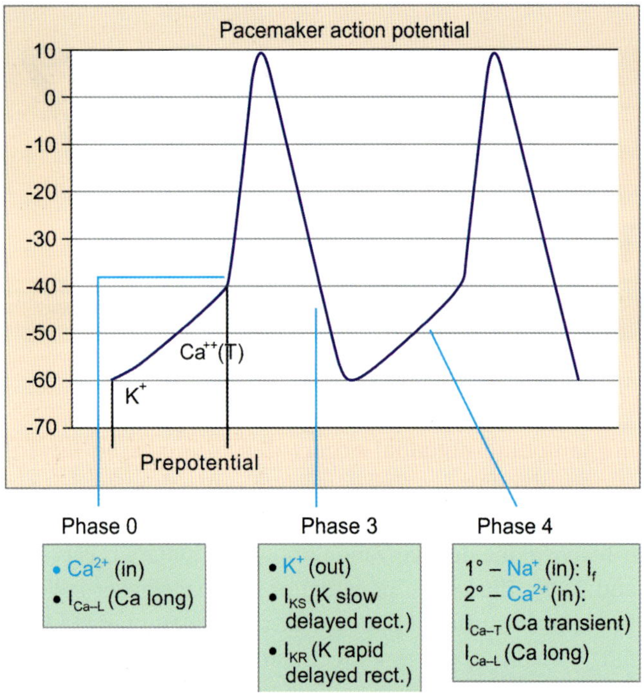

Fig. 27.3: The cardiac pacemaker cell action potential and ion shifts involved in depolarization and repolarization (Image created by Diberri and Silvia3 and posted on Wikipedia Commons. CC).

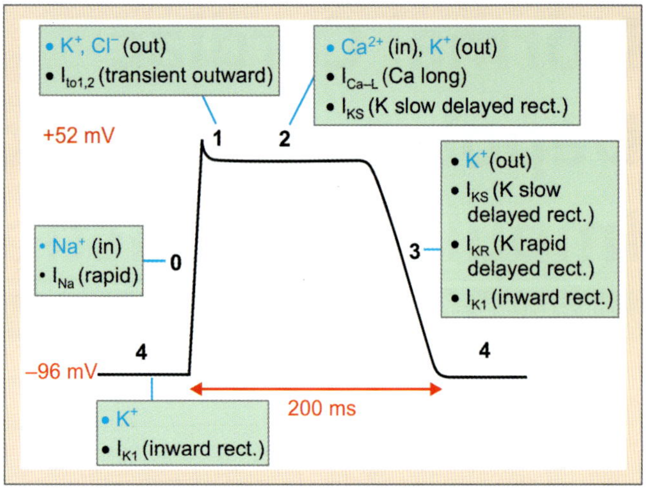

Fig. 27.4: Phases of the cardiac myocyte and ion shifts involved in depolarization and repolarization (Image created by Quasar and Silvia3 and posted on Wikipedia Commons. CC).

This is followed by the plateau or phase 2. This is the longest phase of the action potential and is the result of interplay between inward (Ca^{2+} and late component of Na^+ current) and outward K^+ rectifier (I_{KR} and I_{KS}) currents. During phase 3, inward currents are being inactivated and there is only continuing flow of outward K^+ currents unopposed by any inward current; the cell repolarizes to its resting potential (phase 4). Differences between the action potential of myocytes and of skeletal muscle cells are highlighted in Figures 27.6A to C.

Blockade of inward sodium current causes slowing of impulse propagation throughout the His-Purkinje system and the myocardium, whereas blockade of outward potassium channels causes prolongation of refractoriness.

Different classes of antiarrhythmic agents have different and specific effects on the sodium and potassium channels, and thus affect action potential, depolarization, refractory periods, and repolarization in different manners (Table 27.1).

- Class IA antiarrhythmic drugs (quinidine, procainamide, disopyramide) slow conduction due to sodium channel blockade, and also block potassium channels, resulting in prolongation of both QRS and QT intervals.
- Class IB antiarrhythmic drugs (lidocaine, mexiletine) suppress conduction in ischemic tissue without significantly affecting the conduction properties of healthy tissue. Usually, there is no change in QRS and QT intervals.
- Class IC antiarrhythmic drugs (flecainide, propafenone) cause significant suppression of conduction in His-Purkinje system due to potent sodium channel blocking properties. This results in prolongation of the QRS interval.
- Class II antiarrhythmic drugs are the beta blockers, which decrease the rate of depolarization of the action potential.
- Class III antiarrhythmic drugs (amiodarone, sotalol, dofetilide, dronedarone) block various potassium channels, decreasing the outward transmembrane currents and prolonging the repolarization phase of action potential. This results in prolongation of the QT interval.
- Class IV antiarrhythmic drugs (the calcium channel blockers verapamil and diltiazem) decrease the rate of depolarization of the action potential.

ANATOMY AND FUNCTION OF THE CONDUCTION SYSTEM

The normal conduction system of the heart is shown in Figure 27.6A. The physiological pacemaker of the heart is the sinoatrial (SA) node (Figs. 27.6B and C). Under normal

Table 27.1: Vaughan Williams classification of antiarrhythmic drugs.

Antiarrhythmic drug class	*Ion channel affected*	*Electrophysiologic effect*
I (A, B and C)	Sodium	Slowing of the depolarization (phase 0 of action potential) resulting in suppression of intracardiac conduction; as a result—QRS prolongation
II	Beta adrenergic receptor blockade	Suppression of tissue automaticity (including SA node and AV node); slowing of conduction in the AV node
III	Potassium	Slowing of the repolarization (phase 3 of action potential) Resulting in increase of refractoriness; as a result—QT prolongation
IV	Calcium channel blockade	Suppression of Ca-channel dependent tissue automaticity (including SA node and AV node); slowing of conduction in the AV node

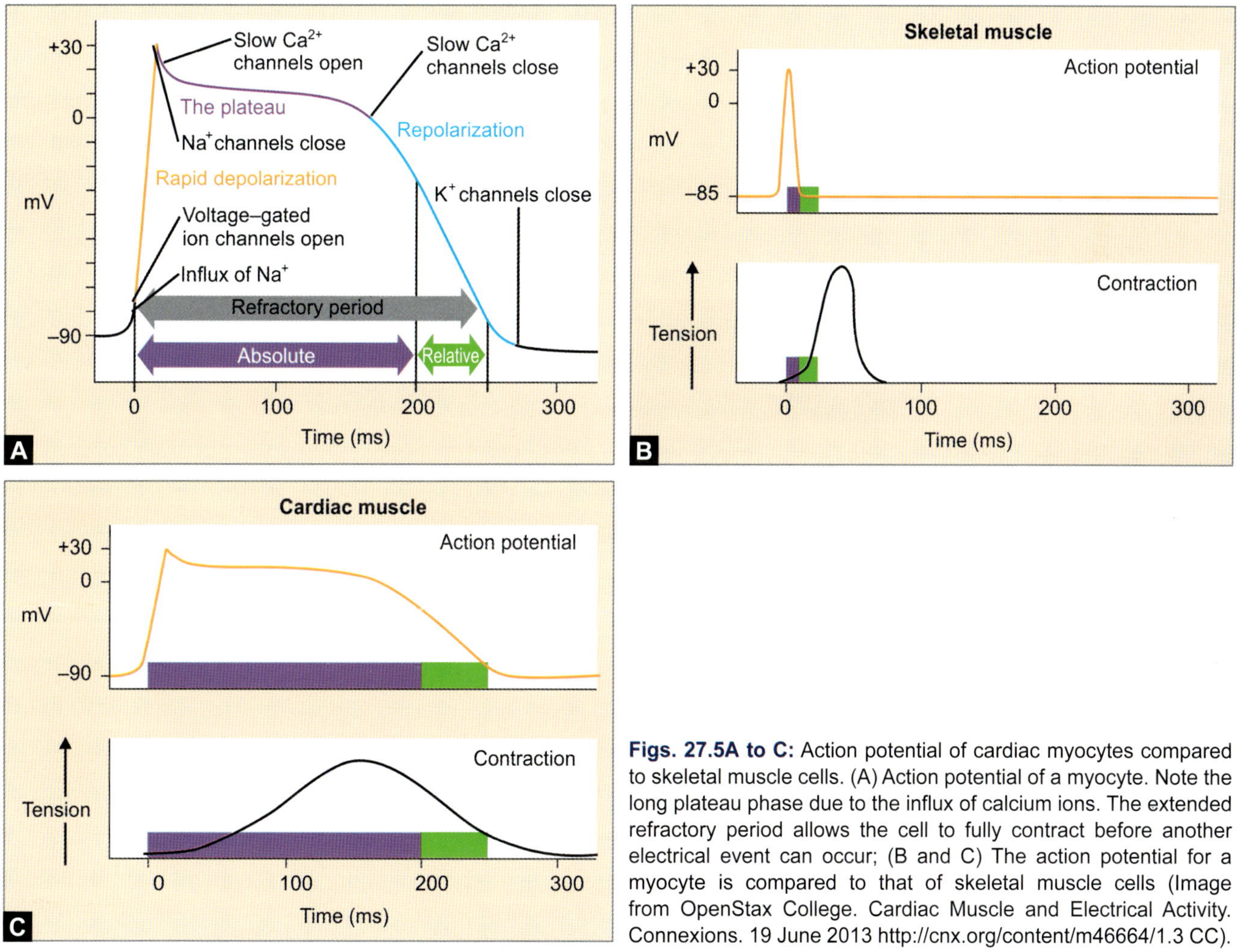

Figs. 27.5A to C: Action potential of cardiac myocytes compared to skeletal muscle cells. (A) Action potential of a myocyte. Note the long plateau phase due to the influx of calcium ions. The extended refractory period allows the cell to fully contract before another electrical event can occur; (B and C) The action potential for a myocyte is compared to that of skeletal muscle cells (Image from OpenStax College. Cardiac Muscle and Electrical Activity. Connexions. 19 June 2013 http://cnx.org/content/m46664/1.3 CC).

physiological conditions, the SA node spontaneously depolarizes 60–100 times each minute. Numerous factors can modulate spontaneous SA node depolarization and lead to sinus bradycardia (Table 27.2) or sinus tachycardia (Table 27.3). The depolarization impulse that arises in the SA node is rapidly propagated to the left atrium through Bachmann's bundle. The depolarization impulse is also propagated to the AV node via specialized *internodal* tracts. Depolarization of the atria is demonstrated in Figure 27.7.

The AV node is anatomically located toward the apex of Koch's triangle (Figs. 27.8A and B). The atria are electrically

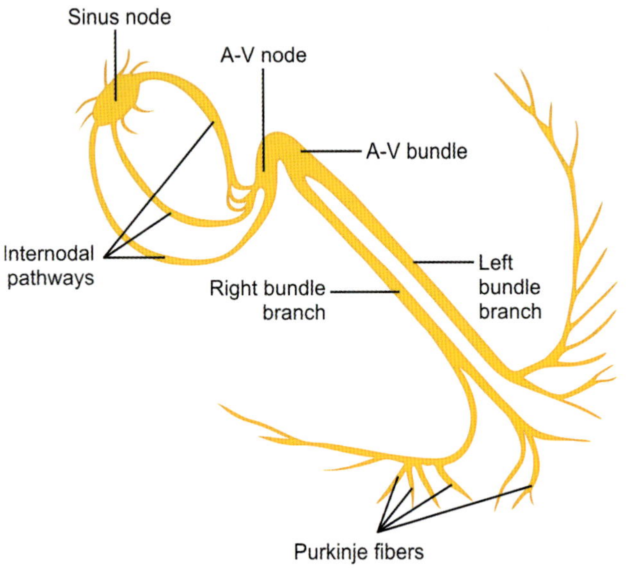

Fig. 27.6A: The conduction system of the heart (Image created by Madhero88 and posted on Wikimedia Commons. CC).

isolated from the ventricles, and normally connected to them only by the atrioventricular (AV) node. Normal delay of conduction from the atria to the ventricles is reflected in part by the PR interval, as discussed below. Factors that prolong conduction through the AV node and can lead to a prolonged PR interval are listed in Table 27.4.

After being propagated through the AV node, the depolarization impulse in conducted toward the apex of the heart down the interventricular septum first by the *bundle of His* and then, after the bundle of His bifurcates, the *left bundle branch* and the *right bundle branch*. The short left bundle branch in turn bifurcates into the *left anterior fascicle* and *left posterior fascicle*. The left posterior fascicle has a dual blood supply, and thus isolated left posterior fascicle block due to coronary artery disease is rare. At the end of this specialized conduction system are numerous *Purkinje fibers*, with branch out to stimulate the myocardial cells to contract. A simplified schematic

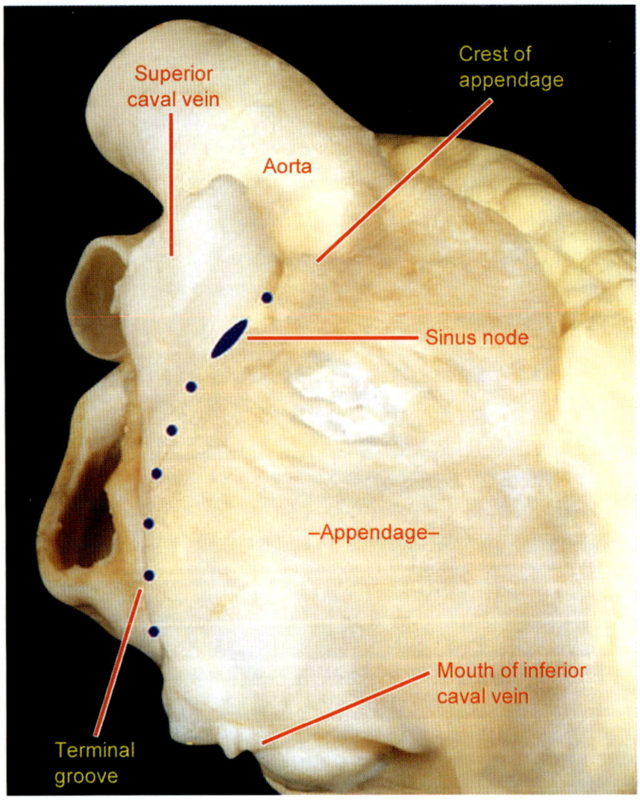

Fig. 27.6B: Right lateral image of the heart showing the anatomic location of the sinoatrial (SA) node. The SA node is a cigar-shaped structure located immediately subepicardially within the terminal grove (Image and legend text courtesy of Dr Robert Anderson, Institute of Genetic Medicine, Newcastle University, United Kingdom).

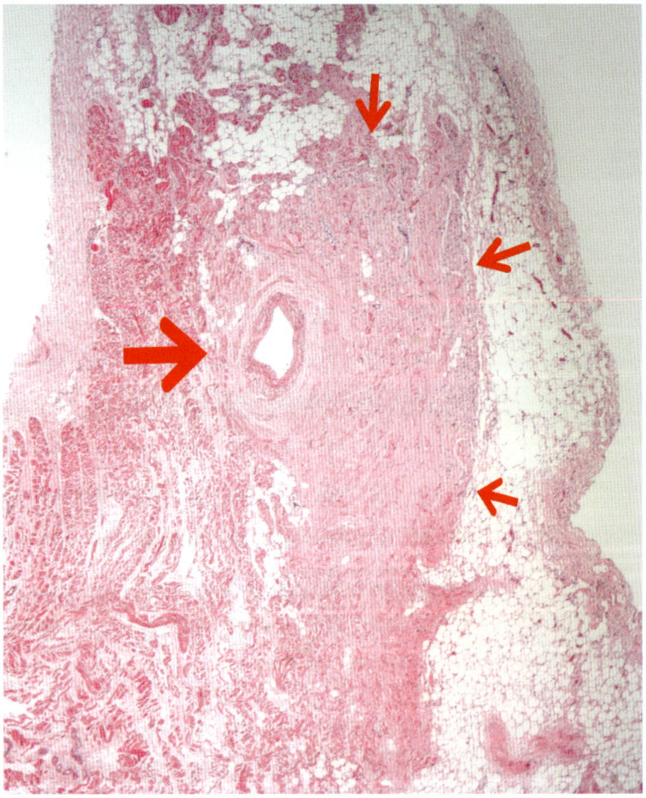

Fig. 27.6C: Histology specimen showing the SA node (arrows) (Image from Nephron posted on Wikimedia Commons).

Table 27.2: Factors associated with sinus bradycardia.

Causes of sinus bradycardia
Intrinsic SA node disease
CNS-mediated increased parasympathetic tone: • Sleep • Increased intracranial pressure
Medications: • Beta blockers • Non-dihydropyridine calcium channel blockers (verapamil, diltiazem) • Digoxin (via increased parasympathetic tone) • Certain antiarrhythmic agents (amiodarone, sotalol, propafenone)
Hypothyroidism
Hypothermia
SA node exit block

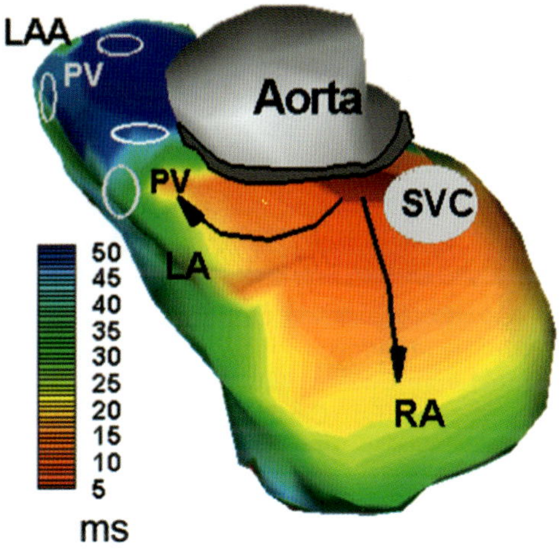

Fig. 27.7: Normal activation sequence of the atria. Image shown in superior-posterior view. Isochrones represent time in milliseconds from initial activation (Image courtesy of Dr Rudy Yoram. Image reproduced with permission from Ramanathan C, et al. Noninvasive electrocardiographic imaging for cardiac electrophysiology and arrhythmia. Published online 14 March 2004; doi: 10.1038/nm1011. CC). (LA: Left atrium; LAA: Left atrial appendage; PV: Pulmonary vein; RA: Right atrium).

of cardiac depolarization is depicted in Figure 27.9A; a more sophisticated computerized simulation of cardiac depolarization is shown in Figure 27.9B.

PHYSIOLOGICAL BENEFITS OF THE EVOLVED CONDUCTION SYSTEM

The specific design of the conduction system has evolved to serve several important functions. The SA node is

Table 27.3: Factors associated with sinus tachycardia.

Causes of sinus tachycardia
CNS-mediated increased sympathetic tone: • Anxiety, fear • Fever • Hypoxemia • Hypotension, hypovolemia or hypoperfusion • Severe anemia
Hyperthyroidism
Medications and drugs: • Sympathomimetics • Beta-agonists • Anticholinergics • Aminophylline • Caffeine • Nicotine • Amphetamines • Cocaine
Pheochromocytoma
Drug withdrawal (beta blockers, clonidine)
SA node reentrant tachycardia

Table 27.4: Causes of prolongation of the PR interval.

Causes of prolongation of the PR interval
Beta blockers
Non-dihydropyridine Ca-channel blockers
Digoxin
Antiarrhythmics: • Amiodarone • Dronedarone • Sotalol • 1C Antiarrhythmic drugs (Flecainide, Propafenone)

subject to both parasympathetic and sympathetic modulation. Relative changes of such modulation, such as with exercise or stress, lead to increase sympathetic tone, decrease parasympathetic tone, and increase in heart rate. Thus, cardiac heart rate, and thus cardiac output, can be readily increased in times of increased systemic oxygen demand.

The AV node has evolved in order to prevent synchronous or near synchronous contraction of the atria and ventricles, which would lead to simultaneous contraction of the upper and lower chambers of the heart. Rather, the delay of impulse conduction in the AV node allows complete emptying of the atria into the ventricles before ventricular systole is initiated.

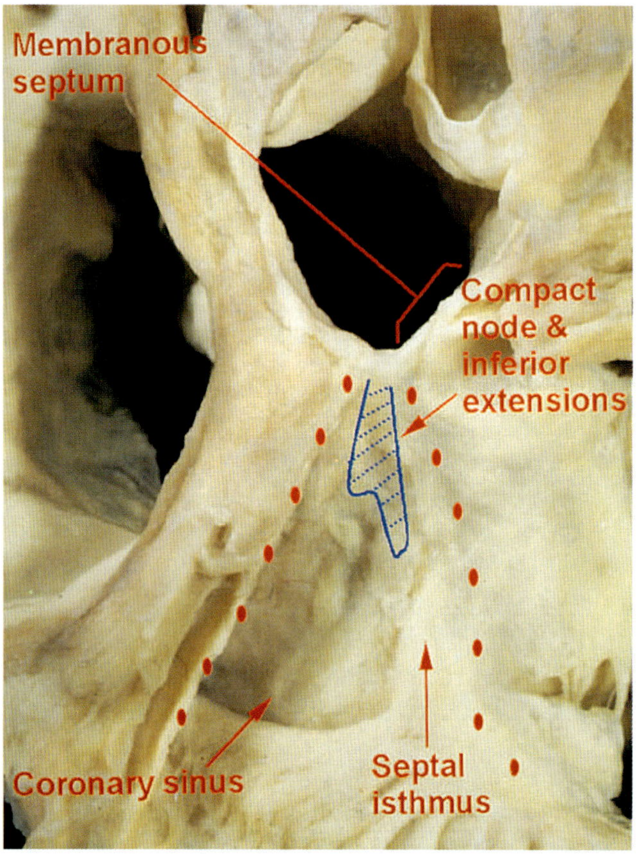

Fig. 27.8A: Location of the AV node (blue hatched area) within the triangle of Koch (Image courtesy of Dr Robert Anderson, Institute of Genetic Medicine, Newcastle University, United Kingdom).

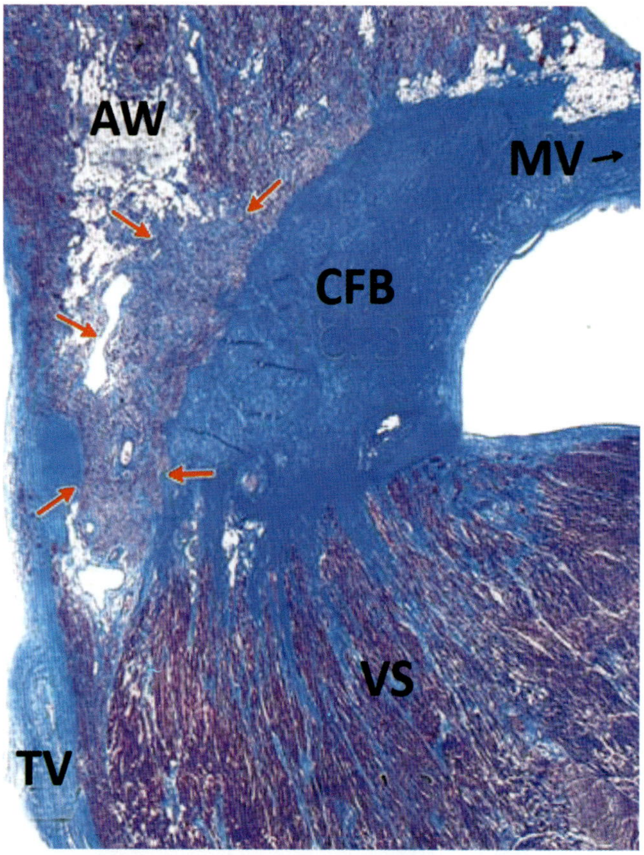

Fig. 27.8B: Microscopic examination of the AV node. At low magnification, the AV node (arrows) is seen abutting the CFB. [Image and legend text from Cheitlin MD, Ursell PC. Cardiac anatomy. In: Chatterjee K et al. (Ed). Cardiology—An Illustrated Textbook. New Delhi, India: Jaypee Brothers Medical Publishers (P) Ltd.]. (AW: Atrial wall; MV: Mitral valve; TV: Tricuspid valve; VS: Ventricular septum; CFB: Central fibrous body).

The AV node also has a property referred to as decremental conduction, which has the protective function in that it prevents very fast ventricular rates during atrial arrhythmias.

The conduction system of the heart has evolved in such a manner as to lead to ventricular contraction beginning from the apex of the heart and then propagating toward the base of the heart. In this manner, ejection of blood from the ventricles begins at the apex, "pushing" blood progressively closer to the semilunar valves and the aorta and pulmonary artery, a more efficient process than simultaneous contraction of all the myocytes in the ventricles. Depolarization impulses reach the papillary muscles slightly before they reach ventricular myocardial cells, with resultant increased tension on the chordae apparatus just prior to myocardial contraction, serving to prevent any mitral regurgitation during the early phase of ventricular systole.

Although as discussed above, there is some slight variation in when different areas of the ventricles begin depolarization, the His-Purkinje system as a whole allows for *near* simultaneous intraventricular and interventricular contraction (Fig. 27.10), a process more efficient and advantageous to what would otherwise be extremely slow and dysynchronous contraction if depolarization impulses only traveled normal ventricular myocyte to myocyte.

Unlike skeletal muscle, myocardial muscle cells have a prolonged action potential. This prolonged action potential maintains myocardial contraction until all ventricular myocytes have contracted, maximizing forward blood flow out the semilunar valves and into the pulmonary and systemic circulations.

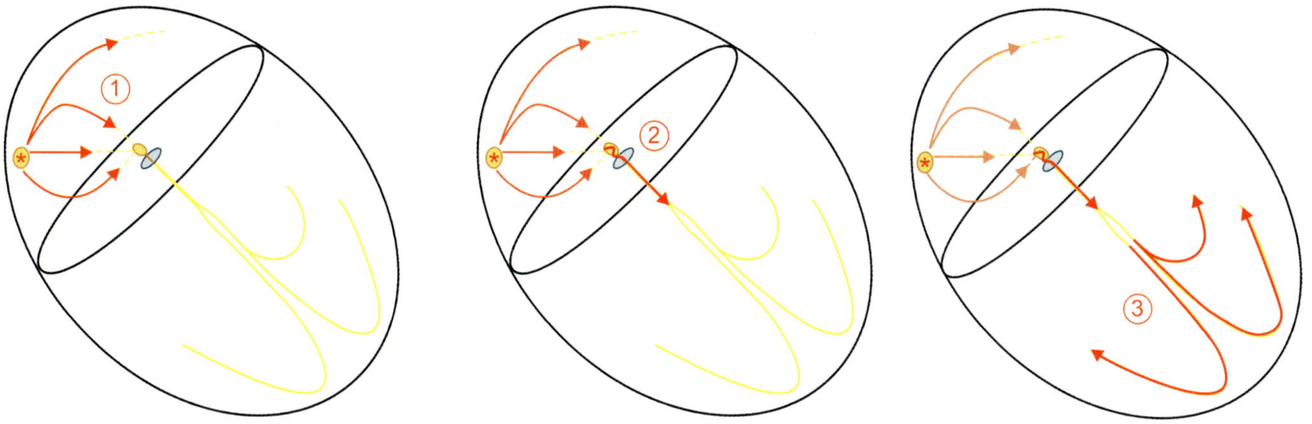

Fig. 27.9A: Simplified schematic of cardiac conduction. (1) The sinoatrial node depolarizes and the depolarization wavefront travels rapidly along the internodal pathways and Bachmann's Bundle, toward the atrioventricular node and the left atrium. (2) As the atrial tissue depolarizes, the depolarization wavefront slows as it travels through the atrioventricular junction. This allows atrial systole to efficiently fill the ventricles. Once through the atrioventricular node the depolarization wavefront rapidly moves through the Bundle of His. (3) Atrial tissue has almost completely repolarized and the tissues in the atrioventricular junction are beginning their repolarization. The depolarization wavefront now spreads rapidly through the right and left bundle branches and into the Purkinje System (Images and legend text courtesy of Christopher Watford, posted on www.sixlettervariable.blogspot.com).

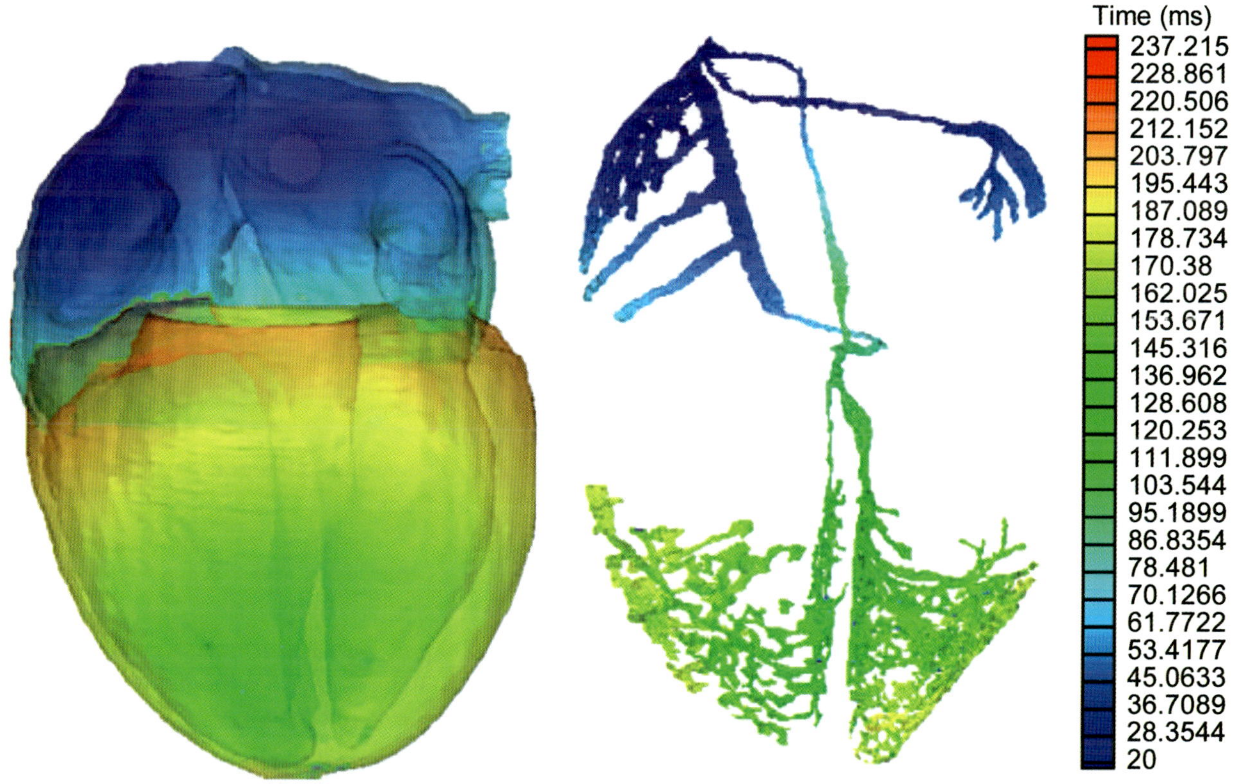

Fig. 27.9B: Simulated normal excitation sequences of the whole human heart. Different colors represent different excitement times, with dark blue representing earliest excitation and red representing latest excitation (Image from Deng D et al. Computational and Mathematical Methods in Medicine Volume 2012, Article ID 891070. doi:10.1155/2012/891070. CC).

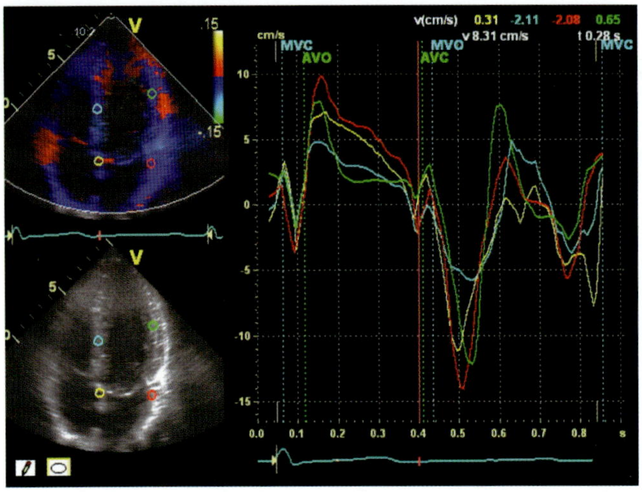

Fig. 27.10: Tissue velocity imaging (TVI), also called tissue Doppler imaging (TDI), of a normal heart. The systolic velocity curves of each wall segment overlap and reach peak systolic velocity at the same time, indicating synchronous depolarization of the left ventricle. http://my.americanheart.org/professional/Councils/Fellowship/Fellowship_UCM_316914_SubHomePage.jsp. [Image from Burns KV, et al. Right ventricular pacing and mechanical dyssynchrony. In: Oraii S (Ed). Electrophysiology—from Plants to Heart. Intechweb.org. CC].

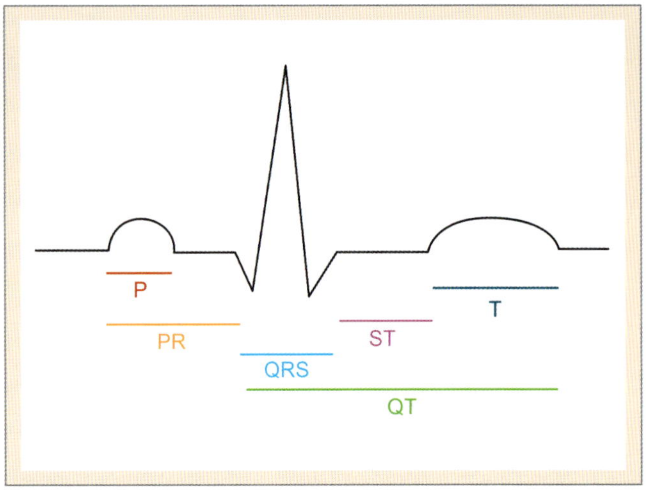

Fig. 27.11: Schematic illustration of the different measured intervals on the surface ECG (Image posted by Dr Rick Sanchez on Wikipedia Commons. CC).

ECG CORRELATES OF DEPOLARIZATION

The surface ECG serves as a crude assessment of impulse initiation and propagation, and of myocyte depolarization and repolarization. Measurement of the duration of P wave and QRS complex, as well as the PR and QT intervals, are used to assess normal conduction and depolarization, or the presence of perturbations of normal conduction, depolarization, or repolarization (Fig. 27.11).

Atrial depolarization is reflected on the surface ECG as the P wave. The normal duration of the P wave is ≤ 120 msec. Perturbations of atrial depolarization, such as with right or left chamber enlargement, are reflected by changes in the P wave morphology or duration as observed in specific leads.

The surface PR interval approximates the time of impulse conduction through the AV node and His-Purkinje system. Normal PR intervals are 120–200 msec. Disease of the AV node or in some cases of the His-Purkinje system is reflected on the surface ECG as a prolonged PR interval. Medications and numerous other factors also lead to a prolonged PR interval (Table 27.4). The presence of accessory bypass tracts, and conduction through such bypass tracts, is reflected on the surface lead by a short (< 120 msec) PR interval.

The QRS width reflects ventricular myocyte depolarization, both the left and right ventricles. Dysfunction of a bundle branch (or both the left anterior and posterior fascicles) leads to right bundle branch block (RBBB) or left bundle branch block (LBBB), reflected on the surface ECG by a widened QRS complex (>120 msec) with distinct morphology. Myocardial disease, such as idiopathic cardiomyopathy or infiltrative disease, can lead to prolonged ventricular depolarization, reflected on the surface ECG as a widened QRS often with neither an RBBB nor an LBBB pattern, and is referred to as *interventricular conduction defect (IVCD)*. Non-specific prolongation of the QRS complex can also occur due to left ventricular hypertrophy, myocardial infarction, hyperkalemia, and antiarrhythmic drugs.

The QT interval, measured from the beginning of the QRS complex to the end of the T wave, reflects, for the most part, ventricular repolarization. When measuring the true QT interval, Bazett's formula is used to "correct" for variation in the heart rate. The formula is given below, where QTc is the corrected QT interval, QT is the measured QT interval, and RR is the RR interval between QRS complexes.

$$QTc = \frac{QT}{\sqrt{RR}}$$

Bazett's formula may under-correct the QT interval at slow heart rates (<60 beats/min) and may over-correct the QT interval at fast heart rates. An alternate formula is Fridericia's correction, which uses the cube root of the RR interval, and is shown below.

$$QTc = \frac{QT}{\sqrt[3]{RR}}$$

Ventricular repolarization and the QT interval may be prolonged due to medications, hypocalcemia, congenital abnormalities, or other factors (Table 27.5).

How depolarization and repolarization of the different tissues and parts of the heart are reflected on the surface ECG are illustrated in Figure 27.12. As discussed in the following chapters, numerous disease processes can lead to abnormalities of normal cardiac depolarization.

Table 27.5: Causes of prolongation of the QT interval.

Causes of QT interval prolongation
Antiarrhythmic agents: • Sotalol • Dofetilide • Azimilide • Amiodarone • Ibutilide • Quinidine • Procainamide
Antidepressant and antipsychotic agents
Methadone
Certain antihistamines (e.g. astemizole)
Macrolide antibiotics
Hypothyroidism
Hypocalcemia
Congenital Long QT Syndrome

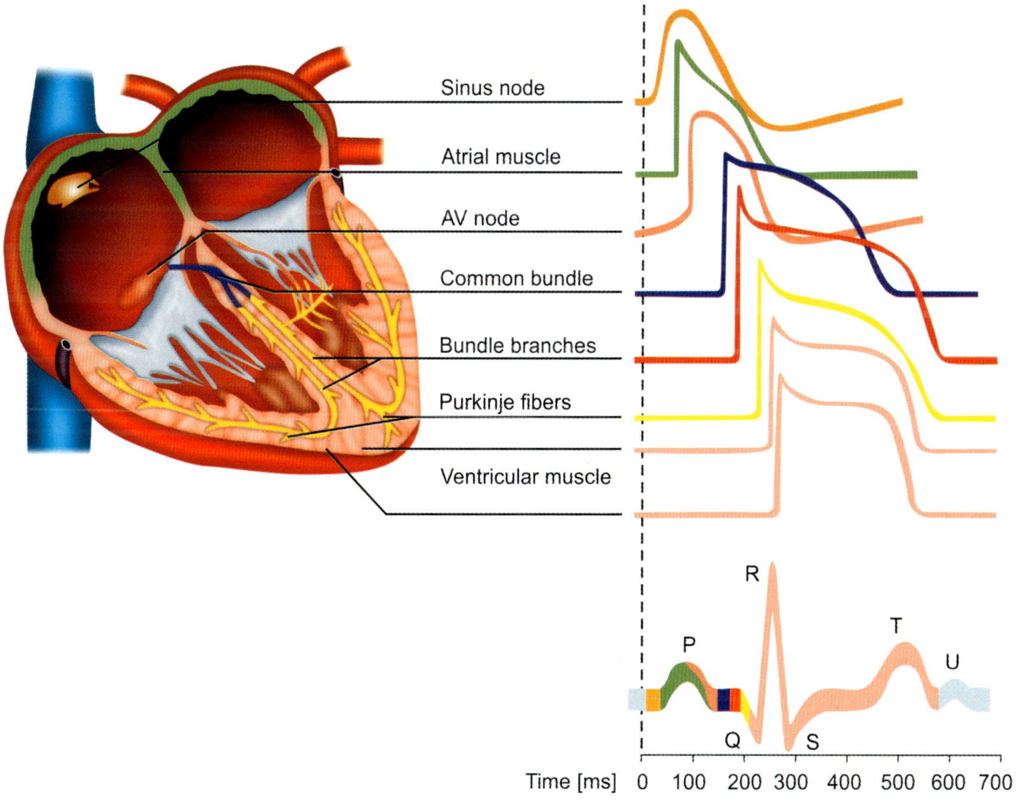

Fig. 27.12: Schematic illustration of how depolarization and repolarization of the different tissues and parts of the heart are reflected on the surface ECG.

REFERENCE

Electrical Conduction System of the Heart. en.wikipedia.org.

Bradyarrhythmias, Conduction Abnormalities, and Heart Block

Philippe R Akhrass, Adam S Budzikowski

INTRODUCTION

Bradycardia is defined conventionally as a heart rate below 60 beats per minute (bpm). The evaluation and management of bradycardia depends on an accurate assessment of the rhythm strip or electrocardiogram (ECG) and proper correlation with the clinical scenario. This correlation is fundamental because bradycardia could be a normal physiological response. On the other hand, it could also be a manifestation of serious disease, such as inferior wall myocardial infarction. It is not unusual for bradycardia to be asymptomatic. However, it may manifest with a spectrum of symptoms including lightheadedness, dizziness, fatigue, exercise intolerance, presyncope, syncope, dyspnea, worsening of angina, and altered mental status. Other symptoms related to the cause of bradycardia could be also manifested like nausea, sweating, or alternating slow and fast heart rate for sick sinus syndrome (SSS).

In the following sections, the bradyarrhythmias and heart block will be discussed in relation to their site (Table 28.1): sinus node related; atrioventricular (AV) junction related; bundle-branch or fascicule related; and finally device related.

Table 28.1: Types of bradyarrhythmias and heart block.

Sinus node related
• Sinus bradycardia
• First-degree sinoatrial (SA) exit block
• Second-degree SA block type I (Wenckebach)
• Second-degree SA block type II
• 2:1 sinoatrial block
• Third-degree SA block
• Sinus arrest
• Chronotropic incompetence
• Sick sinus syndrome
• Tachy-brady syndrome
Atrioventricular (AV) junction related
• First-degree AV block
• Second-degree AV block Mobitz I (Wenckebach)
• Second-degree AV block Mobitz II
• 2:1 AV block and high-degree AV block
• Third-degree AV block
Bundle-branch or fascicule related
• Right bundle branch block
• Left bundle branch block
• Left anterior fascicular block
• Left posterior fascicular block
Device related bradyarrhythmias
• Oversensing
• Failure to capture

SINOATRIAL NODE RELATED BRADYCARDIA

Sinus Bradycardia

Sinus bradycardia is the most commonly encountered type of bradycardia (Fig. 28.1). It is frequently considered a benign finding, but it can be the first manifestation of significant dysfunction of the sinus node. Sinus bradycardia is frequently seen in young patients with normal hearts. It is usually asymptomatic and does not require any intervention. Furthermore, most young well-trained endurance athletes have resting heart rates significantly slower than 60 bpm. No further testing is needed for asymptomatic athletes with structurally normal hearts for sinus bradycardia or even sinus pauses. Other noncardiac causes of sinus bradycardia include increased intracranial pressure, obstructive sleep apnea, and hypothyroidism. The treatment of the underlying cause will usually improve these types of sinus bradycardia.

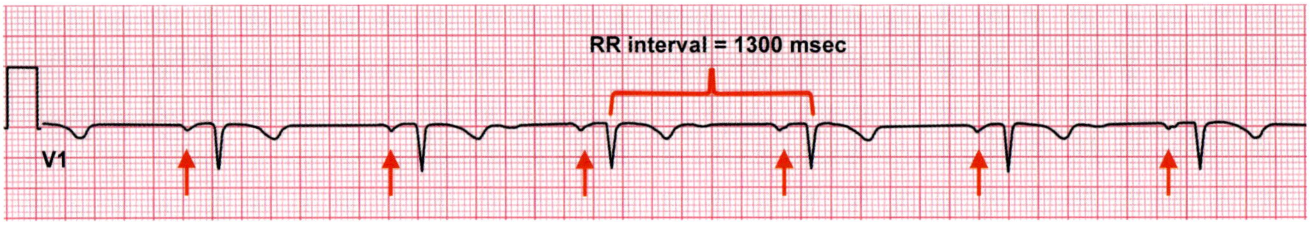

Fig. 28.1: ECG strip demonstrating marked bradycardia at 46 beats per minute. Note that P waves (arrows) are present before each QRS complex and that the RR interval is 1300 msec. Although the rhythm is more likely to be simple sinus bradycardia, it is not possible by surface ECG alone to differentiate between sinus bradycardia and 2:1 sinoatrial block, which could also produce a similar surface ECG tracing.

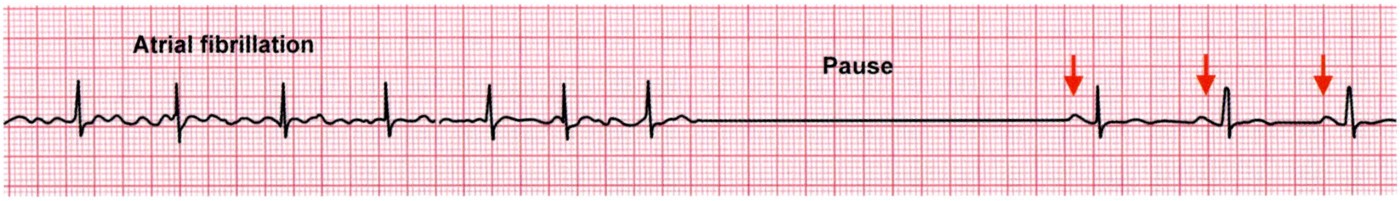

Fig. 28.2: An example of tachy-brady syndrome in a patient with paroxysmal atrial fibrillation and sick sinus syndrome. After the run of atrial fibrillation terminates, there is a long pause before sinus rhythm begins. Arrows point to the P waves present with the resumption of sinus rhythm. [Image from Levine GN (Ed). Arrhythmias 101: The Ultimate Easy-to-Read Introductory Book to Arrhythmias. New Delhi, India: Jaypee Brothers Medical Publishers (P) Ltd; 2013].

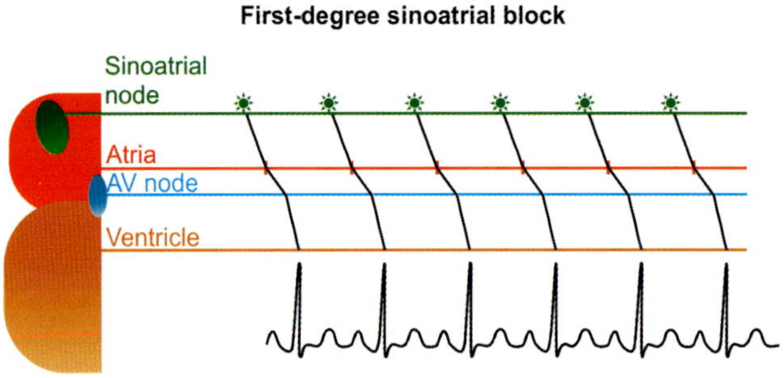

Fig. 28.3: First-degree sinoatrial nodal block. The SA impulse is delayed but eventually reaches the atrium, which depolarizes normally. First-degree sinoatrial nodal block cannot be diagnosed on surface ECG, as the 12-lead surface ECG will appear normal.

Conversely, bradycardia might be a manifestation of electrical disturbance of the heart. In older patients, for example, sinus bradycardia at rest accompanied with symptoms during activity could be due to the inability to increase heart rate on demand, termed *chronotropic incompetence*. A commonly used definition is the inability to increase heart rate to 80–85% of the maximal predicted heart rate during exercise (maximal heart rate = 220 – age).

Sick Sinus Syndrome

Sick sinus syndrome is another entity, most commonly resulting from degeneration and fibrosis of the SA node secondary to aging or other infiltrative and inflammatory diseases, leading to SA node dysfunction. Within the spectrum of the disease the *tachy-brady syndrome* manifests by alternating episodes of sinus bradyarrhythmias and episodes of atrial fibrillation and atrial tachyarrhythmias. Quite commonly, patients with atrial arrhythmias may experience prolonged pauses upon termination of the arrhythmia (Fig. 28.2). The best treatment strategy for these patients is suppression or elimination of atrial arrhythmias.

Depending on the clinical presentation and severity of episodes, patients with chronotropic incompetence and patients with SSS may need implantation of permanent pacemakers. The most common risk factor for the development of SSS is long-standing hypertension.

Sinoatrial Exit Block

Sinoatrial exit block is a form of sinus bradyarrhythmia, where the depolarization of pacemaker cells in the sinoatrial node fails to conduct to the atrial tissue, leading to the absence of P waves on the surface ECG. In first-degree sinoatrial block, the conduction is slowed but reaches the atrial tissue and P wave is present (Fig. 28.3); therefore diagnosis cannot be made on surface ECG. Second-degree SA nodal exit block has two types; in Type I (Wenckebach type), P to P interval shortens gradually

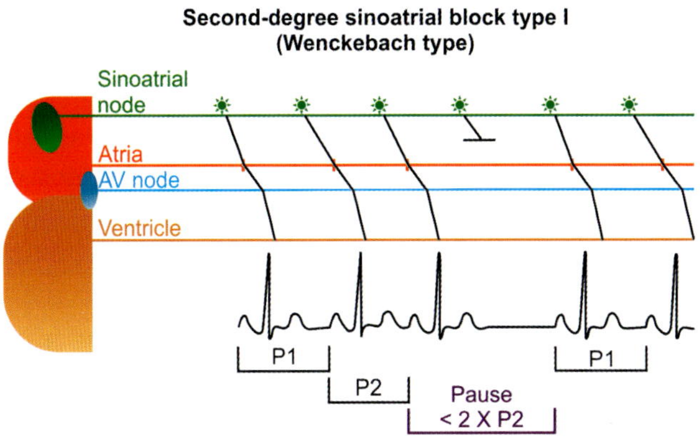

Fig. 28.4: Second-degree type I (Wenckebach type) sinoatrial block. In sinoatrial exit block type I (Wenckebach type), the P to P interval decreases gradually (P2 < P1) prior to a pause, evident by a dropped P wave (pause < 2 x P2). If the pause is longer than 2 times the preceding P to P interval then sinoatrial exit block is excluded.

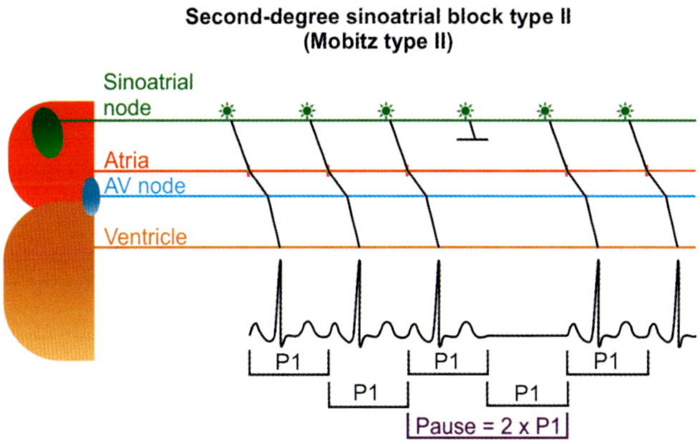

Fig. 28.5: Second-degree type II sinoatrial block. In second-degree sinoatrial exit block type II (Mobitz type II), the P to P interval prior to the dropped P is similar and the pause duration is a multiple of the normal P to P interval.

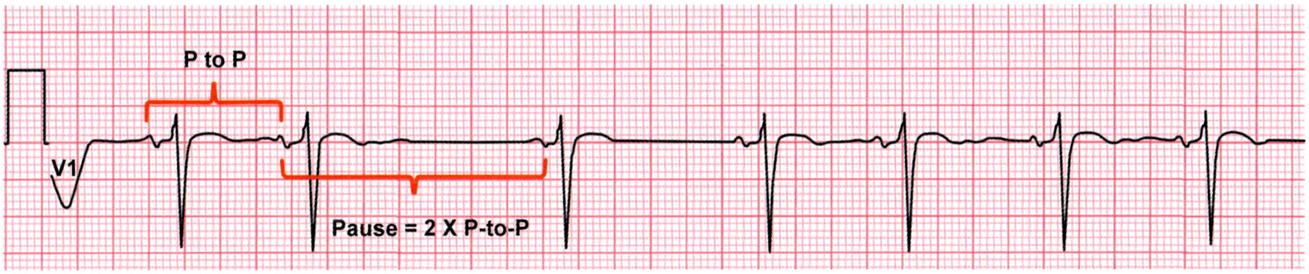

Fig. 28.6: Second-degree type II sinoatrial block. The ECG strip shows a second-degree sinoatrial exit block type II (Mobitz type II) after the first two QRS complexes. The pause is exactly twice the duration of P to P interval.

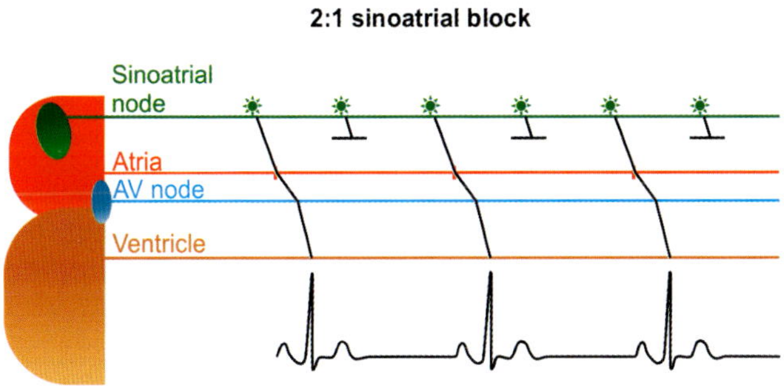

Fig. 28.7: 2:1 sinoatrial exit block. In 2:1 sinoatrial exit block, every other sinoatrial impulse is not conducted to the atrium. 2:1 sinoatrial exit block cannot be differentiated on surface ECG from sinus bradycardia.

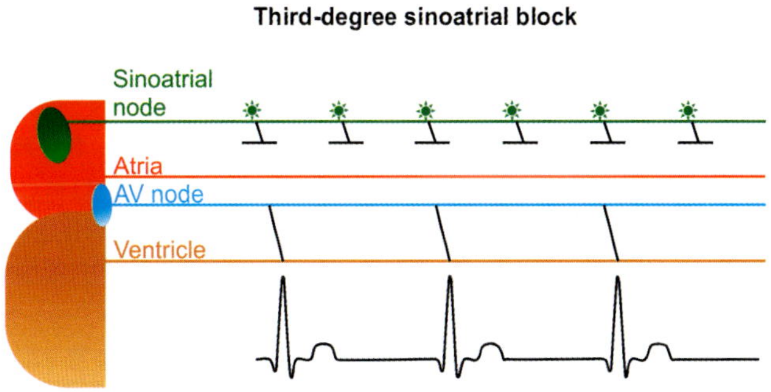

Fig. 28.8: Third-degree sinoatrial exit block. In third-degree sinoatrial exit block, the sinoatrial impulse does not reach the right atrium, therefore, P waves are absent on the surface ECG. Third-degree SA exit block cannot be distinguished on surface ECG from sinus pause or sinus arrest.

prior to a pause, evident by an absent P wave, with pause duration less than two P to P cycles (Fig. 28.4). In type II SA exit block, the P to P interval prior to the absent P is similar, but the pause duration is a multiple of the preceding P to P interval (Figs. 28.5 to 28.7). In third-degree SA nodal exit block, the sinus node pacemaker impulse does not reach the right atrium, consequently P waves will be absent on the surface ECG (Fig. 28.8). Third-degree SA exit block cannot be distinguished on surface ECG from sinus pause, sinus arrest, or atrial standstill.

ATRIOVENTRICULAR NODE RELATED BRADYCARDIA AND HEART BLOCK

Bradycardia or heart block may well occur below the sinus node level, due to dysfunction in the AV node (termed *nodal heart block*) or the His bundle and fascicles (termed infranodal heart block). First-degree AV block is defined by a PR interval > 200 ms (Fig. 28.9). In second-degree AV block Mobitz type I, the PR interval prolongs progressively until QRS is absent (Figs. 28.10 to 28.12). Typically, most of

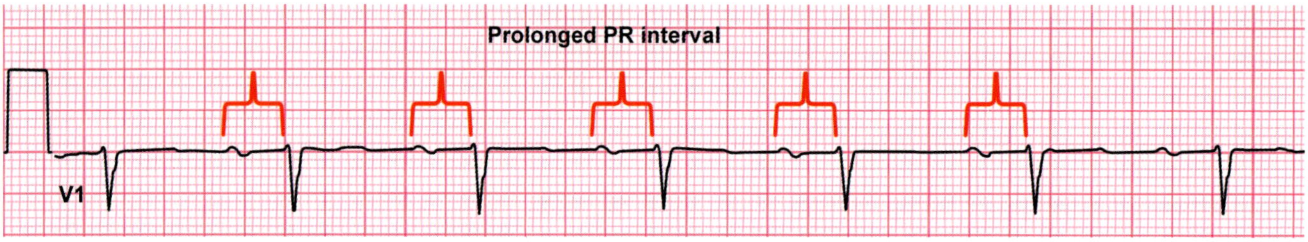

Fig. 28.9: First-degree AV block. The rhythm strip shows a prolonged PR interval at 296 ms.

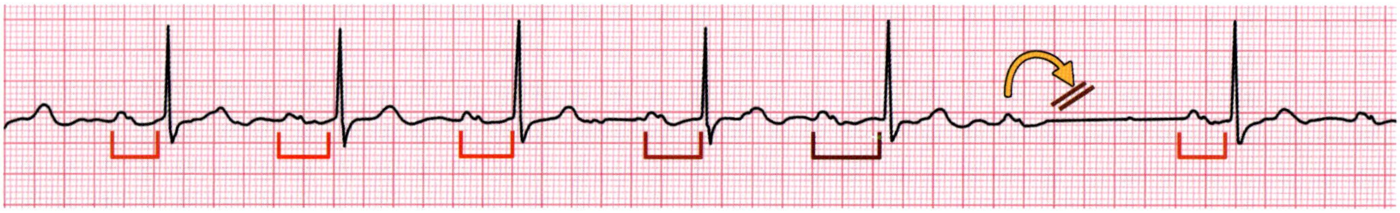

Fig. 28.10: Rhythm strip demonstrating the progressive prolongation of the PR interval before the occurrence of a nonconducted P wave in Mobitz type I second-degree heart block (typical Wenckebach).

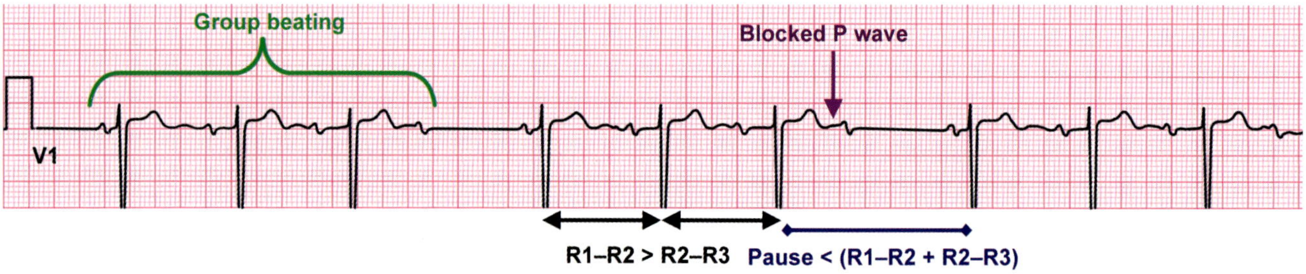

Fig. 28.11: Rhythm strip showing typical second-degree AV block Mobitz type I (typical Wenckebach) characterized by: (1) PR interval progressive prolongation until QRS drops, (2) group beating, (3) PR interval after block shorter than PR before block, (4) decremental lengthening of PR interval leading to progressive shortening of RR interval and (5) pause around dropped P smaller than the sum of any two consecutive R to R intervals.

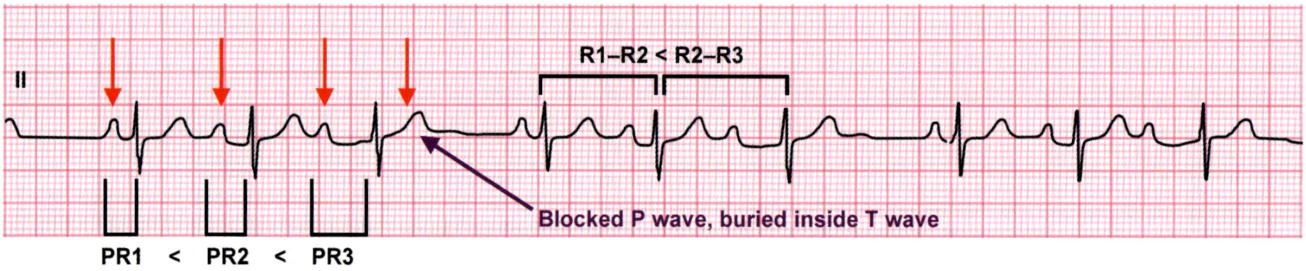

Fig. 28.12: Atypical Wenckebach. This is another ECG that shows second-degree AV block Mobitz type I (Wenckebach). This is deemed "atypical Wenckebach" since the lengthening of the PR interval occurs at decremental increases, leading to progressively shorter RR intervals. In this ECG R2–R3 is longer than R1–R2. Note again the presence of group beating, a feature of second-degree heart block. Arrows point out the P waves in the rhythm strip, with a nonconducted (blocked) P wave buried inside the T wave.

the PR interval prolongation is seen in the first sequence of the cycle, with shortening of the increment of prolongation in subsequent sequences. This results in shortening of the QRS to QRS intervals. In second-degree AV block Mobitz type II the QRS is absent without preceding prolongation in the PR interval (Figs. 28.13A and B). In order to use the Mobitz ECG classification, it is necessary to have two or more conducted P waves. Additionally, Mobitz classification is an ECG definition and although suggestive, it is not always indicative of the site of the block in terms of whether it is nodal or intra-Hisian or infra-Hisian. When distal (below AV node) conduction abnormalities accompany Mobitz type I AV block or when worsening of AV conduction is seen with exercise, this signifies infra-Hisian disease.

2:1 Atrioventricular Block

2:1 AV block is defined by blocked AV conduction every other atrial depolarization and manifest on surface ECG with alternating absence of the QRS (Figs. 28.14 and 28.15). 2:1 AV block may be due to either Wenckebach or to Mobitz type 2 AV block. This usually cannot be discerned from just the 12-lead ECG.

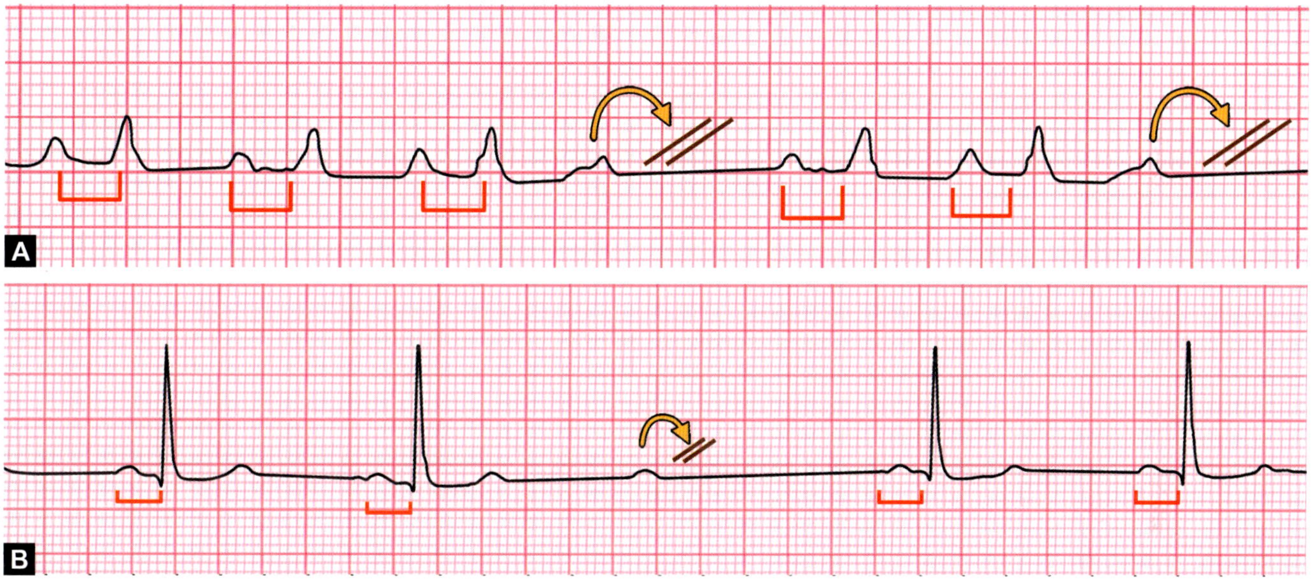

Figs. 28.13A and B: Mobitz type II second-degree AV block. Note that in both rhythm strips, the PR intervals are constant before there is a nonconducted (blocked) P wave.

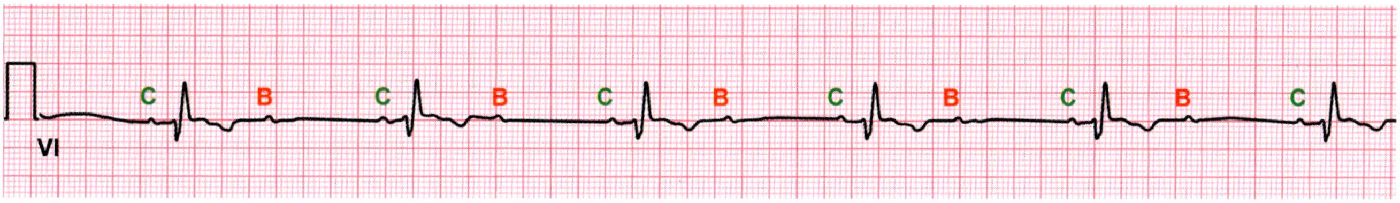

Fig. 28.14: 2:1 AV block. Conducted P waves are marked with (C) while blocked P waves are marked with (B). Only every other P wave is seen as conducted and leading to ventricular depolarization and a resultant QRS complex.

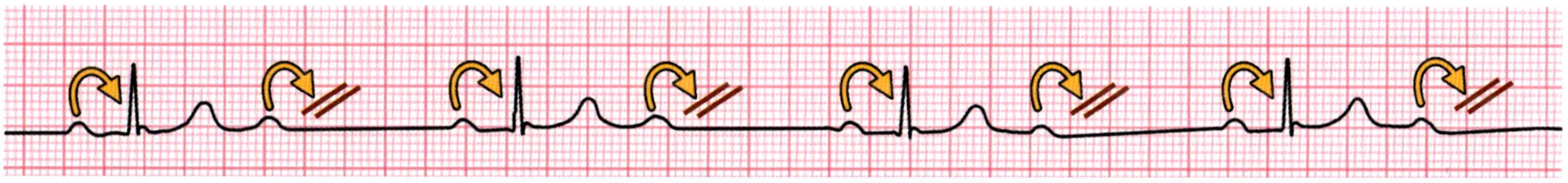

Fig. 28.15: A second example of 2:1 AV block. Based on this surface ECG tracing alone, one cannot distinguish whether the rhythm is Mobitz type I or type II AV block. [Image from Levine GN (Ed). Arrhythmias 101: The Ultimate Easy-to-Read Introductory Book to Arrhythmias. New Delhi, India: Jaypee Brothers Medical Publishers (P) Ltd; 2013].

High-grade Atrioventricular Block

High-grade AV block is defined by AV conduction 3:1 or worse (Fig. 28.16). Third-degree AV block, also referred to as *complete heart block*, occurs when there is no conduction through the AV node with complete dissociation of the atrial and ventricular activity (Figs. 28.17 to 28.19). The escape mechanism can occur anywhere from the AV node

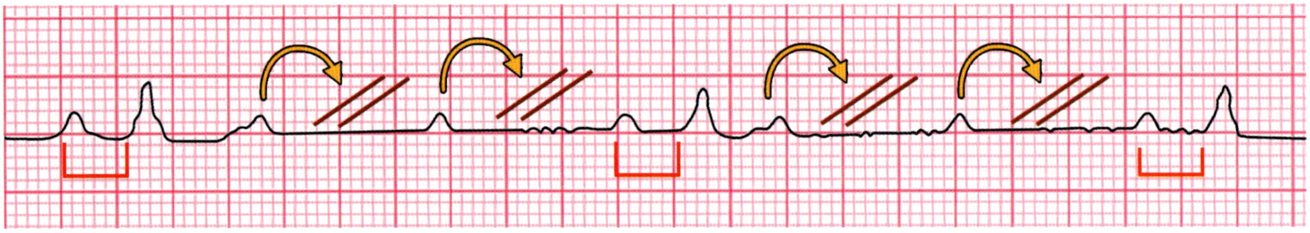

Fig. 28.16: High-grade AV block. There is 3:1 conduction present. In other words, only 1 of 3 P waves are conducted. Levine GN (Ed). Arrhythmias 101: The Ultimate Easy-to-Read Introductory Book to Arrhythmias. New Delhi, India: Jaypee Brothers Medical Publishers (P) Ltd; 2013.

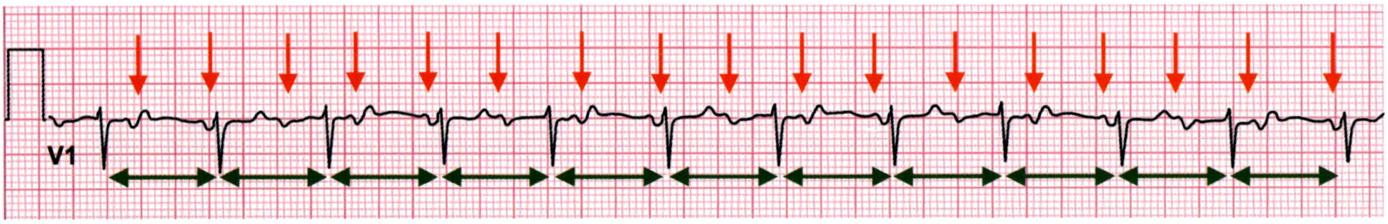

Fig. 28.17: Complete heart block with a junctional escape rhythm. The rhythm strip shows sinus tachycardia (P waves marked with red arrow) with complete heart block and AV dissociation with narrow junctional escape rhythm (constant RR intervals shown in double-headed green arrows).

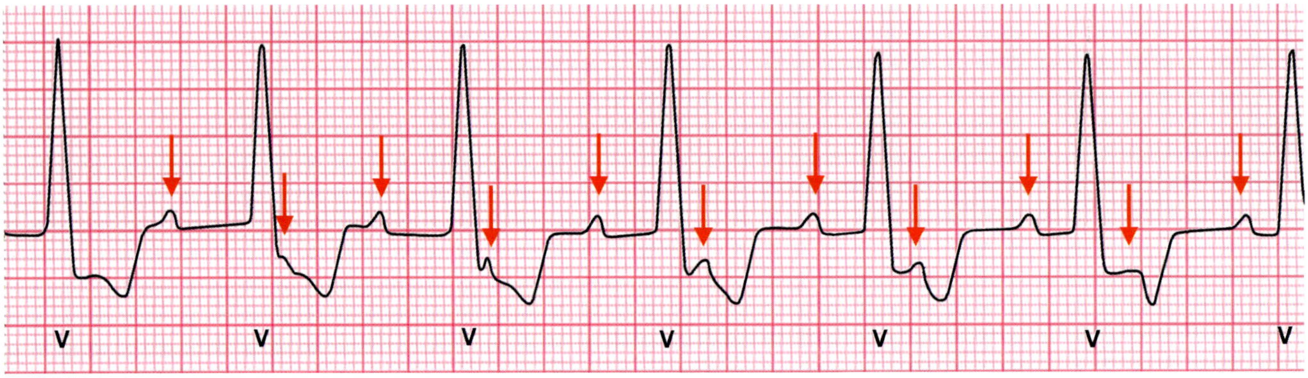

Fig. 28.18: Complete heart block with ventricular escape rhythm. The P waves (arrows) are dissociated from the wide QRS ventricular escape beats (V). The RR interval is constant, consistent with complete heart block and an escape rhythm.

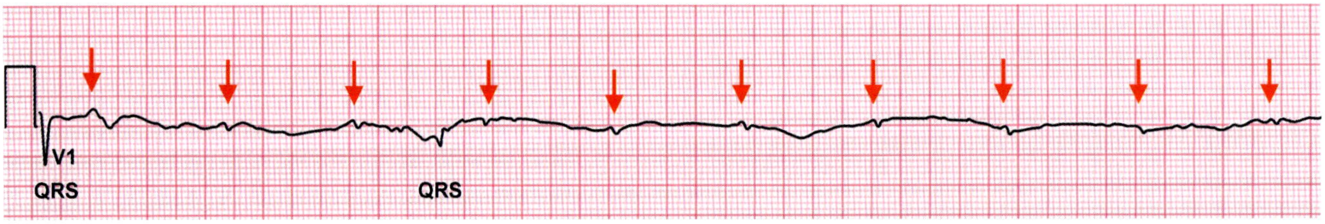

Fig. 28.19: Sinus rhythm (arrows) with complete AV block and absence of AV conduction or any escape rhythm except for two QRS complexes.

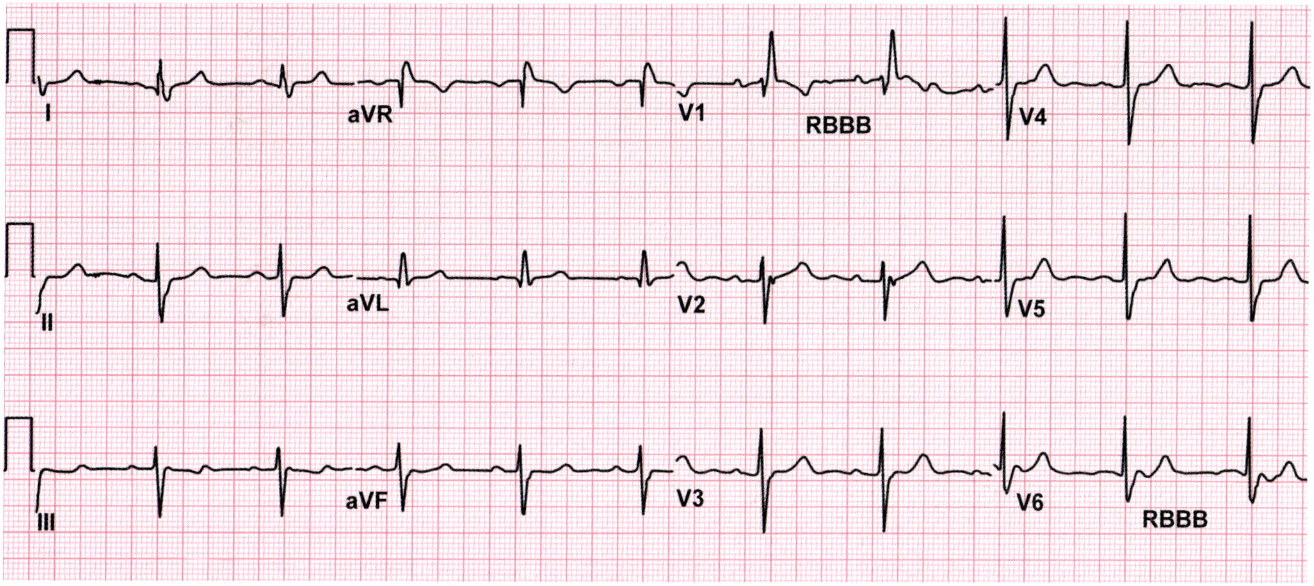

Fig. 28.20: Right bundle branch block (RBBB). The ECG demonstrates a wide QRS complex with an rSr′ pattern in lead V1 and terminal wide S waves in the lateral leads. Also present on the ECG is first-degree AV block (PR = 210 ms) and left anterior fascicular block (QRS axis between –45° and –90°). The ECG findings suggest significant conduction system disease, and this patient developed higher degree AV block several months later, requiring placement of a permanent dual chamber pacemaker.

to the bundle-branches, the Purkinje system, or ventricular myocardium. In general, patients with persistent third-degree AV block will require a permanent pacemaker. Indications for permanent pacemakers in "*asymptomatic*" patients with bradycardia or heart block are reviewed in Table 28.2.

BUNDLE-BRANCH BLOCK, FASCICULAR BLOCKS, AND PACED RHYTHMS

When a conduction abnormality occurs below the His bundle, it may manifest as a *right bundle branch block* (RBBB) (Fig. 28.20), *left bundle branch block* (LBBB) (Fig. 28.21), *left fascicular anterior block* (LFAB) or *left fascicular posterior block* (LFPB). In general, RBBB and LFAB can be seen in the absence of underlying heart disease, while LBBB and LFPB occur in patients with underlying structural heart disease. The conduction defects and depolarization patterns of patients with RBBB or LBBB are illustrated in Figure 28.22. The presence of LBBB leads to dyssynchronous left ventricular contraction (Figs. 28.23 and 28.24). In patients with heart failure and significant left ventricular systolic dysfunction, biventricular pacing may be used to decrease such dyssynchrony.

Ventricular pacemaker rhythms manifest with widened QRS on surface ECG and should not be confused with bundle branch blocks. Right ventricular pacing manifests with a LBBB-like morphology (Fig. 28.25), while biventricular pacing manifests a negative QRS in I and aVL (Fig. 28.26). The QRS morphology will vary greatly with biventricular pacing depending on the position of pacing leads as well as the relative timing of the right ventricular to left ventricular pacing. The presence of pacemaker artifacts or "spikes" does not necessarily imply that the paced impulse actually captures the paced chamber.

DEVICE RELATED BRADYCARDIA

Bradycardia in patients with pacemakers might be the first sign of pacemaker failure or suboptimal programming. *Oversensing* occurs when the pacemaker senses electrical activity different from the native activity and inhibits pacing. Oversensing will lead to underpacing. It is seen when the lead oversenses opposite chamber activity, diaphragmatic and/or pectoral myopotential, artifact caused by a fractured lead, or external electromagnetic interference. *Failure to capture* can also cause bradycardia, whether it is caused by battery depletion, a compromised lead, or changes in threshold due to electrolytes abnormalities, medications or change in tissue characteristics (e.g. fibrosis, infarct).

Table 28.2: Indications for permanent pacemaker in asymptomatic patients according to 2012 ACC/AHA/HRS guidelines. (LOE: Level of evidence).

Class I (should be performed, is recommended)
• 3rd degree or advanced 2nd degree AV block in sinus rhythm with documented periods of a systole > or = 3.0 seconds (LOE = C)
• 3rd degree or advanced 2nd degree AV block in sinus rhythm with any escape rate less than 40 bpm, or with an escape rhythm that is below the AV node (LOE = C)
• 3rd degree or advanced 2nd degree AV block in patients with AF and bradycardia with 1 or more pauses > or = to 5.0 seconds (LOE = C)
• 3rd degree or advanced 2nd degree AV block associated with neuromuscular diseases* (LOE = B)
• Persistent 3rd degree AV block with ventricular rates > 40 bpm if cardiomegaly or LV dysfunction is present or if the site of block is below the AV node (LOE = B)
• Second or third-degree AV block during exercise in the absence of myocardial ischemia (LOE = B)
Class IIa (is reasonable)
• Persistent 3rd AV block with an escape rate > 40 bpm in patients without cardiomegaly (LOE = C)
• Asymptomatic 2nd degree AV block at intra or infra-His levels found at electrophysiological study (LOE = B)
• Asymptomatic 2nd degree AV block type II with a narrow QRS (LOE = B)
Class IIb (may be reasonable)
• Any degree of AV block (including first-degree AV block) in patients with neuromuscular diseases* because there may be unpredictable progression of AV conduction disease (LOE = B)
Class III (not beneficial, should not be performed)
• Not indicated for sinus node dysfunction in asymptomatic patients (LOE = C)
• Not indicated for asymptomatic first-degree AV block (LOE = B)
• Not indicated for asymptomatic 2nd degree AV block type I, at the supra-His (AV node) level (LOE = C)
• Not indicated for AV block that is expected to resolve and is unlikely to recur (e.g. drug toxicity, Lyme disease, or transient increases in vagal tone or during hypoxia in sleep apnea syndrome in the absence of symptoms) (LOE = B)

*Neuromuscular diseases: Myotonic muscular dystrophy, Kearns-Sayre syndrome, Peroneal muscular atrophy and Erb's dystrophy (limb-girdle muscular dystrophy). (AV: Atrioventricular; AF: LOE=C, LOE=B).

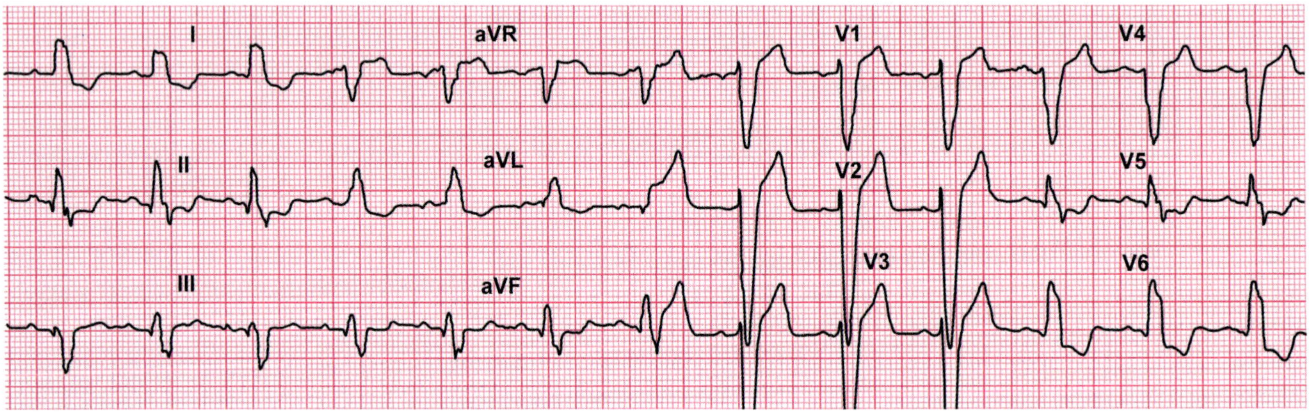

Fig. 28.21: Left bundle branch block (LBBB). 12-lead ECG showing LBBB with a QRS width >120 ms, broad notching or the R wave in the lateral leads (I, aVL, V5 and V6, and ST and T wave repolarization in the opposite direction as the QRS complex).

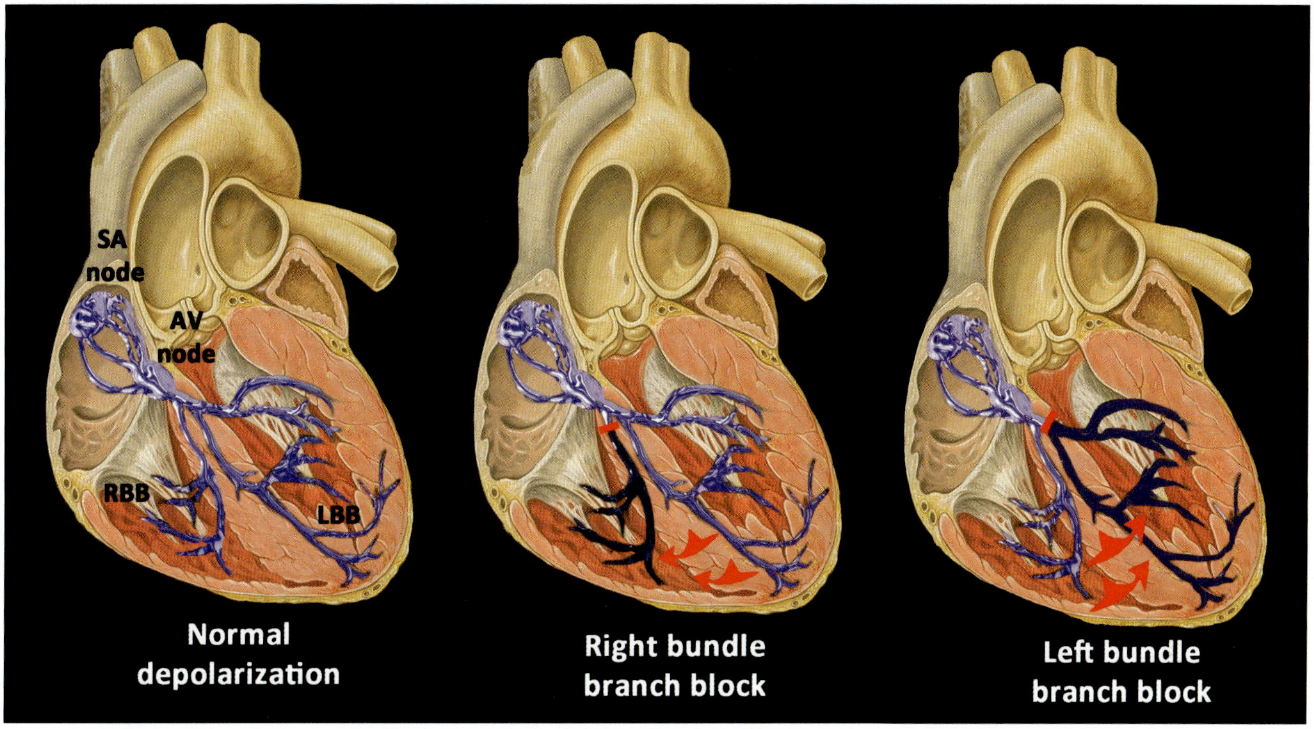

Fig. 28.22: Schematic representation of the conduction system and normal depolarization, depolarization with right bundle branch block, and depolarization with left bundle branch block. Small red rectangles represent block in the conduction system; red arrows represent wavefront of delayed depolarization due to the bundle branch block. (Figures modified from a figure created by J Heuser, posted on Wikimedia Commons, based on an original image by Patrick J Lynch and C Carl Jaffe).

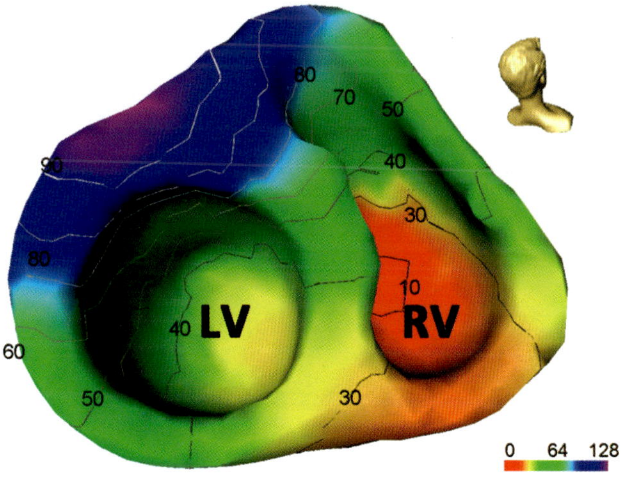

Fig. 28.23: Activation time map in a patient with LBBB. Isochrones are given in milliseconds after first onset of depolarization. Note how depolarization occurs earlier in the right ventricle and only later in the left ventricle. [Image from Seger M, Bernhard Pfeifer and Thomas Berger. Noninvasive imaging of cardiac electrophysiology (NICE). In: Oraii S (Ed). Electrophysiology: From Plants to Heart. InTech; 2012].

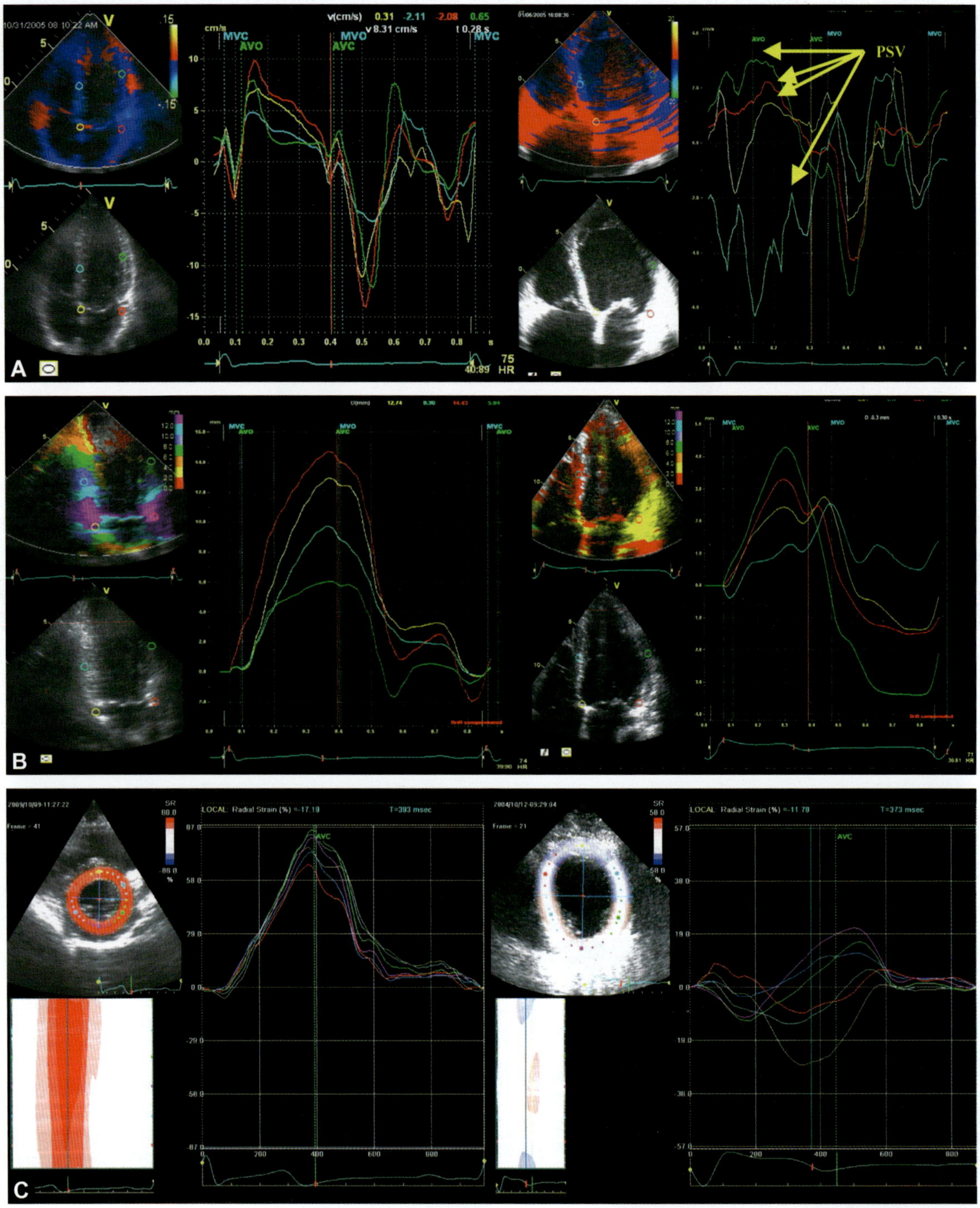

Figs. 28.24A to C: Echocardiography imaging of the heart in the setting of normal depolarization (left panels) and in the setting of conduction abnormalities and dyssynchrony (right panels). (A) Apical four-chamber tissue velocity imaging (TVI) of a normal heart (left panel), and a dyssynchronous heart (right panel.) In the normal heart, the systolic velocity curves of each wall segment overlap and reach peak systolic velocity (PSV) at the same time. In the dyssynchronous heart, peak velocity occurs at different times (marked with arrows in the right panel) for each wall segment; (B) Apical four-chamber tissue tracking (TT) curves of a normal (left panel) and dyssynchronous (right panel) heart. In the normal heart, all wall segments reach peak displacement at the same time, at aortic valve closure. In the dyssynchronous heart, wall segments do not reach peak displacement at the same time, and may reach a peak after aortic valve closure; (C) Speckle tracking echocardiography (STE) images of radial strain in a normal (left panel) and dyssynchronous (right panel) heart. In the normal heart, strain curves overlap, while in the dyssynchronous heart strain patterns are very different for different wall segments. [Images from Burns KV, Gage RM, Bank AJ. Right ventricular pacing and mechanical dyssynchrony. In: Oraii S (Ed). Electrophysiology: From Plants to Heart. InTech; 2012].

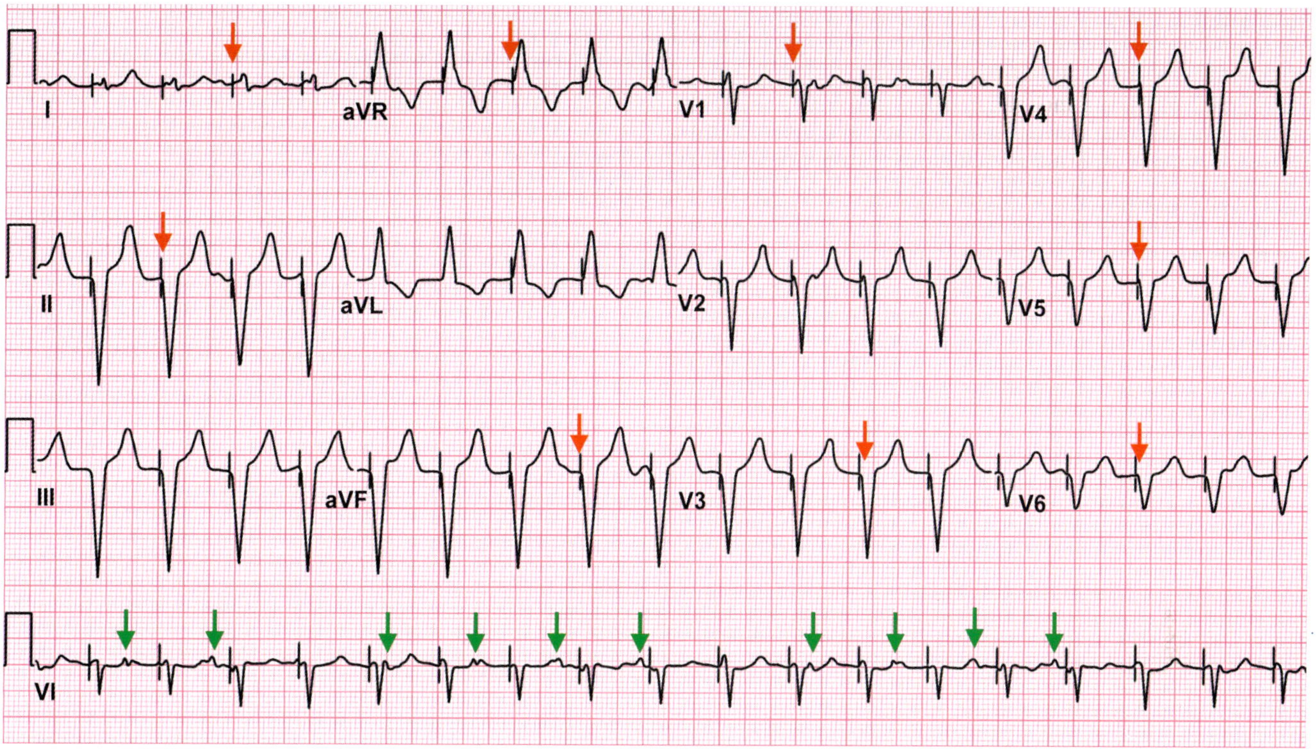

Fig. 28.25: Right ventricular pacing. Right ventricular pacing resulting in a QRS morphology consistent with LBBB. Pacer spikes (red arrows) are clearly visible in almost all leads. The rhythm strip at the bottom of the ECG shows the presence of AV dissociation, with the visible P waves (green arrows) "marching through" and not leading to any native QRS complexes.

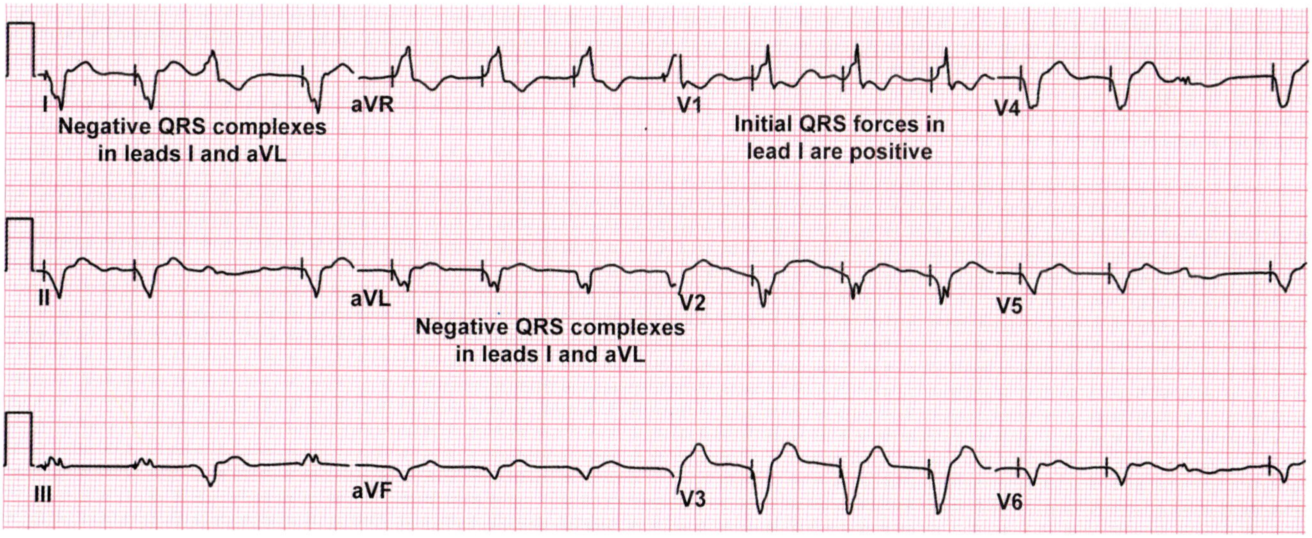

Fig. 28.26: Biventricular pacing. The 12-lead ECG shows biventricular pacing with paced QRS complexes in which the initial forces in lead V1 are positive and in leads I and aVL are more negative. This sequence occurs in group beating. In fact for the advanced, this ECG represents a typical Wenckebach not typical Wenckebach: the reason is that in typical Wenckebach the lengthening of the PR interval occurs at decremental increases, leading to progressively shorter RR interval.

REFERENCES

Epstein AE, DiMarco JP, Ellenbogen KA, et al. 2012 ACCF/AHA/HRS focused update incorporated into the ACCF/AHA/HRS 2008 guidelines for device-based therapy of cardiac rhythm abnormalities: a report of the American College of Cardiology Foundation/American Heart Association Task Force on Practice Guidelines and the Heart Rhythm Society. J Am Coll Cardiol. 2013;61(3):e6-75.

Hiss RG, Lamb LE, Allen MF. Electrocardiographic findings in 67,375 asymptomatic subjects. X. Normal values. Am J Cardiol. 1960;6:200-31.

Lee S, Wellens HJ, Josephson ME. Paroxysmal atrioventricular block. Heart Rhythm. 2009;6(8):1229-34.

Mangrum JM, DiMarco JP. The evaluation and management of bradycardia. N Engl J Med. 2000;342(10):703-9.

Maron BJ, Zipes DP. Introduction: eligibility recommendations for competitive athletes with cardiovascular abnormalities-general considerations. J Am Coll Cardiol. 2005;45(8):1318-21.

Vardas PE, Simantirakis EN, Kanoupakis EM. New developments in cardiac pacemakers. Circulation. 2013;127(23):2343-50.

CHAPTER

29

Atrial Fibrillation

Michael E Field

DEFINITION AND DIAGNOSIS OF ATRIAL FIBRILLATION

Atrial fibrillation (AF) is the most common sustained cardiac rhythm abnormality, and one that increases in prevalence with advancing age. AF is defined as a cardiac arrhythmia with electrocardiogram (ECG) characteristics of: (1) the surface ECG shows irregular RR intervals; (2) absence of distinct P waves; and (3) the atrial cycle length (i.e. the interval between two atrial activations), when visible, is irregular. Coarse AF is sometimes mistaken for atrial flutter or erroneously called "fib-flutter" (Figs. 29.1A to D). Rarely, the occurrence of AF in a patient with a bypass tract (e.g. Wolff-Parkinson-White syndrome) may not be recognized, and the resulting rhythm incorrectly diagnosed as ventricular tachycardia (Fig. 29.1E).

Atrial fibrillation may be classified according to the duration of episodes (Table 29.1). AF is a heterogeneous disorder and can occur in isolation ("lone AF") or in association with structural cardiac disease or non-cardiac diseases (Fig. 29.2). The term "nonvalvular AF" has been applied to individuals with AF who do not have rheumatic mitral valve disease or mechanical heart valve.

The initial diagnosis of AF is based on the history and clinical examination, and is confirmed by ECG, ambulatory rhythm monitoring (telemetry, Holter monitor, event recorders), implanted loop recorder, or cardiac device interrogation (Figs. 29.3A to C). Part of initial evaluation, all patients with AF should have a two-dimensional transthoracic echocardiogram to detect underlying structural heart disease, to assess cardiac function, and to evaluate atrial size. Additional laboratory evaluation should include assessment of serum electrolytes, thyroid, renal, and hepatic function, and a blood count and a chest radiograph if pulmonary disease or heart failure (HF) is suspected.

GENERAL MANAGEMENT OF ATRIAL FIBRILLATION

Management of AF should involve identifying and correcting underlying conditions that may have precipitated the AF. Thereafter, the primary objectives for the management of AF include:

- Prevention of thromboembolism including stroke
- Controlling the heart rate while in AF (*rate control*)
- Controlling symptoms which may include restoring/maintaining sinus rhythm (*rhythm control*)

These objectives are not mutually exclusive objectives. For example, a rhythm control strategy still requires attention to thromboembolism prevention and rate control. The approach must be tailored to the individual patient depending on a number of factors including the burden of symptoms, age, patient preference and comorbidities. An algorithm for the management of the patient with AF is given in Flow chart 29.1.

PREVENTION OF THROMBOEMBOLISM

Atrial fibrillation results in an increased risk of stroke due to formation of left atrial and particularly left atrial appendage (LAA) thrombi (Figs. 29.4A to D, Video 29.1). The risk of thromboembolism varies considerably between patients, and guidelines utilize the $CHADS_2$ and the CHA_2DS_2-VASc point score system, based on clinical characteristics (Table 29.2) to assess the risk of stroke and aid decisions about anticoagulation.

An algorithm for the choice of antithrombotic therapy for AF is shown in Flow chart 29.2. The choice of antithrombotic therapy should be based on the absolute risks of stroke and bleeding and the net clinical benefit in an individual patient. Bleeding risk scores have been developed to quantify hemorrhage risk, including the Hypertension, Abnormal renal/liver function, Stroke,

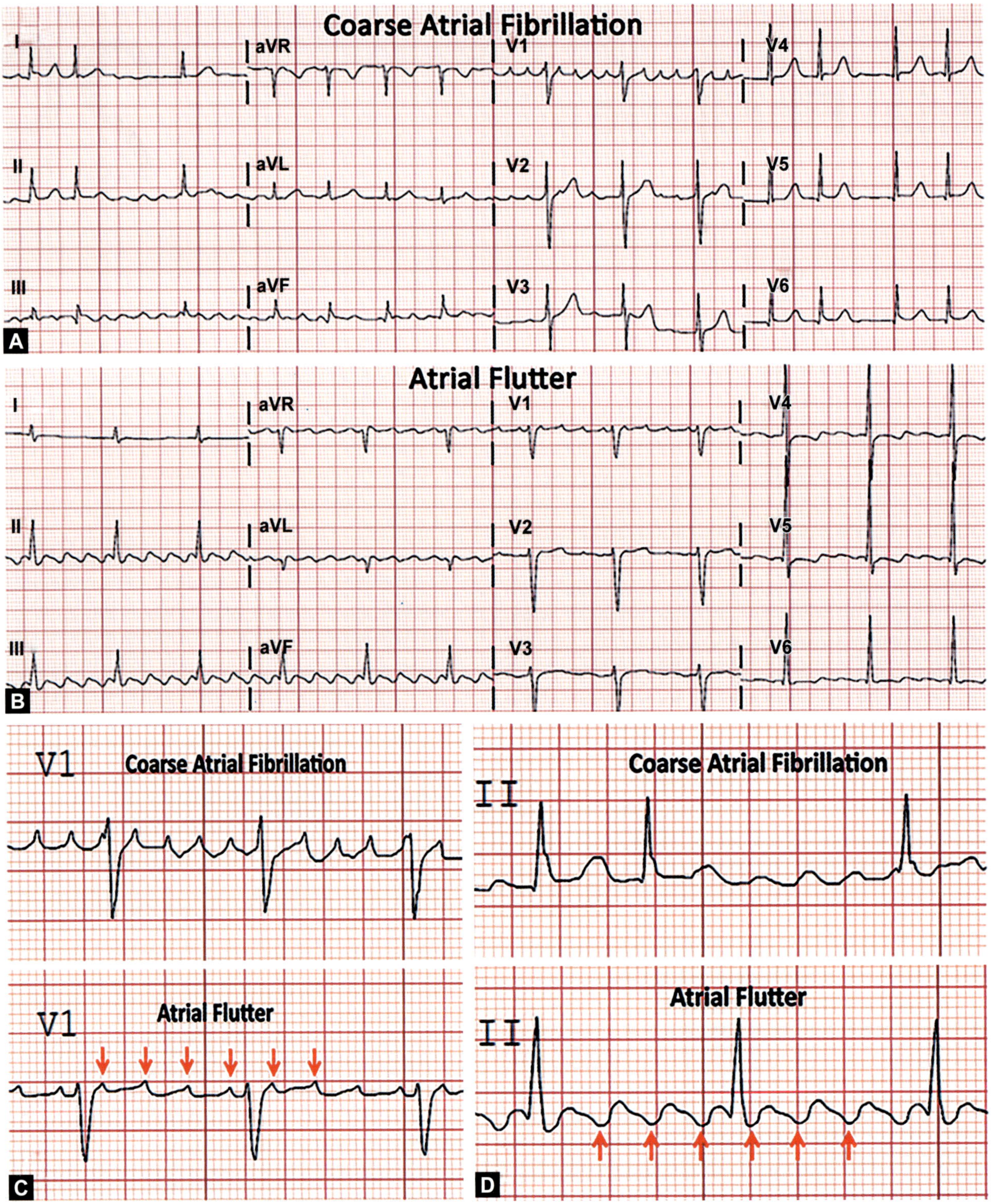

Figs. 29.1A to D: Distinction between coarse atrial fibrillation and atrial flutter. (A) ECG shows coarse atrial fibrillation, which is sometimes mistaken for atrial flutter or erroneously called "fib-flutter" due to the large amplitude waves in lead V1 and II. The atrial activity however is not regular and the morphology is changing making this atrial fibrillation. (B) ECG from a patient with typical atrial flutter demonstrating regular atrial cycle length. (C and D) Direct comparison of the ECG tracings of coarse atrial fibrillation and atrial flutter in leads V1 (C) and II (D) demonstrate the clear difference between coarse fibrillatory waves and regular flutter waves (arrows).

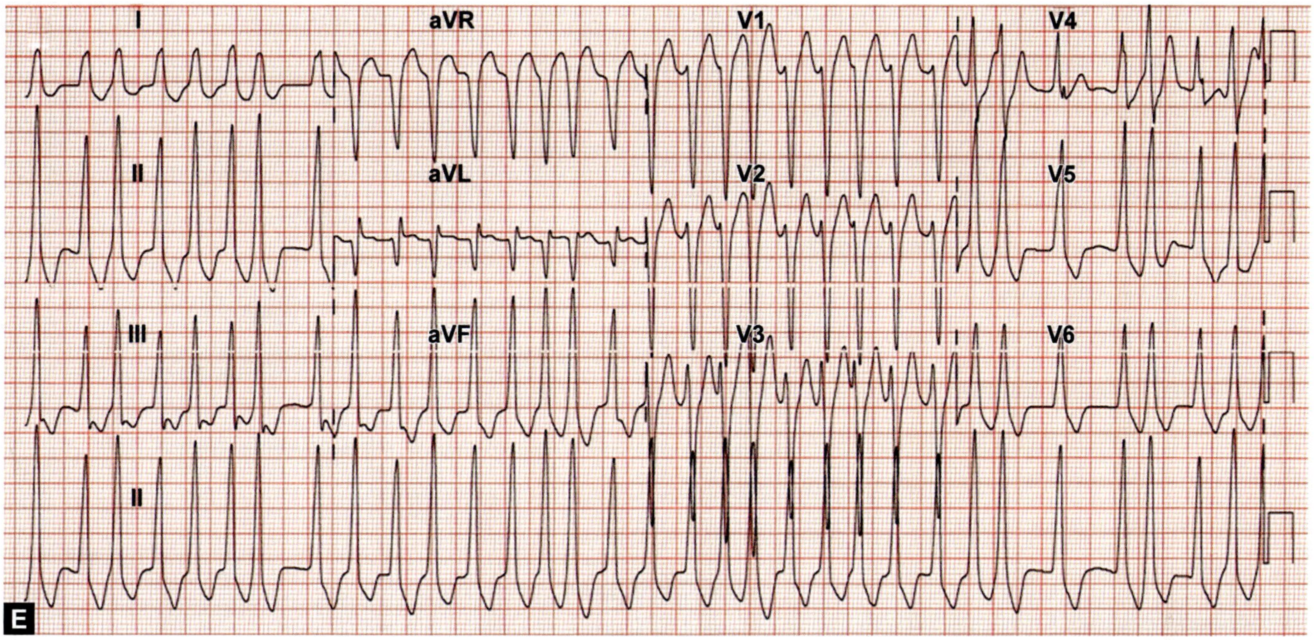

Fig. 29.1E: Atrial fibrillation in a patient with Wolff-Parkinson-White syndrome. There is occasional marked variation in the RR interval, suggestive that the rhythm is atrial fibrillation in a patient with a bypass tract, and not ventricular tachycardia. Also note the changes in the QRS width due to variable degrees of pre-excitation. (Image courtesy of Dr Ed Burns, reproduced from www.lifeinthefastlane.com).

Table 29.1: Atrial fibrillation (AF) definitions. [Adapted from Calkins H, Kuck KH, Cappato R, et al. 2012 HRS/EHRA/ECAS Expert Consensus Statement on Catheter and Surgical Ablation of Atrial Fibrillation: Recommendations for Patient Selection, Procedural Techniques, Patient Management and Follow-up, Definitions, Endpoints, and Research Trial Design. Heart Rhythm. 2012;9(4):632-96].

Term	*Definition*
Paroxysmal AF	AF that terminates spontaneously or with intervention within 7 days of onset
Persistent AF	Continuous AF that is sustained beyond 7 days
Longstanding persistent AF	Continuous AF of >12-month duration
Permanent AF	Permanent AF is used when there has been a joint decision by the patient and clinician to increase further attempts to restore and/or maintain sinus rhythm

Bleeding history or predisposition, Labile International Normalized Ratio, Elderly, Drugs/alcohol concomitantly (HAS-BLED) score (Table 29.3), and are helpful in refining the risk versus benefit ratio of anticoagulant therapy in an individual patient.

The novel oral anticoagulants (NOACs) include the direct thrombin inhibitor dabigatran and factor Xa inhibitors rivaroxaban and apixaban. NOACs offer better efficacy, safety and convenience than warfarin, but may not be chosen due to cost, presence of acute or chronic kidney disease, and concerns over the lack of a reversal agent. The efficacy of stroke prevention with aspirin is weak, with a potential for harm similar to oral anticoagulants. The 2012 European Society of Cardiology (ESC) guidelines have largely limited antiplatelet agents to those who refuse oral anticoagulants.

The LAA is considered to be the site of thrombus in many patients with AF. Surgical excision of the LAA can be considered at the time of cardiac surgery although successful occlusion is highly variable. Several percutaneous closure devices have been developed. These include the WATCHMAN™ device (Boston Scientific, Natick, Massachusetts), which involves insertion of an endocardial plug in the LAA (Figs. 29.5A to C), and the LARIAT device (SentreHeart, Inc., Redwood City, California), which involves using an epicardial snare to tie off the LAA

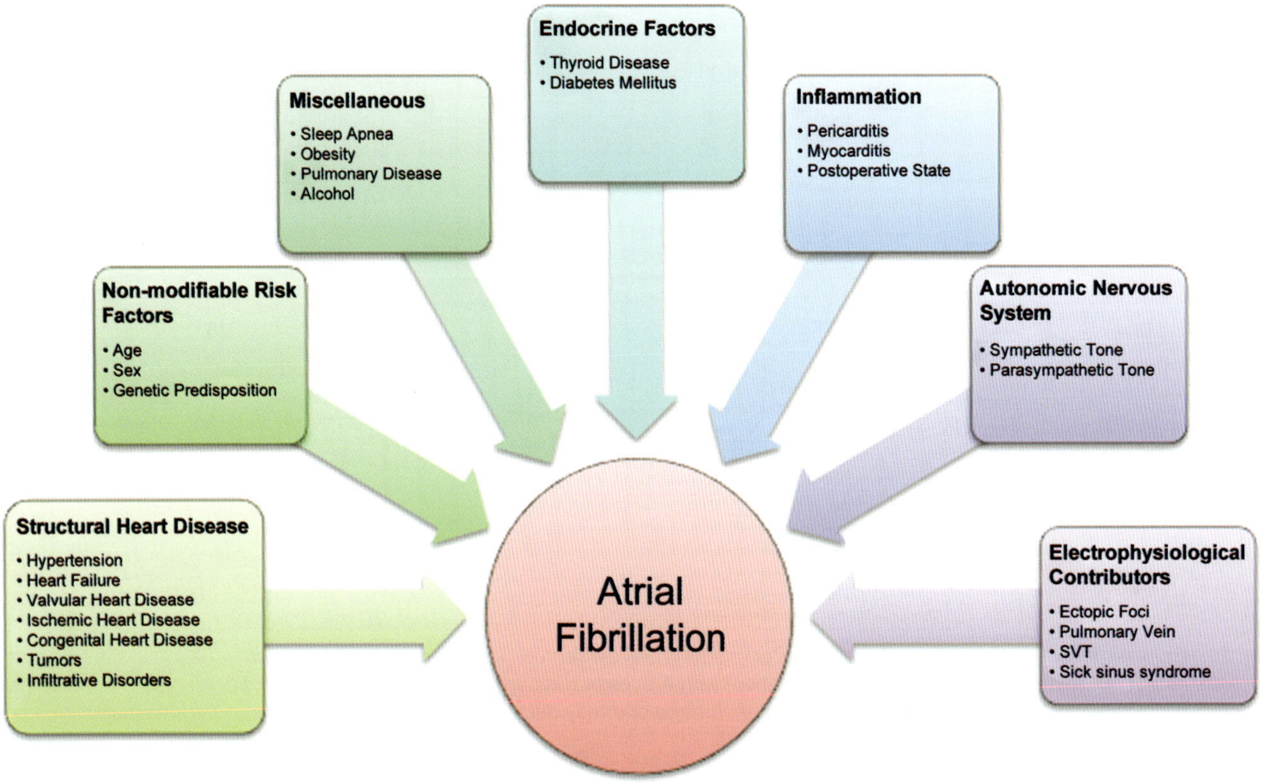

Fig. 29.2: Factors contributing to the development of atrial fibrillation. In the evaluation of a patient with atrial fibrillation, modifiable risk factors should be identified and treated. [Adapted with permission from Lubitz SA, Fischer A, Fuster V. Catheter ablation for atrial fibrillation. BMJ. 2008;336(7648):819-26].

(Figs. 29.6A to F). Closure of the LAA may be considered in patients with a high risk of stroke and contraindications to long-term oral anticoagulation.

RATE CONTROL

A rapid ventricular response in AF can cause symptoms including dyspnea, palpitations, and fatigue. Rate control may reduce symptoms and prevent the development of a tachycardia-mediated cardiomyopathy. The optimal target heart rate for adequate rate control is unknown and probably varies from patient to patient. Previous guidelines indicating low target rates have been challenged by the publication of the Rate Control Efficacy in Permanent Atrial Fibrillation: A Comparison Between Lenient Versus Strict Rate Control II (RACE II) trial, which failed to show a benefit of tighter rate control over more lenient rate control. The choice of pharmacologic agent for rate control of AF is driven by comorbidities (Flow chart. 29.3) and likelihood of drug tolerance, side effects and toxicities in an individual patient.

Atrioventricular (AV) nodal ablation in conjunction with permanent pacemaker implantation effectively controls and regularizes ventricular heart rate and, in selected patients, improves symptoms. AV junction ablation is usually reserved for elderly patients as it leads to pacemaker dependency. With this approach, no rate control medication is required, but anticoagulation to prevent thromboembolization is still required depending on the patient's stroke risk as assessed by the CHA_2DS_2-VASc system.

RHYTHM CONTROL

Long-term AF management may include attempts to restore and maintain sinus rhythm (referred to as a "rhythm control" strategy). Randomized controlled trials comparing outcomes of a rhythm versus rate control strategy have failed to show a superiority of one approach over the other. While an initial rate control strategy is reasonable for many patients (particularly older and asymptomatic patients), it is important to recognize that

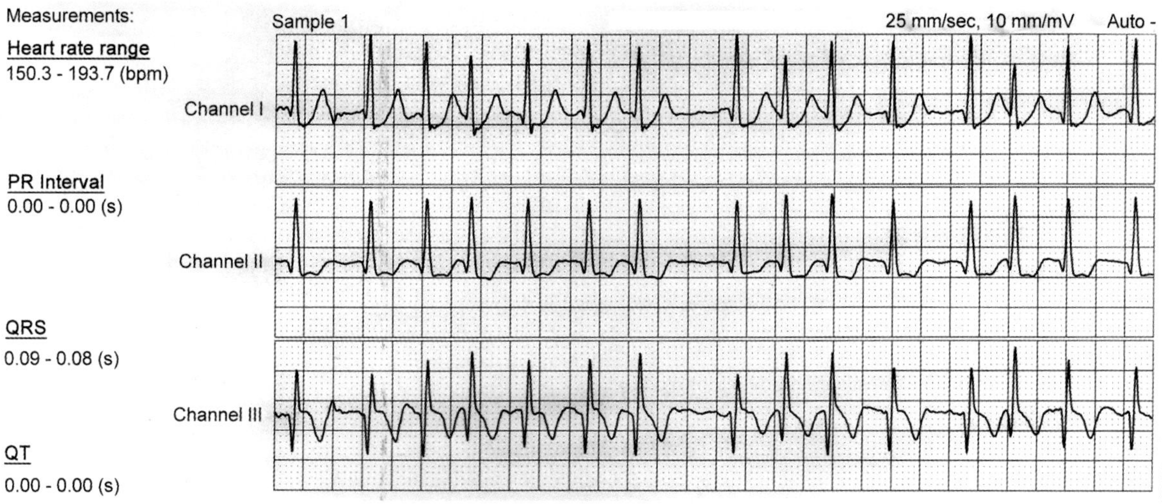

A

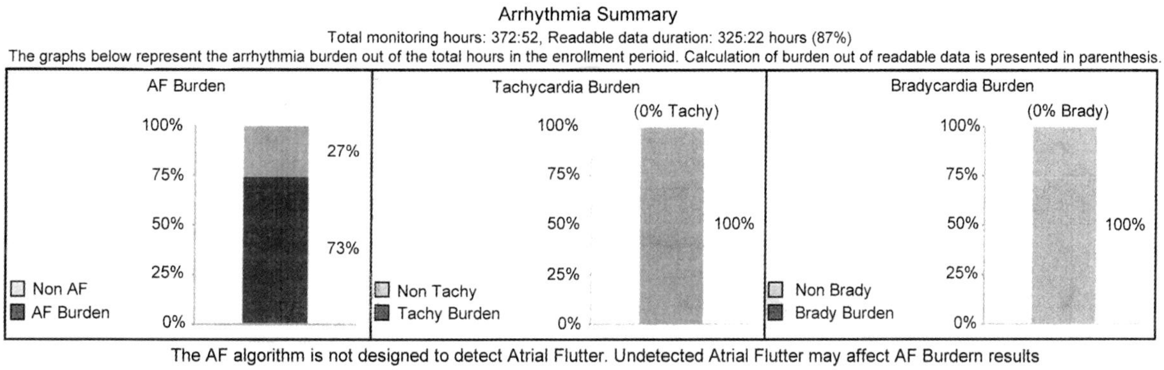

Episodes by Duration	AF	Tachy	Brady
>24 hrs	-	-	-
12-24 hrs	3 events	-	-
1-12 hrs	45 events	-	-
5-60 min	211 events	-	-
1-5 min	21 events	-	-
<1 min	-	-	-

Arrhythmia Statistics		Avg HR	Min HR	Max HR
AF		62 BPM*	23 BPM*	205 BPM*
Tachy		-		-
Brady		-	-	
Pause Quantity	3			

AF Episode	Duration	Heart Rate		Date and Time of Onset	
Longest AF	16:11:50	Avg:	56 BPM	09/24/2013	07:49 pm
Shortest AF	00:01:22	Avg:	79 BPM*	10/03/2013	09:37 am
Fastest AF	04:41:26	Max:	205 BPM	09/30/2013	05:34 am
Slowest AF	06:42:58	Min:	23 BPM	09/25/2013	11:23 pm

B

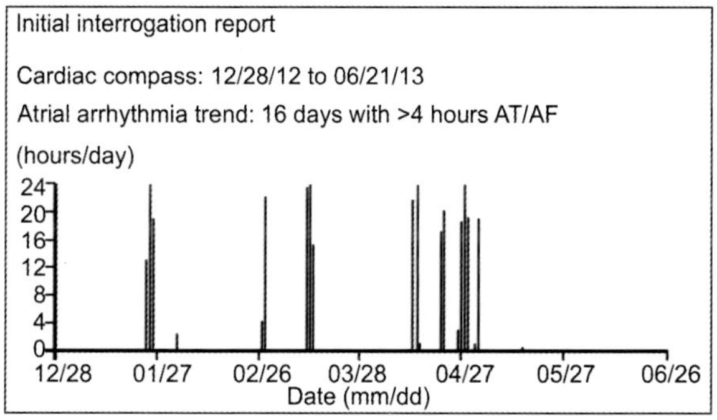

C

Figs. 29.3A to C: Cardiac monitoring for detection of atrial fibrillation (AF). (A) Holter monitor printout of an episode of AF. Frequent episodes of paroxysmal AF can be detected on 24–48-hour Holter monitoring; (B) Summary of a 4-week continuous ambulatory electrocardiogram (ECG) monitor. The summary allows one to determine information such as the duration the patient is in AF, the average, minimum and maximum heart rates, and duration of individual episodes of AF; (C) Infrequent episodes may escape detection on Holter monitor or even on several weeks of ambulatory ECG monitoring. Implantable loop recorders, which provide continuous recordings for up to 3 years, have a high sensitivity for detection of AF and allows characterization of AF burden over time and response to therapy. A sample printout is shown in Figure 29.3C. Each vertical line represents a single day (x-axis) over the course of several months while duration of episode is reflected by the height of the line (y axis from 0 hour to 24 hours).

Flow chart 29.1: General approach to patient with atrial fibrillation (AF). The cascade shown here illustrates the key domains that should be addressed in the work-up of a patient being evaluated for AF. It is necessary to reassess the status of each of these domains at the time of subsequent follow-up visits as well.

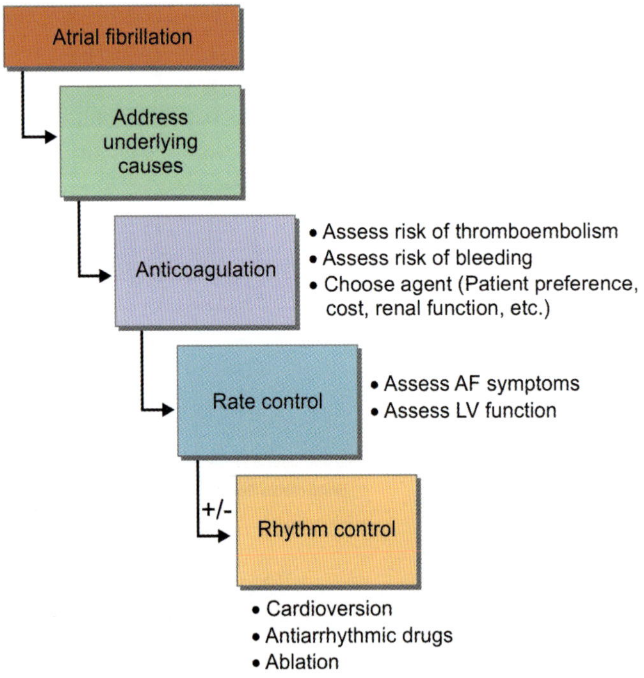

patients enrolled in clinical trials were typically older and relatively asymptomatic. The persistence of AF-related symptoms is the most compelling indication to pursue sinus rhythm. Other factors favoring a rhythm control approach include a high likelihood that sinus rhythm can be restored successfully (and safely), patient preference, younger patient age, presence of a tachycardia-mediated cardiomyopathy, first episode of AF, and AF that is precipitated by an acute illness.

An approach to selecting a rhythm control strategy is shown in Flow chart 29.4. When a rhythm control strategy is chosen, antiarrhythmic drug therapy may be selected to reduce the frequency and duration of symptomatic AF and improve quality of life. Before antiarrhythmic drug therapy is initiated, reversible causes of AF should be identified and corrected. Decisions regarding anticoagulation should be made independent of response to antiarrhythmic drug therapy and instead should be based on the individual patient's stroke risk profile. A number of different antiarrhythmic drugs are available, and selection is based on clinical parameters such as underlying structural disease [HF, significant left ventricular hypertrophy (LVH), and coronary artery disease]. Importantly, safety rather than efficacy should drive drug selection.

The cornerstone of ablation of AF is the isolation of the pulmonary veins (PVs) where discrete potentials around sleeves of myocardium extend into the veins. Haïssaguerre et al. observed in their seminal paper that the PVs serve as the source of AF initiation. This led to the development of PV isolation as a means of treating AF.

An understanding of the anatomy of the left atrium, the PVs and the surrounding structures is critical for understanding the technique of catheter ablation (Figs. 29.7A to D). A pre-procedure cardiac CT or MRI is usually performed to identify variant PV anatomy (Figs. 29.8A and B), including a single left common PV or anomalous PV.

The decision whether to pursue catheter ablation depends on a large number of variables including the type of AF (paroxysmal vs persistent vs longstanding persistent), degree of symptoms, presence of structural heart disease, candidacy for alternative options such as rate control or antiarrhythmic drug therapy, likelihood of complications and patient preference. Ablation is reserved primarily for symptomatic patients refractory to antiarrhythmic medication, although in select patients it may be appropriate as first-line treatment. The indications for catheter ablation of AF are listed in Table 29.4.

In the radiofrequency (RF) ablation procedure, energy is delivered via a steerable ablation catheter advanced into the left atrium via a trans-septal puncture (Figs. 29.9A and B). Intracardiac ultrasound guidance is helpful for guiding trans-septal puncture, identifying the location of PV ostia, and monitoring for complications such as pericardial effusion (Figs. 29.10A and B). A common approach is to isolate the PVs with a wide area circumferential lesion set (Fig. 29.11). A circular electrical mapping catheter is placed into the PV ostium, which can record PV potentials and help to document the endpoint of electrical isolation of the veins (Figs. 29.12A to D).

Alternatively, the cryoballoon technique has been developed as a means of single delivery PV isolation (Figs. 29.13A to D). Cryoballoon for AF is an established alternative to point-by-point RF ablation to achieve PV isolation.

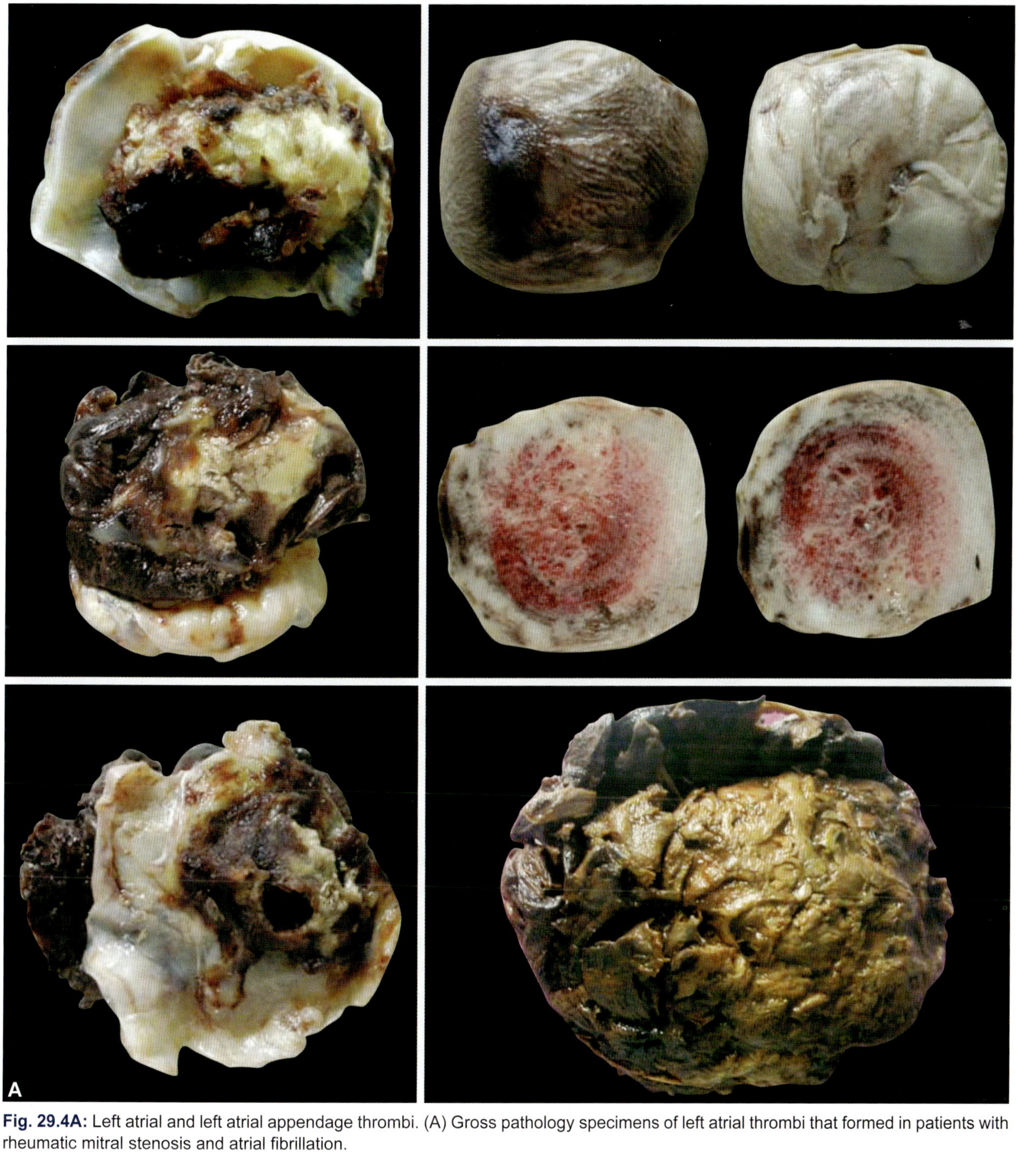

Fig. 29.4A: Left atrial and left atrial appendage thrombi. (A) Gross pathology specimens of left atrial thrombi that formed in patients with rheumatic mitral stenosis and atrial fibrillation.

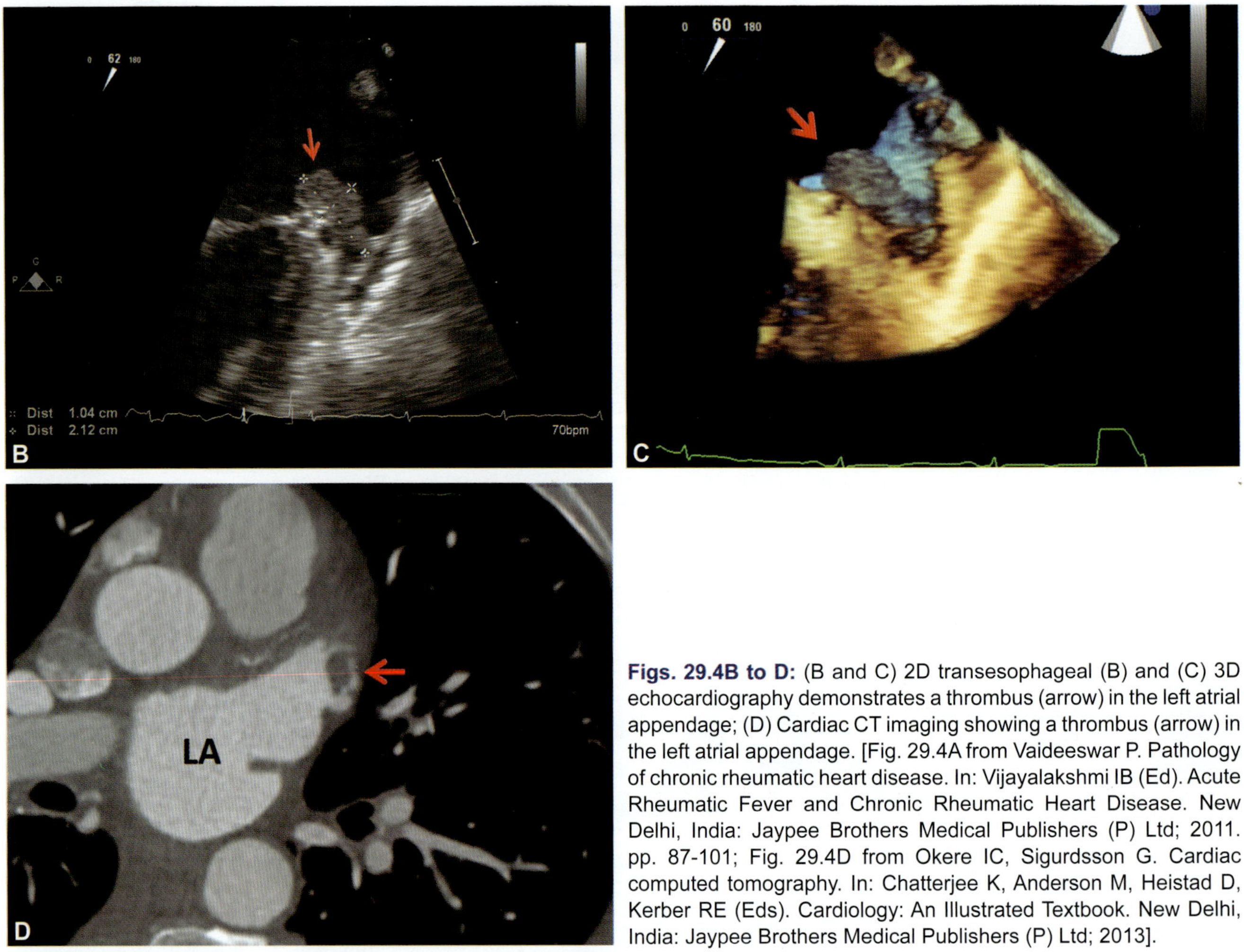

Figs. 29.4B to D: (B and C) 2D transesophageal (B) and (C) 3D echocardiography demonstrates a thrombus (arrow) in the left atrial appendage; (D) Cardiac CT imaging showing a thrombus (arrow) in the left atrial appendage. [Fig. 29.4A from Vaideeswar P. Pathology of chronic rheumatic heart disease. In: Vijayalakshmi IB (Ed). Acute Rheumatic Fever and Chronic Rheumatic Heart Disease. New Delhi, India: Jaypee Brothers Medical Publishers (P) Ltd; 2011. pp. 87-101; Fig. 29.4D from Okere IC, Sigurdsson G. Cardiac computed tomography. In: Chatterjee K, Anderson M, Heistad D, Kerber RE (Eds). Cardiology: An Illustrated Textbook. New Delhi, India: Jaypee Brothers Medical Publishers (P) Ltd; 2013].

Atrial fibrillation catheter ablation is associated with important risks of major complications including an approximately 1% rate of cardiac tamponade and an approximately 1% rate of stroke or transient ischemic attack (TIA). The esophagus is adjacent to the posterior left atrium. Atrium-esophageal fistula (Figs. 29.14A and B) or pericardial-esophageal fistula is a rare but often fatal complication and typically presents about 1–2 weeks after the procedure with dysphagia, unexplained fever, chills, sepsis, and neurological events from septic emboli. PV stenosis (Figs. 29.15A to D) may also present later after the procedure with dyspnea, cough or hemoptysis and require PV dilation or stent (Figs. 29.15A to D).

Research is continuing on questions as to whether an early rhythm control strategy may prevent progression of AF and whether a rhythm control strategy using catheter ablation is superior to current state-of-the-art therapies with either rate control or rhythm control drugs.

Surgical AF ablation has evolved from the original "cut and sew" Maze to various techniques involving RF ablation or cryoablation to achieve PV isolation and, in some cases, perform additional linear lesions and ablate ganglionic plexi on the posterior left atrium. The LAA may also be surgically excluded. Surgical AF ablation may be performed at the time of a cardiac surgery performed for other indications or as a stand-alone procedure (Figs. 29.16A to C).

TACHY-BRADY SYNDROME

Pharmacological attempts at either rate control or rhythm control can be associated with tachy-brady syndrome.

Table 29.2: The CHA_2DS_2-VASc scoring system and the corresponding stroke rate associated with each score. (CHF: Congestive heart failure; LVEF: Left ventricular ejection fraction; TIA: Transient ischemic attack).

Risk factor	*Points*
CHF or LVEF ≤40%	1
Hypertension	1
Diabetes	1
Vascular disease	1
Age 65–74 years	1
Female sex	1
Age ≥ 75 years	2
Stroke/TIA/thromboembolism	2
Maximum score	9

CHA_2DS_2-VASc score	*Stroke rate (%/year)* [a]
0	0%
1	1.3%
2	2.2%
3	3.2%
4	4.0%
5	6.7%
6	9.8%
7	9.6%
8	6.7%
9	15.2%

[a]Adjusted stroke rates based on data Lip GY, Nieuwlaat R, Pisters R, et al. Refining clinical risk stratification for predicting stroke and thromboembolism in atrial fibrillation using a novel risk factor-based approach: the Euro Heart survey on atrial fibrillation. Chest. 2010;137(2):263-72. Actual rates of stroke might vary in contemporary cohorts from these estimates.

Table 29.3: The HAS-BLED Bleeding Risk Score. [Table adapted from Pisters R, Lane DA, Nieuwlaat R, et al. A novel user-friendly score (HAS-BLED) to assess 1-year risk of major bleeding in atrial fibrillation patients: The Euro Heart Survey. Chest. 2010;138(5):1093-100]. (INR: International normalized ratio).

Clinical characteristic	*Points*
Hypertension	1
Stroke	1
Bleeding	1
Labile INRs	1
Elderly (age > 65 years)	1
Abnormal renal and liver function (1 point each)	1 or 2
Drugs or alcohol (1 point each)	1 or 2
Maximum score	9

Flow chart. 29.2: Choice of antithrombotic therapy for atrial fibrillation (AF). The choice of antithrombotic therapy should be based on the absolute risks of stroke and bleeding and the net clinical benefit in an individual patient. Note that females who are age < 65 years and have lone AF (although because of their sex have a CHA_2DS_2-VASc score of 1) are considered low risk and no antithrombotic therapy is recommended. Preference is given to the novel oral anticoagulants (NOACs) over warfarin for most patients. Given the limited efficacy of antiplatelet therapy despite having a bleeding risk, the 2012 European Society of Cardiology (ESC) Guidelines have largely limited antiplatelet agents to those who refuse any oral anticoagulant (OAC) or cannot tolerate anticoagulants for reasons unrelated to bleeding. (Algorithm modified from Camm AJ, Lip GY, De Caterina R, et al. 2012 focused update of the ESC Guidelines for the management of atrial fibrillation: an update of the 2010 ESC Guidelines for the management of atrial fibrillation. Developed with the special contribution of the European Heart Rhythm Association. Eur Heart J. 2012;33(21):2719-47). [AF: Atrial fibrillation; NOAC: Novel oral anticoagulant includes factor Xa inhibitors (rivaroxaban and apixaban) and direct thrombin inhibitor (dabigatran)].

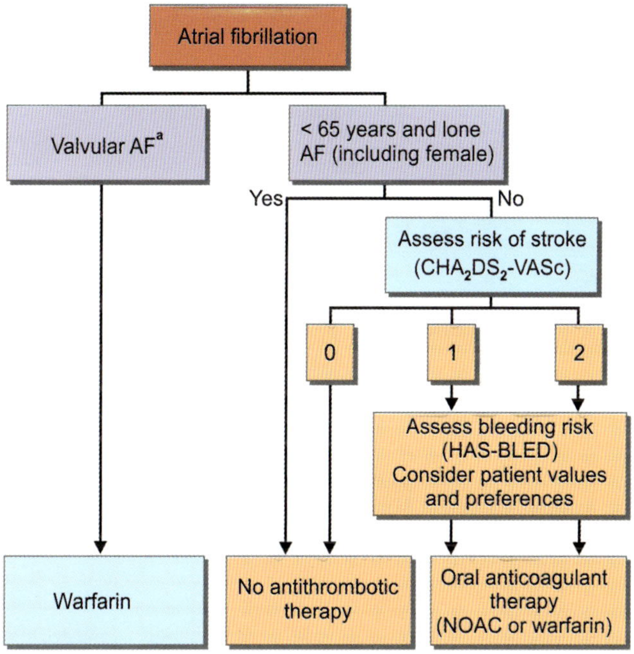

[a]Includes rheumatic valvular disease and prosthetic valves.

The prolonged pause (Fig. 29.17) that may be observed in patients with tachy-brady syndrome results when AF abruptly or spontaneously terminates, and the underlying sinus node is slow to recover (i.e. conversion or off-set pause). Patients in whom a prolonged pause results in symptoms, such as syncope, may require pacemaker implantation.

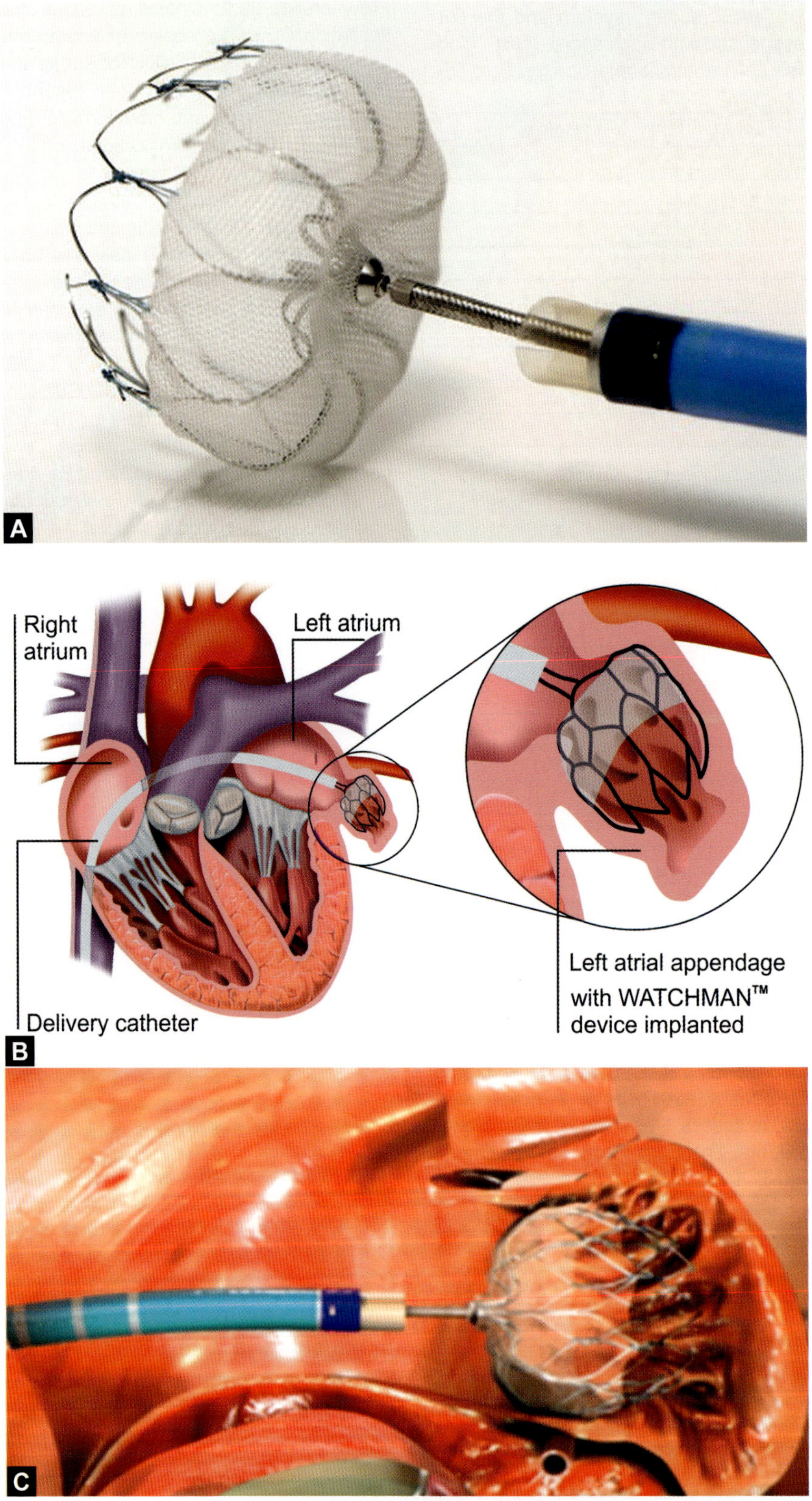

Figs. 29.5A to C: Percutaneous exclusion of the left atrial appendage (LAA) with the WATCHMAN™ LAA closure device. (A) WATCHMAN™ LAA closure device; (B) Schematic of device insertion; (C) Zoomed image of WATCHMAN™ LAA closure deployment in the LAA. (Images courtesy of Boston Scientific).

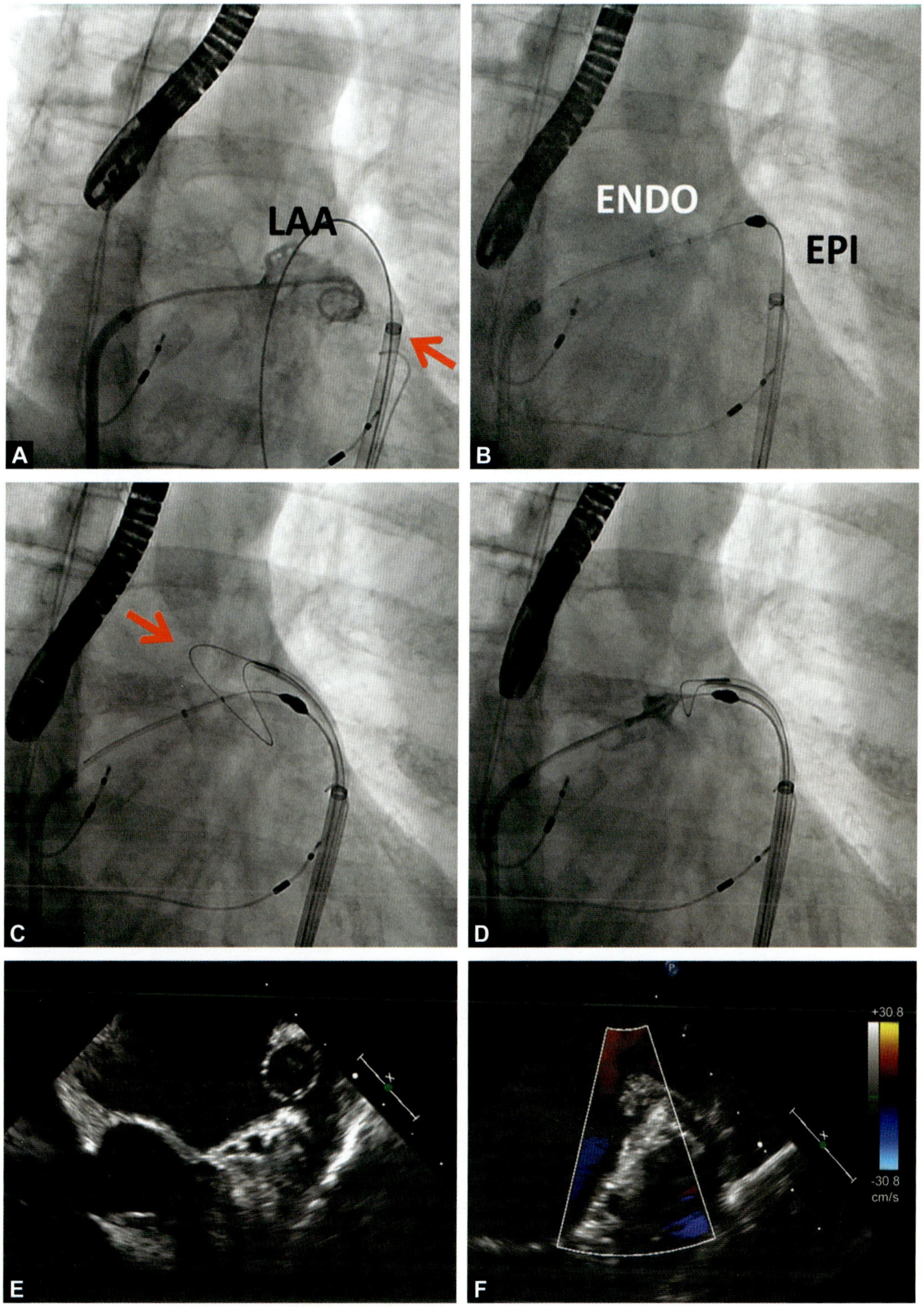

Figs. 29.6A to F: Percutaneous left atrial appendage (LAA) exclusion using a LARIAT® Snare device. (A) Contrast injection from a pigtail catheter placed in the left atrium via a trans-septal puncture delineates the LAA in the left anterior oblique view. The soft-tipped epicardial sheath is in place; (B) The endocardial and epicardial magnet-tipped wires are joined to form the rail for the snare; (C) Epicardial LARIAT® snare is placed at the LAA ostium; (D) The snare is tightened as the LAA is ligated and repeat left atrial angiogram shows exclusion of the LAA; (E) Transesophageal echocardiographic imaging of the LAA at baseline showing an open balloon inside the LAA; (F) Acute lariat exclusion with color Doppler images post suture deployment showing complete closure of the LAA.

Flow chart 29.3: Approach to selecting drug therapy for ventricular rate control of atrial fibrillation. The choice of drugs is based on lifestyle and underlying disease. Small doses of beta 1-selective blockers may be used in patients with chronic obstructive pulmonary disease (COPD) if rate control is not adequate with non-dihydropyridine calcium channel antagonists and digoxin. In rare cases, amiodarone may also be used for rate control in patients who are not candidates or do not respond to other agents. [Image modified from Camm AJ, Lip GY, De Caterina R, et al. 2012 focused update of the ESC Guidelines for the management of atrial fibrillation: an update of the 2010 ESC Guidelines for the management of atrial fibrillation. Developed with the special contribution of the European Heart Rhythm Association. Eur Heart J. 2012;33(21):2719-47].

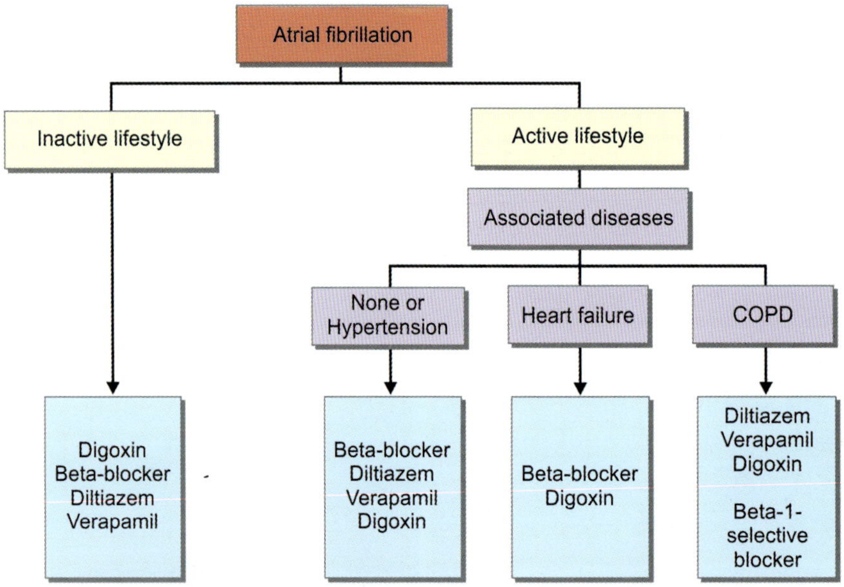

Flow chart 29.4: Antiarrhythmic drugs and atrial fibrillation (AF) ablation for rhythm control in AF. [Image modified from Camm AJ, Lip GY, De Caterina R, et al. 2012 focused update of the ESC Guidelines for the management of atrial fibrillation: an update of the 2010 ESC Guidelines for the management of atrial fibrillation. Developed with the special contribution of the European Heart Rhythm Association. Eur Heart J. 2012;33(21):2719-47]. (AF: Atrial fibrillation; HF: Heart failure).

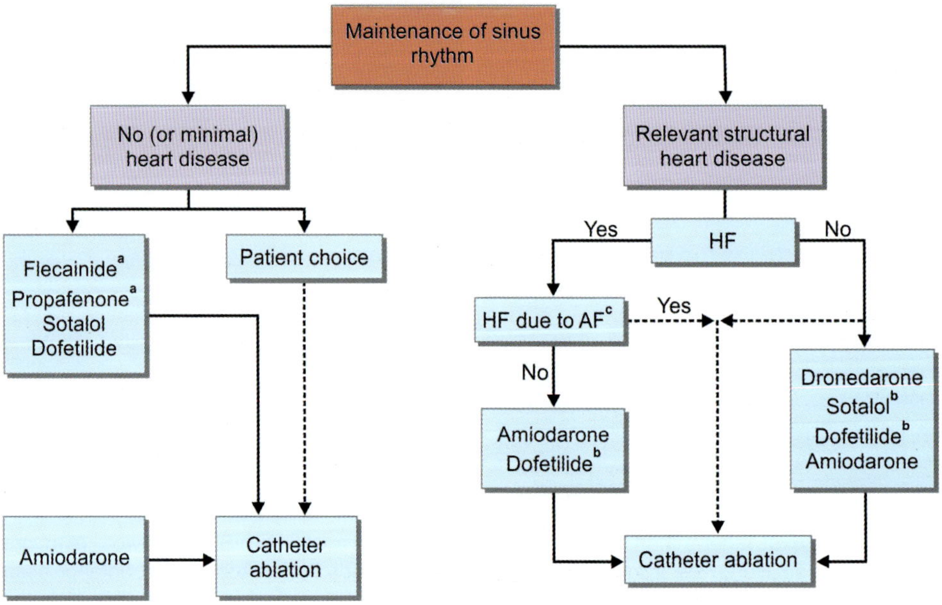

[a]Avoid in coronary heart disease

[b]Not recommended with significant left ventricular hypertrophy (wall thickness > 1.5 cm)

[c]Heart failure due to AF (tachycardiomyopathy).

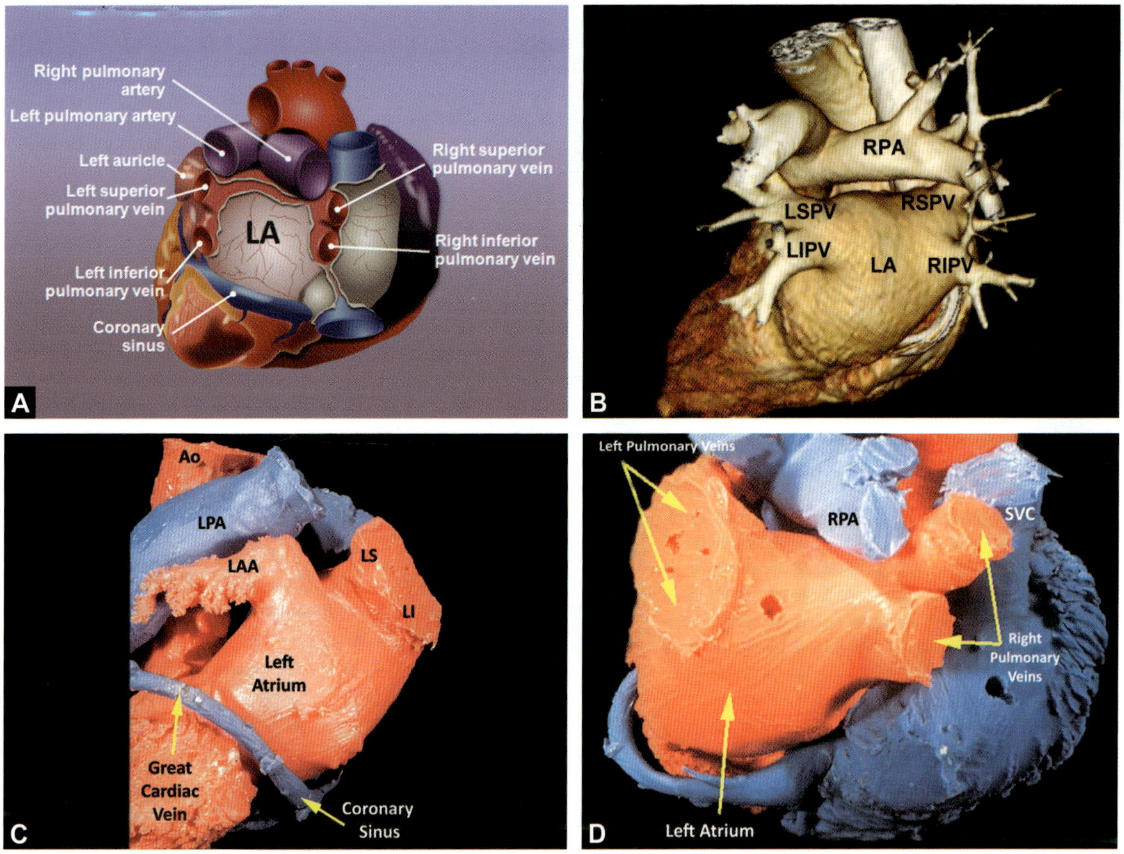

Figs. 29.7A to D: Pulmonary vein (PV) anatomy. (A) Illustration of the left atrium (LA), PVs, and surrounding structures; (B) Corresponding posterior view of a 3D CT scan reconstruction of the heart illustrating relationship of the PVs to the LA and other vascular structures. Typically there are two left-sided and two right-sided PVs as shown here; (C) The endocast viewed from the left lateral aspect shows the relationship of the left atrial appendage (LAA) to the left PVs and the great cardiac vein. The ridge between the LAA and the left superior PV (LS) is a challenging location to get stability during catheter ablation; (D) The endocast viewed from the posterior aspect shows the relationship of the PVs to the other cardiac structures. The right pulmonary artery (RPA) passes immediately above the roof of the LA and the coronary sinus (CS) passes inferior to the inferior wall of the LA. (Images courtesy of Dr Robert Anderson, Institute of Genetic Medicine, Newcastle University, United Kingdom and Medtronic, Inc.). (Ao: Ascending aorta; IVC: Inferior vena cava; LI: Left inferior pulmonary vein; LPA: Left pulmonary artery; LS: Left superior pulmonary vein; RPA: Right pulmonary artery; LA: Left atrium; LIPV: Left inferior pulmonary vein; LSPV: Left superior pulmonary vein; RIPV: Right inferior pulmonary vein; RPA: Right pulmonary artery; RSPV: Right superior pulmonary vein; SVC: Superior vena cava).

Table 29.4: 2012 Heart Rhythm Society (HRS)/European Heart Rhythm Association (EHRA)/European Cardiac Arrhythmia Society (ECAS) expert consensus statement on indications for catheter ablation of atrial fibrillation. [Adapted from data in Calkins H, Kuck KH, Cappato R, et al. 2012 HRS/EHRA/ECAS Expert Consensus Statement on Catheter and Surgical Ablation of Atrial Fibrillation: Recommendations for Patient Selection, Procedural Techniques, Patient Management and Follow-up, Definitions, Endpoints, and Research Trial Design. Heart Rhythm. 2012;9(4):632-96].

Indication for catheter ablation of atrial fibrillation (AF)	*Class*	*Level*
Symptomatic AF refractory or intolerant to at least one Class 1 or 3 antiarrhythmic		
Paroxysmal: Catheter ablation is recommended	I	A
Persistent: Catheter ablation is reasonable	IIa	B
Longstanding persistent: Catheter ablation is reasonable	IIb	B
Symptomatic AF prior to initiation of Class 1 or 3 antiarrhythmic		
Paroxysmal: Catheter ablation is reasonable	IIa	B
Persistent: Catheter ablation may be considered	IIb	C
Longstanding persistent: Catheter ablation may be considered	IIb	C

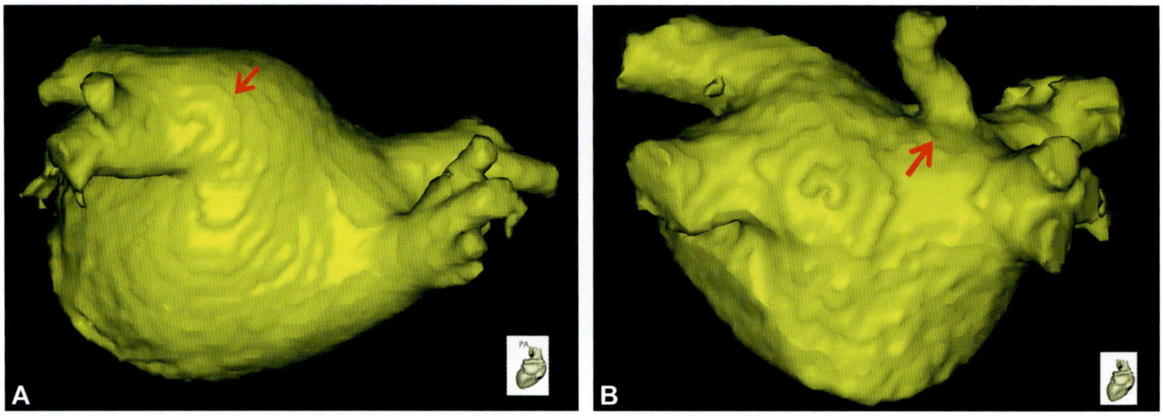

Figs. 29.8A and B: Variations in pulmonary vein (PV) anatomy. (A) The anatomy of the PV varies considerably between patients. A large left common PV (arrow) is shown; (B) Infrequently, there is an accessory PV joining the posterior wall or roof of the LA (arrow). The presence of an anomalous PV would impact the lesion set delivered for ablation and typically CT or magnetic resonance (MR) imaging is performed prior to the atrial fibrillation (AF) ablation procedure.

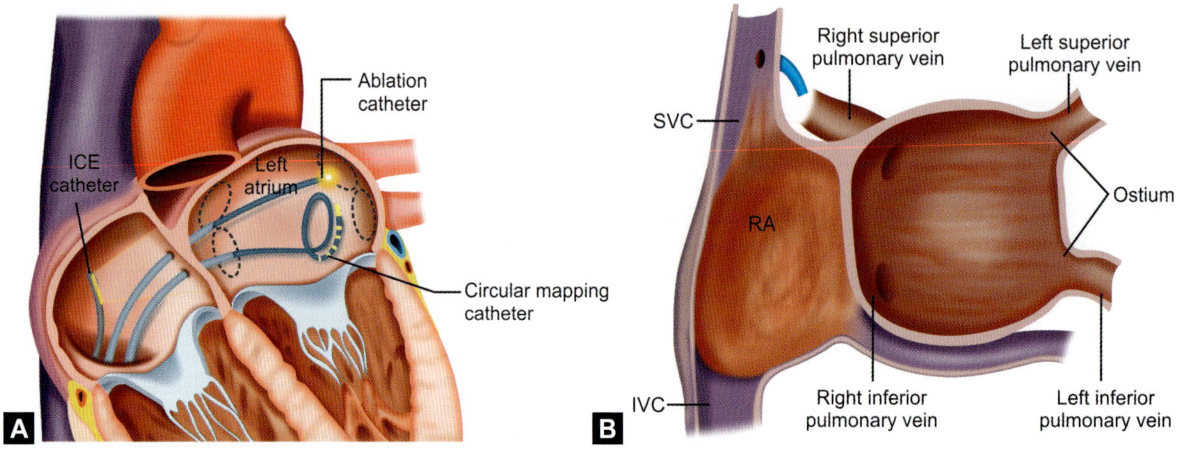

Figs. 29.9A and B: Catheter placement during atrial fibrillation ablation. An ablation catheter and circular mapping catheter is advanced from the femoral vein into the heart and via a trans-septal puncture into the left atrium. An intracardiac echocardiography (ICE) catheter is shown in the image on the left.

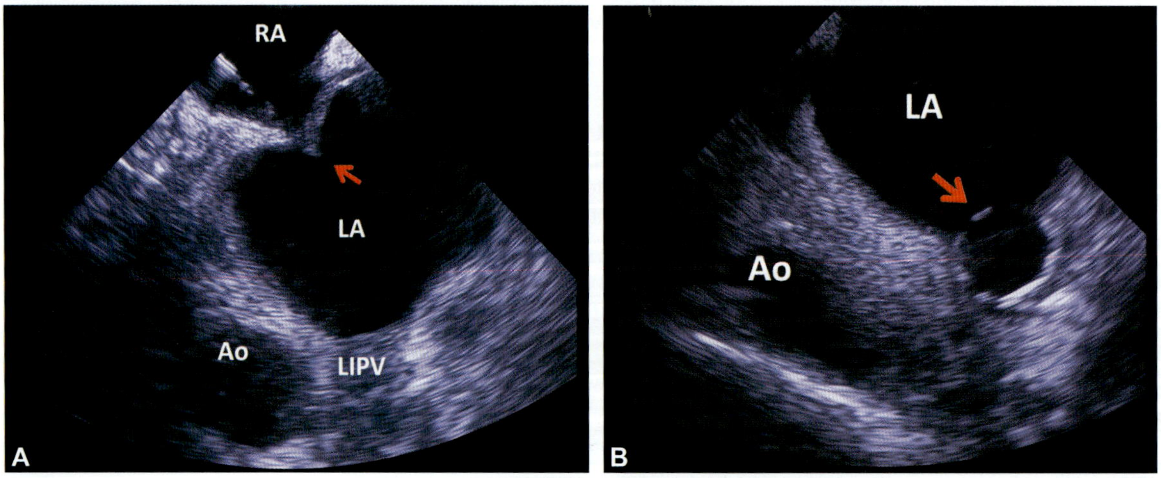

Figs. 29.10A and B: Intracardiac echocardiography (ICE) during catheter ablation for atrial fibrillation. (A) ICE-guided trans-septal puncture demonstrating tenting of the fossa ovalis with the Brockenbrough needle (arrow); (B) Circular mapping catheter (Lasso) is positioned at the ostium of a left common pulmonary vein. (Ao: Ascending aorta; LA: Left atrium; LIPV: Left inferior pulmonary vein; RA: Right atrium).

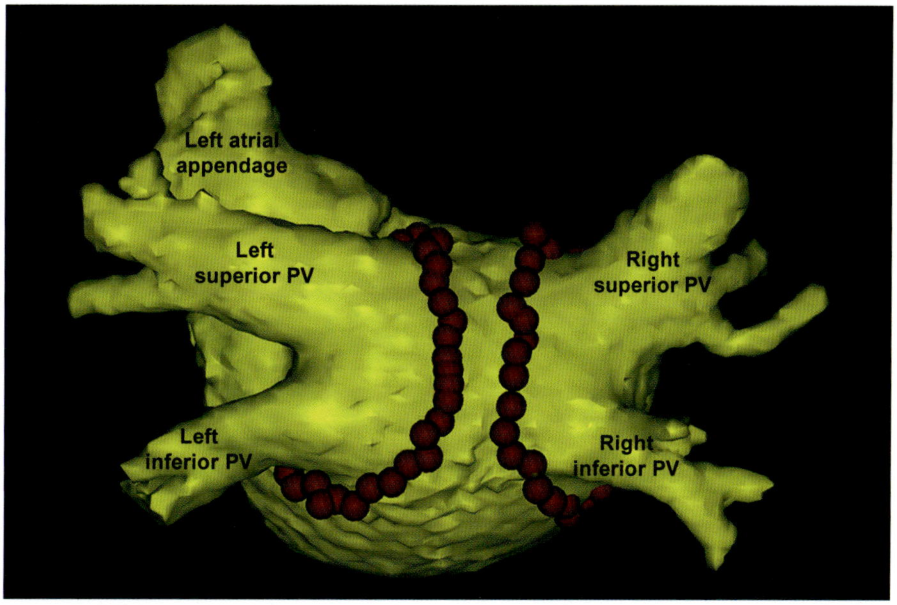

Fig. 29.11: Pulmonary vein isolation lesion set. A standard approach to atrial fibrillation (AF) ablation is to isolate the pulmonary veins. In this case, a wide area circumferential lesion set was performed in which the veins were isolated in pairs on each side. A posteroanterior (PA) view is shown with the lesions (red dots) superimposed on a 3D reconstruction of the left atrium from the pre-procedure cardiac CT scan.

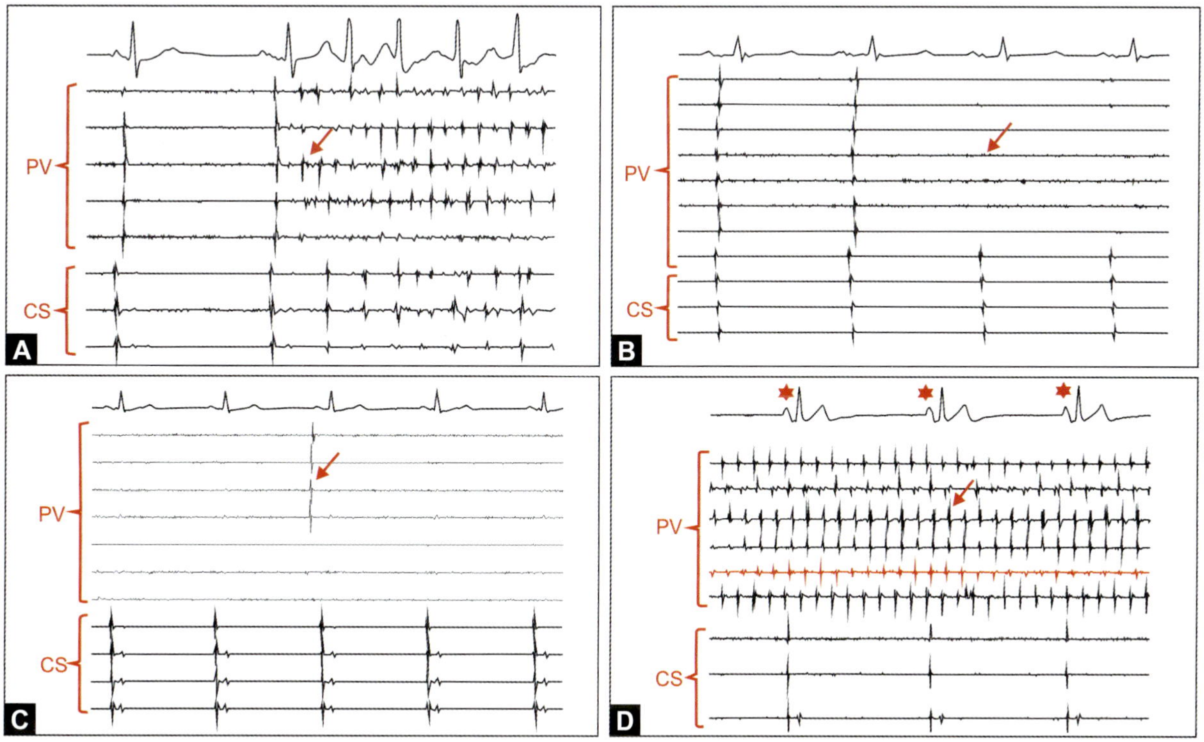

Figs. 29.12A to D: Electrical recordings from the pulmonary veins (PVs). (A) Sinus rhythm is interrupted by the onset of atrial fibrillation preceded by rapid firing from within the PV; (B) The sudden loss of PV electrical activity (arrow) is seen during radiofrequency (RF) ablation due to entrance block into the vein; (C) After PV isolation, spontaneous dissociated firing of the PV tissue may be seen (arrow) indicating that the myocardial vein sleeve is electrically disconnected from the rest of the left atrium and is capable of spontaneous firing; (D) In rare cases, the electrically isolated PV tissue has persistent rapid firing (arrow) while the heart remains in sinus rhythm(*). A single surface lead (lead II) is seen at the top of the tracings. Intracardiac electrograms are obtained from electrodes placed in the PV and coronary sinus (CS).

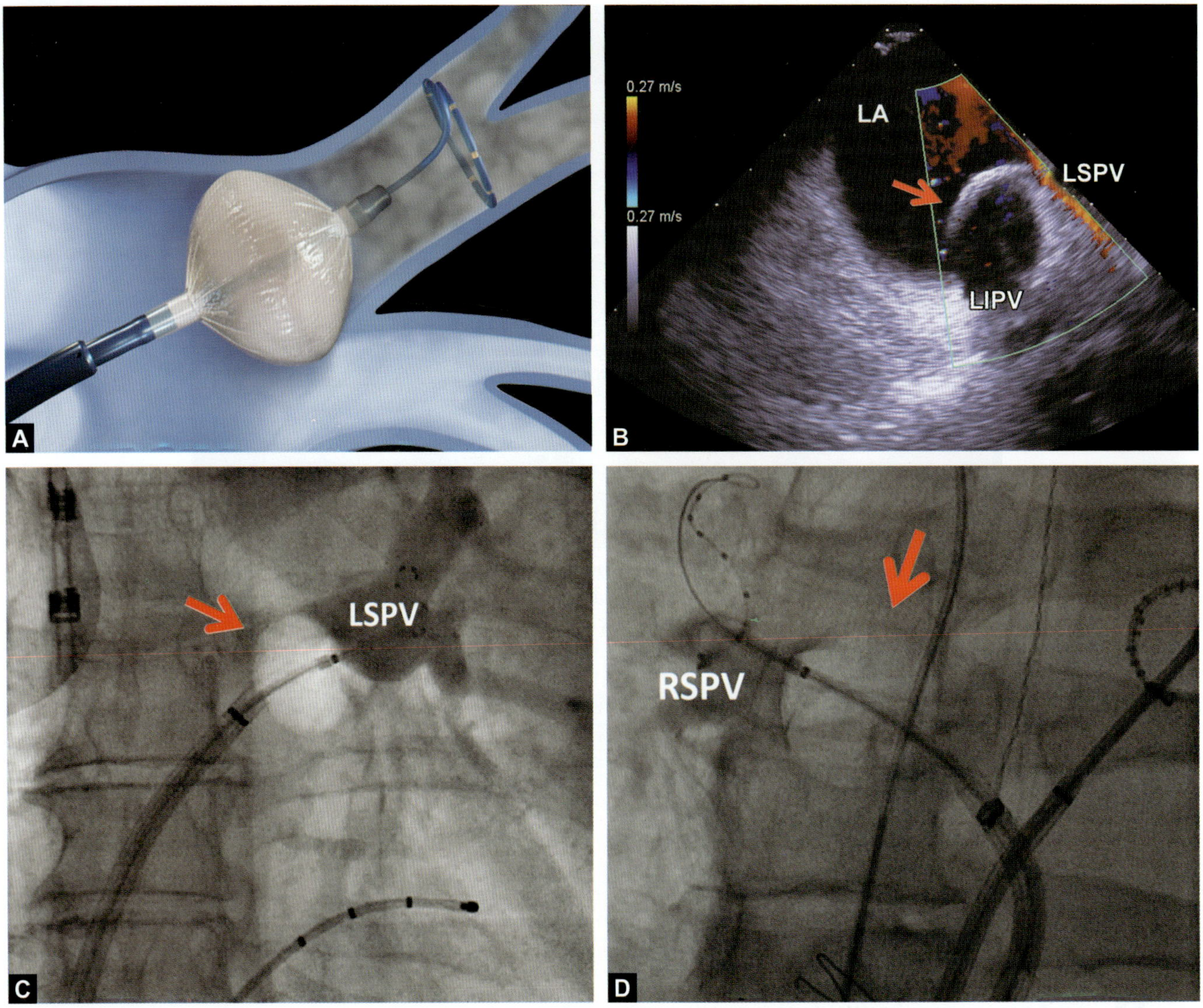

Figs. 29.13A to D: Cryoballoon ablation for atrial fibrillation (AF). (A) The cryoballoon is inflated in the left atrium (LA) and advanced to the ostium of the left superior pulmonary vein (LSPV). During the freeze, areas of tissue contacting the balloon are ablated. A circular mapping catheter is also advanced into the vein via the cryoballoon lumen and can be used to monitor for loss of pulmonary vein (PV) electrical activity during freezes; (B) Intracardiac echocardiography (ICE) is used to verify PV occlusion using color Doppler; The balloon is inflated (arrow) in the left inferior pulmonary vein (LIPV) and no flow from the LIPV is seen indicating good occlusion (an indicator of a successful freeze). A color jet is seen representing flow from the adjacent LSPV in the LA; (C) The cryoballoon is inflated and contrast injection into the LSPV shows complete occlusion. A coronary sinus catheter can also be seen; (D) Right anterior oblique view of the cryoballoon (arrow) in the antrum of the right superior pulmonary vein (RSPV). Contrast injection again demonstrates good occlusion this time of the RSPV. A circumferential "lasso" mapping can also be seen positioned in the LSPV. (Figs. 29.13A and C courtesy of Medtronic, Minneapolis, Minnesota).

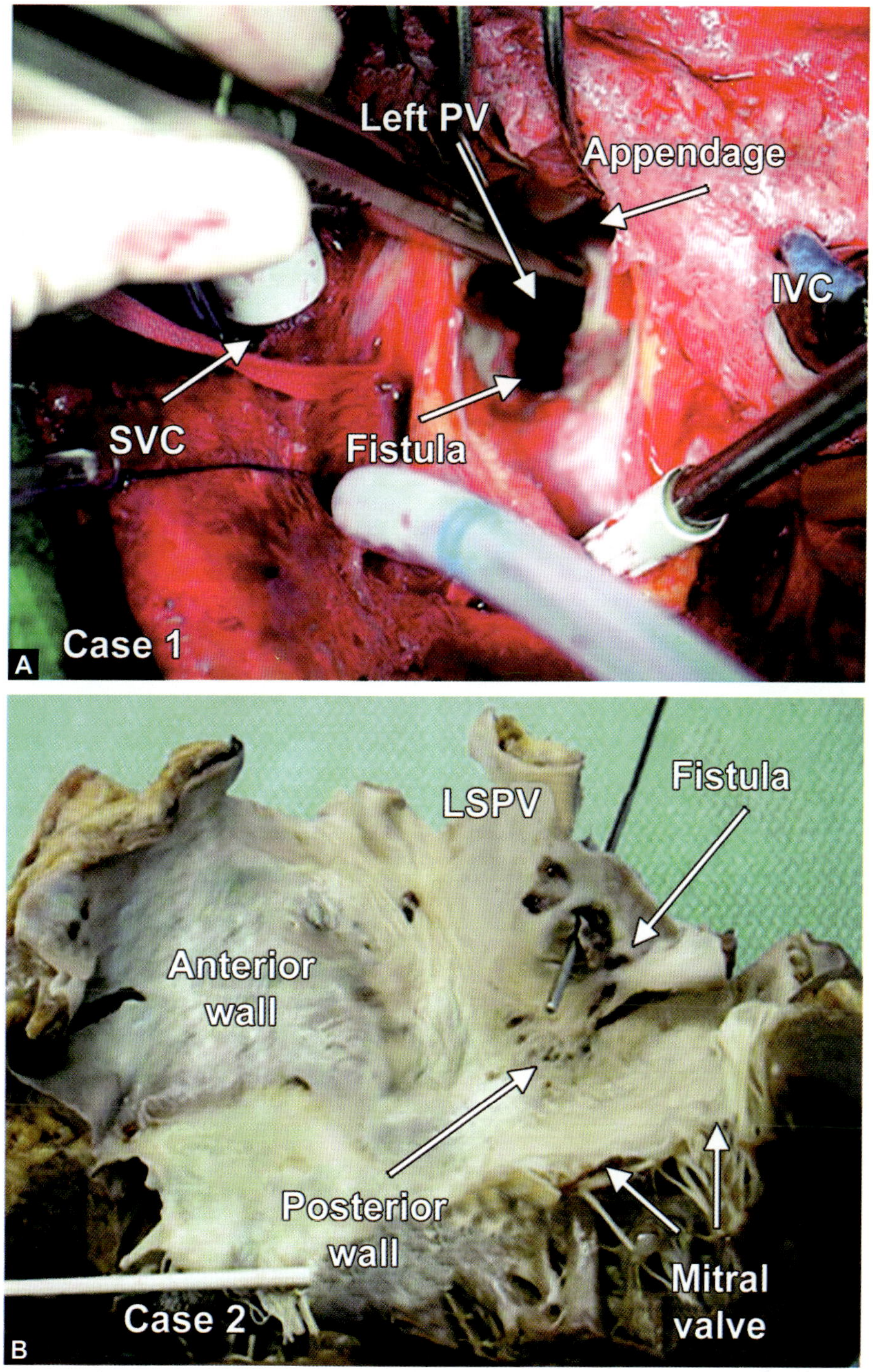

Figs. 29.14A and B: Anatomic demonstration of atrio-esophageal fistulas. (A) Intraoperative photograph taken from patient's right side with head to left, highlighting atrio-esophageal fistula arising medial to left pulmonary vein (PV) ostia; (B) Left atrium (LA) was incised near left superior PV and opened in book fashion, with anterior wall on left and posterior wall on right. Probe passes through fistula, which was on posterior wall near left superior PV. [Image used with permission from Pappone C, Oral H, Santinelli V, et al. Atrio-esophageal fistula as a complication of percutaneous transcatheter ablation of atrial fibrillation. Circulation. 2004;109(22):2724-6]. (IVC: Inferior vena cava; LSPV: Left superior pulmonary vein; SVC: Superior vena cava).

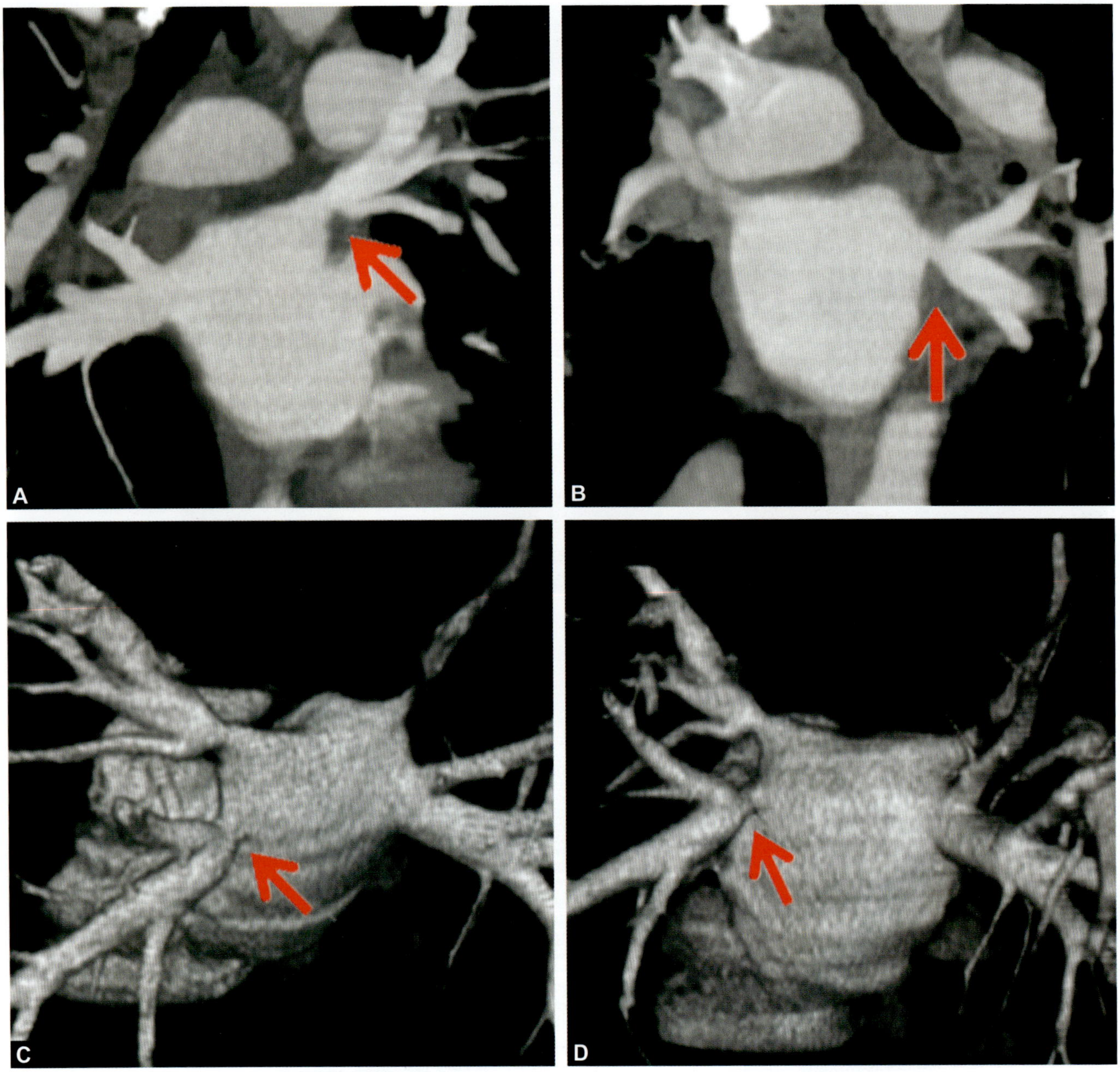

Figs. 29.15A to D: Pulmonary vein stenosis (arrows) seen using CT (A and B) 2D and (C and D) 3D imaging. Pulmonary vein stenosis will not result if ablation delivery is kept proximal to the pulmonary vein ostium. (Image used with permission from Sehar N, Mears J, Bisco S, et al. Anatomic guidance for ablation: atrial flutter, fibrillation, and outflow tract ventricular tachycardia. Indian Pacing Electrophysiol J. 2010;10:339-56).

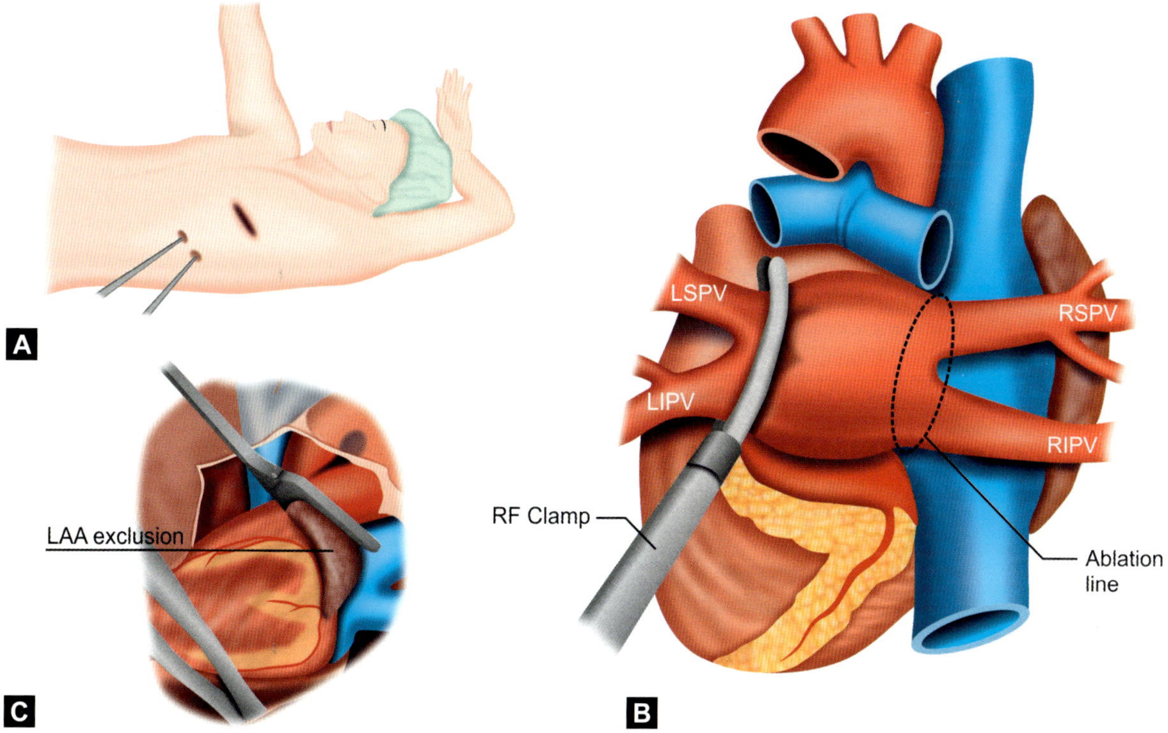

Figs. 29.16A to C: Minimally invasive surgical atrial fibrillation (AF) ablation. (A) Illustration depicts a surgical approach to AF in which the a series of small bilateral incisions is used to gain access to the beating heart; (B) Bipolar radiofrequency energy is delivered via a specialized surgical device at the pulmonary vein-left atrial junctions bilaterally to achieve pulmonary vein isolation; (C) Additionally during the procedure, the left atrial appendage is often surgically excluded using a specialized device.

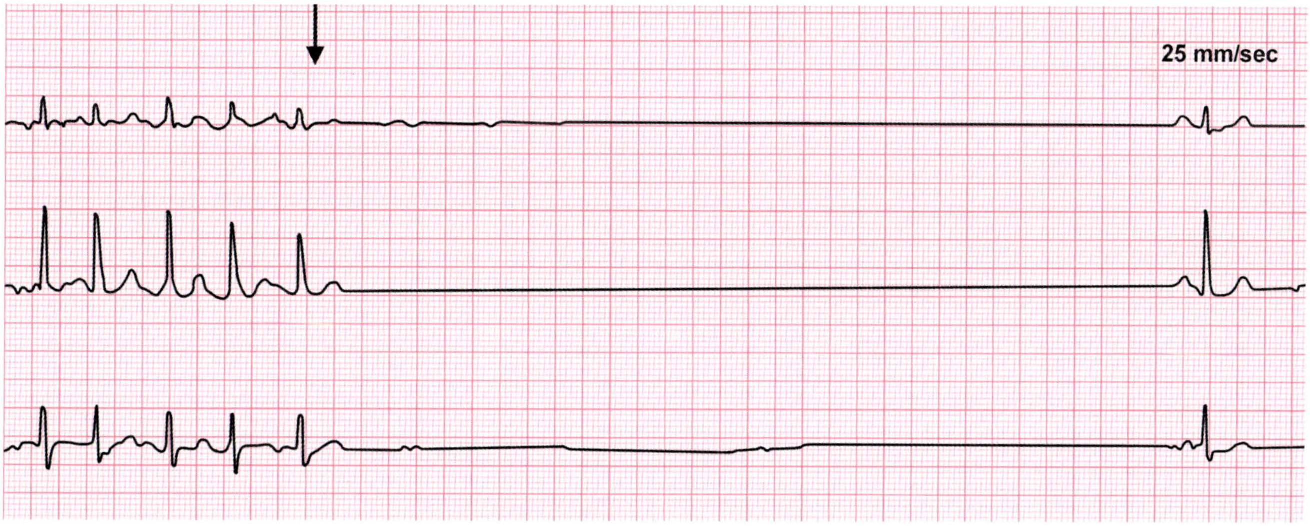

Fig. 29.17: Tachy-Brady syndrome. A prolonged pause results when atrial fibrillation abruptly terminates (arrow) and the underlying sinus node is slow to recover ("conversion" or "off-set" pause). Pharmacological attempts at either rate control or rhythm control can be associated with tachy-brady and the need for pacemaker implantation. [Image from Sullivan RM, Olshansky B, Martins JB, et al. Ambulatory electrocardiographic monitoring. In: Chatterjee K, Anderson M, Heistad D, Kerber RE (Eds). Cardiology: An Illustrated Textbook. New Delhi, India: Jaypee Brothers Medical Publishers (P) Ltd; 2013].

VIDEO LEGEND

Video 29.1: Transesophageal echocardiography (TEE) video clip showing thrombus in the left atrial appendage.

REFERENCES

Calkins H. Catheter ablation to maintain sinus rhythm. Circulation. 2012;125(11):1439-45.

Calkins H, Kuck KH, Cappato R, et al. 2012 HRS/EHRA/ECAS Expert Consensus Statement on Catheter and Surgical Ablation of Atrial Fibrillation: Recommendations for Patient Selection, Procedural Techniques, Patient Management and Follow-up, Definitions, Endpoints, and Research Trial Design. Heart Rhythm. 2012;9(4):632-96.

Camm AJ, Kirchhof P, Lip GY, et al. Guidelines for the management of atrial fibrillation: the Task Force for the Management of Atrial Fibrillation of the European Society of Cardiology (ESC). Eur Heart J. 2010;31(19):2369-429.

Haïssaguerre M, Jaïs P, Shah DC, et al. Spontaneous initiation of atrial fibrillation by ectopic beats originating in the pulmonary veins. N Engl J Med. 1998;339(10):659-66.

Lip GY, Nieuwlaat R, Pisters R, et al. Refining clinical risk stratification for predicting stroke and thromboembolism in atrial fibrillation using a novel risk factor-based approach: the euro heart survey on atrial fibrillation. Chest. 2010;137(2):263-72.

Pisters R, Lane DA, Nieuwlaat R, et al. A novel user-friendly score (HAS-BLED) to assess 1-year risk of major bleeding in atrial fibrillation patients: The Euro Heart Survey. Chest. 2010;138(5):1093-100.

Zimetbaum P. Antiarrhythmic drug therapy for atrial fibrillation. Circulation. 2012;125(2):381-9.

CHAPTER

30

Atrial Flutter

Gregory K Feld, Thomas J McGarry

INTRODUCTION

Typical (or reverse typical) atrial flutter (AFL) (Figs. 30.1 to 30.3), also known as cavotricuspid isthmus (CTI) dependent AFL, is a common atrial arrhythmia, often occurring in association with atrial fibrillation (AF). It can cause significant symptoms and serious adverse effects including embolic stroke, myocardial ischemia and infarction, and, rarely, a tachycardia-induced cardiomyopathy resulting from rapid atrioventricular (AV) conduction.

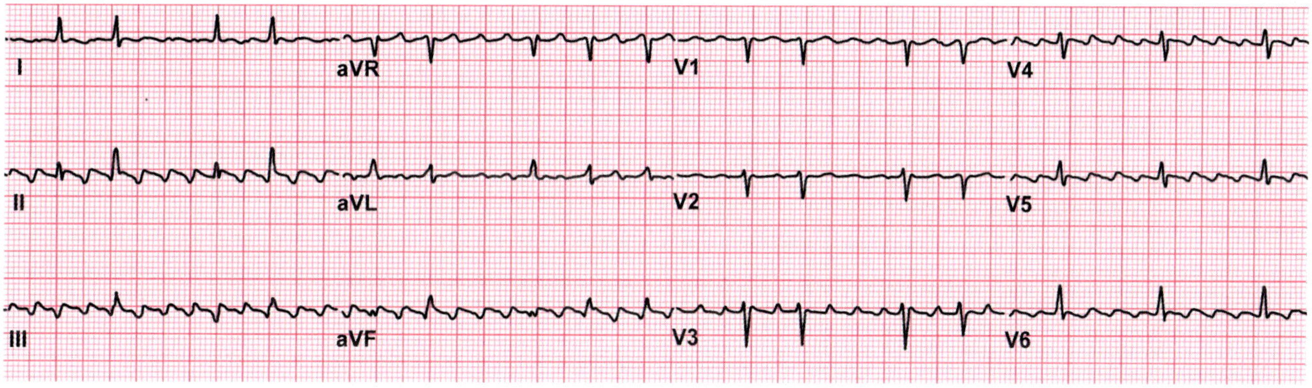

Fig. 30.1A: 12-lead electrocardiogram (ECG) showing typical atrial flutter (AFL). There are "saw-tooth" flutter waves, with negative deflection in the inferior leads. (Image courtesy of Levine GN, MD).

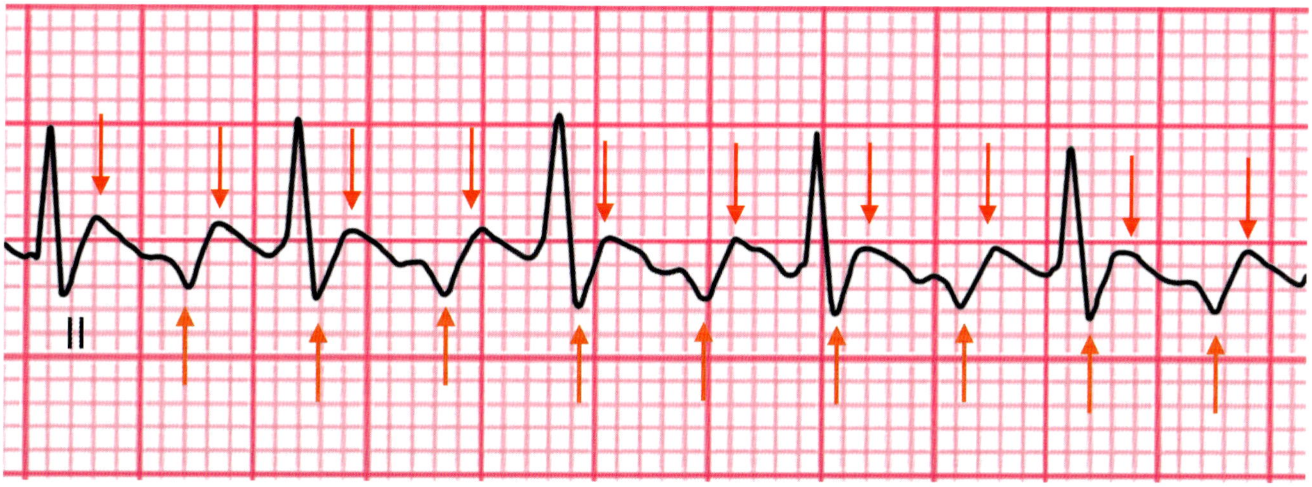

Fig. 30.1B: Rhythm strip of AFL with 2:1 atrioventricular (AV) block, demonstrating the undulating, saw tooth pattern in typical AFL (see arrows). [Image from Levine GN. Arrhythmias 101, 1st edition. New Delhi, India: Jaypee Brothers Medical Publishers (P) Ltd.; 2013].

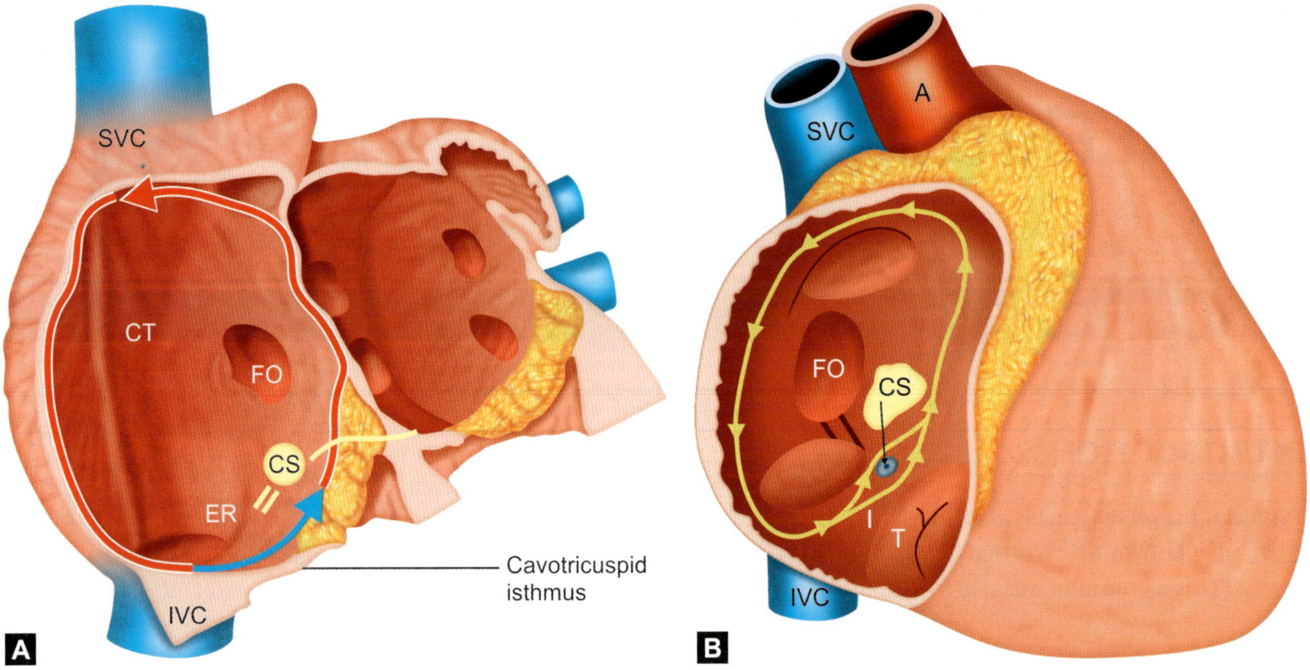

Figs. 30.2A and B: Schematic illustration of the macroreentrant circuit in typical atrial flutter (AFL). (A: Aorta; CS: Coronary sinus; FO: Foramen ovale; I: Atrial isthmus; IVC: Inferior vena cava; SVC: Superior vena cava; T: Tricuspid valve).

The electrophysiologic substrate underlying CTI-dependent AFL has been shown to be due to a combination of slow conduction velocity in the CTI and anatomic and/or functional conduction block along the crista terminalis (CT) and Eustachian ridge (ER). This electrophysiologic milieu produces a long enough reentrant path length, relative to the average tissue wavelength around the tricuspid valve annulus (TVA), to allow for sustained reentry. The triggers of AFL may include premature atrial contractions or nonsustained episodes of AF, which originate most commonly in the left atrium (LA) and pulmonary veins, respectively, and most likely account for the fact that counterclockwise (CCW) CTI-dependent AFL occurs most frequently clinically. CTI-dependent AFL is also relatively resistant to pharmacologic suppression.

As a result of the well-defined anatomic substrate and the pharmacologic resistance of isthmus-dependent AFL, radiofrequency catheter ablation (RFCA) has emerged in the last decade as a safe and effective first-line treatment. Although several procedures have been described for ablating CTI-dependent AFL, the most widely accepted and successful technique is an anatomically-guided approach targeting the CTI. Recent technological developments, including three-dimensional (3-D) electroanatomic mapping and the use of large-tip ablation electrode catheters with high-power generators, and irrigated ablation electrode catheters, have produced almost uniform efficacy without increased risk.

ATRIAL FLUTTER TERMINOLOGY, MECHANISMS, AND ELECTROCARDIOGRAPHIC PATTERNS

Atrial Flutter Terminology

Because of the variety of terms used to describe AFL in humans—including type 1 and type 2 AFL, typical and atypical AFL, CCW and clockwise (CW) AFL, and isthmus-dependent and non-isthmus-dependent AFL—the Working Group of Arrhythmias of the European Society of Cardiology and the North American Society of Pacing and Electrophysiology convened and published a consensus document in 2001 in an attempt to develop a generally accepted standardized terminology for AFL. The consensus was that the widely accepted terms "typical" and "type 1" AFL were most commonly used to describe macroreentrant right atrial tachycardia, utilizing the CTI,

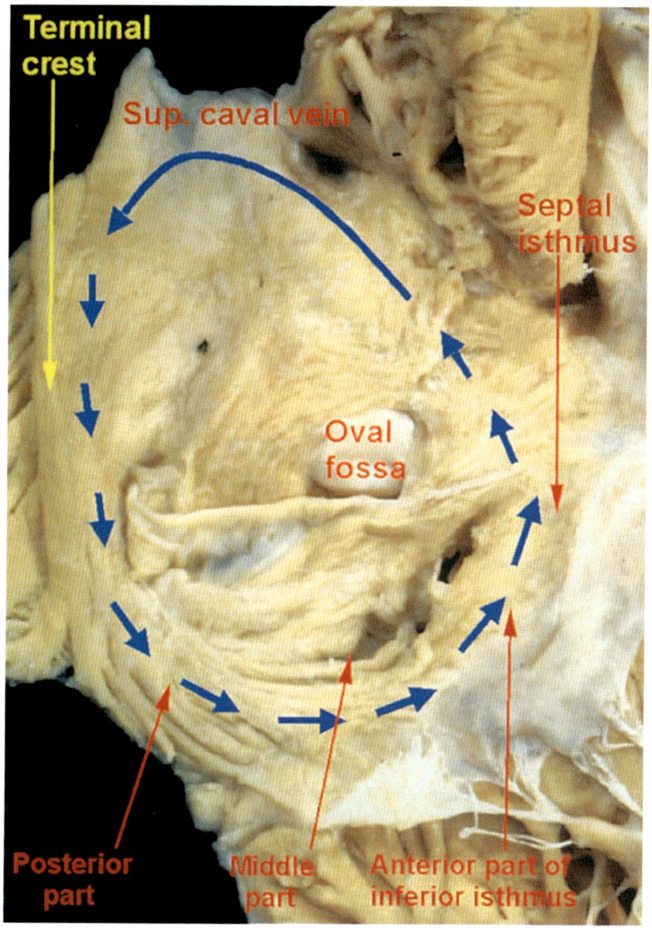

Fig. 30.3: The macroreentrant circuit in typical atrial flutter (AFL), illustrated in a pathological specimen of the right atrium (RA). (Image courtesy of Dr Robert Anderson, Institute of Genetic Medicine, Newcastle University, United Kingdom).

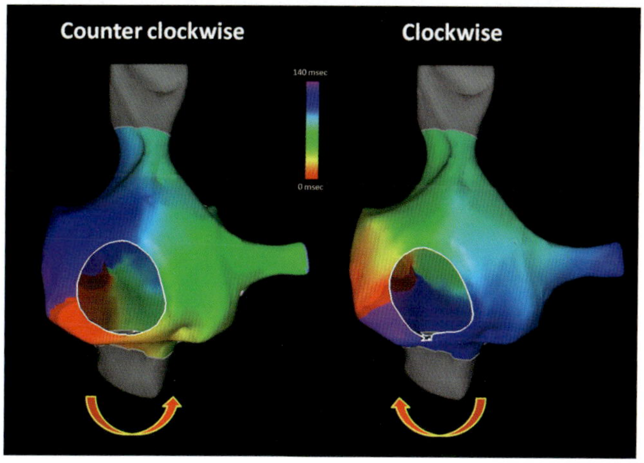

Fig. 30.4: Carto™ three-dimensional (3-D) electroanatomical maps of typical (left panel) and reverse typical (right panel) atrial flutter (AFL). Note the counterclockwise (CCW) activation pattern in typical AFL (left panel) and the clockwise (CW) activation pattern in reverse typical AFL (right panel) in the right atrium (RA). The color red indicates earliest activation and the color purple the latest activation relative to a reference electrogram such as that recorded on the coronary sinus (CS) catheter. (Image courtesy of Levine GN, MD). (CS: Coronary sinus; IVC: Inferior vena cava; RA: Right atrium; SVC: Superior vena cava; TVA: Tricuspid valve annulus).

in either a CCW or a CW direction as visualized from a left anterior oblique perspective (Fig. 30.4). Therefore, the consensus terminology derived from this working group to describe CTI-dependent, right atrial macroreentry tachycardia in the CCW direction is "typical" AFL, and a similar tachycardia in the CW direction is called "reverse typical" AFL. In cases of AFL involving the CTI, 90% of such cases are typical (CCW rotation) flutter (Fig. 30.1A) and 10% of cases are reverse typical (CW rotation) flutter (Fig. 30.5). For the purposes of this book, these two types of typical arrhythmias are referred to specifically as typical and reverse typical AFL when being individually described, but as CTI-dependent AFL when being referred to jointly.

Atypical AFL is used to refer to other types of atrial macroreentrant tachycardias that have reentrant circuits different from that of the CTI in typical AFL. Atypical AFL usually occurs in patients with structural heart disease, including those who have undergone prior heart surgery (particularly congenital heart surgery) or some AF ablation procedures. Such reentrant circuits can develop in other parts of the right atrium (RA), or in the LA. Such macroreentrant circuits can be more challenging to map and treat than typical AFL, and 3-D mapping of the circuit is often utilized.

The term "atrial fibrillation-flutter" is often used to describe a surface electrocardiogram (ECG) that on initial inspection shows "flutter-like" waves but on closer inspection the waves differ in morphology and rate. Electrophysiological studies reveal that in such cases there is usually not a dominant stable circuit, and thus the rhythm should be regarded as more like AF than AFL.

Right Atrial Anatomy and Mechanisms of Isthmus Dependent (Typical and Reverse Typical) Atrial Flutter

Electrophysiologic studies have shown typical and reverse typical AFL to be due to CCW (typical) or CW (reverse typical) macroreentry around the TVA (Fig. 30.6), with

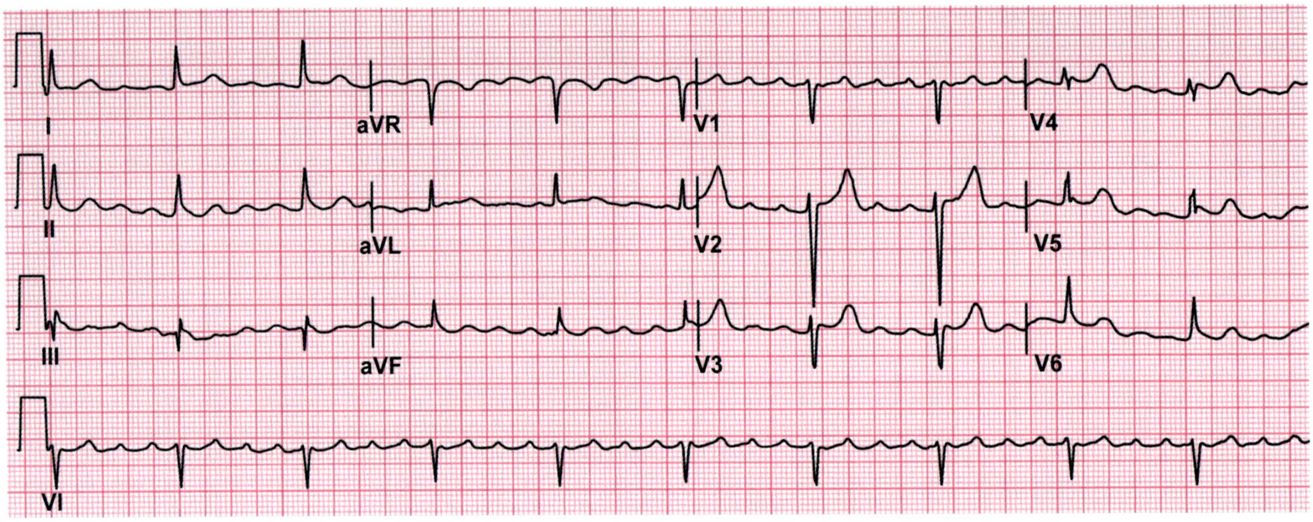

Fig. 30.5: 12-lead electrocardiogram (ECG) of reverse typical atrial flutter (AFL). Note the sine wave appearing F wave pattern, particularly in leads II, III and aVF, the and upright distinct F waves in V1. While the F wave pattern in reverse typical AFL is not diagnostic for an isthmus-dependent flutter, it is nonetheless clearly an AFL as opposed to a coarse atrial fibrillation (AF) or fibrillation-flutter pattern.

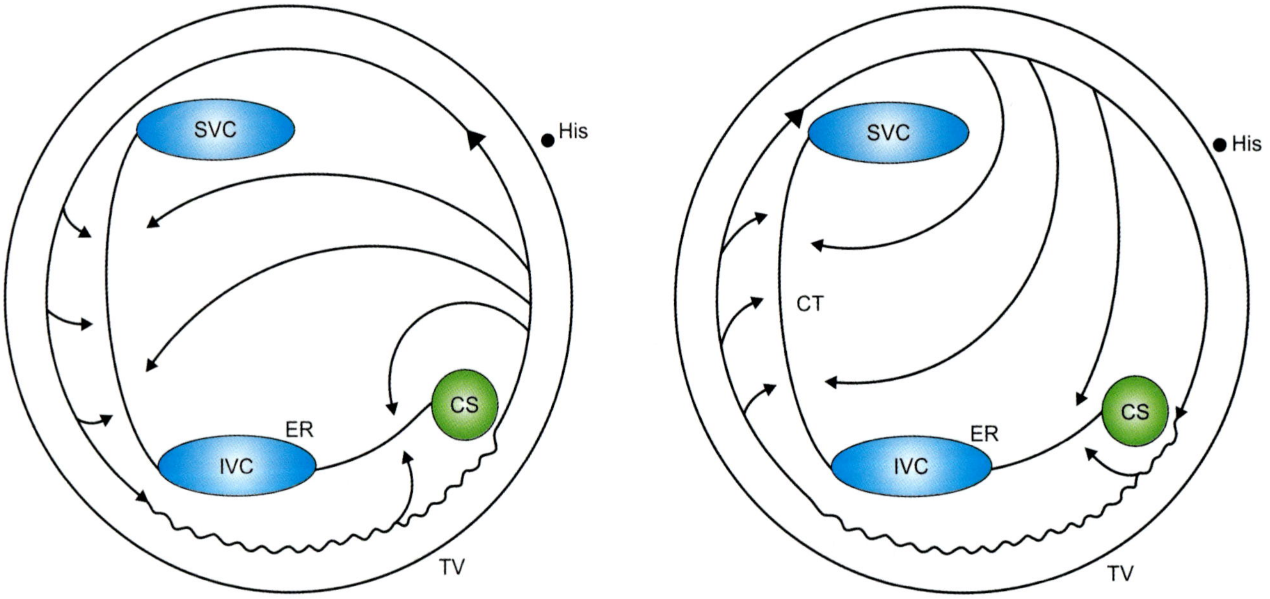

Fig. 30.6: Schematic diagrams demonstrating right atrial activation patterns in typical (left panel) and reverse typical (right panel) forms of cavotricuspid isthmus (CTI)-dependent atrial flutter (AFL). In typical AFL, reentry occurs in a counterclockwise (CCW) direction around the tricuspid valve annulus (TVA), whereas in reverse typical AFL reentry is clockwise (CW). The Eustachian ridge (ER) and crista terminalis (CT) form lines of block, and an area of slow conduction (wavy line) is present in the CTI between the inferior vena cava (IVC) and ER and the TVA. [Image adapted with permission from Feld GK, Srivatsa U, Hoppe B. Ablation of isthmus dependent atrial flutters. In: Huang SS, Wood MA (Eds). Catheter Ablation of Cardiac Arrhythmias. Philadelphia: Elsevier; 2006. pp. 195-218]. (CS: Coronary sinus ostium; His: His bundle; SVC: Superior vena cava; ER: Eustachian ridge; IVC: Inferior vena cava; TV: Tricuspid valve).

an area of slow conduction in the CTI accounting for up to one-third to one-half of the AFL cycle length. The CTI is bounded by the inferior vena cava (IVC) and ER posteriorly and the TVA anteriorly, forming barriers delineating a protected zone in the reentry circuit. Lines of block, including the ER and the CT, along which double potentials are typically recorded during AFL (Figs. 30.7A and B), and an area of slow conduction (i.e. the CTI),

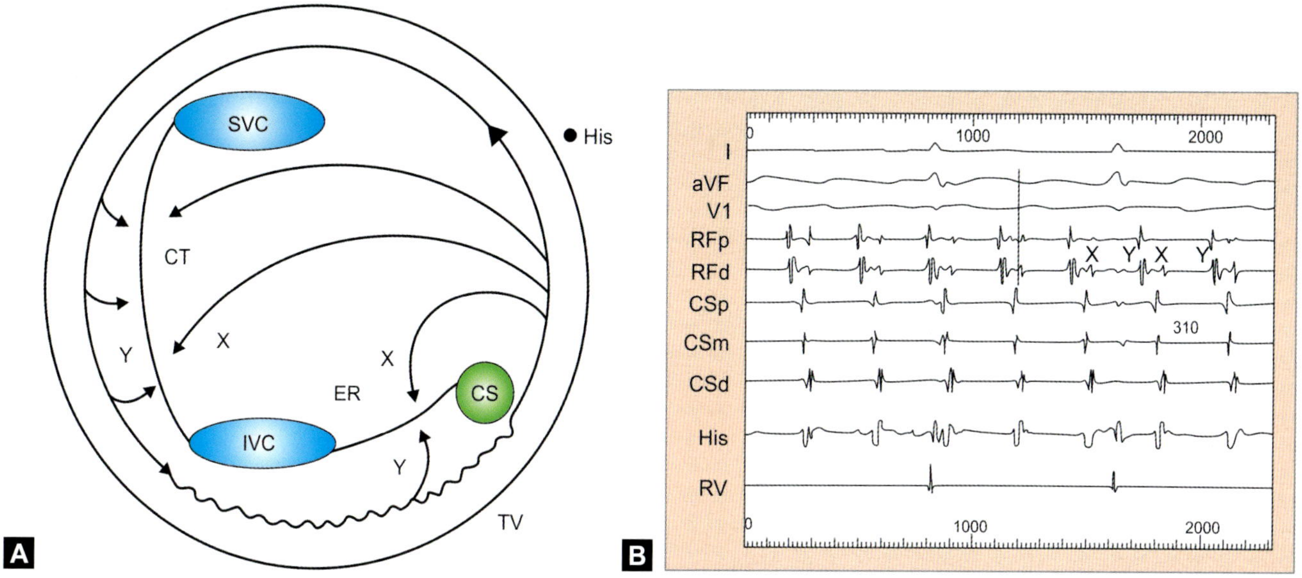

Figs. 30.7A and B: (A) Schematic diagram demonstrating where double potentials (X, Y) are recorded during typical atrial flutter (AFL) along the Eustachian ridge (ER) and crista terminalis (CT); (B) Double potentials recorded from an ablation catheter (RFp&d) positioned at the ER during typical AFL. [Image adapted with permission from Feld GK, Srivatsa U, Hoppe B. Ablation of isthmus dependent atrial flutters. In: Huang SS, Wood MA (Eds). Catheter Ablation of Cardiac Arrhythmias. Philadelphia: Elsevier; 2006. pp. 195-218]. (I, aVF, V1, surface ECG leads; RFp&d: Proximal and distal bipolar recordings from the ablation catheter; CSp-d: Proximal to distal CS electrogram recordings; RV: Right ventricular electrogram recording; SVC: Superior vena cava; CT: Crista terminalis; IVC: Inferior vena cava; ER: Eustachian ridge; His: His bundle; CS: Coronary sinus).

are necessary to establish an adequate path-length for reentry to be sustained and to prevent short circuiting of the reentrant circuit.

The most common clinical presentation of isthmus-dependent AFL is typical AFL, likely triggered by premature atrial contractions originating from the LA or nonsustained AF, which result in CW unidirectional block in the CTI and initiation of CCW macroreentry.

ECG Patterns of Typical (and Reverse Typical) Atrial Flutter

In typical AFL, there is a characteristic inverted saw-tooth F wave pattern in the inferior leads II, III, and aVF. In reverse typical AFL, in contrast, the F wave pattern on the 12-lead ECG is less specific, often with a sine wave pattern in the inferior ECG leads (Figs. 30.8A and B). The F wave pattern on ECG is dependent in part on the activation sequence of the LA, with inverted F waves in the inferior leads in typical AFL the result of activation of the LA initially near the coronary sinus (CS), and upright F waves in the inferior leads in reverse typical AFL resulting from activation of the LA near Bachman's bundle. However, following LA ablation, and even right atrial ablation as in Figures 30.8A and B, the ECG presentation of isthmus-dependent AFL may be significantly different from the characteristic patterns described above.

PHARMACOLOGICAL THERAPY OF ATRIAL FLUTTER

Antiarrhythmic Drug Therapy for Atrial Flutter

Extensive research has been done in the past to determine the most effective pharmacological approach for treatment of AFL. With the determination of the macroreentrant mechanism of CTI-dependent AFL, it was proposed that the class 3 antiarrhythmic drugs, such as sotalol, might be more effective in suppression of CTI-dependent AFL, by prolongation of the atrial action potential duration and effective refractory period by depression of potassium channel activity, compared to the class 1 drugs, particularly the class 1c drugs, which slow conduction velocity by depressing sodium channel activity. While antiarrhythmic drugs have achieved $<50\%$ efficacy over 1–2 years, in most trials for the treatment of AF, efficacy in the treatment of AFL may be higher. For example, using

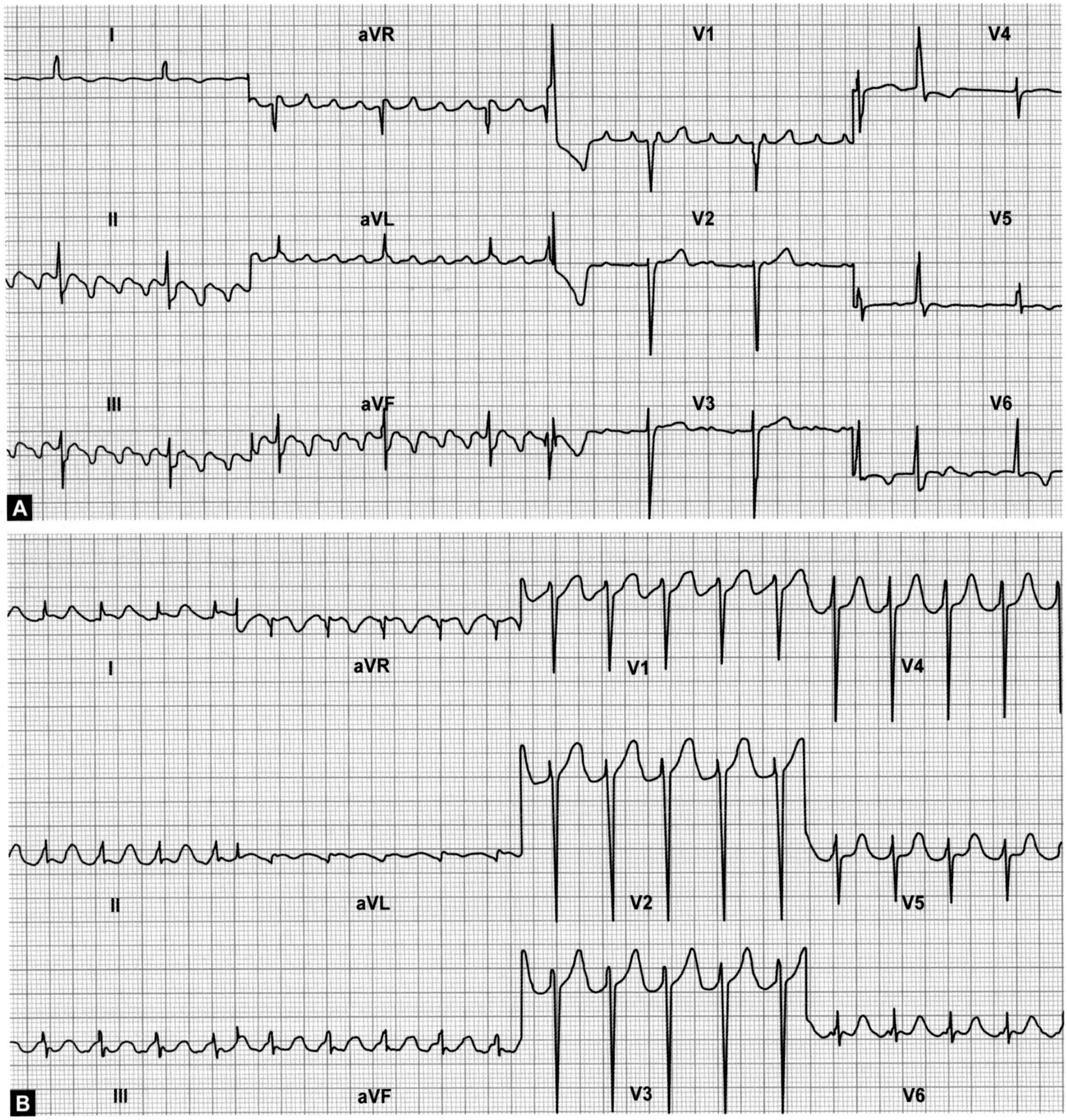

Figs. 30.8A and B: (A) 12-lead electrocardiogram (ECG) recorded during typical atrial flutter (AFL), with typical saw-toothed pattern of inverted F waves in the inferior leads II, III, aVF. (B) 12-lead ECG recorded during reverse typical AFL, with atypical F wave pattern in the inferior leads. [Image adapted with permission from Feld GK, Srivatsa U, Hoppe B. Ablation of isthmus dependent atrial flutters. In: Huang SS, Wood MA (Eds). Catheter Ablation of Cardiac Arrhythmias. Philadelphia: Elsevier; 2006. pp. 195-218].

class 3 antiarrhythmic drugs, the acute conversion of AFL with ibutilide has been reported to be as high as 63%, and the chronic suppression of AFL with N-acetylprocainamide as high as 100%. Most studies however, have not separated out the results of antiarrhythmic drug suppression of AFL and AF, so it is difficult to determine if the newer class 3 antiarrhythmic drugs are more effective for the treatment of AFL compared to AF, and most patients

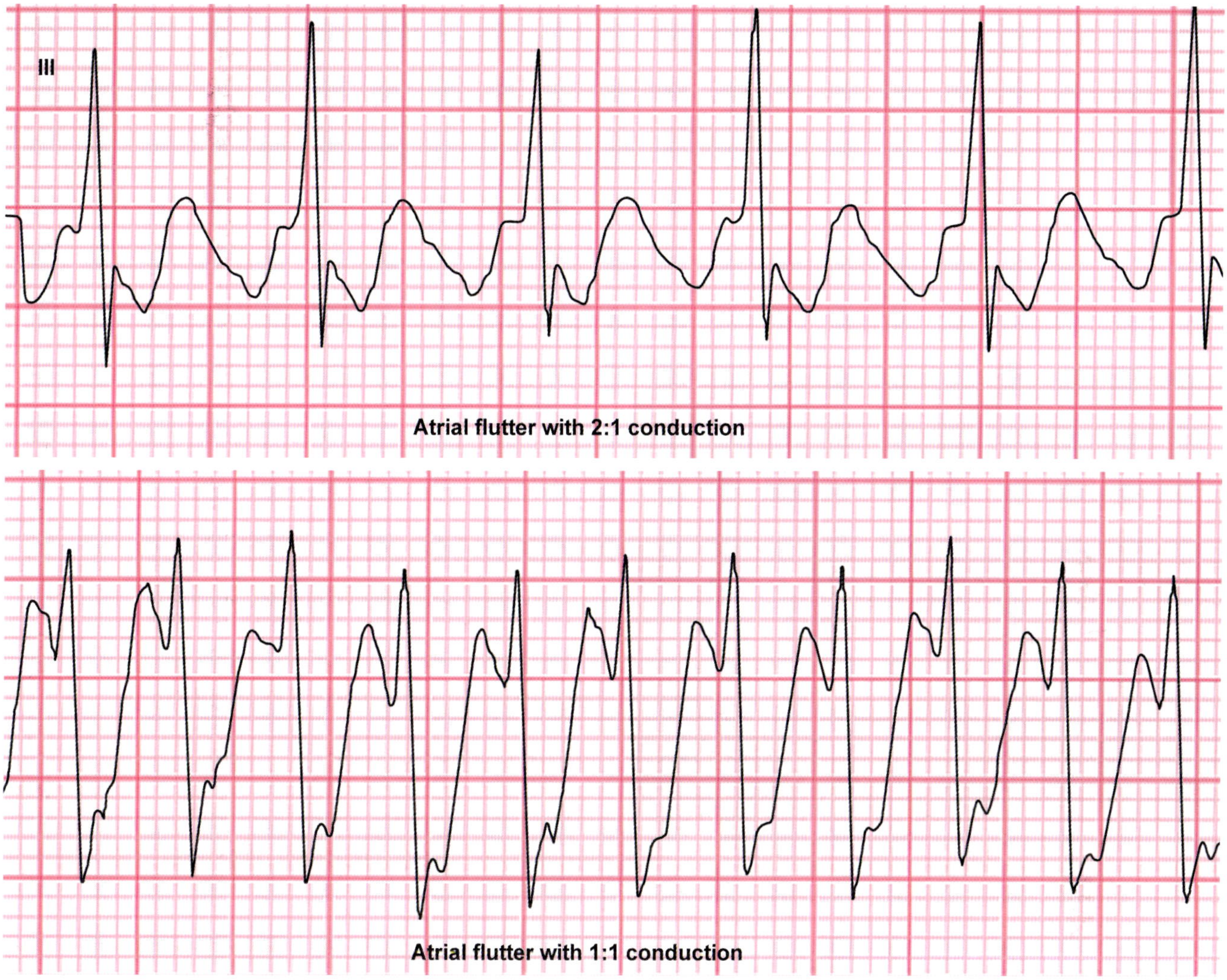

Fig. 30.9: An example of atrial flutter (AFL) with 2:1 conduction (upper panel) that becomes AFL with 1:1 conduction (lower panel). (Image courtesy of Tom Bouthillet).

have both arrhythmias at one time or another. There is also some data to suggest that curative ablation of CTI-dependent AFL as first-line therapy is more cost-effective than antiarrhythmic drug therapy for suppression of AFL.

Rate Control

In patients who require short-term (or in rare cases long-term) control of the ventricular response rate, drugs that slow conduction through the AV node are utilized, including beta-blockers and non-dihydroyridine calcium channel blockers (verapamil and diltiazem). Digoxin is less effective. Initiation of AV-node blocking medications is important in patients treated with certain antiarrhythmic agents (such as procainamide) which slow the flutter rate without significantly blocking AV conduction, because initiation of such antiarrhythmic therapy has the potential to lead to 1:1 conduction and a faster ventricular response rate (Figs. 30.9 and 30.10).

Anticoagulation

There is surprisingly little data on the actual risk of thromboembolism in patients with AFL, as most research has focused on AF. In the past, it was not universally considered necessary to anticoagulate patients with AFL. However, over the past several decades a consensus has been reached that patients with AFL are indeed at risk of thromboembolism, and in general patients with AFL are treated similarly to patients with AF with respect to indications

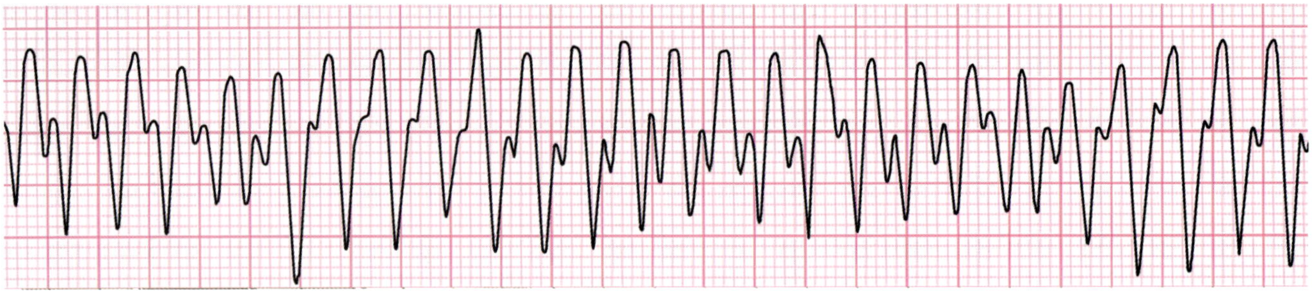

Fig. 30.10: Rhythm strip from a patient with atrial flutter (AFL) who developed 1:1 conduction. (Image courtesy of Levine GN, MD).

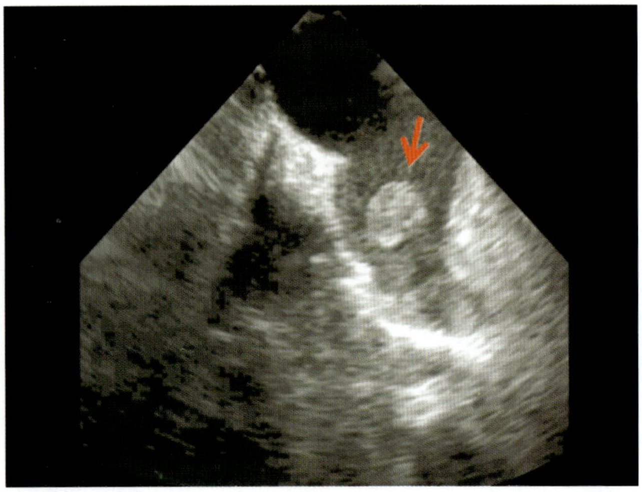

Fig. 30.11: Transesophageal echocardiogram (TEE) in a patient with atrial flutter (AFL) demonstrating a mobile thrombus (arrow) in the left atrial appendage. [Image from Jacob SP. Left atrial thrombosis in rheumatic mitral stenosis. In: Harikrishnan S (Ed). Percutaneous Mitral Valvotomy, 1st edition. New Delhi, India: Jaypee Brothers Medical Publishers; 2012. pp. 382-88].

for anticoagulation. It should be noted, however, that risk assessments systems such as the $CHADS_2$ and $CHADS_2$-VASc systems were developed based on patients with AF, not AFL. As with AF, the target international normalized ratio (INR) for patients on warfarin therapy is 2–3.

Furthermore, anticoagulation is recommended for 3-4 weeks before elective cardioversion of AFL unless precardioversion transesophageal echocardiography is performed to exclude the presence of an atrial thrombus (Fig. 30.11). Anticoagulation is also recommended to be continued for 4 weeks after either cardioversion or CTI ablation therapy.

CARDIOVERSION OF ATRIAL FLUTTER

Typical AFL is a rhythm that usually can be treated when indicated with synchronized cardioversion. The arrhythmia usually only requires 20–50 J, particularly with biphasic devices. As discussed above, the risk of thromboembolism must be considered, and patients are treated with anticoagulation (or precardioversion TEE) before and after cardioversion.

MAPPING AND ABLATION OF ATRIAL FLUTTER

Standard Catheter Mapping of Isthmus-Dependent Atrial Flutter

Despite the characteristic 12-lead ECG pattern, electrophysiologic mapping and entrainment must be performed prior to RFCA of AFL. For standard catheter mapping, multielectrode catheters are typically positioned in the RA, His bundle region, CS, and around the TVA (Fig. 30.12). Recordings obtained during AFL (i.e. spontaneous or induced) are then analyzed to determine the RA activation sequence. Typical or reverse typical AFL is confirmed by observing a CCW or CW activation pattern in the RA around the TVA respectively (Figs. 30.13A and B), and demonstration of concealed entrainment during pacing from the CTI (Figs. 30.14A and B).

Radiofrequency Catheter Ablation of Isthmus-Dependent Atrial Flutter

Radiofrequency catheter ablation of isthmus-dependent AFL is performed with a steerable mapping/ablation catheter inserted via a femoral vein and positioned across the CTI. Catheters with either saline-irrigated ablation electrodes (Thermocool Classic or SF™, Biosense Webster, Diamond Bar, CA; Chili™, Boston Scientific, Natick MA), or large distal ablation electrodes (i.e. 8–10 mm Blazer™, Boston Scientific, Inc., Natick, MA) are preferred for CTI ablation. The preferred target for isthmus-dependent AFL ablation is the CTI (Fig. 30.15A).

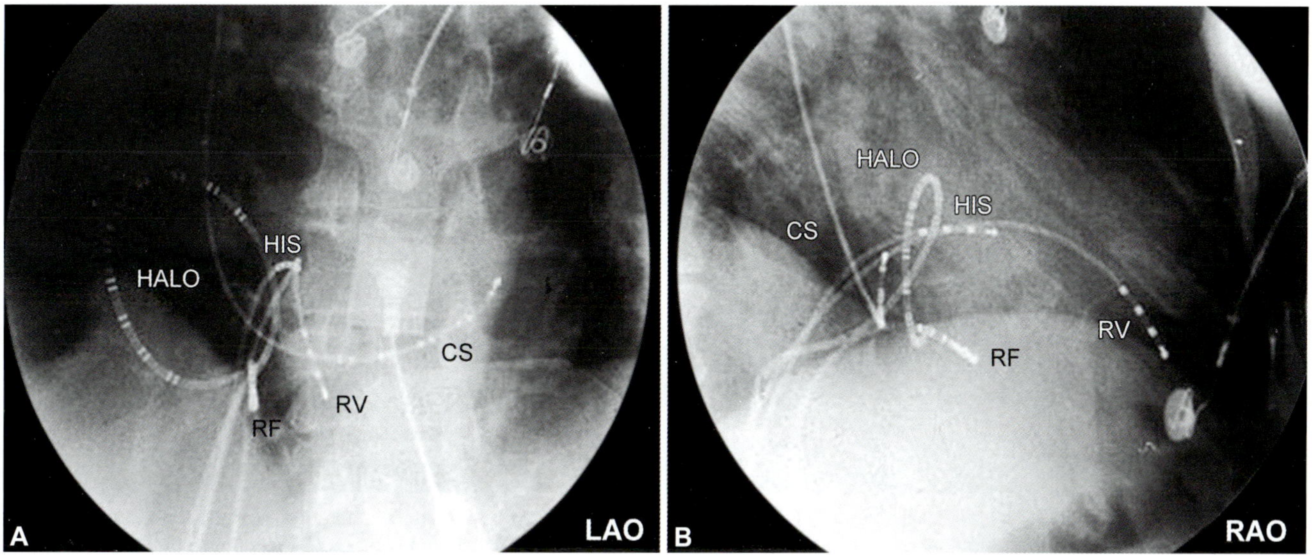

Figs. 30.12A and B: Left anterior oblique (LAO) and right anterior oblique (RAO) fluoroscopic projections showing common intracardiac positions of the right ventricular (RV), His bundle (HIS), coronary sinus (CS), Halo (HALO) and mapping/ablation catheters (RF). [Image adapted with permission from Feld GK, Srivatsa U, Hoppe B. Ablation of isthmus dependent atrial flutters. In: Huang SS, Wood MA (Eds). Catheter Ablation of Cardiac Arrhythmias. Philadelphia: Elsevier; 2006. pp. 195-218].

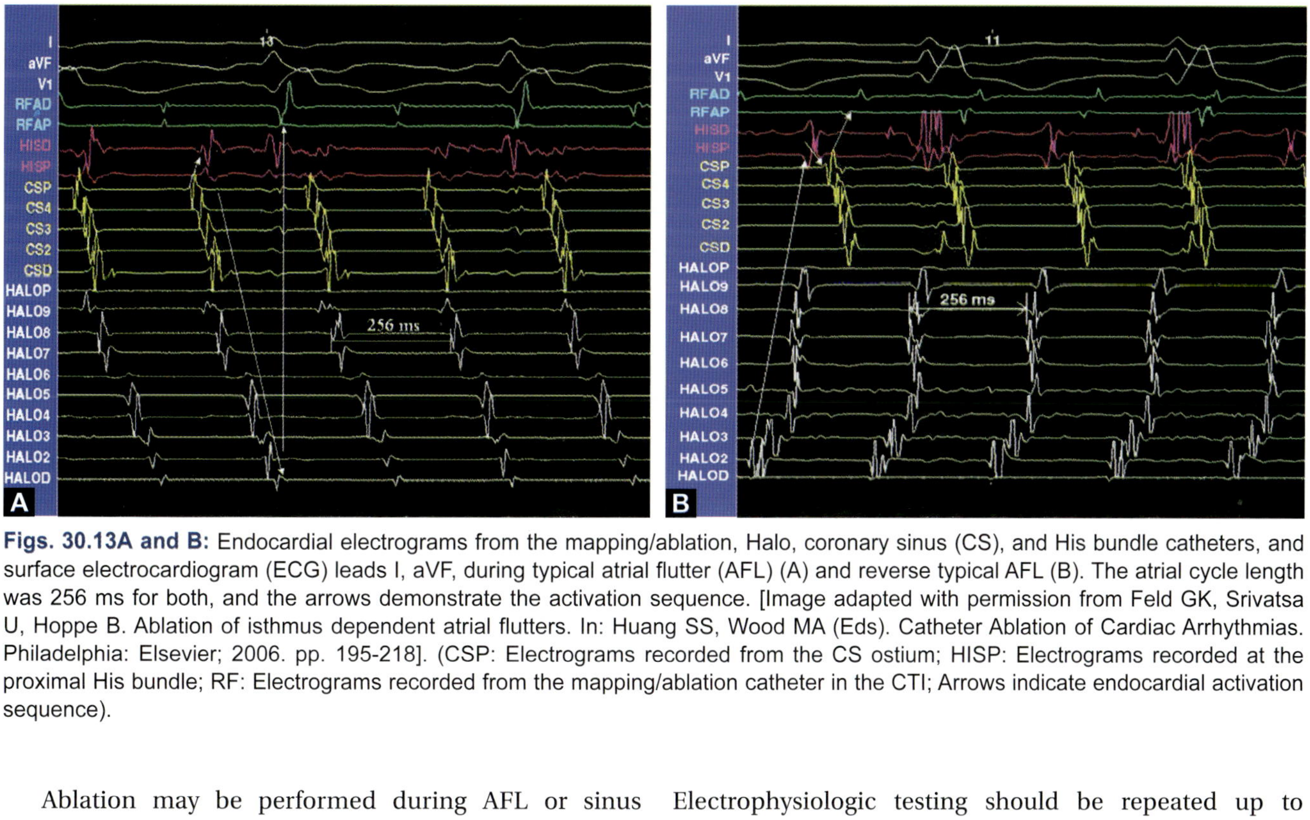

Figs. 30.13A and B: Endocardial electrograms from the mapping/ablation, Halo, coronary sinus (CS), and His bundle catheters, and surface electrocardiogram (ECG) leads I, aVF, during typical atrial flutter (AFL) (A) and reverse typical AFL (B). The atrial cycle length was 256 ms for both, and the arrows demonstrate the activation sequence. [Image adapted with permission from Feld GK, Srivatsa U, Hoppe B. Ablation of isthmus dependent atrial flutters. In: Huang SS, Wood MA (Eds). Catheter Ablation of Cardiac Arrhythmias. Philadelphia: Elsevier; 2006. pp. 195-218]. (CSP: Electrograms recorded from the CS ostium; HISP: Electrograms recorded at the proximal His bundle; RF: Electrograms recorded from the mapping/ablation catheter in the CTI; Arrows indicate endocardial activation sequence).

Ablation may be performed during AFL or sinus rhythm. If performed during AFL, the first endpoint is its termination (Fig. 30.15B). After CTI ablation, electrophysiologic testing is required to ensure the presence of bidirectional conduction block (Figs. 30.16 and 30.17) Electrophysiologic testing should be repeated up to 30–60 minutes after ablation to ensure that bidirectional CTI block persists, and that AFL cannot be re-induced, in order to significantly lower the risk of recurrent AFL during long-term follow-up.

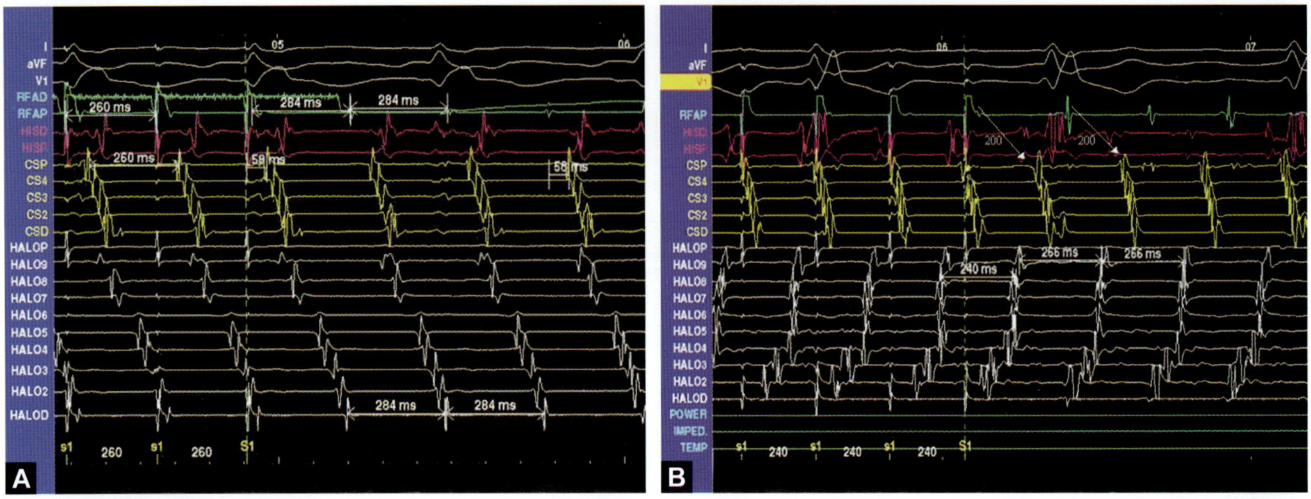

Figs. 30.14A and B: Endocardial electrograms from the RF, Halo, CS, and His bundle catheters, and surface electrocardiogram (ECG) leads I, aVF, and V1, demonstrating concealed entrainment during pacing at the cavotricuspid isthmus (CTI) in typical atrial flutter (AFL) (A) and reverse typical AFL (B). [Image adapted with permission from Feld GK, Srivatsa U, Hoppe B. Ablation of isthmus dependent atrial flutters. In: Huang SS, Wood MA (Eds). Catheter Ablation of Cardiac Arrhythmias. Philadelphia: Elsevier; 2006. pp. 195-218]. (Halo D to Halo P: Bipolar electrograms from the distal to proximal poles of the Halo catheter around the TVA; CSP-D: Bipolar electrograms recorded from the proximal to distal CS catheter electrode pairs; HISP&D: Bipolar electrograms recorded from the proximal and distal His bundle catheter; RFAP&D: Bipolar electrograms recorded from the proximal and distal electrode pairs of the mapping/ablation catheter at the CTI).

Outcomes and Complications of CTI Ablation for Isthmus-Dependent Atrial Flutter

Although early reports of RFCA for AFL revealed recurrence rates up to 20–45%, subsequent studies have demonstrated acute and chronic efficacy in excess of 95% (Table 30.1), although patients with complex CTI anatomy may have higher recurrence rates in long-term follow up.

Radiofrequency catheter ablation for typical AFL is relatively safe, but serious complications can occur, including AV block, cardiac perforation, pericardial tamponade, and thromboembolic events, including pulmonary embolism and stroke. In recent large-scale studies, including those using large-tip ablation catheters and high power generators, major complications have been observed in only 2.5–3.0% of patients.

Computerized 3-D Mapping and Intracardiac Echocardiography Guidance for CTI Ablation

Three-dimensional (3-D) electroanatomical activation mapping systems (Carto™ BioSense-Webster, Diamond Bar, CA, and ESI NavX™, St. Jude, Inc., St. Paul, MN) and noncontact balloon mapping systems (Ensite™, St. Jude, Inc., St. Paul, MN), although not required for isthmus-dependent AFL ablation, are now widely used to map the activation sequence in AFL and the activation sequence after CTI ablation to confirm block (Fig. 30.18). A 3-D mapping system may be particularly useful in difficult cases such as those where prior ablation has failed, those with complex CTI anatomy, or those with surgically corrected congenital heart disease such as an atrial septal defect. Voltage mapping, alone or in combination with activation mapping, may also be helpful to identify areas of thinner muscle in the CTI that may be more easily ablated. Intracardiac echocardiography (ICE) may also be used to identify anatomical variations in the CTI, such as a wide or thickened CTI or deep pouches in the CTI that may make ablation difficult using standard techniques. Visualization of these anatomical variants with ICE may allow the operator to avoid them or to achieve better catheter contact with the CTI, increasing the acute and long-term success rates of ablation (Fig. 30.19).

ATYPICAL FORMS OF ISTHMUS-DEPENDENT ATRIAL FLUTTER

In lower loop reentrant AFL, the activation wavefront spreads through the CT and around the IVC through the

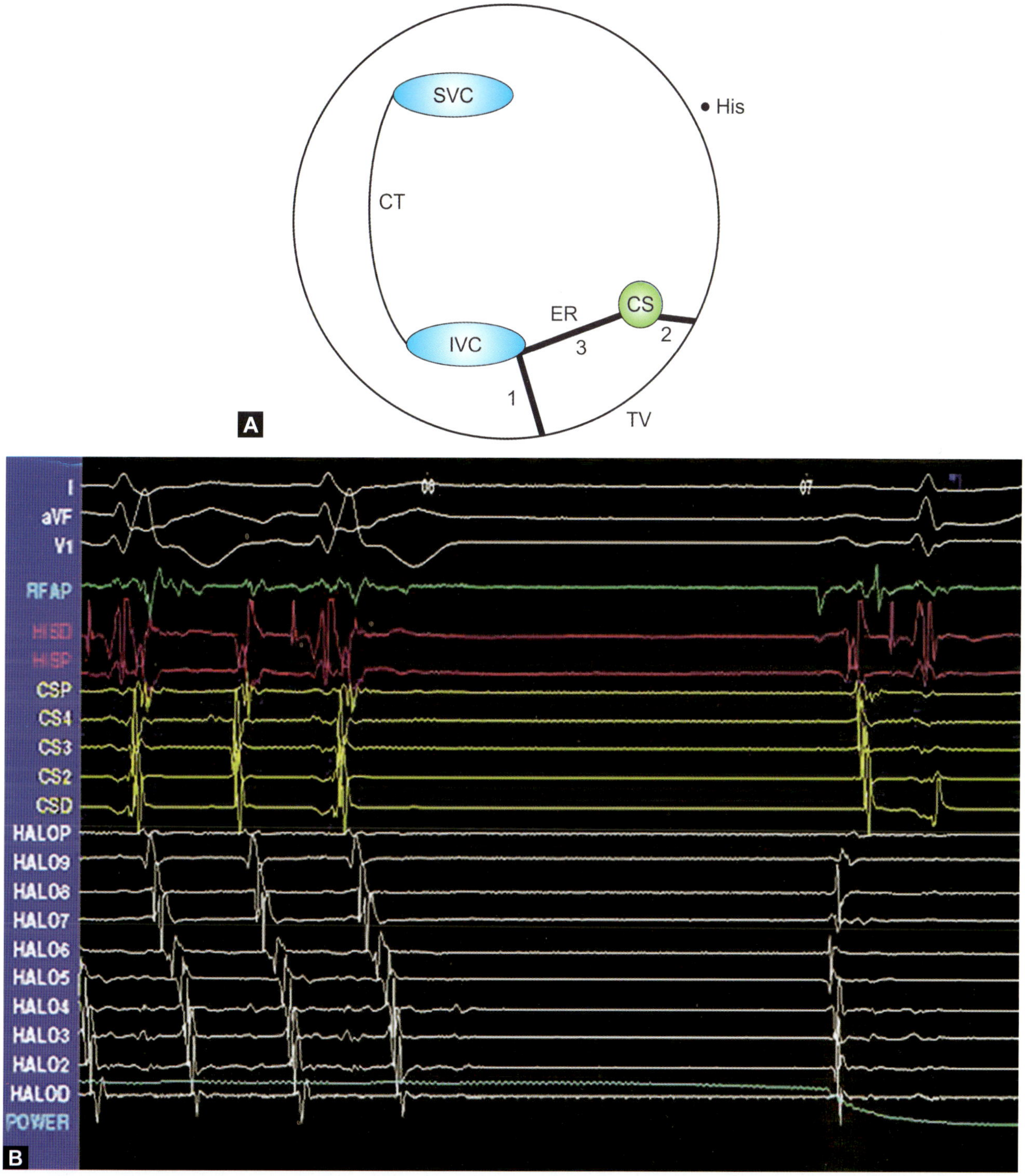

Figs. 30.15A and B: (A) A schematic diagram of the right atrium (RA) demonstrating the potential targets for ablation of cavotricuspid isthmus (CTI)-dependent atrial flutter (AFL). The preferred target for ablation is the CTI. (B) Surface electrocardiogram (ECG) and endocardial electrogram recordings during ablation of the CTI showing termination of AFL. [Image adapted with permission from Feld GK, Srivatsa U, Hoppe B. Ablation of isthmus dependent atrial flutters. In: Huang SS, Wood MA (Eds). Catheter Ablation of Cardiac Arrhythmias. Philadelphia: Elsevier; 2006. pp:195-218]. (I, aVF, V1, surface ECG leads; RFAP: Proximal ablation electrogram; HISP&D: Proximal and distal His bundle electrograms; CSD-P: Distal to proximal CS electrograms; Halo D-P: Distal to proximal Halo catheter electrograms; Imped: Impedance; Temp: Temperature; SVC: Superior vena cava; CT: Crista terminalis; IVC: Inferior vena cava; ER: Eustachian ridge; His: His bundle; CS: Coronary sinus; TV: Tricuspid valve).

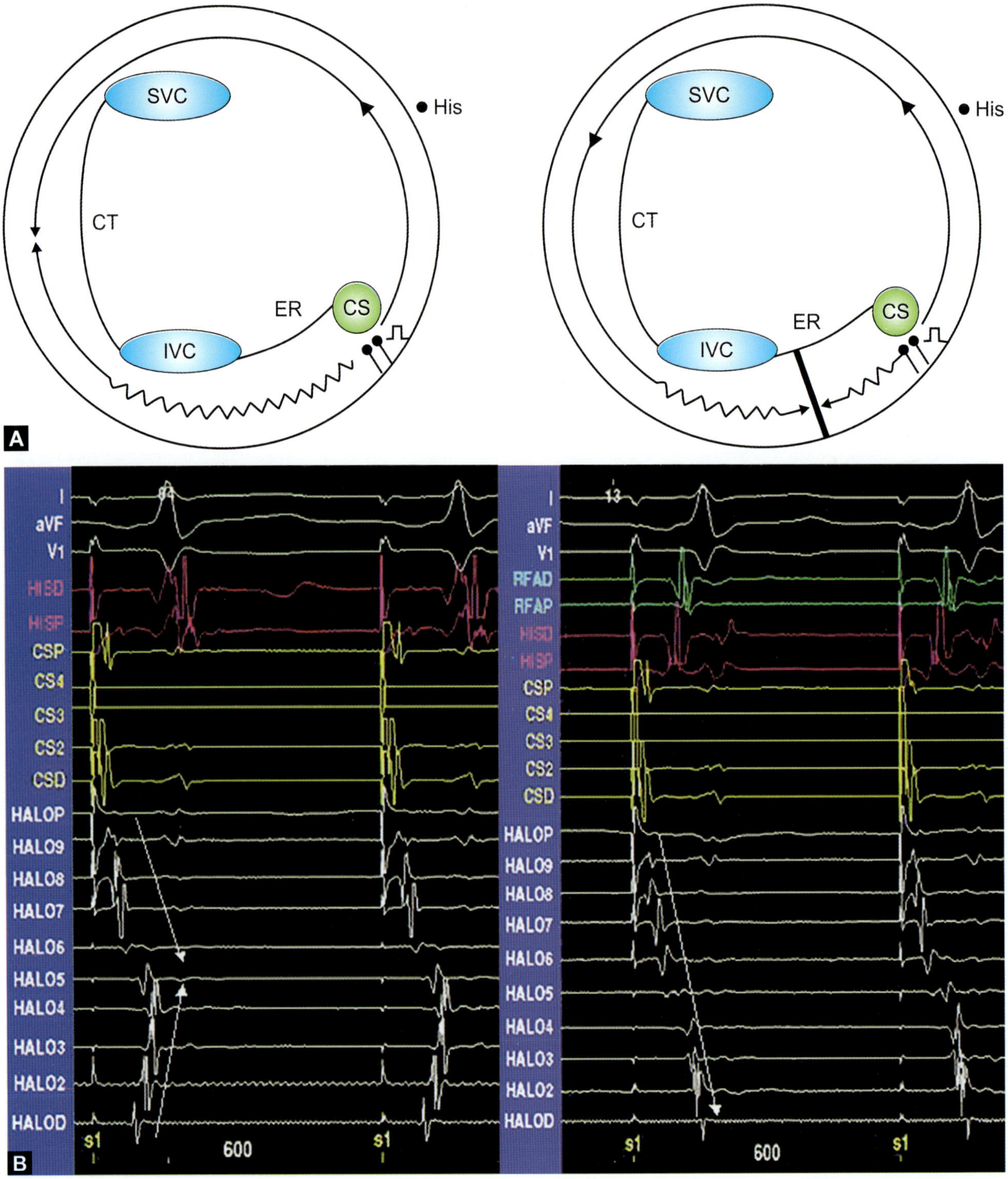

Figs. 30.16A and B: (A) A schematic diagram of the expected right atrial activation sequence during pacing in sinus rhythm from the coronary sinus (CS) ostium before (left panel) and after (right panel) ablation of the cavotricuspid isthmus (CTI). (B) Surface electrocardiogram (ECG) and right atrial endocardial electrograms recorded during pacing in sinus rhythm from the CS ostium before (left panel) and after (right panel) CTI ablation. [Image adapted with permission from Feld GK, Srivatsa U, Hoppe B. Ablation of isthmus dependent atrial flutters. In: Huang SS, Wood MA (Eds). Catheter Ablation of Cardiac Arrhythmias. Philadelphia: Elsevier; 2006. pp. 195-218]. (CT: Crista terminalis; ER: Eustachian ridge; His: His bundle; IVC: Inferior vena cava; SVC: Superior vena cava; CS: Coronary sinus; Arrows indicate endocardial activation sequence).

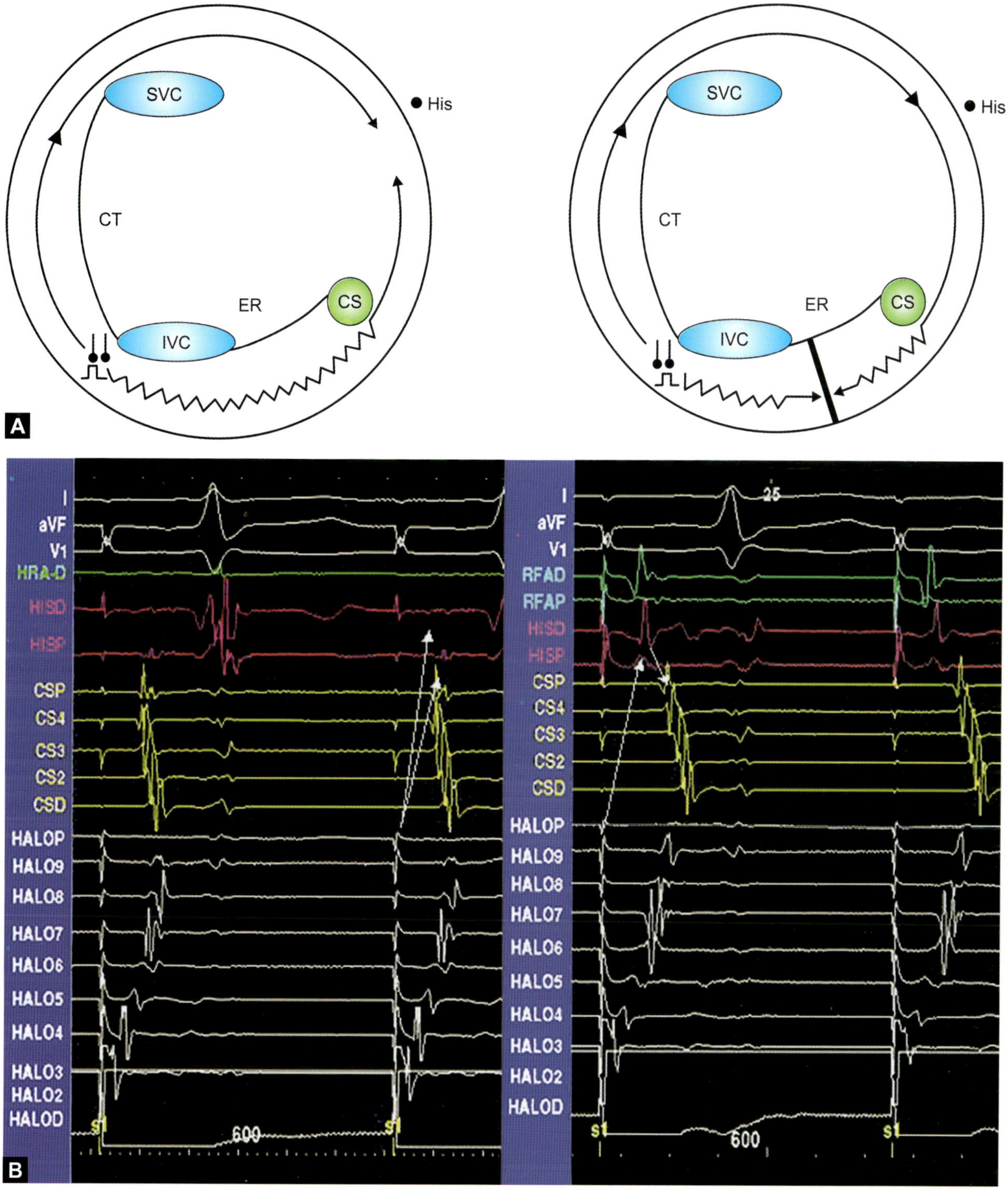

Figs. 30.17A and B: (A) A schematic diagrams of the expected right atrial activation sequence during pacing in sinus rhythm from the low lateral right atrium (RA) before (left panel) and after (right panel) ablation of the cavotricuspid isthmus (CTI); (B) Surface electrocardiogram (ECG) and right atrial endocardial electrograms recorded during pacing in sinus rhythm from the low lateral RA before (left panel) and after (right panel) ablation of the CTI. [Image adapted with permission from Feld GK, Srivatsa U, Hoppe B. Ablation of isthmus dependent atrial flutters. In: Huang SS, Wood MA (Eds). Catheter Ablation of Cardiac Arrhythmias. Philadelphia: Elsevier; 2006. pp. 195-218]. (CT: Crista terminalis; ER: Eustachian ridge; His: His bundle; SVC: Superior vena cava; IVC: Inferior vena cava; CS: Coronary sinus; Arrows indicate endocardial activation sequence).

Table 30.1: Success rates for radiofrequency catheter ablation (RFCA) of atrial flutter (AFL). (N: Number of patients studied; % acute success, termination of AFL during ablation and/or demonstration of bidirectional CTI block following ablation; % chronic success, % of patients in whom type 1 AFL did not recur during follow-up. Acute and chronic success rates are reported as overall results in randomized or comparison studies).

Author	*Year*	*N*	*Electrode length (mm)*	*% Acute success*	*Follow-up (months)*	*% Chronic success*
Feld	1992	16	4	100	4 ± 2	83
Cosio	1993	9	4	100	22 – 18	56
Kirkorian	1994	22	4	86	8 ± 13	84
Fischer	1995	80	4	73	20 ± 8	81
Poty	1995	12	6/8	100	9 ± 3	92
Schwartzman	1996	35	8	100	1 – 21	92
Chauchemez	1996	20	4	100	8 ± 2	80
Tsai	1999	50	8	92	10 ± 5	100
Atiga	2002	59	4 vs cooled	88	13 ± 4	93
Scavee	2004	80	8 vs cooled	80	15	98
Feld	2004	169	8 or 10	93	6	97
Calkins	2004	150	8	88	6	87
Ventura	2004	130	8 vs cooled	100	14 ± 2	98

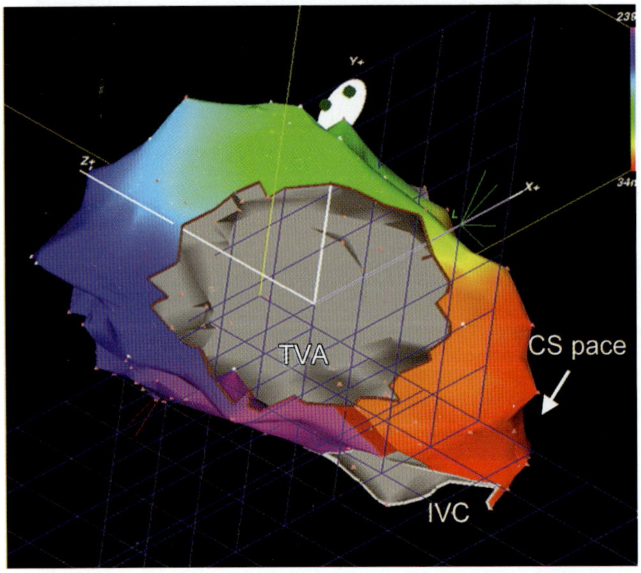

Fig. 30.18: A three-dimensional (3-D) electroanatomical (Carto™) map of the right atrium (RA) is shown in a patient with typical atrial flutter (AFL) after cavotricuspid isthmus (CTI) ablation. Following ablation of the CTI, during pacing from the coronary sinus (CS) ostium, there is evidence of medial to lateral isthmus block as indicated by juxtaposition of orange and purple color in the CTI, indicating early and late activation, respectively, across a line of block. [Image adapted with permission from Feld GK, Birgersdotter-Green U, Narayan S. Diagnosis and ablation of typical and reverse typical (type 1) atrial flutter. In: Wilber D, Packer D, Stevenson W (Eds). Catheter Ablation of Cardiac Arrhythmias: Basic Concepts and Clinical Applications, 3rd edition. Oxford, England: Blackwell Publishing; 2007. pp. 173-92]. (TVA: Tricuspid valve annulus; IVC: Inferior vena cava; CS: Coronary sinus).

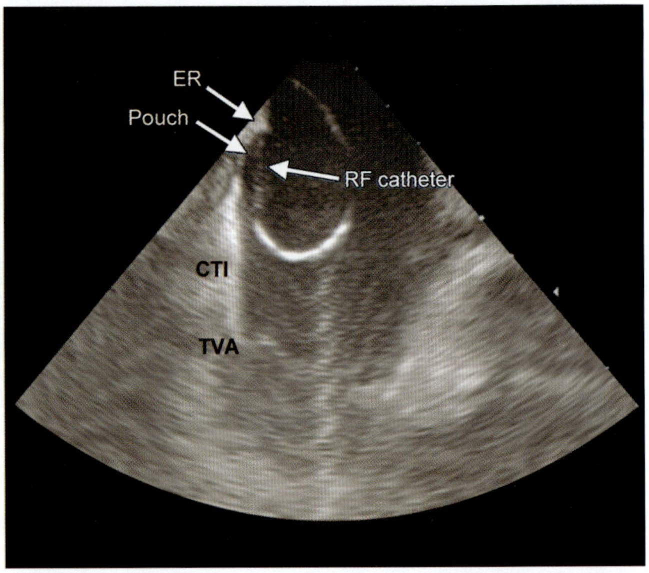

Fig. 30.19: Intracardiac echocardiography (ICE) image of a deep pouch preventing complete cavotricuspid isthmus (CTI) ablation using a standard approach, due to difficulty in achieving adequate contact between the ablation catheter tip and the CTI in the pouch near the Eustachian ridge (ER). Positioning the ablation catheter in the CTI under ICE guidance, with a reverse curl from the inferior vena cava (IVC), such that the ablation electrode was just beneath the ER resulted in improved catheter-tissue contact with complete CTI ablation and bidirectional conduction block. (RF: Radiofrequency; CTI: Cavotricuspid isthmus; TVA: Tricuspid valve annulus; ER: Eustachian ridge).

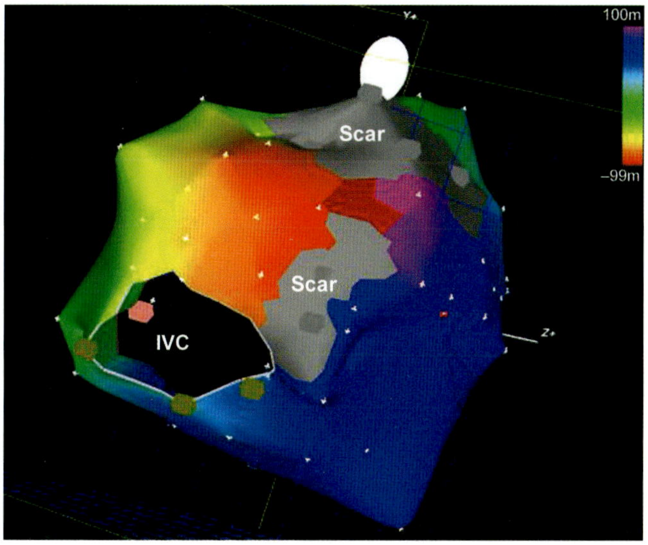

Fig. 30.20: A Carto™ three-dimensional (3-D) activation sequence map (posterior caudal view) is shown in a patient with lower loop reentry. Note that the activation wavefront spreads counterclockwise (CCW) in the right atrium (RA) and horizontally across the crista terminalis (CT) between two (superior and inferior) areas of scarring in the posterior right atrial wall. Ablation between the scarred areas converted this atypical atrial flutter (AFL) into a typical AFL which was ablated at the cavotricuspid isthmus (CTI). [Image adapted with permission from Feld GK, Birgersdotter-Green U, Narayan S. Diagnosis and ablation of typical and reverse typical (type 1) atrial flutter. In: Wilber D, Packer D, Stevenson W (Eds). Catheter Ablation of Cardiac Arrhythmias: Basic Concepts and Clinical Applications, 3rd edition. Oxford, England: Blackwell Publishing; 2007. pp:173-92]. (IVC: Inferior vena cava).

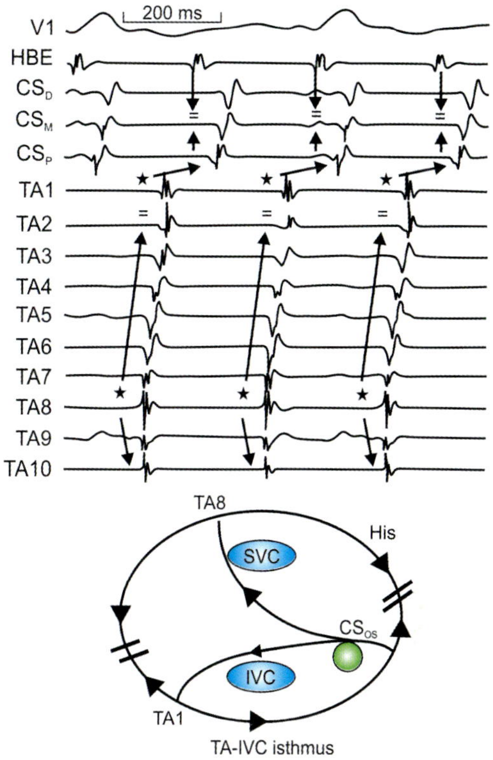

Fig. 30.21: Electrogram and schematic representation of atrial activation in lower loop reentry atrial flutter (AFL). In lower loop reentry, the posterior right atrium (RA) is part of the reentry circuit and wavefronts collide in the lateral RA. The electrograms show multiple collisions at TA1 and TA8 (stars). [Image adapted with permission from Yang Y, Cheng J, Bochoeyer A, et al. Atypical right atrial flutter patterns. Circulation. 2001;103(25):3092-8]. (IVC: Inferior vena cava; SVC: Superior vena cava; TA10: Proximal recording electrodes on Halo catheter near upper septum; TA1: Distal recording electrodes on Halo catheter near lateral aspect of the CTI; CS: Coronary sinus; Arrows indicate endocardial activation sequence).

CTI (Figs. 30.20 and 30.21). This is in contrast to typical AFL, where the CT behaves as a line of block, albeit functional in most cases. Lower loop reentrant AFL may be slowed or terminated by ablation posteriorly along the CT from the superior vena cava to the IVC, but will usually convert to typical AFL and require CTI ablation for cure.

In partial isthmus-dependent flutter, the wavefront bypasses the CTI to enter it laterally and medially in opposite directions, with collisions of the wavefronts near the middle of the CDTI (Fig. 30.22). The CS ostium is activated prematurely, and the tachycardia is not entrained from the CTI itself.

ATYPICAL LEFT ATRIAL FLUTTER

Atypical left AFL is very common after left atrial ablation for AF, usually occurring as a result of development of gaps in lines created during left atrial ablation. Reentry in the LA responsible for atypical AFL may occur for example, around the pulmonary veins through a gap in a line at the roof of the LA, between veins via the anatomical carina between ipsilateral veins, or around the mitral valve annulus. These reentry circuits may be mapped with standard catheter techniques or with 3-D electroanatomical mapping, and ablated with relatively high acute success, but there is a fairly high rate of recurrence of these arrhythmias after ablation, likely due to anatomical differences and differences in ablation methods between the LA and RA.

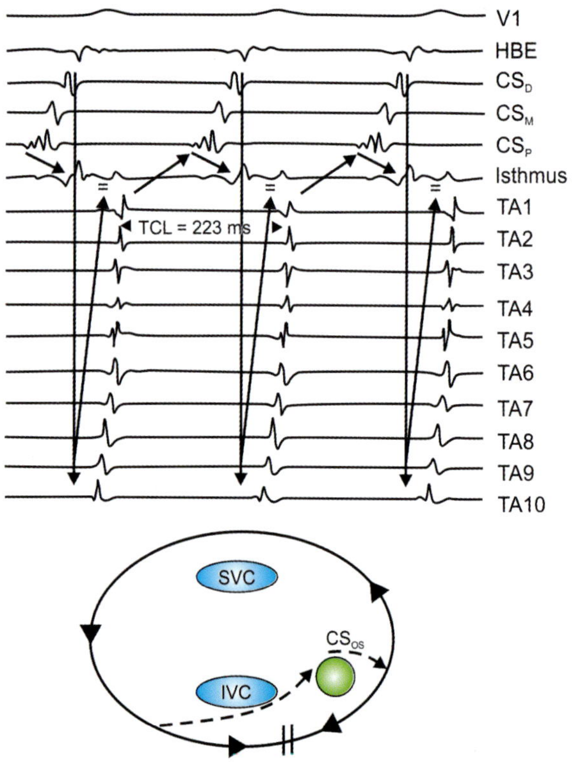

Fig. 30.22: Electrograms and schematic representation of atrial activation in partial isthmus-dependent flutter. In partial isthmus-dependent flutter, the wavefront bypasses the cavotricuspid isthmus (CTI) to enter it laterally and medially. The coronary sinus (CS) ostium is activated prematurely, and the tachycardia is not entrained from the CTI itself. [Image adapted with permission from Yang Y, Cheng J, Bochoeyer A, et al. Atypical right atrial flutter patterns. Circulation. 2001;103(25):3092-8]. (IVC: Inferior vena cava; SVC: Superior vena cava; TA10: Proximal recording electrodes on Halo catheter near upper septum; TA1: Distal recording electrodes on Halo catheter near lateral aspect of the CTI; CS: Coronary sinus; Arrows indicate endocardial activation sequence).

SUMMARY

Atrial flutter is a common atrial and clinically important arrhythmia. Although some aspects of AFL management are similar to AF, it is a distinct arrhythmia that warrants its own management strategy. Mapping of isthmus-dependent AFL can be performed using standard catheter techniques, allowing one to make an accurate diagnosis that will result in successful ablation. RFCA has become a first-line treatment for AFL, with nearly uniform acute and chronic success, and low complication rates.

REFERENCES

Atiga WL, Worley SJ, Hummel J, et al. Prospective randomized comparison of cooled radiofrequency versus standard radiofrequency energy for ablation of typical atrial flutter. Pacing Clin Electrophysiol. 2002;25(8):1172-8.

Calkins H, Canby R, Weiss R, et al. Results of catheter ablation of typical atrial flutter. Am J Cardiol. 2004;94(4):437-42.

Calkins H, Leon AR, Deam AG, et al. Catheter ablation of atrial flutter using radiofrequency energy. Am J Cardiol. 1994;73(5):353-6.

Calkins H. Catheter ablation of atrial flutter: do outcomes of catheter ablation with "large-tip" versus "cooled-tip" catheters really differ? J Cardiovasc Electrophysiol. 2004;15(10):1131-2.

Cauchemez B, Haissaguerre M, Fischer B, et al. Electrophysiological effects of catheter ablation of inferior vena cava-tricuspid annulus isthmus in common atrial flutter. Circulation. 1996;93(2):284-94.

Cha YM, Wales A, Wolf P, et al. Electrophysiologic effects of the new class III antiarrhythmic drug dofetilide compared to the class IA antiarrhythmic drug quinidine in experimental canine atrial flutter: role of dispersion of refractoriness in antiarrhythmic efficacy. J Cardiovasc Electrophysiol. 1996;7(9):809-27.

Chugh A, Latchamsetty R, Oral H, et al. Characteristics of cavotricuspid isthmus-dependent atrial flutter after left atrial ablation of atrial fibrillation. Circulation. 2006;113(5):609-15.

Cosio FG, Goicolea A, Lopez-Gil M, et al. Atrial endocardial mapping in the rare form of atrial flutter. Am J Cardiol. 1990;66(7):715-20.

Cosio FG, Lopez-Gil M, Goicolea A, et al. Radiofrequency ablation of the inferior vena cava-tricuspid valve isthmus in common atrial flutter. Am J Cardiol. 1993;71(8):705-9.

Da Costa A, Mourot S, Romeyer-Bouchard C, et al. Anatomic and electrophysiological differences between chronic and paroxysmal forms of common atrial flutter and comparison with controls. Pacing Clin Electrophysiol. 2004;27(9):1202-11.

Feld G, Wharton M, Plumb V, et al. Radiofrequency catheter ablation of type 1 atrial flutter using large-tip 8- or 10-mm electrode catheters and a high-output radiofrequency energy generator: results of a multicenter safety and efficacy study. J Am Coll Cardiol. 2004;43(8):1466-72.

Feld GK, Fleck RP, Chen PS, et al. Radiofrequency catheter ablation for the treatment of human type 1 atrial flutter. Identification of a critical zone in the reentrant circuit by endocardial mapping techniques. Circulation. 1992;86(4):1233-40.

Feld GK, Mollerus M, Birgersdotter-Green U, et al. Conduction velocity in the tricuspid valve-inferior vena cava isthmus is slower in patients with type I atrial flutter compared to those without a history of atrial flutter. J Cardiovasc Electrophysiol. 1997;8(12):1338-48.

Feld GK, Shahandeh-Rad F. Activation patterns in experimental canine atrial flutter produced by right atrial crush injury. J Am Coll Cardiol. 1992;20(2):441-51.

Feld GK, Nademanee K, Noll E, et al. Oral N-acetylprocainamide compared to quinidine plus digoxin in the chronic suppression of atrial flutter in humans. Cardiovasc Drugs Ther. 1989;3(2):191-8.

Feld GK, Venkatesh N, Singh BN. Pharmacologic conversion and suppression of experimental canine atrial flutter: differing effects of d-sotalol, quinidine, and lidocaine and the significance of changes in refractoriness and conduction. Circulation. 1986;74(1):197-204.

Feld GK, Venkatesh N, Singh BN. Effects of N-acetylprocainamide and recainam in the pharmacologic conversion and suppression of experimental canine atrial flutter: significance of changes in refractoriness and conduction. J Cardiovasc Pharmacol. 1988;11(5):573-80.

Fischer B, Haissaguerre M, Garrigues S, et al. Radiofrequency catheter ablation of common atrial flutter in 80 patients. J Am Coll Cardiol. 1995;25(6):1365-72.

Haissaguerre M, Sanders P, Hocini M, et al. Pulmonary veins in the substrate for atrial fibrillation: the "venous wave" hypothesis. J Am Coll Cardiol. 2004;43(12):2290-2.

Ilg KJ, Kuhne M, Crawford T, et al. Randomized comparison of cavotricuspid isthmus ablation for atrial flutter using an open irrigation-tip versus a large-tip radiofrequency ablation catheter. J Cardiovasc Electrophysiol. 2011;22(9):1007-12.

Jais P, Haissaguerre M, Shah DC, et al. Successful irrigated-tip catheter ablation of atrial flutter resistant to conventional radiofrequency ablation. Circulation. 1998;98(9):835-8.

Kalman JM, Olgin JE, Saxon LA, et al. Activation and entrainment mapping defines the tricuspid annulus as the anterior barrier in typical atrial flutter. Circulation. 1996;94(3):398-406.

Kinder C, Kall J, Kopp D, et al. Conduction properties of the inferior vena cava-tricuspid annular isthmus in patients with typical atrial flutter. J Cardiovasc Electrophysiol. 1997;8(7):727-37.

Kirkorian G, Moncada E, Chevalier P, et al. Radiofrequency ablation of atrial flutter. Efficacy of an anatomically guided approach. Circulation. 1994;90(6):2804-14.

Lee BK, Reyes CM, Hernandez J, et al. Catheter ablation is more cost-effective than cardioversion and drug therapy for first-line treatment of atrial flutter. Heart Rhythm. 2005;2:S1.

Lesh MD, Van Hare GF, Epstein LM, et al. Radiofrequency catheter ablation of atrial arrhythmias. Results and mechanisms. Circulation. 1994;89(3):1074-89.

Lo LW, Tai CT, Lin YJ, et al. Characteristics of the cavotricuspid isthmus in predicting recurrent conduction in the long-term follow-up. J Cardiovasc Electrophysiol. 2009;20(1):39-43.

Mangat I, Tschopp DR, Yang Y, et al. Optimizing the detection of bidirectional block across the flutter isthmus for patients with typical isthmus-dependent atrial flutter. Am J Cardiol. 2003;91(5):559-64.

Okumura K, Plumb VJ, Page PL, et al. Atrial activation sequence during atrial flutter in the canine pericarditis model and its effects on the polarity of the flutter wave in the electrocardiogram. J Am Coll Cardiol. 1991;17(2):509-18.

Olgin JE, Kalman JM, Fitzpatrick AP, et al. Role of right atrial endocardial structures as barriers to conduction during human type I atrial flutter. Activation and entrainment mapping guided by intracardiac echocardiography. Circulation. 1995;92(7):1839-48.

Olgin JE, Kalman JM, Lesh MD. Conduction barriers in human atrial flutter: correlation of electrophysiology and anatomy. J Cardiovasc Electrophysiol. 1996;7(11):1112-26.

Olgin JE, Kalman JM, Saxon LA, et al. Mechanism of initiation of atrial flutter in humans: site of unidirectional block and direction of rotation. J Am Coll Cardiol. 1997;29(2):376-84.

Olshansky B, Okumura K, Hess PG, et al. Demonstration of an area of slow conduction in human atrial flutter. J Am Coll Cardiol. 1990;16(7):1639-48.

Oshikawa N, Watanabe I, Masaki R, et al. Relationship between polarity of the flutter wave in the surface ECG and endocardial atrial activation sequence in patients with typical counterclockwise and clockwise atrial flutter. J Interv Card Electrophysiol. 2002;7(3):215-23.

Poty H, Saoudi N, Abdel Aziz A, et al. Radiofrequency catheter ablation of type 1 atrial flutter. Prediction of late success by electrophysiological criteria. Circulation. 1995;92(6):1389-92.

Saoudi N, Cosio F, Waldo A, et al. Classification of atrial flutter and regular atrial tachycardia according to electrophysiologic mechanism and anatomic bases: a statement from a joint expert group from the Working Group of Arrhythmias of the European Society of Cardiology and the North American Society of Pacing and Electrophysiology. J Cardiovasc Electrophysiol. 2001;12:852-66.

Sawhney N, Anand K, Robertson CE, et al. Recovery of mitral isthmus conduction leads to the development of macro-reentrant tachycardia after left atrial linear ablation for atrial fibrillation. Circ Arrhythm Electrophysiol. 2011;4(6):832-7.

Sawhney N, Anousheh R, Chen W, et al. Circumferential pulmonary vein ablation with additional linear ablation results in an increased incidence of left atrial flutter compared with segmental pulmonary vein isolation as an initial approach to ablation of paroxysmal atrial fibrillation. Circ Arrhythm Electrophysiol. 2010;3:243-8.

Scavee C, Jais P, Hsu LF, et al. Prospective randomised comparison of irrigated-tip and large-tip catheter ablation of cavotricuspid isthmus-dependent atrial flutter. Eur Heart J. 2004;25(11):963-9.

Schwartzman D, Callans DJ, Gottlieb CD, et al. Conduction block in the inferior vena caval-tricuspid valve isthmus: association with outcome of radiofrequency ablation of type I atrial flutter. J Am Coll Cardiol. 1996;28(6):1519-31.

Spach MS, Dolber PC, Heidlage JF. Influence of the passive anisotropic properties on directional differences in propagation following modification of the sodium conductance in human atrial muscle. A model of reentry based on anisotropic discontinuous propagation. Circ Res. 1988;62(4):811-32.

Spach MS, Miller WT, Dolber PC, et al. The functional role of structural complexities in the propagation of depolarization in the atrium of the dog. Cardiac conduction disturbances due to discontinuities of effective axial resistivity. Circ Res. 1982;50(2):175-91.

Stambler BS, Wood MA, Ellenbogen KA, et al. Efficacy and safety of repeated intravenous doses of ibutilide for rapid conversion of atrial flutter or fibrillation. Ibutilide Repeat Dose Study Investigators. Circulation. 1996;94(7):1613-21.

Suzuki F, Toshida N, Nawata H, et al. Coronary sinus pacing initiates counterclockwise atrial flutter while pacing from the low lateral right atrium initiates clockwise atrial flutter. Analysis of episodes of direct initiation of atrial flutter. J Electrocardiol. 1998;31:345-61.

Tada H, Oral H, Sticherling C, et al. Double potentials along the ablation line as a guide to radiofrequency ablation of typical atrial flutter. J Am Coll Cardiol. 2001;38(3):750-5.

Tai CT, Chen SA, Chiang CE, et al. Electrophysiologic characteristics and radiofrequency catheter ablation in patients with clockwise atrial flutter. J Cardiovasc Electrophysiol. 1997; 8(1):24-34.

Tai CT, Haque A, Lin YK, et al. Double potential interval and transisthmus conduction time for prediction of cavotricuspid isthmus block after ablation of typical atrial flutter. J Interv Card Electrophysiol. 2002;7(1):77-82.

Tai CT, Huang JL, Lee PC, et al. High-resolution mapping around the crista terminalis during typical atrial flutter: new insights into mechanisms. J Cardiovasc Electrophysiol. 2004; 15(4):406-14.

Tsai CF, Tai CT, Yu WC, et al. Is 8-mm more effective than 4-mm tip electrode catheter for ablation of typical atrial flutter? Circulation. 1999;100(7):768-71.

Ventura R, Klemm H, Lutomsky B, et al. Pattern of isthmus conduction recovery using open cooled and solid large-tip catheters for radiofrequency ablation of typical atrial flutter. J Cardiovasc Electrophysiol. 2004;15(10):1126-30.

Waldo A, Feld GK. Interrelationships of atrial fibrillation and atrial flutter: mechanisms and clinical implications. J Am Coll Cardiol. 2008;51(8):779-86.

Wann LS, Curtis AB, January CT, et al. 2011 ACCF/AHA/HRS focused update on the management of patients with atrial fibrillation (Updating the 2006 Guideline): a report of the American College of Cardiology Foundation/American Heart Association Task Force on Practice Guidelines. Heart Rhythm. 2011;8(1):157-76.

Yang Y, Cheng J, Bochoeyer A, et al. Atypical right atrial flutter patterns. Circulation. 2001;103(25):3092-8.

Yang Y, Varma N, Badhwar N, et al. Prospective observations in the clinical and electrophysiological characteristics of intra-isthmus reentry. J Cardiovasc Electrophysiol. 2010;21(10): 1099-106.

CHAPTER 31

Wolff-Parkinson-White Syndrome and Atrioventricular Reciprocating Tachycardia

Christopher R Ellis, Arvindh N Kanagasundram

INTRODUCTION AND DEFINITION

In 1930, Louis Wolff, Sir John Parkinson, and Paul Dudley White (Fig. 31.1A) reported on 11 patients with bouts of tachycardias and ECG findings of a short PQ time and a delta wave. Patients with electrophysiological abnormalities that cause these findings and tachyarrhythmias have since been referred to as having Wolff-Parkinson-White (WPW) syndrome. The accessory atrioventricular pathways responsible for these ECG findings and arrhythmias are aberrant muscular connections outside the usual conduction system (Fig. 31.1B).

If the accessory pathway is capable of antegrade conduction, the electrocardiogram can exhibit a short PR interval and a slurred upstroke of the QRS complex known as a delta wave (Figs. 31.2A and B). The PR interval shortening is due to the fact that the accessory pathway bypasses the AV node and "pre-excites" the ventricle. If ventricular

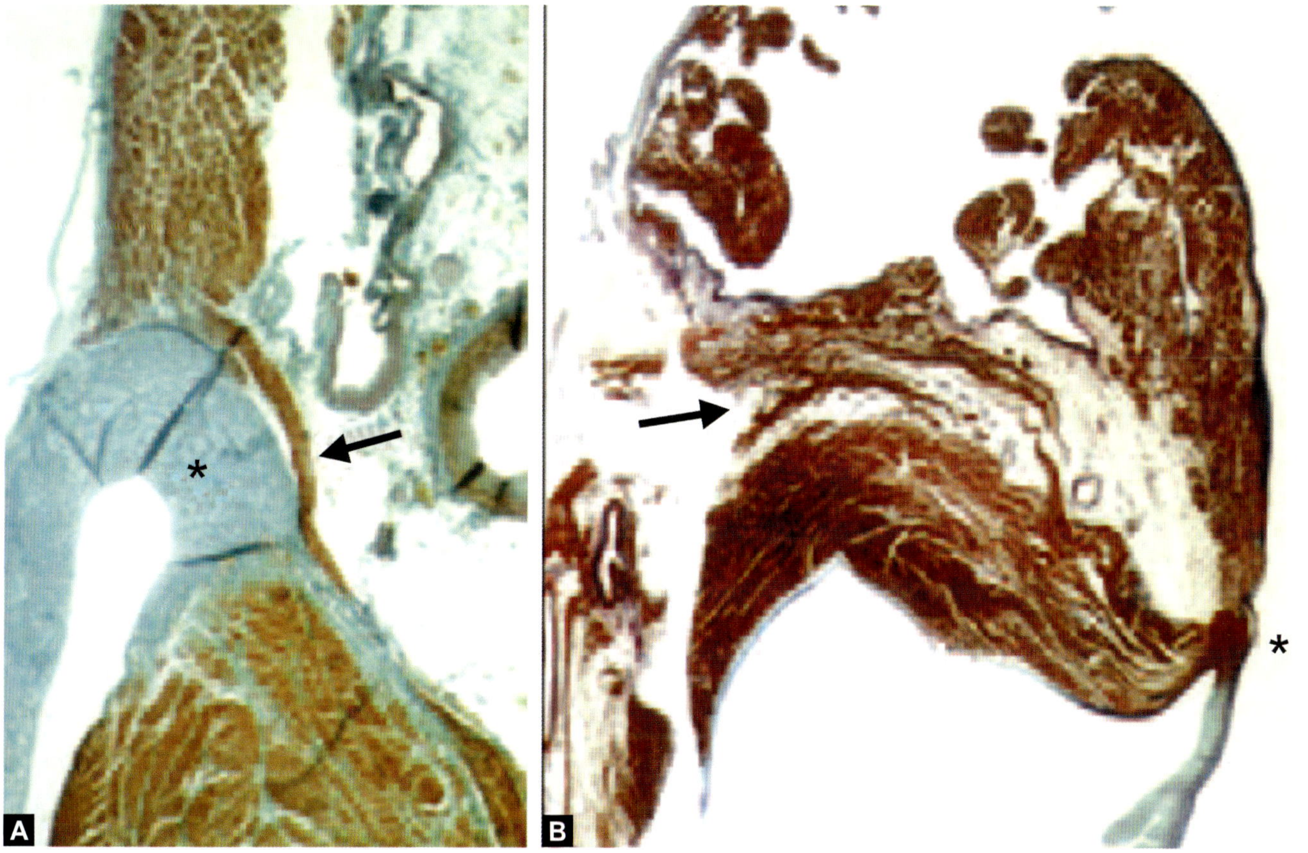

Figs. 31.1A and B: Histological sections demonstrating left (A) and right-sided (B) accessory pathways. (Ho SY. Accessory Atriovetricular Pathways: Getting to the Origins. Circulation. 2008; 117:1502-4).

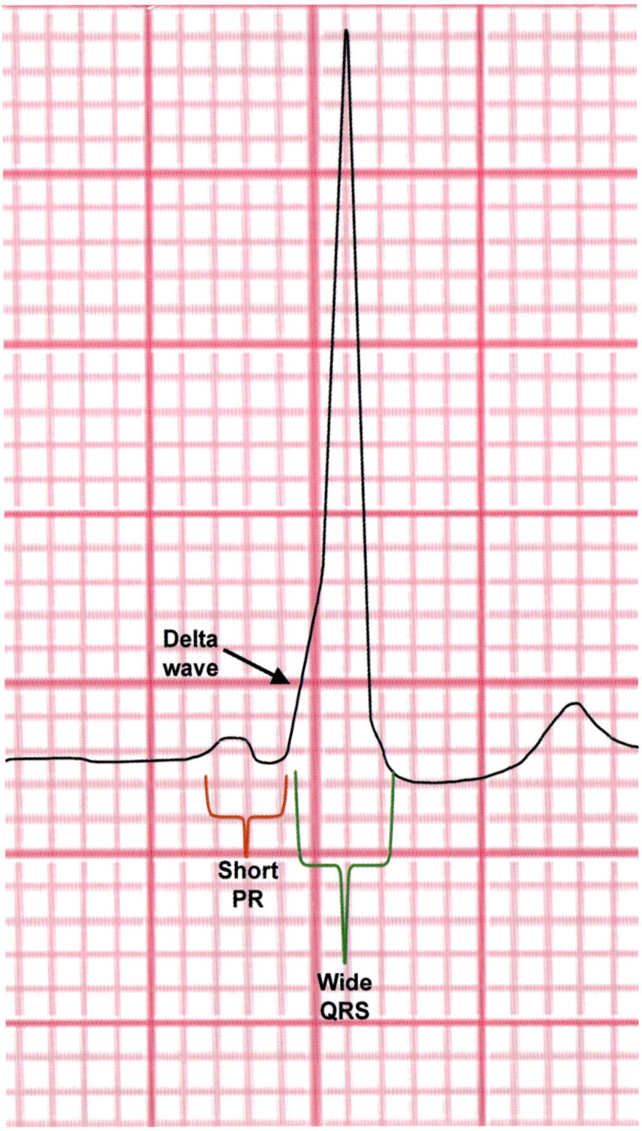

Fig. 31.2A: Characteristic appearance of the ECG in a patient with Wolff-Parkinson-White syndrome and antegrade conduction. ECG shows a short PR interval, delta wave, and wide QRS complex. (Image courtesy of Glenn N Levine, MD).

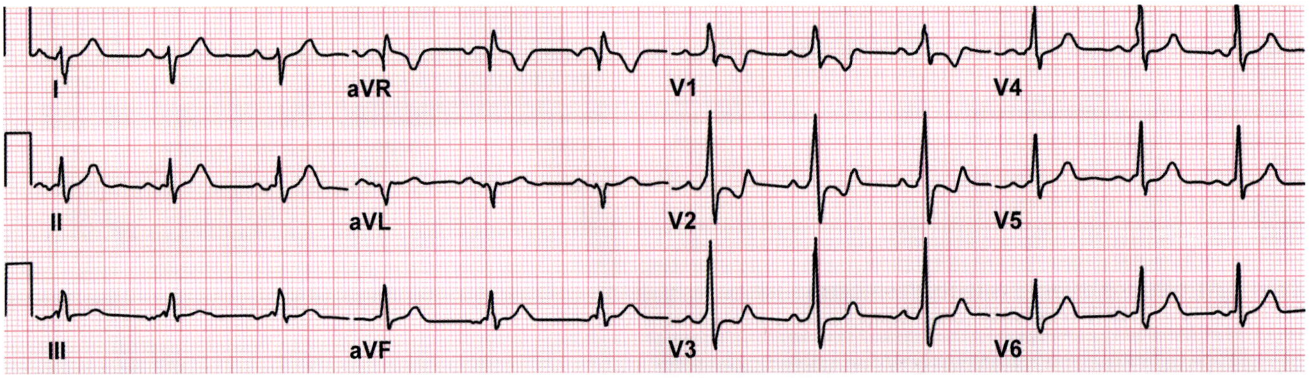

Fig. 31.2B: Manifest pre-excitation. Positive delta wave in V1, positive delta wave in aVF, negative delta wave in aVL, consistent with left lateral free wall accessory pathway.

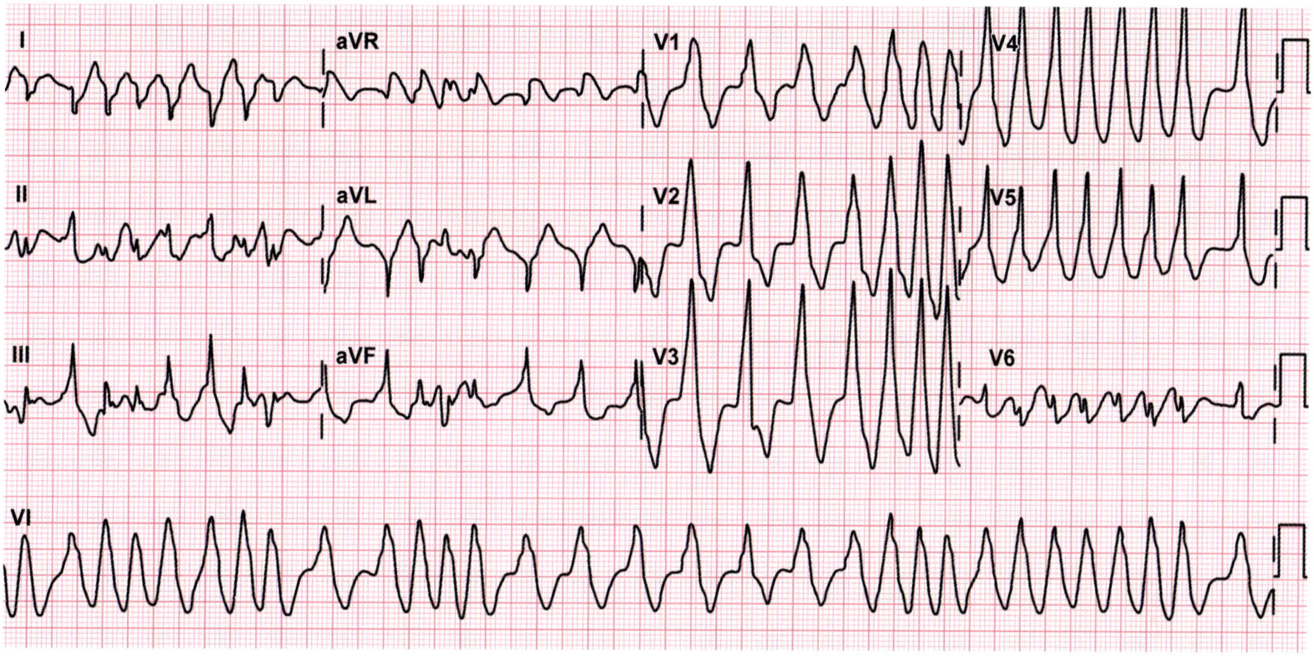

Fig. 31.3: Atrial fibrillation in a patient with a bypass tract (pre-excited atrial fibrillation). Irregular wide complex tachycardia with RBBB pattern and variable QRS duration. Rightward QRS axis, negative delta wave in aVL consistent with a left lateral pathway. (RBBB: Right bundle branch block).

pre-excitation is seen on the resting electrocardiogram, the accessory pathway is termed "manifest". The level of pre-excitation depends on the relative conduction velocity over the accessory pathway (compared with the AV node) and the proximity of the pathway to the sinus node. If the accessory pathway is capable only of retrograde conduction the electrocardiogram during sinus rhythm will exhibit a normal QRS complex, and thus the accessory pathway is termed "concealed".

TERMINOLOGY

Wolff-Parkinson-White syndrome is used to describe patients who have evidence of pre-excitation on electrocardiogram with documented tachycardia. In the absence of arrhythmia the patient is said to have the WPW pattern on electrocardiogram.

CLINICAL PRESENTATION

The presentation of patients with atrioventricular reciprocating tachycardia (AVRT) can include symptoms of palpitations, light-headedness, dyspnea and chest discomfort. Syncope is uncommon with AVRT but can be caused by atrial fibrillation with rapid conduction to the ventricles over the pathway (Fig. 31.3). AVRT usually presents at a younger age in patients without structural heart disease, although it can present at any age.

ANATOMY

Accessory pathways (AP) are typically found straddling the mitral or tricuspid valves and in this case are known as atrioventricular pathways. The majority (~60%) attach along the mitral valve annulus and are known as left "free wall" pathways. The next most common site is along the septal aspect of the tricuspid or mitral valves (~25% right anteroseptal, right posteroseptal or left posteroseptal), followed by the lateral tricupid annulus, coined right "free wall" pathways (~15%) (Figs. 31.4A and B). Congenital anomalies of the coronary sinus may be associated with epicardial accessory pathways located in pouches, or diverticula of the CS branches.

Less frequently, accessory pathways do not insert along the atrioventricular valves. Examples of such connections are atriofasicular (right atrium to distal right bundle; capable of antegrade conduction only), nodoventricular (AV node to right ventricular myocardium), nodofascicular (AV node to specialized conduction tissue) and atrio-nodal (right atrium to the AV node) (Fig. 31.5).

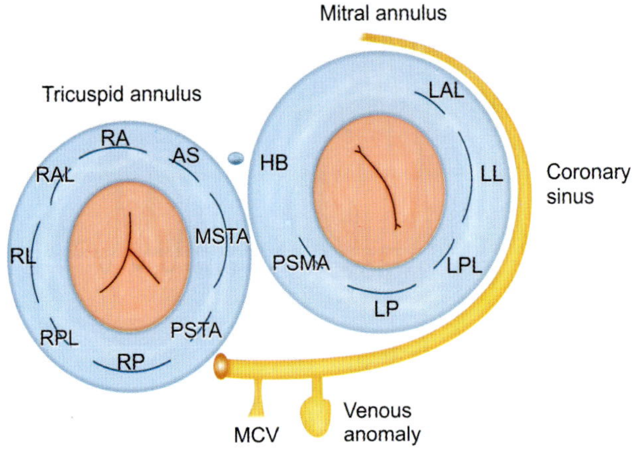

Fig. 31.4A: Anatomic locations of accessory atrioventricular connections. (HB: His bundle; CSOs: Coronary sinus ostium; MCV: Middle cardiac vein; RA: Right anterior; RAL: Right anterolateral; RL: Right lateral; RPL: Right posterolateral; RP: Right posterior; PSTA: Posteroseptal tricuspid annulus; MSTA: Mid-Septal tricuspid annulus; AS: Anteroseptal; PSMA: Posteroseptal mitral annulus; LP: Left posterior; LPL: Left posterolateral; LL: Left lateral; LAL: Left anterolateral).

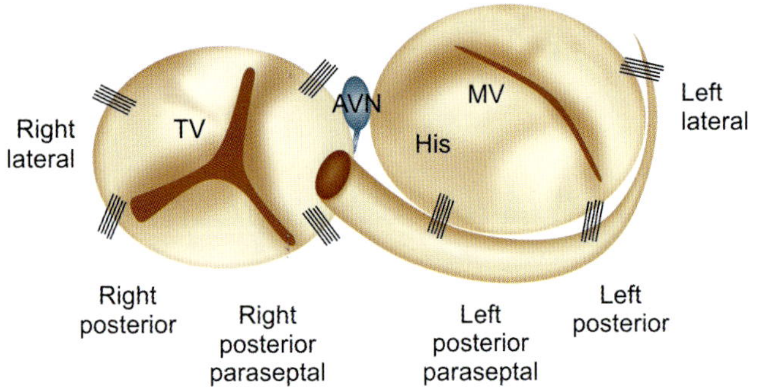

Fig. 31.4B: Schematic illustration of location of accessory pathways in WPW. (WPW: Wolff-Parkinson-White syndrome).

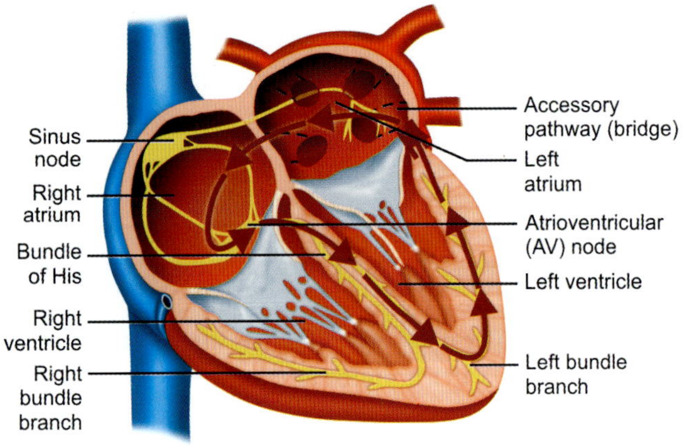

Fig. 31.5: An example of the reentrant circuit in a patient with WPW. (WPW: Wolff-Parkinson-White syndrome).

PATHOPHYSIOLOGY

Atrioventricular reciprocating tachycardia is a macro reentrant tachycardia usually utilizing both the normal conduction of the heart and the accessory pathway. Orthodromic reentrant tachycardia is the more common tachycardia, with antegrade conduction over the AV node and retrograde conduction over the pathway. This results in a narrow complex tachycardia, except for when bundle branch aberrancy is present. Antidromic recriprocating tachycardia is less frequent and occurs with antegrade conduction over the accessory pathway and retrograde conduction over the AV node. This results in a wide complex tachycardia with QRS morphology reflective of the site of ventricular insertion of the pathway (Fig. 31.6).

DIAGNOSIS

When pre-excitation is present, the axis of the delta wave (first 40 ms) (Fig. 31.7) is indicative of the location of the ventricular insertion of the pathway (Flow charts 31.1A to D and Fig. 31.8). Some of the features on electrocardiogram that are indicative of orthodromic reciprocating tachycardia being the mechanism of an arrhythmia include initiation of tachycardia with block in the accessory pathway (Fig. 31.9), a retrograde P wave that comes distinctly after QRS (longer RP relationship) (Fig. 31.10) and QRS alternans. The presence of atrioventricular block or dissociation during tachycardia rules out AVRT being the mechanism of an arrhythmia, as the atria and ventricles are both obligatory parts of the circuit.

INVASIVE ELECTROPHYSIOLOGY TESTING

Intracardiac diagnosis of pre-excitation is a short (<35 ms) or negative HV interval (Fig. 31.11). Evidence of eccentric atrial activation during ventricular pacing is evidence of retrograde conduction over an accessory pathway. Accessory pathway depolarization can be seen as a sharp,

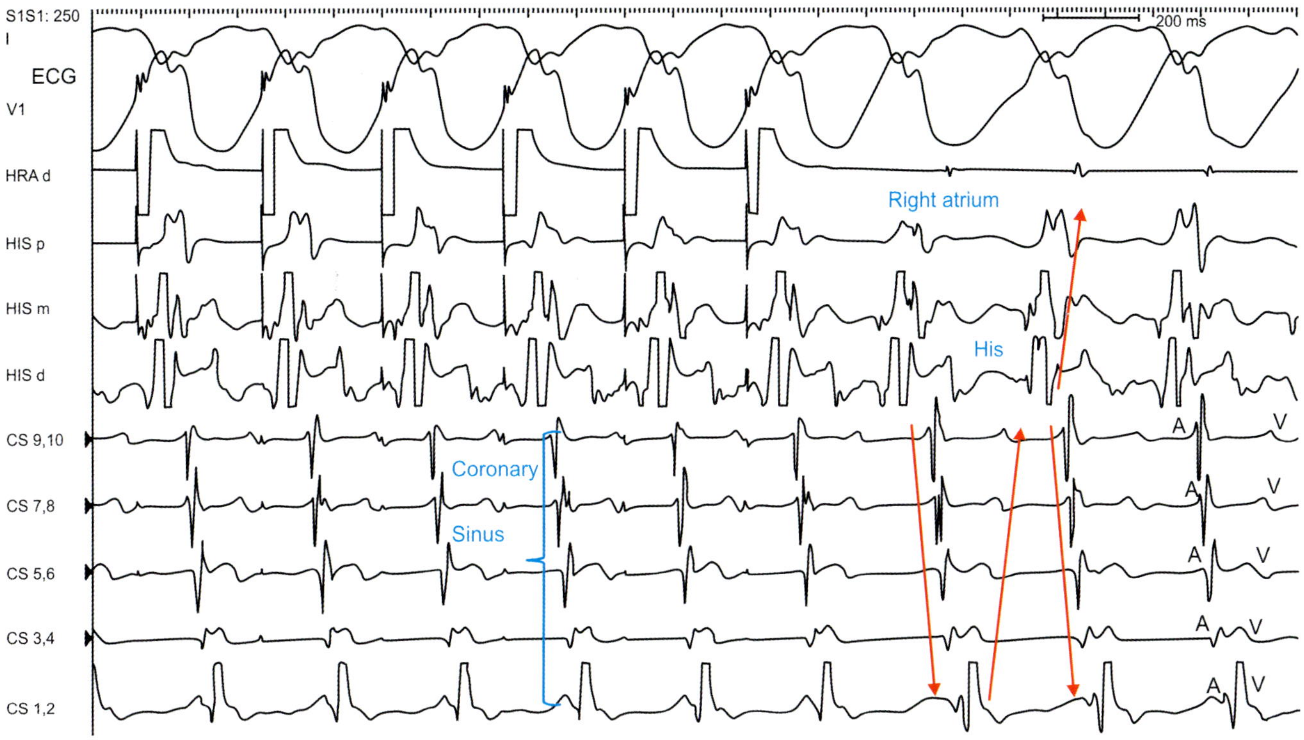

Fig. 31.6: Atrial pacing initiates antidromic AV re-entry tachycardia upon conduction block in the AVN. Regular wide complex right bundle branch (RBB) pattern tachycardia with 1:1 AV relation and eccentric ventricular activation early at lateral coronary sinus, consistent with a left lateral accessory pathway insertion site.

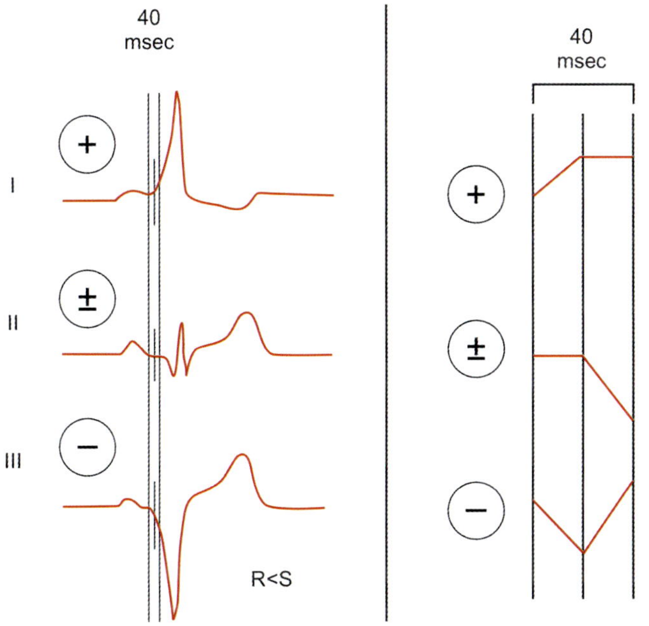

Fig. 31.7: Delta wave polarity for accessory pathway ECG localization.

high frequency deflection between the atrial and ventricular electrograms and precedes the onset of the delta wave (Fig. 31.12). Ventricular entrainment and premature ventricular contractions can be used to distinguish orthodromic reentrant tachycardia from other narrow complex tachycardias.

MANAGEMENT

It is important to identify pathways which can be at high-risk for sudden cardiac death due to rapid conduction to the ventricles over the pathway during atrial arrhythmias. One of the major determinants of the rate of conduction over an accessory pathway is the effective refractory period of the bypass tract. Patients who develop ventricular fibrillation have pathways that have a shorter effective refractory period.

Intermittent pre-excitation refers to abrupt loss of pre-excitation (and prolongation of PR interval) on the same rhythm strip. This correlates with a long effective

Flow chart 31.1A: Stepwise ECG algorithm for accessory pathway ECG localization. (Arruda MS, McClelland JH, Wang X, et al. J Cardiovasc Electrophysiol. 1998:9;2-12).

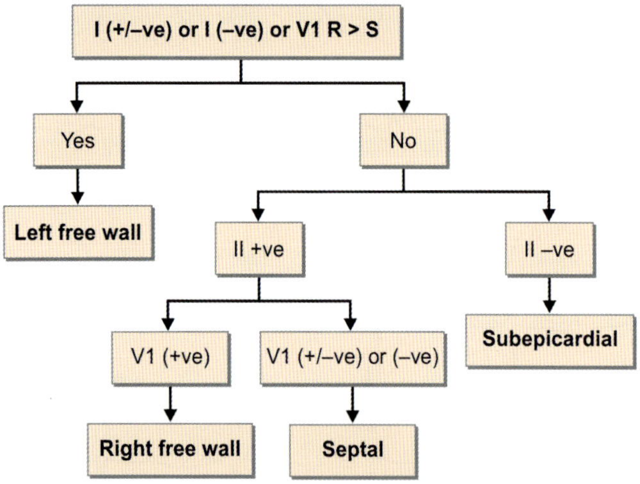

Flow chart 31.1B: Stepwise ECG algorithm for accessory pathway ECG localization. (LP: Left posterior; LPL: Left posterolateral; LL: Left lateral; LAL: Left anterolateral (Arruda MS, McClelland JH, Wang X, et al. J Cardiovasc Electrophysiol. 1998:9;2-12).

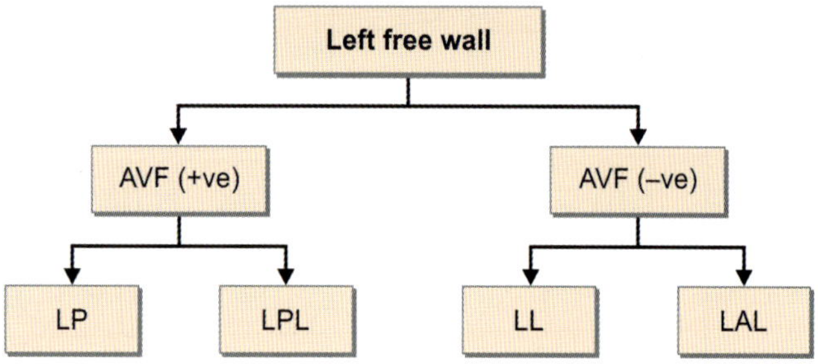

Flow chart 31.1C: Stepwise ECG algorithm for accessory pathway ECG localization. (PSMA: Posteroseptal Mitral annulus; PSTA: Posteroseptal tricuspid annulus; AS: Anteroseptal; MS: Midseptal (Arruda MS, McClelland JH, Wang X, et al. J Cardiovasc Electrophysiol. 1998:9;2-12).

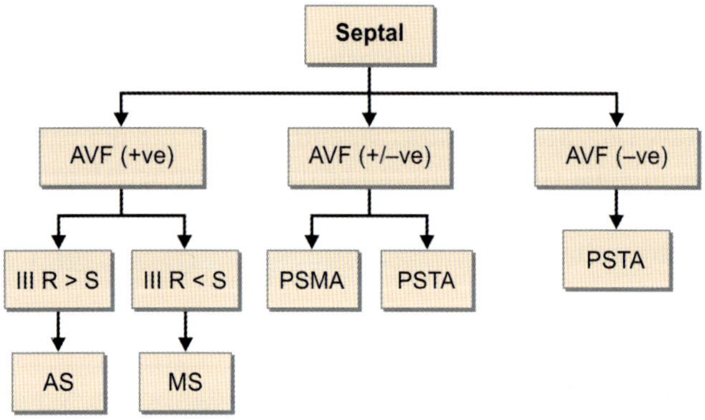

Flow chart 31.1D: Stepwise ECG algorithm for accessory pathway ECG localization. (RA: Right anterior; RAL: Right anterolateral; RL: Right lateral; RP: Right posterior; RPL: Right posterolateral (Arruda MS, McClelland JH, Wang X, et al. J Cardiovasc Electrophysiol. 1998:9;2-12).

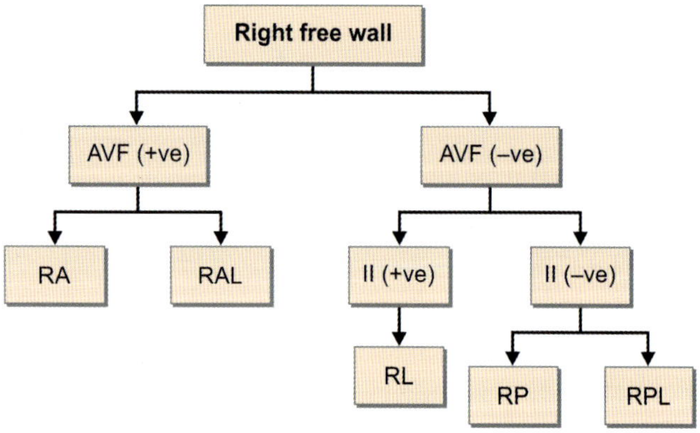

refractory period and is associated with a low-risk of developing sudden death (Fig. 31.13). Exercise testing and antiarrhythmic medications can also be used to identify low-risk pathways by demonstrating antegrade block in the accessory pathway.

During atrial fibrillation in patients with a bypass tract, AV nodal blocking agents should be avoided, and procainamide or amiodarone should be used preferentially (Figs. 31.14A and B). In patients with high-risk pathways or recurrent, AVRT an electrophysiology study with ablation can be a very effective treatment modality. Ideal locations for ablation of accessory pathways is determined by: 1) the earliest site of ventricular insertion during manifest pre-excitation or during antidromic reentrant tachycardia; 2) the earliest site of atrial activation during retrograde AP conduction with ventricular pacing or during orthodromic reentrant tachycardia; and 3) AP potentials (Figs. 31.15 and 31.16).

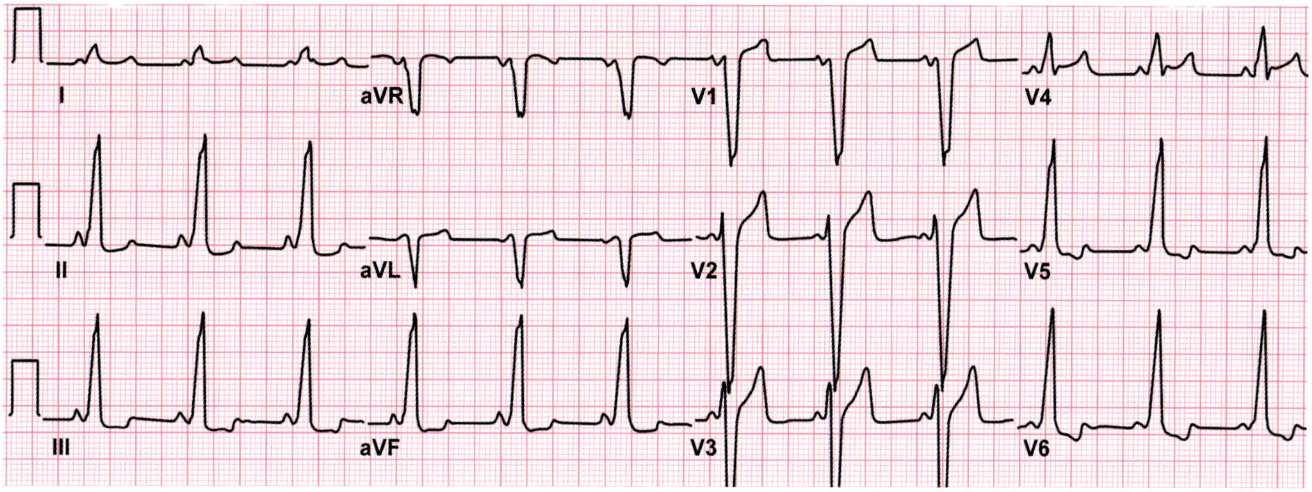

Fig. 31.8: Pre-excitation with negative delta in V1, positive delta in aVF, and R > S in lead III consistent with right anteroseptal accessory pathway.

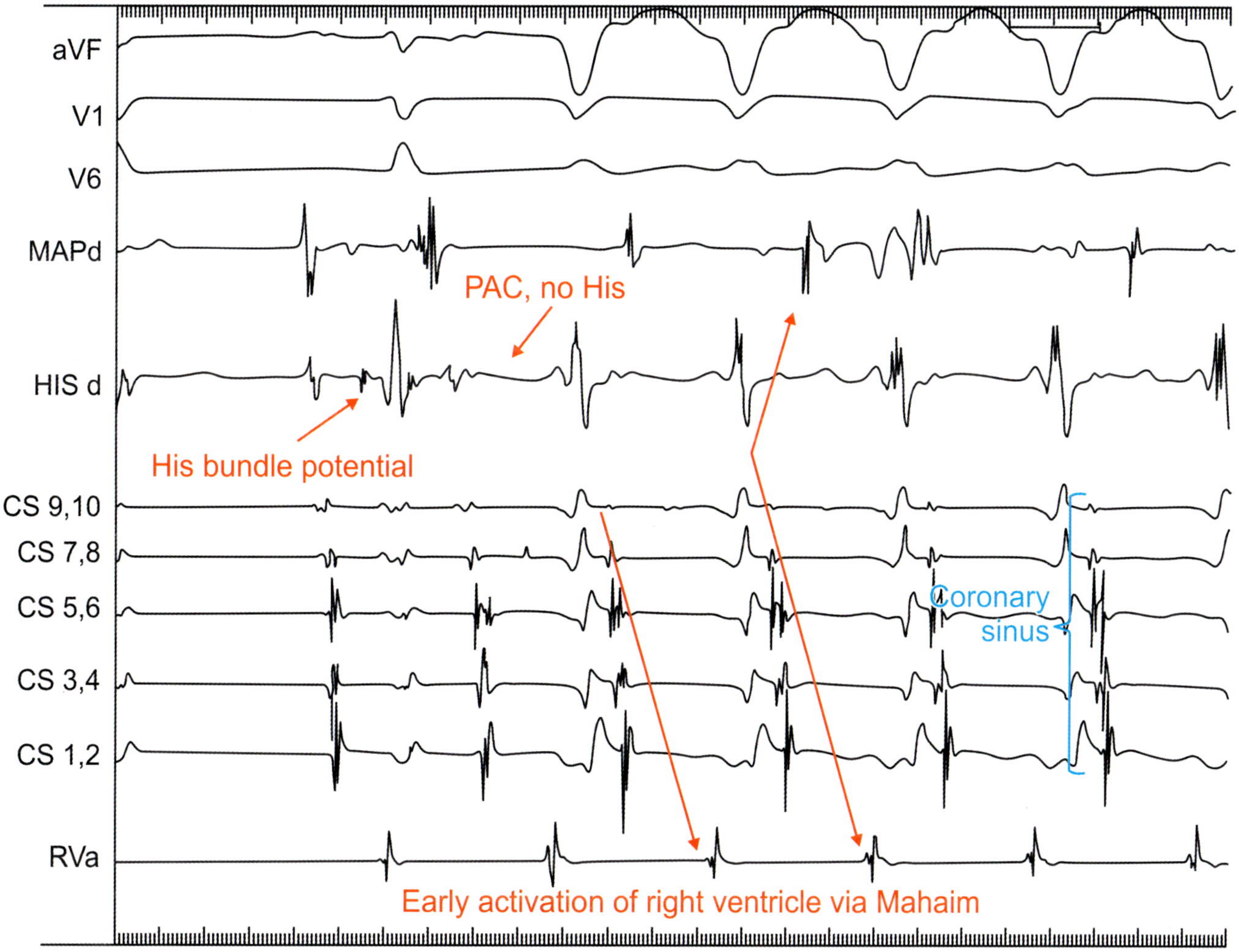

Fig. 31.9: Onset of antidromic AVRT down a Mahaim fiber (atrio-fasicular accessory pathway). Regular wide complex tachycardia with LBBB pattern QRS initiates with a PAC which blocks in the AVN and conducts down the Mahaim. Note loss of His potential at SVT onset. (AVRT: Atrioventricular reciprocating tachycardia; LBBB: Left bundle branch block; PAC: Premature atrial contraction; AVN: atrio-ventricular node; SVT: Supraventricular tachycardia).

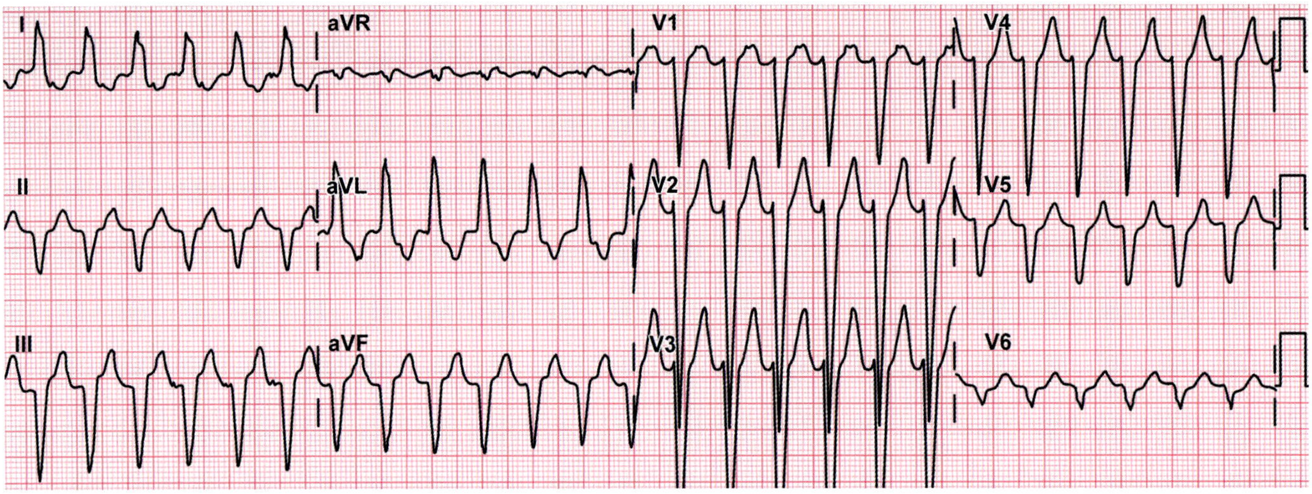

Fig. 31.10: 12-Lead ECG of antidromic AVRT down a Mahaim fiber (atriofasicular accessory pathway). Regular wide complex tachycardia with LBBB pattern QRS and sharp intrinsicoid deflection in V1/V2. Note that P wave comes after QRS. (AVRT: Atrioventricular reciprocating tachycardia; LBBB: Left bundle branch block).

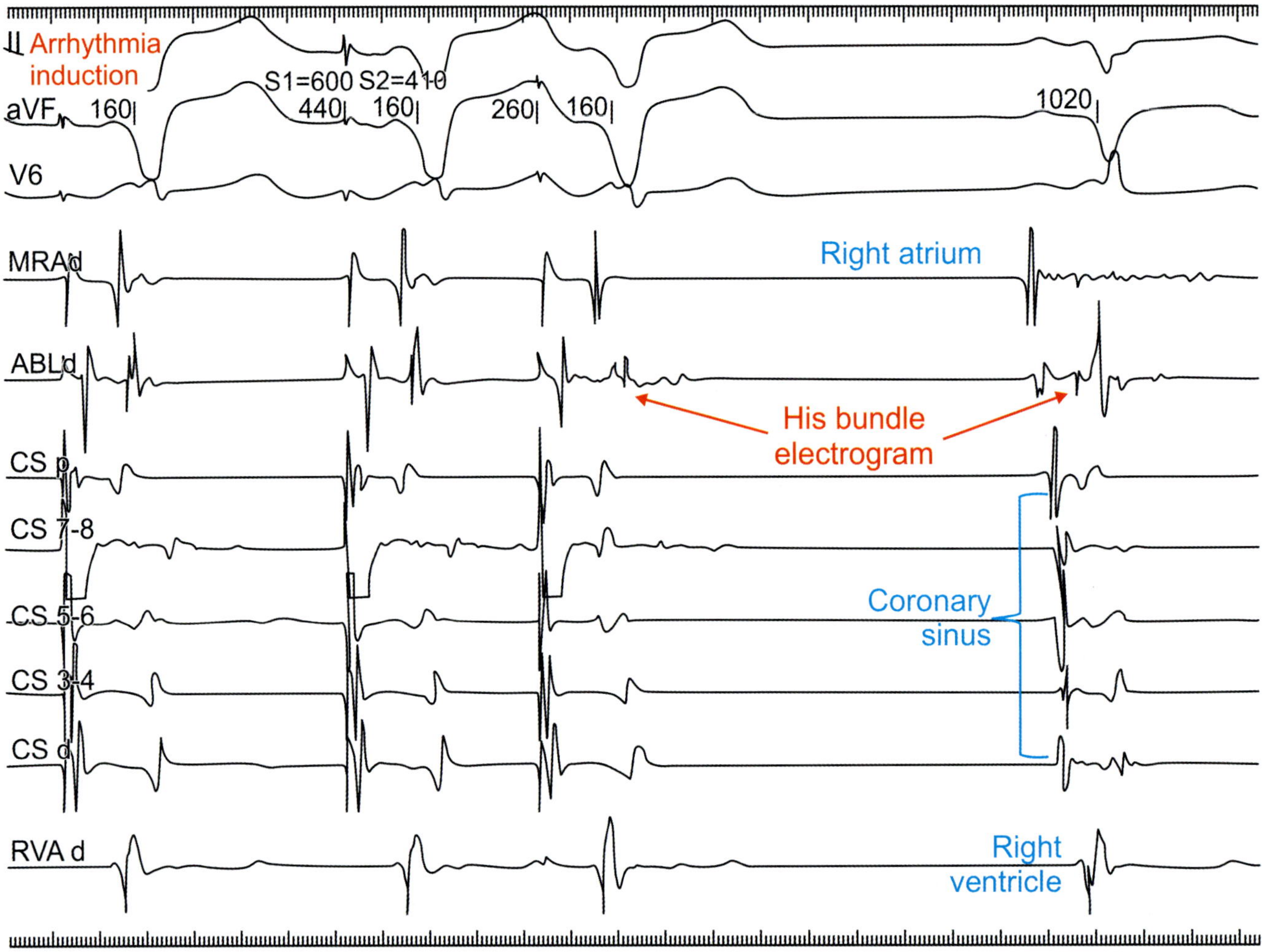

Fig. 31.11: Right posteroseptal accessory pathway. Pacing from CS catheter with premature beat (A1/A2), conducts down both AVN-His and AP. Ablation catheter positioned at His Bundle. His spike occurs 60 ms after QRS onset confirming ventricular pre-excitation. (CS: Coronary sinus; AVN: Atrioventricular node).

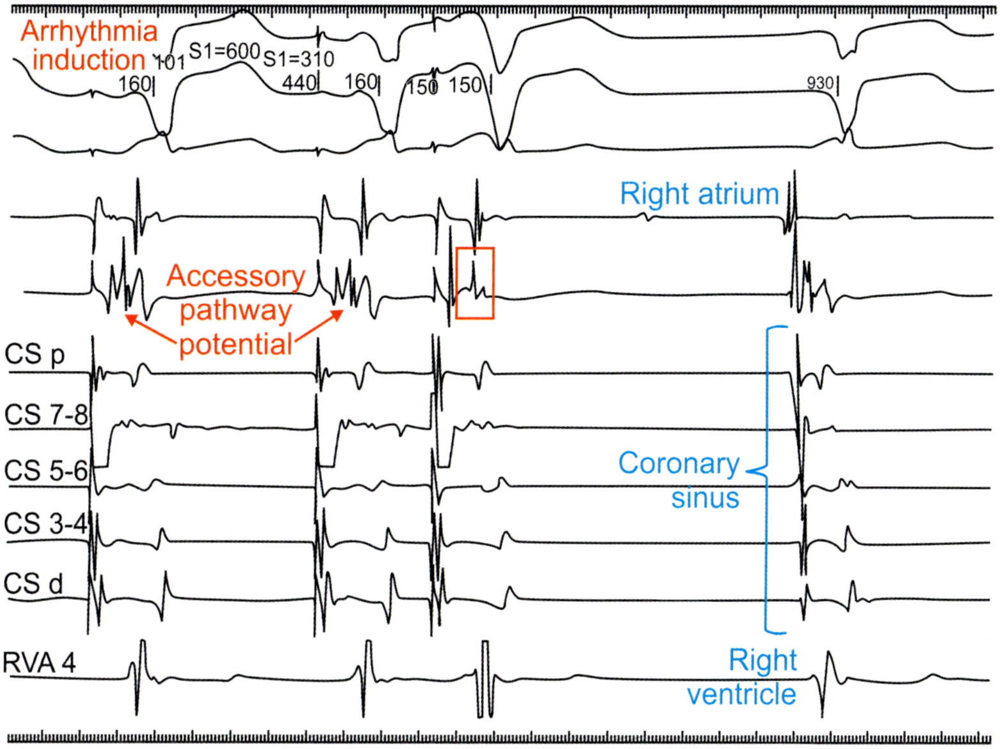

Fig. 31.12: Right posteroseptal accessory pathway. Pacing from CS catheter with premature beat (A1/A2), conducts down AP only revealing AP potential on ablation catheter positioned at accessory pathway. (CS: Coronary sinus; AP: Anteroposterior).

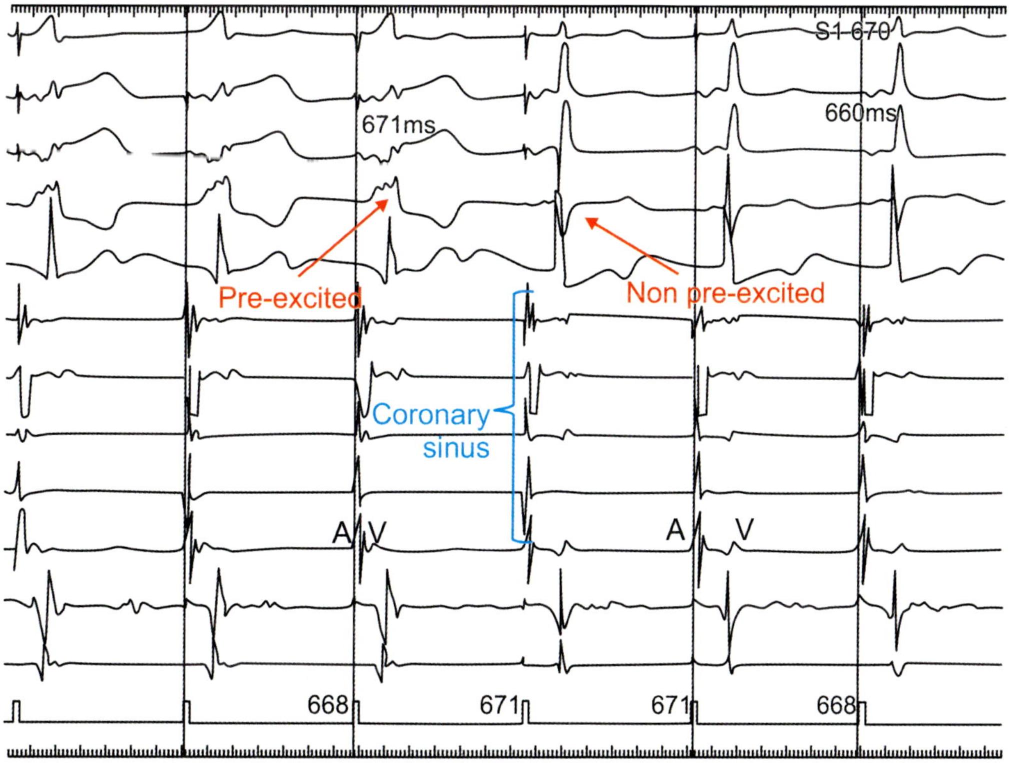

Fig. 31.13: Intermittent antegrade pre-excitation with coronary sinus pacing at fixed rate of 90 bpm. First three beats show left posterolateral AP pattern (AV fusion at coronary sinus), last three beats are abruptly not pre-excited. (AP: Anteroposterior).

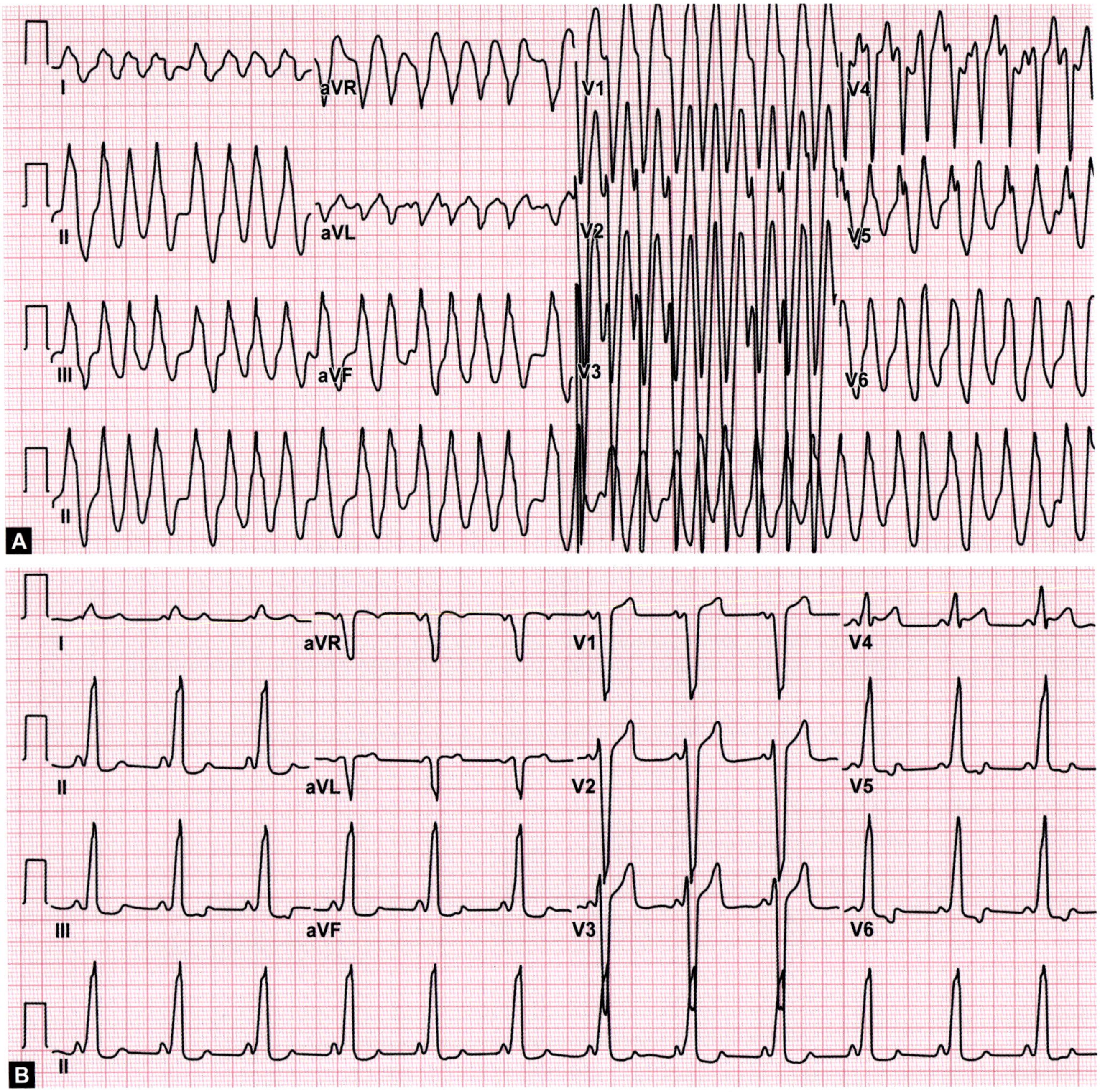

Figs. 31.14A and B: (A) Pre-excited atrial fibrillation with rapid ventricular rate; (B) Sinus rhythm after administration of Procainamide. Pre-excitation pattern consistent with a right anteroseptal pathway.

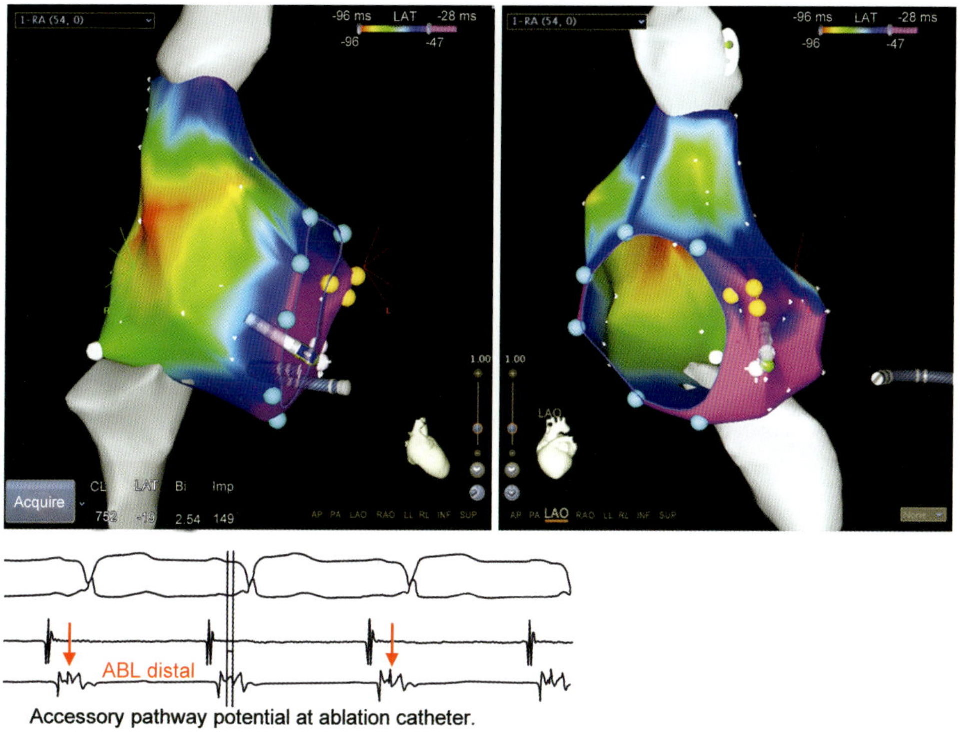

Fig. 31.15: Right posteroseptal accessory pathway location. Orange dots locate compact AVN junction, blue dots locate tricuspid valve. Ablation catheter at pink dot EGM denotes AP potential. (AVN: Atrioventricular node; AP: Anteroposterior).

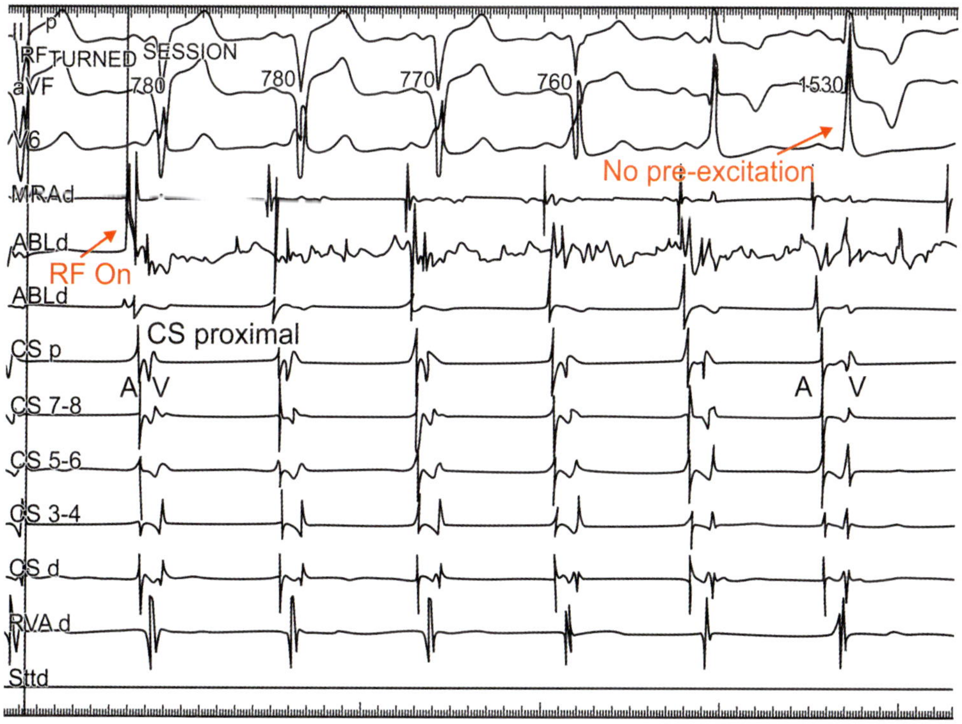

Fig. 31.16: Radio-frequency (RF) ablation of RPS accessory pathway. RF energy application with gradual loss of pre-excitation over 4 sinus beats, then lack of pre-excitation with memory T-wave changes (far right). Note AV interval timing at coronary sinus proximal electrogram. Memory T wave axis is usually similar to the axis of the delta wave during pre-excitation. (RPS: Right posteroseptal; AV: Atriventricular).

REFERENCES

Arruda MS, McClelland JH, Wang X, et al. Development and validation of an ECG algorithm for identifying accessory pathway ablation site in Wolff-Parkinson-White syndrome. J Cardiovasc Electrophysiol. 1998;9(1):2-12.

Blomström-Lundqvist C, Scheinman MM, Aliot EM, et al. ACC/AHA/ESC guidelines for the management of patients with supraventricular arrhythmias--executive summary: a report of the American College of Cardiology/American Heart Association Task Force on Practice Guidelines and the European Society of Cardiology Committee for Practice Guidelines (Writing Committee to Develop Guidelines for the Management of Patients With Supraventricular Arrhythmias). Circulation. 2003;108(15):1871-909.

Chiang CE, Chen SA, Teo WS, et al. An accurate stepwise electrocardiographic algorithm for localization of accessory pathways in patients with Wolff-Parkinson-White syndrome from a comprehensive analysis of delta waves and R/S ratio during sinus rhythm. Am J Cardiol. 1995;76(1):40-6.

Chugh A, Morady F. Atrioventricular Reentry and Variants. In: Zipes D, ed. Cardiac Electrophysiology: From Cell to Bedside, 5th ed. Philadelphia: WB Saunders; 2009:605-12.

de Chillou C, Rodriguez LM, Schläpfer J, et al. Clinical characteristics and electrophysiologic properties of atrioventricular accessory pathways: importance of the accessory pathway location. J Am Coll Cardiol. 1992;20(3):666-71.

Ho SY. Accessory atrioventricular pathways: getting to the origins. Circulation. 2008;117(12):1502-4.

Jackman WM, Wang XZ, Friday KJ, et al. Catheter ablation of accessory atrioventricular pathways (Wolff-Parkinson-White syndrome) by radiofrequency current. N Engl J Med. 1991; 324(23):1605-11.

Klein GJ, Hackel DB, Gallagher JJ. Anatomic substrate of impaired antegrade conduction over an accessory atrioventricular pathway in the Wolff-Parkinson-White syndrome. Circulation. 1980;61(6):1249-56.

Knight BP, Ebinger M, Oral H, et al. Diagnostic value of tachycardia features and pacing maneuvers during paroxysmal supraventricular tachycardia. J Am Coll Cardiol. 2000;36(2): 574-82.

Michaud GF, Tada H, Chough S, et al. Differentiation of atypical atrioventricular node reentrant tachycardia from orthodromic reciprocating tachycardia using a septal accessory pathway by the response to ventricular pacing. J Am Coll Cardiol. 2001;38(4):1163-7.

Morady F. Catheter ablation of supraventricular arrhythmias: state of the art. J Cardiovasc Electrophysiol. 2004;15(1): 124-39.

Nakagawa H, Jackman WM. Catheter ablation of paroxysmal supraventricular tachycardia. Circulation. 2007;116(21): 2465-78.

Peters NS, Rowland E, Bennett JG, et al. The Wolff-Parkinson-White syndrome: the cellular substrate for conduction in the accessory atrioventricular pathway. Eur Heart J. 1994;15(7): 981-7.

Sun Y, Arruda M, Otomo K, et al. Coronary sinus-ventricular accessory connections producing posteroseptal and left posterior accessory pathways: incidence and electrophysiological identification. Circulation. 2002;106(11): 1362-7.

Wellens HJ. Catheter ablation for cardiac arrhythmias. N Engl J Med. 2004;351(12):1172-4.

CHAPTER

32

Atrioventricular Nodal Re-entrant Tachycardia

George D Katritsis, Demosthenes G Katritsis

INTRODUCTION

Atrioventricular nodal re-entrant tachycardia (AVNRT) is the most common regular supraventricular arrhythmia. It is more prevalent in women. AVNRT tends to first appear in youth and the attacks recur throughout life, most commonly as palpitations of sudden onset and offset. Occasionally, certain events, such as physical exercise, emotional upset, indigestion or alcohol consumption, precipitate attacks. Polyuria, probably indicating increased atrial natriuretic peptide (ANP) levels, may be present during or after a prolonged attack. AVNRT may result in atrial fibrillation that usually, although not invariably, is eliminated following catheter ablation of AVNRT.

MECHANISM OF AVNRT

Atrioventricular nodal re-entrant tachycardia is a micro re-entrant arrhythmia that occurs within the AV node (Figs. 32.1A and B). Several models have been proposed to explain the mechanism of the arrhythmia, which still remains elusive. It is postulated that a dual conduction system is present in the AV node, one having a faster conduction time and longer refractory period (fast pathway), the other having a slower conduction time and shorter refractory period (slow pathway) (Figs. 32.2A to C). At a critical coupling interval, the premature impulse blocks in the faster pathway and conducts in the still excitable slow pathway, causing a sudden jump in the AV conduction time. Following that, the impulse returns to the atria, supposedly via the fast pathway, which has then recovered, and an atrial echo beat or sustained tachycardia results (Figs. 32.3 and 32.4). This is the typical form of AVNRT (also called slow-fast AVNRT), in which abnormal (retrograde) P′ waves are constantly related to the QRS and in the majority of cases are indiscernible or very close to the QRS complex (RP′ interval/RR interval < 0.5) (Figs. 32.5 to 32.8). Thus P′ waves are either masked by the QRS complex or seen as a small terminal P′ wave that is not present during sinus rhythm. During electrophysiology study with recordings of atrial, ventricular, bundle of His, and coronary sinus activation, typical slow-fast

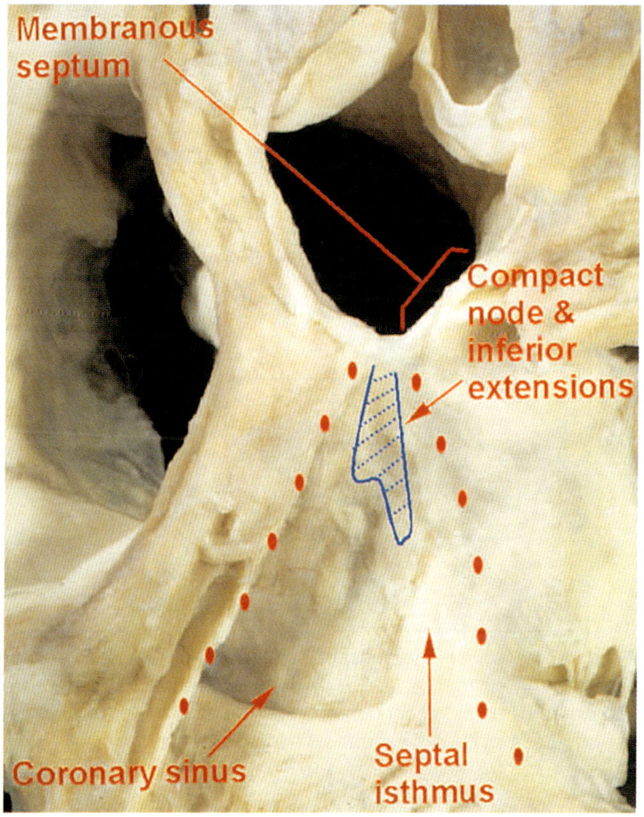

Fig. 32.1A: Location of the AV node (blue hatched area) within the triangle of Koch. (Image courtesy of Dr Robert Anderson, Institute of Genetic Medicine, Newcastle University, United Kingdom).

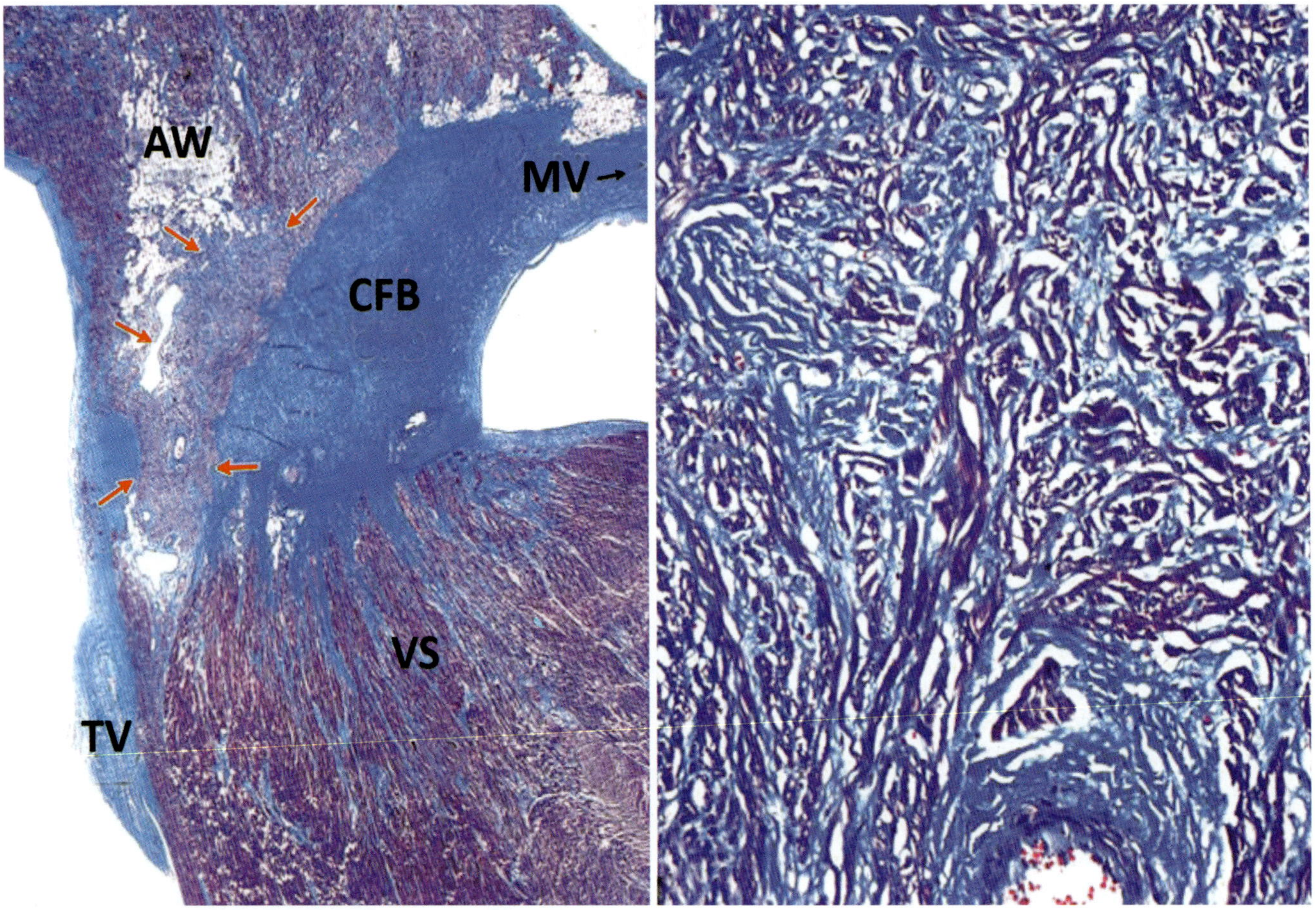

Fig. 32.1B: Microscopic examination of the AV node. At low magnification (left panel), the AV node (arrows) is seen abutting the central fibrous body (CFB). At high magnification (right panel), the narrow-caliber specialized muscle fibers (red in this trichrome stain) appear haphazard in orientation and are separated by collagen (blue). [Image and legend text from Cheitlin MD, Ursell PC. Cardiac anatomy. In: Chatterjee K, Anderson M, Heistad D, Kerber RE. (Eds). Cardiology: An Illustrated Textbook. New Delhi, India: Jaypee Brothers Medical Publishers (P) Ltd.; 2012]. (AW: Atrial wall; MV: Mitral valve; TV: Tricuspid valve; VS: Ventricular septum).

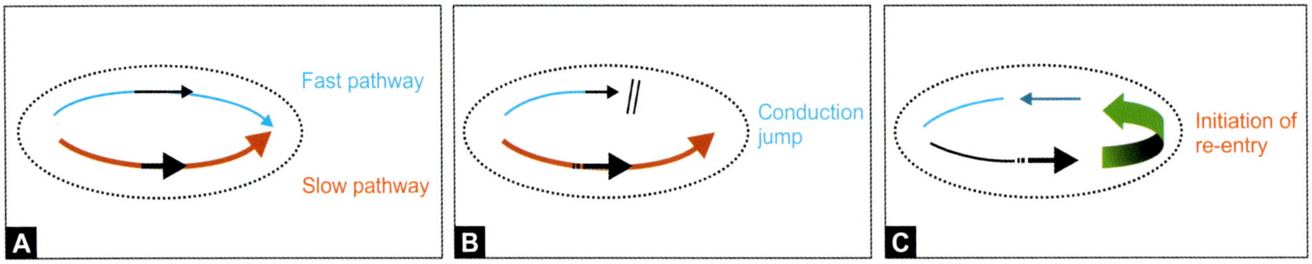

Figs. 32.2A to C: Theoretical depiction of the AV nodal re-entrant circuit. (A) During sinus rhythm, the impulse penetrates both the fast and slow pathway; (B) A premature beat results in conduction block of the fast pathway and propagation through the slow; (C) An earlier impulse encounters more delay in the slow pathway in a way that the blocked fast pathway has recovered when the now retrograde impulse arrives and tachycardia begins.

AVNRT displays simultaneous antegrade ventricular and retrograde atrial activation. AVNRT is a narrow-complex tachycardia, i.e. QRS duration less than 120 ms, unless aberrant conduction, which is usually of the right bundle branch block (RBBB) type, or a previous conduction defect exists. Tachycardia-related ST depression as well as RR

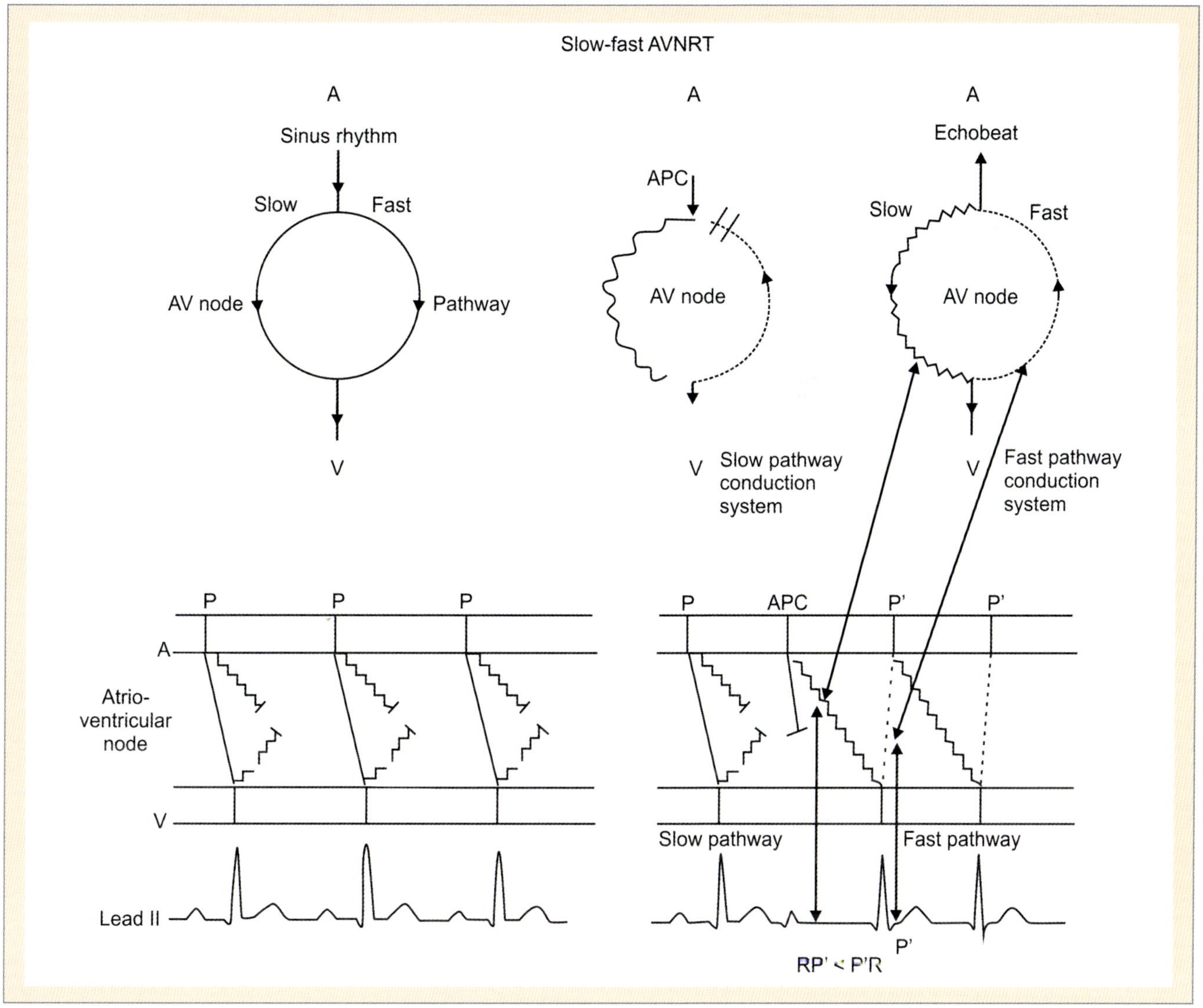

Fig. 32.3: Mechanism of typical slow fast AVNRT. An atrial premature contraction (APC) is blocked in the fast pathway, due to the long refractory period, and conducts through the slow pathway. Once the fast pathway recovers, the impulse from the slow pathway conducts retrograde through the fast pathway, producing an echo beat. If this impulse continues through the slow pathway, it produces slow fast AVNRT. [Image and legend text from Sathish S. Tachyarrhythmias. In: Rao PS, Chugh R (Eds). A Comprehensive Approach to Congenital Heart Diseases. New Delhi, India: Jaypee Brothers Medical Publishers (P) Ltd.; 2013].

interval variation may be seen. Although AV dissociation is usually not seen, it can occur since neither the atria nor the ventricles are necessary for the re-entry circuit (Fig. 32.9).

In 5% of patients with AV nodal re-entry, antegrade conduction is thought to proceed over the fast pathway and retrograde conduction over the slow pathway and may result in an atypical form of AVNRT that may be incessant. This pattern of conduction, as well as the incessant nature, can also be seen in the presence of concealed septal accessory pathways, i.e. pathways that conduct only retrogradely, with decremental properties. In the atypical form of AVNRT, P' waves are clearly visible before the QRS, and the RP' interval is longer than the P'R interval, denoting a "long RP tachycardia" (Fig. 32.10). Two types of atypical AVNRT have been described: fast-slow (Fig. 32.11), and slow-slow (Fig. 32.12) based on electrophysiologic criteria (Table 32.1), but this classification may not be always possible with atypical AVNRT. Thus, for clinical purposes AVNRT should be classified as typical and atypical.

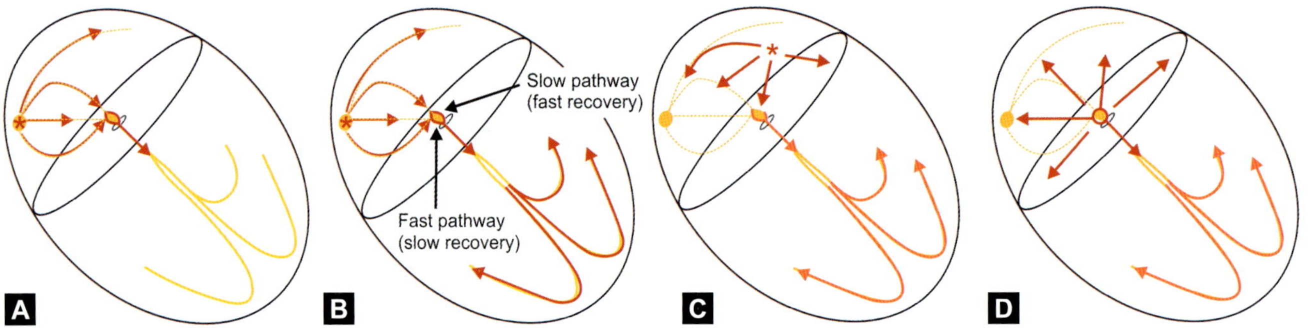

Figs. 32.4A to D: Simplified mechanistic illustration of the initiation of AVNRT. (A) A depolarization impulse originating in the SA node enters an AV node with dual pathways; a slow pathway, which recovers quickly, and a fast pathway, which recovers slowly; (B) Once through the AV node the depolarization wavefront continues through the bundle of His and into the bundle branches and Purkinje fibers as during normal conduction. The slow pathway with its shorter effective refractory period begins recovering quicker than the fast pathway; (C) A depolarization impulse from an atrial premature contraction reaches the slow pathway when it is completely recovered, while the fast pathway is still refractory; (D) As the depolarization impulse from the APC travels down the slow pathway, the fast pathway becomes no longer refractory, and after the depolarization impulse travels down the slow pathway it travels up the fast pathway. The re-entrant circuit is thus initiated. Each rotation of the impulse down the slow pathway and up the fast pathway then leads to depolarization of the ventricles and of the atria. (Images courtesy of Christopher Watford. Images and modified text from Christopher Watford. (2013). (Challenging Tradition: Better Precordial Lead Placement. [Online] Available from www.sixlettervariable.blogspot.com [Access on February 2014]).

Table 32.1: Classification of AVNRT types. The distinction is for categorization only, and not relevant for mechanism or therapy. Atypical AVNRT has been traditionally classified as fast-slow (HA > 70 ms, VA > 60, AH/HA < 1, and AH < 200 ms) or slow-slow (HA > 70 ms, VA > 60 ms, AH/HA > 1, and AH > 200 ms). Not all of these criteria are always met and atypical AVNRT may not be sub-classified accordingly. AH: atrial to His interval, HA: His to atrium interval, VA: interval measured from the onset of ventricular activation on surface ECG to the earliest deflection of the atrial activation on the bundle of His electrogram. (Adapted from Katritsis DG, Josephson ME. Classification of electrophysiological types of atrioventricular nodal re-entrant tachycardia: a reappraisal. Europace. 2013;15(9):1231-40).

	HA	*VA (His)*	*AH/HA*
Typical AVNRT	≤ 70 ms	≤ 60 ms	> 1
Atypical AVNRT	> 70 ms	> 60 ms	Variable

The concept of longitudinally dissociated dual AV nodal pathways that conduct around a central obstacle with proximal and distal connections can provide explanations for many aspects of the electrophysiological behavior of these tachycardias, but several obscure points remain. These pathways have not been demonstrated histologically, the exact circuit responsible for the re-entrant tachycardia is unknown, and critical questions still remain unanswered.

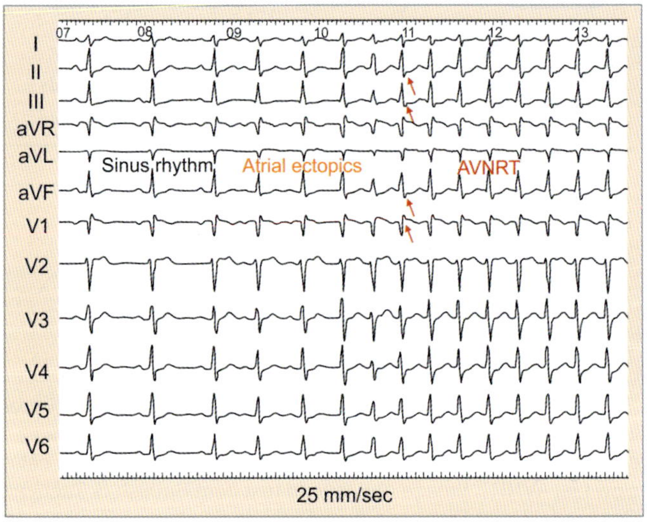

Fig. 32.5: Induction of typical AVNRT by atrial ectopy. The first three beats are sinus beats. The next two are atrial ectopics conducted with a short PR (apparently over the fast pathway). The next atrial ectopic is conducted with a prolonged PR over the slow pathway due to antegrade block of the fast pathway and initiates AVNRT by returning retrogradely through the fast pathway that has recovered. Retrograde P' waves are more prominent in lead V1 and, especially, the inferior leads (arrows). (Modified from Katritsis DG, Camm AJ. Atrioventricular nodal re-entrant tachycardia. Circulation. 2010;122:831-40).

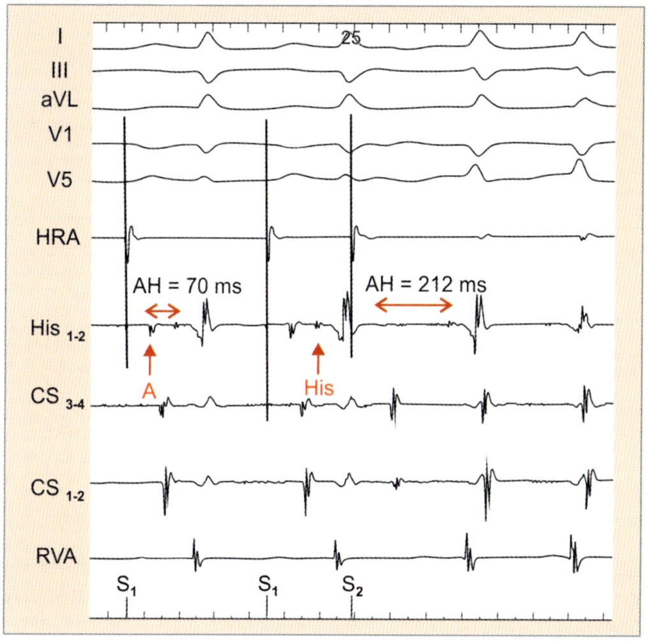

Fig. 32.6: A sudden prolongation of the AH interval in a patient with dual atrioventricular nodal pathways (so-called atrioventricular conduction jump) results in typical (slow-fast) AVNRT induction. During atrial pacing at 400 ms (150 bpm) the AH interval is 70 ms indicating nodal conduction through the fast pathway. At an extrastimulus of 240 ms the AH prolongs to 212 ms thus indicating conduction block to the fast pathway and conduction through the slow one with initiation of tachycardia. Note that ventricular and atrial activations are almost simultaneous during typical, slow-fast AVNRT. (I: ECG lead; III: Lead III of the surface ECG; aVL: Lead aVL of the surface ECG; V1: Lead V1 of the surface ECG; V5: Lead V5 of the surface ECG; HRA: High right atrium; His: Bundle of His; CS: Coronary sinus; RVA: Right ventricular apex).

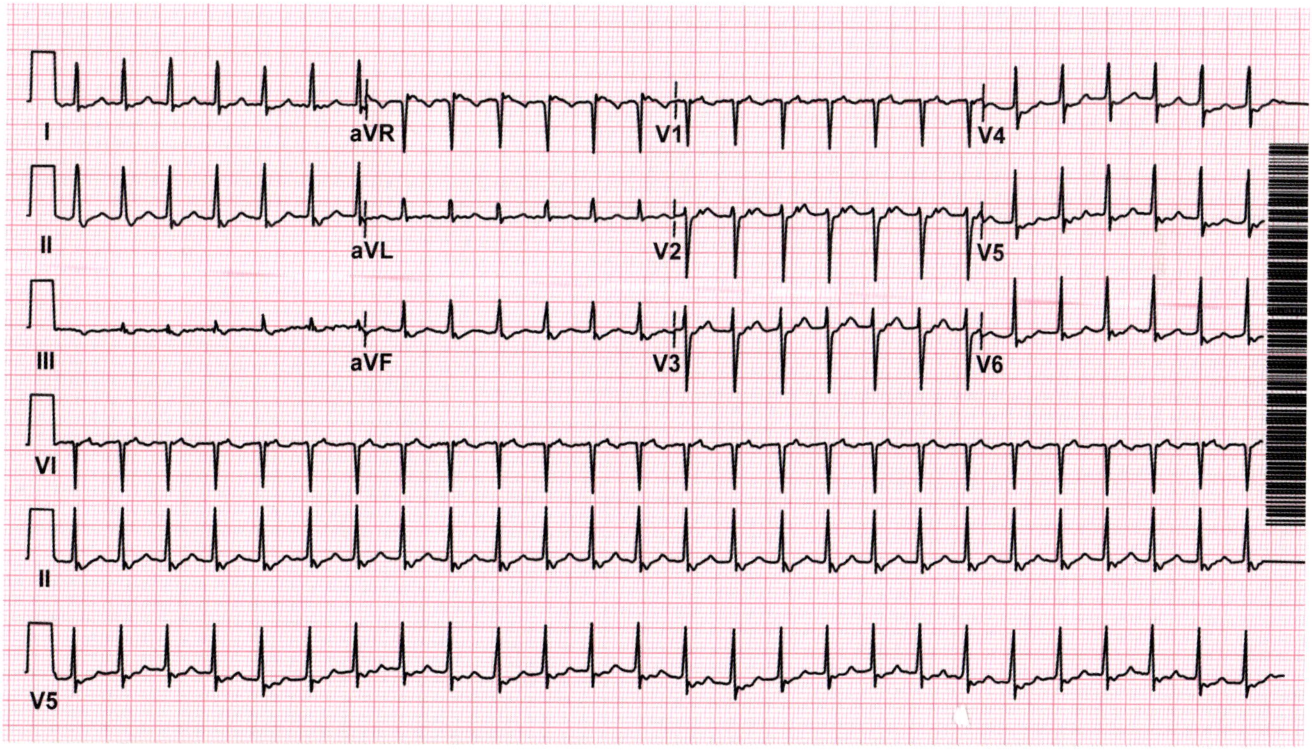

Fig. 32.7: A 12-lead ECG demonstrating typical atrioventricular nodal re-entrant tachycardia with a short RP' interval. Retrograde P waves are visible immediately after the QRS complexes.

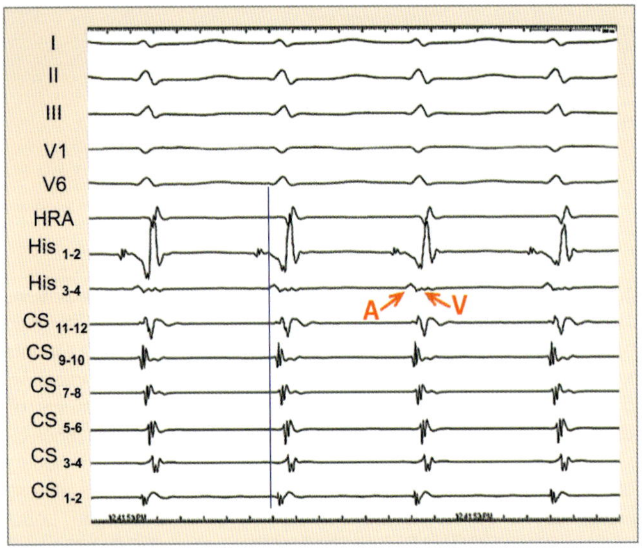

Fig. 32.8: Typical slow-fast atrioventricular nodal re-entrant tachycardia during electrophysiology study. Antegrade ventricular (V) and retrograde atrial activation (A) are almost simultaneously recorded. Usually, but not invariably, earliest retrograde atrial activation is recorded by the bundle of His recording electrode (line). (I: to V6, 12-lead ECG leads; HRA: High right atrium; His: Bundle of His electrogram; CS: Coronary sinus).

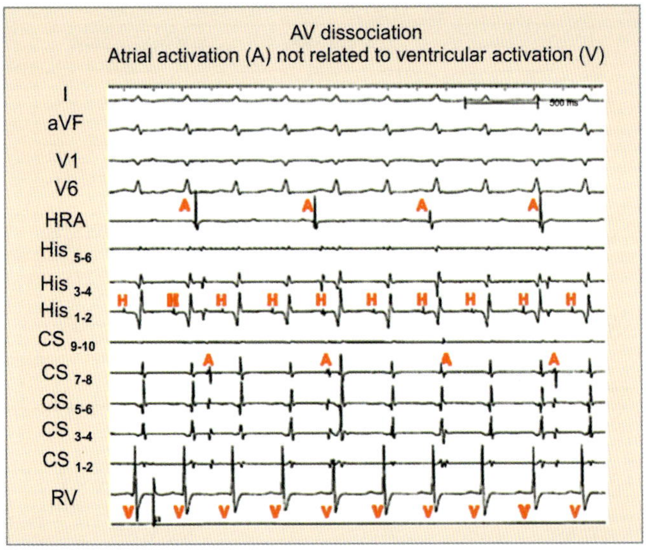

Fig. 32.9: Atrioventricular dissociation during AVNRT. Atrial activation is not related to bundle of His electrograms, and the last A-A interval is not the same with the previous ones. This suggests retrograde block with variable conduction. (Modified from Katritsis DG, Josephson ME. Classification of electrophysiological types of atrioventricular nodal re-entrant tachycardia: a reappraisal. Europace 2013;15:1231-40.

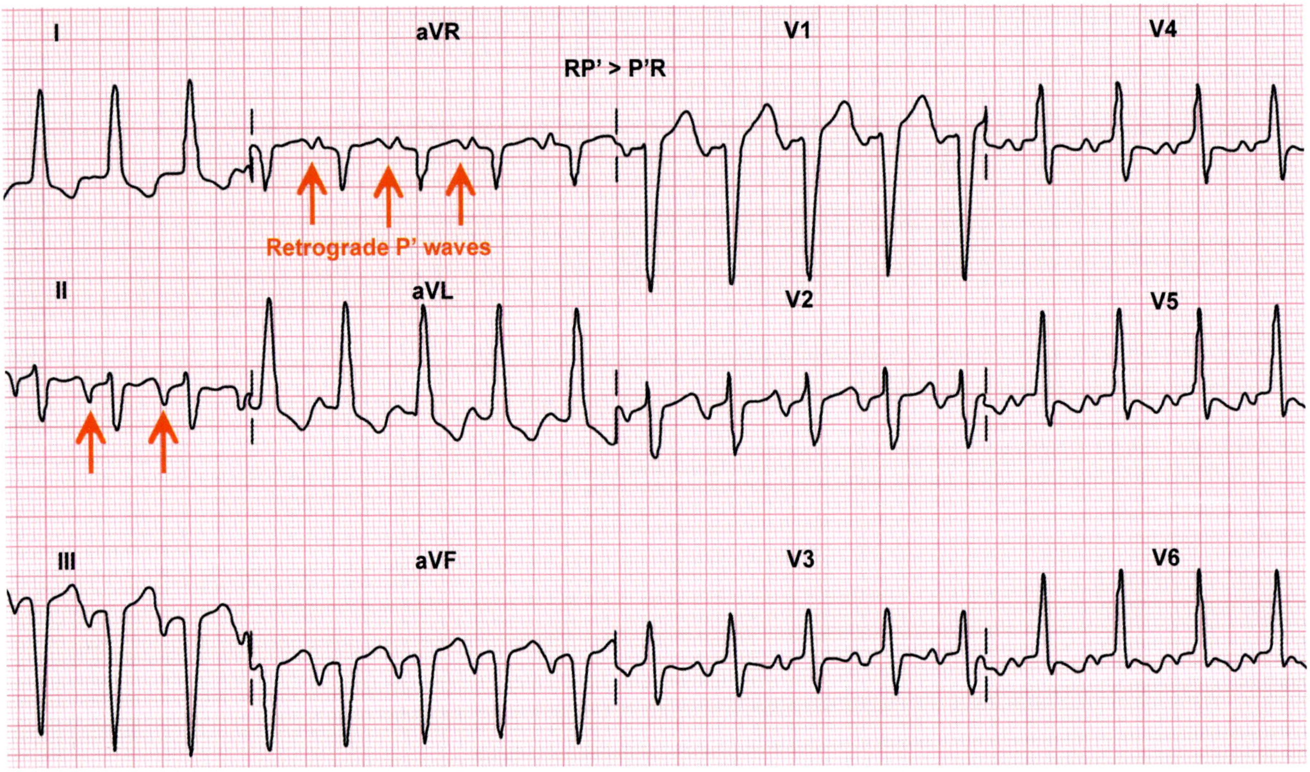

Fig. 32.10: A 12-lead ECG showing "atypical" AVNRT. In the atypical form of AVNRT, P' waves are clearly visible before the QRS, and the RP' interval is longer than the P'R interval, denoting a *"long RP tachycardia"*.

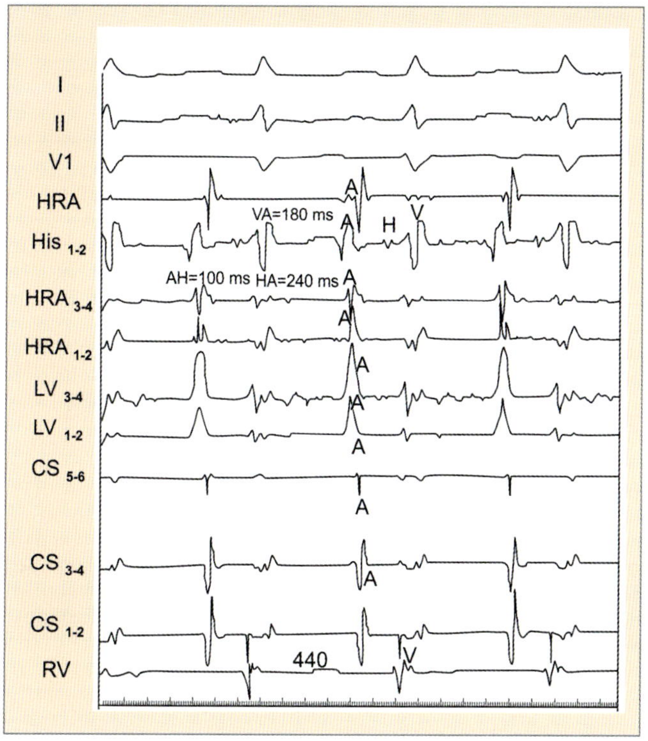

Fig. 32.11: Atypical AVNRT. The form is conventionally fast-slow defined by AH < HA, HA > 70 ms, AH < 200 ms. (Modified from Katritsis DG, Josephson ME. Classification of electrophysiological types of atrioventricular nodal re-entrant tachycardia: a reappraisal. Europace. 2013;15:1231-40). (I: to V6, 12-lead ECG leads; HRA: High right atrium; His: Bundle of His electrogram; CS: Coronary sinus; LV: Electrode at the left side of the septum; RV: Right ventricle).

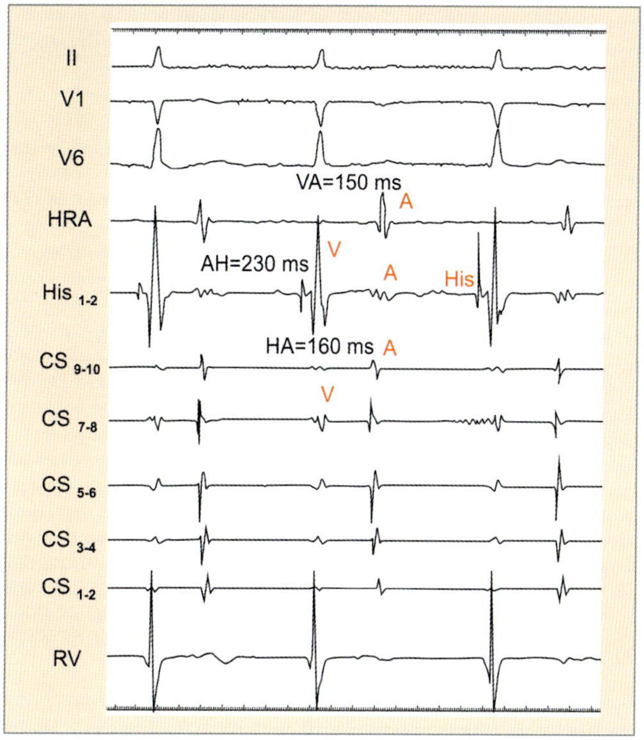

Fig. 32.12: Atypical AVNRT. The form is conventionally slow-slow defined by AH > HA, HA > 70 ms, AH > 200 ms. (Modified from Katritsis DG, Josephson ME. Classification of electrophysiological types of atrioventricular nodal re-entrant tachycardia: a reappraisal. Europace. 2013;15:1231-40).

Consequently, several attempts to provide a reasonable hypothesis based on anatomic or anisotropic models have appeared. Recently, there has been substantial evidence in favor of re-entry in the context of the complex anatomy of the AV node and its atrial extensions. The right and left inferior extensions of the human AV node and the atrio-nodal inputs they facilitate may provide the anatomic substrate of the slow pathway, and a comprehensive model of the tachycardia circuit for all forms of atrioventricular nodal re-entrant tachycardia based on the concept of atrio-nodal inputs has been proposed (Fig. 32.13).

DIFFERENTIATING AVNRT FROM OTHER ARRHYTHMIAS

In the presence of a narrow-QRS tachycardia, AVNRT should be differentiated from atrial tachycardia or orthodromic atrioventricular re-entrant tachycardia (AVRT) due to an accessory pathway (Fig. 32.14). When a wide-QRS tachycardia is encountered and ventricular tachycardia is excluded, the possible diagnoses are AVNRT or atrial tachycardia with aberrant conduction due to bundle branch block, AVNRT with a bystanding accessory pathway, and antidromic AVRT due to an accessory pathway. Aberrant conduction, although rare, can be seen in AVNRT and is usually of the RBBB type. However, cases of left bundle branch block (LBBB) have been reported (Fig. 32.15). Usually, this differentiation requires an electrophysiology study.

TREATMENT OF AVNRT

In acute episodes of AVNRT that do not respond to Valsalva maneuvers, intravenous adenosine is the treatment of choice. Alternatively, a single dose of oral diltiazem (120 mg) and a beta-blocker (i.e. propranolol 80 mg) may be tried. Chronic administration of antiarrhythmic drugs (such as beta-blockers, non-dihydropyridine calcium channel blockers, flecainide or propafenone) may be ineffective

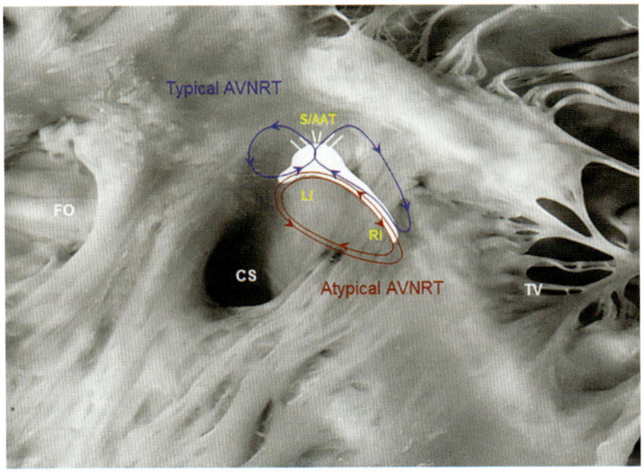

Fig. 32.13: Proposed circuit of AVNRT. During typical AVNRT (slow-fast), right- or left-sided circuits may occur with antegrade conduction through the inferior inputs and retrograde conduction through the superior inputs (S) or the anisotropic atrionodal transitional area (AAT). In atypical AVNRT conduction occurs anterogradely through one of the inferior inputs, left (LI) or right (RI) and retrogradely through the inferior inputs and retrogradely through the other one. Depending on the orientation of the circuit we may record the so-called "fast-slow" or "slow-slow" types. (Modified from Katritsis DG, Becker A. The circuit of atrioventricular nodal re-entrant tachycardia: a proposal. Heart Rhythm. 2007;4:1354-60). (RS: Right superior input; LS: Left superior input; RI: Right inferior input; LI: Left inferior input; CS: Coronary sinus; TV: Tricuspid valve; FO: Foramen ovale).

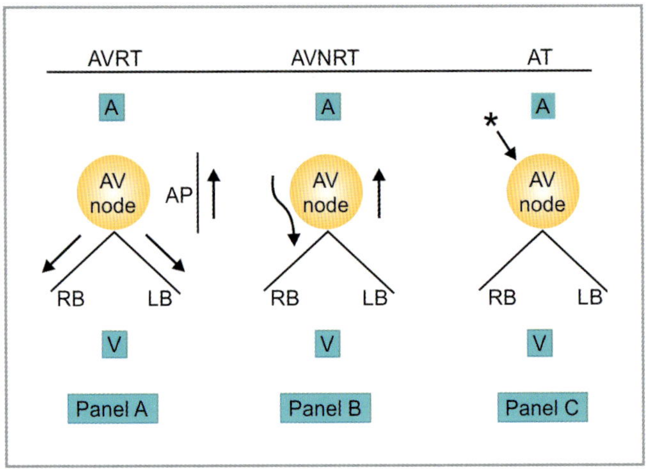

Fig. 32.14: Mechanisms of AV re-entrant tachycardia (AVRT), AV nodal re-entrant tachycardia (AVNRT), and atrial tachycardia (AT). All three arrhythmias may result in a regular narrow complex tachycardia. [Reproduced from Sullivan RM, Li WW, Olshansky B. Supraventricular tachycardia. In: Chatterjee K, Anderson M, Heistad D, Kerber RE. (Eds). Cardiology: An Illustrated Textbook. New Delhi, India: Jaypee Brothers Medical Publishers (P) Ltd.; 2012]. (A: Atria; AP: Accessory pathway; RB: Right bundle branch; LV: Left bundle branch; V: Ventricle).

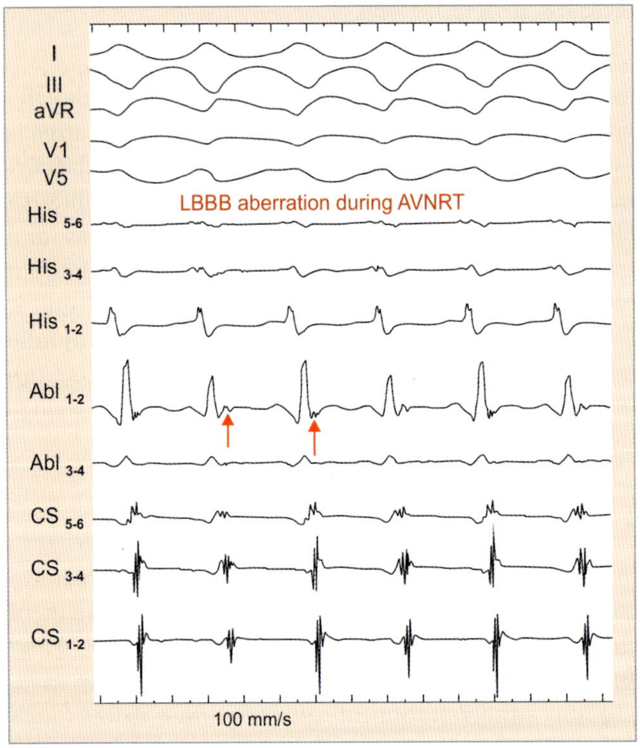

Fig. 32.15: Typical AVNRT conducted with LBBB aberration and with inability to record bundle of His electrograms. Retrograde atrial electrograms are indicated by arrows. (Modified from Katritsis DG, Josephson ME. Classification of electrophysiological types of atrioventricular nodal re-entrant tachycardia: a reappraisal. Europace. 2013;15:1231-40). (I: ECG lead; III: Lead III of the surface ECG; aVR: Lead aVR of the surface ECG; V1: Lead V1 of the surface ECG; V5: Lead V5 of the surface ECG; HRA: High right atrium; His: Bundle of His; CS: Coronary sinus; Abl: Ablation electrode positioned at the area of the slow pathway).

in up to 50% of cases. Thus, catheter ablation is the current treatment of choice. Slow pathway ablation or modification is effective in both typical and atypical AVNRT. This approach offers a success rate of 95%, is associated with a risk of 0.5–1% AV block and has an approximately 4% recurrence rate. Although a <0.6% mortality has been reported in earlier studies, no deaths are seen in recent trials. Advanced age is not a contraindication for slow pathway ablation.

REFERENCES

Katritsis DG, Becker A. The atrioventricular nodal re-entrant tachycardia circuit: a proposal. Heart Rhythm. 2007;4:1354-60.

Katritsis DG, Camm AJ. Atrioventricular nodal re-entrant tachycardia. Circulation. 2010;122:831-40.

Katritsis DG, Josephson ME. Classification of electrophysiological types of atrioventricular nodal re-entrant tachycardia: a reappraisal. Europace. 2013;15(9):1231-40.

CHAPTER

33

Ventricular Arrhythmias

Ramil Goel, Komandoor Srivathsan, Farouk Mookadam

PREMATURE VENTRICULAR COMPLEX

A premature ventricular complex (PVC) is an electrical impulse originating from the ventricular myocardium. Since the PVC depolarization impulse does not propagate through the ventricles using the His-Purkinje pathway of activation of the myocardium, the impulse spreads in a slow, inefficient manner from one myocyte to another, giving rise to a wider ventricular complex (Fig. 33.1). PVCs are usually a sign of diseased myocardium. Myocardial factors associated with PVCs are myocardial hypertrophy, stretch, ischemia and/or injury. Three mechanisms are generally recognized as leading to PVCs:

1. Increased automaticity, whereby a ventricular myocyte can abnormally fire earlier than the next atrial impulse.
2. Triggered activity, whereby the last atrial beat can cause a premature depolarization leading to a PVC.
3. Re-entry, whereby the last atrial beat enters a re-entrant circuit and exit out as a PVC.

In the latter two cases, the PVCs are usually coupled to the preceding beat in a fixed temporal relationship, giving rise to ventricular bigeminy (Fig. 33.2).

While the presence of PVCs is associated with diseased myocardium, PVCs may also be noted in hearts without any structural damage. In such cases, the prognostic significance of such PVCs is unclear. However, while the presence of occasional PVCs does not require any intervention, there is some data to suggest that a very high PVC burden (>10,000–20,000 PVCs/day) may lead to left ventricular systolic dysfunction. The phenomenon is termed PVC-induced cardiomyopathy. In such cases, ablation of the PVC focus can lead to improvement in ejection fraction. PVC ablation may also be warranted when sustained ventricular tachycardia (VT) or ventricular fibrillation (VF) is repetitively triggered by a PVC (Fig. 33.3).

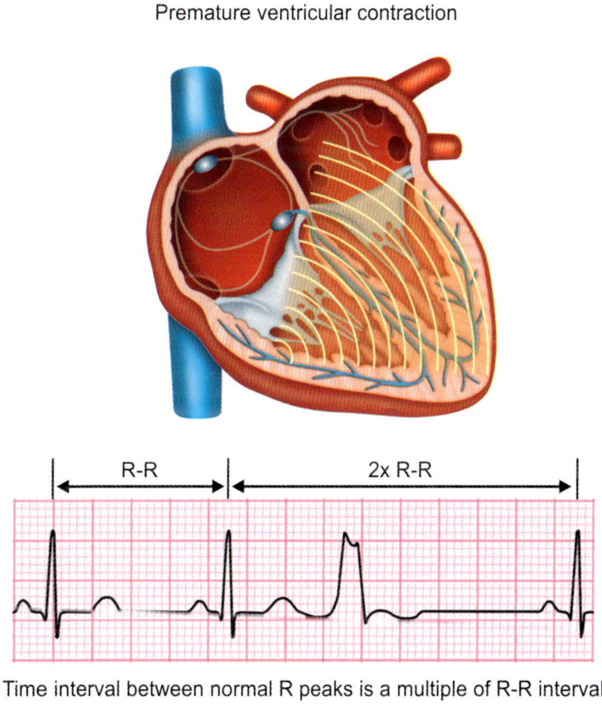

Fig. 33.1: The formation of a premature ventricular complex (PVC) occurs in the right ventricular myocardium. Since the PVC depolarization impulse does not propagate through the ventricles using the His-Purkinje pathway of activation of the myocardium, the impulse spreads in a slow, inefficient manner from one myocyte to another, giving rise to a wider ventricular complex. Note that the subsequent normal sinus beat is two times the R-R interval from the prior normal sinus beat.

VENTRICULAR TACHYCARDIA

Ventricular tachycardia is an arrhythmia that originates in the ventricle (Figs. 33.4 and 33.5). By definition, VT is a series of PVCs more than three beats long at a rate of more than 100/min. It is termed *nonsustained ventricular tachycardia (NSVT)* if its duration is less than 30 seconds and self-terminating. It is termed *sustained VT* if the series

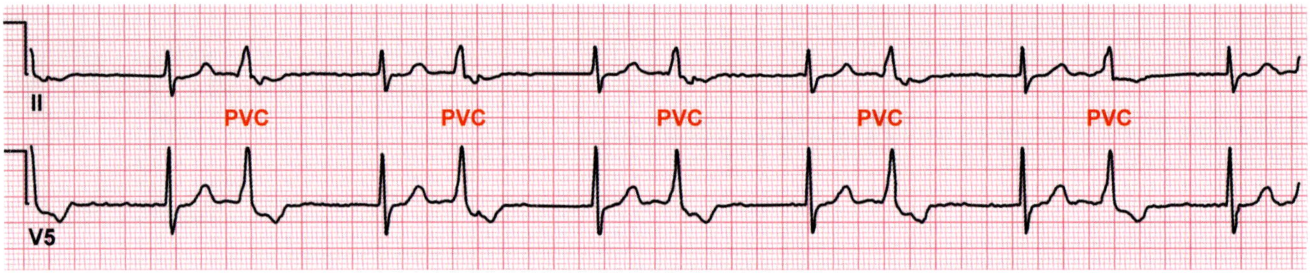

Fig. 33.2: Ventricular bigeminy. Ventricular bigeminy is characterized by a premature ventricular complex (PVC) following every beat of supraventricular origin. This leads to the characteristic pattern of a wide QRS alternating with a normal appearing QRS. Note, however, that if the patient has aberrant conduction through the ventricle (due to a bundle branch block for example), the supraventricular beats may also be wide but usually will have a different morphology compared with the PVCs.

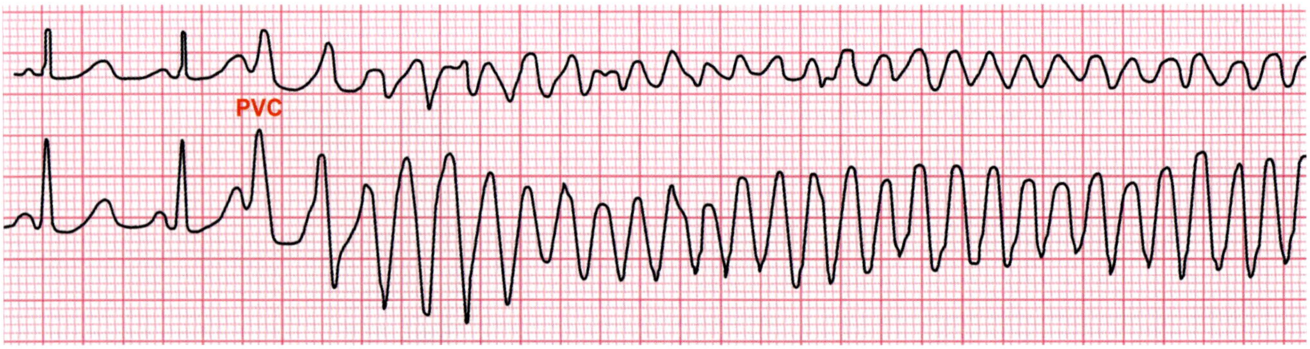

Fig. 33.3: Premature ventricular complex (PVC) triggering ventricular fibrillation.

lasts longer than 30 seconds or is associated hemodynamic instability. Hemodynamic instability may occur because of the loss of AV synchrony and intraventricular dyssynchrony caused by a VT, leading to impairment of cardiac output, particularly in patients with an already-compromised myocardium. Classification of various ventricular arrhythmias are summarized in Table 33.1.

Ventricular tachycardia may also be classified based on QRS complex morphology. The term *monomorphic VT* is used when all QRS complexes are similar in appearance (Figs. 33.6A and B). Monomorphic VT may be due to increased automaticity or due to re-entry. Monomorphic VT typically occurs in a patient with scar from a prior myocardial infarction (MI). Outflow tachycardia (discussed below) also produces a monomorphic VT. When there is significant variation in the QRS morphology, the term *polymorphic VT* is used (Fig. 33.7). Polymorphic VT most commonly occurs in the setting of abnormalities of ventricular muscle repolarization. Most typically, polymorphic VT occurs in the setting of acute myocardial ischemia. When polymorphic VT occurs in the setting of prolonged QT interval, the rhythm is referred to as *torsades de pointes* (discussed below).

As discussed above, there are numerous etiologies for VT. Coronary artery disease may lead to VT through acute ischemia or acute MI, prior MI with scar formation (Figs. 33.8 and 33.9), or aneurysm formation. VT may occur in those with dilated or hypertrophic cardiomyopathies. Electrolyte abnormalities, particularly profound hypokalemia, may predispose to VT. Drug overdose, such as with digoxin (Fig. 33.10), may also precipitate VT. An uncommon but potentially fatal cause of VT is arrhythmogenic right ventricular dysplasia (ARVD) (Figs. 33.11 and 33.12), alternately called arrhythmogenic right ventricular cardiomyopathy (ARVC).

While some patients with VT will have little or no symptoms, VT will more commonly manifest as palpitations (Fig. 33.13), presyncope, chest pain or dyspnea, or overt loss of consciousness.

Ventricular tachycardia must be distinguished from a supraventricular tachycardia (SVT) with aberrancy. The Brugada algorithm is one commonly used method (Flow chart 33.1). Assessment of QRS morphology in leads V1 and V6 (Figs. 33.14A and B) can also be useful to distinguish VT from SVT with wide QRS complexes due to left bundle branch block (LBBB) or right bundle branch block (RBBB).

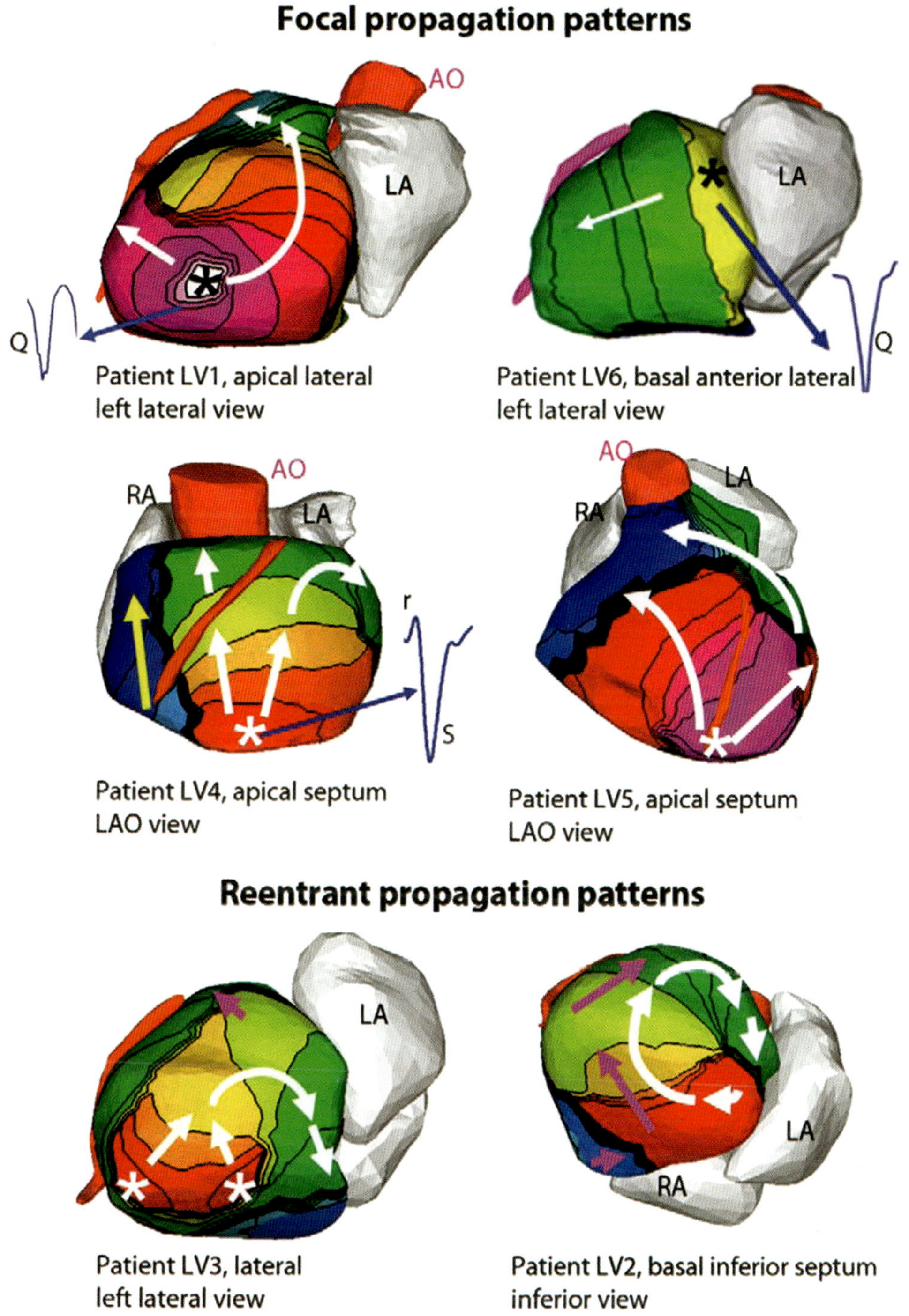

Fig. 33.4: Electrocardiographic imaging imaged propagation patterns, origins, and local electrograms in patients with ventricular tachycardia. The areas of earliest epicardial activation are marked with an asterisk. Top 4 images show focal propagation patterns. Tachycardias that were determined to be focal during EP studies demonstrate radial spread (white arrows) away from the early activation point (asterisk). Yellow arrows indicate later phases of ventricular activation. Bottom 2 images show reentrant propagation patterns. Tachycardias that were determined to be reentrant during EP studies show a rotational activation pattern (white arrows). The description under each image indicates the location of ventricular tachycardia initiation and identifies the displayed view of the heart. [Images courtesy of Dr Yorum Rudy. Images and legend text from Wang Y, Cuculich PS, Zhang J, et al. Noninvasive electroanatomic mapping of human ventricular arrhythmias with electrocardiographic imaging. Sci Transl Med. 2011;3(98):98ra84]. (RA: Right atrium; LA: Left atrium; AO: Aorta; LAD: Left anterior descending coronary artery; RV: Right ventricle; LV: Left ventricle; RVOT: Right ventricular outflow tract).

Table 33.1: Classification of various ventricular rhythms. (PVC: Premature ventricular complex; VT: Ventricular tachycardia).

ECG Finding	***Classification***
Two PVCs in a row	Couplet
Each QRS complex followed by a PVC	Ventricular bigeminy
≥ 3 PVCs in a row, > 30 sec in duration	Nonsustained VT
VT lasting > 30 sec and/or causing hemodynamic instability	Sustained VT
VT with stable QRS morphology	Monomorphic VT
VT with variable QRS morphology	Polymorphic VT
Polymorphic VT occurring in the setting of prolonged QT interval with a "rotating around an axis" appearance	*Torsades de pointes*
Ventricular rhythm with wide QRS complexes at a rate of 250–300 or 250–300 beats/min	Ventricular flutter
Disorganized ventricular electrical activity	Ventricular fibrillation

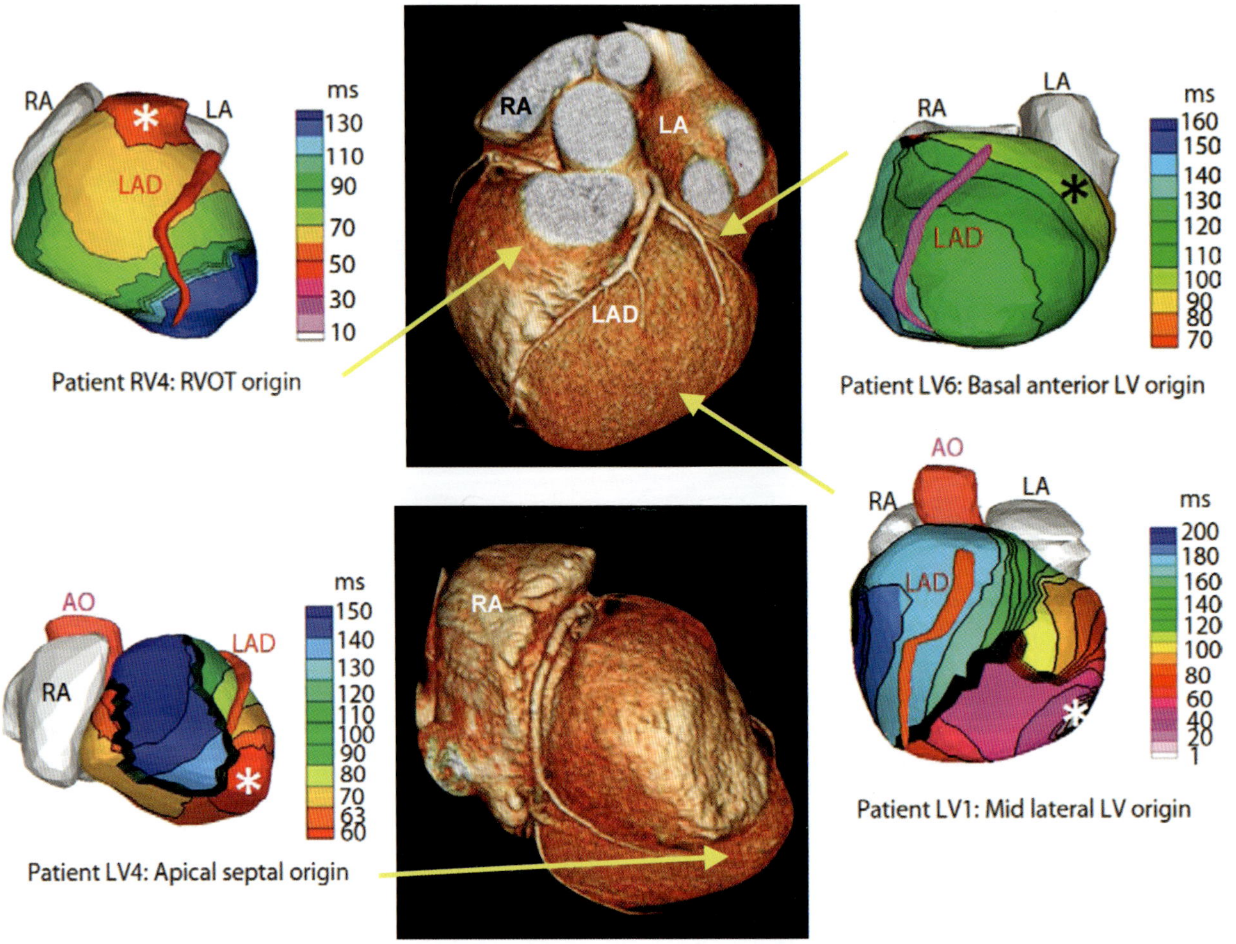

Fig. 33.5: Examples of noninvasive electrocardiographic imaging (ECGI) isochrone maps demonstrating the ventricular tachycardia (VT) site of origin in patients with VT. Epicardial isochrone maps are shown for four patients, with earliest epicardial activation marked with an asterisk. EP study–determined sites of origin are indicated under the ECGI maps. Yellow arrows point to VT origin on a representative CT scan. [Images courtesy of Dr Yorum Rudy. Images and legend text from Wang Y, Cuculich PS, Zhang J, et al. Noninvasive electroanatomic mapping of human ventricular arrhythmias with electrocardiographic imaging. Sci Transl Med. 2011;3(98):98ra84]. (RA: Right atrium; LA: Left atrium; AO: Aorta; LAD: Left anterior descending coronary artery; LV: Left ventricle; RVOT: Right ventricular outflow tract).

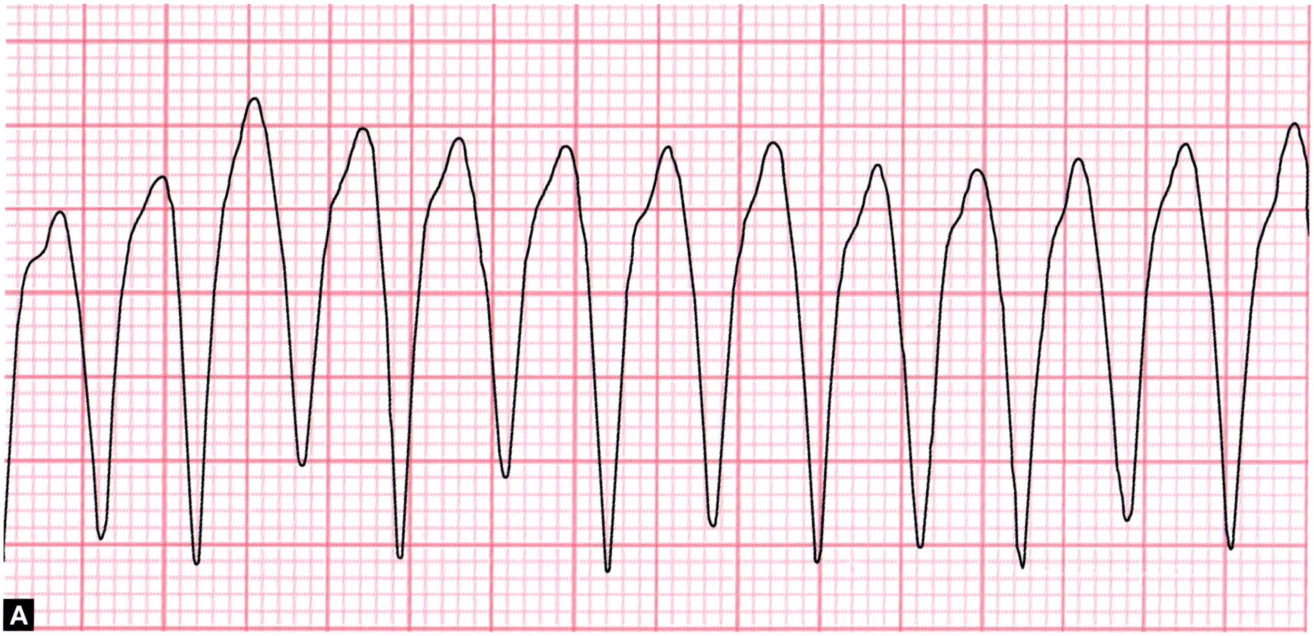

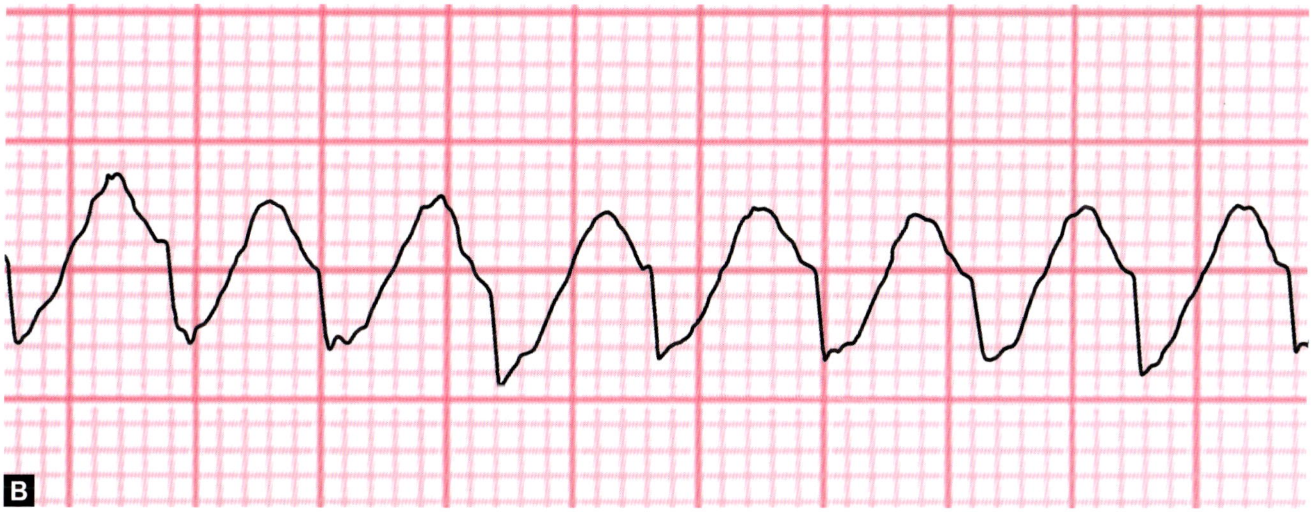

Figs. 33.6A and B: Examples of monomorphic ventricular tachycardia. The QRS complexes have similar morphology.

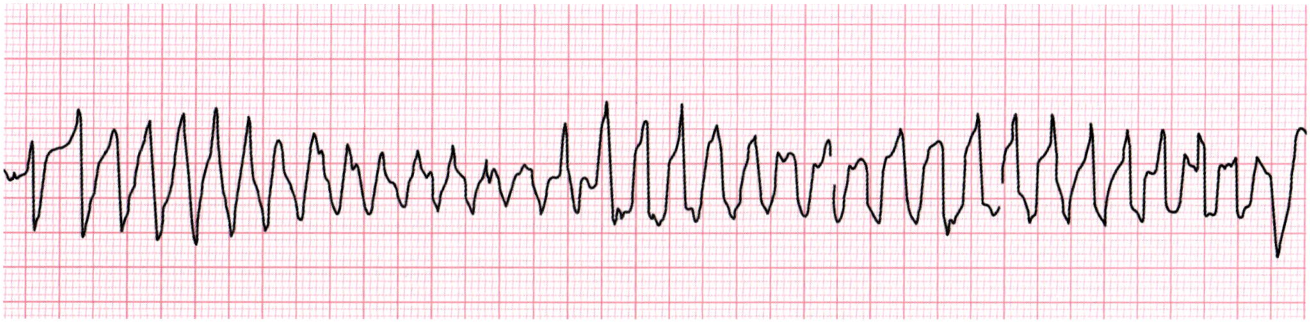

Fig. 33.7: Example of polymorphic ventricular tachycardia. There is variation in the QRS morphology, amplitude, and axis.

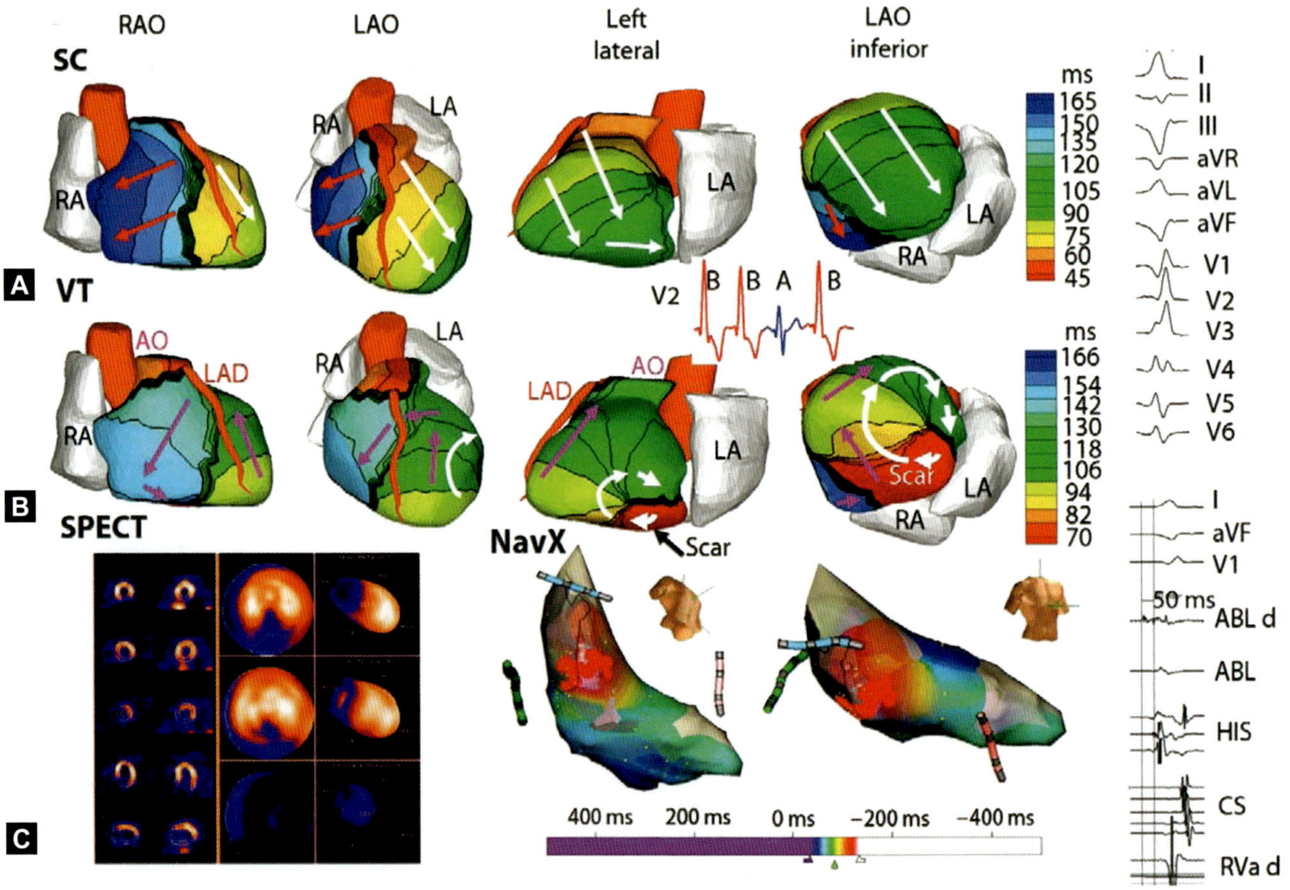

Figs. 33.8A to C: Multimodality assessment of a patient with reentrant ventricular tachycardia due to an inferobasal scar. (A) Electrocardiographic imaging (ECGI) mapping of the activation sequence during a sinus capture (SC) beat (blue beat on the V2 ECG); (B) ECGI mapping of the activation sequence during ventricular tachycardia beats (red on the V2 ECG). White arrows indicate a clockwise lateral loop (left lateral and left anterior oblique inferior views); purple arrows show propagation into the RV in a counterclockwise fashion; (C) (left image) SPECT images showing a scar at the inferobasal LV region (blue); C (right images) Limited invasive endocardial map of VT activation (red, early; blue, late). [Images courtesy of Dr Yorum Rudy. Images and legend text from Wang Y, Cuculich PS, Zhang J, et al. Noninvasive electroanatomic mapping of human ventricular arrhythmias with electrocardiographic imaging. Sci Transl Med. 2011;3(98):98ra84].

Treatment of VT is dependent to some extent on the type of VT, whether it is sustained or not, and what the underlying cause of the VT is. Acute treatment for sustained VT in hemodynamically stable patients includes antiarrhythmic therapy (usually amiodarone) and/or synchronized cardioversion. In hemodynamically unstable patients, treatment is defibrillation. Longer-term management is dictated by clinical setting and patient characteristics. Amiodarone is most commonly used to suppress VT, although use of amiodarone alone [without implantable cardioverter-defibrillator (ICD) implantation] has not been shown to prolong survival, and amiodarone is associated with numerous side effects, including hypothyroidism and hyperthyroidism, elevation of liver function tests (LFTs), and pulmonary fibrosis (Fig. 33.15). Electrophysiology (EP) study and ablation of the isthmus of the VT (the narrowest path in the VT circuit) can effect successful cure of VT in many patients (Figs. 33.16A to C), and should be considered in those not easily treated with antiarrhythmic therapy. Most patients with sustained VT, particularly if it has led to hemodynamic instability or sudden death, will be treated with ICD implantation, unless a clear, reversible and treatable cause of the VT is identified.

Outflow Tract Tachycardia (Right Ventricular Outflow Tachycardia)

A relatively benign form of VT which is better hemodynamically tolerated is *outflow tract tachycardia*. Most commonly, outflow tachycardia is observed in young patients

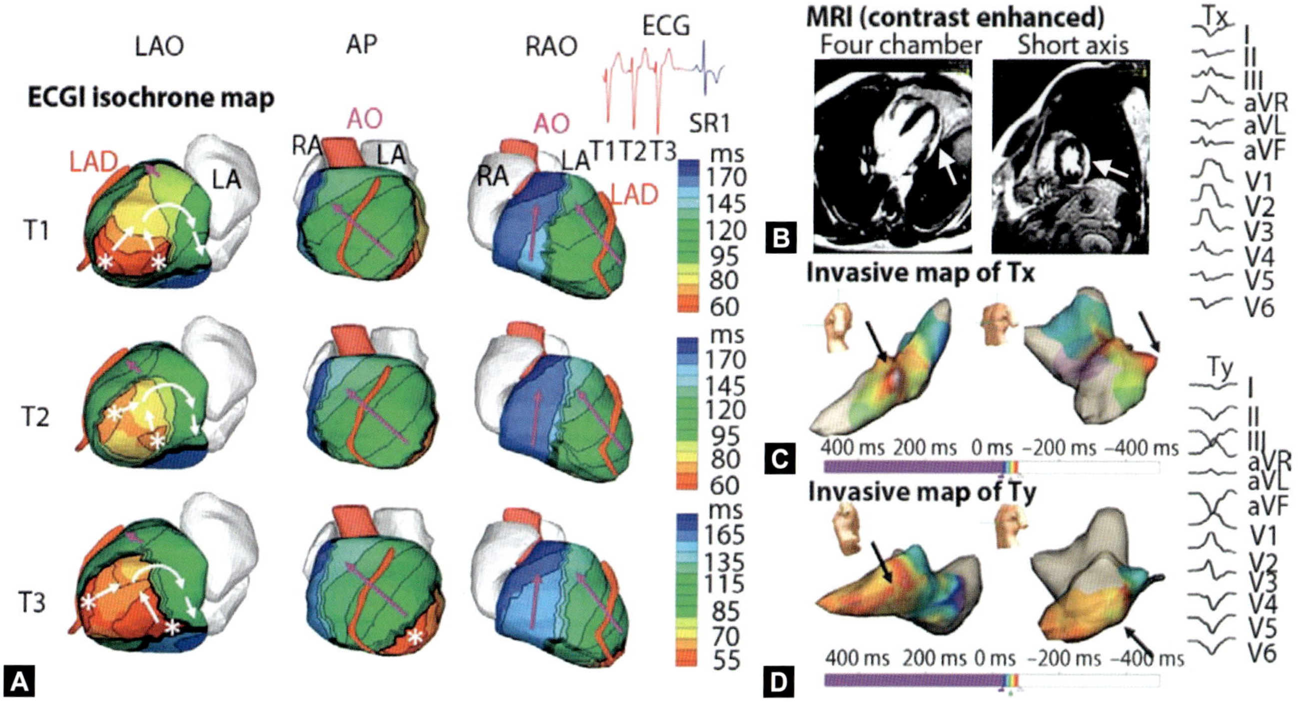

Figs. 33.9A to D: An example of electrocardiographic imaging (ECGI) of reentrant ventricular tachycardia (VT) in lateral wall infiltrative cardiomyopathy (patient LV3). (A) ECGI isochrone map. Activation patterns for three consecutive VT beats (T1, T2, and T3). ECGI identified two distinct areas of early epicardial activation (white asterisks), which differed from beat to beat. The propagation pattern varied somewhat depending on the relative contribution of the two sources, but for all beats, the wavefront turned clockwise and propagated to the left ventricle (LV) lateral base with a high degree of curvature, where it reached a line of block in the inferolateral base. (B) A gadolinium enhanced MRI revealed a patch of myocardial enhancement in the lateral LV (white arrows), consistent with a focal myocarditis or cardiac sarcoid; (C) Invasive electroanatomic map created during the presenting VT (arbitrarily named Tx). The region of earliest activation is shown by black arrows; (D) Invasive electroanatomic map created during a different VT (arbitrarily named Ty) after initial ablation at the site of earliest activation. The earliest activation (black arrows) is shifted more apically. (Right) 12 lead surface ECGs of two VT morphologies (Tx and Ty). [Images courtesy of Dr Yorum Rudy. Images and legend text from Wang Y, Cuculich PS, Zhang J, et al. Noninvasive electroanatomic mapping of human ventricular arrhythmias with electrocardiographic imaging. Sci Transl Med. 2011;3(98):98ra84]. (AP: Anterior-posterior view; SR1: First sinus rhythm beat after VT; RA: Right atrium; LA: Left atrium; AO: Aorta; LAD: Left anterior descending coronary artery; RV: Right ventricle; LV: Left ventricle; RAO: Right anterior oblique; LAO: Left anterior oblique).

with no structural heart disease. Outflow tract tachycardia occurs as a result of triggered activity, related to excessive calcium in the myocardium following the preceding beat. Outflow tract tachycardia most commonly arises from the right ventricle outflow tract (RVOT), and may also arise from the RV infundibulum, RV free wall, posterior aspect of the interventricular septum, or left ventricle outflow tract. Outflow tract arrhythmias usually manifest as frequent PVCs which convert to salvos of VT with exercise, emotional stress, or dietary stimulant use. The ventricular complexes exhibit left bundle branch morphology (Fig. 33.17) and since they come from a superior part of the heart, and have a superior axis giving rise to upright ventricular complexes in the inferior leads (Table 33.1). While the prognosis of outflow tachycardia is generally favorable, outflow tachycardias occasionally can cause symptoms of uncomfortable palpitations and exercise intolerance. In such patients, medical therapy with beta-blockers or nondihydropyridine calcium channel blockers is usually effective. In the occasional patient, catheter ablation of the VT may be required (Fig. 33.18), which has a high rate of cure.

Torsades de Pointes

Polymorphic VT occurring in the setting of a prolonged QT interval is termed *torsades de pointes* (twisting of the points) (Figs. 33.19 and 33.20). Most commonly, torsades occurs when the QT interval is notably prolonged (> 550–600 ms) (Figs. 33.21 to 33.23). Torsades de pointes more commonly develops during periods of bradycardia, when the QT interval is longest. Drugs associated with

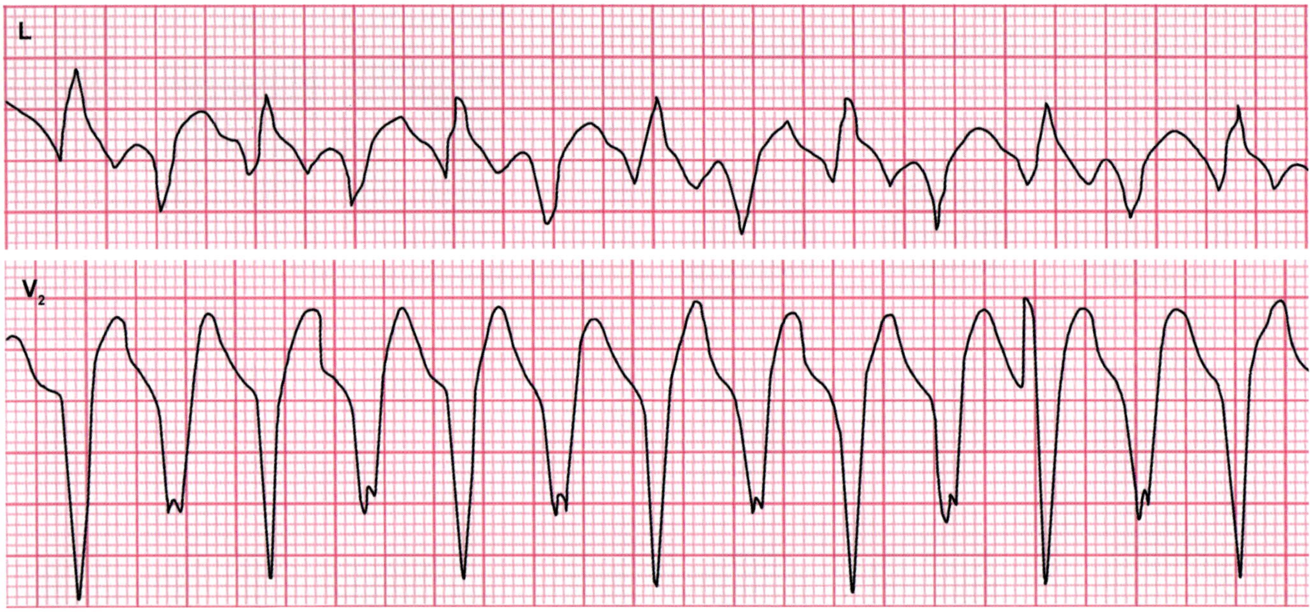

Fig. 33.10: Bidirectional ventricular tachycardia in a patient with digoxin toxicity.

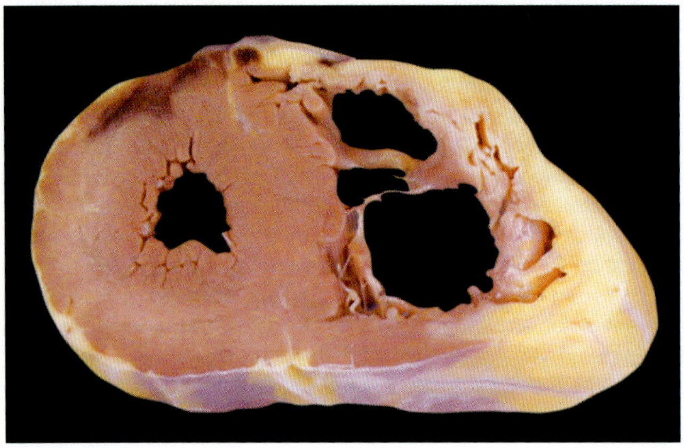

Fig. 33.11: Gross pathology of a patient with arrhythmogenic right ventricular dysplasia showing fatty infiltration of the right ventricle wall.

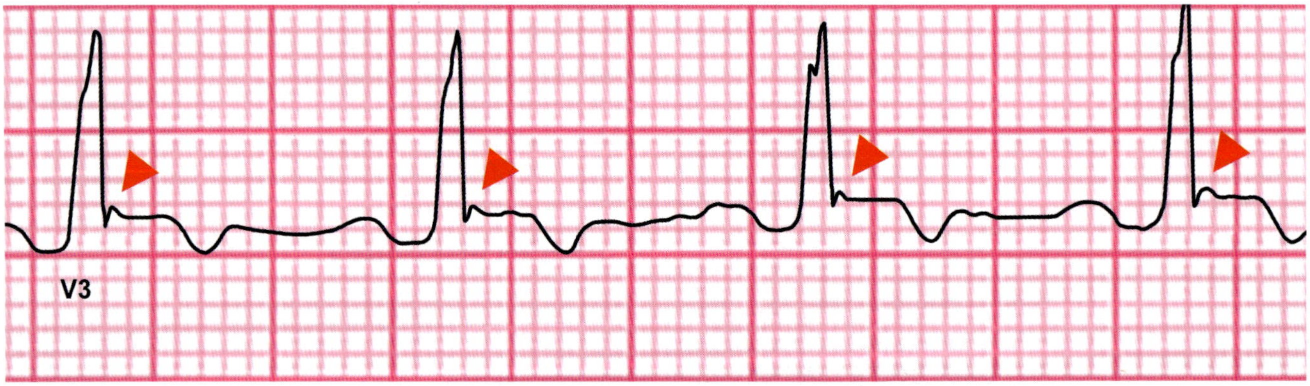

Fig. 33.12: The characteristic ECG findings of arrhythmogenic right ventricular dysplasia (ARVD), which shows a slurred upstroke at the end of the QRS complex in the precordial leads, called the Epsilon wave (arrow). This finding is believed to be due to slowed conduction through fibrofatty myocardium. This finding is quite specific for ARVD but is seldom seen, even in patients with diagnosed ARVD, and its absence does not rule out ARVD. More often seen are T-wave inversions, as are seen in this tracing.

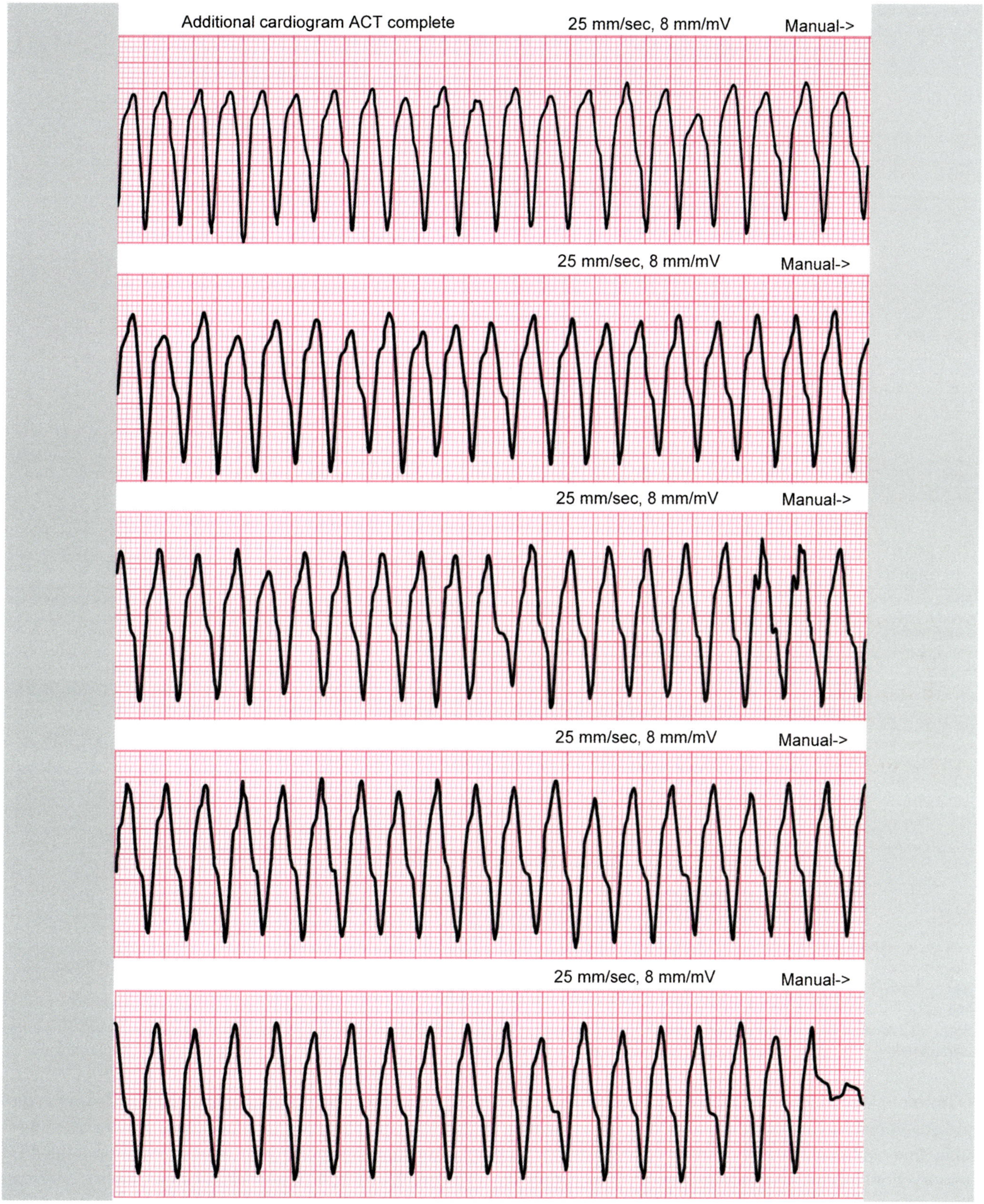

Fig. 33.13: Detection of sustained monomorphic ventricular tachycardia in a patient with episodic palpitations who was undergoing continuous ambulatory ECG monitoring.

Flow chart 33.1: The Brugada algorithm to detect the possible origin of a wide complex tachycardia: ventricular tachycardia (VT) versus supraventricular tachycardia (SVT) with aberrant intraventricular conduction.

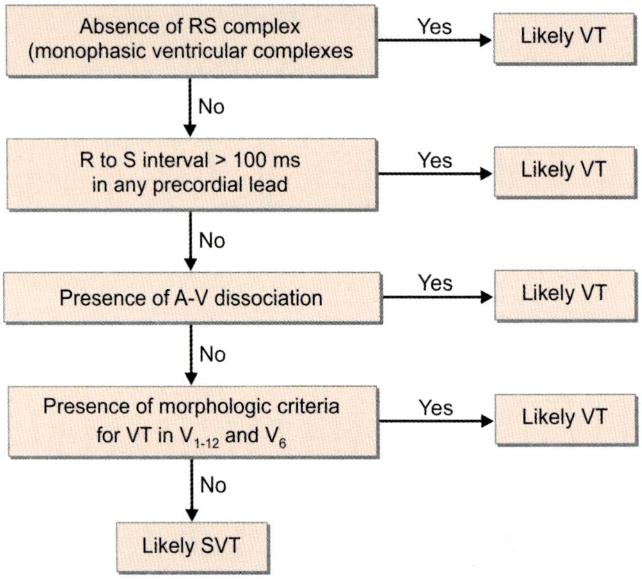

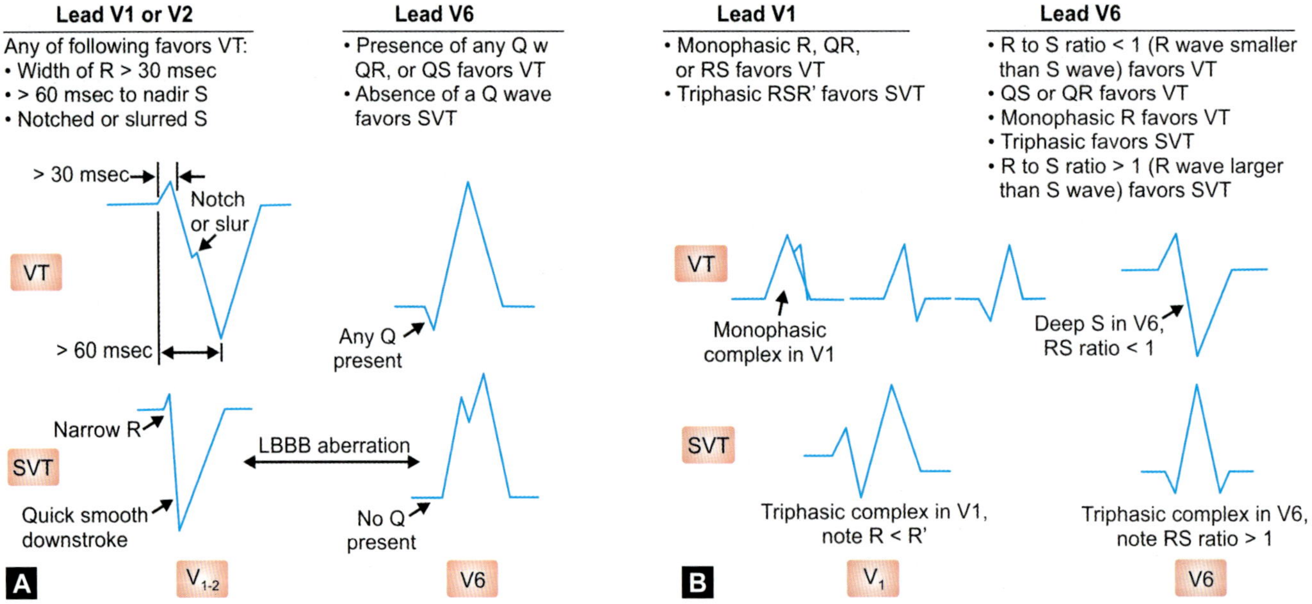

Figs. 33.14A and B: The morphologic criteria which may help distinguish a ventricular tachycardia from supraventricular tachycardia with aberrant conduction when the QRS complex is of (A) left bundle branch morphology or of (B) right bundle branch morphology.

QT prolongation and torsades de pointes include sotalol, amiodarone, ibutilide, encainide, flecainide, procainamide, quinidine, and disopyrimide. Certain antidepressants and antipsychotic agents, particularly if taken in an overdose, can prolong the QT interval and predispose to torsades. Combinations of drugs (e.g. certain antihistamines, antibiotics, antiviral agents, antifungals) which interact via the cytochrome P450 system have also been described as predisposing to torsades de points. Hereditary channelopathies which lead to congenital prolonged QT syndromes include *Jervell and Lange-Nielsen syndrome* (congenitally long QT associated with congenital deafness) and *Romano Ward syndrome* (isolated prolongation of QT interval). Electrolyte abnormalities that have been

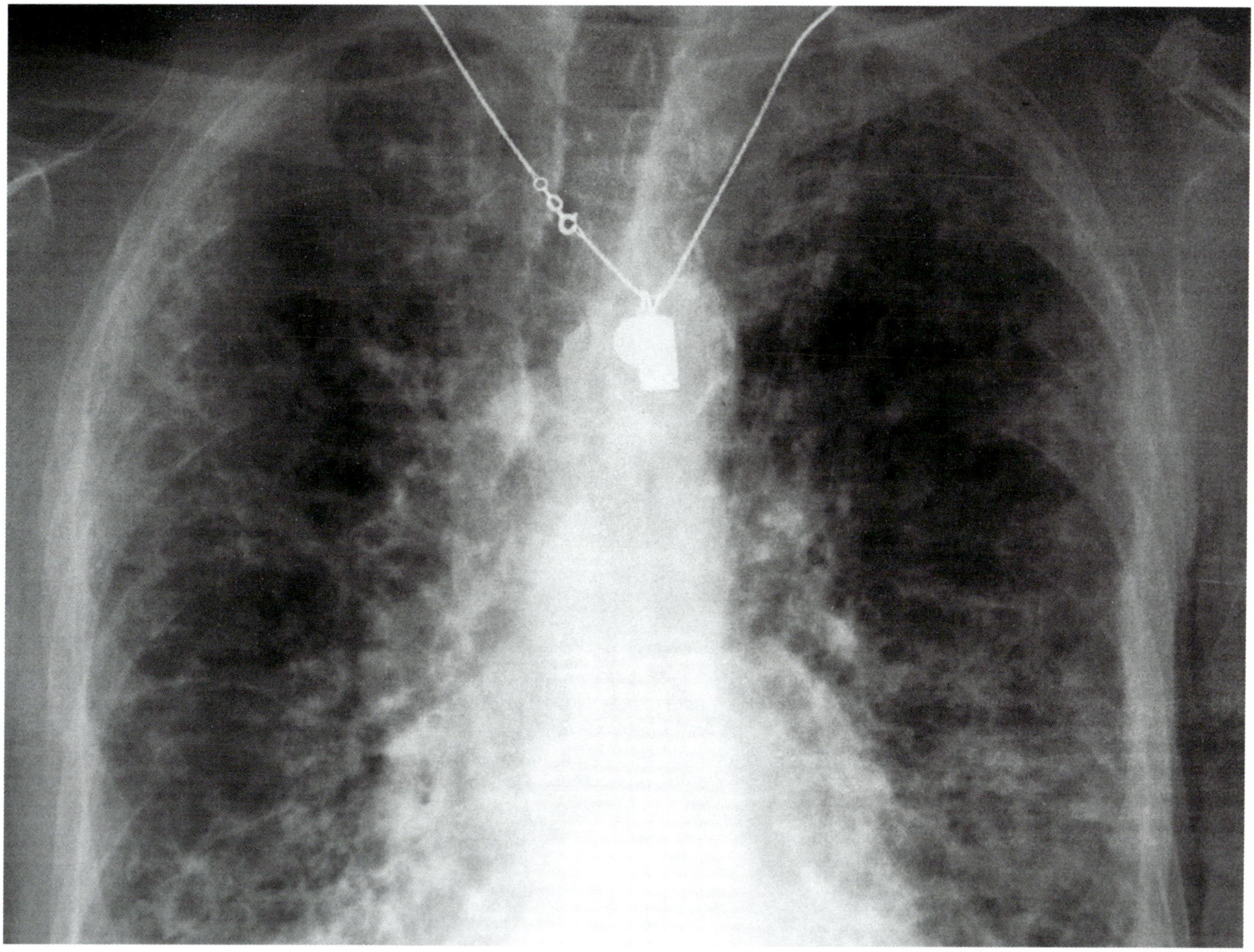

Fig. 33.15: Chest X-ray demonstrating amiodarone-induced pulmonary fibrosis. (Image posted by James Heilman on Wikimedia Commons).

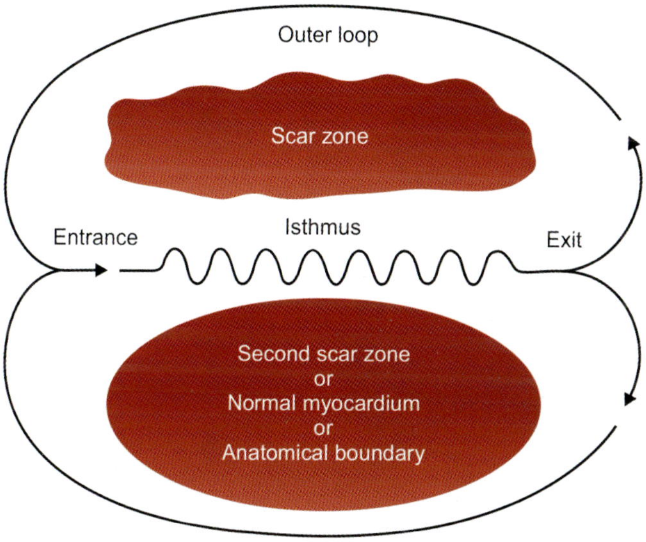

Fig. 33.16A: A schematic of a typical ventricular tachycardia (VT) circuit seen around scarred myocardium (usually seen in ischemic cardiomyopathy). The isthmus may exist between the scar zone and normal myocardium, within or between two scar zones, or between the scar zone and an anatomical boundary such as the mitral valve. The goal of VT ablation in scar related is to create a line of radiofrequency ablation across the isthmus to interrupt the circuit.

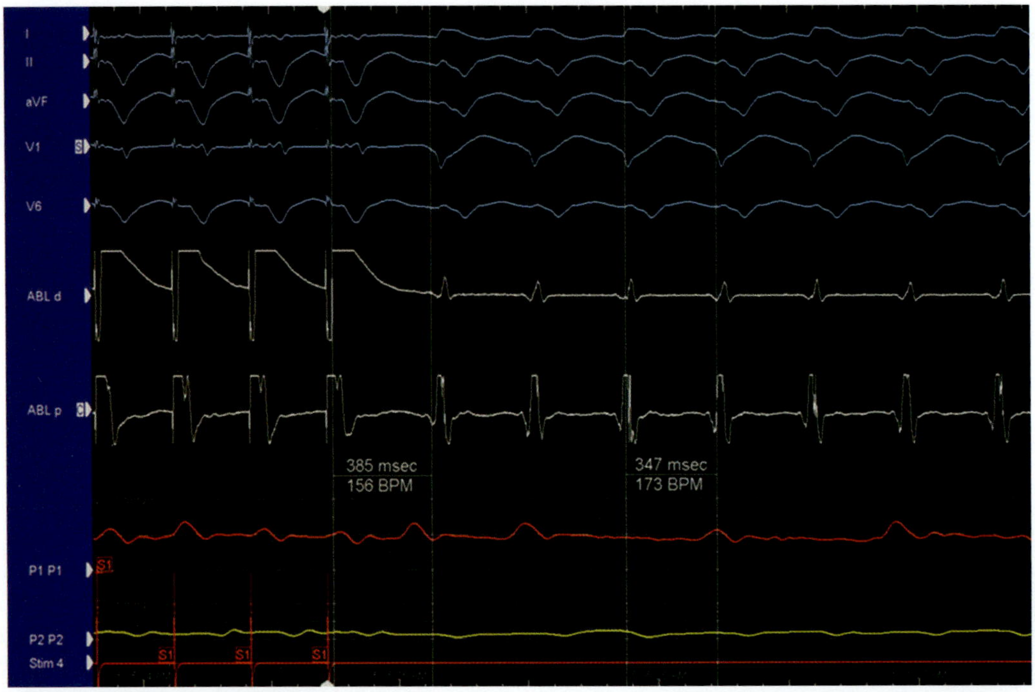

Fig. 33.16B: Intracardiac electrogram tracing showing attempts at entrainment of the ventricular tachycardia (VT) seen in Figure 33.16C during electrophysiology (EP) study. The first third of the tracing shows entrainment of VT whereby it is being sped up by introducing properly timed impulses to the tachycardia circuit at a rate faster than the native VT rate. Entrainment suggests presence of a reentrant circuit and the next goal is to find the narrowest area of the circuit—the isthmus, where ablation can usually terminate the circuit of that specific arrhythmia. The top tracings are regular surface lead EKG which appear wider due to the higher sweep speeds of recording used in the EP lab (at 200 mm/sec instead of 25 mm/sec used for regular EKGs). The channels marked "ABL" are the intracardiac recordings from the site of contact of the ablation catheter with the myocardium.

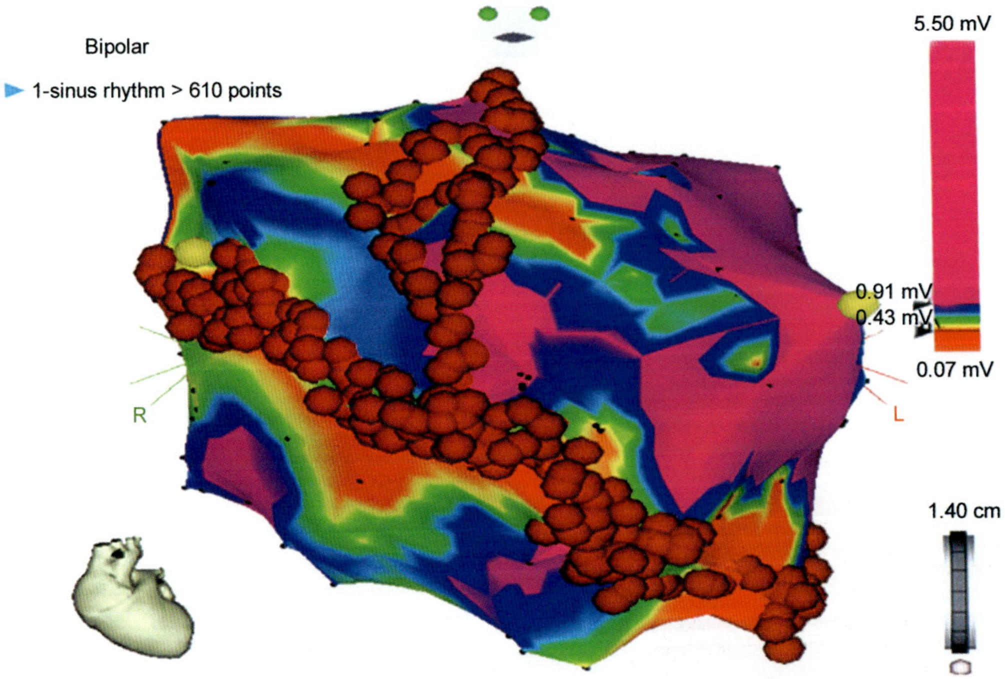

Fig. 33.16C: Ventricular tachycardia ablation study.

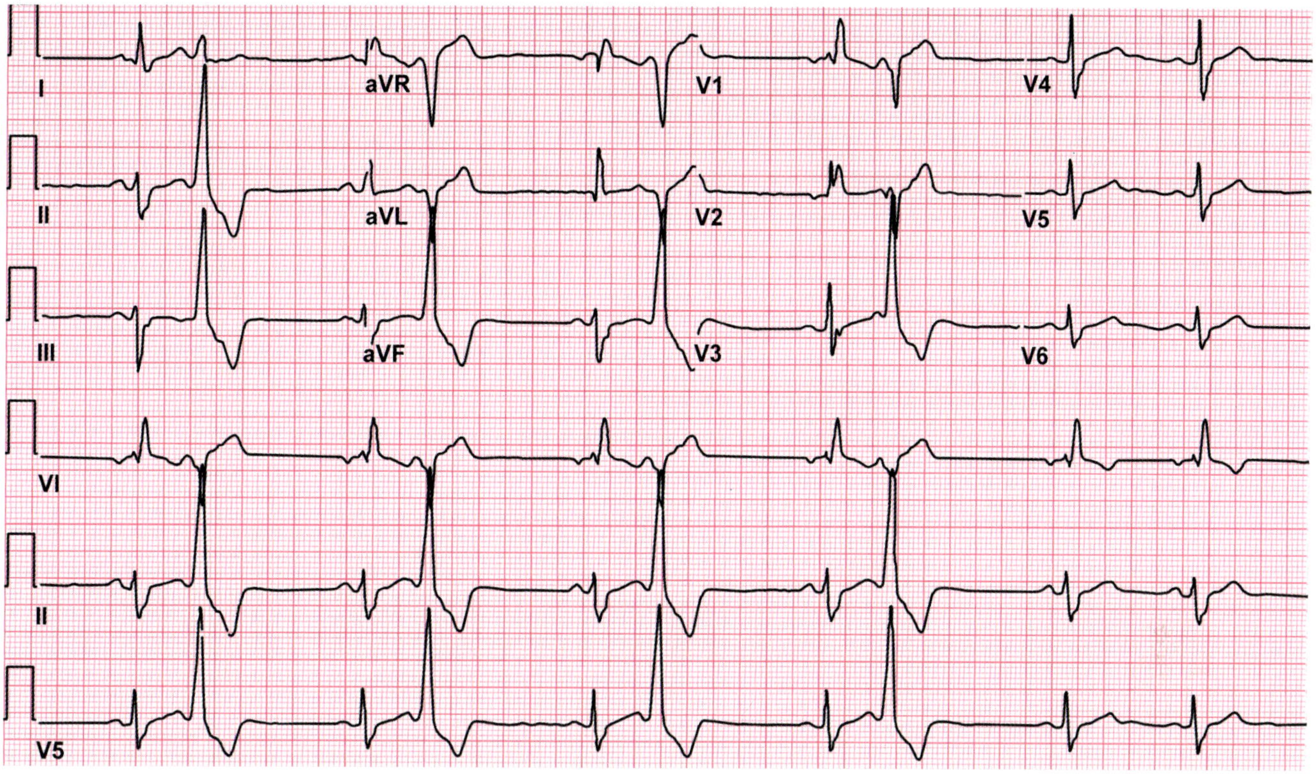

Fig. 33.17: 12-lead ECG showing premature ventricular complexes (PVCs) of right ventricular outflow tract (RVOT) origin in a bigeminal pattern. Note the left bundle branch morphology of the PVCs with upright PVC complexes in the inferior leads suggestive of an inferior axis and superior source of the PVC. Readers may also appreciate that sinus beats show an underlying right bundle branch with left anterior fascicular block. The outflow tract ventricular tachycardias can originate either in the RVOT or the left ventricular outflow tract (LVOT). Usually if the R wave transition happens before or at V2 on the PVC it suggests LVOT origin. An R wave transition at or beyond V4 is generally indicative of RVOT origin.

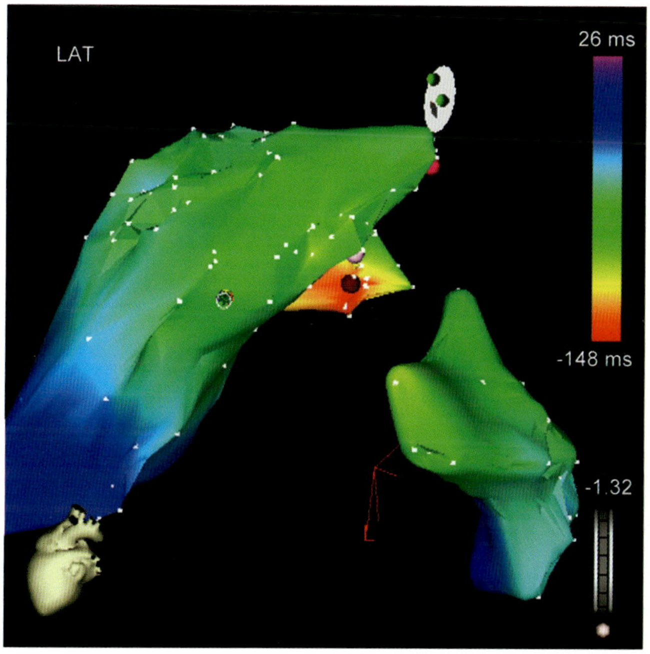

Fig. 33.18: Activation map of an outflow tract ventricular tachycardia which was mapped to the left coronary cusp. This activation map was obtained invasively after mapping the activation sequence of the premature ventricular complex on a shell of the right and left ventricular outflow tracts (seen in the left anterior oblique projection). The red dot was the site of successful ablation.

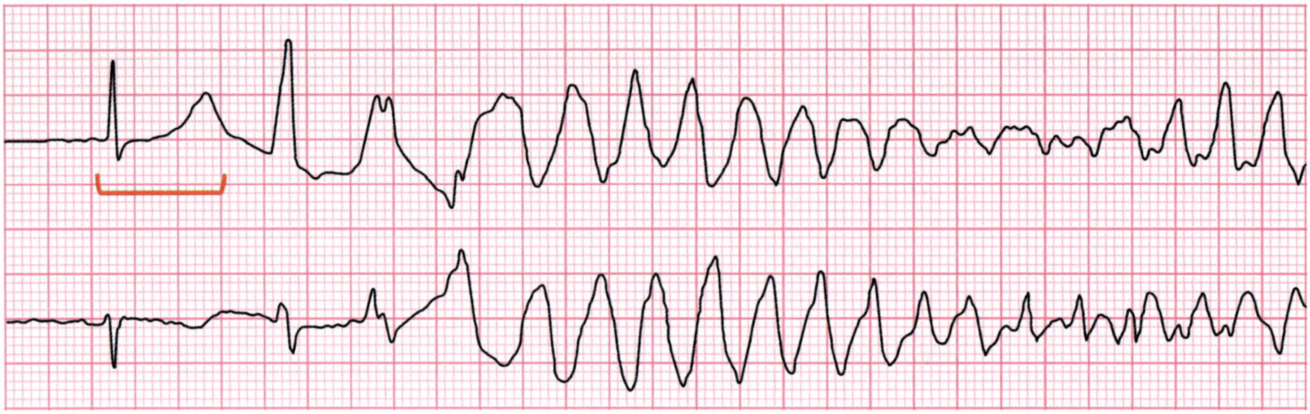

Fig. 33.19: Telemetry tracing of a patient with prolonged QT interval (bracket) who developed *torsades de pointes*.

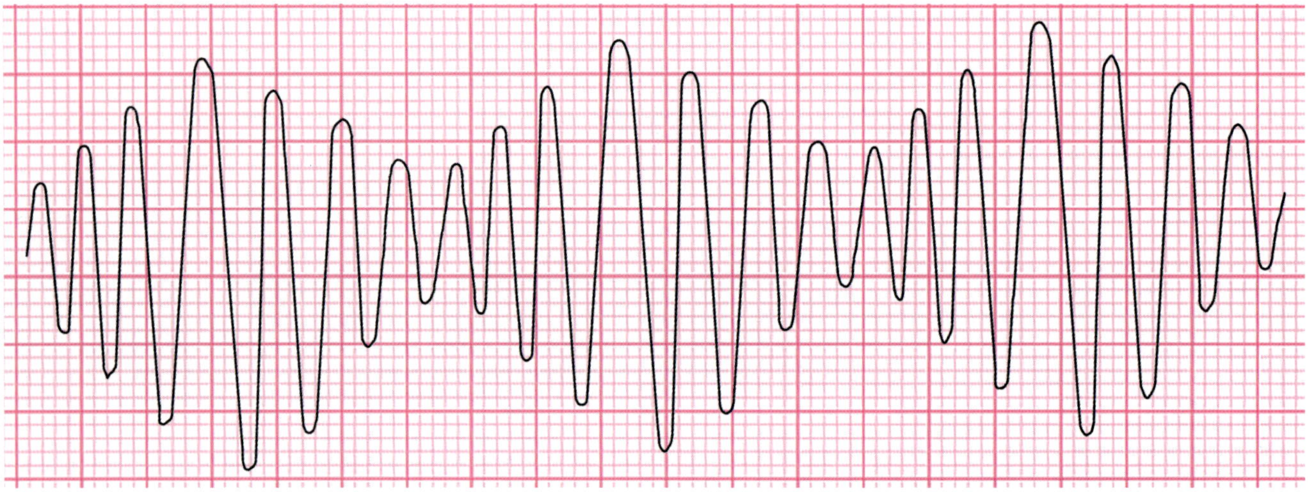

Fig. 33.20: *Torsades de pointes.* Note how the QRS axis seems to "rotate around a point". (Image courtesy of Medtronics, Inc).

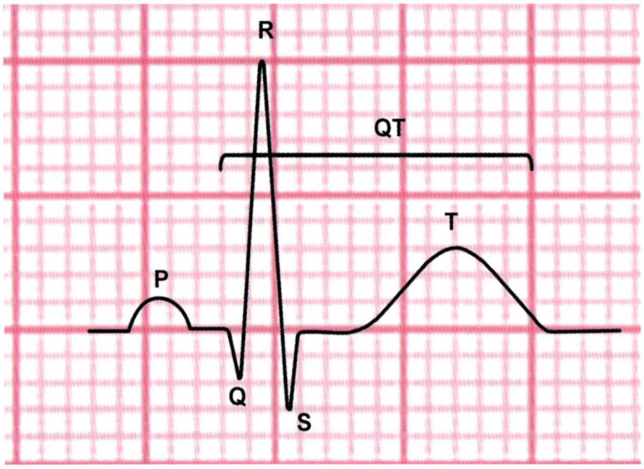

Fig. 33.21: Schematic illustration of a prolonged QT interval. (Image modified from www.medskills.eu).

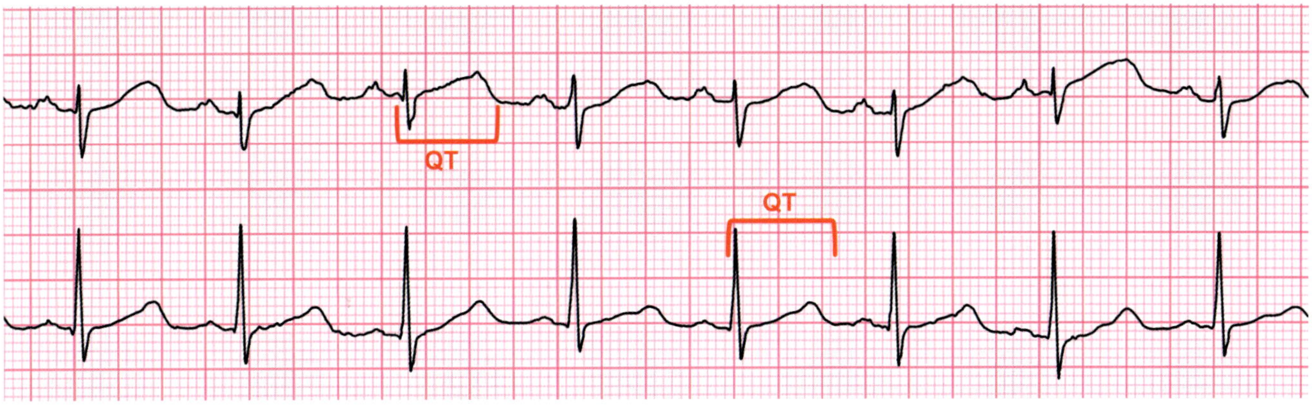

Fig. 33.22: An example of a prolonged QT interval in a patient who developed *torsades de pointes*.

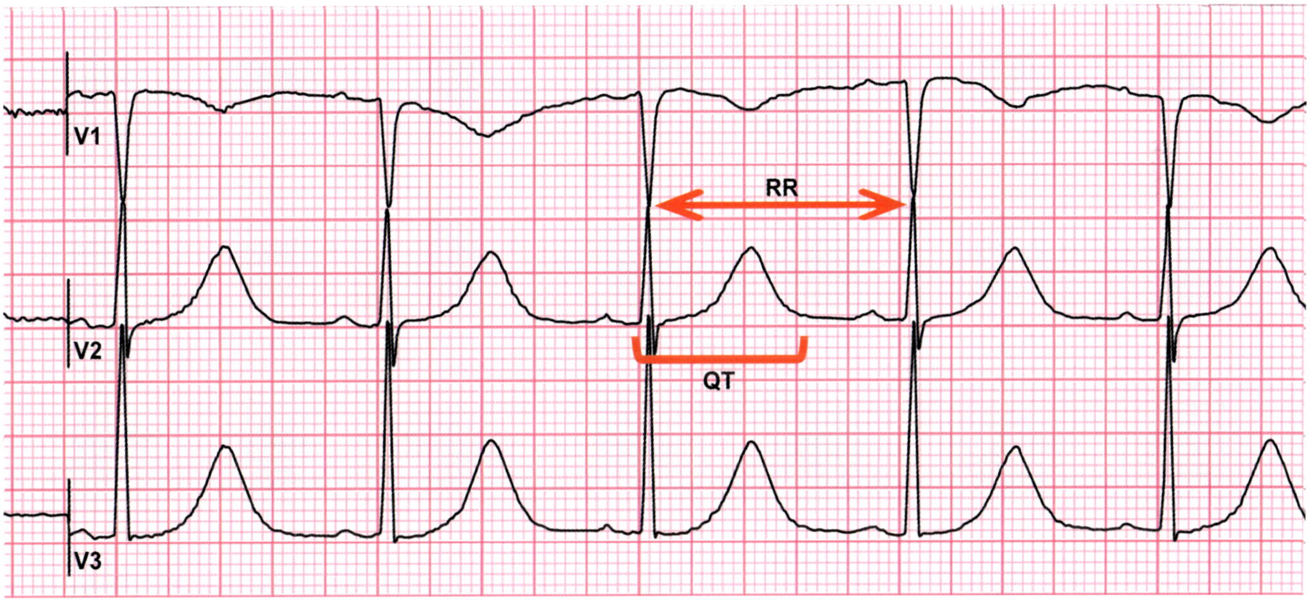

Fig. 33.23: Notably prolonged QT interval due to mediation overdose. Note that the QT interval is clearly greater than half of the R-R interval. (ECG image adapted from ECGpedia).

associated with increased risk of torsades include hypokalemia and hypomagnesemia. Patients who develop sustained torsades de pointes are either hemodynamically unstable or will become hemodynamically unstable shortly. Acute treatment in such cases is defibrillation. Magnesium administration in patients with torsades is also recommended.

Brugada Syndrome

Brugada syndrome is a syndrome associated with the development of potentially fatal episodes of VT in hearts with no apparent structural defect. The classic (though unreliable) finding on the 12-lead ECG of patients with Brugada syndrome is unusual ST-segment elevation in leads V1–V3 (Figs. 33.24 and 33.25).

VENTRICULAR FLUTTER

Ventricular flutter is an unstable rhythm originating in the ventricle. Ventricular flutter is usually defined as a rate between 250 beats/min and 300 beats/min or 250 beats/min and 350 beats/min (Figs. 33.26A and B). Some consider ventricular flutter a possible transition stage between VT and VF. Ventricular flutter results in ineffective ventricular contraction and hemodynamic instability. Treatment

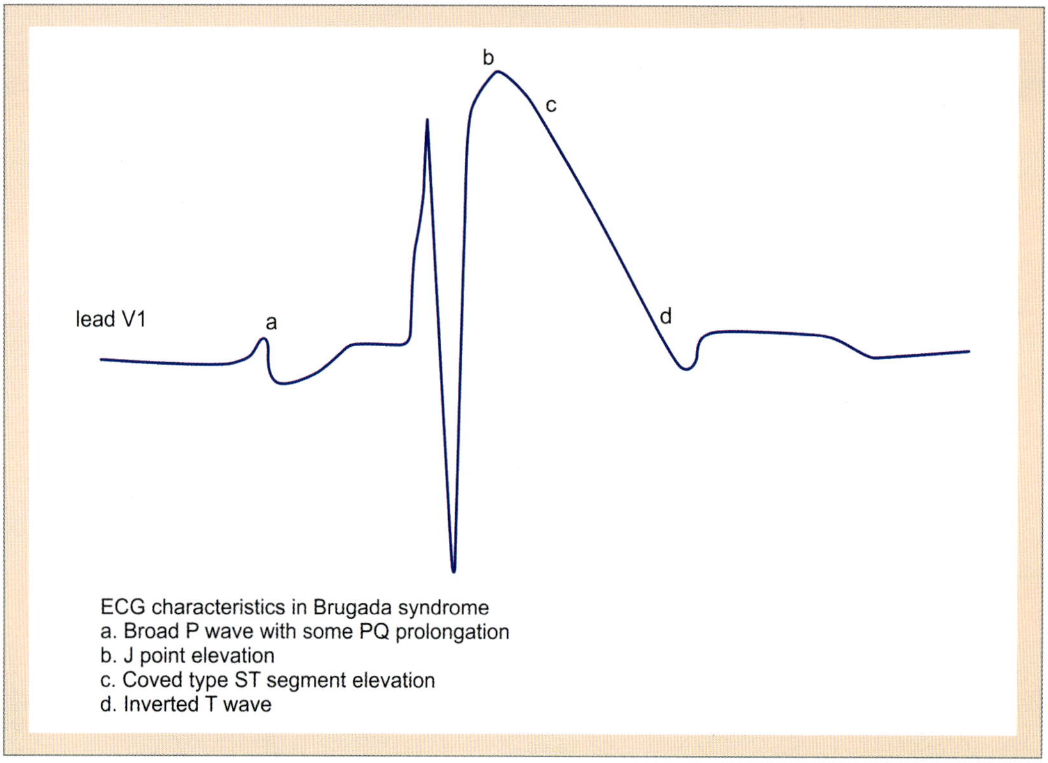

Fig. 33.24: Schematic illustration of the ECG abnormalities observed in Brugada syndrome. (Image from ECGpedia.org).

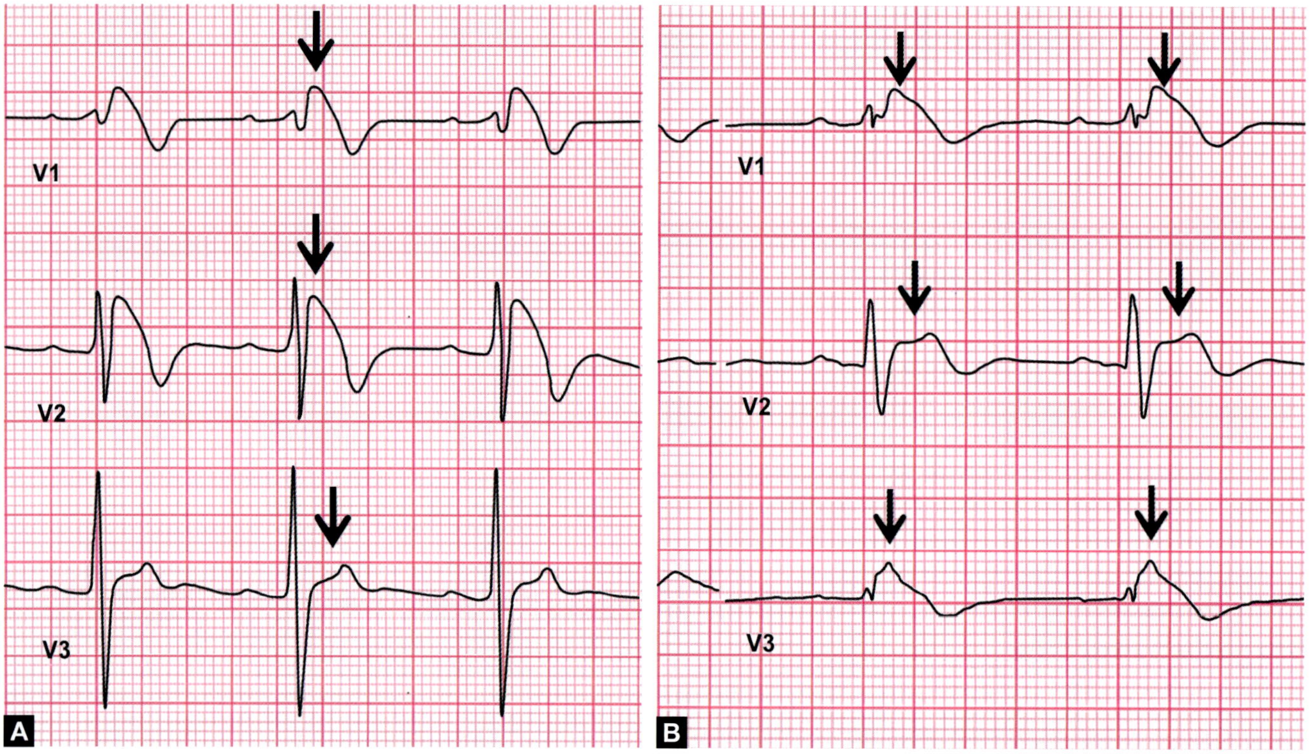

Figs. 33.25A and B: ECG demonstrating several of the unusual ST-elevation patterns (arrows) seen in Brugada syndrome. (Images adapted from ECGpedia.org).

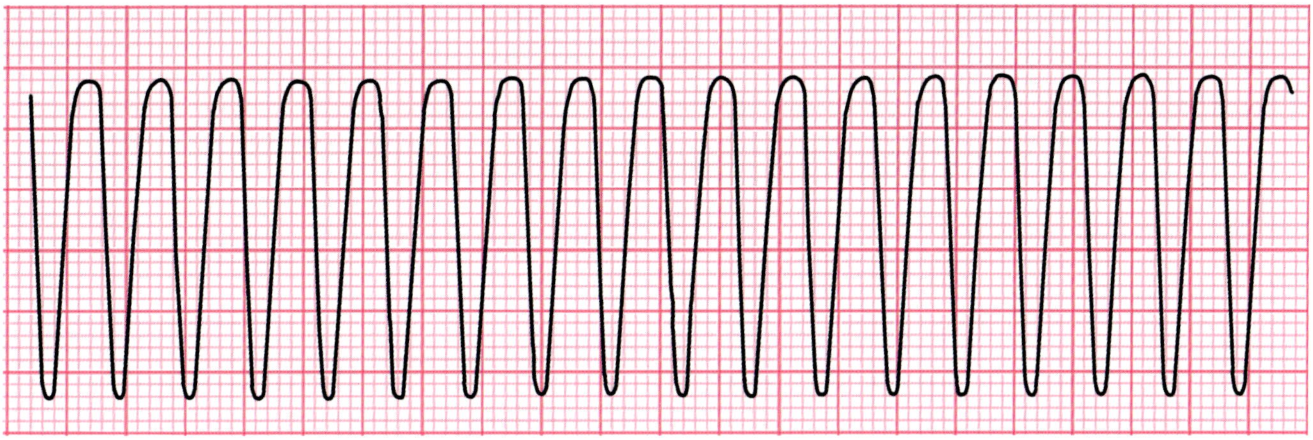

Fig. 33.26A: Rhythm strip showing ventricular flutter at a rate of 280 beats per minute. (Image courtesy of Medtronic, Inc).

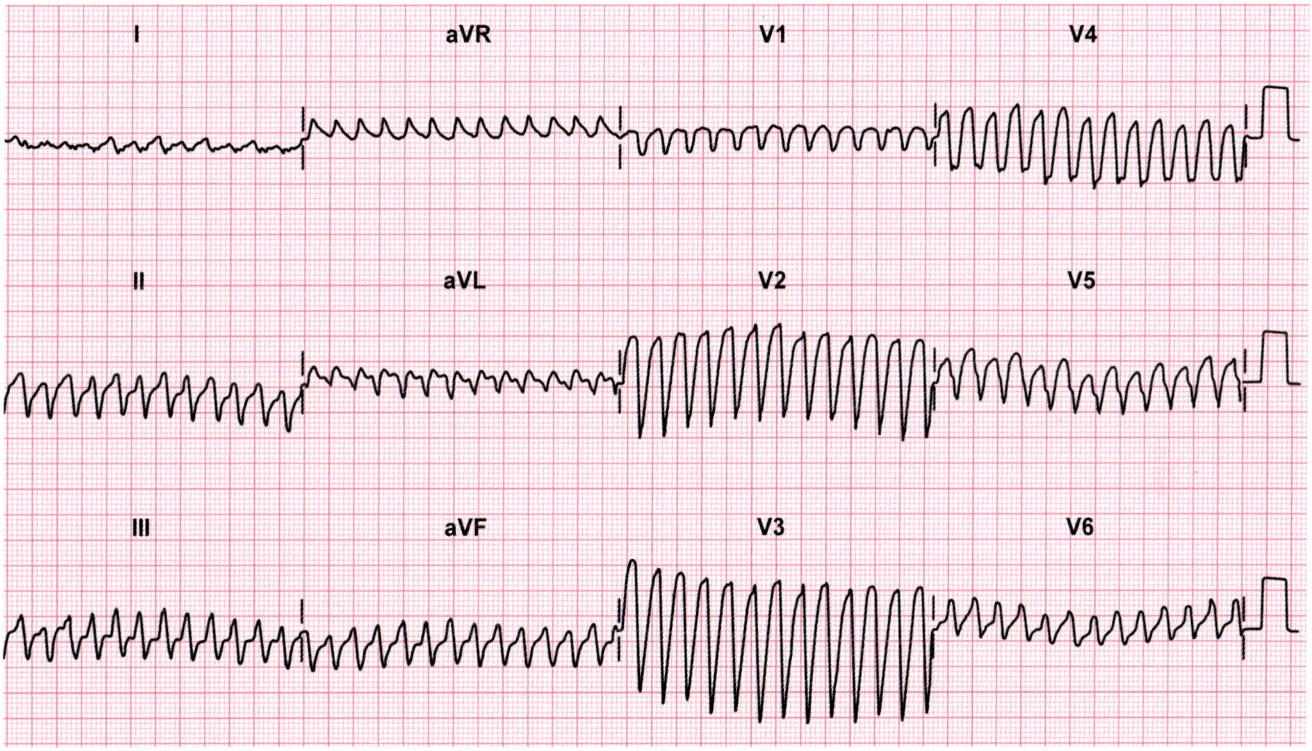

Fig. 33.26B: 12-lead ECG demonstrating ventricular flutter with a ventricular rate of approximately 300 beats per minute.

is usually immediate defibrillation. The spectrum of ventricular arrhythmias is demonstrated in Figure 33.27.

VENTRICULAR FIBRILLATION

Ventricular fibrillation is a fatal ventricular arrhythmia consisting of chaotic ventricular electrical activity, with rates exceeding 300 beats/min (Figs. 33.28 and 33.29). Since there is no organized ventricular mechanical contraction, the cardiac output generated is minimal and thus hemodynamic collapse always ensues. Approximately, 80% of cases of sudden cardiac death have VF as the terminal rhythm.

As a general rule of thumb, earlier VF often has discernable positive and negative deflections on the ECG tracing (so called "coarse VF"). Over time, voltage of the QRS deflections decrease, and "fine VF" is observed (Fig. 33.30).

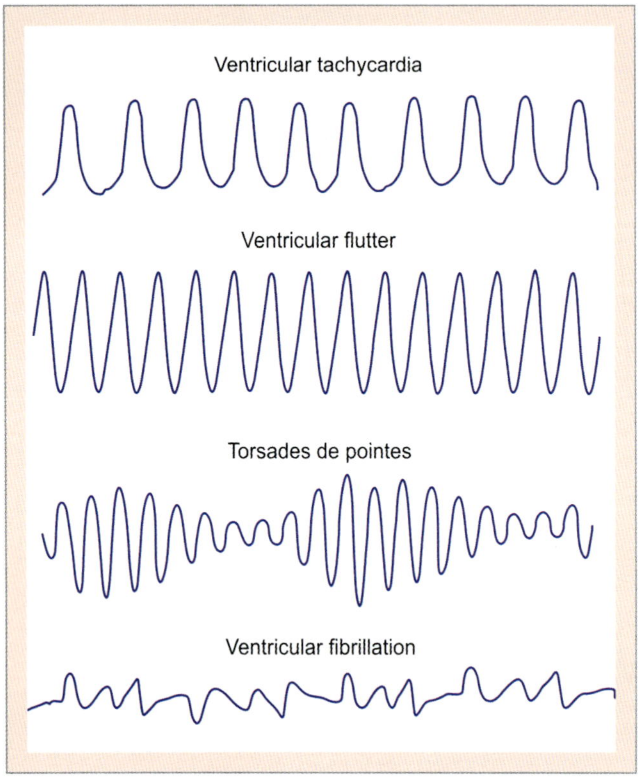

Fig. 33.27: Schematic illustration of the spectrum of ventricular arrhythmias. (Illustration created from tracings adapted from ECGpedia.org).

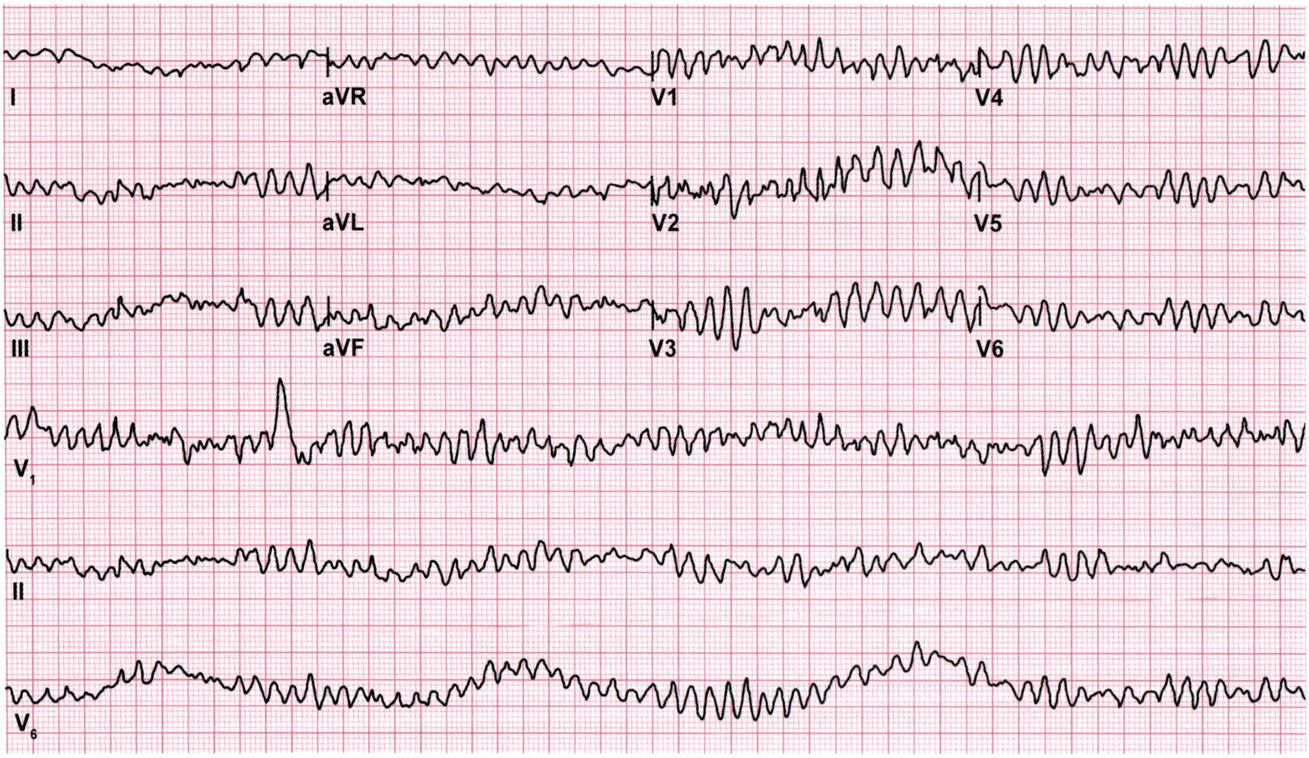

Fig. 33.28: Ventricular fibrillation. (Image posted by Jason E Roedgier, CCT, CRAT on Wikepedia Commons).

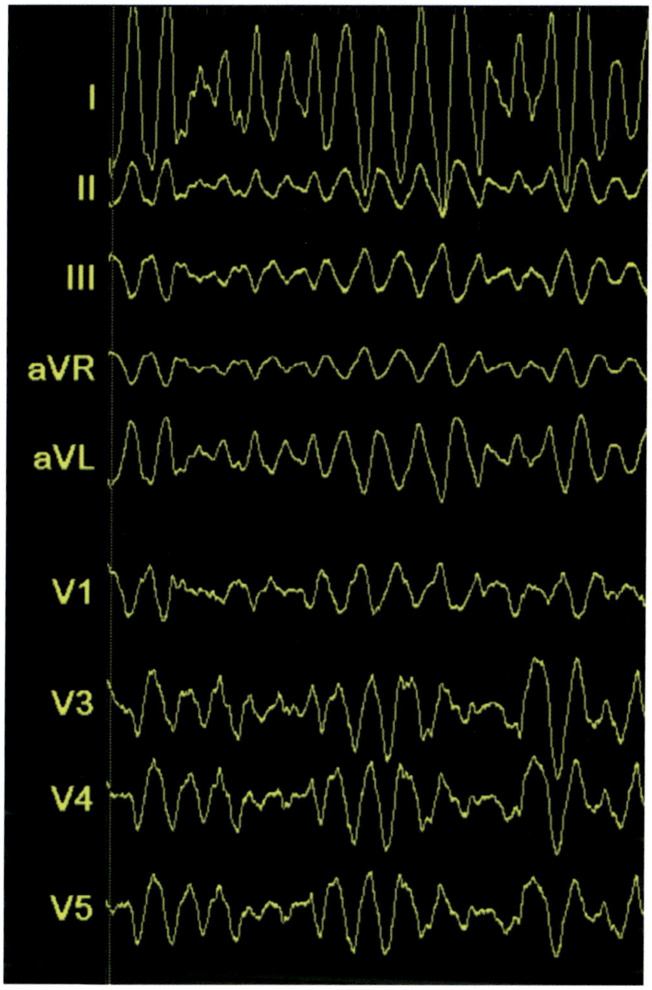

Fig. 33.29: Ventricular fibrillation. [Image from Rosenheck S. Defibrillation shock amplitude, location and timing. In: Harris JJ (Ed). Cardiac Defibrillation—Prediction, Prevention and Management of Cardiovascular Arrhythmic Events. InTech; 2011].

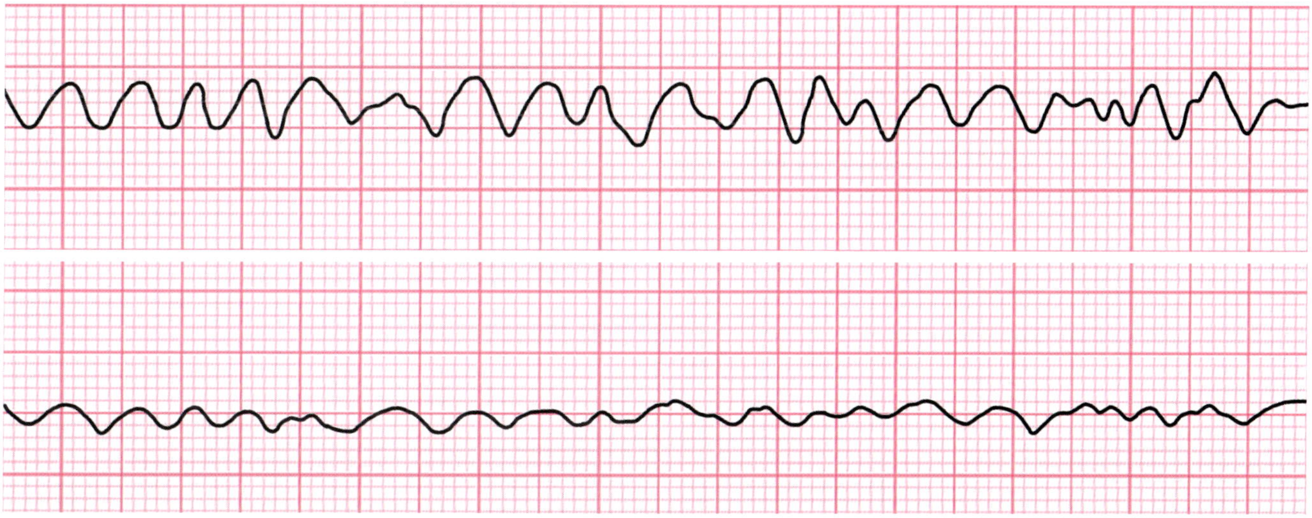

Fig. 33.30: Examples of "coarse" ventricular fibrillation (upper panel) and "fine" ventricular fibrillation (lower panel). Ventricular fibrillation may often first appear as coarse QRS deflections. Over time, the amplitude of deflections may decrease.

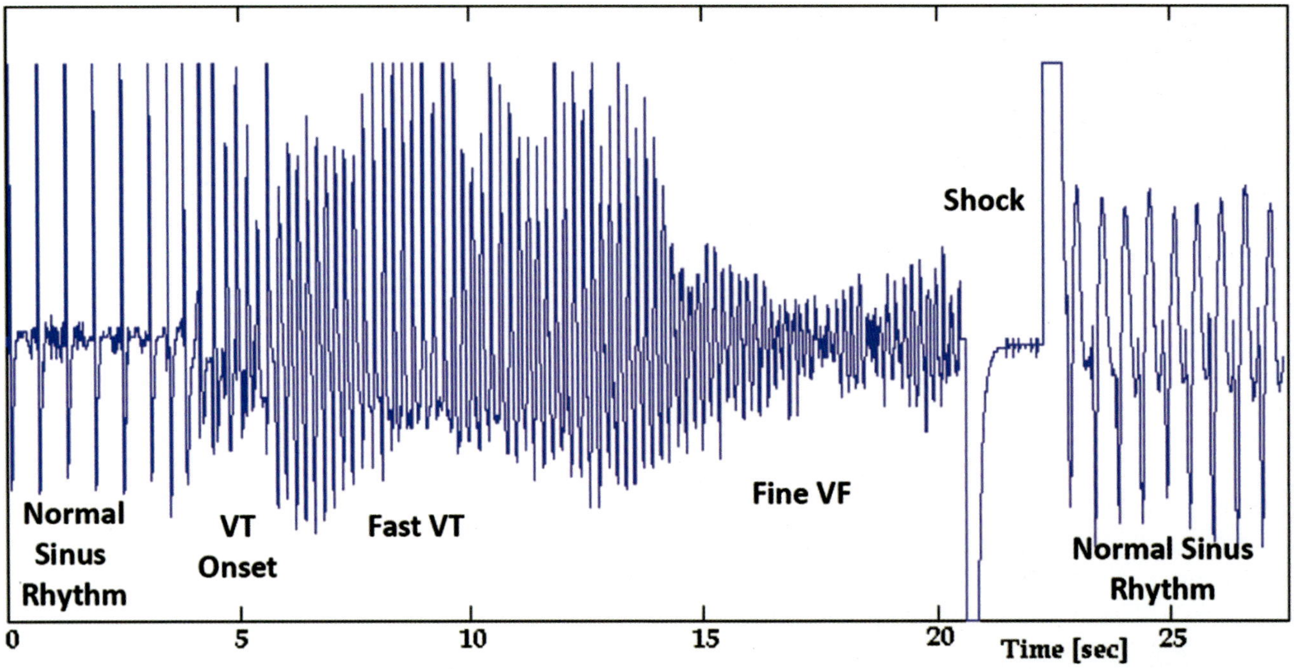

Fig. 33.31: Malignant ventricular tachycardia degenerating into ventricular fibrillation. ICD recording of VT degenerating into VF and reverting to sinus rhythm after appropriate defibrillation. [Image from Casaleggio A, Guidotto T, Malavasi V, et al. Ventricular tachyarrhythmias in implantable cardioverter defibrillator recipients: differences between ischemic and dilated cardiomyopathies. In: Harris JJ (Ed). Cardiac Defibrillation—Prediction, Prevention and Management of Cardiovascular Arrhythmic Events. InTech; 2011].

Ventricular fibrillation most commonly occurs in diseased myocardium, usually as a result of ischemic heart disease. VF may be the manifestation of acute MI leading to out-of-hospital sudden cardiac death in many patients. VF also occurs in those with nonischemic dilated cardiomyopathy, hypertrophic cardiomyopathy, acute myocarditis, electrolyte disturbances, and drug overdoses. VF may also occur as the terminal manifestation of noncardiac disease, such as severe hypoxemia, severe electrolyte disturbances, or severe acidosis. Rarely, there is no discernable cause or detectable underlying pathology, and the term *idiopathic ventricular fibrillation* is used.

Acute treatment is immediate defibrillation—VF rarely terminates spontaneously. Subsequent management includes investigation of underlying cause or predisposing conditions, and often ICD implantation (Fig. 33.31) if a clearly reversible or treatable cause of the VF cannot be determined or achieved.

REFERENCES

Brugada P, Brugada J, Mont L, et al. A new approach to the differential diagnosis of a regular tachycardia with a wide QRS complex. Circulation. 1991;83(5):1649-59.

European Heart Rhythm Association, Heart Rhythm Society, Zipes DP, et al. ACC/AHA/ESC 2006 guidelines for management of patients with ventricular arrhythmias and the prevention of sudden cardiac death: a report of the American College of Cardiology/American Heart Association Task Force and the European Society of Cardiology Committee for Practice Guidelines (Writing Committee to Develop Guidelines for Management of Patients With Ventricular Arrhythmias and the Prevention of Sudden Cardiac Death). J Am Coll Cardiol. 2006;48(5):e247-346.

CHAPTER

34

Pacemakers

Khaled Albouaini

INDICATIONS

Pacing is one of the rapidly advancing subspecialties in cardiology. Numerous pacemakers (Figs. 34.1A to E) and pacemaker leads (Figs. 34.2A to E) are commercially available. In current practice, most patients are treated with a dual chamber pacemaker, with one lead implanted in the right atrial (RA) appendage and one lead implanted in the right ventricular (RV) apex (Figs. 34.3A and B). In patients treated with cardiac resynchronization therapy (CRT), a "left ventricular" lead is also implanted.

American guidelines regarding pacemakers and CRT were published in 2008. The guidelines for CRT were then revised in 2012. In 2013, the European Society of Cardiology published guidelines on cardiac pacing and resynchronization therapy. These guidelines are given in the references section at the end of the chapter. In general, permanent pacemaker implantation is indicated in patients with symptomatic bradycardia due to sinus node dysfunction or advanced atrioventricular (AV) node block, periods of a systole greater than 3–5 seconds, persistent asymptomatic advanced second degree or third degree AV block, and symptomatic chronotropic incompetence. In general, CRT is recommended in patients with depressed left ventricle (LV) systolic (ejection fraction ≤ 30–35%), QRS duration 120–150 ms (particularly if left bundle branch morphology is present), and symptoms of heart failure, although recommendations regarding CRT are continuously evolving.

PACING MODE SELECTION

In selecting the best pacing mode, the physician should take the following into consideration along with the underlying rhythm abnormality: the patient's overall medical status, exercise ability, and chronotropic response to exercise. The vast majority of patients can be treated with one of these pacing modes (with or without rate response): AAIR, VVIR, DDDR. In atrial fibrillation (AF) patients, VVI(R) is the default pacing mode. In patients with sick sinus syndrome (SSS) or AV block, "physiological" dual chamber pacing in the form of DDD(R) is the default pacing mode. However, VVI(R) can be a reasonable choice in the very elderly while AAI(R) is a reasonable choice in patients with SSS with intact AV node conduction. The algorithm in Flow chart 34.1 is suggested by the European guidelines to aid selecting the pacing mode in the most common indications for cardiac pacing; sinus node disease (SND) and AV block.

IMPLANTATION PROCEDURE

After providing informed consent and making sure blood results [e.g. blood counts and international normalized ratio (INR)] are satisfactory, the operator should make sure intravenous (IV) access is obtained on the same side of implantation (usually the left in right handed patients). It is essential to make sure that prophylactic antibiotic is given before making the skin incision. The vast majority of implant procedures are done under local anesthetic as day case procedures. Typically, the procedure takes between 30–60 minutes. Figure 34.4 shows a typical example of disposable pacing implant instruments.

The implanter should be familiar with the venous anatomy (Figs. 34.5A and B) and possible anatomical variations (Fig. 34.6). There are three ways to obtain venous access (Table 34.1), and it is highly recommended that operators should be comfortable and fully trained at performing at least two of them.

Pacemaker leads can be either actively or passively fixed to the targeted cardiac chamber. Active fixations leads are more commonly used, as they are less likely to displace.

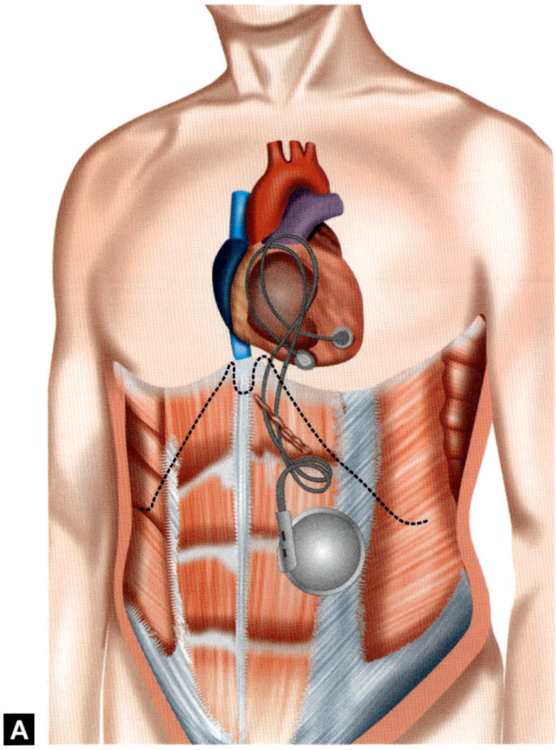

Fig. 34.1A: Example of an early epicardial pacemaker.

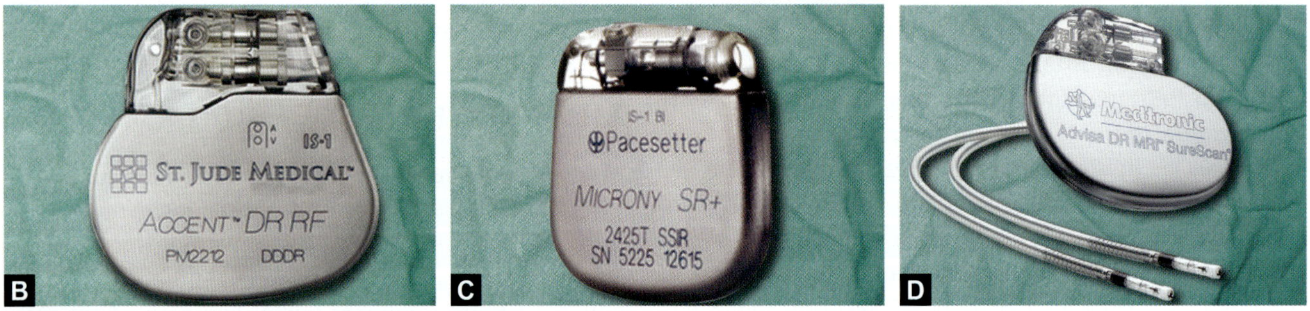

Figs. 34.1B to D: Examples of modern transvenous pacemakers currently used in clinical practice.

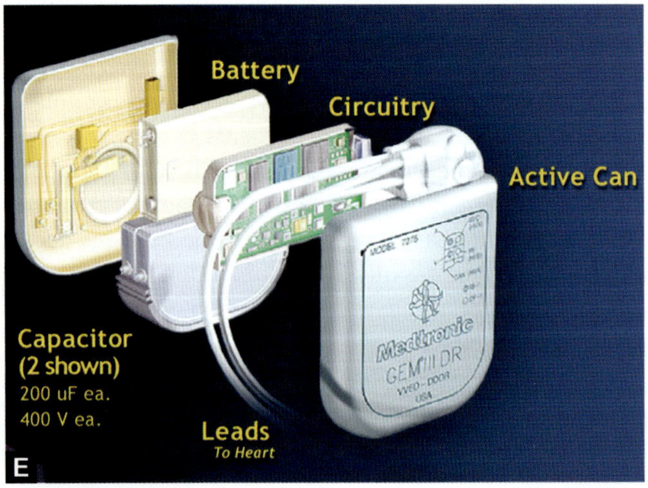

Fig. 34.1E: Composition of a pacemaker. (Image courtesy of Dr Irakli Giorgberidze and Medtronic, Inc.).

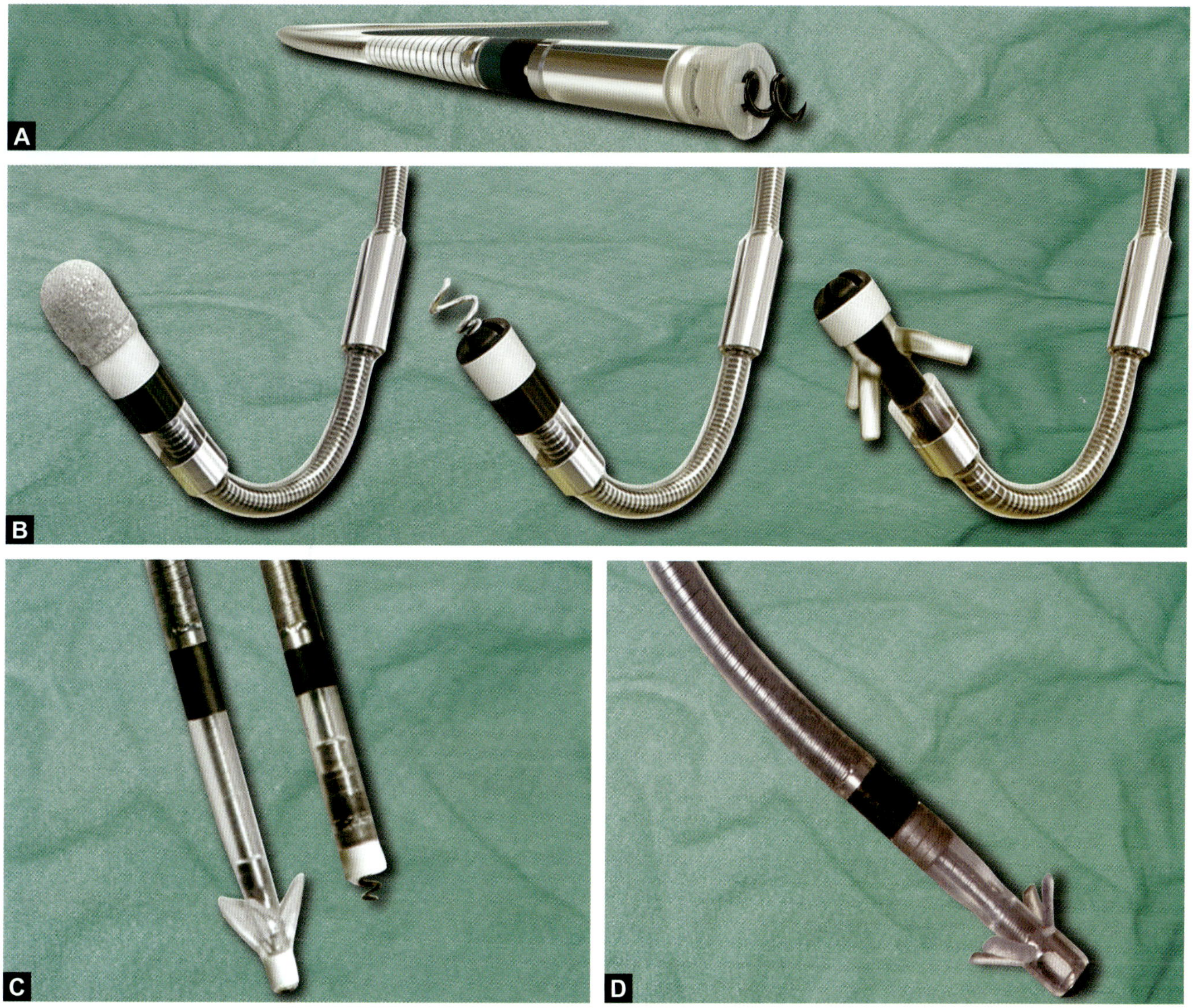

Figs. 34.2A to D: Examples of pacemaker leads. Both active fixation leads (screw at tip) and passive fixation leads (tines at tip) are shown.

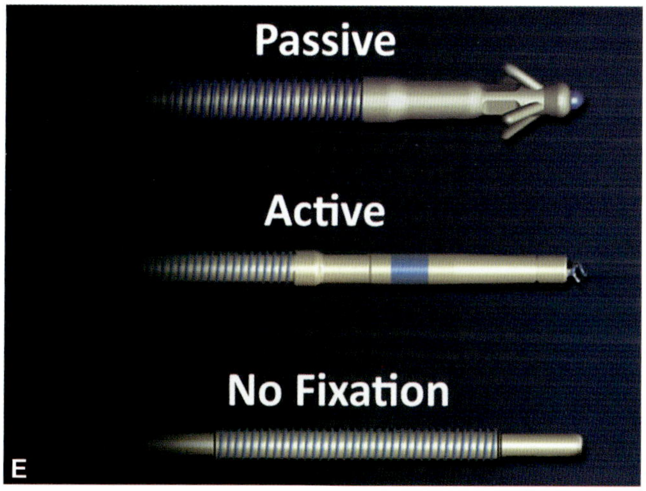

Fig. 34.2E: The difference in leads between passive and active fixation leads, and leads with no fixation device. (Image courtesy of Medtronic, Inc.).

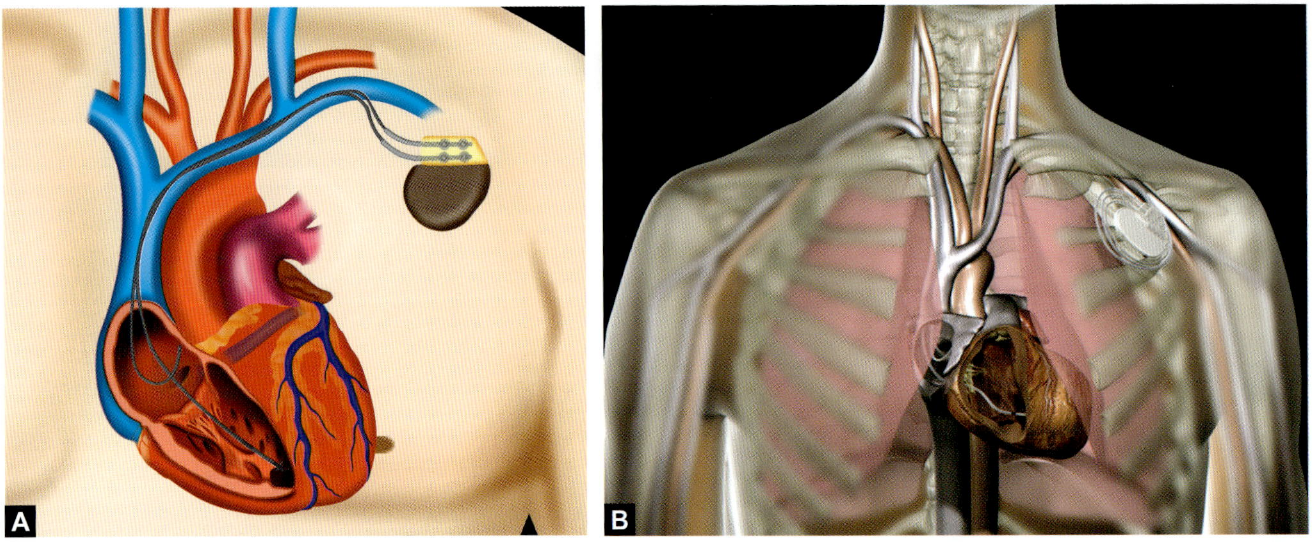

Figs. 34.3A and B: Schematic illustrations of dual chamber pacemakers. One pacemaker lead is implanted into the right atrial appendage and a second pacemaker lead is implanted in the right ventricular apex. (Image 34.3A courtesy of Boston Scientific, Inc.; Image 34.3B courtesy of Medtronic, Inc.).

Flow chart 34.1: Simple algorithm to assist in deciding the best pacing mode in patients with sinus node disease (SND) and atrioventricular (AV) block. (SND: Sinus node disease; AV: Atrioventricular; AF: Atrial fibrillation; AVM: Arteriovenous malformations).

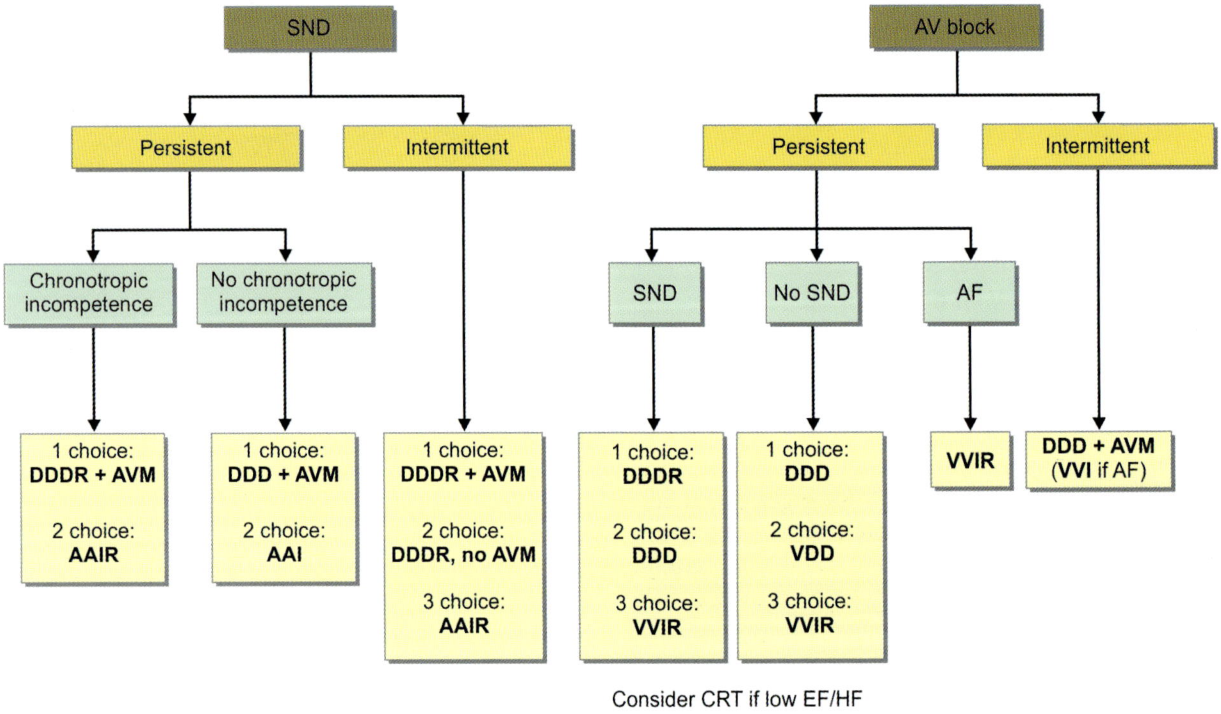

Active fixation leads are mandatory if a non-RV apical site is targeted and are highly desirable in patients with significant tricuspid regurgitation and dilated right ventricle. Some implanters avoid using active fixation atrial leads as they inherently have tendency to cause perforation. The vast majority of pacing leads have the capability to sense and pace in both unipolar and bipolar configuration. Sensing should usually be bipolar to avoid oversensing of muscle potentials (myoinhibition). Pacing can be programmed unipolar (pacing between the active can as an anode

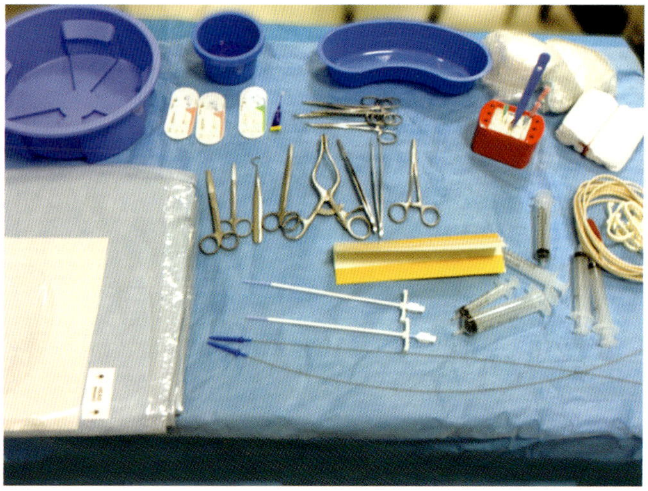

Fig. 34.4: Instruments used to implant a permanent pacing system.

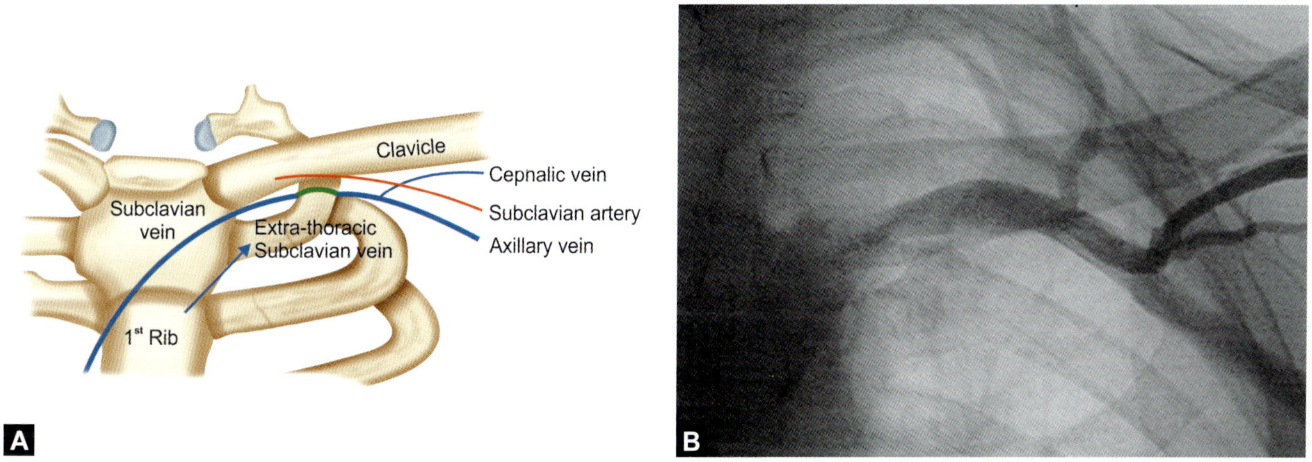

Figs. 34.5A and B: Left sided venogram. (A) Schematic representation of the venogram shown in Figure 34.5B. (B) Venogram demonstrating relevant venous anatomy for cardiac pacemaker lead implantation.

and the tip of the lead as a cathode) so pacing spikes can be visible on the surface ECG. Figures 34.7A and B shows several examples of commonly used programmers.

To target the RV apex, the stilette should be shaped like J to allow the lead to initially go to the right ventricular outflow tract (RVOT) (to make sure one is in the right ventricle). A straight stilette is then used to target the RV apex. More operators in the last few years have been targeting the RVOT septum (Figs. 34.8A and B) as this provides better hemodynamics and is less likely to result in RV pacing-induced left ventricular dysfunction. The sensed R wave should be > 6 mV with a threshold of < 1V.

The atrial lead position in the RA appendage should appear moving similar to a windscreen wiper in postero-anterior (PA) view. The anterior position should be confirmed in right anterior oblique (RAO) view. The sensed P wave should be > 1.5 mV with a threshold < 1.5 V.

The output pulse of both atrial and ventricular leads is programmed with a 3:1 safety margin after implantation and a 2:1 safety margin when the threshold stabilizes (Fig. 34.9). This is usually done at the 6-week follow-up visit in the pacing clinic. Figure 34.10 demonstrates a properly functioning dual chamber pacemaker with atrial and ventricular pacing.

DEVICE FOLLOW-UP

Patients can be discharged on the same day if the wound, pacing check, and chest X-ray (CXR) (Figs. 34.11A and B) are satisfactory. The 6-week visit is important to check the implant site, lead parameters, and to set the output according to threshold. Subsequent 12-monthly check can then be organized. Dizziness can be a result of AV dyssynchrony (pacemaker syndrome) in VVI devices or

Table 34.1: The advantages (in green) and the possible disadvantages (in red) of each venous access used at pacemaker implantation. (SCA: Subclavian artery).

Subclavian vein	*Axillary vein*	*Cephalic vein*
Blindly use anatomical landmarks	Blindly use landmarks or after venography	Under direct vision Not always present
Easy to learn, fast to obtain	Takes longer to learn, fast to obtain	Takes longer to learn, slower to obtain
Can take up to 3 or more leads	Can take up to 3 or more leads	Usually can take 2 leads and rarely 3
If the SCA is accidentally punctured, it is uncompressible	If the axillary artery is accidentally punctured, it is usually compressible	No risk to accidentally puncture the artery
Risk of pneumothorax	Usually no risk of pneumothorax	No risk of pneumothorax
Risk of subclavian crush	No risk of subclavian crush	No risk of subclavian crush
Easier for large subjects	Easier for large subjects	Difficult in large subjects

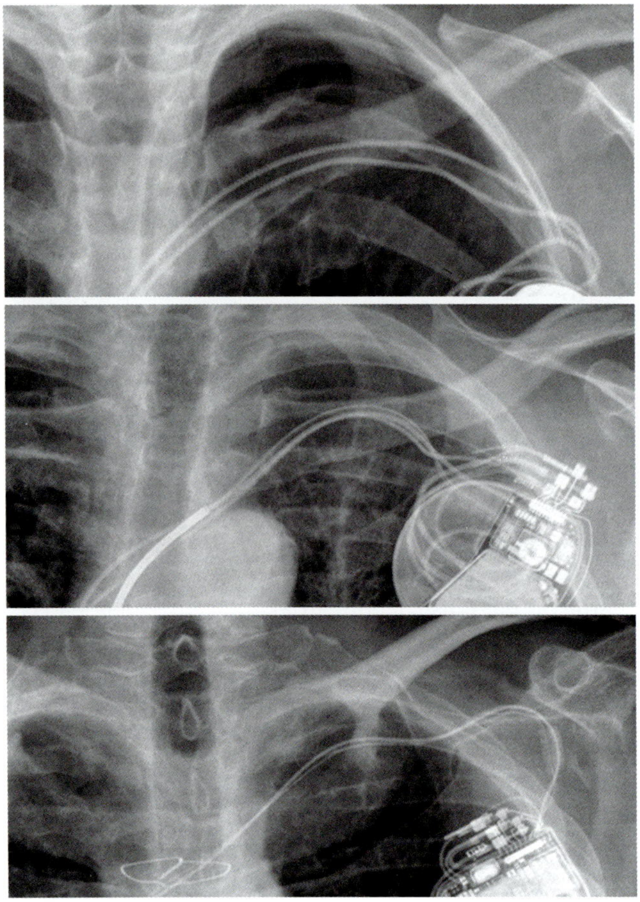

Fig. 34.6: Three different examples demonstrating that the relationship of the vein with the first rib is constant while the relationship of the vein with the clavicle is variable.

due to pacemaker malfunction (Fig. 34.12A), undersensing or oversensing (Fig. 34.12B), loss of capture (such as due to lead fracture, Figs. 34.13A to C), or chronotropic incompetence. Atrial arrhythmias can cause rapid ventricular tracking in DDD mode, if mode switching is not available. Areas of potential malfunction in the pacemaker-lead system are summarized in Figure 34.14.

COMPLICATIONS

Pneumothorax (Fig. 34.15) occurs in 1% of pacemaker implants and is more common in patients with obstructive airways disease. Small size ones (< 15–20 mm) usually resolve spontaneously. Larger ones require aspiration or chest drain insertion. Intrathoracic hematoma is a less likely complication and can be either free in the form of hemothorax or localized (Fig. 34.16). Figure 34.17 reveals a hemopneumothorax.

Pericardial effusion is usually secondary to RV lead perforation (Figs. 34.18 and 34.19). It should be suspected if the patient complains of pericarditic or pleuritic chest pain, high pacing threshold, poor sensing, and absence of injury current. The lead can usually be pulled out without complication.

Atrial fibrillation may occur on positioning the atrial lead. Nonsustained ventricular tachycardia (NSVT), and less likely sustained VT, can occur while positioning the RV lead. These can be treated medically or with direct current (DC) cardioversion, if appropriate.

Low lead impedance (< 250 Ω) immediately after implantation indicates possible damage to the insulation by the scalpel or the needle. High lead impedance (> 1,500 Ω) may indicate that the lead is not pushed deep enough into its port in the header.

Lead displacement can occur during, few days, or even weeks after implantation. It is usually suspected when pacing lead parameters are abnormal. CXR usually confirms macrodisplacement.

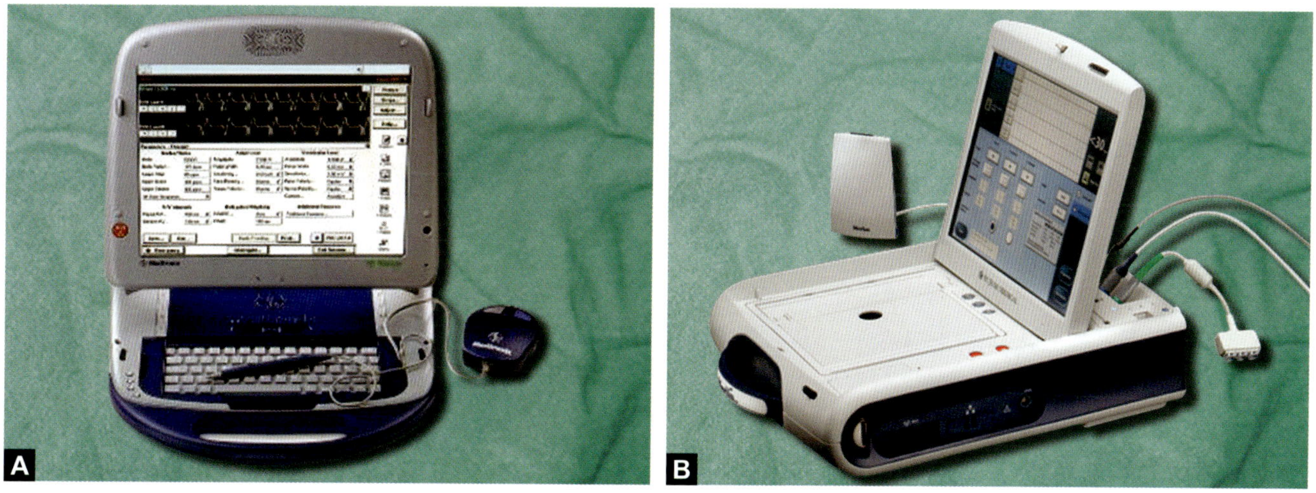

Figs. 34.7A and B: Examples of programmers that can be used at pacemaker implantation and follow-up.

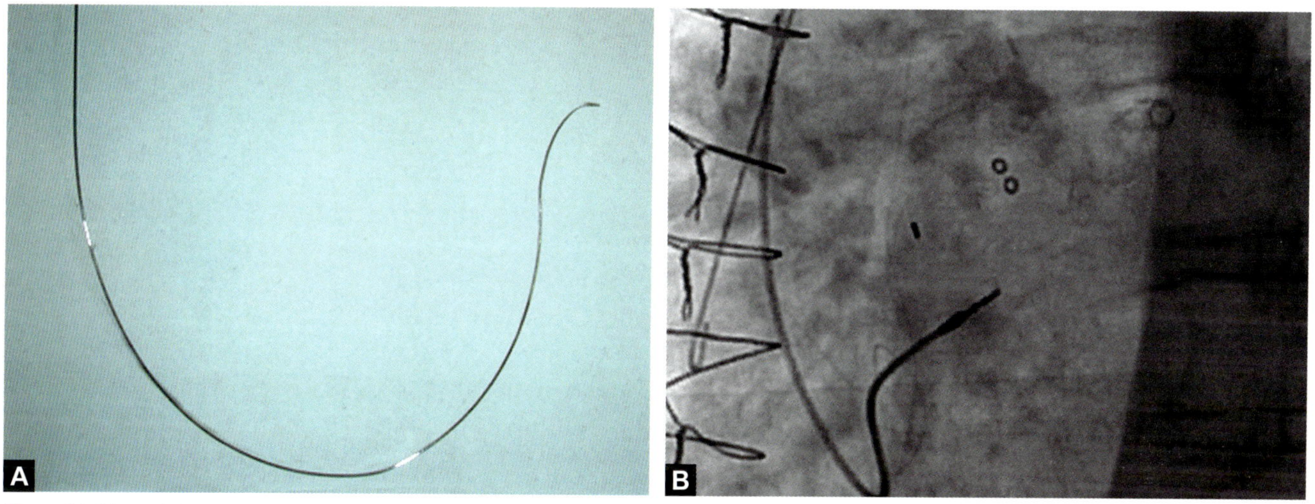

Figs. 34.8A and B: The stilette in Figure 34.8A is shaped to direct the ventricular lead to the right ventricular outflow tract (RVOT) septum. It looks like a left-sided amplatzer catheter with the last 1–2 cm directed posteriorly to target the septal part of the RVOT. The RVOT lead should point to the right side in (LAO) view (Fig. 34.8B) if the RVOT septum is targeted.

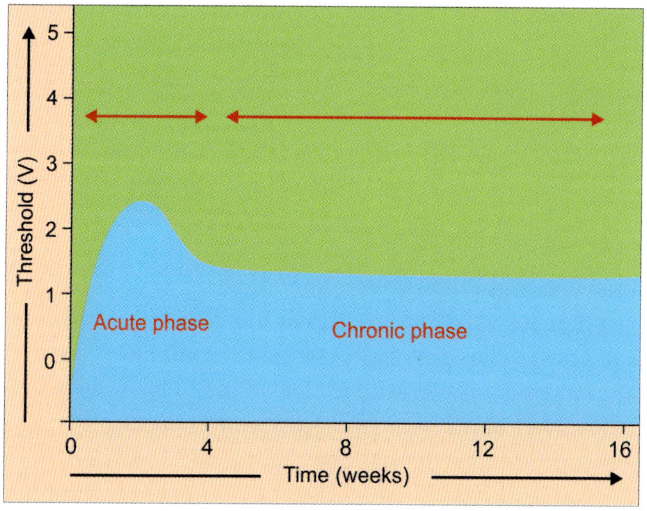

Fig. 34.9: Graph demonstrating that it takes 4–6 week time for the pacing threshold to stabilize. The X-axis represents time from implantation in weeks while the Y-axis represents the pacing threshold in volts.

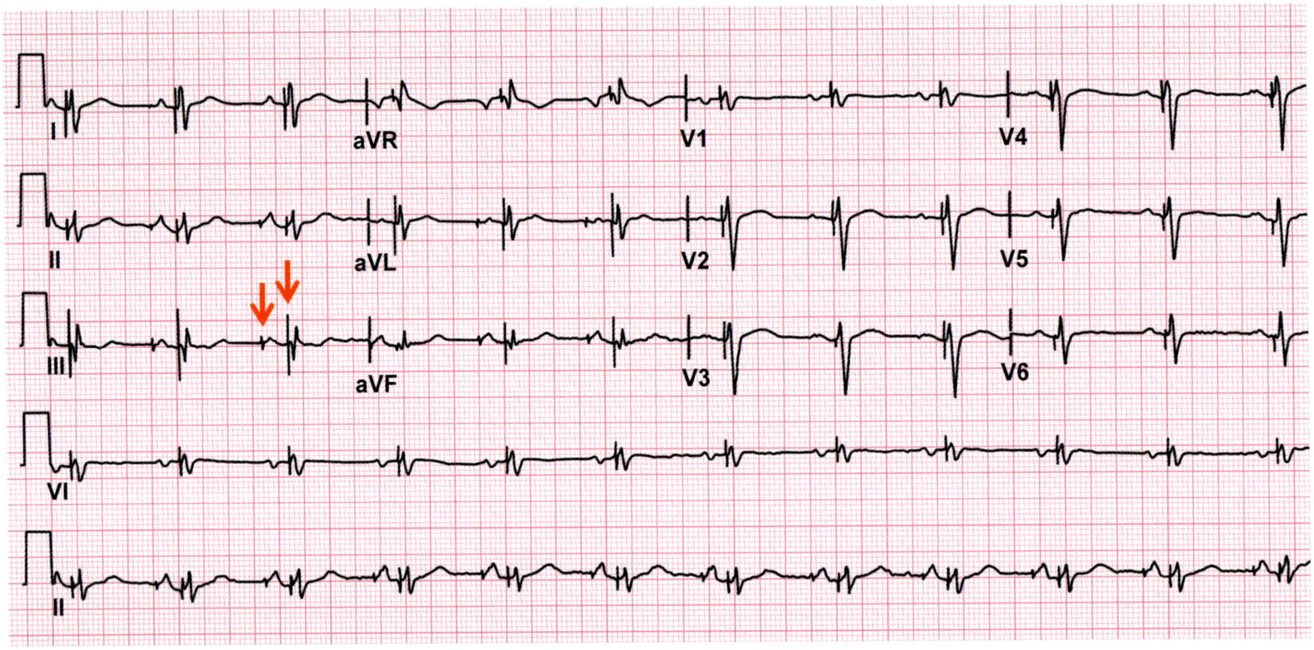

Fig. 34.10: Twelve lead ECG of a patient with dual chamber pacemaker and atrial and ventricular pacing (arrows).

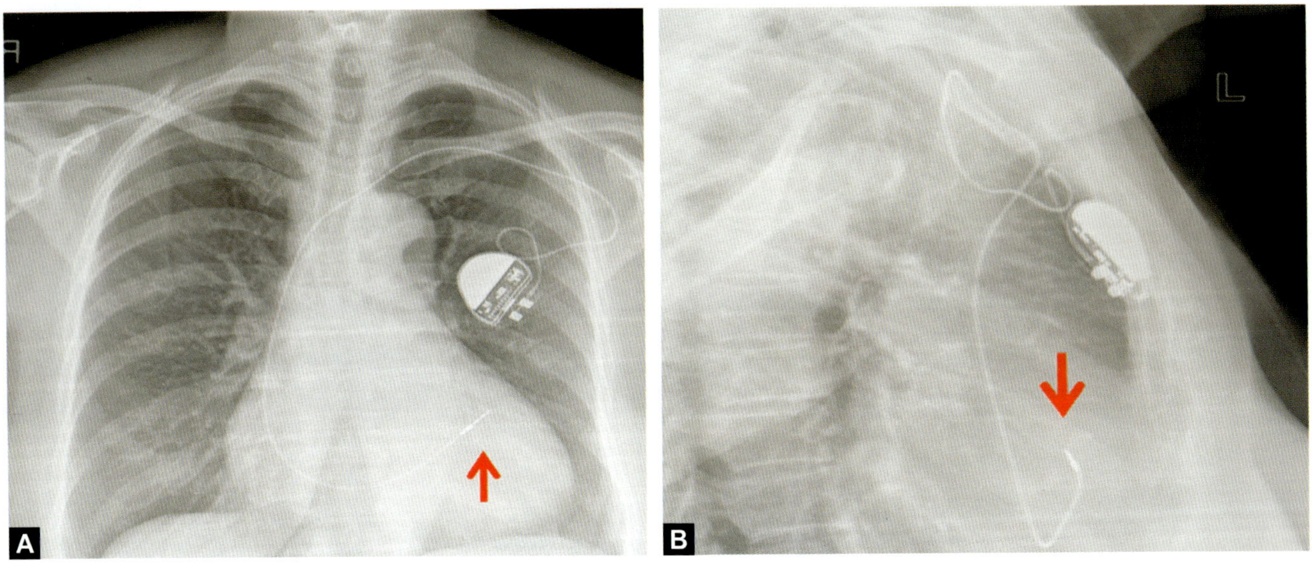

Figs. 34.11A and B: Right ventricular (RV) pacemaker lead implanted in the right ventricular outflow tract (RVOT). (A) Posteroanterior (PA) chest X-ray (CXR) showing the pacing lead actively fixed at the lower border of the RVOT. (B) Lateral CXR showing that the lead is pointing posteriorly toward the septal part of the RVOT.

Small hematoma and site bruising are common after implantation and may take 2–3 weeks to resolve. Large hematoma (Fig. 34.20) can reach a size bigger than a tennis ball and can be very painful. Large hematoma formation increases the risk of infection and may require surgical evacuation.

In addition to pacemaker pocket hematoma, other pocket complications occasionally occur (Figs. 34.21A to D). Infection (Fig. 34.21C) is an uncommon complication. It is usually caused by *Staphylococcus aureus* but *S. epidermidis* can cause late indolent infection. Antibiotics can be attempted if it is confined to the wound only. If the pocket is involved or subsequent sepsis and endocarditis occur, pacemaker explanation is mandatory.

Low lead impedance (<250 Ω), late after implantation, is usually secondary to subclavian crush or trauma, resulting

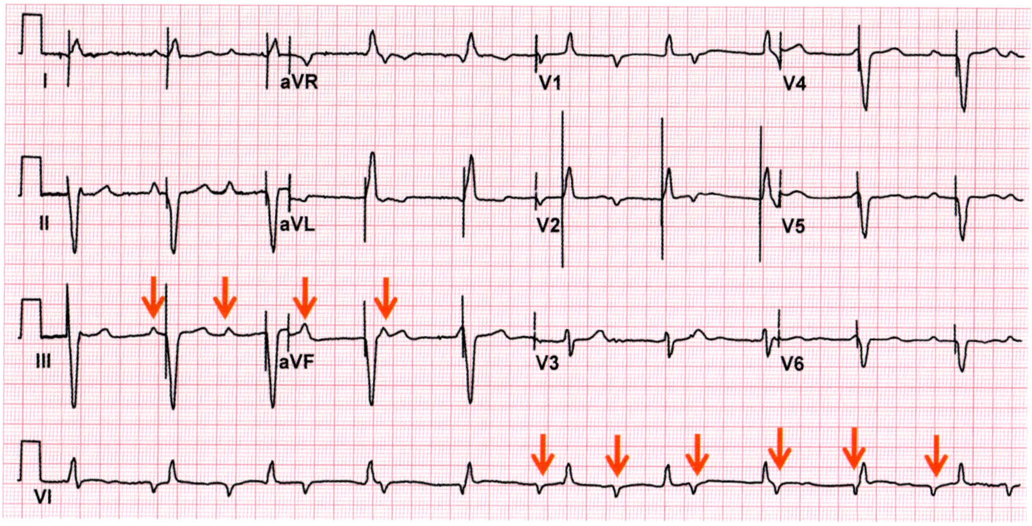

Fig. 34.12A: Pacemaker malfunction. (A) Atrial undersensing. Twelve lead EKG at 6 week follow-up visit to the pacing clinic. This patient had a dual chamber pacemaker for complete heart block and has been complaining of fatigue and shortness of breath for 3 weeks. There is evidence of atrial under sensing (arrows) with subsequent loss of atrioventricular synchrony (pacemaker syndrome). Atrial lead displacement was subsequently confirmed on CXR.

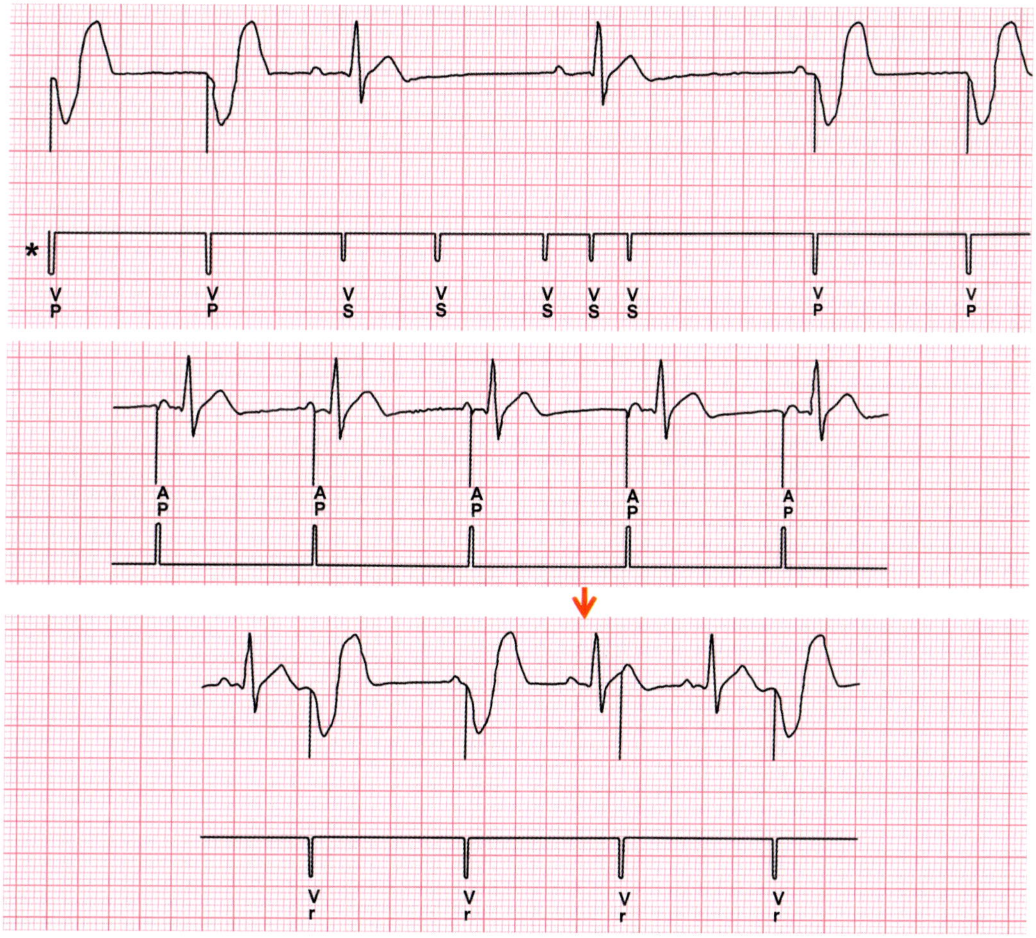

Fig. 34.12B: The top intracardiac electrogram shows evidence of ventricular oversensing as clear from the marker channel (*). The second panel demonstrates undersensing of the second and third sinus beats and, therefore, atrial pacing spikes were delivered. The bottom tracing shows undersensing of the ventricular depolarization (arrow) with subsequent delivery of ventricular pacing spike which does not capture as it falls within the refractory period.

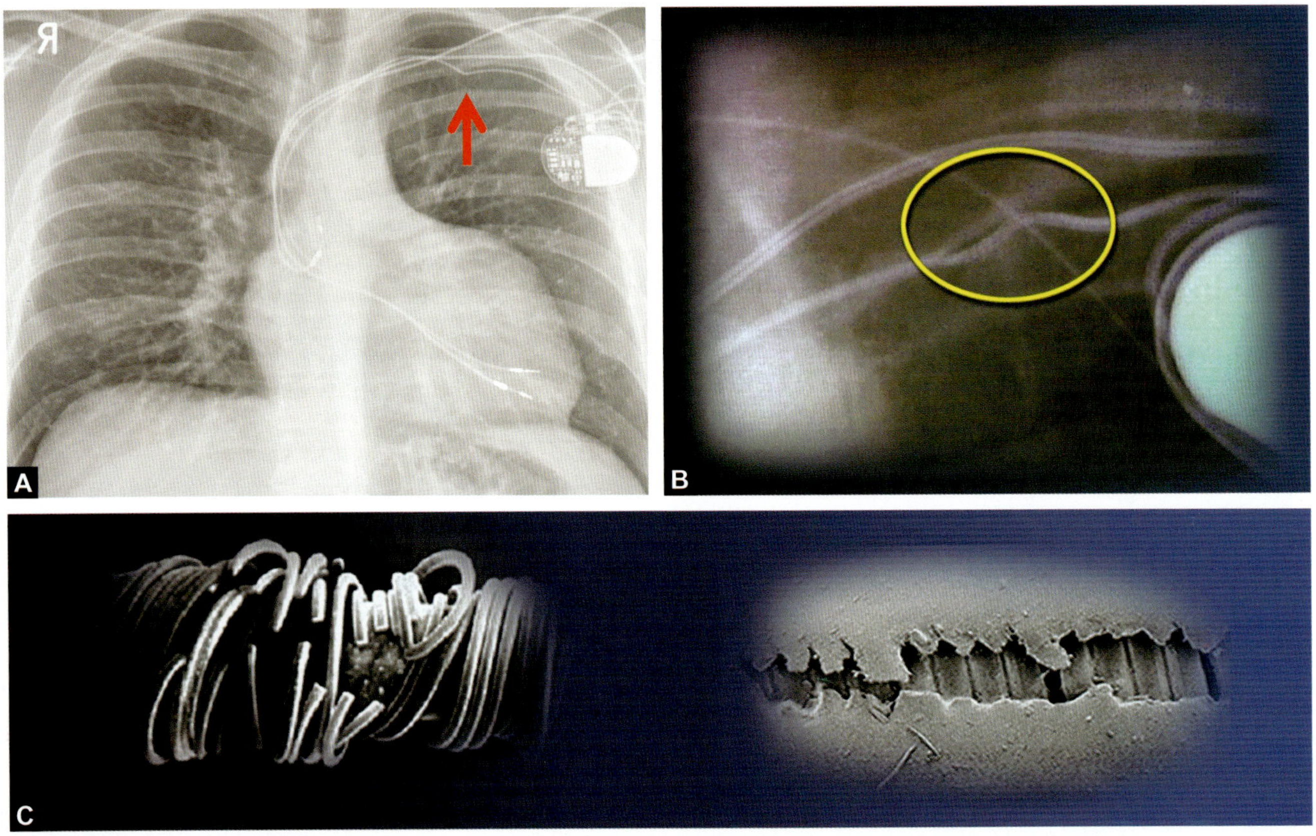

Figs. 34.13A to C: Lead fracture. (A) Typical appearance of pacing lead fracture (arrow) due to subclavian crush, a late complication. This young patient had TGA corrected with a Mustard procedure. Two ventricular leads can be seen in the LV. (B) Zoomed image of a PA chest X-ray demonstrating lead fracture. (C) Microscopic images of lead fracture. (Images 34.13B and C courtesy of Medtronic, Inc.).

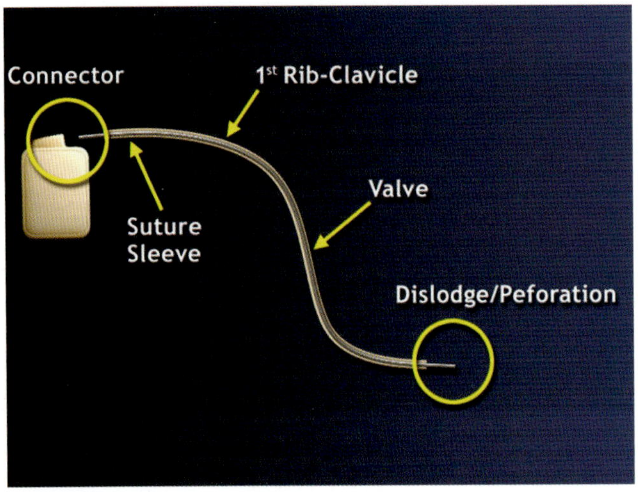

Fig. 34.14: Areas of potential malfunction in the pacemaker-lead system. (Image courtesy of Medtronic, Inc.).

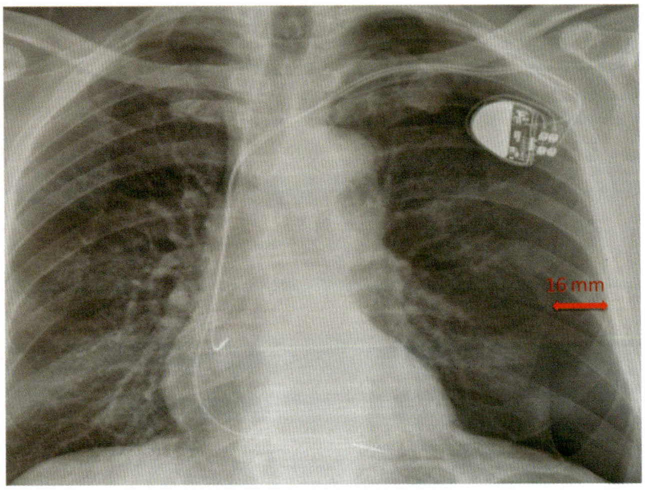

Fig. 34.15: Left-sided pneumothorax after pacemaker implantation. This is usually treated conservatively unless it exceeds 2 cm, in which case aspiration or chest drain is considered.

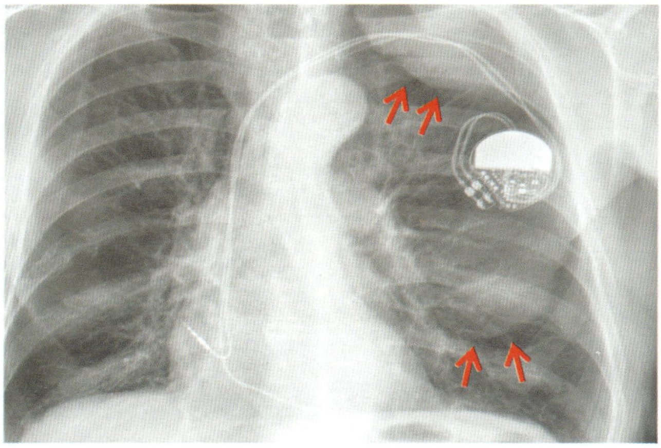

Fig. 34.16: Left-sided intrathoracic hematoma after pacemaker implantation (arrows).

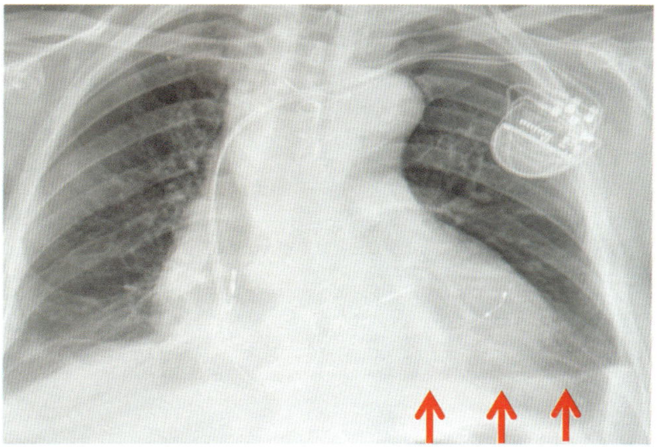

Fig. 34.17: Left-sided hemopneumothorax after biventricular pacemaker implantation (arrows).

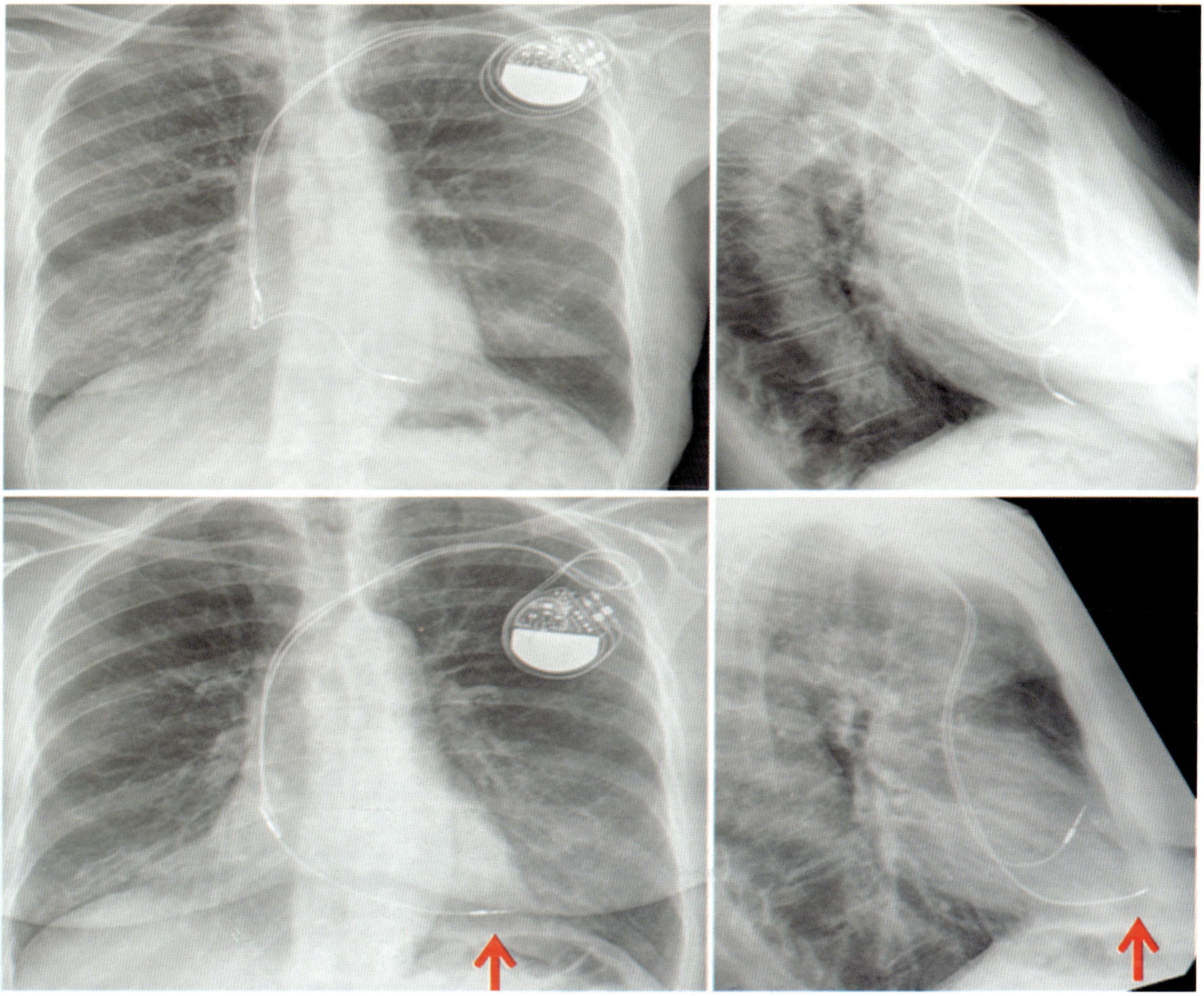

Fig. 34.18: The upper panel PA and lateral chest X-rays were taken a few hours after dual chamber pacemaker implantation. The bottom panel PA and lateral chest X-rays were taken 12 months later in the same patient after the patient developed pericarditic chest pain. The ventricular lead had clearly migrated and perforated (arrows).

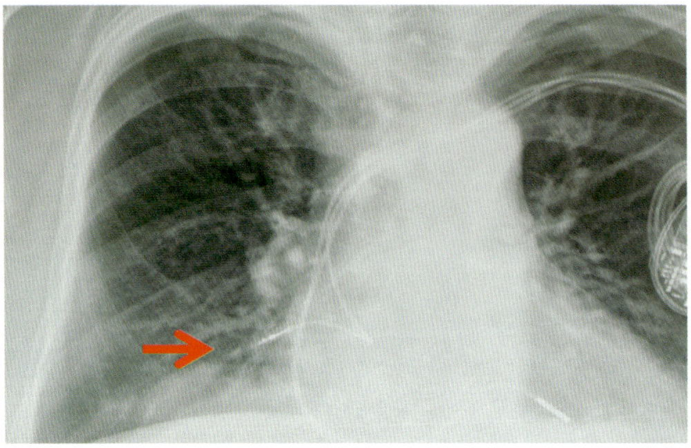

Fig. 34.19: Chest X-ray revealing atrial lead perforation. The lead went through the right atrial wall and can be seen (arrow) outside the cardiac silhouette.

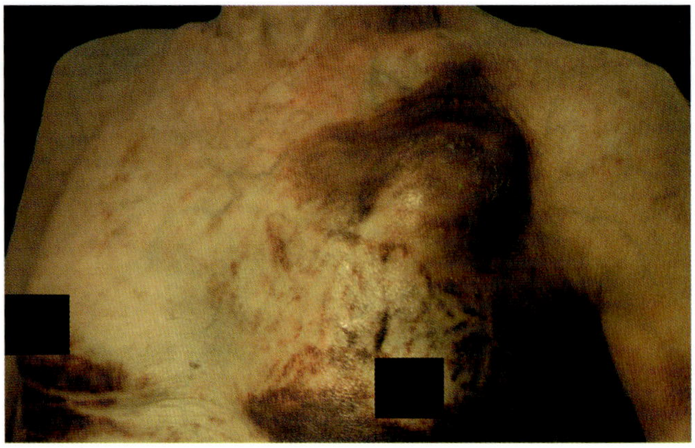

Fig. 34.20: Large hematoma after pacemaker implantation.

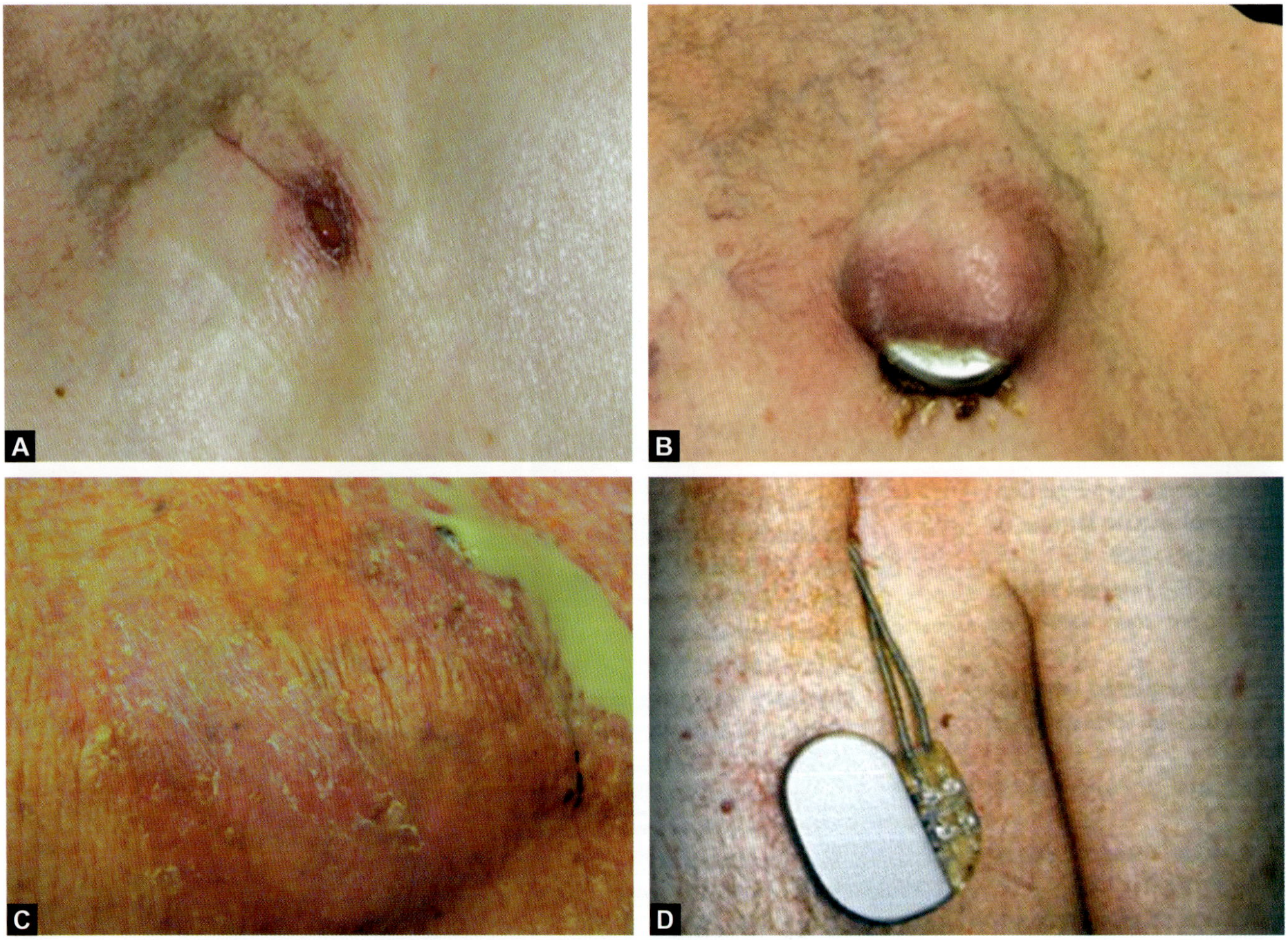

Figs. 34.21A to D: Examples of pacemaker pocket complications. Figure 34.21A shows possible erosion at the corner of the generator which can be a result of a superficial lead or a small pocket. This can clearly introduce infection or develop into a complete erosion, similar to the one in Figure 34.21B where the generator can be clearly seen. Explanation is mandatory if this to happen. Figure 34.21C shows overt infection of the pacemaker pocket with evidence of puss discharge. This can only be treated by explanation. Figure 34.21D shows an extreme example of pacemaker pocket complication in which the pacemaker is no longer contained within the pacemaker pocket. (Image 34.21D courtesy of Dr Irakli Giorgberidze).

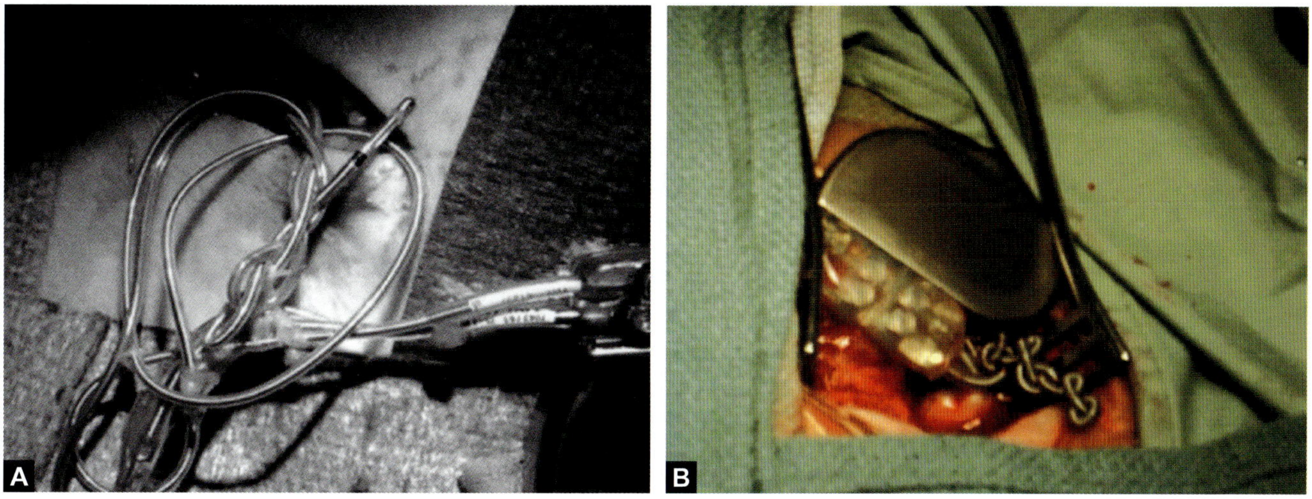

Figs. 34.22A and B: Twiddler's syndrome. Repeated rotation of pacemaker in its subcutaneous pocket leads to pacemaker lead twisting and displacement. This usually happens early after implantation, especially if the pacemaker was placed in the fatty layer rather than the standard pre pectoral position behind the fascia. (Figure 34.22B courtesy of Medtronic, Inc.).

in lead insulation damage. High lead impedance late after implantation is usually related to conductor fracture and can manifest as loss of capture. It is usually confirmed on CXR and can also be a result of the subclavian crush.

Twiddler's syndrome (Figs. 34.22A and B) can result in lead(s) displacement and is usually due to the rotational movements by the patient that cause the generator to flip over and over within the pacemaker pocket.

Pacemaker mediated tachycardia (PMT) can result when a reentrant circuit that involves the pacemaker leads and pacemaker itself occurs (Figs. 34.23A to C). PMT is treated with use of post ventricular atrial refractory period (PVARP).

CARDIAC RESYNCHRONIZATION THERAPY

Cardiac resynchronization therapy may correct AV, interventricular, and intraventricular conduction delays, thereby improving left ventricular contractility. There are two main approaches to achieve LV pacing: the transvenous approach and the surgical approach. The transvenous approach is the preferred approach, with the surgical approach used only when the transvenous approach fails.

The transvenous approach is performed by cannulating the coronary sinus (CS) with a specially designed catheter (Figs. 34.24A to F). These exist in many shapes in order to overcome the surprisingly variable CS anatomy in individual patients. Once the CS is cannulated, a standard balloon occlusion catheter is inserted and a retrograde venography (Fig. 34.24A) is performed using contrast material to enable definition of the cardiac venous anatomy. The LV lead is then positioned (Fig. 34.24B) in the target vein (ideally the posterior, posterolateral, or anterolateral veins) providing satisfactory pacing parameters and stability can be achieved. Figure 34.24C schematically illustrates the position of the pacemaker leads in a patient treated with CRT.

The success rate of the transvenous approach using the currently available tools and techniques is 90–95%. The most common reasons for unsuccessful implants are: inability to access the CS ostium and acute dislodgment. In addition, diaphragmatic twitching secondary to phrenic nerve stimulation can prevent lead placement. In many cases, a compromise between ideal lead position and best attainable stability/pacing parameters is needed. It is essential to document the lead position after the implantation with PA and lateral CXR.

Figures 34.25A to H demonstrates the appearance of the 12 lead ECG with RV lead pacing, LV lead pacing, and biventricular pacing.

SPECIAL CASES

Pacemaker implanters can encounter expected or unexpected challenges. An example of this can be a left-sided superior vena cava (Fig. 34.26), which is the most common congenital venous anomaly in the chest. Although it is prevalent only in 0.3–0.5% of the general population,

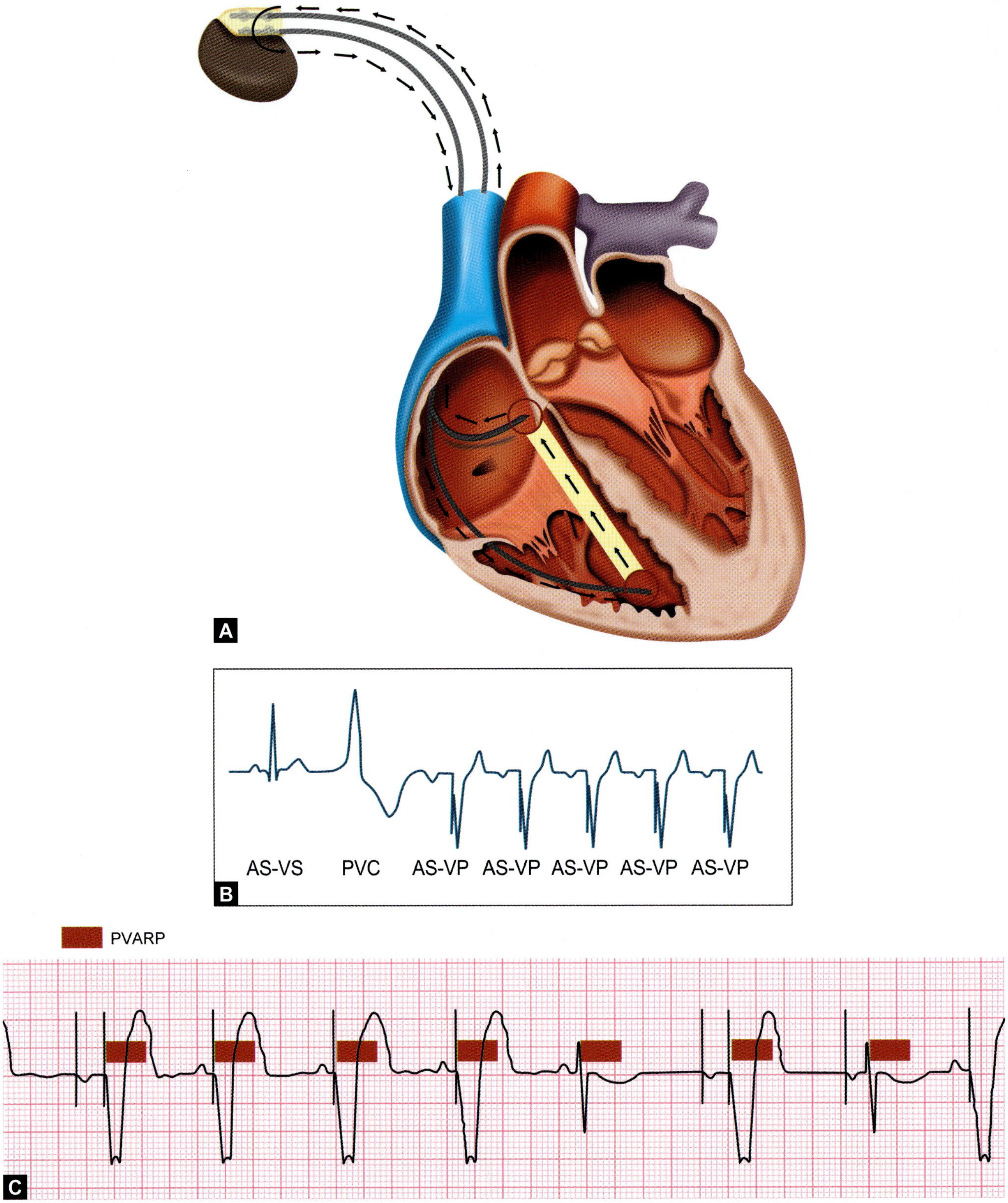

Figs. 34.23A to C: Pacemaker mediated tachycardia (PMT). (A) The effective reentrant circuit involving the pacemaker leads and device itself that occurs in a patient with PMT. (B) PMT triggered by a PVC. (C) The use of postventricular atrial refractory period (PVARP) to prevent PMT. (Images 34.23B and C courtesy of St. Jude Medical). (AS: Atrial sensing; PVC: Premature ventricular contraction; VP: Ventricular pacing; VS: Ventricular sensing).

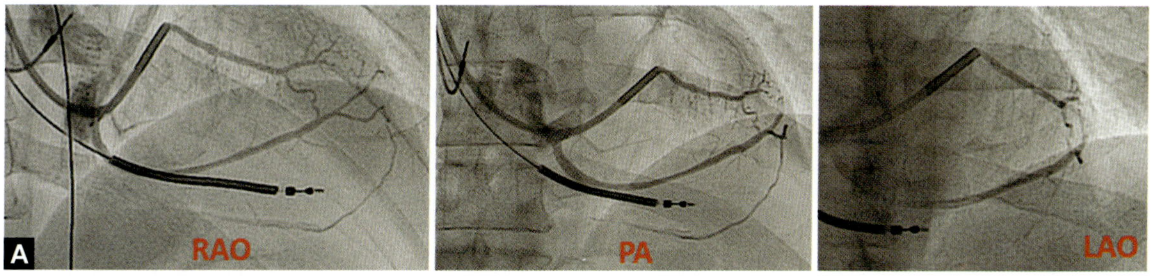

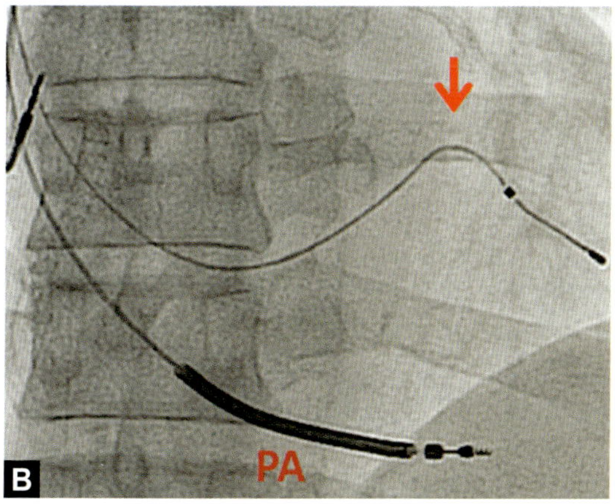

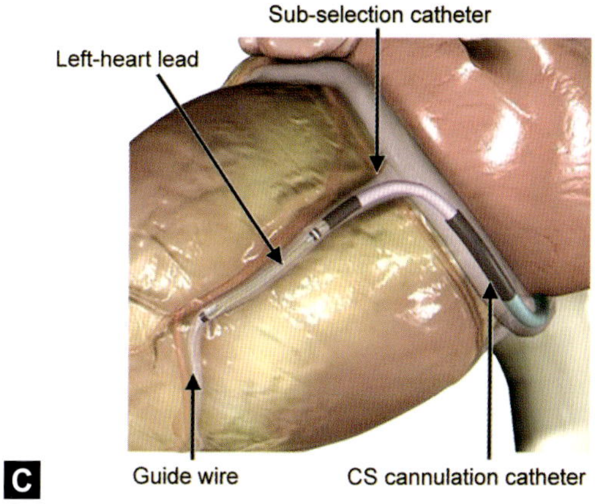

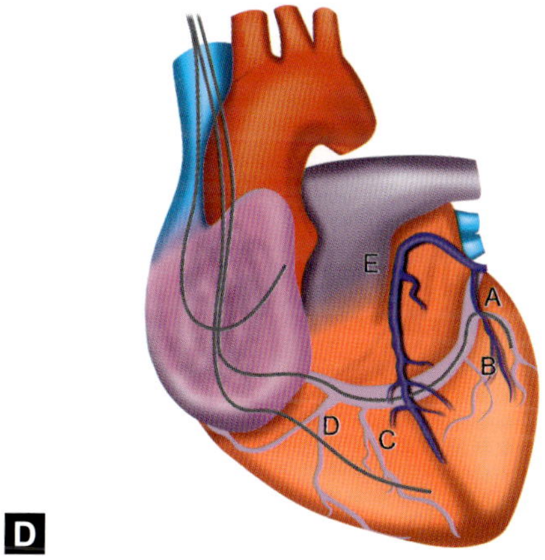

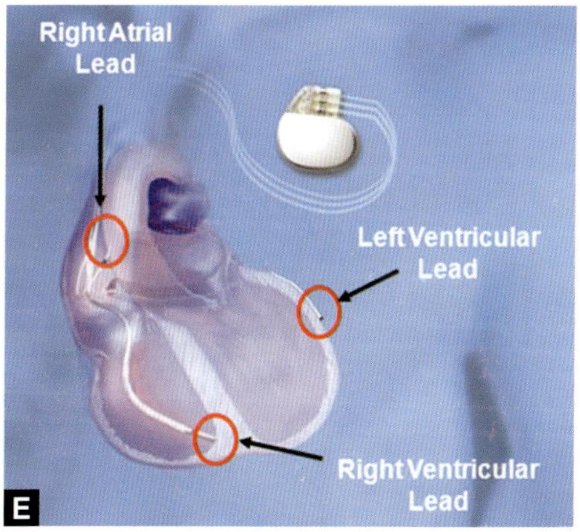

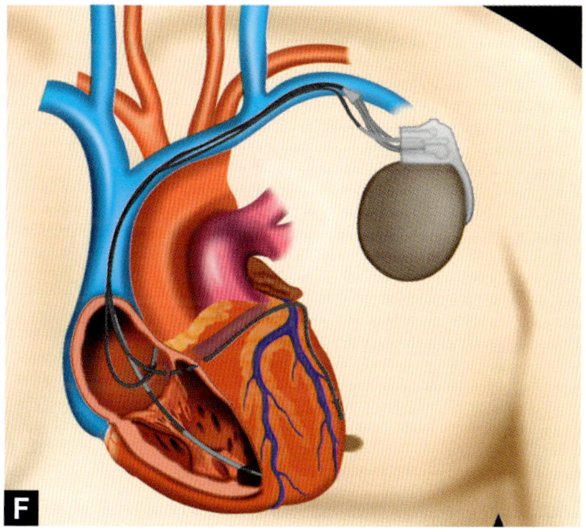

Figs. 34.24A to D: Lead placement and positions in patients treated with cardiac resynchronization therapy (CRT). (A) Retrograde venography is performed using contrast material to enable definition of the cardiac venous anatomy in order to facilitate placement of the left ventricular lead in patients undergoing cardiac resynchronization therapy. Venography should be performed in different views to decide on the optimal lead position. In this example, the catheter has subselected a posterolateral vein; (B) PA chest X-ray demonstrating location of the left ventricular lead (arrow). The pacing/ICD lead in the right ventricle is clearly visible as well. (C) Placement of the left ventricular lead. (D) Coronary vein options for left ventricle lead placement. Preferred options are [A] lateral [marginal] cardiac vein, [B] posterolateral cardiac vein or [C] posterior cardiac vein. Suboptimal lead locations are [D] the middle cardiac vein or [E] the great cardiac vein. (E and F) Schematic illustrations of the position of the pacemaker leads in a patient treated with CRT. (Images 34.24C, D and F courtesy of Medtronic, Inc.; Image 34.24E courtesy of Boston Scientific, Inc.).

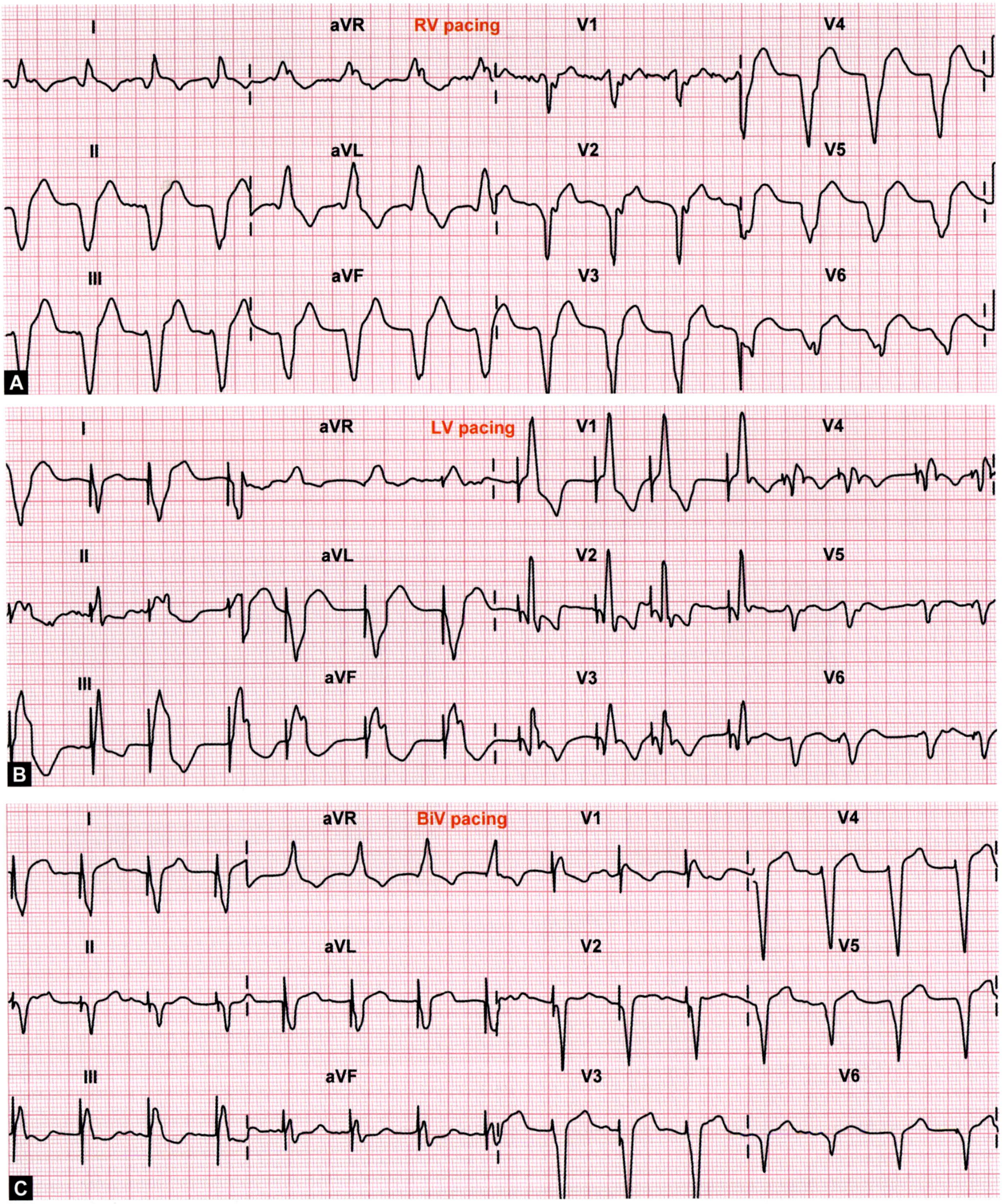

Figs. 34.25A to C: Typical appearance of the twelve lead EKG in the same patient with different pacing configurations. (A) Right ventricular lead pacing, with negative complexes across the precordium and positive deflection in aVL (usually LBBB pattern). (B) Left ventricular pacing, with strongly positive deflection in V1 and negative deflection in aVL (LV pacing with RBBB pattern). (C) Biventricular pacing with narrower QRS complex and negative QRS deflections in leads I and aVL.

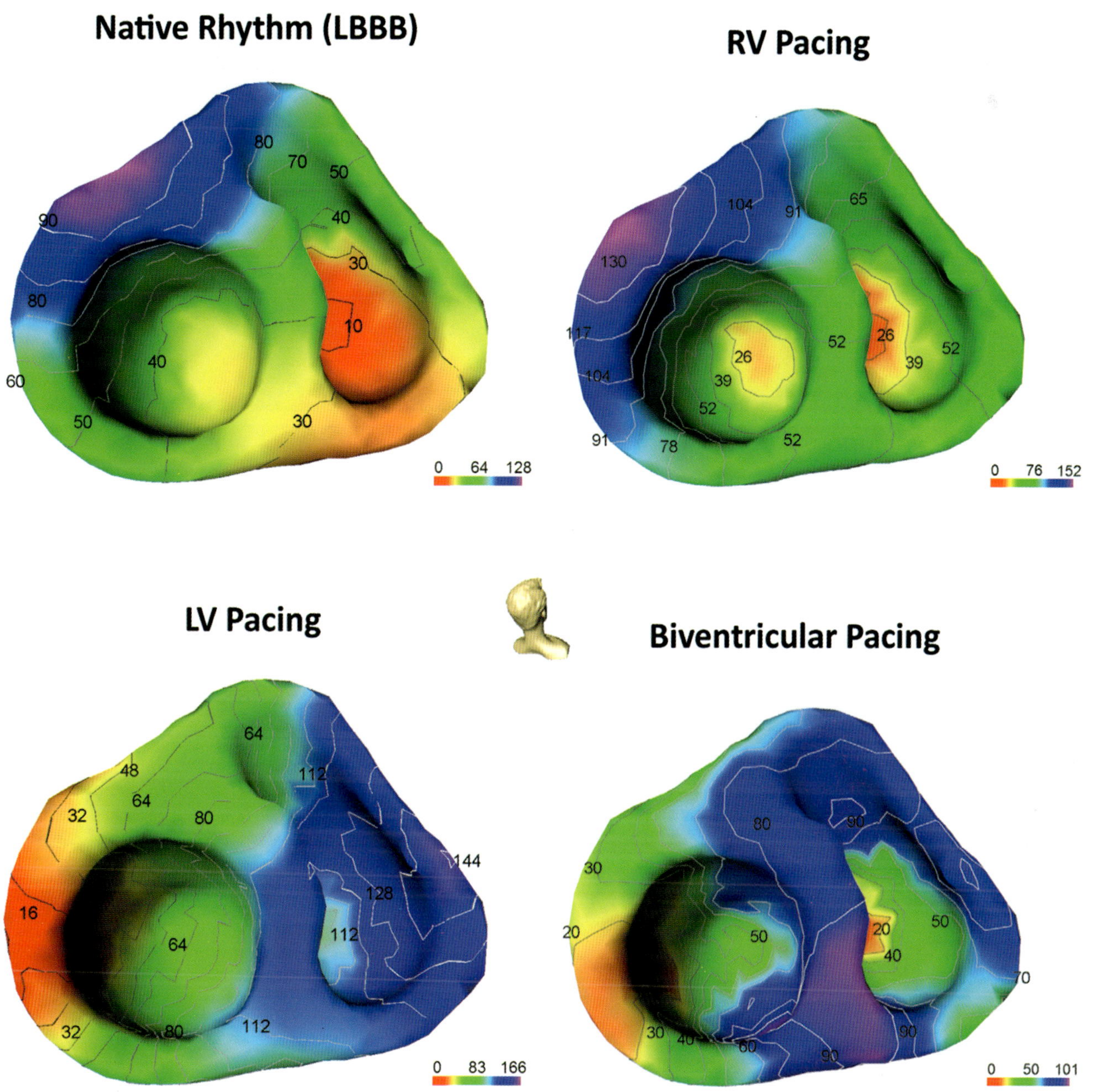

D

Fig. 34.25D: Activation time maps (isochrones given in milliseconds after first onset of depolarization) showing the left and right ventricles of a patient with baseline left bundle branch block who underwent CRT with native depolarization and with different pacing configurations. Red color indicates early electrical activation, blue and purple colors indicate late and very late activation. Note the different scaling of the color maps and the shorter total depolarization time with biventricular pacing. (Image from Seger M, Pfeifer B, Berger T. Noninvasive imaging of cardiac electrophysiology (NICE). In: Oraii S (Ed). Electrophysiology—From Plants to Heart. InTech, 2012).

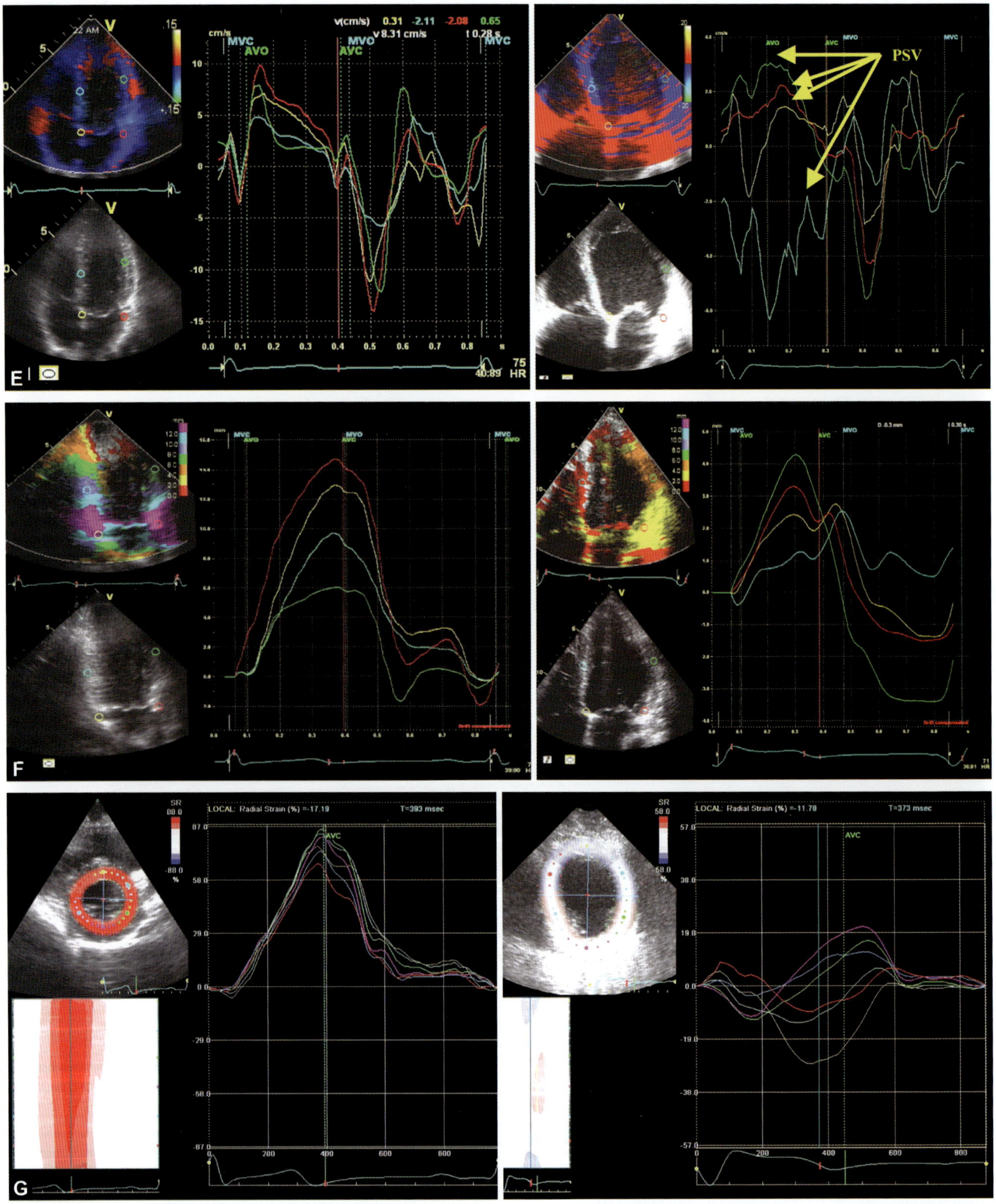

Figs. 34.25E to G: Echocardiographic assessment of ventricular dyssynchrony. (E) Apical four-chamber tissue velocity imaging images of a normal heart (left panel) and a dyssynchronous heart (right panel). (F) Apical four-chamber tissue tracking curves of a normal (left panel) and dyssynchronous heart (right panel). (G) Speckle tracking echocardiography images of radial strain in the normal (left panel) and dyssynchronous (right panel) heart.

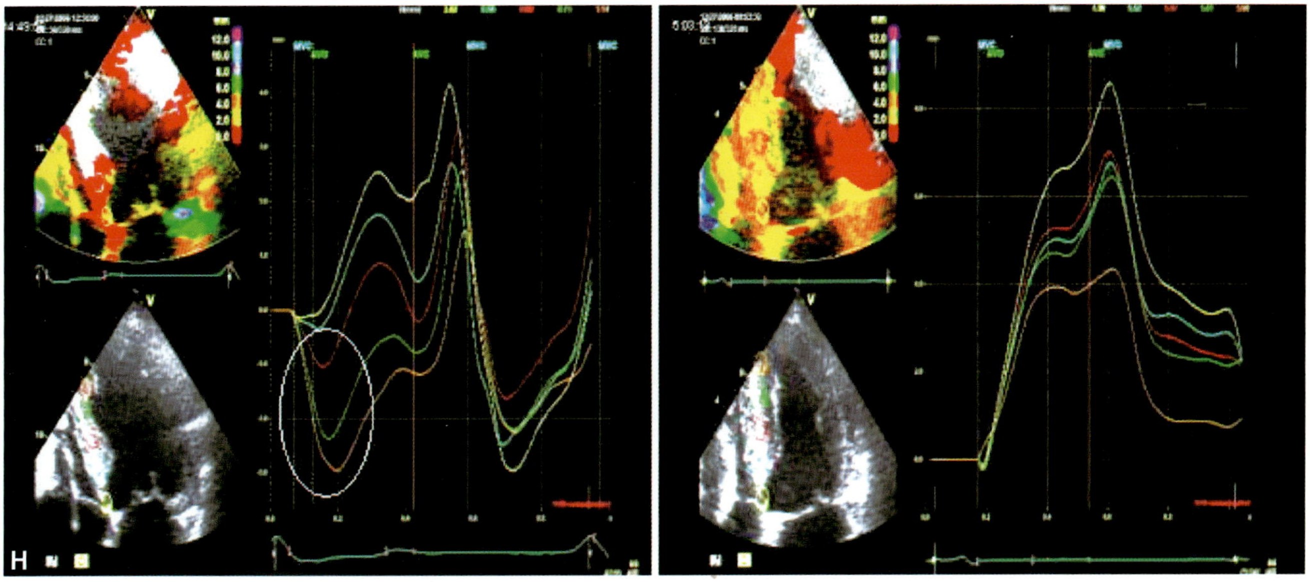

Fig. 34.25H: Intramural dyssynchrony within the septum of a chronically RV-pace patient before (left panel, paradoxical motion circled) and after (right panel) upgrade to CRT. (Images 34.25E to H from Burns KV, Gage RM, Bank AJ. Right ventricular pacing and mechanical dyssynchrony. In: Oraii S (Ed). Electrophysiology—From Plants to Heart. InTech; 2012).

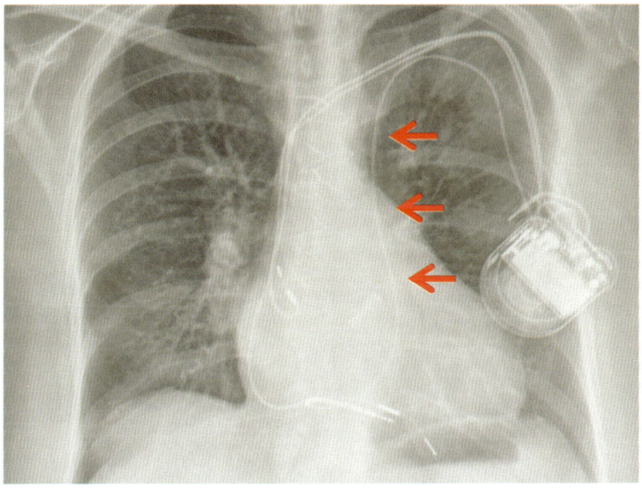

Fig. 34.26: Left-sided superior vena cava (SVC). A newly placed right ventricle (RV) lead is seen in a left-sided SVC (arrows), subsequently entering the RV via the coronary sinus. Older right atrium and RV leads are seen passing through a right-sided SVC, which the patient obviously also has.

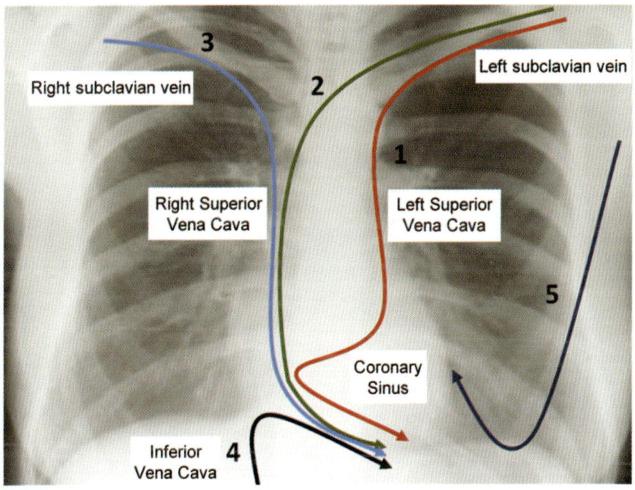

Fig. 34.27: Schematic representation of the possible available options to implant pacing leads in patients with persistent left-sides superior vena cava. (1) Lead is passed from the left subclavian vein through the left superior vena cava (SVC)-coronary sinus-tricuspid valve then right ventricle apex. (2) Lead is passed from the left subclavian vein across to the right SVC through the bridging venous connection between left and right SVCs (one-third of patients with L-SVC have bridging connection). (3) Lead passed from the right subclavian vein through the right SVC (90% of L-CVC patients have SVC duplication). (4) trans- inferior vena cava lead implant. (5) Epicardially implanted lead.

it may be present in 4.3–11% of patients with congenital heart disease. Figure 34.27 shows the available options to pace such patients. Other challenges can be in the form of previous cardiac operations, such as patients who had Mustard or Senning procedures to treat transposition of the great arteries (TGA) (Figs. 34.28A to C).

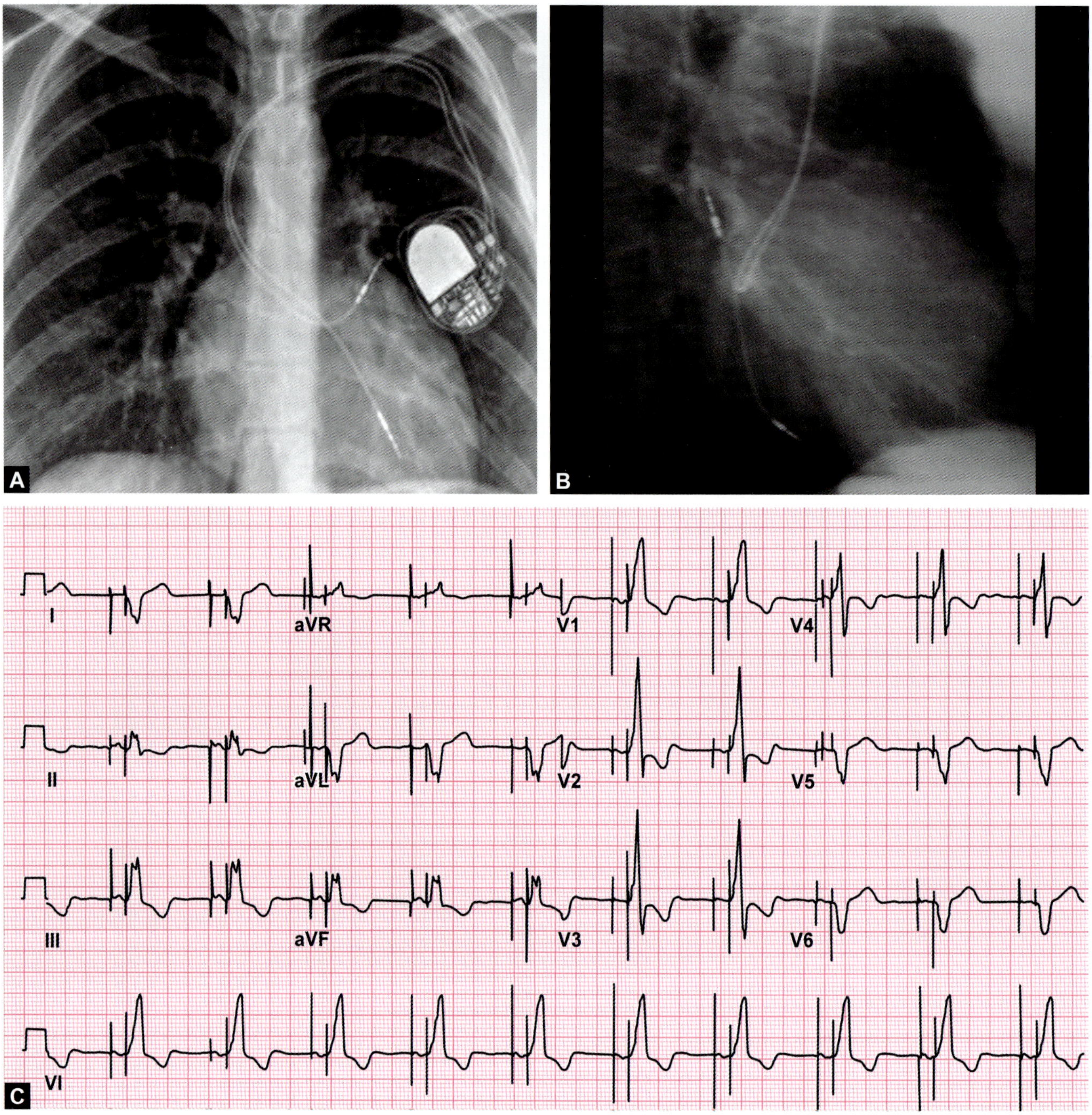

Figs. 34.28A to C: Dual chamber pacing in a patient with a prior Mustard procedure. (A) After a Mustard or Senning procedure, if dual chamber pacing is required, the atrial lead may be passed behind the baffle into the left atrium and actively fixed to the roof of the left atrium. The ventricular lead follows the same route into the left atrium and then advanced across the mitral valve into the left ventricle where it is actively fixed. (B) The lateral chest X-ray confirms the posterior position of both leads in the left atrium and left ventricle. (C) The ECG of the same patient shows right bundle branch block pattern paced ventricular complexes.

REFERENCES

Albouaini K, Alkarmi A, Mudawi T, et al. Selective site right ventricular pacing. Heart. 2009;95(24):2030-9.

Albouaini K, Alkarmi A, Wright DJ. Cardiac resynchronisation therapy: what a hospital practitioner needs to know? Postgrad Med J. 2010;86(1011):12-7.

Burkhardt JD, Wilkoff BL. Interventional electrophysiology and cardiac resynchronization therapy: delivering electrical therapies for heart failure. Circulation. 2007;-115(16):2208-20.

Epstein AE, DiMarco JP, Ellenbogen KA, et al. ACC/AHA/HRS 2008 guidelines for device-based therapy of cardiac rhythm abnormalities: a report of the American College of Cardiology/ American Heart Association Task Force on practice guidelines (Writing committee to revise the ACC/AHA/NASPE 2002 guideline update for implantation of cardiac pacemakers and antiarrhythmia devices): developed in collaboration with the American Association for Thoracic Surgery and Society of Thoracic Surgeons. Circulation. 2008;117:e350.

Tracy CM, Epstein AE, Darbar D, et al. 2012 ACCF/AHA/HRS focused update of the 2008 guidelines for device-based therapy of cardiac rhythm abnormalities: a report of the American College of Cardiology Foundation/American Heart Association Task Force on Practice Guidelines and the Heart Rhythm Society. [corrected]. Circulation. 2012;126:1784.

CHAPTER

Implantable Cardioverter Defibrillators

35

Kevin C Floyd, Lawrence S Rosenthal

INTRODUCTION

Cardiac disease continues to be a leading cause of death worldwide. Approximately 50% of all cardiac deaths are thought to be sudden, and despite improvements in cardiovascular care, this proportion remains constant. Sudden cardiac death (SCD) is defined as an unexpected death due to heart problems, occurring within 1 hour from the start of any cardiac-related symptoms. More commonly, SCD refers to cardiac arrest resulting from life-threatening arrhythmias. Ventricular fibrillation (VF) or hemodynamically unstable ventricular tachycardia (VT) accounts for the majority of patients who experience SCD, and with bradyarrhythmias or asystole accounting for the rest.

If administered rapidly, in patients with VF or unstable VT cardiac defibrillation can prevent death. Despite better availability of automatic external defibrillators, the vast majority of individuals at risk for SCD who suffer from ventricular arrhythmias in the community do not get this treatment in a timely manner and die prior to arrival to a hospital. Even in communities with well-established emergency medical responses and services, survival to hospital discharge is only 5–7%. Thus, a goal of improving survival due to SCD has been to identify high-risk populations and institute therapies to prevent SCD. Implantable cardioverter defibrillators (ICDs) prevent SCD effectively by detecting and terminating fatal arrhythmias within seconds.

EVOLUTION OF THE ICD

The first ICD was implanted in 1980. The first-generation ICDs were large, implanted in the abdomen, and required general anesthesia with a surgical thoracotomy for placement of epicardial leads and patches. By the early 1990s, implantation of ICDs was much facilitated by the introduction of transvenous leads (Fig. 35.1) and the dramatic reduction of ICD size (Figs. 35.2A and B). These allowed for pectoral implantation (Figs. 35.3A and B) without the need for surgical thoracotomy.

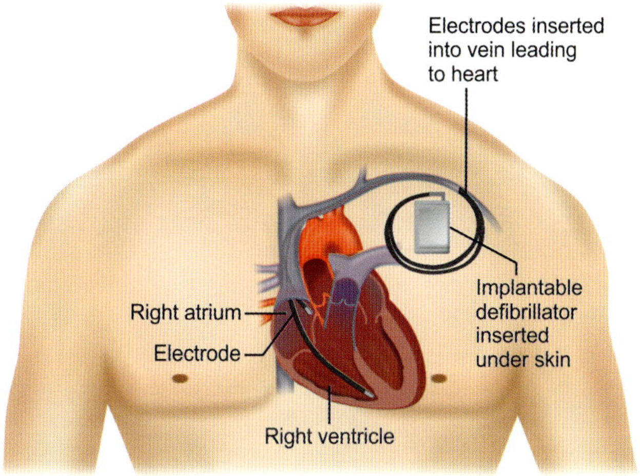

Fig. 35.1: Schematic example of a transvenous implantable cardioverter defibrillator.

In the mid-1990s, the devices became ever smaller with more advanced programmable features. These improvements in form and function prompted several large clinical trials to evaluate the efficacy of such devices as compared with conventional medical therapy in reducing SCD in high-risk patient populations. Data from these studies have shaped our clinical practice in patients with left ventricular (LV) dysfunction.

Current transvenous pacemakers consist of a pulse generator, a pacing/sensing electrode, and a defibrillation electrode. One or more coils are used to deliver the defibrillation shock. The pulse generator contains the battery and sensing, timing and output circuits. As some cases of SCD are believed to be due to bradyarrhythmias, currently

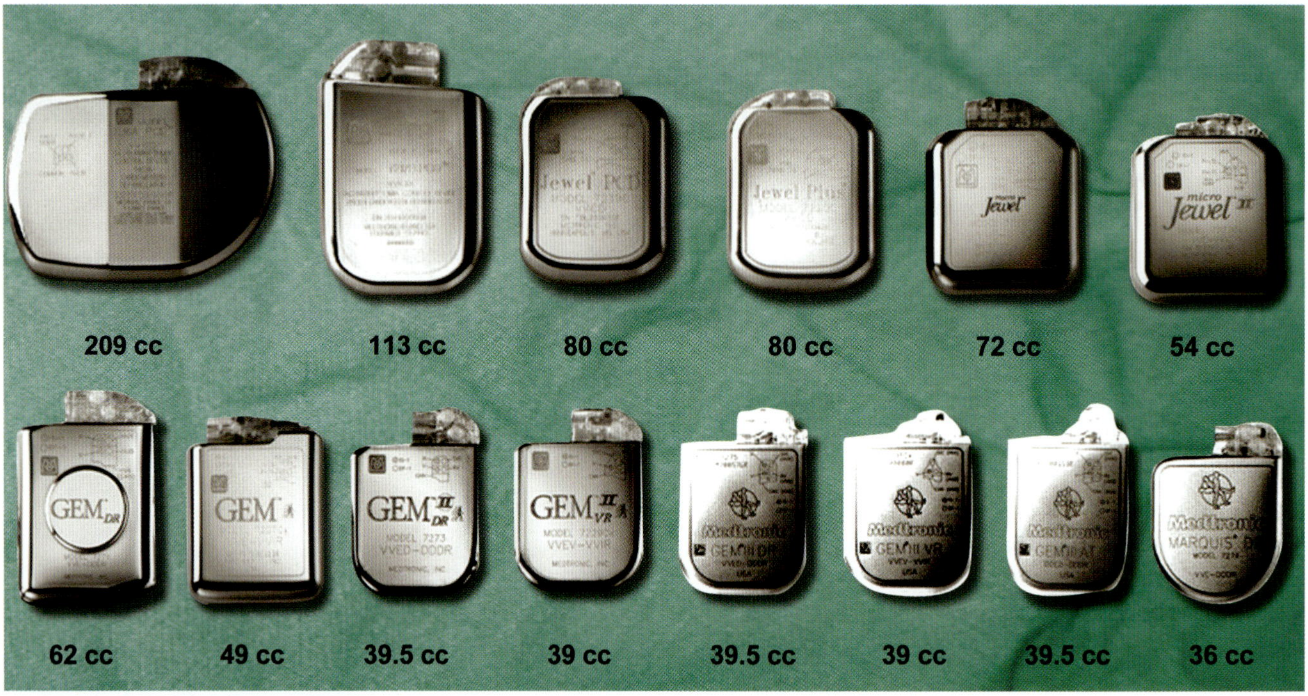

Fig. 35.2A: Examples of implantable cardioverter defibrillators produced over the last several decades, showing the miniaturization of the device over time.

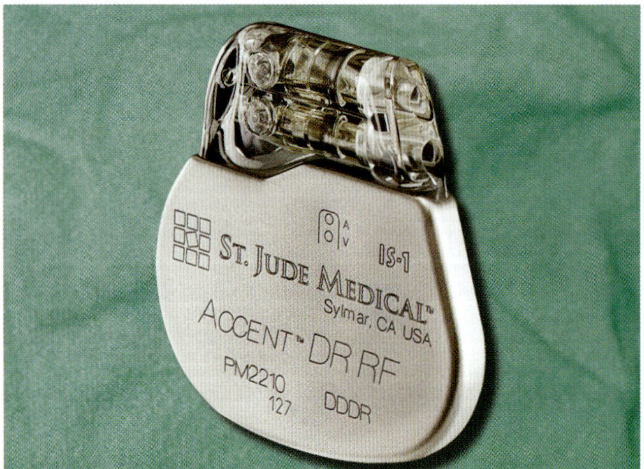

Fig. 35.2B: An example of a current generation implantable cardioverter defibrillator.

manufactured ICDs also have pacing capabilities. With the proven benefits of cardiac resynchronization therapy (CRT) in an overlapping patient population with those at risk for or who have experienced SCD, many ICDs now additionally include CRT capability, and include a lead for ventricular pacing.

A further advance in ICD therapy is the totally subcutaneous ICD (Fig. 35.4). Because the shocking electrode is subcutaneous, rather than intracardiac, the energy required for successful defibrillation is higher than with transvenous ICDs. The device though has been shown to reliably detect and terminated ventricular arrhythmias, and is approved for use by both European and US regulatory agencies.

ICD FOR PRIMARY AND SECONDARY PREVENTION

Secondary prevention refers to the use of an ICD in a patient who has already suffered sustained VT or SCD, and are by definition at risk for further episodes. ICD implantation has been shown in multiple randomized trials to improve survival in such patients, regardless of the underlying structural heart disease. ICD implantation is superior to treatment with antiarrhythmic agents such as amiodarone. ICD implantation for secondary prevention is utilized in patients with ischemic cardiomyopathy, nonischemic cardiomyopathy, hypertrophic cardiomyopathy (HCM), arrhythmogenic right ventricular dysplasia/

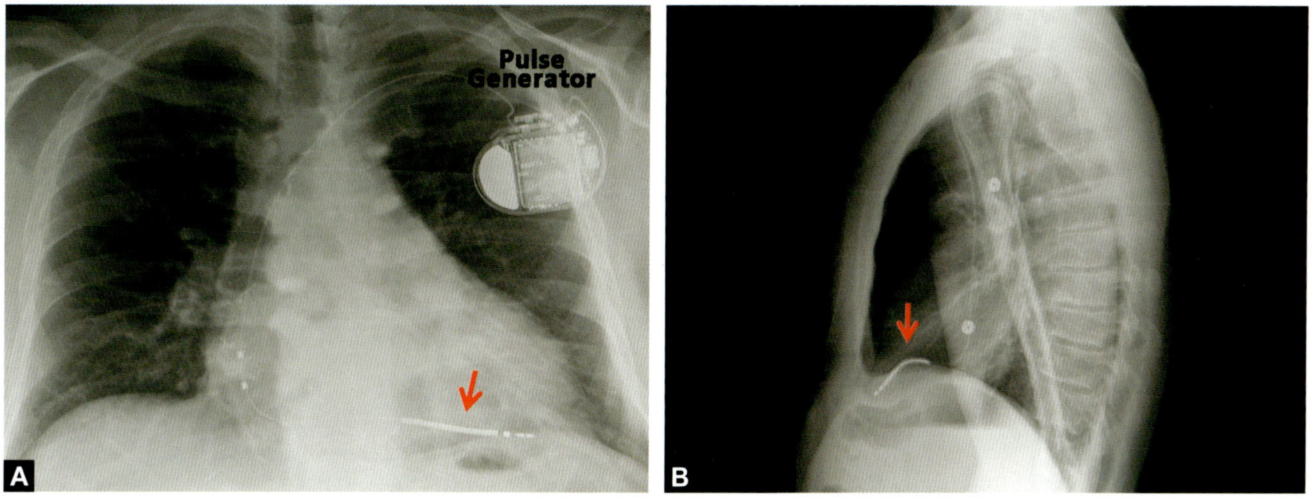

Figs. 35.3A and B: (A) Posteroanterior; and (B) lateral chest X-rays demonstrating the implantable cardioverter defibrillator pulse generator in the pectoral region of the chest and the defibrillation coil (arrows) in the right ventricle.

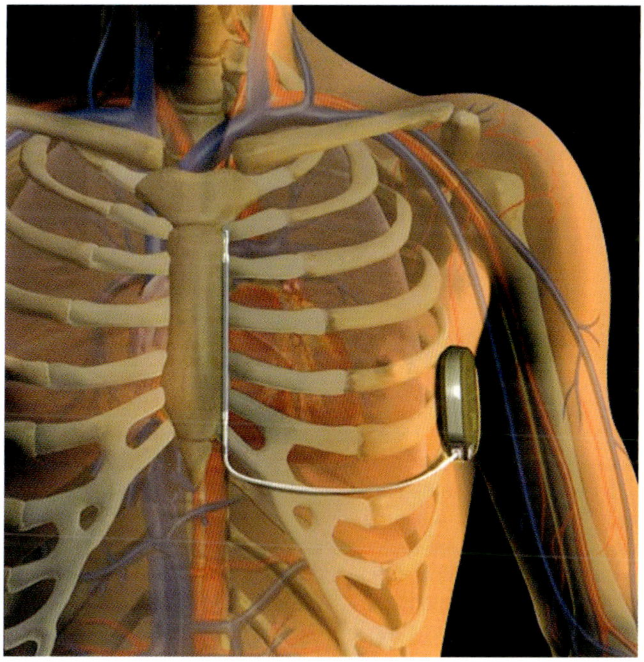

Fig. 35.4: Schematic illustration of the subcutaneous implantable cardioverter defibrillator.

cardiomyopathy (ARVD/C) genetic arrhythmic syndromes (e.g. long QT syndrome), Brugada syndrome, and noncompaction. Recommendations for ICD implantation for secondary prevention have evolved over time, and there are some nuances in recommendations between US and European guidelines. In general, ICD implantation is recommended in those with SCD or sustained VT, unless a clearly reversible cause is identified.

Primary prevention refers to implantation of an ICD in patients who have not suffered SCD or sustained VT but are deemed at high risk of such events. Recommendations on who should receive and who should be considered for primary prevention ICD implantation continue to evolve. In general, such patients include those who have reasonable expectation of meaningful survival for more than 1 year and:

- Left ventricular ejection fraction (LVEF) < 30–35% due to prior myocardial infarction (MI) who are at least 40 days post-MI
- LVEF < 30–35% with nonischemic cardiomyopathy
- LVEF < 40%, nonsustained VT due to prior MI, and inducible VT or sustained VT at electrophysiological study
- HCM or ARVD/C with high risk factors for SCD
- Long-QT syndrome, Brugada syndrome or nonischemic cardiomyopathy and unexplained syncope (a gray area between primary and secondary prevention)
- Chagas disease.

ICD FUNCTION

Current ICDs have both the capability for overdriving pacing of VTs and for defibrillation. With most devices, a heart rate range (or V-V interval) is set in which antitachycardia pacing (ATP) (Figs. 35.5A and B) is employed for ventricular rhythms, and a higher heart rate threshold above which defibrillation (Figs. 35.6 to 35.9) is instead

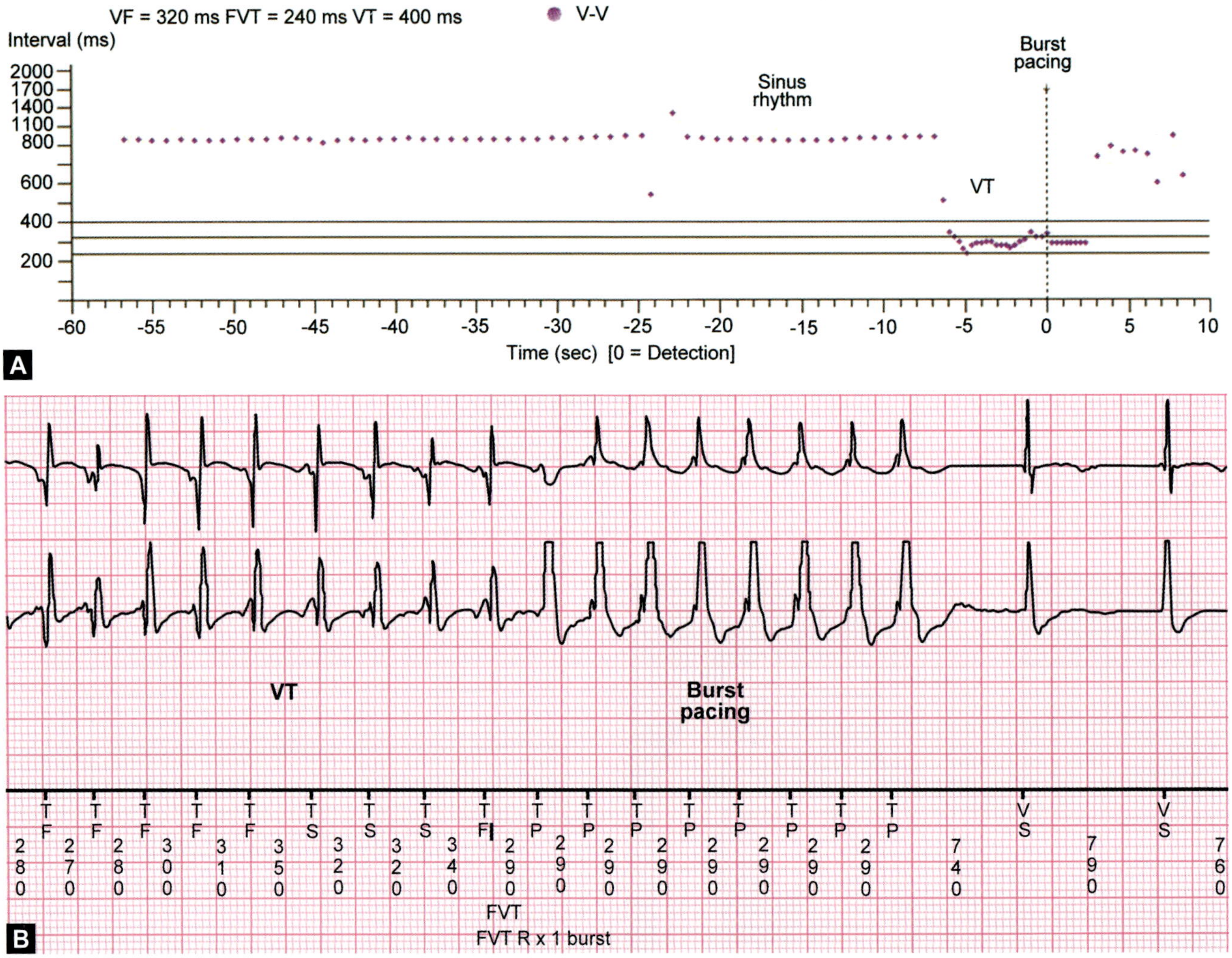

Figs. 35.5A and B: Interrogation of an implantable cardioverter defibrillator (ICD) reveals an episode of fast VT appropriately treated by burst pacing. (A) Interval plot showing the V-V duration (time between QRS impulses) in milliseconds (ms) on the Y axis. During sinus rhythm, the interval is 800 ms, corresponding to a heart rate of 75 bpm. During the episode of fast VT, the V-V interval becomes much shorter and is categorized by the ICD as "fast VT". Burst pacing is initiated. After a short series of burst pacing, the V-T interval again becomes approximately 800 ms, indicating successful termination of the ventricular tachycardia; (B) Intracardiac ECG from the same patient showing the treated arrhythmia. The tracing shows the detected VT, a short series of burst pacing, and termination of the arrhythmia. [Image from Raatikainen MJP, Koivisto UM. Remote monitoring of implantable cardioverter defibrillator therapy. In: Trayanova N (Ed). Cardiac Defibrillation—Mechanisms, Challenges and Implications. Shanghai: InTech; 2011].

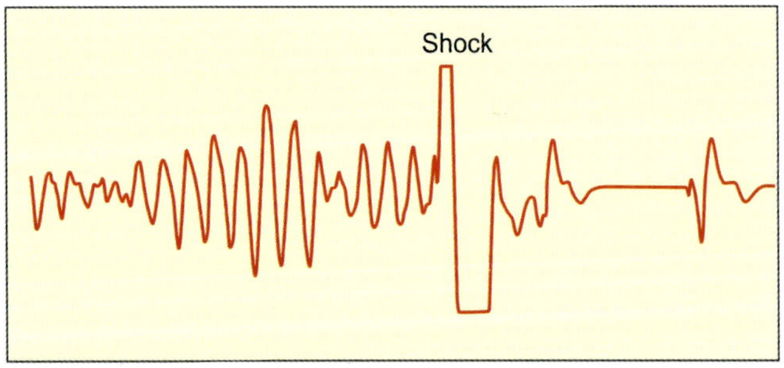

Fig. 35.6: An example of successful implantable cardioverter defibrillator shock in a patient with Torsades de Pointes. [Image from Rosenheck S. Defibrillation shock amplitude, location and timing. In: Harris JJ (Ed). Cardiac Defibrillation Prediction, Prevention and Management of Cardiovascular Arrhythmic Events. Shanghai: InTech; 2011].

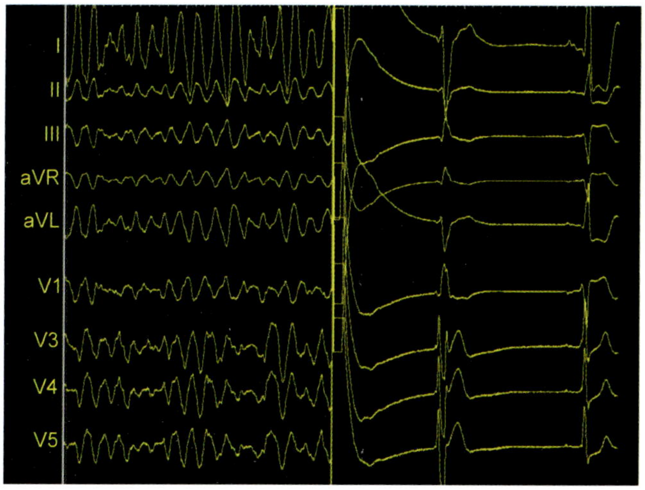

Fig. 35.7: An example of implantable cardioverter defibrillator termination of ventricular fibrillation with an appropriately delivered shock. [Image from Rosenheck S. Defibrillation shock amplitude, location and timing. In: Harris JJ (Ed). Cardiac Defibrillation–Prediction, Prevention and Management of Cardiovascular Arrhythmic events. Shanghai: InTech; 2011].

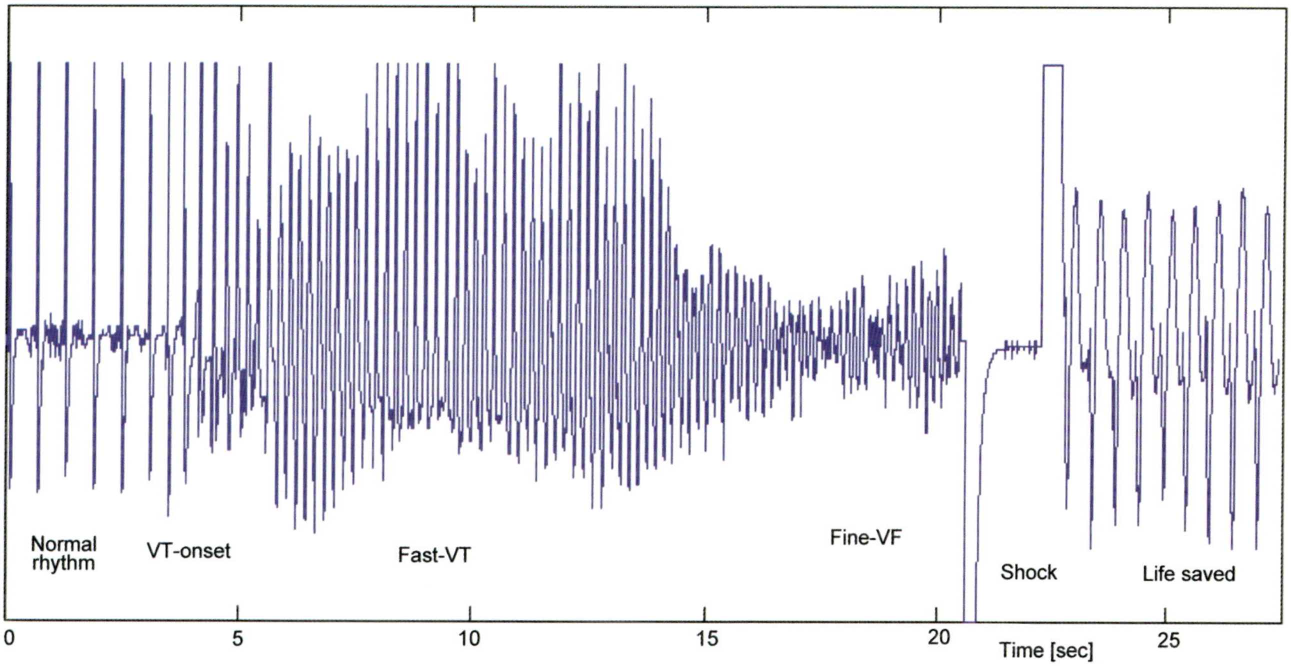

Fig. 35.8: An example of downloaded data from an implantable cardioverter defibrillator. Recording shows the development of malignant ventricular tachycardia which quickly degenerates into ventricular fibrillation. An appropriate shock delivery terminates the arrhythmia. [Image from Casaleggio A, Guidotto T, Malavasi V, et al. Ventricular tachyarrhythmias in implantable cardioverter defibrillator recipients: differences between ischemic and dilated cardiomyopathies. In: Harris JJ (Ed). Cardiac defibrillation–prediction, prevention and management of cardiovascular arrhythmic events. Shanghai: InTech; 2011].

initiated. Numerous programs and algorithms (Figs. 35.10 and 35.11) are utilized to allow the ICD to distinguish ventricular arrhythmias from sinus tachycardia or atrial fibrillation in order to avoid inappropriate ATP or defibrillation.

COMPLICATIONS

Acute or early complications of ICD implantation include pocket infection or hematoma, vessel of cardiac perforation, cardiac tamponade and pneumothorax. Long-term

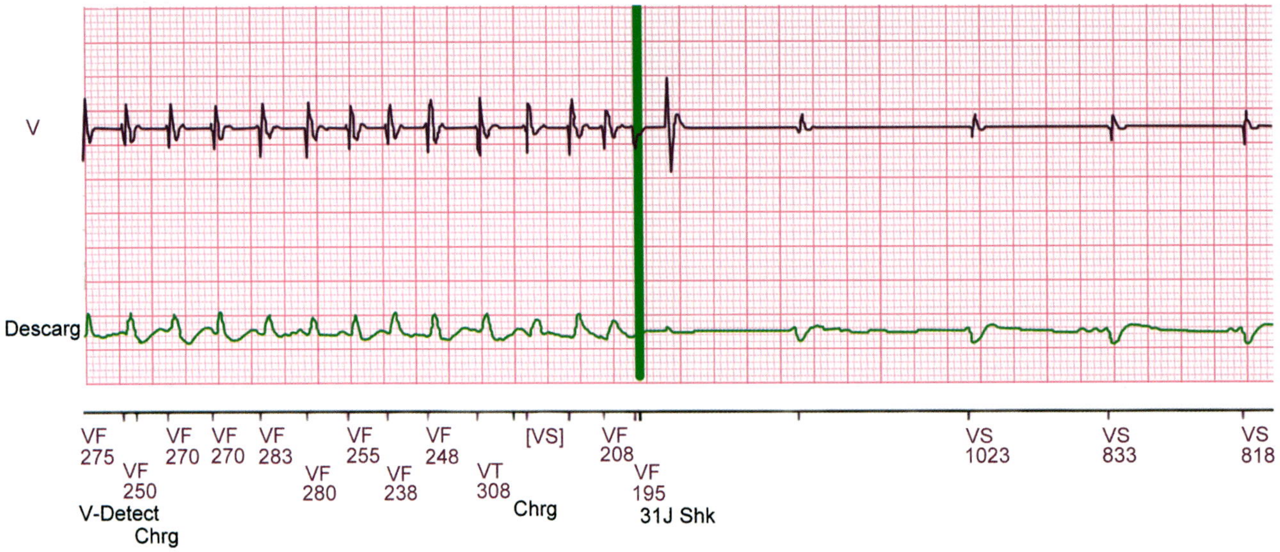

Fig. 35.9: An example of appropriate shock delivery for ventricular fibrillation. [Image from Algarra M, Santiago P, Tercedor L, et al. Implantable-cardioverter defibrillator in pediatric population. In: Trayanova N (Ed). Cardiac Defibrillation–Mechanisms, Challenges and Implications. Shanghai: InTech; 2011].

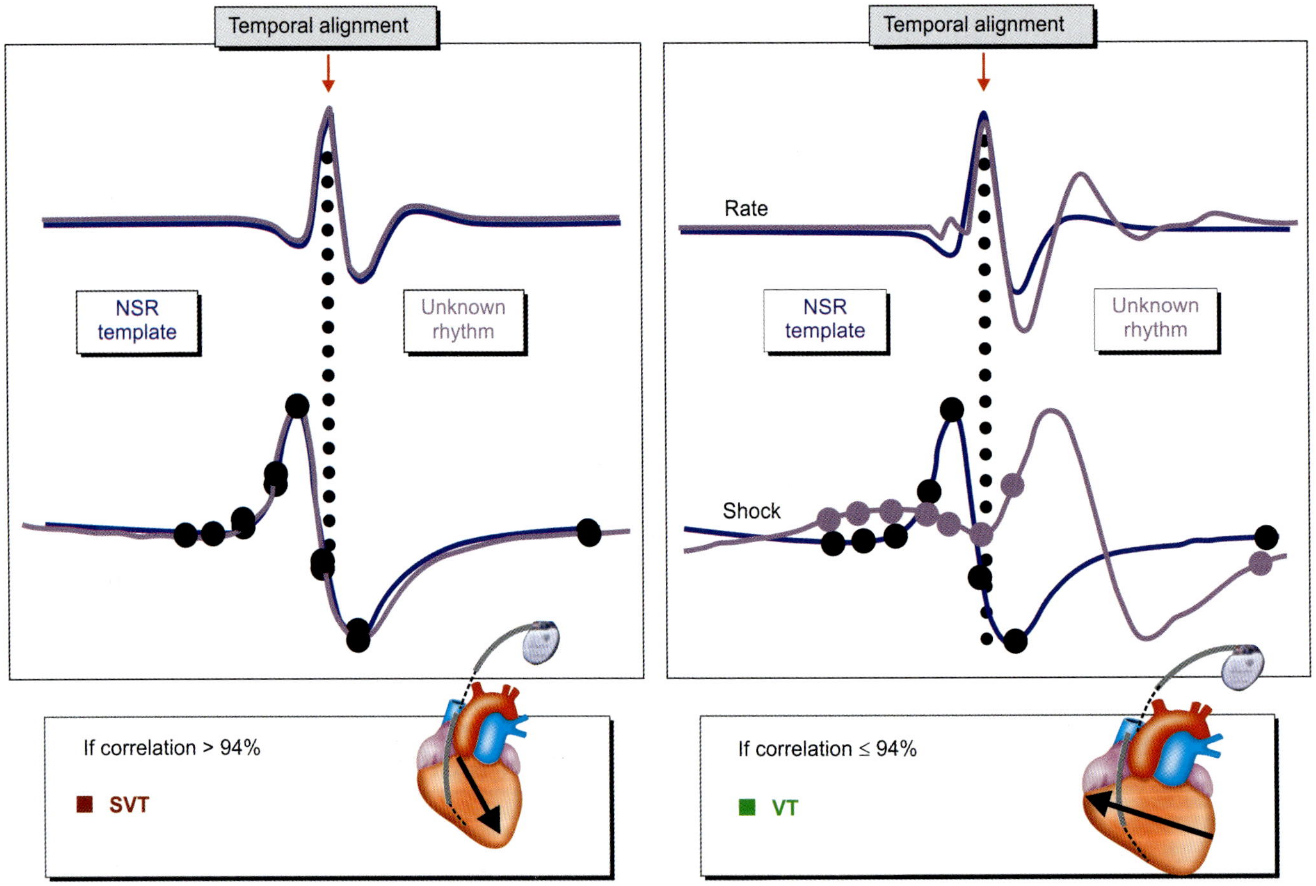

Fig. 35.10: An example of morphology analysis algorithms to allow discrimination between VT and non-VT utilized by defibrillators to avoid inappropriate shocks. [Images from Toquero J, Castro V, Mitroi C, et al. New ways to avoid unnecessary and inappropriate shocks. In: Trayanova N (Ed). Cardiac Defibrillation–Mechanisms, Challenges and Implications. Shanghai: InTech; 2011].

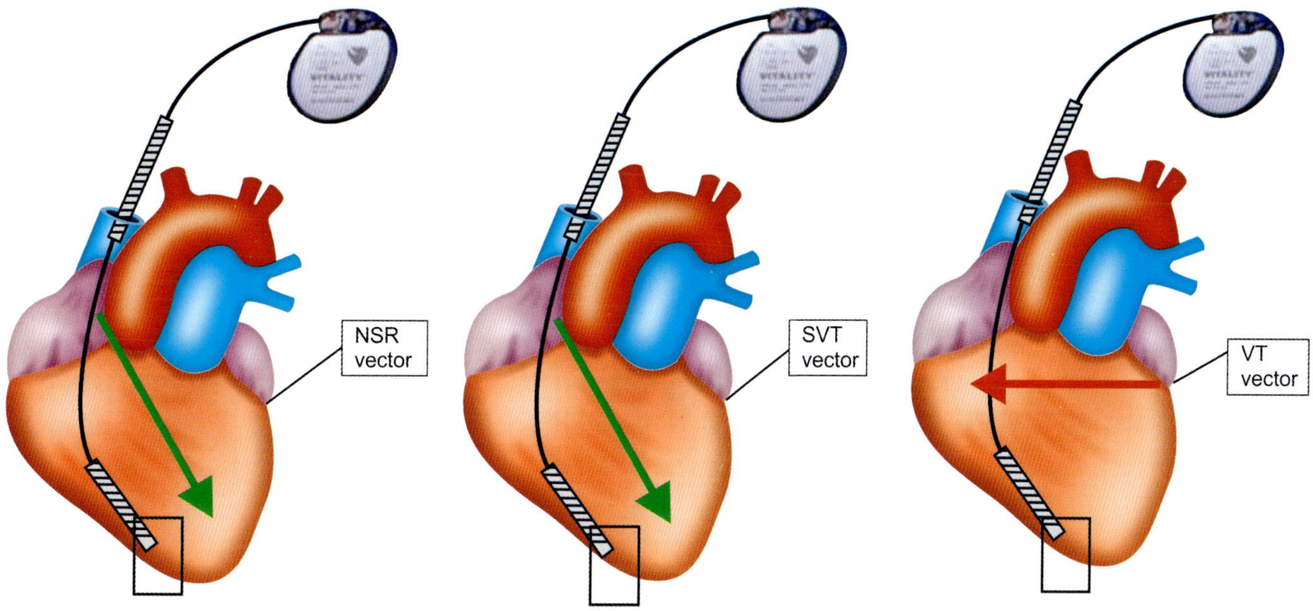

Fig. 35.11: Demonstration of a rhythm discrimination algorithm: discrimination between sinus rhythm and SVT with "normal" vector (green) to a potential VT vector (red). This algorithm is not based on EGM signal but on an internal ECG electrode from device can to RV shock coil and the vena cava shock coil. [Image from Seifert M. Tachycardia discrimination algorithms in ICDs. In: Erkapic D, Bauernfeind T (Eds). Cardiac defibrillation. Shanghai: InTech; 2013].

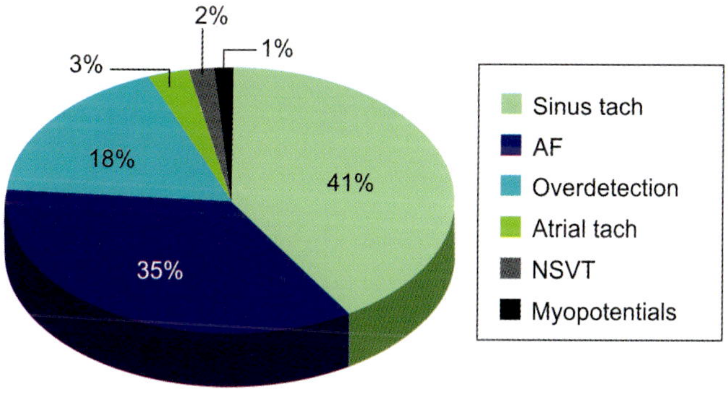

Fig. 35.12: Causes of inappropriate implantable cardioverter defibrillator shocks. [Image from Toquero J, Castro V, Mitroi C, et al. New ways to avoid unnecessary and inappropriate shocks. In: Trayanova N (Ed). Cardiac Defibrillation–Mechanisms, Challenges and Implications. Shanghai: InTech; 2011]. (AF: Atrial fibrillation; NSVT: Nonsustained ventricular tachycardia).

complications include erosion of the pocket by the device, lead infection, lead dislodgment, lead fracture, lead insulation defect and inappropriate shock (Fig. 35.12). Numerous factors can lead to failure to successfully defibrillate (Fig. 35.13). Mechanical interference by the lead with the tricuspid valve can lead to tricuspid regurgitation.

Infants and children present unique challenges to ICD implantation given their small body habitus and given that they will grow over time. In some cases, the device can be implanted subcutaneously, with modification of the usual manner of coil implantation (Figs. 35.14A and B). In very small patients, abdominal implantation will be utilized (Fig. 35.15).

MANAGEMENT OF PATIENTS TREATED WITH ICDs

Periodic monitoring of ICD status is required in patients treated with ICD implantation. Battery life must be monitored; life-expectancy of most ICDs is on the order 5 years or more. Telephonic, internet, and patient-based device interrogation decrease the need for in-person device interrogation (Figs. 35.16 to 35.18).

Both patients treated with ICDs and the patient's spouse or partner have been shown to have fear and anxiety with regard to engaging in certain activities, including sexual activity. Appropriate discussion and counseling of patients and partners is recommended by the American Heart Association and the European Society of Cardiology.

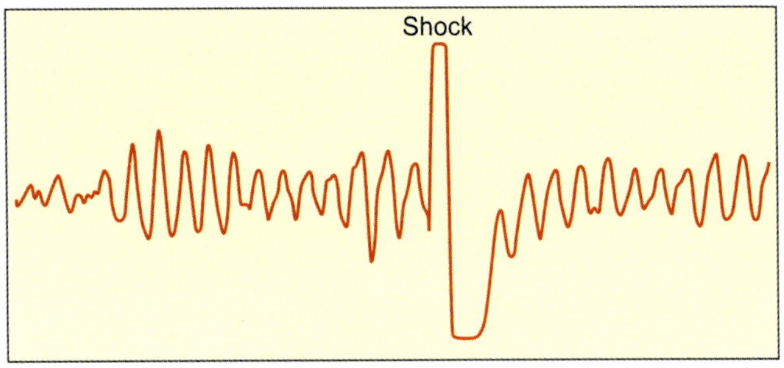

Fig. 35.13: An example of an unsuccessful implantable cardioverter defibrillator shock in a patient with polymorphic ventricular tachycardia. [Image from Rosenheck S. Defibrillation shock amplitude, location and timing. In: Harris JJ (Ed). Cardiac Defibrillation–Prediction, Prevention and Management of Cardiovascular Arrhythmic Events. Shanghai: InTech; 2011].

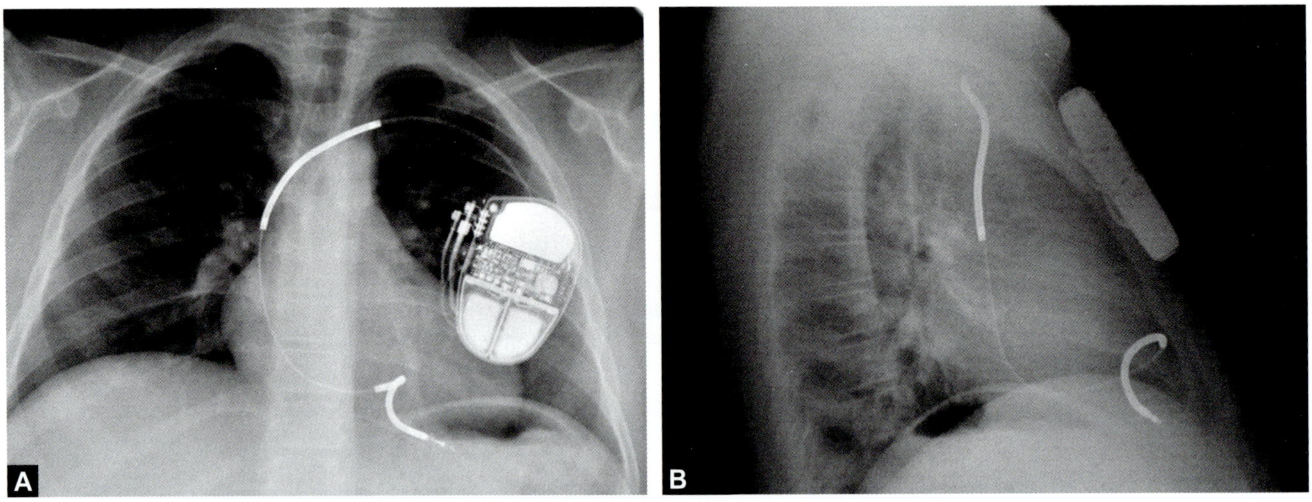

Figs. 35.14A and B: (A) Posteroanterior; and (B) lateral chest X-rays in a 10-year-old patient treated with implantable cardioverter defibrillator (ICD) for Brugada syndrome. Note the positioning and appearance of the leads is different than that in adults treated with ICD. [Image from Algarra M, Santiago P, Tercedor L, et al. Implantable-cardioverter defibrillator in pediatric population. In: Trayanova N (Ed). Cardiac Defibrillation–Mechanisms, Challenges and Implications. Shanghai: InTech; 2011].

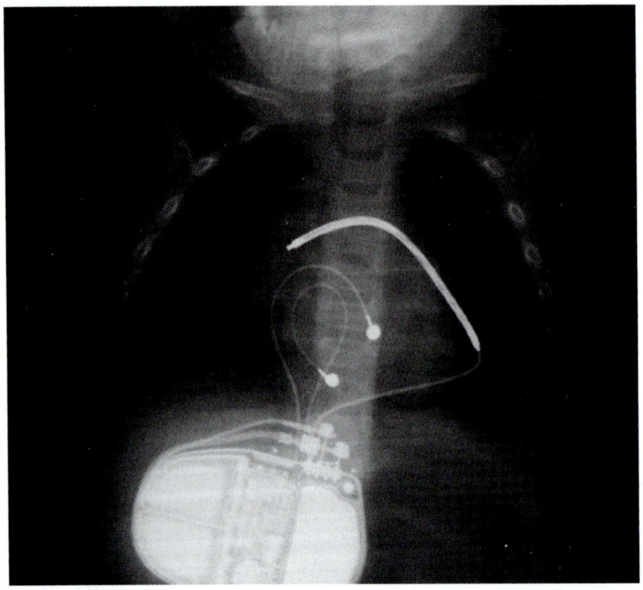

Fig. 35.15: Single-chamber epicardial cardioverter defibrillator in a 2-year-old patient with long QT syndrome. [Image from Algarra M, Santiago P, Tercedor L, et al. Implantable-cardioverter defibrillator in pediatric population. In: Trayanova N (Ed). Cardiac Defibrillation–Mechanisms, Challenges and Implications. Shanghai: InTech; 2011].

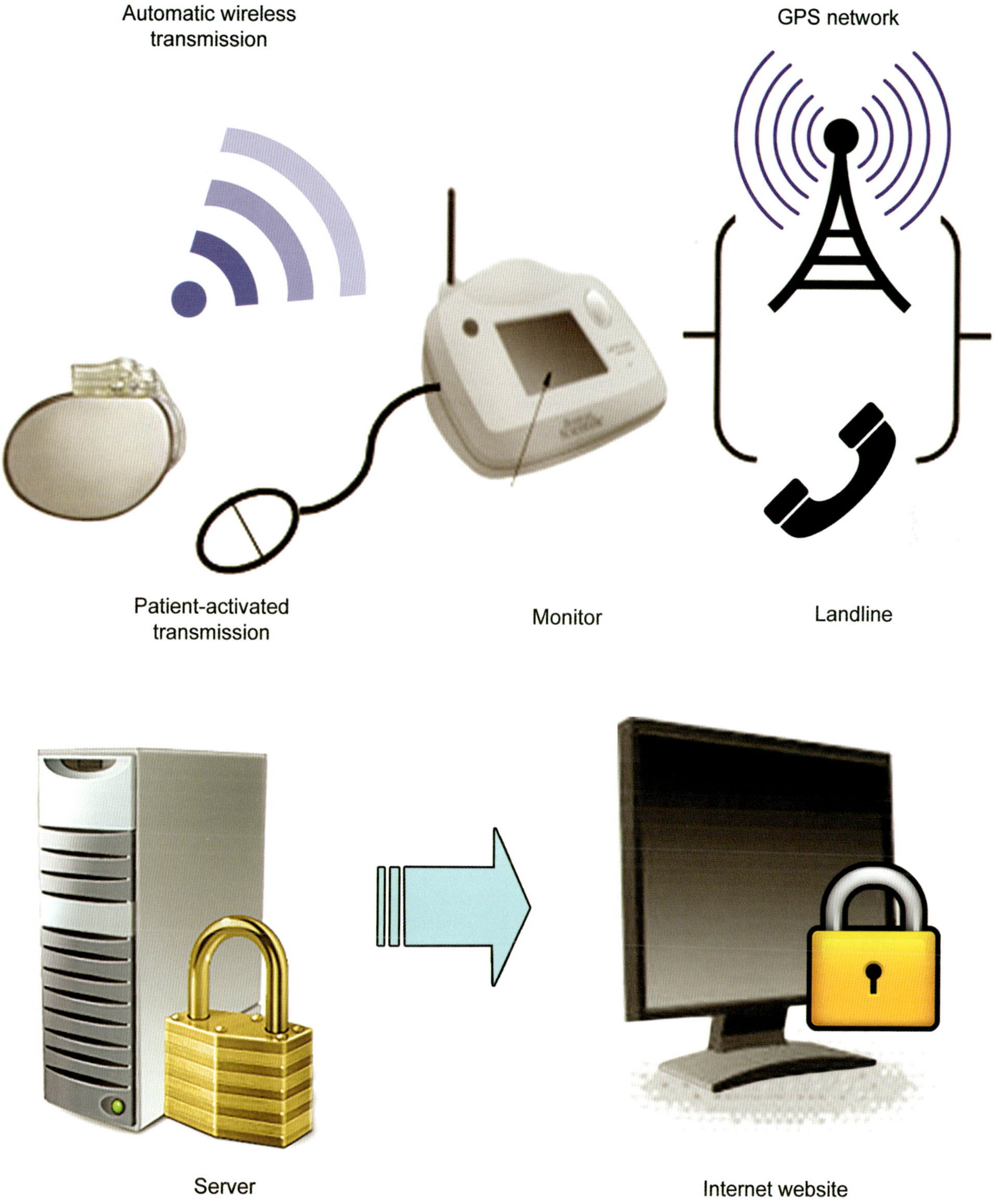

Fig. 35.16: Components of remote monitoring system. Systems differ regarding data transfer, which may require patient's active involvement or is performed wirelessly from the implanted device to a patient monitor. Data from the patient monitor is sent to a central database using either an analog phone landline or via GSM network. The data are accessible to the clinical staff on a secure internet site. [Image from Raatikainen MJP, Koivisto UM. Remote monitoring of implantable cardioverter defibrillator therapy. In: Trayanova N (Ed). Cardiac Defibrillation–Mechanisms, Challenges and Implications. Shanghai: InTech; 2011].

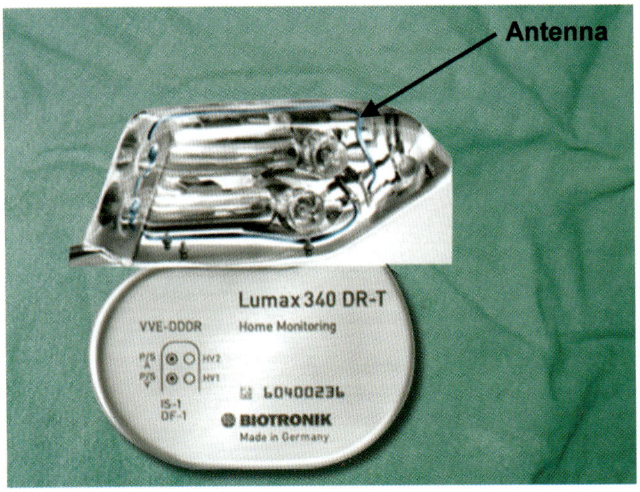

Fig. 35.17: An advanced implantable cardioverter defibrillator with an internal antenna for wireless data transmission to the patient monitor. [Raatikainen MJP, Koivisto UM. Remote monitoring of implantable cardioverter defibrillator therapy. In: Trayanova N (Ed). Cardiac Defibrillation–Mechanisms, Challenges and Implications. Shanghai: InTech; 2011].

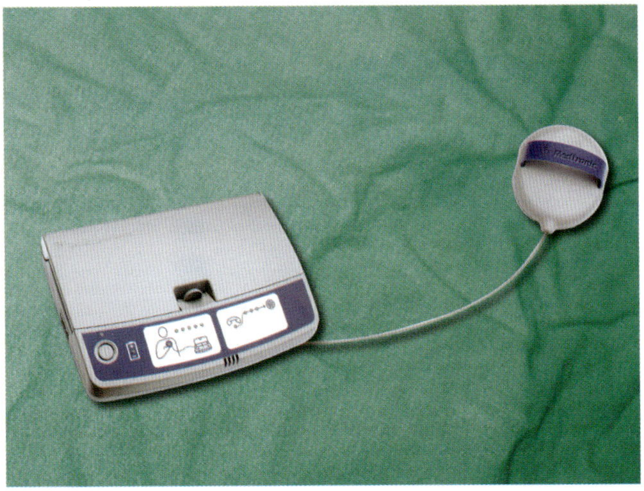

Fig. 35.18: An example of a device for patient home monitoring of the implantable cardioverter defibrillator.

REFERENCES

Bardy GH, Lee KL, Mark DB, et al. Sudden Cardiac Death in Heart Failure Trial (SCD-HeFT) Investigators. Amiodarone or an implantable cardioverter-defibrillator for congestive heart failure. New Engl J Med. 2005;352:225-37.

Bokhari F, Newman D, Greene M, et al. Long-term comparison of the implantable cardioverter defibrillator versus amiodarone: eleven-year follow-up of a subset of patients in the Canadian Implantable Defibrillator Study (CIDS). Circulation. 2004;110: 112-6.

Bristow M, Saxon L, Boehmer J, et al. Cardiac-resynchronization therapy with or without an implantable defibrillator advanced chronic heart failure. N Engl J Med. 2004;350:2140-50.

Buxton AE, Lee KL, Fisher JD, et al. A randomized study of the prevention of sudden death in patients with coronary artery disease. Multicenter unsustained tachycardia trial investigators. N Engl J Med. 1996;335:1933-40.

Connolly SJ, Gent M, Roberts RS, et al. Canadian Implantable Defibrillator Study (CIDS): a randomized trial of the implantable cardioverter defibrillator against amiodarone. Circulation. 2000;101:1297-1302.

Epstein AE, DiMarco JP, Ellenbogen KA, et al. ACC/AHA/HRS 2008 guidelines for device-based therapy of cardiac rhythm abnormalities: a report of the American College of Cardiology/ American Heart Association Task Force on Practice Guidelines (writing committee to revise the ACC/AHA/NASPE 2002 guideline update for implantation of cardiac pacemakers and antiarrhythmia devices). Circulation. 2008;117:e350-e408.

Kuck KH, Cappato R, Siebels J, et al. Randomized comparison of antiarrhythmic drug therapy with implantable defibrillators in patients resuscitated from cardiac arrest: the Cardiac Arrest Study Hamburg (CASH). Circulation. 2000;102:748-54.

Levine GN, Steinke EE, Bakaeen FG, et al. Sexual activity and cardiovascular disease: a scientific statement from the American Heart Association. Circulation. 2012;125(8):1058-72.

Moss AJ, Hall WJ, Cannom DS, et al. Improved survival with an implanted defibrillator in patients with coronary disease at high risk for ventricular arrhythmia. Multicenter automatic defibrillator implantation trial investigators. N Engl J Med. 1996;335:1933-40.

Moss AJ, Zareba W, Hall WJ, et al. Prophylactic implantation of a defibrillator in patients with myocardial infarction and reduced ejection fraction. N Engl J Med. 2002;346:877-83.

Oseroff O, Retyk E, Bochoeyer A. Subanalyses of secondary prevention implantable cardioverter-defibrillator trials: antiarrhythmics versus implantable defibrillators (AVID), Canadian Implantable Defibrillator Study (CIDS), and Cardiac Arrest Study Hamburg (CASH). Curr Opin Cardiol. 2004;19:26-30.

Salukhe TV, Dimopoulos K, Sutton R, et al. Life-years gained from defibrillator implantation: markedly nonlinear increase during 3 years of follow-up and its implications. Circulation. 2004;109:1848-53.

Steinke EE, Jaarsma T, Barnason SA, et al. Sexual counseling for individuals with cardiovascular disease and their partners: a consensus document from the American Heart Association and the ESC Council on Cardiovascular Nursing and Allied Professions (CCNAP). Circulation. 2013;128(18):2075-96.

The Antiarrhythmics versus Implantable Defibrillators (AVID) Investigators: A comparison of antiarrhythmic-drug therapy with implantable defibrillators in patients resuscitated from near-fatal ventricular arrhythmias. N Engl J Med. 1997, 337:1621-3.

Yancy CW, Jessup M, Bozkurt B, et al. 2013 ACCF/AHA guideline for the management of heart failure: a report of the American College of Cardiology Foundation/American Heart Association Task Force on Practice Guidelines. J Am Coll Cardiol. 2013; 62:e147-239.

Zipes DP, Camm AJ, Borggrefe M, et al. ACC/AHA/ESC 2006 guidelines for management of patients with ventricular arrhythmias and the prevention of sudden cardiac death: a report of the American College of Cardiology/American Heart Association Task Force and the European Society of Cardiology Committee for Practice Guidelines (writing committee to develop guidelines for management of patients with ventricular arrhythmias and the prevention of sudden cardiac death). Europace. 2006;8:746-837.

Section 5

Pericardial Disease

Chapters

CHAPTER

Pericarditis

36

Trevor L Jenkins, Brian D Hoit

PERICARDIAL ANATOMY AND FUNCTION

The pericardium is composed of visceral and parietal components. The visceral pericardium is a mesothelial monolayer that adheres firmly to the epicardium, reflects over the origin of the great vessels, and together with a tough, fibrous coat envelops the heart as the parietal pericardium (Figs. 36.1 to 36.3). The pericardial space between these two layers contains up to 50 mL of the pericardial fluid.

The pericardium is not essential for life but the pericardium limits distension and facilitates interaction of the cardiac chambers, prevents excessive torsion and displacement of the heart, minimizes friction, prevents the spread of infection, and equalizes gravitational, hydrostatic, and inertial forces over the surface of the heart.

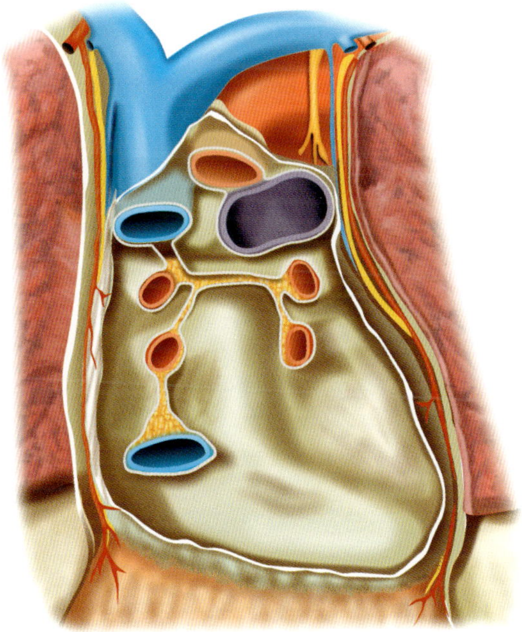

Fig. 36.1: Pericardial anatomy: cross-sectional view of the inferolateral and diaphragmatic pericardium and great vessels. Note both pericardial layers (visceral and parietal) become contiguous about the great vessels producing two potential spaces, the oblique and transverse sinuses. Pericardial recesses are formed at the reflection point joining the two layers.

PERICARDIAL HEART DISEASE

Pericardial heart disease includes only pericarditis (which may be acute, subacute, or chronic; Figs. 36.4 to 36.7)

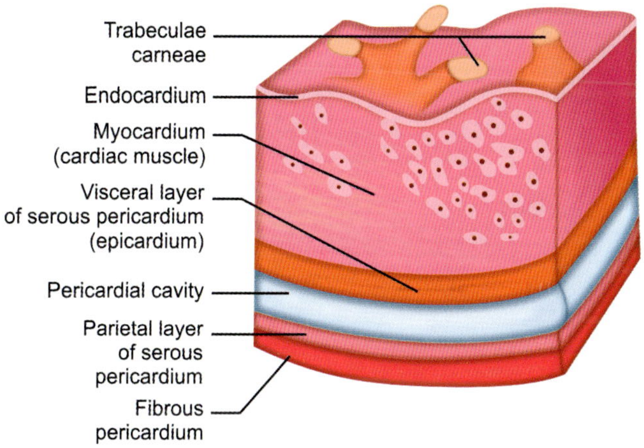

Fig. 36.2: Layers of the pericardium.

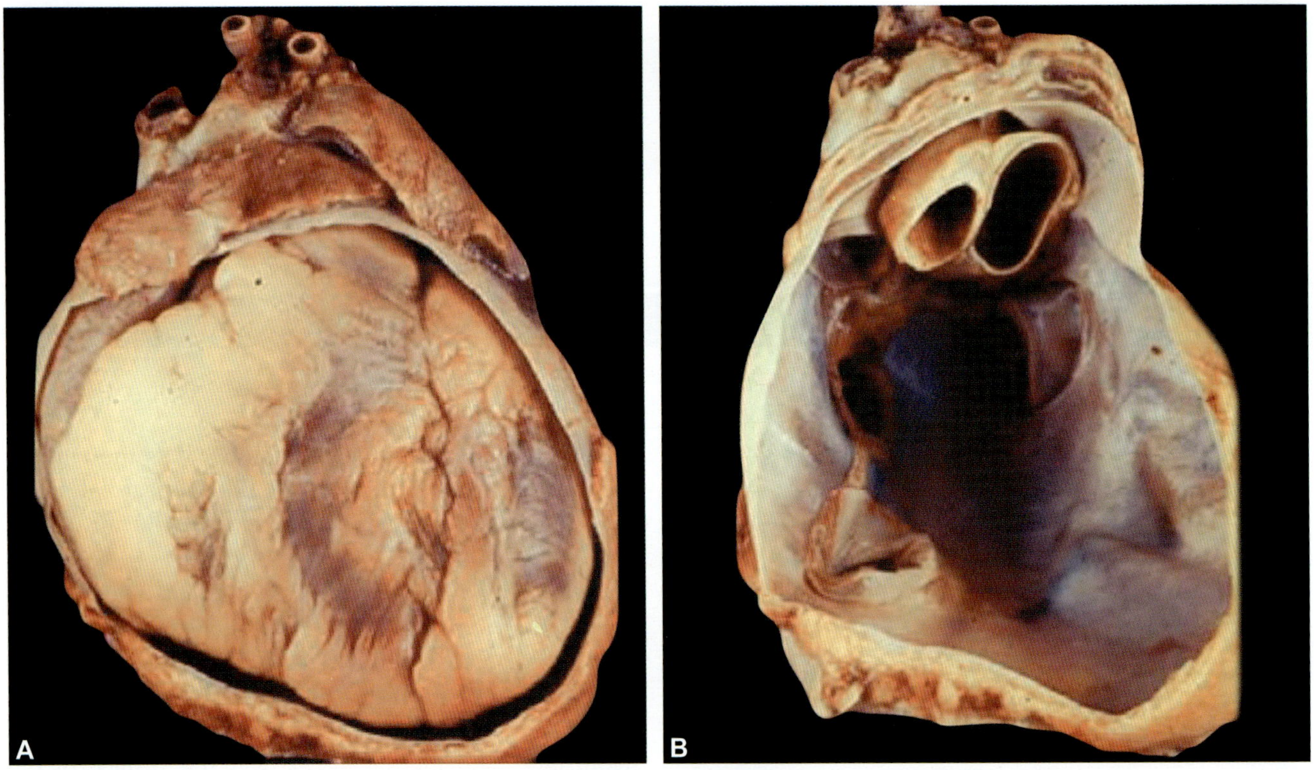

Figs. 36.3A and B: Pathology specimens of normal double-layered pericardium with (A) and without (B) the heart. [Images courtesy of Dr William D Edwards, Mayo Clinic; images published in Khandaker MH, Nishimura RA. Pericardial disease. In: Chatterjee K, Anderson M, Heistad D, Kerber RE (Eds). Cardiology: An Illustrated Textbook. New Delhi, India: Jaypee Brothers Medical Publishers (P) Ltd; 2013].

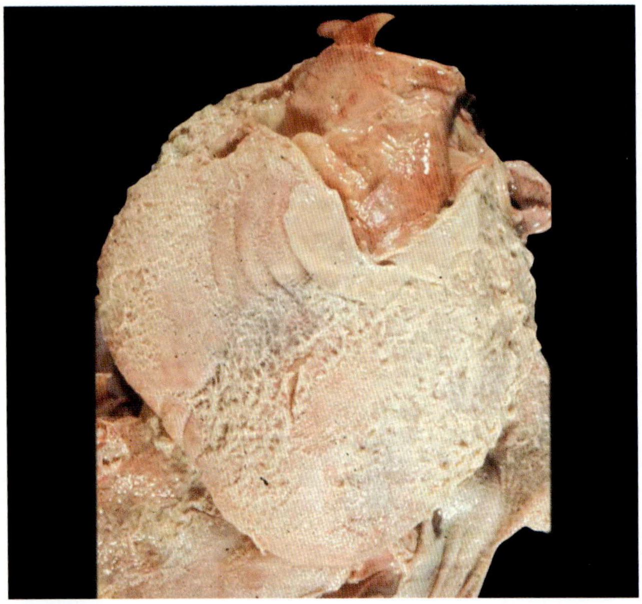

Fig. 36.4: Fibrinous pericarditis. Gross pathology image demonstrated the typical "bread and butter" appearance of fibrinous pericarditis. (Image from the slide collection of the late Dr Charles Kuhn and courtesy of Dr Calvin Oyer, Digital Pathology, Brown Medical School, with permission).

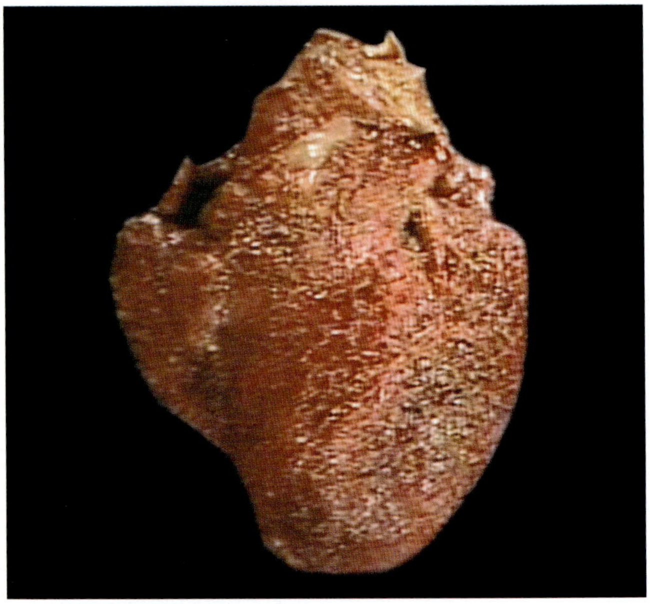

Fig. 36.5: Gross pathology example of pericarditis. [Image from Armed Forces Institute of Pathology (public domain)].

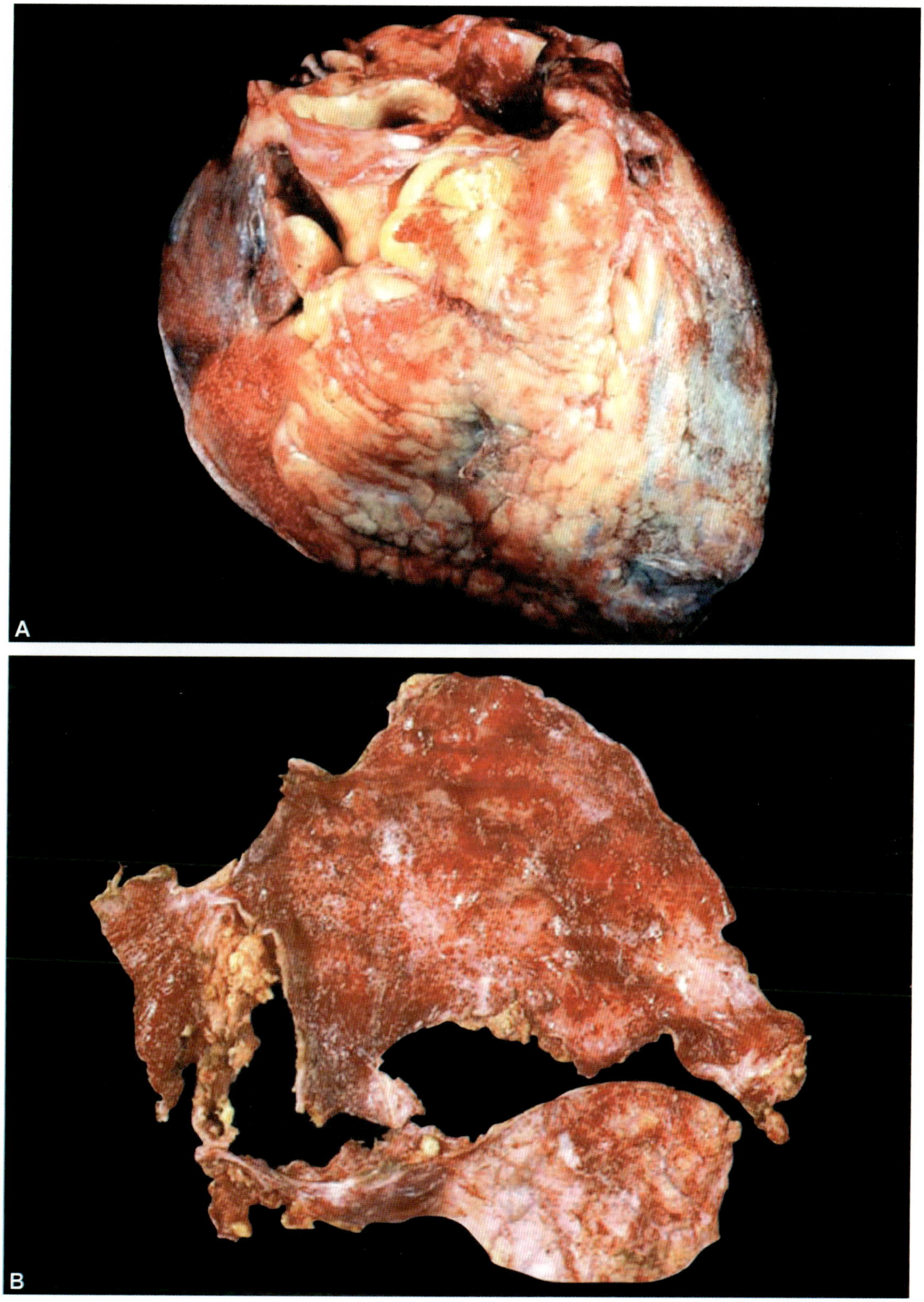

Figs. 36.6A and B: Gross features of relapsing pericarditis. (A) Anterior view of fibrinous pericardium from a patient with relapsing pericarditis; (B) Thickened pericardium post-pericardiectomy from a patient with recurrent pericarditis. [Images courtesy of Dr William D Edwards, Mayo Clinic; images and legend text from Khandaker MH, Nishimura RA. Pericardial disease. In: Chatterjee K, Anderson M, Heistad D, Kerber RE (Eds). Cardiology: An Illustrated Textbook. New Delhi, India: Jaypee Brothers Medical Publishers (P) Ltd; 2013].

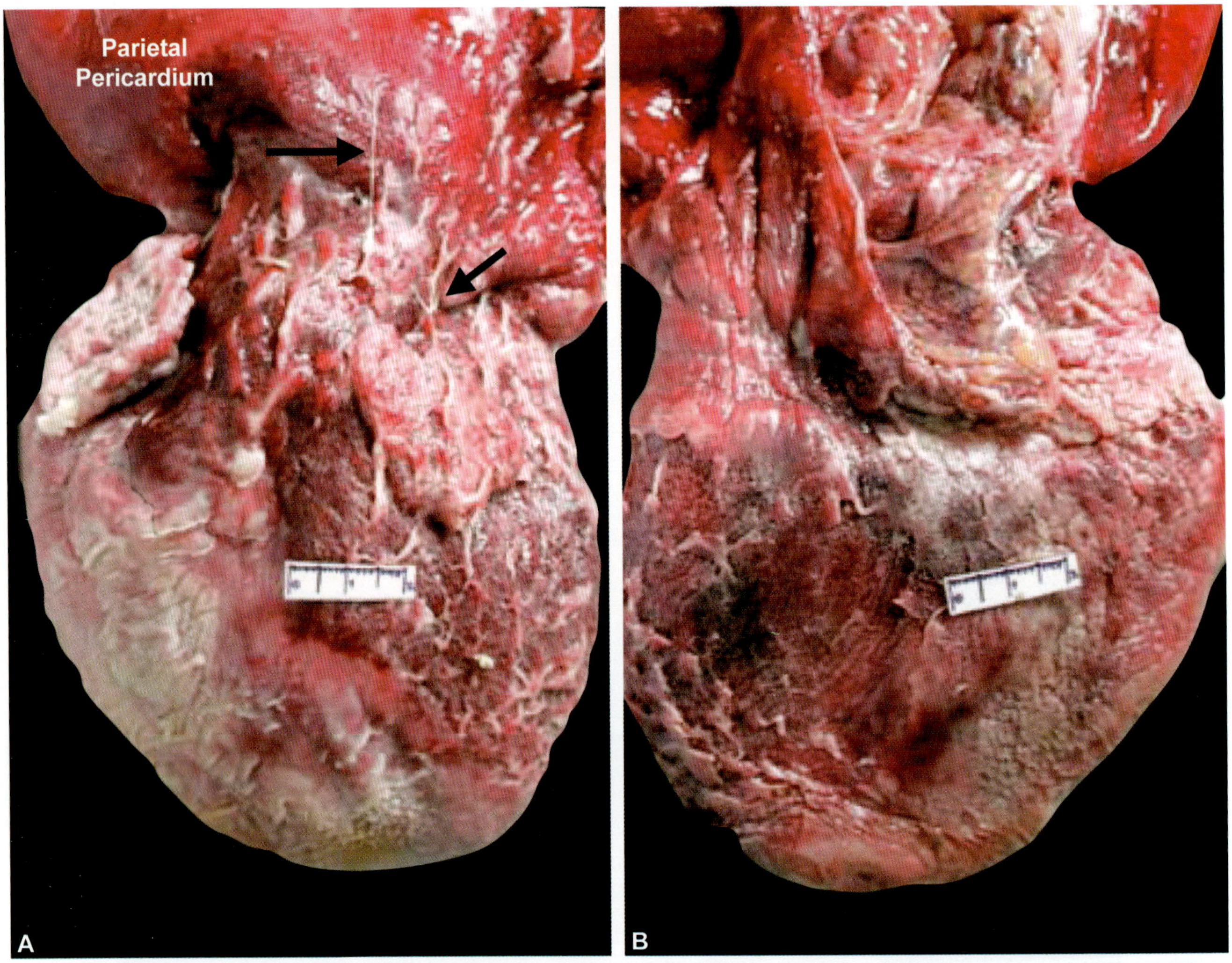

Figs. 36.7A and B: Acute rheumatic pericarditis. Anterior surface (A) and posterior surface (B) with fibrinous/hemorrhagic exudates. There are also delicate adhesions (arrows) between the parietal and visceral pericardium. [Image and legend text from Bharati S, Bharati S. Etiopathogenesis and pathology of carditis in rheumatic fever. In: Vijayalakshmi IB (Ed). Acute Rheumatic Fever and Chronic Rheumatic Heart Disease. New Delhi, India: Jaypee Brothers Medical Publishers (P) Ltd; 2011].

Table 36.1: Etiologies of acute pericarditis. (AIDS: Acquired immunodeficiency syndrome; HIV: Human immunodeficiency virus).

Idiopathic
Infectious (viral, bacterial, mycobacterial, fungal, or AIDS/HIV)
Collagen vascular disease
Neoplastic [primary (mesothelioma), secondary (especially breast, lung, melanoma, lymphoma)]
Radiotherapy
Drugs and toxins
Metabolic (uremic, dialytic, myxedema, amyloidosis)
Post-cardiac injury syndrome (PCIS): Post-myocardial infarction, pericardiotomy, or trauma
Acute injury syndromes (non-PCIS): Myocardial infarction, cardiac surgery, trauma

and its complications, tamponade and constriction. However, despite a limited number of clinical syndromes, the pericardium is affected by virtually every category of disease (Table 36.1). Therefore, the physician is likely to encounter patients with pericardial disease in a variety of settings, either as an isolated phenomenon or as a complication of a variety of systemic disorders, trauma, or certain drugs.

Acute fibrinous or dry pericarditis is a syndrome characterized by typical chest pain, a pathognomonic pericardial friction rub, and specific electrocardiogram (ECG) changes. Symptoms and signs of acute pericarditis are shown in Figure 36.8.

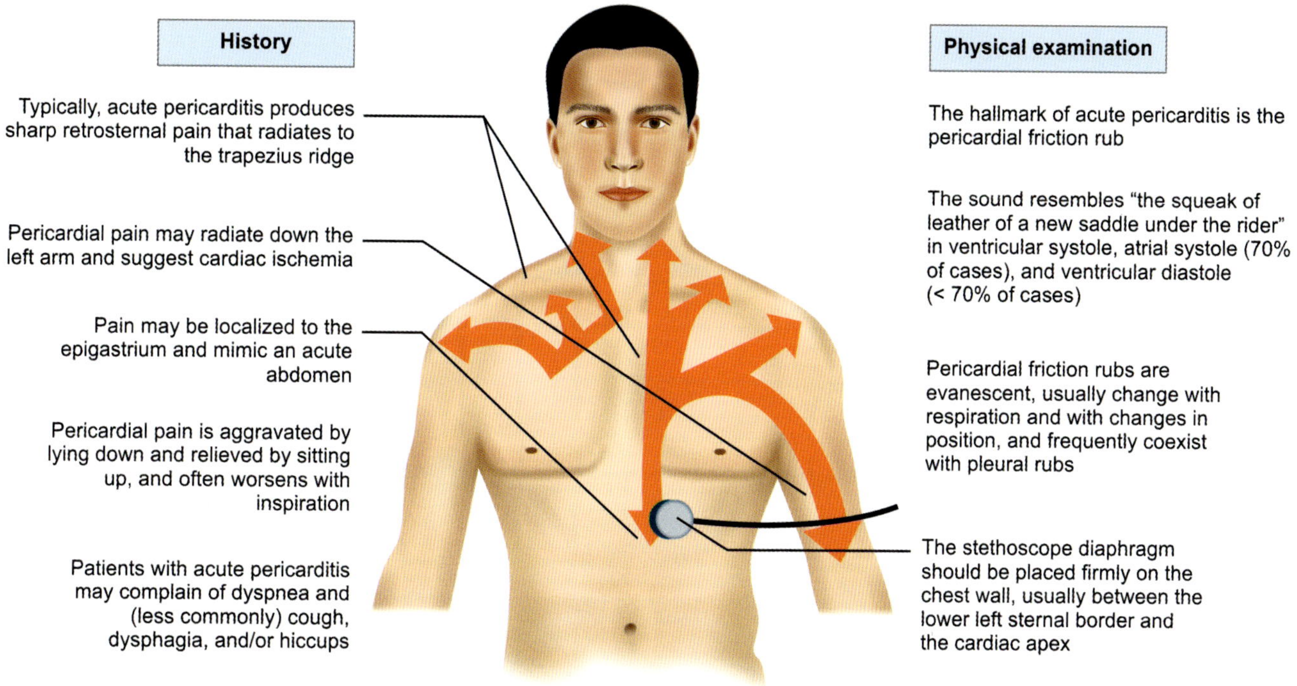

Fig. 36.8: Clinical features of acute pericarditis: symptoms and physical examination. (Adapted from: Clinical features of acute pericarditis: presenting signs and physical exam; reproduced with permission from Hoit BD. Acute pericarditis: diagnosis and differential diagnosis. Hosp Pract. 1991;27:23-43).

EVALUATION OF PATIENTS WITH SUSPECTED PERICARDITIS

The ECG may either confirm the clinical suspicion of pericardial disease or first alert the clinician to the presence of pericarditis. A very early ECG abnormality that may be seen in pericarditis is PR segment depression (Fig. 36.9). More commonly, diffuse ST-segment elevation (Fig. 36.10) is seen. Serial tracings may be needed to distinguish the ST-segment elevations from those caused by acute myocardial infarction (MI) or normal early repolarization, since the ST-T-wave changes in acute pericarditis are diffuse and have characteristic, but variable evolutionary change.

In uncomplicated acute pericarditis, the chest X-ray is generally normal. However, an enlarged cardiac silhouette may be evident because of a moderate or large pericardial effusion (Fig. 36.11).

The use of echocardiography for the evaluation of all patients with suspected pericardial disease was given a class I recommendation by the 2003 Task Force of the American Heart Association (AHA)/American College of Cardiology (ACC)/American Society of Echocardiography (ASE). Echocardiographic identification of pericardial effusion confirms the clinical diagnosis of acute pericarditis (Figs. 36.12 and 36.13, Videos 36.1 to 36.3), but a patient with purely fibrinous acute pericarditis may have a normal echocardiogram. Echocardiography estimates the volume of pericardial fluid, identifies cardiac tamponade, suggests the basis of pericarditis, and documents associated acute myocarditis with congestive heart failure.

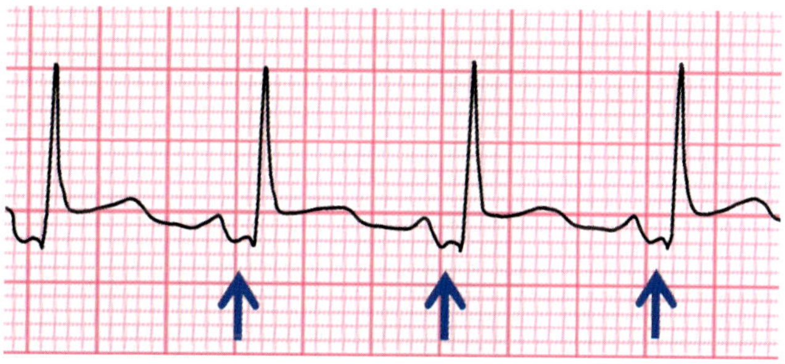

Fig. 36.9: PR-segment depression, an early electrocardiogram (ECG) abnormality that may occasionally be seen in patients with pericarditis.

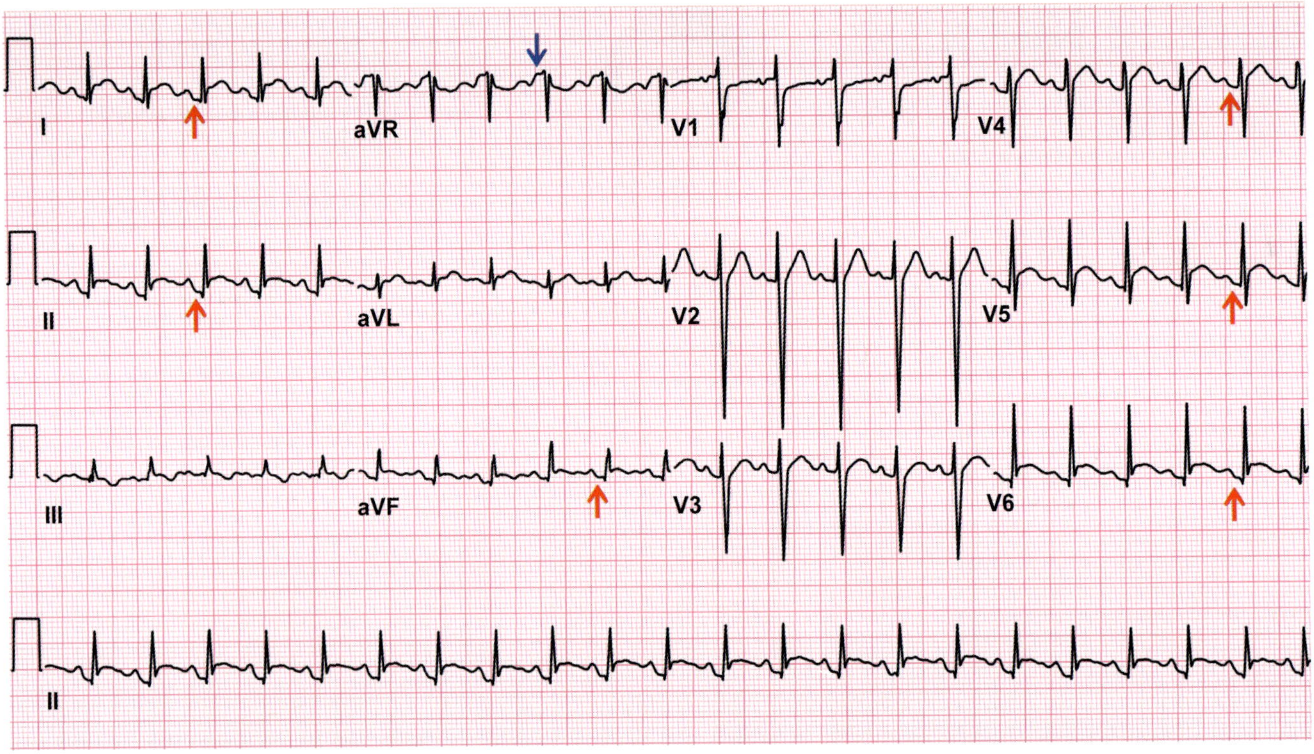

Fig. 36.10: Electrocardiogram (ECG) findings in pericarditis. Diffuse ST-segment elevation, as well as PR-segment depression (red arrows), are present in a non-coronary artery territory distribution. Note that there is reciprocal ST-segment depression and PR-segment elevation (blue arrow) in lead aVR.

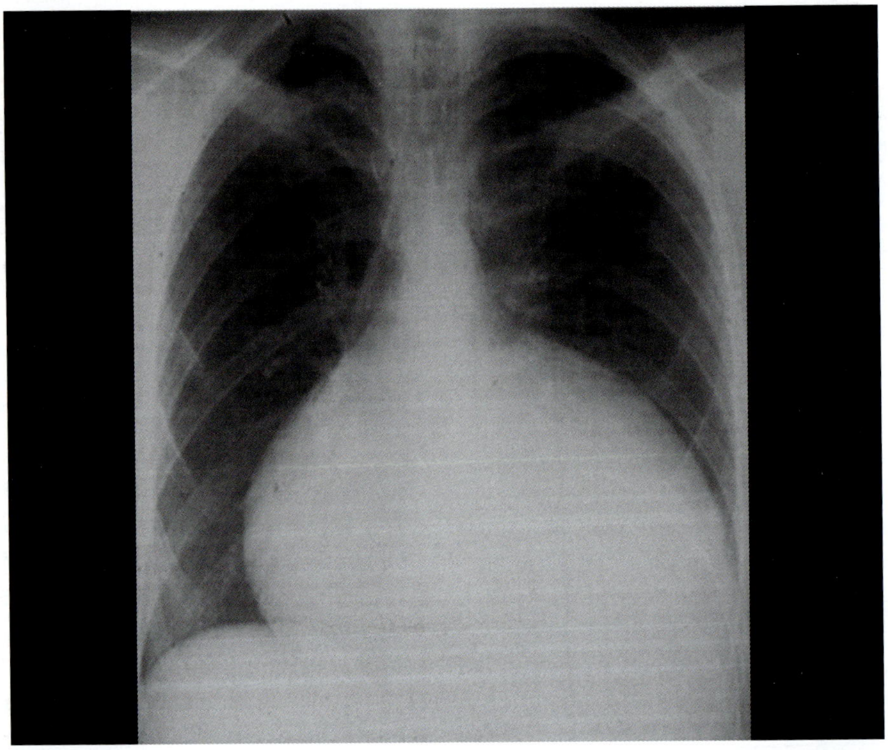

Fig. 36.11: Chest X-ray of a patient with pericarditis demonstrating a "water-bottle" heart, highly suggestive of a large pericardial effusion.

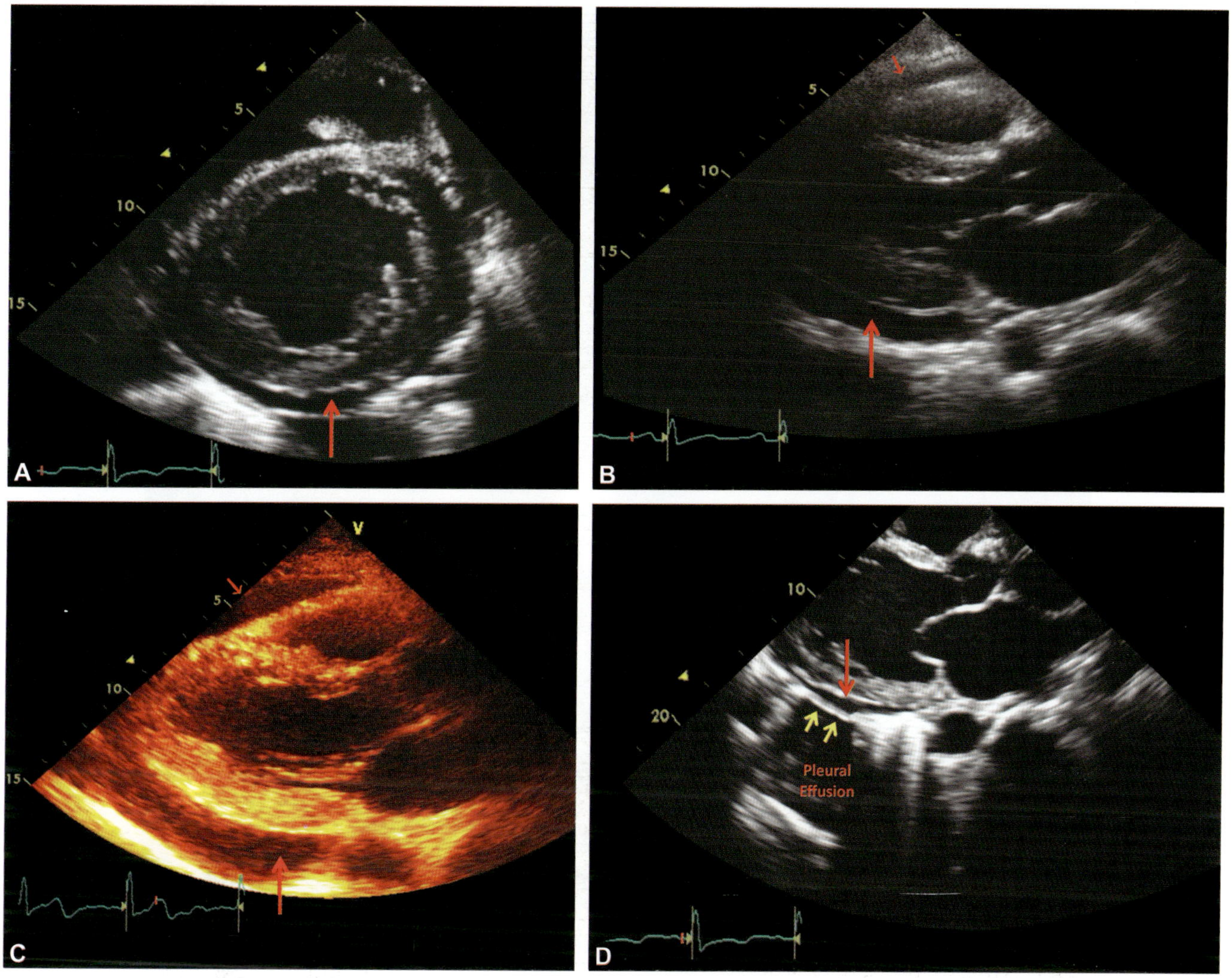

Figs. 36.12A to D: Two-dimensional (2D) echocardiography of pericardial effusions (red arrows) of varying size. Anterior (small red arrows) and posterior (large red arrows) effusions are seen as echo-free spaces of increasing size including (A) small posterior, (B) moderate circumferential, and (C) large circumferential. Figure 36.12D shows a large pleural effusion posterior to a small pericardial effusion with the pericardium visualized as an echogenic linearity between both (yellow arrows). [Reproduced from Jenkins T, Hoit BD. Pericardial disease. In: Nanda NC (Ed). Comprehensive Textbook of Echocardiography. New Delhi, India: Jaypee Brothers Medical Publishers (P) Ltd; 2014].

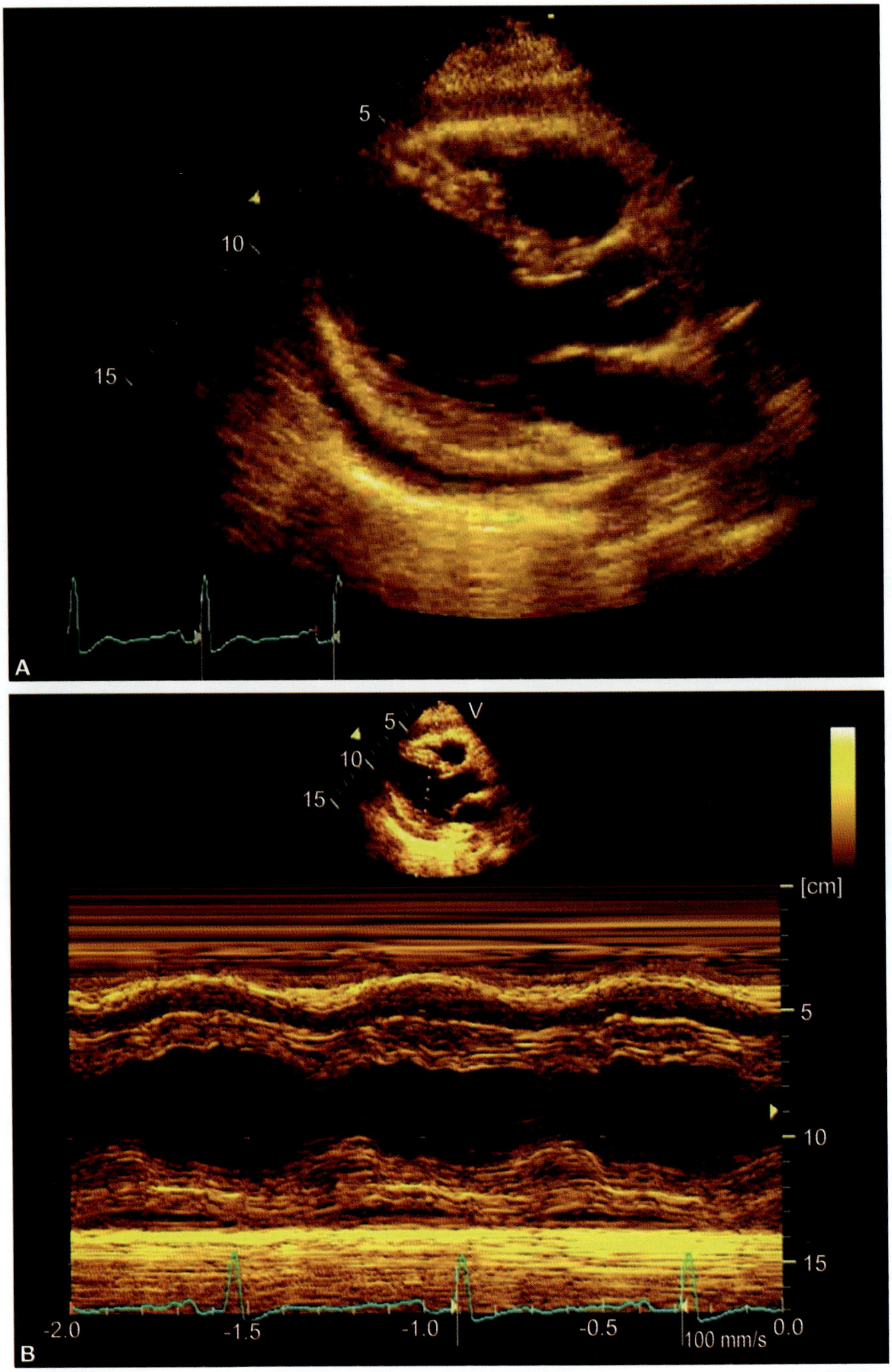

Figs. 36.13A and B: (A) Two-dimensional (2D) echocardiogram and (B) M-mode images of effusive constrictive pericarditis from the parasternal view. [Reproduced from Jenkins T, Hoit BD. Pericardial disease. In: Nanda NC (Ed). Comprehensive Textbook of Echocardiography. New Delhi, India: Jaypee Brothers Medical Publishers (P) Ltd; 2014].

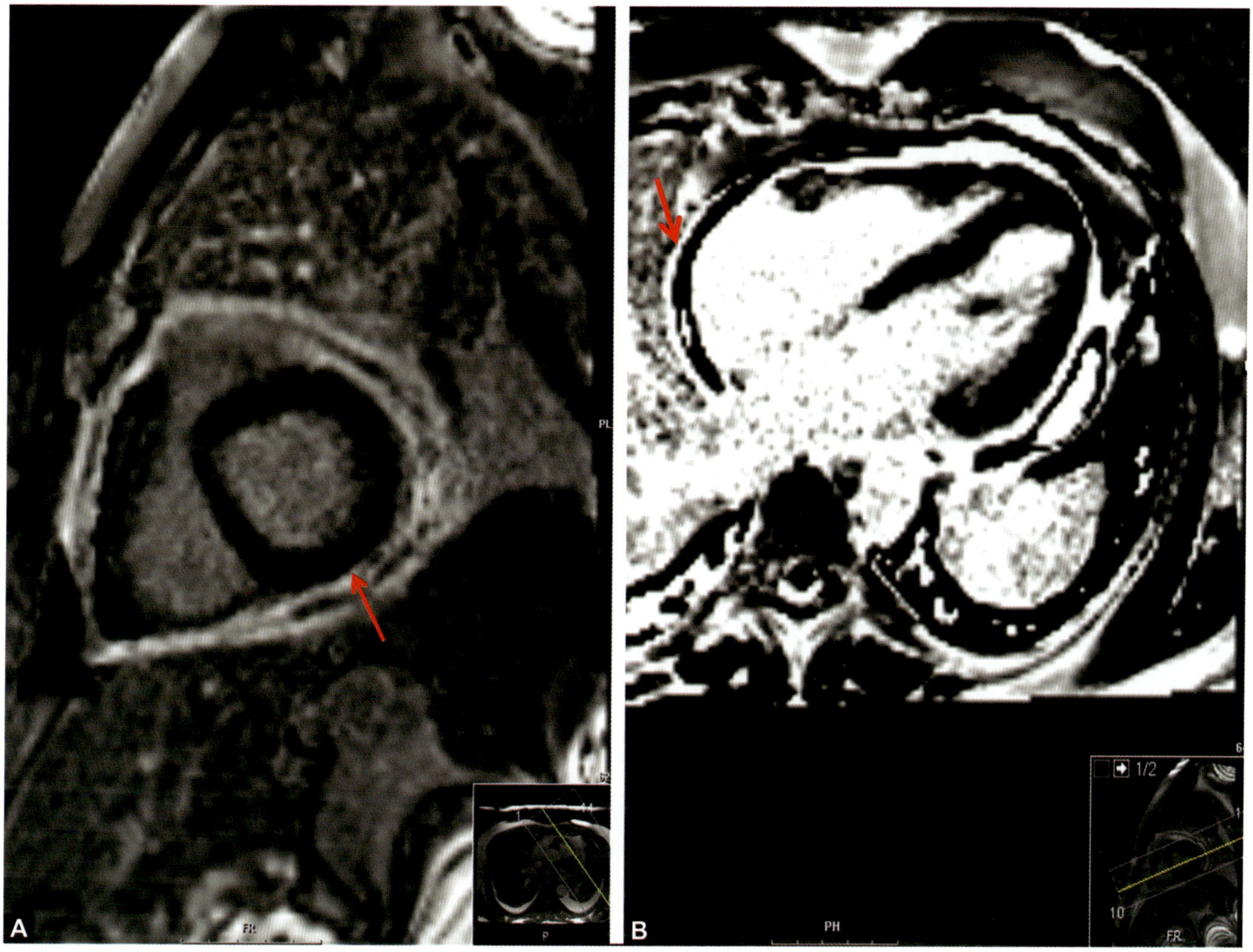

Figs. 36.14A and B: Magnetic resonance imaging (MRI) demonstrating pericardial inflammation in acute pericarditis. Delayed gadolinium-enhancement (DGE) sequences demonstrate diffuse enhancement (arrows) on inversion recovery (A) and phase-sensitive inversion recovery DGE (B) sequences. [Reproduced from Jenkins T, Hoit BD. Pericardial disease. In: Nanda NC (Ed). Comprehensive Textbook of Echocardiography. New Delhi, India: Jaypee Brothers Medical Publishers (P) Ltd; 2014].

Nonspecific blood markers of inflammation, such as the erythrocyte sedimentation rate (ESR), C-reactive protein (CRP) and the white blood cell count, usually increase in cases of acute pericarditis. Patients with extensive epicarditis occasionally have increase in serum cardiac isoenzymes suggestive of acute MI.

Imaging with cardiac magnetic resonance (CMR; Figs. 36.14 to 36.17) or cardiac computed tomography (CCT; Fig. 36.18) should be considered when there are complexities associated with the clinical presentation. They have little role in acute pericarditis but may be considered when the echo is inconclusive and there are ongoing concerns, there is a failure to respond promptly to anti-inflammatory therapy, the presentation is atypical, or when acute pericarditis occurs in the setting of cancer, lung or chest infection, or trauma. A comparison of cardiac imaging modalities in acute and chronic pericarditis are shown in Table 36.2.

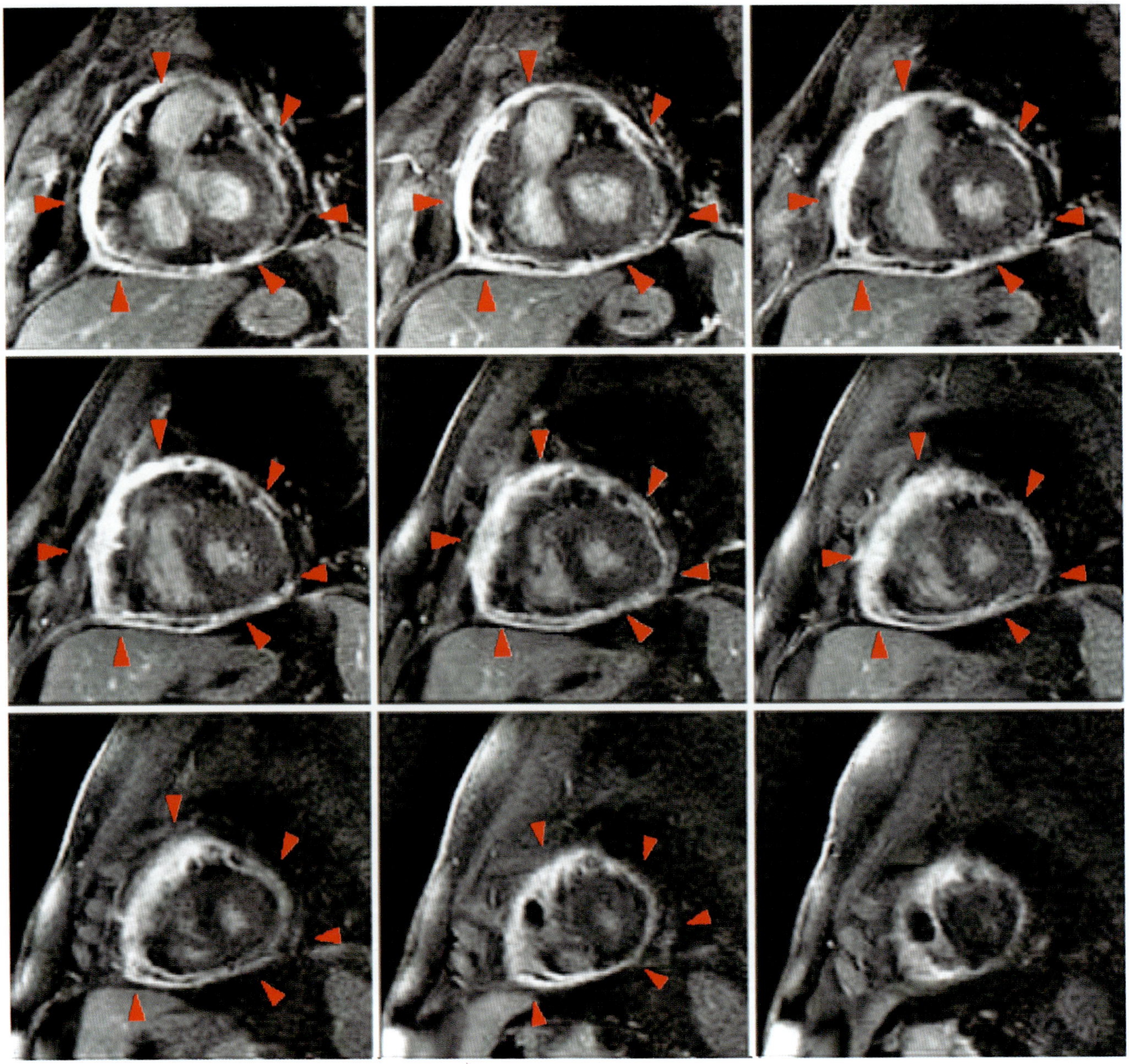

Fig. 36.15: Cardiac MRI of a patient with relapsing pericarditis. Short-axis gadolinium enhancement images demonstrate brightly enhancing pericardium (arrowheads) suggestive of pericardial inflammation. [Image and figure legend from Khandaker MH, Nishimura RA. Pericardial disease. In: Chatterjee K, Anderson M, Heistad D, Kerber RE (Eds). Cardiology: An Illustrated Textbook. New Delhi, India: Jaypee Brothers Medical Publishers (P) Ltd; 2013].

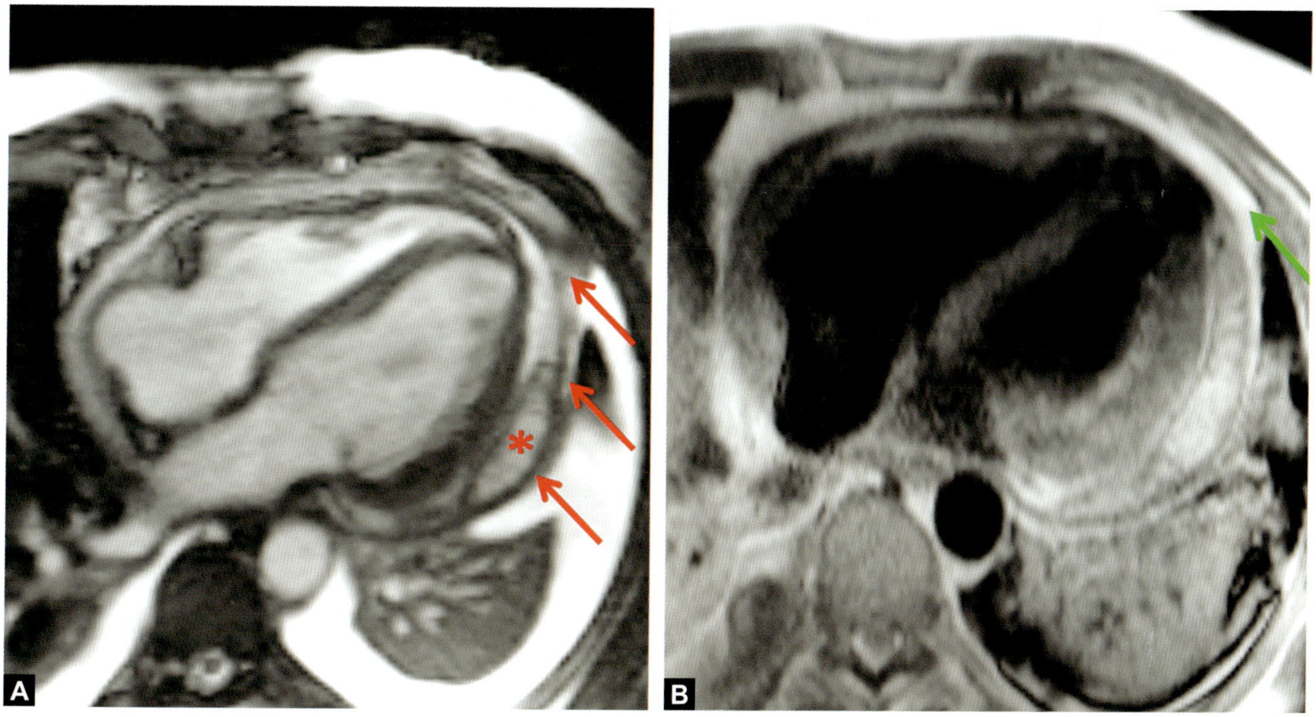

Figs. 36.16A and B: Acute effusive constrictive pericarditis evaluated by cardiac MRI. (A) Steady-state free precession (SSFP) imaging in the 4-chamber view. Note thickened parietal pericardium (red arrows) on SSFP with pericardial loculation (*); (B) T1-weighted black-blood double inversion recovery (T1 black-blood) sequences in the 4-chamber viewing window demonstrates high T1 signal within the pericardium (green arrow) suggestive of an exudative effusion.

TREATMENT OF PERICARDITIS

Treatment of pericardial disease is challenging in that there are few randomized, placebo-controlled trials from which appropriate therapy may be selected and important clinical decisions supported. Tables 36.3A and B summarize the European Society of Cardiology guidelines for the evaluation and management of patients with pericarditis.

Acute pericarditis usually responds to oral nonsteroidal anti-inflammatory drugs (NSAIDs, e.g. aspirin or ibuprofen). Colchicine, either as a supplement to the use of NSAIDs or as monotherapy, is effective for the acute episode, is well-tolerated, and may prevent recurrences. Painful recurrences of pericarditis often respond to NSAIDs but may require corticosteroids. Colchicine should be used with NSAIDs before attempting steroid therapy.

Hospitalization is warranted for many patients who present with an initial episode of acute pericarditis with high-risk features (moderate or large effusions, myopericarditis, elevated temperature, subacute onset, immunosuppression, recent trauma, oral anticoagulant therapy, and aspirin or NSAID failure) to determine the etiology and observe for cardiac tamponade; close follow-up is important in the remainder of patients not admitted to the hospital. Establishing the exact cause of acute pericarditis is an important aspect of management, but considerable judgment must be exercised in deciding whether and how to investigate the possibility of concomitant systemic disease.

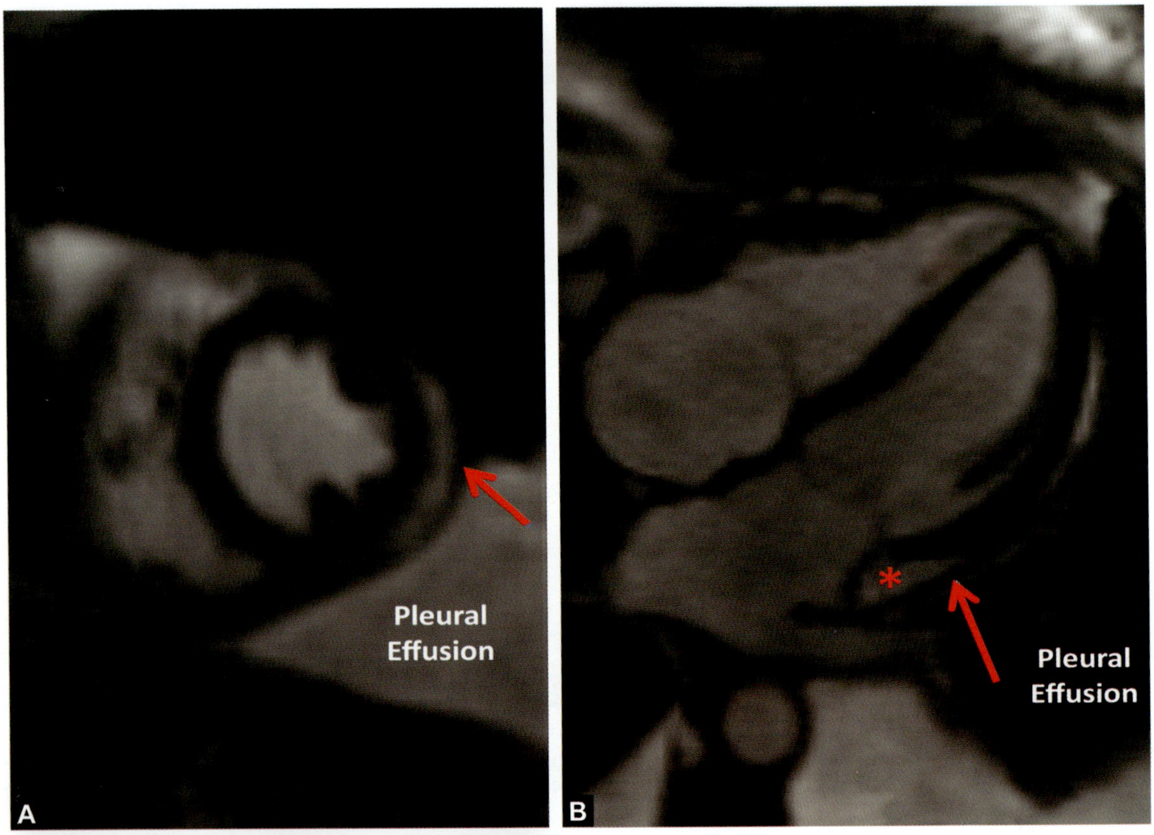

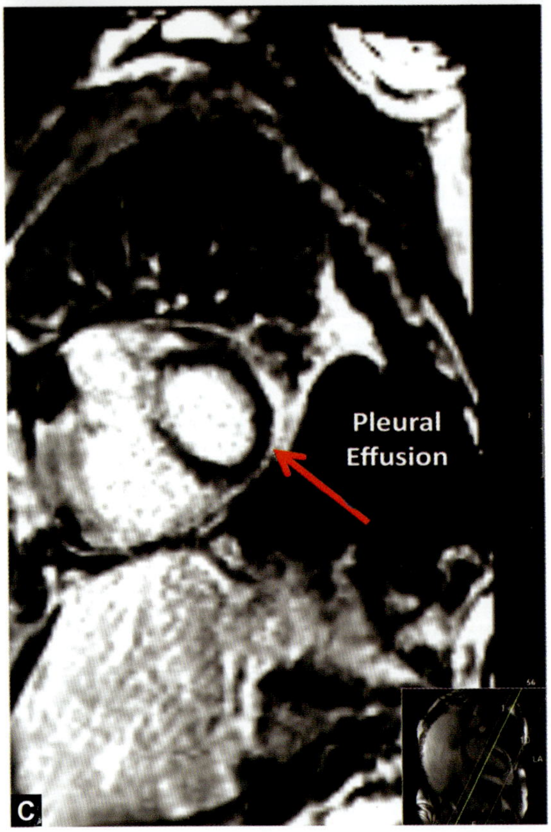

Figs. 36.17A to C: Magnetic resonance imaging (MRI) sequences of chronic constrictive pericarditis including (A) short-axis steady-state free precession (SSFP), (B) 4-chamber SSFP, and (C) phase-sensitive inversion recovery delayed gadolinium-enhancement (DGE) sequence. Chronic pericardial enhancement (arrows) is demonstrated on DGE sequence, implying persistent pericardial inflammation is present. Note large left pleural effusion and small pericardial effusion (*) in the left atrioventricular groove.

Table 36.2: Comparison of cardiac imaging modalities in evaluation of acute and chronic pericarditis. (Modified from Verhaert D, Gabriel RS, Johnston D, et al. The role of multimodality imaging in the management of pericardial disease. Cir Cardiovasc Imaging. 2010;3(3):333-43). (COPD: Chronic obstructive pulmonary disease; ECG: Electrocardiogram; ICD: Implantable cardioverter-defibrillator; TTE: Transthoracic echocardiogram).

	Echocardiography	*Cardiac computed tomography (CCT)*	*Cardiac magnetic resonance imaging (MRI)*
Strengths	• First-line imaging modality for pericardial disease • Low cost • No radiation • Readily available and portable • High temporal resolution • Noninvasive hemodynamic evaluation with Doppler echocardiography	• Anatomic evaluation of entire pericardium • First-choice imaging modality for evaluation of pericardial calcification • Evaluation of extracardiac thoracic structures • Concomitant evaluation of coronary artery anatomy	• Anatomic evaluation of entire pericardium • Evaluation of tissue inflammation with late gadolinium-enhancement (LGE) sequences • Evaluation of tissue edema with T2-weighted imaging sequences • Evaluation of ventricular interdependence on free-breathing sequences
Weaknesses	• Normal pericardium visualization impaired by low signal-to-noise ratio • TTE with limited acoustic viewing windows • Acoustic windows limited by patient body habitus (obesity) or comorbidity (COPD, postoperative state) • Operator dependent image quality acquisition • Calcification less well visualized than CT	• Requires ionizing radiation and iodinated intravenous contrast • Requires breath-holding for image acquisition • Hemodynamically stable patients only • Image quality dependent on ECG-gating (arrhythmia or tachycardia degrades spatial resolution)	• High cost • Time intensive • Less readily available • Requires breath-holding for some sequence acquisition • Hemodynamically stable patients only • Calcification less well visualized than CT • Contraindicated for most types of pacemaker or ICD • Gadolinium contrast contraindicated in patients with advanced kidney disease (glomerular filtration rate < 30 mL/min)

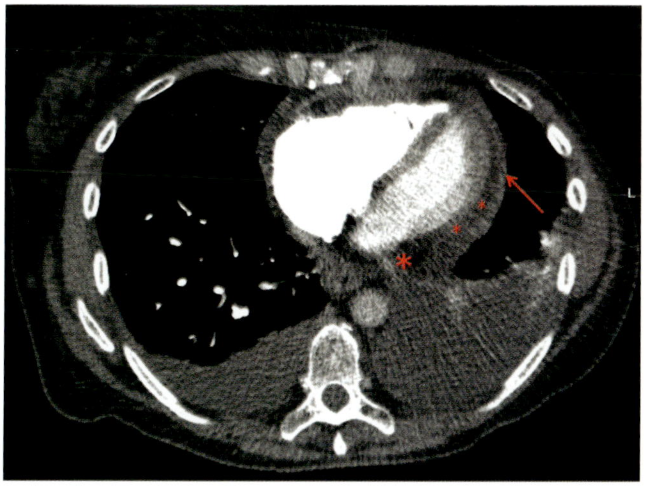

Fig. 36.18: Axial computed tomography (CT) with contrast demonstrates a diffusely thickened pericardium (arrow) and small pericardial effusion (*) in a patient with chronic pericarditis. Note concomitant moderate to large bilateral pleural effusions.

Table 36.3A: Summary of recommendations for acute pericarditis diagnostic evaluation from the European Society of Cardiology (ESC) 2004 guidelines on the diagnosis and management of pericardial heart disease. (CK-MB: Creatine kinase-MB; CRP: C-reactive protein; ESR: Erythrocyte sedimentation rate; LDH: Lactate dehydrogenase; LOE: Level of evidence; MR: Mitral regurgitation; TTE: Transthoracic echocardiogram; WBC: White blood cell).

Class I (is recommended; is beneficial)
• Cardiac auscultation MR (LOE = B)
• Electrocardiogram (LOE = B)
• Echocardiography (TTE) (LOE = B)
• Blood analysis [troponin, CK-MB, ESR, CRP, LDH, leukocyte count (WBC)] (LOE = B)
• Chest X-ray (LOE = B)
Class IIa (is reasonable)
• Cardiac CT or cardiac MRI (LOE = B)

Table 36.3B: Summary of recommendations for acute and chronic pericarditis therapeutic interventions from the European Society of Cardiology (ESC) 2004 guidelines on the diagnosis and management of pericardial heart disease. (LOE: Level of evidence; NSAIDs: Nonsteroidal anti-inflammatory drugs).

Acute Pericarditis
Class I (is recommended; is beneficial)
• NSAIDS (LOE = B)
Class IIa (is reasonable)
• Colchicine (LOE = B)
• Systemic corticosteroids (LOE = B)
Recurrent Pericarditis
Class I (is recommended; is beneficial)
• Colchicine (LOE = B)
Class IIa (is reasonable)
• Systemic corticosteroids (LOE = C)
• Pericardiectomy (LOE = B)
Chronic Pericarditis
Class IIb (can be considered)
• Balloon pericardiotomy or pericardiectomy (LOE = B)

VIDEO LEGENDS

Video 36.1: Parasternal long-axis transthoracic echocardiography (TTE) demonstrating a circumferential pericardial effusion in a patient with pericarditis.

Video 36.2: Pericardial effusion imaged in the parasternal long axis view in a patient with suspected pericarditis.

Video 36.3: Apical 4-chamber transthoracic echocardiography (TTE) in a patient with pericarditis demonstrating a circumferential pericardial effusion.

REFERENCES

Feng D, Glockner J, Kim K, et al. Cardiac magnetic resonance imaging pericardial late gadolinium enhancement and elevated inflammatory markers can predict the reversibility of constrictive pericarditis after antiinflammatory medical therapy: a pilot study. Circulation. 2011;124(17):1830-7.

Hoit BD. Diseases of the pericardium. In: Fuster V, Walsh RA (Eds). Hurst's The Heart, 13th edition. New York: McGraw-Hill; 2011. pp. 1917-39.

Klein AL, Abbara S, Agler DA, et al. American Society of Echocardiography clinical recommendations for multimodality cardiovascular imaging of patients with pericardial disease: endorsed by the Society for Cardiovascular Magnetic Resonance and Society of Cardiovascular Computed Tomography. J Am Soc Echocardiogr. 2013;26(9):965-1012.

Maisch B, Seferović PM, Ristić AD, et al. Guidelines on the diagnosis and management of pericardial diseases executive summary; The Task force on the diagnosis and management of pericardial diseases of the European society of cardiology. Eur Heart J. 2004;25(7):587-610.

Peebles CR, Shambrook JS, Harden SP. Pericardial disease—anatomy and function. Br J Radiol. 2011;84(Spec No 3): S324-37.

Verhaert D, Gabriel RS, Johnston D, et al. The role of multimodality imaging in the management of pericardial disease. Circ Cardiovasc Imaging. 2010;3(3):333-43.

CHAPTER

37

Pericardial Effusion

Faisal F Syed, Nandan S Anavekar, William D Edwards, Jae K Oh

INTRODUCTION

The normal pericardium is a thin, avascular sac which encompasses the heart and a portion of the adjoining great vessels (Fig. 37.1). Its two layers, the visceral and parietal pericardium, are separated by a potential space containing 10–50 mL of lubricating ultrafiltrate.

Pericardial effusion is the accumulation of fluid within the pericardial space (Figs. 37.2 to 37.4, Videos 37.1 to 37.4). The etiology is protean and mainly depends on the epidemiological setting and clinical risk factors (Table 37.1). Most pericardial effusions in the developed world are noninfectious, with common causes including idiopathic, autoimmune, neoplastic, metabolic (especially hypothyroidism and renal failure), infectious, traumatic and, increasingly, iatrogenic pericarditides (after an invasive procedure). In patients living in tuberculosis-endemic regions, a pericardial effusion without apparent cause is likely to be tuberculous until proven otherwise.

HEMODYNAMIC SEQUELAE

With increasing pericardial fluid accumulation, a rising pressure within the pericardial space compresses the

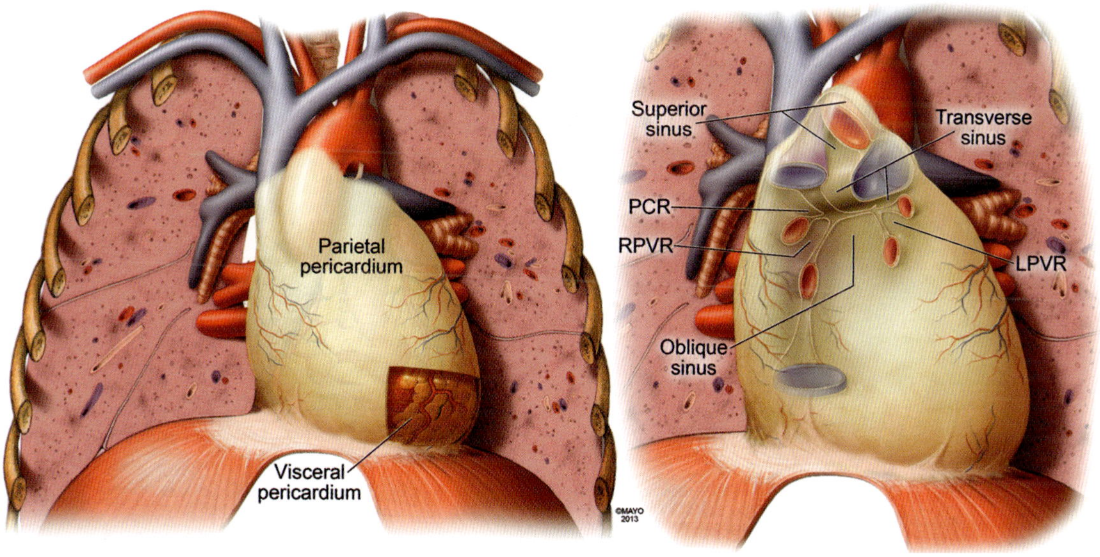

Fig. 37.1: The normal visceral pericardium is a cellular monolayer adherent to the myocardium which reflects onto the fibrous parietal pericardium to form the double-walled pericardial sac (left panel). The fibrous pericardium fuses with the adventitia of the great vessels superiorly and posteriorly, and has ligamentous attachments to the sternum anteriorly and diaphragmatic central tendon inferiorly. Its reflections form potential spaces at the back of the heart known as pericardial sinuses (right panel). In addition to a small amount of pericardial fluid, the pericardial space also houses the coronary vessels, autonomic ganglia, and epicardial fat, which is usually co-localized with the vessels and ganglia, likely serving a protective function. The phrenic nerves travel either side between the pleurae and fibrous pericardium and provide sensory fibers to the pericardium. Knowledge of related anatomy is important to avoid damage to related structures during pericardiocentesis, in particular the pleurae, lungs, internal thoracic vessels, intercostal nerves/vessels, liver, diaphragm, and myocardium.

heart and impairs cardiac filling in diastole, resulting in the syndrome of pericardial tamponade, the hemodynamic hallmarks of which are pulsus paradoxus (a fall in systolic blood pressure > 10 mm Hg with inspiration) and loss of the *y*-descent in the atrial waveform (Figs. 37.5 to 37.7). Intracardiac filling pressures become elevated as a compensatory response such that diastolic cardiac pressures equalize to the level of the increased intrapericardial pressure. With progressive failure of compensatory mechanisms, ventricular stroke volume is reduced, systemic pulse pressure falls, tachycardia develops and subsequently systemic hypotension develops.

The hemodynamic effect of the effusion is determined by its volume, rate of accumulation, and the patient's intravascular volume status, such that a continuum exists between no significant hemodynamic effect, increasing degrees of hemodynamic compensation, and severe tamponade with hypotension (usually with intrapericardial pressure > 15–20 mm Hg). Slowly, accumulative effusions allow for adaptive pericardial changes which blunt intrapericardial pressure elevation, whilst abrupt tamponade can occur when the fluid accumulation is rapid, such as with cardiac perforation or aortic dissection (Fig. 37.8). With intravascular volume depletion, low-pressure tamponade occurs without elevated filling pressures (i.e. normal jugular venous pressure). The effusion may be loculated and exert regional pressure with atypical hemodynamic effects (Figs. 37.9A and B). A typical clinical example is one after a cardiac surgical procedure. Pneumopericardium can also result in tamponade and is usually the result of gas-forming bacterial pericarditis as a result of penetrating trauma, but can be seen early in the evolution of atrial esophageal fistula following atrial fibrillation ablation. Effusive-constrictive pericarditis is seen when a pericardial effusion is associated with constriction of the visceral pericardium, such that intracardiac pressures remain elevated after removal of pericardial fluid and normalization of intrapericardial pressure (Fig. 37.10). This condition is relatively common after pericardiocentesis and often self-limiting, typically resolving within 2–3 months, but a minority of patients can develop chronic constrictive pericarditis.

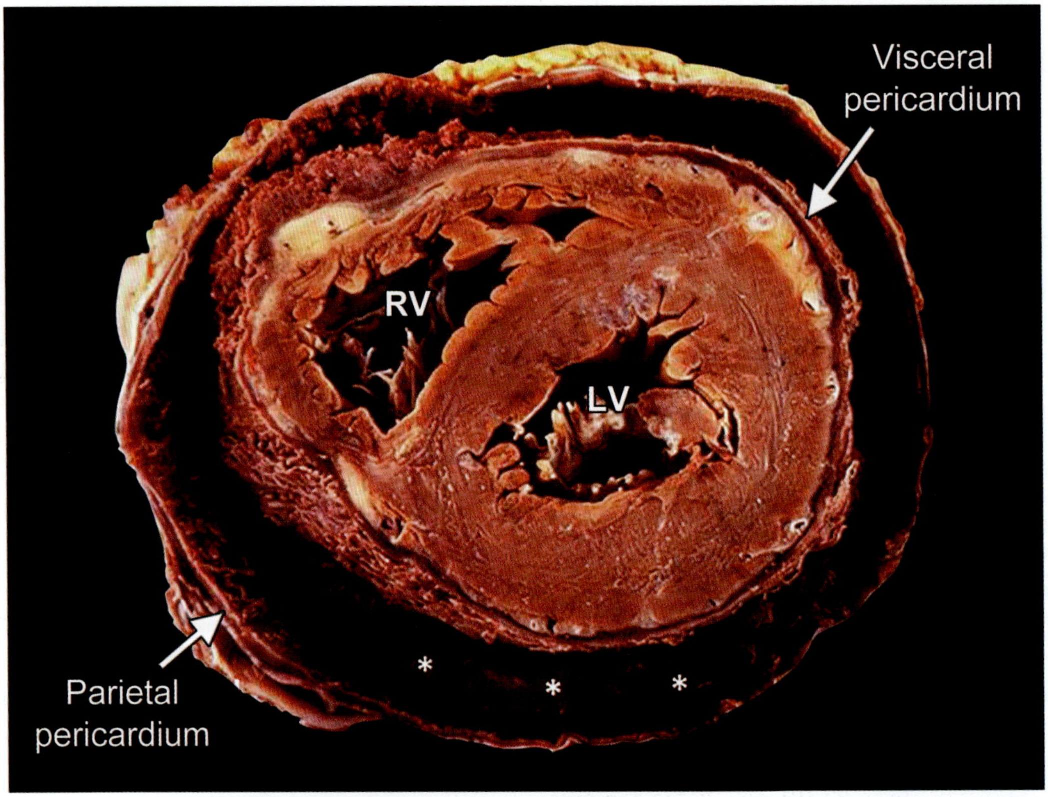

Fig. 37.2: Postmortem specimen demonstrating pericardial effusion (white stars). The gross appearance of the pericardial fluid may vary from serous, serosanguinous, frankly hemorrhagic, purulent or chylous, depending on etiology. Application of Light's criteria is the most reliable method to identify exudative from transudative effusions [whereby an exudate is defined as having one or more of the following: pericardial fluid protein divided by serum protein > 0.5; pericardial fluid lactate dehydrogenase (LDH) divided by serum LDH > 0.6; and/or pericardial fluid LDH level > two-thirds the upper limit of normal for serum LDH].

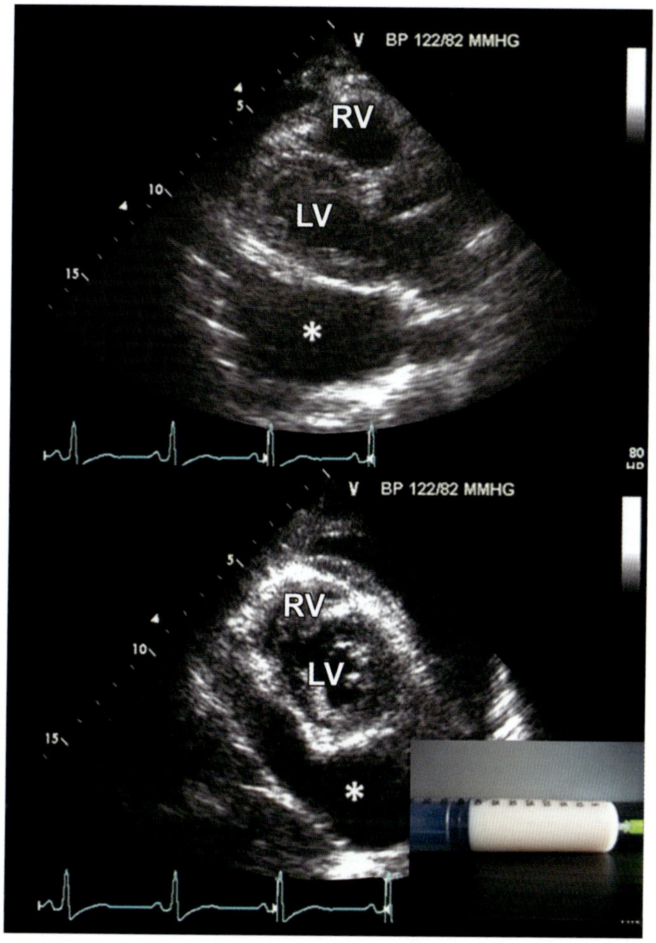

Fig. 37.3: A case of chylous pericardial effusion caused by occlusion of the proximal thoracic duct immediately below the junction of the subclavian and jugular veins. Echocardiography demonstrated a large pericardial effusion (white stars). Approximately 500 mL of milky pericardial effusion were aspirated (right lower inset) and laboratory analysis was consistent with a chylous effusion. The patient was successfully treated with surgical reanastomosis of the thoracic duct to the left internal jugular vein.

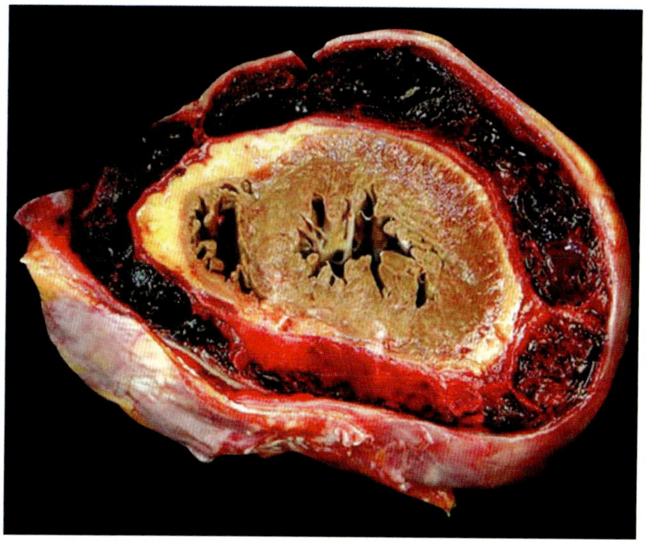

Fig. 37.4: Gross pathology of a patient with hemopericardium. (Image courtesy of Dr William D Edwards, Mayo Clinic. Image and legend text from Khandaker MH, Nishimura RA. Pericardial disease. In: Chatterjee K, Anderson M, Heistad D, Kerber RE (Eds). Cardiology: An Illustrated Textbook. New Delhi, India: Jaypee Brothers Medical Publishers (P) Ltd.; 2012).

APPROACH TO DIAGNOSIS

Larger pericardial effusion may be suspected based on ECG (Figs. 37.11A and B) and chest X-ray (Fig. 37.12) findings. Given its ease of detection, pericardial effusion was the first clinical indication of echocardiography (Fig. 37.13). Currently, echocardiography is the investigational modality of choice as it detects both the presence and size of effusion (Figs. 37.14 and 37.15), its hemodynamic effect (Figs. 37.16 to 37.19), echogenic contents within the pericardium that serve as clues to etiology (Figs. 37.20A to C), and the presence of additional cardiac disease (Figs. 37.21A and B). For example, in acute tamponade from pericardial hemorrhage, such as with aortic dissection or contained cardiac rupture, echocardiography may demonstrate the causative lesion as well as a coagulated mass within the pericardium. Although CT is used in suspected cases of constrictive pericarditis to assess for pericardial thickening, it is generally not indicated for the evaluation of pericardial effusion. However, when an effusion is identified incidentally (Figs. 37.22A to C), the larger field of view offered by CT serves to better evaluate loculated effusions and related structures in the lungs and mediastinum, and may identify an associated neoplasm or infection. Cardiac MRI (Fig. 37.23) is increasingly being used in the evaluation of inflammatory pericardial disease and when an incidental effusion is discovered, it may offer similar additional information.

Evaluation of etiology is best guided by background epidemiology and clinical presentation. Pericardiocentesis is generally indicated for relief of tamponade, chronic (>1 month) large pericardial effusions, or for suspicion of infectious and neoplastic pericardial effusion, with appropriate testing of pericardial fluid. At a minimum, such testing of pericardial fluid includes aerobic and tuberculosis cultures, cytology, cell counts, hemoglobin and chemistry (protein, specific gravity, glucose and lactate dehydrogenase), with additional tests as indicated by the clinical and epidemiological setting. For example, if suspicion for tuberculous pericarditis is high, further

Table 37.1: Etiology of pericardial effusion. (Modified from Imazio M, Adler Y. Management of pericardial effusion. Eur Heart J. 2013;34:1186-97). (EBV: Epstein-Barr virus; CMV: Cytomegalovirus; HBV: Hepatitis B virus; HCV: Hepatitis C virus; HIV: Human immunodeficiency virus; HHV-6: Human herpes virus 6).

Cause	***Examples***
	Infectious
Viral	Echovirus, coxsackievirus, influenza, EBV, CMV, adenovirus, varicella, rubella, mumps, HBV, HCV, HIV, parvovirus B19, HHV-6
Bacterial	*Mycobacterium tuberculosis*, *Coxiella burnetii*, pneumococcus, meningococcus, gonococcus, hemophilus, staphylococci, chlamydia, mycoplasma, legionella, leptospira, listeria
Fungal	Histoplasma, aspergillosis, blastomycosis, candida
Parasitic	Echinococcus, toxoplasma
	Non-infectious
Idiopathic	A proportion of these may be viral
Connective tissue disease	Systemic lupus erythematosus, Sjögren syndrome, rheumatoid arthritis, systemic sclerosis, systemic vasculitides, Behcet syndrome, sarcoidosis, familial mediterranean fever
Pericardial injury syndromes	Postpericardiotomy syndrome, postmyocardial infarction, post-traumatic
Primary neoplastic	Teratoma, mesothelioma, sarcoma, primary cardiac lymphoma, fibrosarcoma, lymphangioma, hemangioma, neurofibroma, lipoma
Secondary metastatic tumors	Lung carcinoma, breast carcinoma, leukemia, lymphoma, melanoma, Kaposi sarcoma, esophageal carcinoma
Metabolic	Renal failure, hypothyroidism, hypoalbuminemia
Trauma	Thoracic injury, esophageal perforation, iatrogenic
Radiation	Cance radiation therapy
Drugs and toxins (lupus-like syndrome)	Procainamide, hydralazine, isoniazid, phenytoin
Hypersensitivity	Hypersensitivity pericarditis with eosinophilia—penicillins
Drug-Induced cardiomyopathy ± pericardial disease	Doxorubicin and daunorubicin
Medications	Minoxidil
Hemodynamic	Heart failure, pulmonary hypertension

tests include adenosine deaminase, interferon-gamma, pericardial lysozyme, and TB-PCR. Pericardial biopsy is generally reserved for persistence without a defined etiology utilizing pericardioscopy or when creating a pericardial window for recurrent tamponade.

In the era of echocardiography, invasive right heart catheterization is now only rarely performed to make the diagnosis of tamponade physiology. The finding of equalization of pressures (Fig. 37.24) in a patient with pericardial effusion is suggestive of tamponade physiology, and characteristic changes in atrial and arterial pressure waveforms should be looked for (Fig. 37.5).

PERICARDIOCENTESIS

The most effective therapy for cardiac tamponade is removal of pericardial fluid. Even a small amount of fluid removal (50–200 mL) is effective in reducing intrapericardial pressure enough to relieve tamponade, although usually the effusion is gradually drained to completion using an indwelling pericardial catheter. Depending on etiology and the clinical circumstance, removal of pericardial fluid can be achieved by percutaneous catheter pericardiocentesis (Fig. 37.25), balloon or surgical pericardiotomy (with creation of a pericardial window) or upon

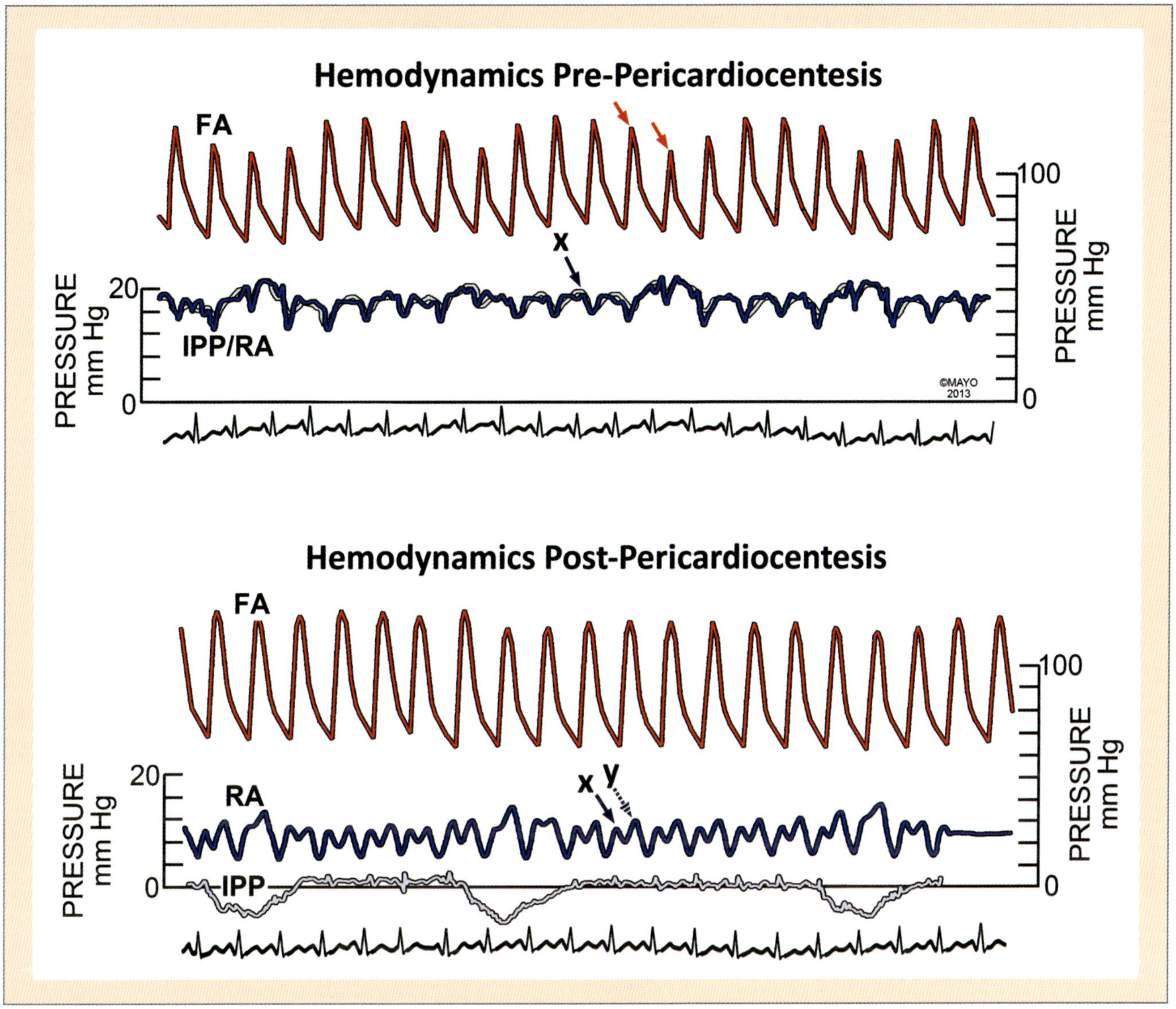

Fig. 37.5: Hemodynamic study in a patient with cardiac tamponade before and (B) after treatment with pericardiocentesis. In tamponade, there is elevation and equalization of right atrial (RA) and intrapericardial pressures (IPP). Although not shown, the pulmonary capillary wedge pressure and pulmonary artery diastolic pressure are also usually equal to within 4–5 mm Hg, cardiac output is reduced, and systemic vascular resistance is elevated. In advanced stages, hypotension is typical, whilst in the early stages of acute tamponade, there may be hypertension due to sympathetic activation. The hemodynamic hallmarks of tamponade are pulsus paradoxus, as observed here in the femoral artery tracing (FA, red arrows), and blunting or loss of the *y* descent in the atrial waveform (absent dashed blue arrow in top tracing). There may also be a more prominent atrial *a* wave in patients in sinus rhythm. The *x* descent (solid blue arrow) is preserved because ventricular systole results in temporary reduction in atrial and IP pressures, with atrial filling becoming restricted to this phase of the cardiac cycle as tamponade progresses. The *y* descent becomes blunted or absent as diastolic ventricular filling is restricted throughout the cardiac cycle by the pericardial fluid ("elastic" form of compression), as compared to constriction in which the *y* descents are prominent because restriction to filling only occurs once the heart exceeds a critical size ("inelastic" form of compression). On account of this, the ventricular diastolic dip and plateau (the "square root" sign), characteristic of pericardial constriction, is not seen in tamponade. Equal elevation of diastolic pressures may also be seen with dilated cardiomyopathy and right ventricular infarction. After pericardiocentesis, the pericardial pressure is normalized and becomes subatmospheric in inspiration, right atrial pressure is reduced with normalization of the *x* descent re-appearance of the *y* descent (dashed blue arrow), and pulsus paradoxus is no longer present. (Modified from Goldstein JA. Cardiac tamponade, constrictive pericarditis, and restrictive cardiomyopathy. Curr Probl Cardiol. 2004;29:503-67).

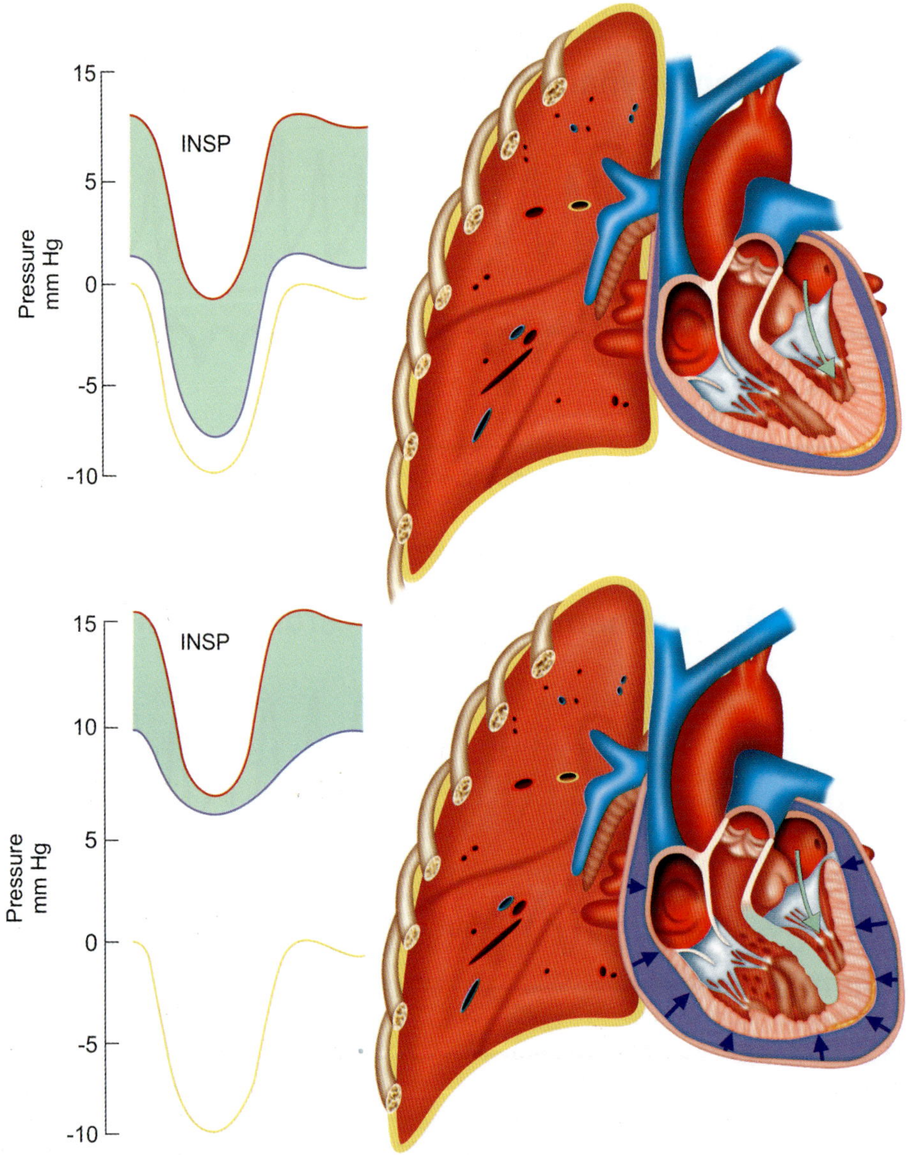

Fig. 37.6: Mechanisms underlying pulses paradoxus, ventricular interdependence and respiratory changes in trans-mitral and trans-tricuspid blood flow velocities. Top Figure represents the situation when an effusion results in no change to normal hemodynamics. Intrathoracic pressure changes (yellow) during normal ventilation are transmitted to both the pericardial space (blue) and pulmonary veins/left atrium (red). Therefore, during normal ventilation, the pressure gradient between the atria and pericardial space (green tracing) and consequently blood flow into the ventricles (green arrow) varies little with ventilation. The translation of these ventilatory changes to beat-beat systolic blood pressure is complex, but in healthy individuals, systolic blood pressure declines no more than 10 mm Hg during quiet inspiration. Bottom Figure represents the situation in tamponade, with pericardial fluid exerting significant pressure on the heart (small blue arrows). Ventilatory changes in thoracic pressures are not transmitted to the pericardial space (i.e. there is disassociation of intrathoracic and intracardiac pressures). With inspiration, a decrease in intrathoracic pressures is transmitted via the pulmonary veins to the left atrium, resulting in decreased left atrial pressure. However, pericardial pressure changes little, such that in inspiration the left atrial-pericardial pressure gradient and consequently left ventricular filling is reduced. Consequently, mitral valve opening is delayed, which lengthens the isovolumic relaxation time (IVRT) and decreases mitral E velocity. Opposite changes on the right occur, with inspiratory augmentation of systemic venous return, increased transtricuspid flow and velocity, and increased right heart volumes. The reduced left ventricular filling in combination with limited expansion of the right ventricular free wall due to the increased intrapericardial pressure results in shift of the interventricular septum to the left in inspiration. These changes in pressure, blood flow velocities, ventricular filling and chamber volumes are reversed in expiration. [Image reproduced with permission from Oh JK, Tajik AJ, Seward JB. Pericardial Diseases. In: Oh JK, Seward JB, Tajik AJ (Eds). The Echo Manual, 3rd edition. Philadelphia: Lippincott Williams & Wilkins; 2006. pp. 289-309]. (INSP: Inspiration).

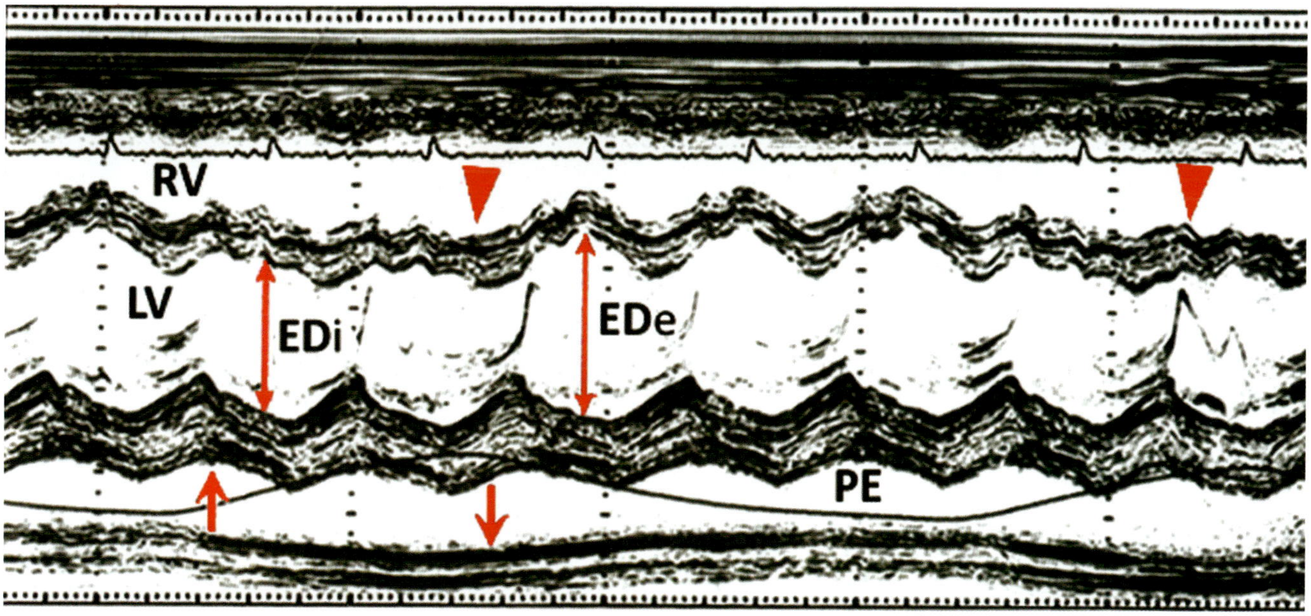

Fig. 37.7: Echocardiographic M-mode recording demonstrating the reciprocal changes in ventricular dimensions with ventilation in tamponade, with simultaneous respirometer tracings at the bottom (undulates up in inspiration and down in expiration). With tamponade, there is interventricular dependence such that the left ventricular (LV) dimension during inspiration (EDi) becomes smaller than with expiration (EDe), whilst the opposite changes occur in the right ventricle (RV). These changes in ventricular dimensions result in shift of the interventricular septum (arrowheads) to the left in inspiration and right in expiration. [Image reproduced with permission from Oh JK, Tajik AJ, Seward JB. Pericardial Diseases. In: Oh JK, Seward JB, Tajik AJ (Eds). The Echo Manual, 3rd edition. Philadelphia: Lippincott Williams & Wilkins; 2006. pp. 289-309]. (PE: Pericardial effusion).

surgical pericardiectomy. Percutaneous catheter pericardiocentesis, on account of being less invasive and less expensive, is the usual treatment of choice and can be performed using the parasternal, subxiphoid or apical approaches. Unless the clinical situation demands an immediate, blind attempt via the subxiphoid approach, echocardiographic or fluoroscopic guidance is used. At Mayo Clinic, pericardiocentesis is almost always performed under echocardiographic guidance, with selection of optimal site of puncture depending on the most significant site of fluid location, distance from transducer and interposed anatomical structures. In 60–70% of the cases, an apical location is optimal for pericardiocentesis. Agitated saline contrast administration is helpful in locating the position of the catheter or needle. At some centers, a right-heart cardiac catheterization is performed at the time of pericardiocentesis to measure right atrial pressure, which is useful in the diagnosis of effusive constrictive pericarditis. However, hemodynamic evaluation by echocardiography, which is equally diagnostic for persistent constrictive features, can avoid the right-heart catheterization.

Potential complications vary depending on technique and include myocardial puncture or laceration, coronary vascular damage, cardiac arrhythmias (usually vasovagal-mediated bradycardia), air embolism, liver or diaphragm laceration, pneumothorax or hemothorax, laceration of the internal thoracic, intercostal, inferior phrenic or subxiphoid fat tissue arteries, puncture of the peritoneal cavity or abdominal viscera, and purulent pericarditis. Reflex left ventricular systolic dysfunction and pulmonary edema can usually be avoided by taking care not to remove too much fluid at once (generally not more than 1 L at a time). In the case of aortic dissection leading to tamponade, pericardiocentesis can lead to further deterioration and is usually avoided unless absolutely necessary to stabilize the patient for emergency surgical aortic repair.

OTHER CONSIDERATIONS IN PATIENTS WITH CARDIAC TAMPONADE

Intravascular volume expansion serves as an adjunctive temporizing therapy in patients in cardiac tamponade, but is not a substitute in itself for therapeutic pericardiocentesis. Mechanical ventilation can lead to further hemodynamic compromise in the patient in cardiac tamponade by increasing intrathoracic pressure and thereby reducing venous return to the right heart.

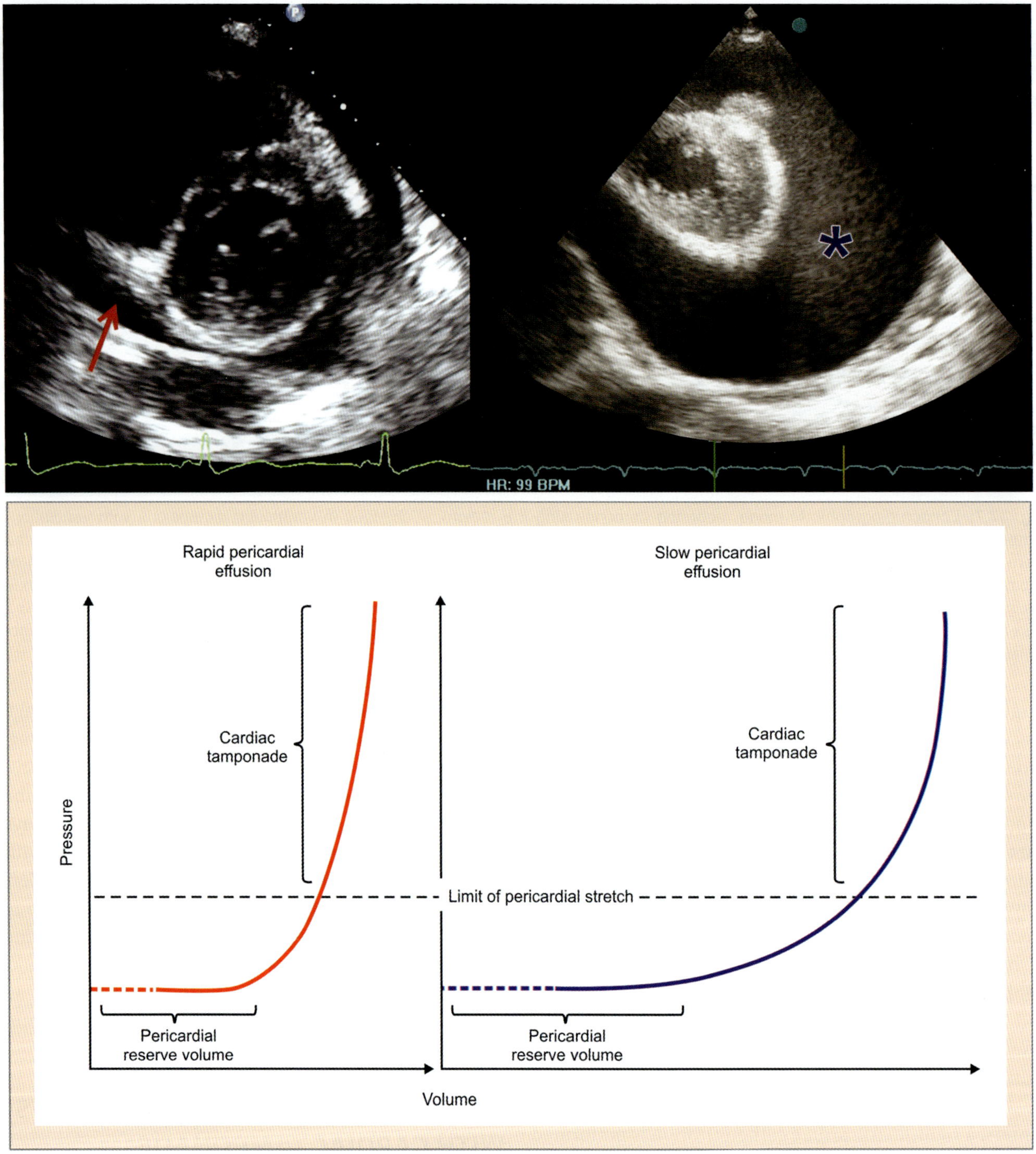

Fig. 37.8: Both echocardiographic images are short-axis views taken from the parasternal window from patients with cardiac tamponade. Left is from a patient who developed acute pericardial effusion (arrow) from right ventricular perforation upon temporary pacemaker wire insertion. Right is from a patient with tuberculous pericarditis which results in gradual pericardial fluid (blue star) accumulation. (Image courtesy of Professor Bongani Mayosi, Department of Medicine, The University of Cape Town, South Africa). Underneath are the representative hemodynamic representations, which indicate that in chronically accumulating effusions, pericardial remodeling allows for greater pericardial reserve volumes and blunts the rise in pericardial pressure. Once the volume exceeds the limit of pericardial stretch, even a small subsequent increase in pericardial fluid result in large increases in pressure. [Adapted from Oh JK, Tajik AJ, Seward JB. Pericardial Diseases. In: Oh JK, Seward JB, Tajik AJ (Eds). The Echo Manual, 3rd edition. Philadelphia: Lippincott Williams & Wilkins; 2006. pp. 289-309].

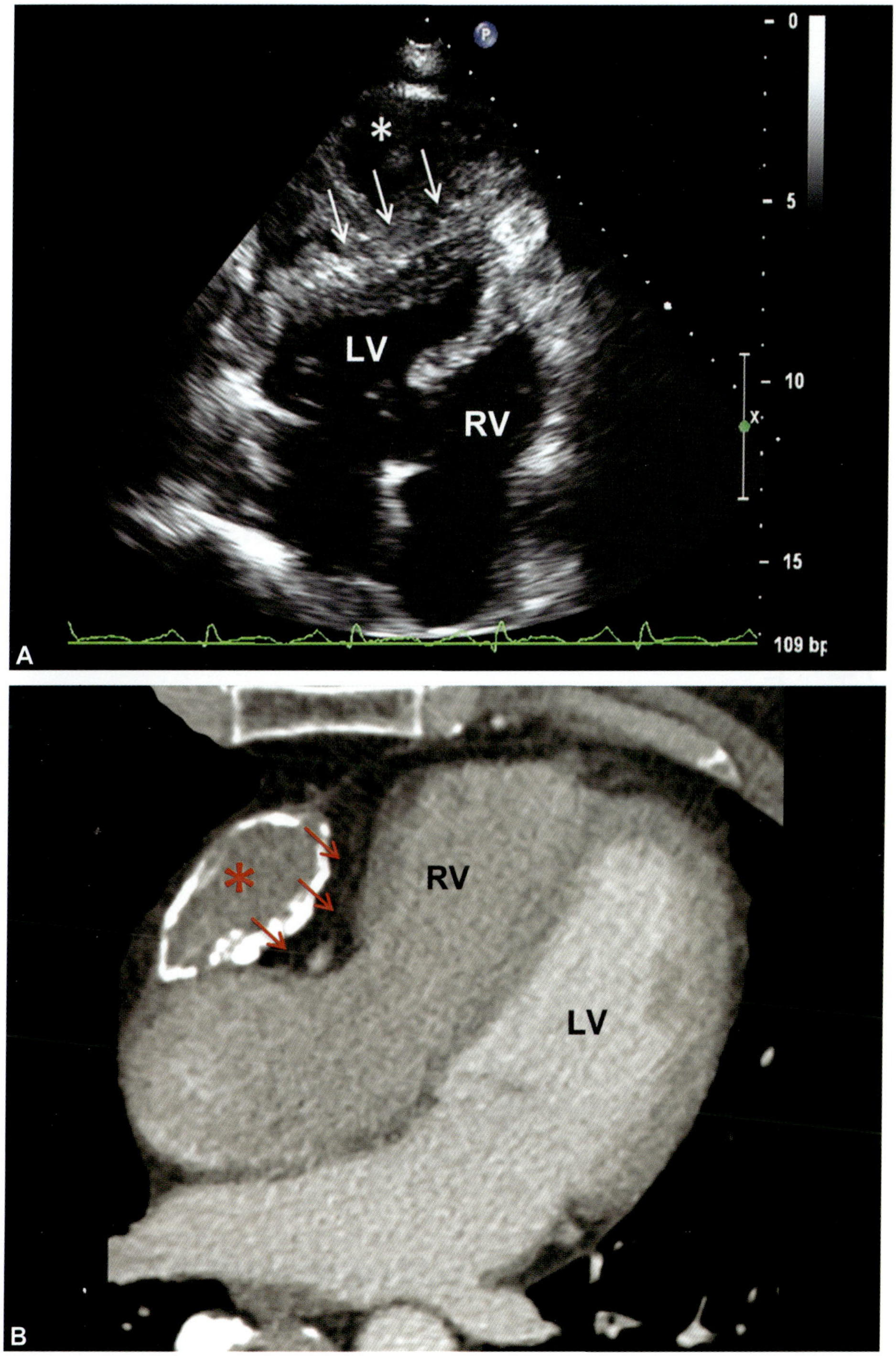

Figs. 37.9A and B: Regional tamponade. (A) Echocardiographic image from apical four-chamber view in a patient with an inhomogeneous mass and loculated effusion which was causing localized compression of the left ventricle (white arrows). Surgical pericardiectomy was performed. Histology demonstrated high-grade angiosarcoma. (B) CT image demonstrating a non-enhancing mass in the pericardium near the right ventricular free wall with peripheral calcification in a patient with a history of precordial trauma, likely represents a calcified hematoma (red star) causing regional tamponade effect on the right ventricle (red arrows). Localized pericardial and intramural hematomas have been known to compress cardiac chambers causing obstructive symptoms. Other scenarios associated with regional tamponade include following cardiac surgery or other postoperative settings. Posteriorly located effusions adjacent to the atria pose challenges for detection by echocardiography and suspected in patients with hemodynamic instability following cardiac surgery. (LV: Left ventricle; RV: Right ventricle).

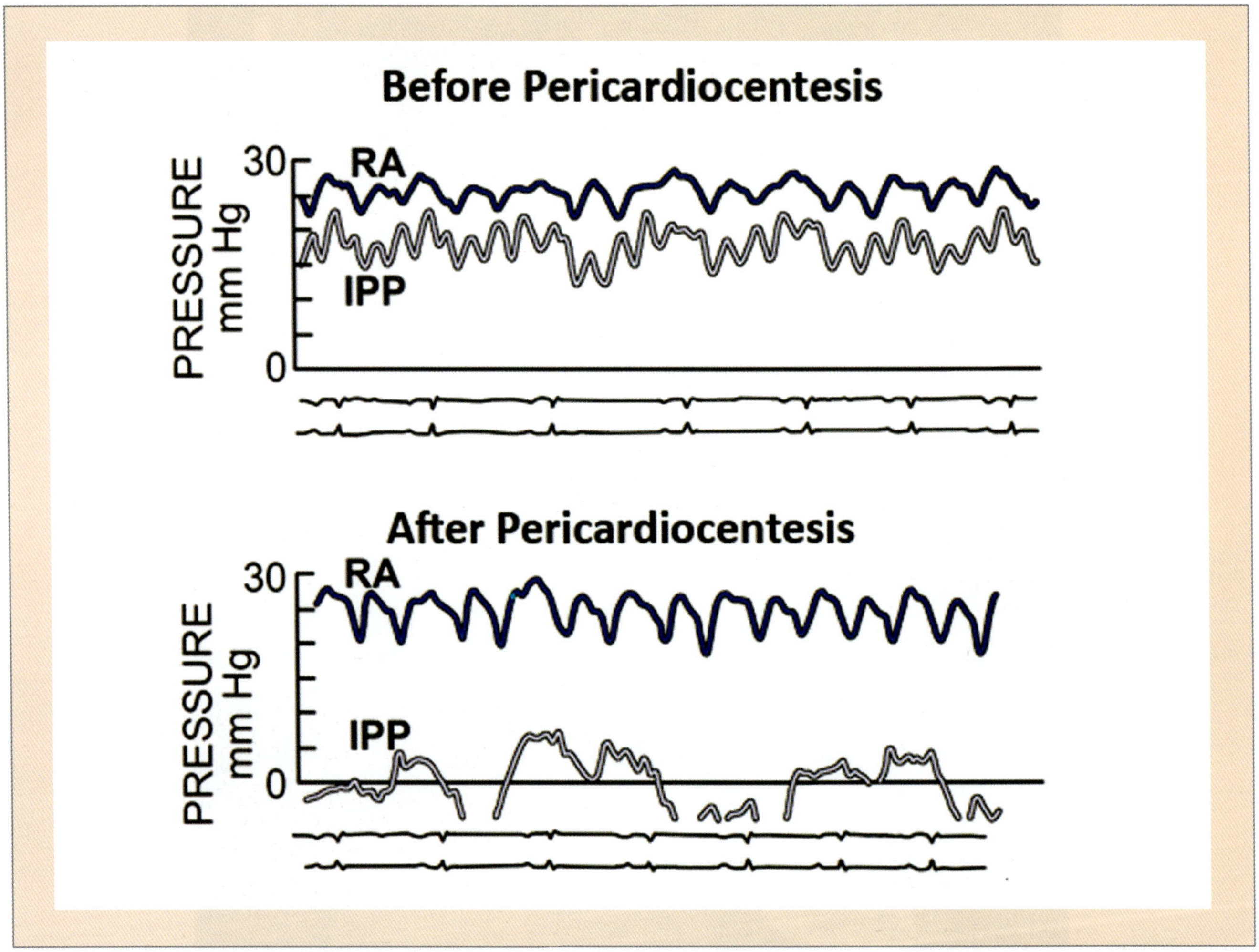

Fig. 37.10: A case of tuberculous effusive-constrictive pericarditis. (Upper panel) Before pericardiocentesis, both right atrial (RA) and intrapericardial pressures (IPP) are elevated. (Lower panel) After pericardiocentesis, IPP is normalized and but the RA pressure is unchanged, because there is constriction at the level of the visceral pericardium. When assessed in this manner (i.e. with simultaneous IPP/RA pressure measurements during pericardiocentesis), approximately 8% of patients with tamponade have underlying effusive-constrictive pericarditis in developed countries, whilst in contemporary series of tuberculous pericarditis in the developing world, the prevalence has been reported at 38%. Clinically, there are no features which reliably distinguish pure effusive from effusive-constrictive disease, although patients may have clinical features of both these entities, for example, with the overt fluid retention and pericardial knock (or early third heart sound) typical of constrictive pericarditis in combination with pulsus paradoxus and jugular venous (JVP) waveform that are seen with tamponade. There are also no specific echocardiographic features, the presence of septal dysmotility and restrictive ventricular filling typical of constrictive pericarditis may be present in addition to the findings of pericardial effusion and chamber collapse that are seen with tamponade. In most patients, however, the diagnosis is suspected when there is persistent JVP elevation after successful pericardiocentesis and confirmed upon repeat hemodynamic echocardiographic assessment when typical findings of constrictive pericarditis are found [abnormal ventricular septal motion due to interventricular dependence, respiratory variation of mitral inflow velocities, late-diastolic flow reversals in the hepatic vein with expiration, and normal or augmented medial early diastolic velocity (e') which is higher than that of the lateral mitral e'].

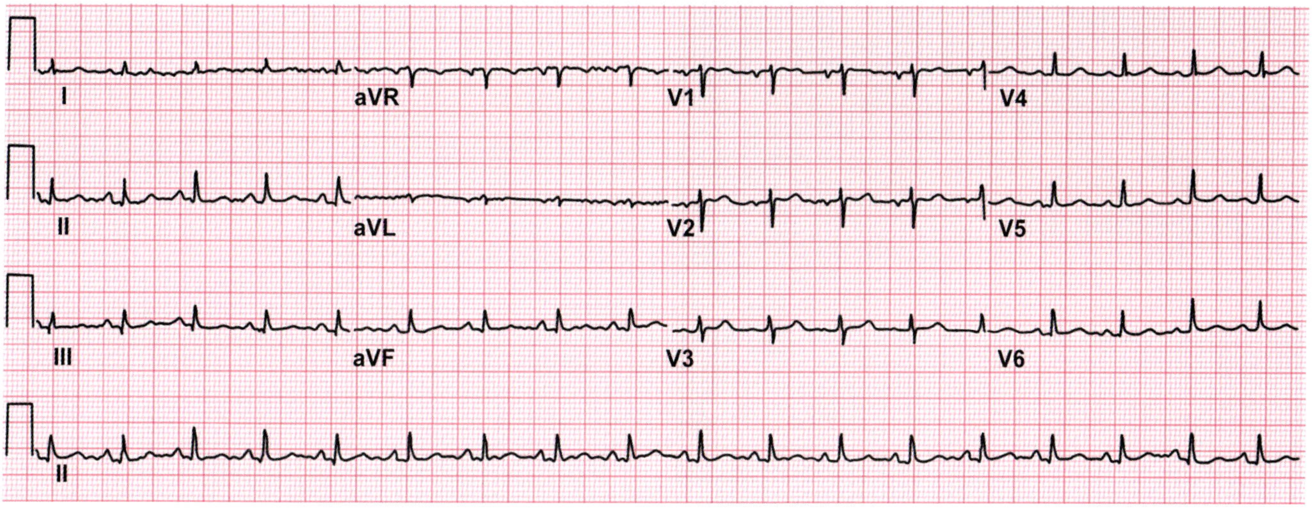

Fig. 37.11A: The electrocardiogram in pericardial effusion. The 12 lead ECG shows the typical findings of microvoltage in both precordial leads (maximum QRS amplitude < 1 mV) and limb leads (maximum QRS amplitude < 0.5 mV). Microvoltage is more common in larger effusions. Different mechanisms have been proposed including increased distance due to the effusion, mechanical effects of the fluid on the myocardium, and reduction of cardiac size and volume. Normalization of QRS voltage may not be immediate upon pericardiocentesis and may take a few days.

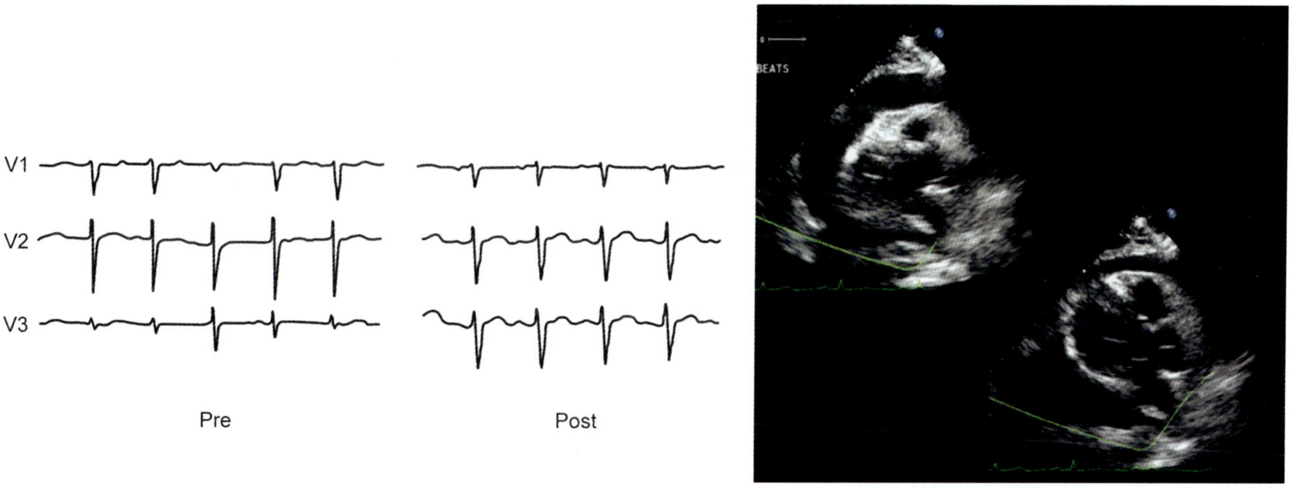

Fig. 37.11B: An example of electrical alternans. Electrical alternans, defined as beat to beat alterations in QRS amplitude or axis, is generally held to be specific but not sensitive for tamponade. It reflects the swinging motion of the heart in pericardial fluid, as demonstrated in the accompanying echocardiographic still frames.

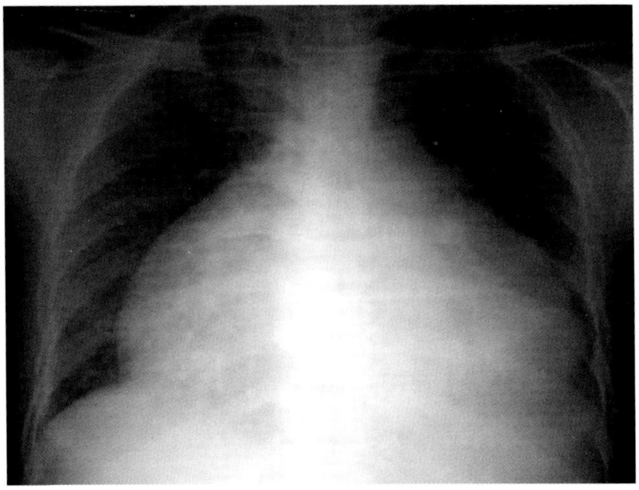

Fig. 37.12: The chest X-ray in a case of tuberculous pericardial effusion. Although in acute tamponade, there are usually no significant findings on chest X-ray, in chronic effusions, the cardiac silhouette starts to enlarge when more than 200 mL of fluid accumulates. Unlike the increased cardiac silhouette that accompanies dilated cardiomyopathy, the heart takes on a globular appearance with a "water-bottle" configuration, and there is paucity of pulmonary vascular markings. In cardiomyopathy, there is usually pulmonary congestion, unless there is associated severe tricuspid regurgitation. Although a number of other specific but insensitive signs have been described upon careful inspection of the chest X-ray in pericardial effusions, the advent of more advanced imaging has generally superseded this modality for confirming the diagnosis. (Image courtesy of Professor Bongani Mayosi, Department of Medicine, The University of Cape Town, South Africa).

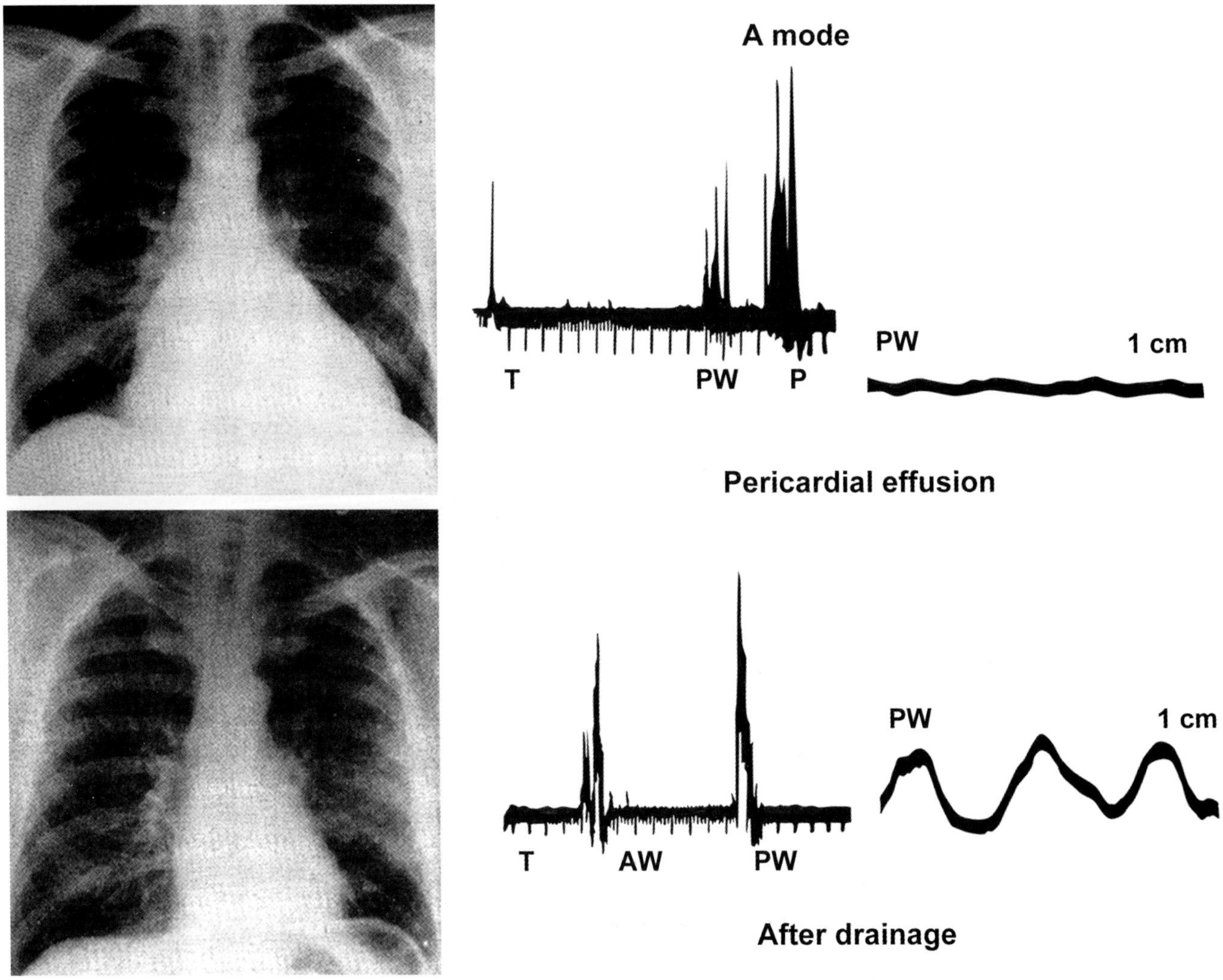

Fig. 37.13: First report of detecting pericardial effusion by echocardiography, using A-mode echocardiography. [Reproduced with permission from Feigenbaum H, Waldhausen JA, Hyde LP. Ultrasound diagnosis of pericardial effusion. JAMA. 1965;191(9):711-4]. (P: Pericardial effusion; PW: Posterior wall of the heart).

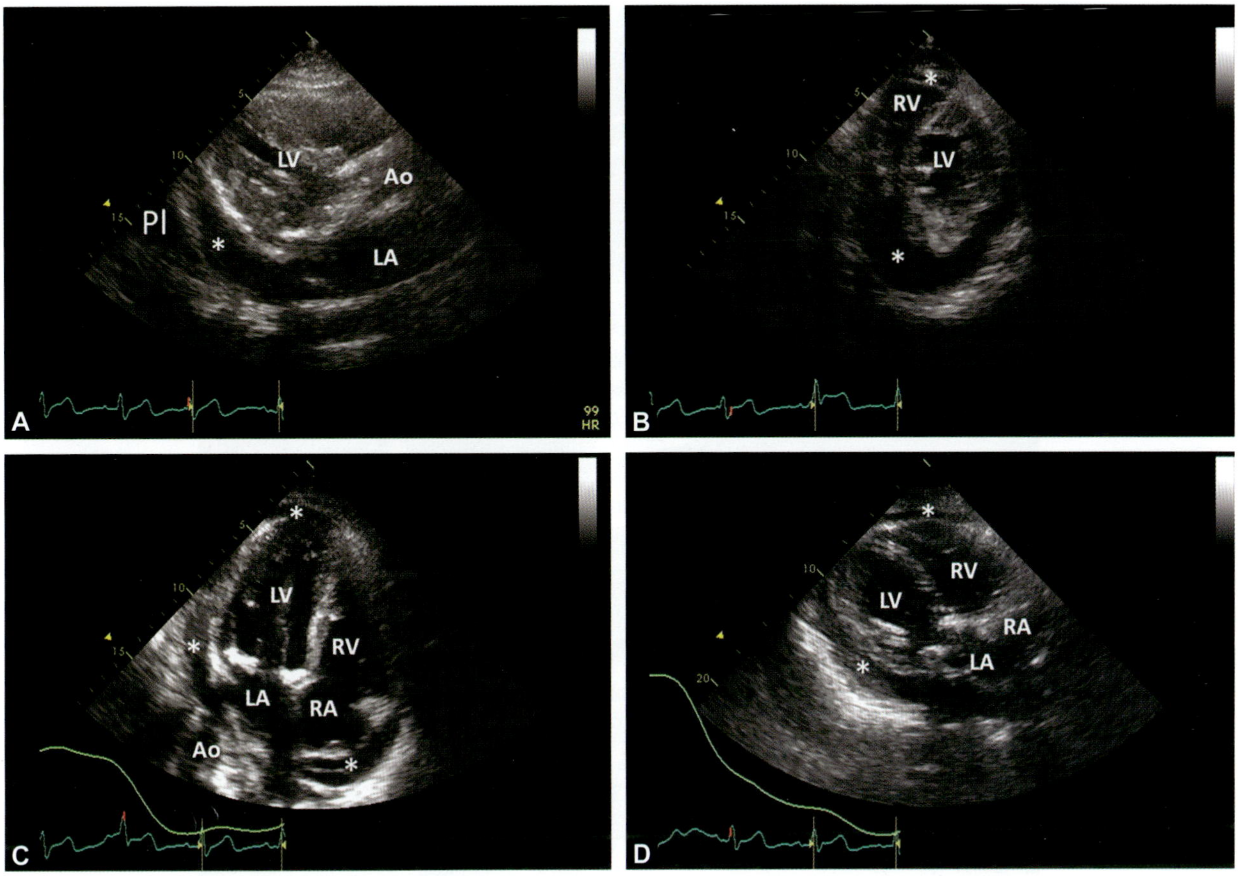

Figs. 37.14A to D: Echocardiographic appearances of a large circumferential pericardial effusion (white star) shown in standard echocardiographic windows: (A) parasternal long axis, (B) parasternal short axis, (C) apical long axis and (D) subcostal. As seen in this example, the effusion is often larger posteriorly due to the effects of gravity, whilst small effusions first become apparent in this location. The size of the effusion can be classified by its maximum depth in diastole (e.g. small < 1 cm, moderate 1–2 cm, large > 2 cm. (Ao: Aorta; LA: Left atrium; LV: Left ventricle; Pl: Pleural effusion; RA: Right atrium; RV: Right ventricle).

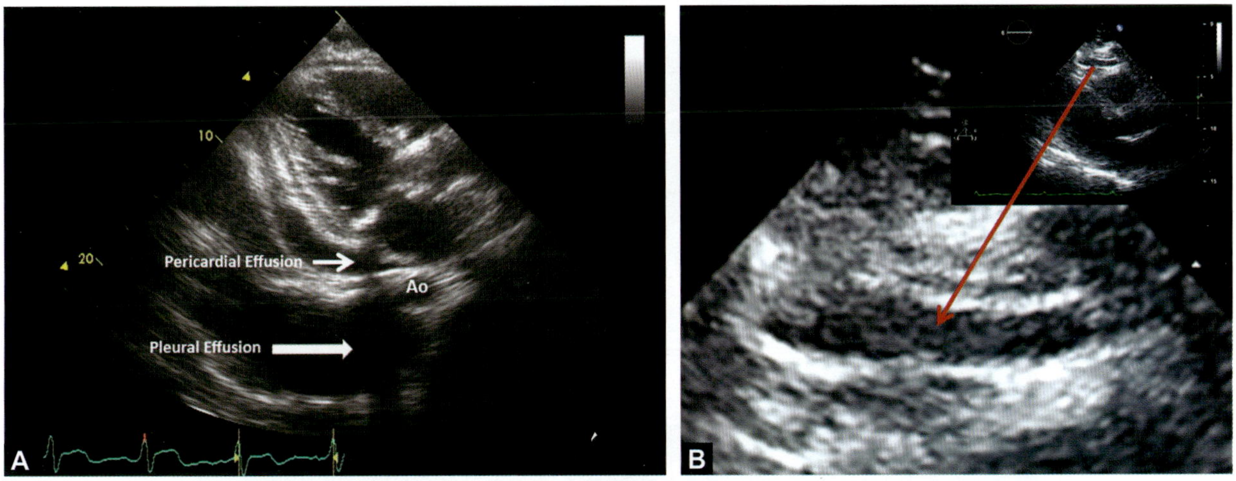

Figs. 37.15A and B: Caveats in the diagnosis of pericardial effusion on echocardiography. Both Figures A and B are standard parasternal long axis views of the heart. (A) Both a pericardial effusion (slim arrow) and pleural effusion (thick arrow) are present. The two effusions can be distinguished in relation to the descending aorta (Ao), an extra-pericardial structure. Pericardial effusions therefore do not pass posterior to this structure, whereas pleural effusion do. (B) A thick layer of epicardial fat mimics pericardial effusion. Clues to this being fat are its "starry night" appearance and fixed dimensions during the cardiac cycle, as opposed to effusions which usually have increased diameter in diastole.

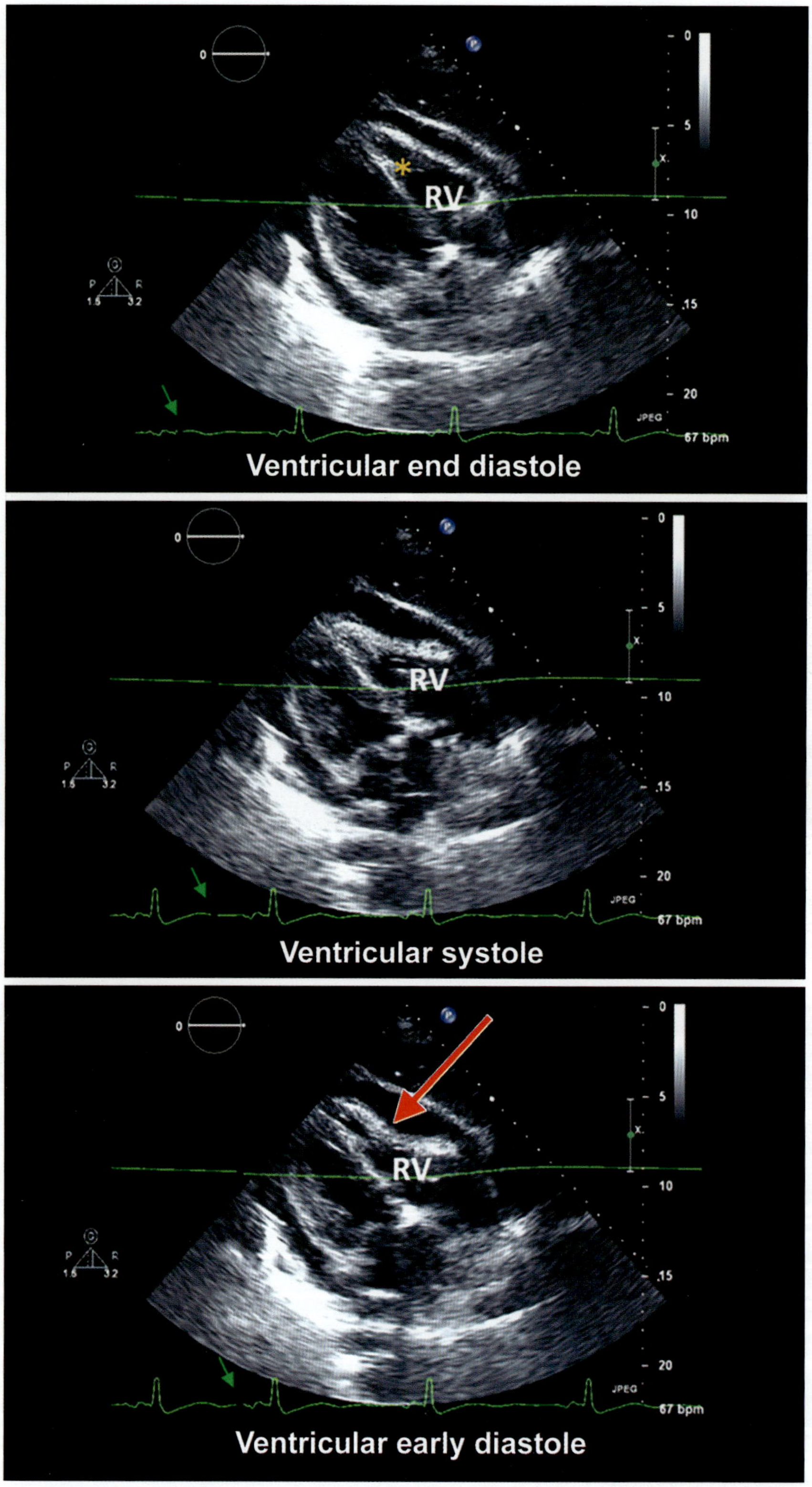

Fig. 37.16A: Right ventricular collapse in cardiac tamponade. Two-dimensional features of tamponade: early diastolic collapse of the right ventricle (arrow), when the intrapericardial pressure exceeds intracavitary pressure. Reported sensitivity is 48–100%, and specificity 72–100%. Note the temporary wire (yellow star) which resulted in right ventricular perforation causing tamponade.(RV: Right ventricle).

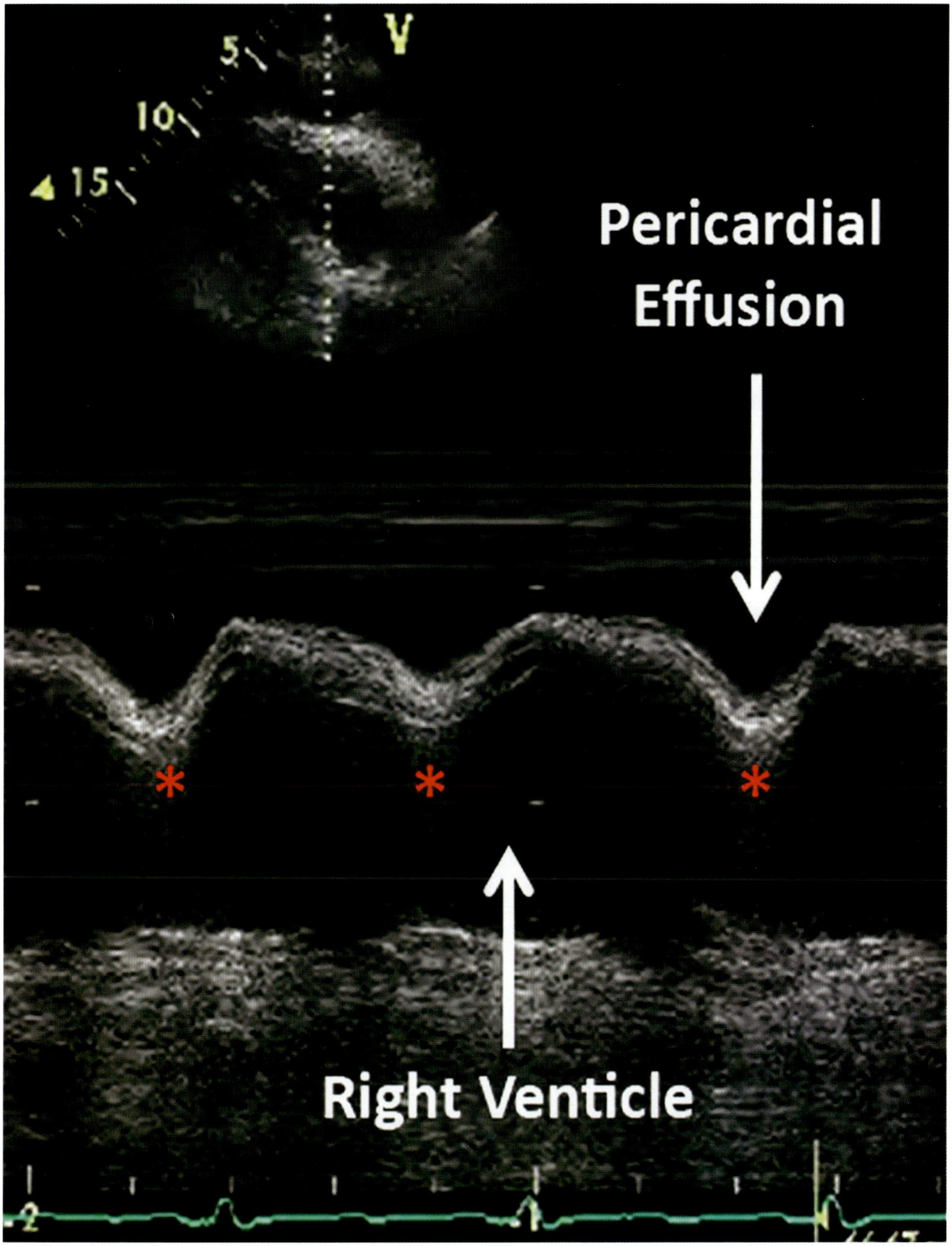

Fig. 37.16B: Right ventricular collapse in cardiac tamponade. Demonstration of right ventricular diastolic collapse (red stars) by M-mode echocardiography. Note the timing of collapse in relation to the cardiac cycle by comparing it to the ECG tracing (green).

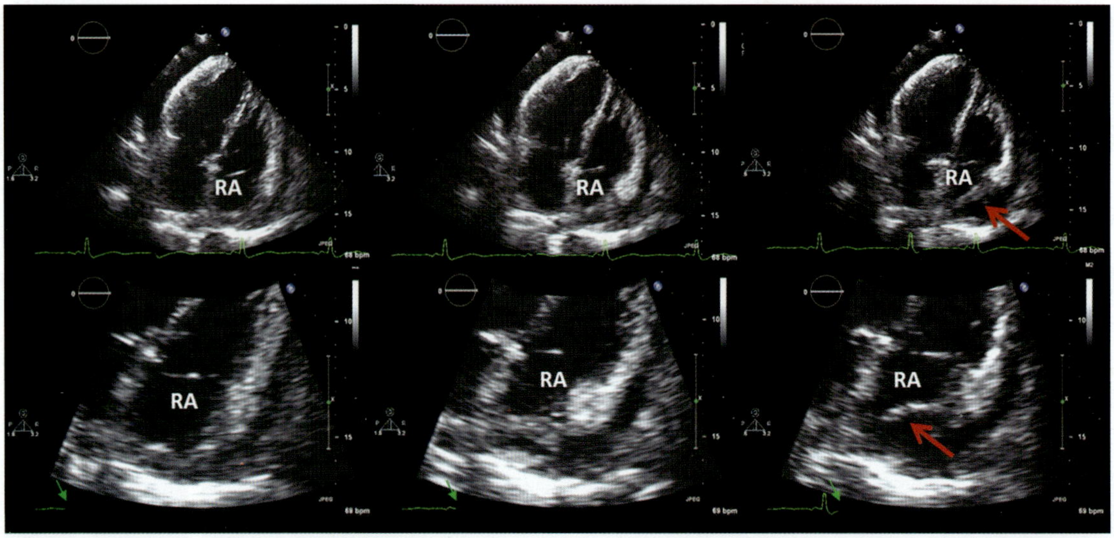

Fig. 37.17: Two-dimensional features of tamponade: right atrial (RA) collapse. This occurs at the time of ventricular systole (atrial diastole), when right atrial pressure falls (x descent) and is exceeded by intrapericardial pressure. In general, this is a more sensitive but less specific sign of tamponade than RV diastolic collapse. However, when the duration of RA collapse exceeds a third of the cardiac cycle, sensitivity is > 90% and specificity 100%. Collapse of the left atrium is rare, but when it occurs, it is highly specific for tamponade. Left ventricular collapse is rare because of the muscular nature of the LV wall. Other two-dimensional findings include ventricular interdependence (see Fig. 37.7) and IVC dilatation (see Fig. 37.18). Note images are displayed using the "Mayo Clinic" format with the right-sided heart chambers on the right of the image display.

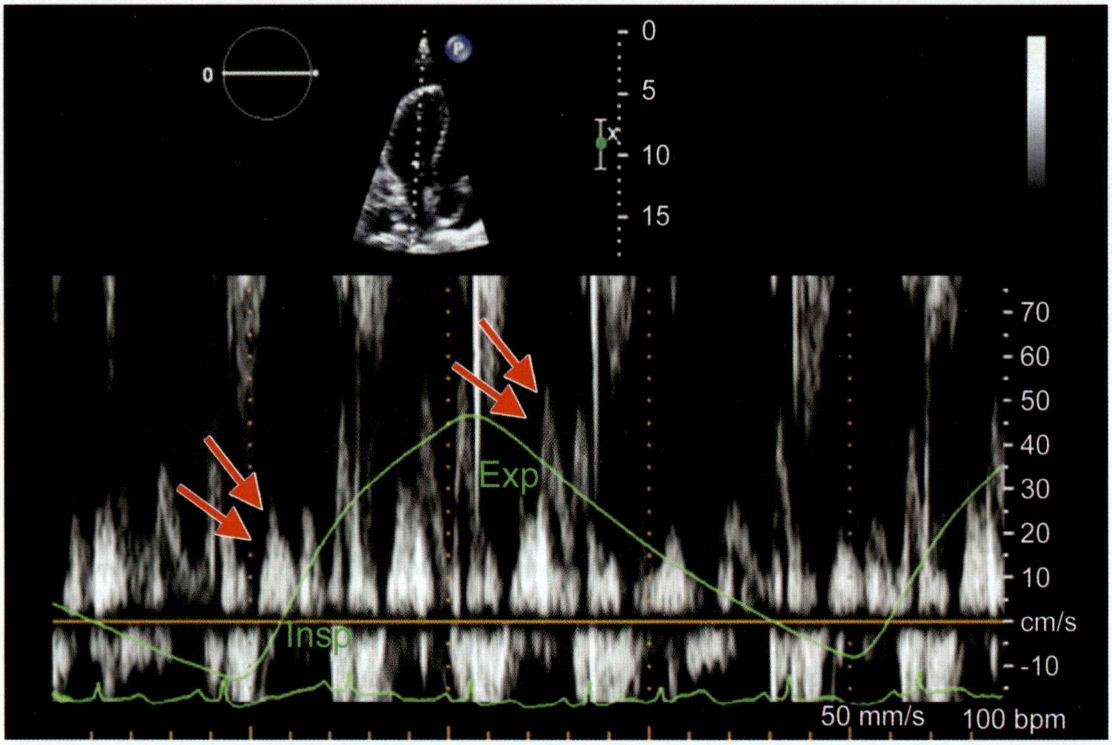

Fig. 37.18: Doppler features of tamponade: transmitral velocities. There is blunted early ventricular filling (reduced initial E velocity), and disassociation between intracardiac and intrathoracic pressures as evidenced by reduced transmitral E velocity (arrows) in inspiration as compared to expiration. The opposite changes occur across the tricuspid valve. Further explanation is provided in Figure 37.3. The Doppler features of cardiac tamponade precede the two-dimensional findings, changes in cardiac output, and changes in blood pressure.

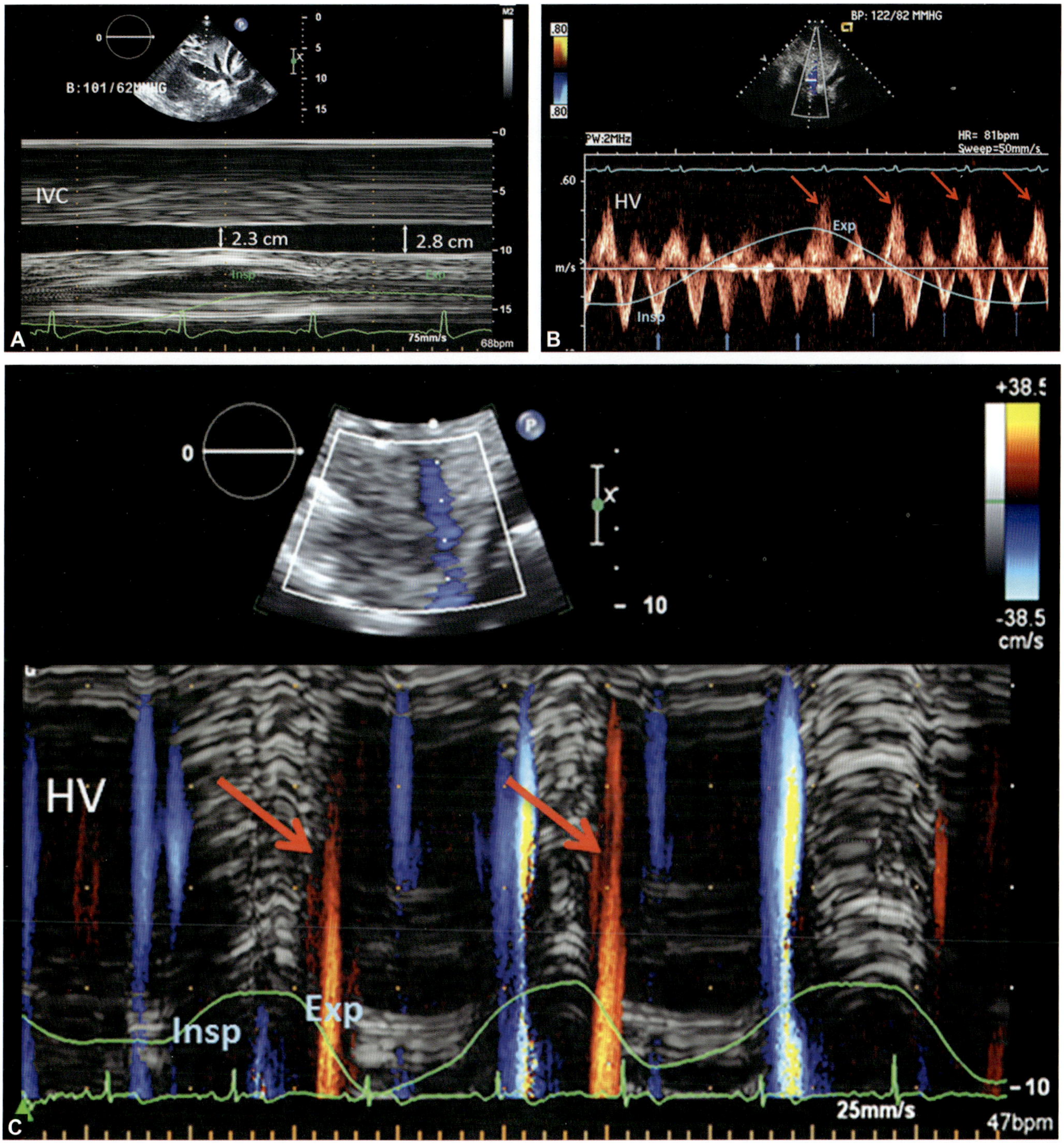

Figs. 37.19A to C: The inferior vena cava and hepatic veins in tamponade. (A) Dilatation of the inferior vena cava to > 2 cm with less than 50% inspiratory collapse is sensitive but not specific; (B) Augmented end-diastolic expiratory flow reversals (red arrows) in the hepatic veins on pulse-waved Doppler of the hepatic veins (red arrow) with reduction of diastolic forward flow velocities in expiration (blue arrows); (C) Demonstration of augmented hepatic vein end-diastolic expiratory flow reversals using color M-mode (red arrows). (IVC: Inferior vena cava; HV: Hepatic veins).

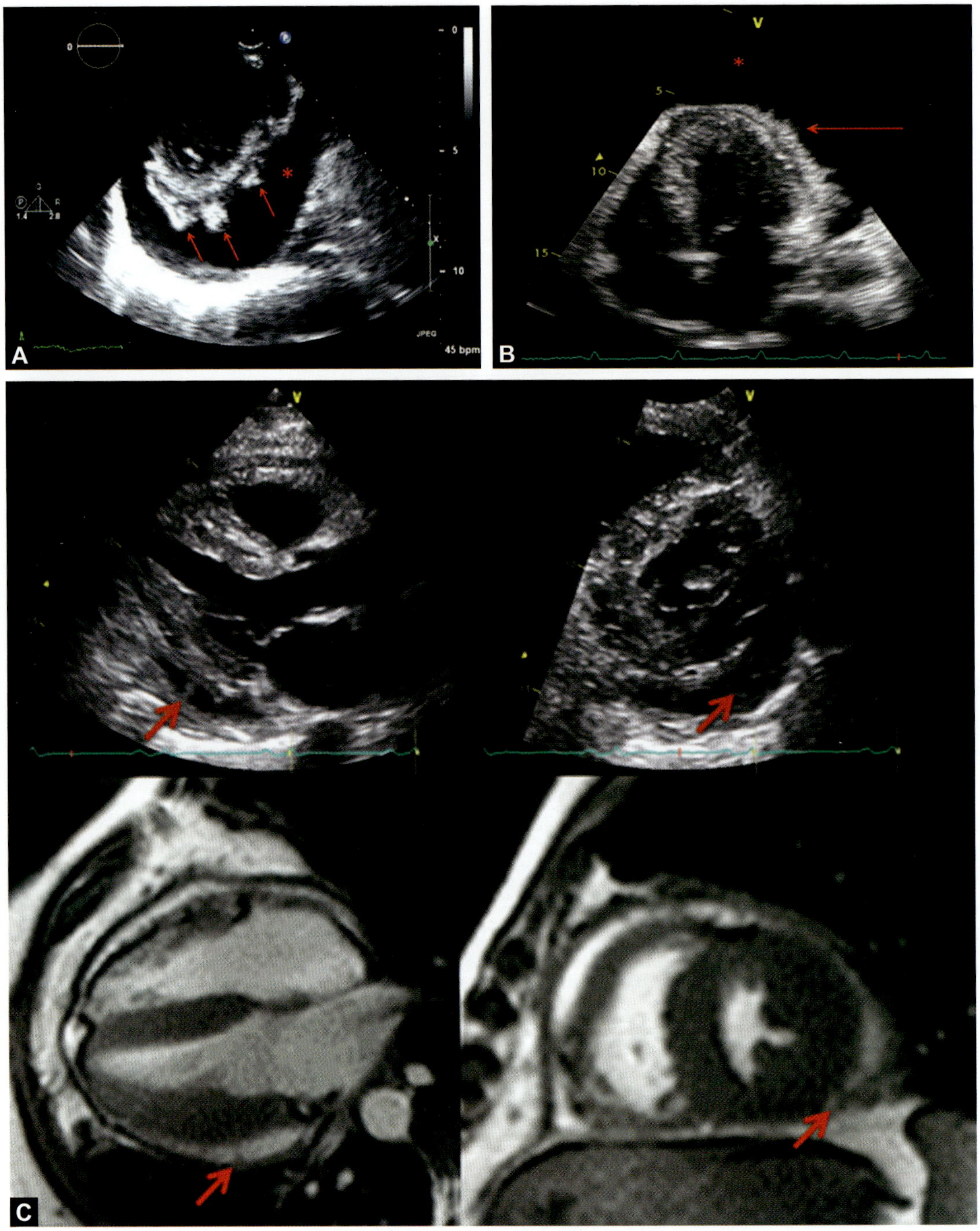

Figs. 37.20A to C: Intrapericardial contents as clues to etiology. (A) Patient with metastatic paraganglioma who was presented with a large pericardial effusion (star) and nodular epicardial lesions (arrows), likely tumor deposits. (B) Typical pericardial findings in a case of tuberculous pericarditis, with a large pericardial effusion (star), and pericardial thickening with shaggy-appearing exudate and fibrin strands (arrow). Although characteristic of tuberculous pericarditis, fibrinous strands with pericardial thickening can also be seen in pericardial effusions from purulent pericarditis, connective tissue disease, malignancy and trauma. (C) Pericarditis due to systemic lupus erythematosus, with loculated pericardial effusion located posterior to the left ventricle, pericardial thickening and fibrin strands traversing the pericardial space (arrows) resulting in septation. Complementary information was obtained from echocardiography (top), which defined the hemodynamic effect of the pericardial disease, and cardiac MRI (bottom, FIESTA images) which allowed precise assessment of areas of fluid loculations, accurately measured pericardial thickness (6 mm in this case, with > 4 mm being abnormal on MRI) and identified any areas of abnormal enhancement suggesting inflammation or fibrosis of the pericardium or myocardium. (For Fig. 37.20B, photo courtesy of Professor Mpiko Ntsekhe, Division of Cardiology, Groote Schuur Hospital, Cape Town, South Africa).

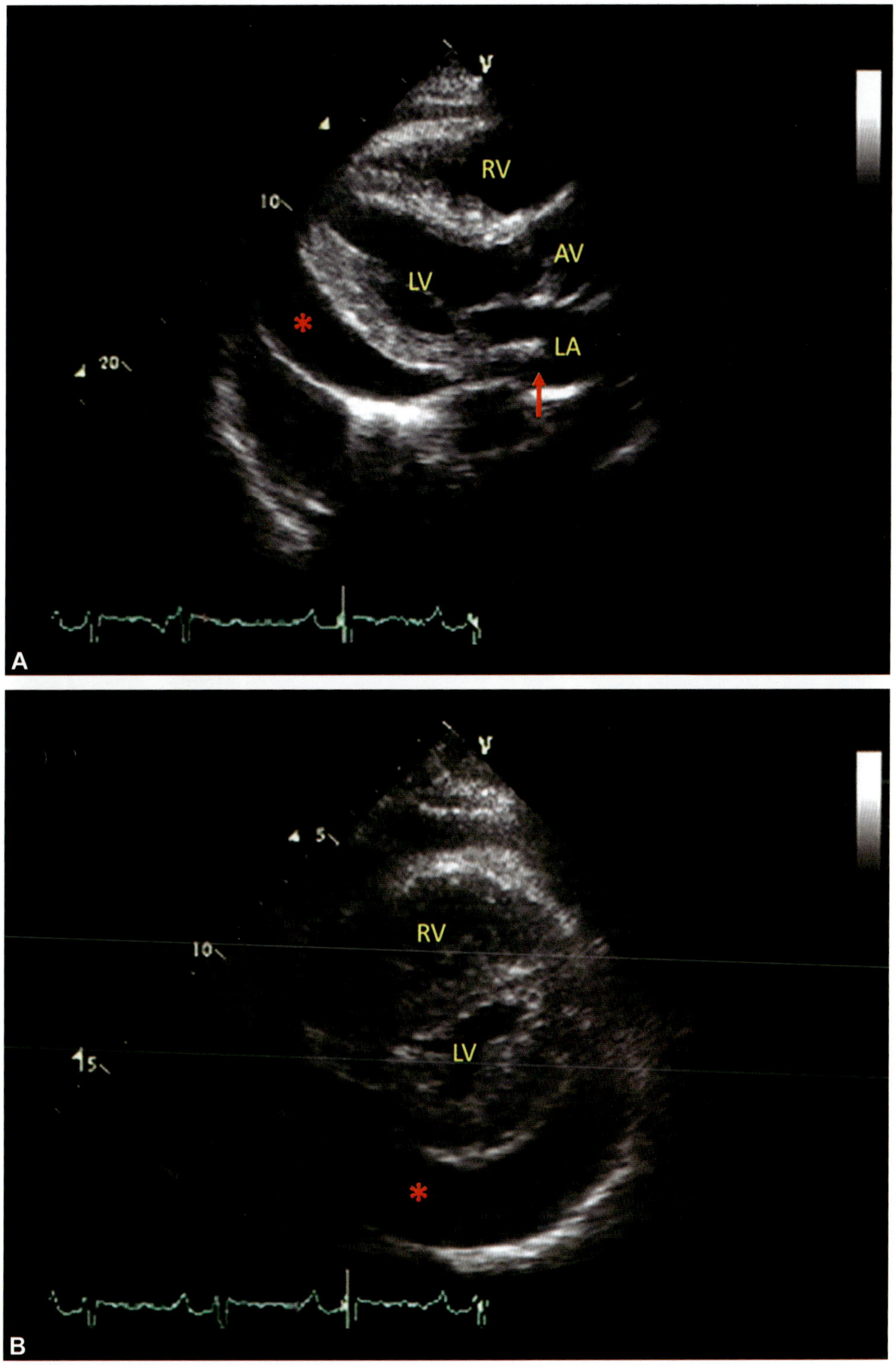

Figs. 37.21A and B: Tamponade in a case of severe pulmonary hypertension with parasternal long-axis (A) and short-axis (B) views, demonstrating right ventricular dilatation and hypertrophy with displacement of the interventricular septum, resulting in a D-shaped left ventricle. The presence of pericardial effusion (star) in pulmonary hypertension is an adverse prognostic sign as it is indicative of severe right atrial pressure elevation. Right ventricular collapse is not a sensitive sign in this setting. However, right and left atrial collapse, transmitral velocity variation with ventilation, and expiratory hepatic flow reversals remain useful features to identify those with tamponade. This case demonstrates left atrial collapse (arrow). (Images courtesy of Dr Garvan Kane and Dr Eric Fenstad, Division of Cardiovascular Diseases, Mayo Clinic, Rochester, MN, USA). (AV: Aortic valve; LA: Left atrial; LV: Left ventricle; RV: Right ventricular).

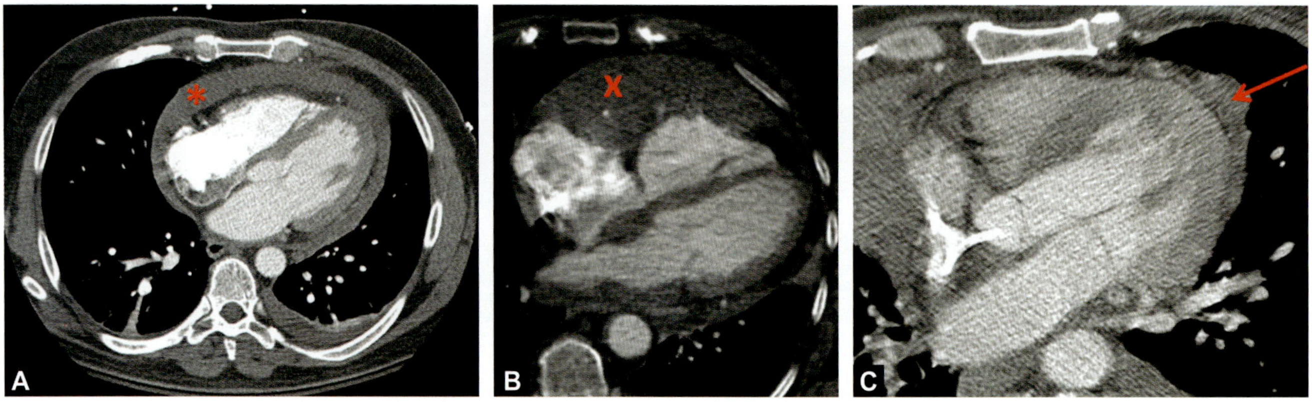

Figs. 37.22A to C: Usefulness of cardiac CT in the evaluation of pericardial effusions. (A) Findings of pericardial effusion (star) on CT. A partial characterization of the nature of the pericardial fluid can be gained through density measurements on CT. In general, pericardial effusions are of low density, but with higher protein content such as with hemorrhage or inflammation/infection, there may be increased attenuation. In general, CT is an excellent modality for identifying loculated effusions and has high sensitive at detecting pericardial calcification. A limitation is that there may sometimes be difficulty in differentiating pericardial thickening from fluid. (B and C) Another advantage of CT is in evaluating masses associated with effusions, such as primary cardiac lymphoma (Fig. 37.22C, red cross) demonstrating an infiltrative pattern of growth involving both the myocardium and the pericardium, and pericardial metastasis from rectal cancer (Fig. 37.22C, red arrow)

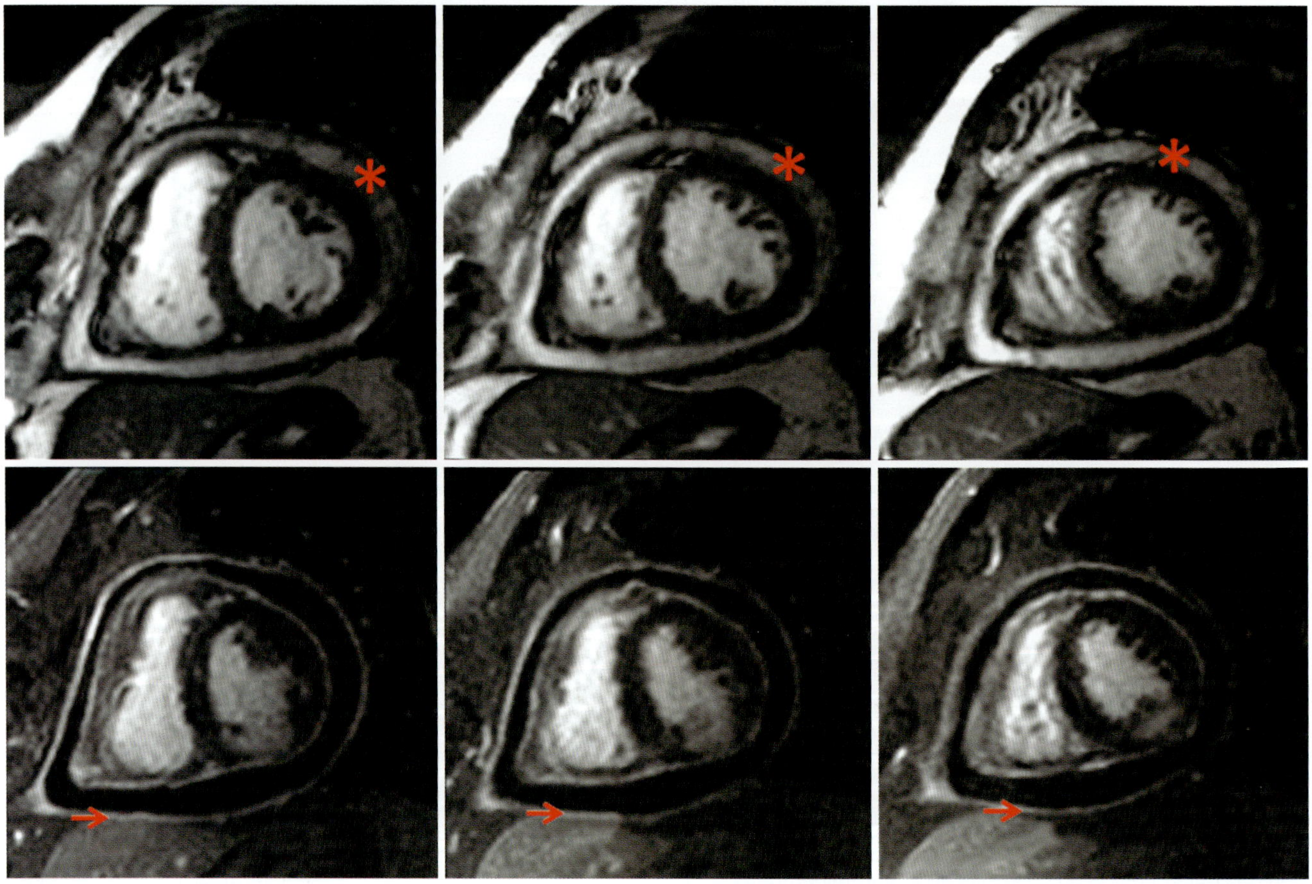

Fig. 37.23: Cardiac MRI images obtained with steady state free procession (top panel of images) and delayed gadolinium enhancement (bottom panel of images), demonstrating effusion (star) and pericardial inflammation (arrow). There is also patchy myocardial delayed gadolinium enhancement. MRI has a superior ability to characterize pericardial effusions and masses with the use of a combination of T1-weighted, T2-weighted, gradient-recalled echo cine sequences and identification of ongoing pericarditis or myocarditis with the use of intravenous gadolinium contrast.

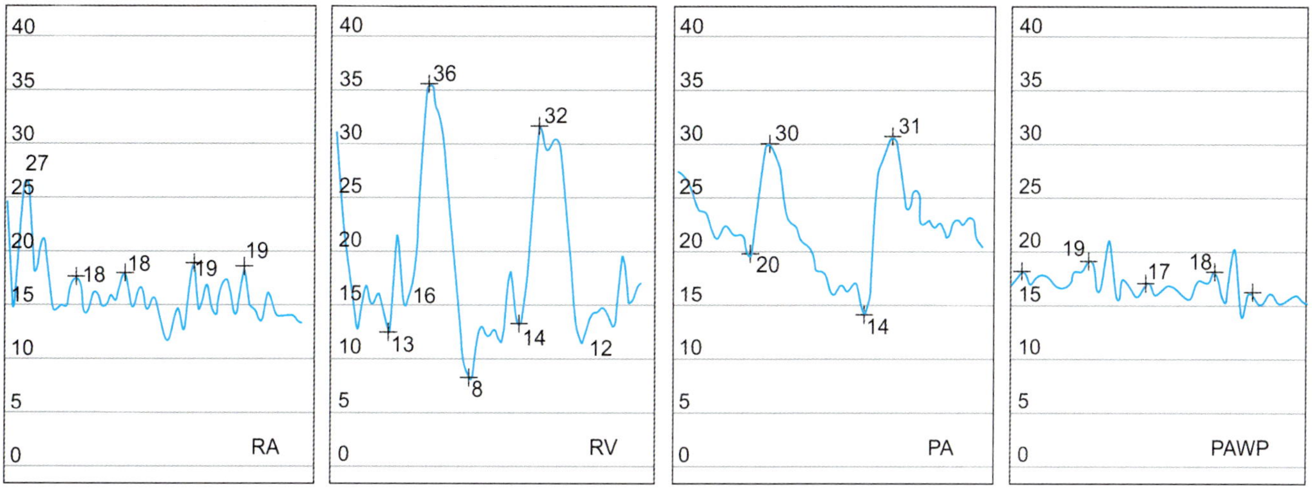

Fig. 37.24: Pressure tracings in a patient with cardiac tamponade. There is equalization of right atrial (RA), right ventricular (RV) diastolic pressure, pulmonary artery (PA) diastolic pressure, and the pulmonary artery wedge pressure (PAWP). The PAWP reflects left atrial pressure. RA of note, intracardiac pressures are clearly elevated. [Image reproduced with permission from Ahmed J, Philippides G. Bedside hemodynamic monitoring. In: Levine GN (Ed). Cardiology Secrets, 4th edition. Philadelphia: Elsevier Saunders; 2013].

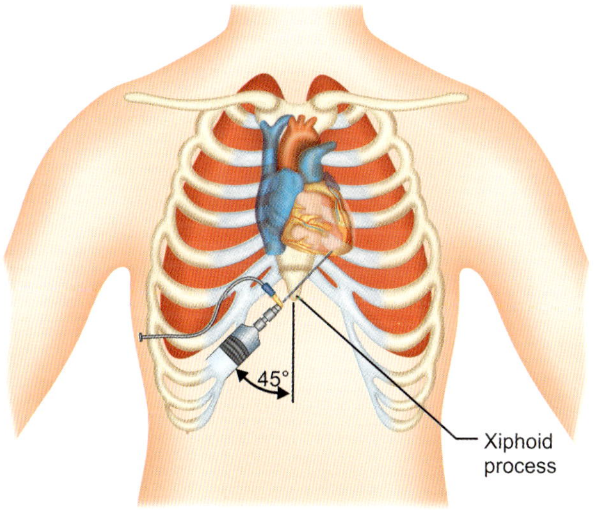

Fig. 37.25: Illustration of a pericardiocentesis procedure. Pericardiocentesis is usually performed under echocardiographic guidance, with selection of optimal site of puncture depending on the most significant site of fluid location, distance from transducer and interposed anatomical structures.

VIDEO LEGENDS

Video 37.1: Parasternal long-axis TTE demonstrating a large circumferential pericardial effusion.

Video 37.2: Circumferential effusion imaged in the parasternal long-axis view.

Video 37.3: Parasternal long-axis transthoracic echocardiogram videoclip showing pericardial effusion with RV collapse.

Video 37.4: Apical 4-chamber TTE showing pericardial effusion with some inversion and compression of the right atrium.

REFERENCES

Bernal JM, Pradhan J, Li T, et al. Acute pulmonary edema following pericardiocentesis for cardiac tamponade. Can J Cardiol. 2007;23:1155-6.

Bruch C, Schmermund A, Dagres N, et al. Changes in QRS voltage in cardiac tamponade and pericardial effusion: reversibility after pericardiocentesis and after anti-inflammatory drug treatment. J Am Coll Cardiol. 2001;38:219-26.

Feng D, Glockner J, Kim K, et al. Cardiac magnetic resonance imaging pericardial late gadolinium enhancement and elevated inflammatory markers can predict the reversibility of constrictive pericarditis after anti-inflammatory medical therapy: a pilot study. Circulation. 2011;124:1830-7.

Fenstad ER, Le RJ, Sinak LJ, et al. Pericardial effusions in pulmonary arterial hypertension: characteristics, prognosis and role of drainage. Chest. 2013;144(5):1530-8.

Goldstein JA. Cardiac tamponade, constrictive pericarditis, and restrictive cardiomyopathy. Curr Probl Cardiol. 2004;29: 503-67.

Grubina R, Cha YM, Bell MR, et al. Pneumopericardium following radiofrequency ablation for atrial fibrillation: insights into the natural history of atrial esophageal fistula formation. J Cardiovasc Electrophysiol. 2010;21:1046-49.

Hoit BD. Pericardial disease. In: Fuster V, Walsh R, Harrington R (Eds). Hurst's The Heart, 13th edition. New York: McGraw Hill Professional; 2010.

Imazio M, Adler Y. Management of pericardial effusion. Eur Heart J. 2013;34:1186-97.

Khandaker MH, Espinosa RE, Nishimura RA, et al. Pericardial disease: diagnosis and management. Mayo Clin Proc. 2010;85: 572-93.

Loukas M, Walters A, Boon JM, et al. Pericardiocentesis: a clinical anatomy review. Clin Anat. 2012;25:872-81.

Melduni RM, Oh JK, Bunch TJ, et al. Reconstruction of occluded thoracic duct for treatment of chylopericardium: a novel surgical therapy. J Vasc Surg. 2008;48:1600-2.

Oh JK, Tajik AJ, Seward JB. Pericardial diseases. In: Oh JK, Seward JB, Tajik AJ (Eds). The Echo Manual, 3rd edition. Philadelphia: Lippincott Williams & Wilkins; 2006. pp. 289-309.

Oh KY, Shimizu M, Edwards WD, et al. Surgical pathology of the parietal pericardium: A study of 344 cases (1993-1999). Cardiovasc Pathol. 2001;10:157-68.

Refaat MM, Katz WE. Neoplastic pericardial effusion. Clin Cardiol. 2011;34:593-8.

Reuter H, Burgess L, van Vuuren W, et al. Diagnosing tuberculous pericarditis. QJM. 2006;99:827-39.

Sorajja P. Invasive hemodynamics of constrictive pericarditis, restrictive cardiomyopathy, and cardiac tamponade. Cardiol Clin. 2011;29:191-9.

Syed FF, Mayosi BM. A modern approach to tuberculous pericarditis. Prog Cardiovasc Dis. 2007;50:218-36.

Syed FF, Ntsekhe M, Mayosi BM, et al. Effusive-constrictive pericarditis. Heart Fail Rev. 2013;18:277-87.

Tsang TS, Enriquez-Sarano M, Freeman WK, et al. Consecutive 1127 therapeutic echocardiographically guided pericardiocenteses: clinical profile, practice patterns, and outcomes spanning 21 years. Mayo Clin Proc. 2002;77:429-36.

CHAPTER

38

Constrictive Pericarditis

Min Pu, Hiroyuki Iwano, William C Little

NORMAL PERICARDIUM

The normal pericardium consists of two layers forming a closed potential space. The visceral pericardium covers the epicardial surface of the heart with a monolayer membrane of mesothelial cells, collagen and elastin. The parietal pericardium is a thin fibrous structure which is about 2 mm thick, surrounding most of the heart. The visceral and parietal pericardium meet around the great arteries and veins at the base of the heart. This area is referred to as the pericardial reflection. The pericardium encloses the right atrium, portions of the superior and inferior vein cava, the right ventricle, the left ventricular (LV) and most of the left atrium (Figs. 38.1A and B).

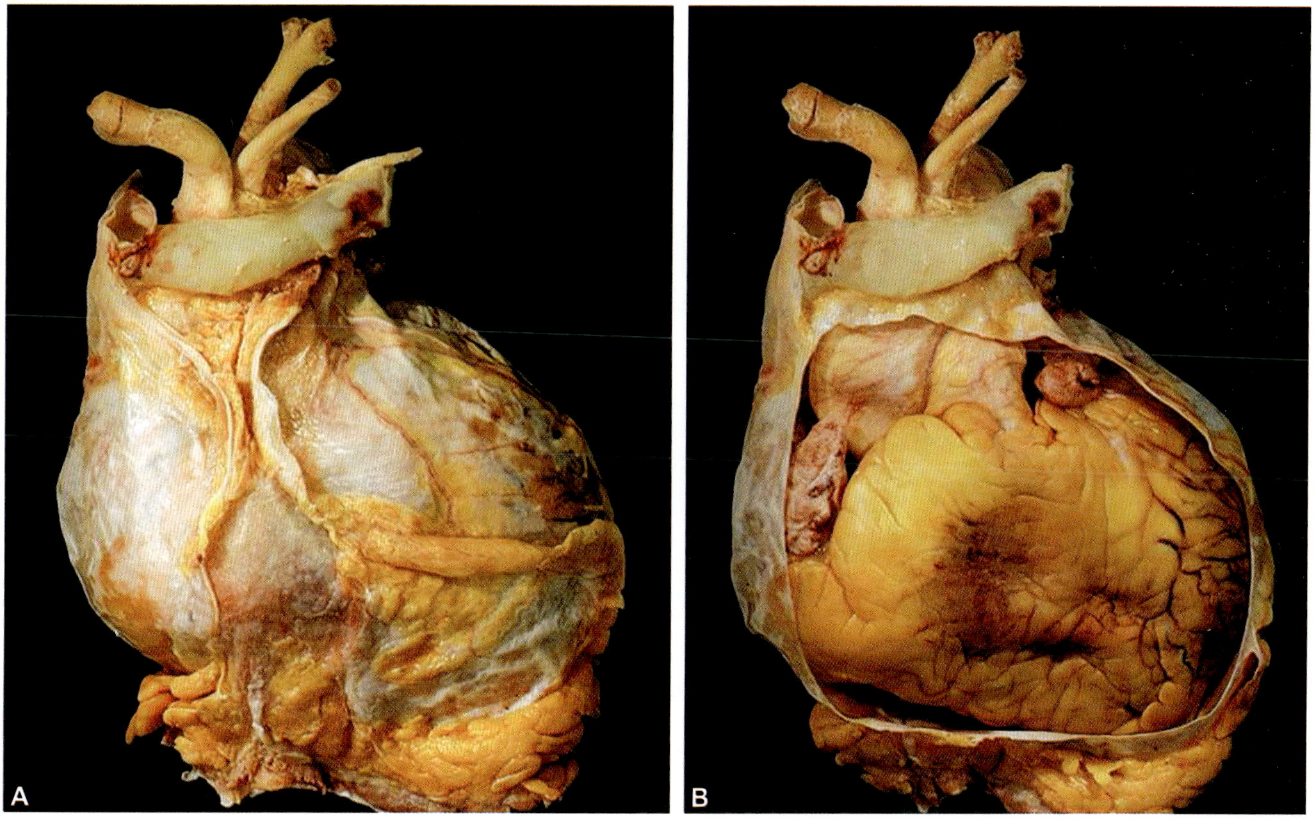

Figs. 38.1A and B: Anatomy of pericardium. (A) Anterior view of the intact parietal pericardial sac; (B) The anterior portion of the pericardial sac has been removed. The proximal segments of the great arteries are in the pericardial space. Rupture of the aortic root caused by aortic dissection could lead tamponade and death. [Klein AL, Abbara S, Agler DA, et al. American Society of Echocardiography clinical recommendations for multimodality cardiovascular imaging of patients with pericardial disease: endorsed by the Society for Cardiovascular Magnetic Resonance and Society of Cardiovascular Computed Tomography. J Am Soc Echocardiogr. 2013;26(9): 965-1012.e15]. (Images with permission from Elsevier).

The space between the visceral and parietal pericardium normally contains a small amount of fluid (5–10 mL), which may be detected by echocardiography. The descending aorta is located posteriorly and outside of the pericardial sac. This anatomic relationship is helpful for differentiating a pericardial effusion from a left pleural effusion. The pericardium anatomically isolates the heart from the lungs, the pleural space and the rest of mediastinum. This may reduce the risk of infection spreading from the lungs into the heart. The pericardium may also have a lubricating function to allow normal movement of the heart (vertical motion, rotation, translation).

CLINICAL PRESENTATION

Pericardial constriction, which is usually the result of longstanding pericardial inflammation, occurs when a scarred, thickened, and/or calcified pericardium impairs cardiac filling, thereby limiting the total cardiac volume (Figs. 38.2A and B). The most frequent causes in the developed world are previous cardiac surgery, chronic idiopathic or viral pericarditis, and mediastinal radiation. In developing countries, tuberculous pericarditis (Fig. 38.3) is a more common cause of constrictive pericarditis. Other less common causes include malignant disease, especially lung cancer, breast cancer, or lymphoma; histoplasmosis; rheumatoid arthritis; and uremia (Table 38.1). However, a specific cause may not be identified in many patients. Constrictive pericarditis is mostly a chronic condition, although subacute and transient cases have been reported. Patients may develop constrictive pericarditis 20 years after the initial radiation therapy.

Patients with pericardial constriction typically present with manifestations of elevated systemic venous pressures and low cardiac output. Because there is equalization of all cardiac pressures (including right and left atrial pressures), systemic congestion is much more marked than pulmonary congestion. Typically, patients develop marked jugular venous distention, hepatic congestion, ascites, and peripheral edema, but their lungs remain clear. The limited cardiac output typically presents as exercise intolerance and may progress to cardiac cachexia with muscle wasting. In longstanding pericardial constriction, pleural effusions, ascites, and hepatic dysfunction may be prominent clinical features. Patients with pericardial constriction are much more likely to have left-sided or bilateral pleural effusions than right-sided effusions. Because longstanding hepatic congestion may lead to the development of cirrhosis with ascites and abnormal liver function, patients may be evaluated for hepatic disease before constrictive pericarditis is recognized. Constrictive pericarditis has many hemodynamic characteristics

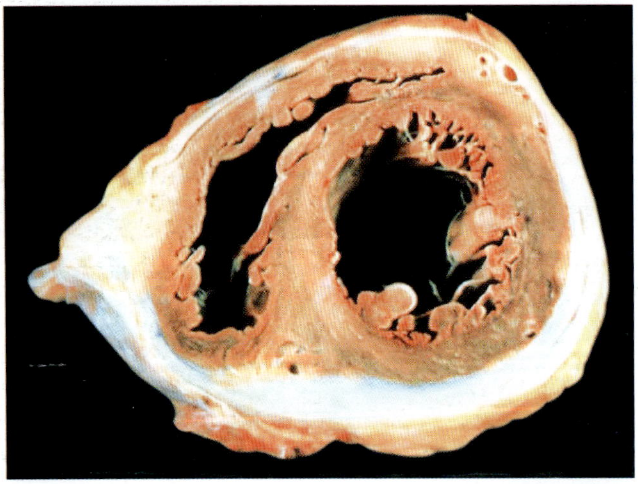

Fig. 38.2A: Gross pathological features of constrictive pericarditis. The pericardium is thickened and calcified and there is fibrosis and adhesion of the pericardial layers. [Image courtesy of Dr William D Edwards, Mayo Clinic. Image and legend text from Khandaker MH, Nishimura RA. Pericardial disease. In: Chatterjee K, Anderson M, Heistad D, Kerber RE (Eds). Cardiology: An Illustrated Textbook, 1st edition. New Delhi, India: Jaypee Brothers Medical Publishers (P) Ltd; 2012. pp. 1489-504].

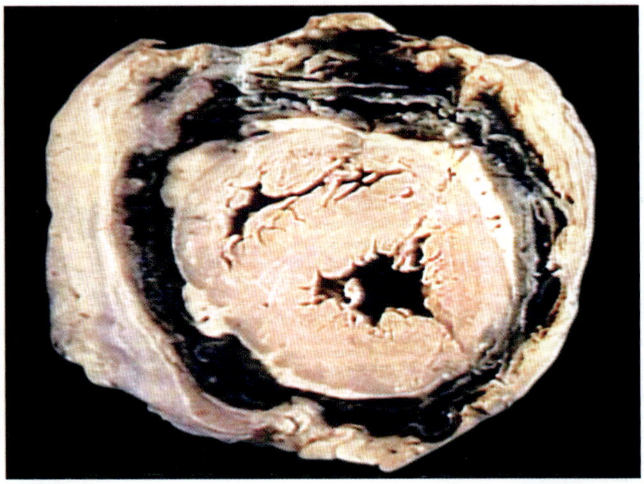

Fig. 38.2B: Gross pathology from a patient with constrictive pericarditis. [Image from Armed Forces Institute of Pathology (public domain)].

similar to those of cardiac tamponade. Many of the clinical features of constriction are also present in patients with restrictive cardiomyopathies.

Table 38.1: Etiologies of constrictive pericarditis.

Idiopathic
Infectious: • Postviral • Tuberculosis • Bacterial (nontubercular)
Postradiation
Neoplastic: • Metastatic tumor • Primary cardiac malignancy
Connective tissue disease
Postcardiac trauma: • Accident • Complication of cardiac procedure
Uremic

DIAGNOSIS

Pericardial constriction should be considered in any patient with unexplained systemic venous congestion. Some patients with constriction may be referred for cardiac imaging without clinical consideration of constrictive pericarditis. Although a simple chest X-ray in a patient with congestion and edema may occasionally suggest that constrictive pericarditis is present, the potential importance of the finding of a calcified pericardium on chest X-ray may not be appreciated unless there is a clinical suspicion of constrictive pericarditis (Figs. 38.4 and 38.5).

Echocardiography is essential in the evaluation of any patient suspected of having constriction. With a fixed pericardial volume (constriction), the left and right ventricles compete for the restrictive pericardial space. Thus an increase in right heart filling during inspiration will reduce the volume of the left heart (ventricular interdependence). Therefore, the dimensions of the right and left ventricles

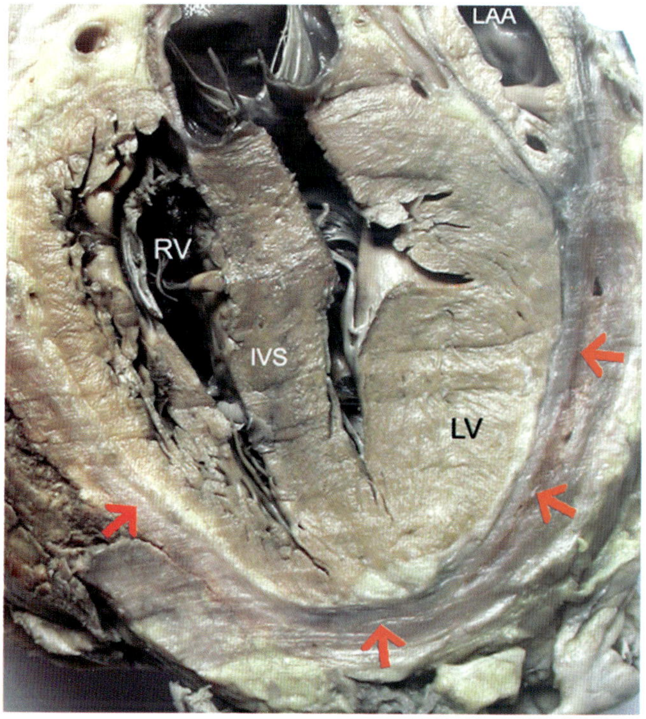

Fig. 38.3: Gross pathology specimen showing thickened pericardium (arrows) in a patient with tuberculous constrictive pericarditis. [Image courtesy of Dr Pradeep Vaideeswar, Department of Pathology (Cardiovascular and Thoracic Division), Seth GS Medical College, Mumbai, India]. (RV: Right ventricular; IVS: Interventricular septum; LV: Left ventricular; LAA: Left atrial appendage).

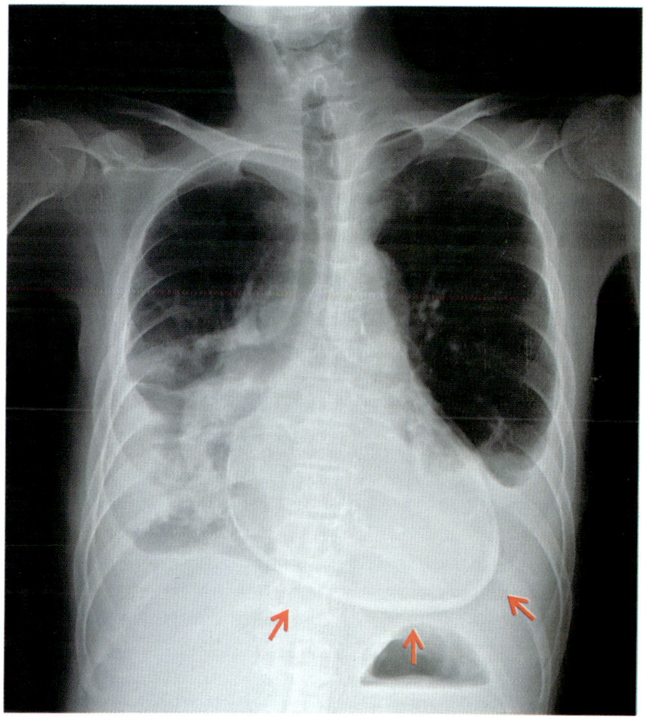

Fig. 38.4: Posteroanterior (PA) chest X-ray demonstrating a heavily calcified pericardium (arrows). This finding can be an early clue that the patient with congestion and edema may have constrictive pericarditis. [Image courtesy of Dr Dae-Won Sohn. Image from Sohn DW. Constrictive pericarditis as a never ending story: what's new? Korean Circ J. 2012;42(3):143-50].

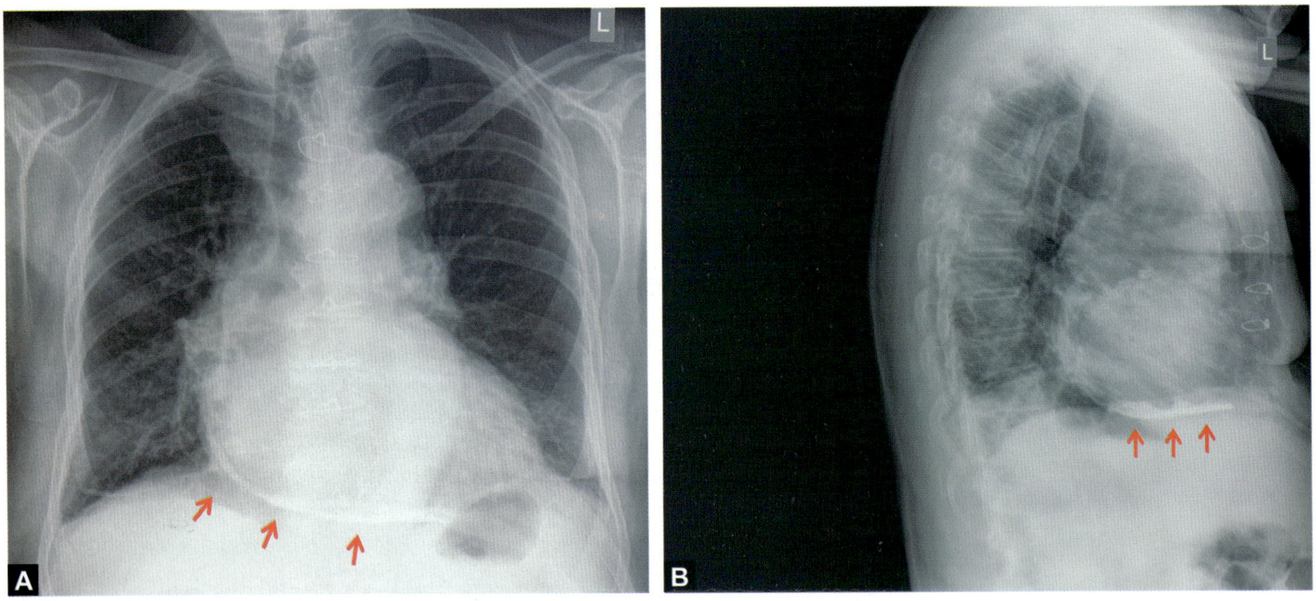

Figs. 38.5A and B: Posteroanterior (PA) (A) and lateral (B) chest X-rays demonstrating heavy calcification (arrows) of the pericardium. (Image posted by Hellerhoff on Wikimedia Commons).

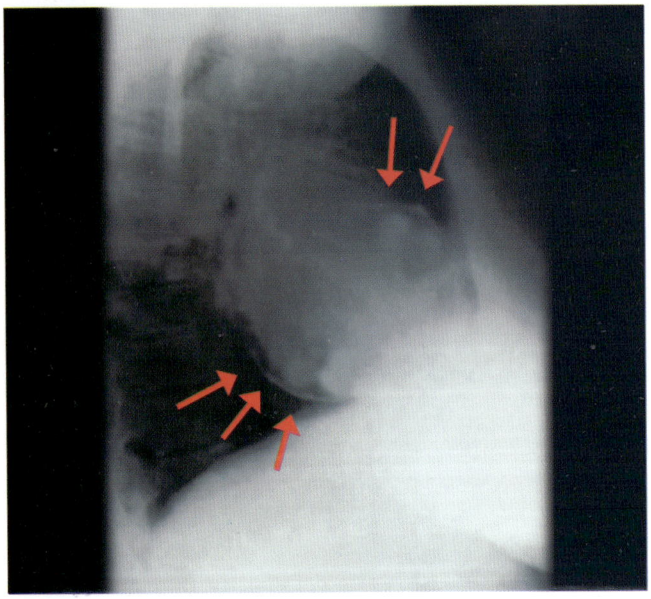

Fig. 38.5C: Lateral chest X-ray showing calcified pericardium (arrows). The relevance of this finding may not be appreciated in a patient with heart failure symptoms unless constrictive pericarditis is considered.

vary with respiration. This ventricular interdependence can be detected by M-mode echocardiography (Fig. 38.6) as an abnormal septal motion in early diastole (septal bounce). A flattened posterior wall in diastole may be noted. Two-dimensional (2D) echocardiography shows that interventricular septum (IVS) moves toward the left ventricle during inspiration, leading to an increase in right ventricular volume and a decrease in the LV volume. During expiration, an increase in chest pressure reduces the return of venous blood flow, leading to a decrease in the right ventricle volume. During this time the IVS is observed bulging towards (into) the right ventricle (Figs. 38.7A and B). The "septal bounce" detected by M-mode and/or 2D echocardiography is often the first echocardiography finding to prompt a sonographer to perform a constrictive pericarditis protocol. Because of the phenomenon of ventricular interdependence, systolic blood pressure may fluctuate with respiration.

Doppler echocardiography plays an important role in the diagnosis of constrictive pericarditis. Doppler examination focuses on changes in flow velocity across the mitral and tricuspid valves, and in the hepatic vein, with respiration. In a normal subject, an increase in tricuspid inflow is usually less than 40% and a decrease in mitral inflow velocity is less than 25% during inspiration. However, in constrictive pericarditis, tricuspid diastolic velocity significantly increases (> 40%) and mitral inflow velocity significantly decreases (> 25%) with inspiration. A decrease in tricuspid flow velocity and an increase in mitral flow velocity are present during expiration (Figs. 38.8A to C). Color M-mode study shows brisk early LV filling, due to an increase in left atrial pressure, in early diastole, and due to restricted filling of the left ventricle in middle and late diastole caused by the pericardial constriction (Fig. 38.9).

The inferior vena cava is dilated due to elevated central venous pressure. Although the dilation of the inferior venous cava lacks the specificity for the diagnosis of

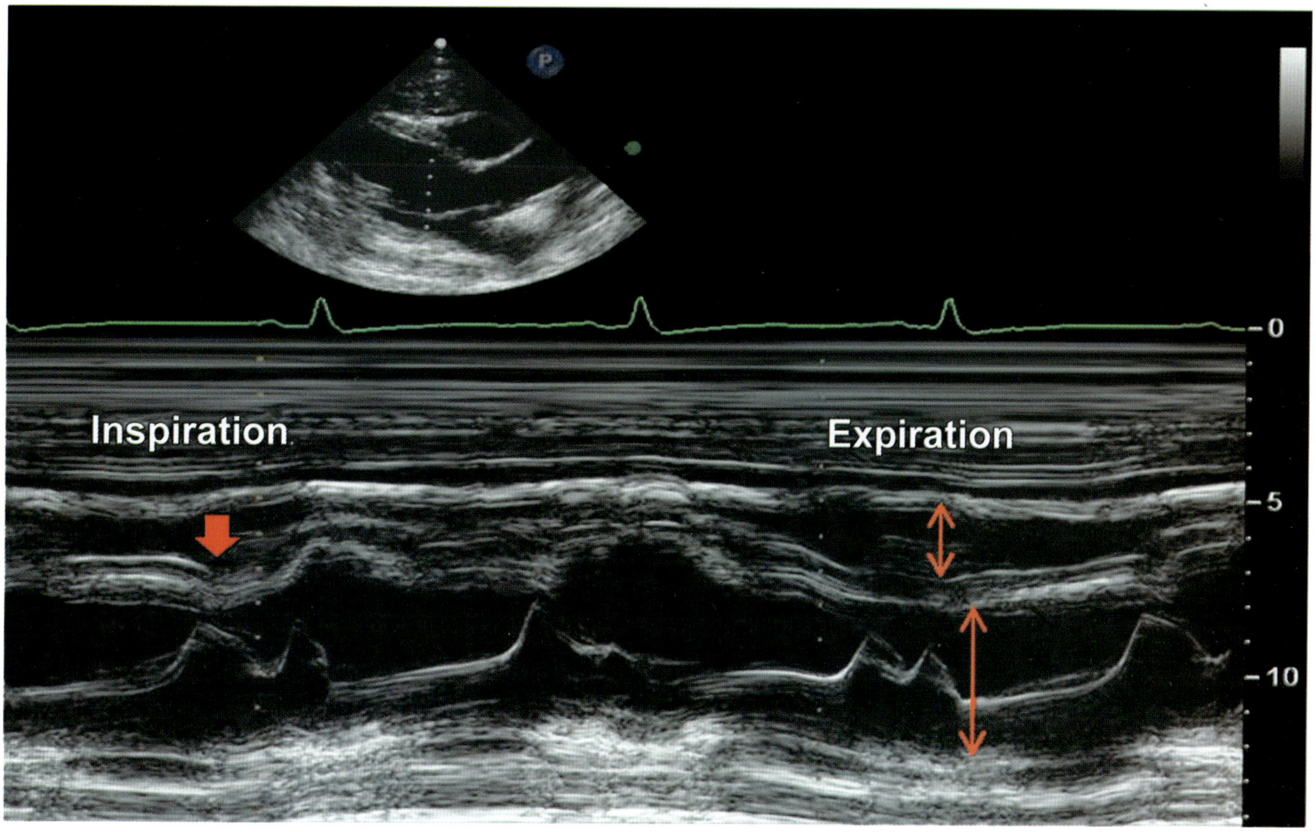

Fig. 38.6: M-mode echocardiographic study of a patient with constrictive pericarditis. Abnormal septal motion and ventricular interdependence were demonstrated. During inspiration, the interventricular septum (IVS) bulges toward the left ventricle (thick arrow) and during expiration, the IVS shifts toward the right ventricle (RV). Interventricular dependence is demonstrated, as during inspiration the RV enlarges as there is an increase in RV volume, while the left ventricular (LV) becomes smaller (thin arrows).

constrictive pericarditis, a normal sized inferior venous cava makes diagnosis of constrictive pericarditis less likely. Significant expiratory hepatic diastolic flow reversal is one of the characteristics of Doppler echocardiographic finding in constrictive pericarditis. This is due to a sudden decrease in right ventricular volume associated with interventricular motion towards the right ventricle during expiration (Fig. 38.10).

In normal hearts, tissue Doppler imaging usually demonstrates a lateral mitral annulus velocity is higher than septal mitral annulus velocity. However, with pericardial constriction, the lateral e′ is usually lower than the septal e′ (Figs. 38.11A and B). The septal e′ is not reduced in constriction but almost always reduced in patients with restrictive cardiomyopathies (Figs. 38.12A to D).

Computed tomography (CT) imaging is useful for the assessment of the pericardium, particularly for assessment of pericardial thickness. Cardiac CT in patients with constrictive pericarditis usually reveals thickened pericardium with or without pericardial calcification. Most patients with pericardial constriction have a thickened pericardium (>2 mm). Thickened pericardium can be global or focal. CT may also reveal pericardial calcification (Figs. 38.13A and B). CT may also be helpful for identifying extrapericardial lesions such as pleural effusion, ascites, or tumor compression. Delineation of detailed pericardial structure, particularly the location and severity of pericardial thickening and calcification, is helpful to the surgeon in surgical plan and risk stratification.

Cardiac magnetic resonance imaging (MRI) is also used for the diagnosis of constrictive pericarditis. As with CT, cardiac MRI may demonstrate thickened pericardium (Fig. 38.14). Cine acquisition may show abnormal interventricular septal motion similar to that seen on echocardiography. Cardiac MRI may also be used for evaluation of pericardial edema and inflammation, or detection of pericardial-myocardial adherence. The American Society of Echocardiography (ASE) recently published clinical recommendation for multimodality cardiovascular imaging for patients with pericardial disease.

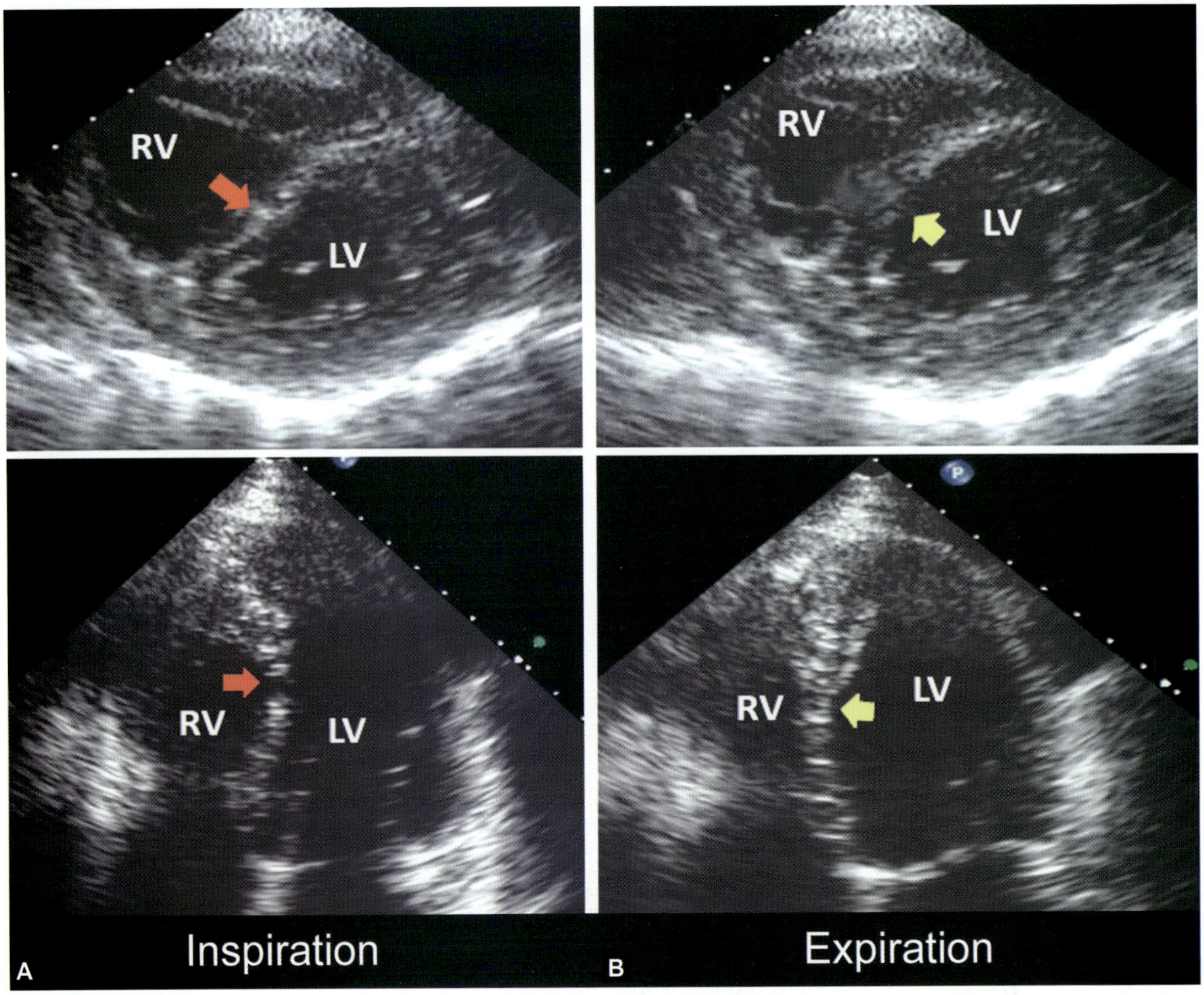

Figs. 38.7A and B: Two-dimensional (2D) echocardiographic study of constrictive pericarditis demonstrating ventricular interdependence. Short-axis images are displayed on the upper figure images, apical four chamber images on the lower figure images. (A) During inspiration, the right ventricular (RV) volume increases, and the interventricular septum (IVS) bulges toward the left ventricular (LV) (red arrows); (B) During expiration, the opposite occurs, and the IVS moves back towards the RV (yellow arrows).

Confirmation of the diagnosis of constrictive physiology may require cardiac catheterization in patients whose noninvasive evaluation is not clear-cut. Traditional invasive hemodynamic findings are the equalized end-diastolic pressures in the right and left ventricles and the "dip and plateau" pattern of LV diastolic pressure (Fig. 38.15). Specific invasive hemodynamic features of pericardial constriction are based on the respiratory variation in ventricular filling; the simultaneous measurement of left and right ventricular pressures demonstrates discordant changes in their systolic pressures.

Invasive hemodynamic assessment may be used when differentiation of constrictive pericarditis from restrictive cardiomyopathy cannot be reliably made based on clinical presentation and image study. Hemodynamic characteristics of constrictive pericarditis include a significant increase in atrial and ventricular pressure, equal diastolic pressures in the right atrium, right ventricle and pulmonary artery, with nearly normal pulmonary wedge pressure. Rapid early ventricular filling (high atrial pressure) with a rapid rise in ventricular diastolic pressure (restriction) results in the "square root" shape of the pressure tracing. Variations of left and right diastolic pressure and systolic pressure associated with respiration are key findings in constrictive pericarditis. The simultaneous measurement of left and right

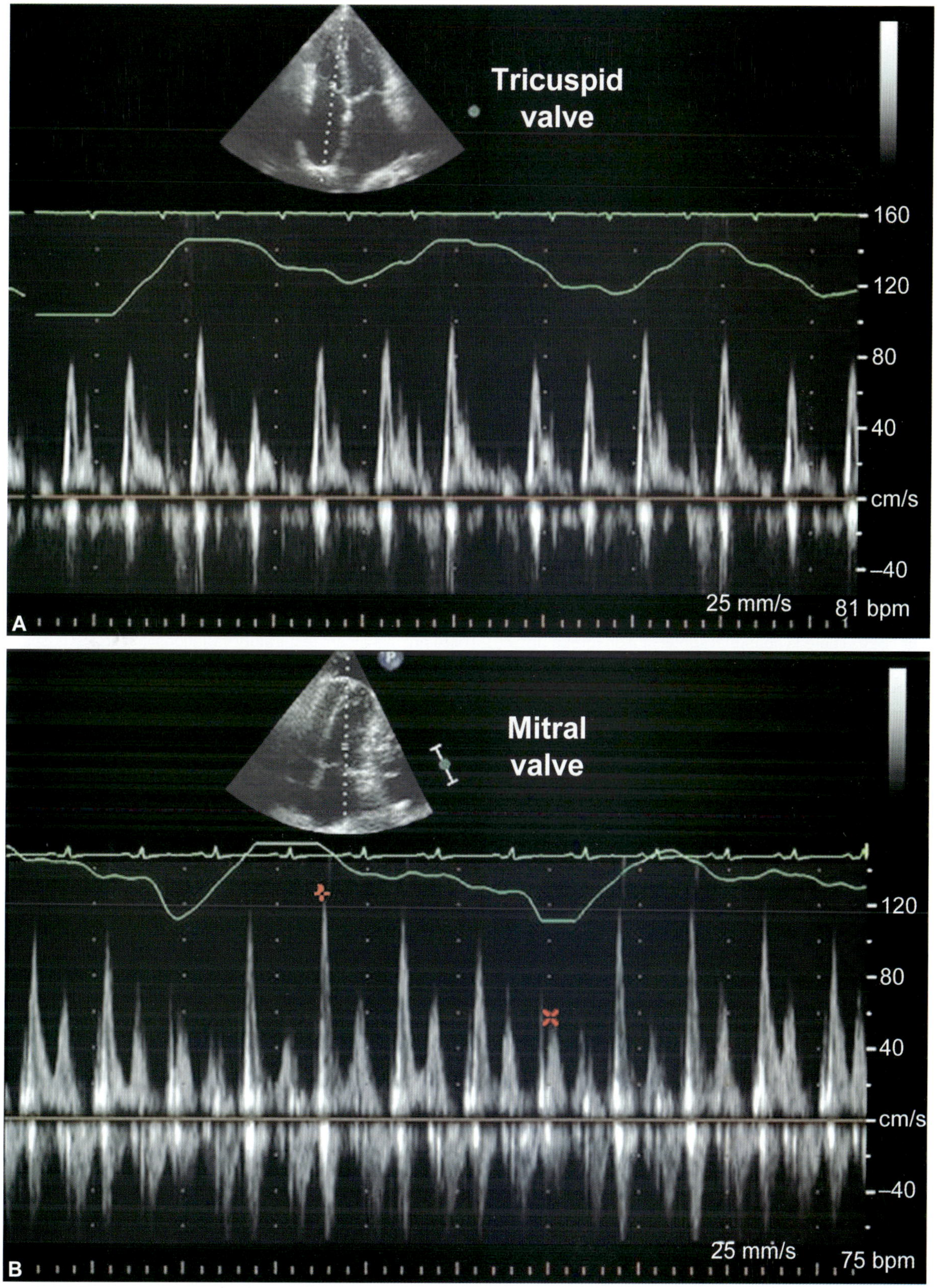

Figs. 38.8A and B: Doppler study of respiratory variation in tricuspid (A) and mitral (B) inflow in constrictive pericarditis. The early diastolic velocity of transtricuspid inflow accelerates during inspiration whereas that of transmitral inflow accelerates during expiration.

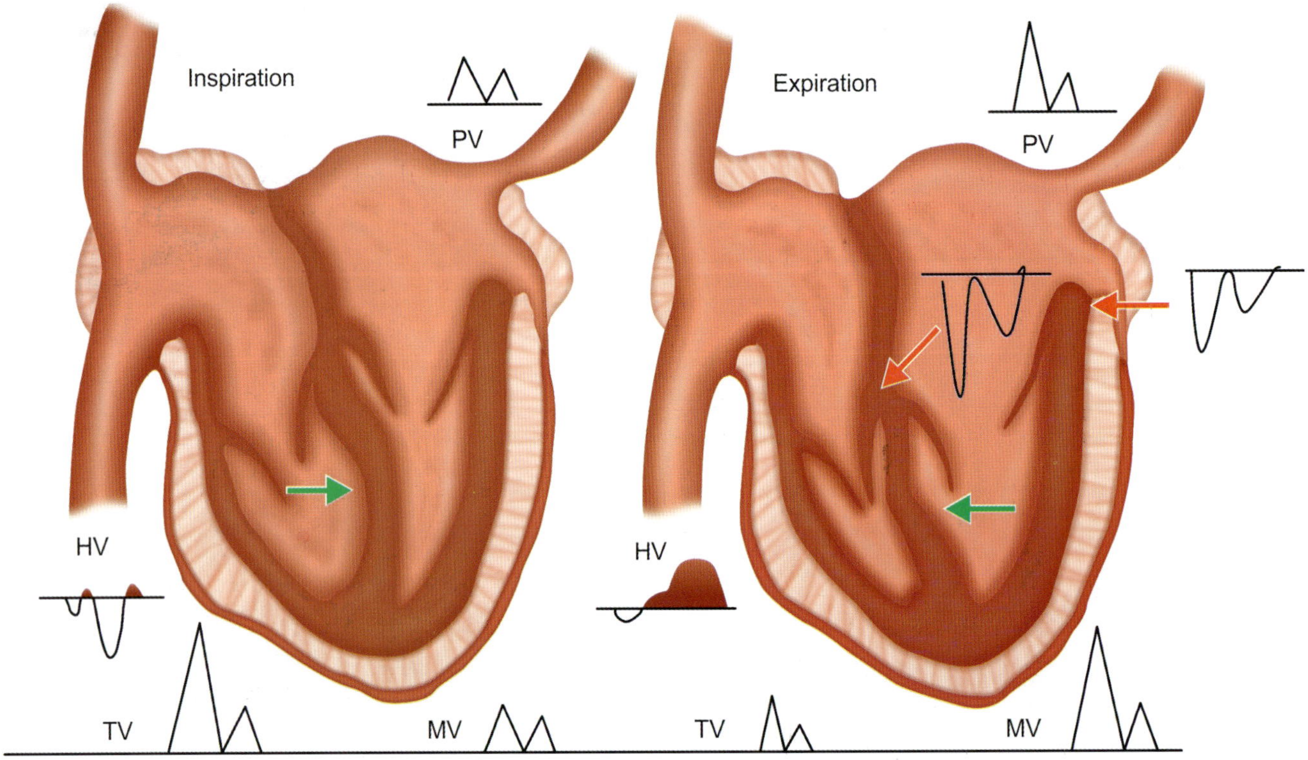

Fig. 38.8C: Diagram of the pathophysiology of constrictive pericarditis. The thickened pericardium (brown hatched areas) limits ventricular filling. There is abnormal septal motion (green arrows). There are significant respiratory variations in mitral, tricuspid, hepatic and pulmonary venous flow velocities. Tissue Doppler imaging shows the early diastolic velocity of the lateral mitral annulus is lower than the early diastolic velocity of the septal mitral annulus (red arrows). (Image courtesy of Shirley Pu). (HV: Hepatic vein; TV: Tricuspid valve; PV: Pulmonary vein; MV: Mitral valve).

ventricular pressures demonstrates discordant changes in their systolic pressures with respiration in constrictive pericarditis. In contrast, the direction of these pressures is concordant (both pressure in left and right sides increase with expiration and decrease with inspiration) in restrictive cardiomyopathy. In addition, restrictive cardiomyopathy is a myocardial disease with a significant reduction in myocardial compliance, which restricts the LV and right ventricular filling from the atria. Therefore, the left and right atria are often significantly dilated. In contrast to constrictive pericarditis, in restrictive cardiomyopathy, left and right ventricular systolic and diastolic function may be decreased. Additionally, left atrial pressure is elevated in restrictive cardiomyopathy and is often normal in constrictive pericarditis.

EFFUSIVE-CONSTRICTIVE PERICARDITIS

Although constrictive pericarditis often occurs at a late stage in pericardial disease, constrictive physiology may sometimes be observed in a patient who still has pericardial effusion. In some patients (< 10%) who present with cardiac tamponade, the elevated right atrial pressure and jugular venous distention do not resolve after removal of the pericardial fluid. In these patients, pericardiocentesis converts the hemodynamics from those typical of tamponade to those of constriction. This syndrome is often defined as an effusive-constrictive pericarditis. The restriction of cardiac filling is due not only to pericardial effusion but also to pericardial constriction, predominantly involving the visceral pericardium. Effusive-constrictive pericarditis most likely represents an intermediate transition from acute pericarditis with pericardial effusion to pericardial constriction. Echocardiographic study in such patients often shows mild or moderate pericardial effusion. However, there is significant ventricular independence characterized by observing obvious respiratory variation in mitral and tricuspid inflows (Figs. 38.16A and B) associated with abnormal septal motion. Effusive-constrictive pericarditis may resolve with medical treatment after several weeks of treatment with an nonsteroidal anti-inflammatory drug (NSAID) or may instead lead to the development of constrictive pericarditis in the future. The time between the effusive-constrictive pericarditis and development of clinical significant constrictive pericarditis may be difficult to predict.

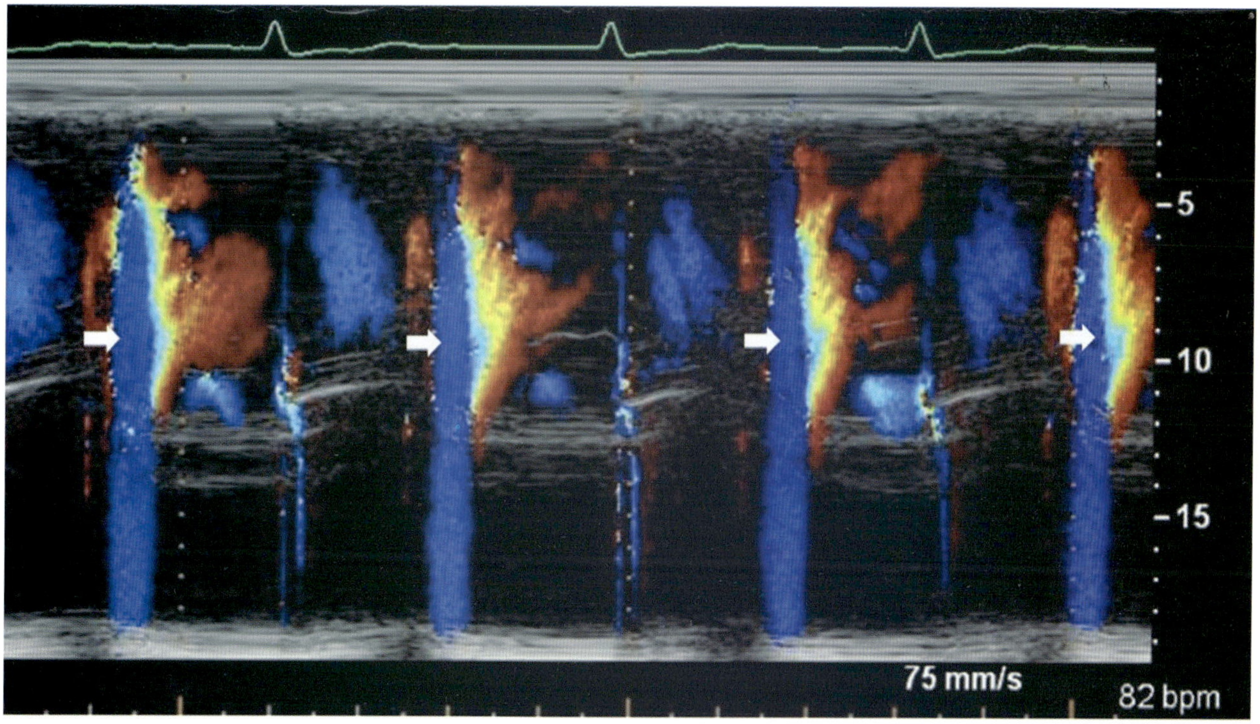

Fig. 38.9: Color M-mode study of mitral inflow in a patient with constrictive pericarditis shows early rapid filling of the left ventricle with color alias (blue and yellow color: arrows).

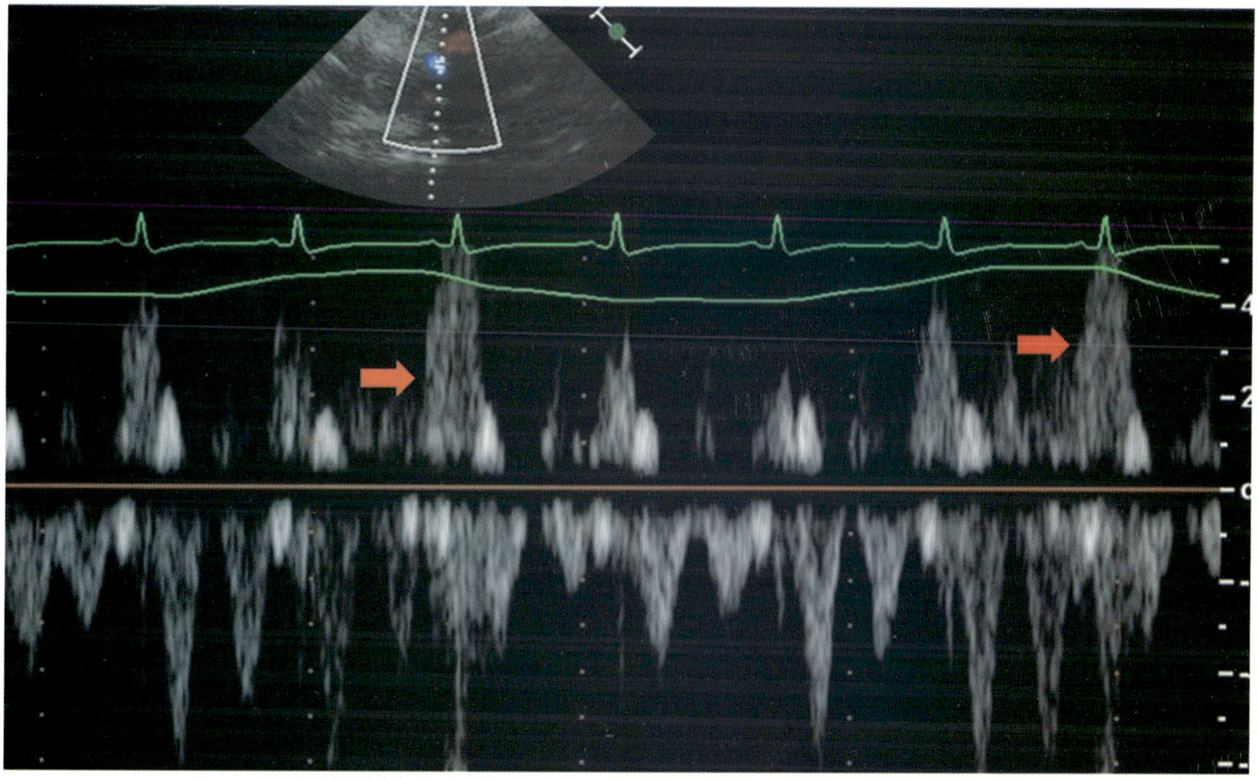

Fig. 38.10: Changes in hepatic venous flow pattern in constrictive pericarditis. Doppler echocardiography study in a patient with constrictive pericarditis shows respiratory variation in hepatic venous flow and significant hepatic venous flow reversal (arrows). During expiration, interventricular septal shifts towards the right ventricle (RV). This leads to a brief increase in RV pressure. In addition, decrease in chest pressure may not transfer to ventricular chambers due to pericardial constriction.

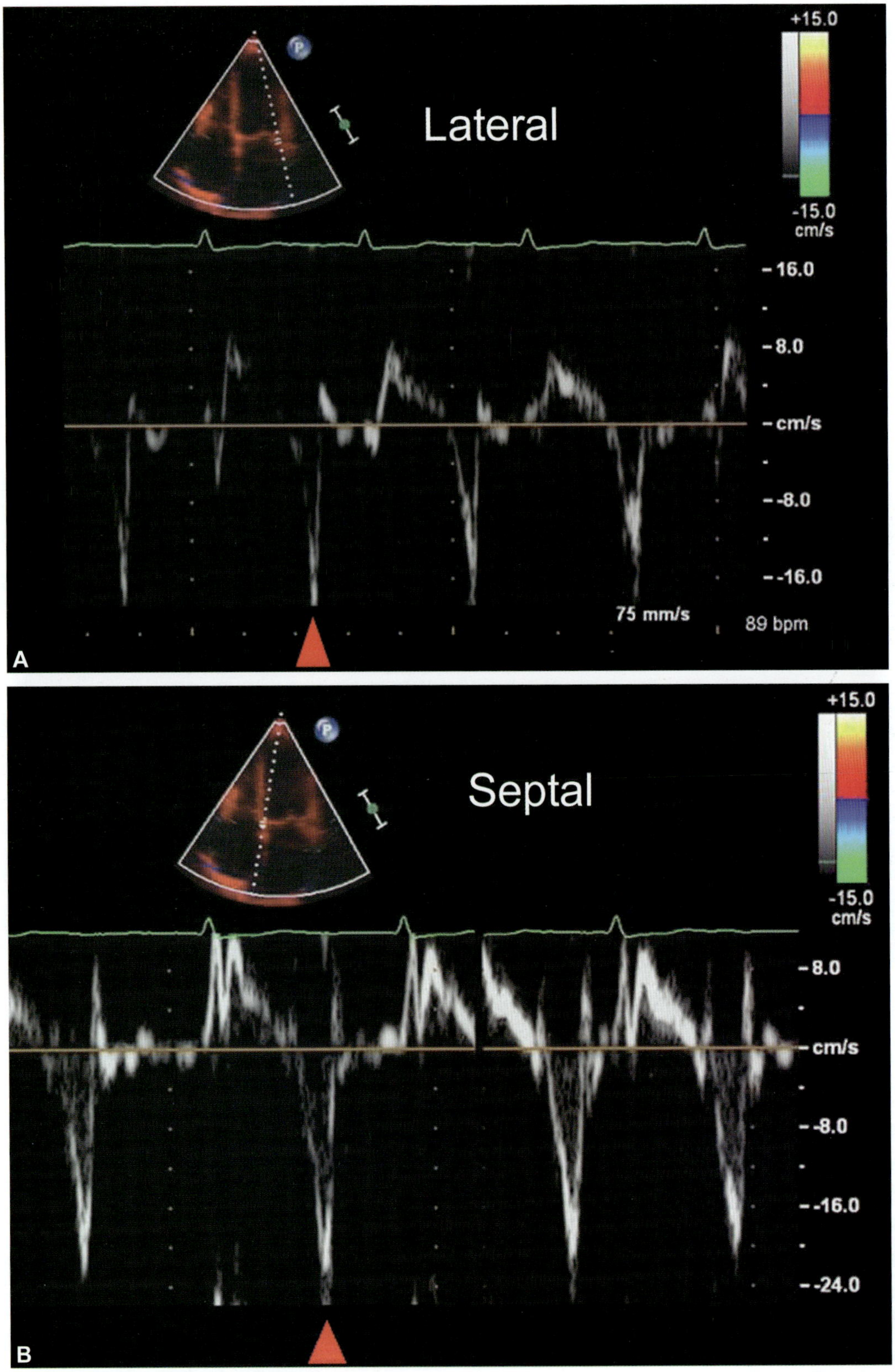

Figs. 38.11A and B: Tissue Doppler imaging study in constrictive pericarditis. Early diastolic velocity (e′) of mitral lateral annulus (top panel) is lower than septal velocity (bottom panel). Note that in contrast to restrictive cardiomyopathy and heart failure with preserved ejection fraction (diastolic heart failure), the tissue Doppler velocities in constrictive pericarditis are normal.

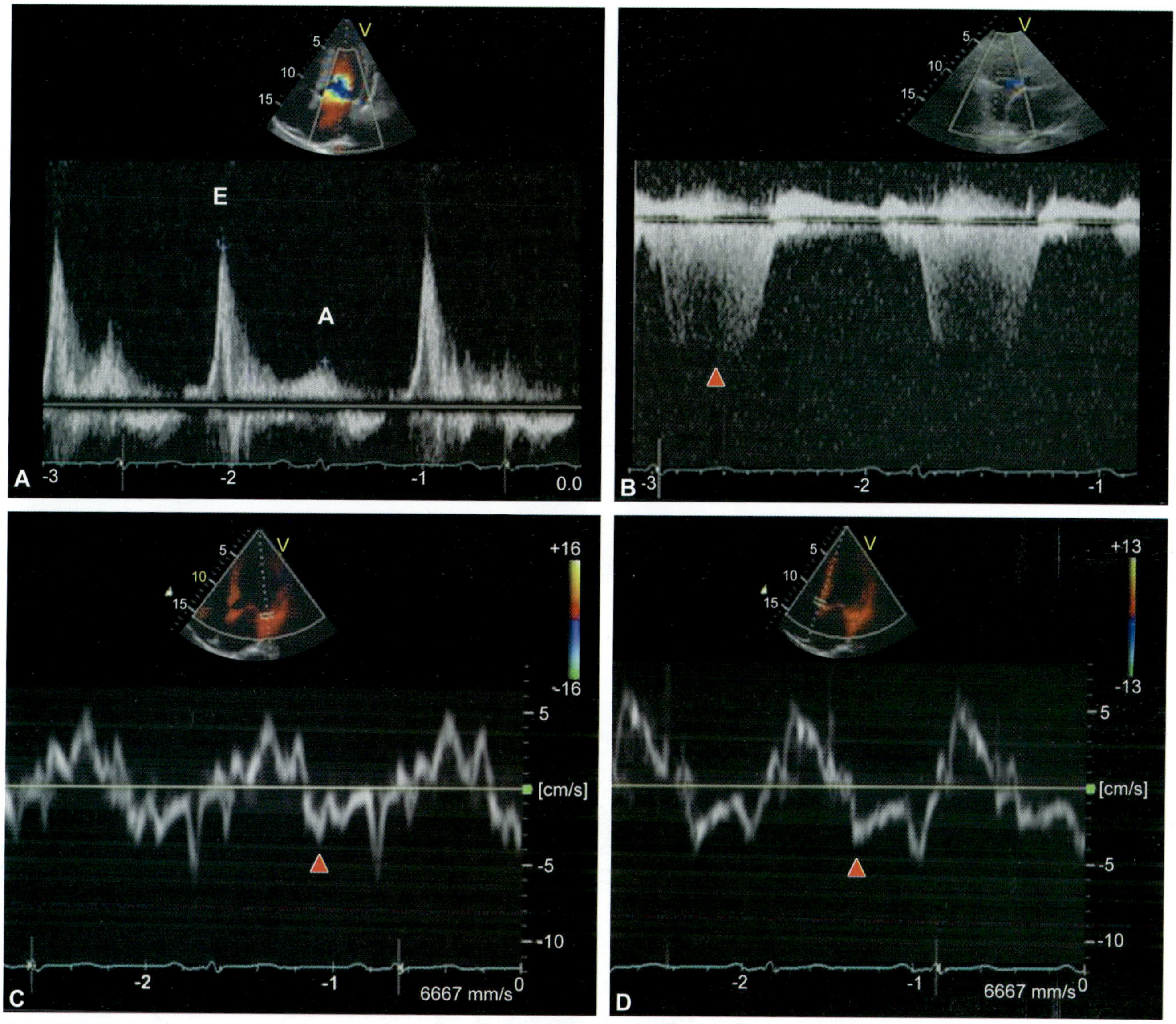

Figs. 38.12A to D: Restrictive cardiomyopathy pathophysiology. Echocardiographic study in a patient with exertional dyspnea, decreased exercise capacity, and preserved left ventricular (LV) systolic function. (A) Pulsed wave spectral Doppler shows a restrictive filling pattern of mitral inflow with E/A ratio of 3.6; (B) Estimated pulmonary systolic pressure is 60 mm Hg (moderate pulmonary hypertension); (C and D) Tissue Doppler imaging demonstrated a significant decrease in both lateral (C) and septal (D) early diastolic mitral annulus velocities. The echocardiographic findings in this study suggest this patient has pathophysiology suggestive of restrictive cardiomyopathy. In contrast with restrictive cardiomyopathy, there is often normal pulmonary artery systolic pressure and normal mitral annulus early diastolic velocity (e') in constrictive pericarditis, as illustrated in Figure 11.

MANAGEMENT OF CONSTRICTIVE PERICARDITIS

The diagnosis of constrictive pericarditis may often involve several diagnostic modalities. Although an increase in C-reactive protein (CRP) and erythrocyte sedimentation rates in acute or subacute constrictive pericarditis may be observed, imaging studies are almost always required to made diagnosis (Figs. 38.17A to F). Patients with the recent development of constriction who have evidence of inflammation (elevated CRP and/or sedimentation rate) may have resolution of constrictive physiology and

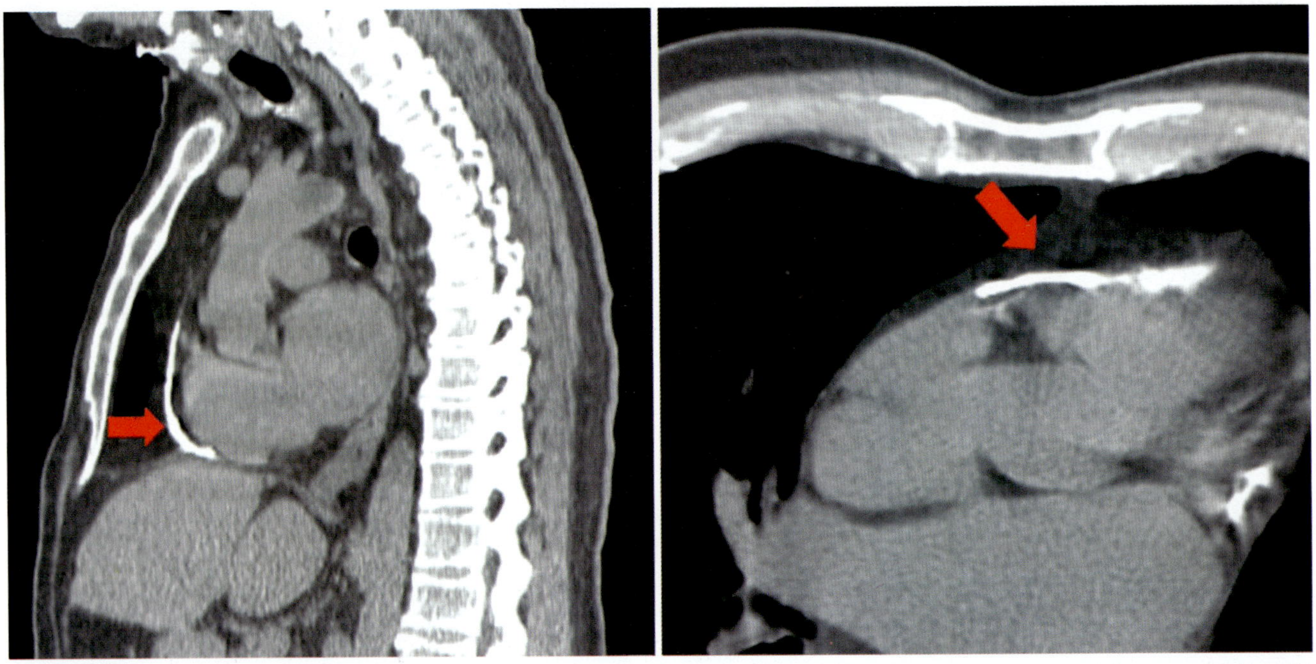

Fig. 38.13A: Pericardial calcification demonstrated by cardiac CT. There is significant calcification of the pericardium around the right ventricular free wall (arrows).

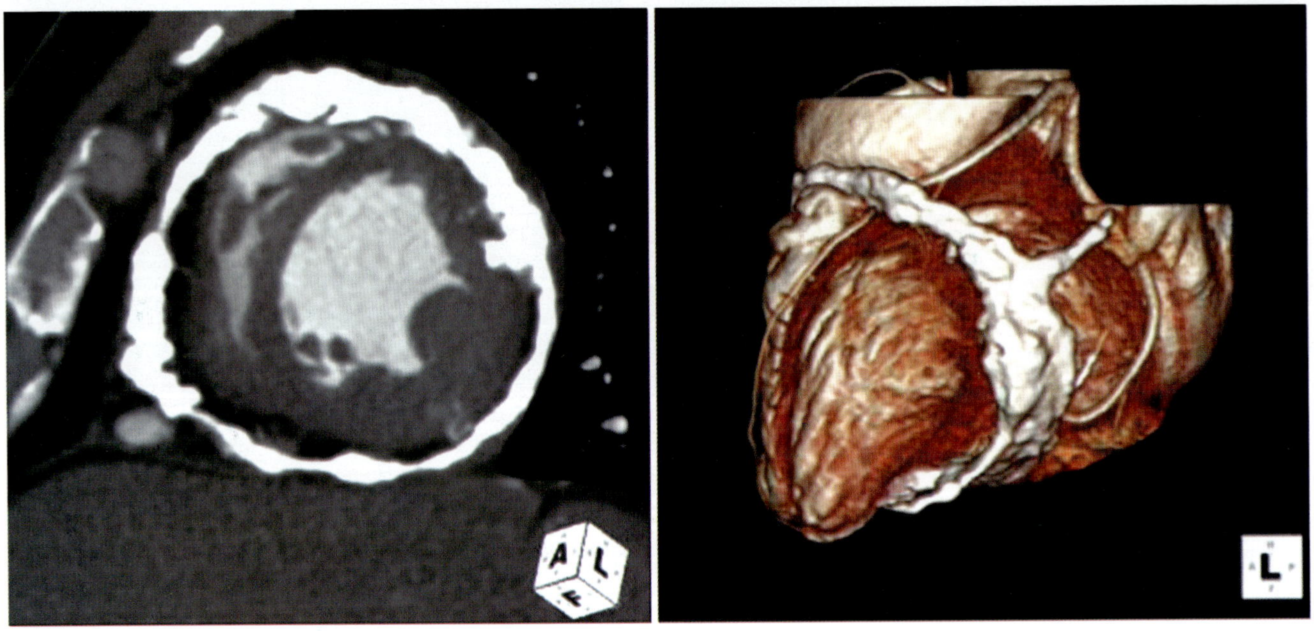

Fig. 38.13B: Cardiac CT imaging demonstrating heavy "eggshell" calcification encircling the heart. Images courtesy of Professor Bong Gun Song, Konkuk University Medical Center. Images and legend text from Song BG et al. Heart in an eggshell calcification: idiopathic calcific constrictive pericarditis. Cardiol Res 2011;2(6):310-12.

symptoms after intensive anti-inflammatory therapy. However, for chronic constrictive pericarditis, treatment of constrictive pericarditis can be challenging. Diuretic therapy may reduce congestion and edema but does not treat the underlying disease. Additionally, too aggressive diuresis may lead to a decrease in cardiac output. Pericardiectomy is the treatment of choice in appropriately selected candidates (Figs. 38.18A to D). However, the procedure is often lengthy and technically challenging, and is associated with a surgical mortality of 5–15%. Additionally, diastology may remain abnormal after the procedure.

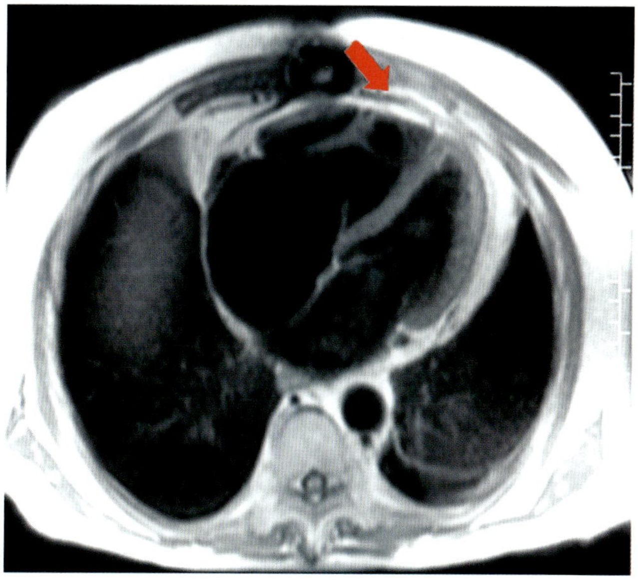

Fig. 38.14: Magnetic resonance imaging (MRI) study of pericarditis. There is significant thickened pericardium anteriorly (arrow). There is artifact caused by metal wires used for closure of the sternum in the prior open heart surgery. (Image courtesy of Dr Brandon Stacey).

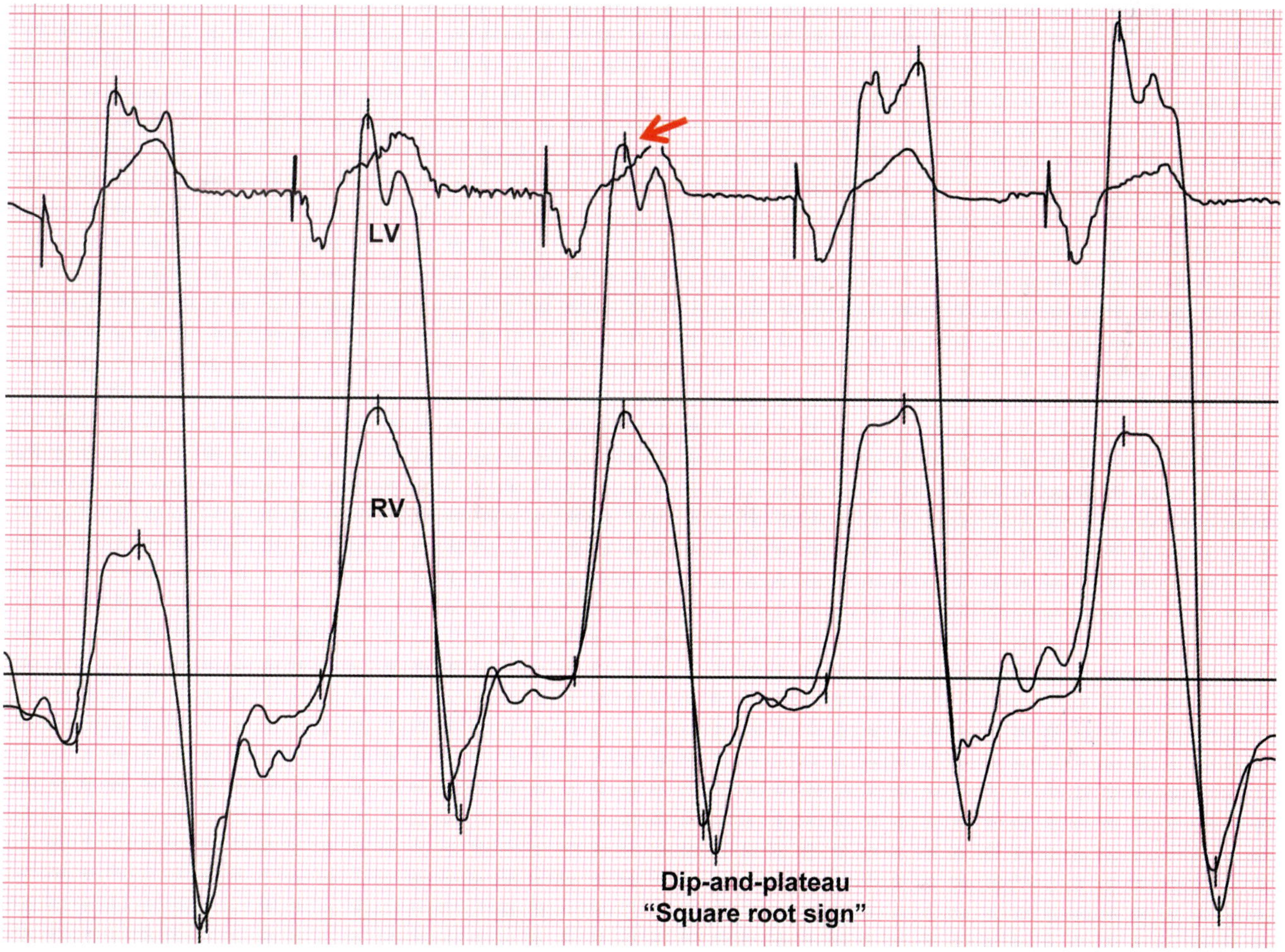

Fig. 38.15: Hemodynamic study of constrictive pericarditis. Simultaneous recording of the left ventricular (LV) and right ventricular (RV) pressures showing a characteristic dip-and-plateau pattern at diastole (square root sign). LV and RV diastolic pressures elevate and show near equilibration. During inspiration, there is a decrease in LV systolic pressure and increase in RV systolic pressure (arrow). In contrast, during expiration, LV systolic pressure increases whereas RV systolic pressure decreases.

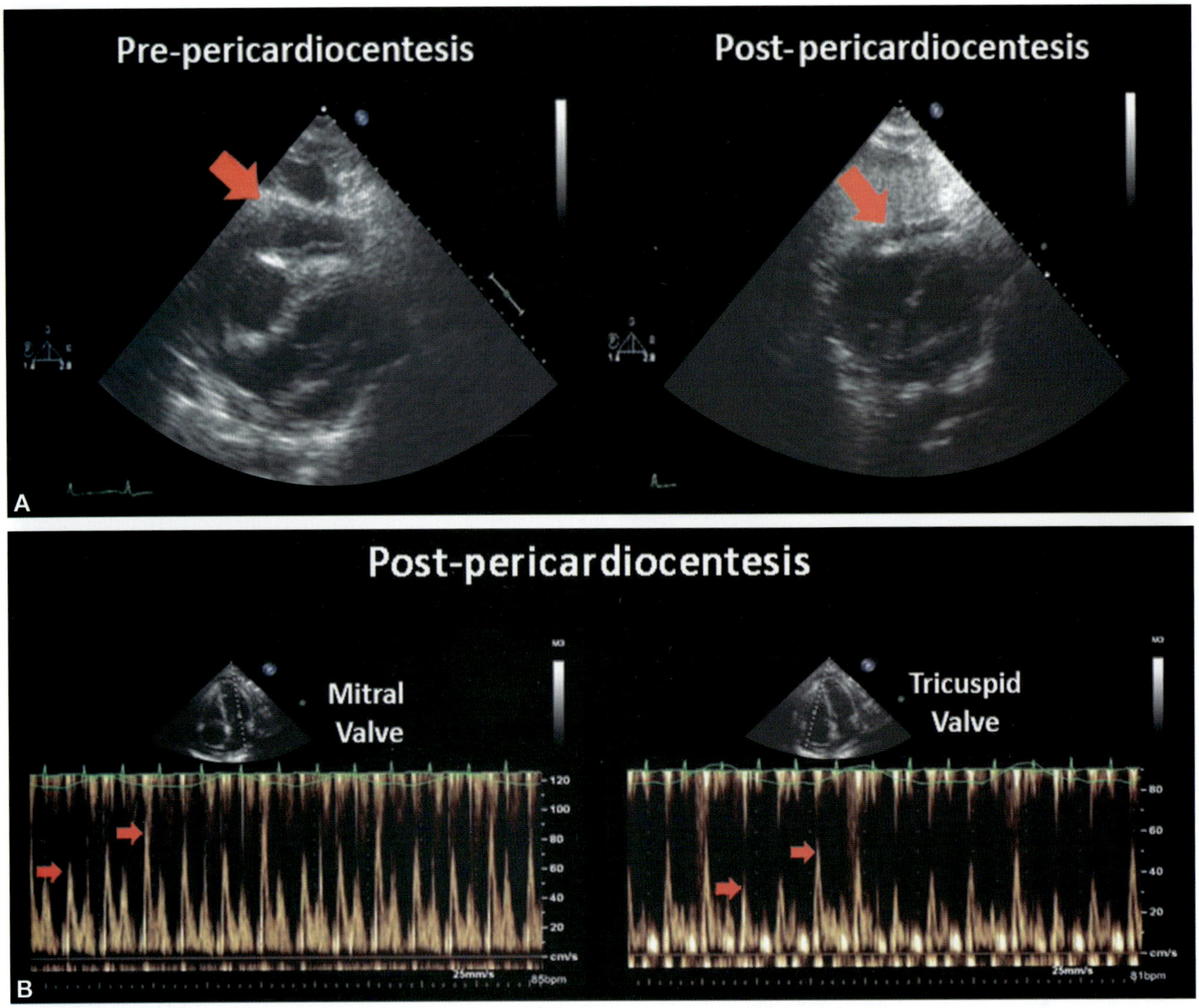

Figs. 38.16A and B: Effusive-constrictive pericarditis. (A) There is a moderate to large pericardial effusion (arrow) prior to pericardiocentesis (left panel). Post-pericardiocentesis (right pane) there is only a small residual pericardial effusion (arrow); (B) Despite pericardiocentesis, Doppler study post-pericardiocentesis demonstrates significant respiratory variation in mitral and tricuspid diastolic flow (arrows).

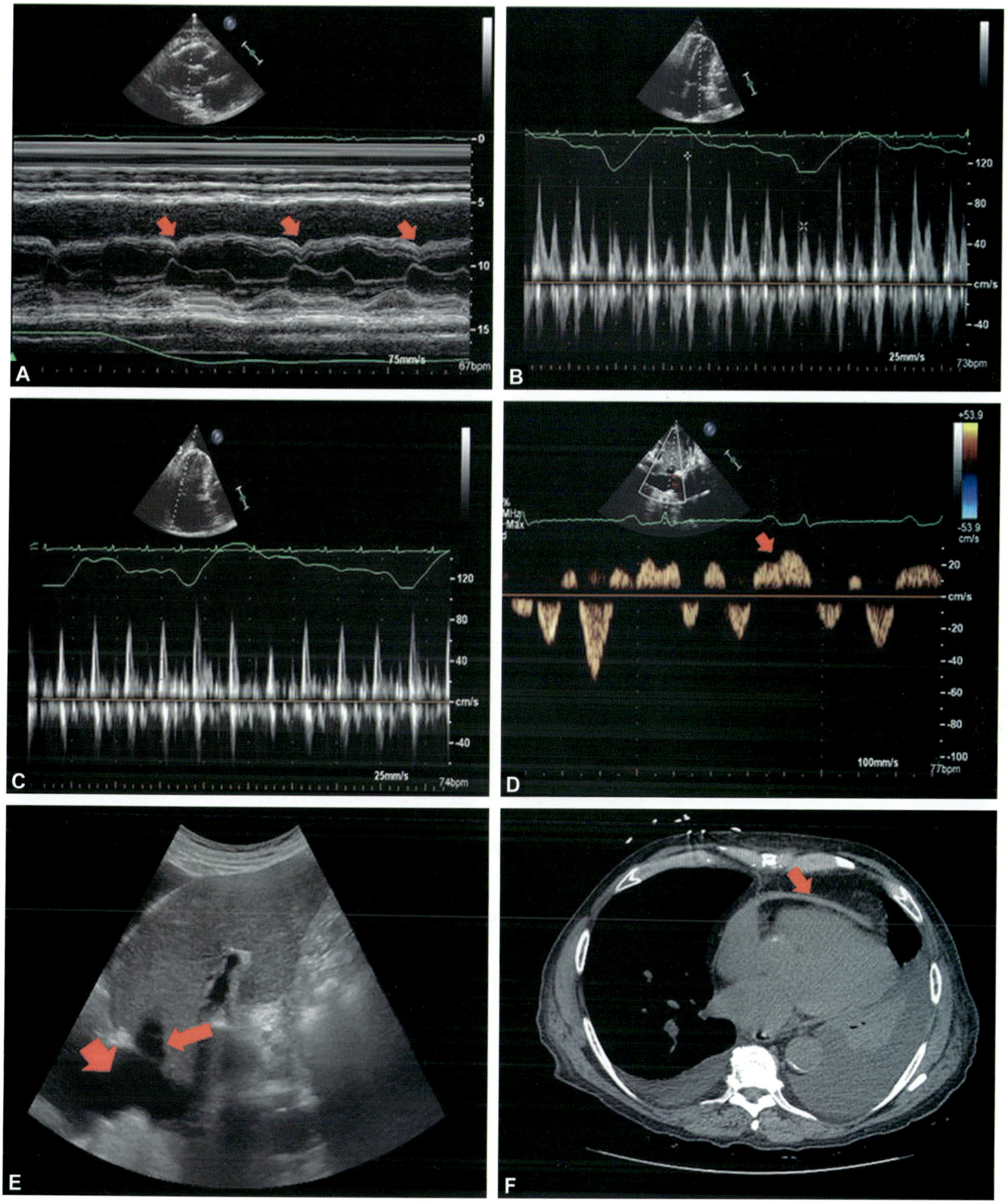

Figs. 38.17A to F: Subacute constrictive pericarditis. Doppler echocardiography study demonstrates abnormal septal bounce (figure A, arrows), significant variation in diastolic mitral and tricuspid flows with respiration (figures B and C), and diastolic hepatic venous flow reversal (figure D, arrow). Abdominal ultrasound (figure E) reveals dilation of the inferior vena cava (thick short arrow) and hepatic vein (thin long arrow) with ascites. Computed tomography (CT) scan (figure F) demonstrates diffuse pericardial thickening (arrow) with a large left pleural effusion. The patient underwent pericardiectomy and pathology demonstrated thickening and fibrosis of the pericardium.

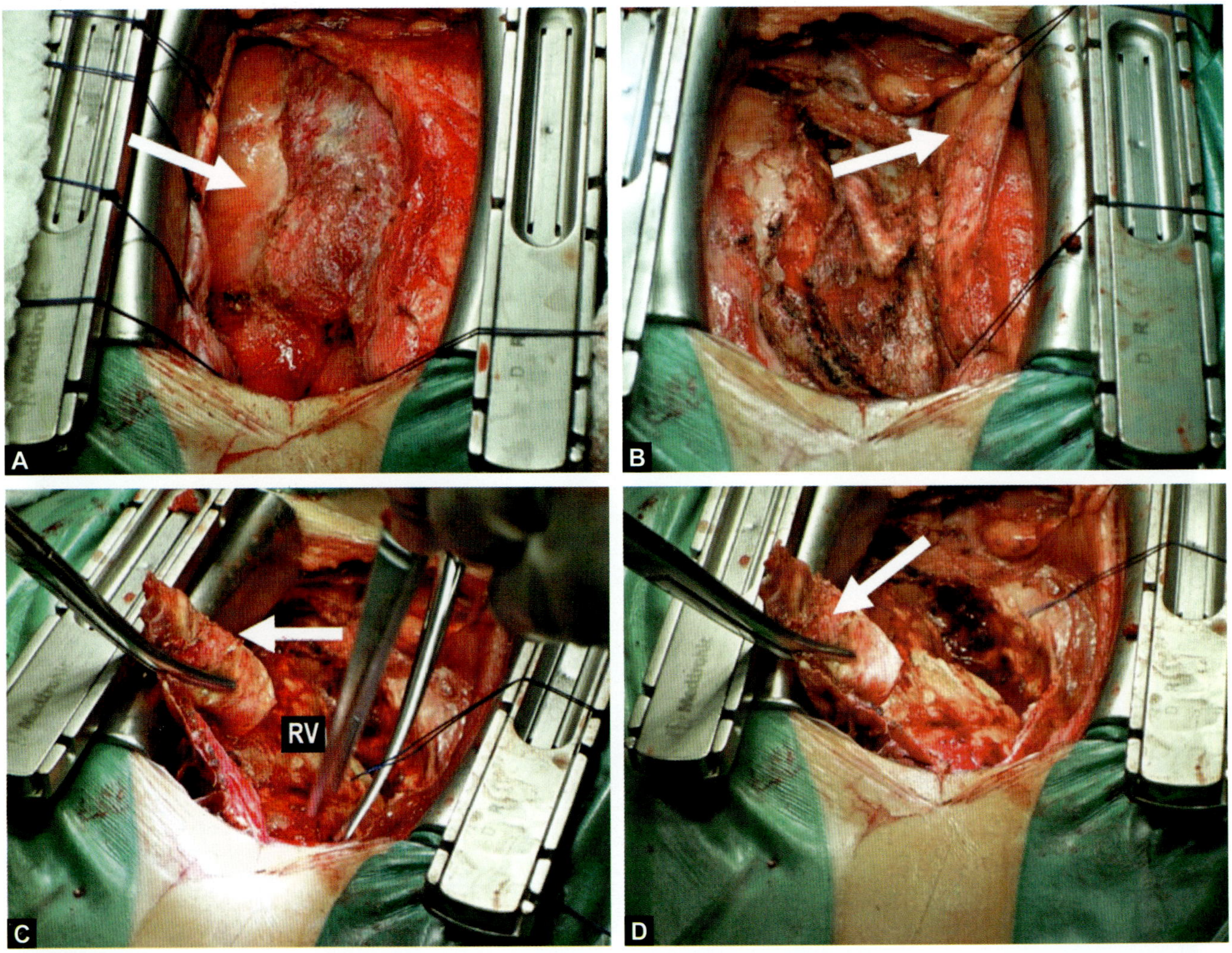

Figs. 38.18A to D: Images of a pericardiectomy in a patient with constrictive pericarditis and a thickened and calcified pericardium (arrows). [Image from Lima MV, Cardoso JN, Cardoso CM, et al. Constrictive pericarditis with extensive calcification. Arq Bras Cardiol. 2011;96(1):e7-10]. (RV: Right ventricular).

REFERENCES

Feng D, Glockner J, Kim K, et al. Cardiac magnetic resonance imaging pericardial late gadolinium enhancement and elevated inflammatory markers can predict the reversibility of constrictive pericarditis after antiinflammatory medical therapy: a pilot study. Circulation. 2011;124(17):1830-7.

Klein AL, Abbara S, Agler DA, et al. American Society of Echocardiography clinical recommendations for multimodality cardiovascular imaging of patients with pericardial disease: endorsed by the Society for Cardiovascular Magnetic Resonance and Society of Cardiovascular Computed Tomography. J Am Soc Echocardiogr. 2013;26(9):965-1012.e15.

Section 6

Congenital Heart Disease

Chapters

- Patent Foramen Ovale
- Atrial Septal Defects
- Ventricular Septal Defect
- Ebstein Anomaly
- Tetralogy of Fallot
- Transposition of the Great Arteries
- Supravalvular and Subvalvular Aortic Stenosis
- Aortic Coarctation
- Patent Ductus Arteriosus

CHAPTER

39

Patent Foramen Ovale

Luc M Beauchesne, John P Veinot

EMBRYOLOGY

Embryologically, the atrial septum is formed by the partial fusion of two walls: the septum primum and the septum secundum (Figs. 39.1A to C). Each septum has an intrinsic defect (the ostium secundum and the foramen ovale, respectively). It is important to understand that, although these two holes do not overlap, a potential passage or channel is present between the two walls which can allow communication between the atria. This interatrial channel is essential for normal fetal physiology (Fig. 39.2). After birth, in most individuals, complete fusion of the septal walls will eventually occur and lead to obliteration of the channel. However, in a significant proportion (25–30% of adults) there will be incomplete fusion and the channel will remain open. This residual channel is called patent foramen ovale (PFO; Figs. 39.3A and B).

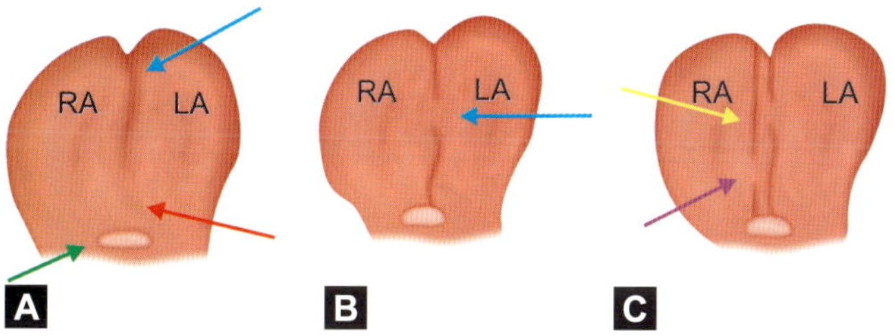

Figs. 39.1A to C: Embryology of the atrial septum. Reviewing the embryology of the atrial septum is important in order to understand the anatomy and physiology of the patent foramen ovale (PFO). (A) The septum primum (blue arrow) progressively comes down from the roof the atria to fuse with the endocardial cushions (green arrow). At one point in the process there is a potential space which has been traditionally termed the ostium primum (red arrow); (B) As the septum primum continues to grow, the ostium primum is obliterated. A new hole, through apoptosis, is formed in the superior pole of the septum primum which is called the ostium secundum (blue arrow); (C) A second membrane comes down on the right side of the septum primum which is called the septum secundum (yellow arrow). Like the septum primum, the septum secundum is an incomplete wall and has a defect which is named the foramen ovale (purple arrow).

DIAGNOSIS OF PATENT FORAMEN OVALE

Clinically, the diagnosis of a PFO is usually made by transthoracic echocardiography (TTE) with the use of color Doppler, peripheral saline contrast injection and the aid of

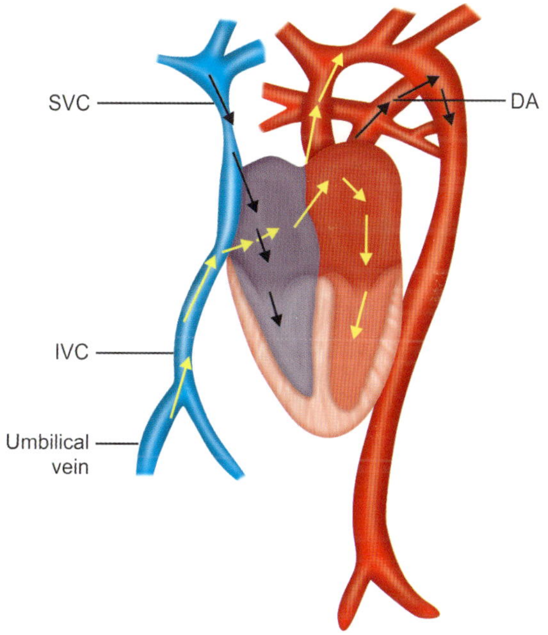

Fig. 39.2: Fetal circulation. The PFO is an essential component of normal fetal cardiac physiology. Oxygenated blood (yellow arrows) from the placenta, is directed by the umbilical vein to the IVC and then to the RA. The blood then streams across the RA and traverses the atrial septum, though the foramen ovale, into the LA, then to the LV and aorta, to the head and upper limbs. Deoxygenated blood (black arrows) arrives from the SVC to the RA where it is streamed across the RA into the RV, then to the main pulmonary artery, then through the DA, to the descending aorta where eventually it will be directed to the placenta for re-oxygenation. (DA: Ductus arteriosus; IVC: Inferior vena cava; LA: Left atrium; LV: Left ventricle; RA: Right atrium; RV: Right ventricle; SVC: Superior vena cava).

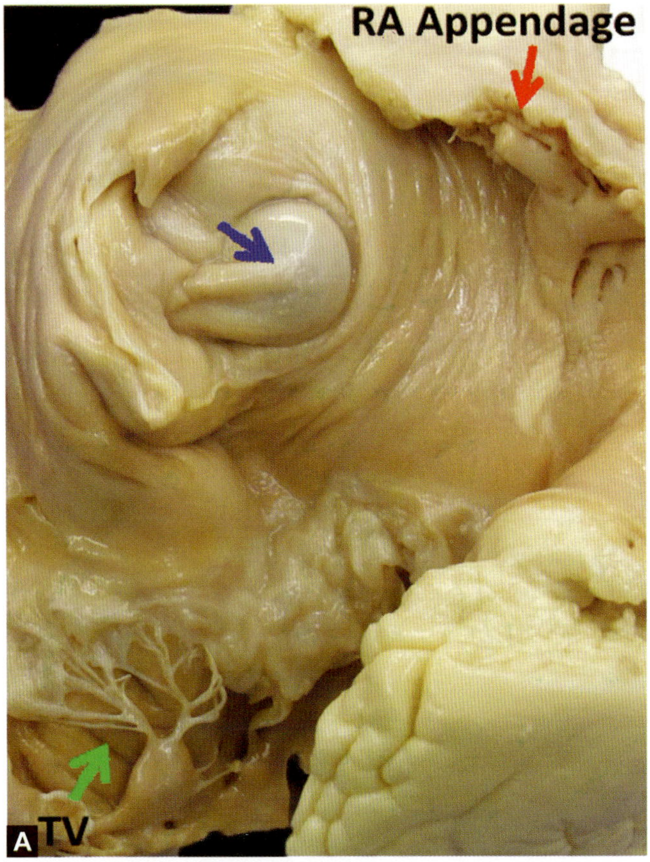

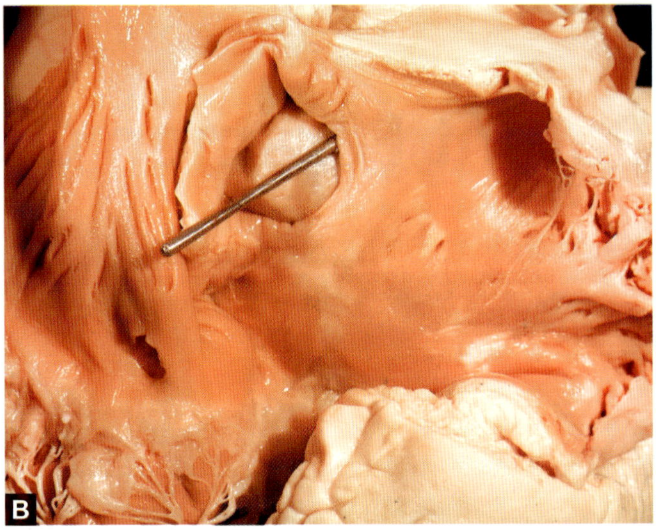

Figs. 39.3A and B: Atrial septum anatomy. (A) Pathological specimen of the right atrium and atrial septum. When looking at the atrial septum from the right side, one can appreciate a slight depression which is named the fossa ovalis. The fossa ovalis represents the foramen ovale of the septum secundum. A rim or limbus surrounds the fossa ovalis. The fossa is obliterated by a membrane (floor of the fossa ovalis, blue arrow) which represents a component of the septum primum. Red arrow: right atrial appendage. Green arrow: tricuspid valve. The potential channel between the two atria can not be appreciated on this image; (B) A probe is seen crossing the atrial septum demonstrating the presence of a patent foramen ovale.

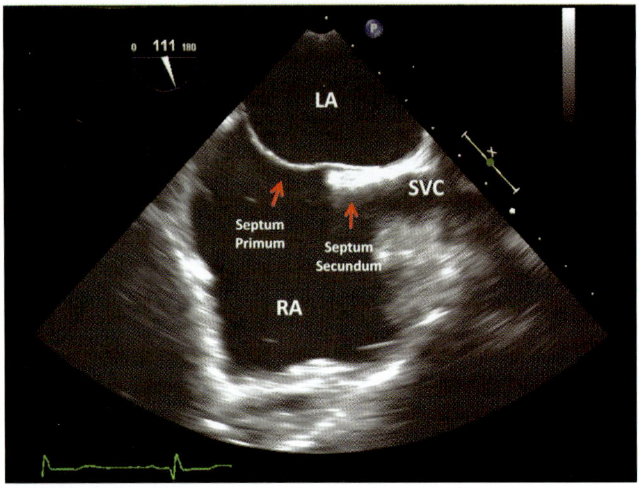

Fig. 39.4: Transesophageal echocardiography (TEE) at 111° rotation, of normal atrial septal anatomy. Note the usual thin membrane septum primum and thicker septum secundum. (LA: Left atrium; RA: Right atrium; SVC: Superior vena cava).

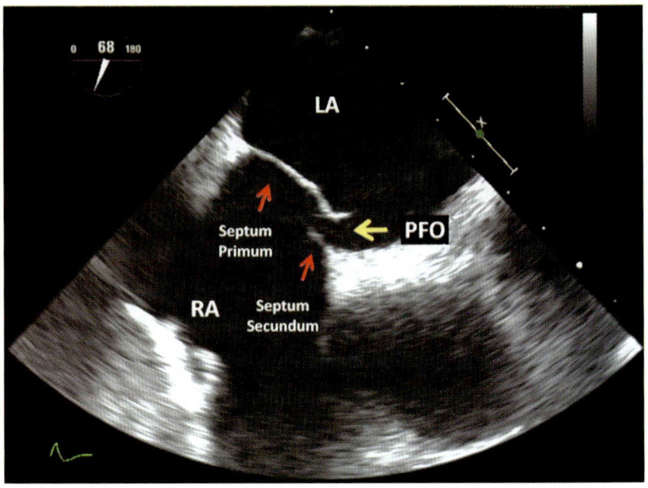

Fig. 39.5: Transesophageal echocardiography (TEE), demonstrating a patent foramen ovale (PFO). (A) TEE, at 68° rotation, view shows a large PFO channel between the septum and septum secundum (yellow arrow). (LA: Left atrium; RA: Right atrium).

maneuvers that transiently increase right-sided pressures (e.g. Valsalva, coughing). The diagnostic sensitivity and characterization of the atrial septal anatomy can be further increased with the use of transesophageal echocardiography (TEE; Figs. 39.4 to 39.9, Videos 39.1 to 39.3). Although transcranial Doppler (TCD) is regarded by many

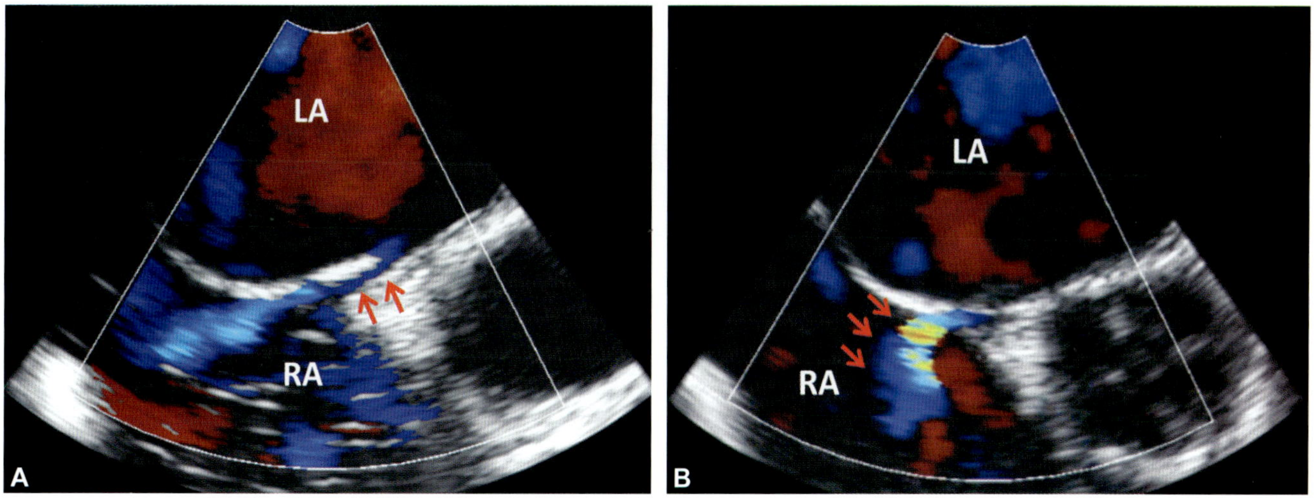

Figs. 39.6A and B: Color Doppler transesophageal echocardiography (TEE) demonstrating patent foramen ovale (PFO) and flow from the left atrium in to the right atrium. (A) The PFO and flow through the PFO is clearly seen (arrows); (B) The jet of flow through the PFO into the right atrium is demonstrated (arrows). (Images courtesy of Glenn N Levine, MD). (LA: Left atrium; RA: Right atrium).

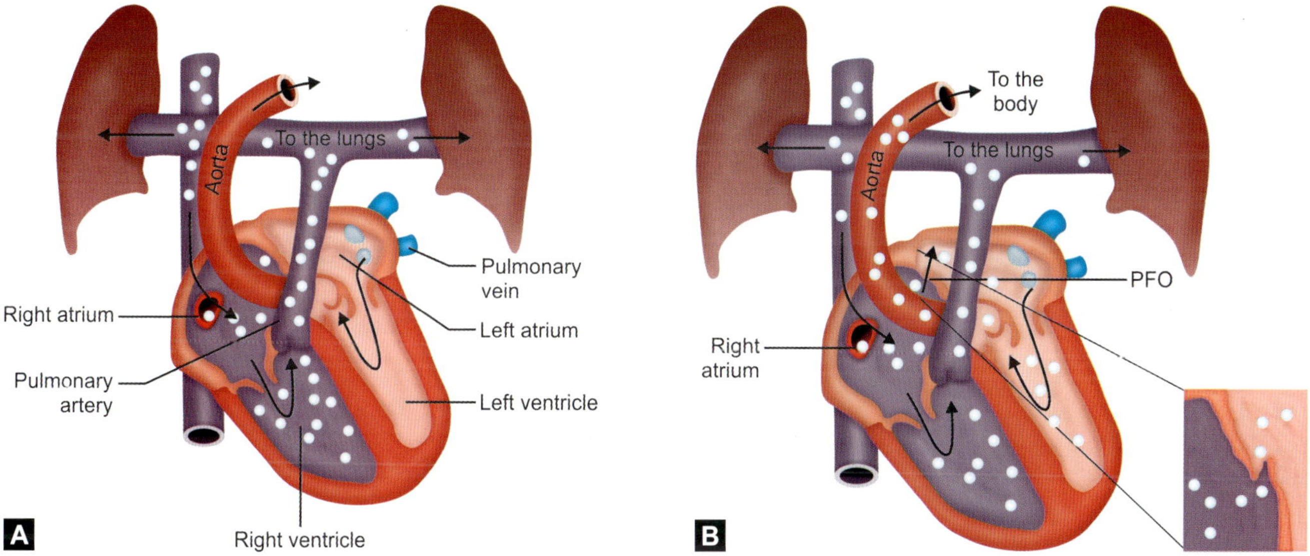

Figs. 39.7A and B: Schematic representation of an agitated saline "bubble" study in the (A) absence and (B) presence of a patent foramen ovale (PFO); (A) With the release phase of the Valsalva maneuver, no bubbles are seen crossing from the right side of the heart in to the left side of the heart; (B) The release phase of the Valsalva results in an increase in right atrial pressure and some flow of blood and bubbles into the left atrium, and subsequently the left ventricle and aorta. [Image adapted from Sykes O, Clark JE. Patent foramen ovale and scuba diving: a practical guide for physicians on when to refer for screening. Extrem Physiol Med. 2013;2(1):10, with permission].

as the best screening method for PFO, it is not clinically available at most centers, and does not allow differentiation from the presence of pulmonary arteriovenous malformations, which can also cause right to left shunting. In many individuals, the portion of the septum primum that forms the floor of the fossa ovalis can be very redundant. On echocardiography, these patients will typically be found to have an atrial septal aneurysm (ASA; Figs. 39.10A and B). Although frequently associated with a PFO, the clinical significance of an ASA is unclear at the present time, and may simply represent a variant of normal atrial septal anatomy.

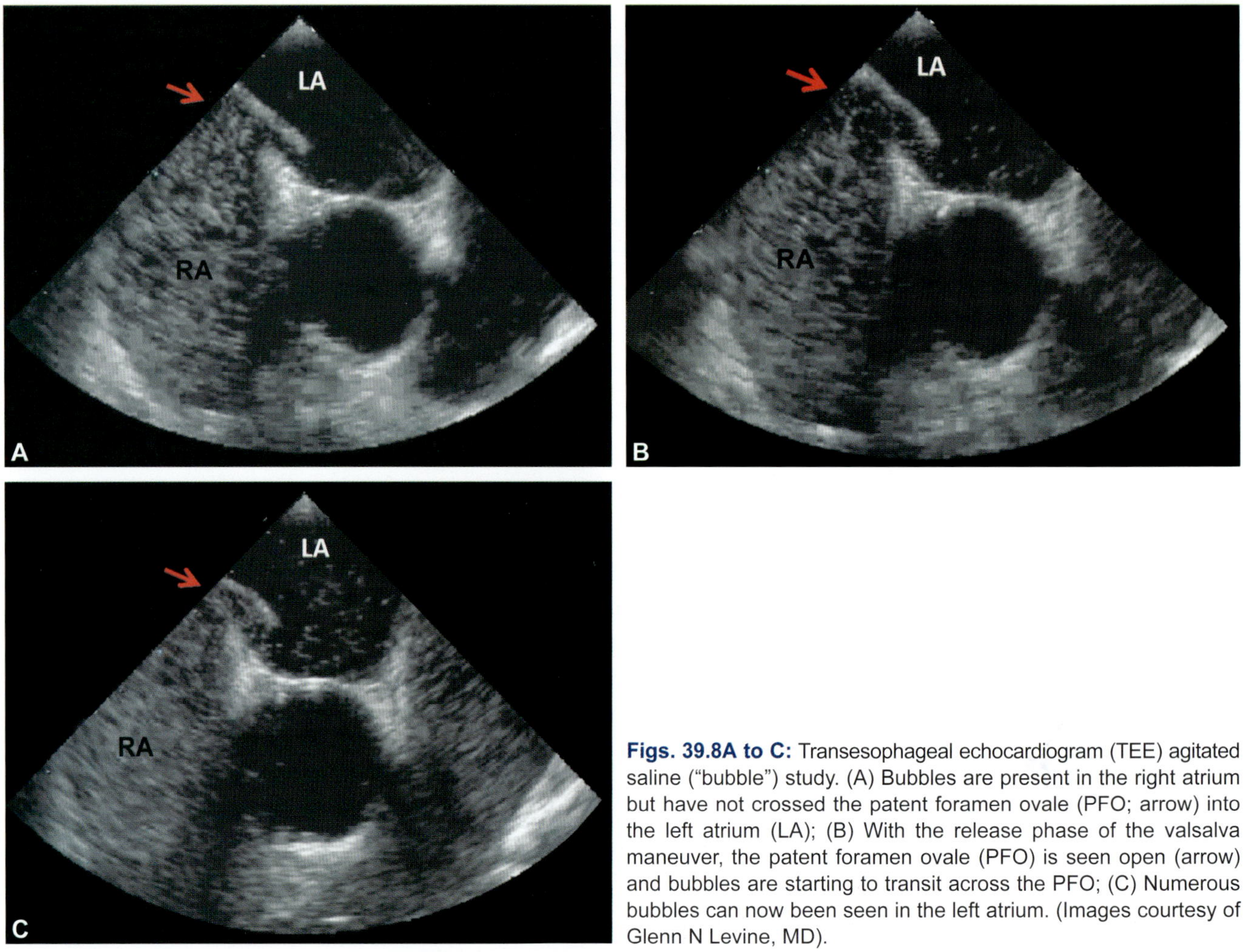

Figs. 39.8A to C: Transesophageal echocardiogram (TEE) agitated saline ("bubble") study. (A) Bubbles are present in the right atrium but have not crossed the patent foramen ovale (PFO; arrow) into the left atrium (LA); (B) With the release phase of the valsalva maneuver, the patent foramen ovale (PFO) is seen open (arrow) and bubbles are starting to transit across the PFO; (C) Numerous bubbles can now been seen in the left atrium. (Images courtesy of Glenn N Levine, MD).

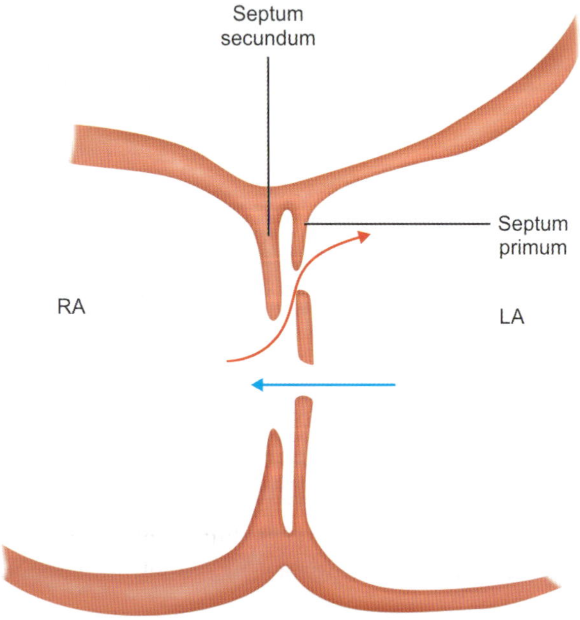

Fig. 39.9: Diagram of the atrial septum contrasting a patent foramen ovale (PFO) from a small secundum atrial septal defect (ASD). The PFO represents a potential channel between the septum primum and septum secundum that can allow for intermittent right to left shunting in circumstances where right atrial pressure exceeds left atrial pressure. A small secundum ASD represents a defect of the septum primum, per se, which creates a substrate for left to right shunting. These two entities may sometimes be difficult to differentiate on transthoracic echocardiogram (TTE) and may require transesophageal echocardiogram (TEE) imaging to sort out, if this is clinically indicated. (LA: Left atrium; RA, Right atrium).

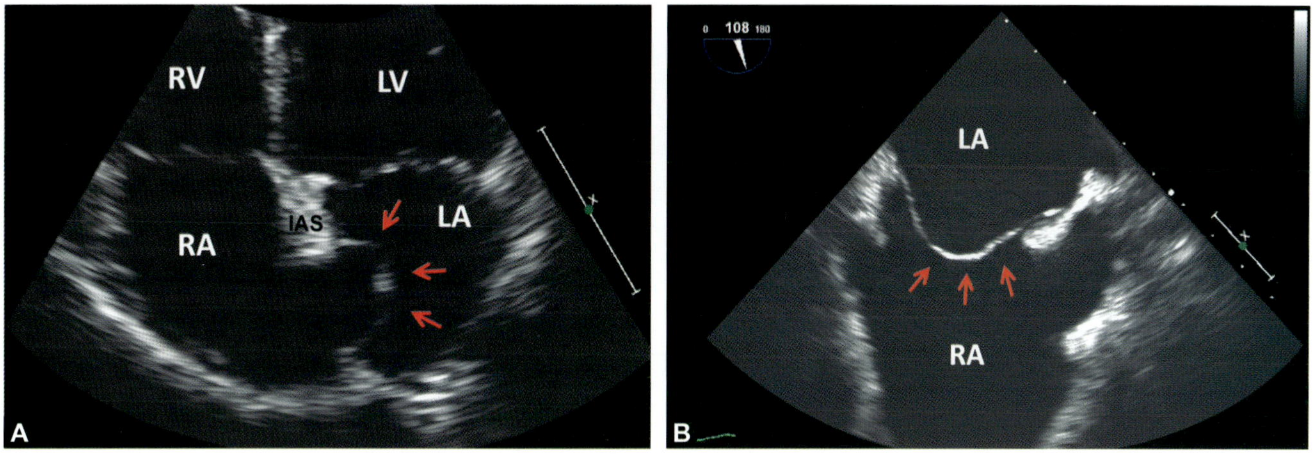

Figs. 39.10A and B: Atrial septal aneurysm (ASA). (A) Transthoracic echocardiogram (TTE) showing large redundant ASA (red arrows) projecting into left atrium; (B) Transesophageal echocardiogram (TEE) of another patient with an ASA. (IAS: Interatrial septum; LA: Left atrium; LV: Left ventricle; RA: Right atrium; RV: Right ventricle).

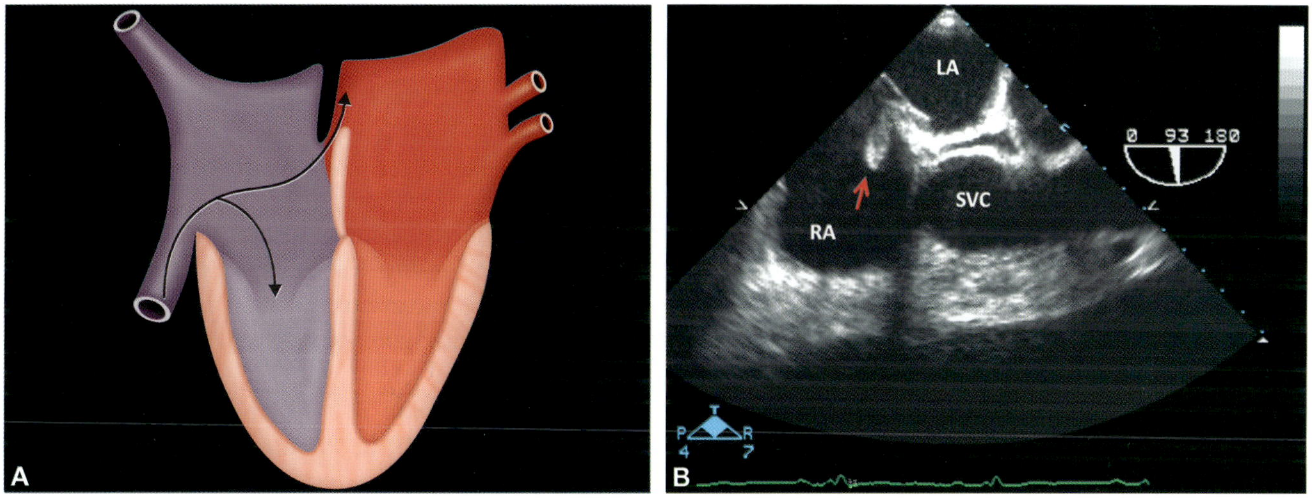

Figs. 39.11A and B: Paradoxical embolus. (A) Diagram showing embolism arising from thrombus from the iliofemoral venous system. A component travels to the pulmonary artery leading to a pulmonary embolus. Another portion "paradoxically" crosses over to the left side of the heart by transiting through a patent foramen ovale (PFO); (B) On these transesophageal echocardiogram (TEE) images a thrombus (arrow) is seen crossing the atrial septum through the PFO. A portion of this thrombus extends into the left atrium (arrow). On further imaging, the patient was documented to have a lower limb deep venous thrombosis (DVT) and evidence of pulmonary embolism. The thrombus was surgically extracted to prevent left sided peripheral embolism. (IVC: Inferior vena cava; LA: Left atrium; RA: Right atrium; RV: Rright ventricle.

Paradoxical Emboli

In the vast majority of individuals, the presence of a PFO is of no clinical significance. However, there continues to be a debate on the possible role of the PFO as a culprit for cryptogenic stroke in young patients. A PFO represents a potential conduit for paradoxical (i.e. right to left) shunting of an embolic fragment arsing from a deep venous thrombus (DVT) and subsequent left-sided embolization. This mechanism has been clinically demonstrated to occur and is reported in several case reports (Figs. 39.11 and 39.12). Several case control and prospective cohort studies on the association between PFO and cryptogenic stroke have been published, but have yielded discordant findings. Even if an association is present, it has been postulated that the PFO may not be causative but simply a marker of underlying left atrial dysfunction, which could lead to atrial fibrillation and left atrial appendage thrombus formation.

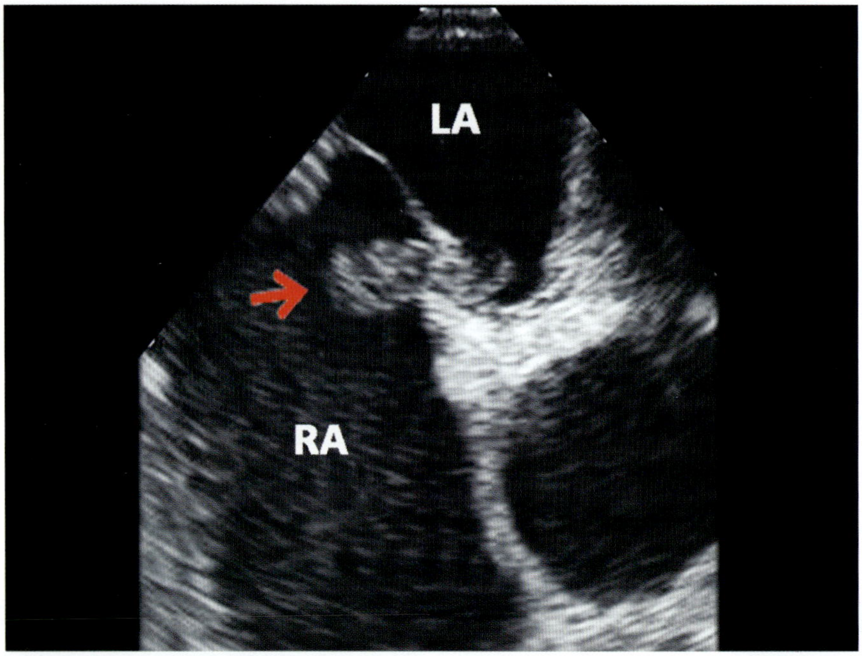

Fig. 39.12: Transesophageal echocardiogram (TEE) showing paradoxical embolus. A thrombus is seen (arrow) crossing a patent foramen ovale. (LA: Left atrium; RA: Right atrium).

PATENT FORAMEN OVALE CLOSURE DEVICES

Over the last two decades, the development of percutaneous devices has led to significant clinical enthusiasm for PFO closure (Figs. 39.13 to 39.16). These devices are relatively easy to use and can be deployed in the catheterization laboratory under fluoroscopy, without the need of general anesthesia. Drawbacks include a real, but small, risk of major complications (pericardial tamponade, embolization, thrombus formation) and persistence of demonstrable right to left shunting in a minority of patients.

Recently, three large, prospective, randomized controlled trials evaluating the benefit of PFO device closure in cryptogenic stroke have been published. Overall, in all three studies, device closure did not show better outcomes when compared to medical therapy. However, the trials were limited by low event rates and signals in the data suggest that some patients may still benefit from PFO closure.

Detailed evaluation by a neurologist should be performed in any patient in whom PFO closure for stroke prevention is being considered. At this point in time, other possible indications for PFO closure are few but can include: unexplained diving related decompression illness, and unusual clinical situations in which there is significant desaturation due to right to left shunting through the PFO (e.g. platypnea-orthodeoxia syndrome, severe right ventricular infarction, left ventricular assist device-associated severe hypoxia).

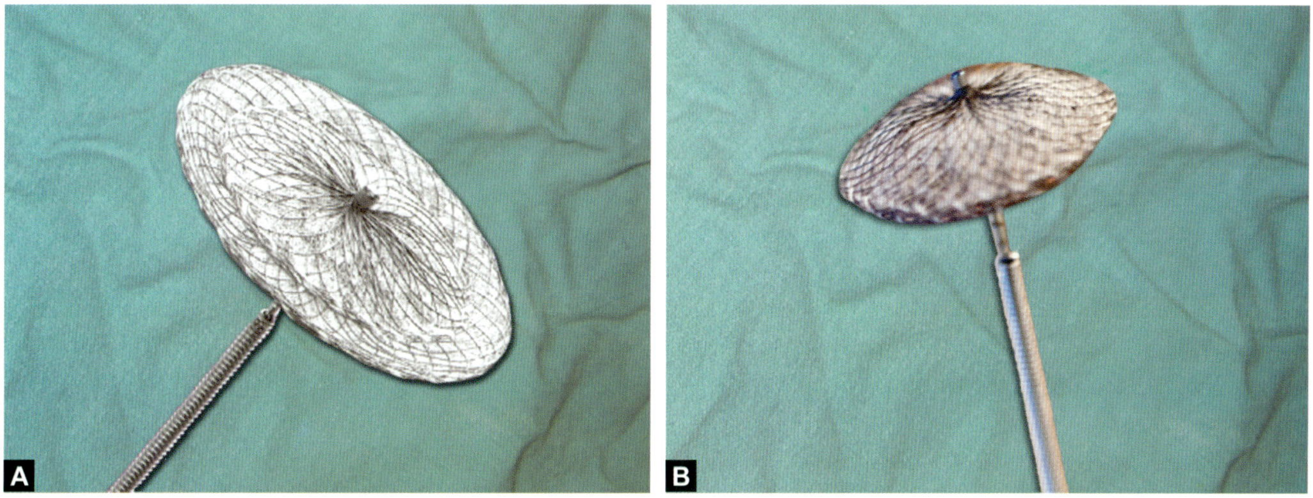

Figs. 39.13A and B: Examples of patent foramen ovale (PFO) occluders.

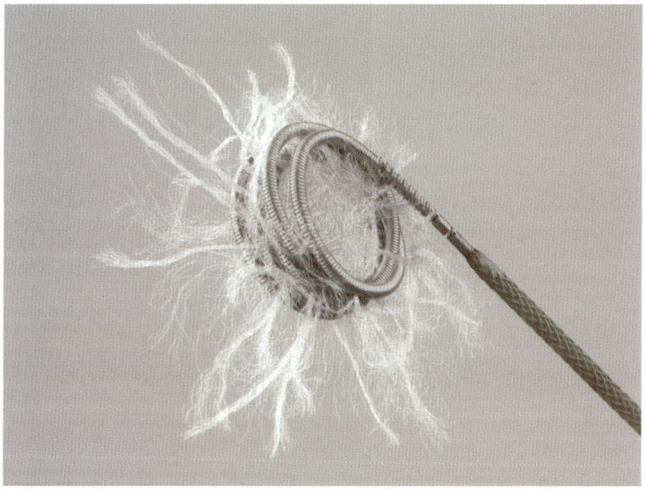

Fig. 39.13C: Patent foramen ovale (PFO) coil occluder. (Image courtesy of and with permission from Cook Medical).

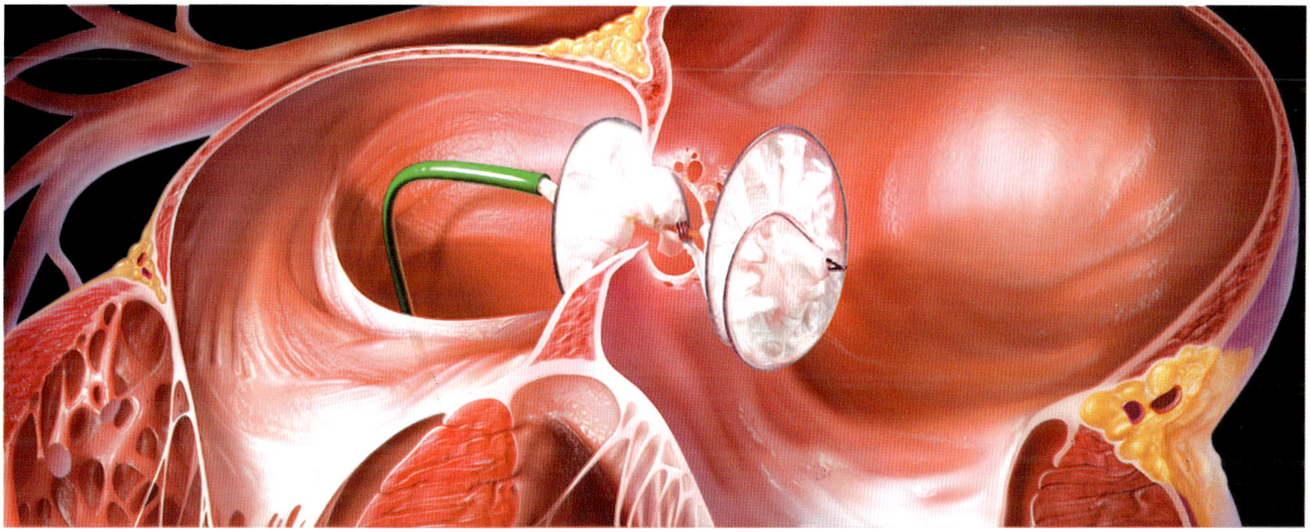

Fig. 39.14: Schematic illustration of a patent foramen ovale (PFO) occluder. (Image courtesy of and with permission from WL Gore & Associates, Inc.).

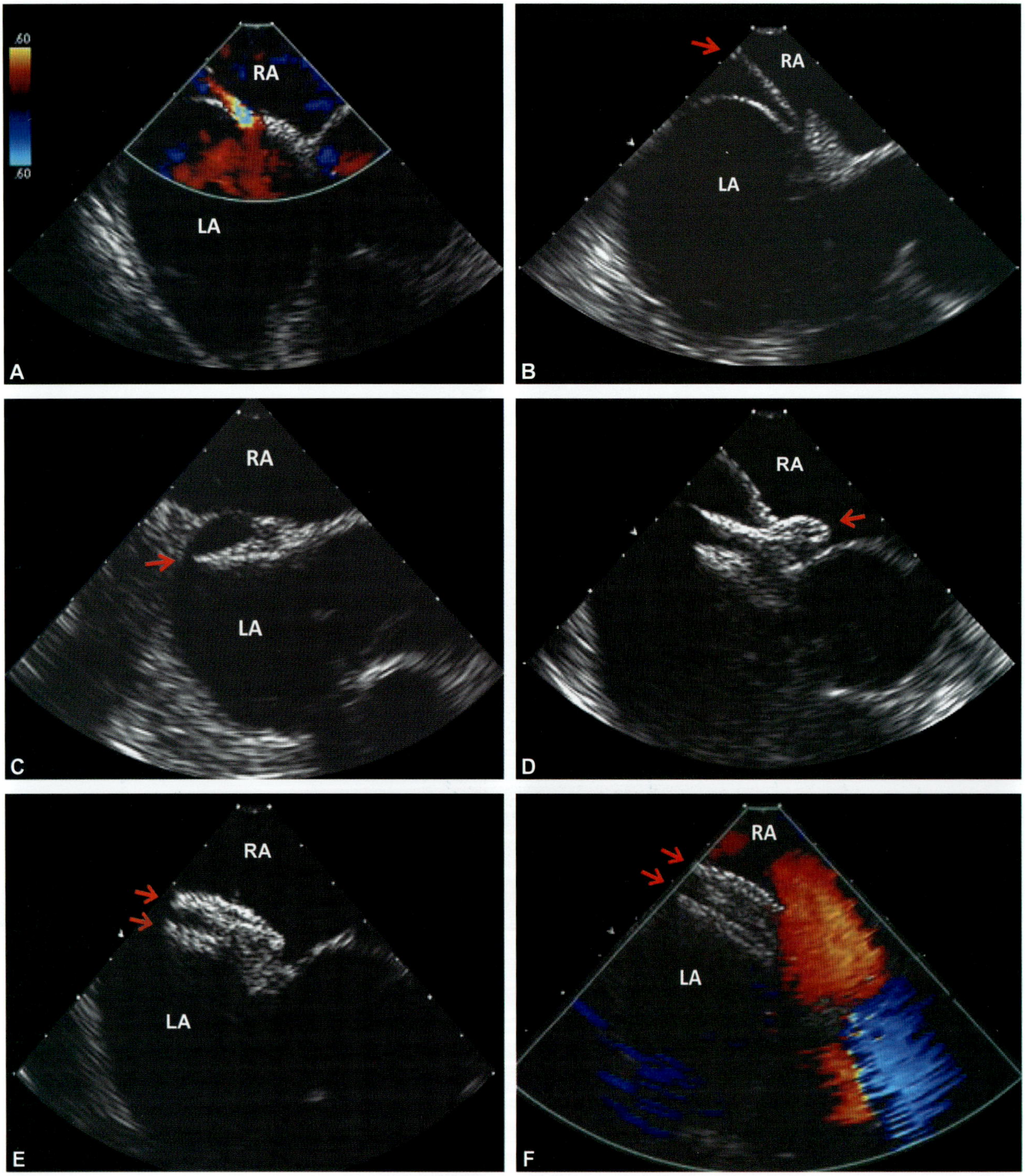

Figs. 39.15A to F: Percutaneous closure of a patent foramen ovale (PFO). (A) Intracardiac echocardiograph (ICE) imaging of PFO with Doppler ultrasound, showing blood flow in the tunnel between the septum primum and septum secundum; (B) ICE imaging of the diagnostic catheter (arrow) engaging and crossing the tunnel between the septum primum and septum secundum; (C) Positioning of the left atrial disk (arrow) under ICE guidance, against the left atrial side of the interatrial septum; (D) Positioning of the right atrial disk (arrow) under ICE guidance, on the right atrial side of the interatrial septum; (E) Deployed PFO occluder (arrows) under ICE imaging; (F) Doppler image of a successfully deployed PFO occluder (arrows) with significant reduction in the interatrial shunt and no obstruction of the superior vena cava flow. [Images and legend text from Daraban N, Reyes M, Smalling RW. Transcatheter occlusion of atrial septal defects for prevention of recurrence of paradoxical embolism. In: Rao PS (Ed). Atrial Septal Defect. InTech; 2012, with permission]. (LA: Left atrium; RA: Right atrium).

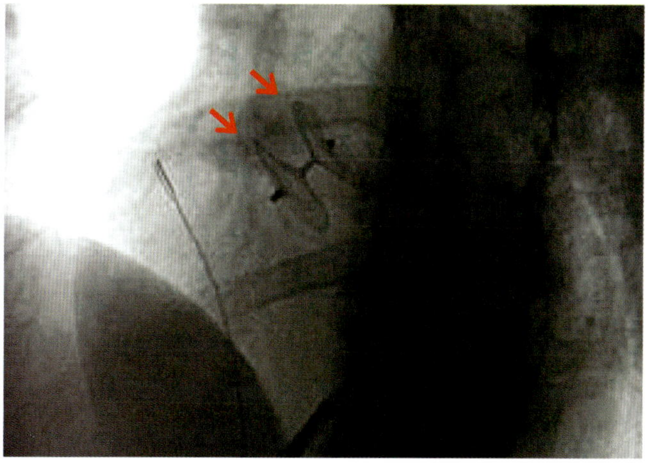

Fig. 39.16: Fluoroscopy image of a fully deployed patent foramen ovale (PFO) occluder (arrows). [Images from Daraban N, Reyes M, Smalling RW. Transcatheter occlusion of atrial septal defects for prevention of recurrence of paradoxical embolism. In: Rao PS (Ed). Atrial Septal Defect. InTech; 2012, with permission].

VIDEO LEGENDS

Video 39.1: Transesophageal echocardiogram (TEE) showing a patent foramen ovale (PFO) with intermittent right to left flow during an agitated saline ("bubble") study. (Video clip courtesy of Glenn N Levine, MD).

Video 39.2: Color Doppler transesophageal echocardiogram (TEE) demonstrating a patent foramen ovale (PFO).

Video 39.3: Color Doppler transesophageal echocardiogram (TEE) showing a patent foramen ovale (PFO) with intermittent left-right flow (intermittent thin blue jet). (Video clip courtesy of Glenn N Levine, MD).

REFERENCES

Carroll JD, Saver JL, Thaler DE, et al. Closure of patent foramen ovale versus medical therapy after cryptogenic stroke. N Engl J Med. 2013;368(12):1092-100.

Furlan AJ, Reisman M, Massaro J, et al. Closure or medical therapy for cryptogenic stroke with patent foramen ovale. N Engl J Med. 2012;366(11):991-7.

Hagen PT, Scholz DG, Edwards WD. Incidence and size of patent foramen ovale during the first 10 decades of life: an autopsy study of 965 normal hearts. Mayo Clin Proc. 1984; 59(1):17-20.

Hara H, Virmani R, Ladich E, et al. Patent foramen ovale: current pathology, pathophysiology, and clinical status. J Am Coll Cardiol. 2005;46(9):1768-76.

Kuch B, Riehle M, von Scheidt W. Hypoxemia from right-to-left shunting through a patent foramen ovale in right ventricular infarction: treatment by revascularization, preload reduction, and, finally, interventional PFO closure. Clin Res Cardiol. 2006; 95(12):680-4.

Landzberg MJ, Khairy P. Patent foramen ovale: when is intervention warranted? Can J Cardiol. 2013;29:890-2.

Loforte A, Violini R, Musumeci F. Transcatheter closure of patent foramen ovale for hypoxemia during left ventricular assist device support. J Card Surg. 2012;27(4):528-9.

Meier B, Kalesan B, Mattle HP, et al. Percutaneous closure of patent foramen ovale in cryptogenic embolism. N Engl J Med. 2013;368(12):1083-91.

Pavlovic M, Buellesfeld L, Meier B. Tools & techniques: PFO/ASD closure. EuroIntervention. 2011;7(3):408-10.

CHAPTER

40

Atrial Septal Defects

Luc M Beauchesne, Carole J Dennie

INTRODUCTION

Atrial septal defects (ASDs) are among the most common congenital heart defects. There are four types of ASDs: the secundum ASD (75%), the sinus venosus ASD (15%), the primum ASD (10%) and the coronary sinus ASD (< 1%) (Figs. 40.1 and 40.2).

SECUNDUM ASD

The secundum ASD, by definition, is a defect in which part of the margin involves the floor of the fossa ovalis of the atrial septum (see the chapter on PFO and the discussion of atrial septal anatomy) (Figs. 40.3 to 40.7, Videos 40.1 to 40.4). The hole can extend from the fossa ovalis into different directions (e.g. posterior versus anterior extension) and can be of various morphologies (round, oval, tear drop). In some cases, there can be multiple secundum ASDs (Fig. 40.8). Secundum ASDs come in different sizes (diameter ranges from 2 mm to 40 mm). As a rule, a hemodynamically significant secundum ASD (i.e. one which will lead to right sided volume overload) is ≥ 10 mm in diameter. Secundum ASDs are typically isolated defects which are not associated with other structural anomalies. Secundum ASDs are frequently first diagnosed in adulthood (even sometimes in elderly patients) with various means of presentation including murmur, abnormal ECG (Fig. 40.9), dyspnea, or even as an incidental finding on imaging (Fig. 40.10).

SINUS VENOSUS ASD

The sinus venosus ASD is located in the posterior part of the atrial septum and does not involve the fossa ovalis (Figs. 40.11 and 40.12). The majority are located superiorly near the superior vena cava (SVC), but they may sometimes be located inferiorly near the IVC (Fig. 40.13).

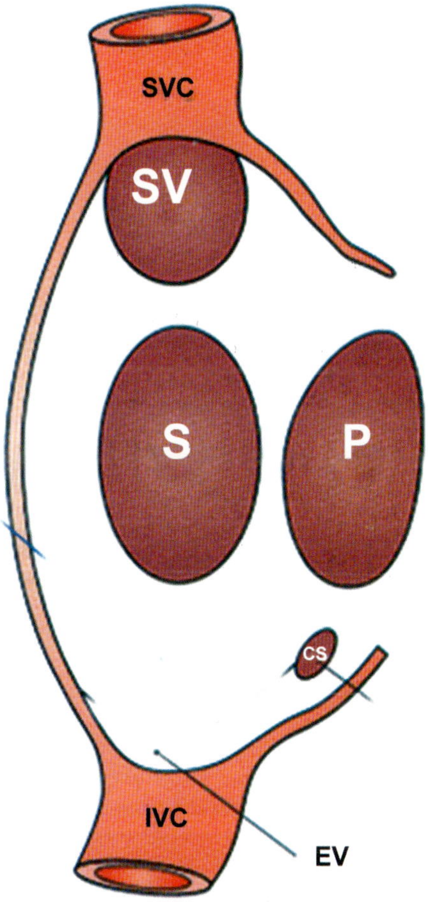

Fig. 40.1: Illustration of the atrial septum, from the right side, demonstrating the location of the different atrial septal defects (ASD). SV: Sinus venosus ASD (superior type), S: secundum ASD, P: Primum ASD, CS: Coronary sinus ASD. The secundum ASD is, by far, the most common of the four.

The defects are invariably significant in size (≥ 10 mm). The majority of sinus venosus ASDs are associated with anomalous connection or drainage of the right sided pulmonary veins (to the right atrium or the SVC) (Fig. 40.14).

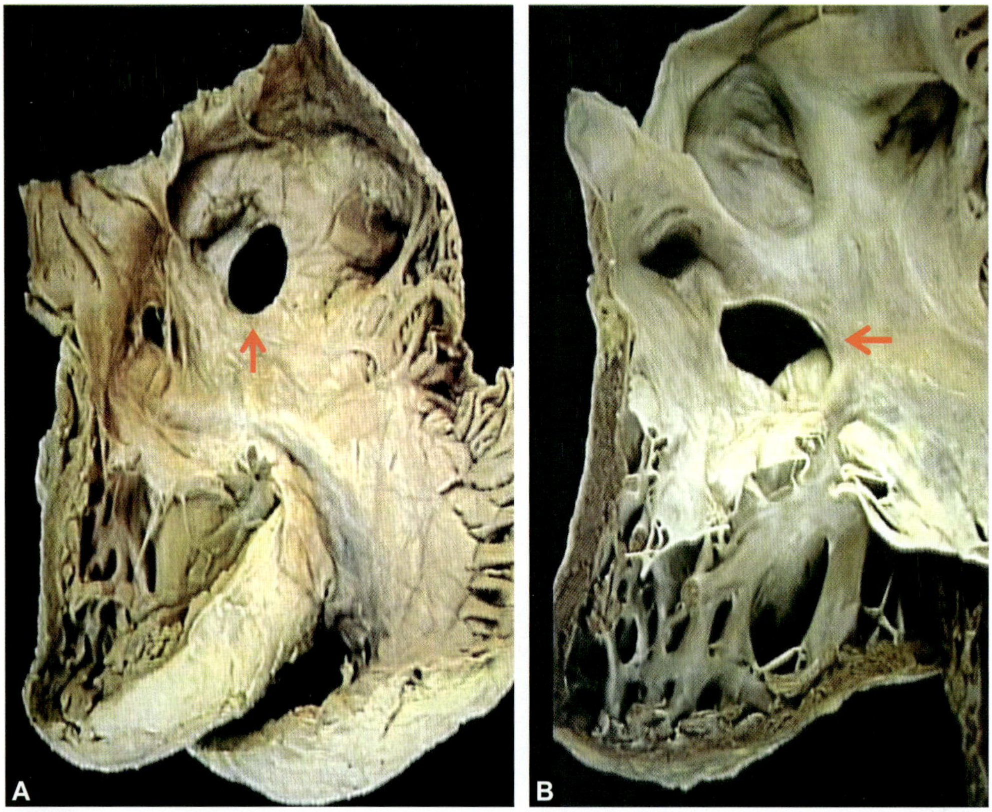

Figs. 40.2A and B: Gross pathology specimens demonstrating ASDs. (A) Secundum ASD. (B) Primum ASD. [Images from Armed Forces Institute of Pathology (public domain images)].

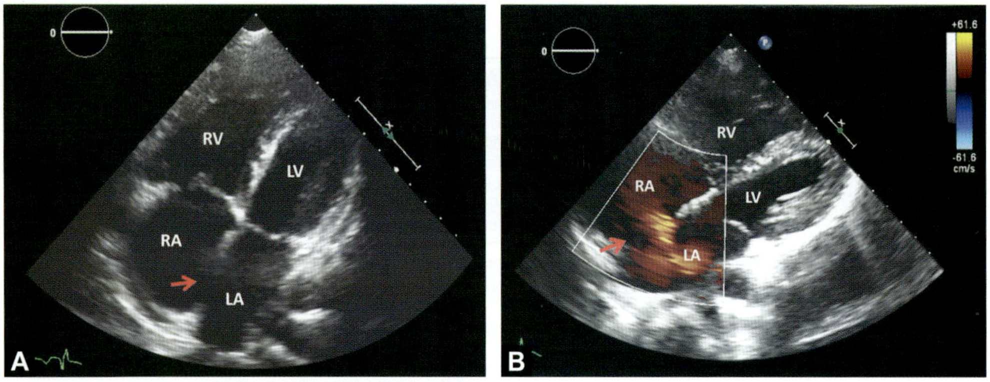

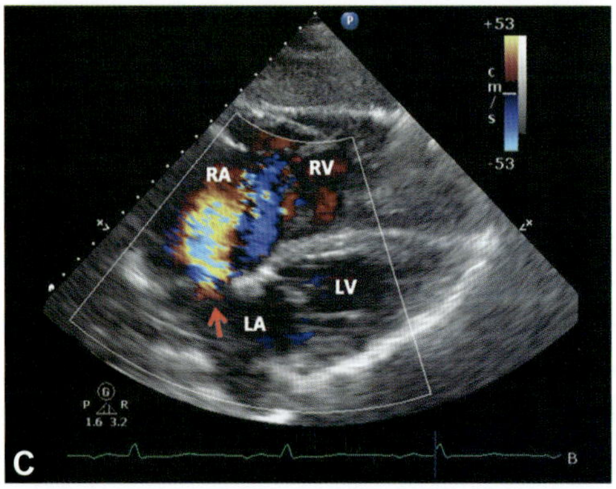

Figs. 40.3A to C: Secundum ASD. (A) Apcial four-chamber transthoracic echocardiographic (TTE) image showing a large defect (arrow) in the interatrial septum. Note that the right atrium (RA) and right ventricle (RV) are dilated; (B) Subcostal view with color Doppler showing left to right shunt (arrow). Note again the dilated RA and RV; (C) Color Doppler subcostal view transthoracic echocardiogram showing relatively high velocity flow across a small restrictive secundum ASD (arrow). Video 40.4 shows the corresponding video of this still image. Image courtesy of Glenn N Levine, MD.

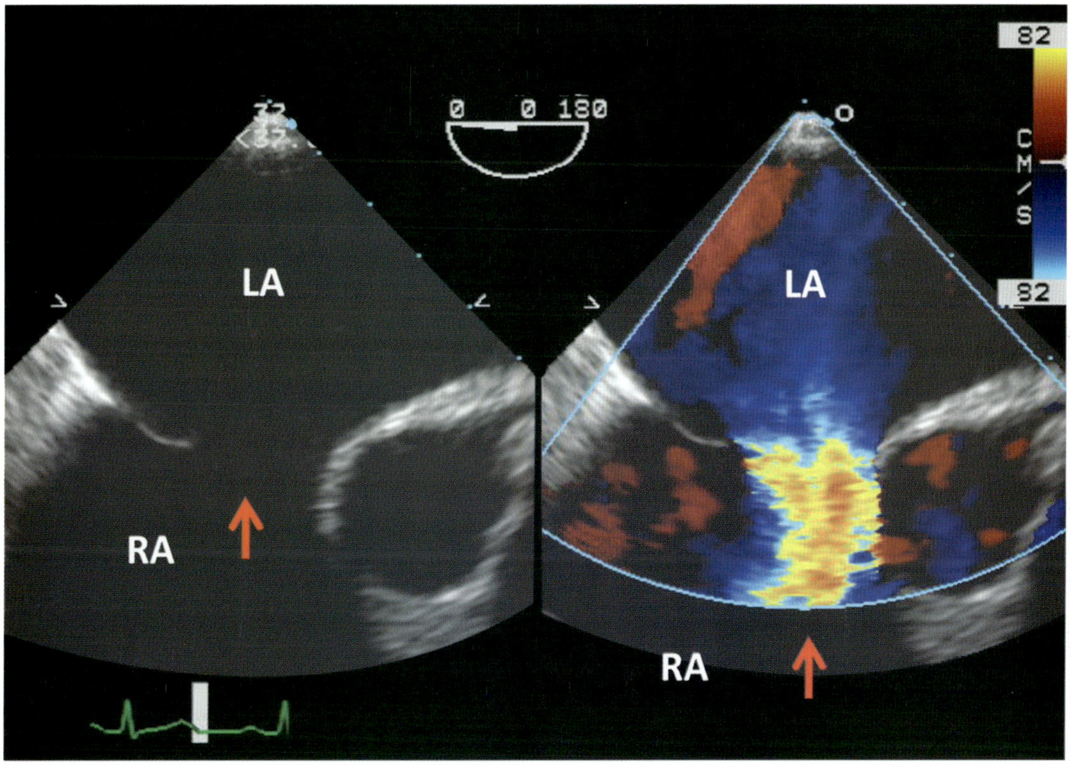

Fig. 40.4: Transesophageal echocardiography of a secundum ASD. The ASD (arrow) is clearly visible in the left panel. In the right panel, color Doppler imaging demonstrates shunt flow (arrow) through the ASD.

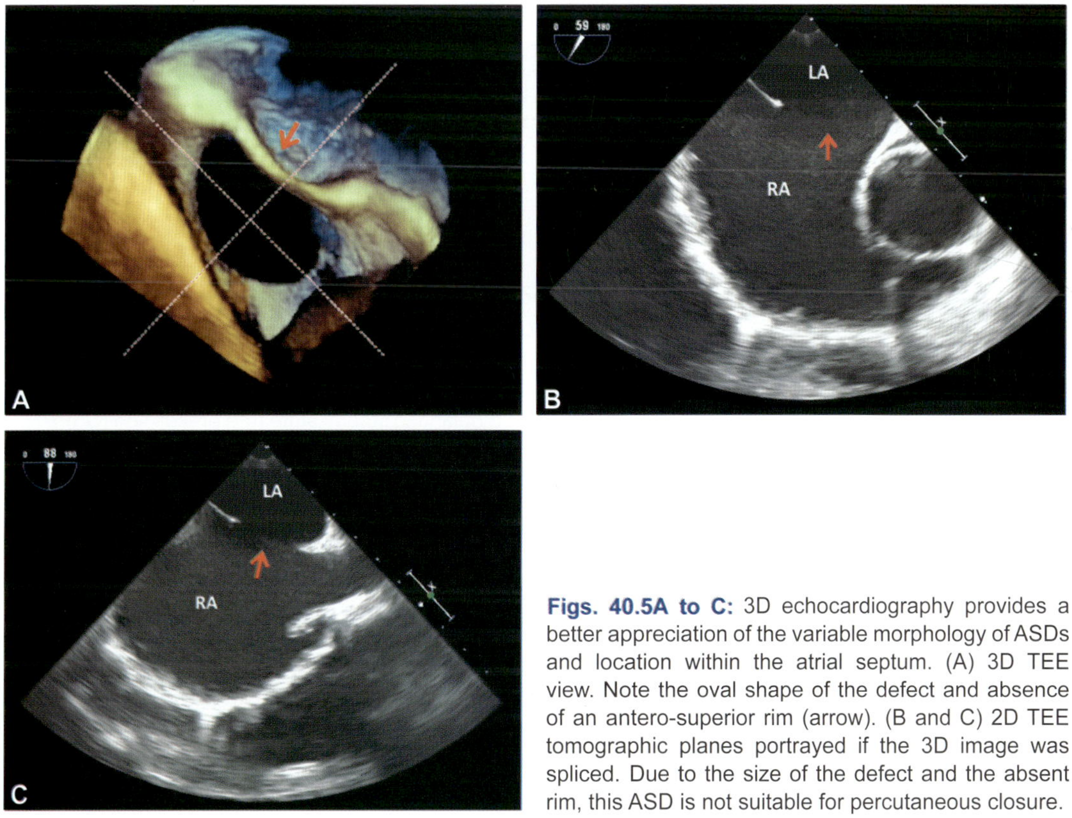

Figs. 40.5A to C: 3D echocardiography provides a better appreciation of the variable morphology of ASDs and location within the atrial septum. (A) 3D TEE view. Note the oval shape of the defect and absence of an antero-superior rim (arrow). (B and C) 2D TEE tomographic planes portrayed if the 3D image was spliced. Due to the size of the defect and the absent rim, this ASD is not suitable for percutaneous closure.

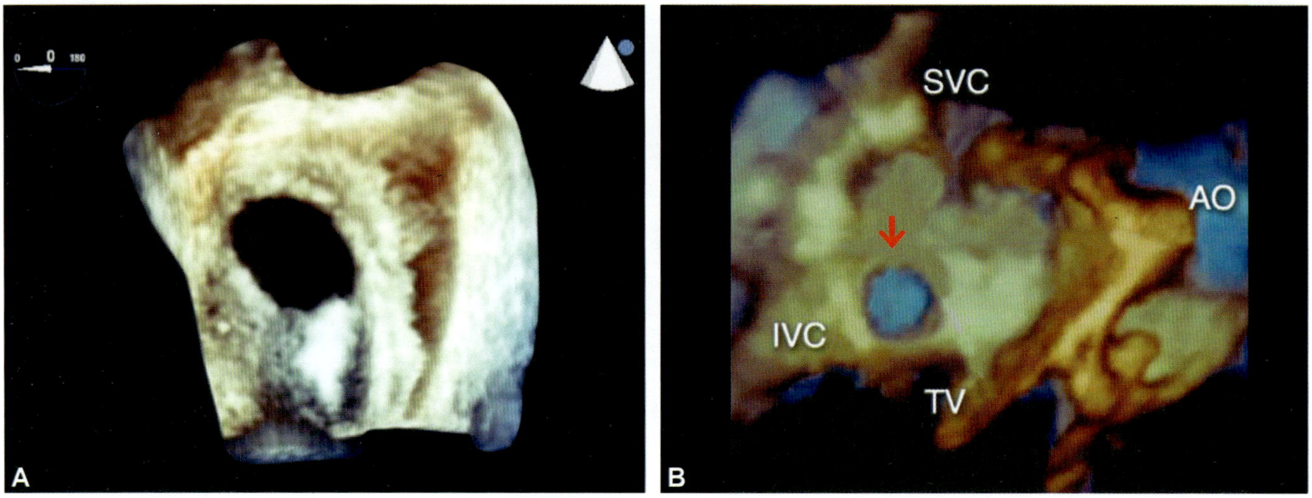

Figs. 40.6A and B: 3D TEE imaging of secundum ASDs. (A) 3D TEE demonstrating the elliptical shape of the ASD. (B) 3D TEE demonstrating a small inferior posterior ASD. [Image 40.6A from Akagi T. Atrial septal defect closure in geriatric patients. In: R PS (ed). Atrial septal defect. Intechopen.com. Image 40.6B from Gonzales I. Role of intracardiac echocardiography (ICE) in transcatheter occlusion of ASDs. In: R PS (ed). Atrial septal defect. Intechopen.com].

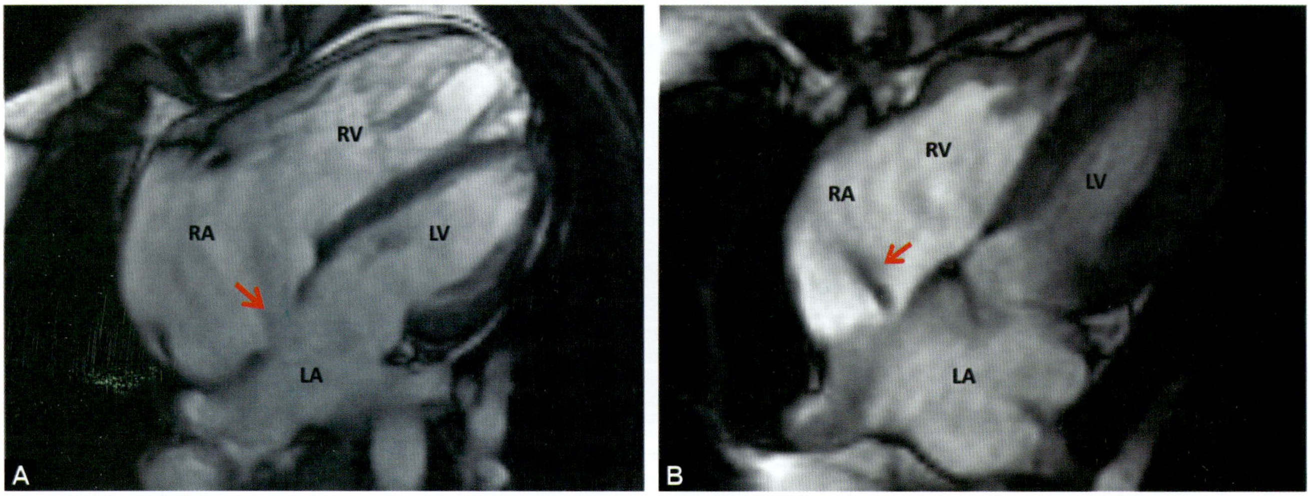

Figs. 40.7A and B: Cardiac MRI images of a segundum ASD. (A) Four-chamber view from a cardiac MRI shows a large secundum ASD. Note the discontinuity of the mid-portion of the interatrial septum (arrow). The right ventricle (RV) and right atrium (RA) are markedly dilated as a result of the left-to-right shunt. (B) Still frame from a balanced steady state free precession (SSFP) MRI sequence (four-chamber view) shows a small ostium secundum defect. Note the dephasing jet (arrow) in the right atrium (RA) as the blood crosses from the left atrium (LA) into the RA through the defect.

It is important to appreciate that sinus venosus ASDs are frequently missed by transthoracic echocardiography (TTE) as they are located in the far field of view. In view of this, any patient who is found to have unexplained right sided enlargement on TTE should have a sinus venosus ASD ruled out. Transesophageal echocardiography (TEE), CT or MRI may be used to achieve this.

PRIMUM ASD

The primum ASD is a defect that is located at the crux of the heart (where the mitral and tricuspid valves attach to the interventricular septum) (Figs. 40.15A and B). Primum ASDs represent a component of atrioventricular septal defects and are typically associated with a cleft of the left

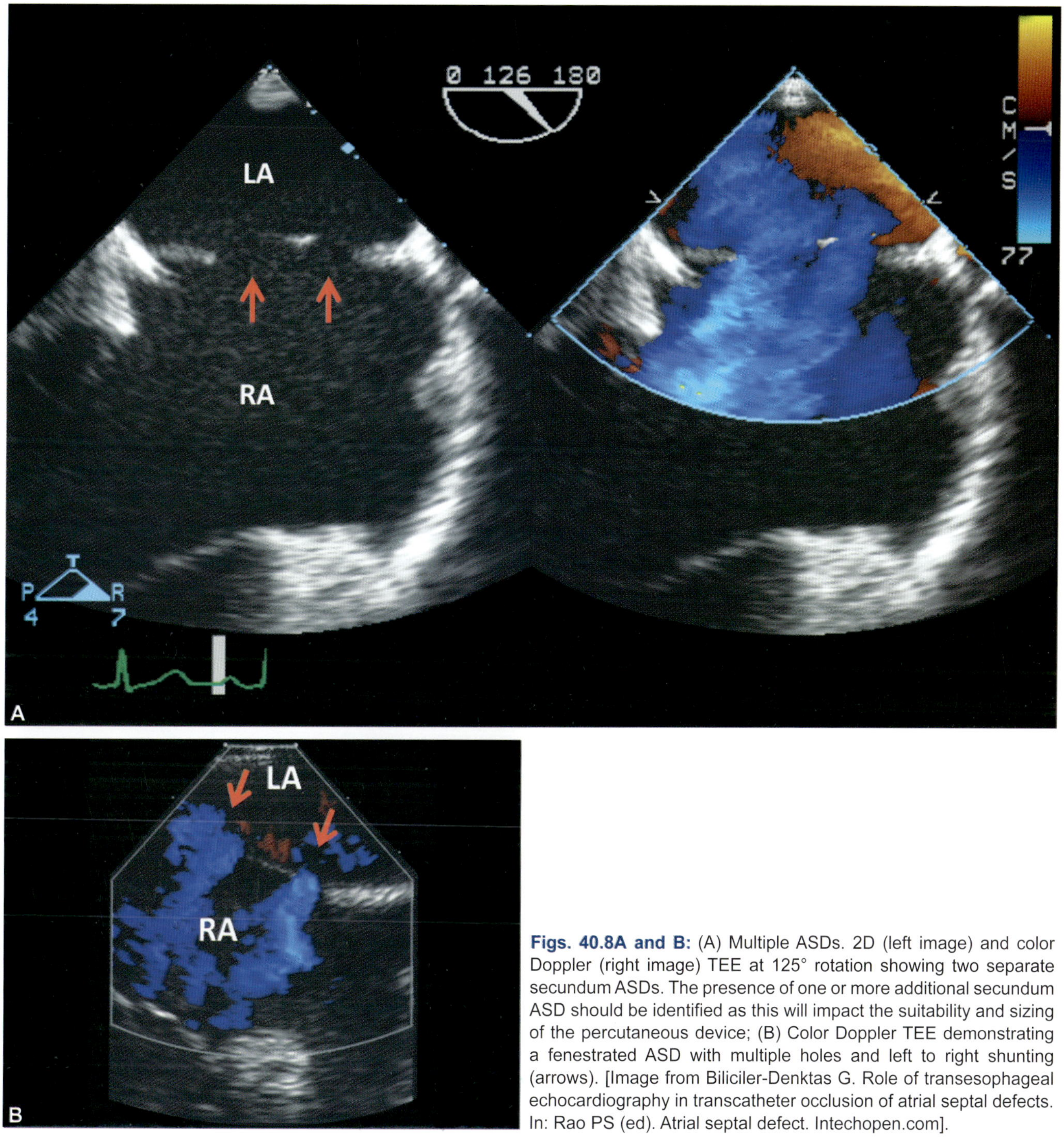

Figs. 40.8A and B: (A) Multiple ASDs. 2D (left image) and color Doppler (right image) TEE at 125° rotation showing two separate secundum ASDs. The presence of one or more additional secundum ASD should be identified as this will impact the suitability and sizing of the percutaneous device; (B) Color Doppler TEE demonstrating a fenestrated ASD with multiple holes and left to right shunting (arrows). [Image from Biliciler-Denktas G. Role of transesophageal echocardiography in transcatheter occlusion of atrial septal defects. In: Rao PS (ed). Atrial septal defect. Intechopen.com].

atrioventricular (mitral) valve, conduction abnormalities (Fig. 40.16) and sometimes a ventricular septal defect (VSD) located near the crux (inlet VSD). Embryologically, atrioventricular septal defects represent an abnormality of endocardial cushion development. Similar to sinus venosus ASDs, primum ASDs tend to be large.

CORONARY SINUS ASD

Somewhat of a misnomer, the coronary sinus ASD is not a defect of the atrial septum per se, but a deficiency of the wall between the left atrium (LA) and the coronary sinus (Figs. 40.17A and B). This results in left to right shunting

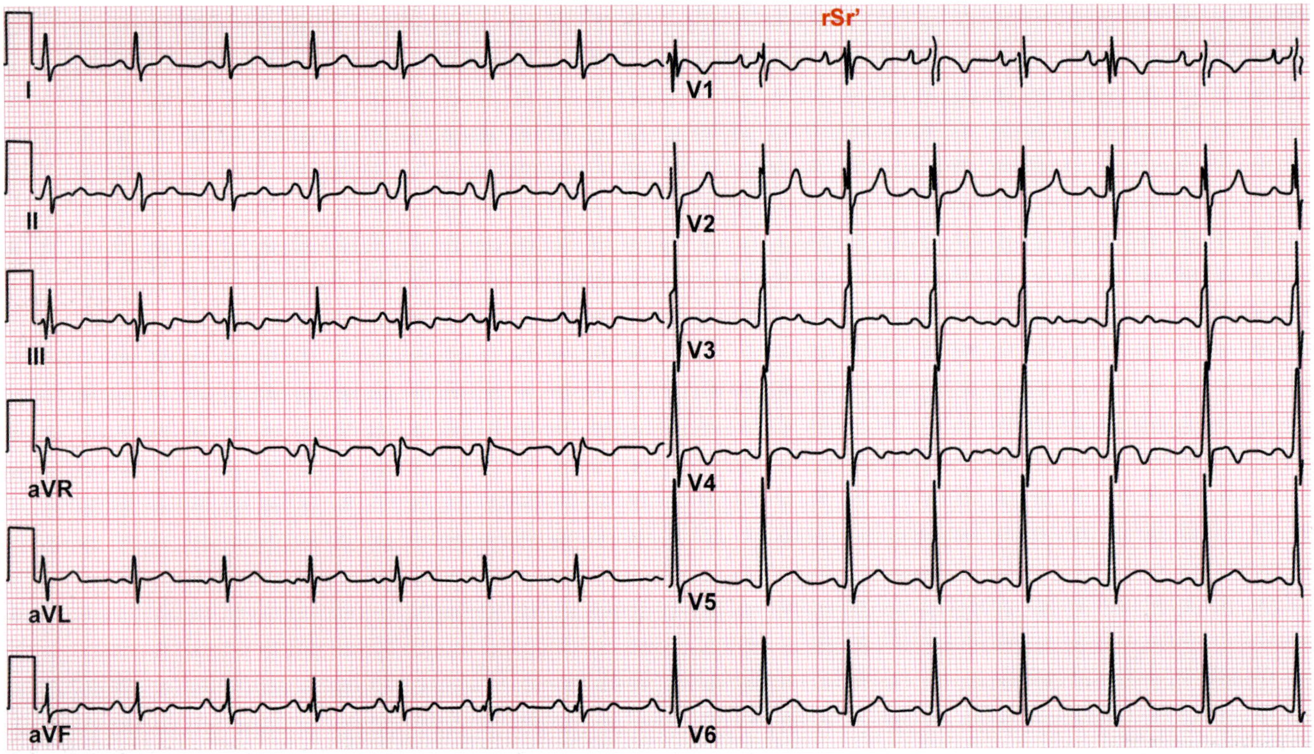

Fig. 40.9: ECG of a patient with a secundum ASD. The rSr' pattern in V1 represents the typical conduction delay due to right ventricular enlargement from the left to right shunt. However, it is important to note that this finding is not specific for ASDs and can be found in many individuals without structural heart disease as a variant of normal.

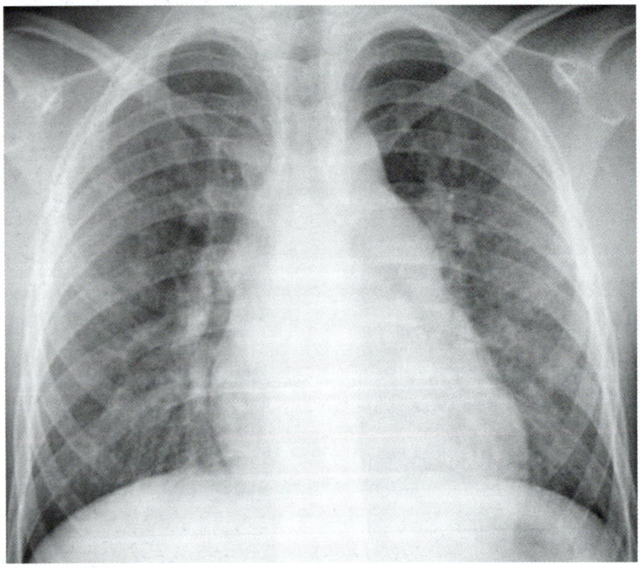

Fig. 40.10: Frontal chest radiograph demonstrates shunt vascularity. Both the central and peripheral vessels are enlarged and visible out to the periphery of the lung. The upper and lower lobe vessels are equally dilated. This is to be contrasted with pulmonary edema, where the upper lobe vessels become dilated but the lower lobe vessels actually become smaller. Also in pulmonary edema, the central pulmonary arteries are not dilated, there are Kerley B lines and the bronchi also become thick-walled (peribronchial cuffing).

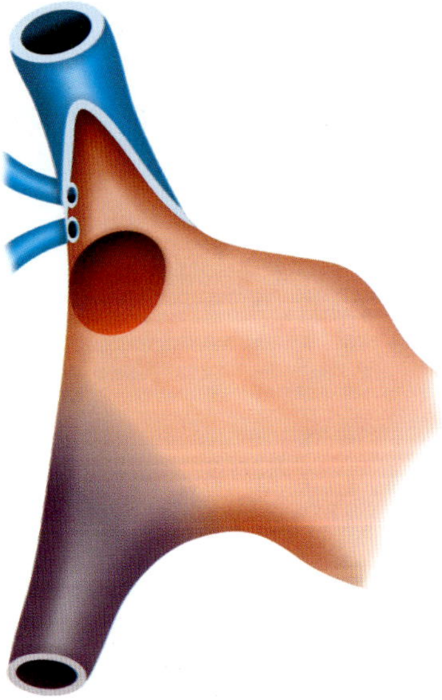

Fig. 40.11: Sinus venosus ASD. This represents the superior subtype which is the most common. Most sinus venosus ASDs are associated with right sided partial anomalous pulmonary vein return which drains either to the right atrium or superior vena cava (as illustrated in this case).

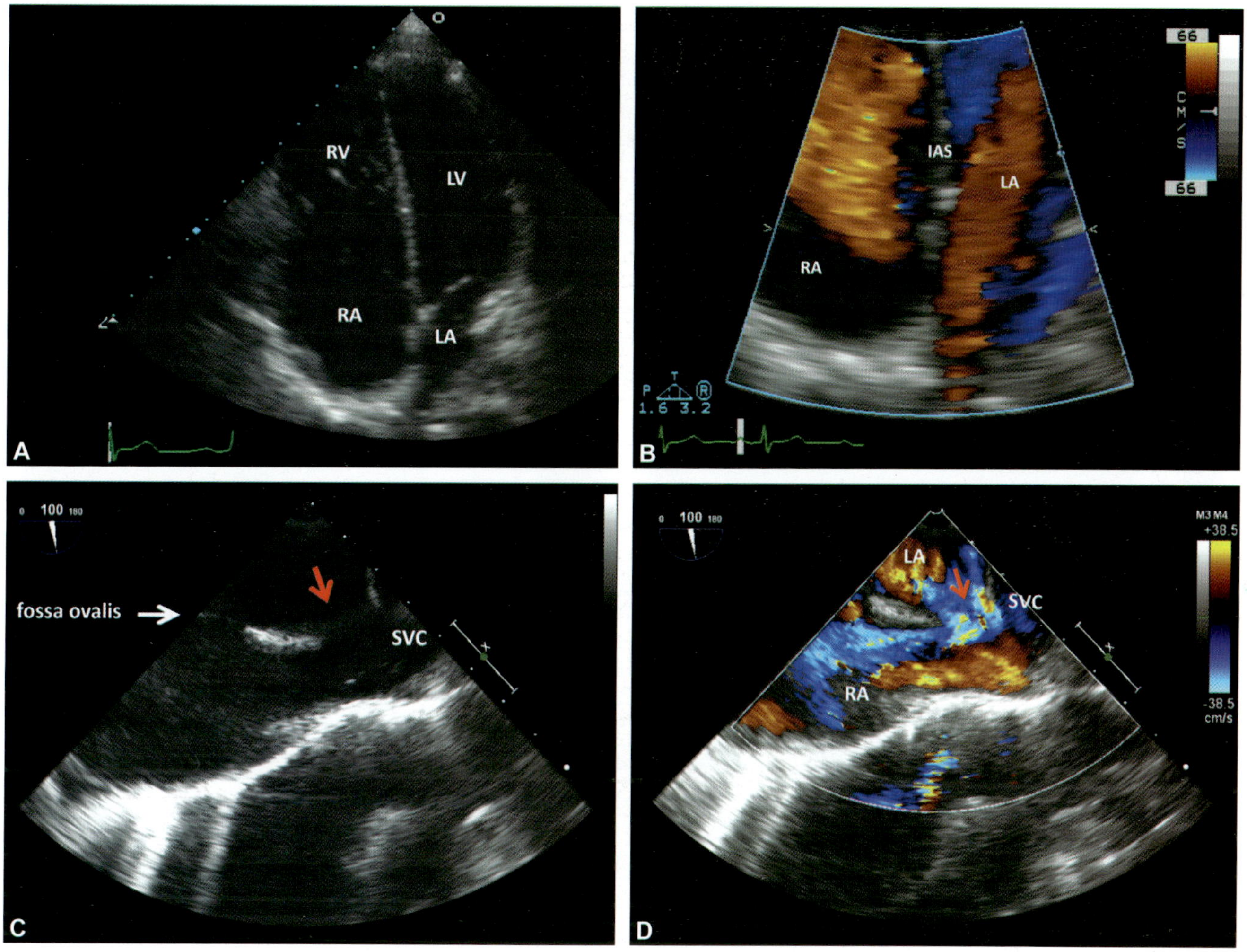

Figs. 40.12A to D: Echocardiographic images of a patient with a sinus venosus ASD. (A) TTE apical four-chamber view showing right-sided enlargement. (B) TTE four-chamber zoomed view with color Doppler. The interatrial septum (IAS) appears intact; (C) TEE at 100° rotation demonstrating a superior type of sinus venosus ASD (red arrow). Note that unlike a secundum ASD the fossa ovalis is intact; (D) TEE at 100° rotation with color Doppler demonstrating left to right shunting (arrow).

from the LA to the coronary sinus, then to the right atrium (RA) through the coronary sinus os. Frequently, coronary sinus ASDs are associated with a persistent left-sided superior vena cava.

COMPLICATIONS OF ASDs

The physiology of all ASDs is the same. Left to right shunting leads to right-sided volume overload. The two determinants of the degree of shunt are the size of the defect and the relative difference in the pulmonary and systemic resistances. With increasing age or systemic hypertension, diastolic dysfunction on the left side can further increase the left to right shunting. Long standing left to right shunt leads to right atrial enlargement, right ventricular enlargement, tricuspid regurgitation, right ventricular dysfunction and pulmonary hypertension. It is important to note that the pulmonary hypertension is mostly due to increased flow rather than elevated pulmonary vascular resistance. This means that in most patients, pulmonary pressure will decrease with closure of the ASD. Another well-documented complication of ASDs is atrial fibrillation due to right atrial dilation. Finally, the presence of an ASD can potentially lead to paradoxical embolus, where a thrombus that originates at the site of a deep venous thrombosis embolizes through the ASD and in to the systemic arterial circulation. Embolic stroke is the most important complication of paradoxical embolus.

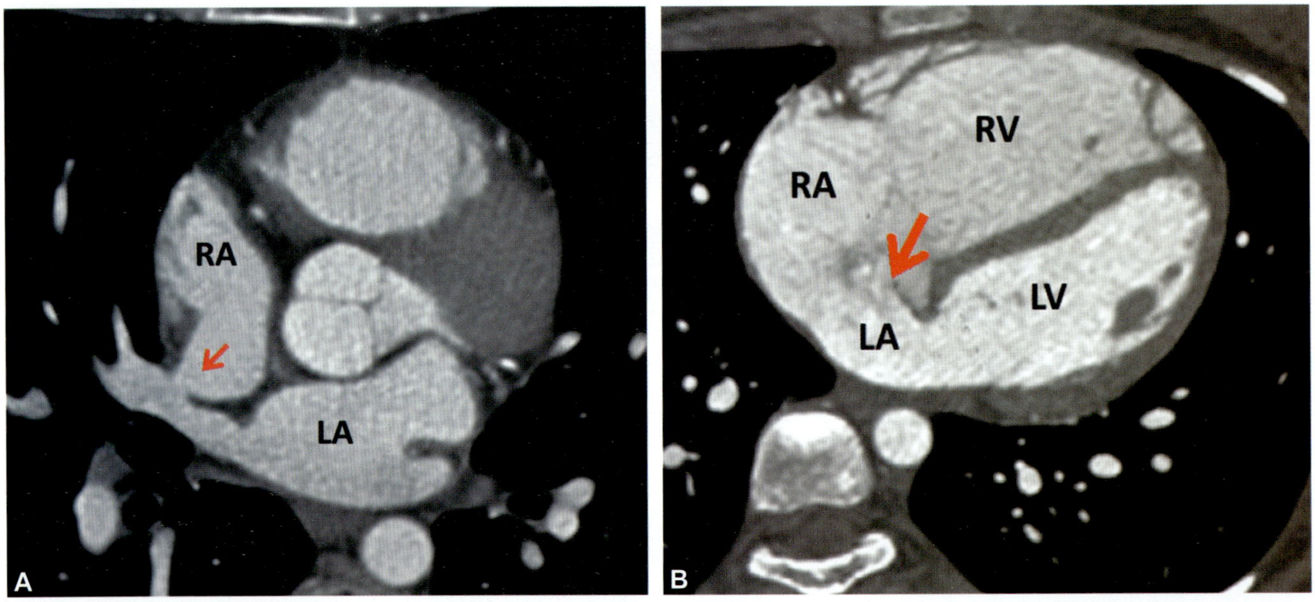

Figs. 40.13A and B: Sinus venosus ASDs imaged on CT scan. (A) Superior sinus venosus ASD (arrow), the more common location of a sinus venosus ASD. (B) Inferior sinus venosus ASD (arrow), the less common location of a sinus venosus ASD. (Image from Kivistö S. Partial anomalous pulmonary venous return and atrial septal defect in adult patients detected with 128-slice multidetector computed tomography. Journal of Cardiothoracic Surgery. 2011;6:126).

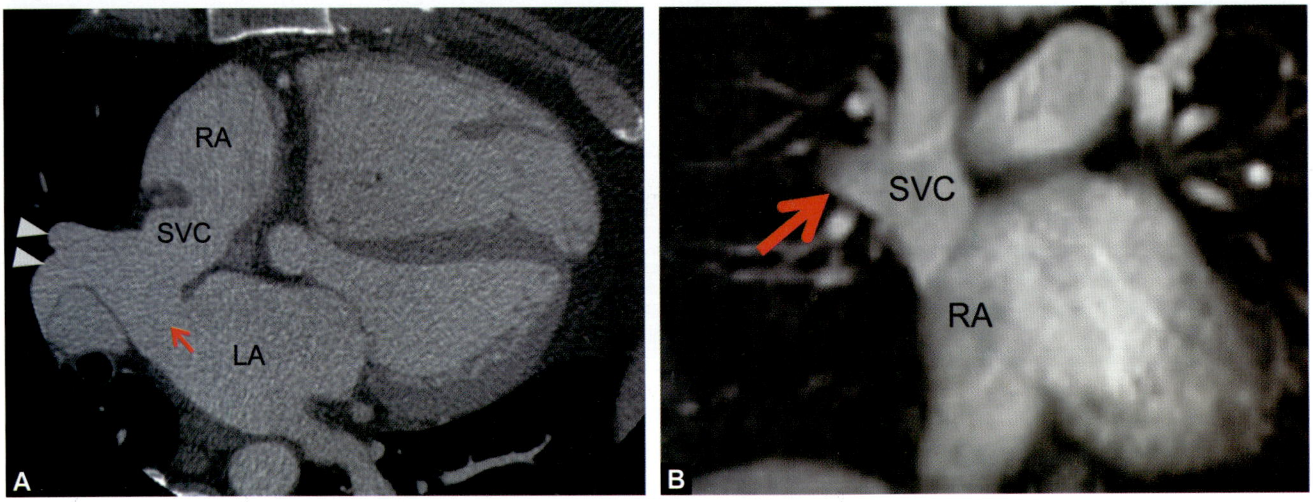

Figs. 40.14A and B: Anomalous pulmonary veins in patients with sinus venosus ASDs. (A) Four-chamber view from a cardiac CT demonstrates anomalous pulmonary venous drainage and sinus venosus defect. Note the absence of the posterior interatrial septum (arrow) at the junction of the superior vena cava (SVC) and the right atrium (RA). Also note the two anomalous veins from the right lung (arrowheads) draining into the SVC rather than the left atrium (LA) at the same level. (B) Coronal VIBE MR sequence post-gadolinium injection in a different patient reveals an anomalous vein (arrow) from the right upper lobe draining into the superior vena cava (SVC) above its junction with the right atrium (RA).

MANAGEMENT OF ASDs

Most ASDs should be closed; exceptions include: small secundum ASDs with no right-sided volume overload, and ASDs in very elderly patients who are asymptomatic.

As a rule, secundum ASDs are now closed percutaneously (Figs. 40.18 and 40.19). A TEE is usually done beforehand to assess the rims, morphology and location of the defect. Intracoronary echocardiography (ICE) is frequently used during the procedure (Fig. 40.20). Serious complications

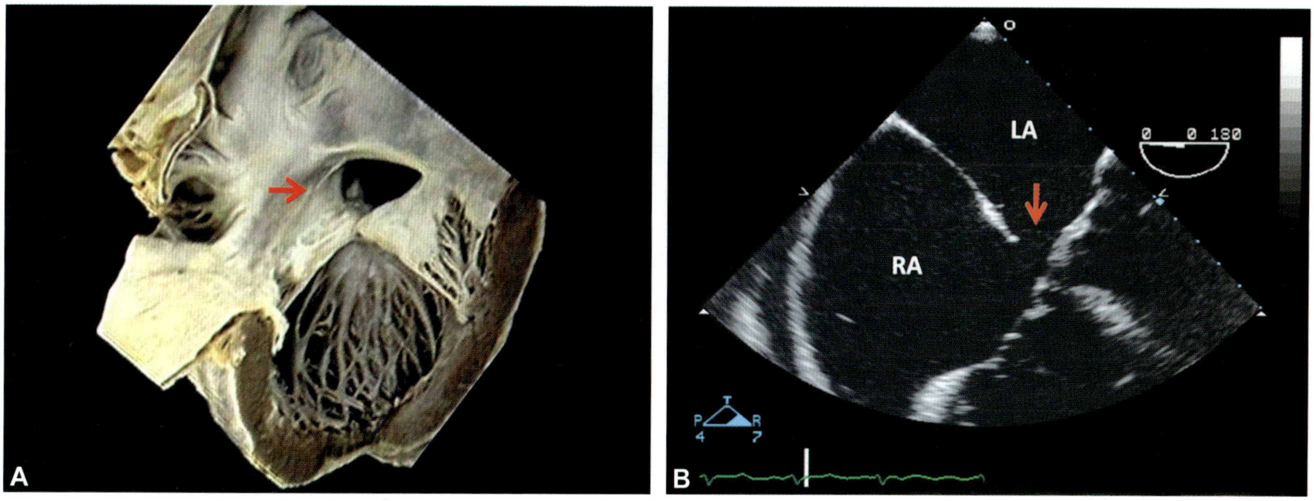

Figs. 40.15A and B: Primum ASD. (A) Gross pathology specimen. (B) TEE four-chamber view at 0° rotation. The defect (red arrow) is located next to the crux of the heart where the atrioventricular valves insert into the inter-ventricular septum. [Image 40.15A from Armed Forces Institute of Pathology (public domain image)].

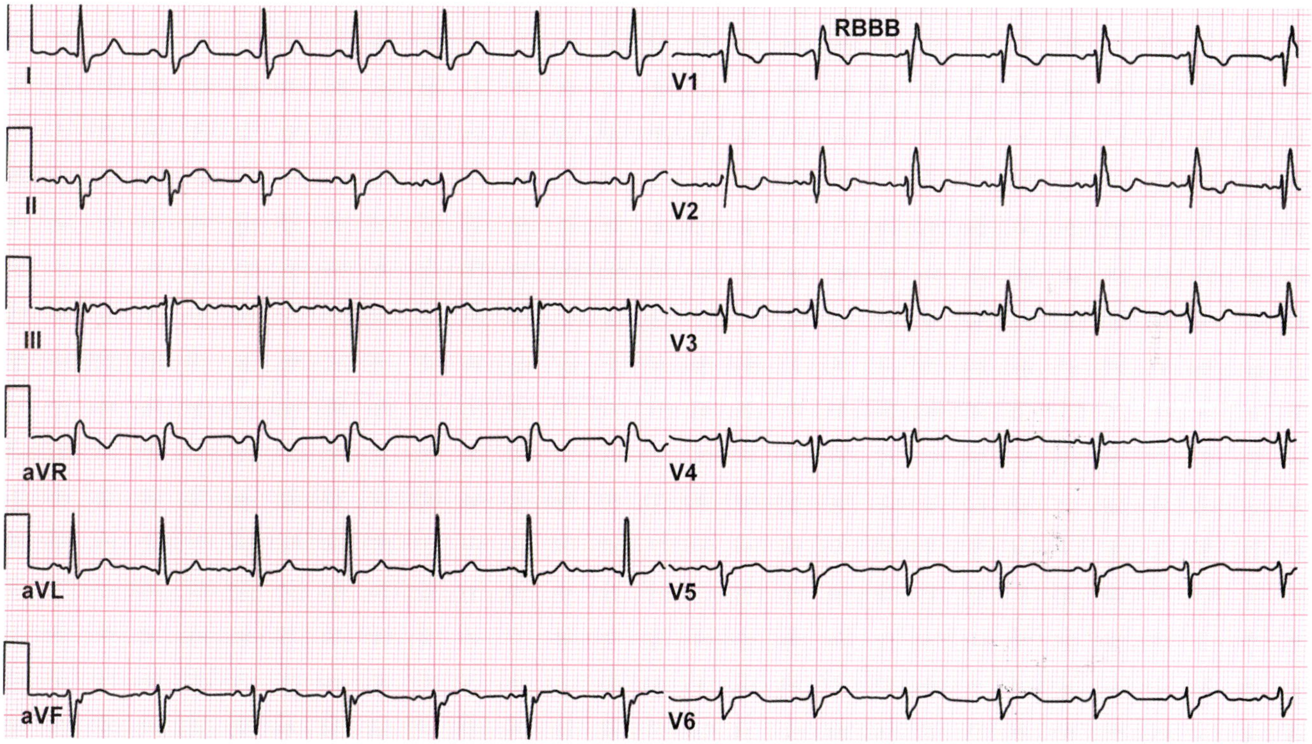

Fig. 40.16: ECG from a patient with a primum ASD. There is an RBBB from RV enlargement secondary to the left to right shunt from the ASD. A left axis deviation (LAD) is invariably present in these patients. The LAD is not due to a left anterior fascicular block (LAFB) but from the associated infero-superior displacement of the AV node that is seen in this cardiac abnormality.
(RBBB: Right Bundle Branch Block).

of percutaneous closure are rare (< 1%) but include perforation of the atrial roof (which will result in pericardial effusion/tamponade), thrombus formation, aorta to RA fistula, and embolization of the device. The device takes a few months to endothelialize. In view of this, low dose aspirin and clopidogrel are prescribed for six months post-procedure. Following the procedure, most patients (including the elderly), will have reverse remodeling [i.e.

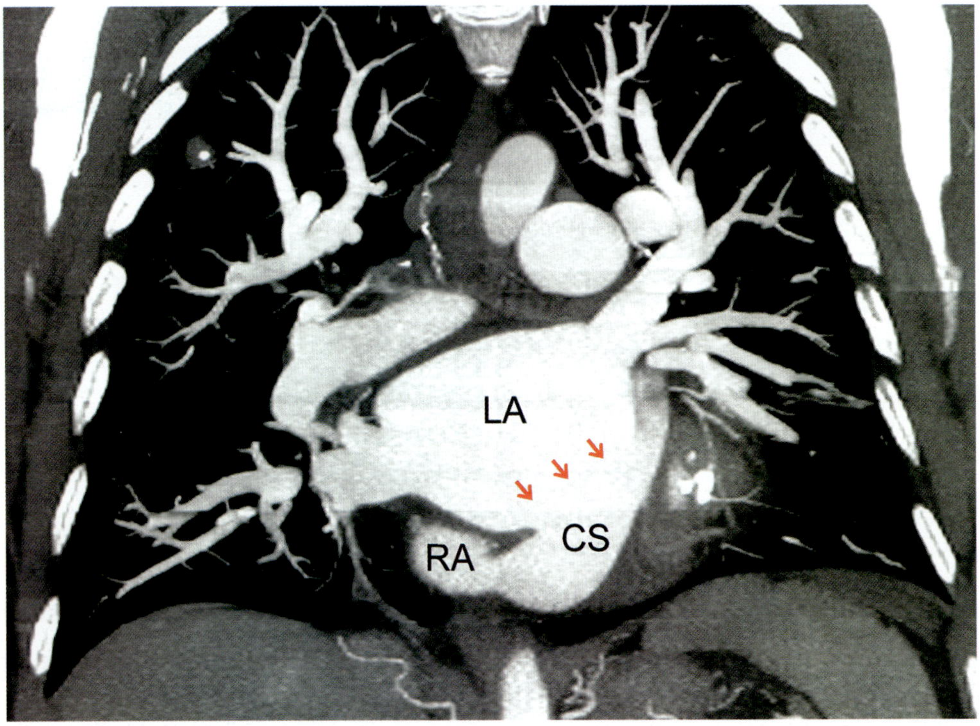

Fig. 40.17A: Coronal oblique maximum intensity projection (MIP) from a cardiac CT shows a coronary sinus defect. The roof of the coronary sinus (CS) is discontinuous (arrows) along the inferior aspect of the left atrium (LA) allowing blood from the LA to flow into the CS and then into the right atrium (RA) thus resulting in a left-to-right shunt.

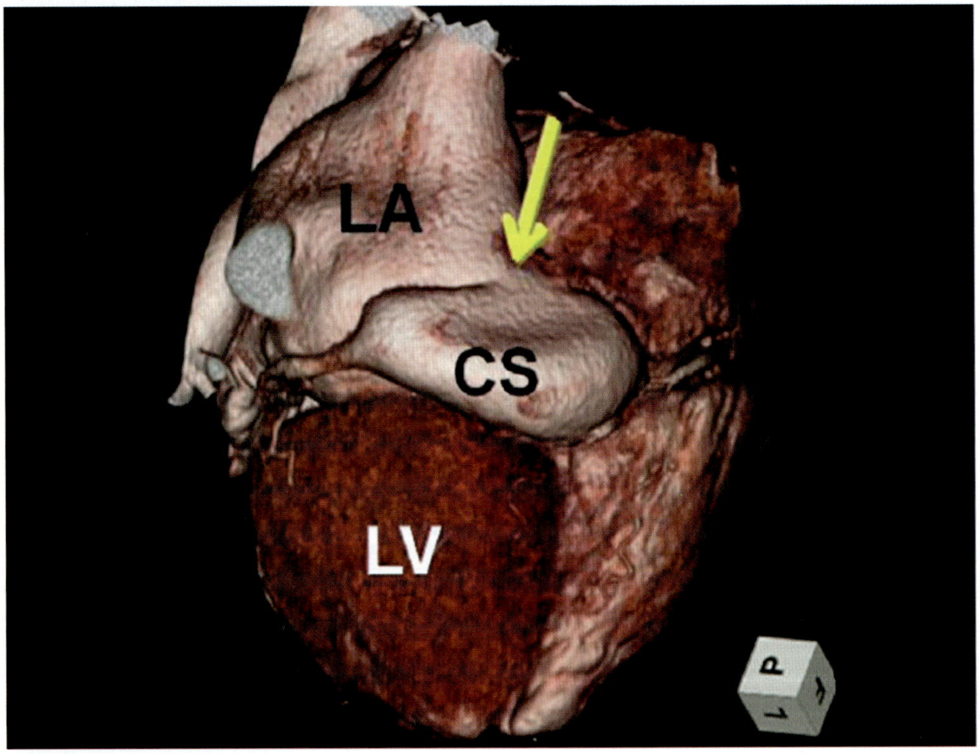

Fig. 40.17B: Volume rendered cardiac CT scan showing dilated, partially unroofed coronary sinus (arrow). (Image from Oyama N, Komuro K, Nambu T, et al. Non-coronary cardiac findings and pitfalls in coronary computed tomography angiography. J Clin Imaging Sci. 2011;1:51. http://www.clinicalimagingscience.org/text.asp?2011/1/1/51/86666).

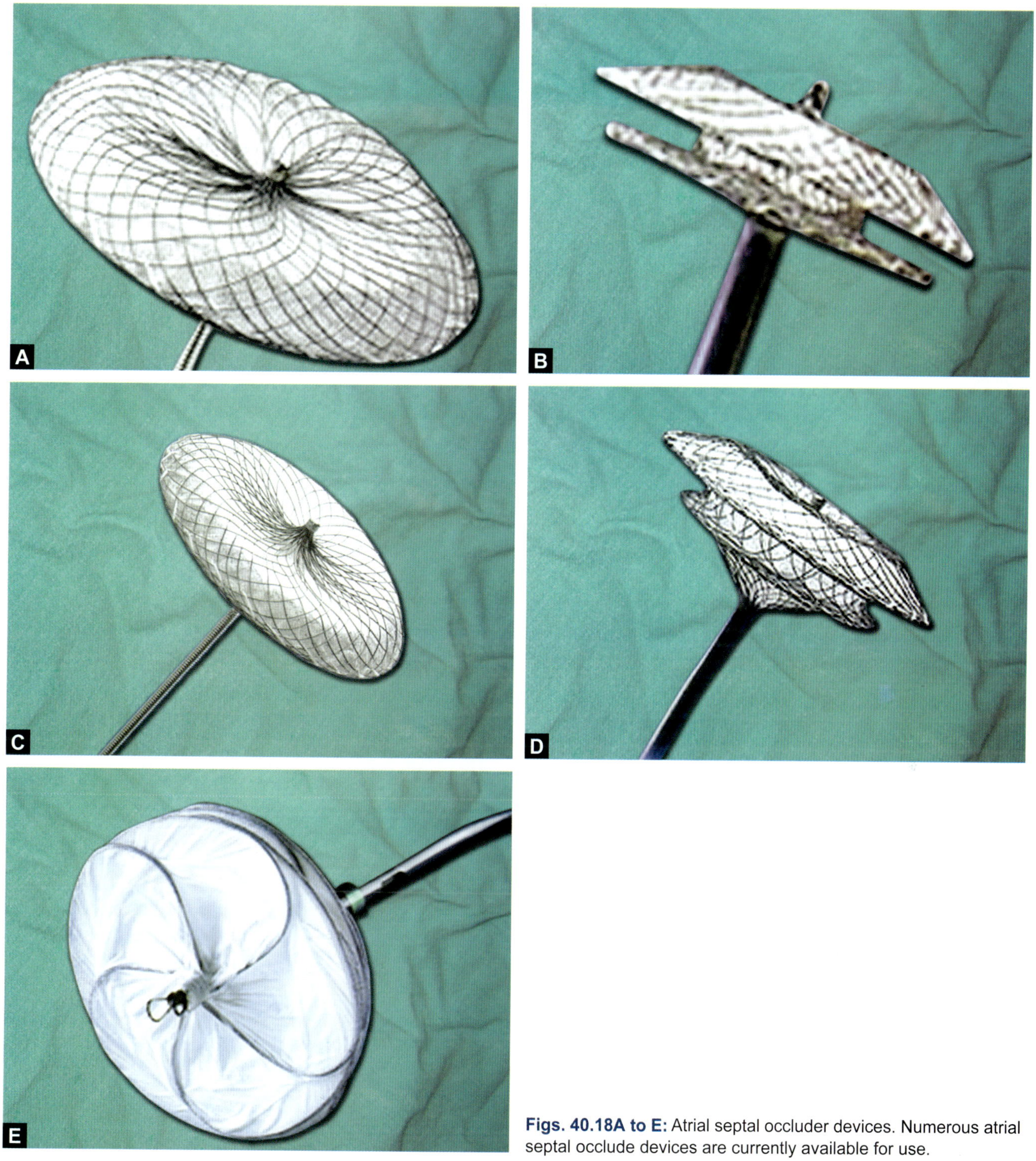

Figs. 40.18A to E: Atrial septal occluder devices. Numerous atrial septal occlude devices are currently available for use.

reduction in RA and right ventricle (RV) size] and improvement in functional capacity. In rare cases, a secundum ASD is not suitable for percutaneous closure (hole too big, poor margins, multiple defects located far apart) and will require surgical correction. Sinus venosus and primum ASDs cannot be closed percutaneously and require surgical closure. In sinus venousus ASDs, a pericardial baffle is placed to re-route anomalous pulmonary venous flow to the LA (Fig. 40.21). For primum ASDs, the hole is closed with a pericardial patch and the associated cleft of the left

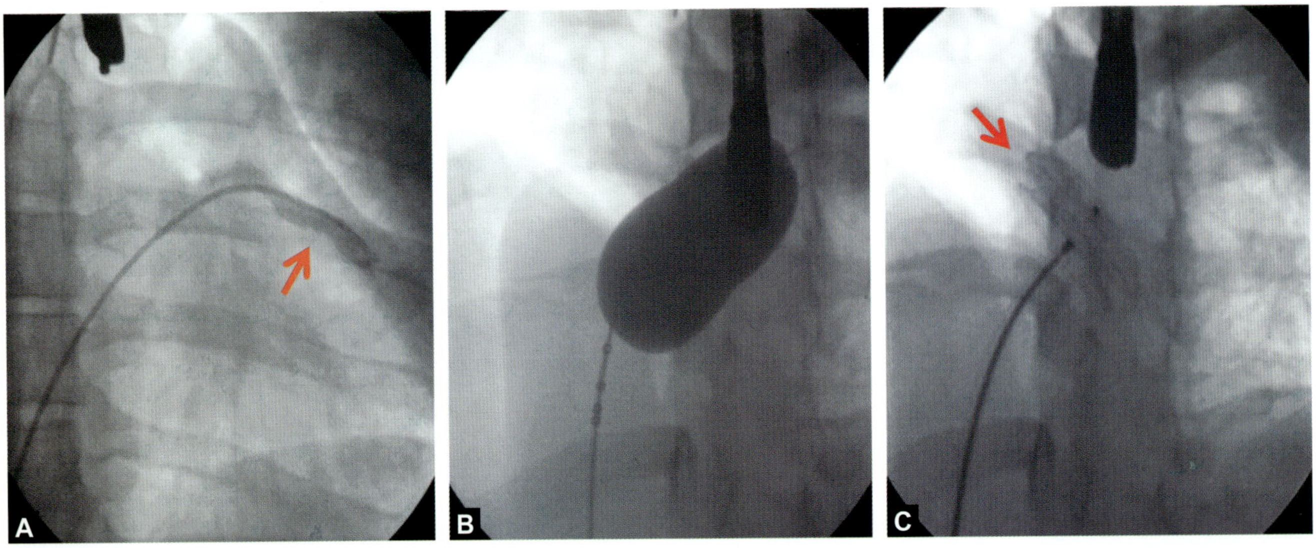

Figs. 40.19A to C: Fluoroscopic images of a percutaneous closure of a secundum ASD under general anesthesia with TEE guidance. (A) The ASD is crossed with an end-hole catheter which is placed in the left upper pulmonary vein (arrow). (B) With the help of an exchange wire, a sizing balloon is placed across the defect and inflated until no flow is seen with TEE imaging. Measurements of the size of the ASD are obtained. (C) An appropriate sized device is positioned. Placement is verified by TEE and if deemed adequate, the device (arrow) is released. Arterial access is not required. In some centers, the procedure is done under local anesthesia with the use of intra-cardiac echocardiography (ICE).

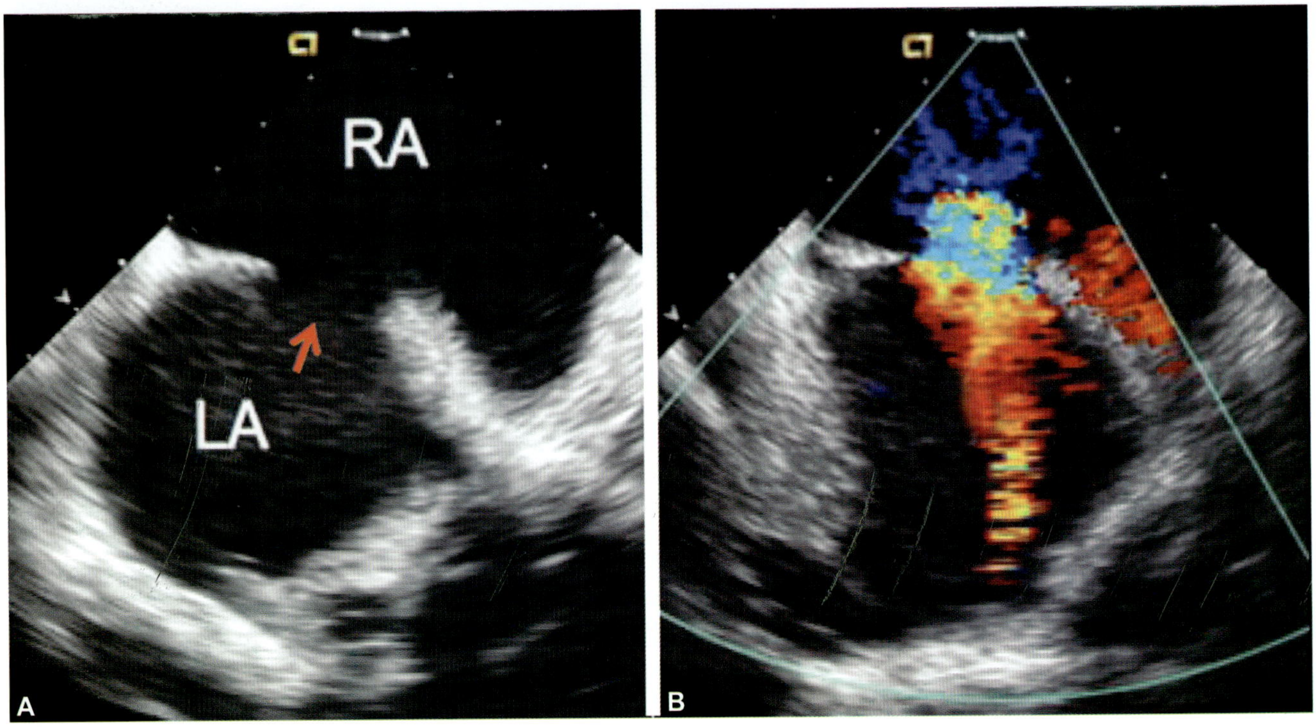

Figs. 40.20A and B: Intracardiac echocardiography (ICE) images of large ASD. (A) 2D image showing the ASD (red arrow). (B) Color Doppler image showing left to right shunting. [Image from Gonzalez I. Role of intracardiac echocardiography (ICE) in transcatheter occlusion of atrial septal defects. In: Rao PS (ed). Atrial septal defect. www.intechopen.com]. (LA: Left atrium; RA: Right atrium).

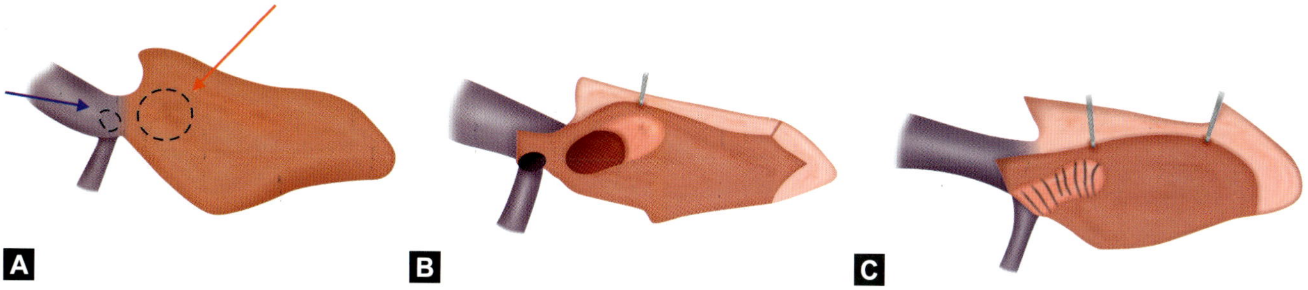

A B C

Figs. 40.21A to C: Surgical repair of a sinus venosus ASD. (A) Surgical view of the right atrium (blue arrow: associated anomalous return of the right upper pulmonary vein to the superior vena cava, red arrow: superior sinus venosus ASD. (B) A right atriotomy has been performed to expose the defects. A patch is being sutured to the ASD. (C) The patch is further sutured to create a baffle to re-route the anomalous pulmonary vein flow to the left atrium.

atrio-ventricular valve is sutured. Coronary sinus ASDs are closed by placement of a patch to obliterate the left atrial to coronary sinus connection.

VIDEO LEGENDS

Video 40.1: Apical four-chamber TTE showing a large secundum ASD. Note that the right atrium and right ventricle are both dilated. Video courtesy of Glenn N. Levine, MD.

Video 40.2: Color Doppler apical four-chamber TTE corresponding to video 40.1, showing left to right flow across a large secundum ASD. Note that the right atrium and right ventricle are dilated, and some tricuspid regurgitation is also present. Video courtesy of Glenn N. Levine, MD.

Video 40.3: Zoomed video of videos 40.1 and 40.2, showing a large secundum ASD with left to right flow. Video courtesy of Glenn N. Levine, MD.

Video 40.4: Subcostal view TTE showing a small restrictive ASD with relatively high velocity left to right flow. Video courtesy of Glenn N. Levine, MD.

REFERENCES

Baumgartner H , Bonhoeffer P , De Groot NM, et al. ESC Guidelines for the management of grown-up congenital heart disease. Eur Heart J. 2010;31:2915-57.

Yared K, Baggish AL, Solis J, et al. Echocardiographic assessment of percutaneous patent foramen ovale and atrial septal defect closure complications. Circ Cardiovasc Imaging. 2009;2(2):141-9.

Humenberger M, Rosenhek R, Gabriel H, et al. Benefit of atrial septal defect closure in adults: impact of age. Eur Heart J. 2011;32:553-60.

Silversides CK, Dore A, Poirier N, et al. Canadian Cardiovascular Society 2009 Consensus Conference on the management of adults with congenital heart disease: shunt lesions. Can J Cardiol; 2010;26:e70-9.

Warnes CA, Williams RG, Bashore TM, et al. ACC/AHA 2008 guidelines for the management of adults with congenital heart disease. Circulation. 2008;118:2395-451.

CHAPTER

41 Ventricular Septal Defect

Elijah H Bolin, Daniel J Penny

INTRODUCTION

Ventricular septal defect (VSD) (Fig. 41.1, Videos 41.1 and 41.2) is the most common form of congenital heart disease when bicuspid aortic valve (AV) is excluded. The highest frequency of VSD is found in neonates in the form of tiny muscular defects located in the trabecular septum. These tiny defects typically disappear within the first year of life. Larger defects and those associated with more complex forms of congenital heart disease (e.g. transposition of the great arteries, Tetralogy of Fallot) do not resolve with time. While VSD is frequently associated with certain chromosomal abnormalities or syndromes, most patients with VSD do not have genetic abnormalities. In those without a defined genetic abnormality or syndrome, the cause is likely multifactorial. This chapter focuses on the anatomic location, pathophysiology, and diagnostic evaluation of isolated VSD.

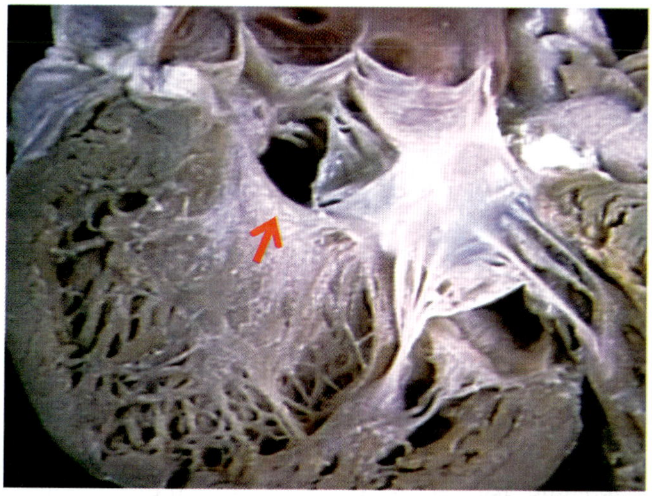

Fig. 41.1: Pathological specimen of a ventricular septal defect (VSD). [Image from Armed Forces Institute of Pathology (public domain)].

TYPES OF VENTRICULAR SEPTAL DEFECT

Three morphologic types of VSD exist: Perimembranous, muscular, and doubly committed and juxta-arterial (Fig. 41.2). Perimembranous defects (Videos 41.3 and 41.4) are the most common type of VSD. The diminutive membranous septum connects the posterior aortic commissure to the anteroseptal tricuspid commissure. All perimembranous defects occupy at least some portion of the membranous septum. Although, also termed "membranous" defects, pathologic specimens show that these defects are almost always larger than the membranous septum itself; therefore, the term "perimembranous" is

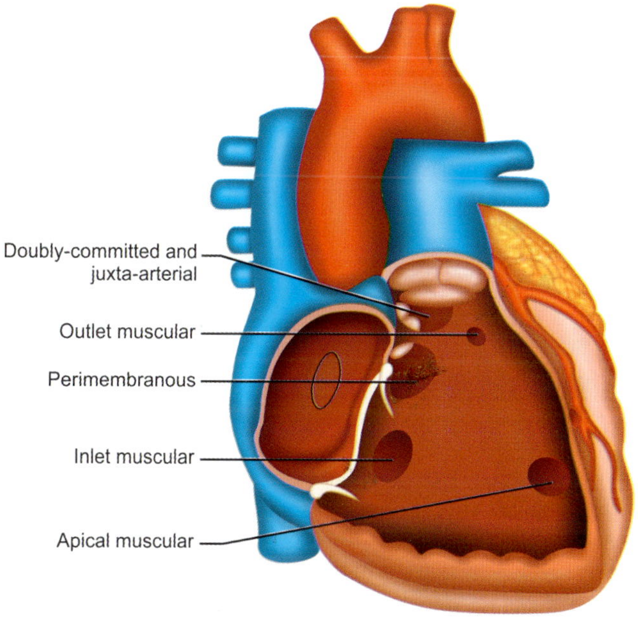

Fig. 41.2: Schematic illustration of the types of ventricular septal defects (VSDs).

preferred. Because of the intimate relationship between the membranous septum and the AV, prolapse of the aortic leaflets may be observed with time, leading to aortic regurgitation. Tricuspid aneurysmal tissue may partially or completely occlude a perimembranous defect. The subendocardial bundle of His and conduction tissues lie just posterior and inferior to perimembranous defects, and are susceptible to injury during surgical repair.

Muscular defects, by definition, are surrounded by muscle. These defects are further described by their location in the interventricular septum: inlet, outlet, or apical. They may also be multiple, as in the case of the so-called "Swiss cheese" septum (Fig. 41.3).

Doubly-committed and juxta-arterial defects (Fig. 41.4) are a third and morphologically distinct category of VSD. Normally, the muscular infundibulum exists as a free-standing sleeve of tissue separating the pulmonary annulus from the base of the heart. However, doubly-committed and juxta-arterial defects border both the aortic and pulmonary annuluses and bring these structures into fibrous continuity. Additionally, there is a muscular rim of tissue posterior and inferior to the defect separating it from the membranous septum, and the tricuspid valve. The bundle of His and conduction tissues are therefore remote, and the surgeon is able to place sutures in the

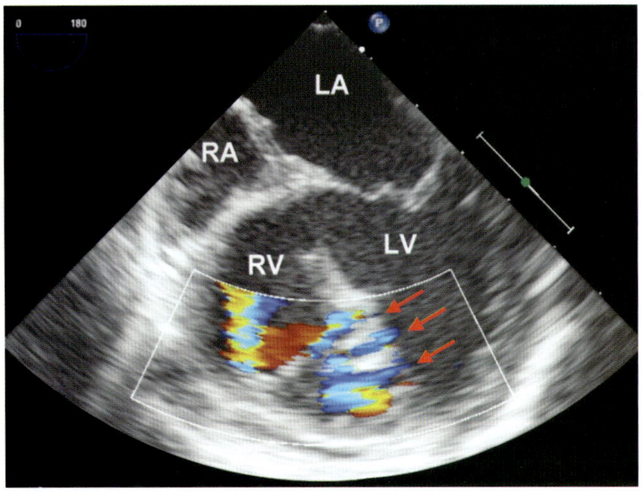

Fig. 41.3: Midesophageal four-chamber view demonstrates multiple muscular ventricular septal defects (VSDs) (arrows). This finding of multiple defects in the septum may be referred to as a "Swiss cheese" septum. [Image from Wang YC, Huang CH. Intraoperative transesophageal echocardiography for congenital heart disease. In: Bajraktari G (Ed). Echocardiography—In Specific Diseases. Intechweb.org.]. (RA: Right atrium; RV: Right ventricle; LA: Left atrium; LV: Left ventricle).

inferior aspect of the defect. When a doubly-committed and juxta-arterial defect extends into the membranous septum, and the inferior muscular rim no longer exists, conduction tissues are again at risk of being injured during surgical intervention.

PATHOPHYSIOLOGY AND CLINICAL MANIFESTATIONS OF VENTRICULAR SEPTAL DEFECT

Ventricular septal defect most commonly causes pathology in three ways: left-to-right shunting causing symptoms of heart failure, chronic left-to-right shunt with resultant pulmonary hypertension and shunt reversal (Eisenmenger syndrome), and aortic insufficiency.

The amount of left-to-right shunting in hearts with VSD can best be understood by considering the relative resistances encountered by blood existing the left ventricle (LV). In the heart without semilunar (aortic or pulmonary) valve stenosis, there are three potential resistors to flow out of the LV: systemic vascular resistance (SVR), VSD, and pulmonary vascular resistance (PVR). PVR and VSD are resistors in series. SVR is a resistor in parallel with both VSD and PVR. As the LV contracts and generates pressure, the amount of pulmonary to systemic blood flow (Qp:Qs) is determined by these three resistors, and symptomatology is in turn determined by Qp:Qs.

Consider first the case of a large VSD. With left ventricular systole, blood may flow out either the VSD or the AV. A large VSD imposes low resistance to flow compared to SVR at the AV. Blood is ejected through the VSD, into the contracting right ventricle (RV), and out the pulmonary valve. The next resistor in series after the large VSD, then, is PVR. In a patient with a large VSD, therefore, Qp:Qs is determined by PVR and SVR, and not the size of the defect.

At the other end of the spectrum is a tiny VSD. Because the radius of the defects is small, the defect imposes a high resistance compared to SVR. Qp:Qs is therefore determined by the defect size, and not PVR. Moderate-sized defects have a variable contribution to Qp:Qs.

A neonate with a large VSD, therefore, will have a Qp:Qs determined by the ratio of PVR to SVR. In the newborn period, infants with a large VSD will not manifest symptoms. This is because PVR is elevated in the neonatal

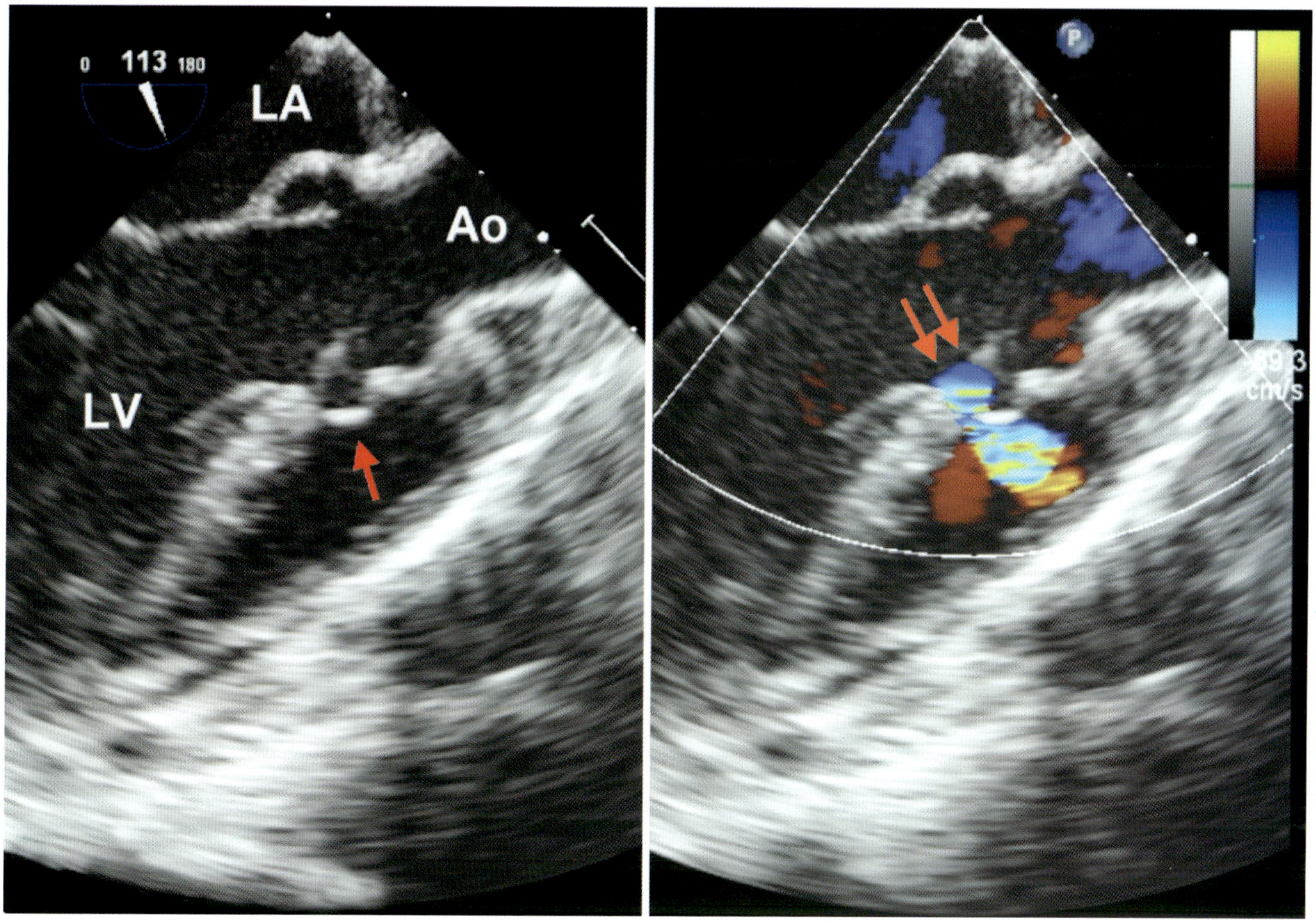

Fig. 41.4: Doubly-committed ventricular septal defect (VSD). Midesophageal long-axis view shows the prolapse of aortic cusp (arrow) and the septal defect (double arrow). [Image from Wang YC, Huang CH. Intraoperative transesophageal echocardiography for congenital heart disease. In: Bajraktari G (Ed). Echocardiography—In Specific Diseases. Intechweb.org.]. (LA: Left atrium; LV: Left ventricle; Ao: Aorta).

period, a residuum of fetal physiology. As PVR drops in the first weeks of life, the ratio of PVR to SVR decreases, and Qp:Qs increases. Qp:Qs can be as much as 4:1 or more, which is to say, for every one cardiac output going to the body, four go to the lungs. A large VSD presents a pressure load to the RV and pulmonary arteries, and a volume load to the pulmonary arteries, left atrium (LA) and LV (Fig. 41.5A). With time, the RV becomes hypertrophied, and the pulmonary arteries, LA, and LV dilate.

Children with large VSD present with progressive signs and symptoms of heart failure and pulmonary congestion, including failure to thrive, difficulty in feeding, diaphoresis, tachypnea, cough, and frequent respiratory infections. Physical examination will reveal retractions, tachycardia, a laterally displaced apical impulse, usually a soft holosystolic murmur, a diastolic rumble, and bilateral crackles.

Children with moderate-sized VSD have varying signs and symptoms of heart failure, based on the size of the VSD and the PVR. The murmur produced by a moderate-sized VSD is typically louder than that of a large defect. This is because a larger pressure gradient develops as the radius of the defect decreases. Small and tiny defects do not cause heart failure and pulmonary congestion. The murmur may be loud in small defects if a significant enough volume of blood crosses the defect, but tend to become softer as the degree of left-to-right shunting is limited by the defect's size.

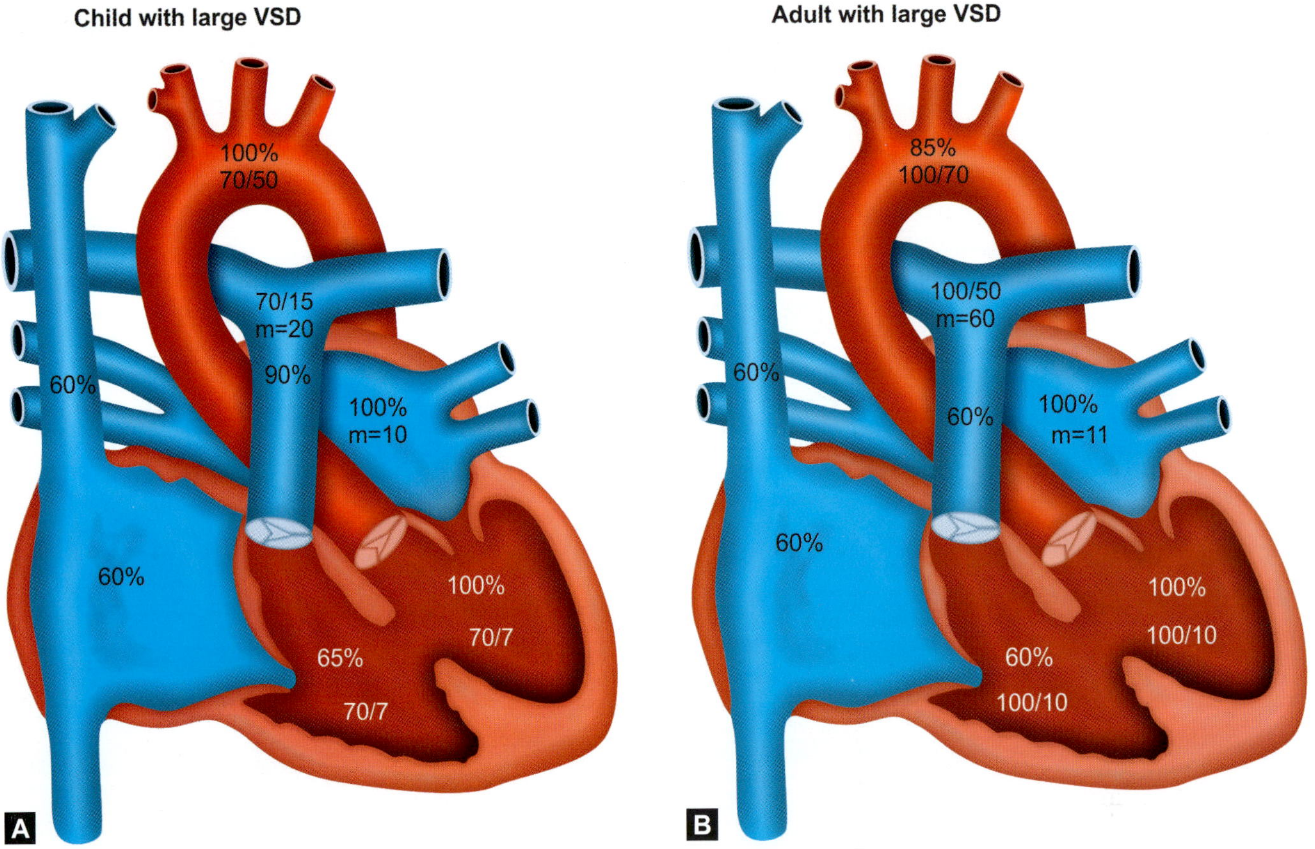

Figs. 41.5A and B: (A) Catheterization diagram depicting a child with a large ventricular septal defect (VSD) and Qp:Qs of 4:1. Using an assumed oxygen consumption of 160 mL/min/m^2, and hemoglobin (Hb) of 11 g/dL, the Fick equation yields pulmonary flow (Qp) of 10.7 L/min/m^2 and pulmonary vascular resistance (PVR) of 0.9 Woods units·m^2; (B) Catheterization diagram of an adult with a large VSD and Eisenmenger syndrome. The Qp:Qs = 0.4:1. Using an assumed cardiac output of 135 cc/min/m^2, and a Hb of 17 g/dL, the Fick equation gives a pulmonary blood flow (Qp) of 1.5 L/min/m^2 and PVR of 33 Woods units·m^2. Numbers with percentages are oxygen saturations. Numbers in black are pressures in mm Hg. M mean pressures in mm Hg.

Eisenmenger syndrome occurs when a left-to-right ventricular level shunt becomes a right-to-left shunt as a result of persistently elevated pulmonary vascular pressure resulting in elevated PVR. Pulmonary hypertension can be the result of increased flow, increased resistance, or both, as described the hydraulic analogy of Ohm's law:

$$\Delta P = Q \times R$$

The change in pressure across the pulmonary vascular bed, or transpulmonary gradient (ΔP), is the product of the flow (Q) through the lungs and the resistance (R) of the pulmonary vasculature. Children with large VSD and low PVR have pulmonary hypertension because of increased flow (Fig. 41.5A). Over time, the pulmonary vascular bed remodels, resulting in inflammation, cell proliferation, vasoconstriction, and fibrosis. These maladaptive changes ultimately lead to irreversible elevation in PVR. Patients with Eisenmenger syndrome, therefore, have pulmonary hypertension because of elevated resistance (Fig. 41.5B). These patients present with cyanosis, clubbing, polycythemia, stroke, and systemic embolism.

Ventricular septal defect may also lead to distortion of the AV. Prolapse of the right coronary cusp may occur in perimembranous, doubly-committed and juxta-arterial, or muscular outlet defects. The amount of prolapse may be enough to occlude the defect. However, significant distortion of the aortic leaflets may also occur with resultant aortic insufficiency, which does not improve after surgical closure of the defect. It is, therefore, recommended that even a small VSD be closed if there is prolapse of an aortic cusp, before insufficiency develops.

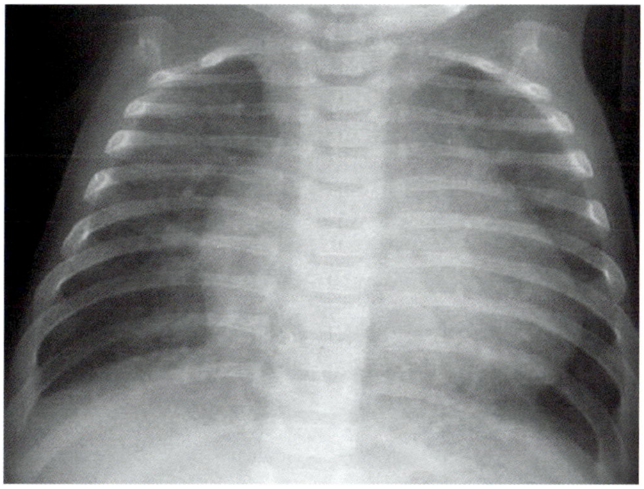

Fig. 41.6: Posteroanterior radiograph demonstrates cardiomegaly and increased pulmonary vascular markings. The thymus gland is also appreciable.

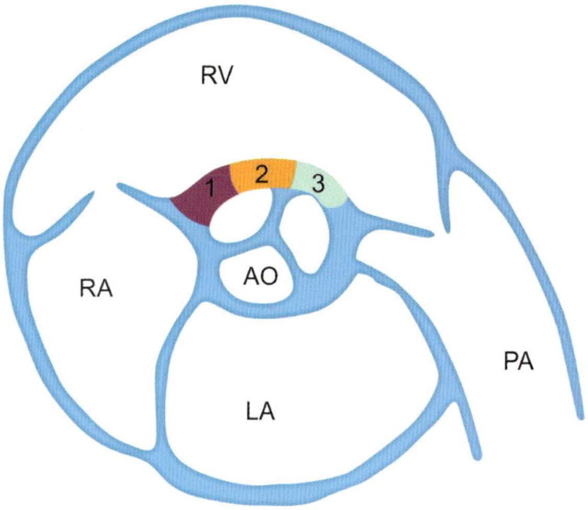

Fig. 41.7: The parasternal short axis is useful for differentiating several types of ventricular septal defect (VSD): (1) perimembranous VSD, (2) muscular outlet VSD, and (3) doubly-committed and juxta-arterial VSDs. (AO: Aorta; RV: Right ventricle; RA: Right atrium; LA: Left atrium; PA: Pulmonary artery).

DIAGNOSTIC EVALUATION

In an infant with a large left-to-right shunt, chest X-ray will show the hallmarks of congestive heart failure, including cardiomegaly and increased pulmonary vascularity (Fig. 41.6).

Echocardiography is currently the diagnostic modality of choice for VSD because of its ease of use, anatomic precision, and minimal side effects. A comprehensive examination is required from multiple scanning windows. Goals of an examination include detailing: the type of defect; the defect's location, rims, number and size; the direction of shunting; right heart pressures; and presence of any semilunar valve override, septal malalignment, tricuspid aneurysmal tissue, aortic cusp prolapse, or aortic insufficiency.

One of the most useful imaging planes for defining VSD is the parasternal short axis (Fig. 41.7). The AV can be thought of as a clock face. Perimembranous defects are typically found between 9 o'clock and 10 o'clock, with the tricuspid valve and AV forming borders of these defects (Fig. 41.8A). Subaortic outlet muscular defects are at 11 to 1 o'clock and are bordered by the AV, but not the tricuspid or pulmonary valves (Fig. 41.8B). Doubly-committed and juxta-arterial defects are at 1 to 3 o'clock, are bordered by the aortic and pulmonary valves, and bring the aortic and pulmonary valves into fibrous continuity (Fig. 41.8C).

In addition to the parasternal short axis, perimembranous defects can be viewed in the parasternal long, apical four chamber, and subcostal imaging planes. In the parasternal long axis, color Doppler will reveal a jet directed toward the probe arising from below the AV into the RV (Fig. 41.9). In the apical window, perimembranous defects can be seen by directing the probe anteriorly until the AV comes into view (Fig. 41.10). The subcostal imaging plane will similarly show a defect with borders along the AV and tricuspid valve (Fig. 41.11).

Muscular defects can be discovered by performing sweeps in multiple imaging planes, including the parasternal long (Fig. 41.12), parasternal short (Fig. 41.13), and apical four chamber (Fig. 41.14). Muscular defects of the inlet septum are best seen in the apical four-chamber view by tilting the transducer posteriorly to bring both atrioventricular valves into view (Fig. 41.15).

Semilunar valve override can occur when a defect results from deviation of the outlet septum. Anterior deviation of the outlet septum leads to VSD and pulmonary stenosis, and is responsible for the constellation of findings in Tetralogy of Fallot. This morphology is demonstrated in the parasternal short (Fig. 41.16) and parasternal long axis (Fig. 41.17). Conversely, posterior deviation of the outlet septum results in VSD and aortic stenosis (Fig. 41.18).

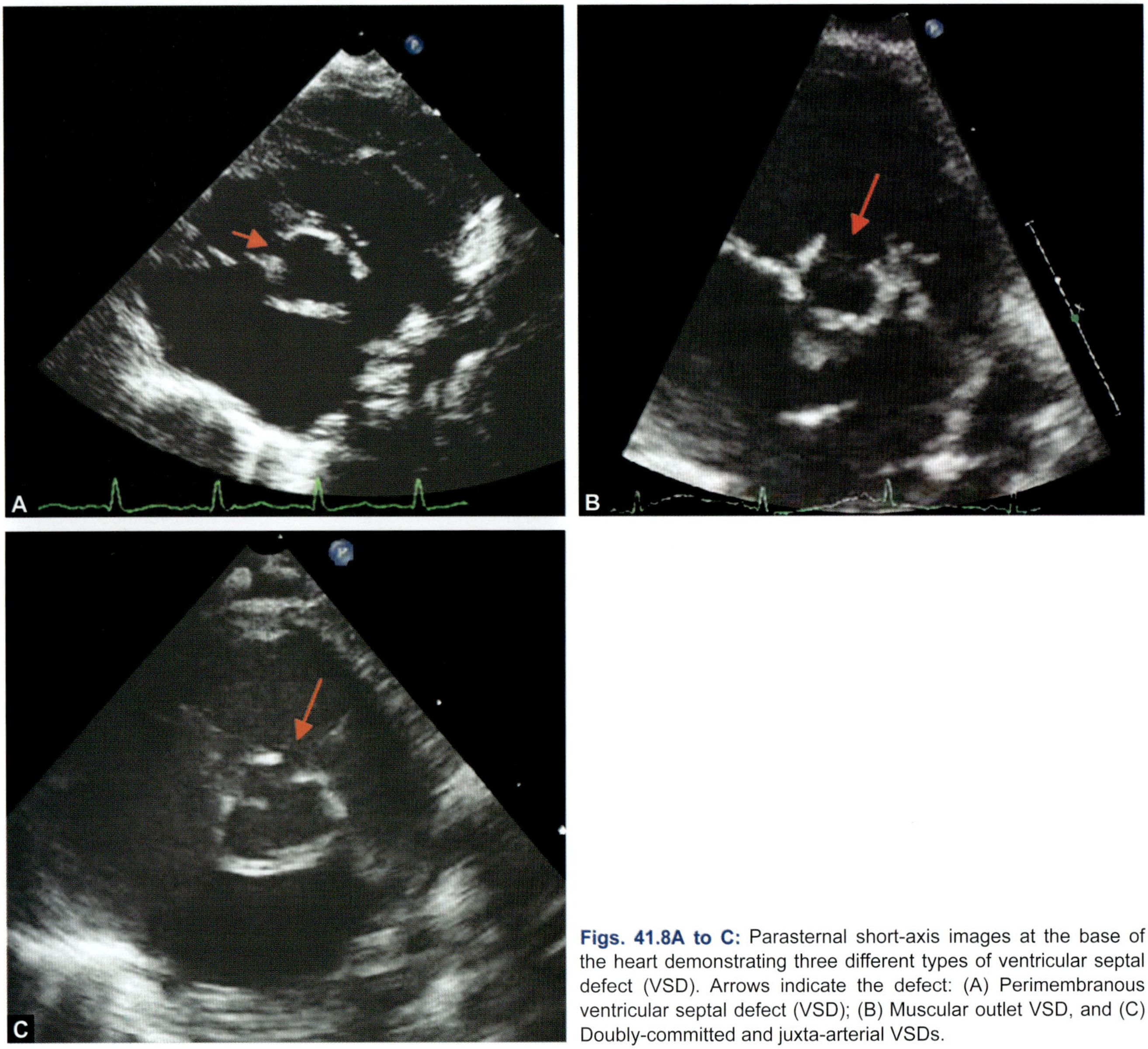

Figs. 41.8A to C: Parasternal short-axis images at the base of the heart demonstrating three different types of ventricular septal defect (VSD). Arrows indicate the defect: (A) Perimembranous ventricular septal defect (VSD); (B) Muscular outlet VSD, and (C) Doubly-committed and juxta-arterial VSDs.

As previously noted, perimembranous, muscular outlet, and doubly-committed and juxta-arterial defects place the aortic cusps at risk for prolapse with subsequent aortic regurgitation (Fig. 41.19). This can be seen in multiple imaging planes of the AV. Aortic prolapse and aortic insufficiency are indications for surgical intervention, even if the defect is closed by AV tissue.

Fetal echocardiography is a sensitive modality for detecting prenatal congenital heart disease, including VSD (Figs. 41.20 and 41.21). Most VSDs, even small ones, can be detected by the experienced sonographer. The same concepts apply to evaluating a fetus with VSD as in a child with VSD; a study should detail the type of defect, location, rims, number, size, direction of shunting, semilunar valve

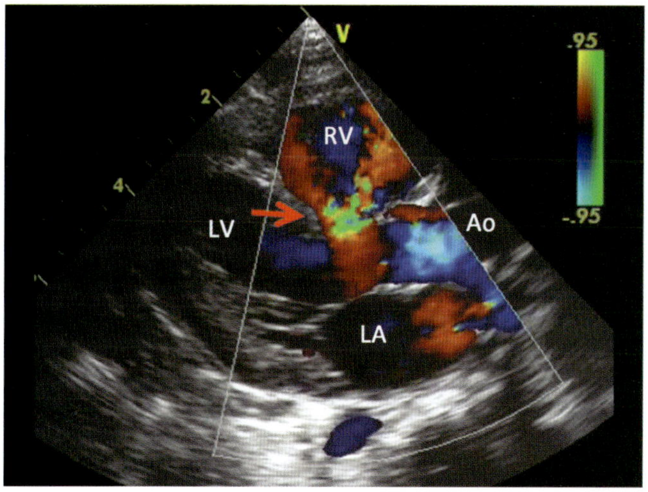

Fig. 41.9: Parasternal long axis with color Doppler showing a perimembranous defect. Red flow directed towards the probe represents a left ventricle (LV) to right ventricle (RV) shunt (arrow). (AO: Aorta; RV: Right ventricle; RA: Right atrium; LA: Left atrium).

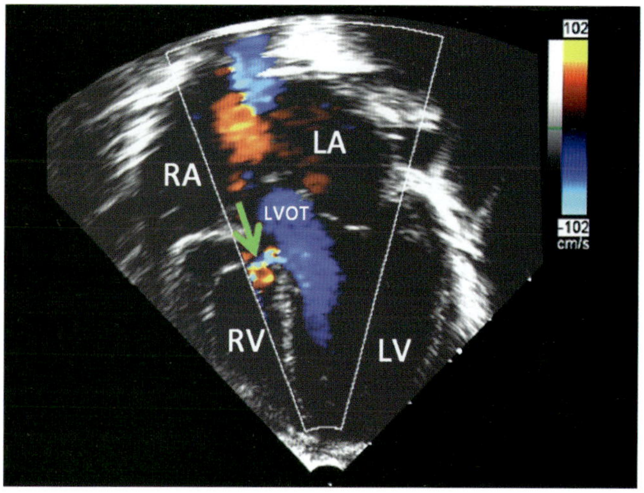

Fig. 41.10: View from the apex directed anteriorly to bring out the left ventricular outflow tract (LVOT, blue jet), and aliasing (arrow) resulting from blood crossing the ventricular septal defect (VSD) into the right ventricle (RV). (RV: Right ventricle; RA: Right atrium; LA: Left atrium; LV: Left ventricle; LVOT: Left ventricular outflow tract).

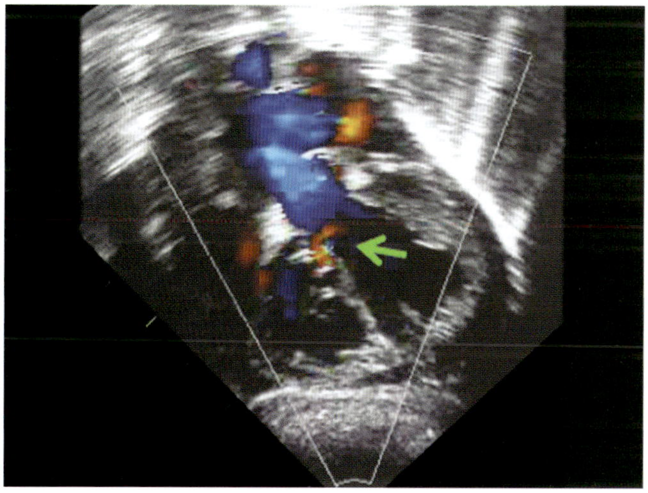

Fig. 41.11: Subcostal view demonstrating a perimembranous ventricular septal defect (VSD) (arrow) partially occluded by tricuspid aneurysmal tissue (arrow).

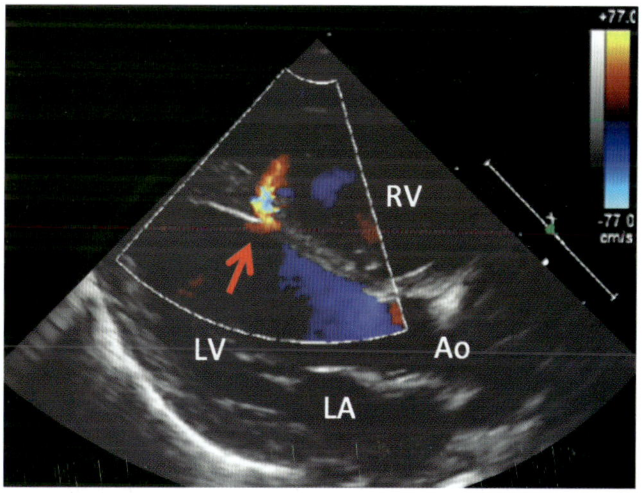

Fig. 41.12: Parasternal long-axis view showing a muscular defect in the trabecular septum with left to right shunting (arrow). (AO: Aorta; RV: Right ventricle; RA: Right atrium; LA: Left atrium).

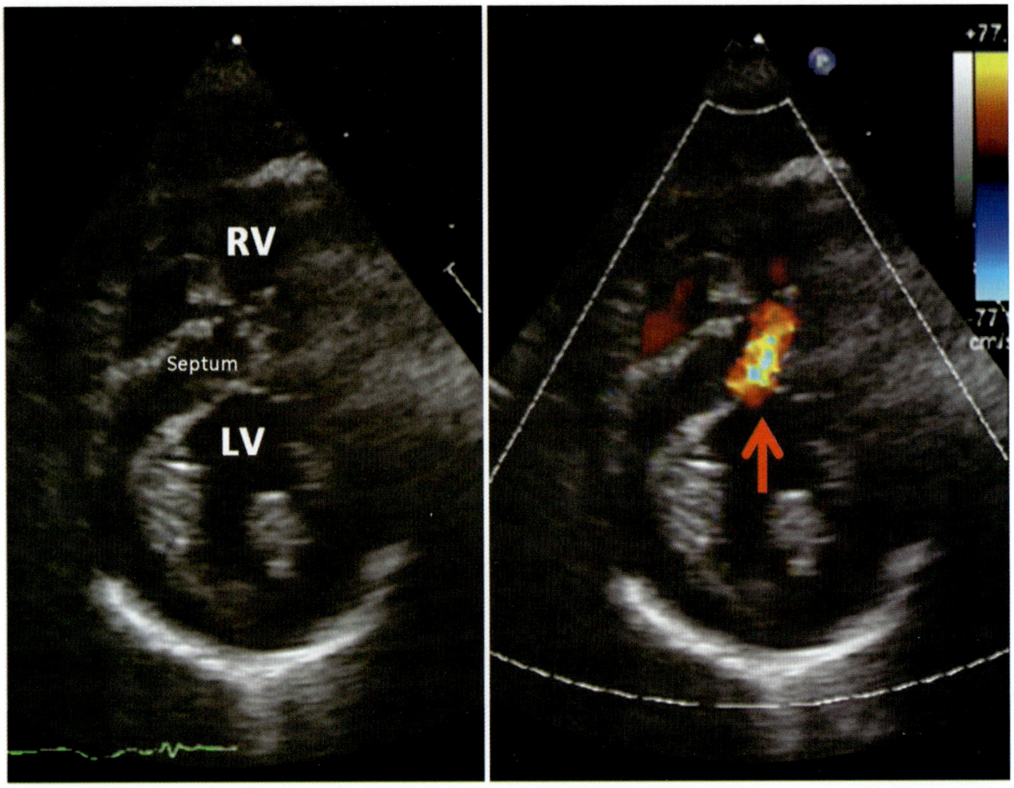

Fig. 41.13: Parasternal short axis of the same patient as in Figure 41.12, again showing a defect (arrow) in the trabecular septum. (RV: Right ventricle; LV: Left ventricle).

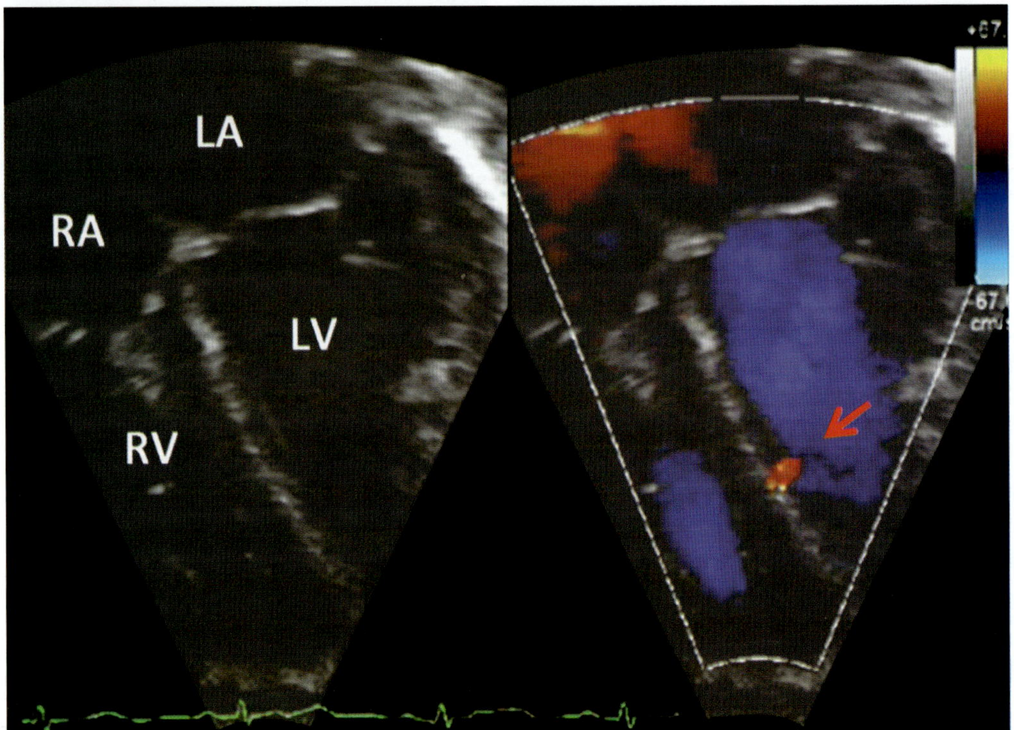

Fig. 41.14: Modified apical view of the same patient as in Figures 41.12 and 41.13, again showing a muscular defect in the trabecular septum. (RV: Right ventricle; RA: Right atrium; LA: Left atrium; LV: Left ventricle).

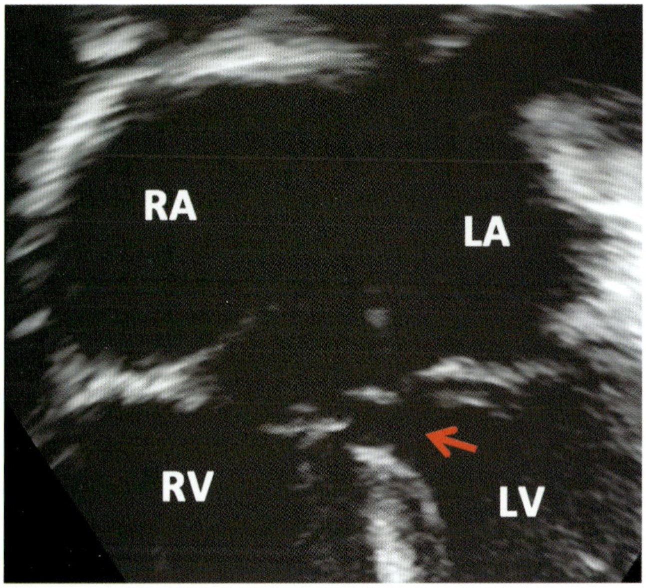

Fig. 41.15: Apical four-chamber view with magnification on the crux of the heart revealing an inlet defect of the muscular septum. There is deficiency (arrow) of the interventricular septum just below the atrioventricular valves. Note that the transducer is tilted posteriorly such that the aortic valve (AV) is not in the imaging plane. (RV: Right ventricle; RA: Right atrium; LA: Left atrium; LV: Left ventricle).

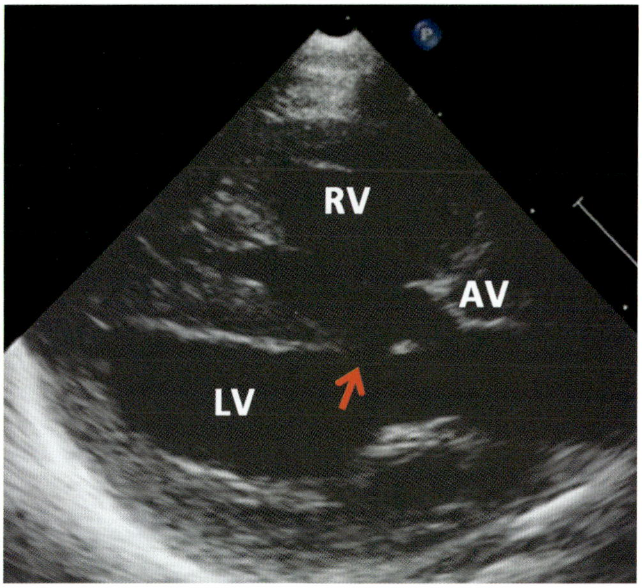

Fig. 41.16: Parasternal long-axis demonstrating ventricular septal defect (VSD) (arrow) with the aortic valve (AV) overriding the interventricular septum in a patient with Tetralogy of Fallot. (RV: Right ventricle; AV: Aortic valve; LV: Left ventricle).

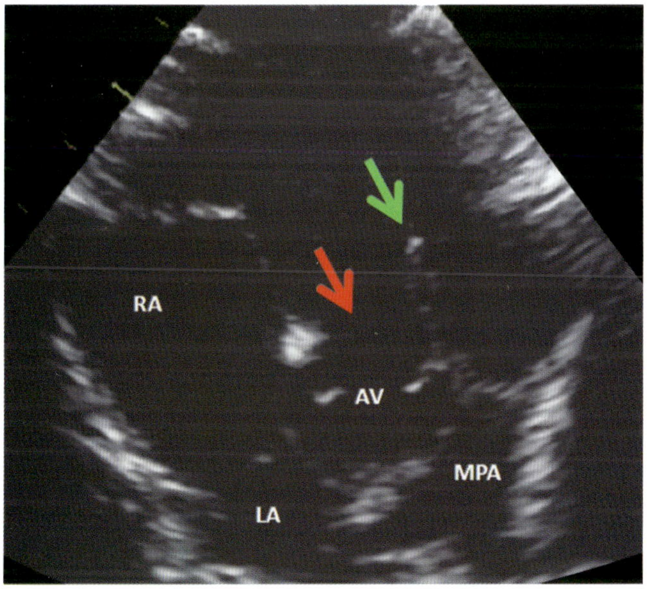

Fig. 41.17: Parasternal short-axis of a patient with Tetralogy of Fallot. There is a large ventricular septal defect (VSD) (red arrow), anterior and superior deviation of the outlet septum (green arrow), and pulmonary stenosis. (RA: Right atrium; LA: Left atrium; MPA: Main pulmonary artery; AV: Aortic valve).

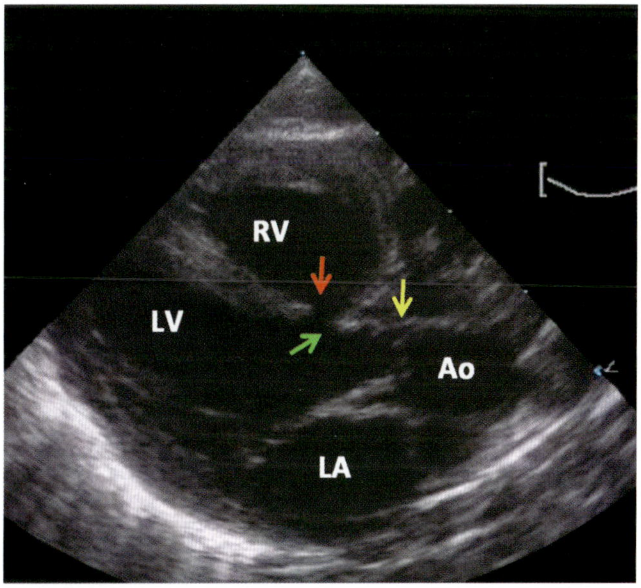

Fig. 41.18: Parasternal long-axis showing ventricular septal defect (VSD) (red arrow) resulting from posterior deviation of the outlet septum (green arrow). There is accompanying aortic stenosis and doming of the aortic leaflets (yellow arrow) in systole. (Ao: Aorta; RV: Right ventricle; LA: Left atrium; LV: Left ventricle).

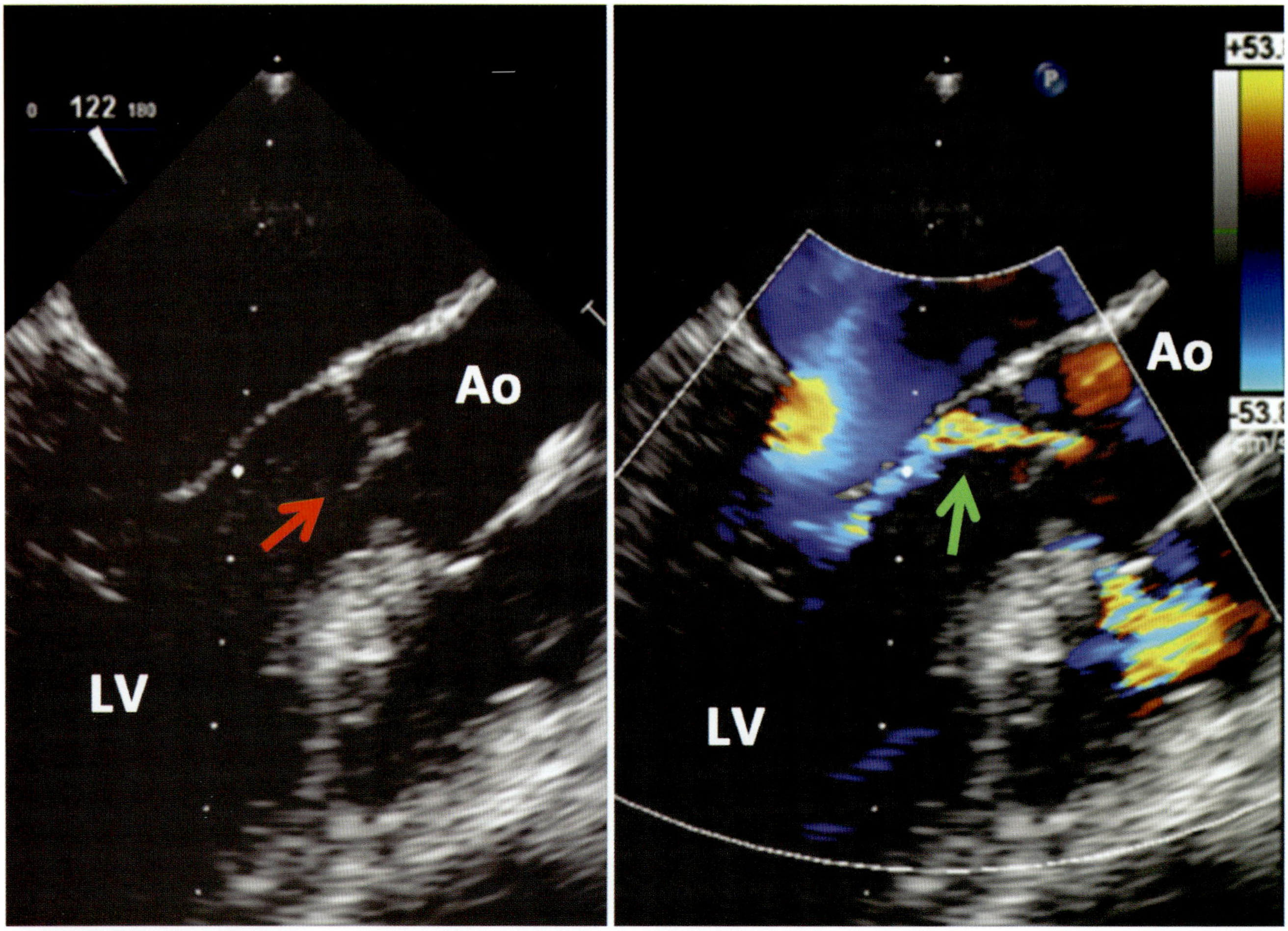

Fig. 41.19: Transesophageal image showing a perimembranous defect partially occluded by a prolapsed anterior aortic cusp (red arrow) and resultant aortic insufficiency (green arrow). (Ao: Aorta; LV: Left ventricle).

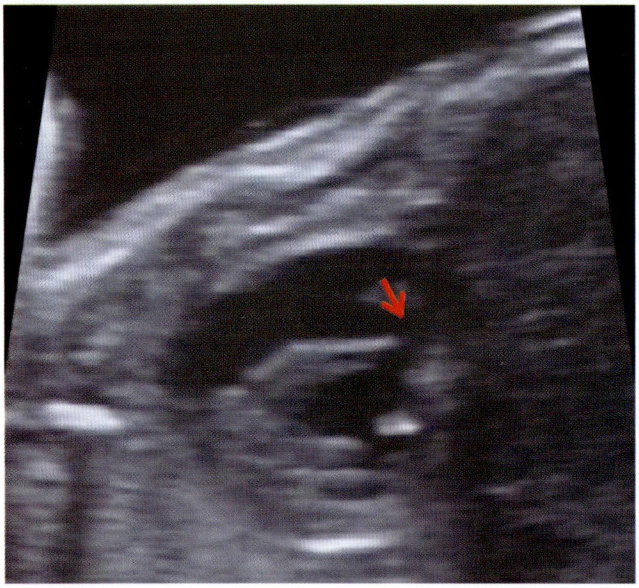

Fig. 41.20: Fetal echocardiogram showing an inlet muscular ventricular septal defect (VSD) in the short axis. Red arrow indicates the defect.

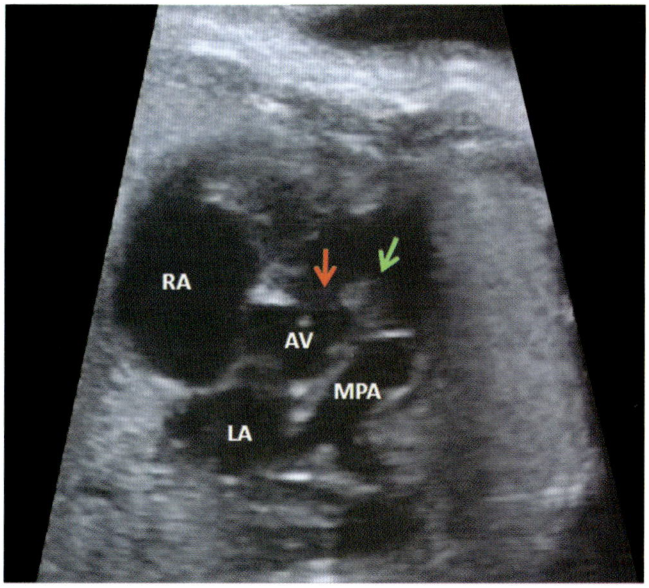

Fig. 41.21: Fetal echocardiogram in the short-axis plane of a patient with Tetralogy of Fallot. There is anterior and superior deviation of the outlet septum (green arrow), and a large ventricular septal defect (VSD) (red arrow). (AV: Aortic valve; LA: Left atrium; MPA: Main pulmonary artery; RA: Right atrium).

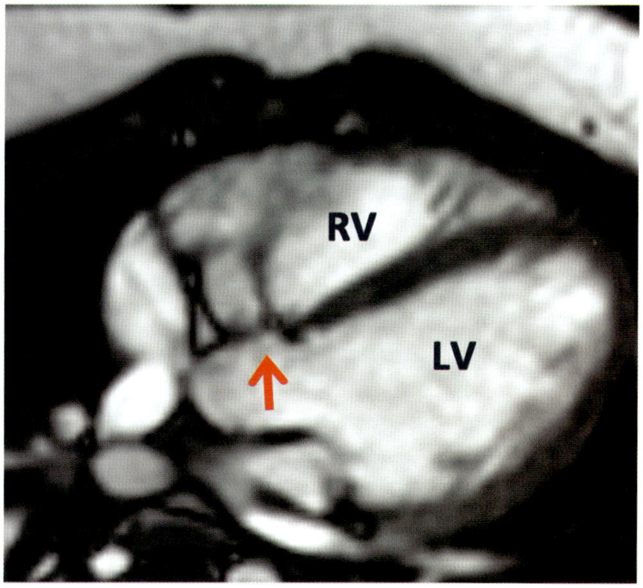

Fig. 41.22: Cardiac magnetic resonance (CMR) imaging balanced turbo field echo (bTFE) four-chamber view of a perimembranous defect. Arrow indicates a dephasing jet of left-to-right shunting across the ventricular septal defect (VSD). Note also there is left ventricular (LV) dilation. (LV: Left ventricle; RV: Right ventricle).

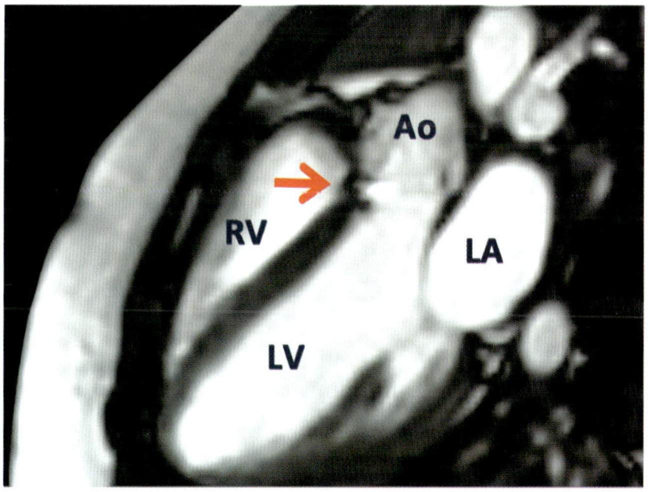

Fig. 41.23: Cardiac magnetic resonance (CMR) imaging balanced turbo field echo (bTFE) in the left ventricular (LV) outflow tract plane of a perimembranous defect (same patient as in Fig. 41.22). Arrow indicates dephasing jet of left-to-right shunting. (LV: Left ventricle; RV: Right ventricle; AV: Aortic valve; LA: Left atrium).

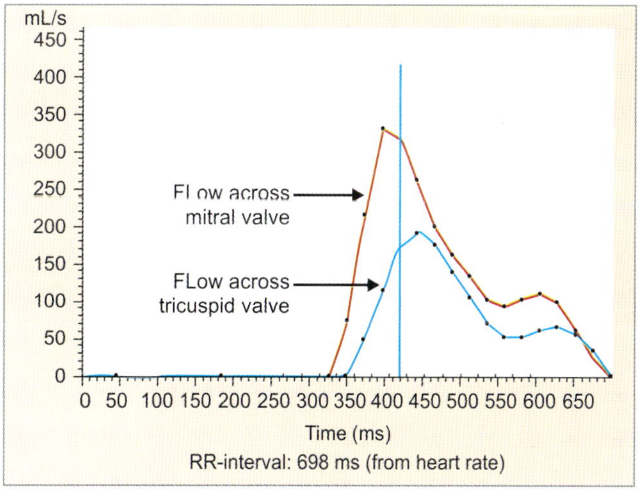

Fig. 41.24: Phase contrast across the atrioventricular valves in the same patient as in Figures 41.22 and 41.23. The red line represents flow across the mitral valve, and the blue line represents flow across the tricuspid valve. There is increased flow across the mitral valve, the pathophysiologic origin of a diastolic rumble heard on auscultation.

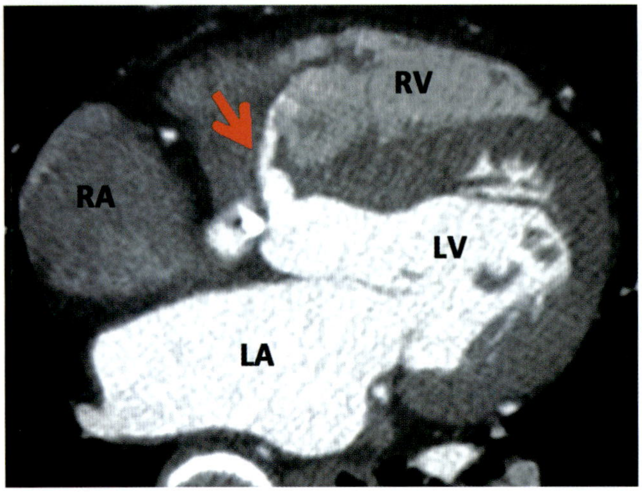

Fig. 41.25: Computed tomography (CT) scan image showing incidental detection of a ventricular septal defect (VSD) (arrow). Iodinated contrast, which appears bright, is seen passing from the left ventricle (LV) in to the right ventricle (RV). [Image from Oyama-Manabe N, Sugaya T, Yamaguchi T, et al. Non-coronary cardiac findings and pitfalls in coronary computed tomography angiography. J Clin Imaging Sci. 2011;1:51. [online]. Available from www.clinicalimagingscience.org/text.asp?2011/1/1/51/86666. (Accessed February, 2014)]. (LV: Left ventricle; RV: Right ventricle; RA: Right atrium; LA: Left atrium).

override, septal malalignment, tricuspid aneurysmal tissue, aortic cusp prolapse, and aortic insufficiency.

Cardiac magnetic resonance (CMR) imaging is rarely indicated in the management of VSD. However, in patients with inadequate echocardiographic imaging planes, CMR can give detailed anatomic and functional assessment (Figs. 41.22 and 41.23). In addition, CMR can measure flow, therefore providing an assessment of Qp:Qs (Fig. 41.24).

Computed tomography (CT) is not a usual imaging modality for assessment of VSD but occasionally may incidentally detect a VSD in a patient undergoing CT for a different indication (Fig. 41.25).

MANAGEMENT OF PATIENTS WITH VENTRICULAR SEPTAL DEFECT

Management of patients with VSD is dependent on factors such as the size and type of the VSD and whether there is dilation of left-sided structures. Mechanical complications, such as prolapse of an AV leaflet, with or without aortic regurgitation and double chamber RV may also be indications for surgical intervention. Additionally, early onset of pulmonary hypertension or failure of PVR to drop in an infant is also an indication for surgical closure in the presence of a moderate-to-large VSD. Neonates with hemodynamically significant VSD and symptoms of congestive heart failure may be placed on anticongestive medications, in particular furosemide, although in the current surgical era, there is no benefit to delaying surgery.

Older patients, who have developed Eisenmenger syndrome as a result of longstanding left-to-right shunting, are difficult to manage and warrant PVR testing in the catheterization laboratory. Eisenmenger patients who are responsive to pulmonary vasodilator therapy may be put forward for surgery, but those patients with fixed PVR should not have their VSD closed, as it will lead to right ventricular failure. It is important to evaluate main pulmonary artery (MPA) and branch pulmonary artery (PA) anatomy for stenosis in patients with purported Eisenmenger syndrome. If MPA or bilateral branch PA stenosis is present, then it is possible that the pulmonary vascular bed was protected over time and the cause of high PA pressures is not due to disease at the pulmonary arteriolar level.

An asymptomatic patient with a small, hemodynamically insignificant VSD is managed conservatively, with appropriate clinical follow-up.

Surgical closure usually involves patch closure through a sternotomy with cardiopulmonary bypass. Defects that are near the apex may be difficult to access through either the AV or semilunar valves and are technically more challenging. As previously mentioned, repair of perimembranous VSD carries a risk of damage to the conduction system.

Transcatheter techniques for VSD closure have evolved over the last several decades. Transcatheter closure is generally limited to patients with a muscular VSD (Figs. 41.26A to D), as there is a risk of damage to conduction tissues.

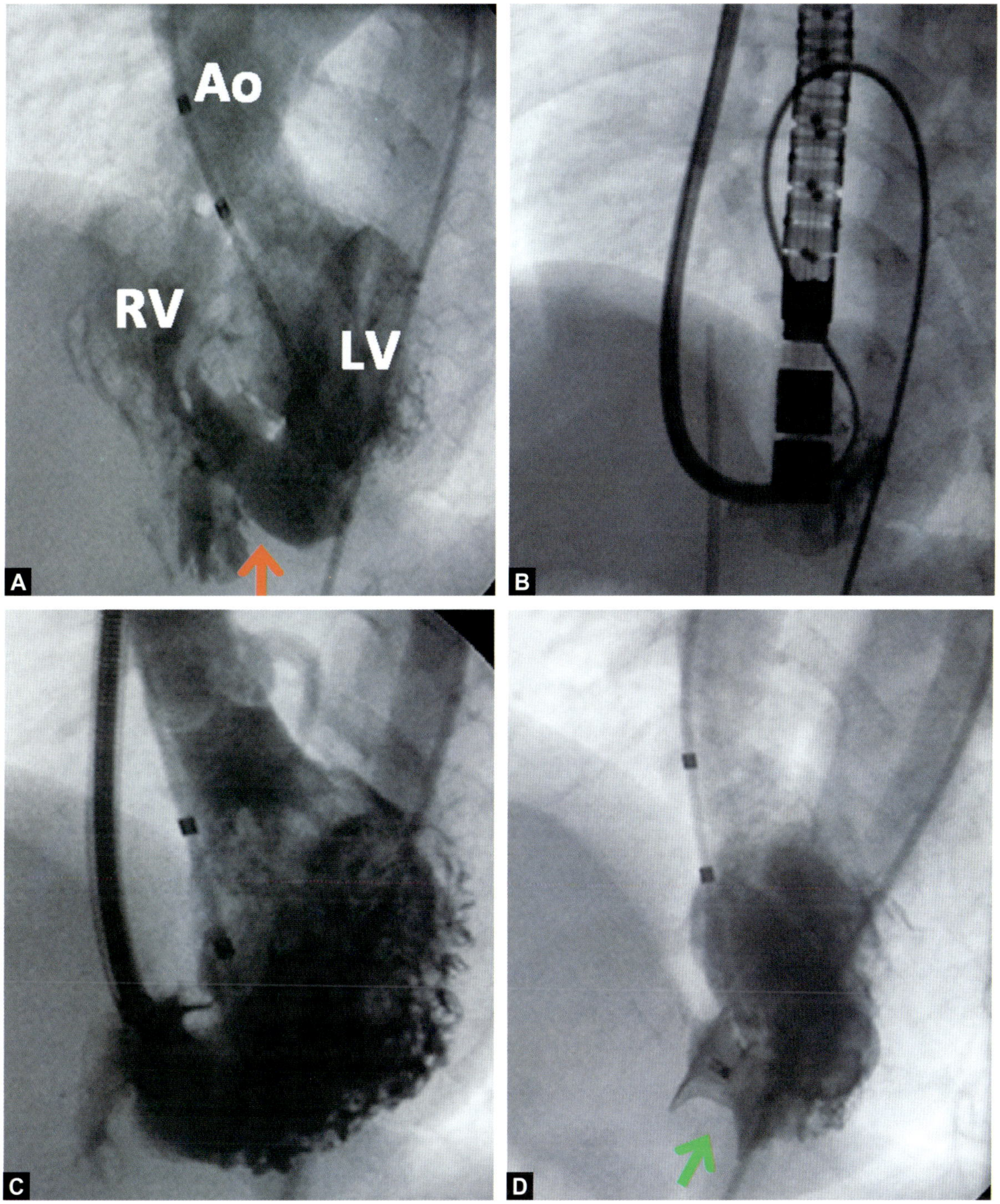

Figs. 41.26A to D: Percutaneous closure of a membranous ventricular septal defect (VSD). (A) Left ventricular (LV) angiogram demonstrating a large apical muscular VSD. The VSD is crossed retrograde from the LV using a Judkins right catheter and a soft tipped wire which is advanced into the main pulmonary artery (MPA). The wire is snared in the MPA from a right internal jugular vein (RIJV) approach and externalized forming an arteriovenous wire loop; (B) The delivery sheath is advanced from the RIJV through the VSD and into the LV. The wire is removed; (C) The defect is measured using transesophageal echocardiographic (TEE) and angiographic measurements and a device 1–2 mm larger than the defect is chosen and advanced through the sheath and deployed across the VSD; (D) The device is released from the delivery system and a repeat angiogram demonstrates appropriate placement of the device within the defect. (Image and legend text from Balzer D. Current status of percutaneous closure of ventricular septal defects. Pediatr Therapeut. 2012;2:2. [online]. Available from dx.doi.org/10.4172/2161-0665.1000112. [Accessed February, 2014]). (LV: Left ventricle; RV: Right ventricle; Ao: Aorta).

VIDEO LEGENDS

Videos 41.1 and 41.2: Magnetic resonance imaging (MRI) video clips demonstrating a ventricular septal defect (VSD) with flow from the left ventricle (LV) to the right ventricle (RV). (Videoclips courtesy of Scott D Flamm, MD).

Video 41.3: Five-chamber transthoracic echocardiography (TTE) demonstrating a perimembranous ventricular septal defect (VSD) with flow from the left ventricle (LV) to the right ventricle (RV). (Video courtesy of Glenn N Levine, MD).

Video 41.4: Short-axis transthoracic echocardiography (TTE) demonstrating a perimembranous ventricular septal defect (VSD). (Video courtesy of Glenn N Levine, MD).

REFERENCES

Benson LN, Yoo SJ, Habshan FA, et al. Ventricular septal defects. In: RH Anderson (Ed). Paediatric Cardiology, 3rd edition. Philadelphia, PA: Elsevier; 2010. pp. 591-624.

Penny DJ, Vick GW. Ventricular septal defect. Lancet. 2011; 377(9771):1103-12.

CHAPTER

42

Ebstein Anomaly

Christine H Attenhofer Jost, Patrick W O'Leary, Joseph A Dearani, Heidi M Connolly

INTRODUCTION

Ebstein anomaly (EA) is a rare type of congenital heart disease (CHD) primarily manifest by abnormalities of the tricuspid valve (TV) and the right ventricle (RV). Figure 42.1 is from the original publication in which Wilhelm Ebstein (Fig. 42.2) demonstrated a clear depiction of the characteristic features of EA. Figure 42.3 schematically depicts EA. Figure 42.4 is a post-mortem cardiac specimen portrayed in a 4-chamber view showing a severe form of EA.

Ebstein anomaly occurs due to abnormal myocardial development with incomplete delamination of the TV leaflets from the underlying myocardium. In EA, the RV is usually dilated and has reduced function. However, the hallmark of the disorder is the TV deformity. Patients with EA have TVs that are apically and anteriorly displaced. This rotates the TV orifice toward the RV outflow tract and impairs the function of the valve, resulting in significant regurgitation. The TV shows the following main characteristics in EA:

- Elongation, tethering (due to short chords or direct myocardial insertions) and occasional fenestrations of the anterior TV leaflet
- Adhesion of the posterior and septal TV leaflets to the underlying myocardium with the functional annulus being apically displaced and consequent "atrialization" of the involved portion of the RV

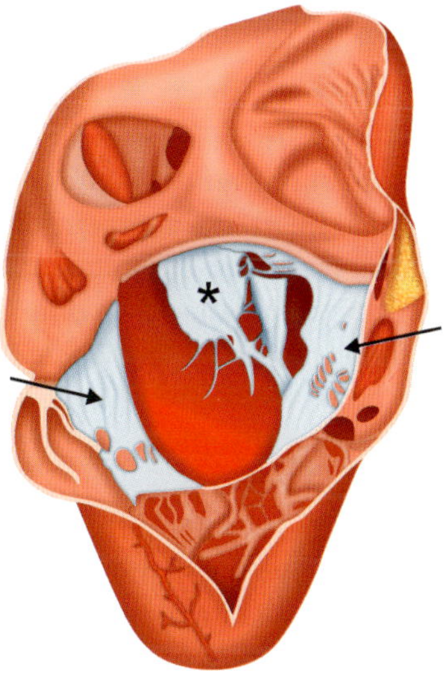

Fig. 42.1: The figure from Ebstein's case report shows right atrium and right ventricle opened along right border beginning at the superior vena cava. This is an example of severe Ebstein anomaly with only a rudimentary septal leaflet (*) and a large, but severely tethered and fenestrated anterior leaflet (black arrows). [Image with permission from Mann RJ, Lie JT. The life story of Wilhelm Ebstein (1836–1912) and his almost overlooked description of a congenital heart disease. Mayo Clin Proc. 1979;54(3):197-204].

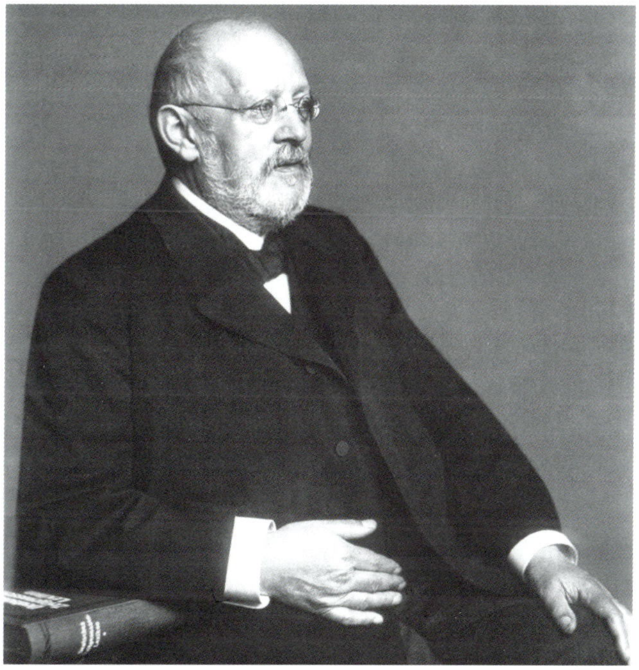

Fig. 42.2: Wilhelm Ebstein. [Image by Nicola Perscheid, published in Photographische Gesellschaft (1906) and posted on Wikipedia Commons].

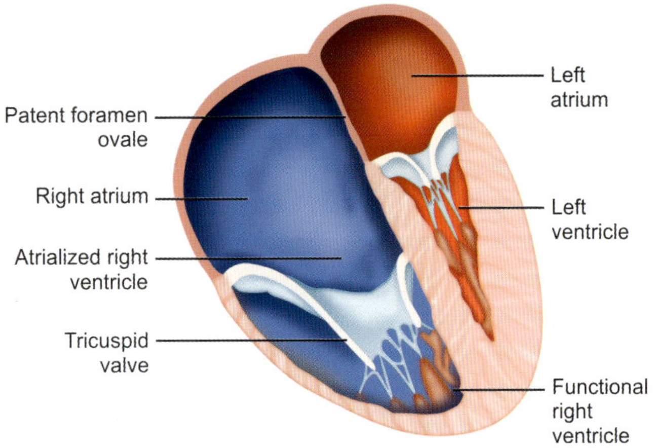

Fig. 42.3: Schematic illustration of Ebstein anomaly.

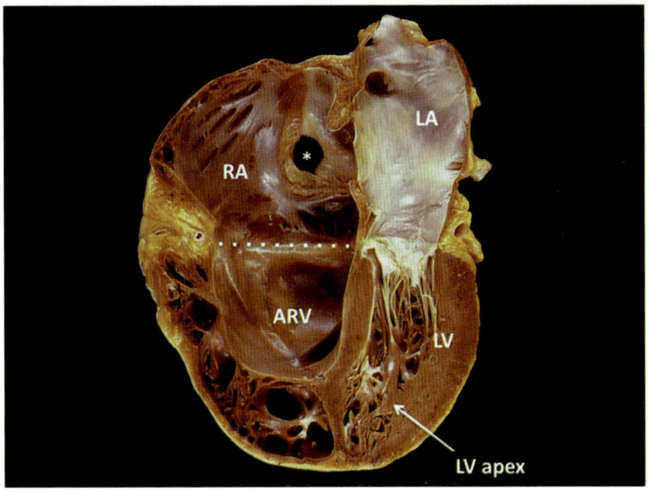

Fig. 42.4: Pathologic image of a heart severely affected by Ebstein anomaly. There is no functional tricuspid valve (TV) tissue present anywhere within this image of the anatomic inflow tract (dashed line indicates the anatomic TV annulus). The mobile segments of the TV are displaced anteriorly and apically and are out of the plane of the image. The right heart is severely enlarged and the anterior TV "leaflet" is adherent to the right ventricle (RV) myocardium, essentially forming the endocardial border of the atrialized right ventricle (ARV). Typical for Ebstein anomaly, the anatomic right atrium (RA) and the ARV are enlarged. The myocardium near the apex of the left ventricle (LV) demonstrates abnormal architecture (white arrow) suggesting non-compaction. (Image courtesy of WD Edwards, MD, Department of Pathology, Mayo Clinic). (LA: Left atrium).

- Secondary dilatation of the right atrioventricular junction (true TV annulus).

Figures 42.5A to D demonstrate features of the explanted TV in EA, illustrating the broad anatomic variation seen in this disorder. Up to 20% of TV leaflets are fenestrated. The left ventricular myocardium may also be abnormal, often showing features that resemble non-compaction.

DIAGNOSIS OF EBSTEIN ANOMALY

Ebstein anomaly can be diagnosed at any age and the age at diagnosis depends largely on the severity of the disorder and the presence/severity of associated anomalies. The most common clinical manifestations of EA are exercise intolerance, cyanosis and atrial arrhythmias. Cyanosis, reduced exercise ability and, in severe cases, heart failure symptoms are related to TV regurgitation and ventricular dysfunction (RV more often than LV). The reduced systemic oxygen level (cyanosis) is related to the right-to-left shunt through an atrial septal defect (ASD) or stretched patent foramen ovale (PFO). The inefficient TV/RV performance and the frequent association of ASD/PFO with EA make this a frequent presenting symptom. In fact, cyanosis with exertion is extremely common in older children and adults with unrepaired EA.

Accessory conduction pathways are common in EA, thus arrhythmias may be the initial presenting symptom. Figures 42.6A and B show two typical electrocardiogram examples of EA with or without an accessory conduction pathway.

The chest radiograph (Figs. 42.7 and 42.8) generally demonstrates features of right heart enlargement in EA. The cardiomegaly reflects right ventricular and right atrial enlargement. Classically, the heart is described as having a "box shape" with decreased pulmonary markings on a frontal chest radiograph, although these findings are nonspecific.

Transthoracic echocardiography is the cardiac imaging method of choice to confirm the diagnosis and assess EA severity. In a normal heart, the septal insertion of the TV is positioned apical to that of the mitral valve. In EA, TV displacement is exaggerated due to incomplete separation (delamination) from the underlying RV myocardium; this is the anatomic hallmark of the disorder. The distance between the two septal insertions can be measured by echocardiography, and in those with EA is 8 mm/m^2 body surface area, or at least 15 mm in the adult. Figures 42.9A (echocardiographic 4-chamber view), and 42.9B [4-chamber view by cardiac magnetic resonance (CMR) imaging] both show examples of the apical displacement of the septal TV leaflet. The most common coexisting CHD seen in those with EA is an ASD or PFO. Such interatrial shunts are present in up to 80% of patients with EA. Other cardiovascular anomalies may also be present in EA (Table 42.1). Figures 42.10 and 42.11 show typical echocardiographic features of moderate EA with a single jet of severe TV regurgitation. In Figure 42.10, the

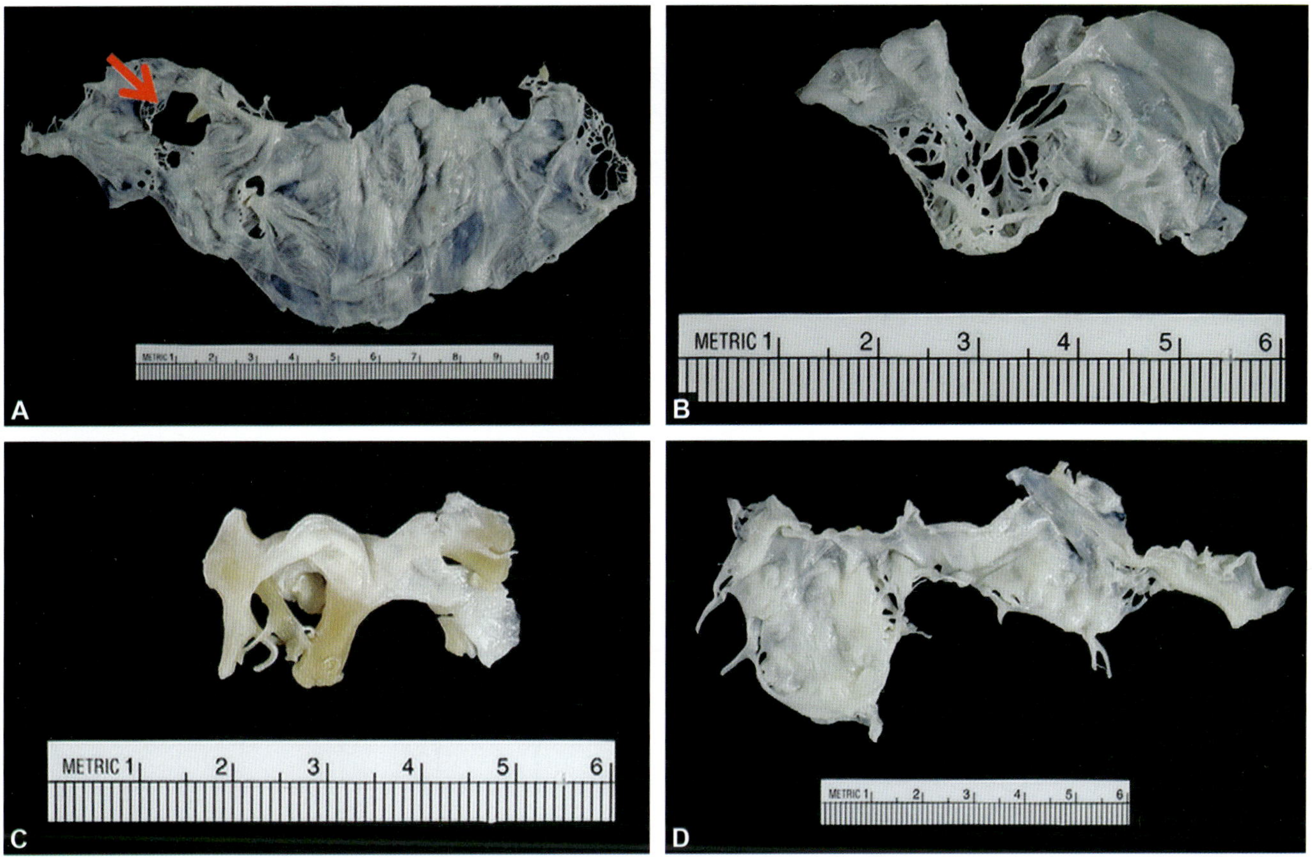

Figs. 42.5A to D: Pathologic variation of tricuspid valve involvement in Ebstein anomaly. (A) Large anterior tricuspid valve leaflet (right atrial aspect), from a 42-year-old male, demonstrates a large fenestration on the left (arrow); (B) Complex web-like malformation from a 16-year old male; (C) Direct insertion of myocardium into leaflet tissue, without intervening tendinous cords (right atrial aspect), from a 10-year-old female; (D) Diffuse leaflet and cordal thickening presumably due to hemodynamic effects of chronic tricuspid regurgitation (right atrial aspect), from a 26-year-old male. [Image with permission from Barbara DW, Edwards WD, Connolly HM, et al. Surgical pathology of 104 tricuspid valves (2000–2005) with classic right-sided Ebstein's malformation. Cardiovasc Pathol. 2008;17(3):166-71].

displacement index was 18 mm (11 mm/m^2 body surface area). Video 42.1 present a typical echocardiographic example of a patient with moderately severe EA showing the apical displacement of the TV leaflet. Figure 42.12 shows a typical echocardiographic example of a patient with EA, with direct muscular insertions into a fenestrated anterior TV leaflet. Multiple tricuspid regurgitation (TR) jets may be due to leaflet fenestrations, to segments of the leaflet that are unsupported by chordae, or to free wall attachments distorting valve closure.

Cardiac magnetic resonance imaging can further delineate anatomic and functional features of EA. Figures 42.13A and B demonstrate a CMR study of a patient with EA—the posterior TV leaflet and tethered anterior leaflet are well visualized. CMR is most frequently utilized to quantitatively assess the degree of RV enlargement and/or measure RV systolic ventricular function.

The right ventricular angiogram (Figs. 42.14A and B) is primarily of historical interest, as this is no longer performed clinically. Echocardiography and magnetic resonance imaging have surpassed angiography as diagnostic imaging techniques for the patient with EA.

MANAGEMENT OF PATIENTS WITH EBSTEIN ANOMALY

Intervention should be considered for EA patients with severe TV regurgitation and associated symptoms, deteriorating exercise capacity, increasing cardiomegaly, cyanosis, enlarging RV, declining RV function or those with paradoxical embolus.

Cardiac surgical interventions can significantly improve the clinical status of patients with EA. Surgical procedures include TV repair or replacement, and ASD closure. In the past, interruption of conduction pathways associated with arrhythmias was performed via surgery, but in the current era these are approached percutaneously by catheter ablation. Plication of the atrialized RV is

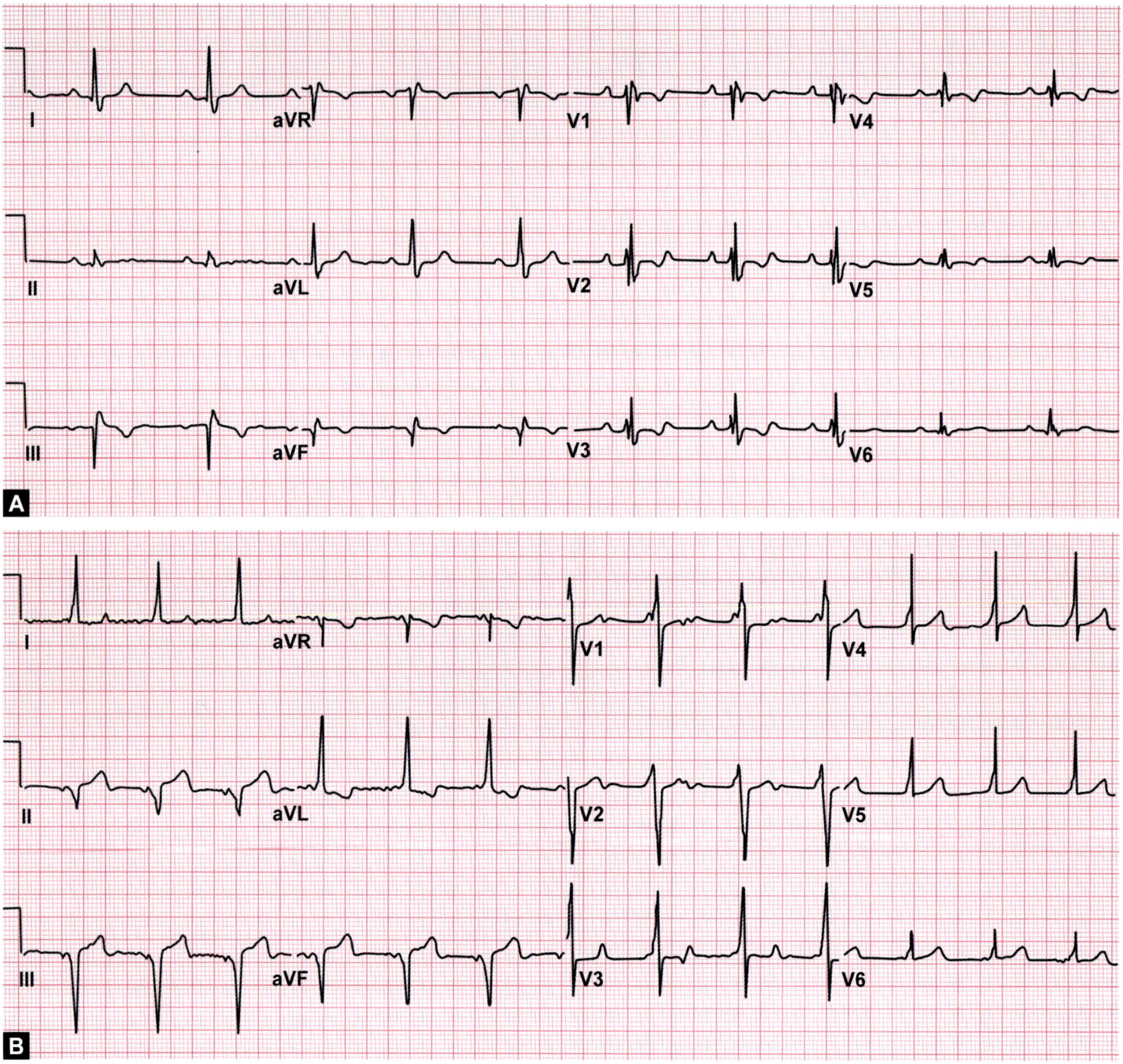

Figs. 42.6A and B: Typical electrocardiogram examples from patients with Ebstein anomaly. (A) Typical electrocardiogram example of a patient with Ebstein anomaly showing bizarre QRS complexes, small R waves and first degree atrioventricular block, but no pre-excitation; (B) Electrocardiogram from a patient with Ebstein anomaly and pre-excitation. Most of the accessory pathways found in patients with Ebstein anomaly are located around the orifice of the malformed tricuspid valve.

done selectively and right reduction atrioplasty is done routinely. A concomitant bidirectional cavopulmonary shunt is reserved for patient with severe right ventricular enlargement or dysfunction.

Leaflet mobility is one of the factors that can help determine whether TV repair is feasible. Anatomic features that are favorable for repair in EA include large mobile anterior TV leaflet (especially at the leading edge) and the presence of some septal leaflet. Assessment of TV repairability is performed by echocardiographic imaging.

Surgical repair for EA historically involved a monocusp repair. In this procedure, the anterior TV leaflet is used to form a functional "monocusp" valve, coapting with the ventricular septum (Figs. 42.15A to G). More recently, a circumferential valve reconstruction has been used ("cone repair"). This is the most common anatomic repair, in

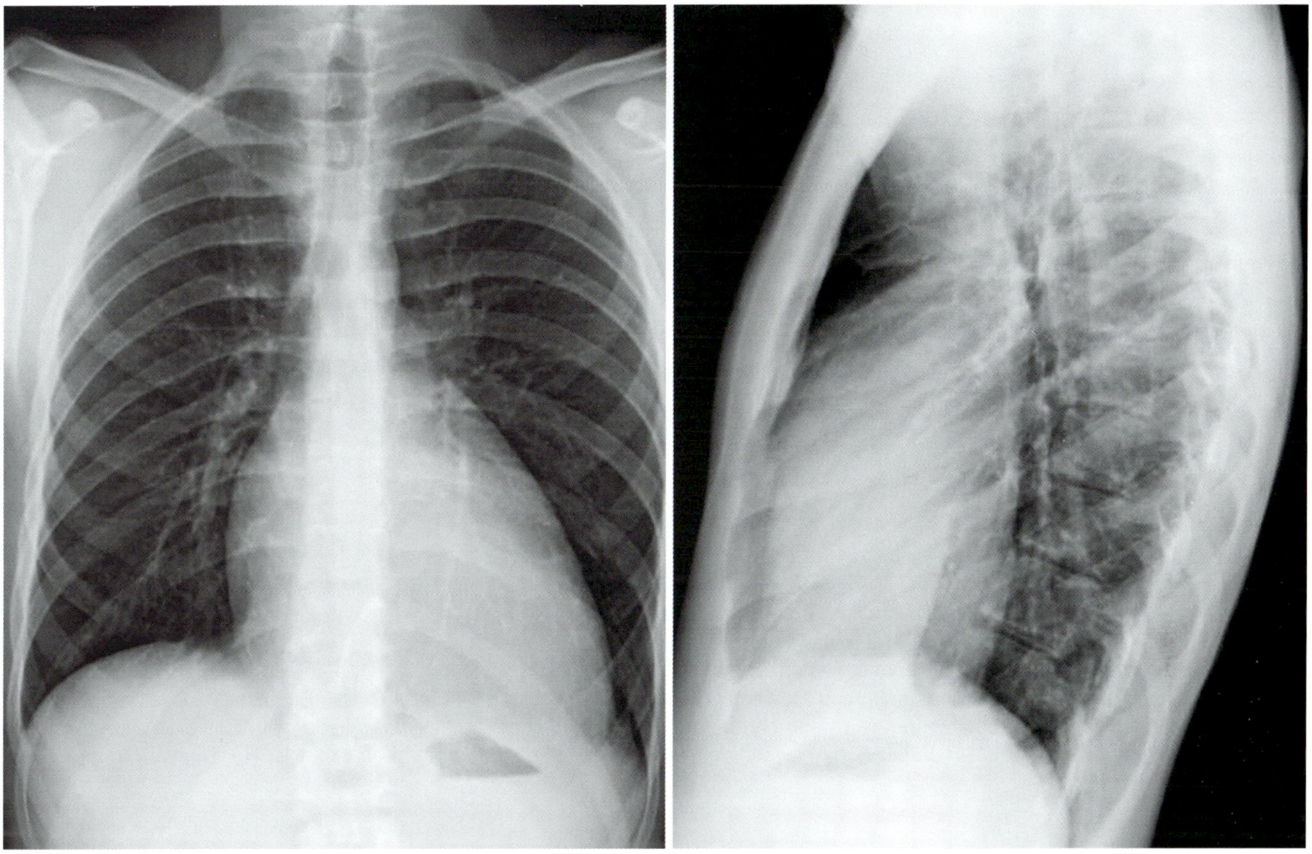

Fig. 42.7: Chest radiograph of a patient with severe Ebstein anomaly. The chest radiograph findings depend on the severity of Ebstein anomaly and the degree of right heart enlargement. This is an example of a patient with severe Ebstein anomaly prior to cardiac surgery.

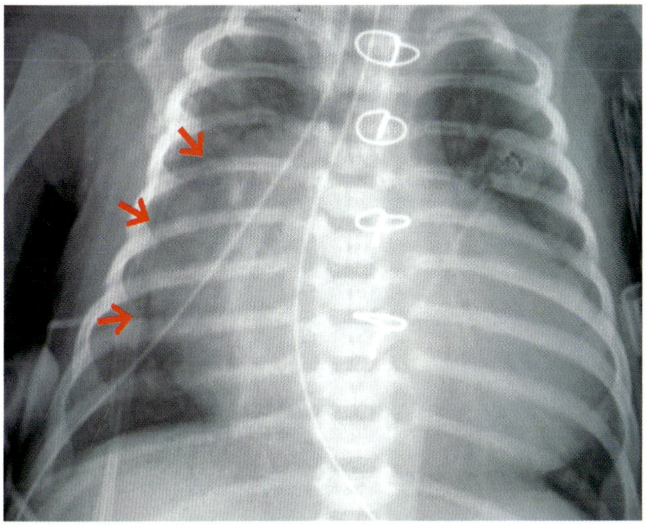

Fig. 42.8: Chest X-ray of a patient with severe Ebstein anomaly demonstrating severe cardiomegaly, primarily due to right atrial enlargement (arrows). [Image from Balaguru D, Rao PS. Diseases of the tricuspid valve. In: Vijayalakshmi IB, Rao PS, Chugh R (Eds). A Comprehensive Approach to Congenital Heart Disease. New Delhi: Jaypee Brothers Medical Publishers; 2013].

Table 42.1: Associated cardiac anomalies in Ebstein anomaly.

Interatrial shunting • Patent foramen ovale • Atrial septal defect
Mitral valve abnormalities • Mitral valve prolapse • Mitral regurgitation
Pulmonary valve abnormalities • Valvular stenosis • Supravalvular stenosis • Pulmonary atresia • Pulmonary regurgitation
Left ventricular non-compaction
Ventricular septal defect
Bicuspid aortic valve
Patent ductus arteriosus
Accessory conduction pathways

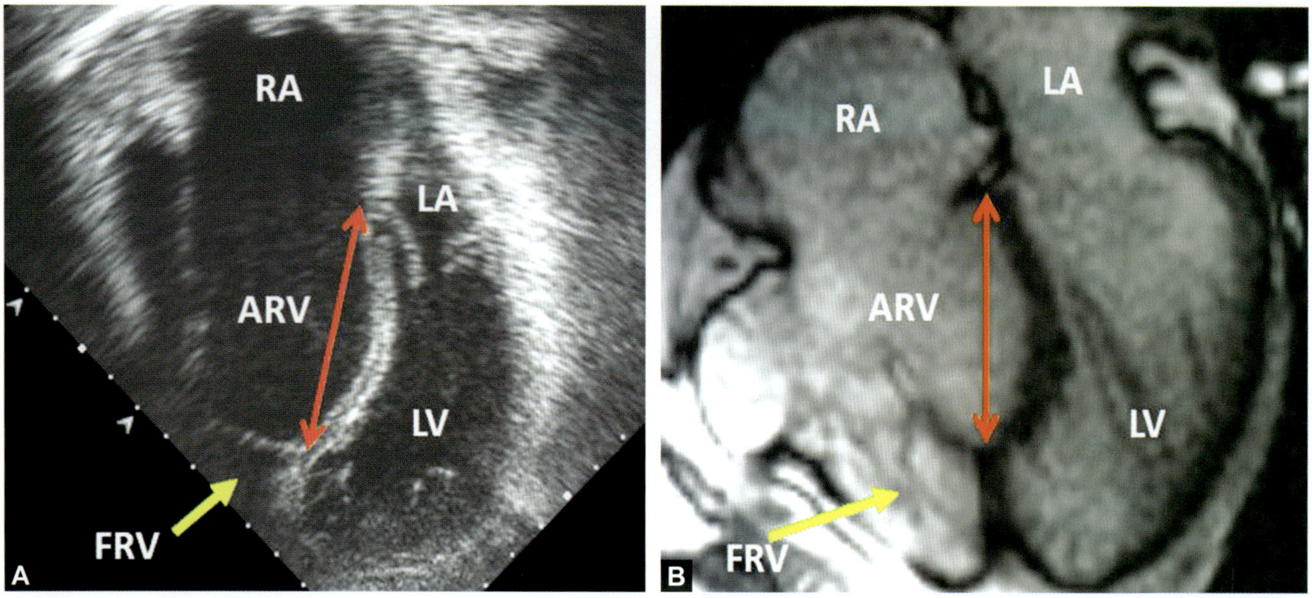

Figs. 42.9A and B: Comparison of equivalent 4-chamber views obtained by (A) transthoracic echocardiogram and (B) cardiac magnetic resonance imaging of a heart with Ebstein anomaly. Solid, single headed yellow arrows point to the functional right ventricle (FRV) in Figures 42.9A and B. Solid, double headed, red arrows point out the apical displacement of the septal tricuspid valve hinge point away from the septal mitral valve insertion. [Image modified with permission from Attenhofer Jost CH, Edmister WD, Julsrud PR, et al. Prospective comparison of echocardiography versus cardiac magnetic resonance imaging in patients with Ebstein's anomaly. Int J Cardiovasc Imaging. 2012;28(5):1147-59]. (ARV: Atrialized right ventricle; LA: Left atrium; LV: Left ventricle; RA: Right atrium).

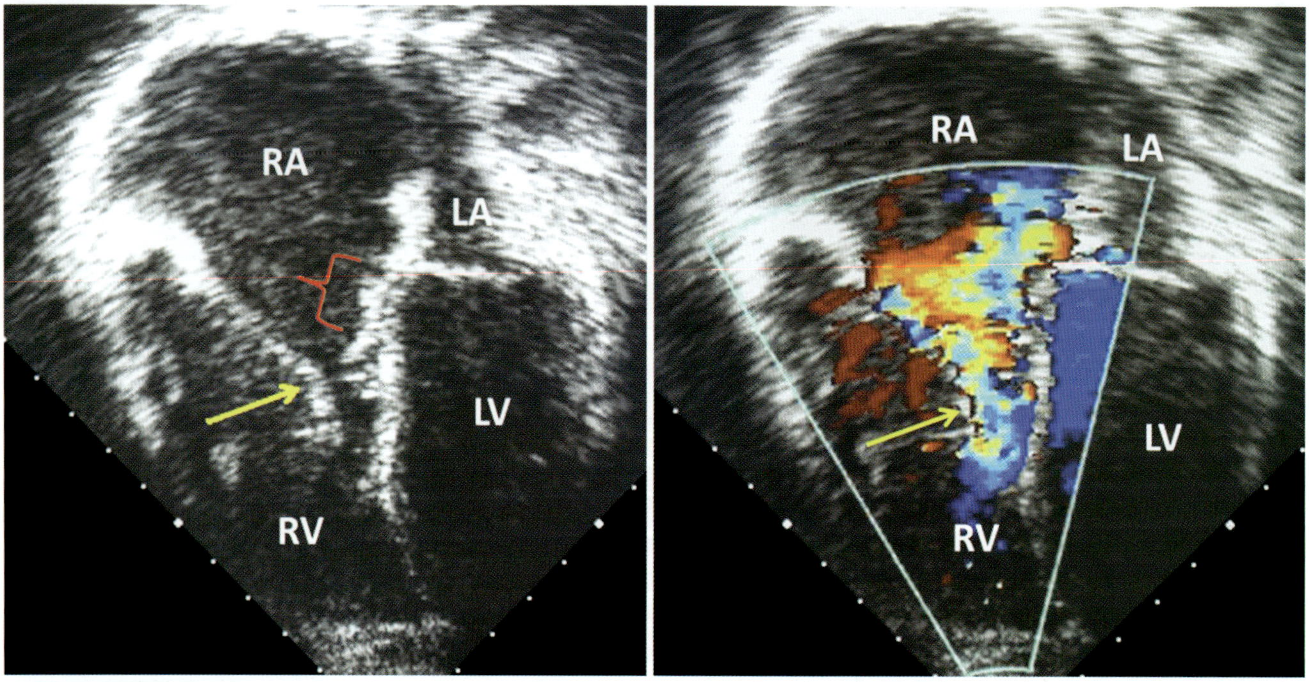

Fig. 42.10: Transthoracic echocardiogram in a patient with typical Ebstein anomaly demonstrated in apex down format. Two-dimensional echocardiogram (left panel) and color-flow Doppler imaging (right panel) in a patient with moderate severity Ebstein anomaly. Note apical displacement of the septal tricuspid valve leaflet (25 mm or 18 mm/m^2 body surface area). The displacement is outlined by the red bracket in the left panel. Tricuspid valve regurgitation originates from the area where the components of the tricuspid valve do not coapt during systole (arrows). (LA: Left atrium; LV: Left ventricle; RA: Right atrium; RV: Right ventricle).

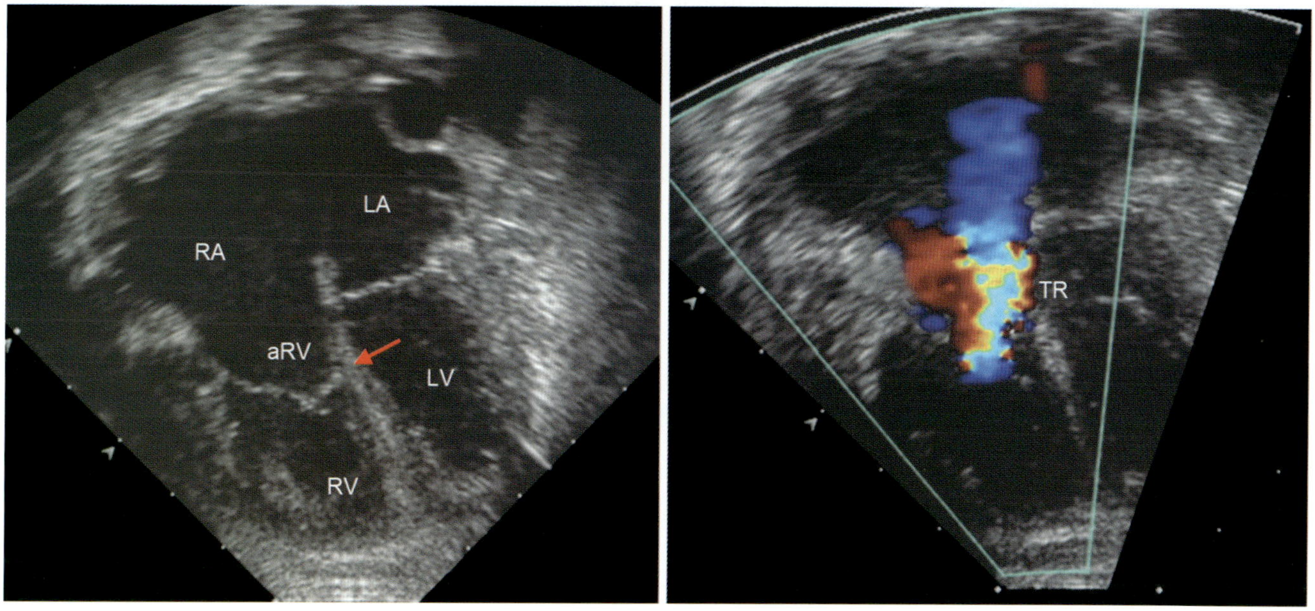

Fig. 42.11: Similar example to Figure 42.10 demonstrating Ebstein anomaly with apical displacement of the septal tricuspid valve leaflet (arrow) and moderate tricuspid regurgitation (TR). [Image from Balaguru D, Rao PS. Diseases of the tricuspid valve. In: Vijayalakshmi IB, Rao PS, Chugh R (Eds). A Comprehensive Approach to Congenital Heart Disease. New Delhi, India: Jaypee Brothers Medical Publishers (P) Ltd; 2013]. (aRV: Aatrialized right ventricle; LA: Left atrium; LV: Left ventricle; RA: Right atrium; RV: Right ventricle).

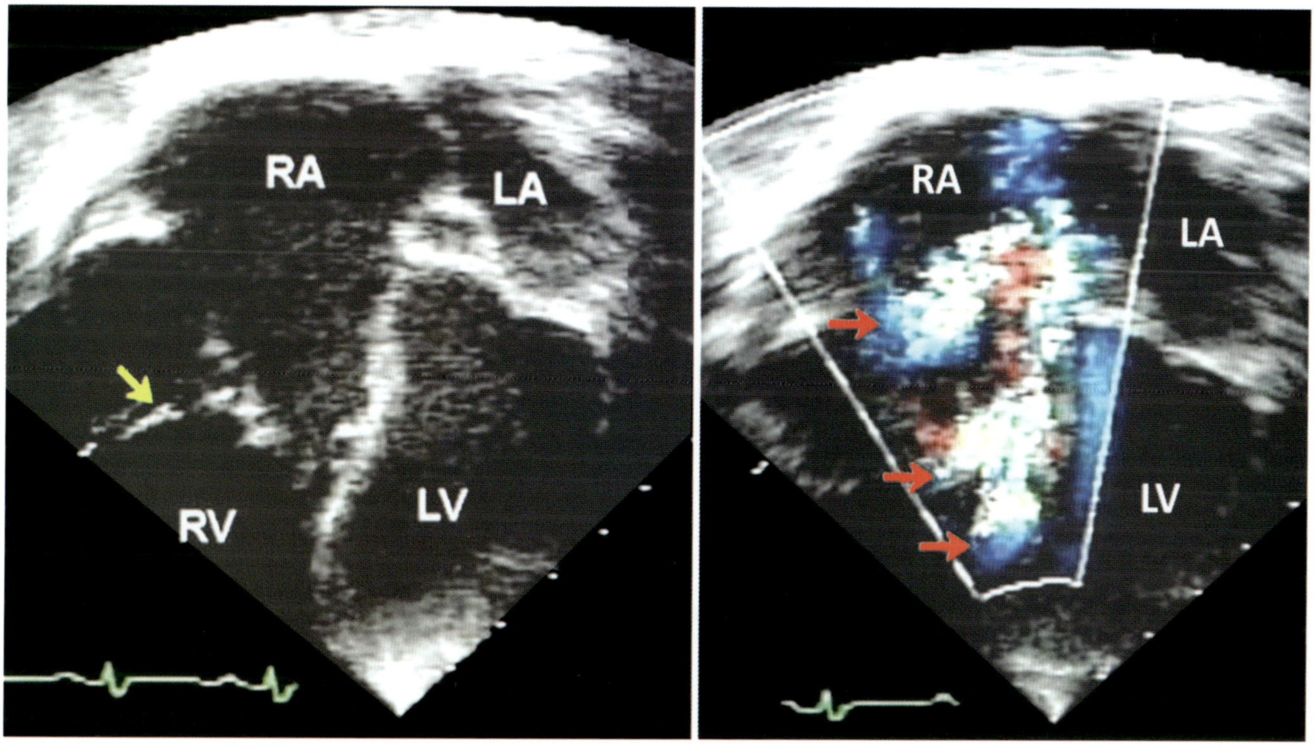

Fig. 42.12: Transthoracic echocardiogram in a patient with tricuspid valve fenestrations related to Ebstein anomaly. Left panel shows an example of moderately severe Ebstein anomaly. The yellow arrow points to a direct muscular insertion of a free wall papillary muscle into the anterior tricuspid valve leaflet. Right panel shows color Doppler examination, demonstrating multiple fenestrations in the anterior leaflet, causing at least three separate jets of tricuspid regurgitation (red arrows). The limited mobility and the multiple points of tricuspid regurgitation make this valve suboptimal for repair. (LA: Left atrium; LV: Left ventricle; RA: Right atrium; RV: Right ventricle).

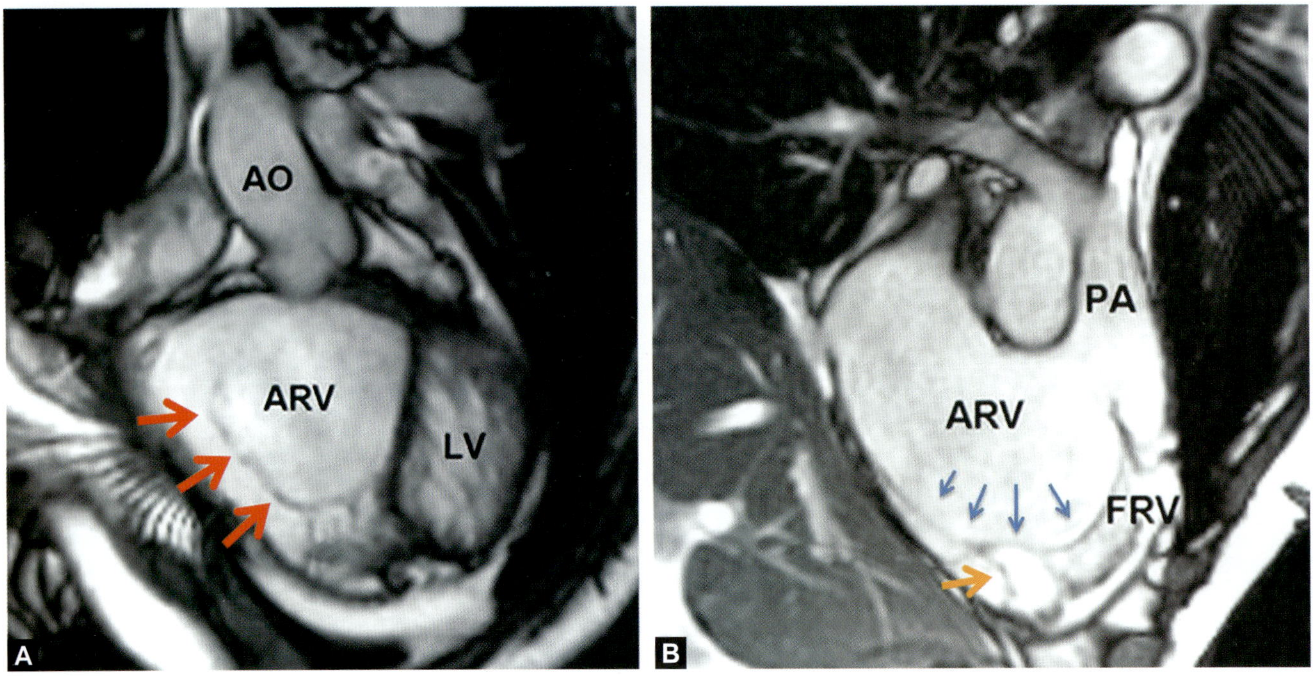

Figs. 42.13A and B: Cardiac magnetic resonance images of a patient with Ebstein anomaly. (A) Oblique transaxial image plane, which transects the ventricles (apex pointing inferiorly) and the great arteries superiorly, showing delineation of the tethered posterior and anterior leaflets (red arrows); (B) Oblique sagittal image plane image demonstrating the inflow, apex, and outflow portions of the right ventricle. Example of severe tethering (orange arrow) and adhesion of the anterior leaflet (blue arrows). [Image adapted with permission from Attenhofer Jost CH, Edmister WD, Julsrud PR, et al. Prospective comparison of echocardiography versus cardiac magnetic resonance imaging in patients with Ebstein's anomaly. Int J Cardiovasc Imaging. 2012;28(5):1147-59]. (AO: Aorta; ARV: Atrialized right ventricle; FRV: Functional right ventricle; LV: Left ventricle; PA: Pulmonary artery).

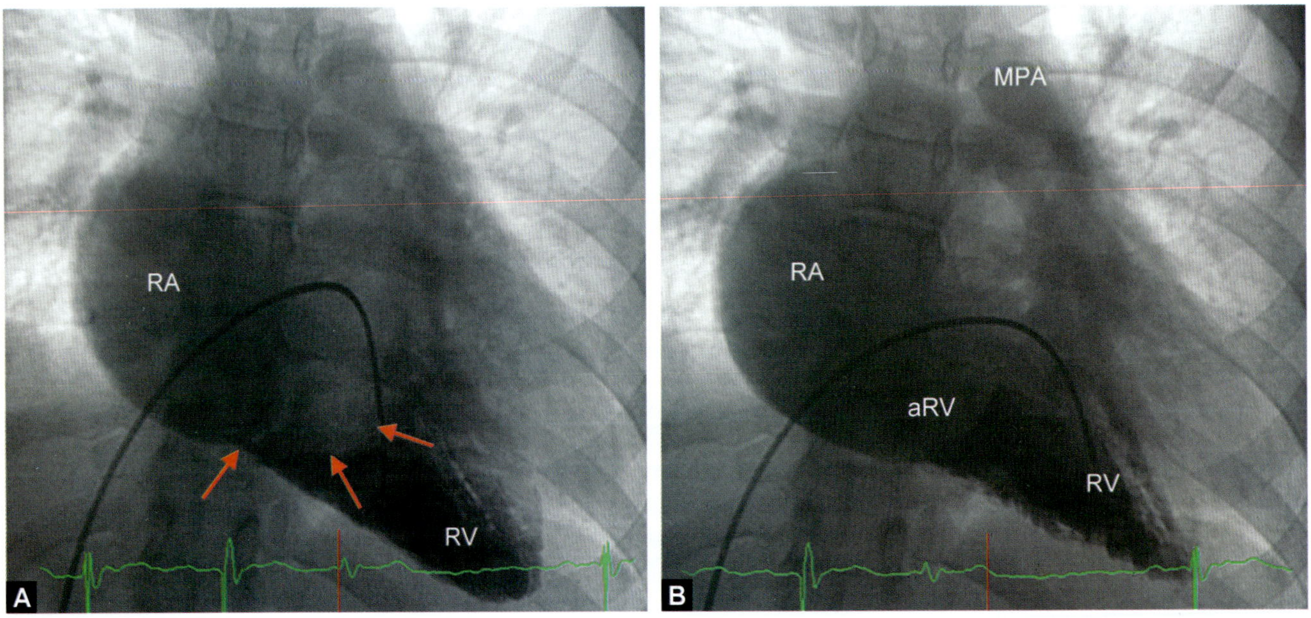

Figs. 42.14A and B: Right ventricular angiogram in posteroanterior view from an adolescent with Ebstein anomaly. (A) Tricuspid valve regurgitation leads to opacification of an enlarged right atrium (RA). The true tricuspid valve annulus and attachment of the displaced tricuspid valve leaflets (arrows) are shown; (B) In a subsequent cine frame, atrialized right ventricle (aRV) is shown. [Images and legend text from Balaguru D, Rao PS. Diseases of the tricuspid valve. In: Vijayalakshmi IB, Rao PS, Chugh R (Eds). A Comprehensive Approach to Congenital Heart Disease. New Delhi, India: Jaypee Brothers Medical Publishers (P) Ltd; 2013]. (MPA: Main pulmonary artery; RV: Right ventricle).

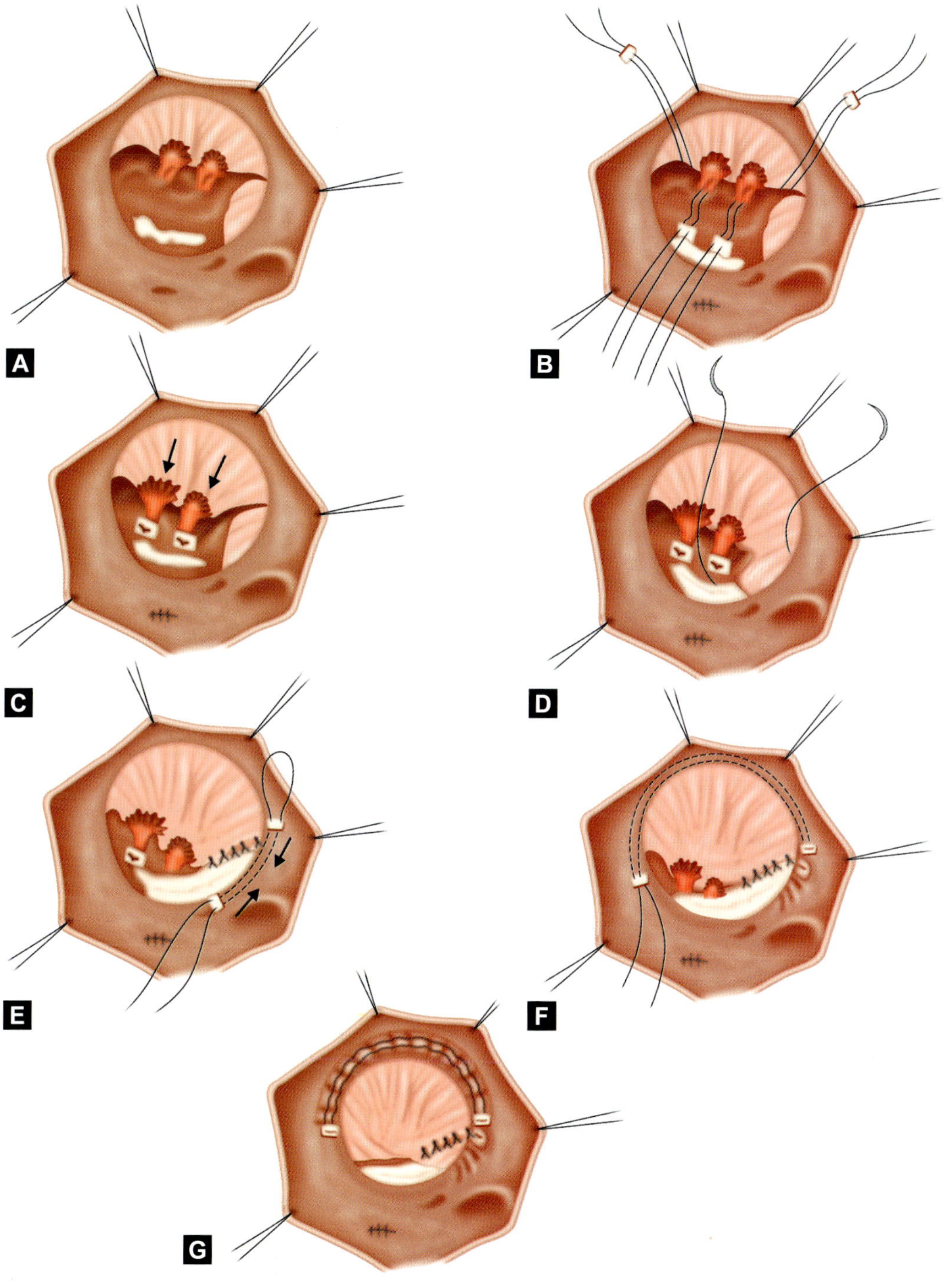

Figs. 42.15A to G: Schematic demonstrating classic monocusp repair. This repair was described by Dr GK Danielson. (A) Two papillary muscles arise from the free wall of the right ventricle, with short chordal attachments to the leading edge of the anterior leaflet. The septal leaflet is diminutive. The posterior leaflet is not well formed and is adherent to the underlying endocardium. A small patent foramen ovale is present; (B and C) The base of each papillary muscle is moved toward the ventricular septum at the appropriate level with horizontal mattress sutures backed with felt pledgets. The patent foramen ovale is closed by direct suture; (D) The posterior angle of the tricuspid orifice is closed by bringing the right side of the anterior septum down to the septum and placating the nonfunctional posterior leaflet in the process; (E) A posterior annuloplasty is performed to narrow the diameter of the tricuspid annulus; (F) An anterior purse-string annuloplasty is performed to further narrow the tricuspid annulus; (G) Completed repair that allows the anterior leaflet to function as a monocuspid valve. (Image adapted with permission from Dearani JA, Danielson GK. Tricuspid valve repair for Ebstein's anomaly. Oper Tech Thorac Cardiovasc Surg. 2003:188-92).

which the atrioventricular junction is surrounded by 360 degrees of mobilized leaflet tissue that is reanchored at the true annulus. The thorough mobilization (surgical delamination) of available leaflet tissue has greatly expanded the percentage of EA patients that can have successful TV repair (Figs. 42.16 to 42.18).

Long-term clinical and echocardiographic follow-up is recommended for all patients with EA.

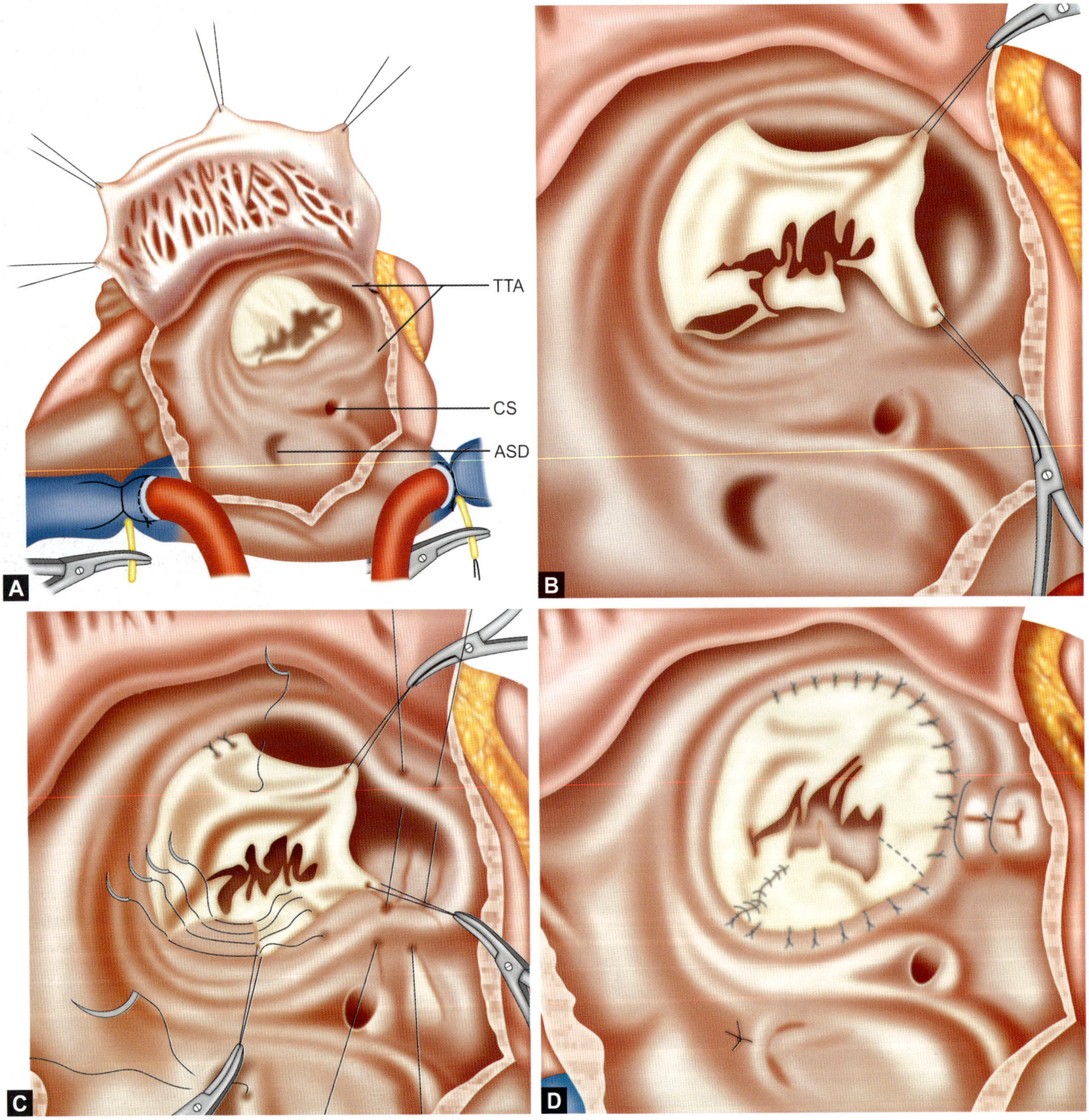

Figs. 42.16A to D: Schematic demonstrating operative steps of the cone procedure for Ebstein anomaly repair. (A) Opened right atrium showing displacement of the tricuspid valve; (B) Detached part of the anterior and posterior tricuspid valve leaflet forming a single piece; (C) Clockwise rotation of the posterior leaflet edge to be sutured to the anterior leaflet septal edge and plication of the true tricuspid annulus; (D) Complete valve attachment to the true tricuspid annulus and closure of the atrial septal defect. [Image adapted with permission from da Silva JP, Baumgratz JF, da Fonseca L, et al. The cone reconstruction of the tricuspid valve in Ebstein's anomaly. The operation: early and midterm results. J Thorac Cardiovasc Surg. 2007;133(1):215-23]. (ASD: Atrial septal defect; CS: Coronary sinus; TTA: True tricuspid annulus)

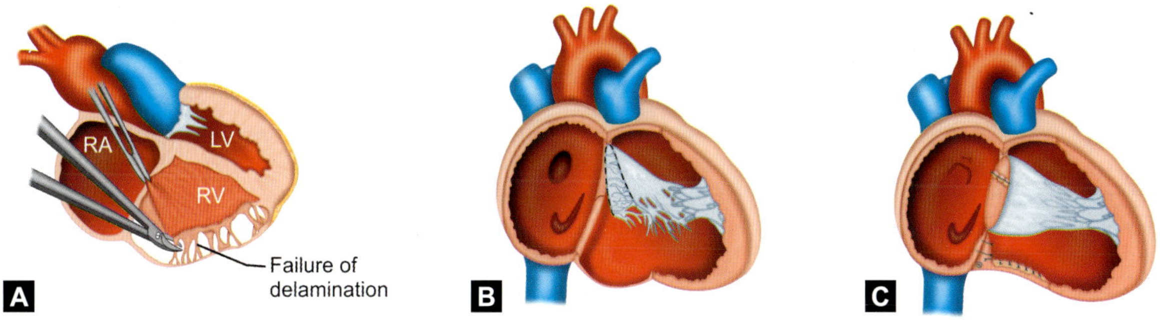

Figs. 42.17A to C: Schematic of Ebstein pathology and subsequent cone type repair. The three panels illustrate cone reconstruction in Ebstein anomaly (EA) from a different point of view. (A) The adherent segments of the tricuspid valve tissue being separated from the anatomic annulus and the underlying right ventricular (RV) myocardium; (B) The sheet of tricuspid tissue after it has been released. This tissue is used to create a cone, often attaching the anterior leaflet to the remnants of the septal leaflet (see suture line in the right panel); (C) Once the cone is created, the base is attached to the atrioventricular junction, restoring the hinge points to a nondisplaced position. When dilated, thin or dyskinetic, the atrialized RV is reduced in size by internal plication from the "apex-to-base". The annuloplasty reduces the size of the true tricuspid annulus to the appropriate size of the reconstructed cone. Placement of a flexible annuloplasty ring is performed routinely when somatic growth is complete or when there is no concern about tricuspid stenosis. [Image reproduced with permission from Dearani JA, Danielson GK. Tricuspid valve repair for Ebstein's anomaly. Oper Tech Thorac Cardiovasc Surg. 2003:188-92]. (LV: Left ventricle; RA: Right atrium).

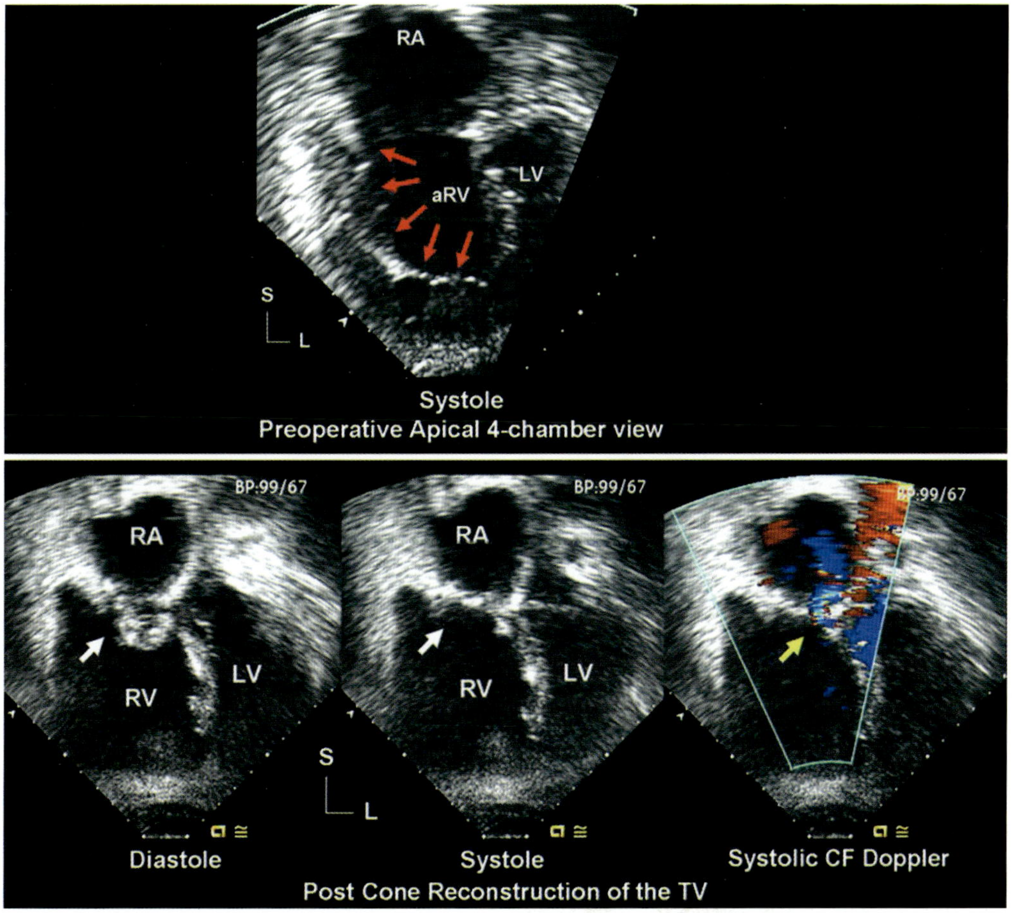

Fig. 42.18: Preoperative and postoperative transthoracic echocardiographic images of a patient with Ebstein anomaly, before and after cone repair. This apex down transthoracic echocardiogram demonstrates features of Ebstein anomaly with pronounced tethering of the anterior tricuspid valve leaflet preoperatively (red arrows, top panel). Following successful cone type of repair (bottom panel), the echocardiographic images demonstrate improved anterior tricuspid valve leaflet mobility (white arrows, lower left and middle panels) and minimal tricuspid valve regurgitation by color Doppler (yellow arrow; lower right panel). (ARV: Atrialized right ventricle; LV: Left ventricle; RA: Right atrium; RV: Right ventricle).

VIDEO LEGEND

Video 42.1: MRI in the 4-chamber projection demonstrating Ebstein anomoly.

REFERENCES

Attenhofer Jost CH, Connolly HM, Dearani JA, et al. Ebstein's anomaly. Circulation. 2007;115(2):277-85.

Attenhofer Jost CH, Connolly HM, Warnes CA, et al. Noncompacted myocardium in Ebstein's anomaly: initial description in three patients. J Am Soc Echocardiogr. 2004;17(6):677-80.

Attenhofer Jost CH, Edmister WD, Julsrud PR, et al. Prospective comparison of echocardiography versus cardiac magnetic resonance imaging in patients with Ebstein's anomaly. Int J Cardiovasc Imaging. 2012;28(5):1147-59.

Barbara DW, Edwards WD, Connolly HM, et al. Surgical pathology of 104 tricuspid valves (2000-2005) with classic right-sided Ebstein's malformation. Cardiovasc Pathol. 2008;17(3):166-71.

Brown ML, Dearani JA, Danielson GK, et al. The outcomes of operations for 539 patients with Ebstein anomaly. J Thorac Cardiovasc Surg. 2008;135(5):1120-36.

da Silva JP, Baumgratz JF, da Fonseca L, et al. The cone reconstruction of the tricuspid valve in Ebstein's anomaly. The operation: early and midterm results. J Thorac Cardiovasc Surg. 2007;133(1):215-23.

Dearani JA, Danielson GK. Tricuspid valve repair for Ebstein's anomaly. Oper Tech Thorac Cardiovasc Surg. 2003:188-92.

Mann RJ, Lie JT. The life story of Wilhelm Ebstein (1836-1912) and his almost overlooked description of a congenital heart disease. Mayo Clin Proc. 1979;54(3):197-204.

Martinez RM, O'Leary PW, Anderson RH. Anatomy and echocardiography of the normal and abnormal tricuspid valve. Cardiol Young. 2006;16:4-11.

Warnes CA, Williams RG, Bashore TM, et al. ACC/AHA 2008 guidelines for the management of adults with congenital heart disease: a report of the American College of Cardiology/American Heart Association Task Force on Practice Guidelines (Writing Committee to Develop Guidelines on the Management of Adults With Congenital Heart Disease). Developed in Collaboration With the American Society of Echocardiography, Heart Rhythm Society, International Society for Adult Congenital Heart Disease, Society for Cardiovascular Angiography and Interventions, and Society of Thoracic Surgeons. J Am Coll Cardiol. 2008;52(23):e143-263.

CHAPTER 43

Tetralogy of Fallot

Gruschen R Veldtman, Ryan Allen Moore, Peace C Madueme, Gary D Webb

EPIDEMIOLOGY AND GENETICS OF TETRALOGY OF FALLOT

Tetralogy of Fallot (TOF) has an incidence of 0.5 per 1,000 live births. It is the most common complex congenital cardiac malformation, accounting for between 5% and 7% of congenital heart defects. During adult life, it compromises approximately 2.9% of all congenital heart disease.

Fifty to sixty percent of cases of TOF have no known genetic cause or association. 20% have a chromosomal abnormality. In 10–20% of cases, there is a single gene mutation and in 10% of cases, a de novo copy number variant.

Genetic syndromes associated with TOF include CHARGE syndrome (coloboma, heart defect, atresia of the choanae, retarded growth and development, genital hypoplasia, ear anomalies/deafness), 22q11 deletion syndrome, Alagille syndrome, and trisomy 21, 18, and 13.

The primary and secondary heart fields (Fig. 43.1), developing at approximately 3 weeks of gestation in humans, are the precursors to the developing heart tube. Disruption of the right side of the secondary heart field, or interference with signaling at this stage leads to development of TOF in experimental mouse models. Blunting of fibroblast growth factor 8 or neurotrophin 3 signaling, for example, or mutation or microdeletion of JAGGED1 (also associated with Alagille syndrome) results in pulmonary stenosis, pulmonary atresia, double outlet RV and TOF. Approximately 10–15% of Alagille syndrome patients will have TOF.

FUNCTIONAL AND SURGICAL ANATOMY OF TETRALOGY OF FALLOT

The four seminal features of TOF (Figs. 43.2 to 43.5) relate to presence of the following abnormal anatomic features which are discussed below:

Muscular Outlet Septum

The muscular OS, also known as infundibular septum, is deviated in an anterior and cephalad fashion. This displacement, together with hypertrophied muscular bands that connect the OS and the anterior limb of the septal band to the anterior wall of the subpulmonary infundibulum, and the frequent presence of a stenotic bicuspid pulmonary valve, create the composite RVOT stenosis observed in TOF (Figs. 43.6 and 43.7).

Perimembranous Outlet Ventricular Septal Defect

A perimembranous outlet ventricular septal defect (VSD) (Figs. 43.8A and B) is commonly cradled between the anterior and posterior limbs of the septal band. The muscular OS forms its superior margin. Posteriorly and inferior are the areas of fibrous continuity between the medial aspect of the anterosuperior leaflet of the tricuspid valve and the right coronary cusp of the aortic valve, as well the fibrous continuity between the mitral and aortic valve. The defect may be doubly committed, and may also be entirely muscular, located in the infundibular septum.

Overriding Aorta

The aortic valve overrides the VSD to varying degrees and, indeed, in some may have predominant origin from the RV (double outlet RV) causing associated muscular separation of the fibrous continuity between the mitral and aortic valve leaflets.

Right Ventricular Hypertrophy

There is secondary hypertrophy of the RV (Fig. 43.9), and this includes hypertrophy of the septoparietal trabeculations, which contribute to the RVOT obstruction.

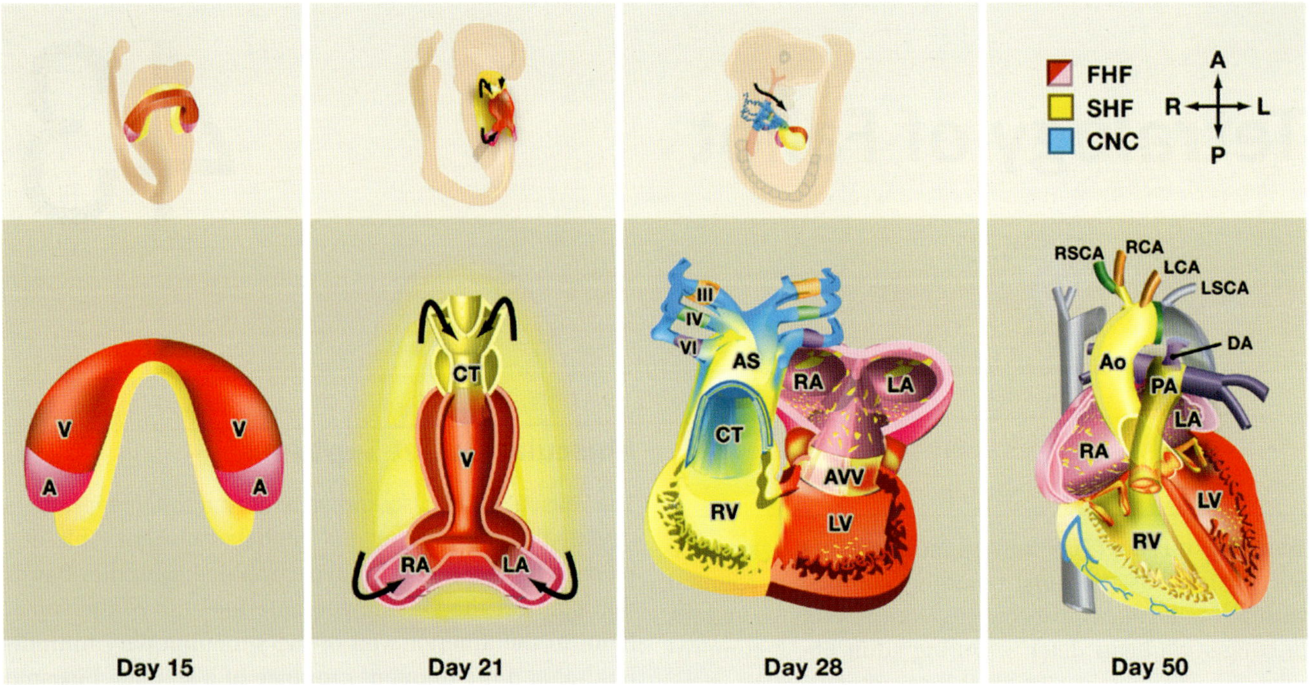

Fig. 43.1: Mammalian heart development. Oblique views of whole embryos and frontal views of cardiac precursors during human cardiac development are shown. First panel on the left shows first heart field (FHF) cells form a crescent shape in the anterior embryo with second heart field (SHF) cells medial and anterior to the FHF. Second panel shows SHF cells lie dorsal to the straight heart tube and begin to migrate (arrows) into the anterior and posterior ends of the tube to form the right ventricle (RV), conotruncus (CT), and part of the atria (A). Third panel shows following rightward looping of the heart tube, cardiac neural crest (CNC) cells also migrate (arrow) into the outflow tract from the neural folds to septate the outflow tract and pattern the bilaterally symmetric aortic arch arteries (III, IV, and VI). Fourth (far right) panel shows eptation of the ventricles, atria, and atrioventricular valves (AVV) results in the four-chambered heart. [Image courtesy of Dr Deepak Srivastava. Image from Srivastava D. Making or breaking the heart: from lineage determination to morphogenesis. Cell. 2006;126(6):1037-48]. (V: Ventricle; LV: Left ventricle; LA: Left atrium; RA: Right atrium; AS: Aortic sac; Ao: Aorta; PA: Pulmonary artery; RSCA: Right subclavian artery; LSCA: Left subclavian artery; RCA: Right carotid artery; LCA: Left carotid artery; DA: Ductus arteriosus).

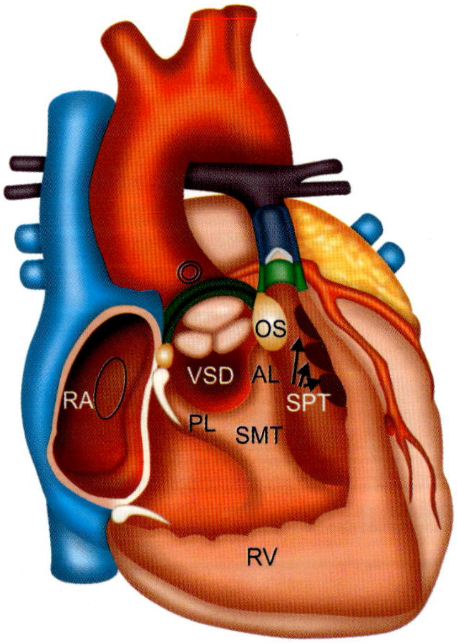

Fig. 43.2: Functional and surgical anatomy of Tetralogy of Fallot (TOF). The right atrium (RA) and right ventricle (RV) have been exposed to demonstrate the relevant anatomy. The ventricular septal defect (VSD) is cradled between the anterior limb (AL) and posterior limb (PL) of the septomarginal trabeculum (SMT). There is anterocephalad deviation of the outlet septum (OS), and hypertrophy of the septoparietal bands (SPT) contributing to the characteristic outflow tract obstruction. The pulmonary valve is commonly bicuspid and there may be varying degrees of underdevelopment of the pulmonary arteries and pulmonary vascular bed.

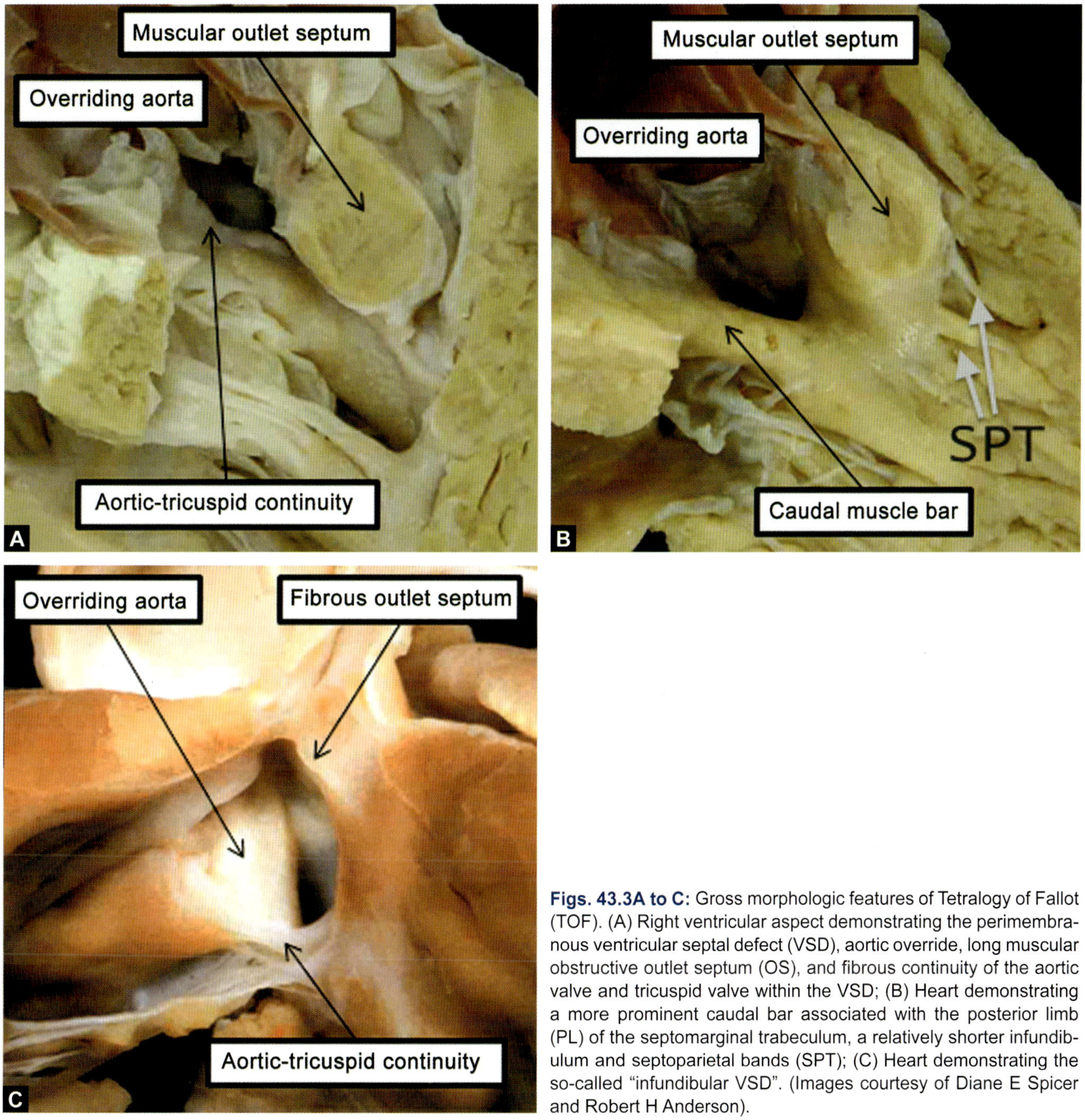

Figs. 43.3A to C: Gross morphologic features of Tetralogy of Fallot (TOF). (A) Right ventricular aspect demonstrating the perimembranous ventricular septal defect (VSD), aortic override, long muscular obstructive outlet septum (OS), and fibrous continuity of the aortic valve and tricuspid valve within the VSD; (B) Heart demonstrating a more prominent caudal bar associated with the posterior limb (PL) of the septomarginal trabeculum, a relatively shorter infundibulum and septoparietal bands (SPT); (C) Heart demonstrating the so-called "infundibular VSD". (Images courtesy of Diane E Spicer and Robert H Anderson).

ASSOCIATED LESIONS WITH TETRALOGY OF FALLOT

Several important lesions and findings are associated with TOF. Atrioventricular septal defect occurs in approximately 1.7% of cases of TOF. Aortopulmonary collateral arteries (Fig. 43.10) may coexist with TOF, even in the absence of complete atresia of the pulmonary valve. The collaterals rarely develop on the side of a patent ductus arteriosus (DA). Anomalous coronary arteries are seen in 5–12% of cases of TOF. Most commonly, the left anterior descending (LAD) originates from the right coronary artery; left main coronary artery arising from the right carotid artery (RCA), and the RCA originating from the left main coronary artery or from the LAD, are also seen (Figs. 43.11A and B). Right aortic arch occurs in approximately 25% of cases of TOF (Fig. 43.12).

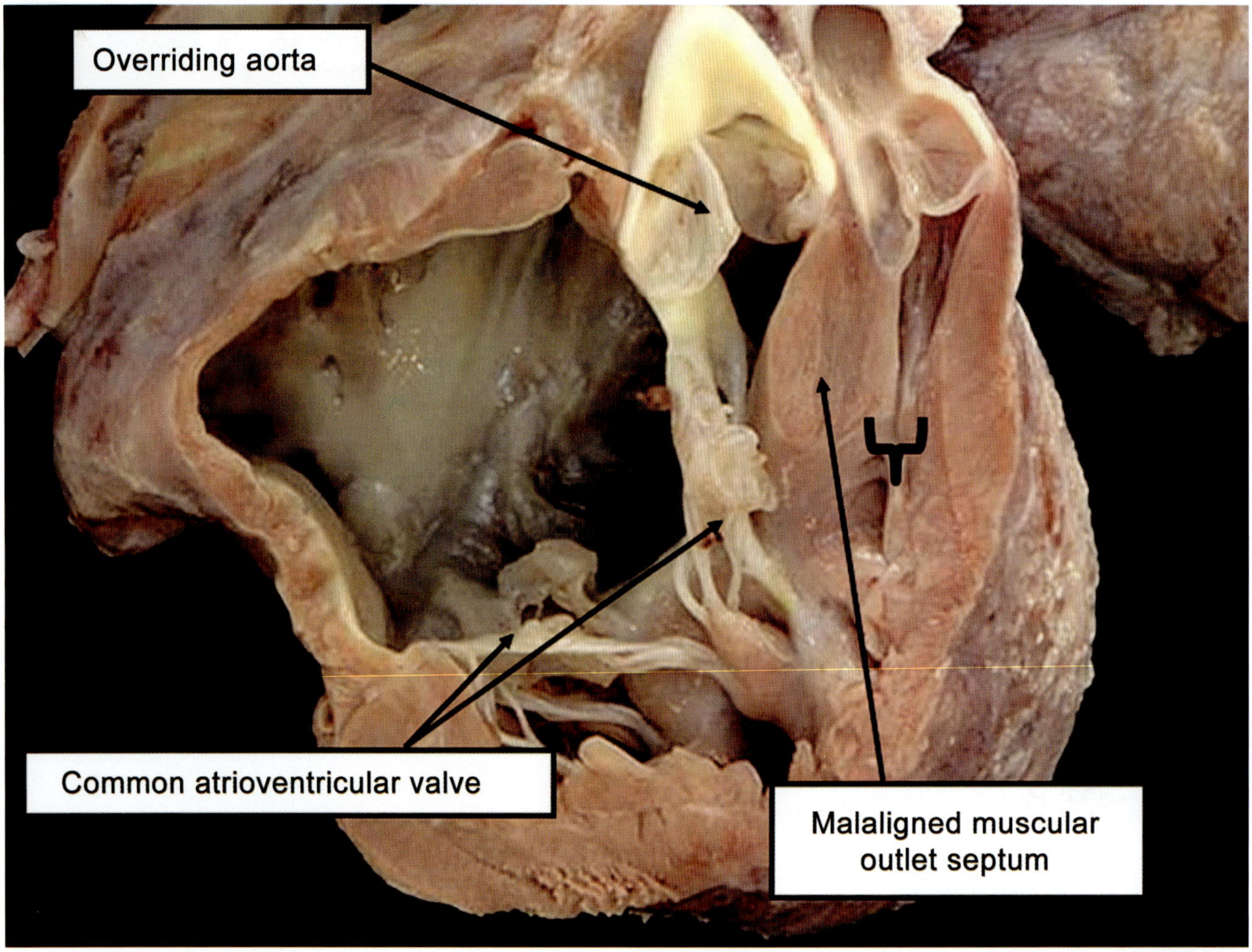

Fig. 43.4: Morphologic features of common atrioventricular valve (AVV) associated with Tetralogy of Fallot (TOF). The malaligned outlet septum (OS) remains a constant feature. The common AVV demonstrates fibrous continuity with the aortic valve. (Image courtesy of Diane E Spicer and Robert H Anderson).

Developmental abnormalities of the pulmonary vascular bed in patients with TOF including focal pulmonary artery (PA) stenosis (Figs. 43.13 and 43.14), generalized PA hypoplasia, discontinuous pulmonary arteries, or a generally decreased pulmonary vascular bed, are well described in TOF. The intracinar pulmonary arteries may also be smaller and reduced in number. In patients with longer standing arterial shunts, the pulmonary vascular bed may be further reduced due to medial and intimal overgrowth and obliteration of the vessel lumen. When hypoplastic pulmonary arteries are present (Fig. 43.15), aortopulmonary arteries may be present. The proximal pulmonary arteries in a minority of patients require a combination of surgical and percutaneous intervention in an attempt to rehabilitate the pulmonary arteries (Fig. 43.16).

The pulmonary arterial wall is markedly abnormal in many patients with TOF. These findings include elastic tissue fragmentation, medionecrosis, fibrosis, and cyst-like formation (Figs. 43.17A to F). Such changes are associated with high characteristic impedance and abnormally low compliance. This contributes to right ventricular dilation and dysfunction through adverse ventriculo-arterial coupling.

SURGICAL INTERVENTION FOR TETRALOGY OF FALLOT

Surgical interventions for TOF have evolved over the past eight decades. The first palliative surgery was the creation of a Blalock-Taussig-Thomas shunt (BTTS) (Fig. 43.18), in 1945, in which a subclavian to PA connection was created. This was followed by Lord Brock's closed technique of right

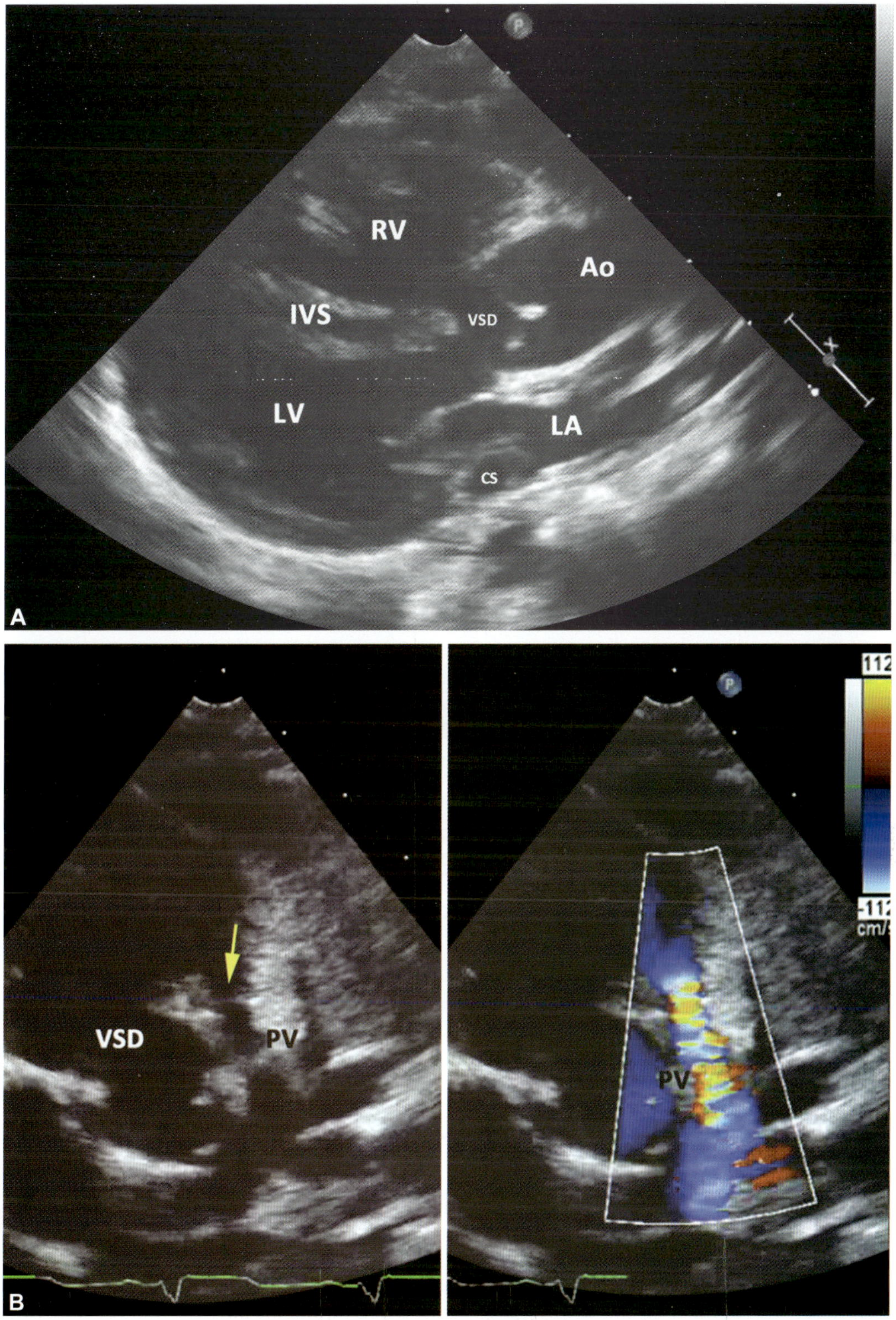

Figs. 43.5A and B: Echocardiographic features of unrepaired Tetralogy of Fallot (TOF). (A) Parasternal long-axis view demonstrating left ventricle (LV), interventricular septum (IVS), left atrium (LA) overriding aorta (Ao), right ventricle (RV) and enlarged coronary sinus (CS) due to an associated left superior caval vein, ventricular septal defect (VSD); (B) Short-axis view demonstrating the VSD, infundibular stenosis (yellow arrow) due to a combination of anterior deviation of the outlet septum (OS), the presence of septoparietal bands and a stenotic pulmonary valve (PV). The right panel demonstrates color flow Doppler indicating obstruction starting well below the level of the pulmonary valve.

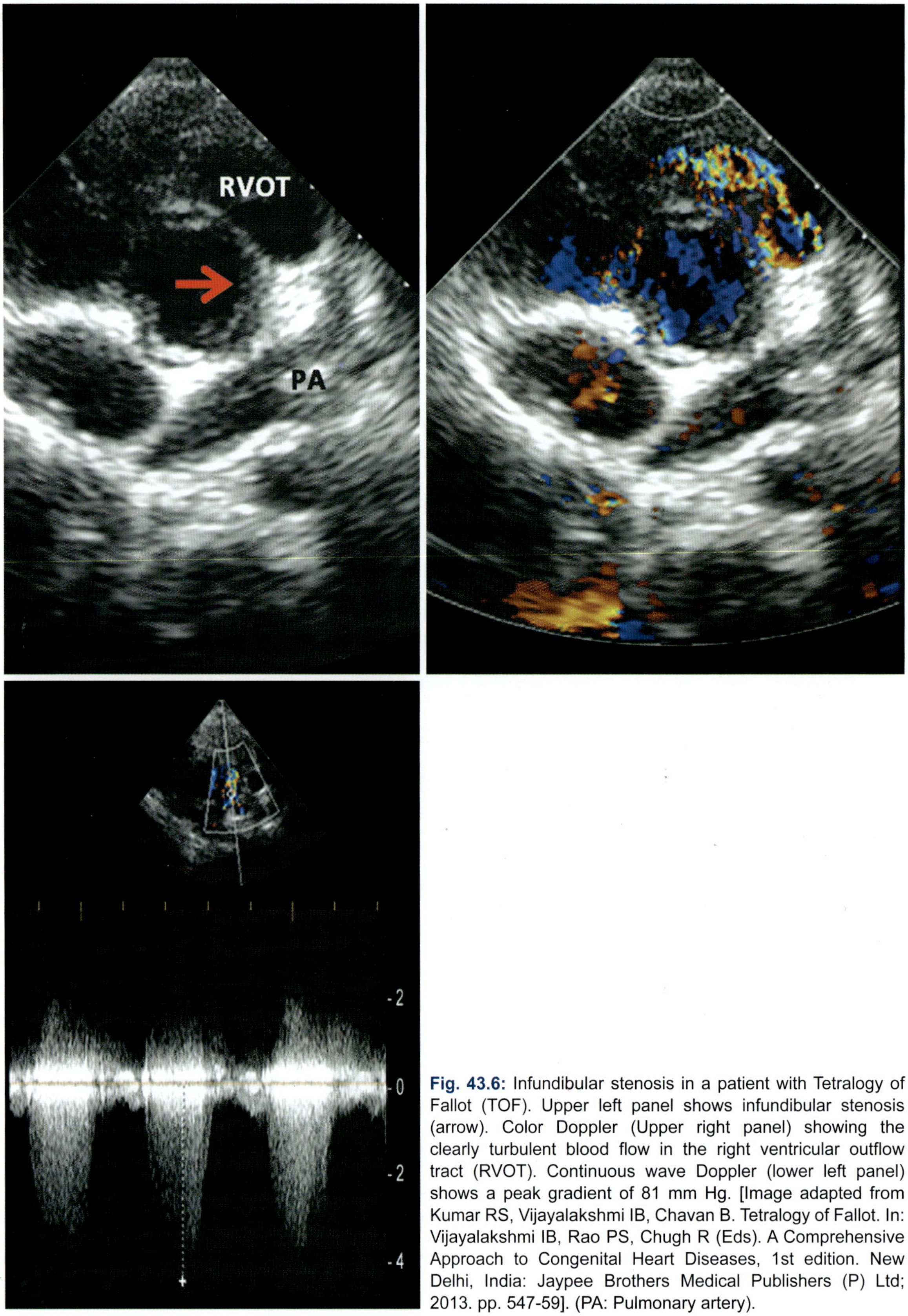

Fig. 43.6: Infundibular stenosis in a patient with Tetralogy of Fallot (TOF). Upper left panel shows infundibular stenosis (arrow). Color Doppler (Upper right panel) showing the clearly turbulent blood flow in the right ventricular outflow tract (RVOT). Continuous wave Doppler (lower left panel) shows a peak gradient of 81 mm Hg. [Image adapted from Kumar RS, Vijayalakshmi IB, Chavan B. Tetralogy of Fallot. In: Vijayalakshmi IB, Rao PS, Chugh R (Eds). A Comprehensive Approach to Congenital Heart Diseases, 1st edition. New Delhi, India: Jaypee Brothers Medical Publishers (P) Ltd; 2013. pp. 547-59]. (PA: Pulmonary artery).

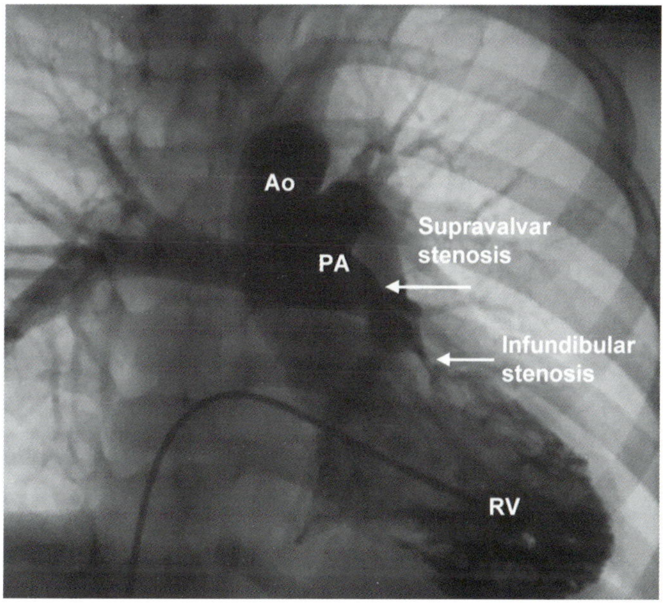

Fig. 43.7: Right ventricular angiogram in frontal view shows trabeculated right ventricle (RV) with simultaneous opacification of aorta (Ao) and pulmonary artery (PA) with severe infundibular stenosis and pulmonary valvar and supravalvar stenosis. [Image and legend text from Kumar RS, Vijayalakshmi IB, Chavan B. Tetralogy of Fallot. In: Vijayalakshmi IB, Rao PS, Chugh R (Eds). A Comprehensive Approach to Congenital Heart Diseases, 1st edition. New Delhi, India: Jaypee Brothers Medical Publishers (P) Ltd; 2013. pp. 547-59].

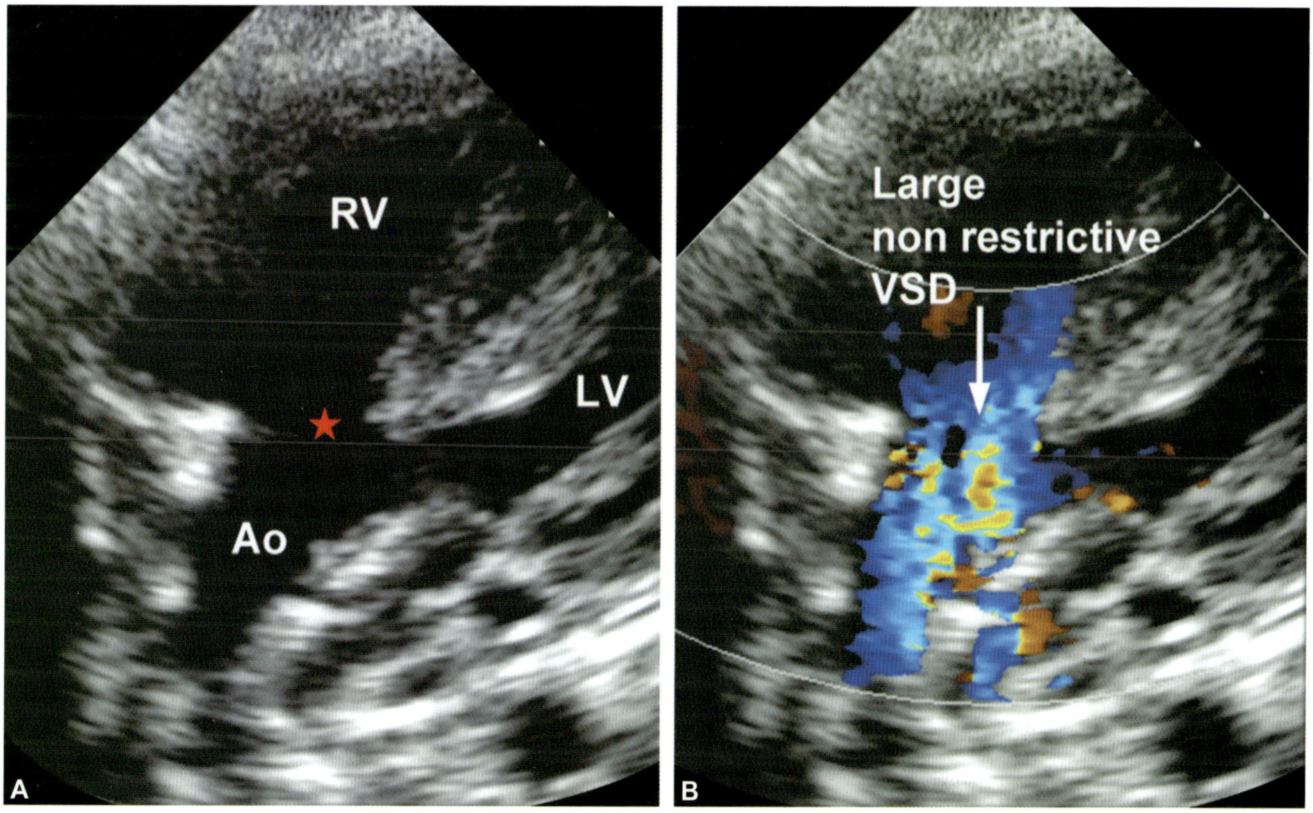

Figs. 43.8A and B: Echocardiography in Tetralogy of Fallot (TOF). (A) Five-chamber view shows large ventricular septal defect (VSD) (red star) between the right ventricle (RV) and left ventricle (LV), and overriding aorta (Ao). (B) Color Doppler echocardiography of same image shows bidirectional shunt across the VSD. [Image and legend text from Kumar RS, Vijayalakshmi IB, Chavan B. Tetralogy of Fallot. In Vijayalakshmi IB, Rao PS, Chugh R (Eds). A Comprehensive Approach to Congenital Heart Diseases, 1st edition. New Delhi, India: Jaypee Brothers Medical Publishers (P) Ltd; 2013. pp. 547-59].

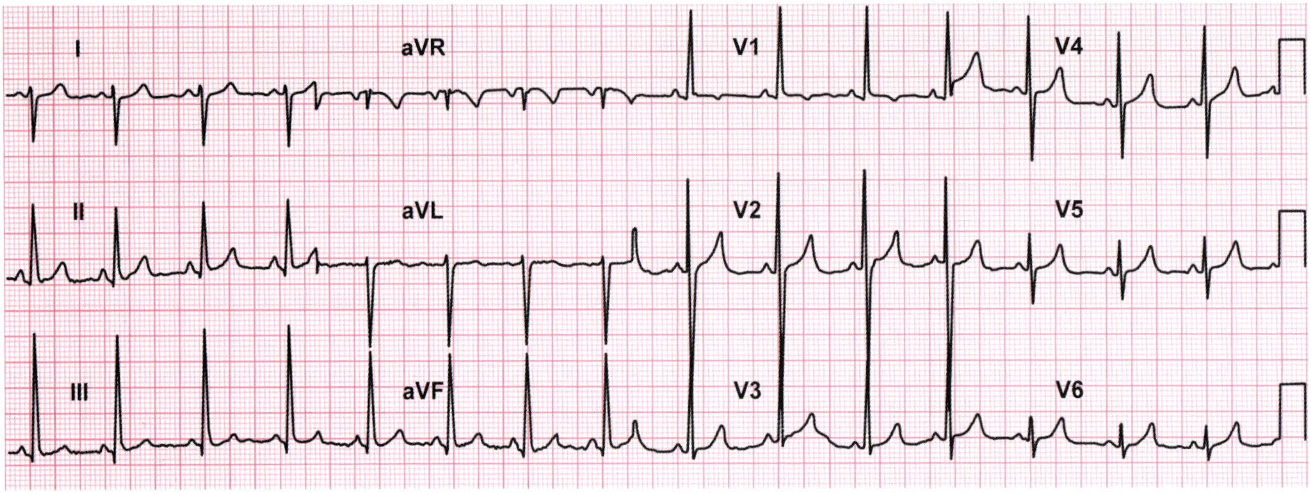

Fig. 43.9: Electrocardiography in Tetralogy of Fallot (TOF) shows right-axis deviation and a tall R wave in V1, indicative of right ventricular hypertrophy (RVH). There is also a typical sudden transition in V2 with deep S wave. [Image and legend text from Kumar RS, Vijayalakshmi IB, Chavan B. Tetralogy of Fallot. In: Vijayalakshmi IB, Rao PS, Chugh R (Eds). A Comprehensive Approach to Congenital Heart Disease, 1st edition. New Delhi, India: Jaypee Brothers Medical Publishers (P) Ltd; 2013. pp. 547-59].

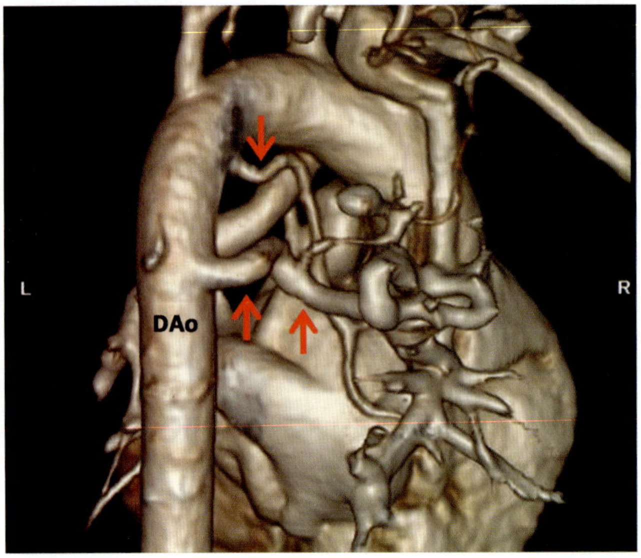

Fig. 43.10: Tetralogy of Fallot (TOF) with major aortopulmonary collaterals (arrows). Three-dimensional (3-D) rendered magnetic resonance imaging (MRI) depicts major aortopulmonary collateral arteries (red arrows) from the descending aorta (DAo), communicating with the native pulmonary arteries.

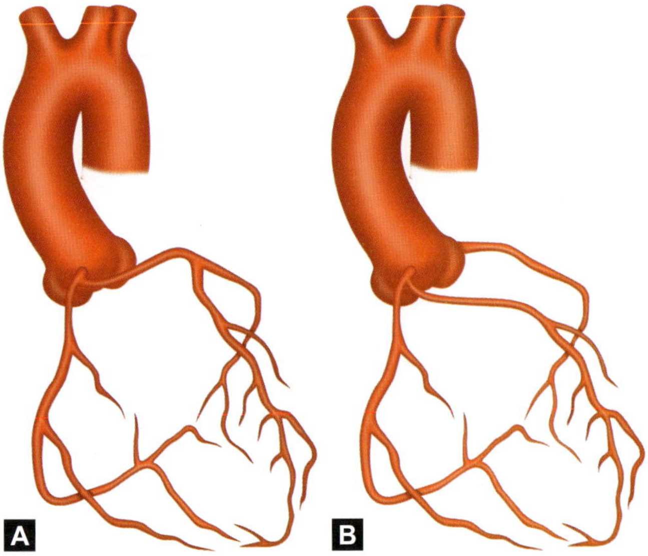

Figs. 43.11A and B: Several of the most common and surgically important coronary arterial anomalies seen in Tetralogy of Fallot (TOF). (A) Single common coronary artery arising from the right sinus, with the left coronary system crossing the right ventricular outflow tract (RVOT); (B) Left anterior descending (LAD) artery arising from the right coronary artery and crossing the right ventricular outflow tract.

ventricular infundibular resection, with use of Brock's valvulotome that either "punched" or created bioptome-like resection of the obstructing muscle. The first open heart repair by Lillehei and Varco was achieved in 1954 and established the technique of VSD closure and relief of RVOT obstruction (Figs. 43.19 and 43.20).

Further important milestones in the evolution of surgical repair include transatrial repair, first reported by Allen Hudspeth in 1963, where the VSD was closed through the right atrial incision, although did not become standard practice until much later. The first reports on repairs in infants were in the 1970s. Changing

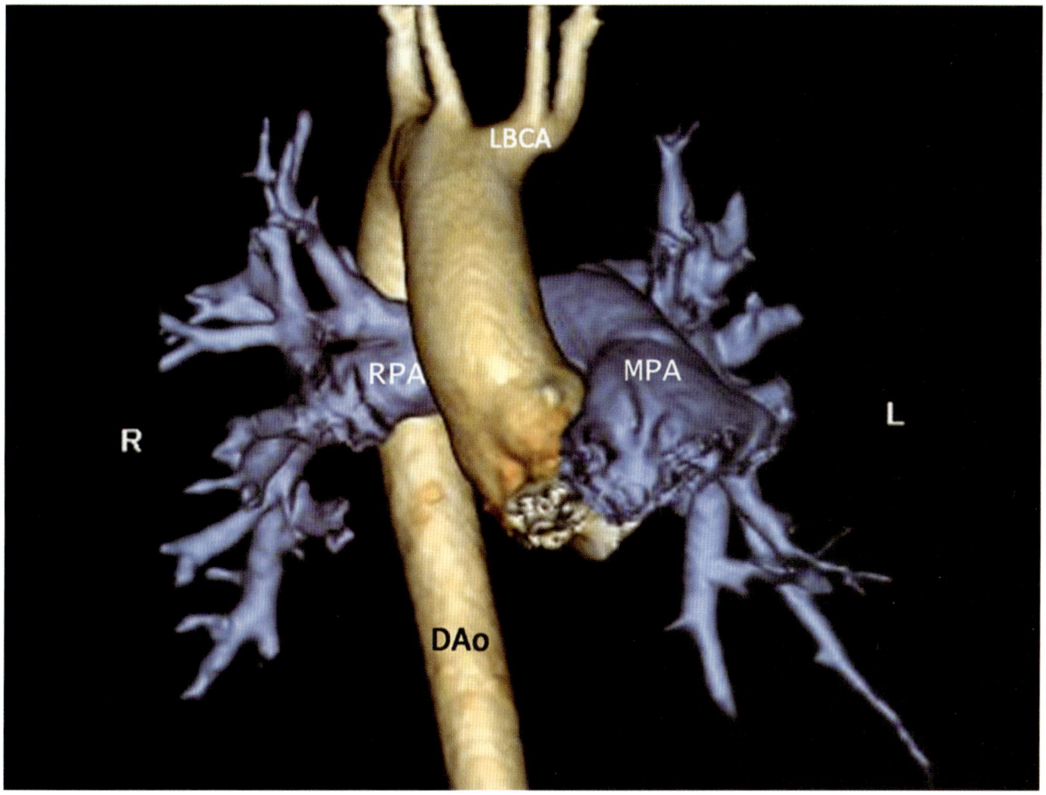

Fig. 43.12: Right aortic arch. The aorta arches over the right main bronchus and right pulmonary artery (RPA). Characteristically, the first branch that arises from the aorta is the left brachiocephalic artery (LBCA). (PMA: Main pulmonary artery; DAo: Descending aorta; S: Subclavian artery).

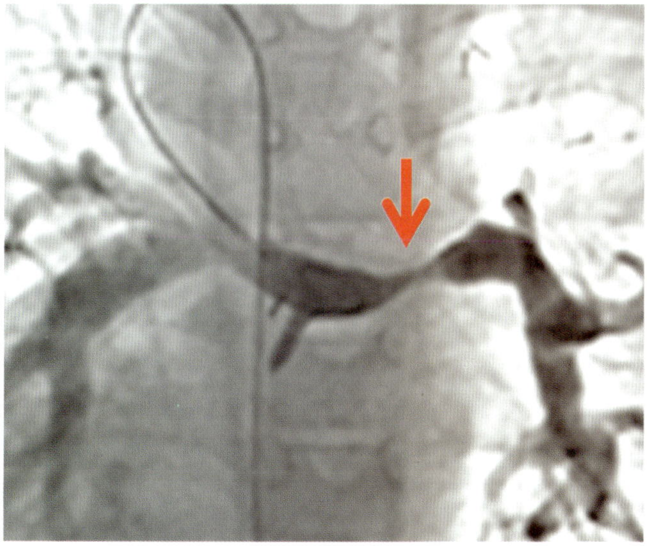

Fig. 43.13: Pulmonary angiogram demonstrating stenosis of the left pulmonary artery (LPA) (arrow). [Image from Kumar RS, Vijayalakshmi IB, Chavan B. Tetralogy of Fallot. In: Vijayalakshmi IB, Rao PS, Chugh R (Eds). A Comprehensive Approach to Congenital Heart Diseases, 1st edition. New Delhi, India: Jaypee Brothers Medical Publishers (P) Ltd; 2013. pp. 547-59].

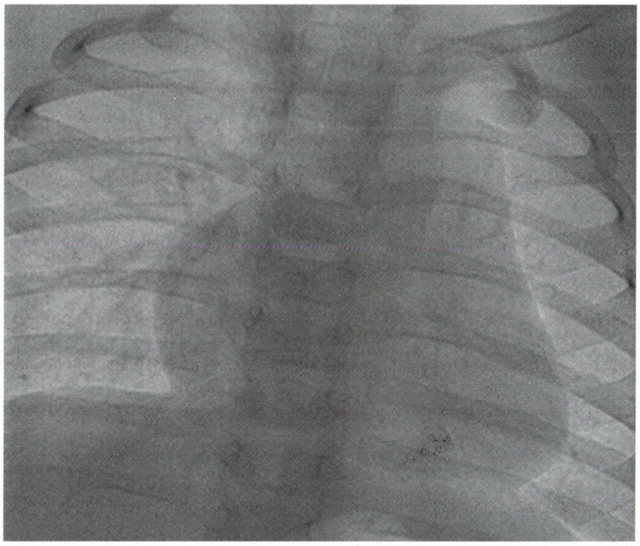

Fig. 43.14: Fluoroscopic image of 4 months infant Tetralogy of Fallot (TOF) with absent left pulmonary artery (LPA), shows oligemia in right lung and absent vascular markings in left lung. [Image and legend text from Hedge M, Vijayalakshmi IB. Role of radiography in congenital heart diseases. In: Vijayalakshmi IB, Rao PS, Chugh R (Eds). A Comprehensive Approach to Congenital Heart Diseases, 1st edition. New Delhi, India: Jaypee Brothers Medical Publishers (P) Ltd; 2013. pp. 190-202].

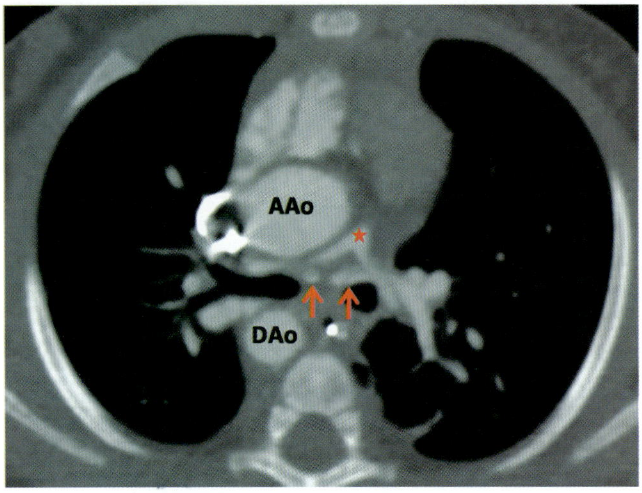

Fig. 43.15: Hypoplastic pulmonary arteries. Computerized tomography (CT) demonstrating confluent bilateral pulmonary arteries that are profoundly hypoplastic (star). There are additionally aortopulmonary collateral vessels supplying both lungs (arrows). Notice the pronounced bilateral pulmonary hypoperfusion, i.e. very little vasculature in both lung fields. In this instance, the pulmonary arterial hypoplasia was associated with Tetralogy of Fallot (TOF) with pulmonary atresia. (AAo: Ascending aorta; DAo: Descending aorta).

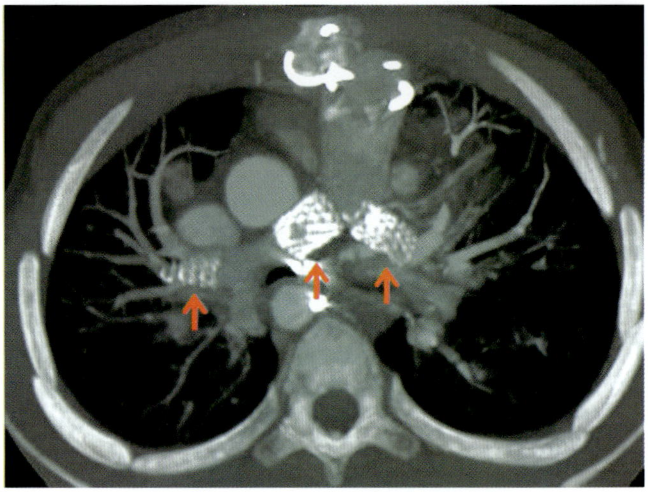

Fig. 43.16: Computerized tomography (CT) demonstrating bilateral proximal stent implantation as well distal right pulmonary stent implant (arrows). This patient has had multiple percutaneous interventions on multilevel stenosis in both pulmonary arteries. There is also evidence of extensive calcification in the right ventricular outflow tract (RVOT) which contains a homograft.

understanding of the role of residual RVOT obstruction in allowing greater preservation of RV function allowed for greater conservation of native pulmonary valve tissue, infundibular functional elements, and therefore minimized the use of transannular patching (TAP), and minimized the size of patches. The most ideal approach nowadays is, therefore, to use none or as little patch material as is possible in the outflow tract and accept a degree of residual obstruction.

LATE COMPLICATIONS IN PATIENT WITH TETRALOGY OF FALLOT

Aortic Root Dilation

Aortic root dilation (Fig. 43.21) occurs at a frequency of approximately 15% during adult life. Aortic regurgitation is frequently associated with this dilation, but is seldom more than mild to moderate. There are only a few reported cases of this aortic root dilation leading to rupture or dissection, and these cases occurred only in aortic diameters greater than 6 cm. Despite this relative scarcity of aortic wall complications, histologically these aortic walls have similar appearances to Marfan syndrome (Fig. 43.22), and tumor growth factor (TGF) beta signaling anecdotally also appears to play a role similar to fibrillin-1 mutations. Interestingly, similar changes, albeit to a lesser degree, have been demonstrated in the pulmonary arteries of unrepaired TOF and in fetuses with TOF, suggesting that there may be genetic predetermination in association with the hemodynamic perturbation. These changes include elastic tissue fragmentation, medionecrosis, fibrosis, and cyst-like formation.

Right Ventricular Outflow Tract Pathology

Right ventricular outflow tract pathology includes regurgitation, stenosis, aneurysmal transformation, and calcification. Such failure of the RVOT constitutes the most common reason for late surgical reintervention. A good understanding of the surgical technique performed at primary repair is important to appreciating the late functional anatomy and arrhythmia risk. Such factors include the size of RVOT incision, transannular extension of incision, TAP and the exact nature of material used, and the placement of the homograft, heterograft or mechanical prostheses in the pulmonary valvar position. Figure 43.23 depicts morphologic variations in the RVOT late after repair.

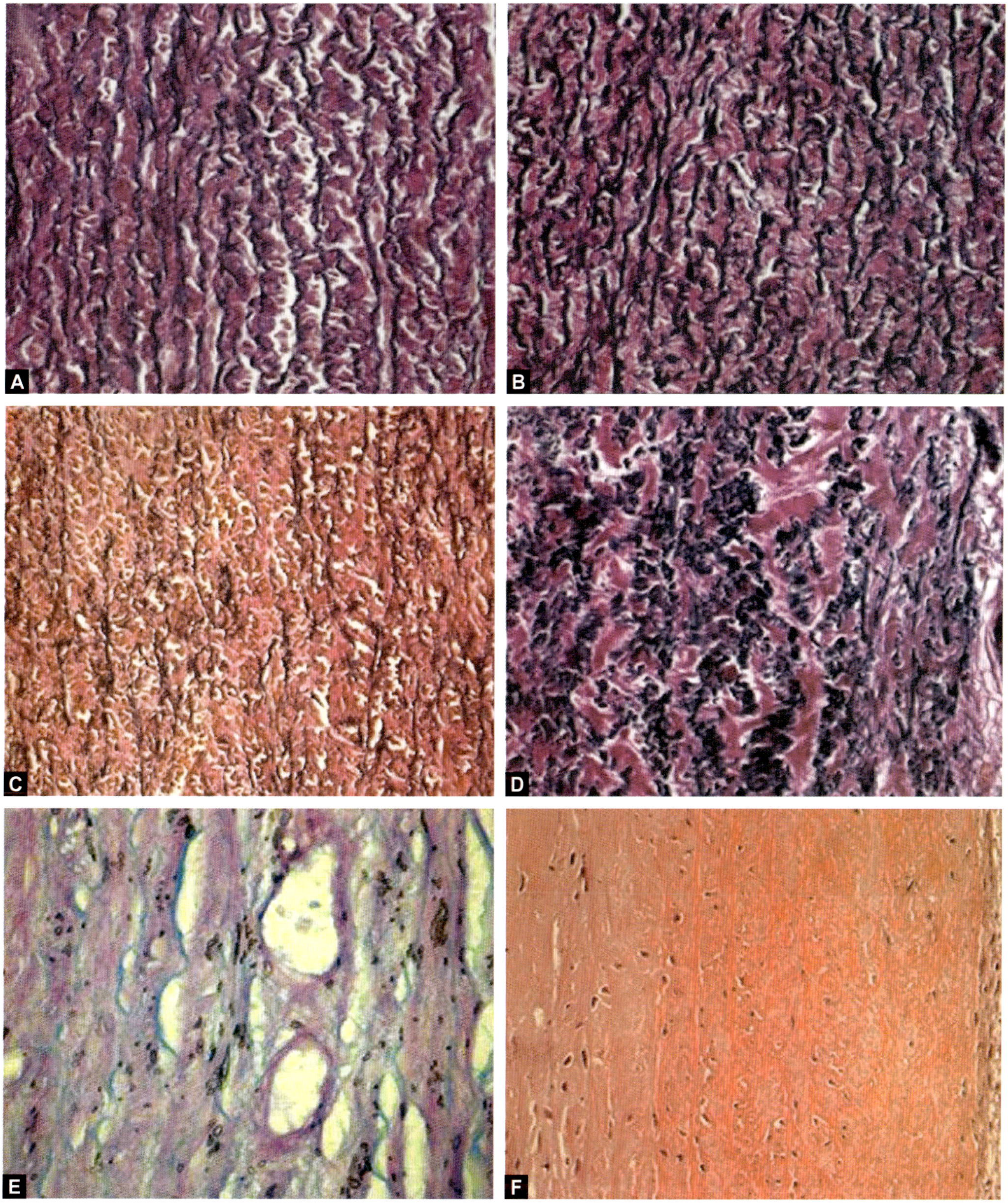

Figs. 43.17A to F: Elastic tissue configuration (ETC) and histological abnormalities from the pulmonary trunk of Tetralogy of Fallot (TOF) specimens. (A) Aorta-like ETC in an infant; (B) Transitional ETC; (C) Adult pulmonary ETC; (D) Hypotensive ETC with grade 3 fibrosis; (E) Grade 3 cyst-like formation (adult); (F) Grade 3 medionecrosis.

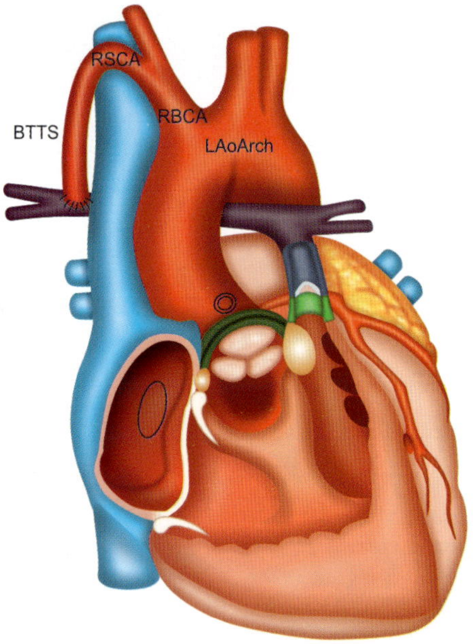

Fig. 43.18: Classical Blalock-Taussig-Thomas shunt (BTTS). The cartoon demonstrates unrepaired Tetralogy of Fallot (TOF) with a surgically down turned right subclavian artery (RSCA) to the right pulmonary artery (RPA) prior to its bifurcation to the upper lobe, the so-called classical BTTS. Right brachiocephalic artery (RBCA) with left-sided aortic arch (LAoArch).

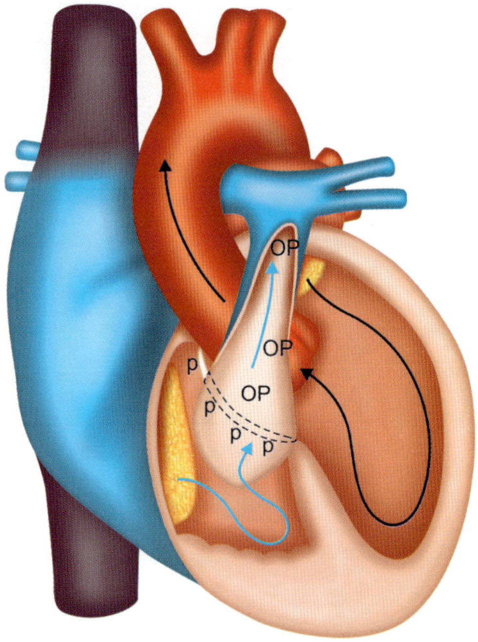

Fig. 43.19: Surgical repair of Tetralogy of Fallot (TOF). Surgical repair is achieved by patch closure of the ventricular septal defect (p), and by placement of a patch in the right ventricular outflow tract (RVOT). The outflow tract patch (OP) can be quite variable, with only a tiny patch in the area above or below the pulmonary valve, or it can extend to or beyond the bifurcation of the pulmonary arteries. The size of the patch is judged by the degree of hypoplasia/and or stenosis of the RVOT, main pulmonary artery, and or branch pulmonary arteries. The most desirable repairs have the least amount of patch material in the outflow, and have a degree of residual outflow stenosis.

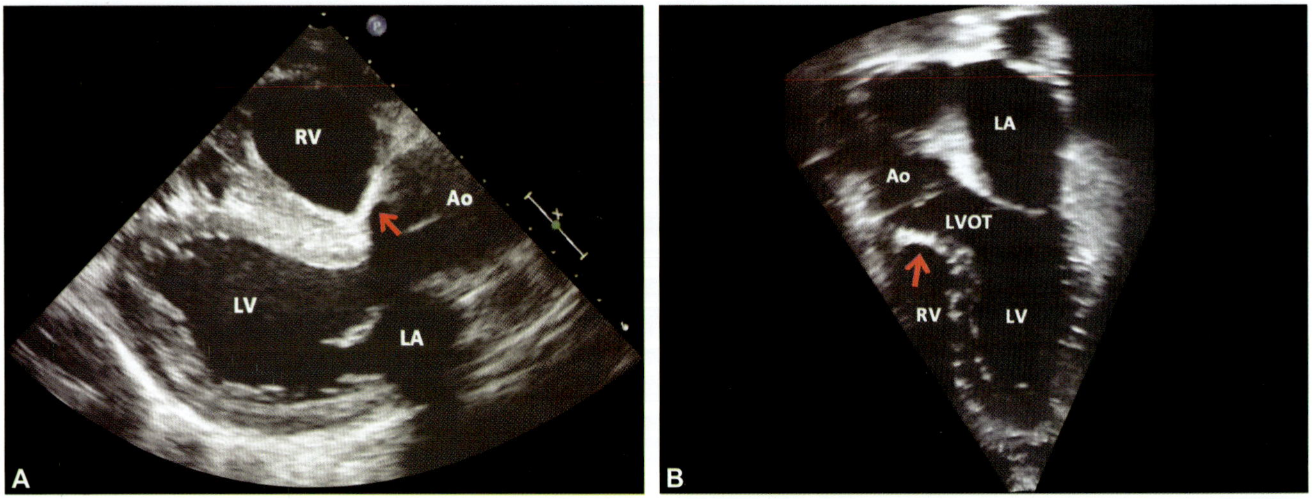

Figs. 43.20A and B: Two-dimensional echocardiography demonstrating surgically repaired Tetralogy of Fallot (TOF). Parasternal long axis (A) and apical five-chamber (B) views clearly show the ventricular septal defect (VSD) patch (arrow). Note that the aorta (Ao) still overrides the native ventricular septum. (LA: Left atrium; LV: Left ventricle; RV: Right ventricle; LVOT: Left ventricular outflow tract).

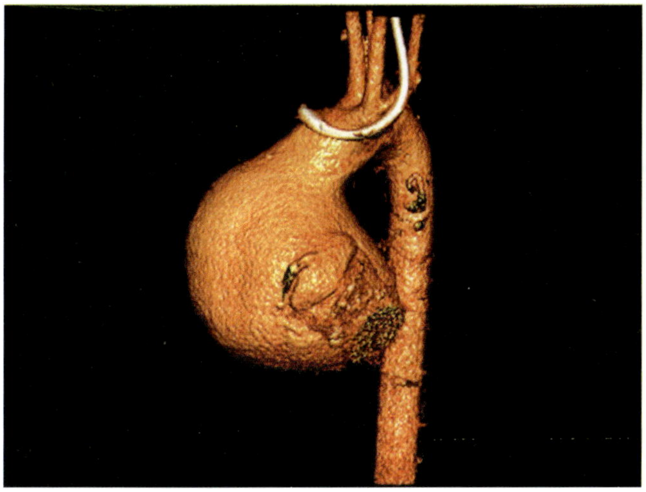

Fig. 43.21: Volume rendered three-dimensional computerized tomography (CT) image demonstrating aortic root aneurysm in Tetralogy of Fallot (TOF). This image was obtained from a 27 years male with TOF with double outlet right ventricle (RV). [Image reproduced with permission from Cleuziou J, Mayr N, Schreiber C, et al. Giant aortic aneurysm 18 years after repair of double-outlet right ventricle with pulmonary stenosis. Ann Thorac Surg. 2006;82(5):e31-2].

Pulmonary Regurgitation

The most common reason for late RVOT failure is pulmonary regurgitation (Figs. 43.24A and B, Video 43.1). Pulmonary regurgitation may be limited by the presence of outflow stenosis and/or a "restrictive" RV. Smaller restrictive RVs tolerate pulmonary regurgitation better.

Pulmonary regurgitation is often a progressive lesion. Current guidelines suggest that pulmonary valve replacement should be performed when the right ventricular end-diastolic volume index is ≥150–160 cc/m^2 and/or right ventricular end-systolic volume index is ≥ 70–80 cc/m^2 in order to prevent irreversible right ventricular dysfunction. These recommendations are based on the ability of the RV to remodel following the insertion of a competent pulmonary valve.

LATE INTERVENTION ON THE RIGHT VENTRICULAR OUTFLOW TRACT

A number of surgical options are currently available for regurgitant and/or stenotic lesions of the RVOT. These include replacement of the incompetent pulmonary valve with a homograft, or a large range of xenografts (Fig. 43.25). It is especially in the case of percutaneous interventions for the operator to be aware of the type of bioprosthesis already in place in the RVOT, as this informs the approach to the intervention. Careful preprocedural evaluation for possible arrhythmias should be included in the assessment.

For suitable outflow tracts, percutaneous or perventricular implants have now become the treatment of choice for suitable anatomic substrates, based on size, shape, and distensibility of the outflow tract, and the nature and topography of the epicardial coronary arteries relative to the stenotic RVOT. For suitable individuals, however, the percutaneously implanted valves provided excellent relief of not only pulmonary regurgitation but also conduit stenosis. Indeed, it is now a widely accepted practice that surgeons will, at the time of first pulmonary valve replacement, institute a bioprosthesis that is suitable for percutaneously delivered therapy. Currently, the upper size that the Melody valve can be deployed to is 22 mm, and 26 mm for the Edwards sapiens valve.

In Europe, bioinjectable valves are also being used that are "injected" through the RV free wall directly into position across the RVOT. This approach is utilized for outflow tracts that are too large for the current percutaneous devices. Under development currently is the "infundibular reducer" which will extend the spectrum of lesions treatable percutaneously for enlarged RVOTs.

RISK ASSESSMENT IN ADULTS WITH TETRALOGY OF FALLOT

The annual risk of sudden cardiac death is of the order of 0.5% per year in repaired TOF during adult life. Risk stratification assessment includes an appreciation of the following parameters: pulmonary regurgitation, tricuspid regurgitation, right ventricular dysfunction, left ventricular dysfunction, left ventricular end-diastolic pressure (EDP), and history of previously documented ventricular tachycardia or ventricular fibrillation. Patients with left ventricular dysfunction appear to have the highest risk of sudden cardiac death, with a hazard ratio of 1.3 per mm Hg of EDP elevated above 12 mm Hg. Treatment should consist of a combination of correcting the hemodynamic problem(s) as well as consideration for primary ventricular tachycardia ablation and/or implantation of a cardioverter-defibrillator.

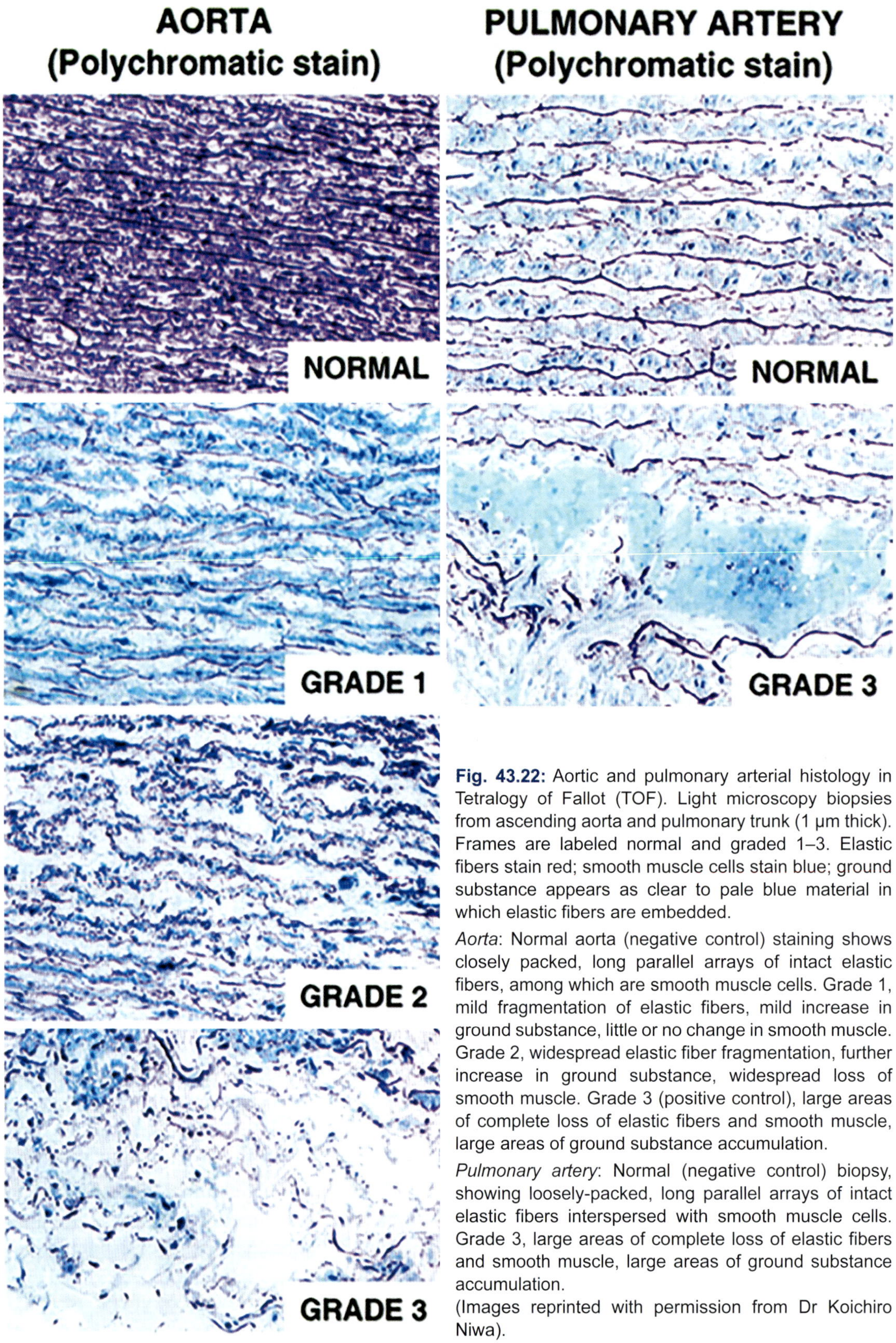

Fig. 43.22: Aortic and pulmonary arterial histology in Tetralogy of Fallot (TOF). Light microscopy biopsies from ascending aorta and pulmonary trunk (1 µm thick). Frames are labeled normal and graded 1–3. Elastic fibers stain red; smooth muscle cells stain blue; ground substance appears as clear to pale blue material in which elastic fibers are embedded.

Aorta: Normal aorta (negative control) staining shows closely packed, long parallel arrays of intact elastic fibers, among which are smooth muscle cells. Grade 1, mild fragmentation of elastic fibers, mild increase in ground substance, little or no change in smooth muscle. Grade 2, widespread elastic fiber fragmentation, further increase in ground substance, widespread loss of smooth muscle. Grade 3 (positive control), large areas of complete loss of elastic fibers and smooth muscle, large areas of ground substance accumulation.

Pulmonary artery: Normal (negative control) biopsy, showing loosely-packed, long parallel arrays of intact elastic fibers interspersed with smooth muscle cells. Grade 3, large areas of complete loss of elastic fibers and smooth muscle, large areas of ground substance accumulation.

(Images reprinted with permission from Dr Koichiro Niwa).

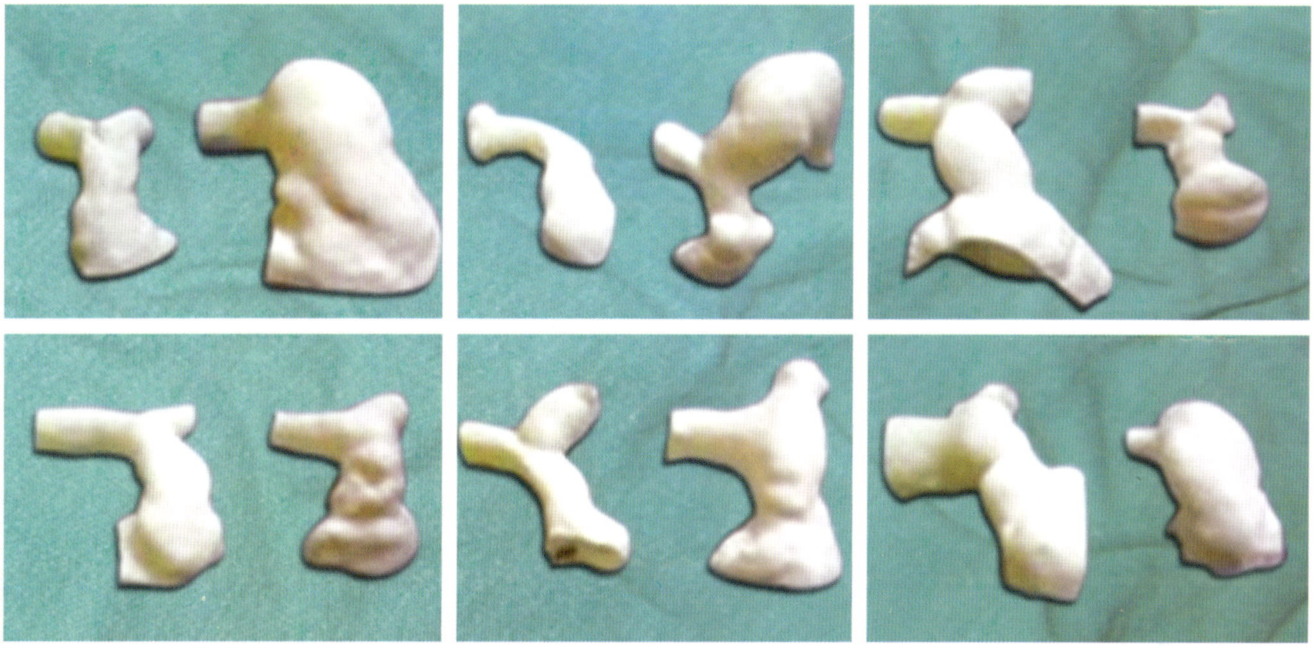

Fig. 43.23: Morphologic variation of the right ventricular outflow tract (RVOT) late after surgery. The series of images demonstrate the enormous range of anatomic variability in the RVOT ranging from stenosed and hypoplastic outflows to aneurysmal transformation. The series also demonstrates variability in branch pulmonary anatomy origin and proximal pulmonary arteries. (Images courtesy of Dr Andrew Taylor, Great Ormond Street Children's Hospital, London).

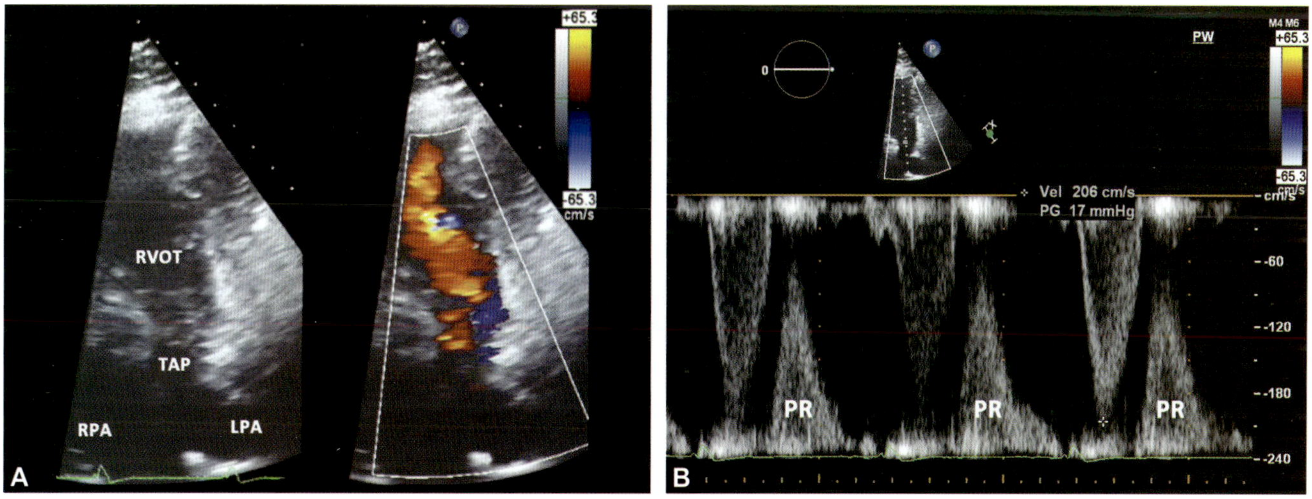

Figs. 43.24A and B: Echocardiographic features of severe pulmonary regurgitation. (A) Left panel shows a parasternal short-axis view demonstrating an aneurysmal outflow tract due to a transannular patch (TAP). Right panel color Doppler imaging demonstrates severe pulmonary regurgitation; (B) Pulse wave Doppler signal in the main pulmonary artery demonstrates unobstructed forward flow, as well as low velocity regurgitation. There is forward flow in the pulmonary artery coincident with atrial contraction consistent with the so-called restrictive right ventricle (RV). The pulmonary regurgitant (PR) signal stops well before the onset of pulmonary artery forward flow, consistent with severe regurgitation. A pressure half-time < 100 ms is generally considered an indication of severe pulmonary regurgitation. (RVOT: Right ventricular outflow tract; LPA: Left pulmonary artery; RPA: Right pulmonary artery).

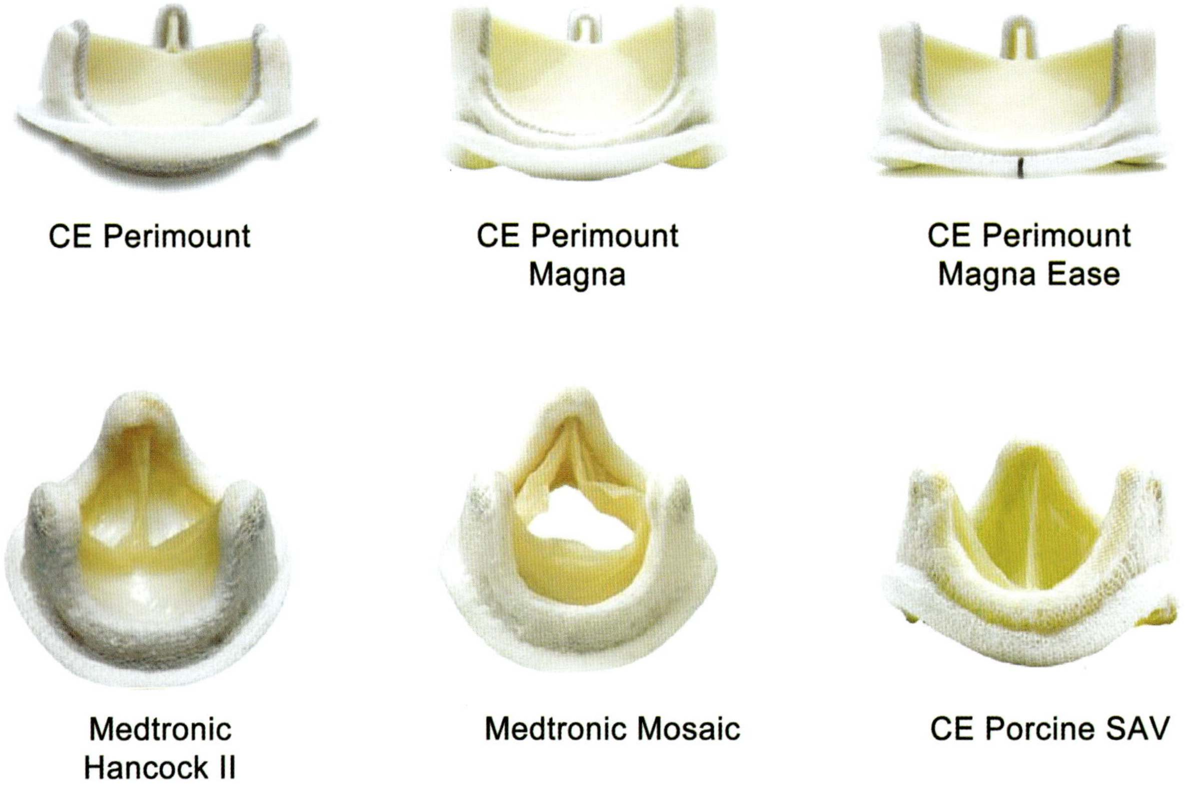

Fig. 43.25: Xenografts—examples of stented porcine and bovine bioprosthetic valves that are used in the right ventricular outflow tracts (RVOTs). [Images reprinted with permission from Piazza N, Bleiziffer S, Brockmann G, et al. Transcatheter aortic valve implantation for failing surgical aortic bioprosthetic valve: from concept to clinical application and evaluation (part 2). JACC Cardiovasc Interv. 2011;4(7):733-42].

SUMMARY

Tetralogy of Fallot has characteristic anatomic features that can be summarized by the presence of anterocephalad deviation of the OS, the presence of a ventricular septal defect and aortic override. Surgical repair has undergone continuous evolution and currently emphasizes conservation of the RV. Late outcomes are frequently defined by the development of RVOT failure, the most common of which is due to pulmonary regurgitation. The interaction of abnormal pulmonary compliance with the RV modulates the progression of adverse RV remodeling and dysfunction dictating the timing of surgical or catheter reintervention. Risk stratification for sudden cardiac death is important. In this context, an appreciation of not only right heart parameters but especially left ventricular dysfunction is essential for better understanding of late risk.

VIDEO LEGEND

Video 43.1: Severe pulmonary regurgitation in a patient with repaired Tetralogy of Fallot (TOF). Blue coloration demonstrates forward flow toward the branch pulmonary arteries and red flow demonstrates regurgitation toward the right ventricle (RV).

REFERENCES

Apitz C, Webb GD, Redington AN. Tetralogy of Fallot. Lancet. 2009;374(9699):1462-71.

Bassett AS, Hodgkinson K, Chow EW, et al. 22q11 deletion syndrome in adults with schizophrenia. Am J Med Genet. 1998; 81(4):328-37.

Beauchesne LM, Warnes CA, Connolly HM, et al. Prevalence and clinical manifestations of 22q11.2 microdeletion in adults with selected conotruncal anomalies. J Am Coll Cardiol. 2005; 45(4):595-8.

Bertranou EG, Blackstone EH, Hazelrig JB, et al. Life expectancy without surgery in tetralogy of Fallot. Am J Cardiol. 1978;42 (3):458-66.

Brock RC. Direct cardiac surgery in the treatment of congenital pulmonary stenosis. Ann Surg. 1952;136(1):63-72.

Di Felice V, Zummo G. Tetralogy of Fallot as a model to study cardiac progenitor cell migration and differentiation during heart development. Trends Cardiovasc Med. 2009;19(4):130-5.

Bédard E, McCarthy KP, Dimopoulos K, et al. Structural abnormalities of the pulmonary trunk in tetralogy of Fallot and potential clinical implications: a morphological study. J Am Coll Cardiol. 2009;54(20):1883-90.

Ferraz Cavalcanti PE, Sá MP, Santos CA, et al. Pulmonary valve replacement after operative repair of tetralogy of Fallot: meta-analysis and meta-regression of 3,118 patients from 48 studies. J Am Coll Cardiol. 2013;62(23):2227-43.

Inuzuka R, Seki M, Sugimoto M, et al. Pulmonary arterial wall stiffness and its impact on right ventricular afterload in patients with repaired tetralogy of Fallot. Ann Thorac Surg. 2013;96(4):1435-41.

Karl TR. Tetralogy of Fallot: a surgical perspective. Korean J Thorac Cardiovasc Surg. 2012;45(4):213-24.

Khairy P, Harris L, Landzberg MJ, et al. Implantable cardioverter-defibrillators in tetralogy of Fallot. Circulation. 2008;117(3): 363-70.

Lillehei CW, Varco RL, Cohen M, et al. The first open heart corrections of tetralogy of Fallot. A 26-31 year follow-up of 106 patients. Ann Surg. 1986;204(4):490-502.

Luijnenburg SE, Helbing WA, Moelker A, et al. 5-year serial follow-up of clinical condition and ventricular function in patients after repair of tetralogy of Fallot. Int J Cardiol. 2013; 169(6):439-44.

Niwa K, Perloff JK, Bhuta SM, et al. Structural abnormalities of great arterial walls in congenital heart disease: light and electron microscopic analyses. Circulation. 2001;103(3):393-400.

Piazza N, Bleiziffer S, Brockmann G, et al. Transcatheter aortic valve implantation for failing surgical aortic bioprosthetic valve: from concept to clinical application and evaluation (part 2). JACC Cardiovasc Interv. 2011;4(7):733-42.

Rabinovitch M, Herrera-deLeon V, Castaneda AR, et al. Growth and development of the pulmonary vascular bed in patients with tetralogy of Fallot with or without pulmonary atresia. Circulation. 1981;64(6):1234-49.

Redington AN, Oldershaw PJ, Shinebourne EA, et al. A new technique for the assessment of pulmonary regurgitation and its application to the assessment of right ventricular function before and after repair of tetralogy of Fallot. Br Heart J. 1988;60(1):57-65.

Srivastava D. Making or breaking the heart: from lineage determination to morphogenesis. Cell. 2006;126(6):1037-48.

CHAPTER

Transposition of the Great Arteries

44

Paula Martins

INTRODUCTION, TERMINOLOGY, AND ANATOMY

Transposition of the great arteries (TGA) is a congenital heart defect that occurs in approximately 20–30 per 100,000 live births, being more prevalent in the offspring of diabetic mothers. TGA can be subcategorized as dextro-transposition of the great arteries (d-TGA) and congenitally corrected-transposition of the great arteries (cc-TGA).

Morphologically, d-TGA is characterized by concordant atrioventricular and discordant ventriculoatrial connections (Figs. 44.1 to 44.3). That is, the atriums and ventricles retain their normal configuration and position, but the great arteries are transposed, arising from the incorrect ventricle. The aorta emerges from the morphological right ventricle (mRV) and pulmonary trunk (PT) from the morphological left ventricle (mLV). d-TGA, particularly in the absence of other congenital abnormalities, produces cyanosis, as the pulmonary and systemic circulations function in parallel, rather than in series. Oxygenated blood returning from the lungs enters the left atrium, passes to the mLV, and then is pumped through the pulmonary artery (PA) back to the lungs, while deoxygenated blood returning from the systemic veins enters the right atrium, passes to the mRV, and then is pumped through the aorta to the systemic arteries (Fig. 44.4).

In cc-TGA, less correctly referred to as levo-transposition of the great arteries (l-TGA) or ventricular inversion by there is both discordant atrioventricular and discordant ventriculoatrial connections (Figs. 44.5 to 44.14). The result of this is that deoxygenated venous blood flows through the morphological right atrium (mRA) into the

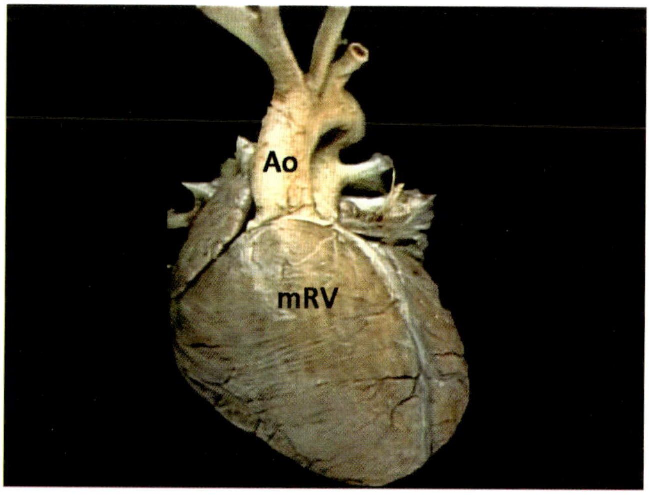

Fig. 44.1: Gross specimen of a heart with dextro-transposition of the great arteries (d-TGA). The aorta (Ao) is visualized arising from what is the morphological right ventricle (mRV). [Image from Armed Force Institute of Pathology (public domain)].

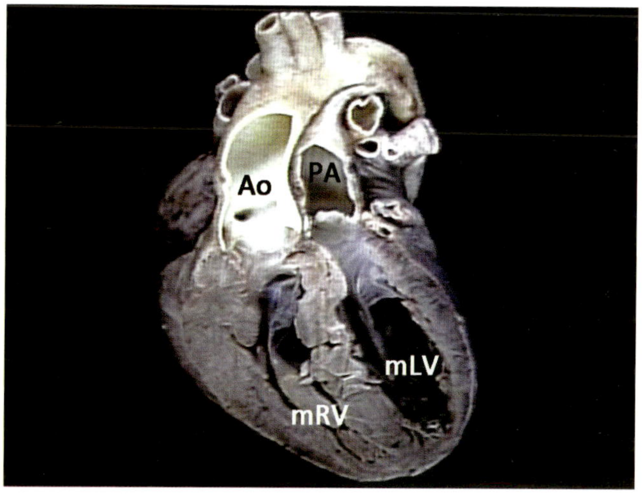

Fig. 44.2: Cut-away gross pathology demonstrating dextro-transposition of the great arteries (d-TGA). The aorta (Ao) is seen arising from the morphological right ventricle (mRV) and the pulmonary artery (PA) is seen arising from the morphological left ventricle (mLV).

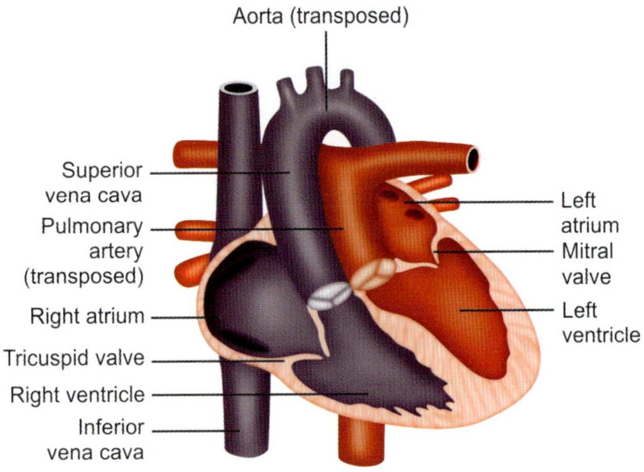

Fig. 44.3: Schematic illustration of dextro-transposition of the great arteries (d-TGA). The aorta (Ao) emerging from the morphological right ventricle (mRV) and the pulmonary trunk (PT) or main pulmonary artery (MPA) arises from the morphological left ventricle (mLV).

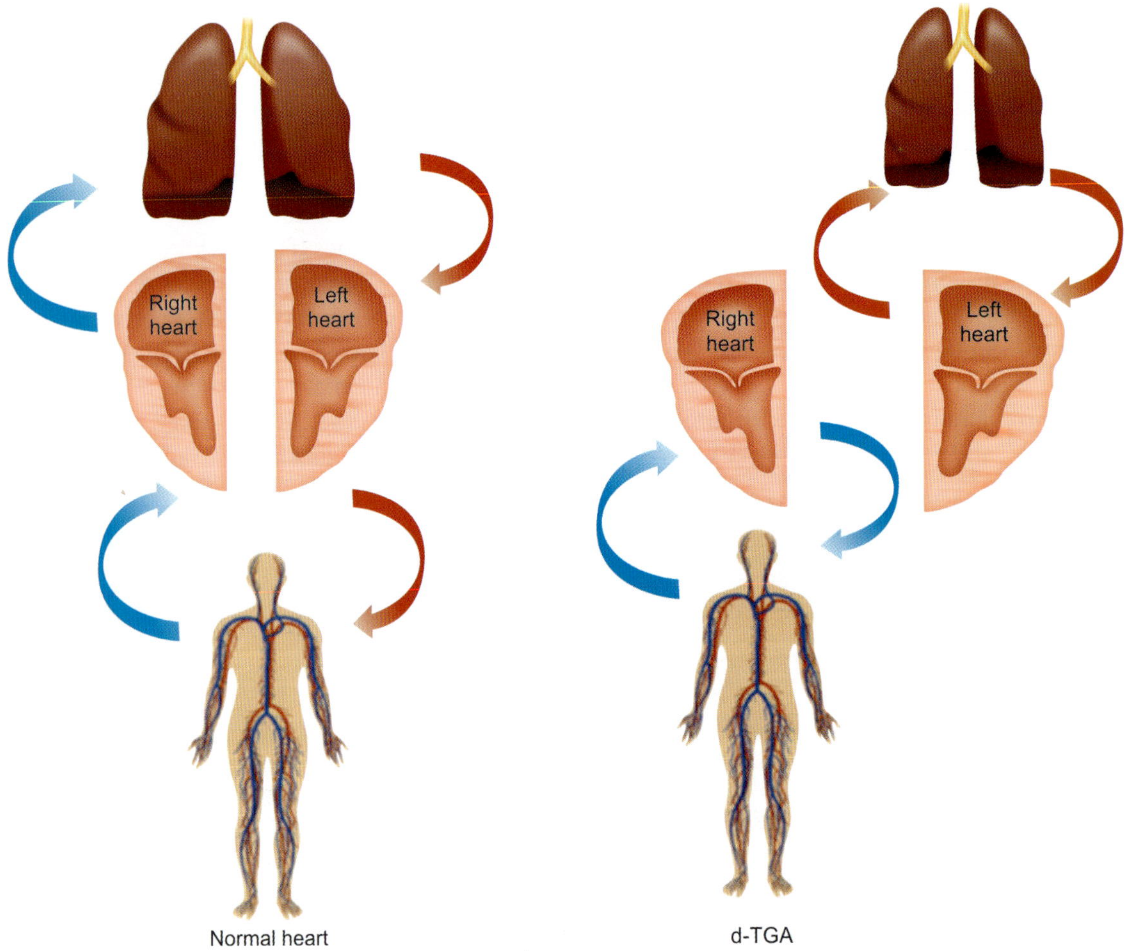

Fig. 44.4: Pathophysiology of the pulmonary and systemic circulations, both in the normal heart (left panel) and in dextro-transposition of the great arteries (d-TGA) (right panel). In a normal heart, the deoxygenated blood (blue arrows) from the systemic veins is received by the right cardiac chambers, and pumped to the lungs. After passing through the pulmonary alveoli, the blood already enriched in oxygen (red arrows), goes back to the heart, but now to the left-sided chambers. There, the left ventricle will be responsible to propel the recently oxygenated blood to the systemic arterial bed. This cycle involves two different circulations (the pulmonary and the systemic circulations) organized in series. In d-TGA the two circulations function in parallel, rather than in series. Oxygenated blood (red arrows) is mostly confined to the pulmonary circulation and to the left heart; whereas deoxygenated blood (blue arrows) recirculates in the systemic vessels and right heart. Without proper mixing among these two circuits, prolonged survival is not feasible.

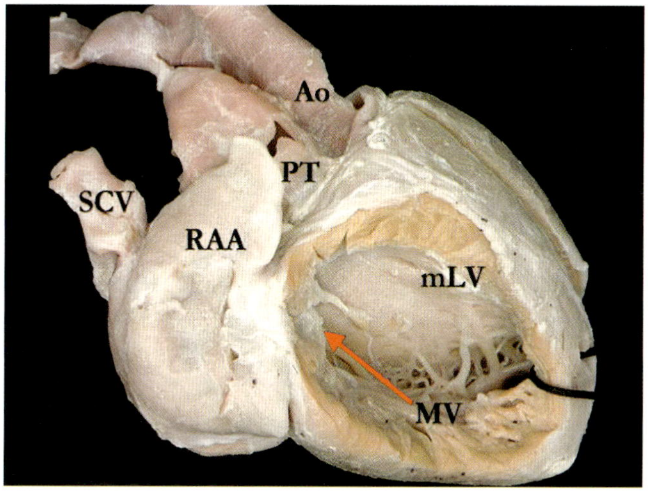

Fig. 44.5: Gross pathology specimen of congenitally corrected-transposition of the great arteries (cc-TGA). The morphological right atrium (mRA), with its characteristic right atrial appendage (RAA), is connected to a morphological left ventricle (mLV) across the mitral valve (MV), with the ventricle then connected to the pulmonary trunk (PT). Note the smooth septal surface of the ventricle. (Image and legend text from Wallis G, Debich-Spicer D, Anderson RH. Congenitally corrected transposition. Orphanet J Rare Dis. 2011;6:22). (Ao: Aorta; SCV: Superior caval vein).

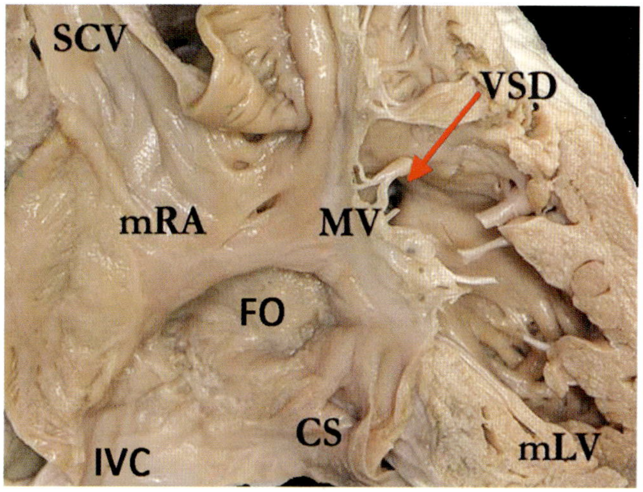

Fig. 44.6: Gross pathology specimen of congenitally corrected-transposition of the great arteries (cc-TGA). The superior caval vein (SCV) and inferior caval vein (IVC) are connected to the morphological right atrium (mRA), which in turn empties through the mitral valve (MV) to the morphological left ventricle (mLV) and thence to the pulmonary trunk (PT). (Image and legend text from Wallis G, Debich-Spicer D, Anderson RH. Congenitally corrected transposition. Orphanet J Rare Dis. 2011;6:22). (CS: Coronary sinus; VSD: Ventricular septal defect; FO: Fossa ovalis).

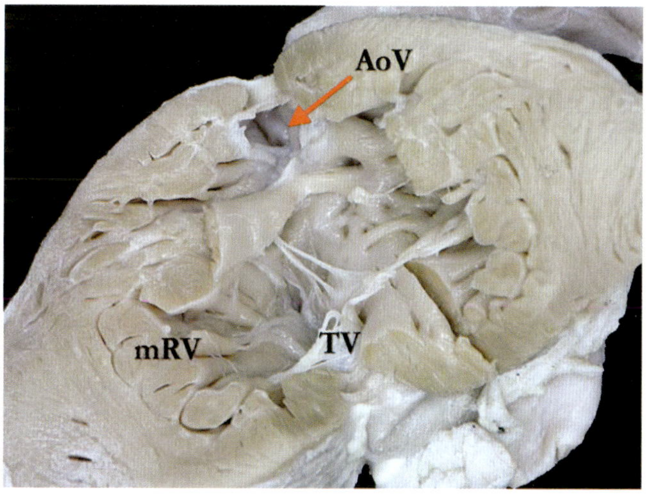

Fig. 44.7: Gross pathology specimen of congenitally corrected-transposition of the great arteries (cc-TGA). The morphological left atrium (mLA) connected to the morphological right ventricle (mRV) across the tricuspid valve (TV), with the ventricle giving rise to the aortic valve (AoV). The ventricle possesses coarse trabeculations, with the leaflets of the tricuspid. (Image and legend text from Wallis G, Debich-Spicer D, Anderson RH. Congenitally corrected transposition. Orphanet J Rare Dis. 2011;6:22).

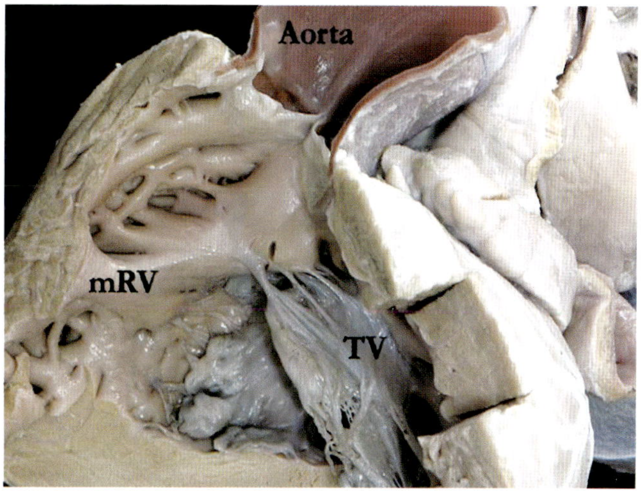

Fig. 44.8: Heart from a patient with congenitally corrected-transposition of the great arteries (cc-TGA). Note how the aorta (Ao) is supported by a complete muscular infundibulum above the coarsely trabeculated morphological right ventricle (mRV), the infundibulum interposing between the hinges of the aortic and tricuspid valves (TVs). (Image and legend text from Wallis G, Debich-Spicer D, Anderson RH. Congenitally corrected transposition. Orphanet J Rare Dis. 2011;6:22).

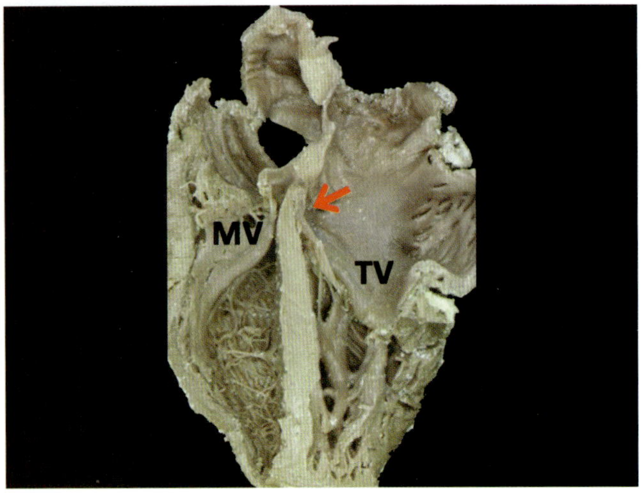

Fig. 44.9: Heart from a patient with congenitally corrected-transposition of the great arteries (cc-TGA). Note the reversed offsetting of the attachments of the leaflets of the atrioventricular valves to the septum (arrow), with the mitral valve (MV) on the right side attached appreciably higher than the tricuspid valve (TV) on the left side. (Image and legend text from Wallis G, Debich-Spicer D, Anderson RH. Congenitally corrected transposition. Orphanet J Rare Dis. 2011;6:22).

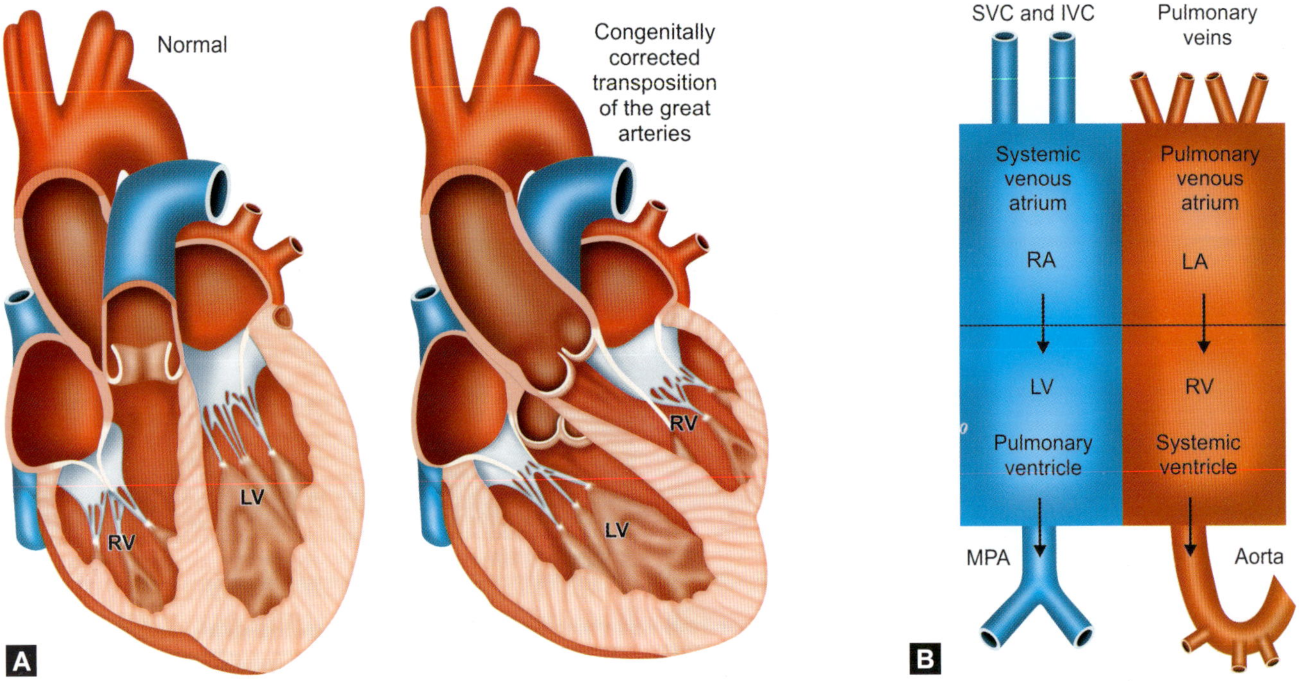

Figs. 44.10A and B: (A) Schematic illustration of congenitally corrected-transposition of the great arteries (cc-TGA). The left panel shows normal cardiac anatomy. The right panel shows cc-TGA. Deoxygenated blood from the inferior vena cava (IVC) and superior vena cava (SVC) returns to the morphological right atrium (mRA) and flows into the morphological left ventricle (mLV) and into the pulmonary artery (PA) [seen underneath the right ventricular outflow tract and aorta (Ao)]. Oxygenated blood from the lungs enters the morphological left atrium (mLA) and flows into the morphological right ventricle (mRV) and then out the Ao to the systemic arteries; (B) Schematic illustration of blood circulation in cc-TGA. [Image from Flack EC, Kaushik N, Graham TP. Congenitally corrected transposition of the great arteries. In: Vijayalakshmi IB, Rao PS, Chugh R (Eds). Comprehensive Approach to Congenital Heart Diseases, 1st edition. 2013. pp. 625-38]. (LA: Left atrium; LV: Left ventricle; MPA: Main pulmonary artery; RA: Right atrium; RV: Right ventricle).

mLV and into the PA. Oxygenated blood flows through the morphological left atrium (mLA) into the mRV and into the aorta.

In 50% of cases of d-TGA, concordant atrioventricular with discordant ventriculoatrial connections is the only abnormal finding, and the condition is described as simple TGA. By contrast, in complex d-TGA, other cardiovascular anomalies are present, namely ventricular septal defect (VSD), left ventricular outflow tract obstruction, aortic arch defects and anomalous coronary patterns (Fig. 44.15). All these anatomical variants should be considered during imaging studies, as they can determine both the prognosis and respective therapeutic options.

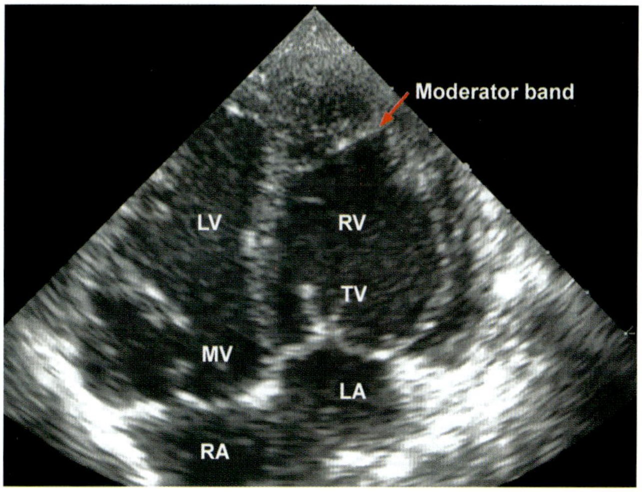

Fig. 44.11: Transthoracic echocardiogram (apical four-chamber view) in congenitally corrected-transposition of the great arteries (cc-TGA) shows the inferior hinge point of the left-sided atrioventricular valve [tricuspid valve (TV)] opening into a morphological right ventricle (RV). In comparison, the superior level of the right-sided atrioventricular valve [mitral valve (MV)] hinge point is seen, as well as valvular attachments to a papillary muscle within the morphological left ventricle (LV). [Image from Flack EC, Kaushik N, Graham TP. Congenitally corrected transposition of the great arteries. In: Vijayalakshmi IB, Rao PS, Chugh R (Eds). Comprehensive Approach to Congenital Heart Diseases, 1st edition. 2013. pp. 625-38].

PRENATAL DIAGNOSIS OF d-TGA

Preferably, d-TGA should be identified *prenatally* during the second trimester obstetric ultrasound examination (Fig. 44.16). Its diagnosis during fetal life remains a challenge, mainly due to the frequent normality of the apical and subcostal four-chamber view. In order to improve detection, the sonographer should pay particular attention to *the ventricular outflow tract views* and assure that the great arteries, at their origins, crossover at right angles. In transposition, this does not occur, and the two arteries will have *a parallel course* with the branching artery (PA) arising from the mLV. Further details can be appreciated in the three-vessel view, where only two vessels, the superior caval vein (SCV) and the aorta, can be identified. In the short-axis view, the PT does not assume its typical configuration, namely, as an anterior and longitudinal structure that wraps around the aorta. Instead, it presents as a circular vessel adjacent to the aorta.

POSTNATAL DIAGNOSIS OF d-TGA

When prenatal diagnosis is not available, signs and symptoms soon after birth raise the suspicion of cardiac disease. The clinical hallmark of transposition is cyanosis refractory to oxygen therapy, as a result of the hypoxemic status created by the parallel circuit, where the systemic venous return is not adequately oxygenated. However, in the presence of a large VSD and in the absence of obstructive lesions, signs of congestive heart failure (e.g. tachypnea, tachycardia, diaphoresis, poor weight gain, gallop rhythm, hepatomegaly) may be observed.

Electrocardiogram (ECG) findings in d-TGA are often nonspecific. In TGA, the PA is usually positioned right of its normal location. This and other factors lead to narrowing of the superior mediastinum. The chest X-ray of a patient with d-TGA may thus show a narrowed superior mediastinum and a cardiac silhouette with a "egg of side" or "egg on a string" appearance (Fig. 44.17). This finding, however, is not specific for TGA.

The diagnosis of TGA is usually made by echocardiography (Fig. 44.18). The echocardiographic images obtained in the long parasternal and subcostal views demonstrate the discordant ventriculoatrial connections, as well as the parallel trajectory of the aorta and PT at their origins. In the short-axis view, the aorta usually assumes an anterior position in relation to the PA. Associated lesions and coronary anomalies should be identified and described in order to better plan the surgical approach.

More advanced diagnostic techniques (Fig. 44.19), such as computed tomography (CT), magnetic resonance imaging (MRI) or cardiac catheterization, are seldom necessary (Table 44.1), although sometimes used as adjunctive imaging modalities.

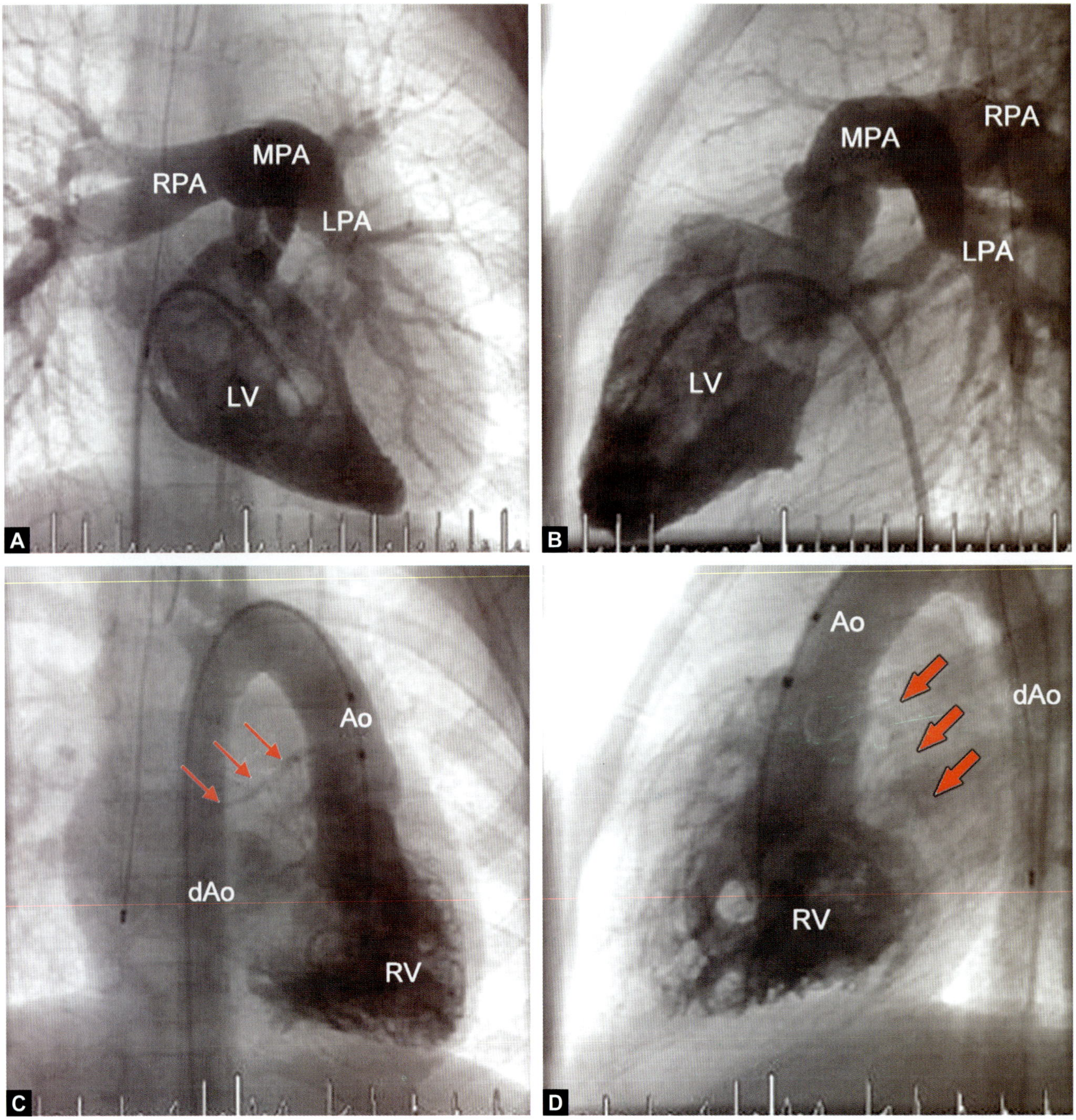

Figs. 44.12A to D: Cardiac catheterization of unrepaired 4-year-old congenitally corrected-transposition of the great arteries (cc-TGA) patient: (A) Morphological left ventricle (mLV), anterior-posterior projection. A catheter is positioned antegrade from the inferior vena cava (IVC) and into the right-sided mLV. Contrast fills the LV, main pulmonary artery (MPA) and pulmonary arteries (PA). There is discrete subvalvular pulmonary stenosis and thickened pulmonary valve leaflets. (B) Lateral projection. Contrast from the LV flows through the posteriorly positioned, stenotic LV outflow tract, across the pulmonary valve, and fills the pulmonary arteries. (C) Morphological right ventricle (mRV), anterior-posterior projection. A catheter is positioned retrograde in the aorta (Ao) and into the left-sided mRV. Contrast fills the trabeculated RV, the Ao and descending aorta (dAo). Closed-arrows indicate the circumflex artery. The left anterior descending (LAD) coronary artery is not seen in this still frame image. (D) Lateral projection. Contrast fills the RV, AAo, and dAo. Bold arrows indicate the course of the right coronary artery (RCA). [Image from Flack EC, Kaushik N, Graham TP. Congenitally corrected transposition of the great arteries. In: Vijayalakshmi IB, Rao PS, Chugh R (Eds). Comprehensive Approach to Congenital Heart Diseases, 1st edition. 2013. pp. 625-38]. (LPA: Left pulmonary artery; RPA: Right pulmonary artery).

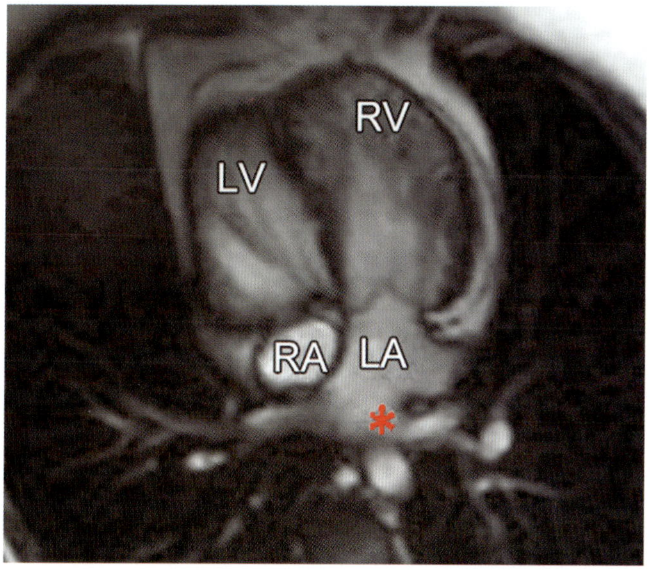

Fig. 44.13A: Axial oblique, T2-weighted cardiac magnetic resonance image (cMRI) of the cardiac four-chamber view in a congenitally corrected-transposition of the great arteries (cc-TGA) patient with levocardia. The right atrium (RA) empties into a right-sided, smooth-walled, morphological left ventricle (mLV). A star (*) labels the entrance of a left pulmonary vein into the left atrium (LA), which empties into a trabeculated, left-sided, morphological right ventricle (mRV). [Image from Flack EC, Kaushik N, Graham TP. Congenitally corrected transposition of the great arteries. In: Vijayalakshmi IB, Rao PS, Chugh R (Eds). Comprehensive Approach to Congenital Heart Diseases, 1st edition. 2013. pp. 625-38].

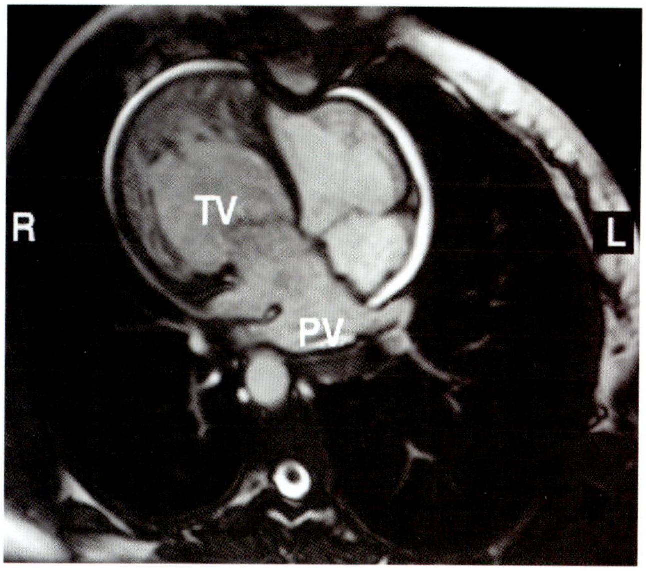

Fig. 44.13B: MRI of a patient with cc-TGA shows a right-sided heart with the apex pointing to the right. The pulmonary veins (PV) are seen entering the LA, with the tricuspid valve (TV) guarding the junction with the coarsely trabeculated systemic mRV. (Image and legend text from Wallis G, Debich-Spicer D, Anderson RH. Congenitally corrected transposition. Orphanet J Rare Dis. 2011; 6:22).

MANAGEMENT OF PATIENTS WITH d-TGA

The initial management of affected newborns faced with severe hypoxemia aims at improving intercirculatory mixing. To avoid closure of the arterial duct, an intravenous infusion of *prostaglandin E1* is started. However, this is frequently insufficient to achieve an acceptable oxygenation of the systemic blood. In these cases, a *balloon atrial septostomy* (Rashkind procedure) is carried out (Figs. 44.20 and 44.21). As this procedure enlarges the existing atrial septal defect, shunting is increased at atrial level.

The definitive treatment is surgical. The procedure of choice is the *arterial switch* operation (Figs. 44.22 and 44.23), also known as the Jatene procedure, and should be performed during the first month of life. It involves sectioning the aorta and PT at their origins, with the distal extremities being reattached to the concordant ventricle. The coronary arteries are also removed from their original location and reimplanted in the neo-aorta. This technique allows both an anatomical and a physiological correction, which translates in good long-term survival rates (89.3% at 15 years) and in low reintervention rates (6% at 10 years).

Some morphological features (complex coronary anatomy or left ventricular outflow tract obstruction not properly relieved by resection) may preclude the use of the arterial switch operation. Other surgical options in these settings imply that the repair will be done either at an atrial level (*Mustard* or *Senning* operations) (Fig. 44.24) or at ventricular level (Rastelli, REV or Nikaidoh's) if a sufficiently large VSD is present.

MANAGEMENT OF PATIENTS WITH cc-TGA

Since patients with simple cc-TGA have "congenitally corrected" transposition and are thus not cyanotic, the condition may not cause symptoms for decades, and the diagnosis may not be made until imaging studies are performed on the patient and the condition is recognized by an imaging specialist with familiarity or expertise in congenital heart disease.

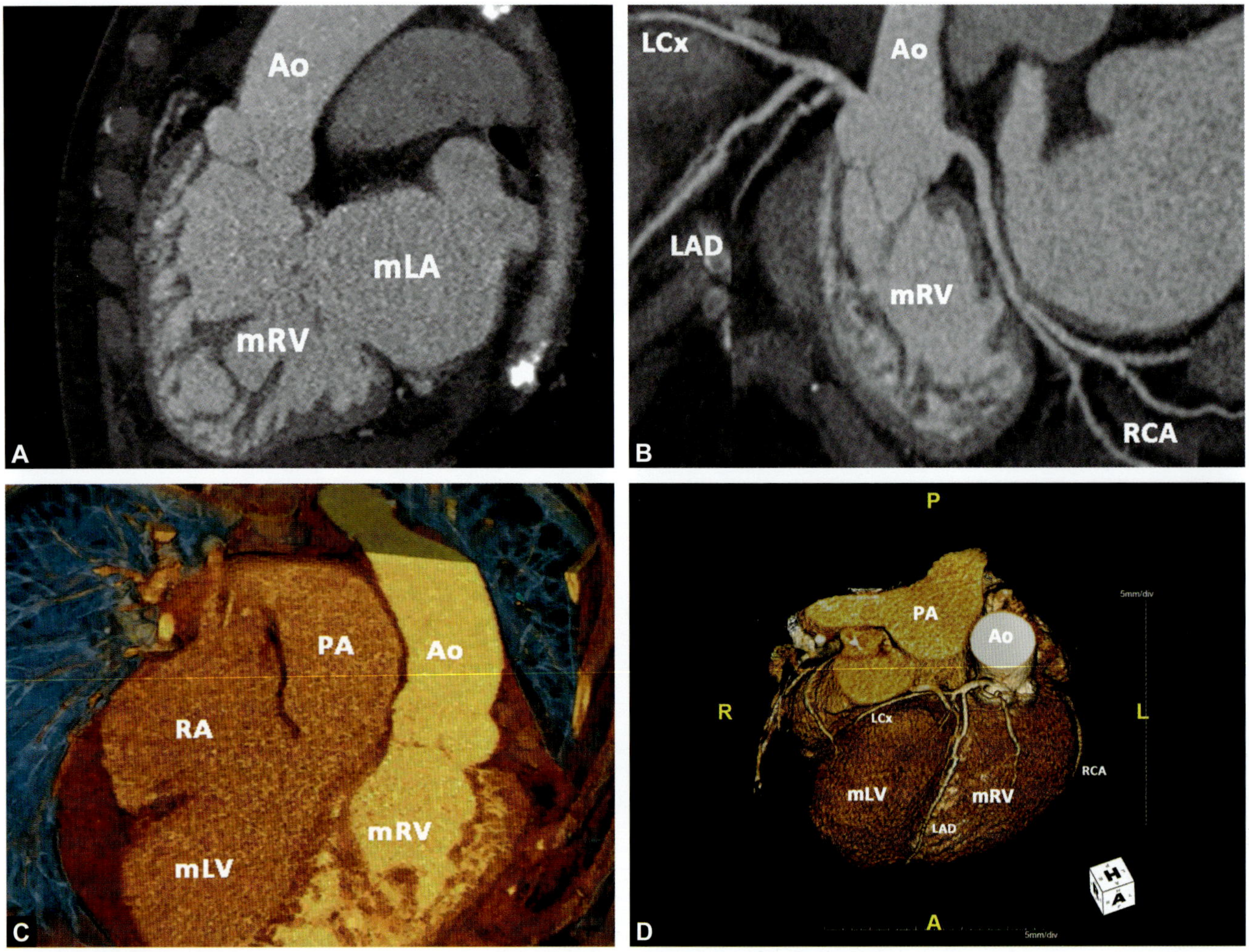

Figs. 44.14A to D: Computed tomography (CT) images of congenitally corrected-transposition of the great arteries (cc-TGA). (A) Maximum intensity projection (MIP) image showing the morphological left atrium (mLA) connecting to the morphological right ventricle (mRV), which in turn connects to the aorta (Ao); (B) Curved multiplanar reformation image demonstrating the course of the left anterior descending (LAD), left circumflex (LCx), and right coronary arteries (RCAs) in a patient with cc-TGA; (C) CT demonstrating the "congenitally corrected" connections of the ventricles to the great arteries; (D) Three-dimensional volume-rendered image showing the origin and course of the coronary arteries in cc-TGA. (Images courtesy of Dr Heon Lee, Soonchunhayng University Hospital Bucheon, Republic of Korea).

The ECG of patients with cc-TGA may have some characteristic though nonspecific findings (Fig. 44.25). Due to the mirror-imaged arrangement of the bundle branches in the presence of left-handed ventricular topology, the initial activation of the ventricles will be from right to left, represented in the ECG by Q waves in the right precordial leads, and an absent Q wave in the left precordial leads.

Over time, there is right ventricular hypertrophy and eventual RV failure, as the mRV fatigues having to contend with systemic afterload. Common presenting symptoms are dyspnea or fatigue. Symptomatic patients are most commonly treated supportively, primarily with diuretic agents and sometimes with afterload reduction or inotropic therapy. In some patients, a "double switch" procedure of the great arteries will be performed.

In contrast to simple cc-TGA (Fig. 44.26), complex cc-TGA may lead to symptoms in the early postnatal period or in childhood, depending on the nature, degree and number of accompanying congenital defects. Right-to-left or bidirectional shunts may produce cyanosis. Management of such patients is complex, and may include temporizing surgeries or percutaneous procedures, or more definitive surgical procedures.

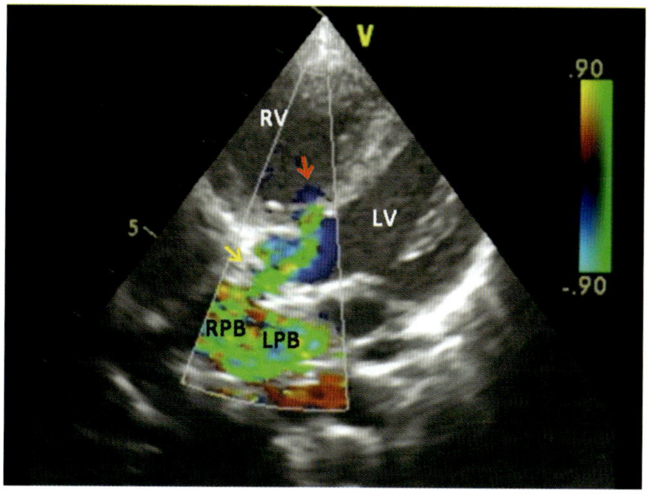

Fig. 44.15: Complex d-TGA. Color Doppler image from a subcostal outlet view of complex transposition with ventricular septal defect (red arrow) and pulmonary stenosis (yellow arrow). Note the turbulent blood flow (green) in the pulmonary trunk and its branches, as result of the subjacent stenosis. (LPB: Left pulmonary branch; LV: Left ventricle; RPB: Right pulmonary branch; RV: Right ventricle).

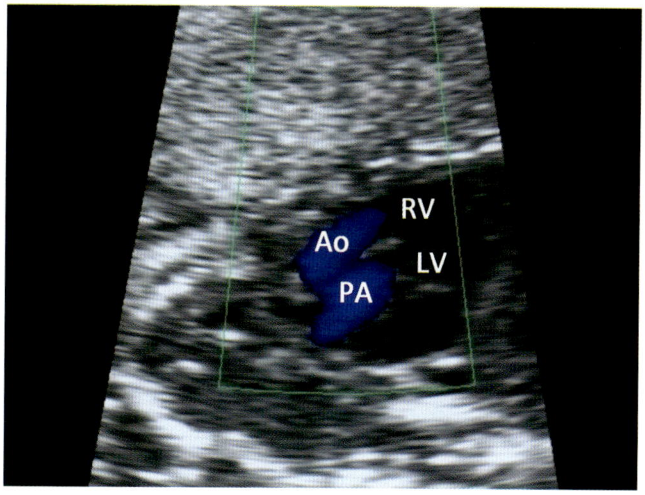

Fig. 44.16: Fetal echocardiogram in simple dextro-transposition of the great arteries (d-TGA). This second-trimester echocardiogram demonstrates the parallel arrangement of the great arteries in their origin, which is characteristic of transposition. (Ao: Aorta; LV: Left ventricle; PA: Pulmonary artery; RV: Right ventricle).

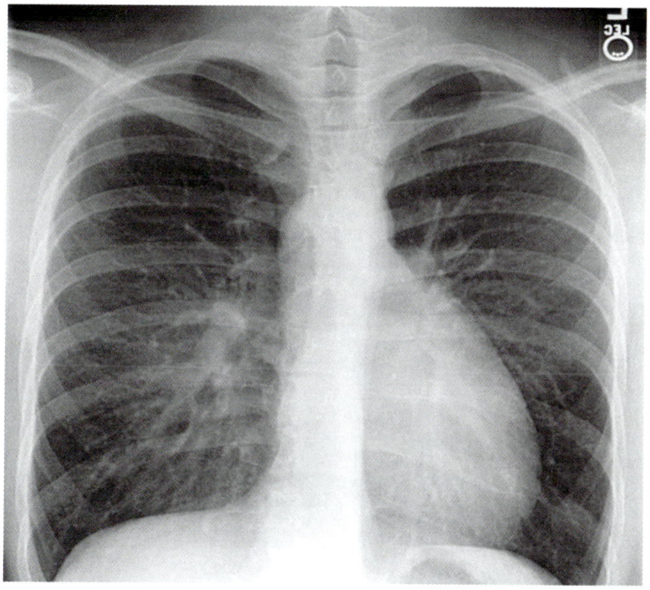

Fig. 44.17: Chest X-ray of a patient with dextro-transposition of the great arteries (d-TGA) showing the characteristic "egg on side" sign. In d-TGA, the pulmonary artery (PA) is positioned right of its normal location. This and other factors lead to narrowing of the superior mediastinum and the "egg on side" or "egg on a string" appearance. (Image posted by Madhero88 on Wikimedia Commons).

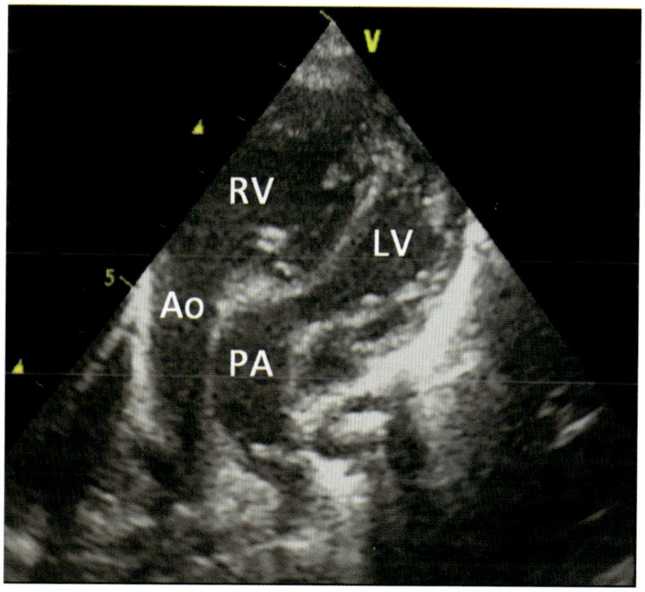

Fig. 44.18: Dextro-transposition of the great arteries (d-TGA) visualized in the subcostal echocardiographic view. Note the parallel course of the pulmonary trunk (PT) and aorta (Ao) as they arise from the discordant ventricle. (LV: Left ventricle; PA: Pulmonary artery; RV: Right ventricle).

Table 44.1: Summary of the data provided by the different diagnostic examinations, other than echocardiogram (ECG). (VSD: Ventricular septal defect; CT: Computed tomography; MRI: Magnetic resonance imaging).

Diagnostic Method	***Information Provided***
Electrocardiogram (ECG)	Nonspecific: • Rightward deviation of the QRS complex axis • Criteria of right ventricular hypertrophy
Chest radiography	Nonspecific: • Narrowed superior mediastinum • Cardiac silhouette with an egg-shaped appearance • In the presence of a large VSD, cardiomegaly with increased pulmonary vascular markings
Cardiac catheterization, MRI or CT imaging	May clarify certain anatomical and hemodynamical aspects. For example: • Coronary anatomy • Characterization of residual postoperative lesions

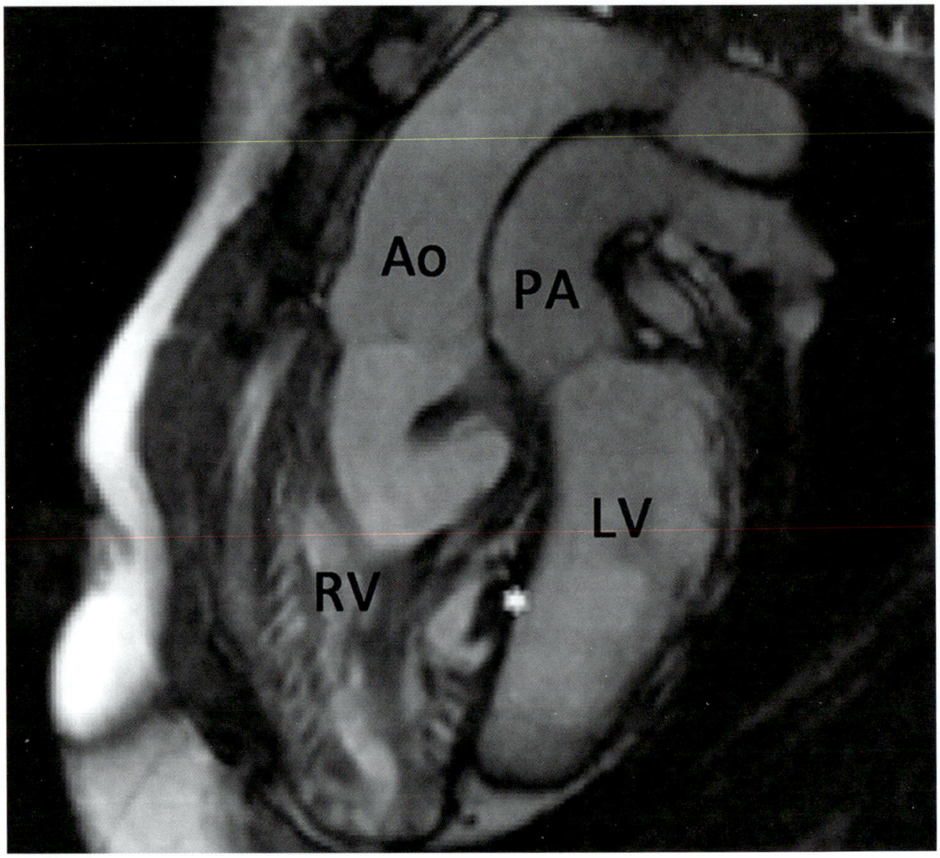

Fig. 44.19: TGA after atrial switch operation with Mustard procedure. A: The aorta (AO) is positioned anteriorly and arises from the hypertrophied, morphologically RV. The pulmonary artery (PA) is positioned posteriorly and arises from the LV, which is smaller and has less myocardial mass. The septum (*) is pertrudes into the LV due to increased RV pressure. Image from Steinmetz M et al. Non-invasive imaging for congenital heart disease—recent progress in cardiac MRI. J Clin Exp Cardiology 2012. S8:008. doi: 10.4172/2155-9880.S8-008.

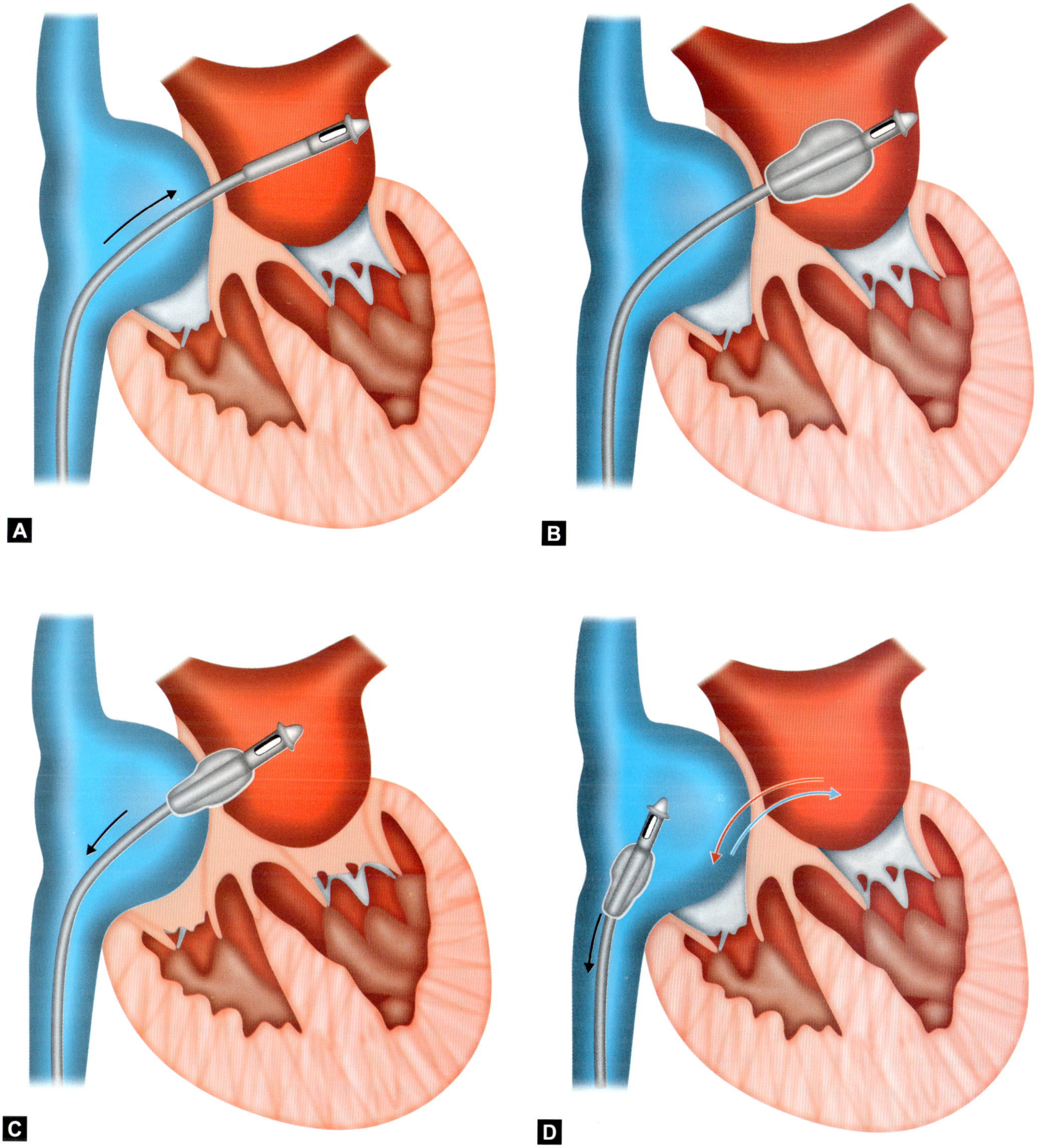

Figs. 44.20A to D: Balloon atrial septostomy. Schematic drawing that shows a balloon-tipped catheter being placed in the left atrium (LA), via the oval foramen and inflated. The catheter is then pulled back into the right atrium (RA), tearing the atrial septum.

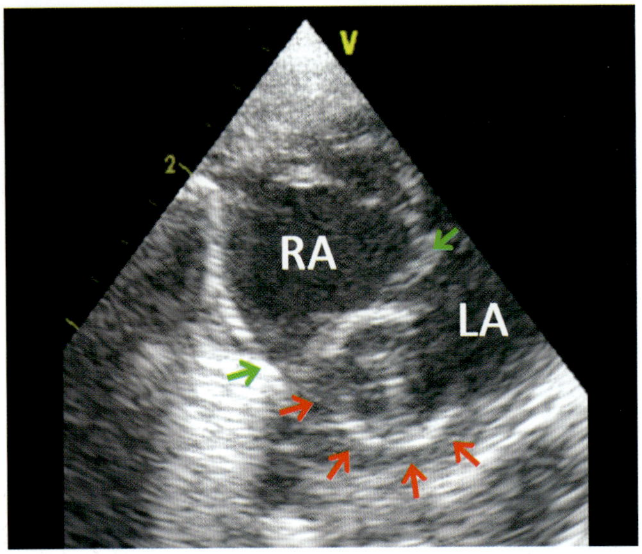

Fig. 44.21: Balloon atrial septostomy in a patient with dextro-transposition of the great arteries (d-TGA). Subcostal image during an echo-guided procedure that shows the balloon inflated in the left atrium (LA) (red arrows) before being pulled back across the atrial septum (green arrows) into the right atrium (RA).

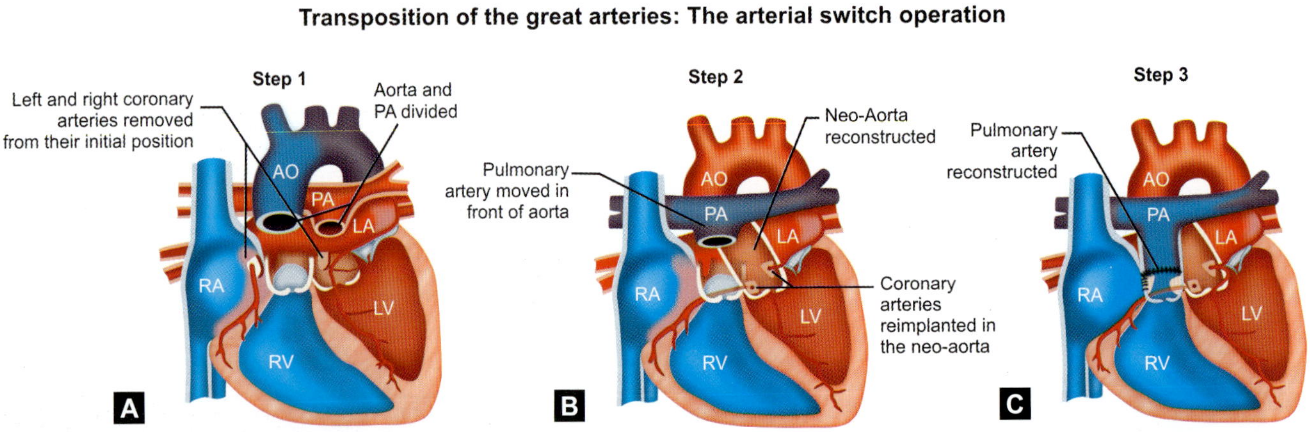

Figs. 44.22A to C: Arterial switch operation. Schematic drawing that highlights the most important steps of the arterial switch: sectioning of aorta (Ao) and pulmonary trunk (PT), reattaching the great arteries to the concordant ventricle, and reimplantation of the coronary arteries.

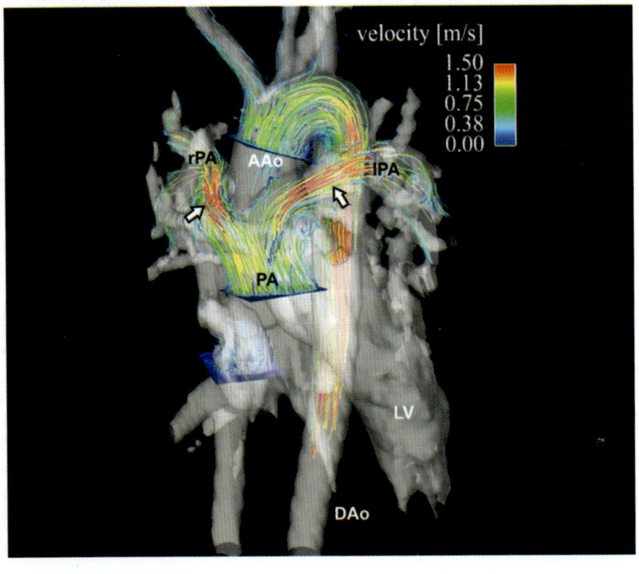

Fig. 44.23: Three-dimensional cine velocity acquisition in a patient with transposition of the great arteries (TGA) corrected by an arterial switch procedure showing the postsurgical course of the pulmonary arteries, straddling the aorta. The three-dimensional pathlines represent systolic flow from emitter planes in the ascending aorta (AAo) and main pulmonary artery (MPA). Flow acceleration with peak velocities greater than 1.5 m/s in left pulmonary artery (LPA) and right pulmonary artery (RPA) can be seen (white arrows) whereas the flow pattern in the aorta (Ao) was normal. (Image from Markl M, Kilner PJ, Ebbers T. Comprehensive four-dimensional velocity mapping of the heart and great vessels by cardiovascular magnetic resonance. J Cardiovasc Magn Reson. 2011;13:7).

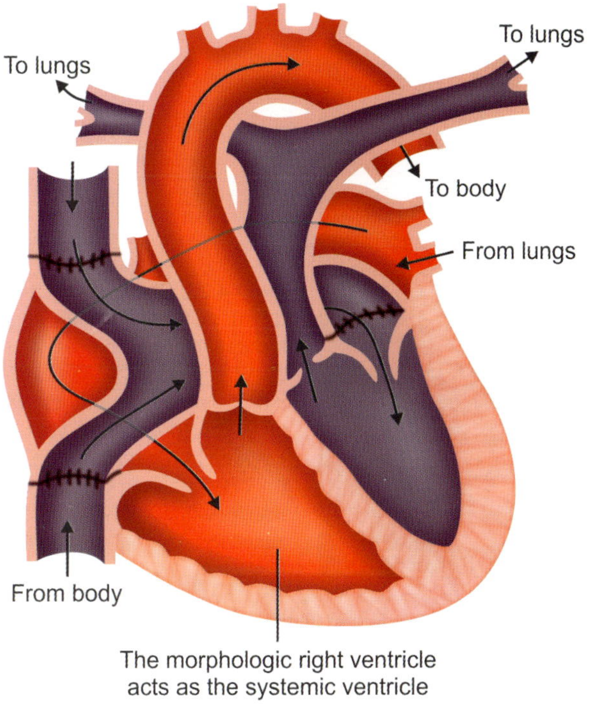

Fig. 44.24: In the Mustard or Senning operations, a baffle is created that shunts systemic venous blood returning via the superior vena cava (SVC) and inferior vena cava (IVC) into the morphological left ventricle (mLV), which is then pumped into the pulmonary arteries (PA) to the lungs. The procedure also shunts oxygenated blood returning from the lungs via the pulmonary veins (PV) into the morphological right ventricle (mRV), where it is then pumped into the aorta (Ao) and the systemic arterial circulation. These procedures were performed before the adoption of the arterial switch procedure, and may still be necessary in some patients in whom morphological features preclude the use of the arterial switch operation.

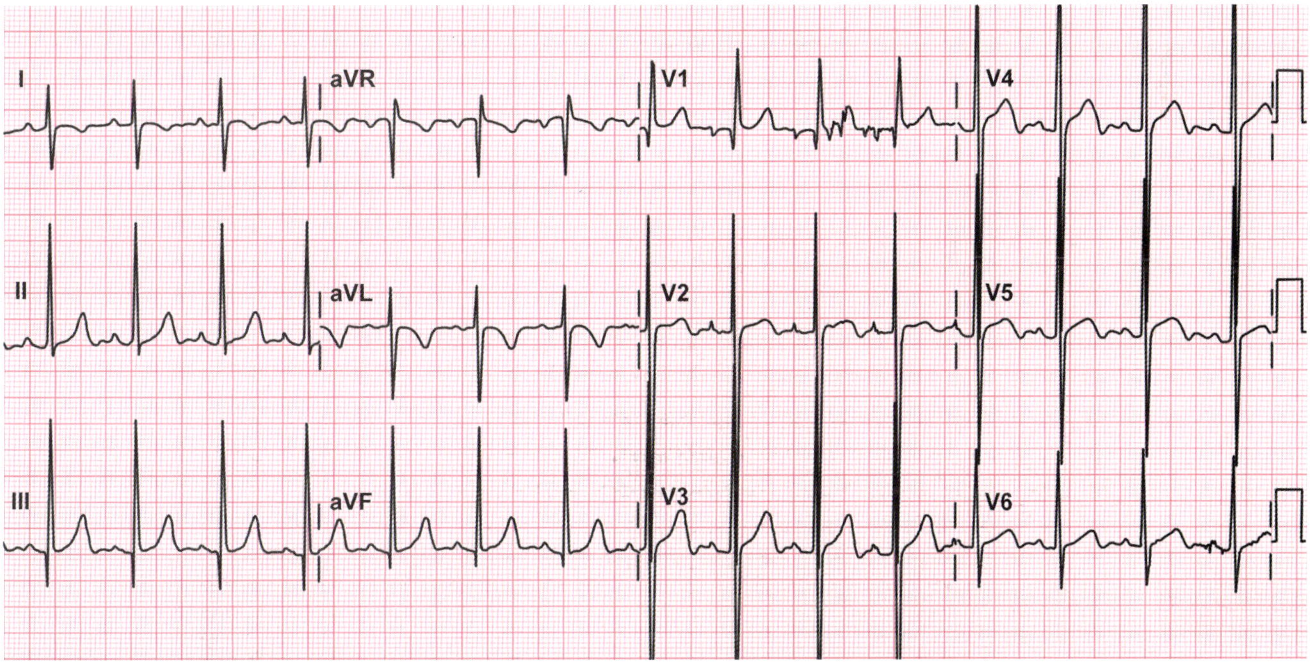

Fig. 44.25: Electrocardiogram (ECG) in corrected transposition of the great arteries (TGA). Due to the mirror-imaged arrangement of the bundle branches in the presence of left-handed ventricular topology, the initial activation of the ventricles will be from right to left, represented in the ECG by Q waves in the right precordial leads, and an absent Q wave in the left precordial leads. (Image and legend text from Wallis G, Debich-Spicer D, Anderson RH. Congenitally corrected transposition. Orphanet J Rare Dis. 2011;6:22).

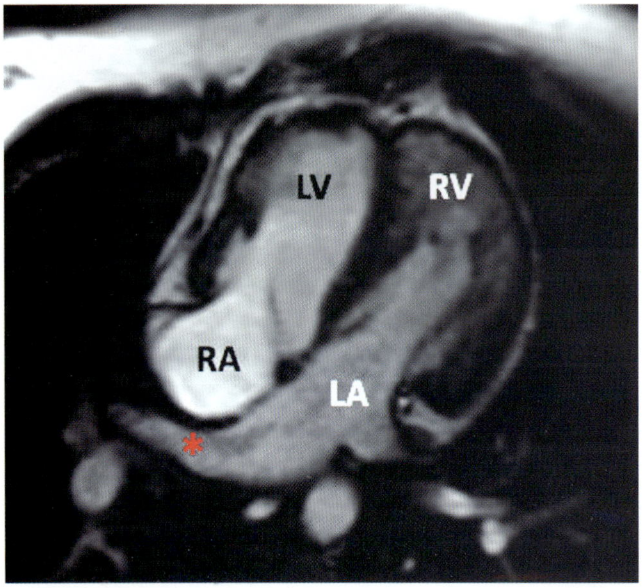

Fig. 44.26: Oblique cut T2-weighted magnetic resonance imaging (MRI) of four-chamber cardiac view of congenitally corrected-transposition of the great arteries (cc-TGA) patient with levocardia. The right atrium (RA) empties into a right-sided, smooth-walled, morphologic left ventricle (mLV). A star (*) labels the entrance of a right pulmonary vein (PV) into the left atrium (LA), which empties into a trabeculated, left-sided, morphologic right ventricle (mRV). [Image from Flack AC, Graham TP. Congenitally corrected transposition of the great arteries. In: Rao PS (Ed). Congenital Heart Disease—Selected Aspects. InTech]. (LV: Left ventricle; RV: Right ventricle).

REFERENCES

de Koning WB, van Osch-Gevers M, Ten Harkel AD, et al. Follow-up outcomes 10 years after arterial switch operation for transposition of the great arteries: comparison of cardiological health status and health-related quality of life to those of the a normal reference population. Eur J Pediatr. 2008;167(9):995-1004.

Ferguson EC, Krishnamurthy R, Oldham SA. Classic imaging signs of congenital cardiovascular abnormalities. Radiographics. 2007;27(5):1323-34.

International Society of Ultrasound in Obstetrics and Gynecology, Carvalho JS, Allan LD, et al. ISUOG Practice Guidelines (updated): sonographic screening examination of the fetal heart. Ultrasound Obstet Gynecol. 2013;41(3):348-59.

Marino B, Corno A, Carotti A, et al. Pediatric cardiac surgery guided by echocardiography. Established indications and new trends. Scand J Thorac Cardiovasc Surg. 1990;24(3):197-201.

Martins P, Castela E. Transposition of the great arteries. Orphanet J Rare Dis. 2008;3:27.

Martins P, Tran V, Price G, et al. Extending the surgical boundaries in the management of the left ventricular outflow tract obstruction in discordant ventriculo-arterial connections—a surgical and morphological study. Cardiol Young. 2008;18(2):124-34.

Tworetzky W, McElhinney DB, Brook MM, et al. Echocardiographic diagnosis alone for the complete repair of major congenital heart defects. J Am Coll Cardiol. 1999;33(1):228-33.

Wallis G, Debich-Spicer D, Anderson RH. Congenitally corrected transposition. Orphanet J Rare Dis. 2011;6:22.

CHAPTER

Supravalvular and Subvalvular Aortic Stenosis

45

Glenn N Levine, Luc M Beauchesne

Supravalvular and subvalvular aortic stenosis (SAS) are both, along with valvular aortic stenosis, types of left ventricular outflow obstruction. Supravalvular and SAS share many of the physiological characteristics and symptomatology of valvular aortic stenosis. It is important to recognize and distinguish the three types of left ventricular obstructive diseases (Table 45.1).

SUPRAVALVULAR AORTIC STENOSIS

Supravalvular aortic stenosis (SVAS) is usually a congenital defect in which there is focal or diffuse narrowing of the ascending aorta beyond the sinus of Valsalva. In many patients, SVAS is due to a mutation in or deletion of the *ELN* gene, which is involved in production of the protein elastin. This form of SVAS is part of Williams syndrome. Other forms of SVAS include a non-Williams familial subtype or sporadic type; SVAS may also occasionally be seen in patients with familial hypercholesterolemia.

There are three anatomic types (Figs. 45.1A to C) of SVAS: (1) an "hourglass" type; (2) diffuse narrowing of the ascending aorta; and (3) a discrete membrane above the aortic valve. Representative images of SVAS are shown in Figures 45.2 to 45.9.

Outflow obstruction leads to concentric left ventricular hypertrophy. Since the origins of the coronary arteries are proximal to the obstruction, the coronary arteries are subject to high systolic pressures, become tortuous and dilated, and may develop premature atherosclerosis. The outflow obstruction may in cases also partially or completely obstruct the coronary ostia.

Table 45.1: Distinguishing features of subvalvular aortic stenosis, valvular aortic stenosis, and supravalvular aortic stenosis. (Table adapted from Vijayalakshmi IB, Vimala J. Left ventricular outflow tract obstruction. In: Vijayalakshmi IB, Rao PS, Chugh R (Eds). Comprehensive Approach to Congenital Heart Disease. New Delhi, India: Jaypee Brothers Medical Publishers (P) Ltd.; 2013).

Feature	*Subvalvular Aortic Stenosis*	*Valvular Aortic Stenosis*	*Supravalvular Aortic Stenosis*
Face	Normal	Normal	"Elfin"
Pulse	Normal to anacrotic	Normal to anacrotic (parvus et tardus)	Right radial/brachial > left radial/brachial
Apical impulse	Heaving	Heaving	Heaving
Ejection click	Uncommon	Present in bicuspid valve stenosis	Absent
Ejection systolic murmur	Left second and third intercostal spaces	Right first intercostal space, radiating to carotids	Right first and second intercostal spaces, radiating to right carotid
Early diastolic murmur	Common	May be present	Uncommon
Transthoracic echocardiography findings	Subaortic membrane or tunnel with gradient and aortic regurgitation	Aortic valve thickening	Hourglass appearance or membrane in aorta with gradient
Angiography	Gradient and aortic regurgitation, visible membrane	"Prussian helmet" appearance	Narrowing in ascending aorta

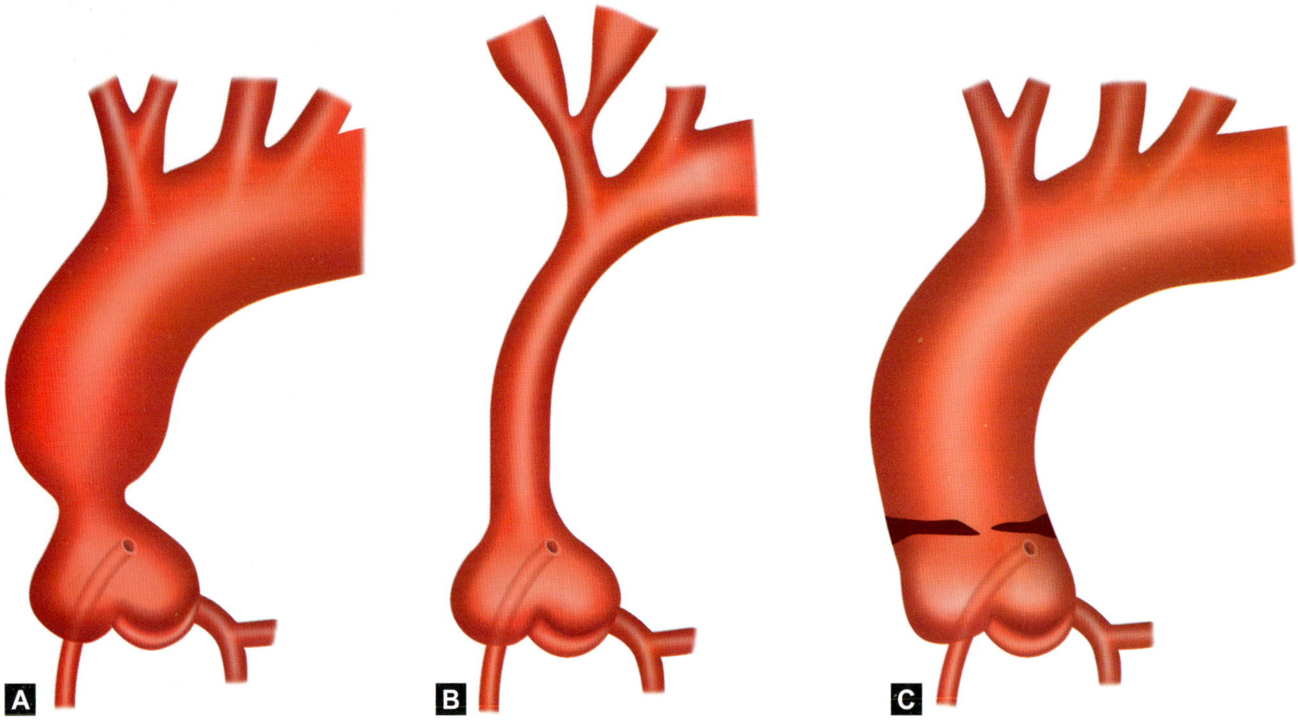

Figs. 45.1A to C: Types of supravalvular aortic stenosis. (A) Hourglass type; (B) Diffuse narrowing of the ascending aorta; (C) Discrete membrane above the aortic valve. (Image and legend text from Vijayalakshmi IB, Vimala J. Left ventricular outflow tract obstruction. In: Vijayalakshmi IB, Rao PS, Chugh R (Eds). Comprehensive Approach to Congenital Heart Disease. New Delhi, India: Jaypee Brothers Medical Publishers (P) Ltd.; 2013).

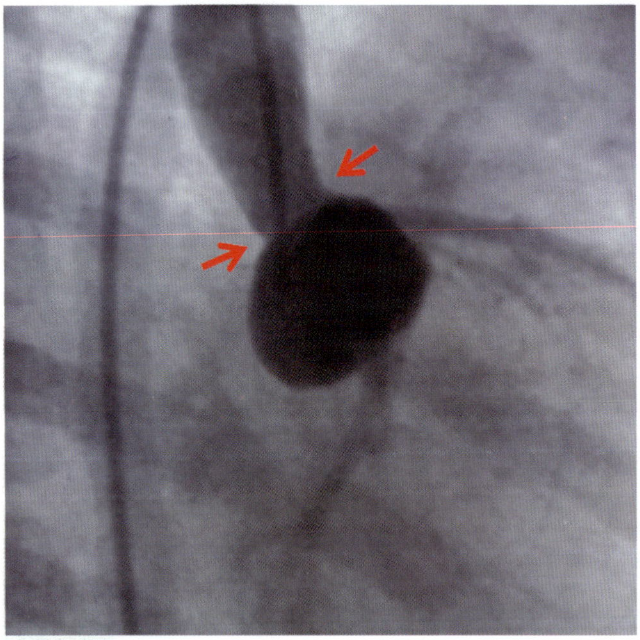

Fig. 45.2A: Aortic root angiogram demonstrating supravalvular aortic stenosis (arrows). Note the "hourglass" appearance. (Image and legend text from Vijayalakshmi IB, Vimala J. Left ventricular outflow tract obstruction. In: Vijayalakshmi IB, Rao PS, Chugh R, (Eds). Comprehensive Approach to Congenital Heart Disease. New Delhi, India: Jaypee Brothers Medical Publishers (P) Ltd.; 2013).

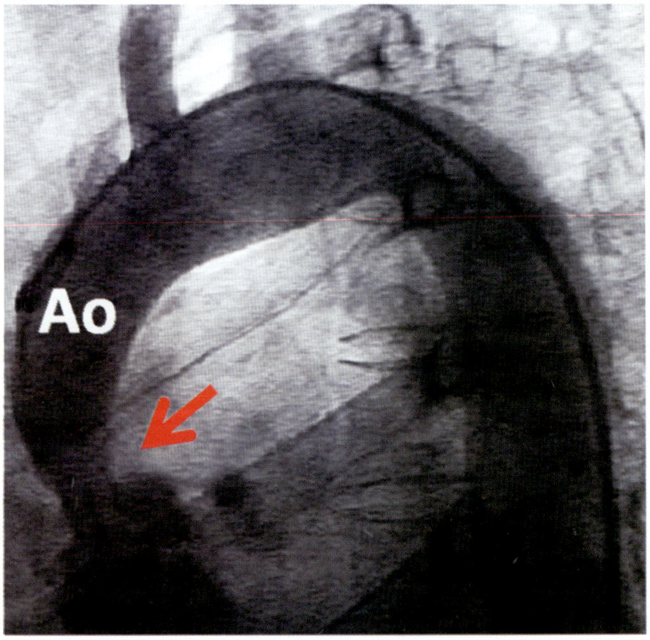

Fig. 45.2B: Angiogram demonstrating supravalvular aortic stenosis (arrow). (Image from Ferlan G, De Pasquale C, Losito C, et al. Diffuse supravalvular aortic stenosis: surgical repair in adulthood. Cardiol Res Pract. 2009;2009:976190). (Ao: Aorta).

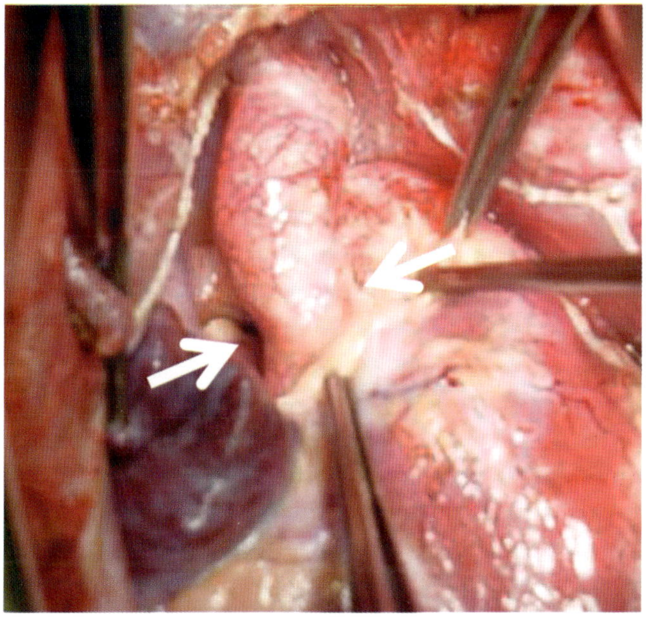

Fig. 45.3: Intraoperative image of supravalvular aortic stenosis (arrows). [Image from Bonini RC, Palazzi EM, Chaccur P, et al. Supravalvular aortic stenosis surgical repair using modified Sousa's technique. Rev Bras Cir Cardiovasc. 2010;25(2):253-6].

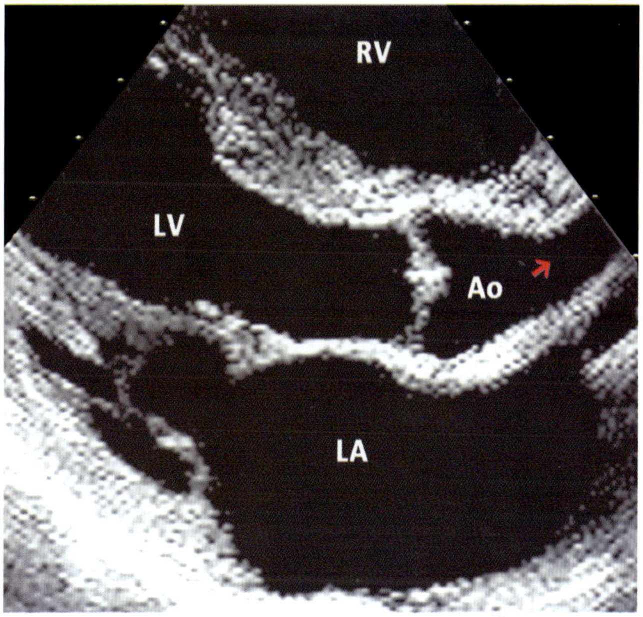

Fig. 45.4: Parasternal long-axis transthoracic echocardiogram showing supravalvular aortic stenosis with diffuse narrowing of the aorta (arrow). [Image and legend text from Vijayalakshmi IB, Vimala J. Left ventricular outflow tract obstruction. In: Vijayalakshmi IB, Rao PS, Chugh R (Eds). Comprehensive Approach to Congenital Heart Disease. New Delhi, India: Jaypee Brothers Medical Publishers (P) Ltd.; 2013]. (Ao: Aorta; LA: Left atrium; LV: Left ventricle; RV: Right ventricle).

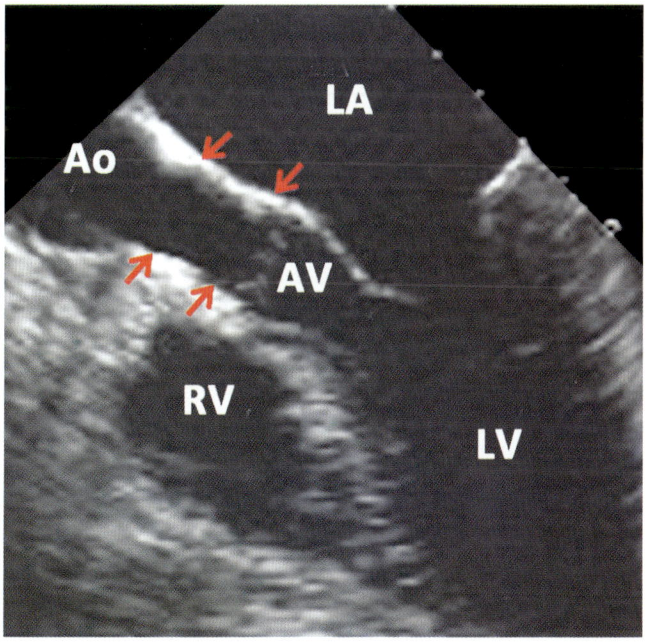

Fig. 45.5: Transesophageal echocardiogram of tubular hypoplasia of the ascending aorta. (Image from Espinola-Zavaleta N, Muñoz-Castellanos L, Kuri-Nivon M, et al. Aortic obstruction: anatomy and echocardiography. Cardiovascular Ultrasound. 2006;4:36). (Ao: Aorta; AV: Aortic valve; LA: Left atrium; LV: Left ventricle; RV: Right ventricle).

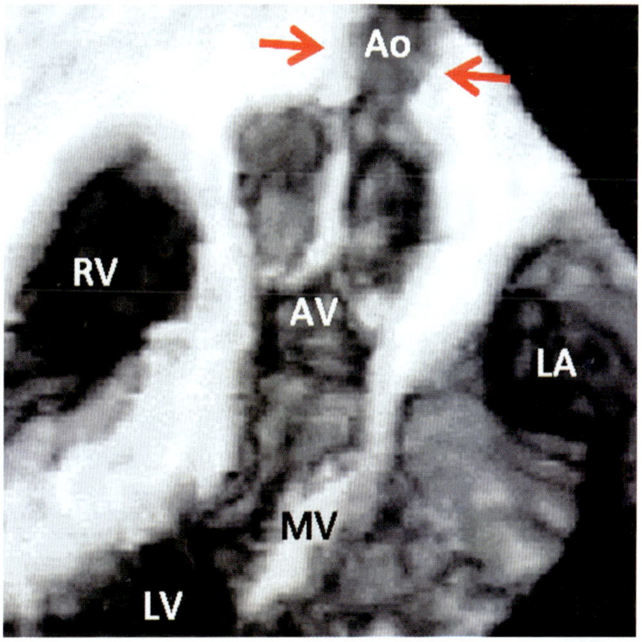

Fig. 45.6: Three-dimensional transesophageal image of supravalvular aortic stenosis (arrows). (Image from Espinola-Zavaleta N, Muñoz-Castellanos L, Kuri-Nivon M, et al. Aortic obstruction: anatomy and echocardiography. Cardiovascular Ultrasound. 2006;4:36). (Ao: Aorta; AV: Aortic valve; LA: Left atrium; LV: Left ventricle; MV: Mitral valve; RV: Right ventricle).

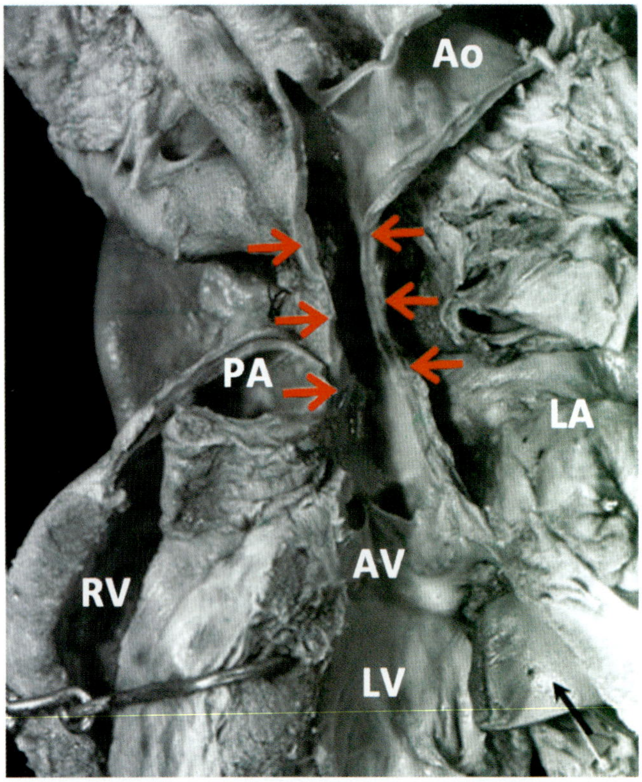

Fig. 45.7: Gross pathology specimen of tubular hypoplasia of the ascending aorta (arrows). (Image from Espinola-Zavaleta N, Muñoz-Castellanos L, Kuri-Nivon M, et al. Aortic obstruction: anatomy and echocardiography. Cardiovascular Ultrasound. 2006;4:36). (Ao: Aorta; AV: Aortic valve; LA: Left atrium; LV: Left ventricle; RV: Right ventricle; PA: Pulmonary artery).

Patients may initially come to medical attention from recognition of a heart murmur. The systolic ejection murmur is heard in the right upper sternal area and can be mistaken for the murmur of aortic stenosis. Pulses and blood pressure are typically greater in the right arm, as due to a Coandă effect, the poststenotic blood flow jet preferentially is directed toward the brachiocephalic artery. Symptomatology usually develops in the first several decades of life. Symptoms may include exertional dyspnea, angina, and syncope, symptomatology similar to that of valvular aortic stenosis.

Initial workup of patients with suspected SVAS is transthoracic echocardiography (TTE). A comprehensive evaluation is critical in identifying SVAS. Of note, spectral Doppler examination may show a higher gradient than catheter-measured gradients. Transesophageal echocardiography can usually provide greater anatomic information than TTE. CT and MRA examinations may also be used to better define the exact anatomic abnormalities.

Surgical intervention is recommended in patients with symptoms and/or Doppler mean gradient of > 50 mm Hg. Asymptomatic patients with lower gradients can be managed conservatively.

SUBVALVULAR AORTIC STENOSIS

Subvalvular aortic stenosis, also referred to as subaortic stenosis, is due to mechanical obstruction of left ventricular outflow (Figs. 45.10 to 45.15). Although classified as a form of congenital heart disease, SAS is seldom present at birth. It is usually a progressive process that is thought to be secondary to abnormal underlying left ventricular outflow tract geometry. Important to pet owners, SAS is a frequent disease in many breeds of dogs.

There are three basic recognized types of SAS: (1) discrete membrane; (2) fibromuscular ridge; and (3) diffuse fibromuscular tunnel-like obstruction.

Approximately half of patients with SAS have other associated congenital heart defects such as bicuspid aortic valve, aortic coarctation, ventricular septal defect, or patent ductus arteriosus.

Physical examination is notable for a systolic ejection murmur best heard at the left sternal border. A palpable left parasternal and/or carotid thrill is often present. A diastolic murmur due to aortic regurgitation may be present.

Progressive obstruction from SAS leads to concentric hypertrophy. Interventricular septal bulging may develop, further exacerbating the obstruction. Valvular dysfunction, particularly aortic regurgitation, is common. Aortic regurgitation is thought to be related to chronic damage to the aortic valve from a high velocity jet.

As with valvular aortic stenosis, the most common symptoms are dyspnea on exertion, angina, and presyncope or syncope.

Transthoracic echocardiography remains the workhorse for initial evaluation of patients with suspected SAS. Not infrequently, with TTE the subaortic membrane is not well visualized and transesophageal echocardiography (TEE) is required to further define the anatomy.

Conservative therapy is usually recommended in patients with peak-to-peak or Doppler mean gradients of < 30 mm Hg who are asymptomatic and have no left ventricular dilation, dysfunction or progressively increasing aortic regurgitation. Surgery (Fig. 45.16) is usually recommended in those with peak gradients ≥ 50 mm Hg or mean gradients ≥ 30 mm Hg.

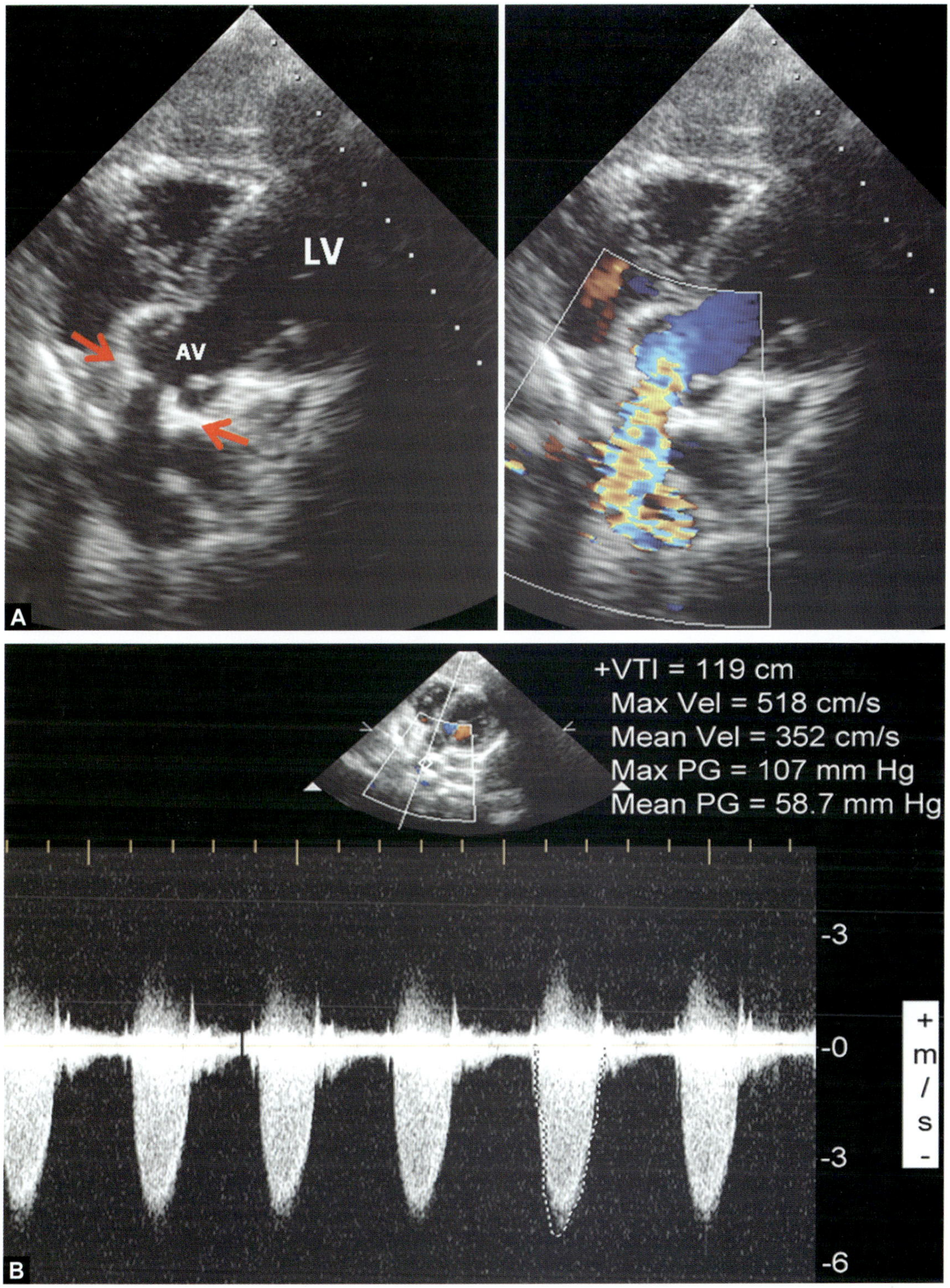

Figs. 45.8A and B: Apical five-chamber transthoracic echocardiography demonstrating a discrete membrane causing supravalvular aortic stenosis. (A) The discrete membrane (arrows) is seen just above the aortic valve (AV). Color Doppler demonstrates turbulent flow across and beyond the membrane; (B) Continuous wave (CW) Doppler demonstrates a maximum velocity across the membrane of 5.18 cm/s, translating into a peak transmembrane gradient of 107 mm Hg. (Image and legend text adapted from Vijayalakshmi IB, Vimala J. Left ventricular outflow tract obstruction. In: Vijayalakshmi IB, Rao PS, Chugh R (Eds). Comprehensive Approach to Congenital Heart Disease. New Delhi, India: Jaypee Brothers Medical Publishers (P) Ltd.; 2013).

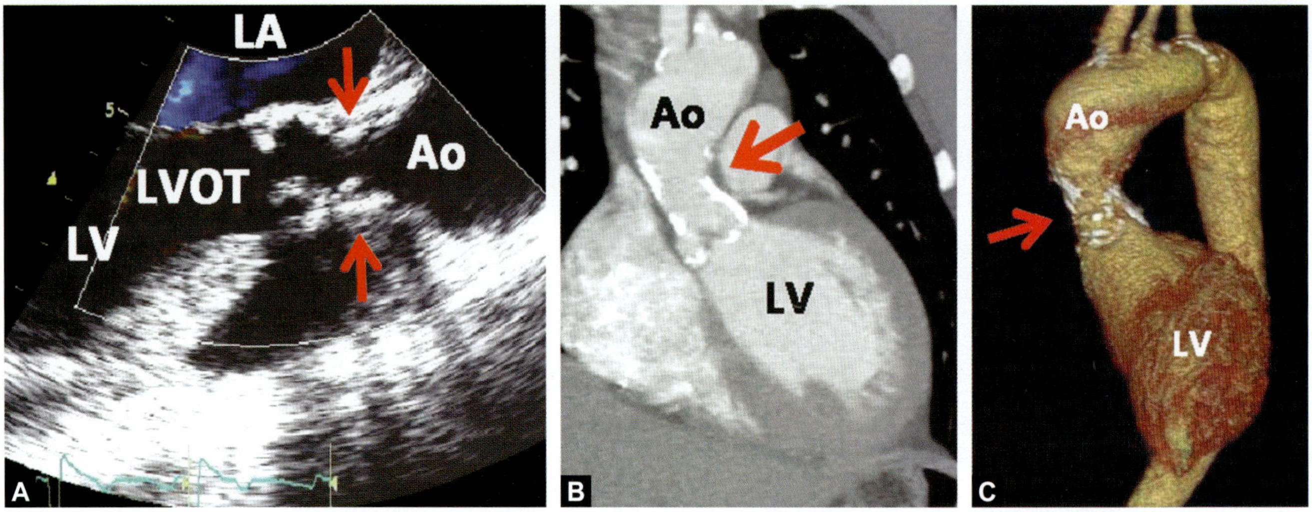

Figs. 45.9A to C: An uncommon form of supravalvular aortic stenosis (arrows) in a 46-year-old patient with familial hypercholesterolemia. There is atheroma and calcification in the proximal ascending aorta. (A) Transesophageal long-axis view; (B) Maximum intensity projection (MIP) CT image; (C) Volume rendered CT image. (Image from Akturk F, Yalçın AA, Ertürk M, et al. Valvular and supravalvular aortic stenosis secondary to familial hyperlipidemia. J Cardiovasc Dis Diagn. 2013;1:1). (Ao: Aorta; LA: Left atrium; LV: Left ventricle; LVOT: Left ventricular outflow tract).

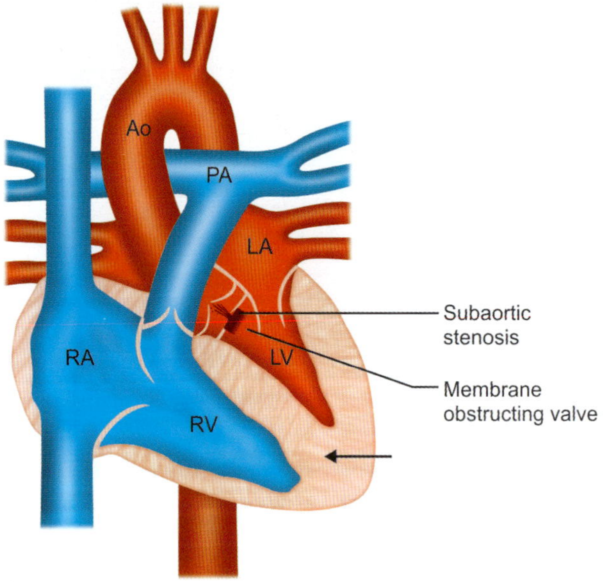

Fig. 45.10: Schematic illustration of subvalvular stenosis. (Ao: Aorta; LA: Left atrium; LV: Left ventricle; RA: Right atrium; RV: Right ventiricle; PA: Pulmonary artery).

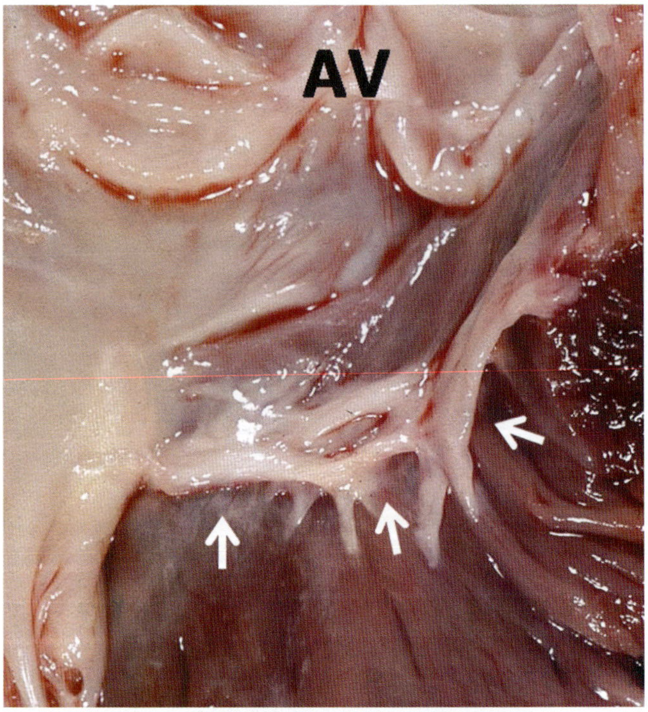

Fig. 45.11: Gross pathology image demonstrating a subvalvular membrane (arrows) below the aortic valve (AV). (Image courtesy of Dr Kathrin Glatz, Universitätsspital Basel, Switzerland. Image from Pathorama website www.pathorama.ch. Dr Glatz and the website retain copyright of this image).

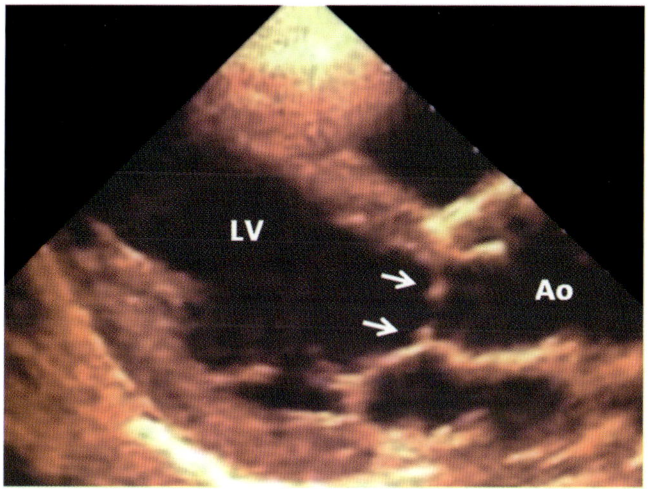

Fig. 45.12A: Parasternal long-axis transthoracic echocardiogram demonstrating a discrete subaortic membrane (arrows) just below the aortic valve. (Image and legend text from Vijayalakshmi IB, Vimala J. Left ventricular outflow tract obstruction. In: Vijayalakshmi IB, Rao PS, Chugh R (Eds). Comprehensive Approach to Congenital Heart Disease. New Delhi, India: Jaypee Brothers Medical Publishers (P) Ltd.; 2013).

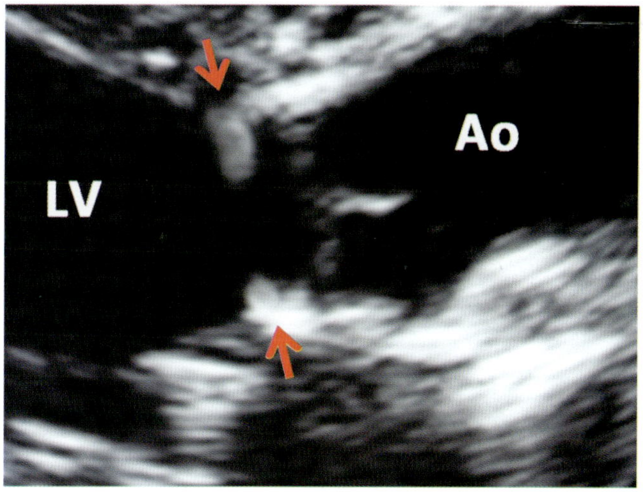

Fig. 45.12B: Transthoracic parasternal long image showing a subaortic membrane (arrows).

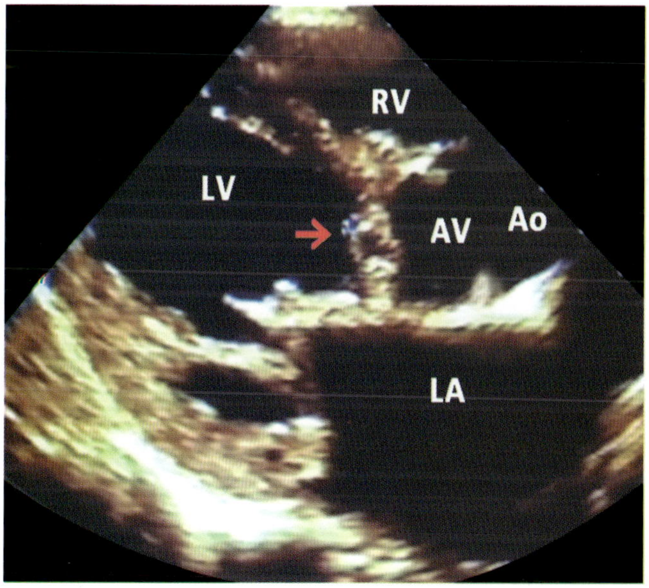

Fig. 45.13: Parasternal long-axis transthoracic echocardiogram in a young child showing severe subaortic stenosis caused by a dense fibromuscular collar (arrow). There is a narrow orifice and severe obstruction (gradient 114 mm Hg). (Image and legend text from Vijayalakshmi IB, Vimala J. Left ventricular outflow tract obstruction. In: Vijayalakshmi IB, Rao PS, Chugh R (Eds). Comprehensive Approach to Congenital Heart Disease. New Delhi, India: Jaypee Brothers Medical Publishers (P) Ltd.; 2013).

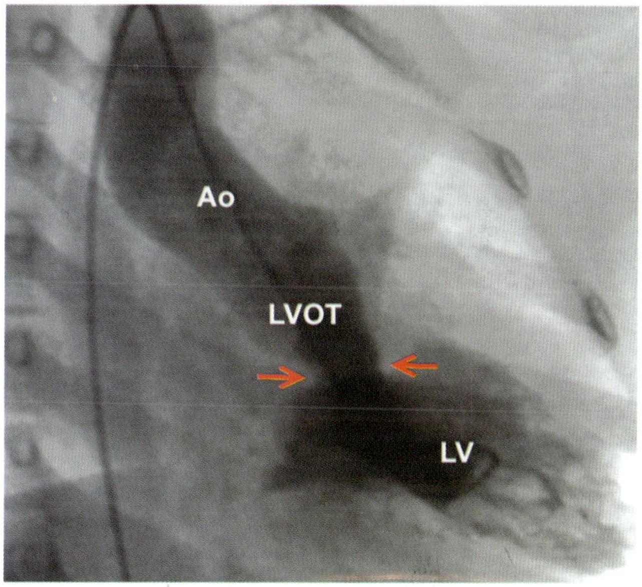

Fig. 45.14: Left ventriculography demonstrating subaortic obstruction (arrows). Systolic LV pressure was 190 mm Hg and systolic pressure above and just below the aortic valve was 114 mm Hg. (Image and legend text from Vijayalakshmi IB, Vimala J. Left ventricular outflow tract obstruction. In: Vijayalakshmi IB, Rao PS, Chugh R (Eds). Comprehensive Approach to Congenital Heart Disease. New Delhi, India: Jaypee Brothers Medical Publishers (P) Ltd.; 2013).

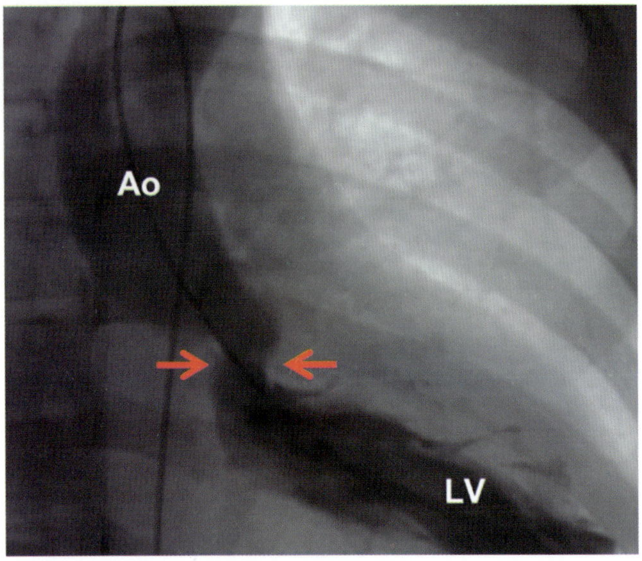

Fig. 45.15: Ventriculogram from a patient with subvalvular aortic stenosis (arrows). [Image from Vijayalakshmi IB, Vimala J. Left ventricular outflow tract obstruction. In: Vijayalakshmi IB, Rao PS, Chugh R (Eds). Comprehensive Approach to Congenital Heart Disease. New Delhi, India: Jaypee Brothers Medical Publishers (P) Ltd.; 2013].

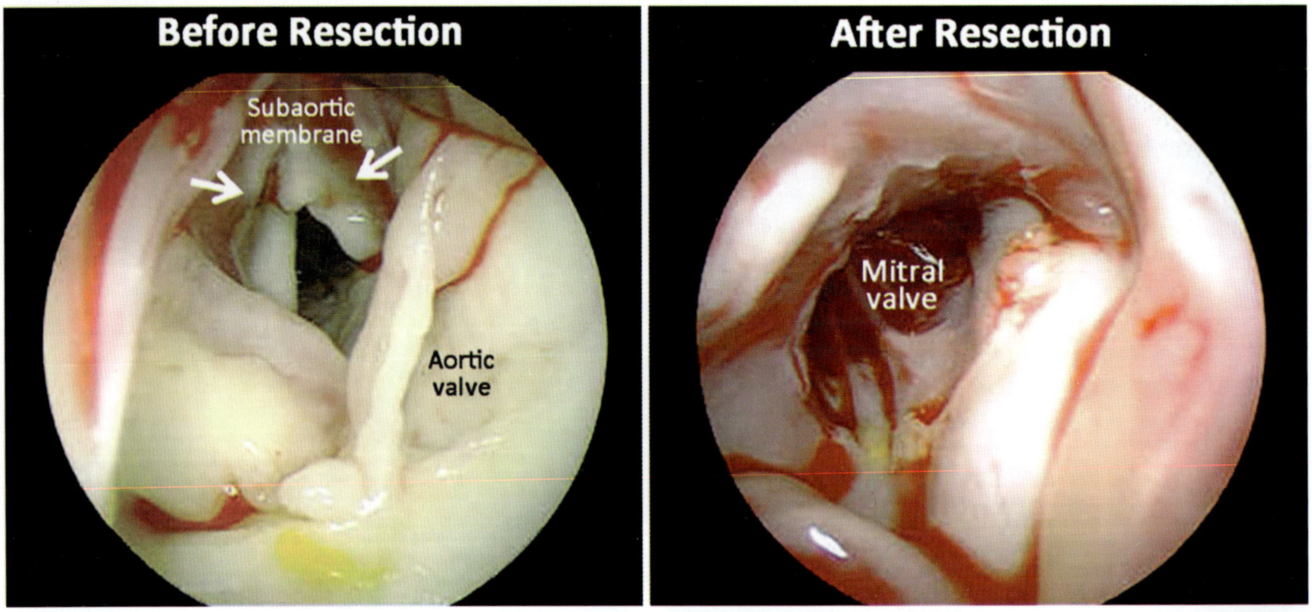

Fig. 45.16: Surgeon's view of subvalvular membrane before and after resection. (Image courtesy of Owen White and CardioAccess, Inc. Image from CardioAccess website http://www.cardioaccess.com/OpImages/Diagrams/diagSM.html).

Importantly for those who care for adults with congenital heart disease, although initial surgical success rates are excellent, 20% of patients will have some long-term recurrence of outflow obstruction. Progressive aortic regurgitation can also happen in some postoperative patients.

CHAPTER

46

Aortic Coarctation

Unnati H Doshi, P Syamasundar Rao

INTRODUCTION

Coarctation of the aorta is a congenital cardiac anomaly in which there is narrowing of the proximal thoracic aorta (Figs. 46.1 to 46.5, Video 46.1). The aortic coarctation may be discrete or a long segment of the aorta may be narrowed. It is commonly associated with varying degrees of hypoplasia of the transverse aortic arch and isthmus of the aortic arch (Fig. 46.6). The coarctation may rarely involve the abdominal aorta and, in such cases, it may be a variant of Takayasu's arteritis (Figs. 46.7 and 46.8).

Typically, the narrowing is seen distal to the origin of the left subclavian artery, around the point of insertion of the ductus arteriosus, and is aptly described as juxtaductal; the previously used terms such as preductal (infantile) and postductal (adult) are not warranted. Pathologic examination demonstrates localized medial and intimal thickening of the coarcted segment that forms a posterior infolding; the so-called "posterior shelf" or it may be a membranous curtain-like structure with a central or eccentric opening.

Coarctation of the aorta accounts for 5–8% of all congenital heart defects and has a slight male preponderance in older patients. Associated anomalies are listed in Table 46.1; bicuspid aortic valve is most frequent and is seen in two-thirds of the neonates and in one-third of older patients. Approximately, 35% of patients with Turner syndrome have coarctation of the aorta.

Coarctation is an important and treatable cause of systemic arterial hypertension. The theories postulated to explain hypertension are (1) development of higher blood pressure to overcome the mechanical obstruction, and (2) activation of the rennin-angiotensin system secondary to decreased renal blood flow. Over time, these patients tend to develop left ventricular hypertrophy as well as collateral vessels that connect the areas above with those below the level of the coarctation.

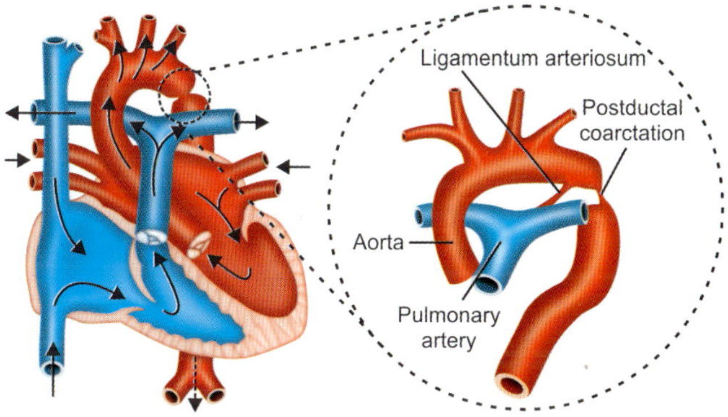

Fig. 46.1: Artist's rendition of the aortic arch and heart from a posterolateral view demonstrating aortic coarctation (highlighted), slightly distal to the origin of the left subclavian artery. (DAo: Descending aorta; LA: Left atrium; LCC: Left common carotid artery; LSCA: Left subclavian artery; RA: Right atrium; RINN: Right innominate artery; RV: Right ventricle).

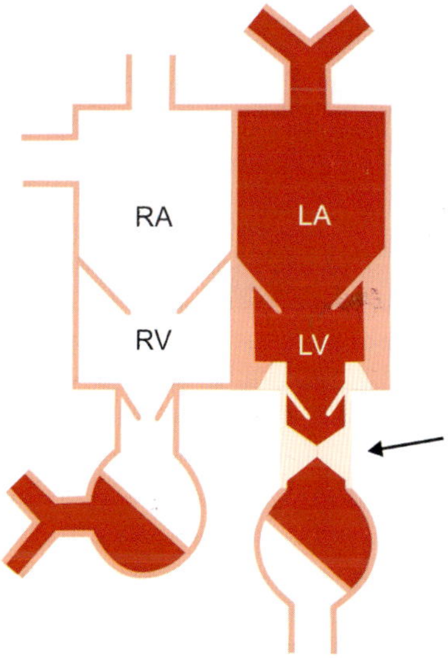

Fig. 46.2: Box diagram of the heart illustrating hypertrophy of the left ventricle (LV) and coarctation (arrow).

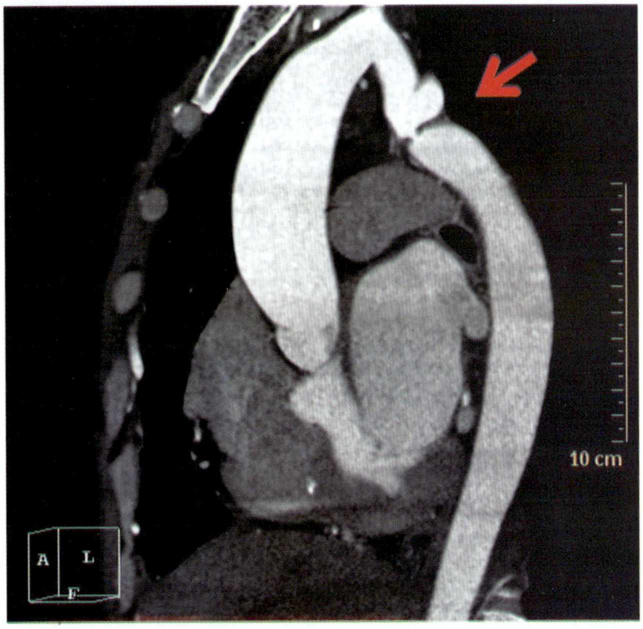

Fig. 46.3: Two-dimensional maximum intensity projection (MIP) image of severe aortic coarctation (arrow). (Image courtesy of Dr Cafer Zorkun).

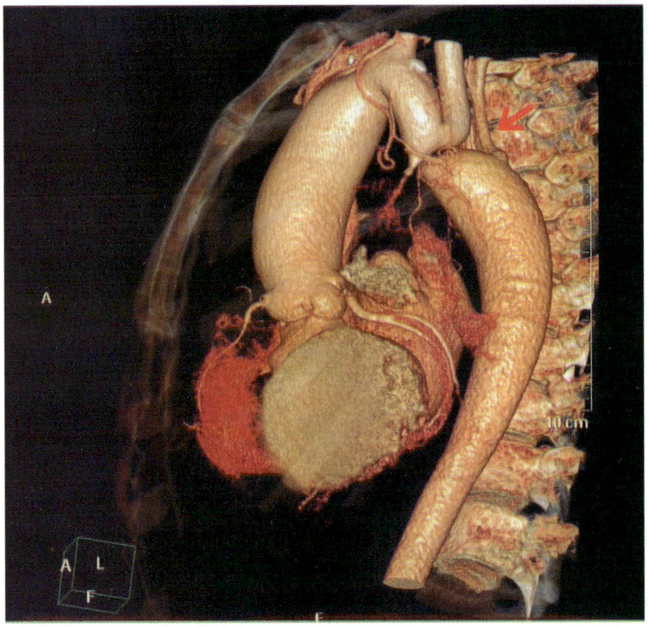

Fig. 46.4: Three-dimensional CT image of aortic coarctation (arrow). (Image courtesy of Dr Cafer Zorkun).

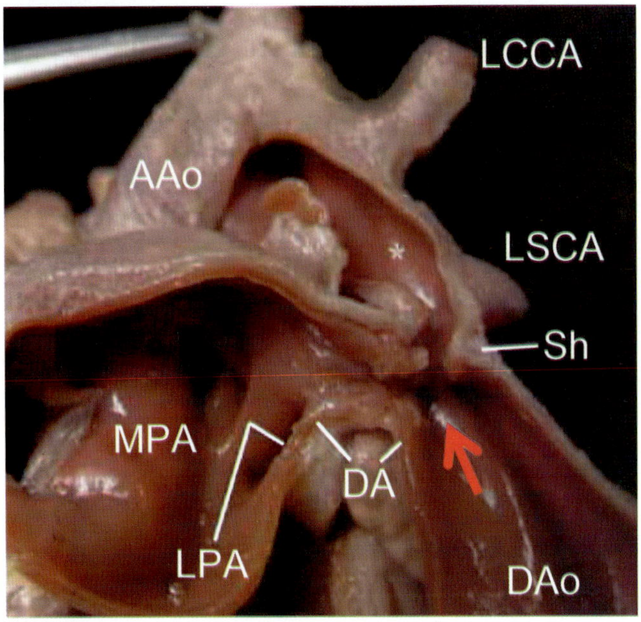

Fig. 46.5: Dissected gross pathology image showing a discrete aortic coarctation (arrow). The posterior shelf (Sh) is seen just distal to the left subclavian artery. The ductus arteriosus is opposite the posterior shelf. Note the fleshy, corrugated appearance of the ductus tissue, completely different from either the main pulmonary artery (MPA) or the descending aorta (DAo). The distal arch (*) is mildly narrow. [Image and legend text from Romth A, Pluchinotta FR, Porayette P, et al. Congenital heart defects in adults: a field guide for cardiologists. J Clin Exp Cardiolog. 2012;(Suppl 8). pii: 007]. (AAo: Ascending aorta; DA: Ductus arteriosus; DAo: Descending aorta; LPA: Left pulmonary artery; LSCA: Left subclavian artery; MPA: Main pulmonary artery).

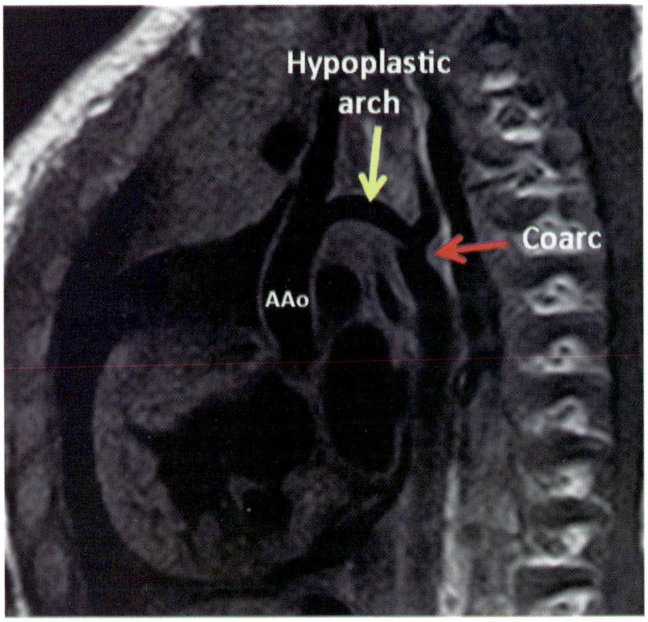

Fig. 46.6: Magnetic resonance imaging study of the aortic arch demonstrating coarcted (Coarc) segment (red arrow) and a hypoplastic aortic arch (yellow arrow). (AAo: Ascending thoracic aorta).

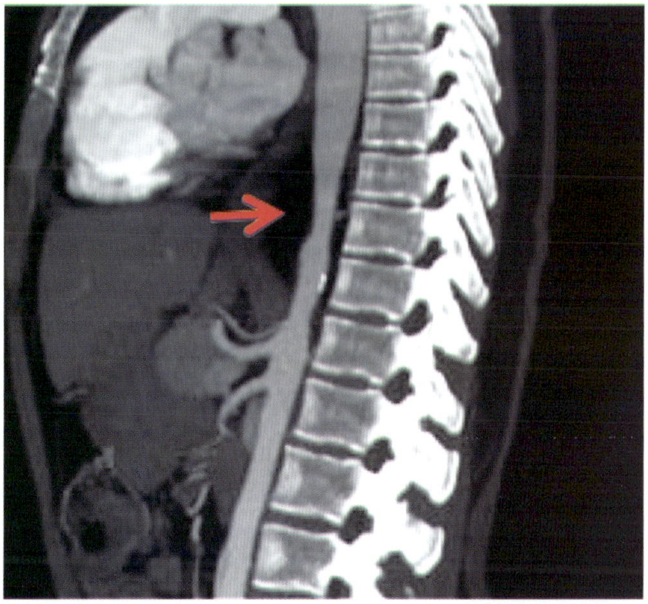

Fig. 46.7: Narrowing of the descending aorta (arrow) due to Takayasu's arteritis. (Image from Konopka C, Braun SK, Machado G. Takayasu's arteritis and Crohn's disease: an unusual association. J Vasc Bras. 2009;8:4).

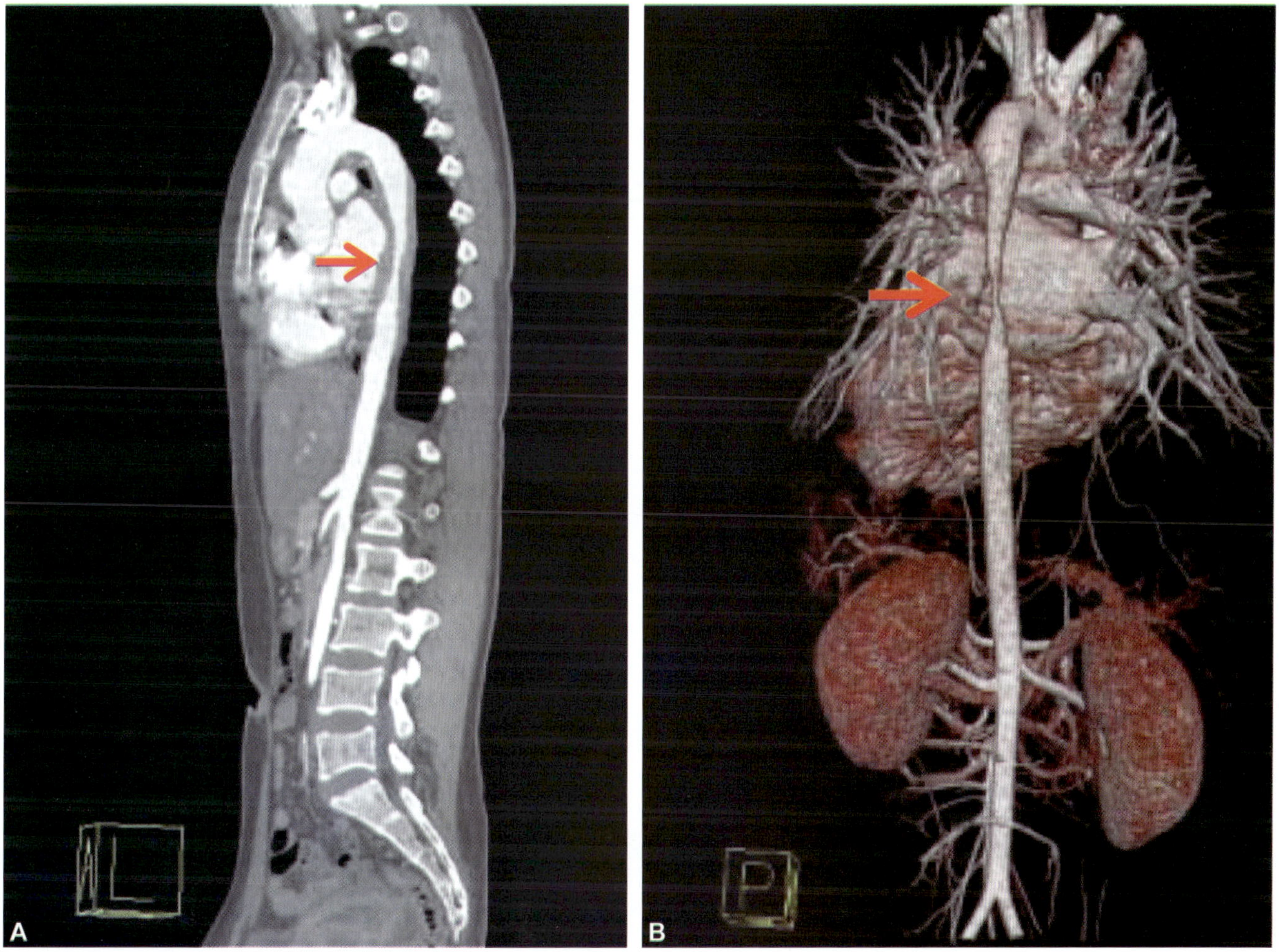

Figs. 46.8A and B: Two-dimensional and three-dimensional CT scan images demonstrating stenosis (arrow) of the descending thoracic aorta in a patient with Takayasu's arteritis. Note the thickened aortic wall visible in the two-dimensional image (left panel). [Bao N. Aortic isthmus arteritis: report of one case. Cardiol Res. 2011;2(6):301-3].

CLINICAL FEATURES

The most common mode of presentation in older children, adolescents and adults is hypertension and/or a systolic murmur detected on routine examination. The diagnosis can be made by findings of delayed or absent femoral arterial pulses as well as an arm-to-leg systolic blood pressure difference of more than 20 mm Hg in favor of arms (Fig. 46.9). It is important that blood pressures are obtained in both arms and either leg because the site of coarctation may involve the origin of the left subclavian artery or an aberrant right subclavian artery arises distal to coarctation. Other findings on examination may include increased left ventricular impulse, thrill in the suprasternal notch, an ejection systolic click [due to associated bicuspid aortic valve (Fig. 46.10)] and an ejection systolic murmur at the right upper sternal border. A continuous murmur may be heard in the left interscapular region due to flow across the coarcted segment or on the back due to collateral vessels. Rare modes of presentation in untreated adult coarctation patients are premature coronary artery disease or aortic dissection. In neonates and young infants, signs of congestive heart failure due to associated defects or sudden closure of the ductus arteriosus are the presenting features.

Table 46.1: Cardiac defects associated with aortic coarctation.

Bicuspid aortic valve
Aortic stenosis
Patent ductus arteriosus (usually seen in neonates and infants)
Ventricular septal defect (usually seen in neonates and infants)
Mitral valve anomalies
Complex, cyanotic congenital heart defects (usually seen in neonates and infants)*
Cerebral aneurysms

*Transposition of the great arteries, Taussig-Bing anomaly, double-inlet left ventricle, tricuspid atresia with transposition of the great arteries and hypoplastic left heart syndrome.

LABORATORY STUDIES

Chest X-Ray and Electrocardiograph

Laboratory investigations such as chest X-ray and ECG may be abnormal, but are not diagnostic. Chest X-ray findings include rib notching (Figs. 46.11 and 46.12) due to collateral vessels and abnormal contour of the localized aortic indentation on a frontal film giving the "figure of 3" sign. Neonates and infants may have cardiomegaly either due to associated defects or due to myocardial dysfunction. ECG may be normal but may show left ventricular hypertrophy with or without strain pattern.

Echocardiogram

Echocardiographic studies provide an adequate assessment in most cases of aortic coarctation. The normal aortic arch can easily be shown in suprasternal echocardiographic views (Figs. 46.13A and B) in normal individuals.

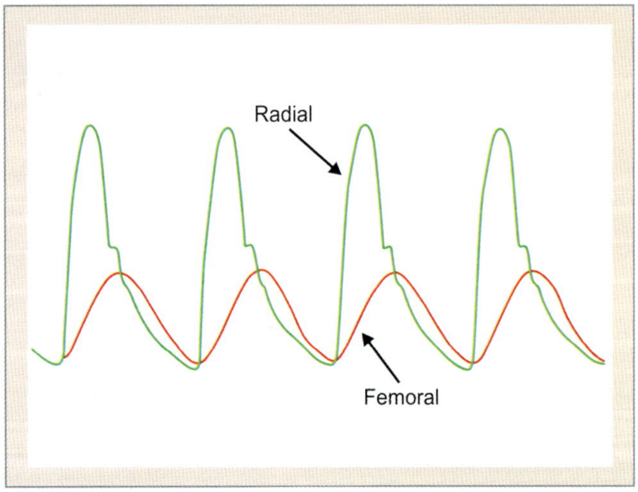

Fig. 46.9: Illustration of simultaneous radial and femoral artery blood pressure tracings in a patient with aortic coarctation. Note the delayed and markedly diminished femoral artery arterial pressure.

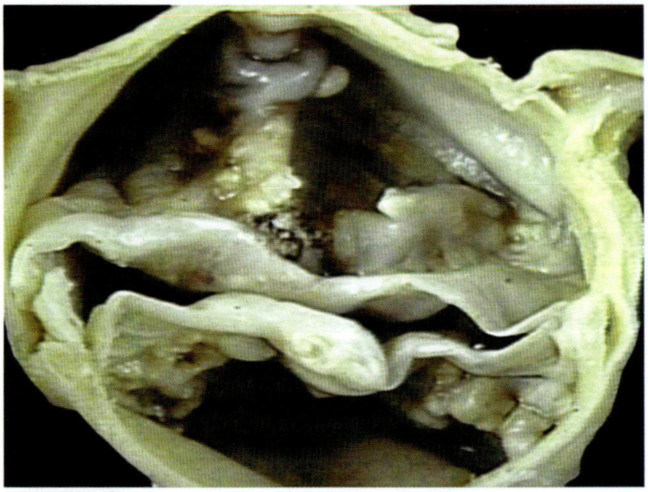

Fig. 46.10: Gross pathology specimen of a bicuspid aortic valve. Bicuspid aortic valve is a frequent finding in patients with aortic coarctation. (Image from Armed Forces Institute of Pathology, Washington, DC, USA).

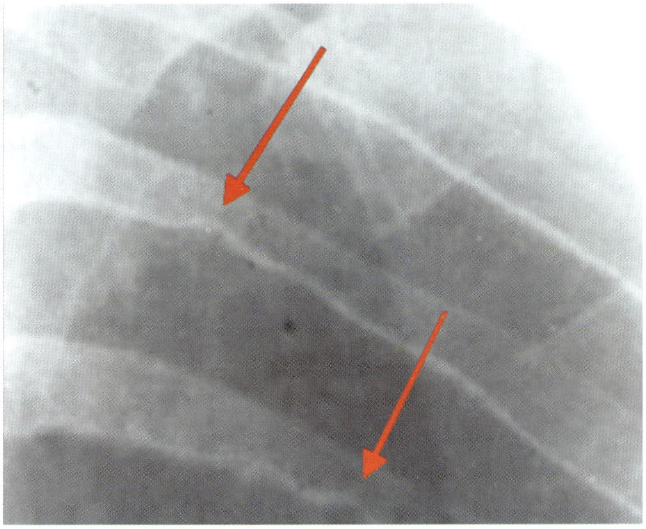

Fig. 46.11: Zoomed chest X-ray image illustrating examples of rib notching (arrows) in a patient with aortic coarctation. [Image from Hedge M, Vijayalakshmi IB. Role of radiography in congenital heart diseases. In: Vijayalkshmi IB, Rao PS, Chug R (Eds). Comprehensive Approach to Congenital Heart Disease. New Delhi, India: Jaypee Brothers Medical Publishers (P) Ltd; 2013].

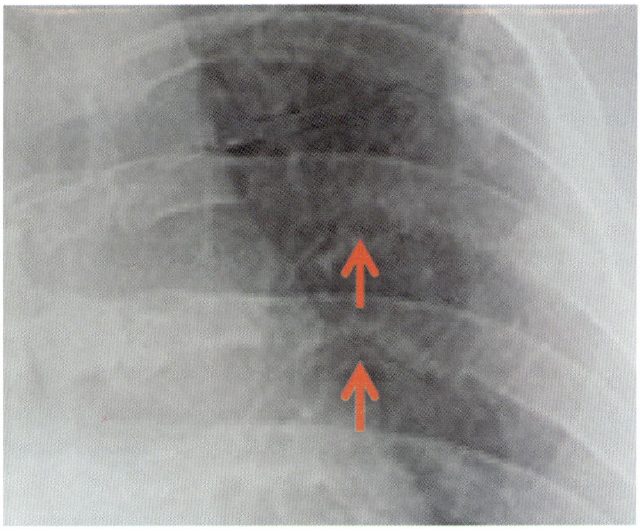

Fig. 46.12: Rib notching (arrows) as a result of intercostals artery hypertrophy as a means of collateral circulation in aortic coarctation.

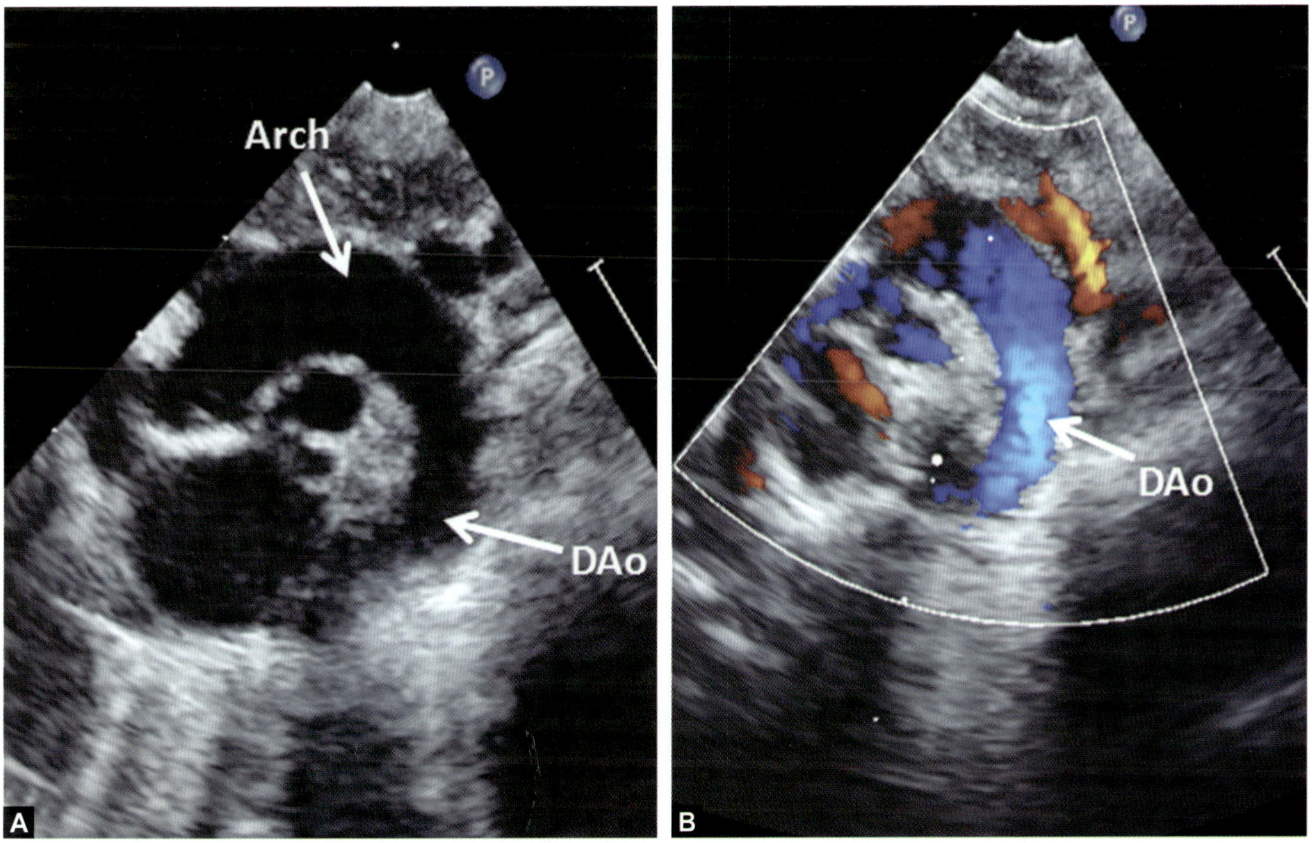

Figs. 46.13A and B: Selected echo video frames from suprasternal notch view in a normal child illustrating the aortic arch (Arch) and wide-open descending thoracic aorta (DAo) both by (A) 2D imaging and (B) color flow mapping.

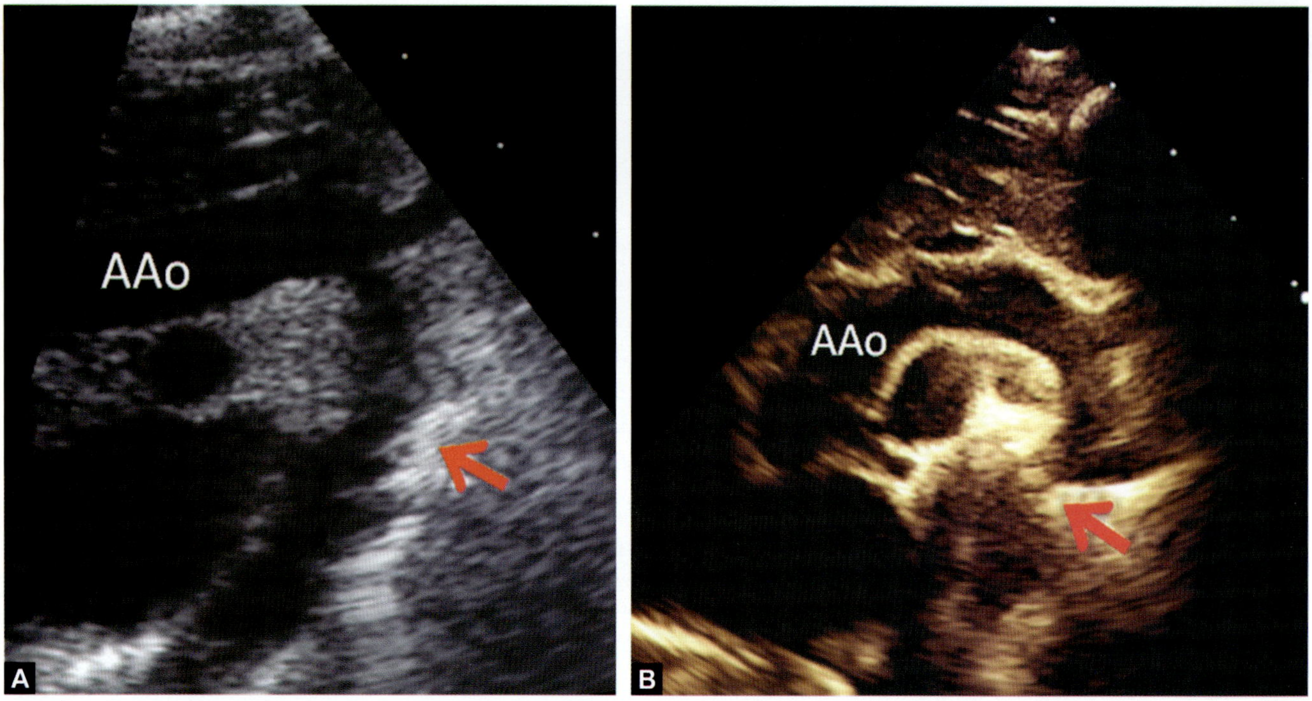

Figs. 46.14A and B: (A) Selected video frame from suprasternal notch view demonstrating aortic coarctation (arrow). Note slightly dilated descending aorta distal to coarctation site; (B) Different background color was used in another patient, also demonstrating coarctation (arrow). (AAo: Ascending thoracic aorta).

Two-dimensional imaging obtained from the suprasternal notch view is useful in demonstrating narrowed or coarcted aortic segment (Figs. 46.14A and B) as well as the aortic arch abnormalities, if any. Color-flow Doppler mapping shows color flow acceleration (Fig. 46.15) at the site of coarctation. Pulse wave Doppler interrogation reveals a jump in the peak flow velocity from the proximal segment to the segment distal to coarctation (Figs. 46.16A and B). Continuous wave Doppler interrogation across the stenotic segment should be performed to obtain maximal velocity (Fig. 46.17). Pulse Doppler sampling of abdominal aorta from subcostal view shows damped trace (Figs. 46.18A and B) suggestive of coarctation.

Peak instantaneous pressure gradient (ΔP) may be calculated by using the modified Bernoulli equation:

$$\Delta P = 4\,(V_2^{\,2} - V_1^{\,2})$$

where ΔP is pressure gradient, V_1 is proximal Doppler flow velocity and V_2 is distal Doppler flow velocity.

The calculated gradient is more likely to be accurate in the presence of pandiastolic extension of the Doppler signal. We recommend using this formula instead of the conventional formula:

$$\Delta P = 4V^2$$

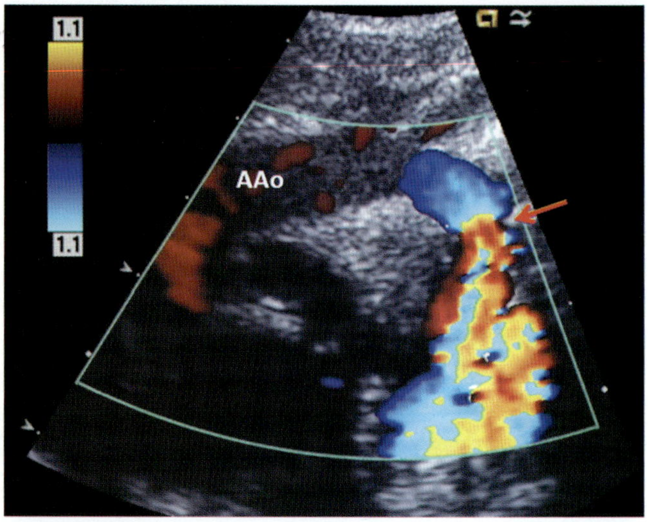

Fig. 46.15: Selected video frame from suprasternal notch view with color flow mapping demonstrating flow acceleration at the level of aortic coarctation (arrow). (AAo: Ascending thoracic aorta).

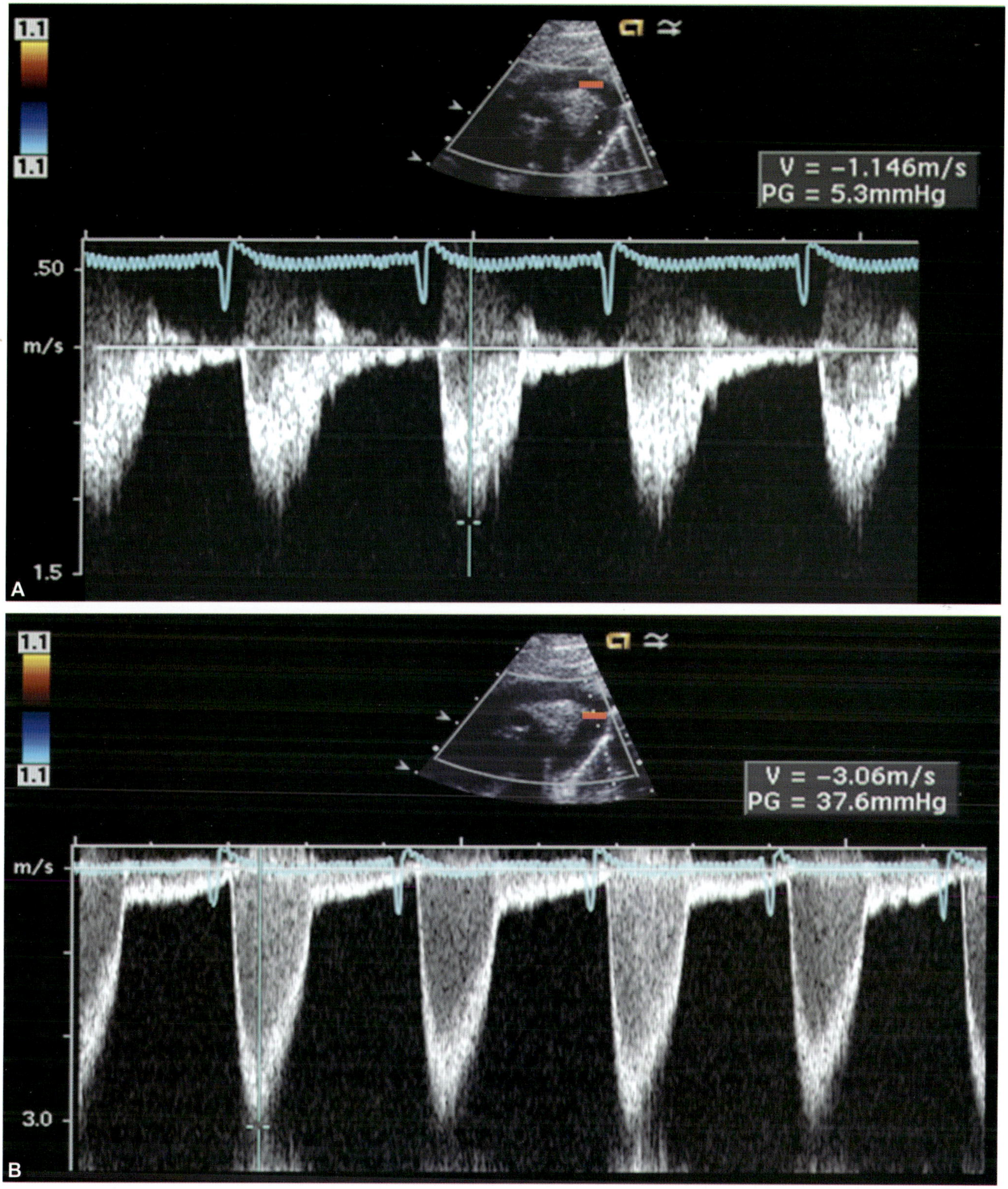

Figs. 46.16A and B: (A) Selected video frames from suprasternal notch view with pulse Doppler sampling (cursor highlighted red) in the distal aortic arch; (B) When sample volume (cursor highlighted red) is moved to just below the level of coarcted segment, marked increase in Doppler velocity is found, suggesting significant aortic obstruction.

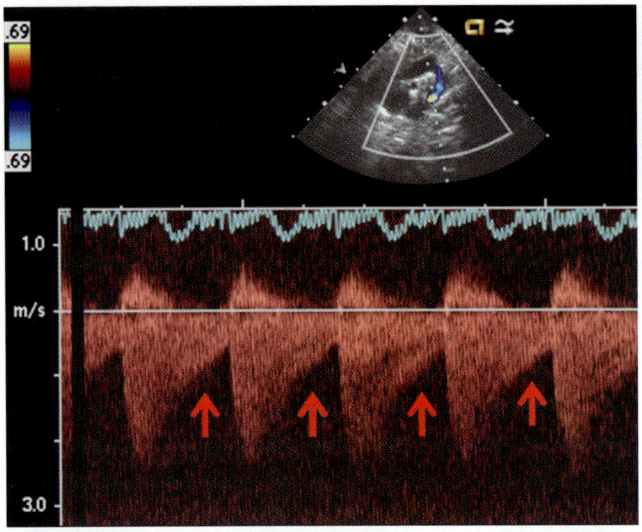

Fig. 46.17: Continuous wave Doppler sampling from suprasternal notch view demonstrating pan-diastolic extension of Doppler signal (arrows) suggesting severe coarctation.

Echo-Doppler studies are also useful in detecting associated defects such as bicuspid aortic valve (Figs. 46.19 and 46.20), mitral valve abnormalities and other defects.

Other Imaging Studies

Other imaging modalities such as magnetic resonance imaging (MRI) (Fig. 46.9), magnetic resonance angiography (MRA) (Figs. 46.21 to 46.26) and multidetector computed tomography (CT) angiography (Fig. 46.27) may be useful, if echocardiographic studies do not provide adequate information. Three-dimensional reconstruction may show the anatomy, including the aortic stenosis and collateral channels, clearly. These studies may provide high quality images and may be used to better define the anatomy, especially in cases with complex anatomy.

Cardiac Catheterization and Angiography

Cardiac catheterization and selective cineangiography are not necessary for diagnosis because the clinical and echocardiographic studies provide the diagnosis with relative ease. However, such procedures are an integral part of catheter interventions. When performed, pressure pullback tracing (Figs. 46.28A and B) reveals a peak to peak systolic pressure gradient greater than 20 mm Hg across the coarcted segment and aortic arch cineangiograms demonstrate the aortic arch anatomy (Fig. 46.29), aortic narrowing (Figs. 46.30 to 46.32) and distribution of collateral vessels. Additional selective angiograms may be performed to demonstrate or exclude other abnormalities found on echocardiographic studies.

MANAGEMENT OF AORTIC COARCTATION

Treatment is indicated in virtually all patients with coarctation of the aorta. Indications for intervention are congestive heart failure and/or hypertension. Congestive heart failure, particularly seen in neonates and infants, may be managed with conventional anticongestive therapies, such as diuretics and digitalis. Hypertension is better managed with relief of the aortic obstruction rather than with antihypertensive medications.

Treatment options include surgical repair, balloon angioplasty and stent placement. There is no consensus with regard to which is the ideal therapy and such selection differs from one institution to the other.

Surgery

In general, surgical repair is an initial therapy of choice in neonates and young infants, and in patients with other major congenital heart defects, such as large patent ductus arteriosus or ventricular septal defect that require concurrent surgical intervention. Older patients with (1) long-segment coarctation, and (2) complete or almost complete occlusion of the coarcted segment with inability to pass a guide wire or catheter across it, are also candidates for surgery. Since the introduction of surgery in the 1940s, various surgical strategies have been used for coarctation repair. The type of surgical repair depends upon the age of the patient, arch anatomy, and surgeons' preference. In general, discrete coarctation is repaired using resection of the coarcted segment with end-to-end anastomosis (Fig. 46.33). In cases with aortic arch hypoplasia or long- segment coarctation, an extended isthmoplasty and, rarely, prosthetic tube grafts (Fig. 46.34), left subclavian flap aortoplasty and prosthetic patch aortoplasty have been used. However, the latter two techniques have higher risk of complications, such as effecting growth potential of left upper extremity with subclavian flap procedure and high incidence of late aneurysms with prosthetic patch technique (Fig. 46.35), and are not generally recommended.

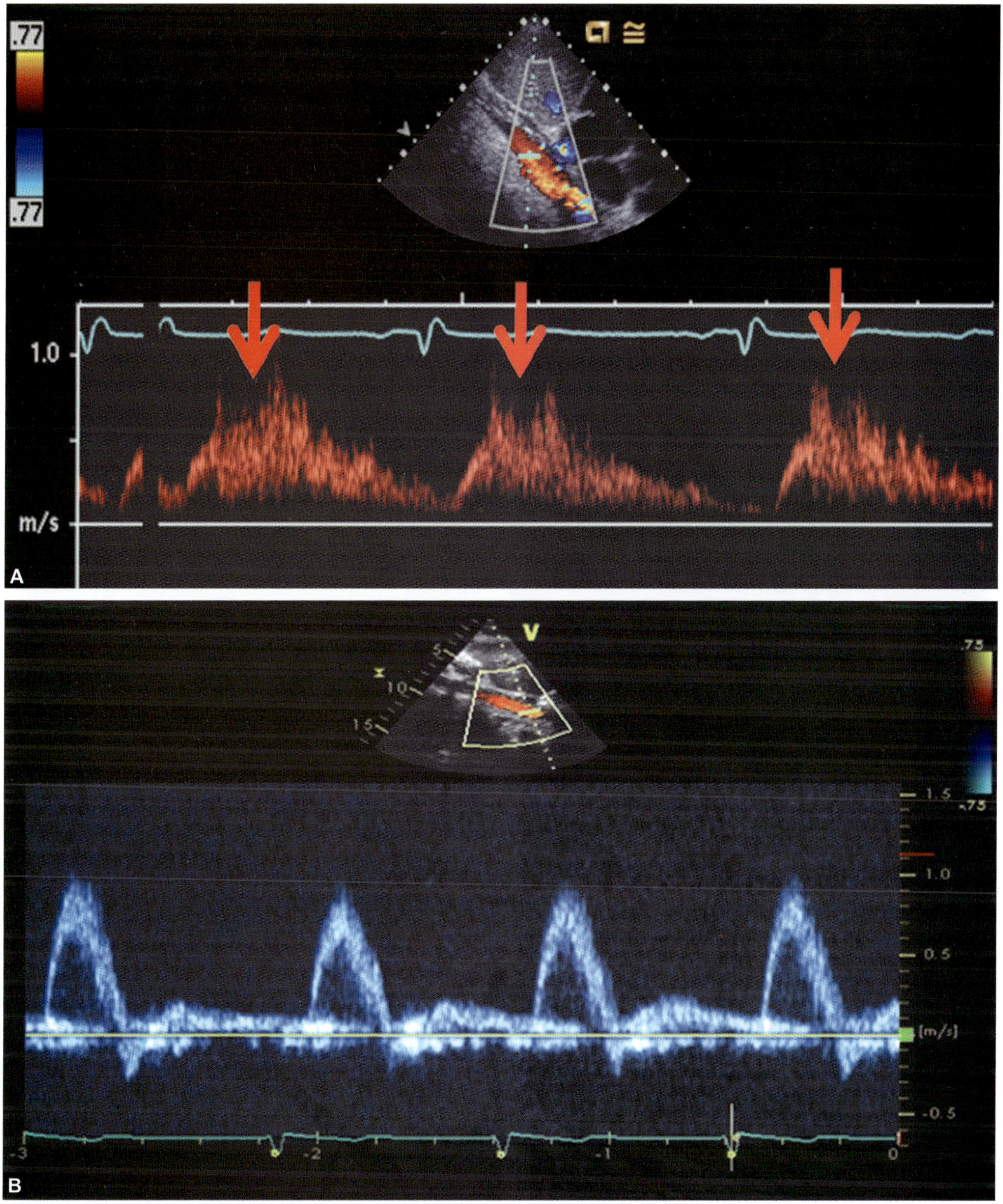

Figs. 46.18A and B: (A) Pulse Doppler sampling of abdominal aorta from subcostal view shows damped velocity envelopes (arrows) suggestive of coarctation; (B) this is in contradistinction to normal Doppler pattern in a patient without coarctation.

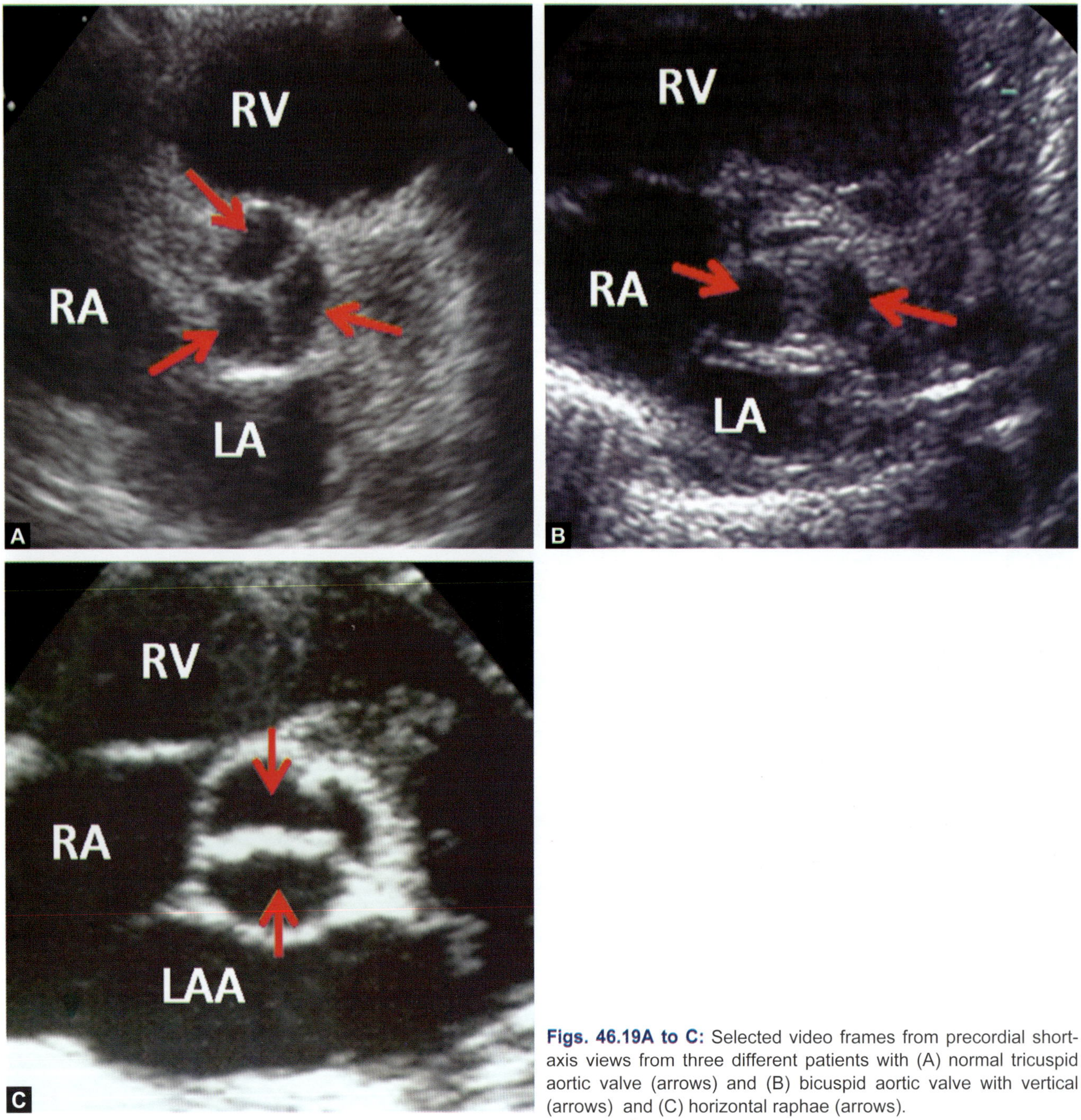

Figs. 46.19A to C: Selected video frames from precordial short-axis views from three different patients with (A) normal tricuspid aortic valve (arrows) and (B) bicuspid aortic valve with vertical (arrows) and (C) horizontal raphae (arrows).

Balloon Angioplasty

Balloon angioplasty of native coarctation is used as first-line therapy at some institutions. Because of high recurrence in neonates and young infants, it is no longer used for these subsets of patients. Infants older than 3–6 six months and children with discrete coarctation are good candidates for balloon angioplasty. The procedure involves placing the selected balloon angioplasty catheter across the aortic coarctation and inflating the balloon with diluted contrast material (Figs. 46.36A and B); the size of the balloon selected should be two or more times the diameter of the coarcted segment, but no larger than the size of the descending aorta at the level of the diaphragm. Immediate results are excellent with good relief of the pressure gradient (as shown in Figs. 46.28A and B),

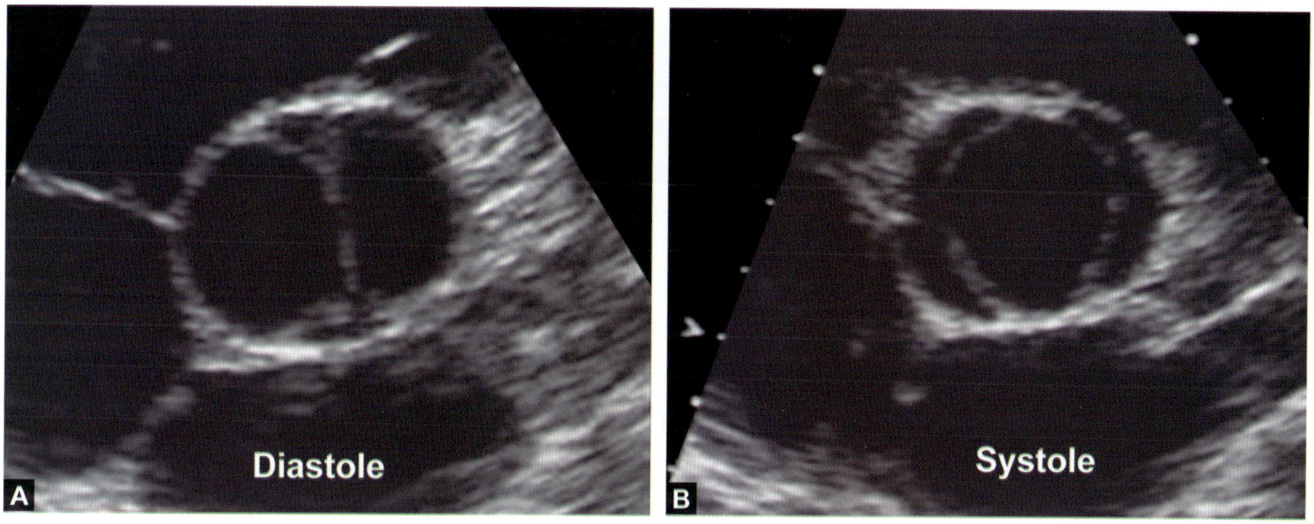

Figs. 46.20A and B: Bicuspid valve in a patient with aortic coarctation imaged during (A) diastole and (B) systole. (Image from Mordi I, Tzemos T. Bicuspid aortic valve disease: a comprehensive review. Cardiol Res Pract. 2012;2012:196037).

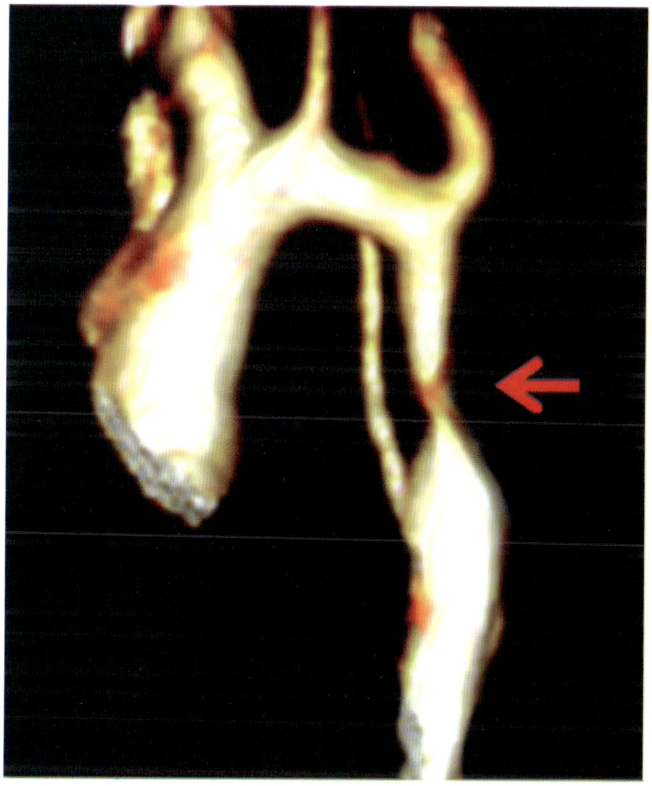

Fig. 46.21: MRI demonstrating aortic coarctation (arrow). [Image from Bentham J, Wilson N. Coarctation of the aorta. In: Vijayalakshmi IB, Rao PS, Chug R (Eds). Comprehensive Approach to Congenital Heart Disease. New Delhi, India: Jaypee Brothers Medical Publishers (P) Ltd; 2013].

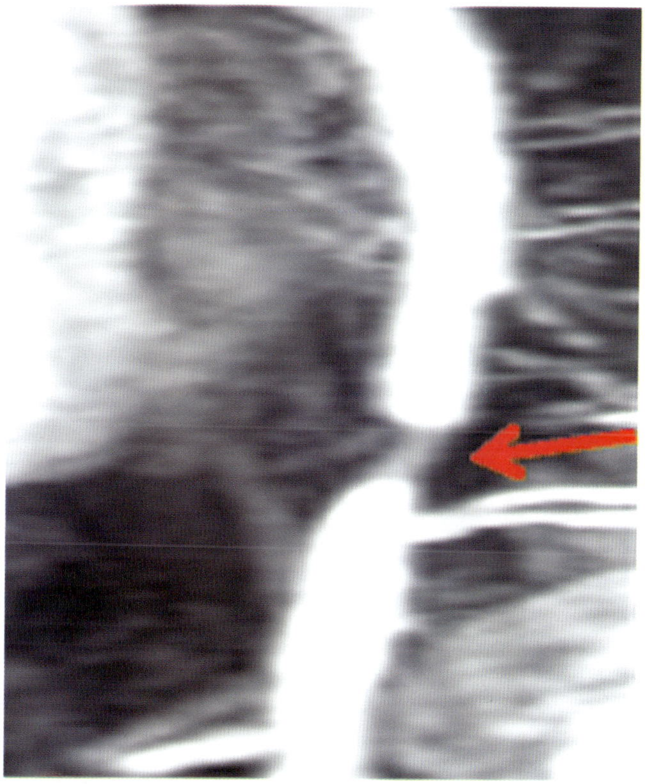

Fig. 46.22: Magnetic resonance angiography image showing severe stenosis of the lower thoracic descending aorta (arrow). This is likely to be related to Takayasu's arteritis.

improved angiographic diameter (Figs. 46.37A and B), and reduction in Doppler gradient (Figs. 46.38A and B). Long-term results (Fig. 46.39) are encouraging.

Recoarctation, defined as peak-to-peak systolic pressure gradient in excess to 20 mm Hg with or without angiographically demonstrable narrowing, may occur after

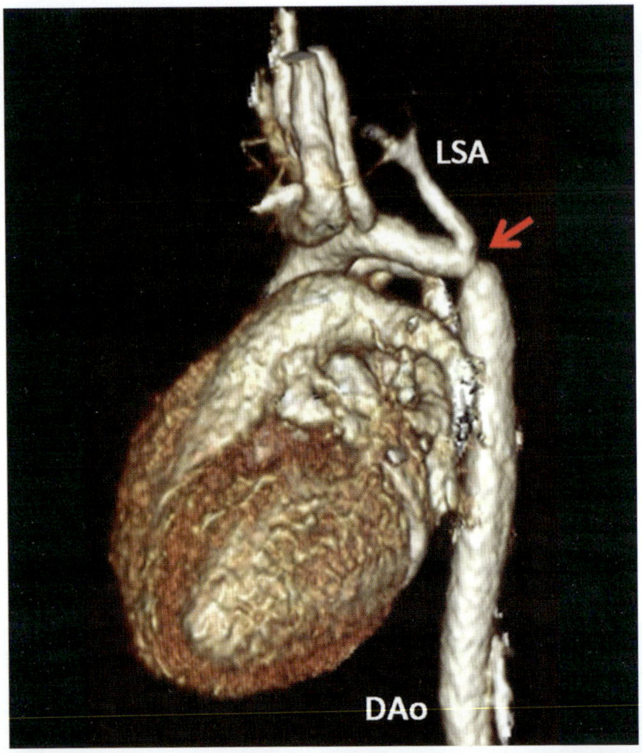

Fig. 46.23: Three-dimensional reconstruction showing coarctation (arrow) of the aorta, with good visualization of the aortic arch and descending aorta (DAo). (Image courtesy of Dr Siddharth Jadhav). (DAo: Descending thoracic aorta; LSA: Left subclavian artery).

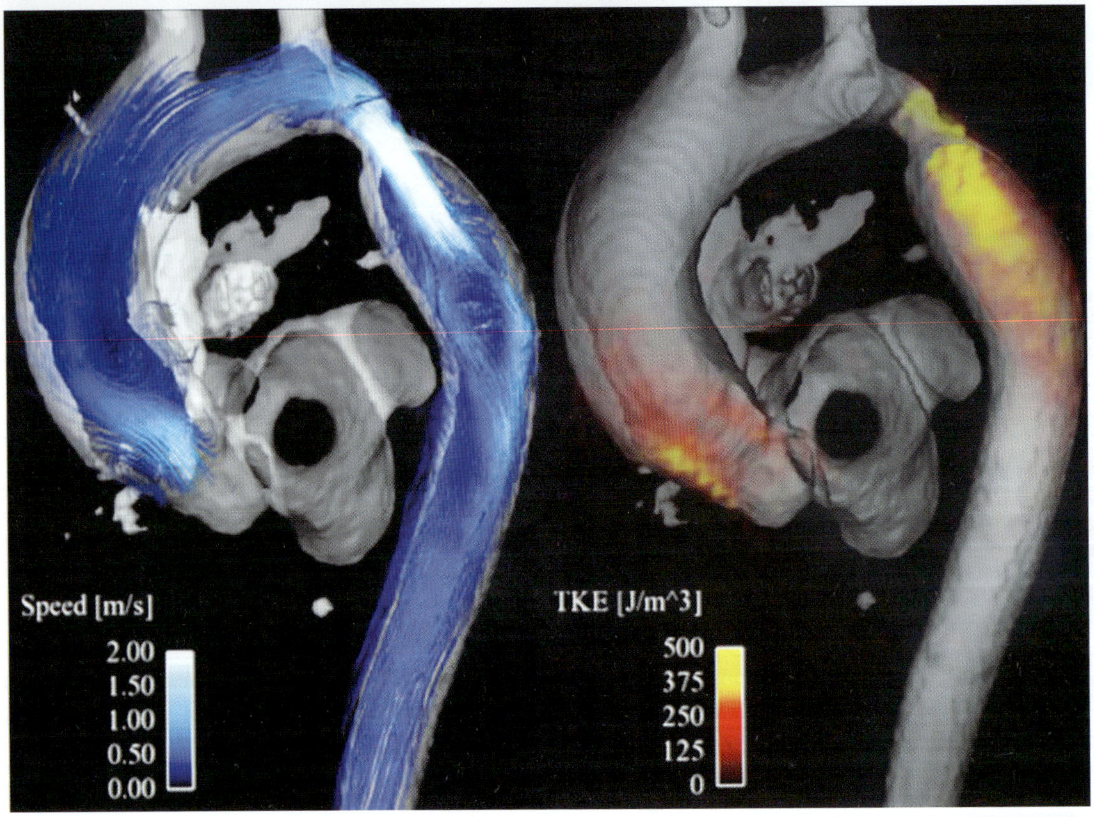

Fig. 46.24: MRI showing streamline visualization of blood flow (left) and volume rendering of turbulence intensity (turbulent kinetic energy, TKE) (right) at peak systole in a patient with an aortic coarctation distal to the left subclavian artery. [Image from Markl M, Kilner PJ, Ebbers T. Comprehensive four-dimensional velocity mapping of the heart and great vessels by cardiovascular magnetic resonance. J Cardiovasc Mag Res. 2011;13:7].

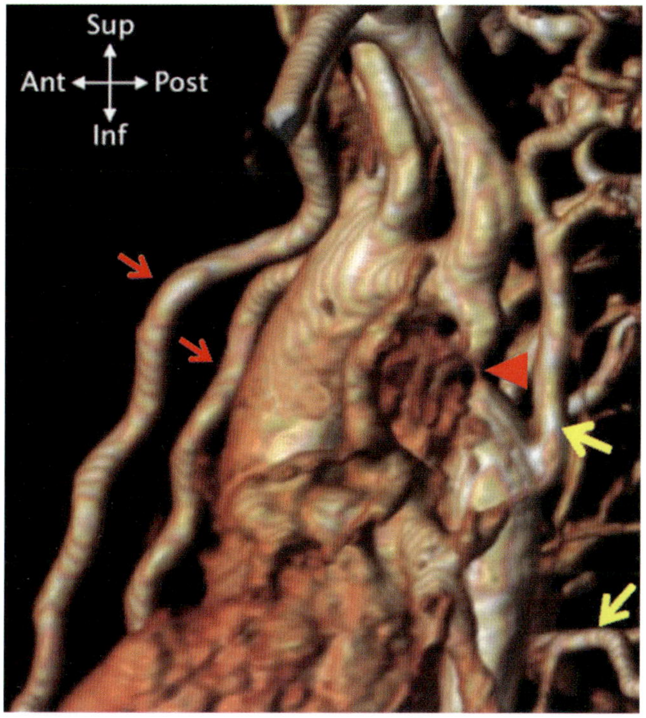

Fig. 46.25: Left lateral view of a three-dimensional reconstruction from a magnetic resonance angiography in an adult with severe coarctation (red arrowhead). MRI demonstrates the large collateral vessels (yellow arrows) and the dilated internal mammary arteries (red arrows). [Image and legend text from Romth A, Pluchinotta FR, Porayette P, et al. Congenital heart defects in adults: a field guide for cardiologists. J Clin Exp Cardiol. 2012;(Suppl 8). pii: 007]. (AAo: Ascending aorta).

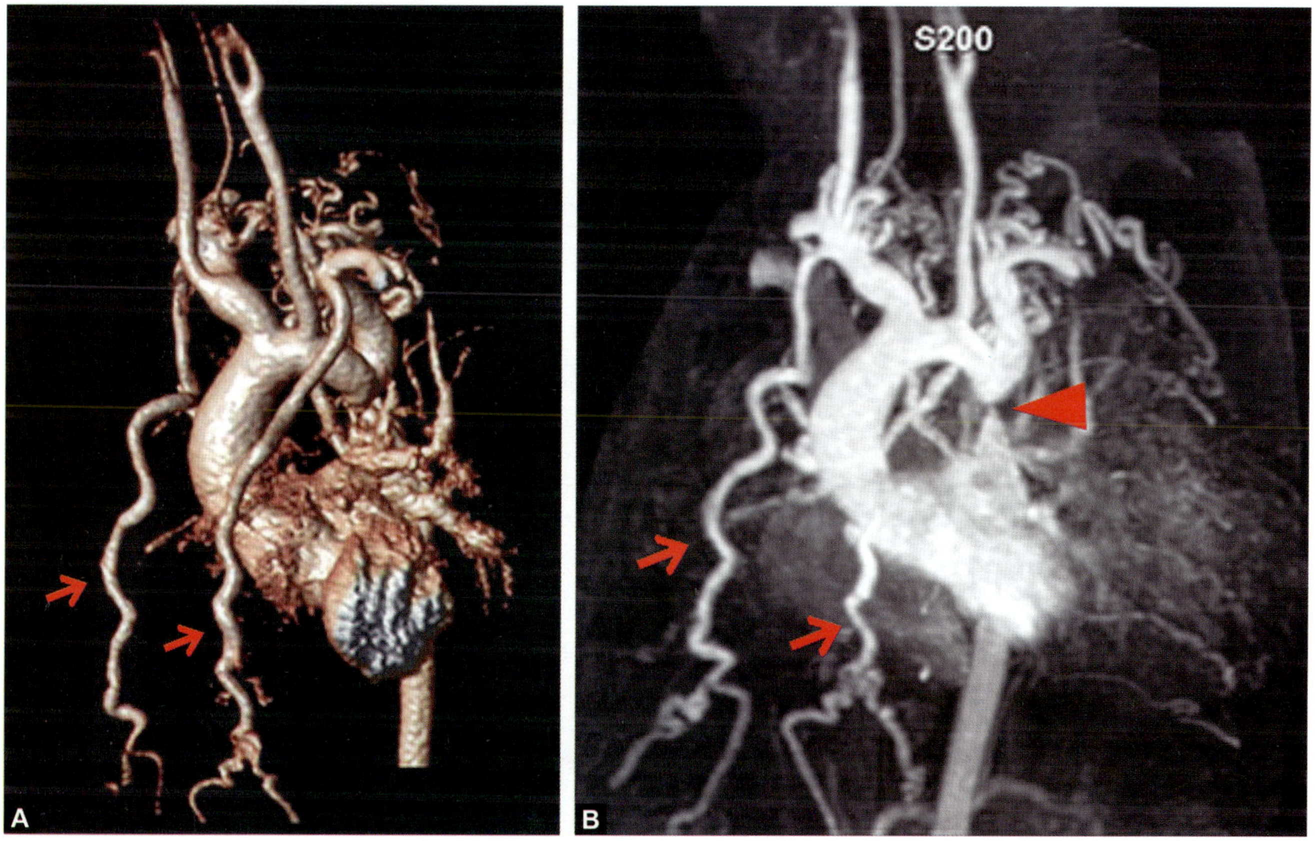

Figs. 46.26A and B: (A) Three-dimensional and (B) late gadolinium MRI images of aortic coarctation (arrowhead) demonstrating extensive collateralization, particularly of the left and right internal mammary arteries (arrows). [Image courtesy of BJM Mulder, EE van der Wall. Image reproduced from Luijendijk P, et al. Percutaneous treatment of native aortic coarctation in adults. Neth Heart J. 2011;19:436-9].

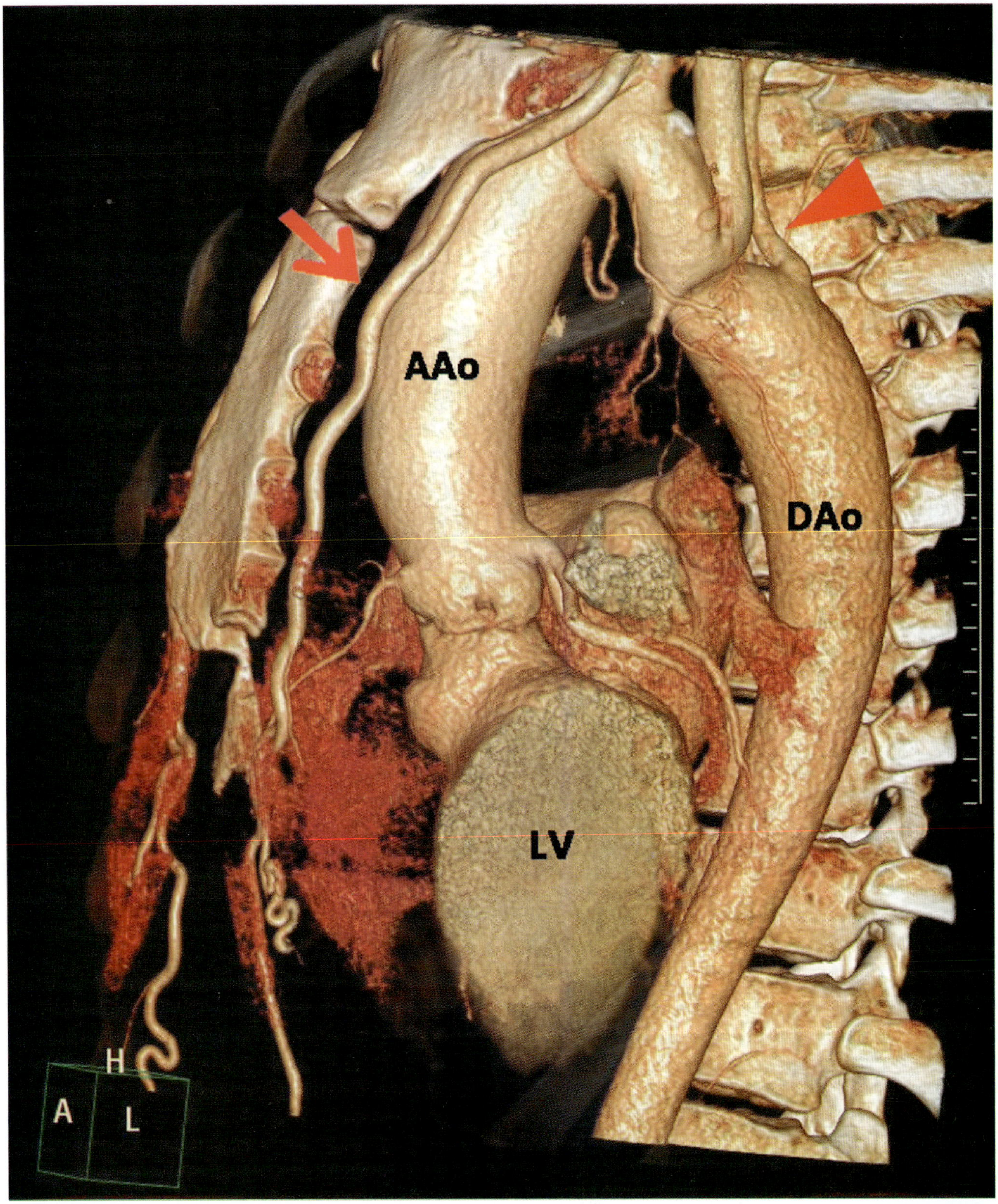

Fig. 46.27: Three-dimensional CT imaging of a patient with aortic coarctation (red arrowhead) demonstrating collateral flow through the left internal mammary artery (LIMA, red arrow). (Image courtesy of Dr Cafer Zorkun). (AAo: Ascending thoracic aorta; DAo: Descending thoracic aorta; LV: Left ventricle).

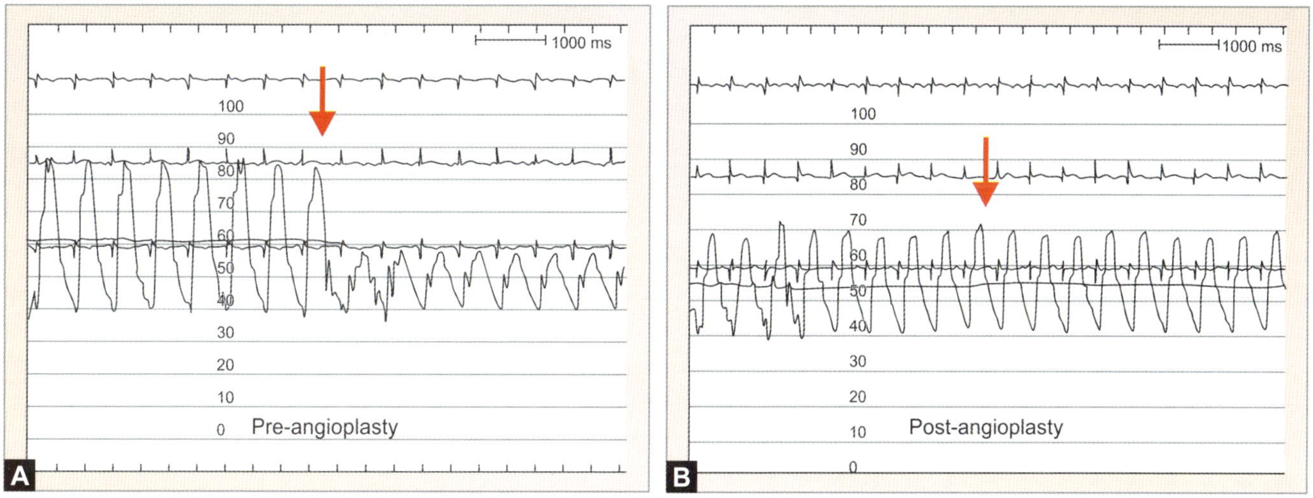

Figs. 46.28A and B: (A) Pressure pullback tracing across coarctation of the aorta (arrows) prior to and (B) immediately after balloon angioplasty demonstrating complete disappearance of the pressure gradient.

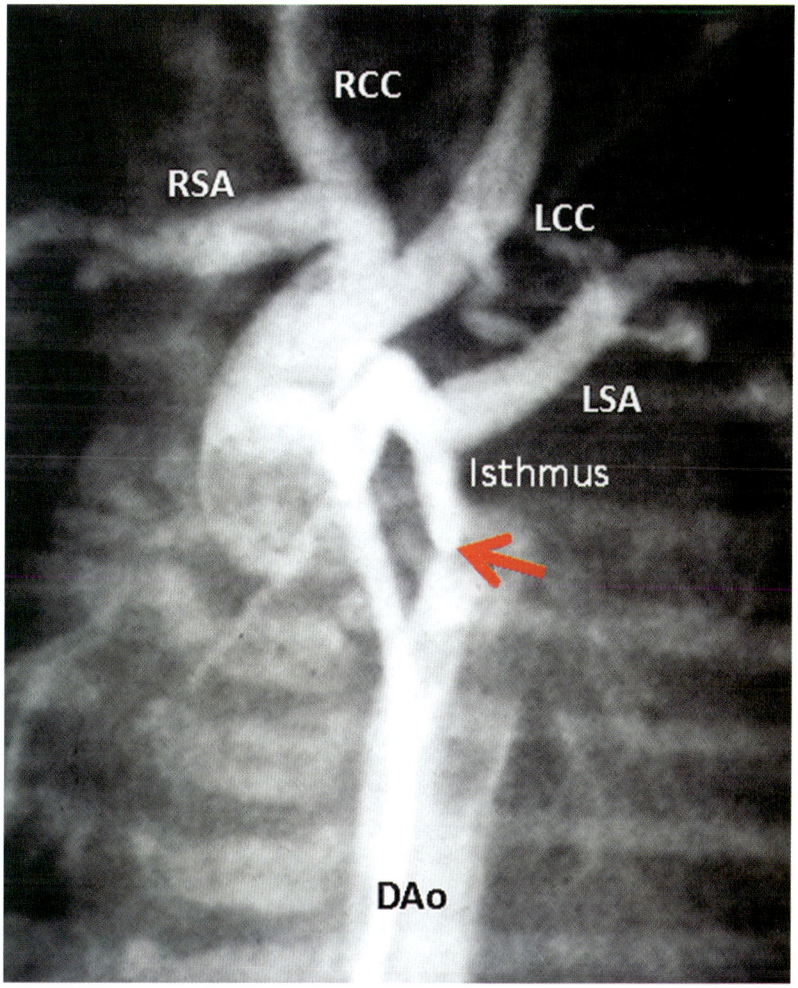

Fig. 46.29: Selected cineangiographic frame from the aortic arch in posteroanterior view in a neonate demonstrating marked hypoplasia of the distal aortic arch and isthmus (Isthmus) with additional discrete narrowing (arrow). (DAo: Descending thoracic aorta; LCC: Left common carotid artery; LSA: Left subclavian artery; RCC: Right common carotid artery; RSA: Right subclavian artery).

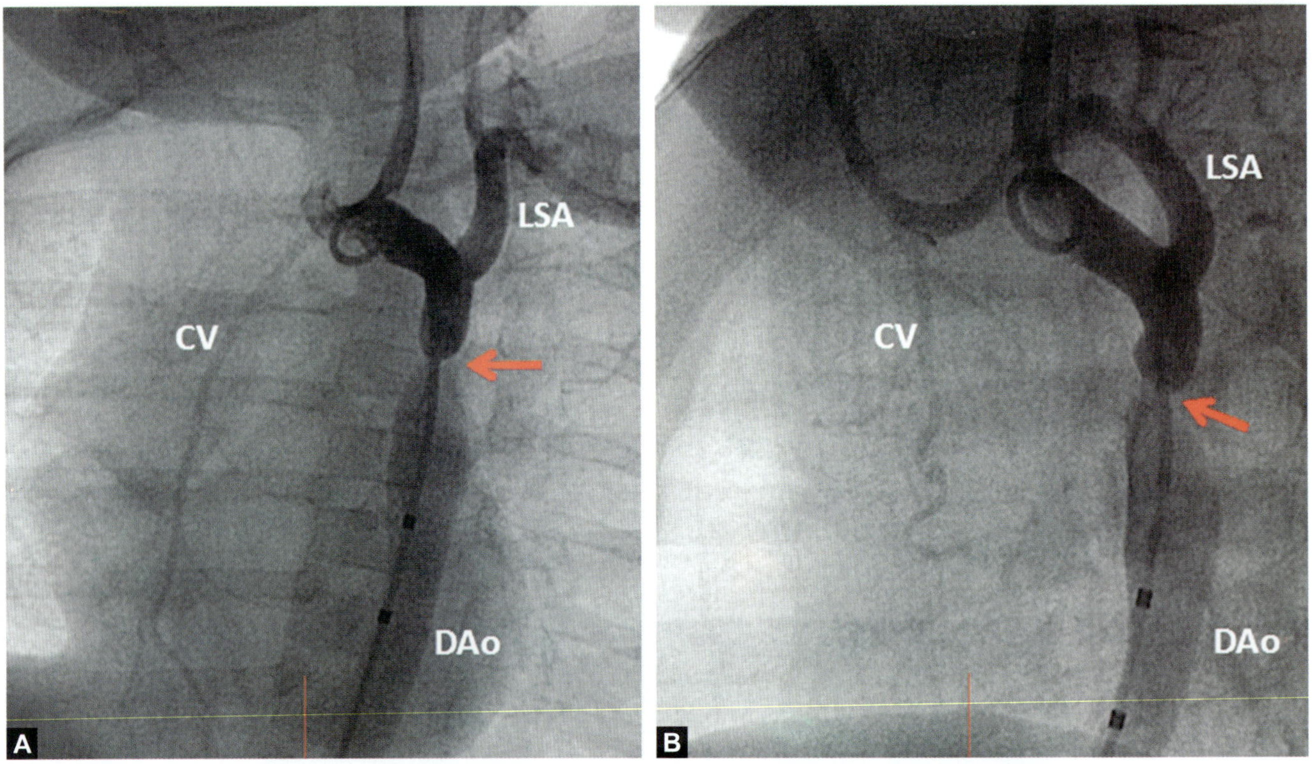

Figs. 46.30A and B: Selected cineangiographic frames from the aortic arch in an infant in 20° (A) left anterior oblique and (B) straight lateral projections demonstrating severe aortic coarctation (arrow). Note mild hypoplasia of the distal aortic arch and isthmus. A small collateral vessel is also seen. (CV: Collateral vessel; DAo: Descending thoracic aorta; LSA: Left subclavian artery).

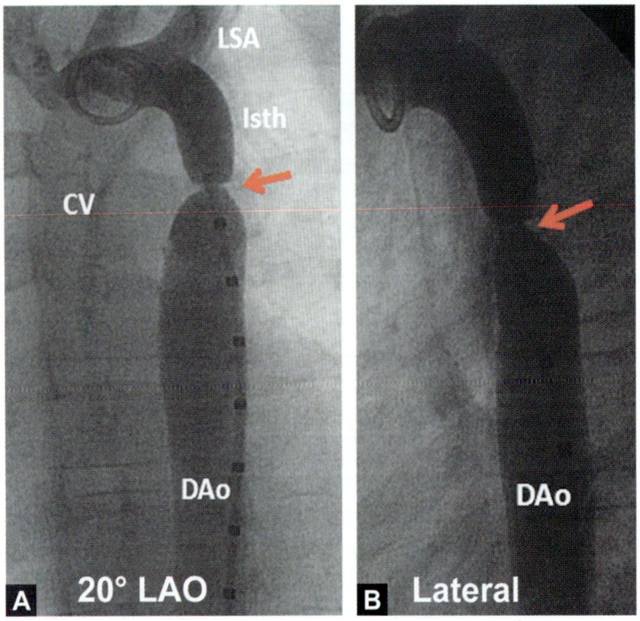

Figs. 46.31A and B: Selected cineangiographic frames from the aortic arch in an adolescent in 20° (A) left anterior oblique and (B) straight lateral projections demonstrating severe aortic coarctation (arrow). Note mild hypoplasia of the isthmus (Isth). A small collateral vessel is also seen. (CV: Collateral vessel; DAo: Descending thoracic aorta; LSA: Left subclavian artery).

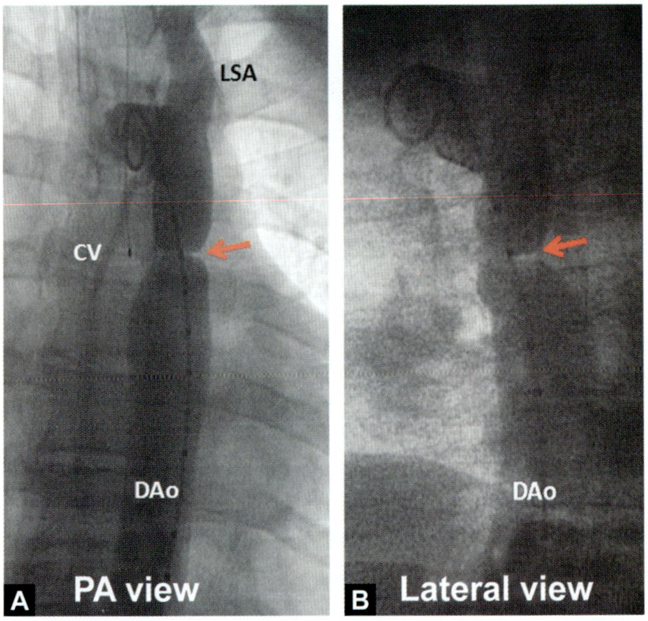

Figs. 46.32A and B: Selected cineangiographic frames from the aortic arch in an adult in (A) posteroanterior and (B) straight lateral projections demonstrating severe aortic coarctation (arrow). Note eccentricity of the coarctation segment in the lateral view. A small collateral vessel (CV) is also seen. (CV: Collateral vessel; DAo: Descending thoracic aorta; LSA: Left subclavian artery).

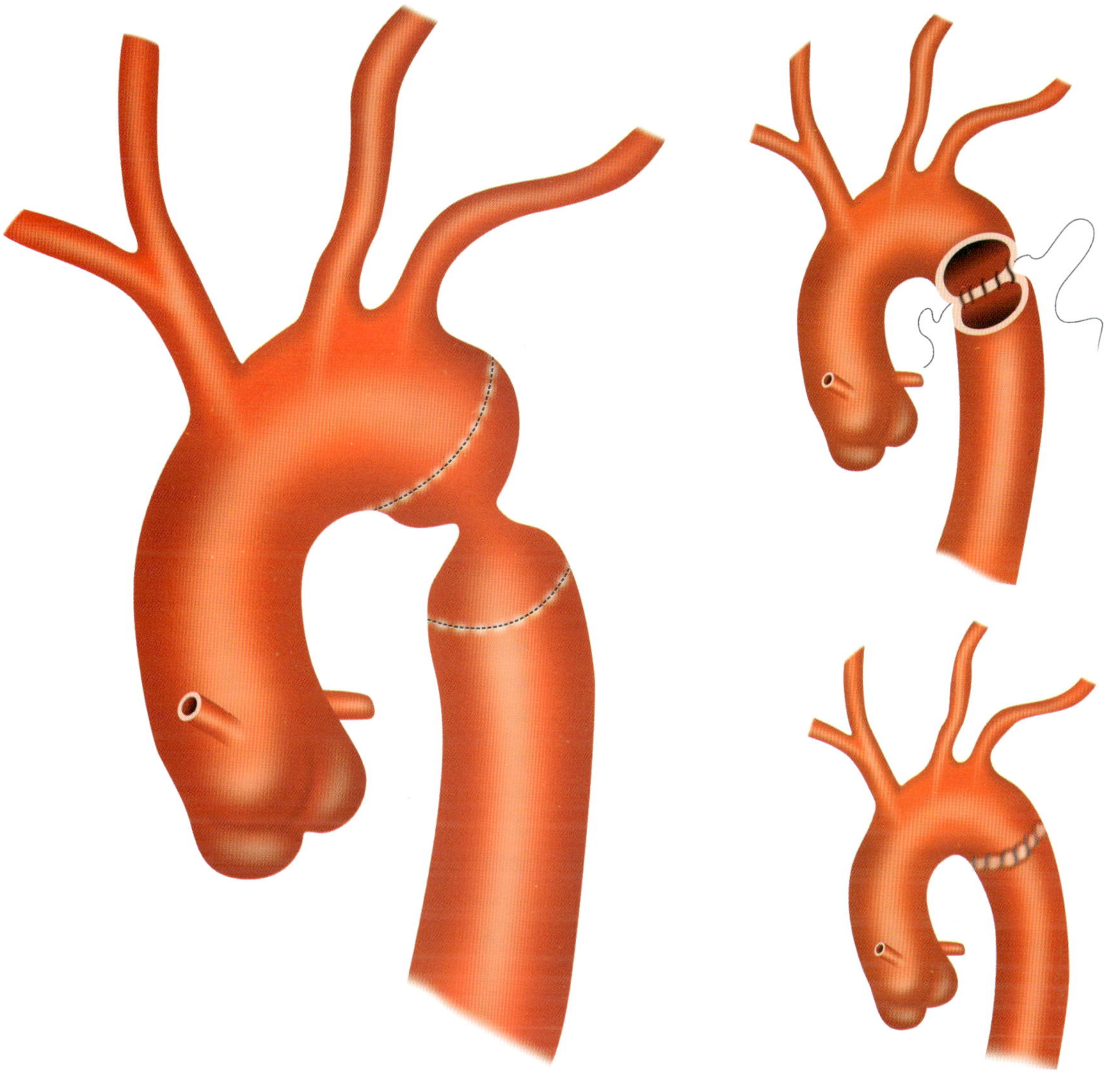

Fig. 46.33: Schematic illustration of surgical treatment of aortic coarctation with direct end-to-end anastomosis.

surgical intervention. The incidence of recoarctation is higher in younger patients than in older patients. There is a general consensus that balloon angioplasty is the first-line of therapy in patients with postoperative recoarctation of the aorta. An example of good immediate and follow-up result is shown in Figures 46.40A to C.

Intravascular Stents

Stents have advantage over balloon angioplasty because of prevention of elastic recoil of the vessel wall and their ability to compress the intimal flaps against the vessel wall. Another advantage is prevention of aneurysms due to scaffolding of a weakened aortic wall by the stent. Due to issues related to growth and need for large sheaths for implantation, intravascular stents are not recommended for infants and young children, and are generally used only in adolescents and adults, especially in patients with (1) long-segment coarctation, (2) associated isthmus or arch hypoplasia, (3) tortuous coarctation with malalignment of proximal with distal aortic segment, or (4) recoarctation or aneurysm formation after initial surgical repair or balloon angioplasty. The procedure involves hand crimping the stent onto a balloon, usually a balloon-in-balloon (BIB) catheter, positioning the balloon/stent assembly across the site of coarctation, and successive inflation of inner and outer balloons with fluoroscopic and angiographic monitoring (Figs. 46.41 to 46.43). Covered stents may be useful in highly selected patients with aortic coarctation.

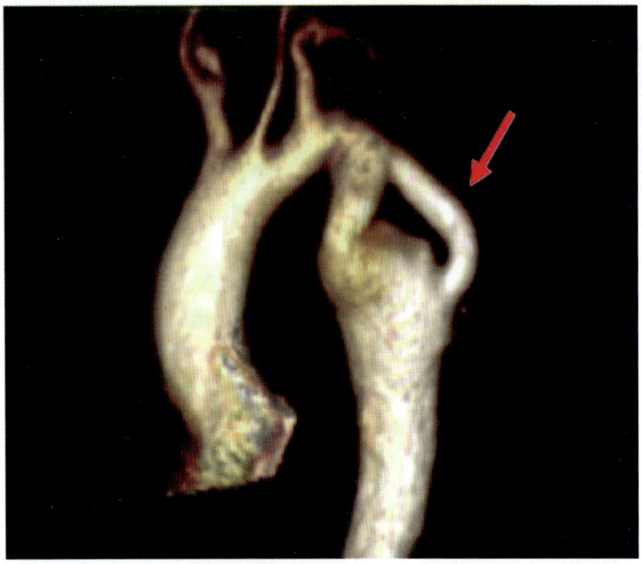

Fig. 46.34: Three-dimensional, contrast-enhanced MR angiogram showing aortic arch hypoplasia and coarctation with a "jump" by-pass graft posteriorly (arrow). (Image and legend text from Ntsinjana HN, Hughes ML, Taylor AM. The role of cardiovascular magnetic resonance in pediatric congenital heart disease. J Cardiovasc Mag Res. 2011;13:51).

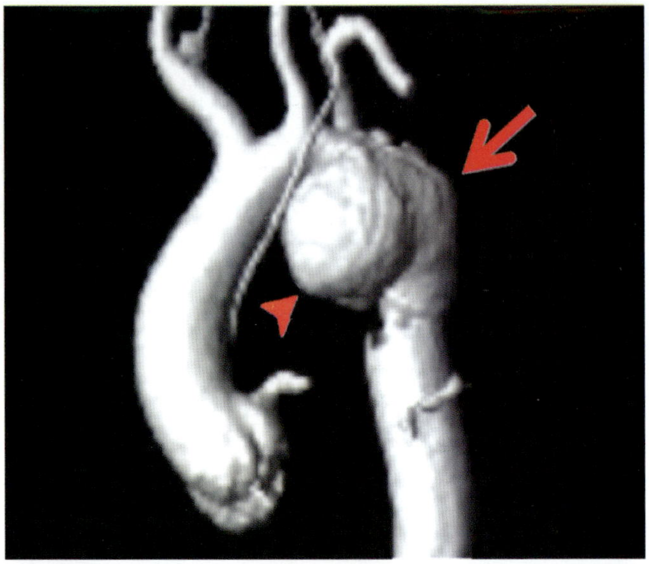

Fig. 46.35: Three-dimensional contrast-enhanced magnetic resonance angiogram showing large pseudoaneurysm (arrowhead) after previous patch angioplasty repair. The true lumen is shown posteriorly (arrow). (Image and legend text from Ntsinjana HN, Hughes ML, Taylor AM. The role of cardiovascular magnetic resonance in pediatric congenital heart disease. J Cardiovasc Mag Res. 2011;13:51).

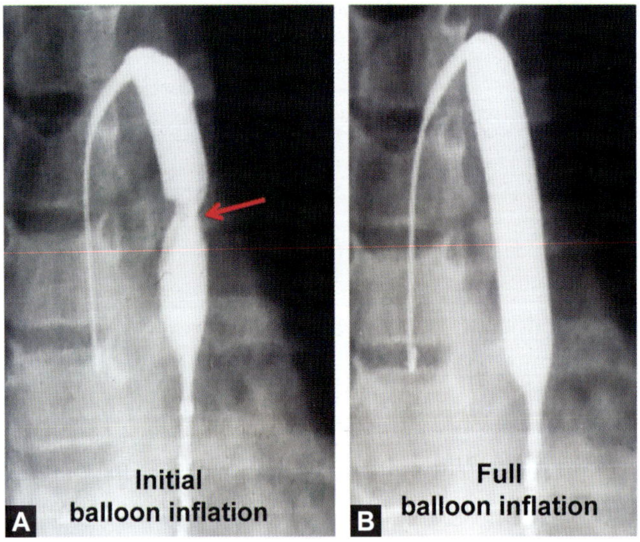

Figs. 46.36A and B: Selected cinefluorographic frames in posteroanterior projection demonstrating an angioplasty balloon across the aortic coarctation with waisting (arrow) of the balloon (A) during the initial phases of balloon inflation. (B) After full balloon inflation, the waist has completely disappeared.

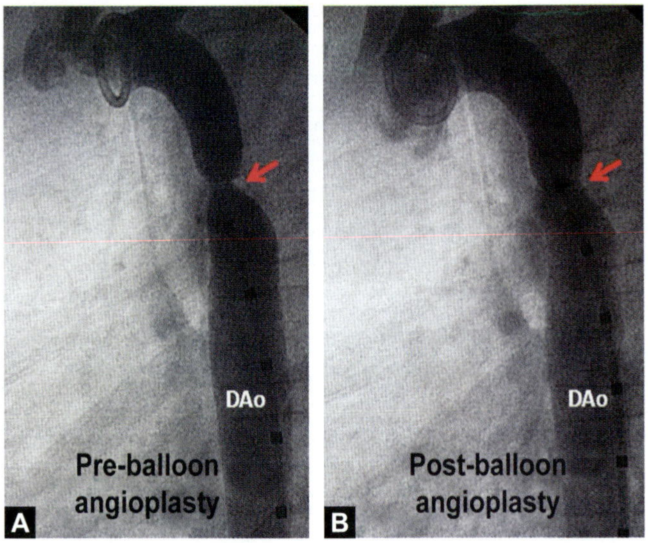

Figs. 46.37A and B: Selected aortic arch cineangiographic frames in straight lateral projection demonstrating narrowed coarcted aortic segment (arrow) prior to balloon angioplasty (A) which improved (B) following balloon angioplasty.

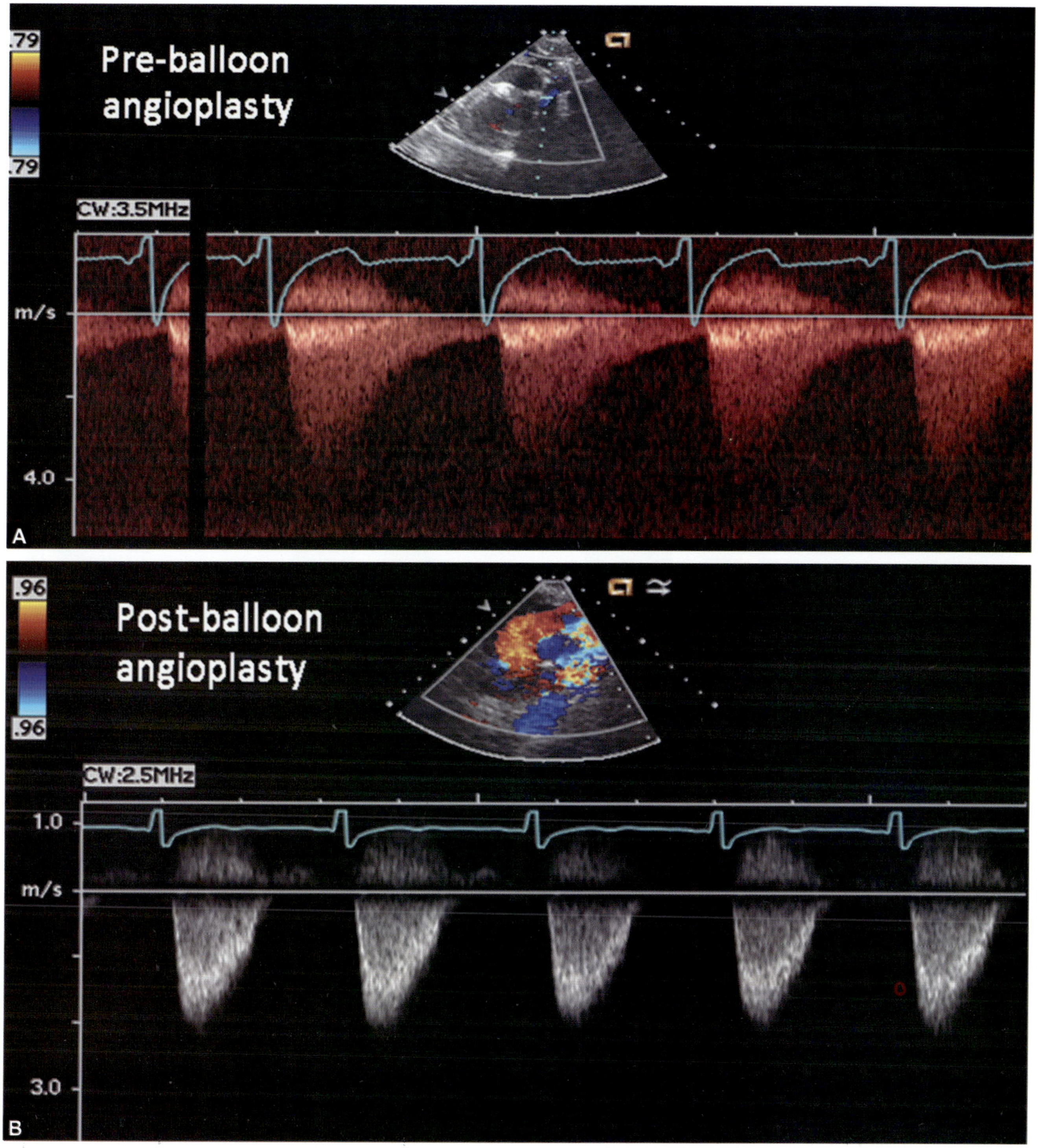

Figs. 46.38A and B: Continuous wave Doppler sampling from suprasternal notch view demonstrating pandiastolic extension of Doppler signal suggesting severe coarctation (A) which has markedly improved (B) after balloon angioplasty. Note the peak Doppler velocity decreased from 4.0 m/s to 2.0 m/s and more importantly, the diastolic extension of the Doppler flow velocity is no longer present.

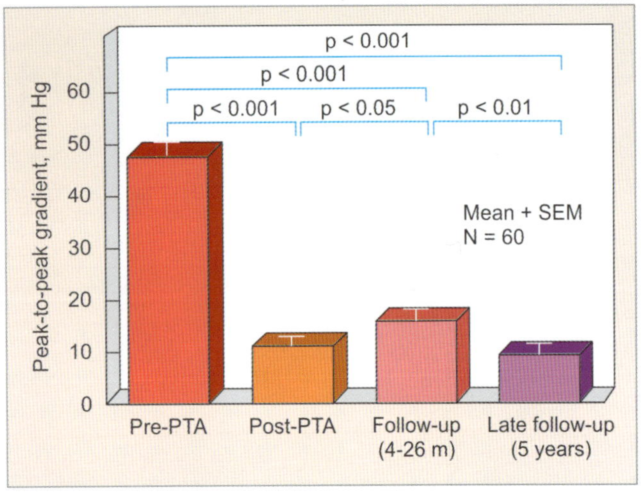

Fig. 46.39: Bar graph presenting immediate and follow-up results after balloon angioplasty of coarctation of the aorta. A significant decrease in the gradient following balloon angioplasty is achieved. The gradient increases slightly at a mean follow-up of 14 months (range, 4–26 months). However, these values continue to be significantly lower than preangioplasty values. At late follow-up at a median of 5 years after balloon angioplasty, arm-leg peak pressure difference by blood pressure measurement is significantly lower than catheterization measured peak gradients prior to balloon angioplasty and those obtained at intermediate-term follow-up. Mean + standard error of mean (SEM) are shown. 'N' indicates the number of patients undergoing balloon angioplasty. (PTA: Percutaneous transluminal angioplasty).

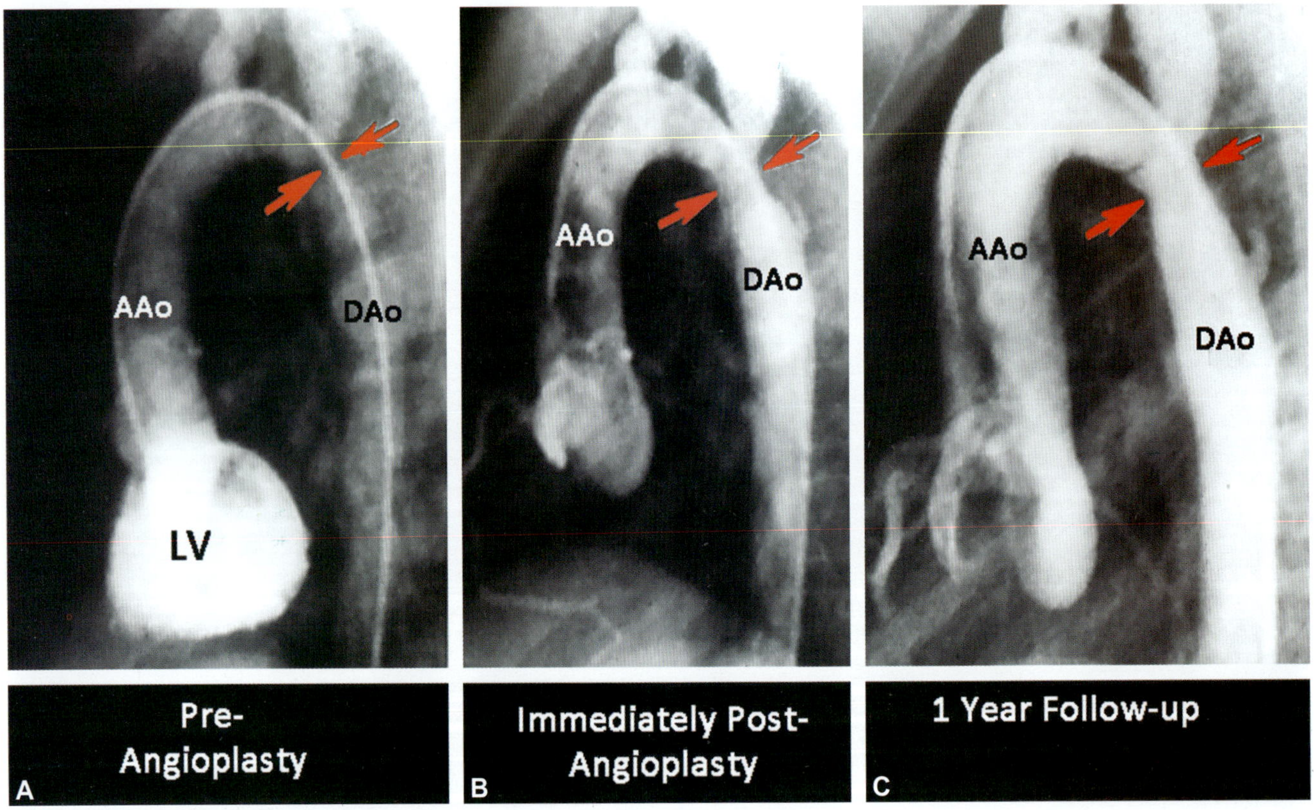

Figs. 46.40A to C: Selected cine frames from angiograms of a child with postsurgical recoarctation (A) prior to, (B) immediately following, and (C) 1 year after balloon angioplasty. Note that the coarcted aortic segment (arrows) improved markedly after angioplasty (Fig. 46.40B) which remains improved at follow-up (Fig. 46.40C). (AAo: Ascending thoracic aorta; DAo: Descending thoracic aorta; LV: Left ventricle).

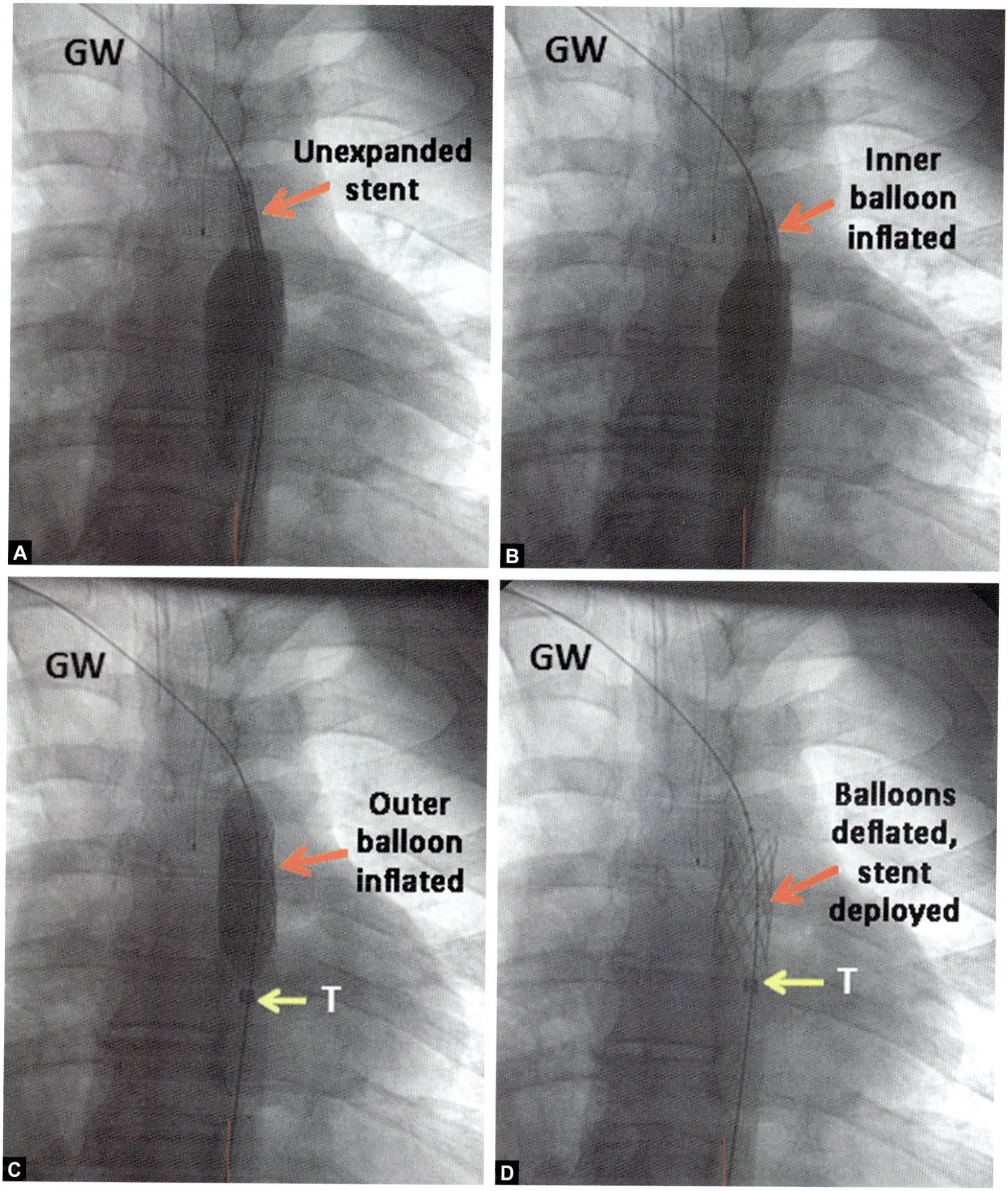

Figs. 46.41A to D: Selected cineangiographic frames demonstrating stent deployment across the aortic coarctation using a balloon-in-balloon catheter. (A) The position of an unexpanded stent following inflation of the (B) inner and (C) outer balloons and (D) after balloon deflation are shown. The deployed stent (arrow) is shown in Figure 46.41D. The guide wire is positioned in the right subclavian artery in an attempt to keep the stent straight. (GW: Guide wire; T: Tip of the delivery sheath).

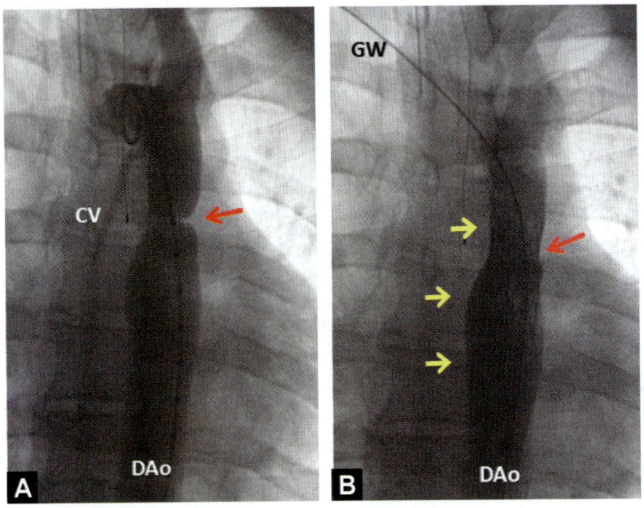

Figs. 46.42A and B: Selected cineaortographic frames demonstrating severe aortic coarctation (A) prior to and (B) immediately after stent (yellow arrows) deployment. Red arrows indicate the location of the coarcted segment. The collateral vessel seen prior to stent is no longer seen after stent placement. (CV: Collateral vessel; DAo: Descending thoracic aorta; LSA: Left subclavian artery; GW: Guide wire).

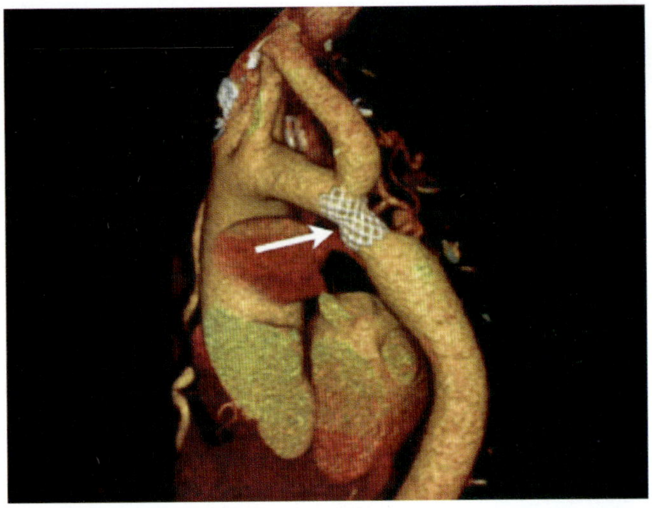

Fig. 46.43: Three-dimensional contrast-enhanced CT angiogram showing deployed, mildly narrowed bare metal stent (arrow) that partially overlies the left subclavian artery origin. (Image and legend text from Ntsinjana HN, Hughes ML, Taylor AM, et al. The role of cardiovascular magnetic resonance in pediatric congenital heart disease. J Cardiovasc Mag Res. 2011;13:51).

Table 46.2: Summary of considerations for therapy selection in patients with aortic coarctation.

Age	*Anatomy of the Coarctation*	*Mode of Intervention*
Neonates and infants < 6 months	Irrespective of anatomy	Surgery*
Infants and young children	Postsurgical recoarctation	Balloon angioplasty
Children older than 6 months and adults	Discrete native coarctation	Balloon angioplasty
Older children, adolescents and adults	Long-segment coarctation or significant isthmic hypoplasia	Stent placement**
Older children, adolescents and adults	Postsurgical recoarctation, post-balloon recoarctation and aneurysms after surgical or balloon therapy	Stent placement**

*Balloon angioplasty is an excellent alternative to surgery in critically ill babies, particularly in those in whom avoidance of anesthesia or aortic cross clamping required for surgery is thought to be beneficial in the overall management. Such circumstances include infants with shock-like syndrome, severe myocardial dysfunction and "hypertensive" cardiomyopathy, prior spontaneous cerebral hemorrhage, severely compromised ventricular function and biliary atresia babies awaiting liver transplantation.
**Bare metal stents are adequate for most patients. Covered stents maybe required in rare situations.

SUMMARY OF MANAGEMENT

While there is no consensus, some generalizations may be made with regard to treatment of aortic coarctation: management by surgery in neonates and young infants, balloon angioplasty in children and stents in adolescents and adults, taking the anatomy of the coarctation into account (Table 46.2).

VIDEO LEGEND

Video 46.1: CT demonstrating aortic coarctation. (Video courtesy of Scott D Flamm).

REFERENCES

Beekman RH. Coarctation of the aorta. In: Allen HD, Shaddy RE, Driscoll DJ, Feltes TF, (Eds). Moss and Adams' Heart Disease in Infants, Children and Adolescents. Philadelphia: Wolters Kluwer/Lippincott Williams and Wilkins; 2013:1044-60.

Doshi AR, Rao PS. Coarctation of aorta-management options and decision making. Pediatr Therapeut. 2012;S5:006.

Forbes TJ, Kim DW, Du W, et al. CCISC investigators. comparison of surgical, stent, and balloon angioplasty treatment of native coarctation of the aorta: an observational study by the CCISC (congenital Cardiovascular Interventional Study Consortium). J Am Coll Cardiol. 2011;58:2664-74.

Qureshi SA. Use of covered stents to treat coarctation of the aorta. Korean Circ J. 2009;39:261-3.

Rao PS, Carey P. Doppler ultrasound in the prediction of pressure gradients across aortic coarctation. Am Heart J. 1989;118: 299-301.

Rao PS, Galal O, Smith PA, et al. Five-to-nine-year follow-up results of balloon angioplasty of native aortic coarctation in infants and children. J Am Coll Cardiol. 1996;27:462-70.

Rao PS, Seib PM. (2012). Coarctation of the aorta. [online] eMedicine website. Available from emedicine.medscape.com/article/895502-overview. [Accessed February, 2014].

Rao PS. Coarctation of the aorta. Current Cardiol Reports. 2005;7: 425-34.

Rao PS. Stents in the management of aortic coarctation in young children (Editorial). J Am Coll Cardiol. 2009;2: 884-6.

Rao PS. Stents in the management of congenital heart disease in the pediatric and adult patients. Indian Heart J. 2001;53: 714-30.

Sahu R, Rao PS. Transcatheter stent therapy in children: an update. Pediatr Therapeut. 2012;S5:001.

Siblini G, Rao PS, Nouri S, et al. Long-term follow-up results of balloon angioplasty of postoperative aortic recoarctation. Am J Cardiol. 1998;81:61-7.

CHAPTER

Patent Ductus Arteriosus

47

David A Parra, Ann Kavanaugh-McHugh

INTRODUCTION

Patent ductus arteriosus (PDA) (Figs. 47.1 to 47.5), when found in isolation, may be an important abnormality relevant to both pediatric and adult cardiologists. A hemodynamically significant PDA can be associated with both short- and long-term pathophysiological and pathological cardiac sequelae. Treatment for most PDAs consists of percutaneous, or in some cases, open surgical, closure.

EMBRYOLOGY AND FUNCTION OF THE DUCTUS ARTERIOSUS

The ductus arteriosus is a crucial structure during fetal life. This vascular structure forms from the sixth aortic arches (Fig. 47.6). The proximal portions of these arches give rise to the proximal left and right branch pulmonary arteries. Most commonly, in the setting of a left aortic arch, the ductus arteriosus forms from the distal portion of the left sixth aortic arch. This vessel arises just beyond the origin of the left subclavian artery and inserts into the main pulmonary artery near the origin of the left pulmonary artery. In the setting of a right aortic arch, the ductus most commonly arises from the left subclavian or left innominate artery and also inserts on the left pulmonary artery (Fig. 47.7). Alternatively, the ductus can arise from the right aortic arch, distal to the right subclavian, entering the right pulmonary artery. Bilateral ductuses are rare but may also occur.

In utero, the ductus carries the majority of the right heart output (Figs. 47.8 and 47.9), 55% of the cardiac combined output, beyond the high resistance pulmonary circuit, to the fetal systemic circulation and to the placenta. Factors responsible for ductal patency in utero include the high pressure within the ductus, and the vasodilatory effects of prostaglandins produced both locally within the ductus and by the placenta, as well as other vasodilatory substances including carbon monoxide and nitric oxide, produced locally by the ductal tissue. Prenatal closure may occur, most commonly in the setting of use of non-steroidal anti-inflammatory agents, and is associated with in utero right heart failure.

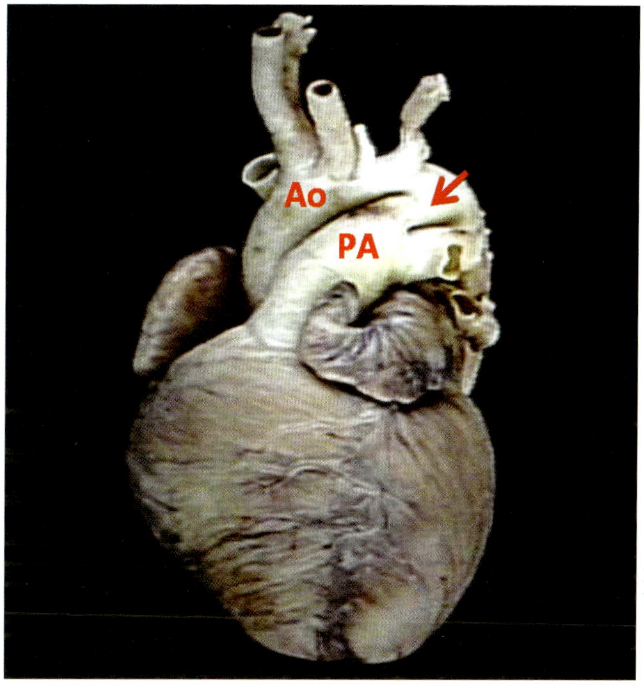

Fig. 47.1: Example of a patent ductus (arrow) which conducts blood flow between the aorta (Ao) and Pulmonary artery (PA).

DUCTAL CLOSURE AND PERSISTENCE

After birth, ductal closure is triggered in all but a small number of term newborns. There is a decrease in the intraluminal pressure within the ductus and a decrease in

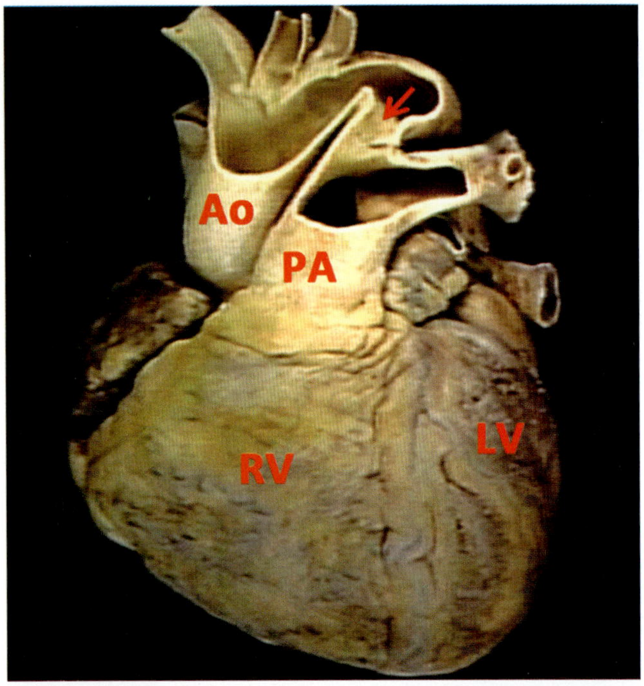

Fig. 47.2: Cut-away gross pathology specimen of a patent ductus arteriosus (arrow). [From Armed Forces Institute of Pathology (public domain)]. (Ao: Aorta; LV: Left ventricle; PA: Pulmonary artery; RV: Right ventricle).

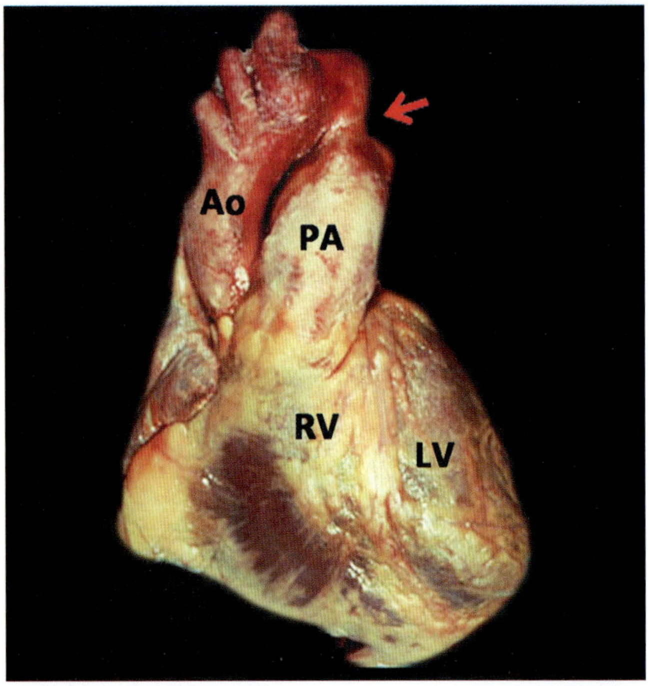

Fig. 47.3: Autopsy specimen demonstrating a patent ductus arteriosus (arrow). (Ao: Aorta; LV: Left ventricle; PA: Pulmonary artery; RV: Right ventricle).

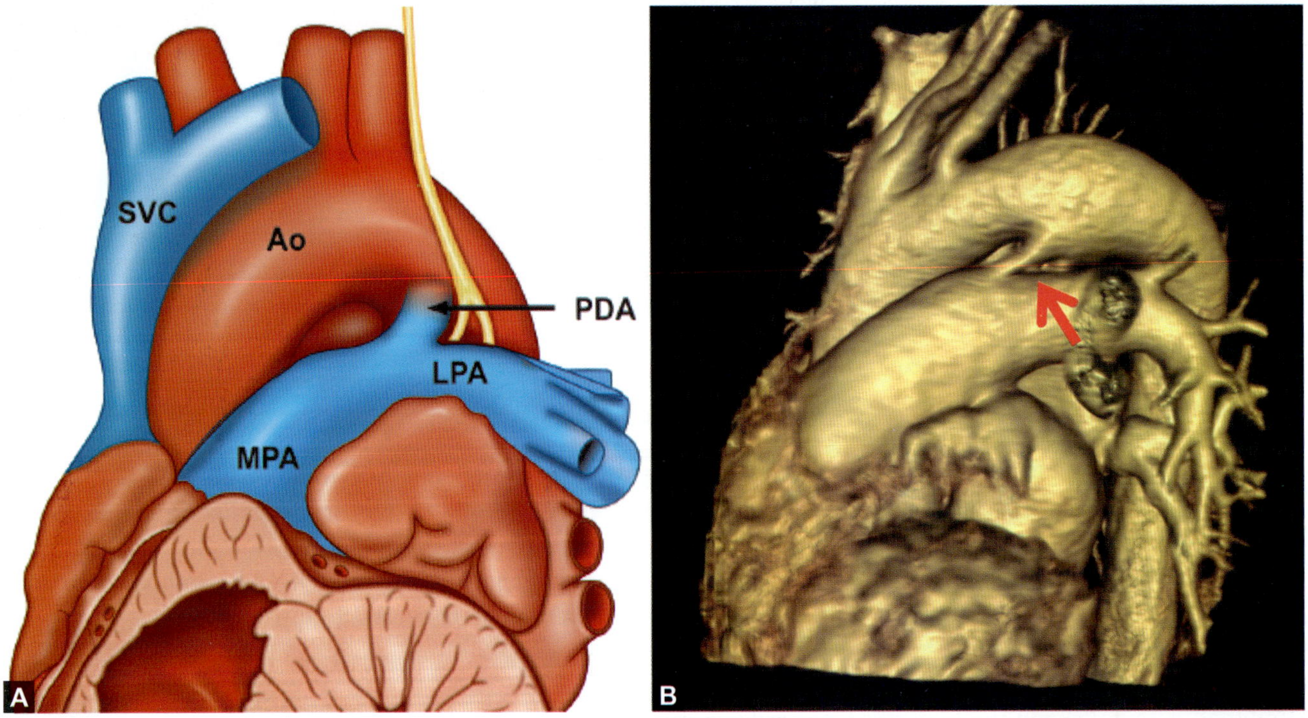

Figs. 47.4A and B: Patent ductus arteriosus (PDA). Diagrammatic representation of the ductus arteriosus (A) and comparable magnetic resonance angiogram (MRA) 3D rendering (B) illustrating the usual course of the ductus (arrow) and its surrounding structures. [Diagrammatic representation (A) from Arora R, Vijayalakshmi IB. Patent ductus arteriosus. In: Vijayalakshmi IB, et al. (Ed). A Comprehensive Approach to Congenital Heart Diseases. New Delhi, India: Jaypee Brothers Medical Publishers (P) Ltd; 2013, with permission]. (SVC: Superior vena cava; Ao: Aorta; MPA: Main pulmonary artery; LPA: Left pulmonary artery).

prostaglandin-mediated vasodilation (due to a reduction in prostaglandin-sensitive receptors within the ductal tissue, an increase in metabolism of prostaglandin within the lungs, and a reduction in circulating prostaglandins with separation from the placenta). In addition, the postnatal increase in PaO_2 triggers a cascade of changes within the ductal tissue, including smooth muscle depolarization, and the release of vasoconstrictors and growth factors that promote smooth muscle constriction, intimal proliferation, and eventual permanent closure of the ductus.

The incidence of persistence of the ductus is approximately 80 in 100,000 live births. Persistence of the ductus may occur in association with genetic syndromes, or may be attributable to other genetic factors. Environmental

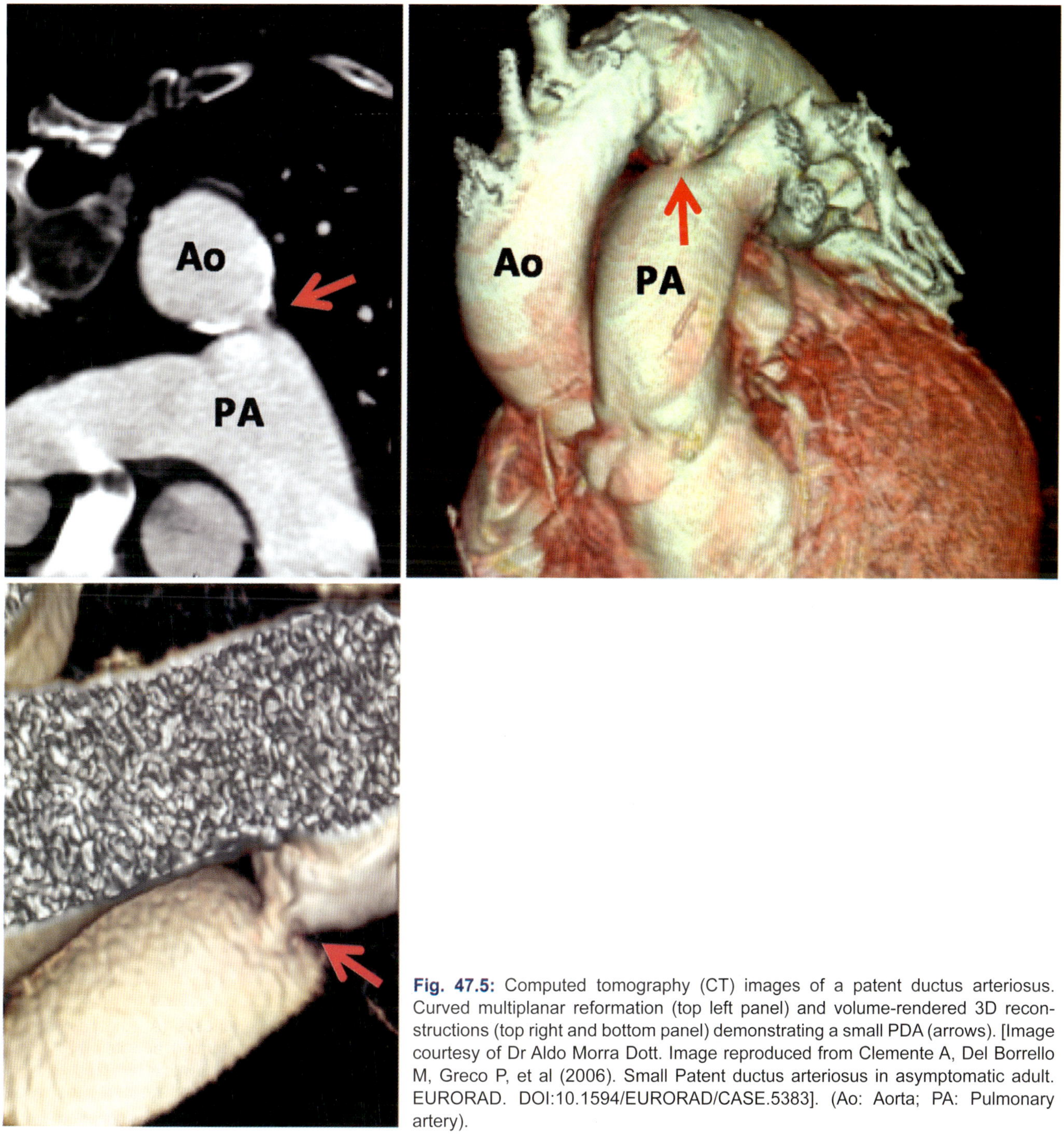

Fig. 47.5: Computed tomography (CT) images of a patent ductus arteriosus. Curved multiplanar reformation (top left panel) and volume-rendered 3D reconstructions (top right and bottom panel) demonstrating a small PDA (arrows). [Image courtesy of Dr Aldo Morra Dott. Image reproduced from Clemente A, Del Borrello M, Greco P, et al (2006). Small Patent ductus arteriosus in asymptomatic adult. EURORAD. DOI:10.1594/EURORAD/CASE.5383]. (Ao: Aorta; PA: Pulmonary artery).

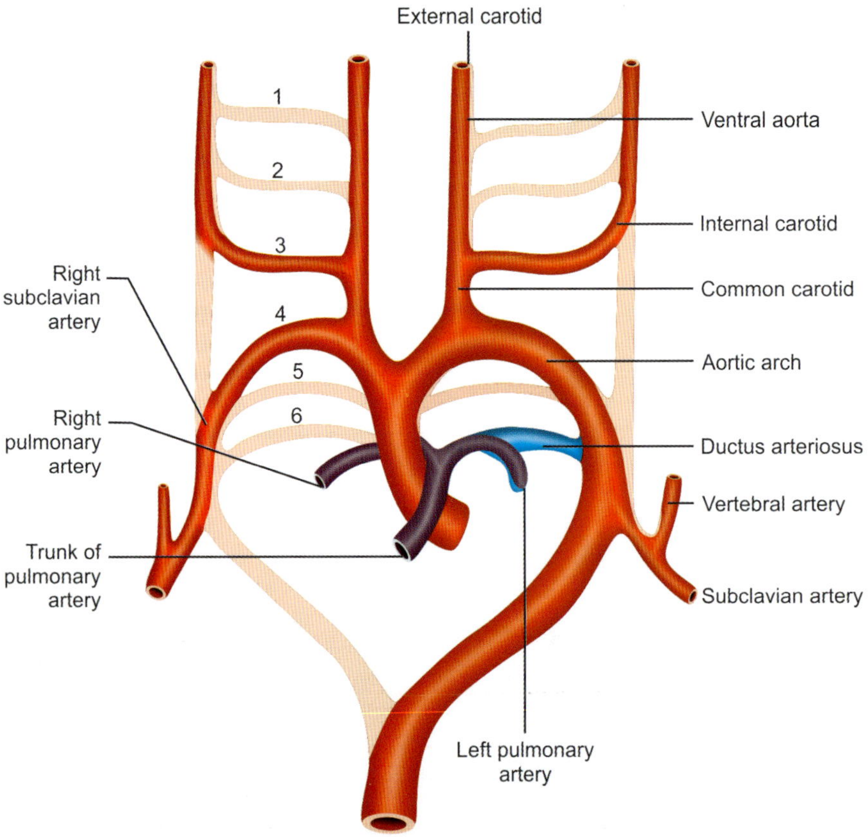

Fig. 47.6: Schematic illustration of the six arches and the embryologic origins of the ductus arteriosus.

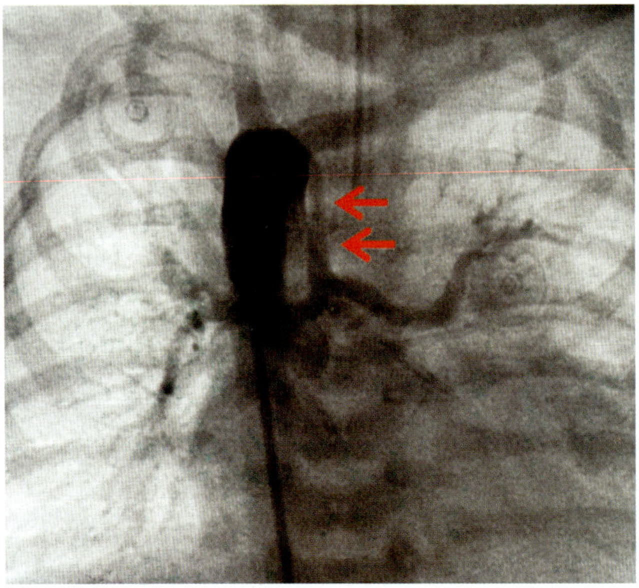

Fig. 47.7: Angiographic image in a patient with right aortic arch. Contrast fills the aorta and the brachiocephalic arteries. The ductus arteriosus is seen originating from the first leftward branch of the right aortic arch (arrows), and descends parallel to the aorta, filling confluent hypoplastic branch pulmonary arteries in this infant with pulmonary atresia.

factors, including prenatal infection with rubella, may also be implicated. Preterm infants are far more likely to have persistent patency of the ductus arteriosus, with a 65% incidence of PDA in infants born at less than 30 weeks of gestation. This increased incidence is attributable to increased sensitivity to vasodilating agents including prostaglandin, nitric oxide and endothelin, and a decreased sensitivity of the oxygen-responsive pathways for smooth muscle constriction in this population.

When the ductus persists, there is considerable variability in size and in geometry. The Krichenko classification (Figs. 47.10 and 47.11) is commonly used to describe the range of anatomic variations seen in the isolated PDA. As ductal closure progresses from the pulmonary insertion of the ductus to its aortic end, the majority of ductuses are funnel shaped, tapering to a larger ductal ampulla. The funnel-shaped ductus may also be broad with a "window" appearance (Krichenko types A and B). Other ductuses may be tubular (Krichenko type C), have multiple constrictions (Krichenko type D), or have elongated configurations with constriction near the pulmonary insertion (Krichenko type E).

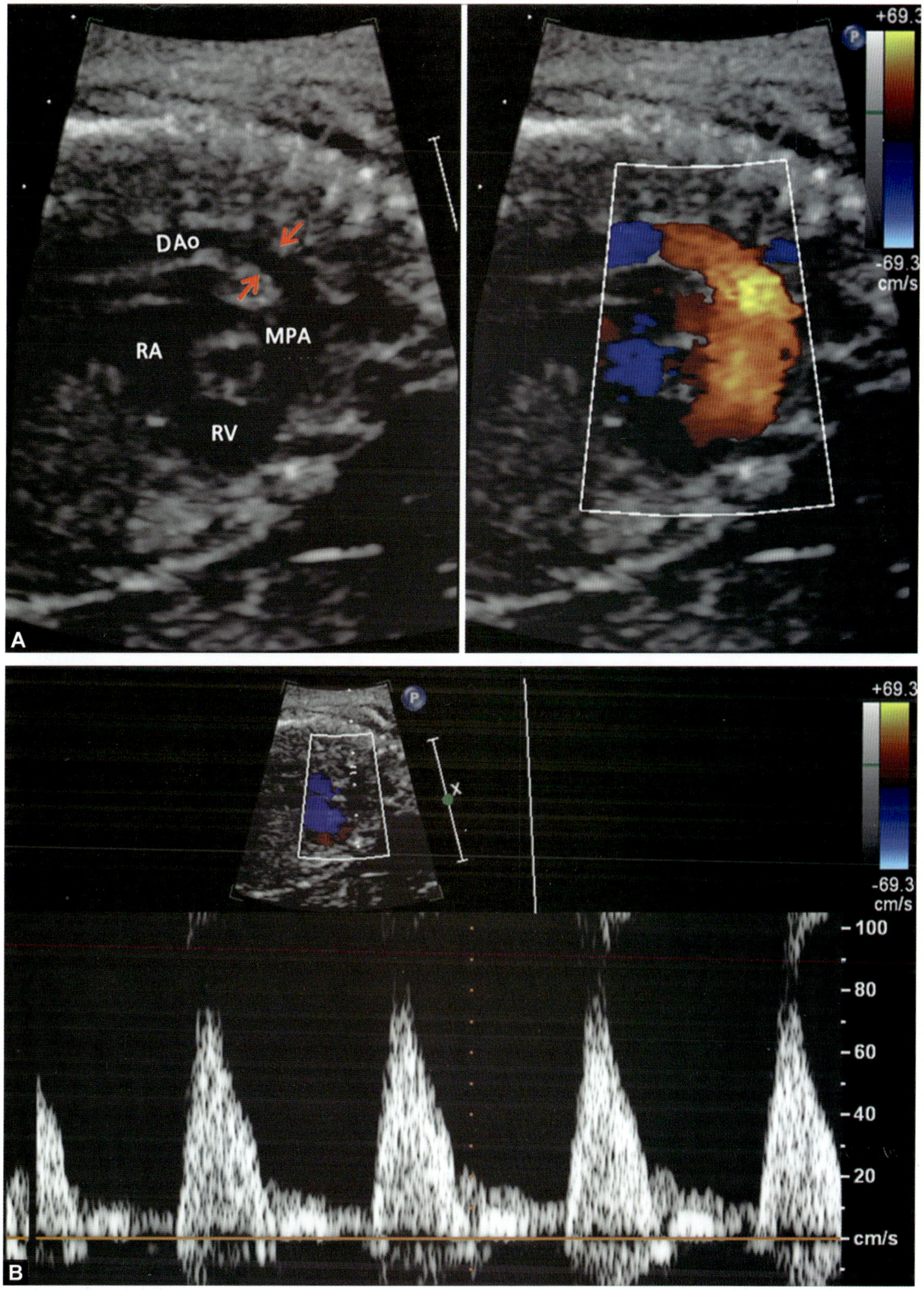

Figs. 47.8A and B: Fetal echocardiogram of the fetal ductal arch at 26 and 5/7 weeks of gestation. (A) 2D and color flow mapping; The arrows depict the ductus arteriosus; (B) Pulsed Doppler demonstrates the normal Doppler waveforms showing low velocity right to left flow with both systolic and diastolic components. (MPA: Main pulmonary artery; RA: Right atrium; RV: Right ventricle; DAo: Descending aorta).

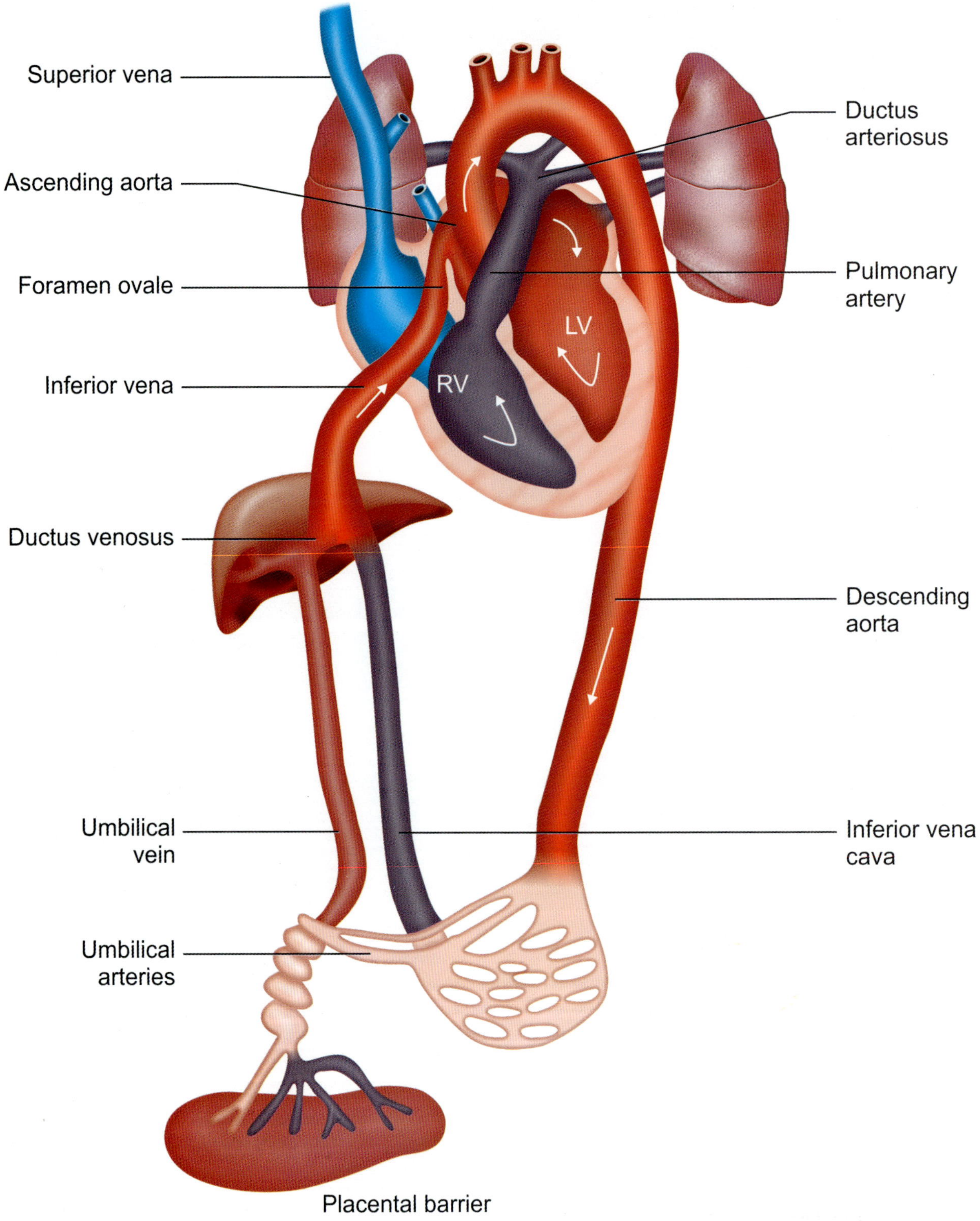

Fig. 47.9: Schematic illustration of the fetal circulation. [From Narasimhan C, Vijayalakshmi IB. In: Vijayalakshmi IB, et al. (Ed). A Comprehensive Approach to Congenital Heart Diseases. New Delhi, India: Jaypee Brothers Medical Publishers (P) Ltd; 2013, with permission].

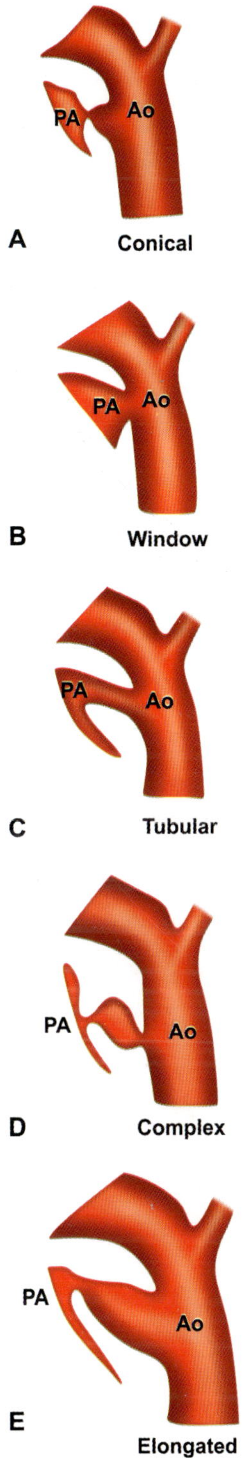

Fig. 47.10: Schematic and angiographic types of patent ductus arteriosus (PDA) based on the Krichenko classification. [From Arora R, Vijayalakshmi IB. Patent ductus arteriosus. In: Vijayalakshmi IB, et al (Ed). A Comprehensive Approach to Congenital Heart Diseases. New Delhi, India: Jaypee Brothers Medical Publishers (P) Ltd; 2013, with permission].

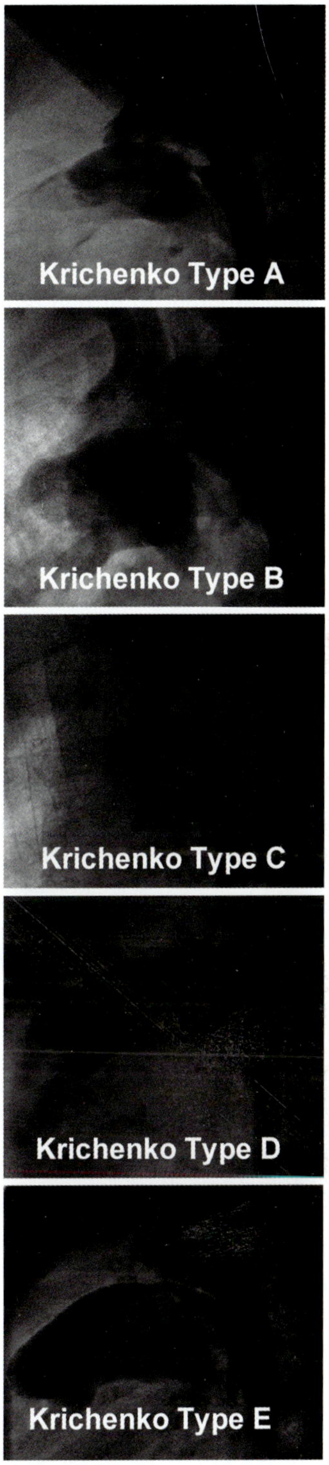

Fig. 47.11: Sample angiograms of the five types of ductuses using the Krichenko classification with. From top to bottom: Krichenko Type A ductus: funnel shaped with large ductal ampulla. Krichenko Type B ductus: short and broad ductus, also referred to as a "window" type ductus. Krichenko Type C ductus: tubular ductus. Krichenko Type D: complex with multiple constrictions. Krichenko Type E: elongated ductus with proximal constriction, remote from the anterior border of the trachea. (Angiographic images courtesy of Dr Thomas Doyle).

The ductus may also be "reverse oriented" (Fig. 47.12) in lesions associated with decreased pulmonary blood flow in utero; the finding of a reverse-oriented ductus denotes an increased likelihood of need for intervention in the perinatal period. In this setting, the ductus descends initially as it arises from the aorta, taking a course which has a concave orientation toward the head, before ascending to its insertion on the pulmonary artery. This appearance is very different from that of the orientation of the normal ductus which, like the aorta, takes a course which is concave toward the feet.

An unusual variant is that of a ductal aneurysm (Fig. 47.13), which may be seen on prenatal or postnatal imaging. These aneurysms most commonly are asymptomatic and resolve spontaneously. Potential complications include thrombus formation with extension into the pulmonary arteries or aorta, thromboembolic events including cerebral infarction, spontaneous rupture, compression of adjacent structures, erosion into airways, and symptoms related to persistent ductal patency.

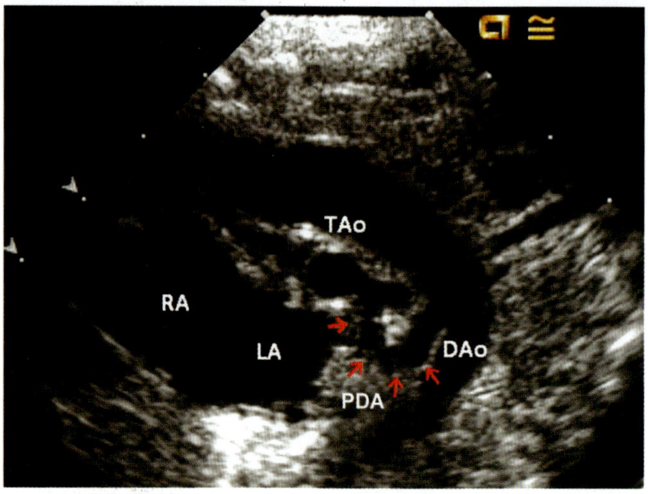

Fig. 47.12: Two-dimensional echocardiographic image of a reverse oriented ductus. In this image, obtained from a suprasternal imaging window, the ductus (arrows) takes a course which is concave toward the head, an inverted orientation to the usual "concave toward the feet" orientation of the normal ductus. (RA: Right atrium; LA: Left atrium; PA: Pulmonary artery; TAo: Transverse aorta; DAo: Descending aorta; PDA: Patent ductus arteriosus).

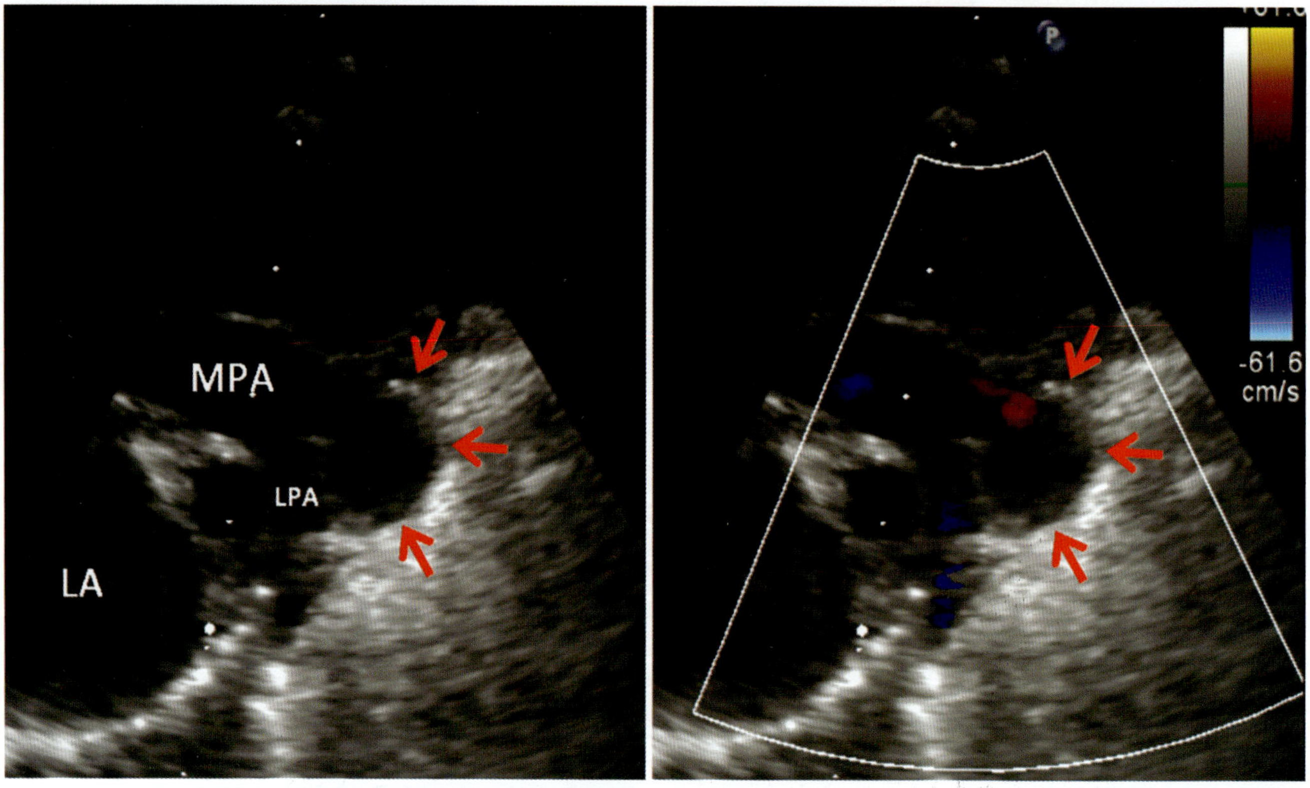

Fig. 47.13: Paired echocardiographic images with or without color flow mapping showing an aneurysm of the ductus (arrows). (MPA: Main pulmonary artery; LPA: Left pulmonary artery; LA: Left atrium).

In the setting of an otherwise normal cardiovascular system, the hemodynamic significance of the ductus arteriosus depends on the degree of shunting. The magnitude of left to right shunting across the ductus arteriosus is dependent on three major factors: size (diameter and length) of the ductus, which regulates its resistance; the pressure differential between the aorta and the pulmonary artery; and the balance of resistances in the systemic and pulmonary circulations. The physiologic features associated with the left to right shunting will also depend on the ability of the myocardium to deal with the extra volume load associated with the shunt. In mature infants and older children, with normal physiology consistent with decreased pulmonary vascular resistance and higher systemic arterial pressure, the size of the communications plays a very important role. A small PDA is likely of no hemodynamic significance, but is associated with the risk of infective endarteritis. A large PDA will have increased left-to-right shunt, and if left untreated, cause pulmonary overcirculation and eventually pulmonary vascular disease (Figs. 47.14A and B).

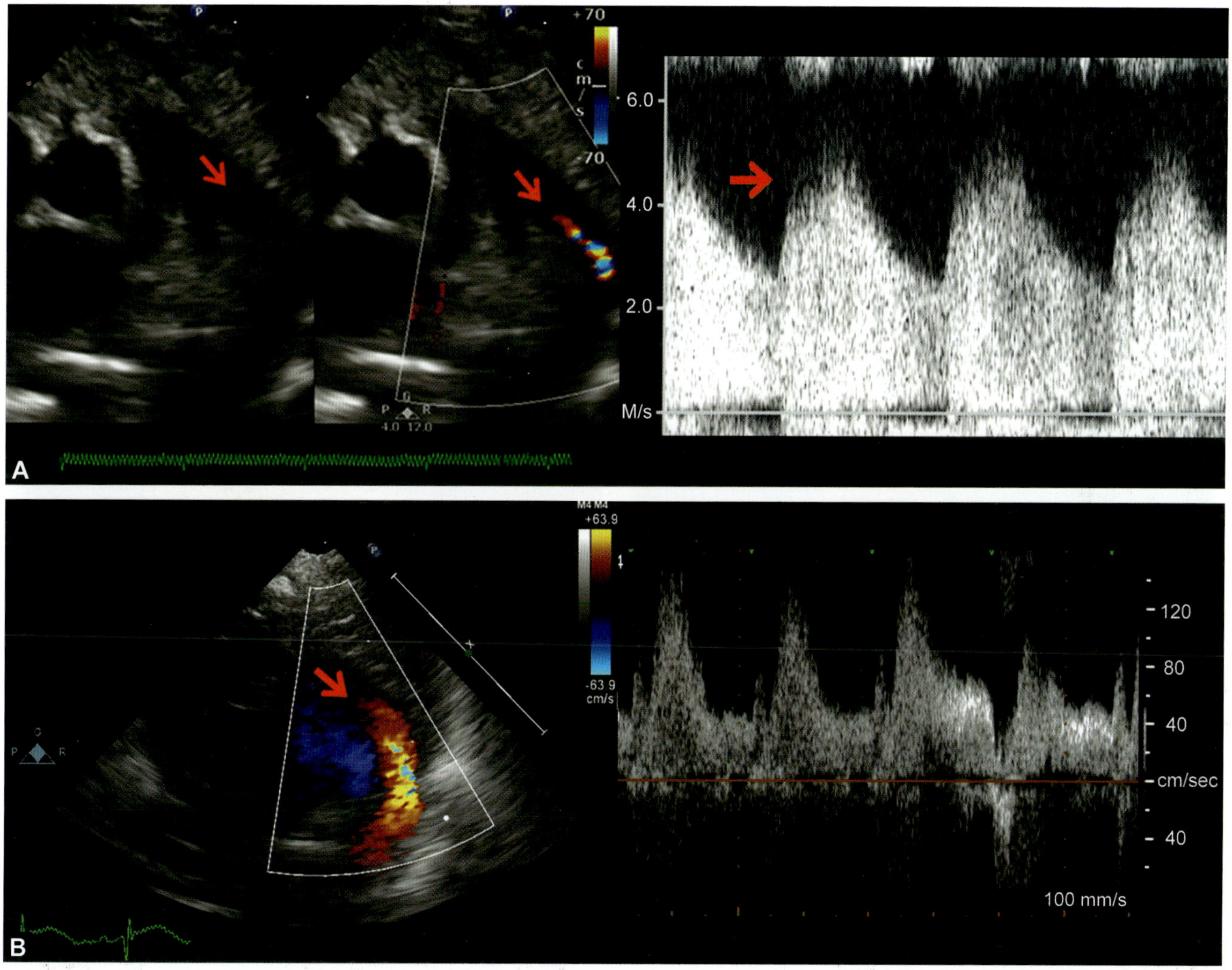

Figs. 47.14A and B: Echocardiographic images of the ductus obtained from the short-axis view color flow mapping (arrows) and with spectral Doppler interrogation: (A) Small ductus arteriosus with continuous left-to-right shunt and a restrictive Doppler pattern characterized by a high flow velocity (over 4 m/sec) consistent with low pulmonary artery pressure; and (B) Large ductus arteriosus with left-to-right shunt with continuous low velocity Doppler signal consistent with elevated pulmonary artery pressure.

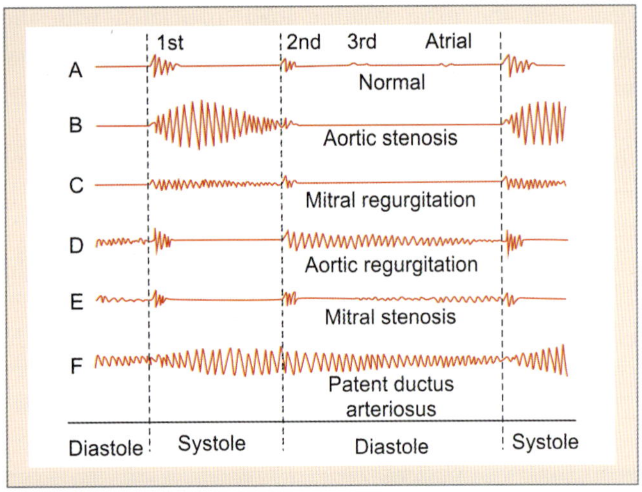

Fig. 47.15: The continuous murmur that may be heard on auscultation in a patient with patent ductus arteriosus (PDA). Note in contrast to valvular lesions, the murmur may be present in both systole and diastole. (Image posted by Madhero88 on Wikipedia).

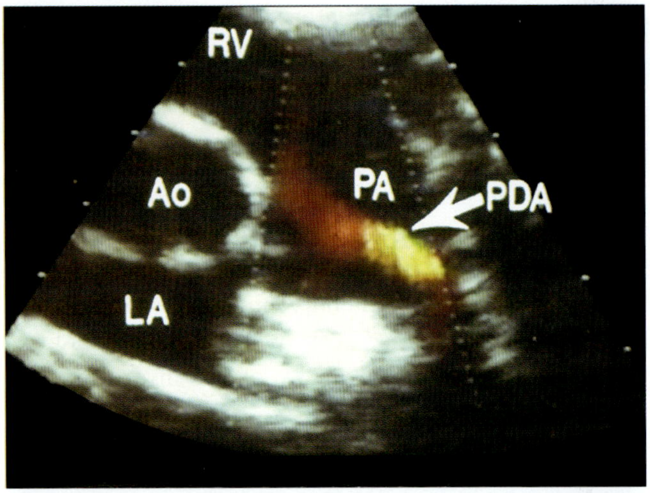

Fig. 47.16: Color Doppler flow mapping of the main pulmonary artery (PA) in a parasternal short-axis view demonstrating the flow (arrow) of the patent ductus arteriosus (PDA). [From Rao PS. Congenital heart defects—a review. In: Rao PS (Ed). Congenital Heart Disease—Selected Aspects. Intechweb.org., with permission]. (Ao: Aorta; LA: Left atrium; RV: Right ventricle).

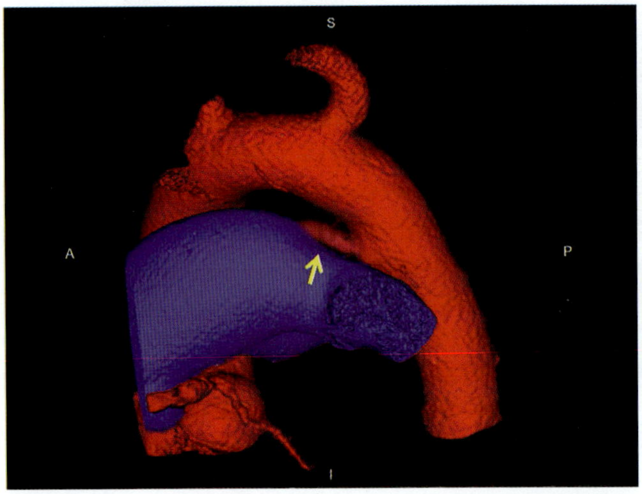

Fig. 47.17A: Contrast-enhanced computed tomography (CT) scan showing patent ductus arteriosus (PDA) (arrow) running from the aorta (shaded red) to the pulmonary artery (shaded blue). (Image courtesy of Glenn N Levine, MD).

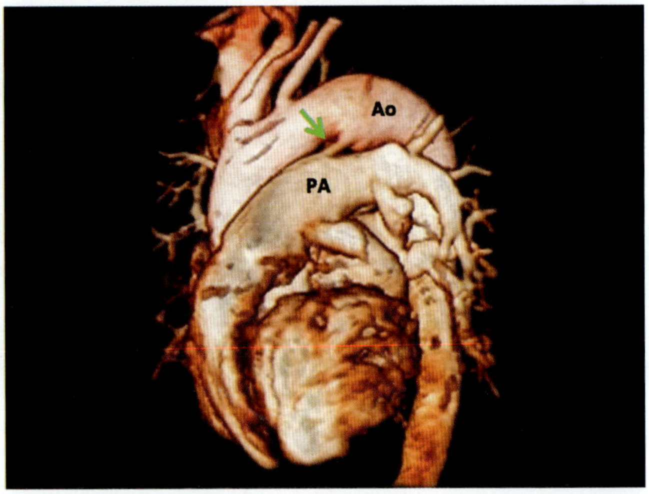

Fig. 47.17B: Magnetic resonance angiogram showing PDA (arrow). (Ao: Aorta; PA: Pulmonary artery).

EVALUATION OF PATENT DUCTUS ARTERIOSUS

In children and adults, the presence of a PDA may first be raised by the finding of a continuous, "machine like", murmur (Fig. 47.15). In the newborn period, the ductus may be silent or characterized by a murmur audible in systole only. In some patients, the PDA may only be incidentally discovered on echocardiography or during the evaluation of a symptomatic patient.

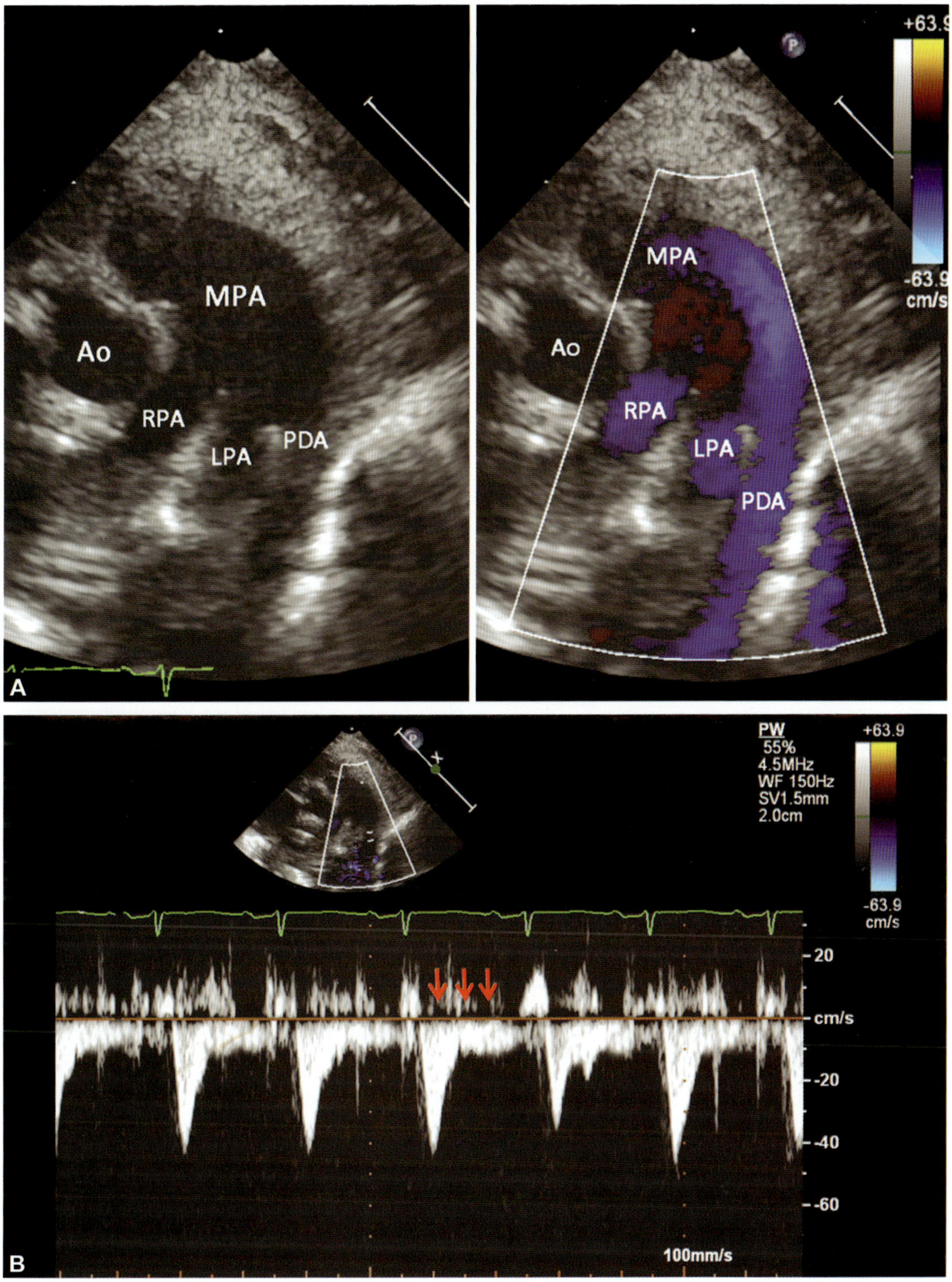

Figs. 47.18A and B: Two-dimensional, color Doppler, and spectral Doppler imaging of a patent ductus arteriosus (PDA) in an infant with severe pulmonary hypertension. (A) Paired two-dimensional echocardiographic images obtained from a short-axis parasternal imaging window with and without color flow mapping. Color flow mapping demonstrates systolic antegrade flow in the main pulmonary artery, the branch pulmonary arteries, and the patent ductus arteriosus; (B) Pulsed Doppler interrogation of ductus arteriosus shows systolic and diastolic antegrade flow (arrows) within the ductus. (Ao: Aorta; MPA: Main pulmonary artery; RPA: Right pulmonary artery; LPA: Left pulmonary artery; PDA: Patent ductus arteriosus).

Most commonly, echocardiography is used to assess the timing and direction of ductal flow, and provides significant information regarding the pulmonary artery pressure. The direction of shunting can be demonstrated by color flow mapping (Fig. 47.16). Rarely, in the older teenager and adult population, other imaging modalities such as computed tomography (CT) (Fig. 47.17A) or magnetic resonance imaging (MRI) (Fig. 47.17B) are needed. Echocardiographic spectral and continuous wave Doppler can be used to demonstrate the characteristic continuous flow pattern with peak late systolic velocity; pulmonary artery pressure can be estimated using the modified Bernoulli equation. Two-dimensional echocardiography may also demonstrate associated left-sided chamber enlargement in the setting of a significant left-to-right shunt.

In the setting of abnormally elevated pulmonary vascular resistance, particularly seen in infants with respiratory distress syndrome from birth, or in patients with pulmonary hypertension from other etiologies, the direction of shunting at the ductus may be bidirectional or even exclusively right to left. Echocardiographic evaluation is again central to evaluation and diagnosis. In the setting of severely elevated pulmonary vascular resistance, color flow mapping and pulsed Doppler demonstrate continuous right to left flow that peaks in early systole (Figs. 47.18A and B).

MANAGEMENT OF PATENT DUCTUS ARTERIOSUS

Closure of the ductus arteriosus is indicated in symptomatic patients with significant left-to-right shunt, those with left-sided volume overload or with reversible pulmonary artery hypertension. Ductal closure is contraindicated in patients whose pulmonary or systemic blood flow is dependent on the presence of a ductus, or in those with pulmonary artery hypertension either severe or irreversible.

The small, "nonhemodynamically" significant ductus arteriosus should still be closed in order to prevent the possibility of bacterial endarteritis.

Surgical closure of the ductus was first performed by Robert Gross in 1939 and over the years it has technically improved and is a safe procedure in even extremely low-birth-weight infants. The surgical closure of the ductus arteriosus is performed through a lateral thoracotomy and is accomplished by ligation and division of the vessel. Less invasive surgical approaches avoid the trauma associated with a thoracotomy incision; video-assisted thoracotomy (VAT) closes the ductus with one or several surgical clips. Surgery continues to be the treatment of choice for infants and for children with very large ductuses.

Percutaneous closure of the ductus arteriosus in the cardiac catheterization laboratory was first reported in 1967 and is now the preferred method in infants and children larger than 6 kg. Device closure of the ductus is traditionally performed with either coil occlusion or placement of an Amplatzer device occluder (Figs 47.19A to F). Coil occlusion is effective and cost effective; however, complications such as coil embolization or residual shunting have been reported. The Amplatzer device occluder is the most commonly used device for the closure of moderate or large size ductuses in older children and adults. The choice of either Amplatzer device closure (Fig. 47.20) or coil occlusion (Fig. 47.21) depends not only on the size of the ductus, but also on the configuration and anatomy of the ductus; the Amplatzer is best suited for the conical ductus with a narrowest segment toward the pulmonary artery.

Catheter intervention to maintain the patency of the ductus arteriosus in the setting of congenital heart defects where the ductus is the source for either systemic or pulmonary blood flow is now being performed more frequently in infants. Stenting the pulmonary artery became possible with the advent of coronary stents in the 1990s. Percutaneous stent implantation has since evolved, and may be used to maintain the patency of the ductus arteriosus to secure flow in infants with inadequate pulmonary blood supply, sometimes obviating the need for surgical stent placement. Stent implantation is also used to secure antegrade systemic blood flow from the right ventricle in infants undergoing hybrid Norwood palliation (Fig. 47.22).

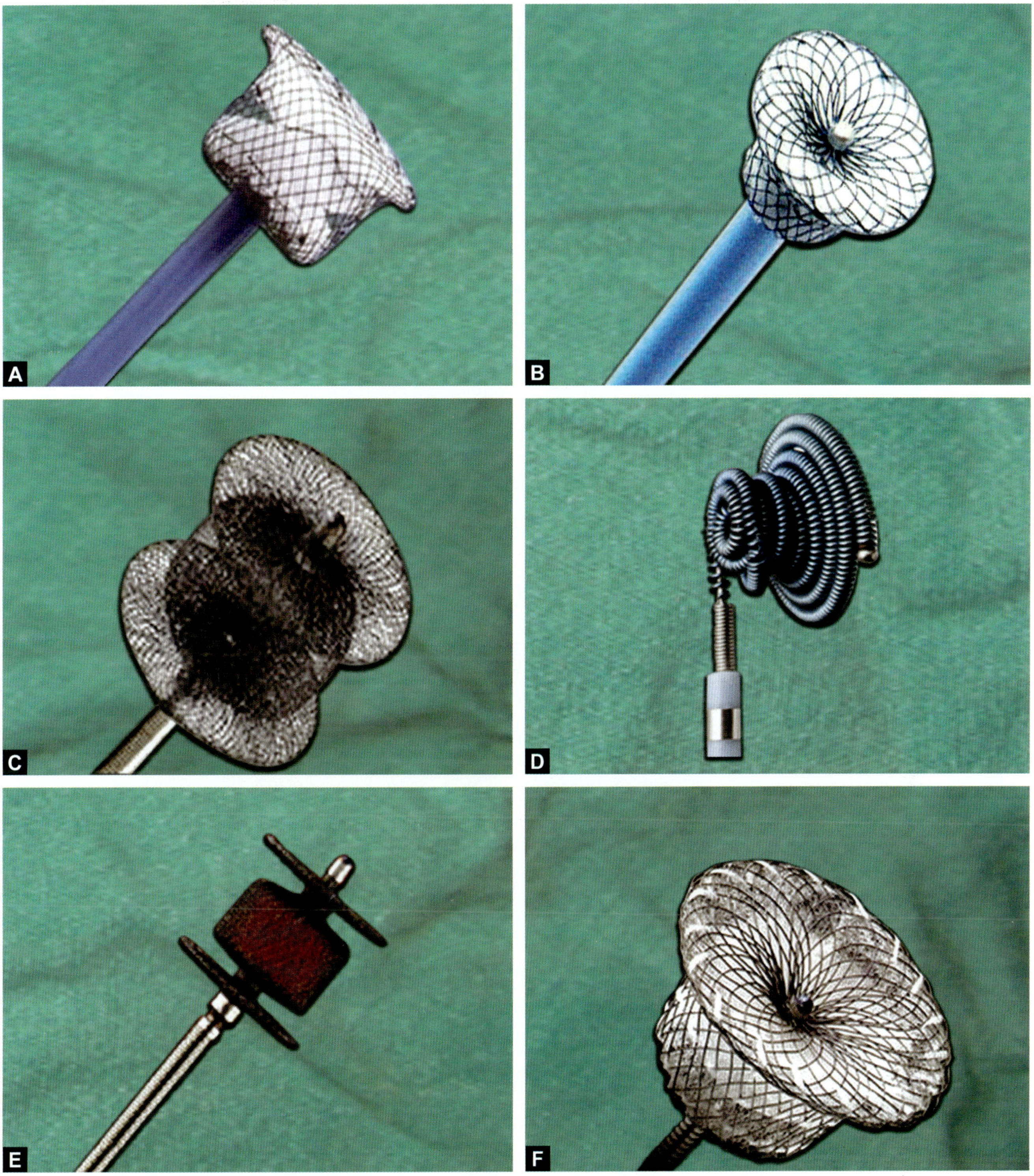

Figs. 47.19A to F: Sample of percutaneous closure devices used to close a patent ductus arteriosus (PDA).

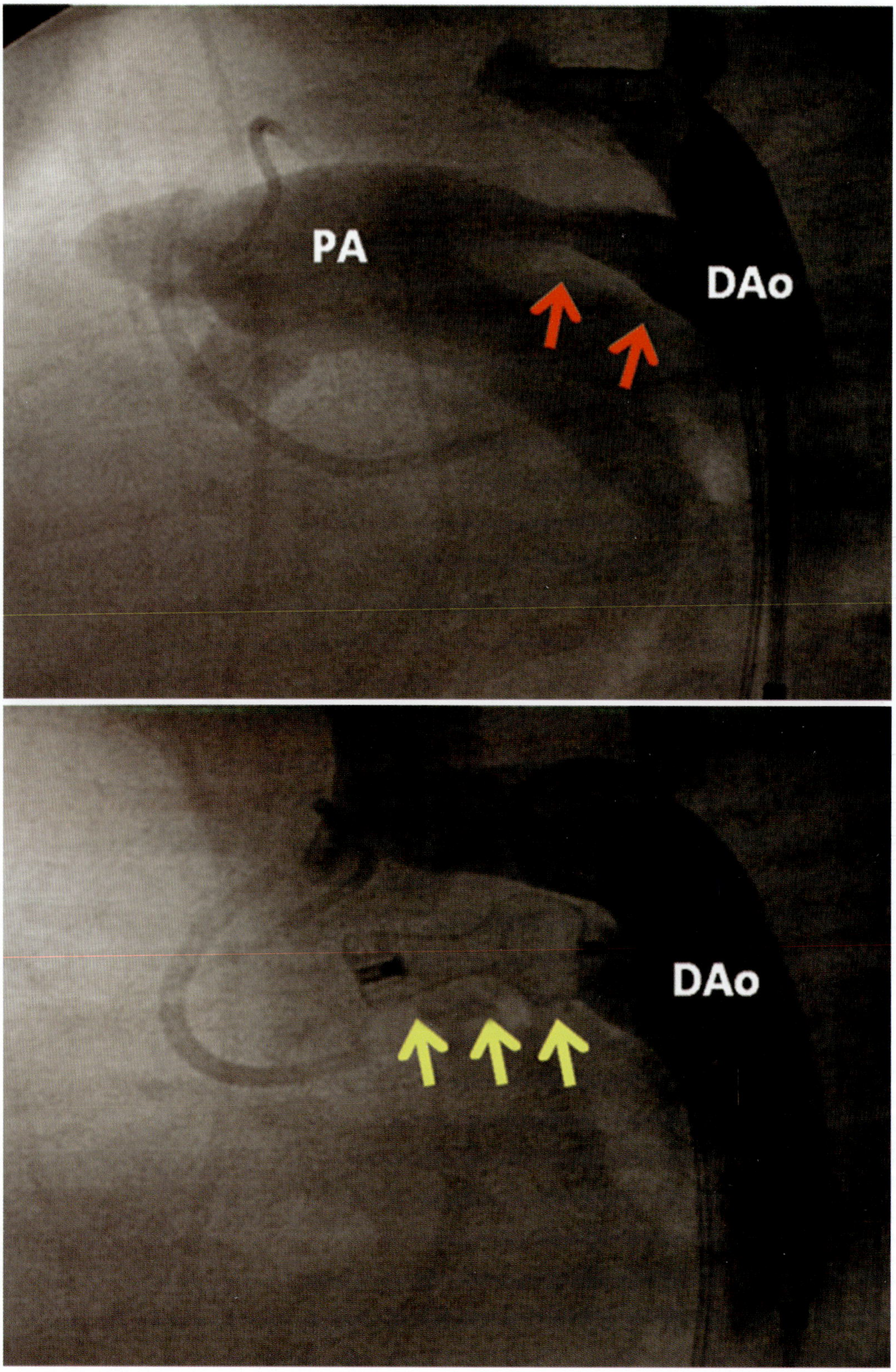

Fig. 47.20: Cine frames taken in the lateral view demonstrating a medium to large-sized patent ductus arteriosus (PDA) (red arrows) which was occluded with an Amplatzer duct occluder (yellow arrows). There is dense opacification (top panel) of the PDA and main pulmonary artery (PA) prior to occlusion and no opacification following occlusion (bottom panel). (DAo: Descending Aorta). [From Rao PS. Congenital heart defects—a review. In: Rao PS (Ed). Congenital Heart Disease—Selected Aspects. Intechweb.org., with permission].

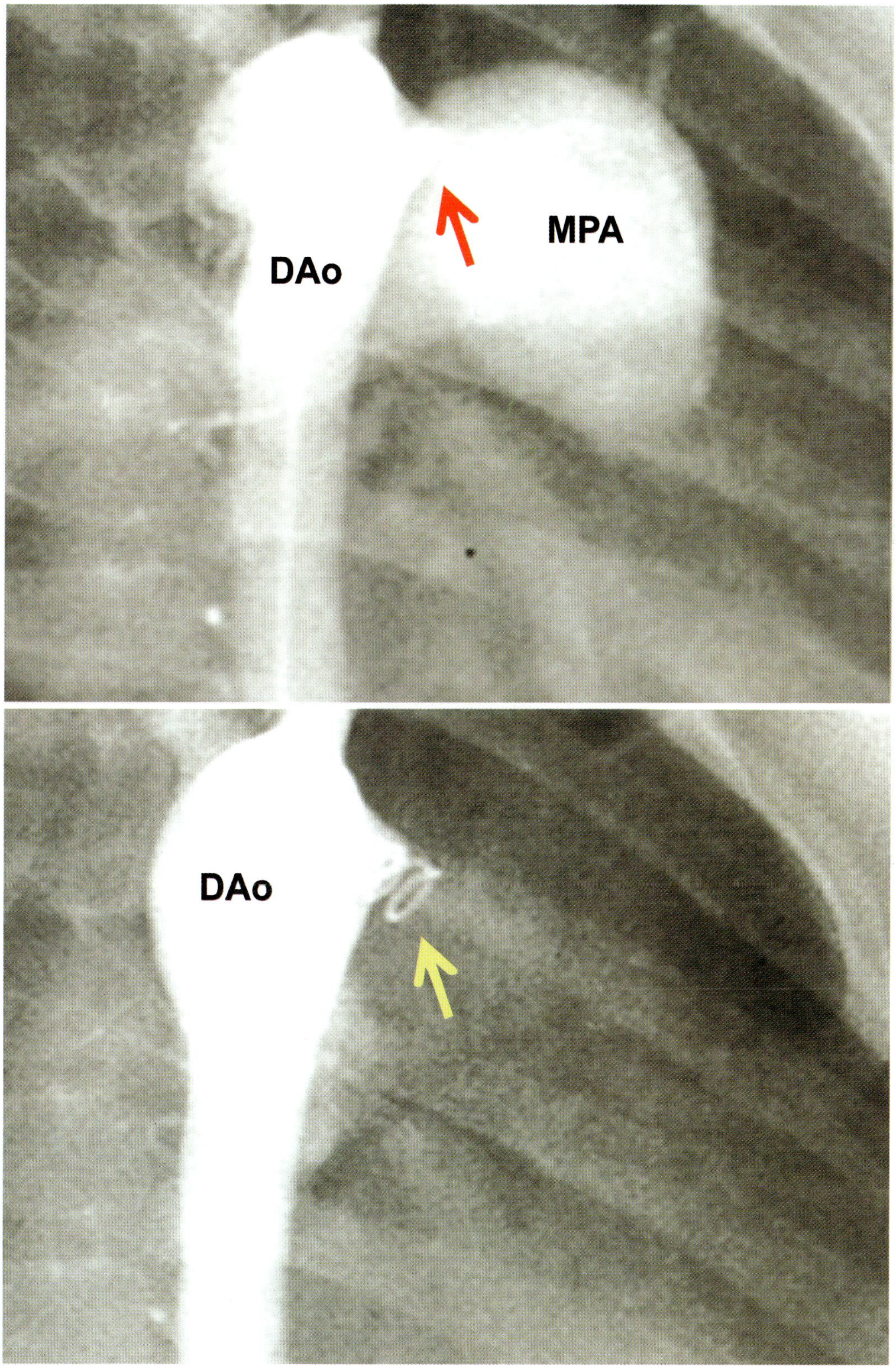

Fig. 47.21: Cine frame images taken in the right anterior oblique view demonstrating a small to medium-sized PDA (red arrow) occluded with a Gianturco coil (yellow arrow). There is dense opacification of the main pulmonary artery (MPA) prior to occlusion (top panel) and no opacification following occlusion with the (bottom panel). (DAo: Descending aorta). [From Rao PS. Congenital heart defects—a review. In: Rao PS (Ed). Congenital Heart Disease—Selected Aspects. Intechweb.org., with permission].

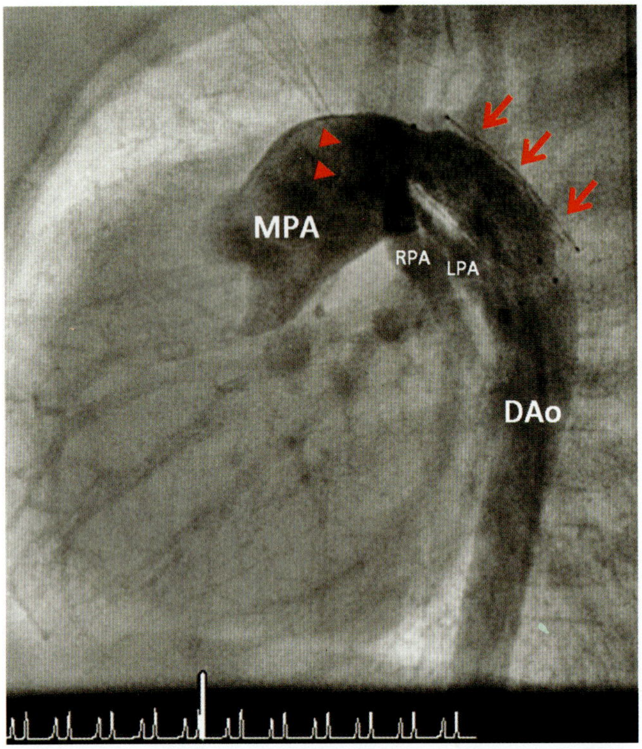

Fig. 47.22: Pulmonary arteriogram with ductal stent (large arrows) in position in an infant with hypoplastic left heart syndrome post hybrid Norwood. The main pulmonary artery, banded branch pulmonary arteries, stented ducts and descending aorta are densely opaque with contrast. There is also less dense opacification of the hypoplastic ascending aorta (small arrows) transverse aorta and brachiocephalics, and native aortic isthmus. (DAo: Descending aorta; LPA: Left pulmonary artery; MPA: Main pulmonary artery; RPA: Right pulmonary artery).

REFERENCES

Antonucci R, Bassareo P, Zaffanello M, et al. Patent ductus arteriosus in the preterm infant: new insights into pathogenesis and clinical management. J Matern Fetal Neonatal Med. 2010; 23(Suppl. 3):34-7.

Clyman RI. Mechanisms regulating the ductus arteriosus. Biol Neonate. 2006;89(4):330-5.

Dyamenahalli U, Smallhorn JF, Geva T, et al. Isolated ductus arteriosus aneurysm in the fetus and infant: a multi-institutional experience. J Am Coll Cardiol. 2000;36(1):262-9.

Giroud JM, Jacobs JP. Evolution of strategies for management of the patent arterial duct. Cardiol Young. 2007;17(Suppl. 2):68-74.

Gournay V. The ductus arteriosus: physiology, regulation, and functional and congenital anomalies. Arch Cardiovasc Dis. 2011;104(11):578-85.

Hinton R, Michelfelder E. Significance of reverse orientation of the ductus arteriosus in neonates with pulmonary outflow tract obstruction for early intervention. Am J Cardiol. 2006; 97(5):716-9.

Hoffman JI, Kaplan S. The incidence of congenital heart disease. J Am Coll Cardiol. 2002;39(12):1890-900.

Kutty S, Zahn EM. Interventional therapy for neonates with critical congenital heart disease. Catheter Cardiovasc Interv. 2008;72(5):663-74.

Moore P, Brook M, Heyman M. Patent ductus arteriosus. In: Heart Disease in Infants, Children and Adolescents, 6th edition. Philadelphia: Lippincott Williams & Wilkins; 2001. pp. 653-69.

Schneider DJ. The patent ductus arteriosus in term infants, children and adults. Semin Perinatol. 2012;36(2):146-53.

Schneider DJ, Moore JW. Patent ductus arteriosus. Circulation. 2006;114(17):1873-82.

Section 7

Peripheral Vascular Disease

Chapters

CHAPTER

48

Peripheral Arterial Disease

Carlos F Bechara, George T Pisimisis

INTRODUCTION

A highly developed network of arteries supplies oxygenated blood to the peripheral legs and arms (Figs. 48.1 to 48.3). Numerous disease processes, most notably atherosclerosis, can lead to stenosis and occlusion (Fig. 48.4) of these arteries, and is termed peripheral arterial disease (PAD). PAD affects more than eight million people in the United States alone, and tens of millions of persons worldwide. PAD is defined by an ankle-brachial index (ABI) of less than 0.9 at rest. Most patients with PAD of the lower extremity either are asymptomatic or have claudication or pain with walking. Most patients with claudication can be managed medically and with lifestyle modification. Patients considered with critical limb ischemia (CLI) includes those with tissue loss and rest pain.

Atherosclerosis is the most common cause of PAD. Modifiable risk factors for atherosclerotic PAD are smoking (strongest association), diabetes, hypertension, and hyperlipidemia. Other risk factors that cannot be controlled are increasing age and ethnicity. PAD incidence increases with age and in non-Hispanic African Americans.

Symptoms and their severity depend on level and extent of disease (Table 48.1). Several classification schemes have been used to categorize symptomatology (Tables 48.2 and 48.3). Since the process is chronic, symptomatology is influenced by the presence and degree of collateral pathway, and by the patient's cardiac reserve (oxygen delivery and carrying capacity). Patients with single level arterial disease, such as iliac artery occlusion, typically present with buttock, thigh or calf claudication. Patients with multilevel arterial disease, typically present with either rest pain or tissue loss. A noninvasive arterial duplex (Fig. 48.5) is a valuable test to perform on these patients. It provides information on the extent of the disease (Fig. 48.6, Table 48.4), and serves as a baseline for future comparisons, especially postintervention. Initial evaluation of the patient should take into consideration not only atherosclerotic peripheral vascular disease as the cause of a patient's symptoms, but other disease processes (Table 48.5) that can often mimic or be mistaken for some of the symptoms of PAD.

AORTOILIAC OCCLUSIVE DISEASE

Figures 48.7 and 48.8 show the distal aorta and iliofemoral arteries both schematically, and as they appear with advanced imaging modalities. Typically, patients with aortoiliac occlusive disease (AIOD) (Figs. 48.9 and 48.10) are in their fifties and present with buttock, thigh or calf claudication. They usually develop large collaterals (Figs. 48.11A and B), compensating for the occlusion. Any low-flow state or disruption in the collateral pathway can lead to acute limb ischemia requiring emergency surgery. Computed tomographic angiography (CTA) has replaced angiography, since it is noninvasive and yields high-quality images. Arterial duplex is a noninvasive test that is also useful in identifying iliac arterial disease. Intravascular ultrasound (IVUS) is an adjunctive tool used during endovascular intervention. IVUS is useful to measure vessel diameter, to assess stent apposition, and to image improvement in arterial lumen with stenting or angioplasty.

Indication for surgery is life-limiting claudication, rest pain, tissue loss (Fig. 48.12) and distal embolization (blue toe syndrome) (Fig. 48.13). Guidelines for treatment were established by the Transatlantic Intersocietal Commission (TASC). For AIOD with stenosis, percutaneous intervention (Figs. 48.14A to D) using the retrograde femoral

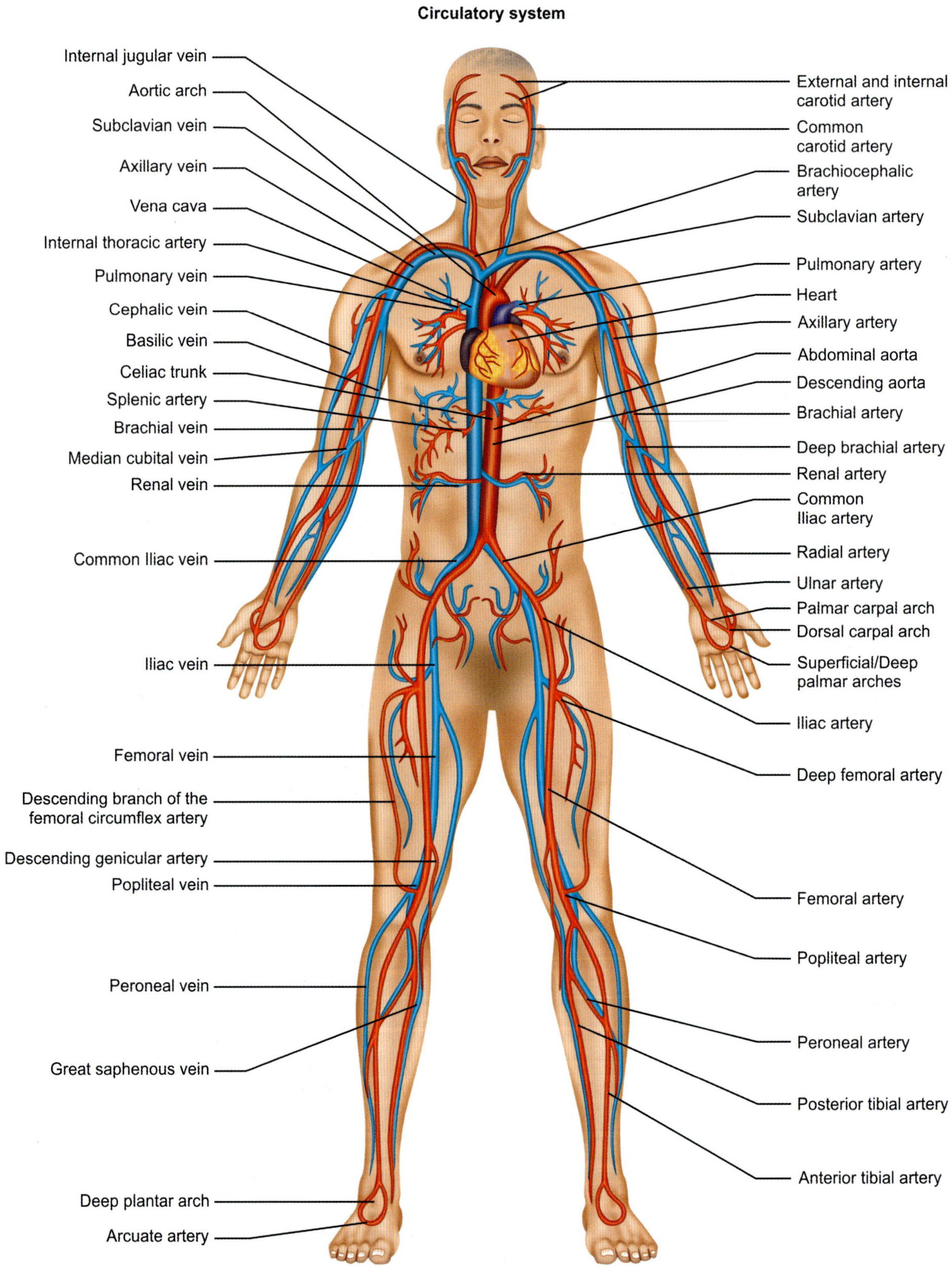

Fig. 48.1: Schematic illustration of the peripheral, central, and cerebral arteries.

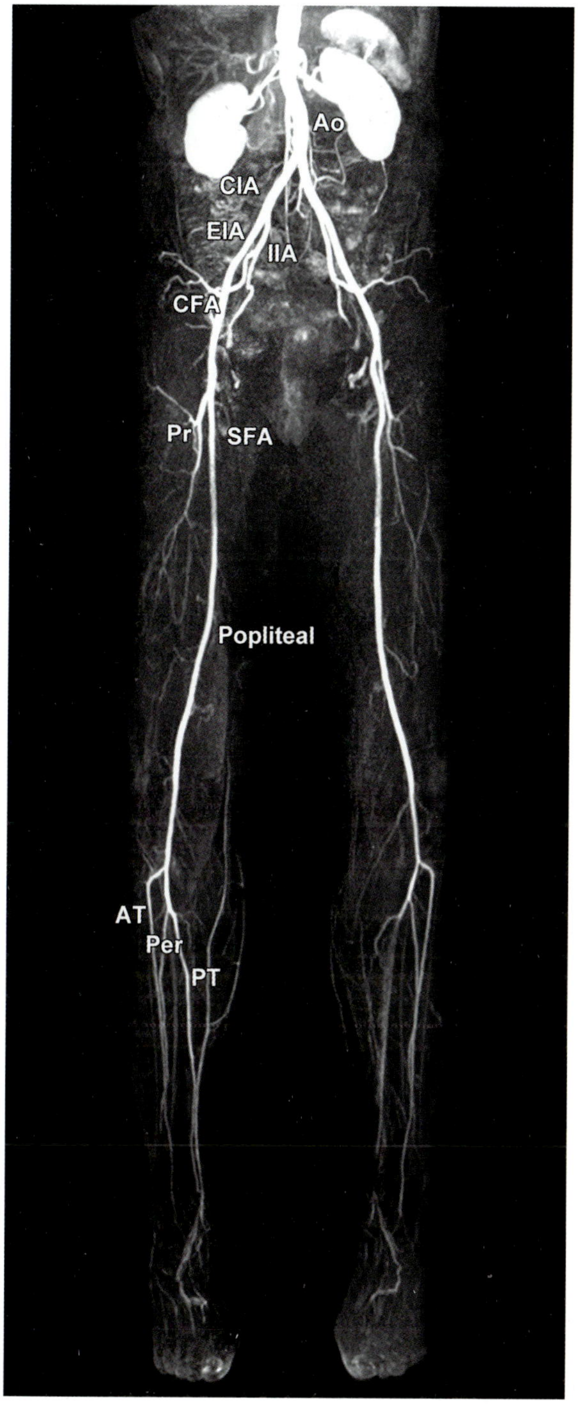

Fig. 48.2: Magnetic resonance angiography of the distal aorta and lower extremities. [Image from Ong MM, Hausotter K, Pilz LR, et al. Steady state vascular imaging with extracellular gadobutrol: evaluation of the additional diagnostic benefit in patients who have undergone a peripheral magnetic resonance angiography protocol. J Cardiovasc Magn Reson. 2013;15(1):97]. (From cranial to caudal: Ao: Aorta; CIA: Common iliac artery; EAI: External iliac artery; IIA: Internal iliac artery; CFA: Common femoral artery; SFA: Superficial femoral artery; Pr: Profunda artery/deep femoral artery; AT: Anterior tibial artery; Per: Peroneal artery; PT: Posterior tibial artery).

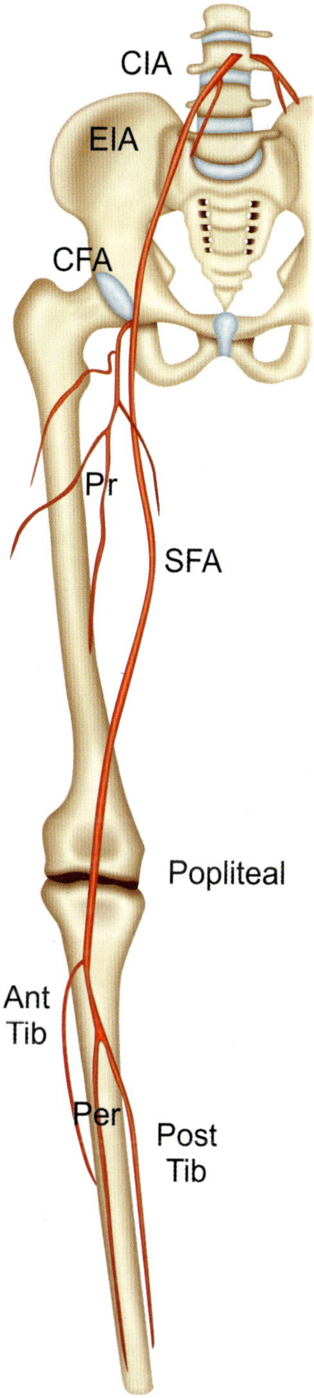

Fig. 48.3: Schematic illustration of the arteries of the lower extremity. [Image from Chavhan G, Jankharia B (Eds). Cross Sectional Anatomy CT and MRI, 1st edition. New Delhi, India: Jaypee Brothers Medical Publishers (P) Ltd.; 2012]. (From cranial to caudal: Ao, aorta; CIA, common iliac artery; EAI, external iliac artery; IIA, internal iliac artery; CFA: Common femoral artery; SFA: Superficial femoral artery; Pr: Profunda artery/deep femoral artery; AT: Anterior tibial artery; Per: Peroneal artery; PT: Posterior tibial artery).

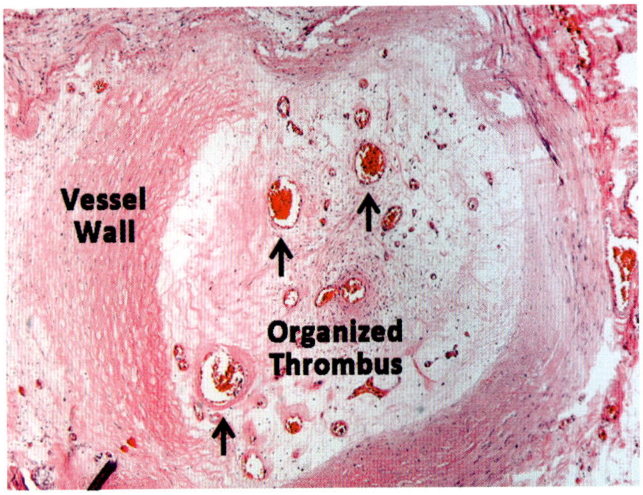

Fig. 48.4: Histology specimen of an occluded artery of the lower leg. The lumen is occluded by an old organized thrombus. Scattered areas of recanularization (arrows) are visible. (Image created by Patho and posted on Wikimedia Commons).

Table 48.1: Usual area of ischemia and claudication with obstructive peripheral arterial disease (PAD).

Area of obstruction	*Anatomic location of ischemia and symptoms*
Aorta or iliac artery	Buttock, hip, thigh
Femoral arteries or branches	Thigh, calf
Popliteal artery	Calf, ankle, foot
Tibial and peroneal arteries	Foot

approach is usually utilized (Figs. 48.15A and B). For iliac artery occlusion, an antegrade approach is often utilized (Figs. 48.16A to D), either from the contralateral femoral artery or the brachial artery. For long segment occlusion in patients who are good surgical candidates, arterial bypass is usually performed (Figs. 48.17 to 48.19).

FEMOROPOPLITEAL OCCLUSIVE DISEASE

The femoropopliteal arteries (Figs. 48.20 and 48.21) are one of the most common areas affected by atherosclerosis that results in intermittent claudication. Patients with femoropopliteal occlusive disease (Figs. 48.22 and 48.23) should be treated conservatively with medical management to control their atherosclerotic risk factors. Symptoms not only depend on location and severity of the

Table 48.2: Summary of the Fontaine scheme for classification of peripheral arterial disease (PAD).

Stage	*Symptoms*
I	Asymptomatic
IIa	Mild claudication
IIb	Moderate-severe claudication–
III	Ischemic rest pain
IV	Ulceration or gangrene

Table 48.3: Summary of the Rutherford scheme for classification of peripheral arterial disease (PAD).

Grade	*Category*	*Symptoms*
0	0	Asymptomatic
I	1	Mild claudication
I	2	Moderate claudication
I	3	Severe claudication
II	4	Ischemic rest pain
III	5	Minor tissue loss
IV	6	Ulceration or gangrene

disease, but also on the presence (or absence) of collateral vessels such as the geniculate arteries (Figs. 48.24A and B). When there is lifestyle-limiting claudication, intervention is warranted, especially after smoking cessation and risk factor modification has been accomplished. Intervention can be done by endovascular means or with open surgery (Fig. 48.25).

There is a wide variety of options for endovascular intervention such as atherectomy devices, balloon angioplasty, stenting, and recently, the addition of antiproliferative drugs to stents and balloons, such as paclitaxel. With surgery, the use of a vein bypass is usually preferred, since it is associated with better long-term patency. The vein bypass can be reversed or left in place (in situ bypass). Surveillance is important to maintain stent or bypass patency (Fig. 48.26). For recurrent stenosis in the bypass anastomosis, endovascular therapy can be used, usually with excellent long-term results.

TIBIAL OCCLUSIVE DISEASE

There are three vessels that provide blood supply to the foot: the anterior tibial, peroneal and posterior tibial

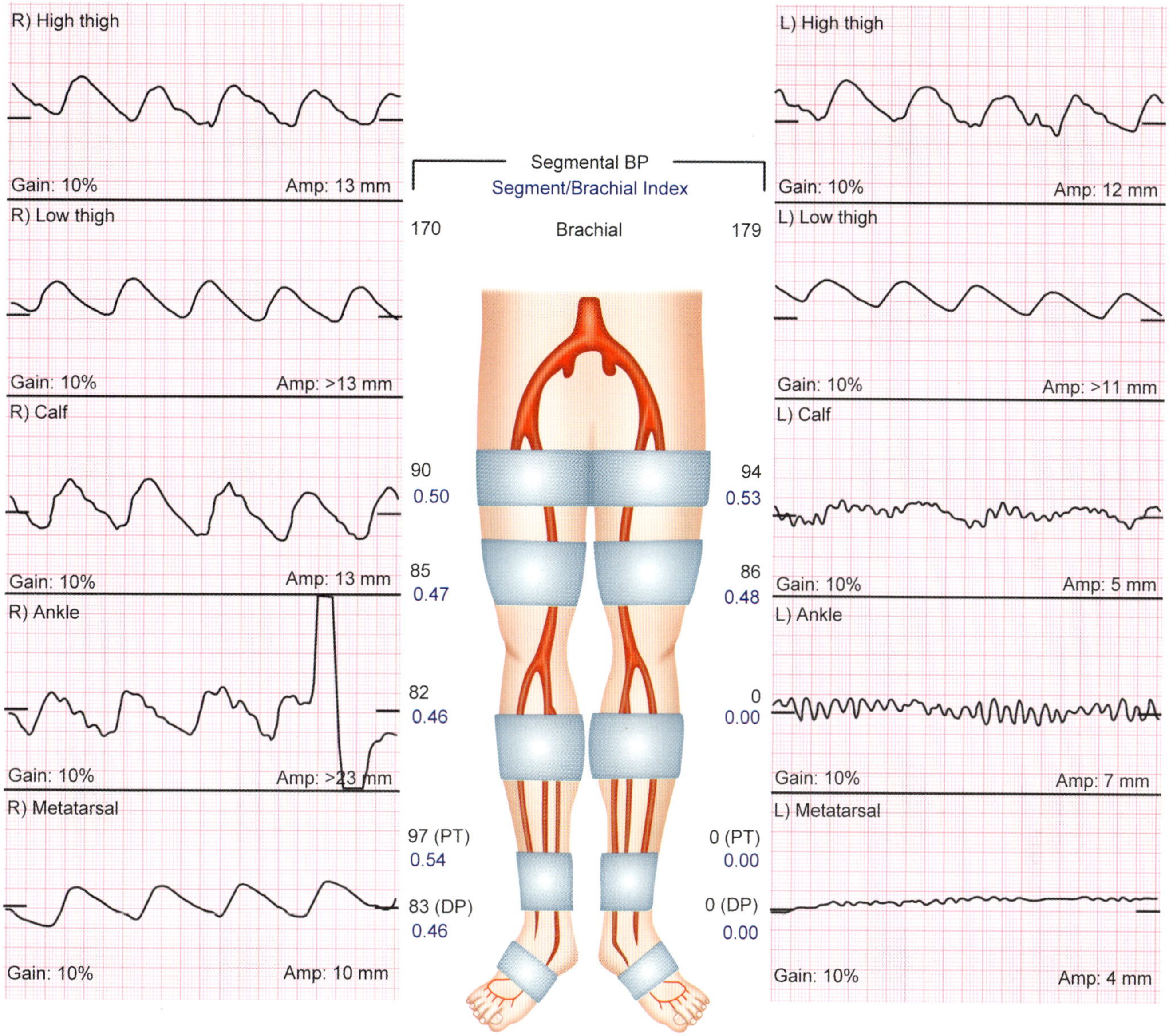

Fig. 48.5: Technique and tracings in determining the ankle-brachial index (ABI). Study demonstrates absent arterial flow in the left posterior tibial and dorsalis pedis arteries. [Image from Al-Sahfie T, Suman P. Aortoiliac occlusive disease. In: Yamanouchi D (Ed). Vascular Surgery. InTech. 2012. pp. 1-37].

arteries (Fig. 48.27). These vessels are sometimes referred to as trifurcation vessels, but in reality they rarely originate at the same level. Many patients who have even only one of these three vessels patent will not have symptoms. However, when tibial occlusive disease is present in conjunction with hemodynamically significant lesions in the iliac arteries or femoropopliteal arteries, tissue loss and risk of limb loss are often present. Such patients with multilevel disease can be treated with a hybrid procedure to provide inflow to the wound to heal. Similar to femoropopliteal occlusive disease, there is a wide variety of options for endovascular intervention, and periodic surveillance is warranted to maintain long-term patency and limb salvage. Patients with diabetic foot infection may benefit from restoration of arterial flow, but often require complex (Fig. 48.28) or repeated intervention.

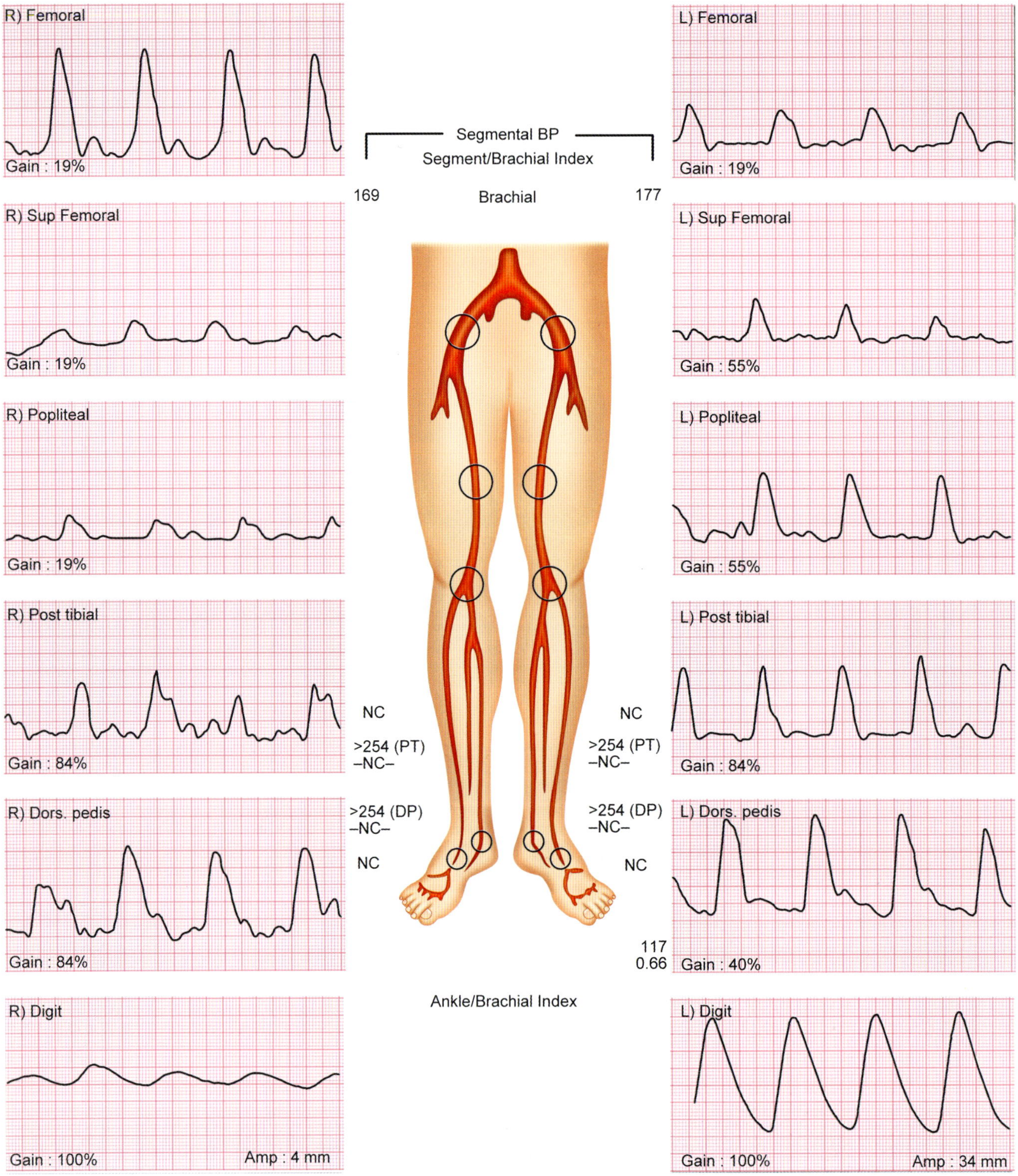

Fig. 48.6: Duplex ultrasound of bilateral lower extremity showing diffuse arterial disease. Note that in this patient, the tibial vessels were noncompressible (NC), causing falsely elevated ankle-brachial indices (ABIs). Toe pressure measurement is crucial for such cases.

Table 48.4: Interpretation of ankle-brachial index (ABI) values.

Ankle-brachial index (ABI) value	*Interpretation*
> 1.2	Abnormal vessel hardening
1.0–1.3	Normal
0.9–1.0	Acceptable
0.8–0.9	Some arterial disease
0.5–0.8	Moderate arterial disease
< 0.5	Severe arterial disease

Table 48.5: Differential diagnosis of disease processes that may mimic some of the symptoms of peripheral arterial disease (PAD).

• Nerve route compression
• Spinal stenosis
• Hip arthritis
• Bakers cyst
• Foot or ankle arthritis
• Venous claudication
• Chronic compartment syndrome

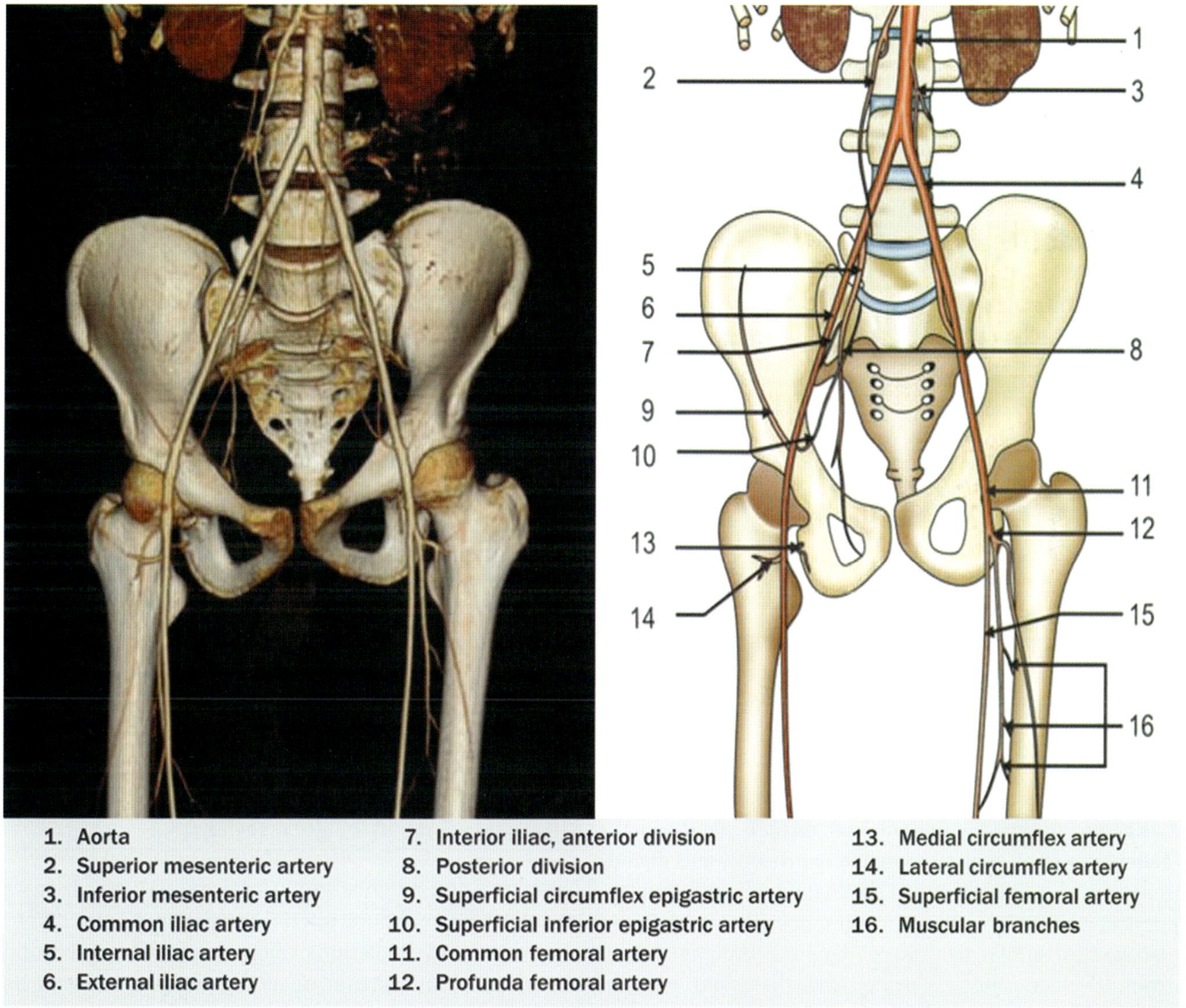

Fig. 48.7: Three-dimensional volume-rendered computed tomography (CT), and corresponding schematic illustration of the distal aorta and lower extremity arteries. [Image from Chavhan G, Jankharia B (Eds). Cross Sectional Anatomy CT and MRI, 1st edition. New Delhi, India: Jaypee Brothers Medical Publishers (P) Ltd; 2012].

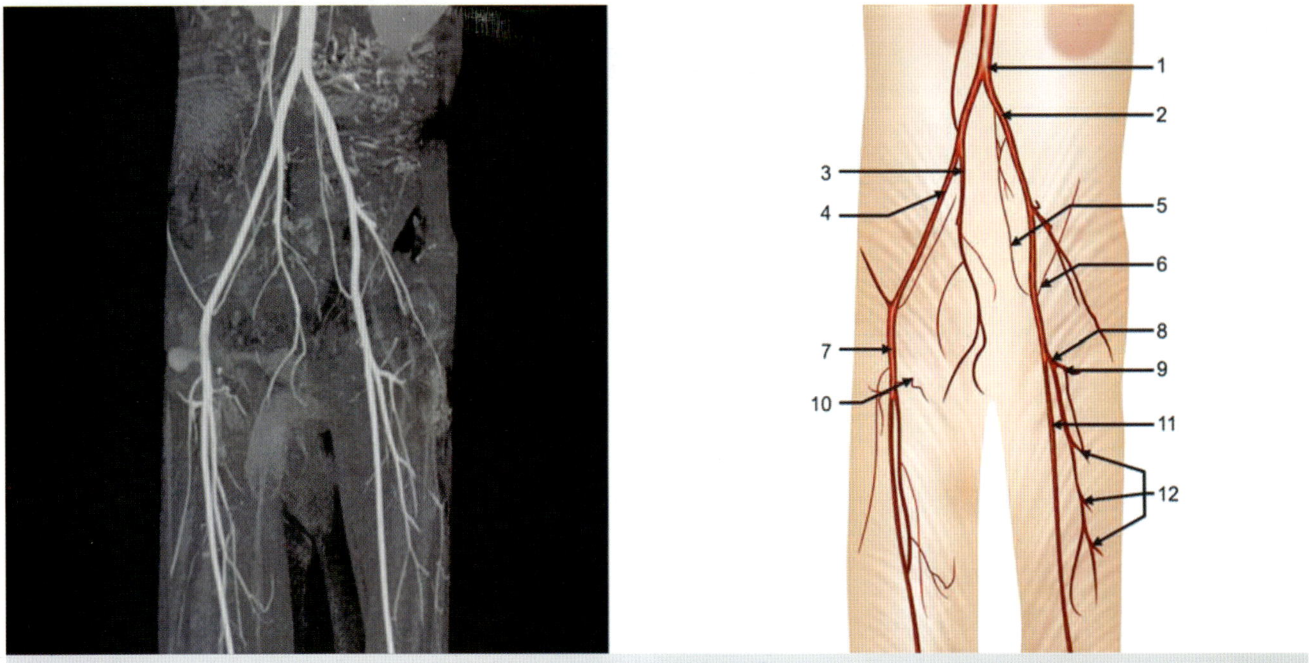

1. Aorta
2. Common iliac artery
3. Internal iliac artery
4. External iliac artery
5. Superficial inferior epigastric artery
6. Superficial circumflex epigastric artery
7. Common femoral artery
8. Profunda femoral artery
9. Lateral circumflex artery
10. Medial circumflex artery
11. Superficial femoral artery
12. Muscular branches

Fig. 48.8: Magnetic resonance imaging (MRI) and corresponding schematic illustration of the distal aorta and lower extremity arteries. [Image from Chavhan G, Jankharia B (Eds). Cross Sectional Anatomy CT and MRI, 1st edition. New Delhi, India: Jaypee Brothers Medical Publishers (P) Ltd; 2012].

UPPER EXTREMITY PERIPHERAL ARTERIAL DISEASE

Symptomatic upper extremity PAD is much less common than symptomatic disease of the lower extremities. Causes of upper arterial disease can include atherosclerosis, systemic inflammatory processes and arteritis, Buerger's disease, connective tissue diseases, fibromuscular dysplasia, and trauma. Symptoms may include claudication, "subclavian steal" with presyncope or syncope, and digital ischemia or necrosis. Initial evaluation, in addition to physical examination, may include upper extremity Doppler studies, similar to those obtained to evaluate lower extremity claudication. Imaging, when indicated, can be via contrast-enhanced computed tomography (CT) scan, magnetic resonance angiography, or invasive angiography (Figs. 48.29 to 48.32). Depending on the cause of an anatomy, percutaneous or surgical intervention is often utilized for treatment (Figs. 48.33A and B). Risk factor modification is implemented for secondary prevention.

NON-ATHEROSCLEROTIC PERIPHERAL ARTERY DISEASE

Numerous non-atherosclerotic focal and systemic diseases can affect the peripheral arterial circulation. A comprehensive review and discussion of all these processes is beyond the scope of this chapter. Several processes, that may be relevant to the reader, are briefly discussed below.

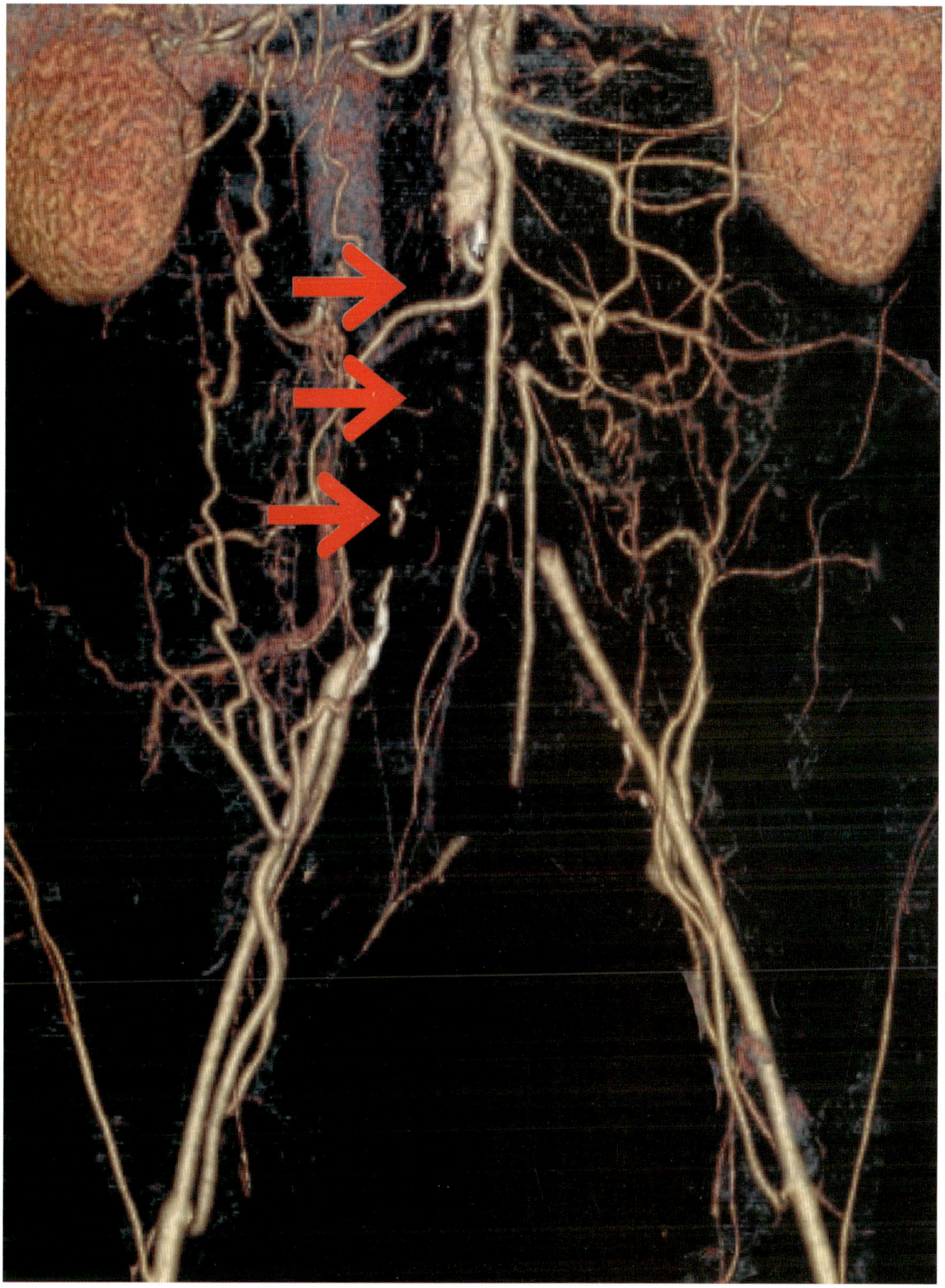

Fig. 48.9: Contrast-enhanced computed tomography (CT) showing complete occlusion of the distal abdominal aorta and proximal iliac arteries (arrows). [Image from Al-Sahfie T, Suman P. Aortoiliac occlusive disease. In: Yamanouchi D (Ed). Vascular Surgery. InTech. 2012. pp. 1-37].

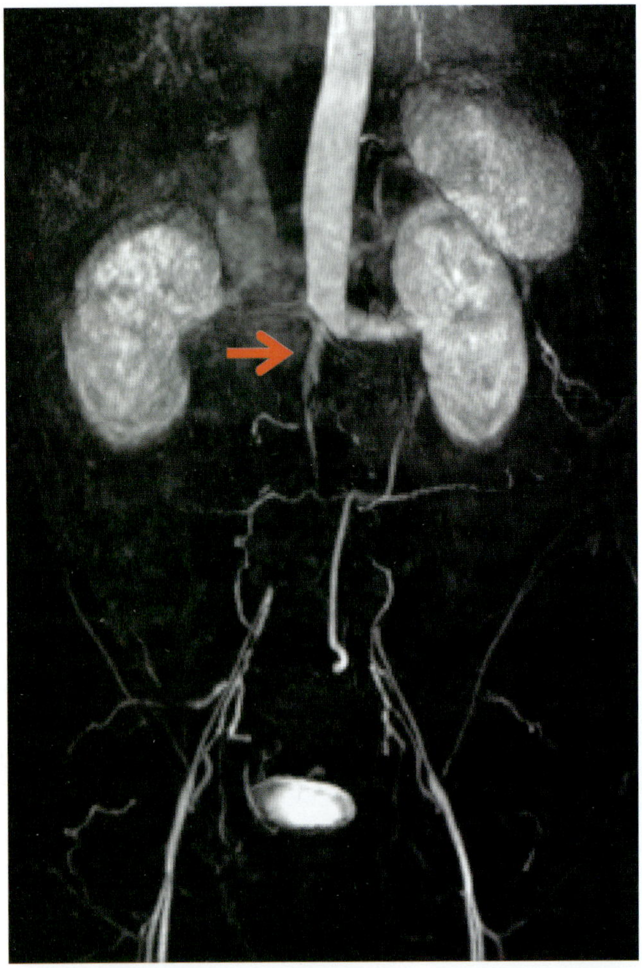

Fig. 48.10: Magnetic resonance angiogram (MRA) demonstrating aortoiliac occlusive disease with complete occlusion (arrow) of the distal abdominal aorta and proximal iliac arteries. [Image from Al-Sahfie T, Suman P. Aortoiliac occlusive disease. In: Yamanouchi D (Ed). Vascular Surgery. InTech. 2012. pp. 1-37].

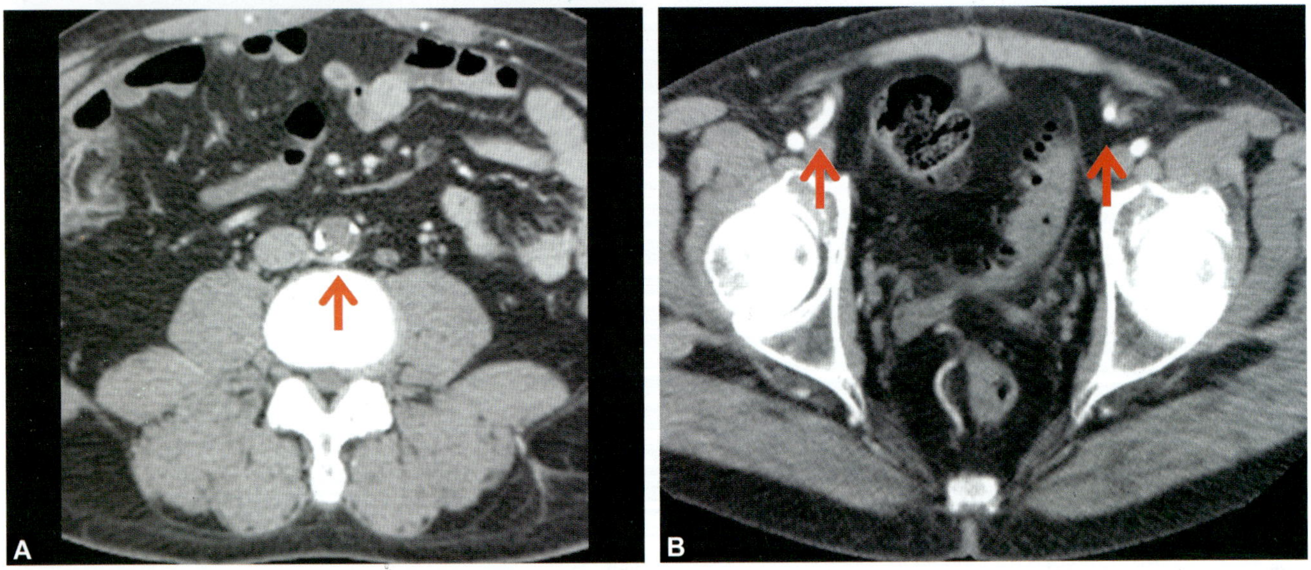

Figs. 48.11A and B: Computed tomographic angiography (CTA) of a patient with occlusion of the distal aorta. (A) Contrast-enhanced axial CTA at the level of the distal aorta shows no contrast in the aorta; (B) Axial image obtained more caudal demonstrates large collaterals via the inferior epigastric arteries (arrows).

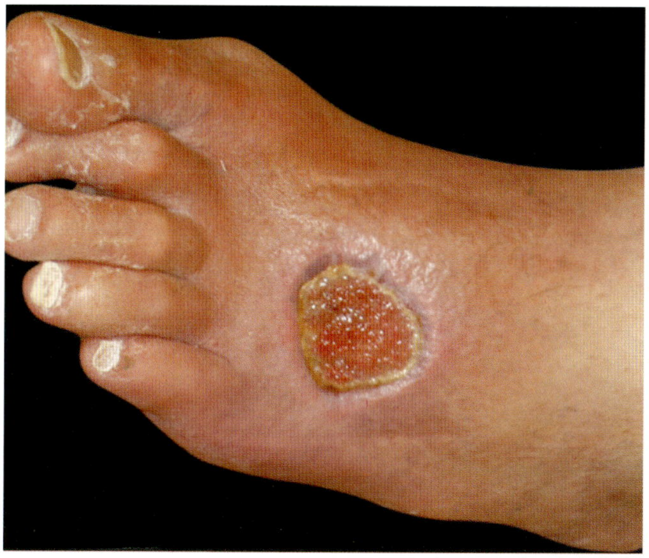

Fig. 48.12: Image from a patient with tissue loss and toe pressure of only 21 mm Hg that required an iliac stent and a bypass to heal this wound.

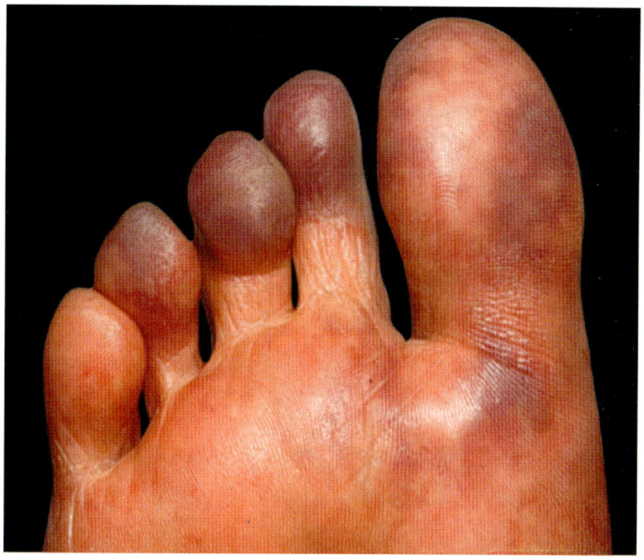

Fig. 48.13: Blue toe syndrome due to cholesterol emboli from the aorta. [Image from Garcia-Borbolla M. Complications of cardiac catheterization. In: Kiraç SF (Ed). Advances in the Diagnosis of Coronary Atherosclerosis. InTech. 2011. pp. 149-68].

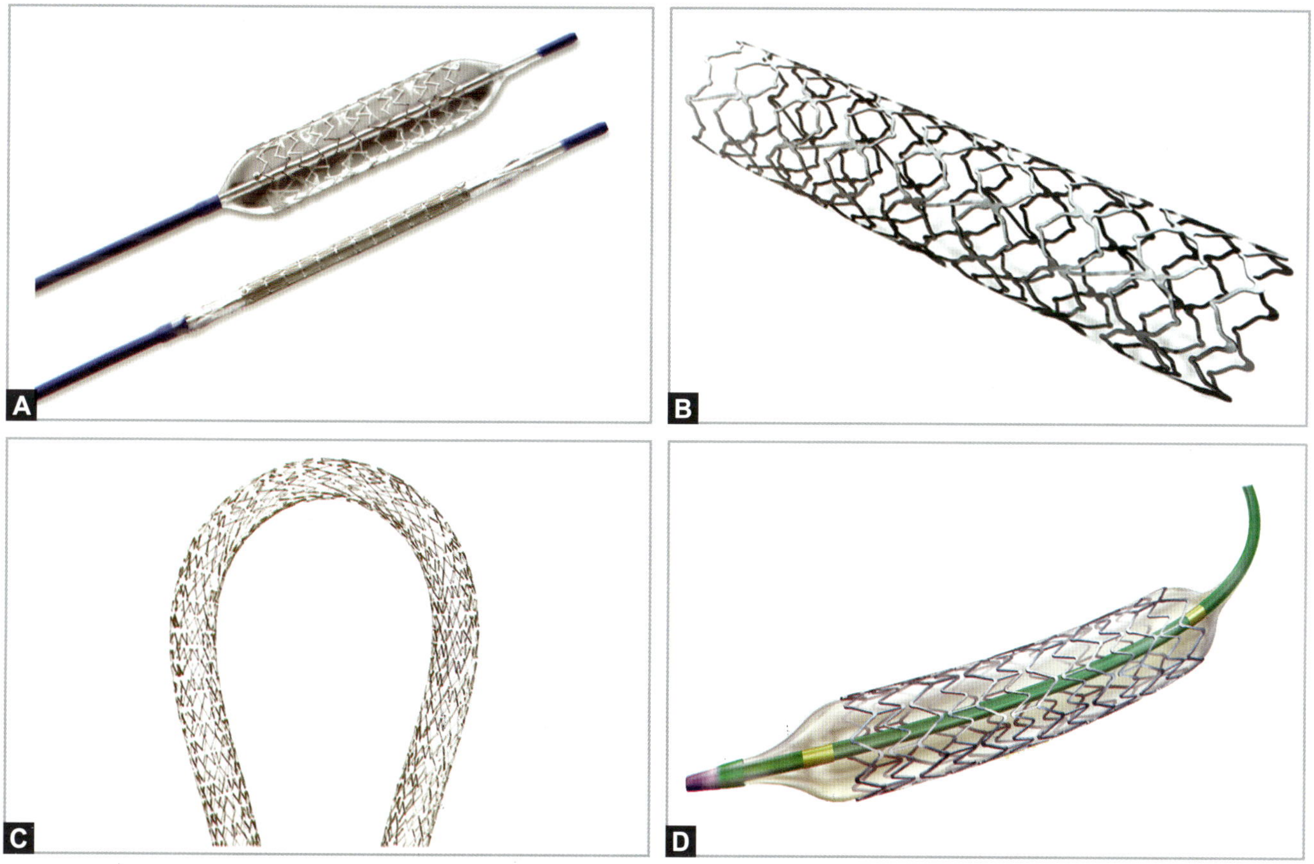

Figs. 48.14A to D: Examples of peripheral stents used in the treatment of peripheral arterial disease (PAD).

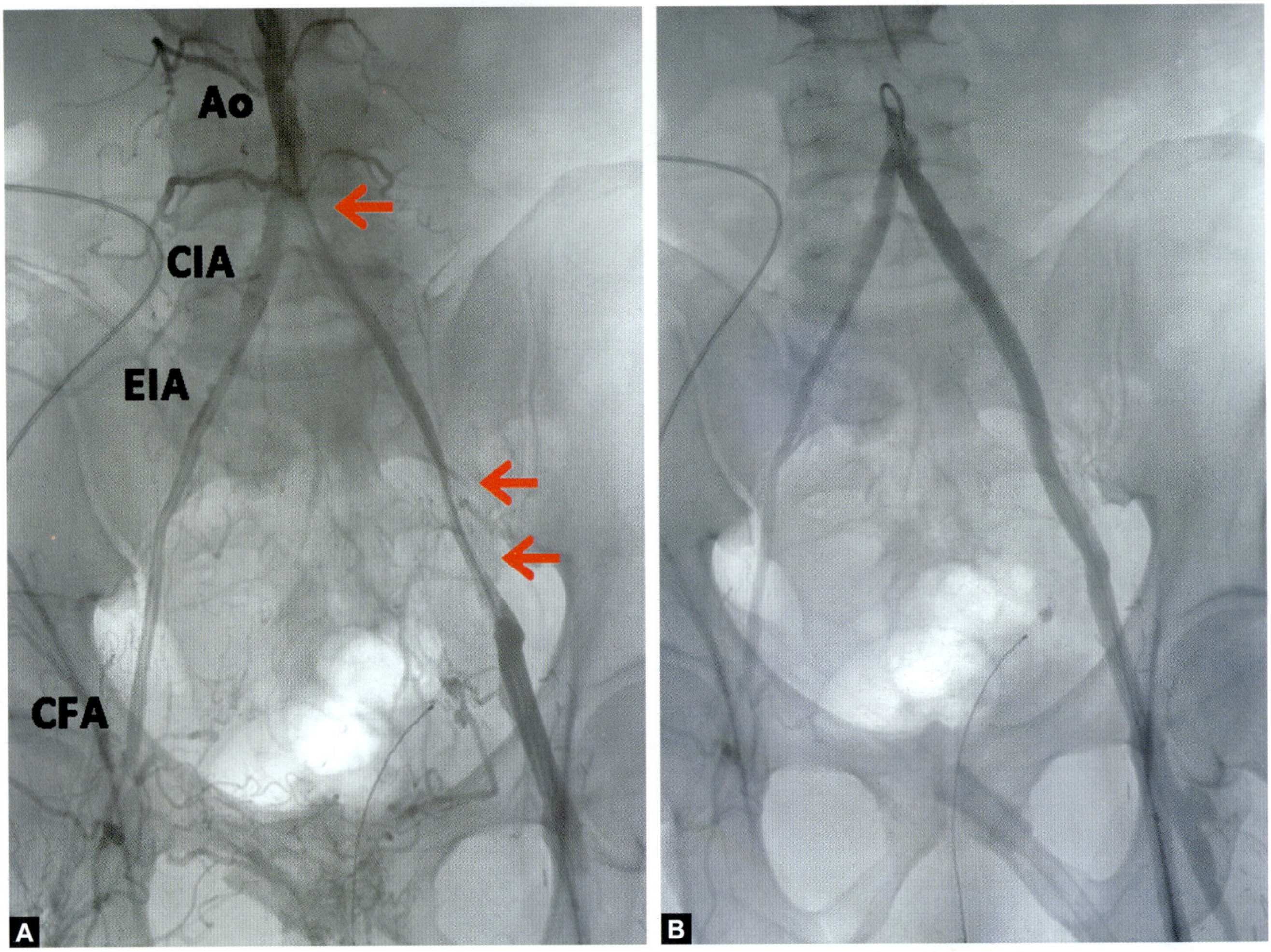

Figs. 48.15A and B: (A) A diffusely diseased iliac artery (arrows) treated with (B) retrograde peripheral stent implantation. (Ao: Aorta; CIA: Common iliac artery; EIA: External iliac artery; CFA: Common femoral artery).

Thromboangiitis Obliterans

Thromboangiitis obliterans (Buerger's disease) is recurring progressive inflammation, and thrombosis of small and medium arteries and veins associated with smoking. The disease typically affects males between 20 years and 40 years of age. Patients present with distal extremity ischemia, either claudication or pain at rest. Imaging studies reveal areas of stenosis or occlusion (Figs. 48.34 and 48.35). Smoking cessation may slow progression of the disease. Drug therapy may decrease symptoms.

Takayasu's Arteritis

Takayasu's arteritis is a form of vasculitis that primarily affects the aorta and large arteries (Figs. 48.36 and 48.37). The disease was actually first described by an ophthalmologist, Dr Mikito Takayasu (Fig. 48.38). The disease most commonly affects young or middle-aged women of Asian descent. Pathologically, there is granulomatous inflammation, intimal fibrosis and vessel narrowing.

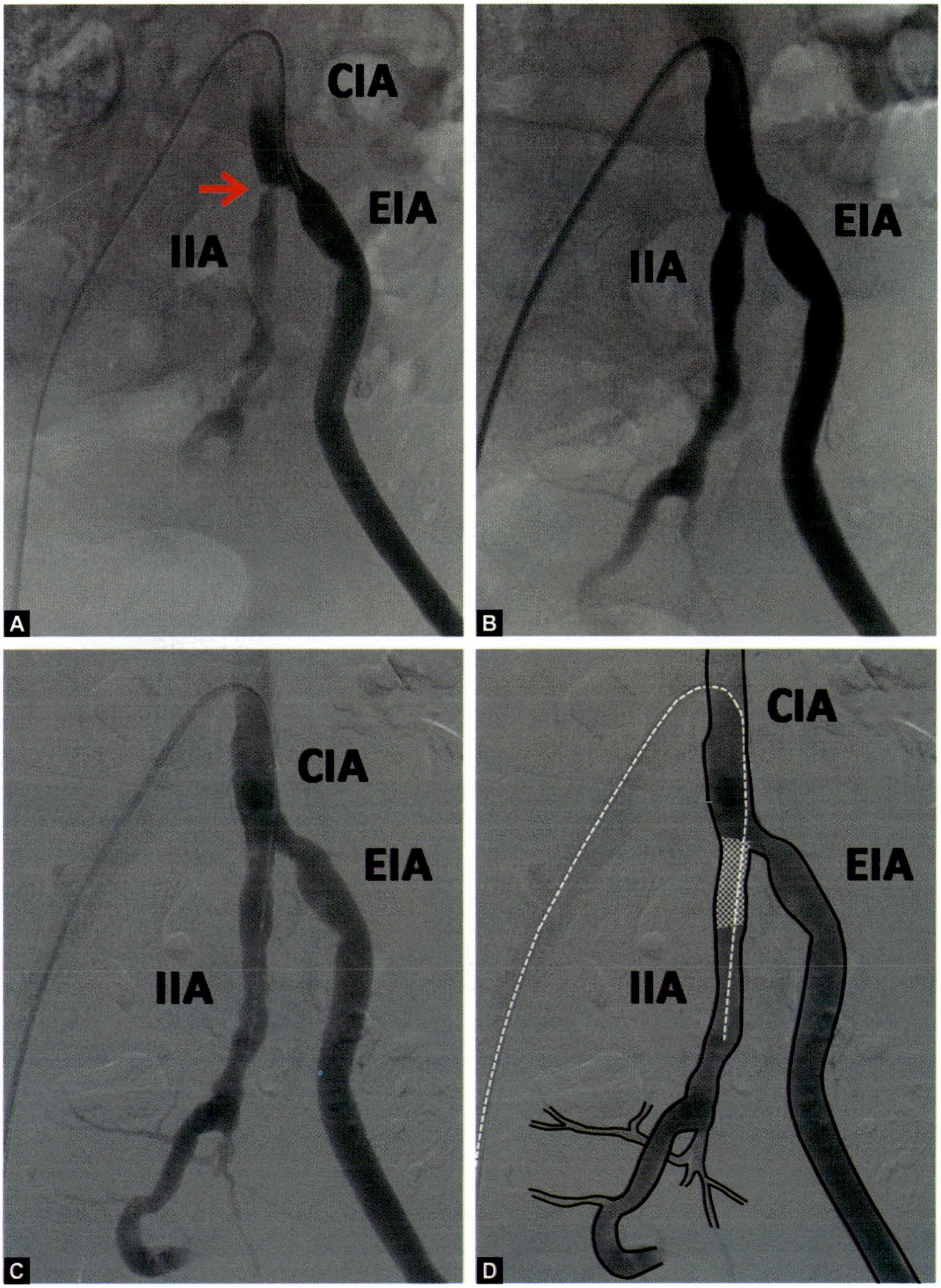

Figs. 48.16A to D: Treatment of an ostial internal iliac artery (IIA) stenosis in a patient with buttock claudication. An antegrade approach was used from the contralateral side. [Image from Prince JF, Smits ML, van Herwaarden JA, et al. Endovascular treatment of internal iliac artery stenosis in patients with buttock claudication. PLoS One. 2013;8(8):e73331]. (CIA: Common iliac artery; EIA: External iliac artery).

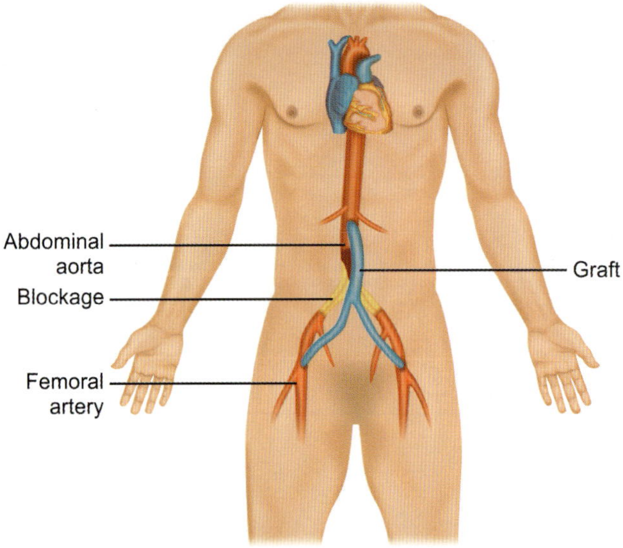

Fig. 48.17: Schematic illustration of an aortobifemoral artery (aorta-bifem) surgical bypass in aortoiliac peripheral vascular disease. Schematic illustration of axillary-femoral and femoral-femoral (fem-fem) surgical bypasses in aortoiliac peripheral vascular disease. This technique is used less frequently than the aorta-bifem technique.

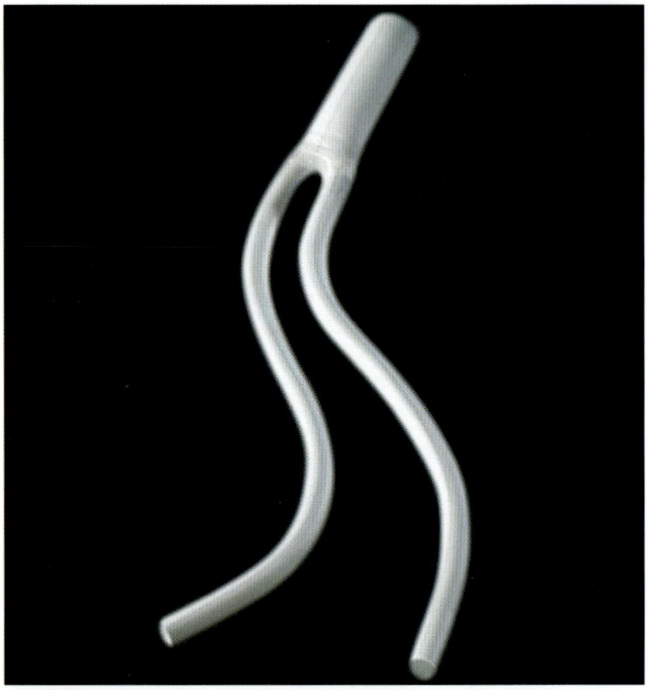

Fig. 48.18: Example of a Gore-Tex graft used in aortobifemoral artery (aorta-bifem) bypass surgery.

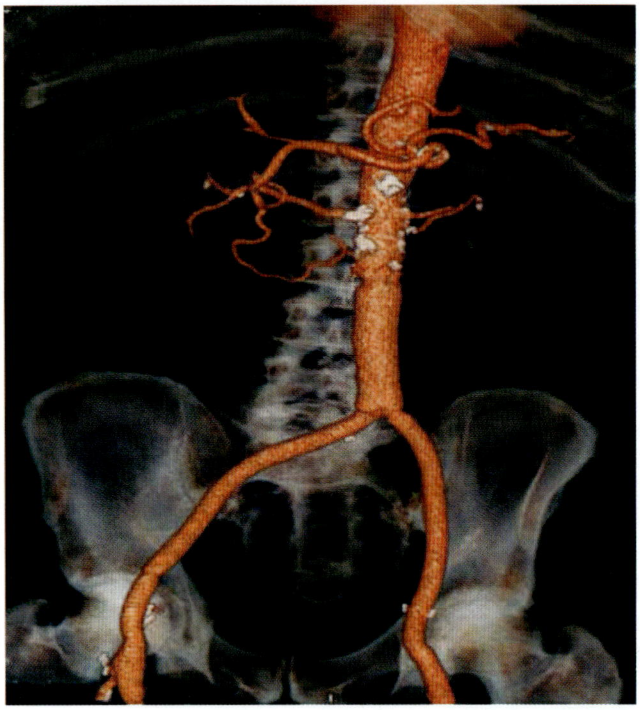

Fig. 48.19: Volume-rendered computed tomography (CT) scan of an aortobifemoral artery bypass. [Image from Dulbecco E, Camporrotondo M, Blanco G, et al. In situ reconstruction with bovine pericardial tubular graft for aortic graft infection. Rev Bras Cir Cardiovasc. 2010;25(2):249-52].

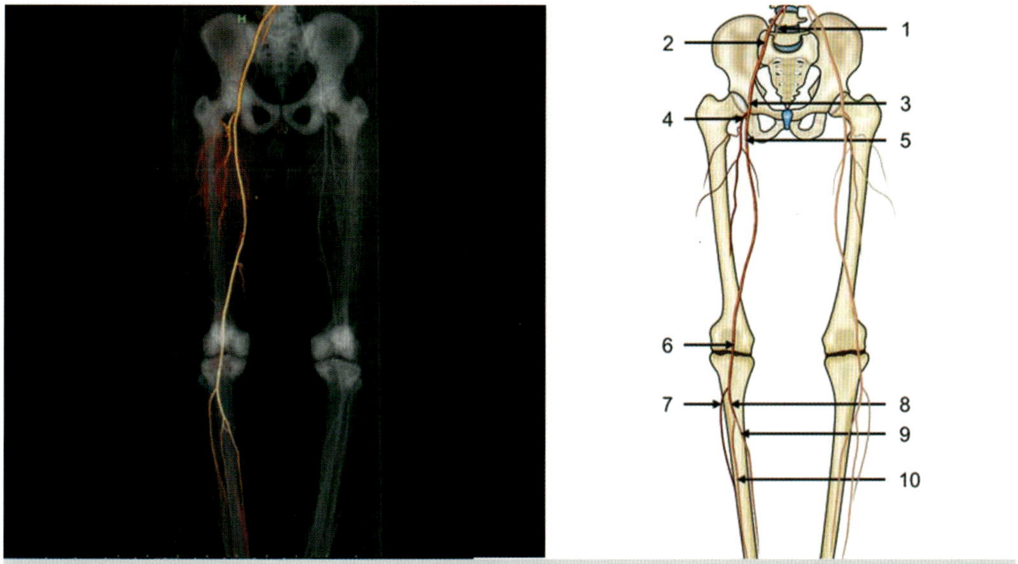

1. Internal iliac artery
2. External iliac artery
3. Common femoral artery
4. Profunda femoral artery
5. Superficial femoral artery
6. Popliteal artery
7. Anterior tibial artery
8. Tibioperoneal trunk
9. Posterior tibial artery
10. Peroneal artery

Fig. 48.20: Three-dimensional volume-rendered computed tomography (CT) and corresponding schematic illustration of the arteries of the leg. [Image from Chavhan G, Jankharia B (Eds). Cross Sectional Anatomy CT and MRI, 1st edition. New Delhi, India: Jaypee Brothers Medical Publishers (P) Ltd; 2012].

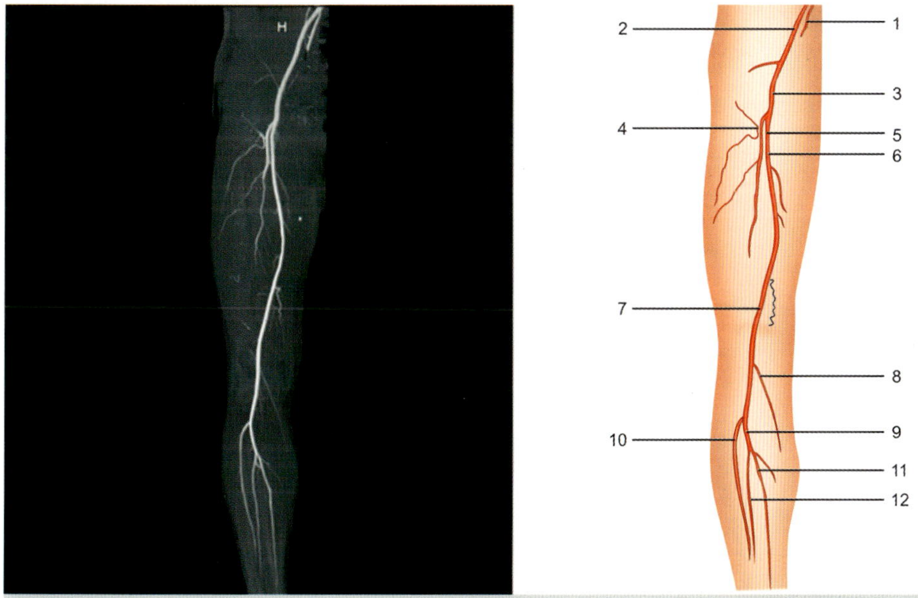

1. Internal iliac artery
2. External iliac artery
3. Common femoral artery
4. Lateral circumflex artery
5. Profunda femoral artery
6. Superficial femoral artery
7. Popliteal artery
8. Genicular branch
9. Tibioperoneal trunk
10. Anterior tibial artery
11. Posterior tibial artery
12. Peroneal artery

Fig. 48.21: Magnetic resonance imaging (MRI) and corresponding schematic illustration of the arteries of the leg. [Image from Chavhan G, Jankharia B (Eds). Cross Sectional Anatomy CT and MRI, 1st edition. New Delhi, India: Jaypee Brothers Medical Publishers (P) Ltd; 2012].

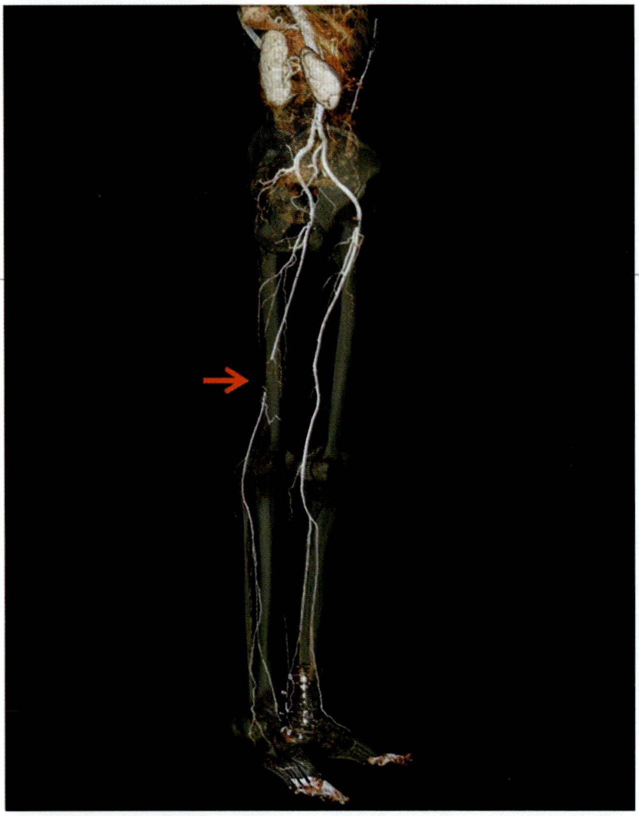

Fig. 48.22: Three-dimensional reconstruction of computed tomography (CT) angiogram demonstrating occlusion (arrow) of the superficial femoral artery (SFA) with reconstitution of flow distally. [Image from Kobayashi L, Coimbra R. Vascular trauma: new directions in screening, diagnosis and management. In: Yamanouchi D (Ed). Vascular Surgery. InTech. 2012. pp. 39-72].

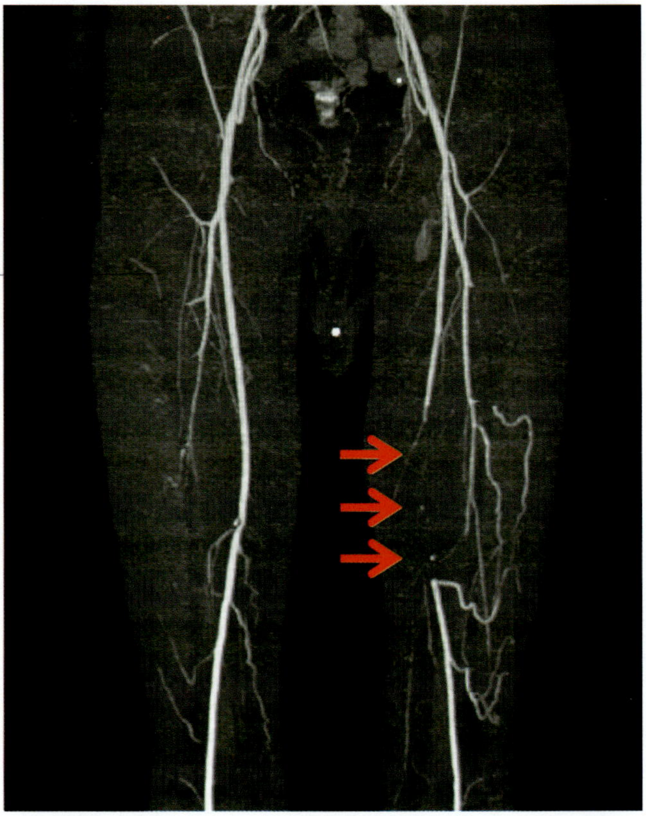

Fig. 48.23: Magnetic resonance imaging (MRI) demonstrating arterial occlusion (arrows) in the superficial femoral artery (SFA) with collateral flow to the more distal lower extremity. [Image from Al-Sahfie T, Suman P. Aortoiliac occlusive disease. In: Yamanouchi D (Ed). Vascular Surgery. InTech. 2012. pp. 1-37].

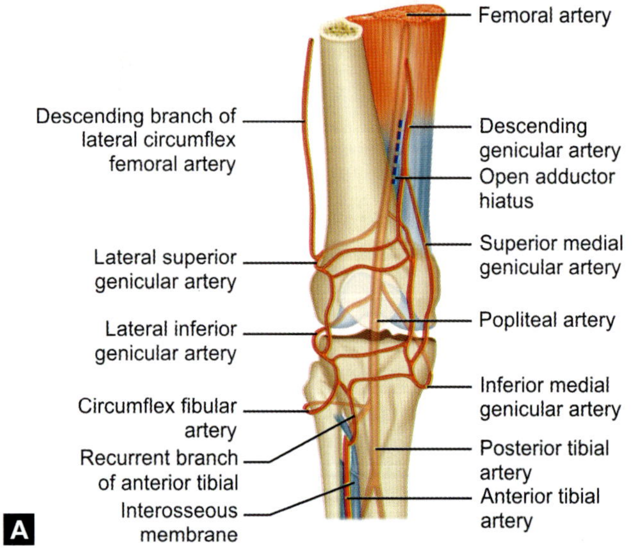

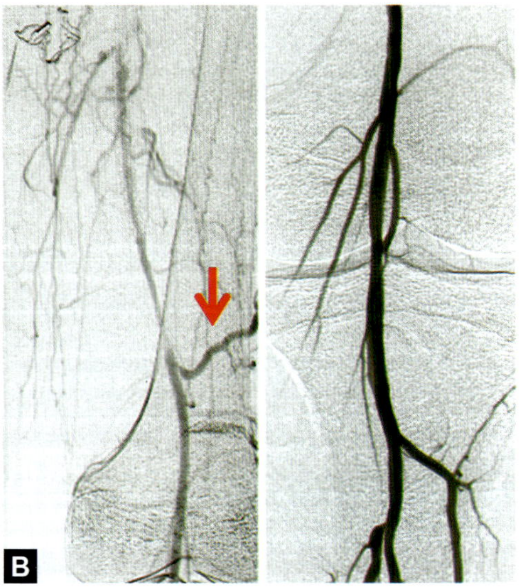

Figs. 48.24A and B: (A) Schematic illustration of the geniculate circulation, which often provides collateral flow in patients with femoropopliteal arterial occlusive disease; (B) Femoropopliteal peripheral arterial disease and geniculate collateral flow. Left panel shows femoropopliteal occlusion with geniculate collateral flow (arrow). Right panel shows arterial circulation after balloon angioplasty and stent implantation.

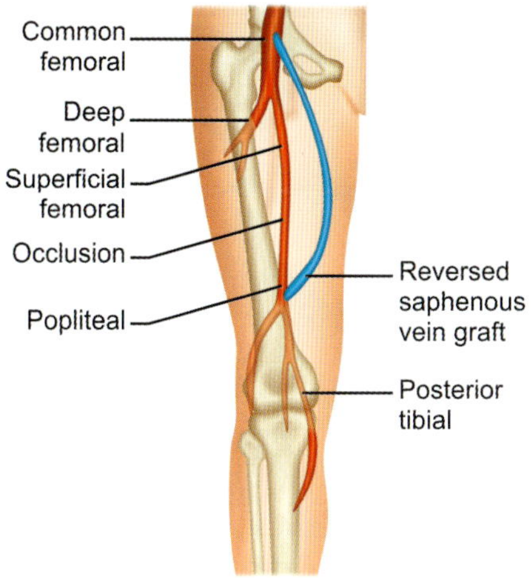

Fig. 48.25: Schematic illustration of a femoral-popliteal bypass for femoropopliteal occlusive arterial disease.

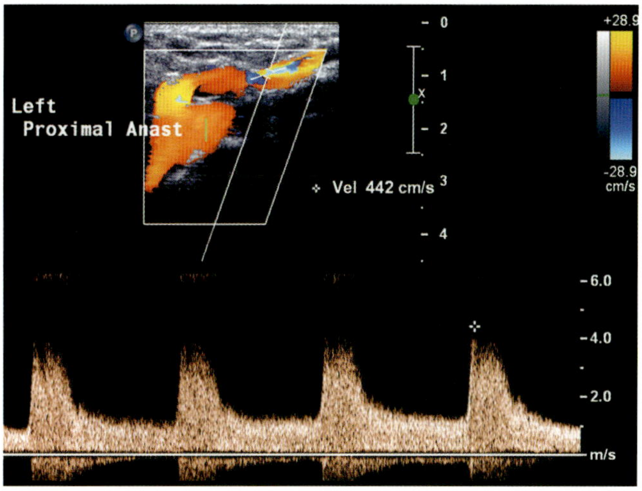

Fig. 48.26: Postoperative ultrasound surveillance of a bypass graft shows high-grade stenosis in the proximal vein bypass anastomosis (442 cm/s). The lesion was treated with balloon angioplasty.

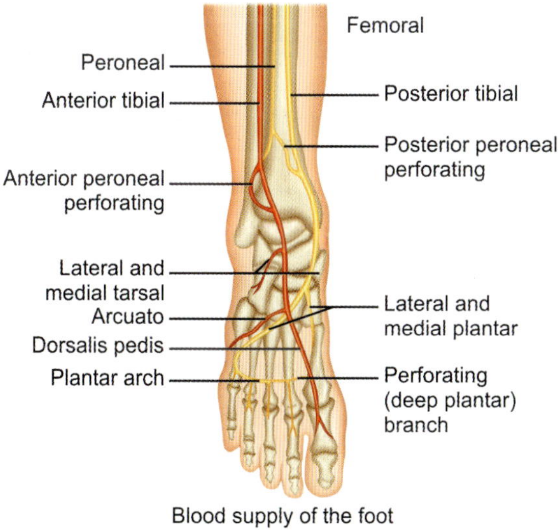

Fig. 48.27: Schematic illustration of the arteries of the lower leg and foot.

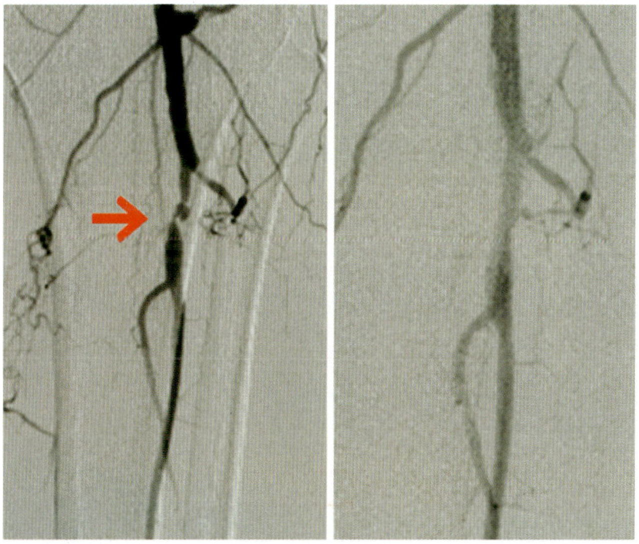

Fig. 48.28: Angiogram showing tibioperoneal trunk lesion (left panel, arrow) successfully treated with laser atherectomy followed by balloon angioplasty (right panel).

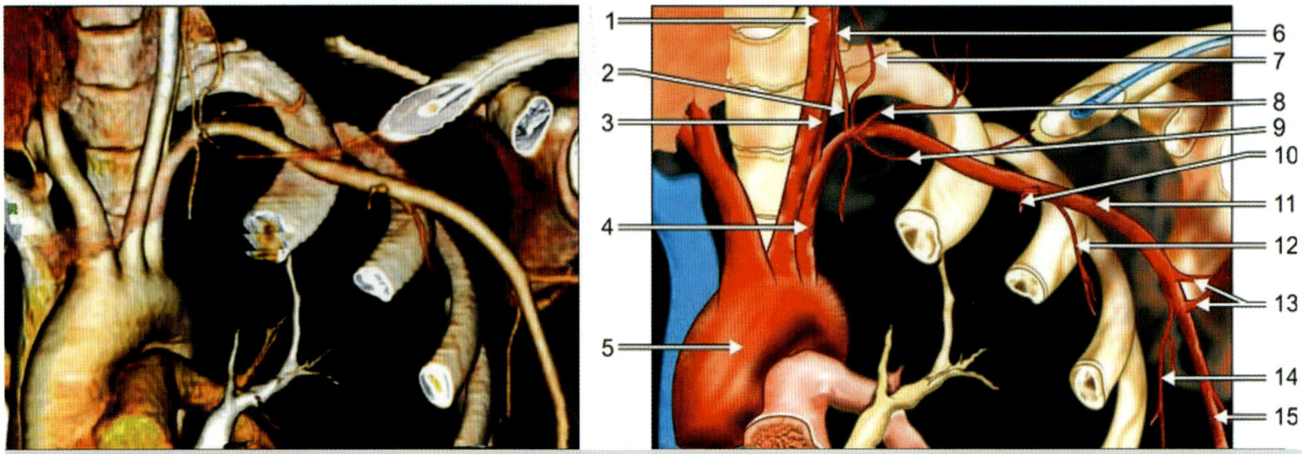

1. Left carotid artery
2. Thyrocervical trunk
3. Left vertebral artery
4. Left subclavian artery
5. Arch of aorta
6. Inferior thyroid artery
7. Transverse cervical artery
8. Costocervical trunk
9. Suprascapular artery
10. Superior thoracic artery
11. Axillary artery
12. Lateral thoracic artery
13. Circumflex humeral arteries
14. Subscapular artery
15. Brachial artery

Fig. 48.29: Three-dimensional volume-rendered computed tomography (CT) and corresponding schematic illustration of the aortic arch and upper extremity arteries. [Image from Chavhan G, Jankharia B (Eds). Cross Sectional Anatomy CT and MRI, 1st edition. New Delhi, India: Jaypee Brothers Medical Publishers (P) Ltd; 2012].

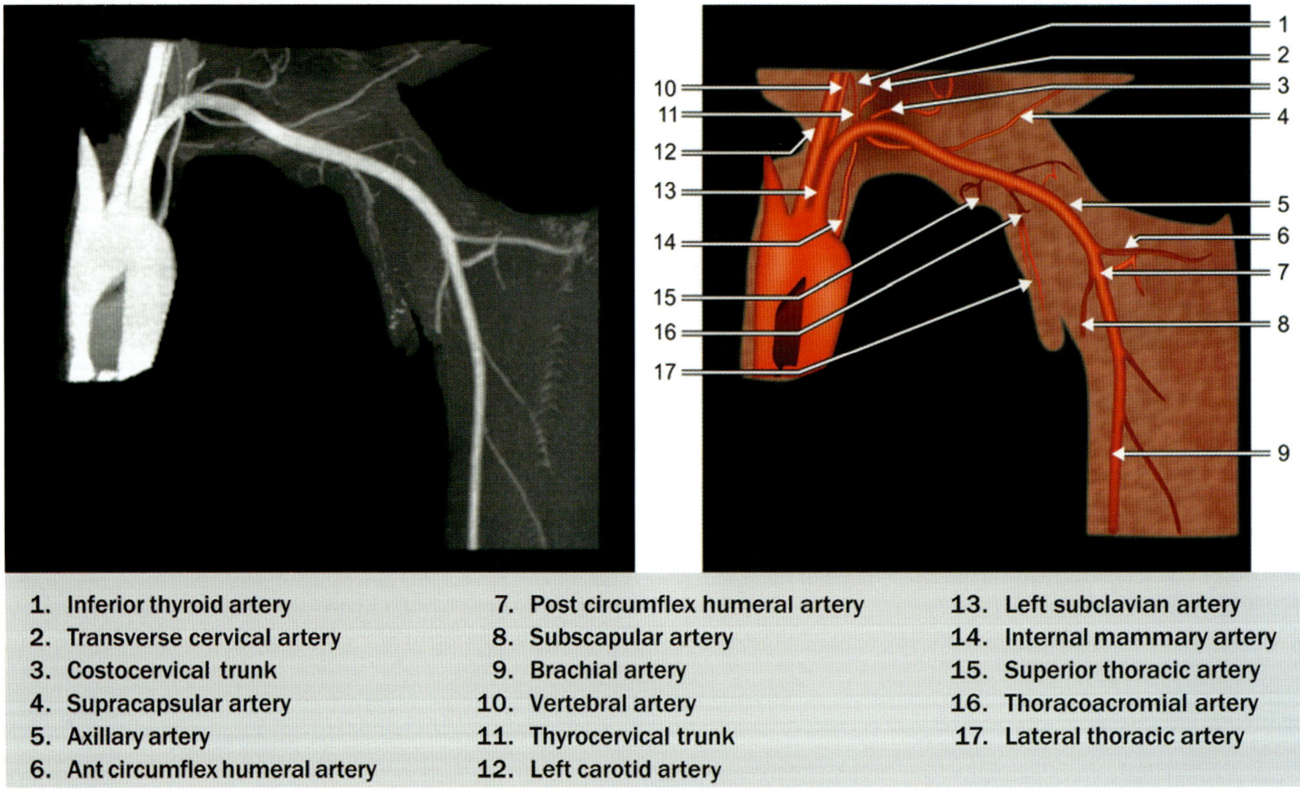

1. Inferior thyroid artery
2. Transverse cervical artery
3. Costocervical trunk
4. Supracapsular artery
5. Axillary artery
6. Ant circumflex humeral artery
7. Post circumflex humeral artery
8. Subscapular artery
9. Brachial artery
10. Vertebral artery
11. Thyrocervical trunk
12. Left carotid artery
13. Left subclavian artery
14. Internal mammary artery
15. Superior thoracic artery
16. Thoracoacromial artery
17. Lateral thoracic artery

Fig. 48.30: Magnetic resonance imaging (MRI) and corresponding schematic illustration of the upper extremity arteries. [Image from Chavhan G, Jankharia B (Eds). Cross Sectional Anatomy CT and MRI, 1st edition. New Delhi, India: Jaypee Brothers Medical Publishers (P) Ltd; 2012].

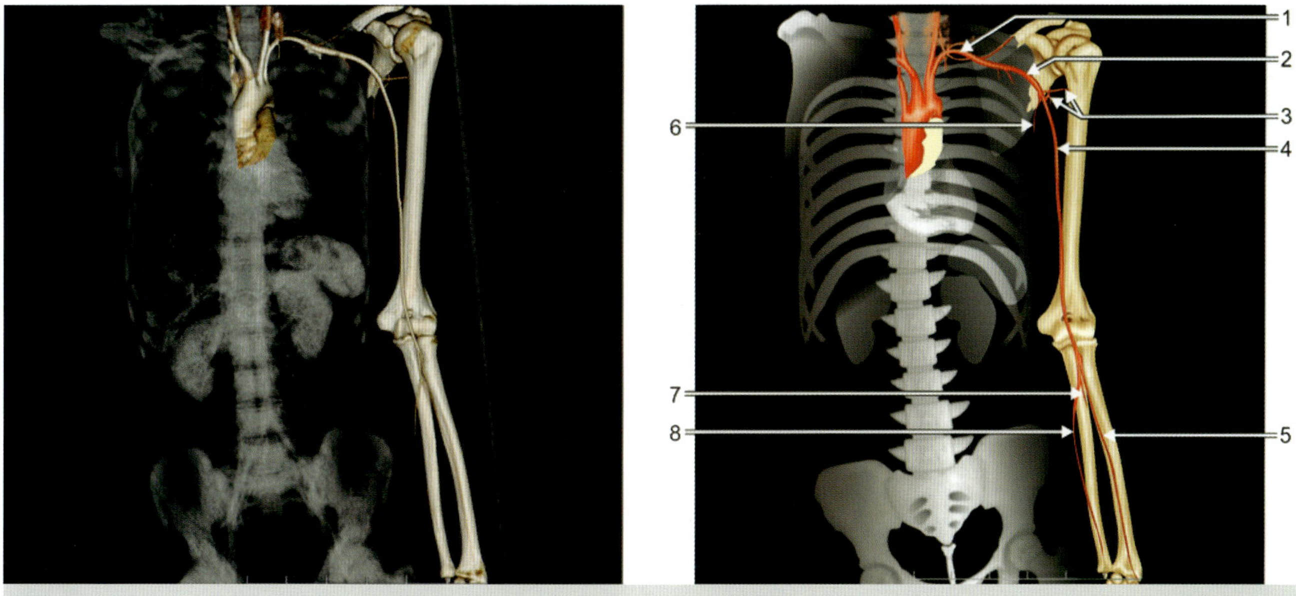

1. Subclavian artery
2. Axillary artery
3. Circumflex humeral artery
4. Brachial artery
5. Radial artery
6. Subscapular artery
7. Interosseous artery
8. Ulnar artery

Fig. 48.31: Three-dimensional volume-rendered computed tomography (CT) and corresponding schematic illustration of the upper extremity arteries. [Image from Chavhan G, Jankharia B (Eds). Cross Sectional Anatomy CT and MRI, 1st edition. New Delhi, India: Jaypee Brothers Medical Publishers (P) Ltd; 2012].

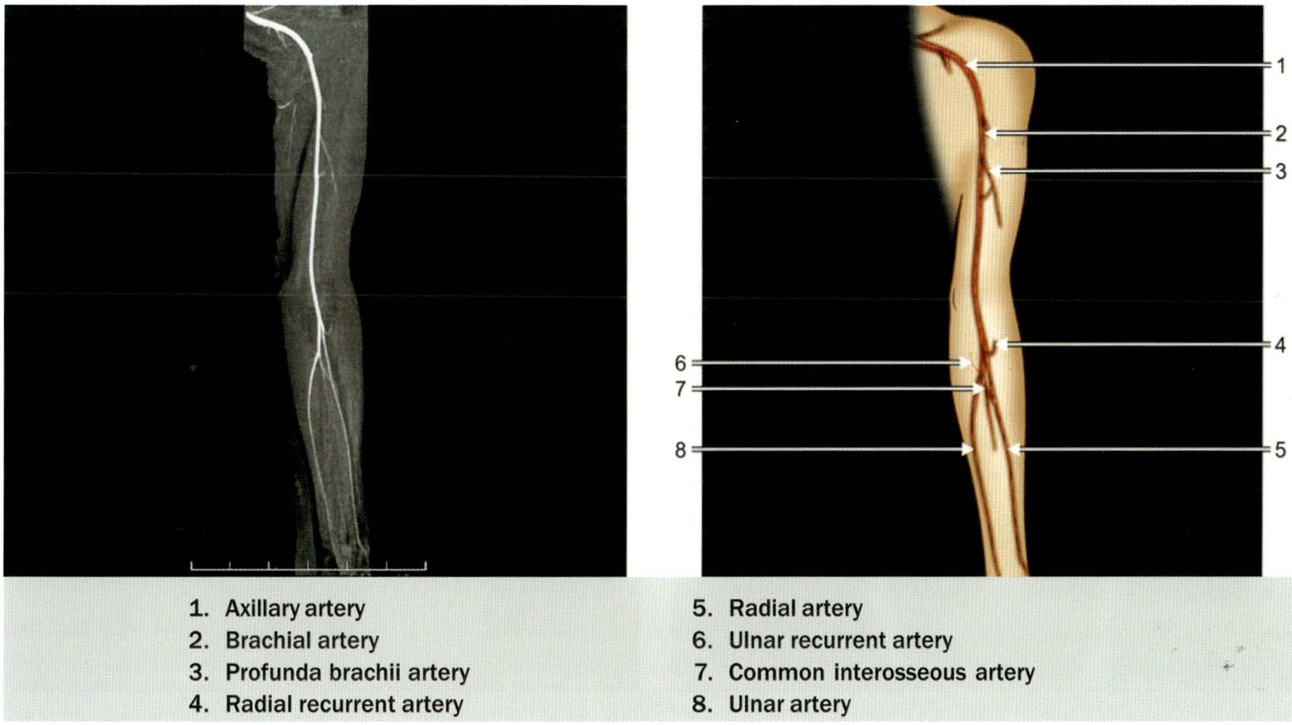

1. Axillary artery
2. Brachial artery
3. Profunda brachii artery
4. Radial recurrent artery
5. Radial artery
6. Ulnar recurrent artery
7. Common interosseous artery
8. Ulnar artery

Fig. 48.32: Magnetic resonance imaging (MRI) and corresponding schematic illustration of the upper extremity arteries. [Image from Chavhan G, Jankharia B (Eds). Cross Sectional Anatomy CT and MRI, 1st edition. New Delhi, India: Jaypee Brothers Medical Publishers (P) Ltd; 2012].

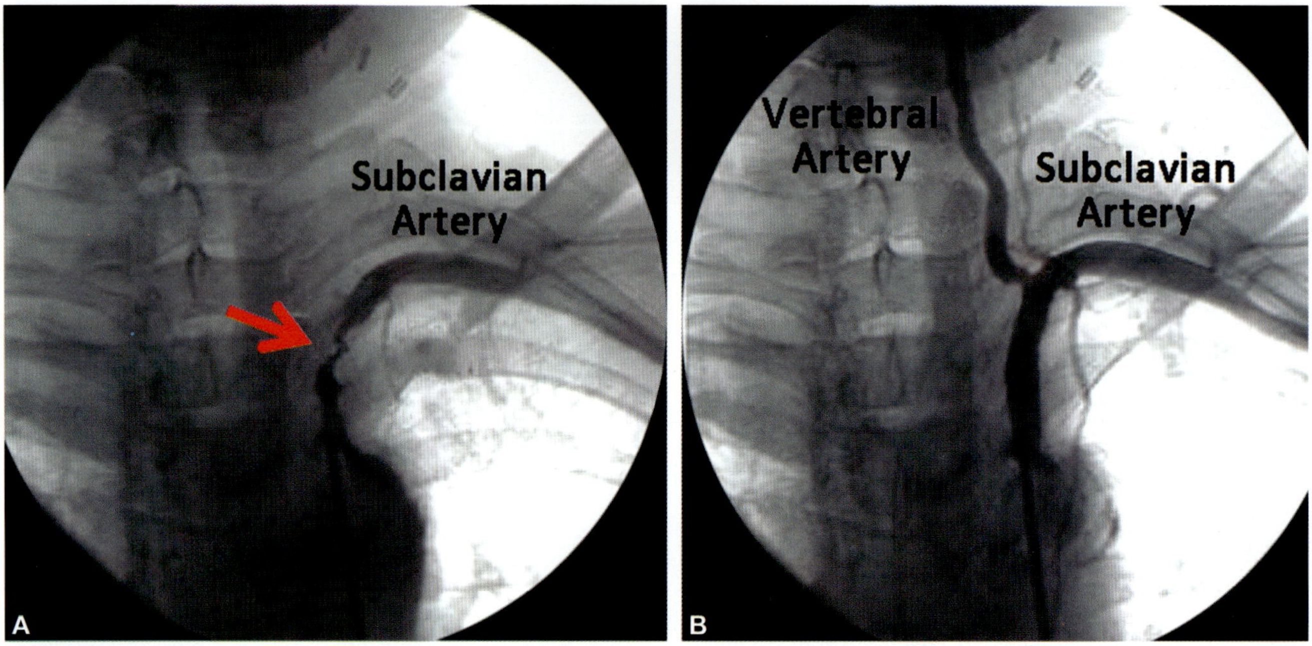

Figs. 48.33A and B: Angiogram in an elderly patient with left arm claudication and severe dizziness. (A) Selective angiogram of the left subclavian artery demonstrates severe proximal stenosis (arrow) and no flow into the left vertebral artery. (B) After stenting of the stenosis, there is now flow visualized in the vertebral artery. [Image from Haddadian B, et al. Peripheral vascular and cerebrovascular disease. In: Chatterjee K, Anderson M, Heistad D, Kerber RE (Eds). Cardiology—An Illustrated Textbook, 1st edition. New Delhi, India: Jaypee Brothers Medical Publishers (P) Ltd; 2012. pp. 1145-65].

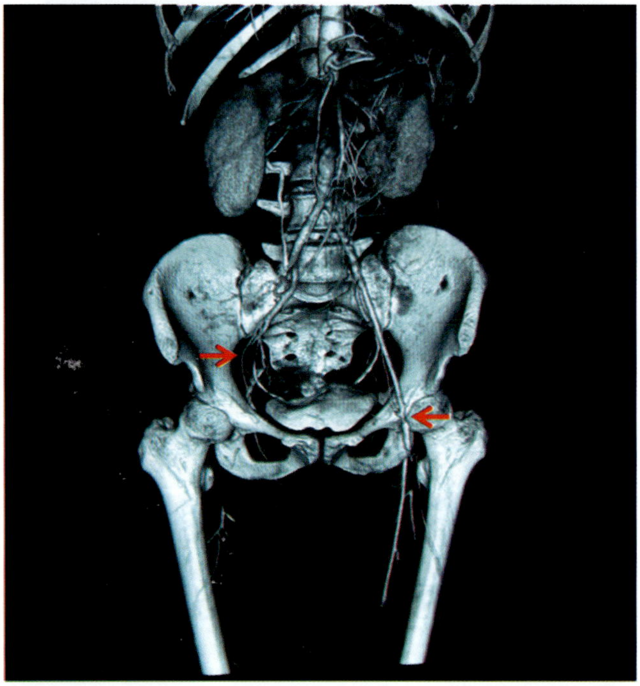

Fig. 48.34: Computed tomography (CT) angiogram of a patient with thromboangiitis obliterans. There is complete occlusion of the right and stenosis of the left femoral artery (arrows). (Image created by Milorad Dimic, MD and posted on Wikipedia).

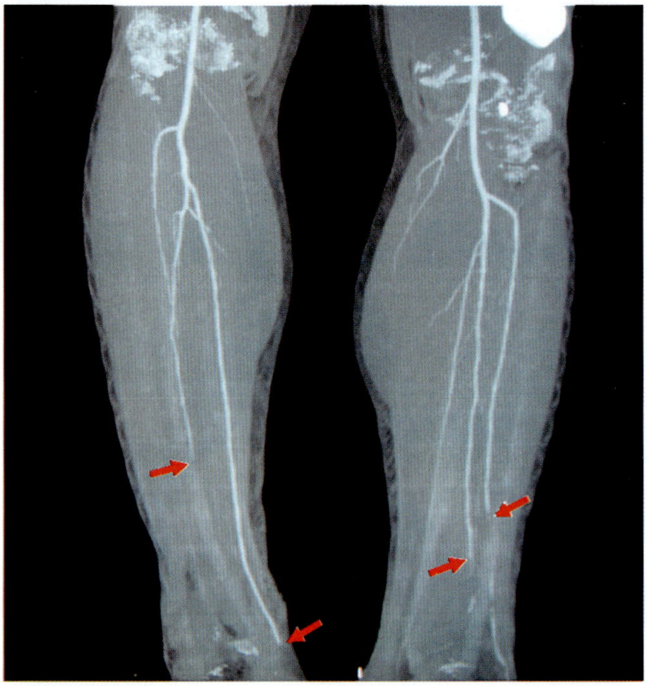

Fig. 48.35: Angiogram of the distal lower extremities in a patient with thromboangiitis obliterans. There are numerous areas of vessel occlusion (arrows). (Image created by Milorad Dimic, MD and posted on Wikipedia).

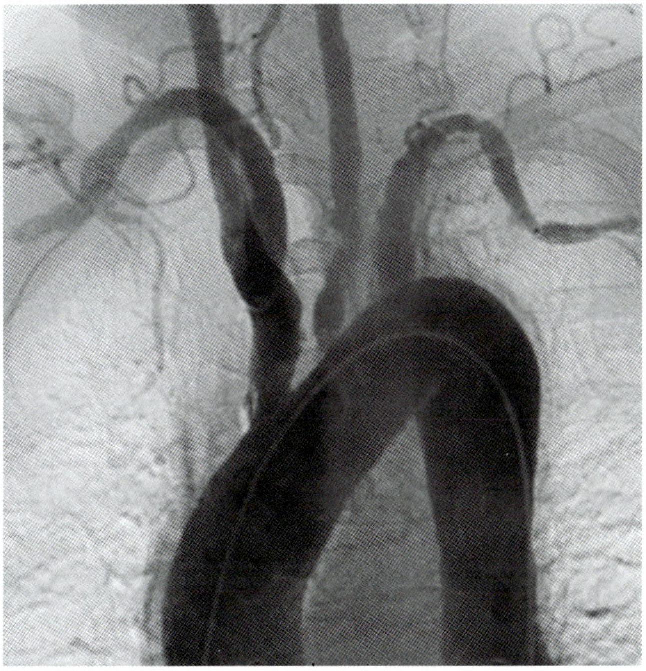

Fig. 48.36: Left anterior oblique (LAO) aortogram in a patient with Takayasu's arteritis. There are multiple areas of stenosis in the great vessels. (Public domain image posted on Wikipedia).

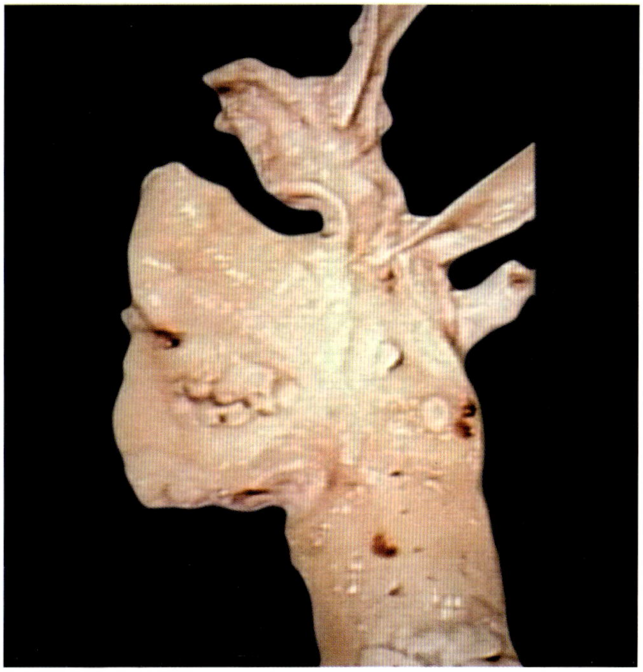

Fig. 48.37: Gross pathology specimen from a patient with Takayasu's arteritis, demonstrating disease involvement of the aortic arch and origin and proximal portions of the great vessels. (Image from Armed Forces Institute of Pathology).

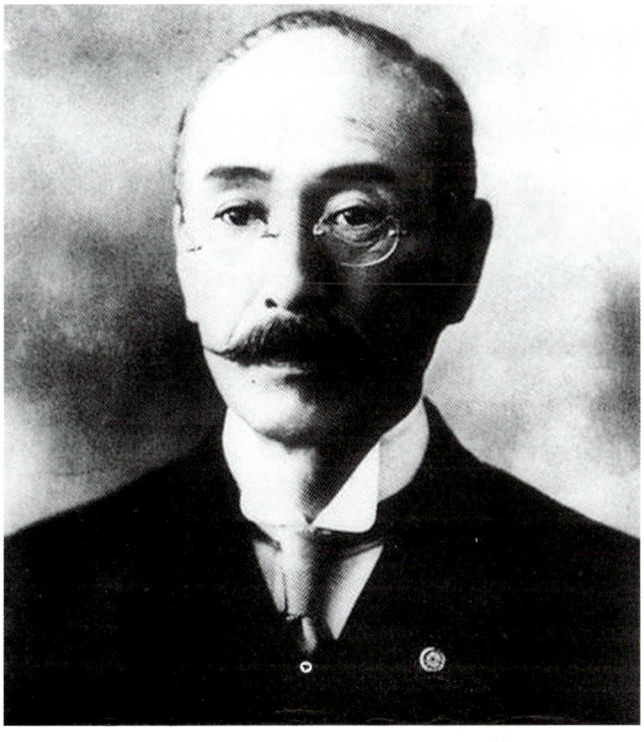

Fig. 48.38: Mikito Takayasu, circa 1910. (Image posted on Wikipedia).

REFERENCES

Allison MA, Criqui MH, McClelland RL, et al. The effect of novel cardiovascular risk factors on the ethnic-specific odds for peripheral arterial disease in the Multi-Ethnic Study of Atherosclerosis (MESA). J Am Coll Cardiol. 2006;48(6):1190-7.

Antoniou GA, Chalmers N, Georgiadis GS, et al. A meta-analysis of endovascular versus surgical reconstruction of femoropopliteal arterial disease. J Vasc Surg. 2013;57(1):242-53.

Barshes NR, Chambers JD, Cohen J, et al. Cost-effectiveness in the contemporary management of critical limb ischemia with tissue loss. J Vasc Surg. 2012;56(4):1015-24.e1.

Bradbury AW, Adam DJ, Bell J, et al. Bypass versus Angioplasty in Severe Ischaemia of the Leg (BASIL) trial: an intention-to-treat analysis of amputation-free and overall survival in patients randomized to a bypass surgery-first or a balloon angioplasty-first revascularization strategy. J Vasc Surg. 2010;51(5 Suppl): 5S-17S.

Hennrikus D, Joseph AM, Lando HA, et al. Effectiveness of a smoking cessation program for peripheral artery disease patients: a randomized controlled trial. J Am Coll Cardiol. 2010;56(25):2105-12.

Hirsch AT, Haskal ZJ, Hertzer NR, et al. ACC/AHA 2005 Practice Guidelines for the management of patients with peripheral arterial disease (lower extremity, renal, mesenteric, and abdominal aortic): a collaborative report from the American Association for Vascular Surgery/Society for Vascular Surgery, Society for Cardiovascular Angiography and Interventions, Society for Vascular Medicine and Biology, Society of Interventional Radiology, and the ACC/AHA Task Force on Practice Guidelines (Writing Committee to Develop Guidelines for the Management of Patients With Peripheral Arterial Disease): endorsed by the American Association of Cardiovascular and Pulmonary Rehabilitation; National Heart, Lung, and Blood Institute; Society for Vascular Nursing; TransAtlantic Inter-Society Consensus; and Vascular Disease Foundation. Circulation. 2006;113(11):e463-654.

Norgren L, Hiatt WR, Dormandy JA, et al. Inter-Society Consensus for the Management of Peripheral Arterial Disease (TASC II). J Vasc Surg. 2007;45(Suppl S):S5-67.

Ouriel K. Peripheral arterial disease. Lancet. 2001;358(9289): 1257-64.

Rooke TW, Hirsch AT, Misra S, et al. 2011 ACCF/AHA focused update of the guideline for the management of patients with peripheral artery disease (updating the 2005 guideline): a report of the American College of Cardiology Foundation/ American Heart Association task force on practice guidelines. J Am Coll Cardiol. 2011;58:2020-45.

CHAPTER

49

Carotid Artery Disease

Gerd Brunner, George T Pisimisis, Vijay Nambi

CAROTID ARTERY ANATOMY

The carotid arteries are the major arteries that supply the head, the neck and the brain (Figs. 49.1 to 49.6, Video 49.1). Typically, the carotid artery has four major segments: the common carotid artery (CCA), the bulb, the external carotid artery (ECA) and the internal carotid artery (ICA). The right common carotid originates from the brachiocephalic trunk, which in turn originates from the aortic arch and divides into the right subclavian artery and the right CCA, while the left CCA originates directly from the aortic arch. In the neck, the CCA (at the level of approximately the fourth cervical vertebra) becomes the bulb and then bifurcates into the ECA and the ICA. Typically the ICA has no branches in the neck while the ECA branches and supplies the face and the neck (Figs. 49.7A to D). Coiling of the left carotid artery (Fig. 49.8), though it may lead to increased detected velocities on Doppler imaging, is a normal variant.

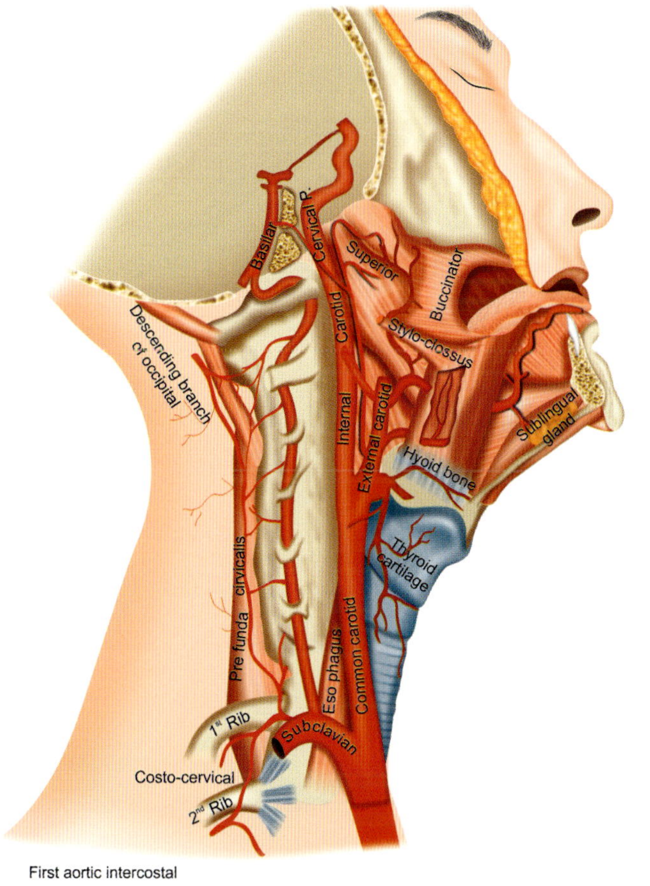

Fig. 49.1: Anatomy of the carotid artery, as classically described. (Image by Henry Gray, posted on Wikimedia Commons).

Carotid Artery Disease

Like most other blood vessels in humans, the carotid artery is prone to various disease processes including atherosclerosis, vasculitis, fibromuscular dysplasia (FMD) and dissection.

Of the various disease processes, atherosclerosis, with a predilection to the carotid bifurcation, remains the most important pathology of the carotid artery and the leading cause of stroke (Figs. 49.9 and 49.10). Similar to coronary artery disease, traditional cardiovascular risk factors are all strongly associated with carotid atherosclerosis. However, unlike acute coronary syndromes, most strokes occur from plaque rupture and embolization, and not thrombosis.

IMAGING OF CAROTID ARTERY DISEASE

The superficial location of the carotid artery makes it easily accessible for evaluation, both clinically and using imaging. All standard imaging modalities including ultrasound, computed tomography (CT), magnetic resonance

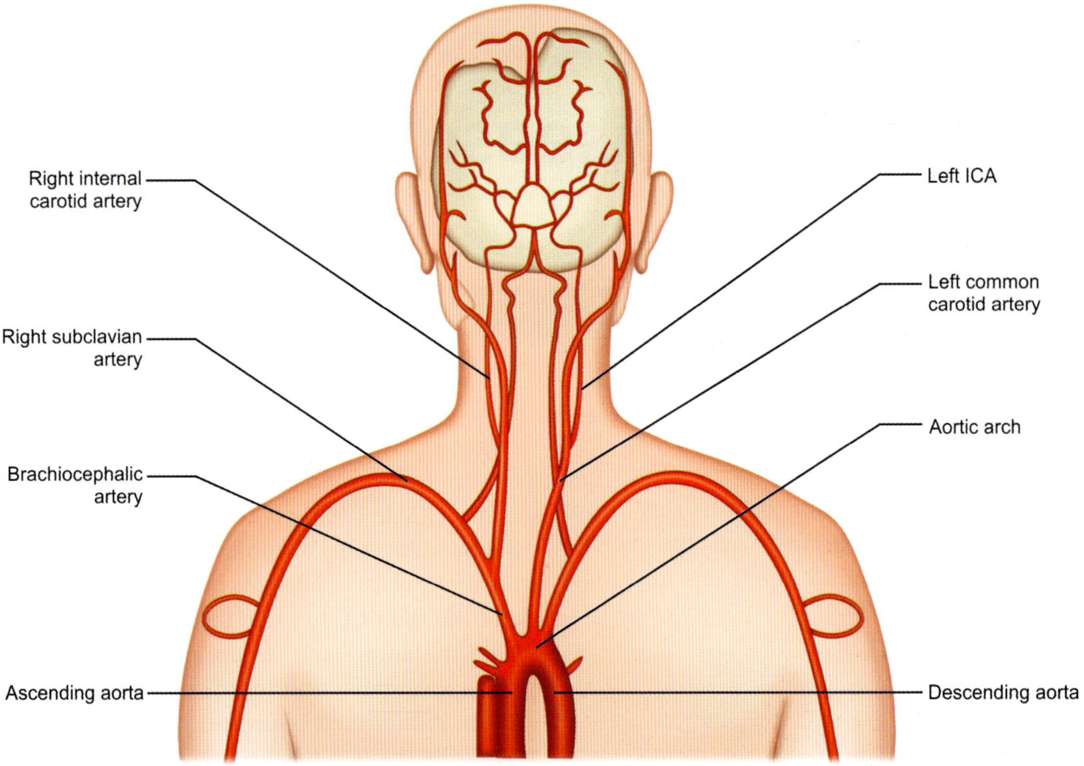

Fig. 49.2: Schematic illustration of the aortic arch and the origins of the carotid arteries.

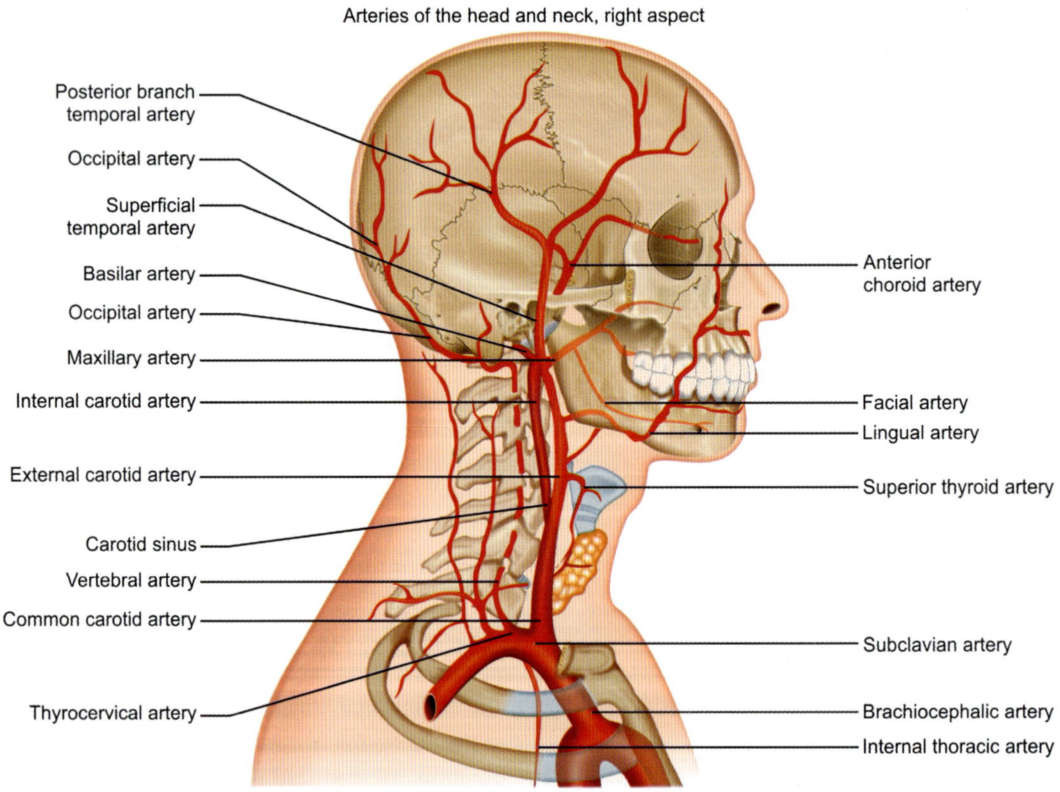

Fig. 49.3: Schematic illustration from the lateral view of the carotid artery.

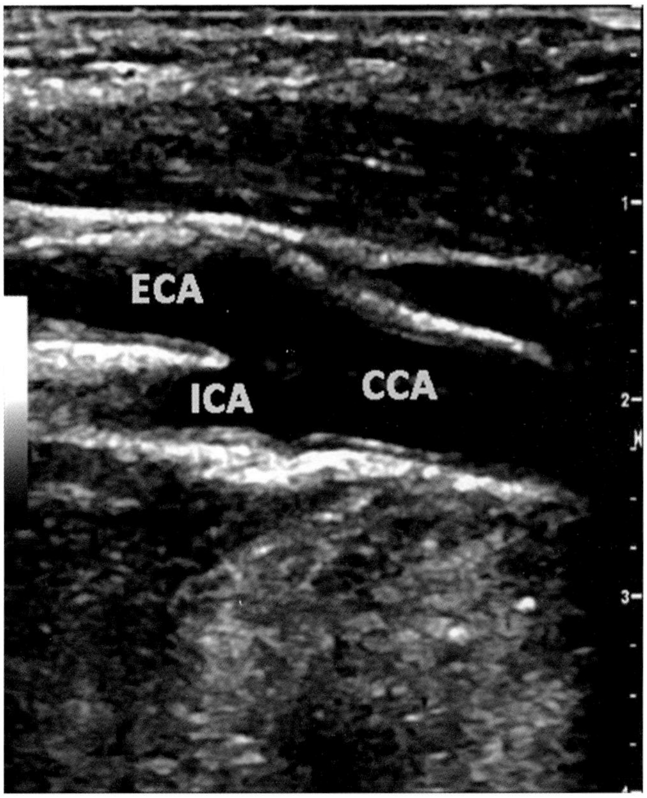

Fig. 49.4: A normal carotid artery as visualized with two-dimensional ultrasound in the "tuning-fork view". (CCA: Common carotid artery; ECA: External carotid artery; ICA: Internal carotid artery).

imaging (MRI) and invasive angiography are useful in the evaluation of carotid artery pathology (Figs. 49.11 to 49.14). Due to the relative safety and high throughput, ultrasound remains the first diagnostic test of choice in a patient where there is clinical concern for carotid artery pathology. Ultrasound imaging of the carotid artery, in fact, provides clues into the general cardiovascular health of the individual. Measurement of the intima-medial thickness (Fig. 49.15) and assessment of plaque presence has been evaluated as a methodology to help stratify cardiovascular risk in an individual and as a research tool. Additionally, local measurement of arterial stiffness using distensibility (Fig. 49.16) or strain (Fig. 49.17) of the carotid artery can also be useful both clinically and as a research tool.

Carotid ultrasound (as with echocardiography) uses both the two-dimensional (2D) and Doppler information to help in the evaluation of degree of carotid stenosis. Several criteria exist in helping grade the severity of stenosis (Table 49.1); in general, local validation of any of the criteria used is recommended.

Computed tomography and MRI provide excellent anatomic information and have significantly reduced the need for invasive angiography. MRI (especially in the research setting) has the additional value of providing insight into the plaque morphology (i.e. identifying high risk or rupture prone plaque).

MANAGEMENT OF ATHEROSCLEROTIC AND NON-ATHEROSCLEROTIC CAROTID ARTERY DISEASE

For symptomatic carotid artery stenosis of < 50% and for asymptomatic patients with carotid stenosis of < 60%, the main stay of treatment is medical therapy. Carotid artery stenosis of > 50% is considered a cardiovascular disease risk equivalent, i.e., treatment goals for risk factors are similar to when one already has cardiovascular disease.

For symptomatic carotid stenosis of > 50% the main stay of treatment is revascularization. Studies have shown that surgery, in appropriately selected patients without high surgical risk, results in a moderate risk reduction for stroke in patients with 50–70% carotid artery stenosis and a significant risk reduction for stroke in patients with > 70% stenosis of the carotid artery, given that the surgical risk is acceptable. In current practice, revascularization strategies include both carotid endarterectomy (CEA) (Figs. 49.18 and 49.19) and percutaneous stent implantation (Figs. 49.20 to 49.24).

Revascularization of asymptomatic subjects is more controversial, especially, given most of the studies that have evaluated this topic compared surgery to very modest contemporaneous medical therapy, which did not include guideline-directed medical therapies such as statins. Typically, for asymptomatic patients there is only a mild benefit for 60–80% carotid stenoses and only a moderate benefit for > 80% stenoses, and this provided that surgery can be performed with low complication rates. Additional ongoing research may further clarify the potential benefit, if any, of revascularization versus guideline-directed medical therapy in asymptomatic patients.

Even in patients who do undergo revascularization, secondary prevention remains a critical part of patient management, with blood pressure control (the risk factor with the strongest association with stroke), lipid therapy, smoking cessation, control of diabetes, and antiplatelet therapy.

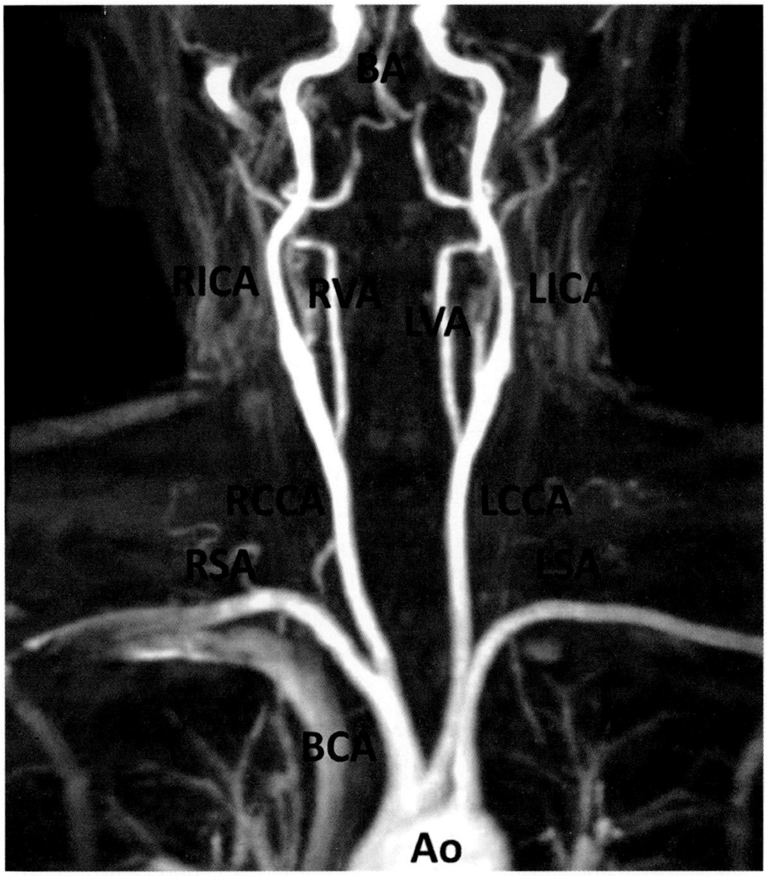

Fig. 49.5: Magnetic resonance imaging (MRI) of the carotid arteries. (Image created by Ofir Glazer and posted on Wikipedia). (Ao: Aorta; BA: Basilar artery; BCA: Brachiocephalic artery; LCCA: Left common carotid artery; LICA: Left internal carotid artery; LSA: Left subclavian artery; LVA: Left vertebral artery; RCCA: Right common carotid artery; RICA: Right internal carotid artery; RSA: Right subclavian artery; RVA: Right vertebral artery).

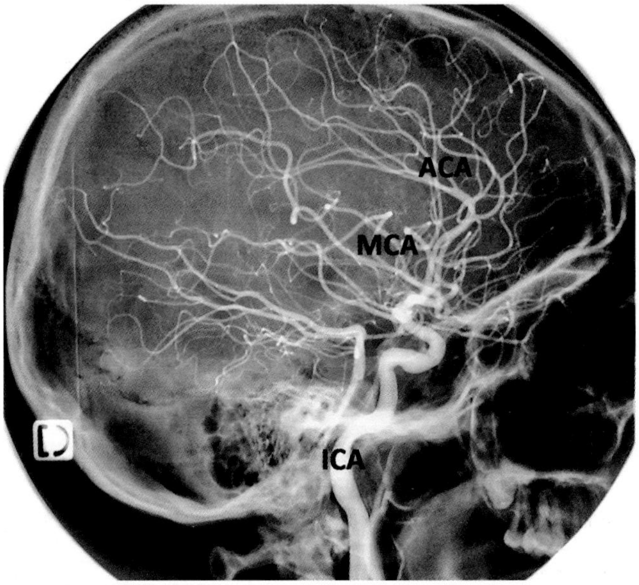

Fig. 49.6: Angiography of the carotid artery and the cerebral vasculature. At its terminus, the internal carotid artery (ICA) divides to form the middle cerebral artery (MCA) and the anterior cerebral artery (ACA). (Image made by Dr Michel Royon and posted on Wikimedia Commons).

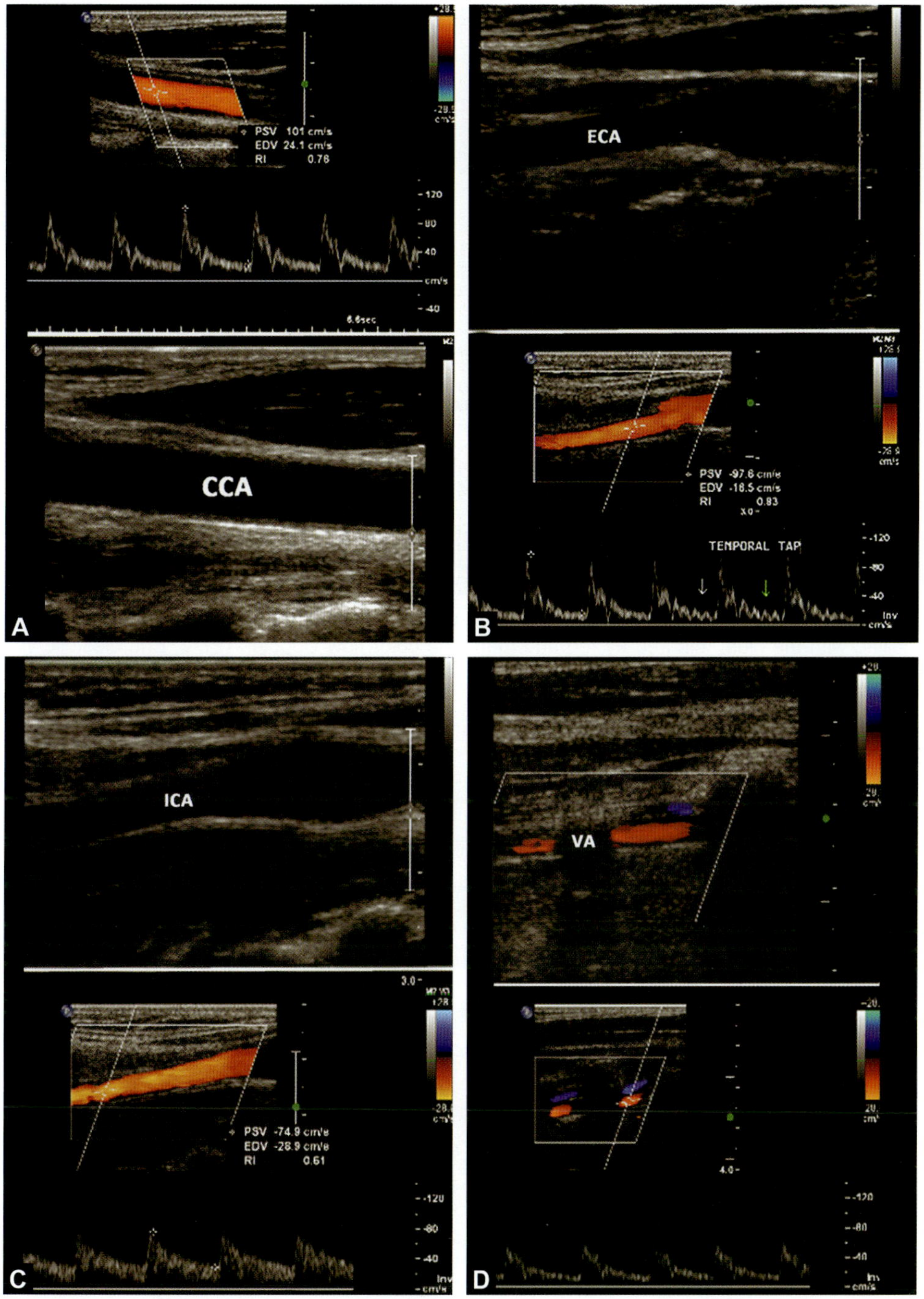

Figs. 49.7A to D: (A) Common carotid arteries (CCA) of a healthy individual: the CCA waveform is typically a combination of both the external carotid artery (ECA) and internal carotid artery (ICA). (B) The ECA and Doppler in a healthy individual: Note the diminished flow in diastole. Also note the "temporal" or "temple tap" where tapping the temporal artery in the face results in the characteristic changes as seen in the figure due to the reflection of the tap onto the artery. While the temporal tap is helpful in distinguishing the ECA from the ICA, presence of a branch is the best way to differentiate the two arteries. (C) ICA of a healthy individual: note the "low" resistive waveform with flow both in systole and diastole and a clean spectral window below the tracing. Blood vessels that feed organs that constantly (systole and diastole) require blood supply (example brain and kidneys) display low resistive signals. Absence of diastolic flow may suggest distal occlusion. (D) Normal vertebral artery flow in a healthy individual: the vertebral arteries (VA) are typically imaged between the transverse processes of the vertebral body (hence the "dropout"). Typically, signals are low resistive (systolic and diastolic flows). Also note (as in this Figure) in vascular ultrasound imaging, red does not always mean toward the probe and blue away from the probe. In this image as noted from the color scale to the right of the image, blue flow is toward the probe while red is away from the probe. (EDV: End diastolic velocity; PSV: Peak systolic velocity; RI: Resistive index).

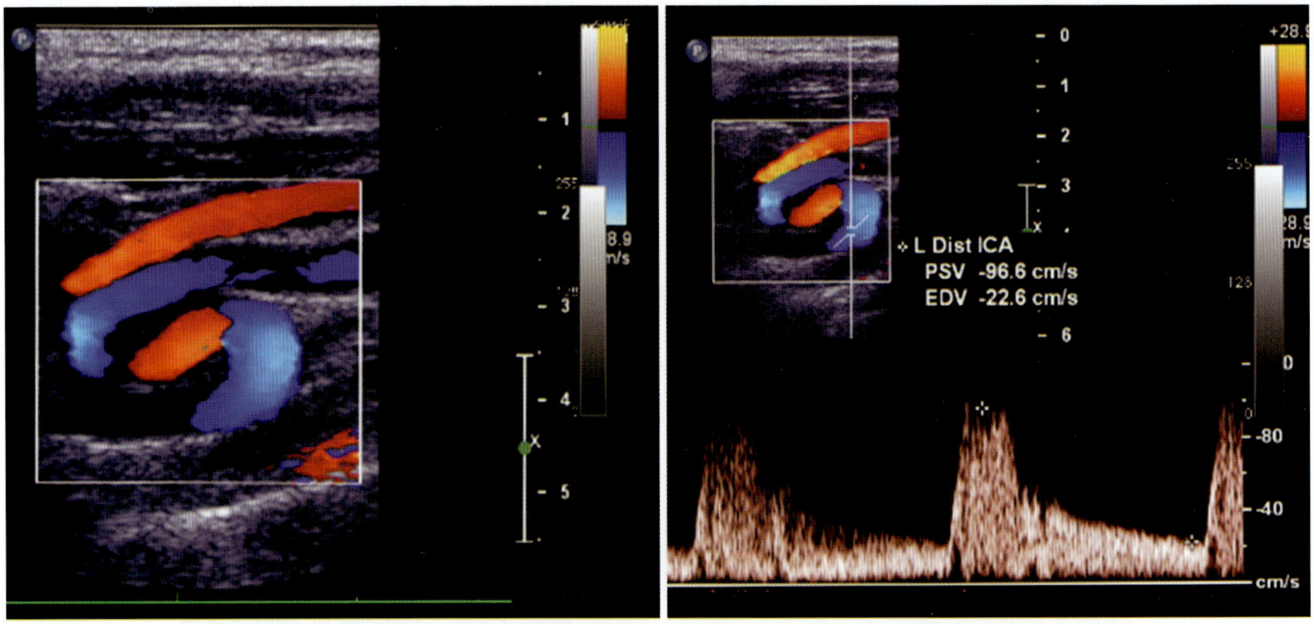

Fig. 49.8: Coiling of the left carotid artery, a normal variant, can sometimes lead to increased velocities. The color Doppler nicely demonstrates the coiling with the blue, followed by red and then blue color flow Doppler. (EDV: End diastolic velocity; ICA: Internal carotid artery; PSV: Peak systolic velocity).

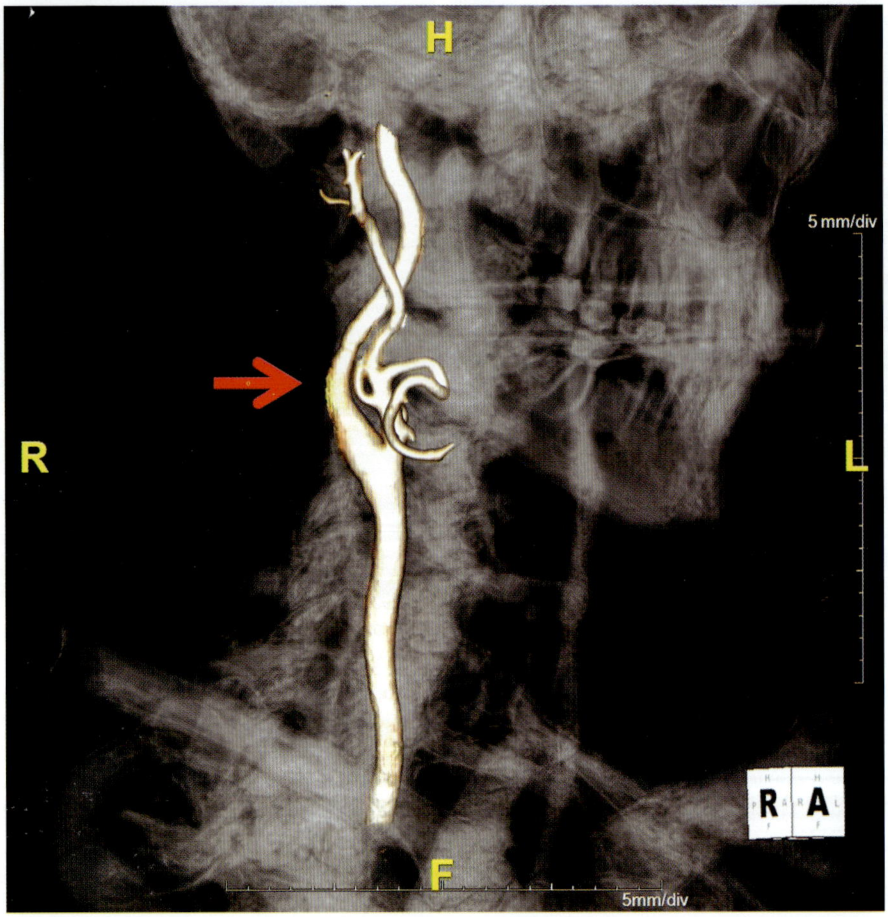

Fig. 49.9: Visualization of an internal carotid artery (ICA) early plaque development (arrow).

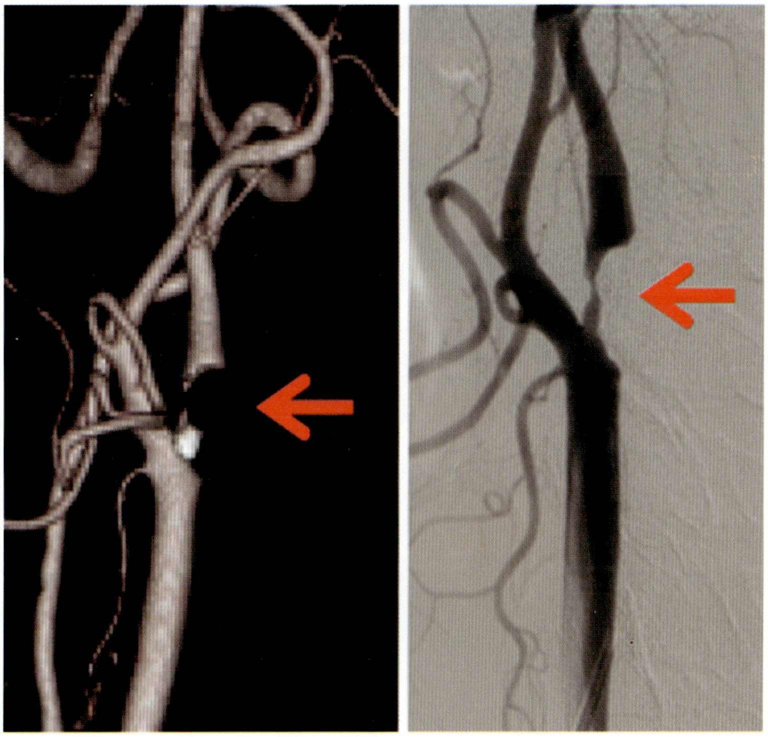

Fig. 49.10A: A three-dimensional rendering of severe left internal carotid artery (LICA) stenosis (arrow) on computed tomography (CT) scan (left panel) and angiography (right panel); note that the external carotid artery (ECA) has branches while the internal carotid artery (ICA) does not have any branches in the proximal segments. [Image from Yokoi Y. Angiography for peripheral vascular intervention. In: Forbes T (Ed). Angioplasty, Various Techniques and Challenges in Treatment of Congenital and Acquired Vascular Stenosis. InTech].

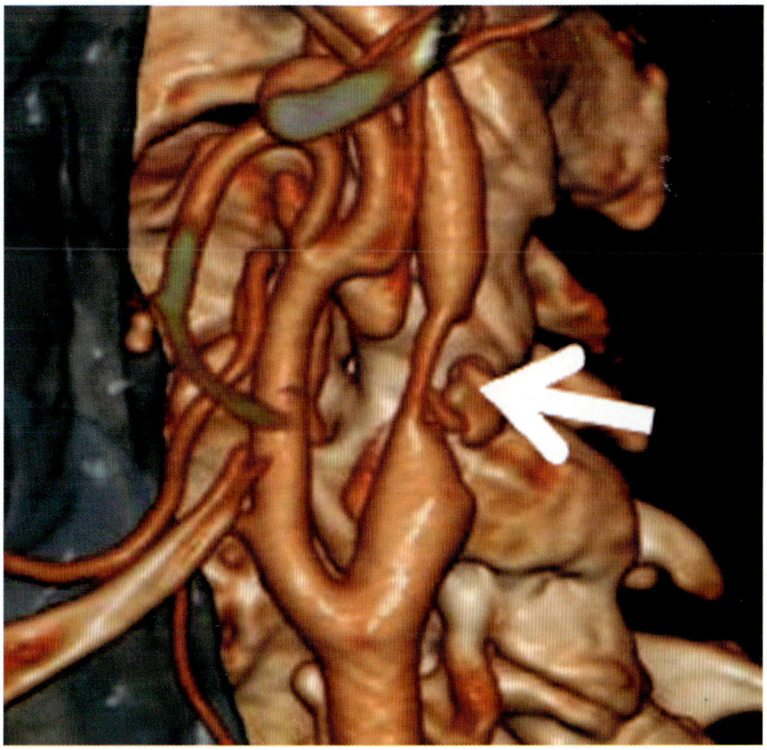

Fig. 49.10B: Volume-rendered CT angiogram demonstrating a tight ICA stenosis (arrow).

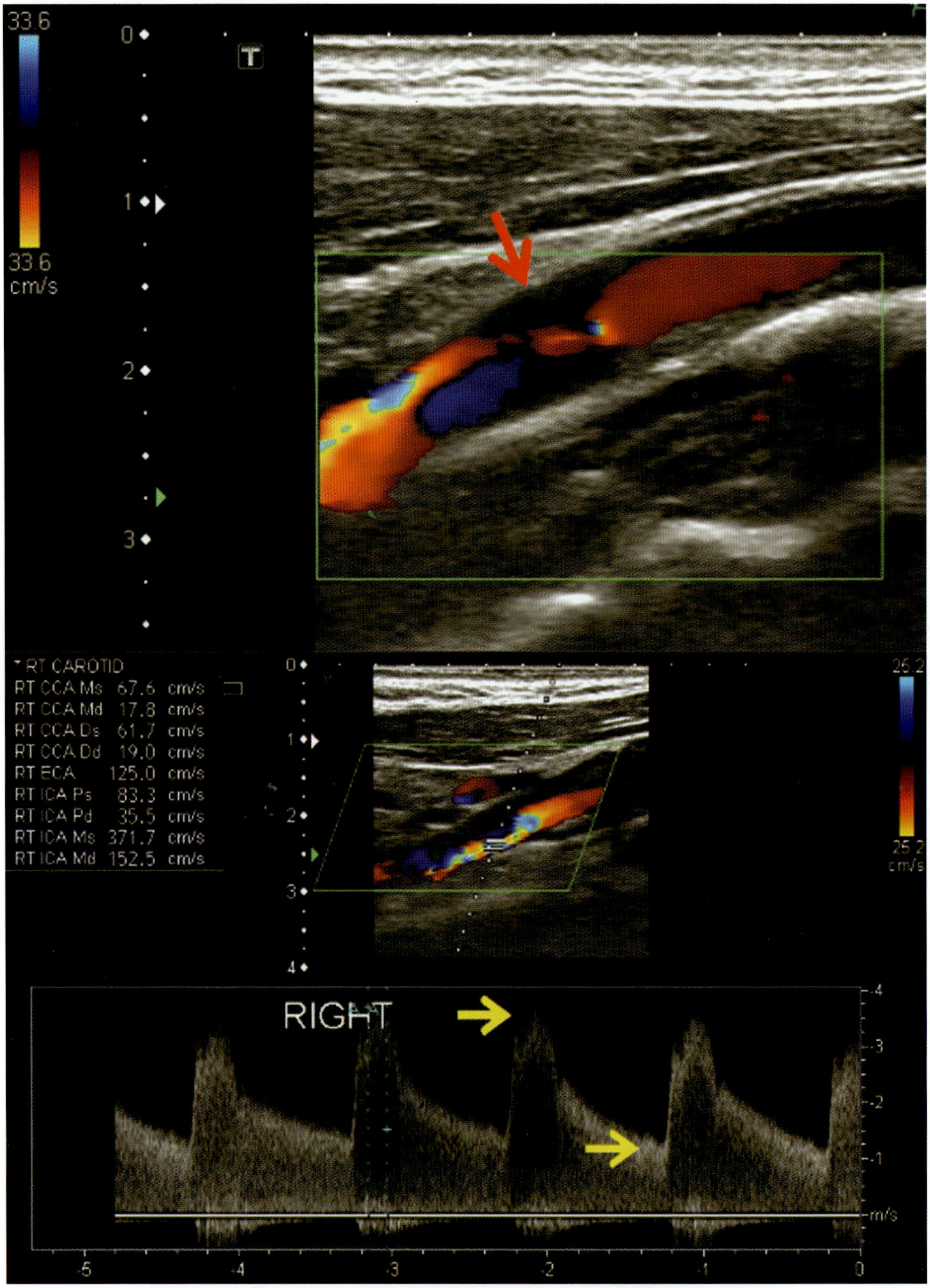

Fig. 49.11: Color two-dimensional and Doppler examination of severe carotid artery stenosis (red arrow in top panel). Note the increased end-systolic and end-diastolic velocities (EDVs) (yellow arrows in bottom panel) which are the criteria (in combination) that are suggestive of significant carotid artery stenosis (> 80% stenosis). Blood velocities are superimposed in red and blue colors indicating flow toward and away from the transducer.

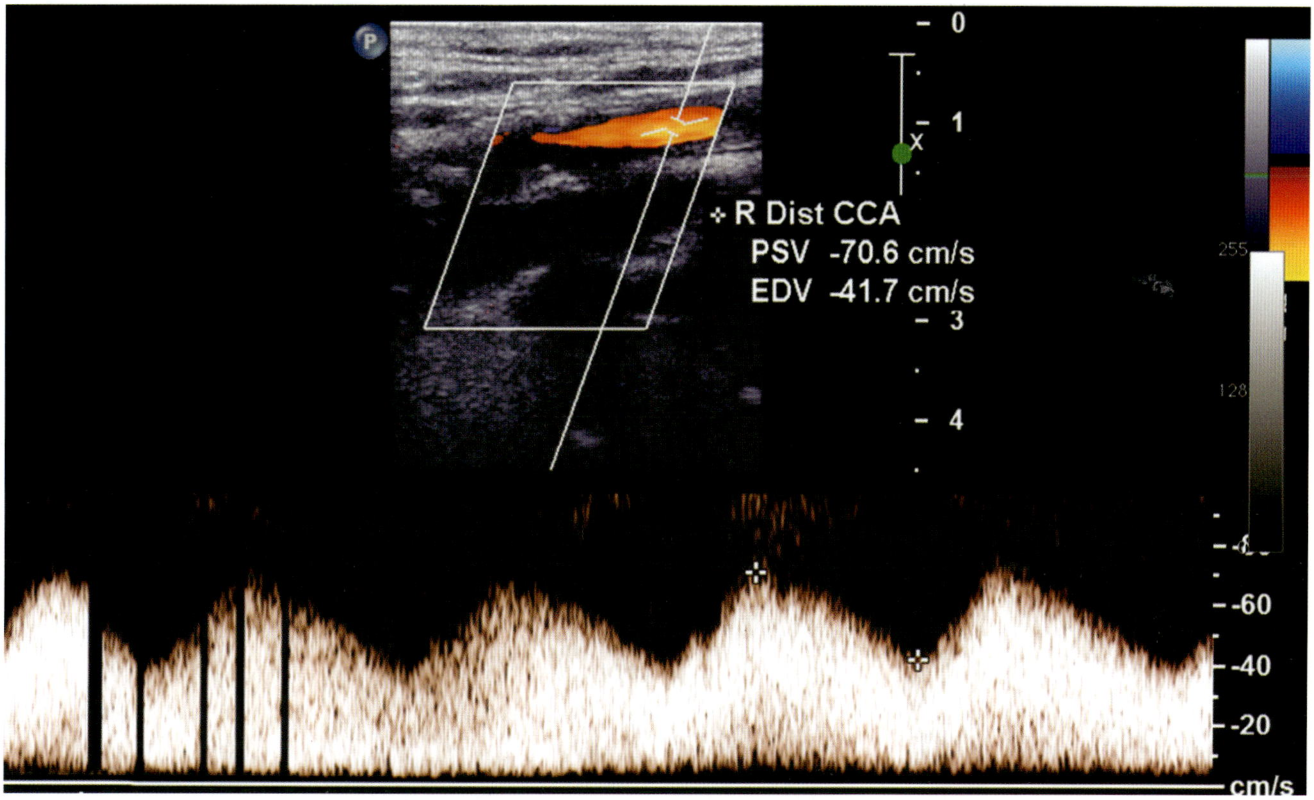

Fig. 49.12: Stenosis in the right distal common carotid artery (CCA): notice the "parvus et tardus" waveform with slow rise of pulse and increased diastolic velocities. (EDV: End-diastolic velocity; PSV: Peak systolic velocity).

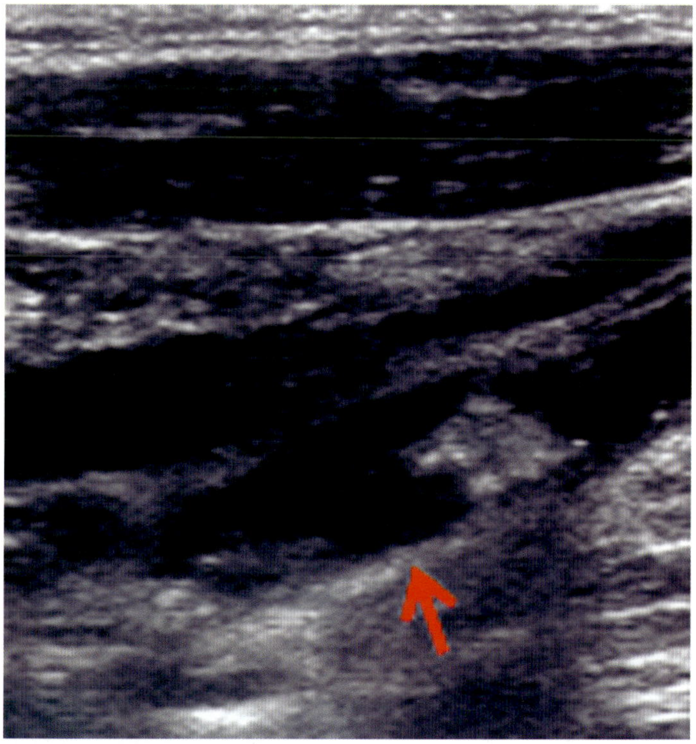

Fig. 49.13: Ulceration in the left internal carotid artery (arrow).

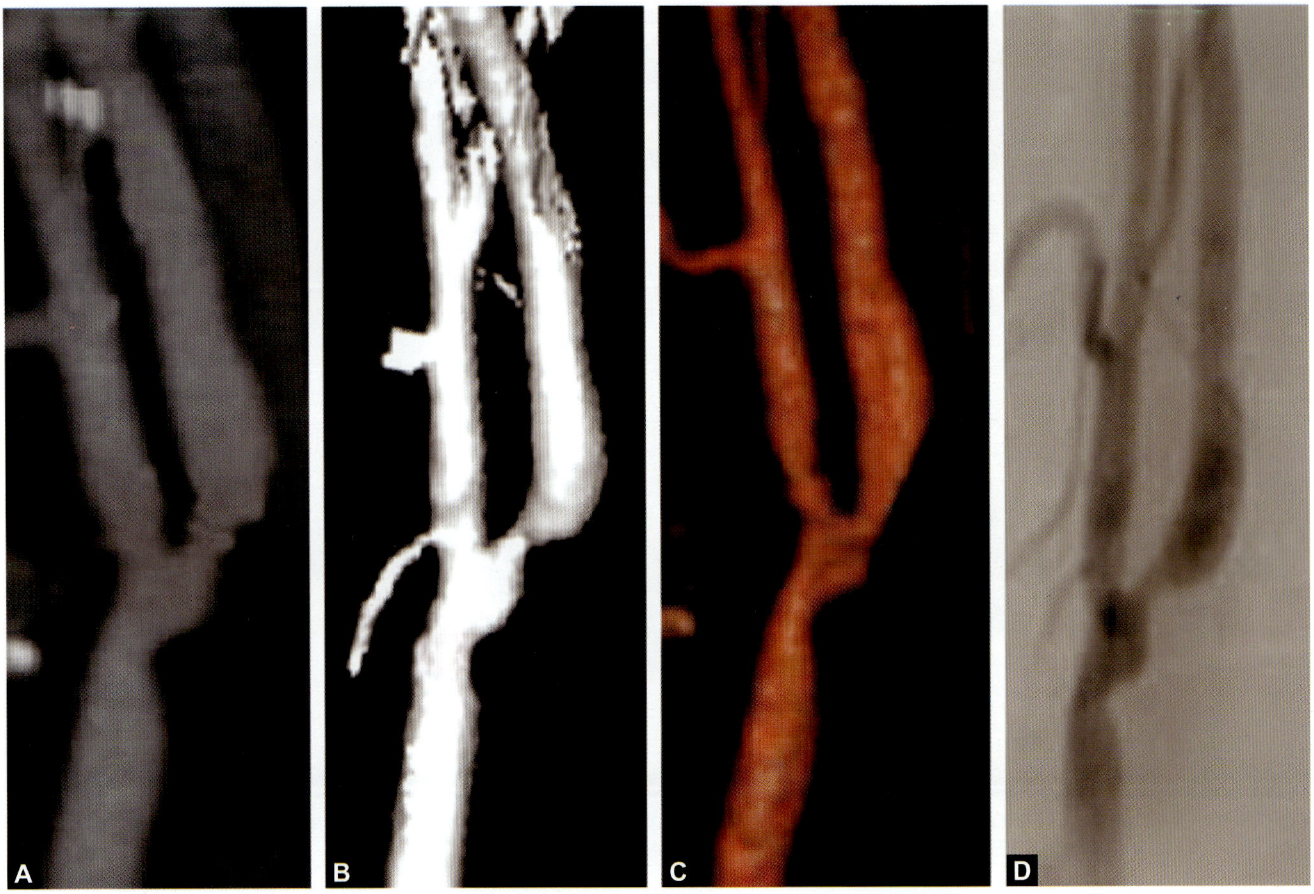

Figs. 49.14A to D: Left common carotid artery (LCCA) and left internal carotid artery (LICA) stenosis: (A) Maximum intensity projection (MIP) computed tomography (CT) image; (B) Shaded surface display (SSD) CT image; (C) Volume-rendered CT image; and (D) Digital subtraction angiography image showing moderate stenosis of distal CCA and proximal ICA. [Image from Khandelwal N, Singh P, Sameer V. Advances of computed tomography technology. In: Khandelwal N, Chowdhury V, Gupta AK (Eds). Diagnostic Radiology: Neuroradiology Including Head and Neck Imaging, 3rd edition. New Delhi, India: Jaypee Brothers Medical Publishers (P) Ltd; 2010. pp. 36-45].

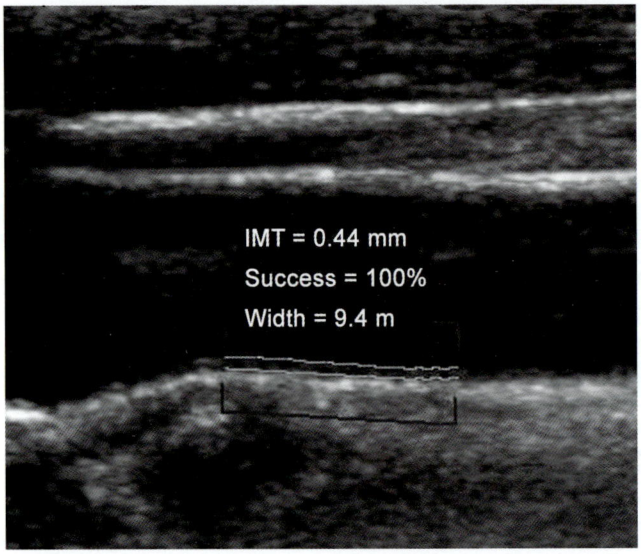

Fig. 49.15: Carotid intima-media thickness (C-IMT) is measured using B-mode ultrasound at the far wall of the common carotid artery (CCA).

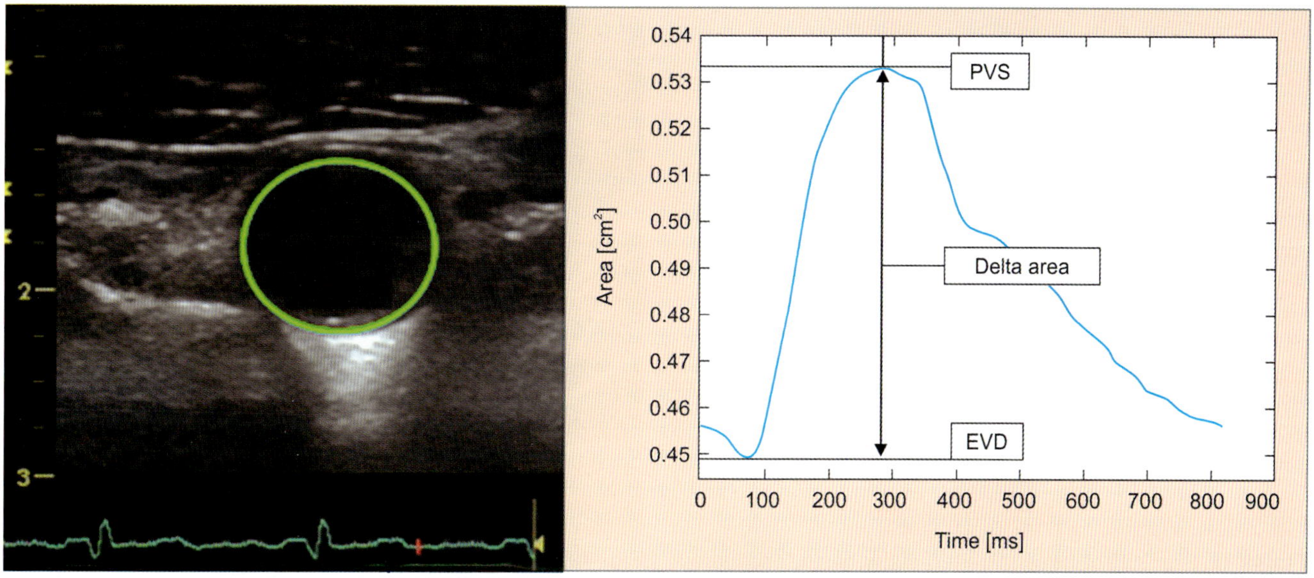

Fig. 49.16: Assessment of carotid artery distensibility. Carotid artery distensibility is a measure of arterial stiffness, which has been associated with risk factors for cardiovascular disease. (PVS: Peak vascular systole; EVD: End vascular diastole).

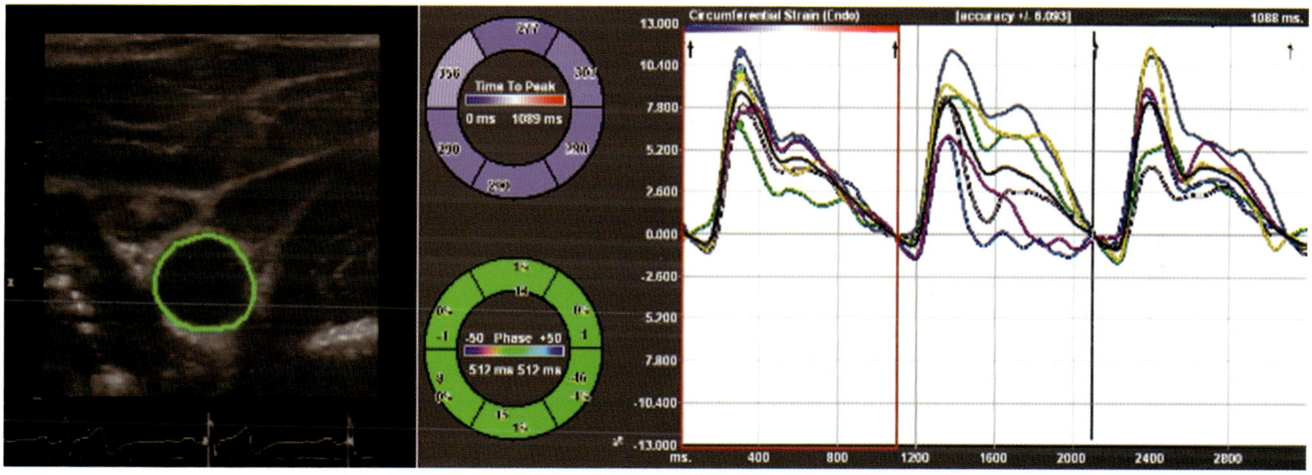

Fig. 49.17: Carotid artery strain analysis. Left panel shows the lumen contour in green of the common carotid artery (CCA) which is tracked over the cardiac cycle. Right panel shows the circumferential strain for several segments of the carotid artery shown in the left panel.

Table 49.1: Summary of criteria used to estimate the degree of stenosis based on carotid ultrasound examination. In borderline cases, additional criteria are utilized. Each laboratory needs to validate its own criteria.

Internal carotid artery (ICA) and peak vascular systole (PVS)	*ICA and end vascular diastole (EVD)*	*Plaque estimate*	*Stenosis range*
< 125 cm/s	< 40 cm/s	NA	Normal
< 125 cm/s	< 40 cm/s	< 50%	< 50%
125–230 cm/s	40–100 cm/s	> 50%	50–69%
> 230 cm/s	> 100 cm/s	> 50%	70% to near occlusion
NA	NA	Visible, no detectable lumen	Total occlusion

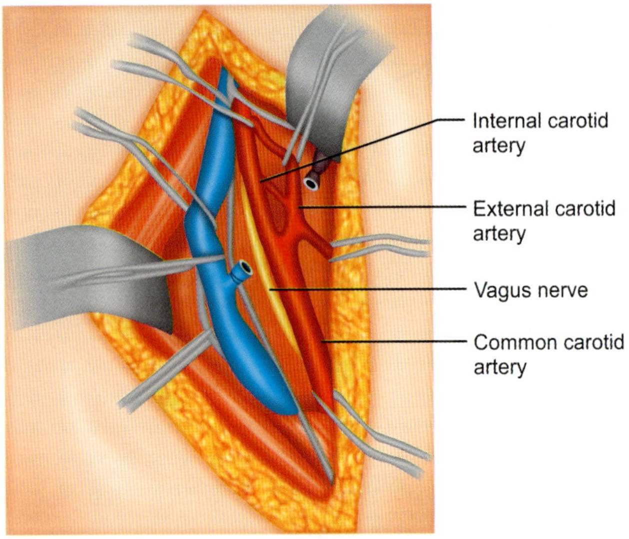

Fig. 49.18: Exposure of the carotid artery during carotid endarterectomy (CEA). [Image from Basu S. Surgical exposure of vessels. In: Khanna AK, Puneet (Eds). Manual of Vascular Surgery, 1st edition. New Delhi, India: Jaypee Brothers Medical Publishers; 2010. pp. 35-83].

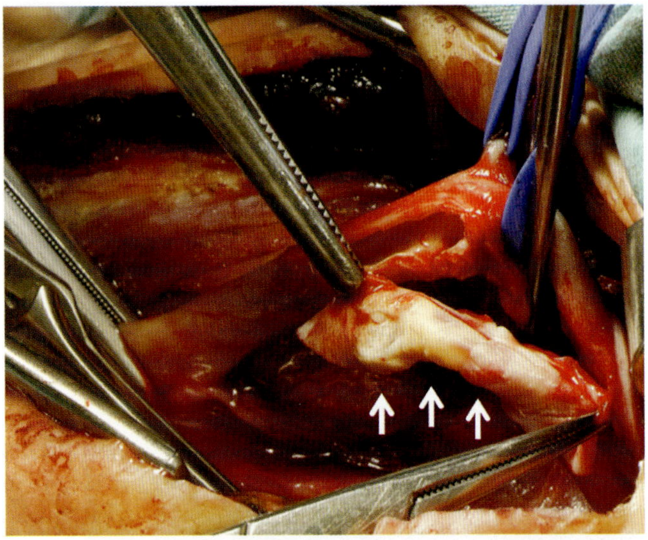

Fig. 49.19: Operative room image of a carotid endarterectomy (CEA) procedure. The excised plaque (arrows) is visualized. [Image from Radak D, Tanasković S. Eversion carotid endarterectomy in patients with near-total internal carotid artery occlusion—diagnostic modalities, indications and surgical technique. In: Yamanouchi D (Ed). Vascular Surgery. InTech. 2012. pp. 73-84].

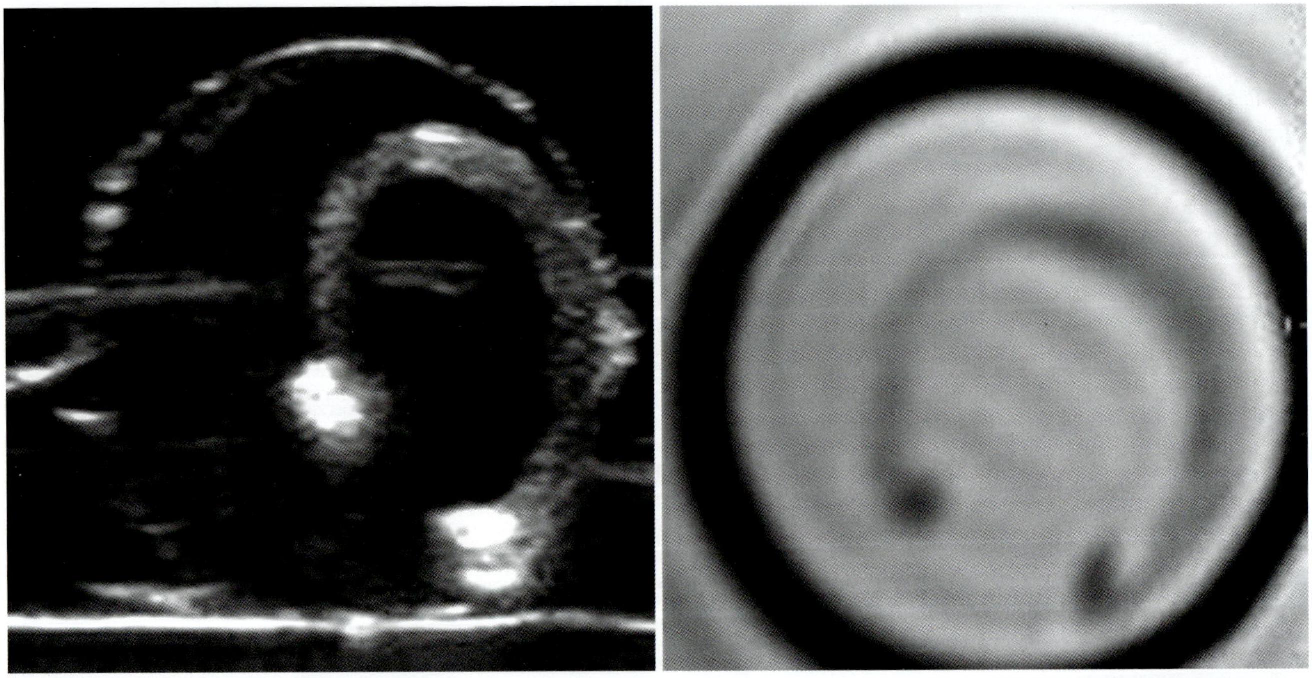

Fig. 49.20: Real-time B-mode ultrasound scans of a carotid endarterectomy (CEA) tissue. Tissue embedded in an agarose gel bed for ultrasound imaging, note the faint circular pattern. Left panel shows a cross-sectional view on ultrasound, whereas the right panel shows the matched magnetic resonance imaging (MRI) slice.

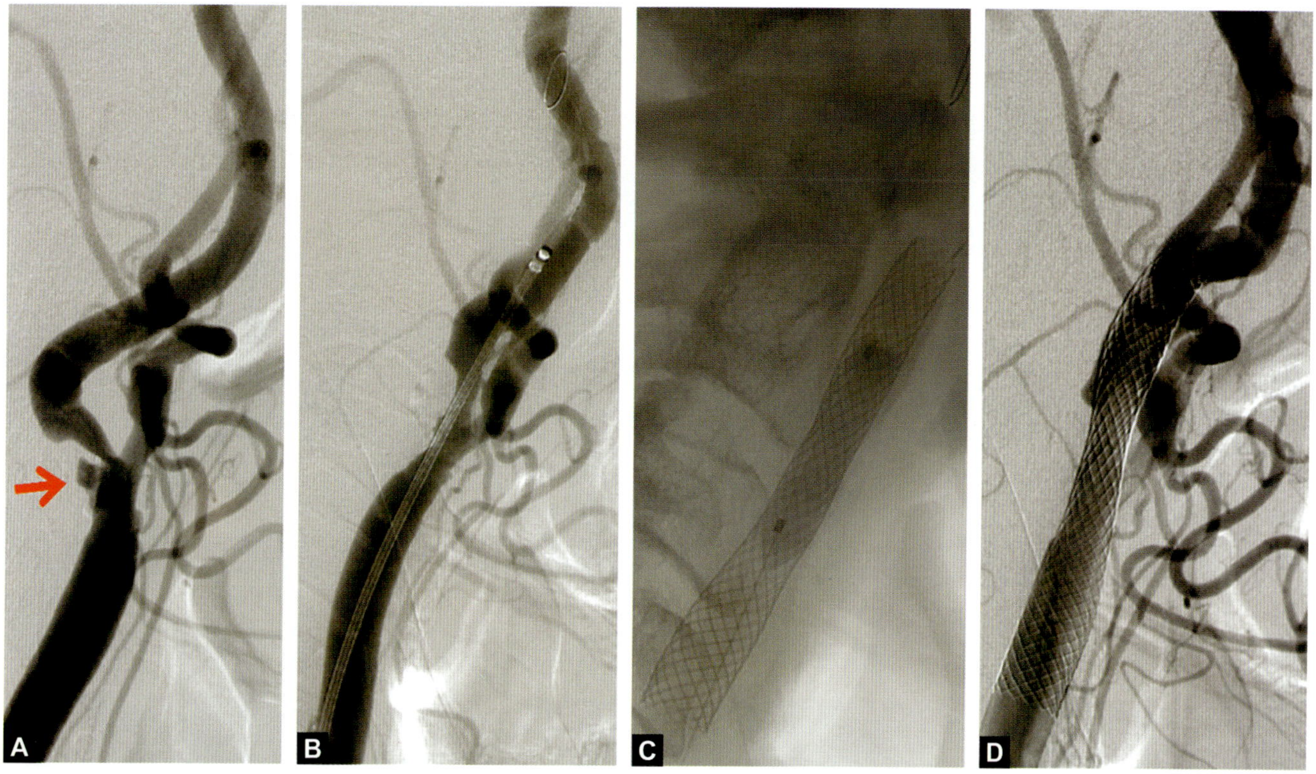

Figs. 49.21A to D: Stenting of a proximal internal carotid artery (ICA) stenosis with a self-expanding stent. (A) Stenosis predilation (arrow). (B) Placement of the self-expanding stent. (C) Postdilation of the deployed stent. (D) Final angiogram showing the deployed postdilated stent. (Image from Myouchin K, Takayama K, Taoka T, et al. Carotid Wallstent placement difficulties encountered in carotid artery stenting. Springerplus. 2013;2:468).

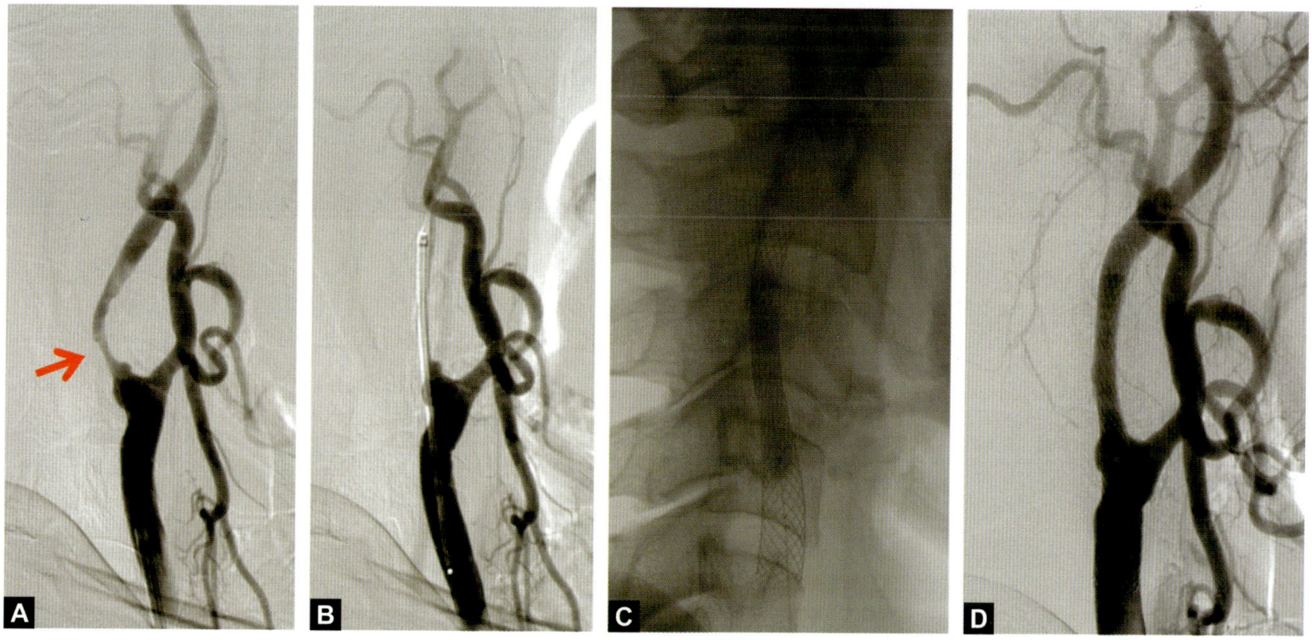

Figs. 49.22A to D: Treatment of a complex right internal carotid stenosis (arrow) with a self-expanding stent. (A) Stenosis predilation (arrow). (B) Placement of the self-expanding stent. (C) Postdilation of the deployed stent. (D) Final angiogram showing the deployed postdilated stent. (Image from Myouchin K, Takayama K, Taoka T, et al. Carotid Wallstent placement difficulties encountered in carotid artery stenting. Springerplus. 2013;2:468).

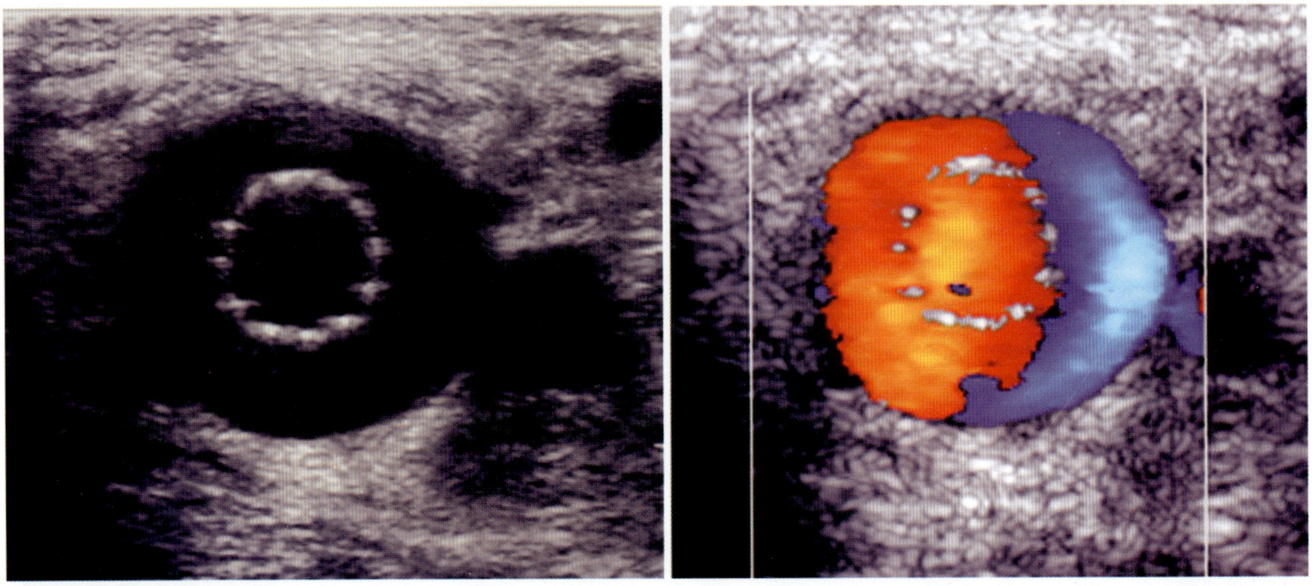

Fig. 49.23: Ultrasound of a left carotid artery treated with endovascular stent implantation. Note that the stent clearly appears undersized and/or underdeployed.

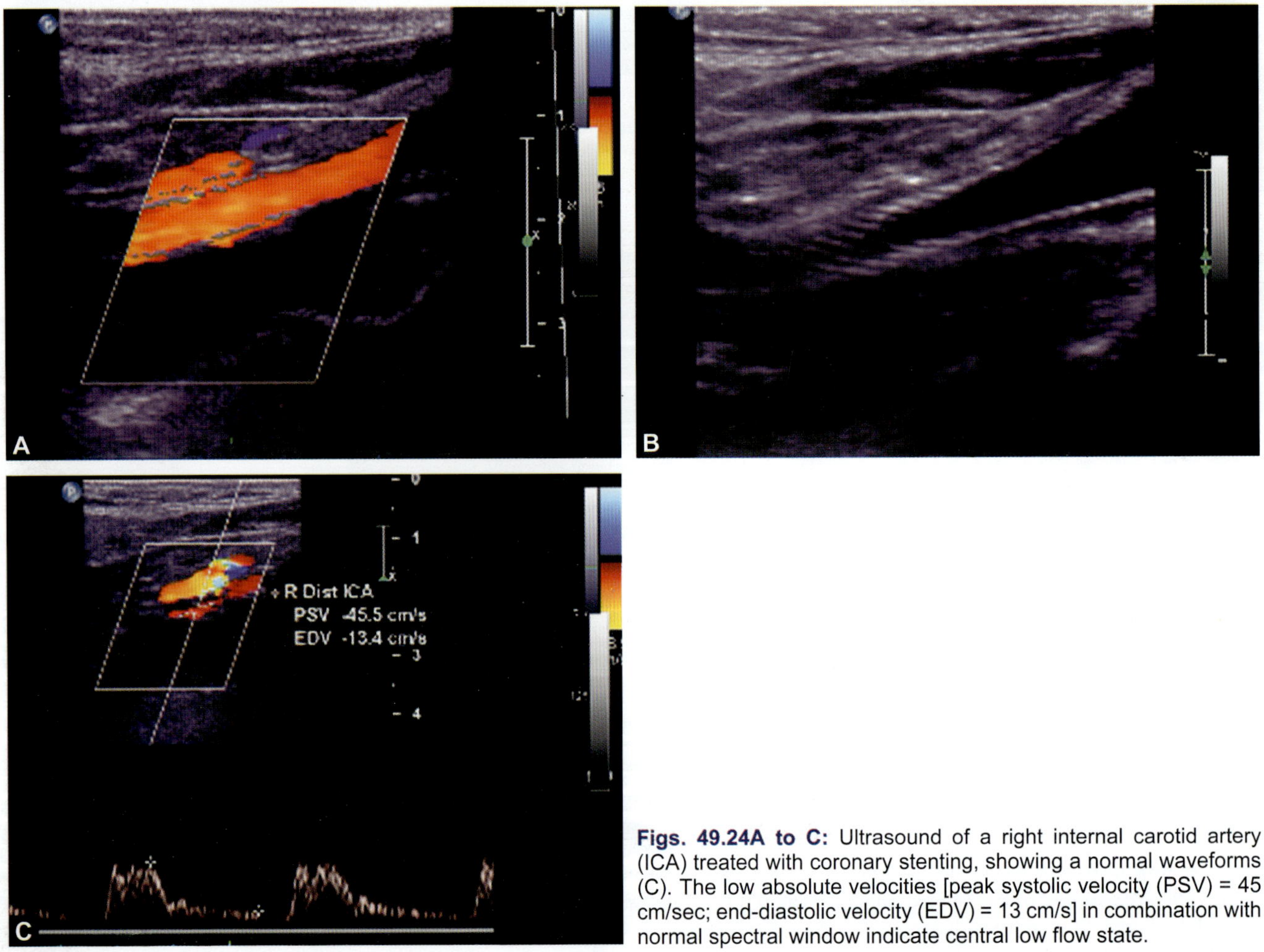

Figs. 49.24A to C: Ultrasound of a right internal carotid artery (ICA) treated with coronary stenting, showing a normal waveforms (C). The low absolute velocities [peak systolic velocity (PSV) = 45 cm/sec; end-diastolic velocity (EDV) = 13 cm/s] in combination with normal spectral window indicate central low flow state.

NON-ATHEROSCLEROTIC CAROTID ARTERY DISEASE

Other disease states such as carotid artery dissection (Figs. 49.25A and B) and FMD are uncommon but are important causes of stroke to recognize, especially in younger individuals. Carotid artery dissection typically presents with unilateral headache/Horner's syndrome and stroke, and is treated with anticoagulation or antiplatelet therapy.

Fibromuscular dysplasia (Figs. 49.26 and 49.27) is more prevalent in women, has atypical presentations and is usually managed conservatively when asymptomatic. Symptomatic disease is generally managed with antiplatelet therapy and percutaneous angioplasty.

Carotid body tumor or paragangliomas (Figs. 49.28 to 49.30) are highly vascular tumors that may develop at the carotid bifurcation, resulting in the bifurcation to be "splayed" out.

Carotid artery aneurysm (Figs. 49.31 and 49.32) is a rare finding which increases the risk of cerebral embolism, transient ischemic attack, or major stroke.

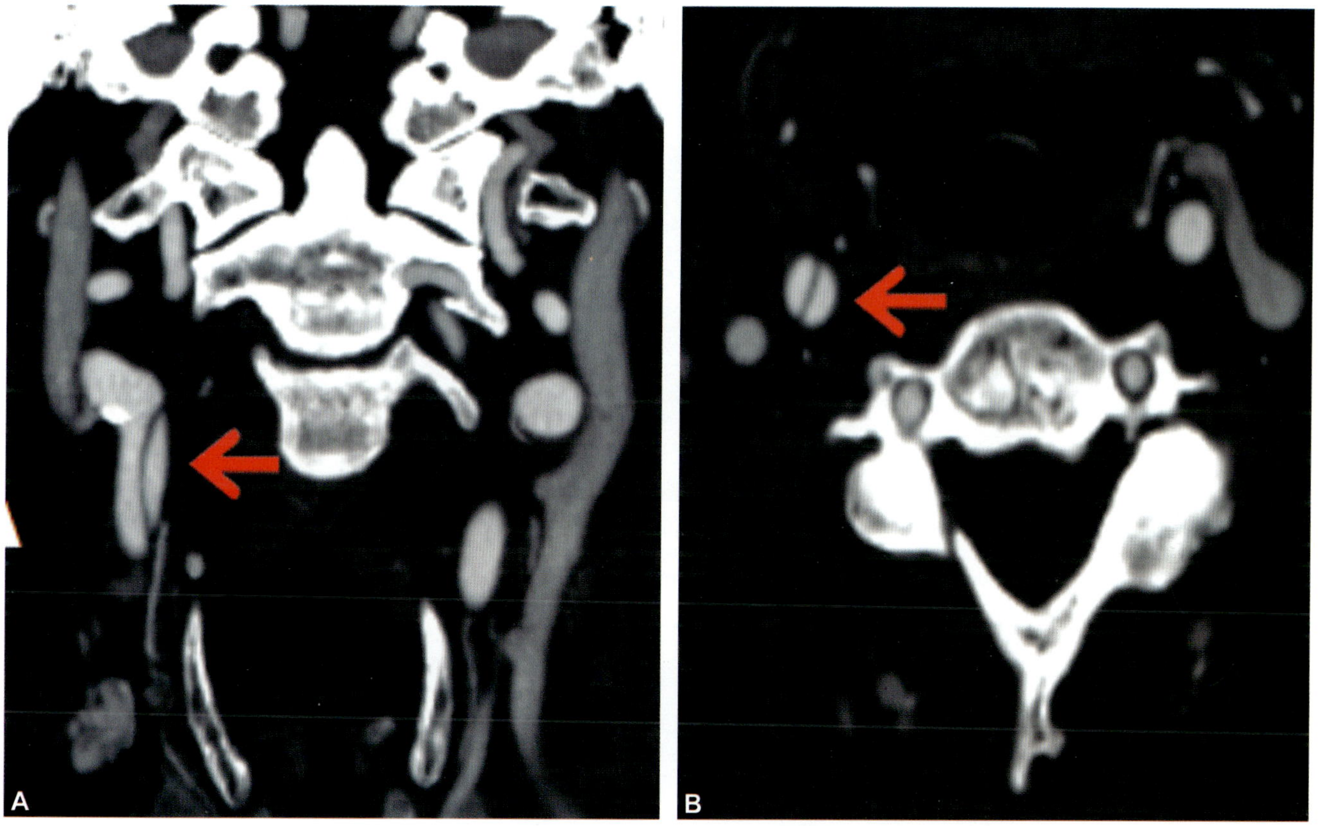

Figs. 49.25A and B: Contrast-enhanced computed tomography (CT) angiography demonstrating dissection of the right carotid artery. A dissection flap (arrow) is clearly visible in both the (A) coronary and (B) axial images. Carotid artery dissections are typically treated with anticoagulation or antiplatelet therapy.

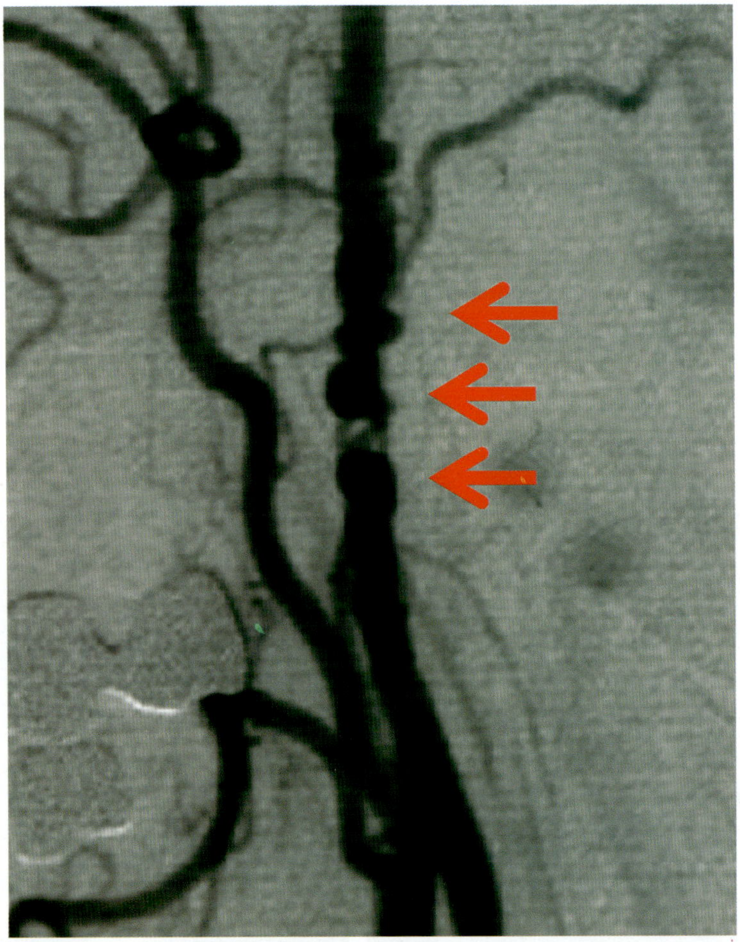

Fig. 49.26: Angiogram of the internal carotid artery (ICA) showing the "string-of-beads" sign (arrows) in a patient with recurrent transient ischemic attacks, found to have fibromuscular dysplasia of the carotid artery. (Image from Arning C, Grzyska U. Color Doppler imaging of cervicocephalic fibromuscular dysplasia. Cardiovasc Ultrasound. 2004;2:7).

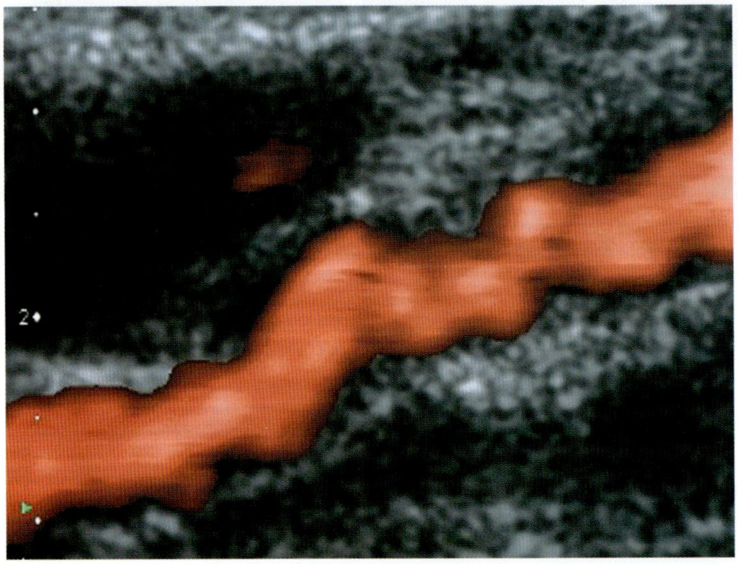

Fig. 49.27: Power Doppler examination showing "string-of-beads" sign in the same patient with fibromuscular dysplasia of the carotid artery. (Image from Arning C, Grzyska U. Color Doppler imaging of cervicocephalic fibromuscular dysplasia. Cardiovasc Ultrasound. 2004;2:7).

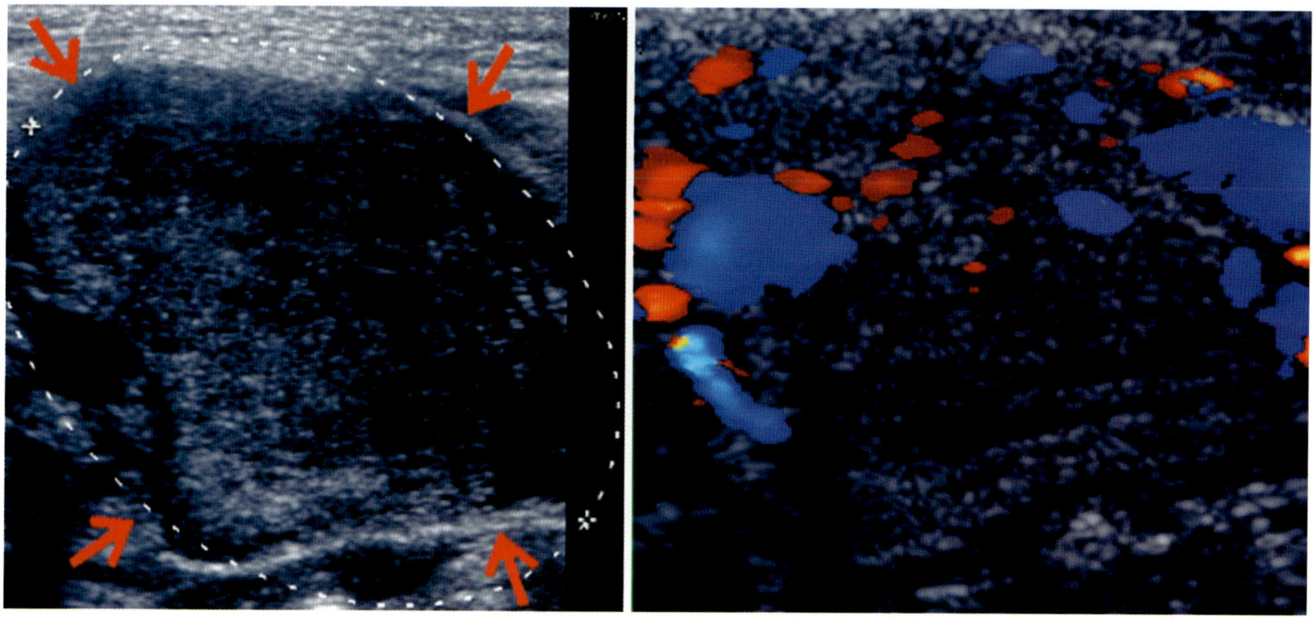

Fig. 49.28: Ultrasound images demonstrating a left carotid body tumor (paraganglioma; arrows). On the right panel, blood velocities are superimposed in red and blue colors indicating flow toward and away from the transducer.

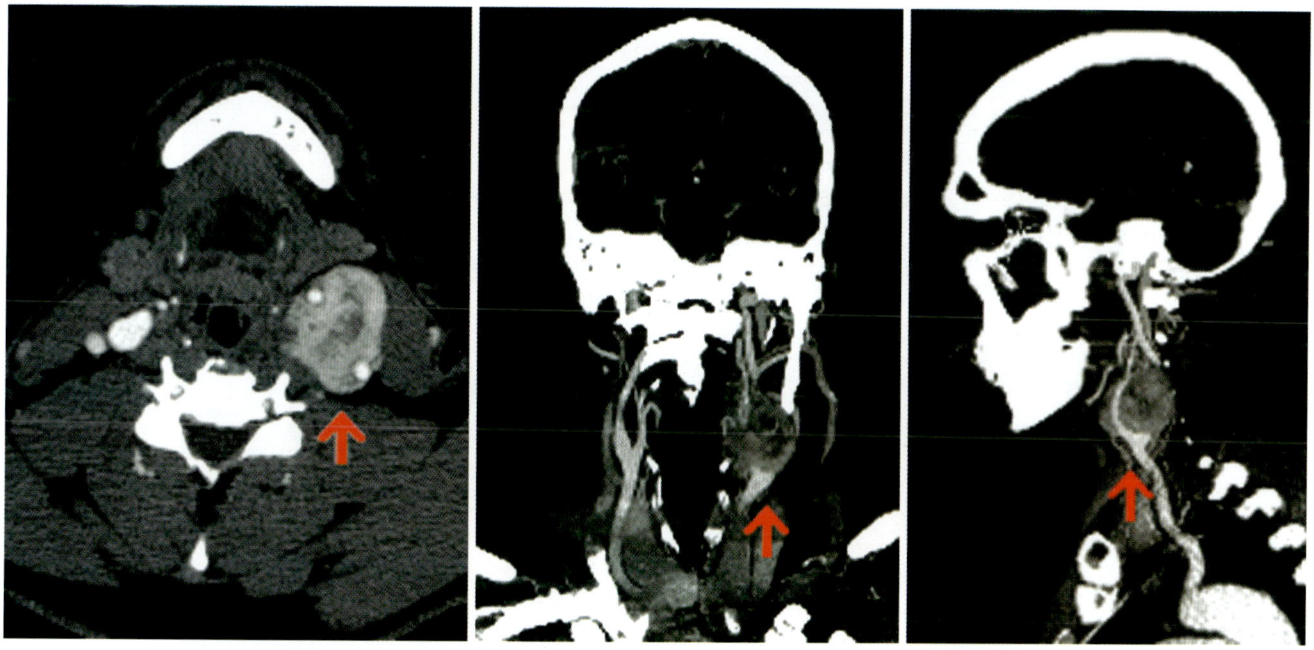

Fig. 49.29: Axial, coronal and sagittal computed tomography (CT) images showing left carotid body tumor (paraganglioma; arrow).

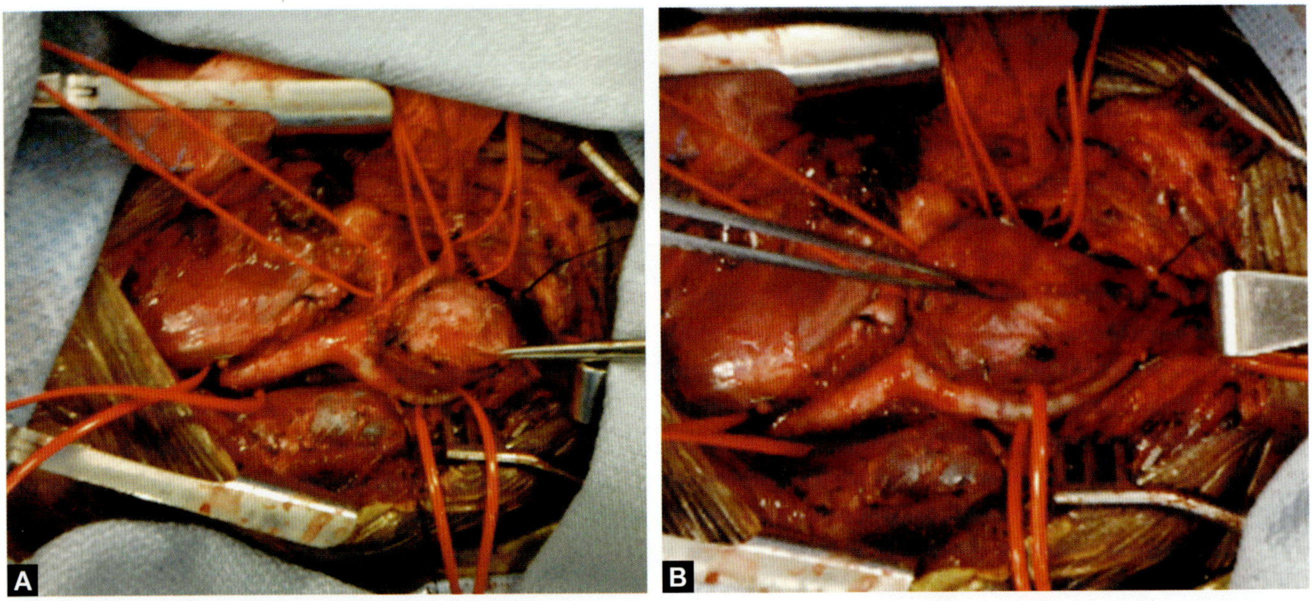

Figs. 49.30A and B: Operative room images of a carotid body tumor. A carotid body tumor or paragangliomas is a highly vascular tumor that typically arises at the carotid bifurcation resulting in the bifurcation to be "splayed" out. Usually benign, symptomatic tumors are treated with surgical removal or intravascular embolization.

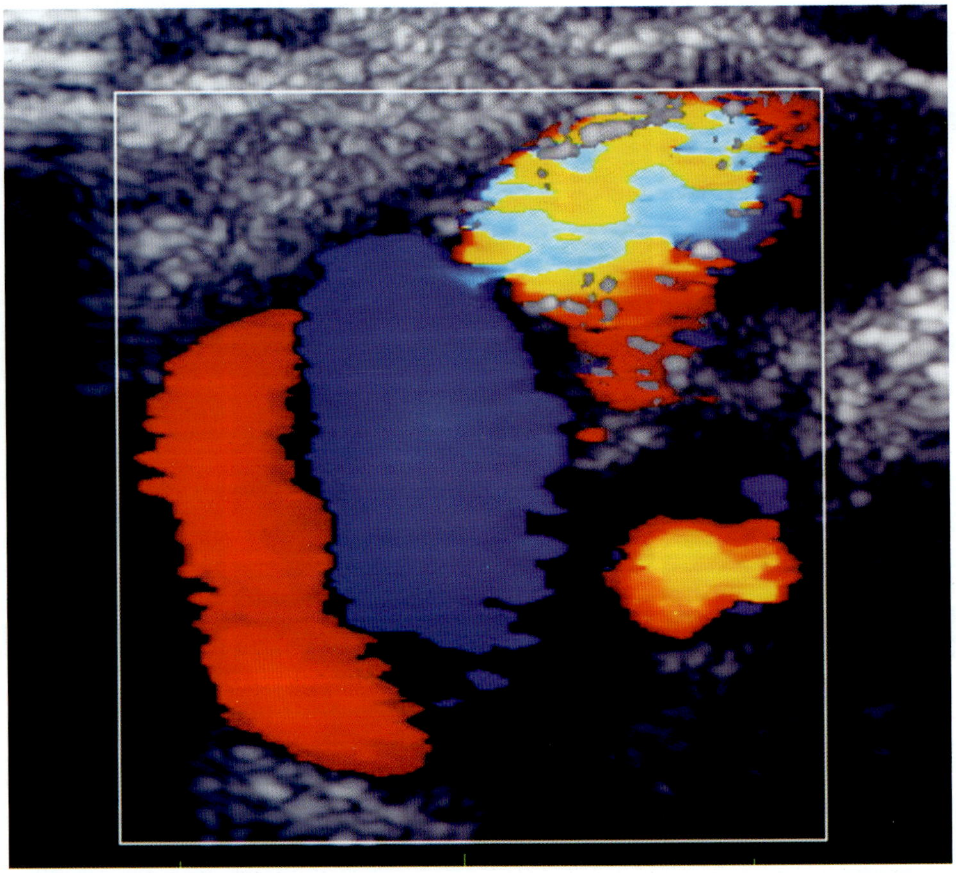

Fig. 49.31: Color Doppler ultrasound of a carotid artery aneurysm. There is turbulent flow (mosaic color) within the aneurysm.

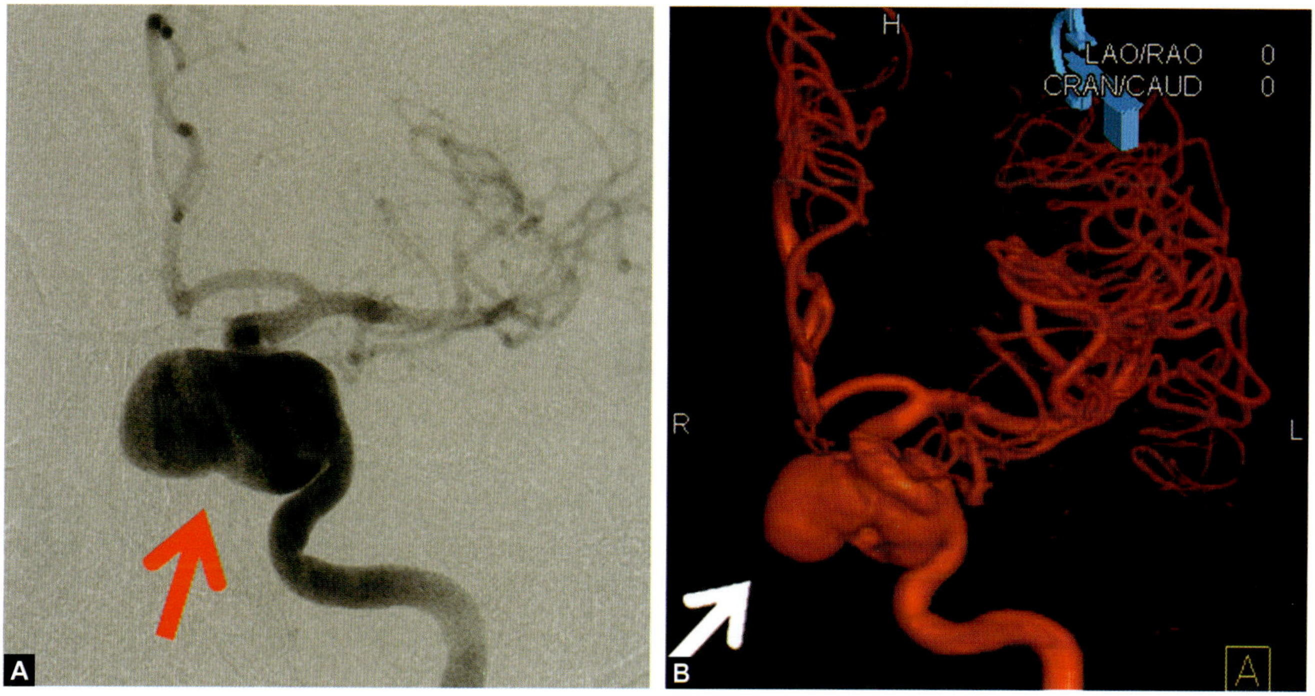

Figs. 49.32A and B: (A) Digital subtraction angiography (red arrow) and (B) colorized images of an internal carotid aneurysm (white arrow). (Image from Kloss BT, Patel R, Sullivan AM. Intracranial internal carotid aneurysm causing diplopia. Int J Emerg Med. 2011;4:56).

ACKNOWLEDGMENTS

The authors acknowledge the contributions The Methodist DeBakey Heart and Vascular Center, Houston Methodist Hospital.

GB was supported by an AHA Beginning Grant-in-Aid-award (13 B GIA 16720014) and by the caroline Wiess Law Fund for Molecular Medicine.

VIDEO LEGEND

Video 49.1: Three-dimensional (3D) computed tomography (CT) reconstruction of the carotid arteries.

REFERENCES

Barnett HJ, Taylor DW, Eliasziw M, et al. Benefit of carotid endarterectomy in patients with symptomatic moderate or severe stenosis. North American Symptomatic Carotid Endarterectomy Trial Collaborators. N Engl J Med. 1998;339(20):1415-25.

Endarterectomy for asymptomatic carotid artery stenosis. Executive Committee for the Asymptomatic Carotid Atherosclerosis Study. JAMA. 1995;273(18):1421-8.

Furie KL, Kasner SE, Adams RJ, et al. Guidelines for the prevention of stroke in patients with stroke or transient ischemic attack: a guideline for healthcare professionals from the American Heart Association/American Stroke Association. Stroke. 2011;42(1):227-76.

Goldstein LB, Bushnell CD, Adams RJ, et al. Guidelines for the primary prevention of stroke: a guideline for healthcare professionals from the American Heart Association/American Stroke Association. Stroke. 2011;42(2):517-84.

Grotta JC. Clinical practice. Carotid stenosis. N Engl J Med. 2013;369 (12):1143-50.

Halliday A, Mansfield A, Marro J, et al. Prevention of disabling and fatal strokes by successful carotid endarterectomy in patients without recent neurological symptoms: randomised controlled trial. Lancet. 2004;363(9420):1491-502.

Jaff MR. Carotid artery disease and stroke. In: Rooke TW, Sullivan TM, Jaff MR (Eds). Vascular Medicine and Endovascular Interventions, 1st edition. Columbia Madison, USA: Blackwell Futura; 2007. pp. 212-20.

North American Symptomatic Carotid Endarterectomy Trial Collaborators. Beneficial effect of carotid endarterectomy in symptomatic patients with high-grade carotid stenosis. N Engl J Med. 1991;325(7):445-53.

Randomised trial of endarterectomy for recently symptomatic carotid stenosis: final results of the MRC European Carotid Surgery Trial (ECST). Lancet. 1998;351(9113):1379-87.

CHAPTER

50

Aortic Aneurysm

Eric M Isselbacher, David M Dudzinski, Brian Ghoshhajra

INTRODUCTION

Aneurysms of the aorta (Figs. 50.1 to 50.4) are often asymptomatic or may cause a variety of symptoms and signs depending on the aneurysm size and location. True aneurysms are more common and involve bulging out of three layers of the vessel wall, whereas pseudoaneurysms result from a focal rupture of the aortic media that is contained by either the adventitia or structures adjacent to the aorta (Fig. 50.5). Most aortic aneurysms are fusiform, or radially symmetric in shape. Saccular aneurysms, which have asymmetric bulging of the aortic wall, are much less common and may reflect a focal inflammatory or traumatic etiology. The overall prevalence of abdominal aortic aneurysms is ~3% after the age of 50 years and ~6% after the age of 65 years, with approximately a 10:1 male to female predominance. Abdominal aneurysms most often involve the infrarenal segment. Thoracic aneurysms are less common, with a prevalence of ~3% by autopsy studies, and a 2:1 male to female ratio; the ascending aorta is the segment most often involved (Fig. 50.2).

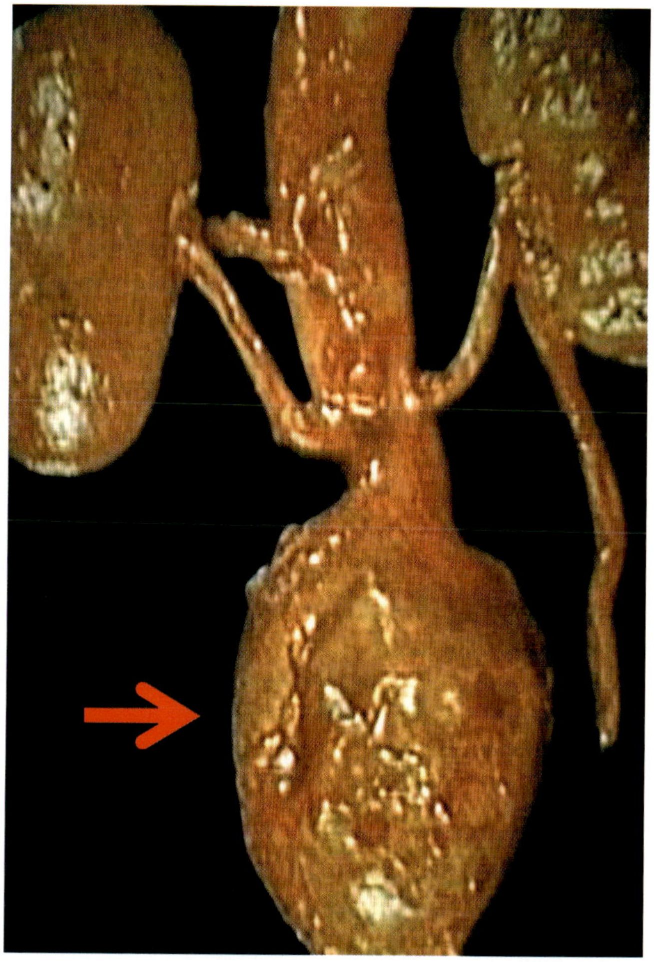

Fig. 50.1: Gross pathology specimen of an abdominal aortic aneurysm. (Image from Armed Forces Institute of Pathology).

PATHOGENESIS OF AORTIC ANEURYSM FORMATION

The pathogenesis of aortic aneurysms is multifactorial and includes hereditary and acquired factors. Smoking is the dominant etiology and risk factor for abdominal aortic aneurysm, while a history of hypertension is the most common risk factor for thoracic aortic aneurysm. Atherosclerosis of the intima may result both in impaired vessel homeostasis and a weakening of elastic fibers, but the key pathophysiologic processes in aneurysm formation occur within the vessel media. Oxidative stress and dyslipidemia result in aortic smooth muscle cell injury, upregulation of proteases (including matrix metalloproteinases), and the release of chemokines that recruit inflammatory cells to the vessel wall. Direct cytotoxicity against structural proteins like elastin and apoptosis of smooth muscle

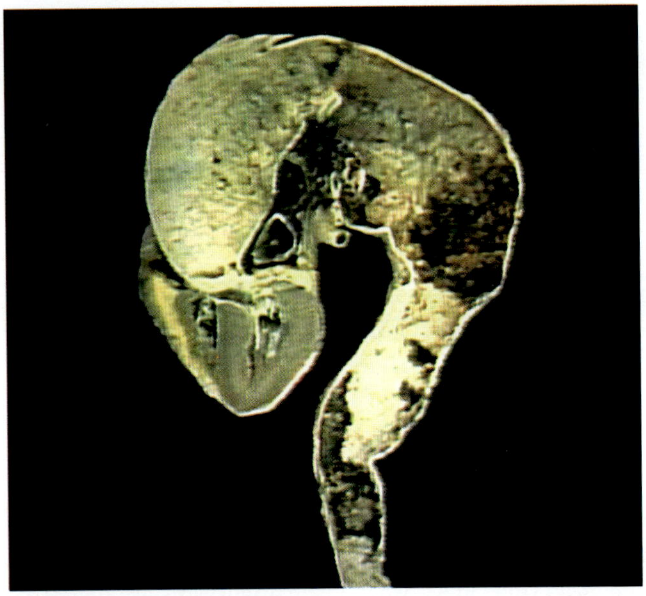

Fig. 50.2A: Gross pathology specimen of a massive thoracic aortic aneurysm. Note that the size of the aneurysm dwarfs that of the heart. (Image from Armed Forces Institute of Pathology).

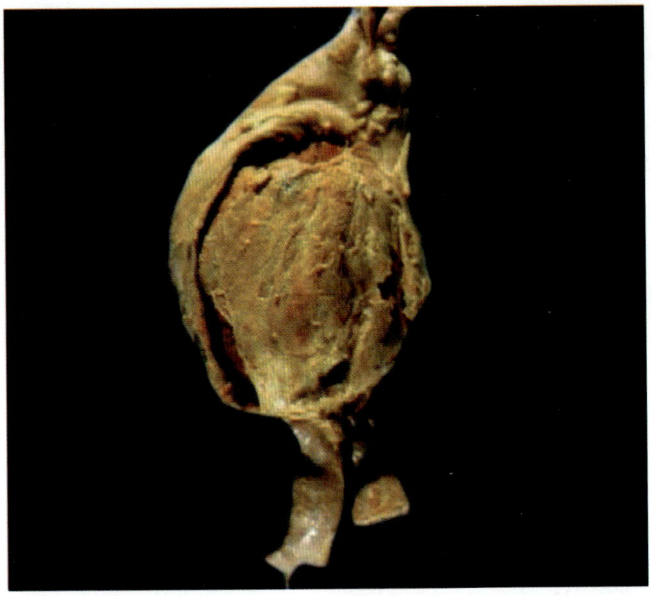

Fig. 50.2B: Gross pathology specimen of a fusiform abdominal aortic aneurysm. (Image from Armed Forces Institute of Pathology).

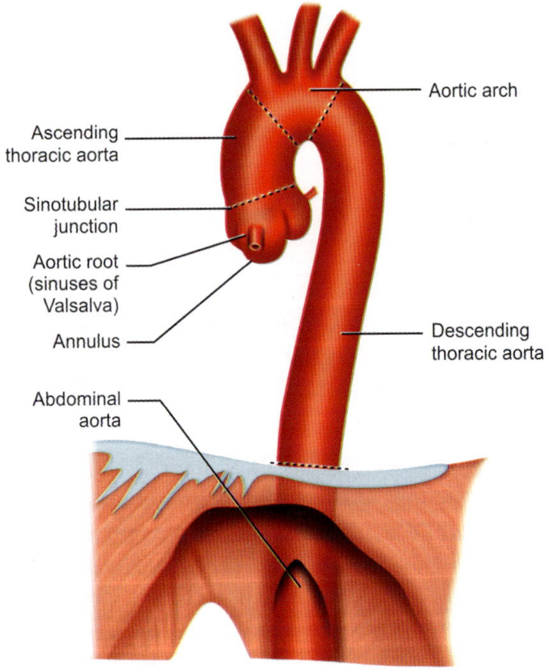

Fig. 50.3: Thoracic aortic anatomy and the prevalence of aneurysm by location. About 60% of thoracoabdominal aortic aneurysms arise in the proximal aorta (aortic root and/or ascending aorta) and about 40% in the descending aorta. About 10% of aneurysms will involve multiple segments of the aorta; aortic arch aneurysms are commonly contiguous with aneurysms of the ascending aorta, and aneurysms of the descending thoracic aorta may extend into the abdominal aorta to form "thoracoabdominal" aneurysms. (©Massachusetts General Hospital Thoracic Aortic Center, used with permission).

cells each contribute to a reduction in the integrity of the aortic media. Reduced wall thickness then leads to aortic dilatation, in accordance with the law of LaPlace. The histology of ascending thoracic aortic aneurysms is typically that of medial degeneration (Fig. 50.6), with fragmentation and destruction of the elastic fibers, apoptosis of smooth muscle cells, and deposition of proteoglycan in the media. The gross pathology of aortic aneurysms is illustrated in Figures 50.4 and 50.5.

There is an increased prevalence of aortic aneurysms among the first-degree relatives of individuals with aneurysms, suggesting underlying heritable bases. Genetic techniques have identified candidate genes in aortic aneurysm syndromes, including those encoding for the TGF-beta receptor in Loeys-Dietz syndrome, fibrillin-1 in Marfan syndrome, and collagen 3A in Ehlers-Danlos syndrome. Although not likely a monogenic disorder, bicuspid aortic valve is associated with connective tissue abnormalities and medial degeneration of the thoracic aorta, resulting in clinical associations with ascending aortic aneurysm, aortic coarctation, and dissection. Other candidate genes in aortic aneurysm formation are those encoding for arterial wall structural (e.g. actin and myosin) and matrix proteins, immunomodulators, and proteases and their inhibitors. Additionally, bacterial or mycobacterial infection, aortitis (e.g. giant cell arteritis, Takayasu arteritis), and trauma may predispose to aortic aneurysms.

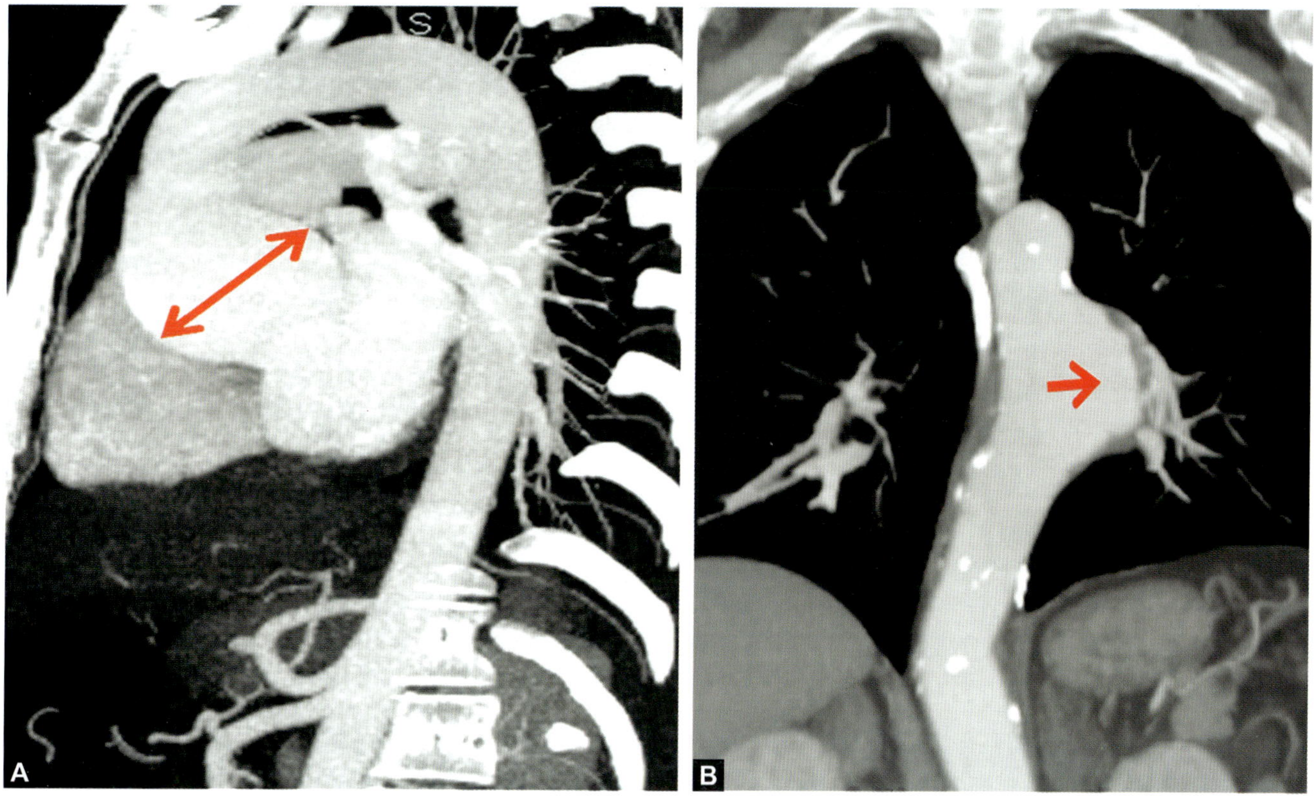

Figs. 50.4A and B: The morphology of aortic aneurysms. (A) A sagittal reformat of a CTA in a patient with a fusiform aneurysm of the aortic root. Note that the aneurysm bulges symmetrically to both sides (arrow) relative to the lumen of the normal aorta. (B) A coronal reformat of a CTA in a patient with a saccular aneurysm of the descending thoracic aorta. Note that the aneurysm bulges only to one side (arrow) relative to the lumen of the normal aorta.

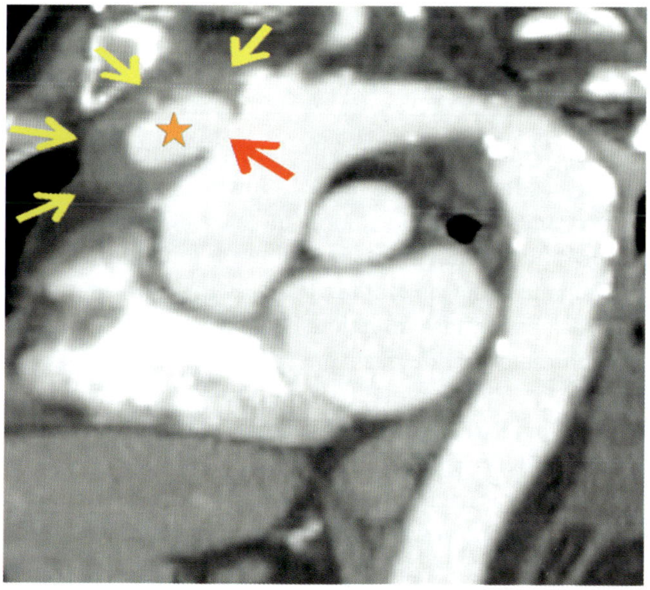

Fig. 50.5: A sagittal reformat of a CTA in a patient with a pseudoaneurysm (orange star) of the distal ascending aorta. Note that there is a defect in the aortic wall (red arrow) leading to a collection outside the lumen of the aneurysm. The pseudoaneurysm is lined with mural thrombus (small yellow arrows).

EARLY DETECTION AND SYMPTOMATOLOGY

Aortic aneurysms are often clinically silent until incidentally discovered on an imaging study obtained for other indications. Some abdominal aortic aneurysms can be detected by palpation during physical examination, whereas thoracic aortic aneurysms are not palpable. The mass effect from an abdominal aneurysm may result in lower back or hypogastric pain of a gnawing quality, or obstruct the gastrointestinal lumen, ureters, or lower extremity vessels. Analogously, the mass effect from a large thoracic aortic aneurysm may produce chest or back pain, or produce signs and symptoms from impingement upon the trachea, esophagus, recurrent laryngeal nerve, or superior vena cava. Aortic root dilatation can also impair aortic valve coaptation, resulting in an aortic insufficiency that may result in an audible diastolic murmur or, when severe, signs and symptoms of heart failure. Unfortunately, many aneurysms go undetected until the occurrence of aortic dissection or rupture.

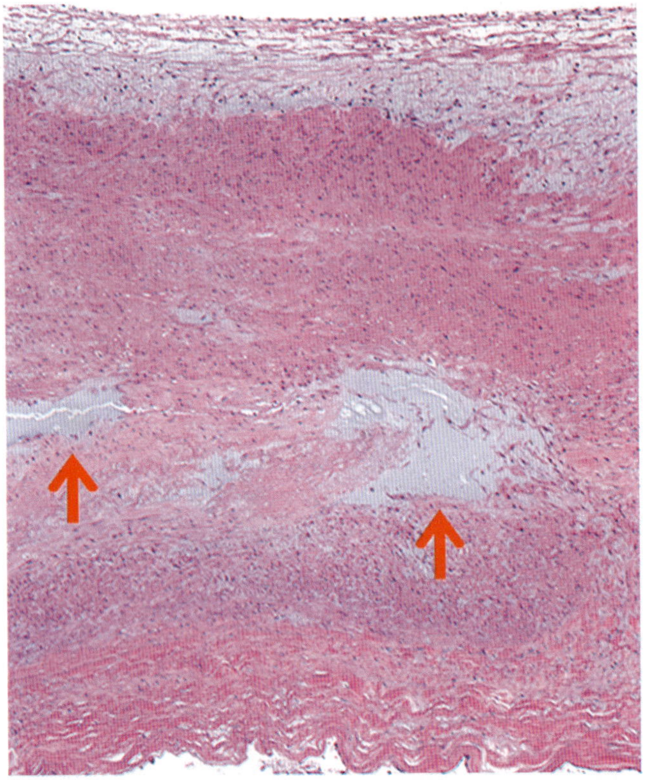

Fig. 50.6: Histologic section with hematoxylin and eosin staining of a cross-section of aorta wall. This cross-section of the aortic wall is oriented with the intima at the top. There is intimal hyperplasia. Medial degeneration is manifested by the pools of eosinophilic (blue) proteoglycan-rich extracellular matrix material (arrows) deposited within the media. Medial degeneration is a classic histopathologic finding in thoracic aorta aneurysms.

AORTIC ANEURYSM IMAGING

While history and physical examination may yield clues to the presence of an aortic aneurysm, formal diagnosis relies on non-invasive imaging studies. Although chest radiography (Figs. 50.7 and 50.8) may offer indirect evidence of thoracic aortic dilatation, chest radiography is not recommended as a diagnostic test to exclude or to size thoracic aortic aneurysms.

Ultrasonography has emerged as the most practical method for infrarenal abdominal aneurysm detection and surveillance (Fig. 50.9), and the United States Preventive Services Task force recommends ultrasonographic screening for abdominal aortic aneurysm in all males age between 65 years and 74 years, who have ever smoked.

Both abdominal and thoracic aortic aneurysms may be imaged and sized by computed tomography angiography (CTA) (Figs. 50.10 and 50.11) and magnetic resonance imaging (MRI) (Figs. 50.12 and 50.13). CTA requires exposure to radiation and iodinated contrast material, but it provides a precise definition of aneurysm anatomy including morphology, calcification, mural thrombus (Figs. 50.14A and B), and branch vessel anatomy, and it permits accurate monitoring of incremental size changes over time. The use of MRI avoids the risks of radiation and iodinated contrast material, and produces excellent images of the thoracic or abdominal aorta; however, MRI is often less readily available than CTA, and the MRI examination may be lengthy. The aorta is often cut off-axis on axial imaging, which results in falsely large diameters (Figs. 50.15A to G). Therefore, in order to report accurate aortic diameters on either CTA or MRI, a true cross sectional plane—orthogonal to the main axis of the aorta—must be identified and measured.

Transthoracic echocardiography (TTE) can reliably image the aortic root and proximal ascending aorta (Figs. 50.16A to F) and, consequently, TTE is often preferred to screen and follow patients with Marfan syndrome given their predilection for aortic root aneurysms. However, TTE visualizes only parts of the arch, descending thoracic, and abdominal aorta, depending on the patient's anatomy.

NATURAL HISTORY OF AORTIC ANEURYSMS

The natural history of all aortic aneurysms is to expand radially, with a rate of growth that depends on aneurysm etiology, location, and size. Once detected, aortic aneurysms must be followed longitudinally by surveillance images studies (CTA, MRA, ultrasound, or TTE, as appropriate) to define changes in aortic diameter and ultimately guide decisions about the timing of aortic repair. At a large enough size, an aortic aneurysm can rupture or dissect, and thus criteria for aneurysm repair are based on reaching the size thresholds associated with significantly increased risk (Fig. 50.17). In general, aortic repair is recommended when ascending thoracic aortic aneurysms reach a diameter of 5.5 cm, descending thoracic aortic aneurysms reach 6.0 cm, thoracoabdominal

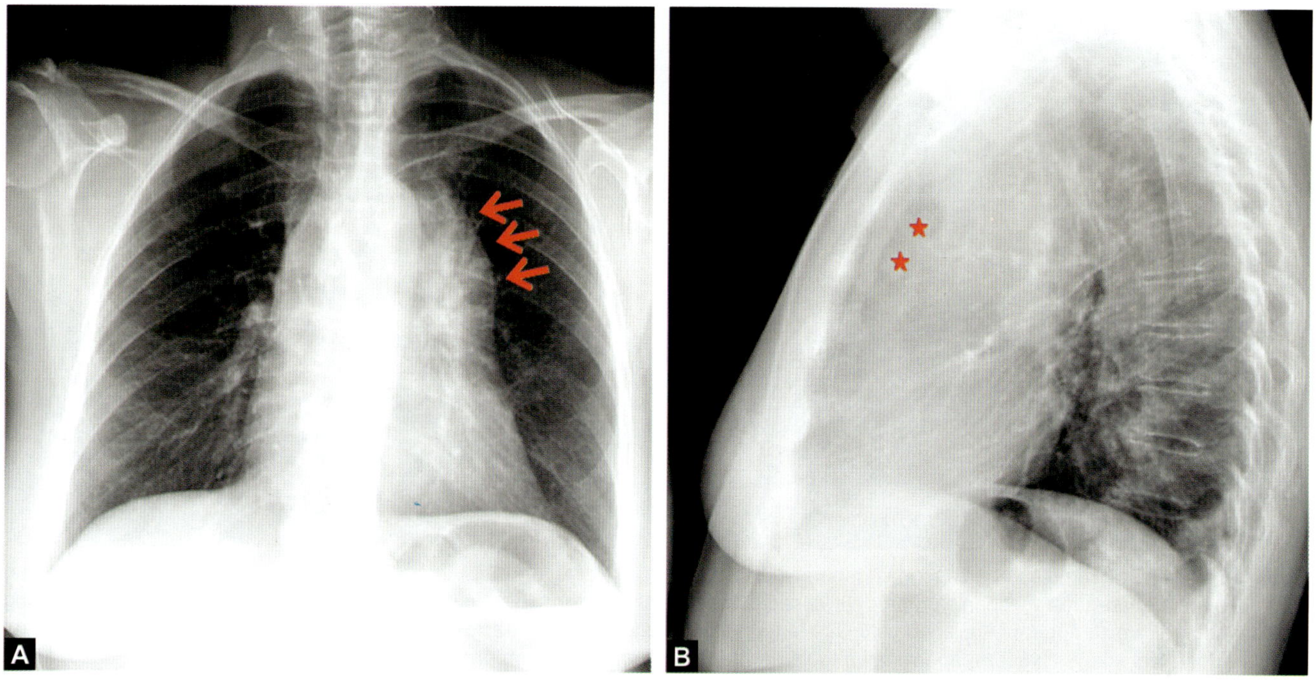

Figs. 50.7A and B: A thoracic aortic aneurysm detected on chest radiography. (A) The posteroanterior view showing a widened mediastinal silhouette (arrows) due to dilatation of the descending thoracic aorta; (B) The lateral view shows a reduced retrosternal space (*), which is due to a dilated ascending thoracic aorta displacing the lung that normally occupies the space.

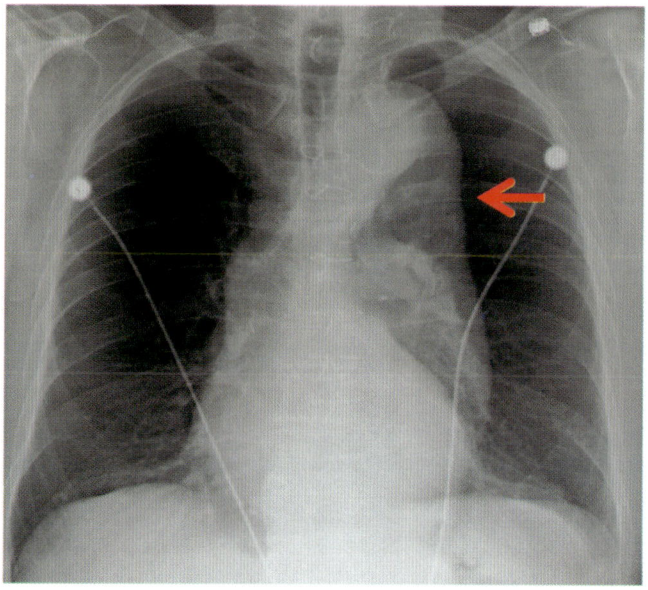

Fig. 50.8: Posteromedial chest X-ray demonstrating a widened mediastinum in a patient with thoracic aortic aneurysm. The arrow marks the lateral border of the aorta. (Image posted by James Heilman, MD, on Wikimedia Commons).

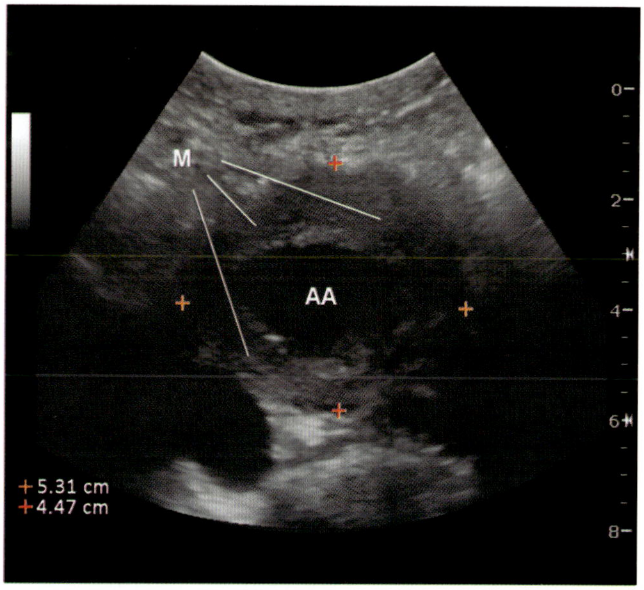

Fig. 50.9: Abdominal ultrasound of an abdominal aortic aneurysm performed as a screening test for a 65-year-old male smoker. Shown is a transverse grayscale ultrasound image of the infrarenal aorta (AA) demonstrating an abdominal aortic aneurysm measuring 4.7 × 5.3 cm in maximal diameter. The exact orientation of the probe and aorta cannot be discerned from the image. Extensive mural thrombus (M) is present circumferentially; note that measurement of aortic diameter should be made from one aortic wall to the opposite wall (+) and not from the luminal surface of the thrombus. The patient underwent open surgical aneurysm repair.

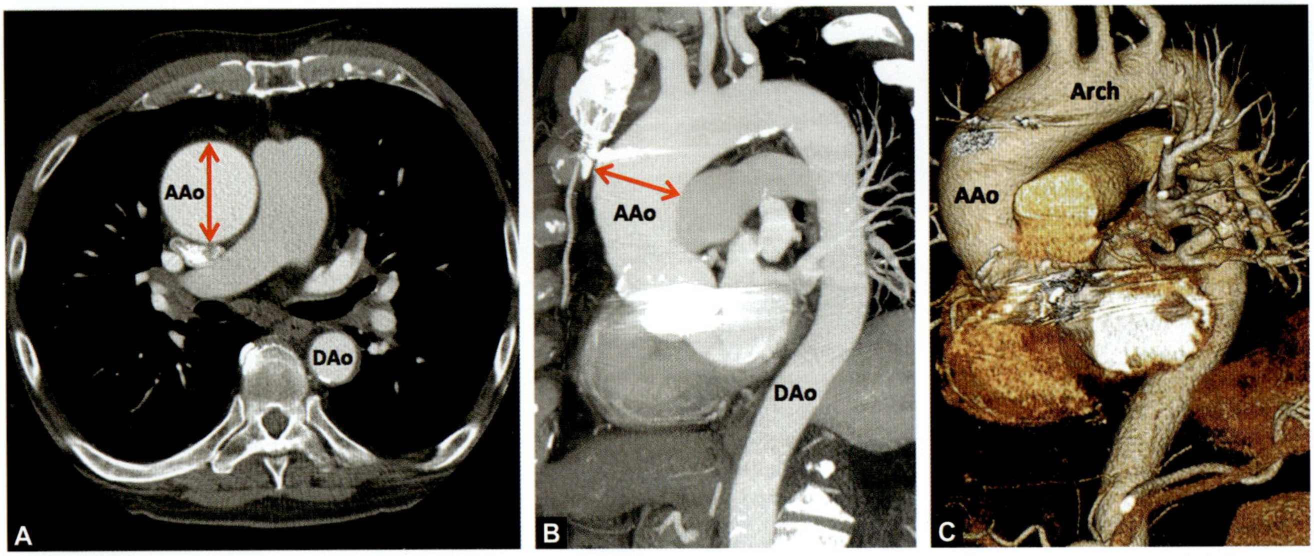

Figs. 50.10A to C: Examples of an ascending thoracic aortic aneurysm in several CTA image formats from a 68-year-old patient who had previously undergone mechanical aortic valve replacement surgery for a bicuspid aortic valve. (A) Axial image demonstrating an ascending thoracic aortic (AAo) aneurysm. The aneurysm measures 5.4 cm (arrow) at the level of pulmonary artery bifurcation. Note that on axial images, vessel dimensions should be measured in a plane perpendicular to the axis of the aorta. The descending thoracic aorta (DAo) measures 2.8 cm. (B) A maximum-intensity projection (MIP) double-oblique "candy cane" view through the aortic arch that demonstrates an ascending thoracic aortic (AAo) aneurysm with a maximal diameter of 5.5 cm (arrow). By rendering bright pixels in a sub-selected "slab" volume of the acquisition, a view analogous to an angiographic image can be depicted, which allows visualization of all branches in a single image. This view however can obscure dissection flaps if the slab thickness is too large. Note that the descending aorta (DAo) is normal is size. (C) Three-dimensional volume-rendered image of the ascending thoracic aortic (AAo) aneurysm with excellent definition of the arch anatomy.

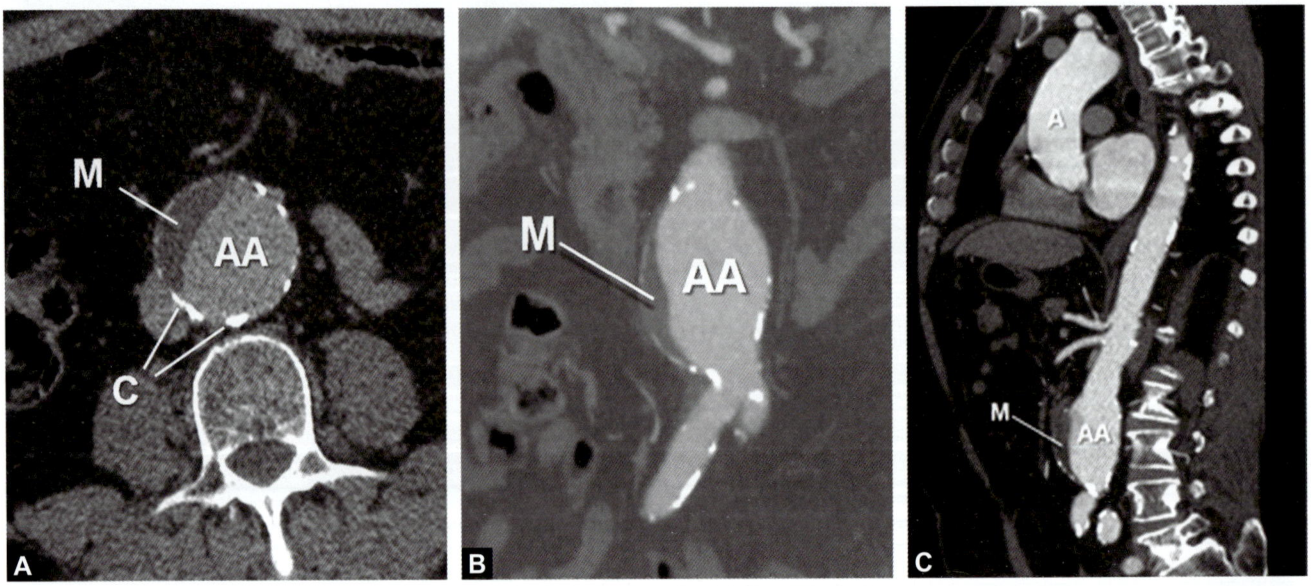

Figs. 50.11A to C: Examples of a CTA demonstrating an abdominal aortic aneurysm in a 76-year-old male smoker with dyslipidemia and hypertension. (A) An axial image demonstrating a 5.6 cm abdominal aneurysm (AA) with mural thrombus (M) and wall calcification (C); (B) A coronal section depicting the superior and inferior extent of the aneurysm. Again evident is the mural thrombus; (C) A sagittal section shows the abdominal aneurysm. Imaging findings suggested the patient was an appropriate candidate for EVAR.

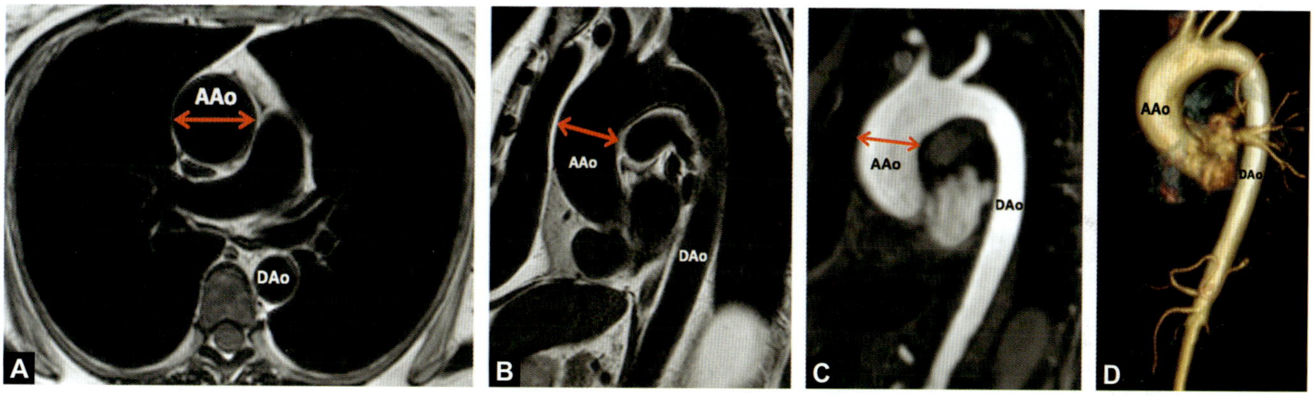

Figs. 50.12A to D: Examples of an ascending thoracic aortic aneurysm on MRI in a 72 year woman (double-headed arrow). (A) An axial image using the "black-blood" technique that demonstrates a 4.3 cm ascending aorta (AAo), which is clearly dilated in comparison with the relatively small descending aorta (DAo). The "black-blood" technique derives a tissue signal from non-moving structures like the vessel walls and fixed anatomy, whereas blood moving perpendicular to the imaging plane renders no signal within vessel lumens, such as the ascending aorta, descending aorta, or pulmonary artery. This technique can yield fine anatomic detail without the use of intravenous contrast media, although scan times are relatively longer than when performing contrast-enhanced MRI. (B) A "candy cane" projection image from a "black-blood" sequence; (C) A "candy cane" projection image from a contrast-enhanced MR angiogram (MRA) sequence. The aortic lumen has an appearance similar to that produced by contrast-enhanced CTA; (D) A three-dimensional volume-rendered image from a contrast-enhanced MRA sequence of the thoracic and abdominal aorta with excellent definition of the anatomy the arch and visceral branches.

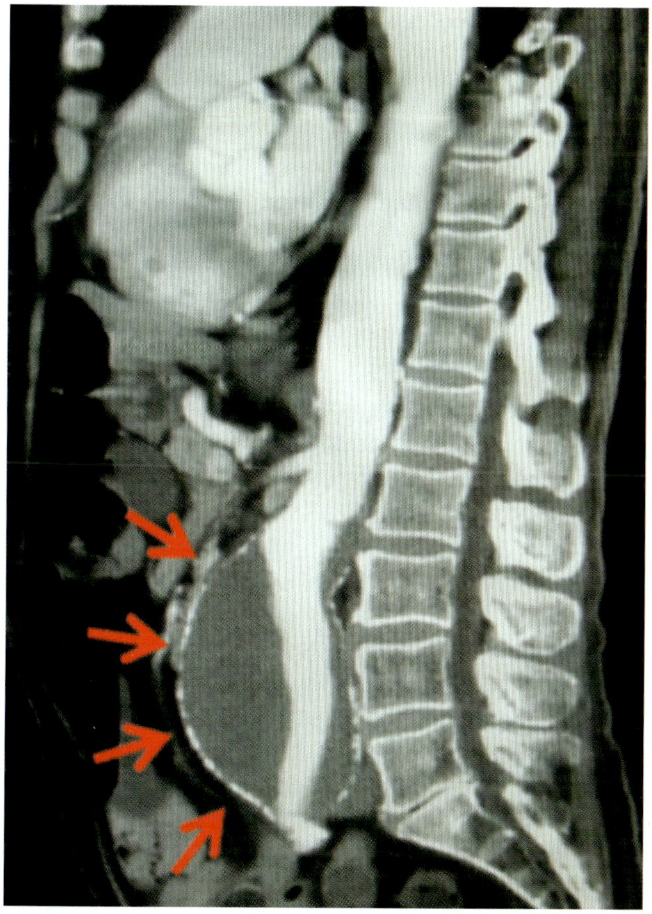

Fig. 50.13: Sagittal MRI demonstrating large abdominal aortic aneurysm (arrows) the extensive mural thrombus. (Image posted by glitzygueen00 on Wikimedia Commons).

aneurysms reach 5.5–6.0 cm, and infrarenal abdominal aortic aneurysms reach 5.5 cm,. These criteria are by no means absolute, and the clinician should entertain smaller thresholds in patients of smaller body habitus, in women (particularly as regards abdominal aneurysms), in patients having cardiac surgery for another indication, in patients with symptoms attributable to the aneurysm, and when rate of aneurysm growth exceeds 0.5 cm/year. Additionally, there are lower thresholds for thoracic aneurysms of particular etiologies, such as 5.0 cm in the setting of Marfan syndrome or bicuspid aortic valve and 4.4 cm (by CT) in patients with Loeys-Dietz syndrome.

MEDICAL THERAPY FOR PATIENTS WITH AORTIC ANEURYSMS

The goal of medical therapy is to reduce the rate of aneurysm growth by reducing risk factors and vascular wall stress (i.e., arterial pressure and dP/dt) (Figs. 50.18 and 19). Beta blockers are used to reduce dP/dt, and other antihypertensive agents are used to reduce arterial pressure. At least for thoracic aortic aneurysms, the target heart rate is often 60 bpm or less and the systolic blood pressure is often 110–120 mm Hg or less. Due to effects on the TGF-β pathway, angiotensin converting enzyme inhibitors and angiotensin receptor antagonists may exert pleiotropic benefits in the treatment of aortic aneurysm, with studies suggesting reduced risk of abdominal aortic aneurysm rupture and, in Marfan syndrome, of thoracic aortic

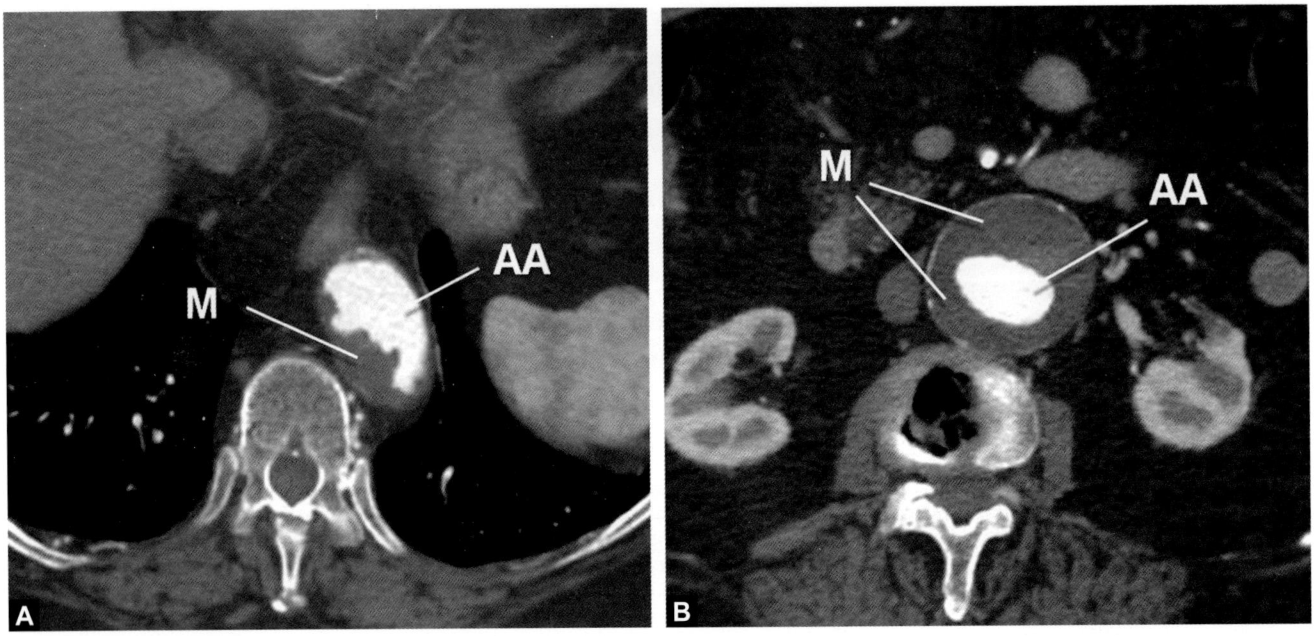

Figs. 50.14A and B: Axial CTA of an abdominal aortic aneurysm (AA) in an 86-year-old woman with uncontrolled hypertension, hyperlipidemia, and a 100 pack-year smoking history. (A) CTA at the level of the diaphragm demonstrates a mildly dilated aorta that is lined with mural thrombus (M) that is irregular and protrudes into the lumen; (B) CTA at the level of the renal arteries demonstrates a 6.1 cm thoracoabdominal aneurysm lined circumferentially with mural thrombus. The patient underwent open thoracoabdominal aortic aneurysm repair.

aneurysm growth. In general, an antiatherosclerotic strategy is prudent, including tobacco cessation, reduction of low density lipoprotein (LDL) levels with statin therapy, and control of hypertension.

SURGICAL AND PERCUTANEOUS TREATMENT OF AORTIC ANEURYSMS

The classic open surgical technique of aneurysm repair involves aneurysmectomy and replacement of diseased aorta with a tubular synthetic graft (Figs. 50.20A to C). Various grafts are available to accommodate branch vessel anatomy (Figs. 50.21A and B). When the aortic root is involved, aortic grafting may require replacement of the aortic valve with a composite valve-aortic graft or, when possible, the valve may be preserved using a valve-sparing root repair (Fig. 50.22). The surgical approach for ascending thoracic and arch aneurysms is via a median sternotomy, whereas the approach for descending thoracic aneurysms is via left thoracotomy, which is associated with significant morbidity; descending aortic repair also carries a significant risk of spinal cord ischemia. Abdominal aneurysm surgery is typically approached by a midline incision.

In recent years endovascular techniques (Figs. 50.23 and 50.24) have presented an attractive alternative to the traditional open surgical approaches for both thoracic and abdominal aortic aneurysms. Endovascular aortic aneurysm repair (EVAR) is a technique of fluoroscopically-guided percutaneous deployment of an endovascular stent within the aneurysm so as to exclude it from the rest of the aortic circulation. EVAR has been most studied for abdominal aortic aneurysms and descending thoracic aortic aneurysms, with multiple randomized trials for the former and registry and meta-analysis data for the latter. Careful patient selection is essential for successful EVAR, as overall aneurysm size, tortuosity, calcification, mural thrombi, and proximal and distal stent graft "landing zone" anatomy all may preclude the procedure. The advantages of EVAR over open repair include reduced peri-procedural morbidity and lower 30-day mortality, but the long-term durability of EVAR does not appear to be as good as an open surgical repair.

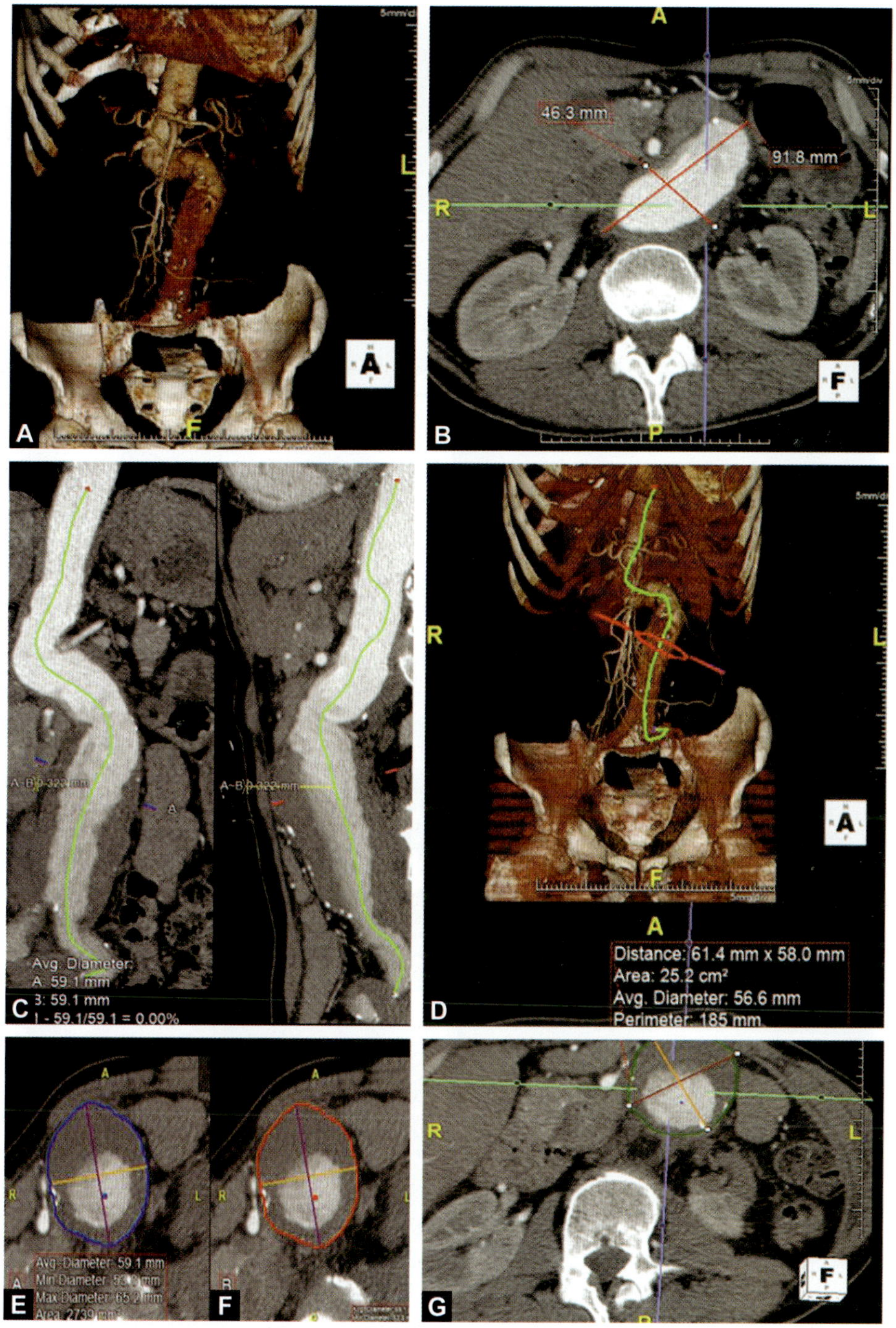

Figs. 50.15A to G: The importance of obtaining true cross-sectional images when determining aortic diameter. (A) Volume-rendered three-dimensional CTA image of a patient with a 6 cm abdominal aortic aneurysm demonstrates a markedly tortuous aorta with an axis that becomes virtually horizontal as it crosses the diaphragm; (B) Axial image demonstrating how the aneurysm is cut off axis and becomes oval and elongated in shape, which can lead to a significant overestimate of its true diameter if measured in this plane. In this image, the aneurysm could appear to be greater than 9 cm in size; (C) Aortic diameter measurements taken from axial images will not be accurate unless the dimensions are measured in a true cross-section, defined as perpendicular to the longitudinal axis or "axis of flow," depicted here as the green line; (D) Obtaining a true short-axis image (the red plane) with a double-oblique orientation results cross-sectional slices of the aorta on which accurate dimensions can be measured, as shown in figures E, F, and G. (E to G) Double oblique images slices that demonstrate that the true maximal aortic diameter is 6.1 cm. Note that the luminal diameter, which is only up to 3.8 cm, is much smaller than the outer diameter. The luminal diameter would be the only portion visible if the aneurysm was imaged using catheter-based angiography, and thus would significantly underestimate the outer luminal diameter.

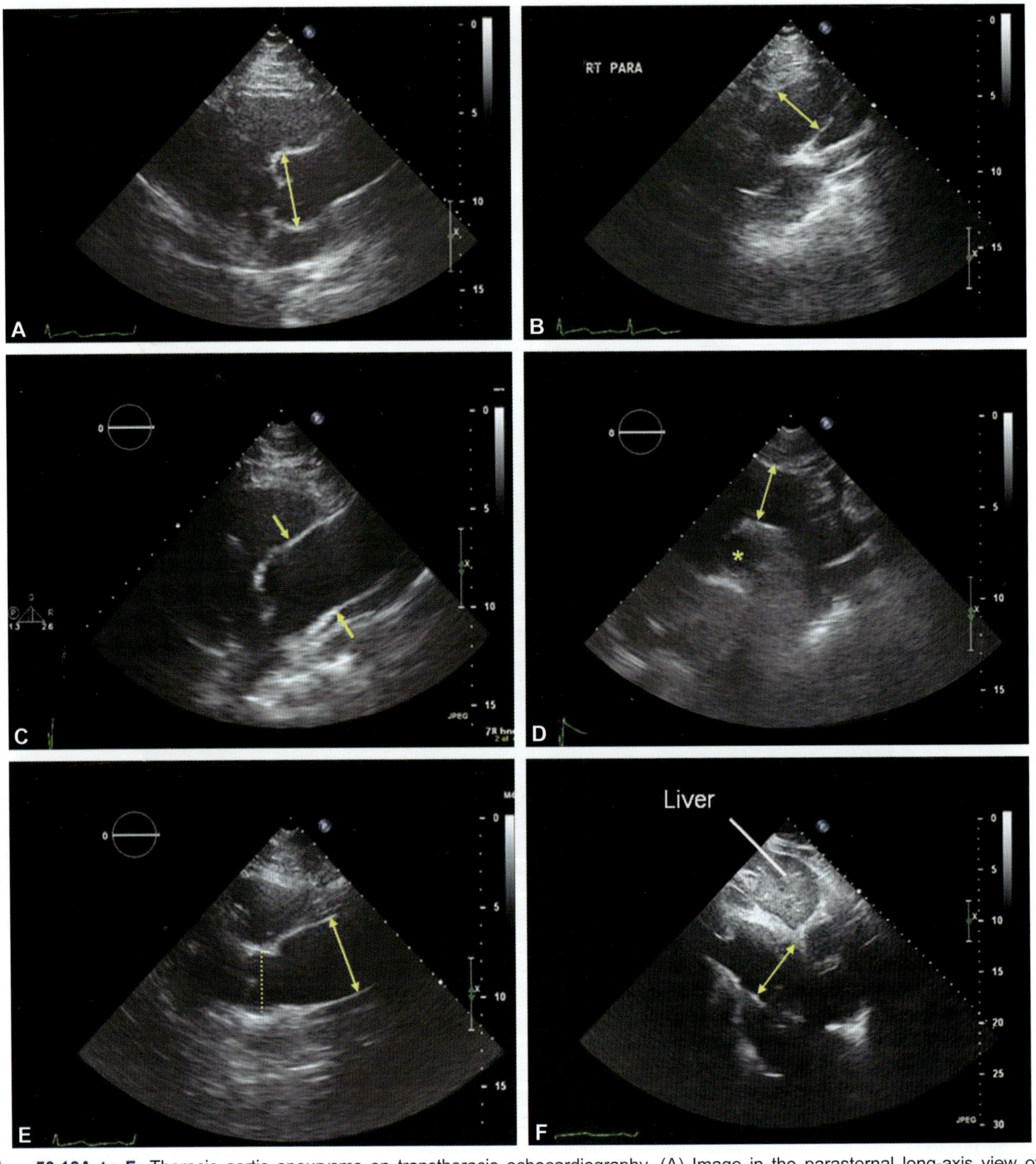

Figs. 50.16A to F: Thoracic aortic aneurysms on transthoracic echocardiography. (A) Image in the parasternal long-axis view of a 58-year-old man with a bicuspid aortic demonstrating a dilated aortic root at 43 mm (double-headed arrow); (B) Right parasternal view of the same patient showing a mildly dilated ascending aorta at 37 mm (double-headed arrow); (C) Image in the parasternal long axis view of a 46-year-old man with a bicuspid aortic valve demonstrating effacement of the sinotubular junction (arrows) due to symmetric dilatation of both the aortic root and the ascending aorta, which measure 46 mm and 45 mm, respectively; (D) View from the suprasternal notch in the same patient showing dilatation of the distal ascending aorta (double-headed arrow); also shown in cross-section is the right pulmonary artery (*); (E) Parasternal long-axis view of a 49-year-old man with a bicuspid valve who has a normal aortic root (dotted line) and a dilated ascending aorta of 44 mm (double-headed arrow); (F) Image in the subcostal view showing a 6.5 cm suprarenal thoracoabdominal aortic aneurysm (arrow) in a 69-year-old female with coronary artery disease, stroke, emphysema, hypertension, and dyslipidemia who presented with persistent epigastric pain. Her aneurysm was repaired with a combined open and endovascular approach. Note that each image the measurement of the aortic diameter is made on an axis that is perpendicular to the longitudinal or flow axis of the aorta at that level.

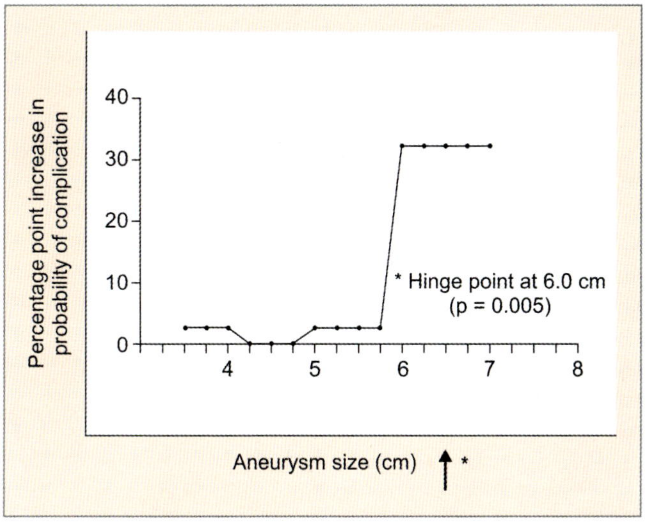

Fig. 50.17: Risk of complication (rupture, dissection, or death) of thoracic aortic aneurysms vs aortic diameter. There is a marked increase in risk when the diameter approaches 6.0 cm. (Adapted from Elefteriades JA. Natural history of thoracic aortic aneurysms: indications for surgery, and surgical versus nonsurgical risks. Ann Thorac Surg. 2002;74:S1877-80. Used with permission).

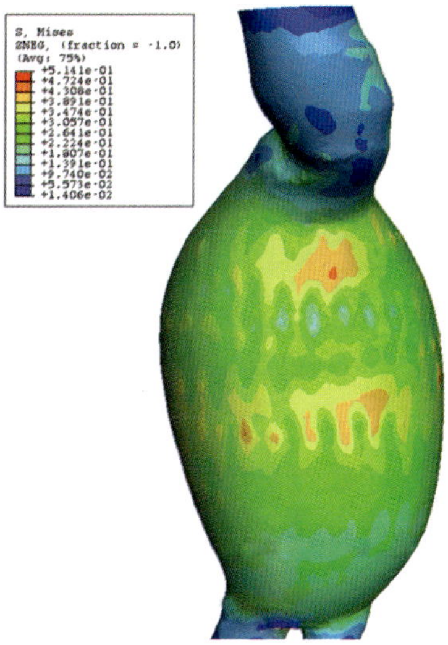

Fig. 50.18: Wall stress mapping throughout an aortic aneurysm wall. Red color depicts peak wall stress locations; blue color represents sites of lowest wall stress. (Image from Georgakarakos E and Ionnou CV. Pathophysiology of abdominal aortic aneurysm rupture and expansion: new insights on an old problem. In Grundmann RT (ed). Etiology, pathogenesis and pathophysiology of aortic aneurysms and aneurysm rupture. Intechweb.org).

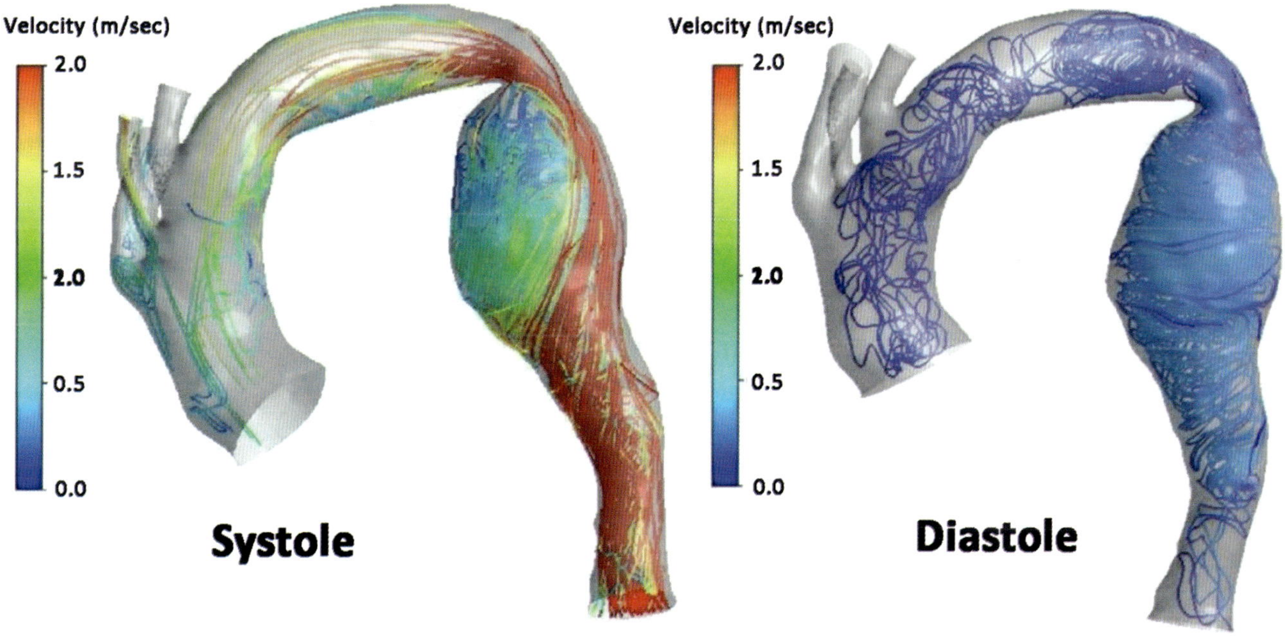

Fig. 50.19: Streamline of blood flow at systole and diastole in aortic aneurysm. [Image from Gao F et al. Numerical simulation in aortic arch aneurysm. In Grundmann RT (ed). Etiology, pathogenesis and pathophysiology of aortic aneurysms and aneurysm rupture. Intechweb.org].

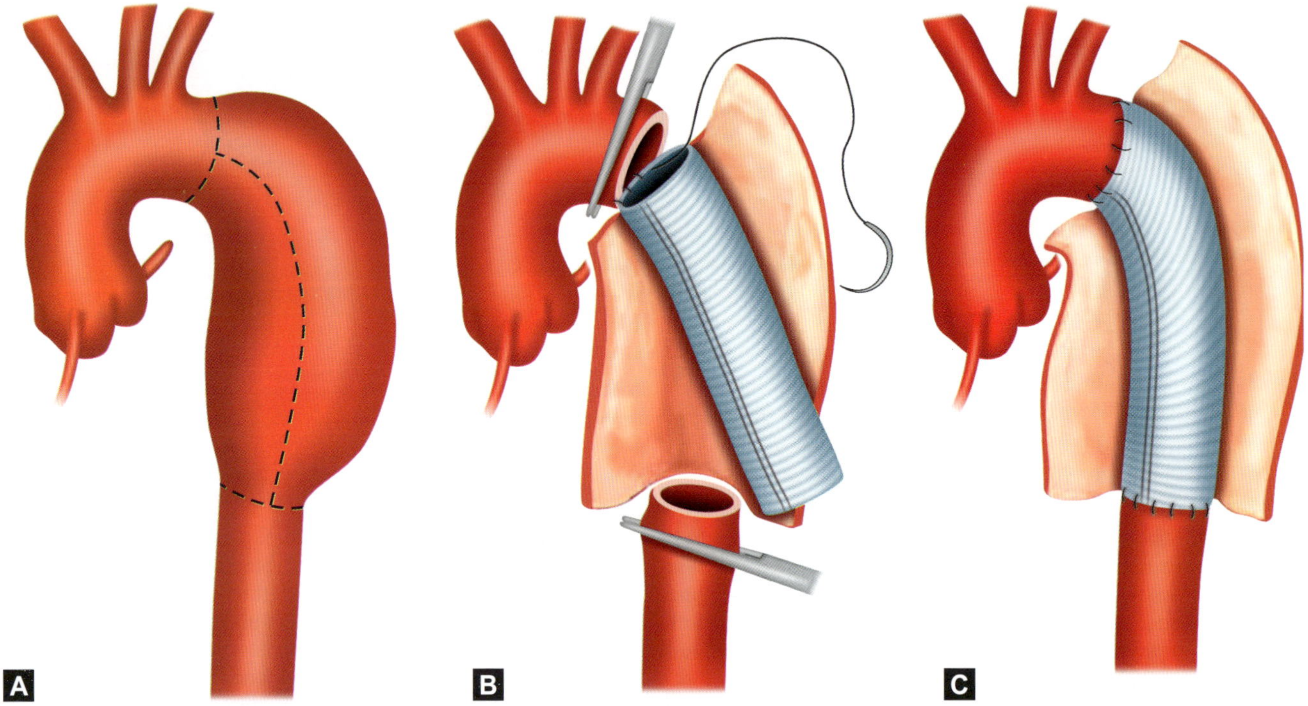

Figs. 50.20A to C: Schematic of open surgical repair of a descending thoracic aortic aneurysm, with and aortotomy (A) and replacement of the aneurysmal aortic segment with an interposition prosthetic tube graft (B). In most cases the surgeon will then wrap the prosthetic tube graft with the native aorta (C) in order to reduce adhesions and the incidence of dangerous fistulae, i.e. aortoesophageal or aorto-bronchial fistulae. (©Massachusetts General Hospital Thoracic Aortic Center, used with permission).

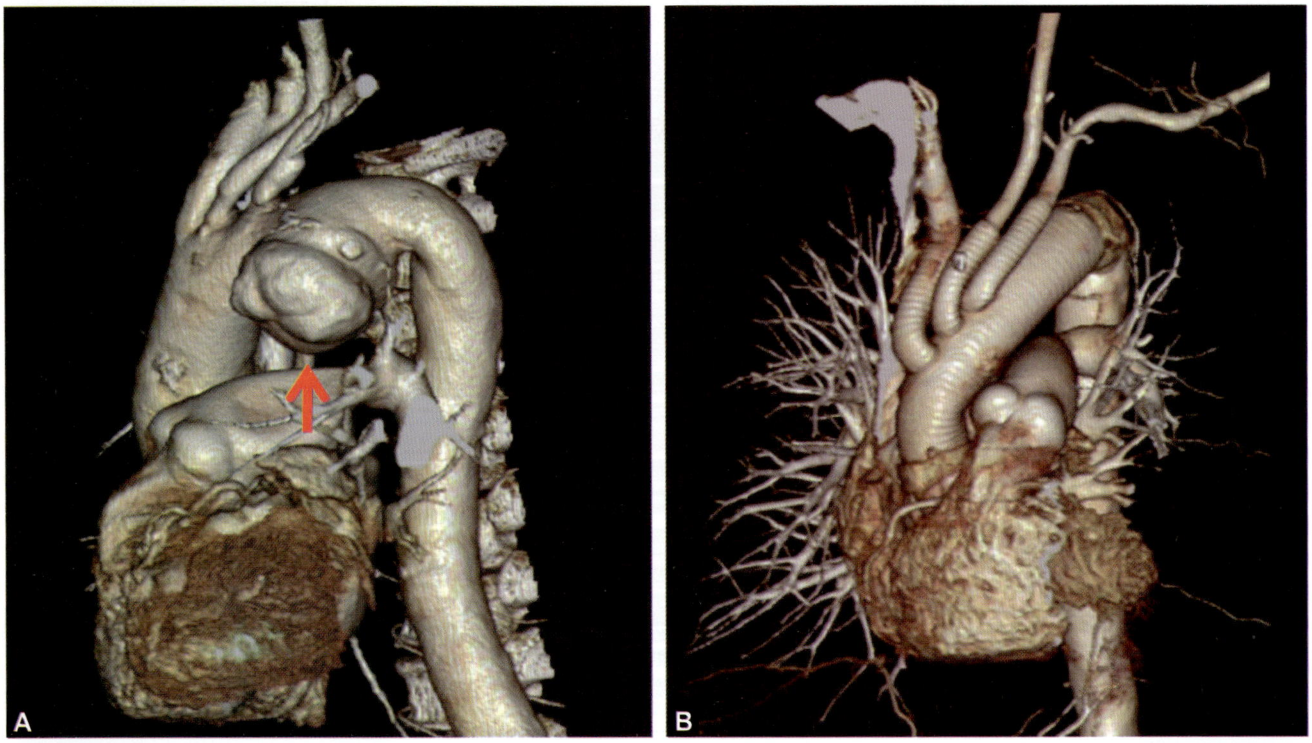

Figs. 50.21A and B: Volume rendered CT images of a distal arch aneurysm (arrow) of the thoracic aorta (A) and postoperative CT image showing the repaired arch with a sealed quadrifurcated Dacron graft (B). [Image from Suzuki T and Asai T. Fast-track total arch replacement. In Firstenberg MS (ed). Principles and practice of cardiothoracic surgery. Intechweb.org].

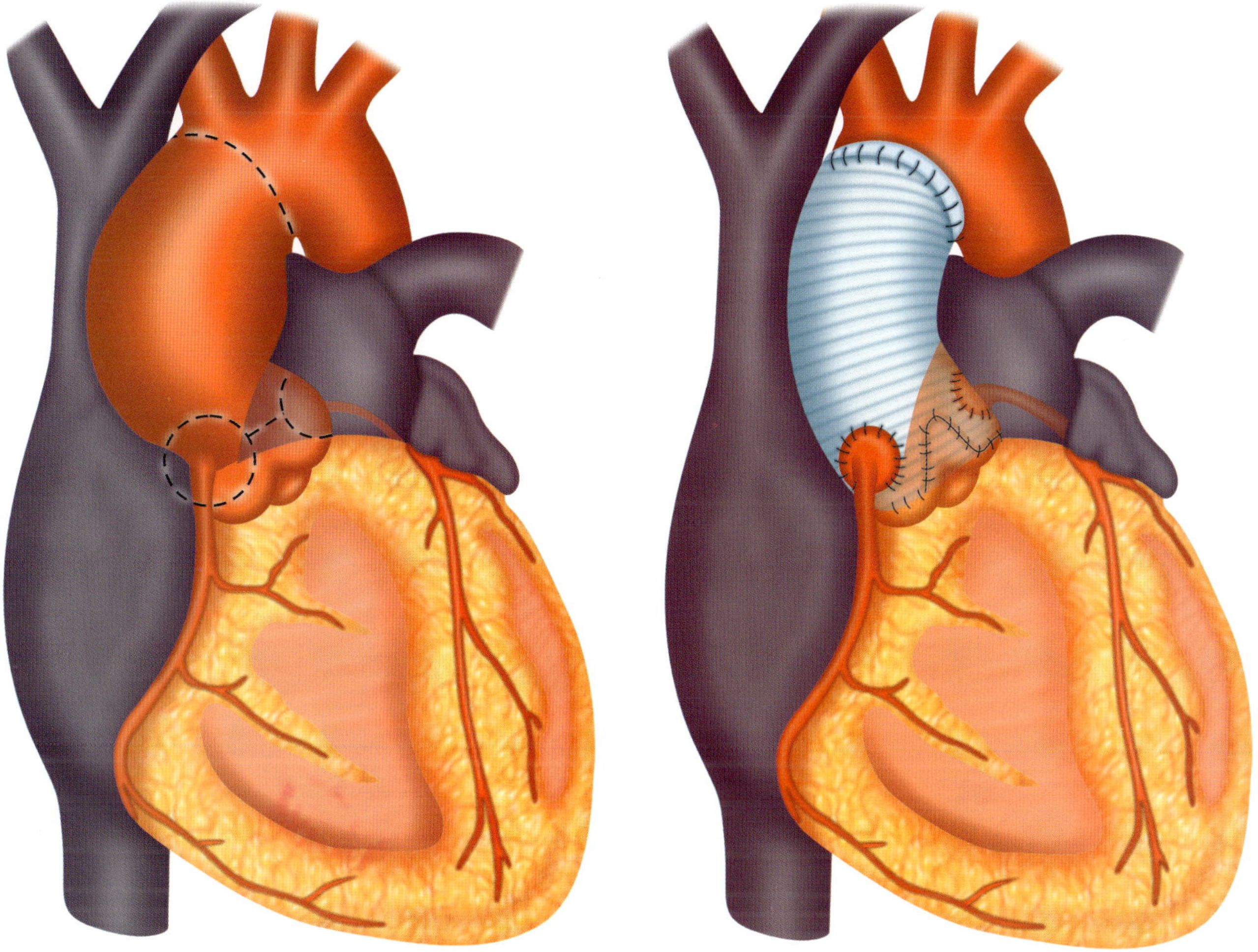

Fig. 50.22: Valve-sparing root repair. When the aortic root is dilated but the aortic valve is otherwise structural normal, rather than sacrifice the aortic valve by performing a composite aortic graft (a prosthetic valve implanted into a tube graft), the aortic root is excised and the native aortic valve is resuspended from within the prosthetic graft in a normal anatomic configuration. The ostial of the coronary arteries are excised from the native aorta as buttons of tissue that are then reimplanted into the prosthetic graft. (©Massachusetts General Hospital Thoracic Aortic Center, used with permission).

Following EVAR, patients may experience endoleaks, reflecting incomplete exclusion of the aneurysm cavity from the aortic circulation (Fig. 50.25). Accordingly, patients who undergo EVAR require frequent post-procedural surveillance imaging (e.g. at 1, 6, and 12 months) and have a 10% higher requirement for re-interventions compared with those who undergo open surgical repair. Therefore, EVAR may be most appropriate option for patients who have comorbidities that increase their risk of open surgery and can comply with the requisite post-EVAR imaging and follow-up.

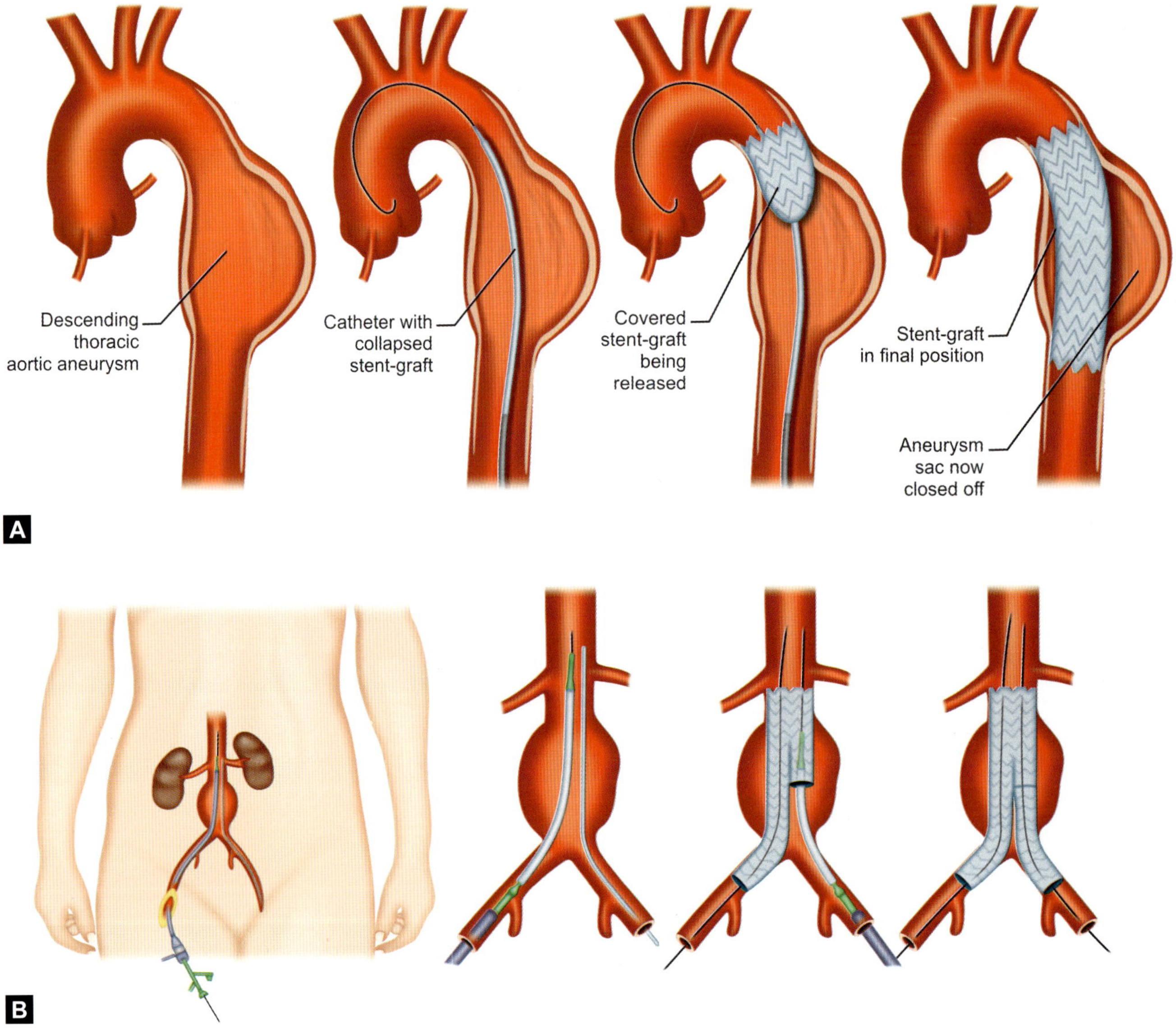

Figs. 50.23A and B: Schematic of endovascular repair of a thoracic (TEVAR) and an abdominal (EVAR) aortic aneurysm. (A) In TEVAR, an unexpanded stent-graft is placed transfemoral and advanced across the aneurysm. The proximal segment is expanded and fixed, followed by the distal end. The blood then flows through the graft, excluding the aneurysmal segment from the circulation. (©Massachusetts General Hospital Thoracic Aortic Center, used with permission). (B) In EVAR, the aneurysm typically extends to the aortic bifurcation, so the stent-graft is designed with arms that extend into each common iliac artery. First, the unexpended stent-graft is advanced transfemorally across the aneurysm and its proximal end is expanded and fixed. Then the attached branch graft is deployed within the ipsilateral common iliac artery. Then, a second branch stent-graft is advanced over a wire from the contralateral side, fixed within the stent-graft, and then deployed within the contralateral common iliac artery. (Images courtesy of and with permission from Mayo Foundation for Medical Education and Research. All rights reserved. Mayo Clinic retains copyright ownership of these images).

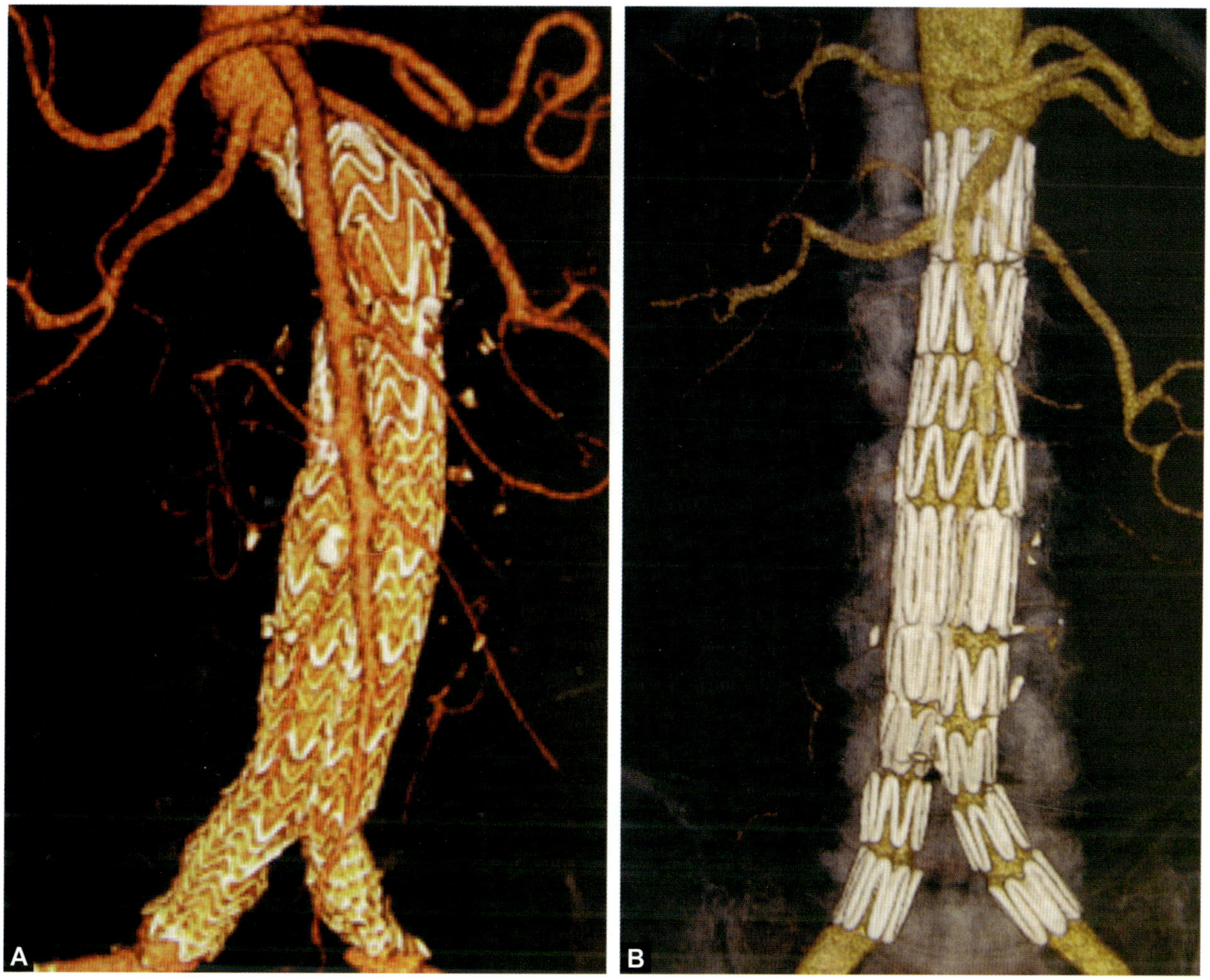

Figs. 50.24A and B: Three-dimensional CT reconstructions showing examples of bifurcating endovascular stent grafts in patients who underwent EVAR for abdominal aortic aneurysms. [Images from Mendonca CT, et al. Endovascular treatment of abdominal aortic aneurysms in high-surgical-risk patients. J Vasc Bras. 2009;8(1):56-64].

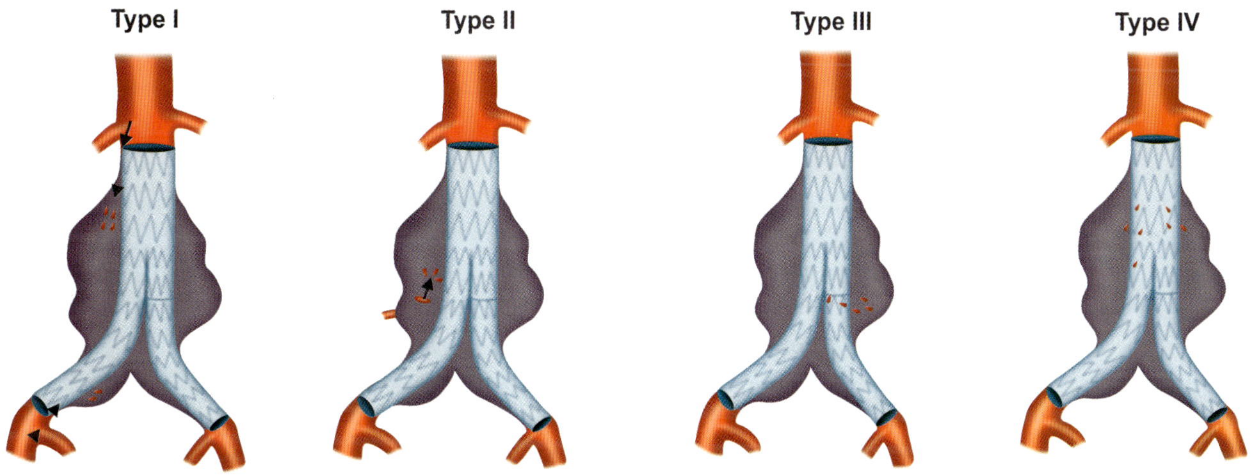

Fig. 50.25: Types of endoleaks. Endoleaks complicate successful deployment of endovascular stent-grafts and result in persistent blood flow within the aneurysm sac. The origin of the blood is either from an imperfect seal at proximal or distal anastomosis (type I), due to retrograde flow from aortic branch vessels into the aneurysm sac (type II), via a structural defect in the endovascular graft or connection with another graft (type III), or due to blood leaking leak through the graft material itself (type IV).

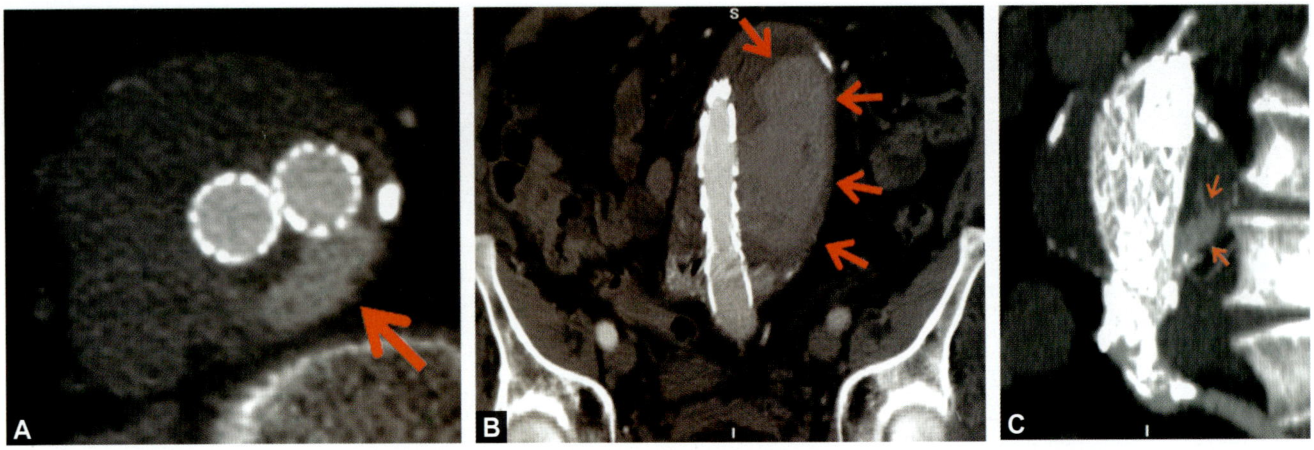

Figs. 50.26A to C: Axial (A), coronal (B), and sagittal (C) images of contrast-enhanced CT studies showing endoleak (arrows) in patients with infrarenal abdominal aortic aneurysms treated with EVAR. (Images courtesy of Dr Benjamin Y. Cheong, Texas Heart Institute).

REFERENCES

Coady MA, Ikonomidis JS, Cheung AT, et al. Surgical management of descending thoracic aortic disease: Open and endovascular approaches. Circulation. 2010;121:2780-804.

De Bruin JL, Baas AF, Buth J, et al. Long-term outcome of open or endovascular repair of abdominal aortic aneurysm. N Engl J Med. 2010; 362:1881-9.

Greenhalgh RM, Powell JT. Endovascular repair of abdominal aortic aneurysm. N Engl J Med. 2008;358:494-501.

Hirsch AT, Haskal ZJ, Hertzner NR, et al. ACC/AHA 2005 Practice Guidelines for the management of patients with peripheral arterial disease (lower extremity, renal, mesenteric, and abdominal aortic). Circulation. 2006;113:e463-654.

Hiratzka LF, Bakris GL, Beckman JA, et al. ACCF/AHA/AATS/ACR/ASA/SCA/SCAI/SIR/STS/SVM guidelines for the diagnosis and management of patients with thoracic aortic disease. Circulation. 2010;121:e266-369.

Isselbacher EM. Thoracic and abdominal aortic aneurysms. Circulation. 2005;111:816-28.

Jackson RS, Chang DC, Freischlag JA. Comparison of long-term survival after open vs endovascular repair of intact abdominal aortic aneurysm among Medicare beneficiaries. JAMA. 2012; 307:1621-8.

Jagadesham VP, Scott DJA, Carding SR. Abdominal aortic aneurysms: An autoimmune disease? Trends in Molecular Medicine. 2008;14:522-9.

Rooke TW, Hirsch AT, Misra S, et al. 2011 ACCF/AHA Focused update of the guideline for the management of patients with peripheral artery disease (updating the 2005 guideline): A report of the American College of Cardiology Foundation/American Heart Association task force on practice guidelines. Circulation. 2011;124:2020-45.

United Kingdom EVAR Trial Investigators, Greenhalgh RM, Brown LC, et al. Endovascular versus open repair of abdominal aortic aneurysm. N Engl J Med. 2010;362:1863-71.

United Kingdom EVAR Trial Investigators. Endovascular repair of aortic aneurysm in patients physically ineligible for open repair. N Engl J Med. 2010;362:1872-80.

Weintraub NL. Understanding abdominal aortic aneurysm. N Engl J Med. 2009;361:1114-6.

CHAPTER

51

Aortic Dissection

Alan C Braverman

INTRODUCTION

Acute aortic dissection is a highly lethal condition requiring prompt diagnosis and urgent therapy. Classical aortic dissection and its variants (aortic intramural hematoma) and penetrating atherosclerotic ulcer (PAU) typically present with acute, severe chest and/or back pain. Risk factors include heritable diseases of the aorta, such as Marfan syndrome and familial thoracic aortic aneurysm syndromes, bicuspid aortic valve, hypertension, aortitis, and aortic trauma, as well as conditions causing excess sheer force in the aorta. Aortic imaging utilizing contrast computed tomography, transesophageal echocardiography, and magnetic resonance imaging is highly accurate in diagnosing aortic dissection. Evaluation of suspected acute aortic dissection includes considering dissection in patients: at high risk for dissection; with high-risk pain features; or high-risk examination findings to enhance identification and expedite aortic imaging. Multiple clinical syndromes are associated with aortic dissection, including aortic regurgitation, heart failure, cardiac tamponade, stroke and other malperfusion syndromes, depending upon the fate of the aorta and its branches. Type A (or ascending) aortic dissection requires emergency cardiac surgery, while type B (or descending) aortic dissection is managed medically unless complications occur. Thoracic endovascular aortic repair (TEVAR) is now the preferred management for most complications of type B dissection. Long-term follow-up involves surveillance of the aorta, medical therapy to control blood pressure, and lifestyle modifications to lessen risk for future aortic events.

ACUTE AORTIC SYNDROMES

Acute aortic syndromes include classic aortic dissection, aortic intramural hematoma, and penetrating atherosclerotic aortic ulcer (Fig. 51.1A). Each of these processes may present with acute chest or back pain and lead to complications including aortic rupture, hemopericardium, or malperfusion. In classic aortic dissection, accounting for 80–90% of acute aortic syndromes, an intimal tear allowing blood to enter the aortic wall (Figs. 51.1B and 51.1C, Video 51.1) propagates variable distances in the aorta (Fig. 51.2). The underlying pathology associated with dissection is often cystic medial degeneration (Figs. 51.3A and B).

Aortic intramural hematoma (IMH), present in 5–15% of acute aortic syndromes, is due to spontaneous rupture of the vasa vasorum leading to bleeding in the aortic wall without evidence of an intimal flap. Circumferential aortic wall thickening or crescentic wall thickening is the imaging hallmark (Figs. 51.4A to D). While acute aortic IMH may resorb spontaneous with medical therapy, classic aortic dissection often occurs after acuteIMH.

Penetrating atherosclerotic aortic ulcer (PAU) is a condition in which an atherosclerotic plaque penetrates through the intima into the media leaving an "ulcer-like" crater in the aortic wall (Figs. 51.5A and 51.5B). This may be associated with intramural hematoma, pseudoaneurysm, a thick-walled dissection flap, or embolization. Penetrating atherosclerotic aortic ulcers are more common in the arch and descending aorta than in the ascending aorta and affect elderly patients with diffuse atherosclerosis.

Aortic dissections are classified using the DeBakey or Stanford Classification, depending upon whether the ascending aorta is involved and the extent of the dissection (Fig. 51.6 and Table 51.1). Dissections involving the ascending aorta require emergency surgery, whereas descending aortic dissections are managed medically unless complications occur. Ascending aortic dissection is most common in patients in the age group of 50s and 60s, while descending aortic dissections more commonly affect older individuals. Dissections are classified as acute

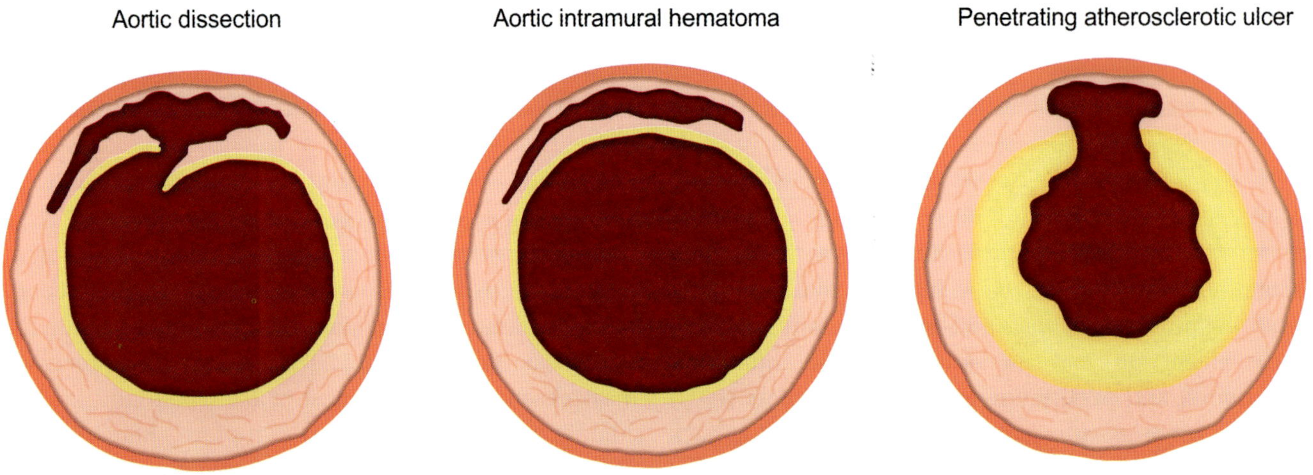

Fig. 51.1A: Acute aortic syndromes. (left panel) Classic aortic dissection. There is a tear in the intima with blood entering the media and a dissecting cleavage plane propagating for variable distances anterograde (and occasionally retrograde) throughout the aortic wall. (middle panel) Aortic intramural hematoma (IMH). A spontaneous hemorrhage of the vasa vasorum leads to bleeding within the media in the absence of an intimal tear or intimal flap. (right panel) Penetrating atherosclerotic aortic ulcer (PAU). An ulcerated aortic plaque ruptures into the media leading to an outpouching or ulceration in the aortic wall. This may be associated with intramural hematoma formation, pseudoaneurysm, or a focal, thick walled aortic dissection. [Reproduced with permission from Braverman AC, Thompson R, Sanchez L. Diseases of the Aorta, Chapter 60. In: Bonow RO, Mann DL, Zipes DP, Libby P, (Eds). Braunwald's Heart Disease, 9th Edition, pp. 1309-1337, Philadelphia, USA: Elsevier; 2011].

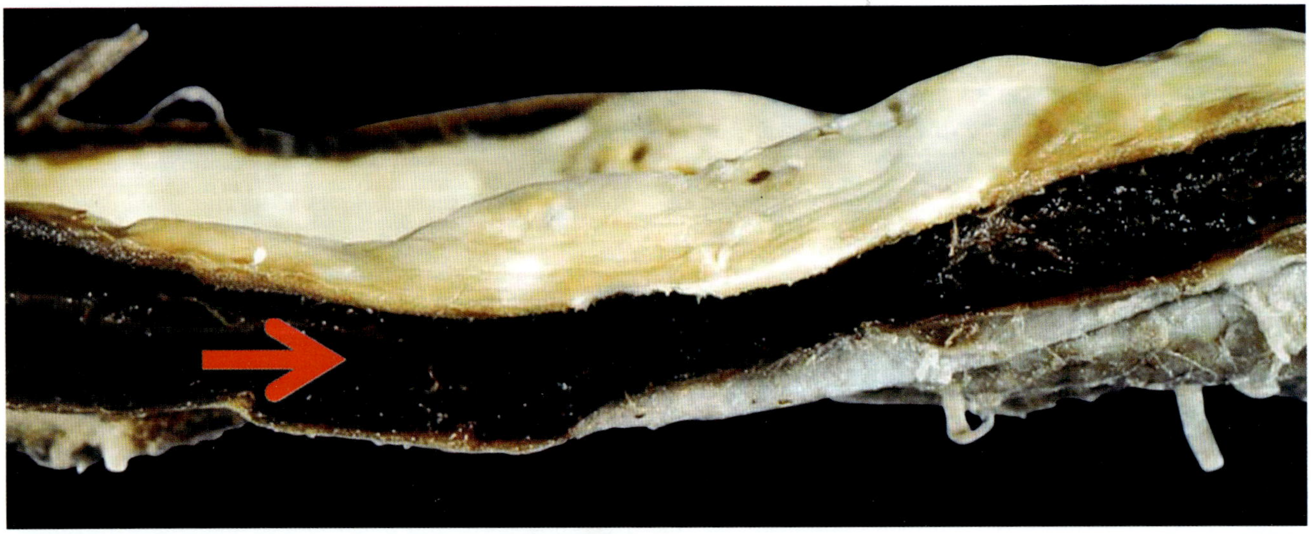

Fig. 51.1B: Gross pathology specimen of aortic dissection. An intimal tear allows blood to enter the aortic wall. There is delamination of the tunica media (arrow) and a false lumen partially filled with blood. [Image and legend text from Clinicopathologic Session Case 5/2000—a 73-year-old woman with retrosternal pain but no obstructive coronary artery lesion on coronary angiography (Instituto do Coracao of Hospital das Clinicas—FMUSP—Sao Paulo). Arq. Bras. Cardiol. vol. 75 n.4 São Paulo Oct. 2000. http://dx.doi.org/10.1590/S0066-782X2000001000008. CC].

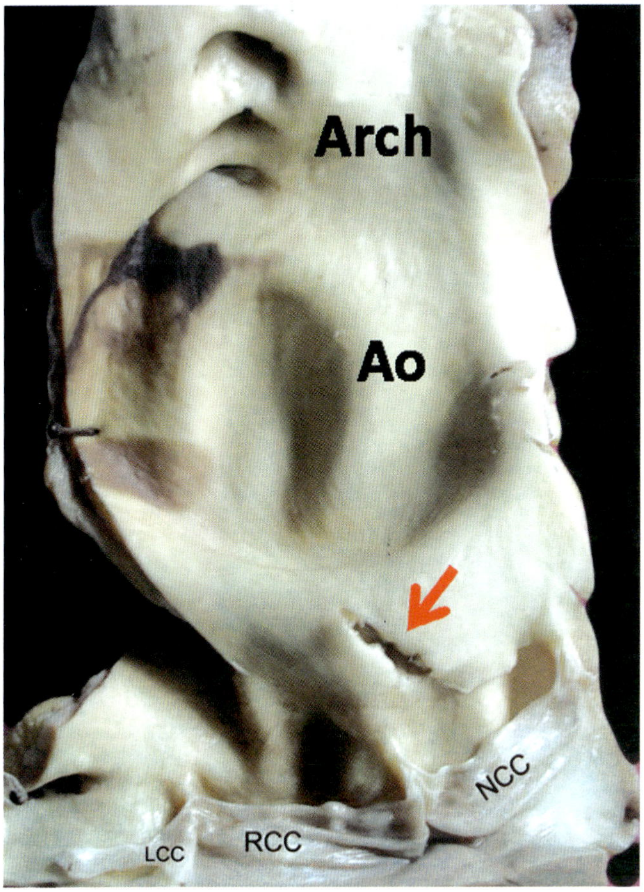

Fig. 51.1C: Gross pathology specimen from a patient with type II aortic dissection demonstrating the area of intimal tear (arrow). [Image courtesy of Pradeep Vaideeswar, Professor (Additional), Department of Pathology, (Cardiovascular & Thoracic Division), Seth GS Medical College, Mumbai, India]. (Ao: Aorta; LCC:Left coronary cusp; RCC:Right coronary cusp; NCC:Noncoronary cusp).

when present for less than 2 weeks, subacute when present for 2–6 weeks, and chronic when present for more than 6 weeks. The highest risk of death from aortic dissection is within the first hours and days after onset.

The underlying causes for aortic dissection are diseases affecting the integrity of the aortic wall or leading to increased aortic wall sheer forces (Table 51.2). Hypertension is present in 75% of patients who suffer aortic dissection, and heritable disorders including Marfan syndrome and familial thoracic aortic aneurysm syndromes, bicuspid aortic valve disease, aortic manipulation, and aortitis are important causes.

DIAGNOSIS OF AORTIC DISSECTION

Acute, abrupt-onset and severe chest and/or back pain is the most common symptom in aortic dissection. A wide

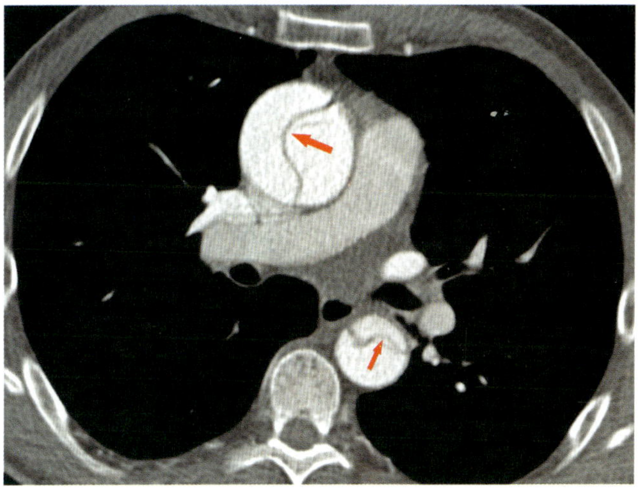

Fig. 51.2: Contrast CT scan of acute type A aortic dissection. The ascending aorta is dilated and a complex dissection flap is visualized in the ascending (arrow) and descending aorta (arrow). [Reproduced with permission from Braverman AC. Diseases of the Aorta. In: Braunwald's Heart Disease, 10th Edition. Mann DL, Bonow RO, Zipes DP, Libby P, (Eds). Philadelphia, USA: Elsevier; 2014. (In press)].

spectrum of clinical syndromes may result due to complications or regions of vascular insufficiency (Table 51.3). The physical examination may demonstrate pulse deficits or aortic regurgitation, but these findings have a low sensitivity for acute dissection.

Diagnosing aortic dissection requires a high index of suspicion. A focused evaluation for underlying risk factors associated with aortic dissection, high-risk pain features, and high-risk physical examination findings will enhance recognition and expedite imaging in acute aortic dissection. The chest X-ray may suggest aortic disease due to abnormal aortic contour, mediastinal widening or displaced intimal calcium (Fig. 51.7). However, a normal chest X-ray is present in 10–20% of acute dissection. The electrocardiogram is usually normal or has nonspecific findings, unless coronary artery malperfusion leads to ischemia or infarction. The D-dimer level is elevated in most patients presenting within the several hours of acute classic aortic dissection and can be a very important clue in diagnosis. A normal D-dimer has a high negative predictive value in acute classic aortic dissection. Because D-dimer may not be elevated in aortic IMH or PAU, one cannot rely on this marker in all cases of suspected acute aortic syndrome.

Contrast computed tomography (CT) scan, transesophageal echocardiogram (TEE), and magnetic resonance imaging (MRI) all have high sensitivity and specificity

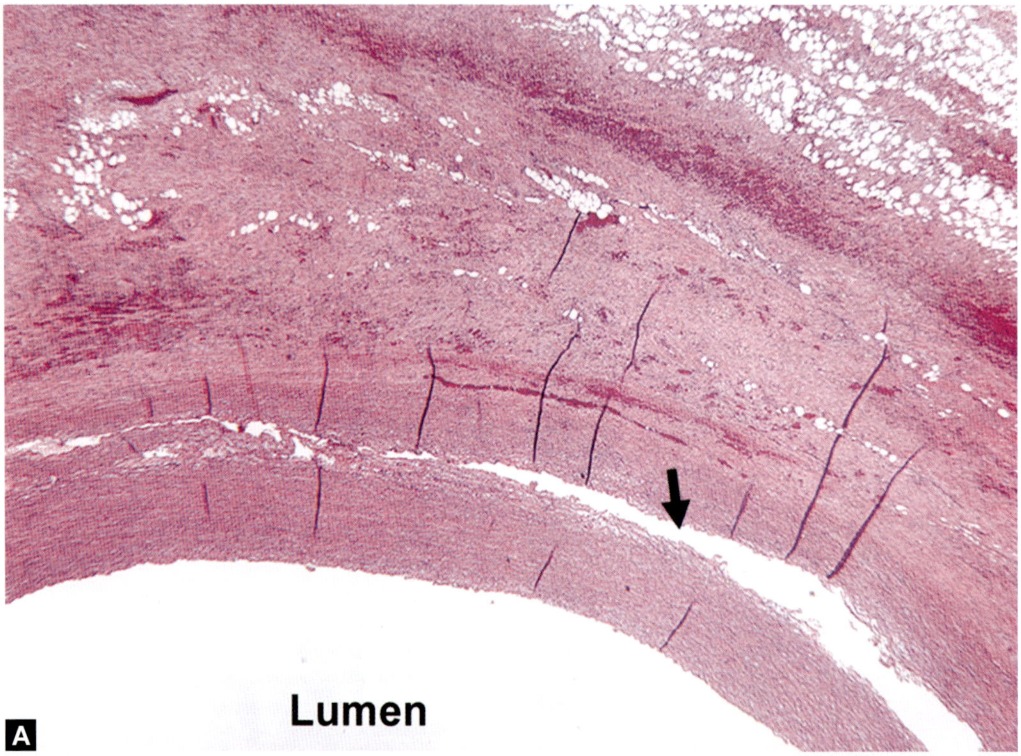

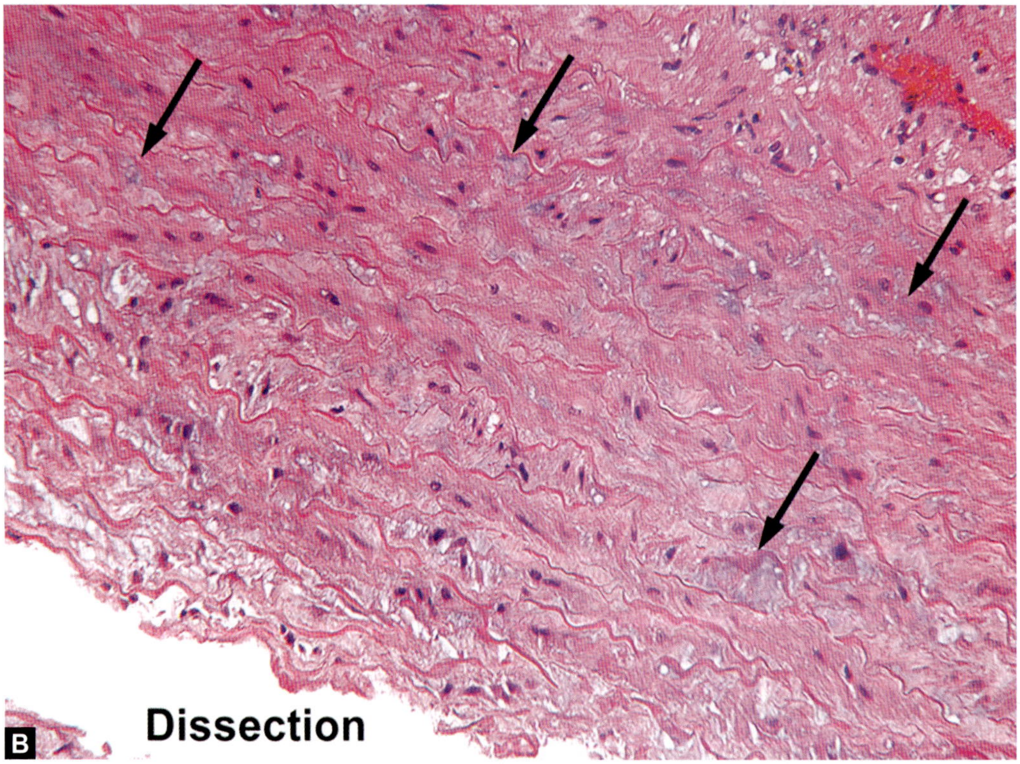

Figs. 51.3A and B: Pathology of acute aortic dissection. (A) Light microscopic view of the aorta in a patient with aortic dissection. The lumen is labeled. There is a cleavage plane in the media demonstrating the small false lumen (black arrow); (B) Hematoxylin and eosin stain (20x) of the aorta with arrows pointing to areas of cystic medial degeneration (staining blue) in a patient with acute type A aortic dissection (labeled). [Modified with permission from Braverman AC. Diseases of the Aorta. In: Braunwald's Heart Disease, 10th Edition. Mann DL, Bonow RO, Zipes DP, Libby P, (Eds). Philadelphia, USA: Elsevier; 2014. (In press)].

(typically > 95%) for acute dissection. Contrast CT is usually the first test performed due to its wide availability and rapid image acquisition (Fig. 51.8). Iodinated contrast must be used in order to visualize the dissection flap and true and false lumens. While transthoracic echocardiogram (TTE) may demonstrate aortic dissection (Videos 51.2 and 51.3), the sensitivity of TEE is much greater (Figs. 51.9A to C) (Video 51.4). Magnetic resonance imaging (Fig. 51.10) is generally less available emergently and takes longer than CT, thus, is not usually the first test performed. Aortography is used mainly in endovascular therapy of dissection complications.

Complications of aortic dissection are related to acute aortic regurgitation, aortic rupture, cardiac tamponade, neurologic and malperfusion syndromes. Thus, many different clinical syndromes may result from acute aortic dissection (Table 51.3).

COMPLICATIONS OF AORTIC DISSECTION

Aortic regurgitation complicates 40–75% of cases of acute type A aortic dissection (Figs. 51.11 and 51.12) (Video 51.3). Multiple mechanisms are responsible for aortic regurgitation complicating aortic dissection including: (a) incomplete leaflet coaptation due to annular or aortic root dilatation; (b) distortion of aortic leaflets or leaflet prolapse caused by the dissection flap interfering with commissural support; (c) dissection flap prolapse across the aortic valve; and (d) underlying aortic valve abnormalities, including bicuspid aortic valve.

Malperfusion of aortic branch vessels (Figs. 51.11 to 51.13) in acute dissection may be caused by the dissection flap involving the branch vessel directly (static obstruction), prolapse of the intimal flap across the orifice

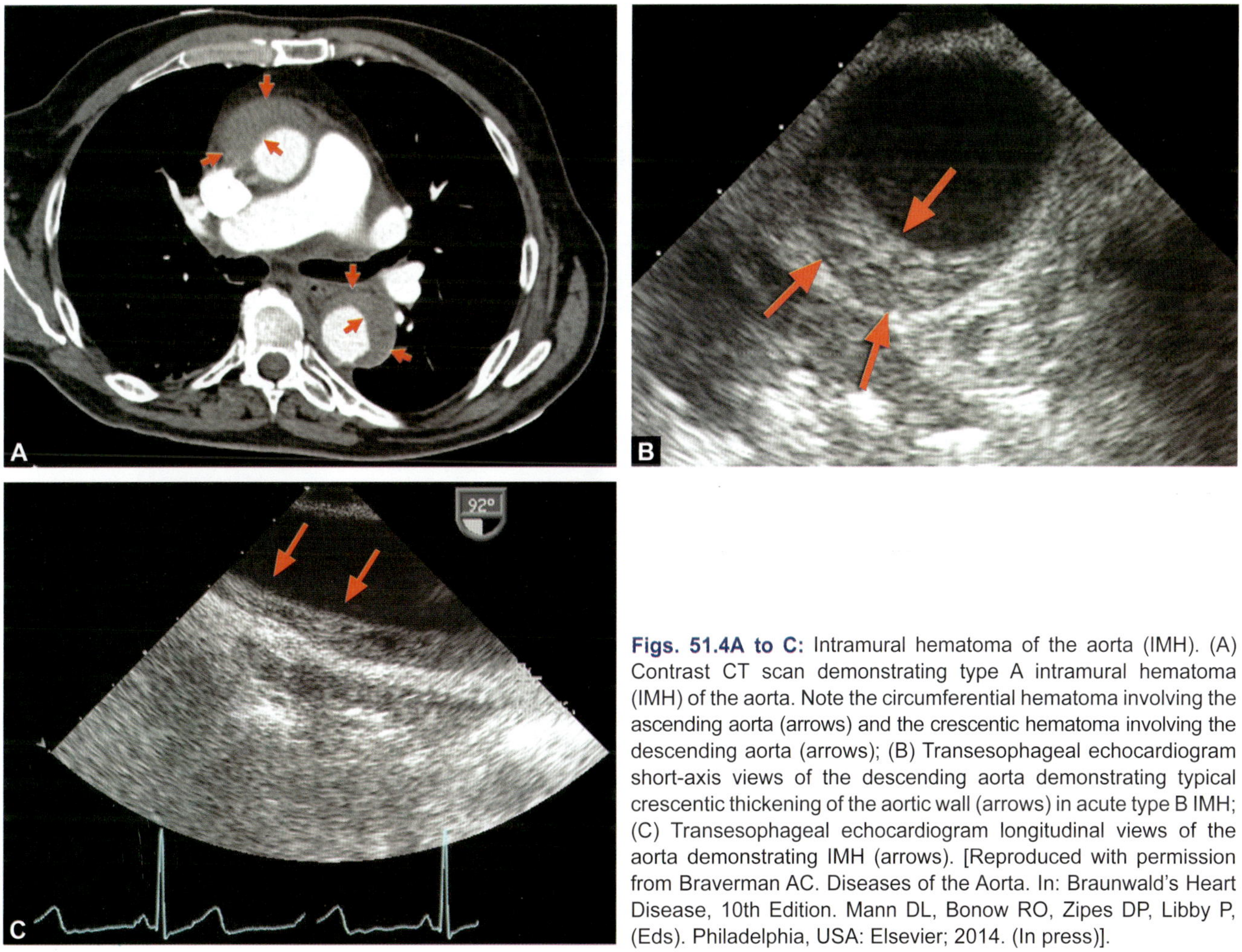

Figs. 51.4A to C: Intramural hematoma of the aorta (IMH). (A) Contrast CT scan demonstrating type A intramural hematoma (IMH) of the aorta. Note the circumferential hematoma involving the ascending aorta (arrows) and the crescentic hematoma involving the descending aorta (arrows); (B) Transesophageal echocardiogram short-axis views of the descending aorta demonstrating typical crescentic thickening of the aortic wall (arrows) in acute type B IMH; (C) Transesophageal echocardiogram longitudinal views of the aorta demonstrating IMH (arrows). [Reproduced with permission from Braverman AC. Diseases of the Aorta. In: Braunwald's Heart Disease, 10th Edition. Mann DL, Bonow RO, Zipes DP, Libby P, (Eds). Philadelphia, USA: Elsevier; 2014. (In press)].

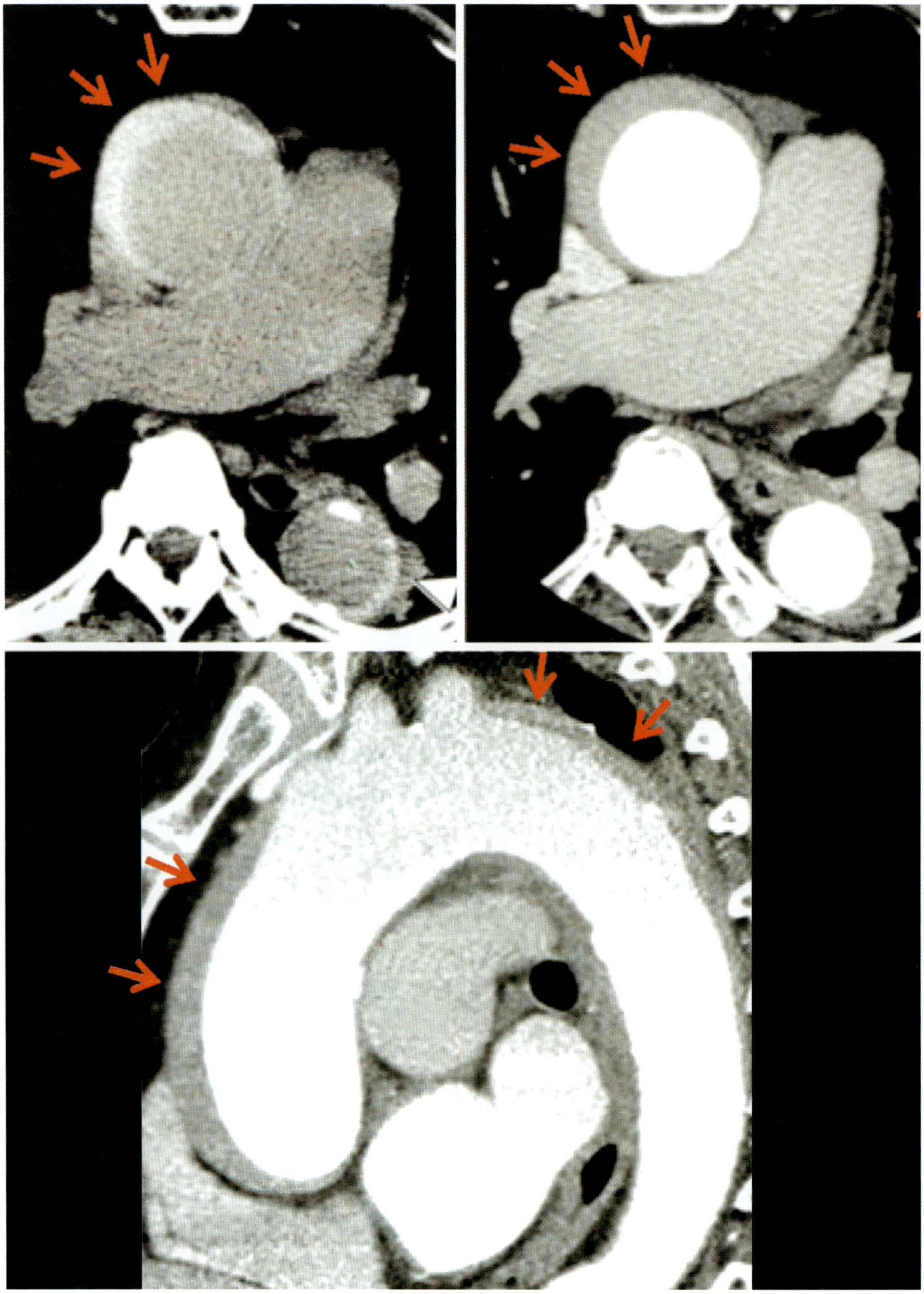

Fig. 51.4D: Computed tomography scan demonstrating intramural hematoma of the thoracic aorta. Top left panel shows noncontrast CT scan, with the crescent-shaped IMH (arrows) appearing brighter due to hematoma formation. Right and bottom panels show axial and oblique sagittal MPR contrast-enhanced images. The IMH is visualized involving the entire thoracic aorta (arrows). (Images courtesy of Dr Takuya Ueda, Department of Radiology, St. Luke's International Hospital, Chuo-ku Tokyo, Japan. Image from Ueda T et al. A pictorial review of acute aortic syndrome: discriminating and overlapping features as revealed by ECG-gated multidetector-row CT angiography. Insights into imaging. 10.1007/s13244-012-0195-7).

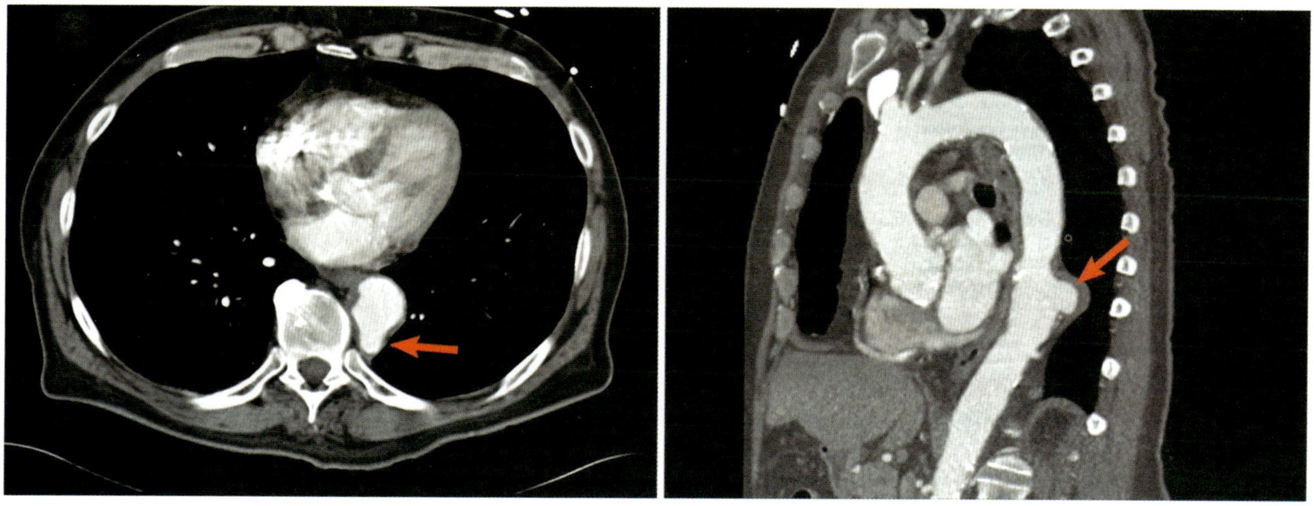

Fig. 51.5A: Contrast CT scan demonstrating an acute penetrating atherosclerotic aortic ulcer (PAU). Axial image (left image) demonstrates the typical focal outpouching of the aortic ulcer (arrow). Sagittal image, (right image) demonstrates the penetrating ulcer (arrow) with associated intramural hematoma. Symptomatic PAU has an increased risk of aortic rupture and is often amenable to endovascular repair.

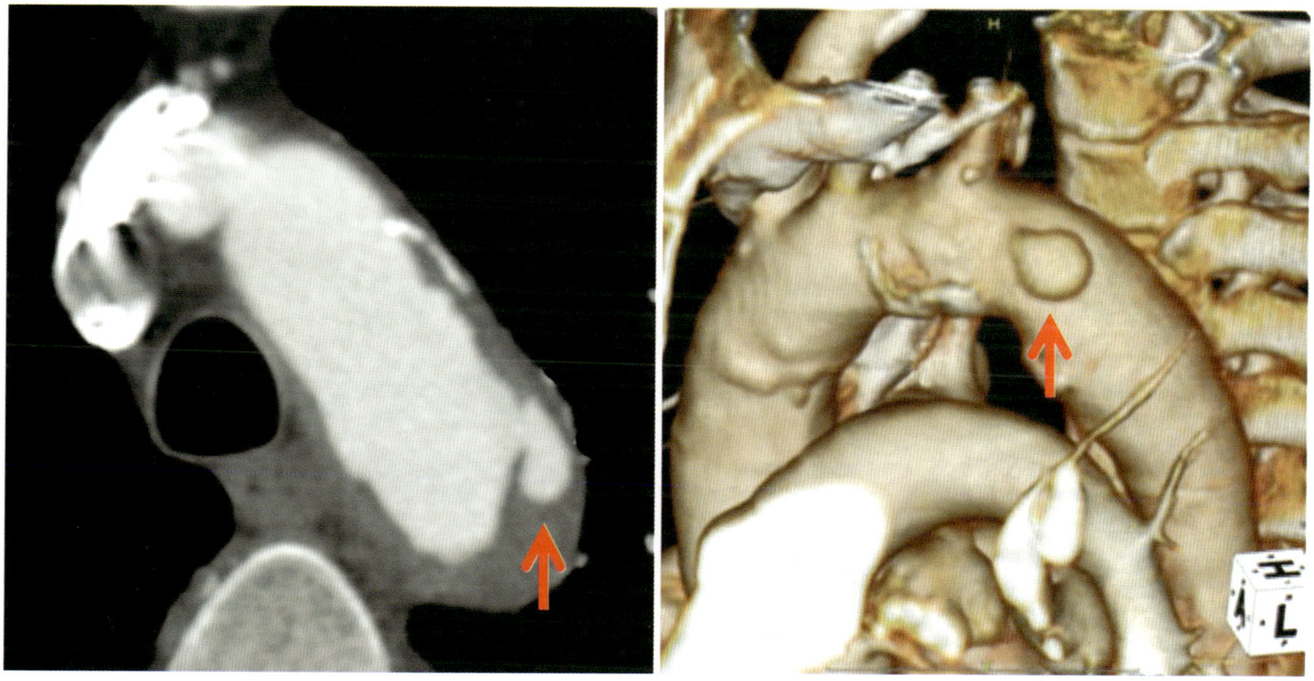

Fig. 51.5B: Penetrating atherosclerotic aortic ulcer. (Left panel) Axial ECG-gated CTA demonstrates the ulcerative lesion (arrow) into the aortic media, which shows associated hemorrhage. (Right panel) 3D-VR image depicts the crater-like ulceration (arrow) on the aortic arch.

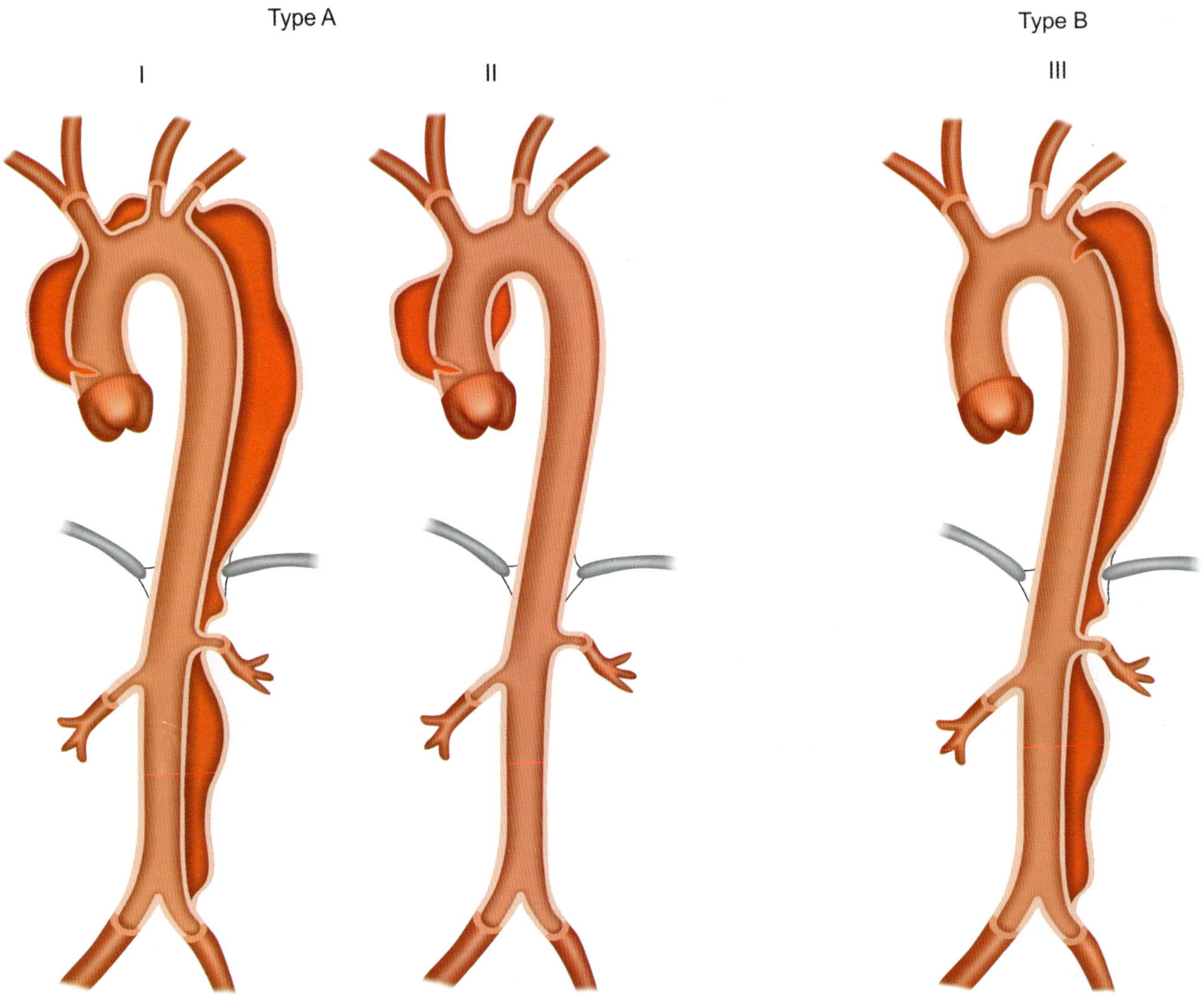

Fig. 51.6: Classification schemes of acute aortic dissection. (Reproduced with permission from Braverman AC. Aortic Dissection. Prompt Diagnosis and Emergency Treatment are Critical. Cleve Clin J Med. 2011;78:1695-1704).

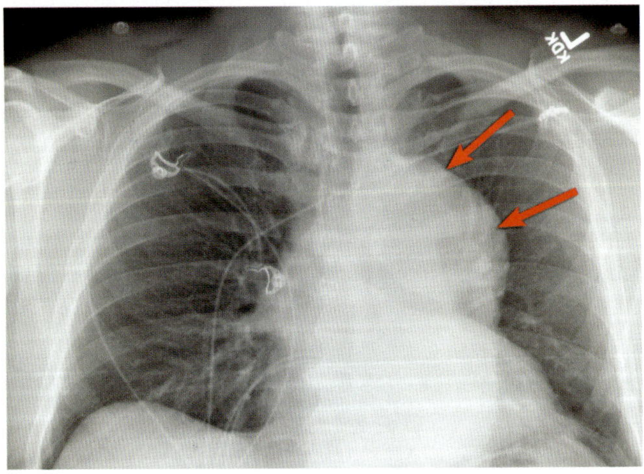

Fig. 51.7: Chest radiograph in acute type A aortic dissection demonstrating a widened mediastinum and enlargement of the ascending and descending aortic shadows (arrows). It is important to remember that in acute aortic dissection a normal chest X-ray is present in ~15% of cases.

Table 51.1: Classification of aortic dissection according to the DeBakey and Stanford Classification systems.

DeBakey Classification	
Type I	Dissection originates in the ascending aorta and extends at least to the aortic arch and often to the descending aorta (and beyond)
Type II	Dissection originates in the ascending aorta and is confined to this segment
Type III	Dissection originates in the descending aorta, usually just distal to the left subclavian artery, and extends distally
Stanford Classification	
Type A	Dissection involves the ascending aorta (with or without extension into the descending aorta)
Type B	Dissection does not involve the ascending aorta

Table 51.2: Risk factors for aortic dissection. Modified with permission from Braverman AC. Diseases of the Aorta. In, Mann DL, Bonow RO, Zipes DP, Libby P Braunwald's Heart Disease, 10th Edition. Philadelphia, USA: Elsevier; 2014. (In press). (IABP: Intraaortic balloon pump; CABG: Coronary artery bypass surgery; AVR: Aortic valve replacement; TEVAR: Thoracic endovascular aortic repair; TAVR: Transcatheter aortic valve replacement.

Hypertension
• Genetically Triggered Thoracic Aortic Aneurysm Diseases – Marfan syndrome – Loeys-Dietz syndrome – Familial thoracic aortic aneurysm/dissection – Vascular Ehlers-Danlos syndrome
• Congenital Heart Disease/Syndromes – Bicuspid aortic valve – Coarctation of the aorta – Tetralogy of Fallot – Turner Syndrome
• Trauma (Blunt or Iatrogenic) – Catheter, stent, IABP – CABG, AVR, aortic surgery, TEVAR, TAVR – Motor vehicle accident
• Atherosclerosis – Penetrating atherosclerotic ulcer
Cocaine/Methamphetamine use
• Aortitis (Inflammatory/Infectious) – Giant cell arteritis, Behçet's disease – Takayasu's arteritis – Syphilis
Pregnancy (with underlying aortopathy)
Weightlifting (with underlying aortopathy)

Table 51.3: Clinical syndromes associated with acute aortic dissection.

Cardiovascular	Cardiac arrest Aortic regurgitation Congestive heart failure Coronary ischemia Myocardial infarction Cardiac tamponade Pericarditis
Pulmonary	Pleural effusion Hemothorax Hemoptysis (aortotracheal or aortobronchial fistula)
Renal	Acute renal failure Renovascular hypertension Renal ischemia or infarction
Neurologic	Stroke Transient ischemic attack Paraparesis/paraplegia Encephalopathy Coma Spinal cord syndrome Ischemic neuropathy
Gastrointestinal	Mesenteric ischemia/infarction Pancreatitis Hemorrhage (from aortoenteric fistula)
Peripheral Vascular	Upper or lower extremity ischemia
Systemic	Fever

[Modified with permission from Braverman AC. Diseases of the Aorta. In: Mann DL, Bonow RO, Zipes DP, Libby P. Braunwald's Heart Disease, 10th Edition. Elsevier/Philadelphia. (In press)].

of the artery (dynamic obstruction), compression of the artery by an expanded false lumen, arterial thrombosis due to slow flow, or cardiogenic failure and low-flow state. Renal artery obstruction occurs in 5–10% cases and may lead to refractory hypertension (Fig. 51.14). Branch vessel malperfusion may resolve after treating acute type A dissection surgically or may require focused endovascular or open repair. Neurologic complications include ischemic stroke, spinal cord malperfusion, syncope and ischemic peripheral neuropathy; many of these symptoms are transient.

Cardiac tamponade (Fig. 51.15), one of the most common causes of death in acute dissection, complicates approximately 20% of acute type A aortic dissections. These patients may present with hypotension, transient

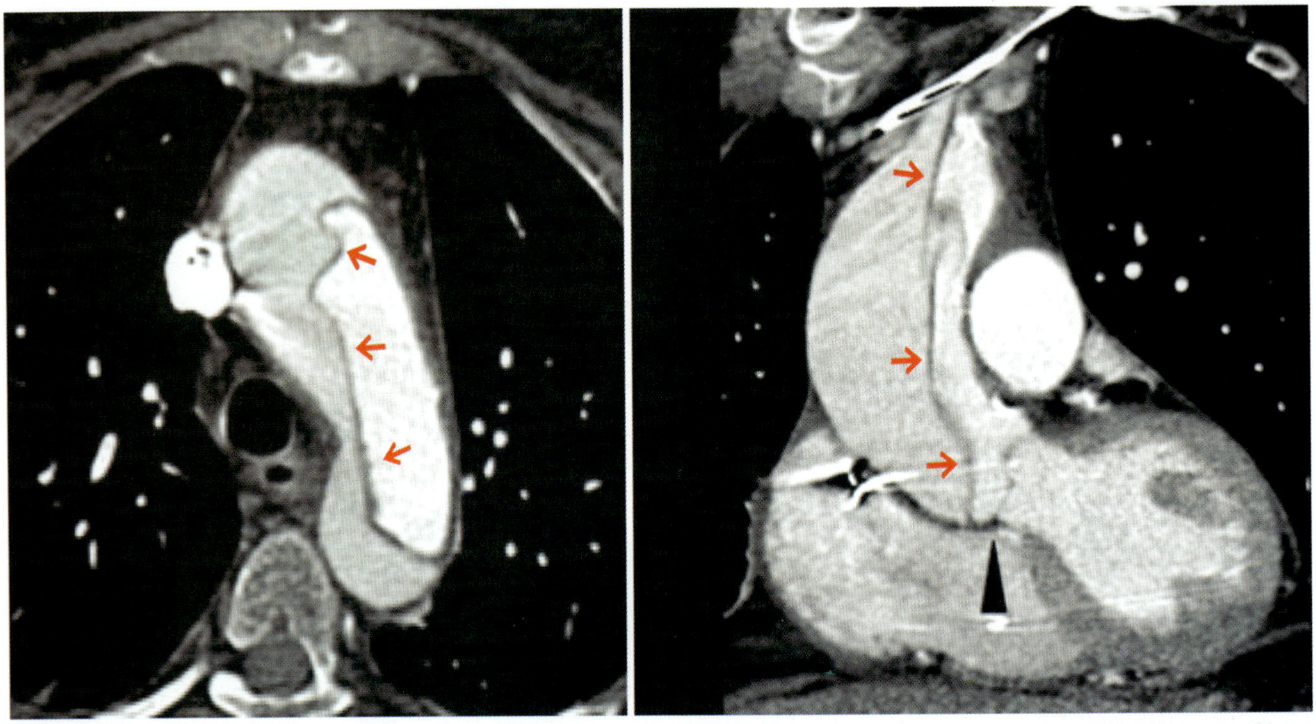

Fig. 51.8: Contrast-enhanced CT images of aortic dissection. The dissection flap is clearly visualized (arrows) extending down into the aortic root and involving the aortic valve apparatus. The true lumen appears brighter in these images as in this case there is a greater concentration of contrast in true lumen. (Images courtesy of Dr Takuya Ueda, Department of Radiology, St Luke's International Hospital, Chuo-ku Tokyo, Japan. Image from Ueda T et al. A pictorial review of acute aortic syndrome: discriminating and overlapping features as revealed by ECG-gated multidetector-row CT angiography. Insights into imaging. 10.1007/s13244-012-0195-7).

syncope, or mental status changes. Pericardiocentesis in this setting has resulted in recurrent bleeding into the pericardium and sudden death. Emergency surgery is recommended for tamponade complicating acute type A dissection. Aortic rupture may cause a slow leak or "contained rupture" (Figs. 51.16 and 51.17), or may lead to sudden hemodynamic collapse, cardiac tamponade, or exsanguination.

MANAGEMENT OF PATIENTS WITH AORTIC DISSECTION

Type A aortic dissection requires emergency surgery to prevent rupture and coronary malperfusion, correct aortic regurgitation, and restore flow into the true lumen, and if possible, obliterate the distal false channel (Figs. 51.18 and 51.19). This surgery is technically challenging and the use of felt and plegeted sutures secure the friable aortic wall (Figs. 51.20A and B); arch vessels may require grafts (Fig. 51.21).

Type B aortic dissection is treated medically unless complications such as rupture (Figs. 51.22A to C) or malperfusion develop. If emergency open surgery is required, the morbidity and mortality rate is very high. Thoracic endovascular aortic repair has a lower acute risk than open repair in this setting and is currently used for most complications of acute type B dissection (Figs. 51.22 and 51.23).

Long-term follow-up after dissection includes evaluation for underlying aortopathy in the patient and first-degree relatives, blood pressure control, lifestyle modification, and long-term aortic imaging. Many patients will require subsequent treatment for aneurysmal enlargement after aortic dissection (Figs. 51.24A to C).

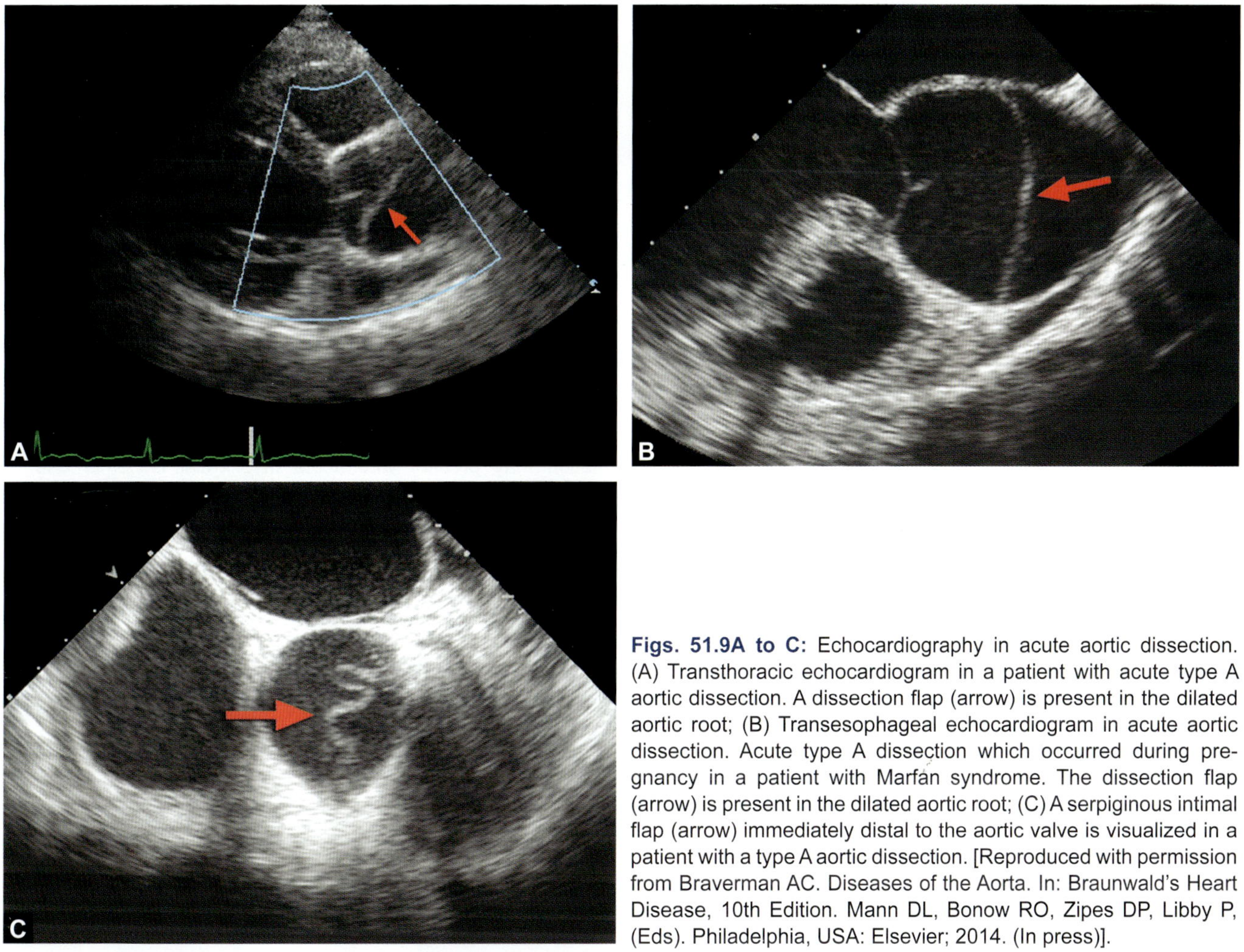

Figs. 51.9A to C: Echocardiography in acute aortic dissection. (A) Transthoracic echocardiogram in a patient with acute type A aortic dissection. A dissection flap (arrow) is present in the dilated aortic root; (B) Transesophageal echocardiogram in acute aortic dissection. Acute type A dissection which occurred during pregnancy in a patient with Marfan syndrome. The dissection flap (arrow) is present in the dilated aortic root; (C) A serpiginous intimal flap (arrow) immediately distal to the aortic valve is visualized in a patient with a type A aortic dissection. [Reproduced with permission from Braverman AC. Diseases of the Aorta. In: Braunwald's Heart Disease, 10th Edition. Mann DL, Bonow RO, Zipes DP, Libby P, (Eds). Philadelphia, USA: Elsevier; 2014. (In press)].

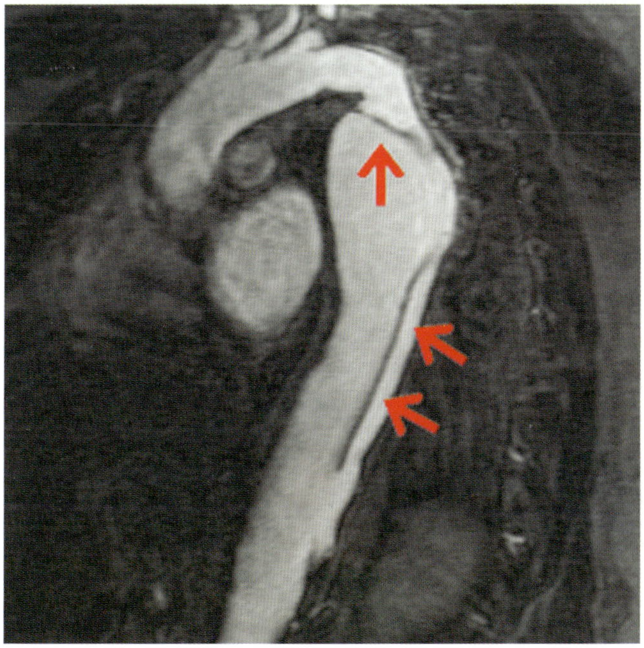

Fig. 51.10: Coronal MRI image demonstrating a Stanford type B (DeBakey type III) aortic dissection (arrows). (Image courtesy of Dr Lars Grenacher, posted on Wikimedia Commons).

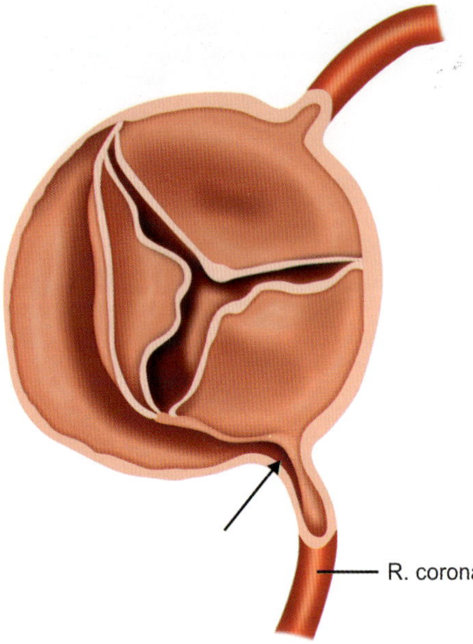

Fig. 51.11: Aortic regurgitation complicating acute type A aortic dissection. The dissection flap distorts the normal aortic leaflet alignment causing malcoaptation of the valve leaflets and aortic regurgitation. In this example, the dissection flap extends into the ostium of the right coronary artery (arrow). This presentation may present with acute myocardial ischemia due to coronary artery malperfusion. [Reproduced with permission from Braverman AC, Thompson R, Sanchez L. Diseases of the Aorta, Chapter 60. In: Bonow RO, Mann DL, Zipes DP, Libby P, (Eds). Braunwald's Heart Disease, 9th Edition, pp. 1309-1337. Philadelphia, USA: Elsevier; 2011].

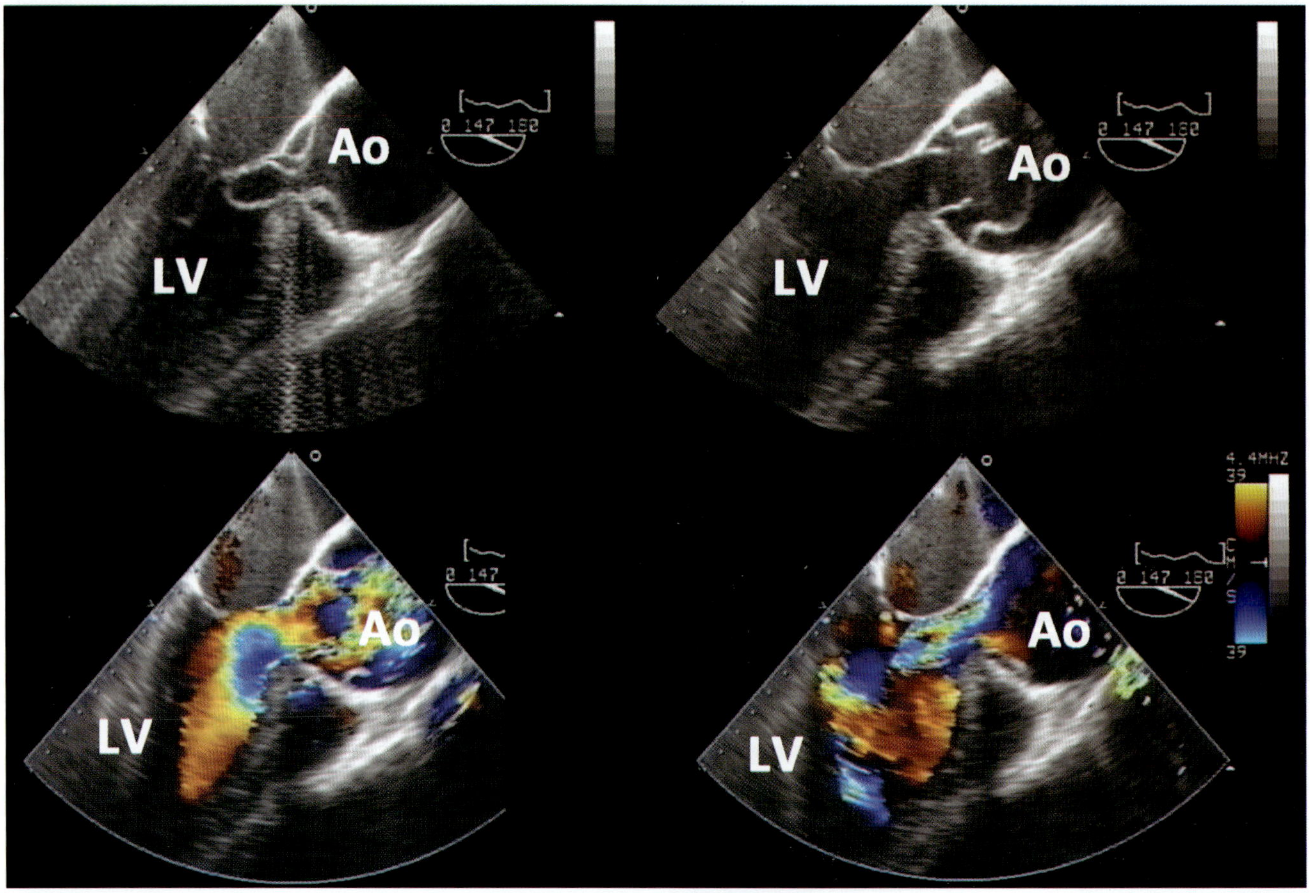

Fig. 51.12: Transesophageal echocardiogram images of aortic dissection flap involving the aortic root, and resultant severe aortic regurgitation. The patient presented with acute coronary syndrome and ST-segment elevation on the ECG, due to malperfusion of the coronary circulation. [Image from D'Aloia A et al. A type A aortic dissection mimicking an acute myocardial infarction. Cardiol Res. 2012;3(2):94-96. CC].

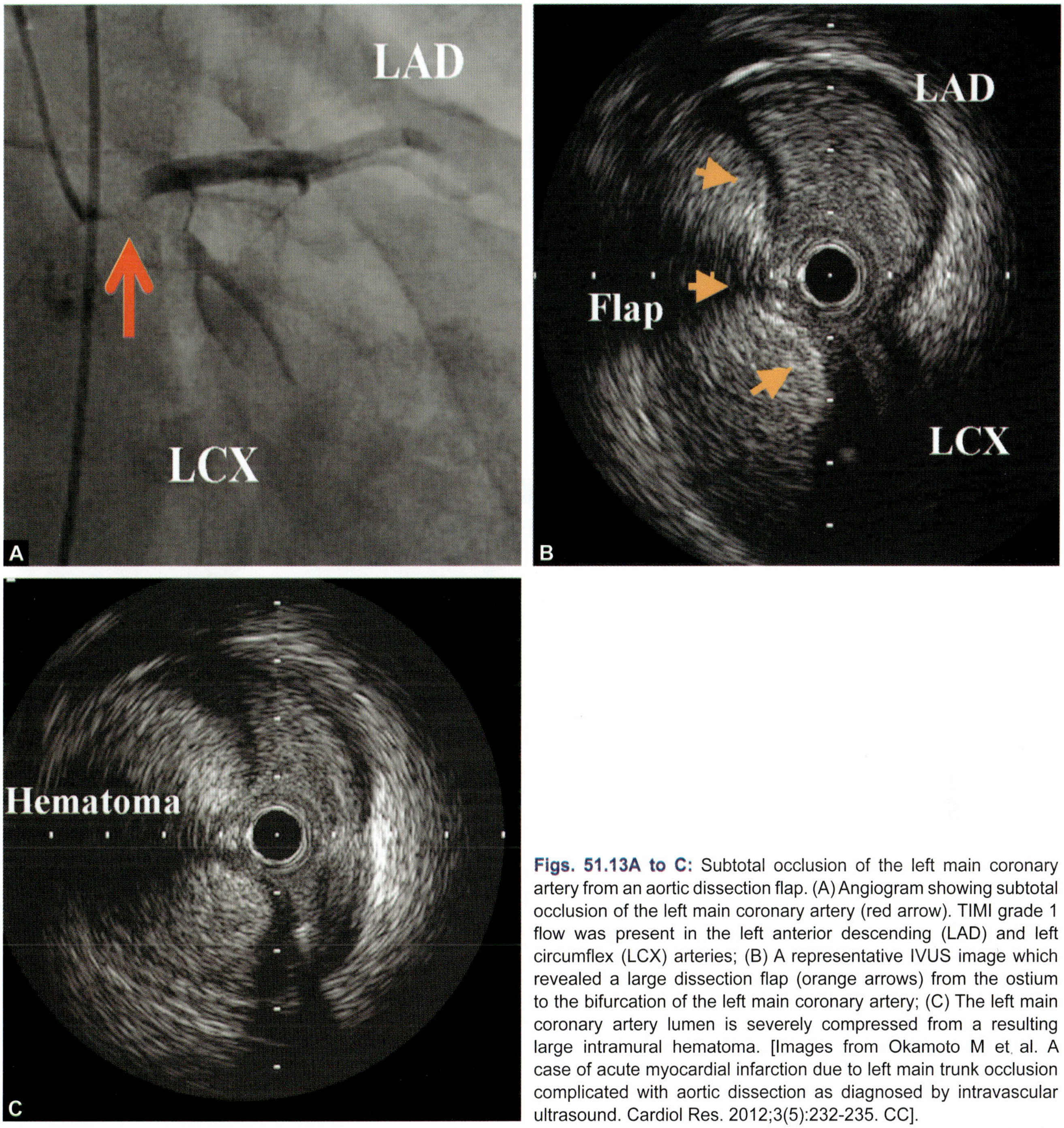

Figs. 51.13A to C: Subtotal occlusion of the left main coronary artery from an aortic dissection flap. (A) Angiogram showing subtotal occlusion of the left main coronary artery (red arrow). TIMI grade 1 flow was present in the left anterior descending (LAD) and left circumflex (LCX) arteries; (B) A representative IVUS image which revealed a large dissection flap (orange arrows) from the ostium to the bifurcation of the left main coronary artery; (C) The left main coronary artery lumen is severely compressed from a resulting large intramural hematoma. [Images from Okamoto M et al. A case of acute myocardial infarction due to left main trunk occlusion complicated with aortic dissection as diagnosed by intravascular ultrasound. Cardiol Res. 2012;3(5):232-235. CC].

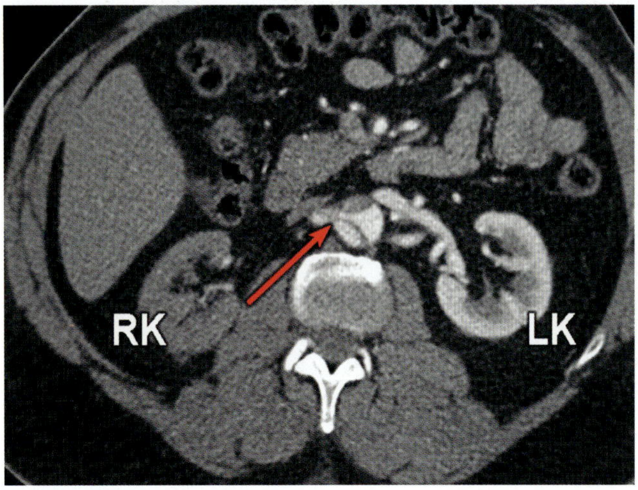

Fig. 51.14: Contrast CT scan demonstrating malperfusion of the right kidney (RK) due to acute aortic dissection. The dissection flap extends into the right renal artery (arrow). The left kidney (LK) demonstrates normal perfusion and opacification, while the right kidney (RK) has poor perfusion with contrast consistent with malperfusion. Renal artery malperfusion may be associated with refractory hypertension and may be amenable to endovascular repair. [Reproduced with permission from Braverman AC. Diseases of the Aorta. In: Braunwald's Heart Disease, 10th Edition. Mann DL, Bonow RO, Zipes DP, Libby P, (Eds). Philadelphia, USA: Elsevier; 2014. (In press)].

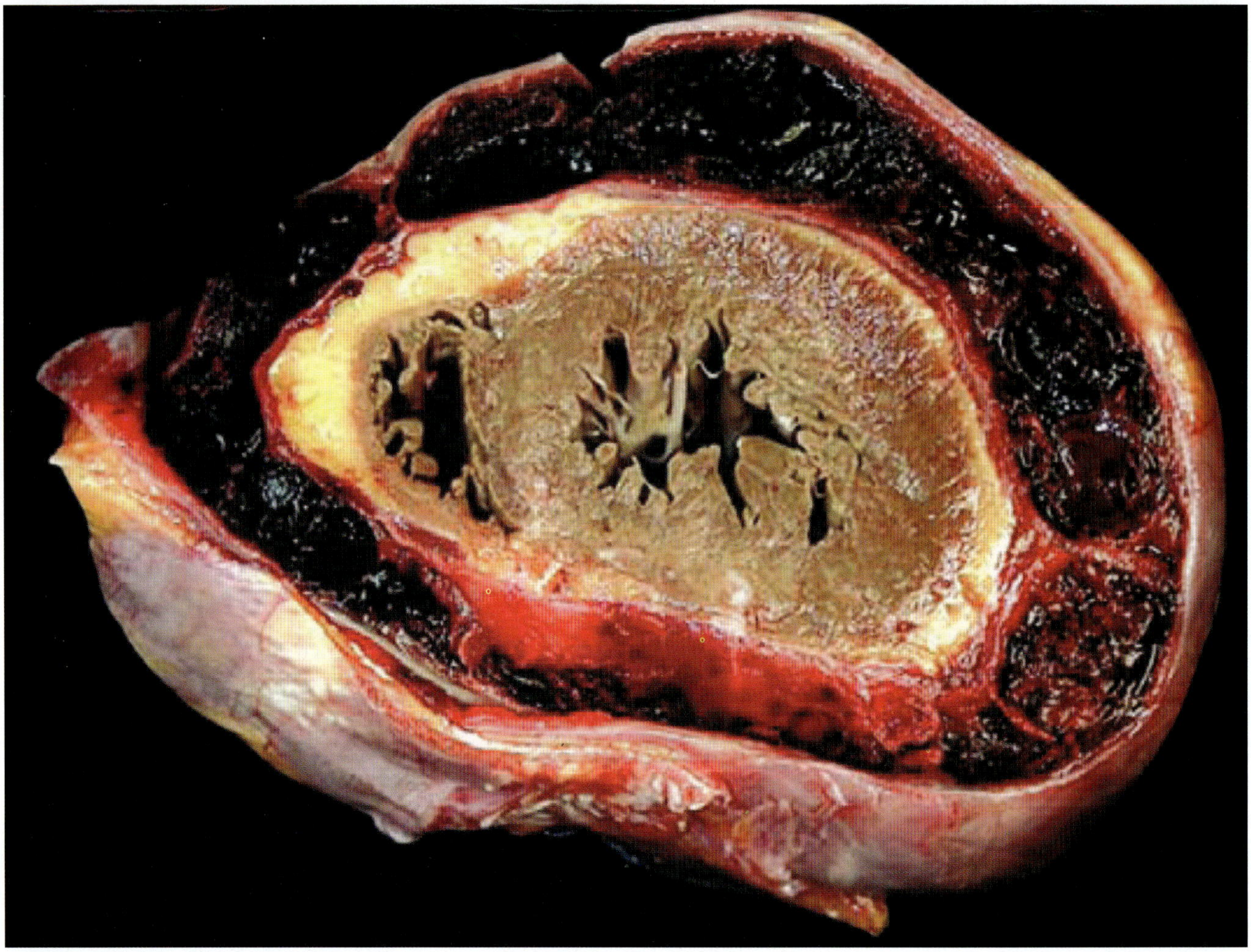

Fig. 51.15: Gross pathology of a patient with hemopericardium. [Image courtesy of Dr William D. Edwards, Mayo Clinic. Image and legend text from Khandaker MH and Nishimura RA. Pericardial disease. In: Chatterjee K et al. (Eds). Cardiology—an illustrated textbook. New Delhi, India: Jaypee Brothers Medical Publishers (P) Ltd.].

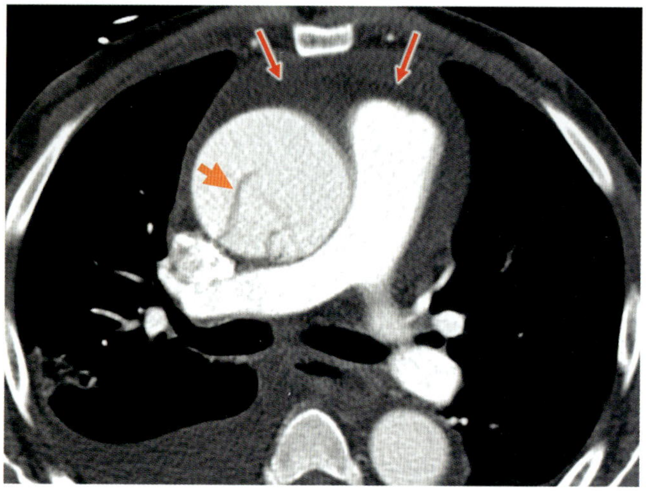

Fig. 51.16: Complicated acute type A aortic dissection. Contrast CT scan of an acute type A aortic dissection with mediastinal rupture. The red arrows point to mediastinal hematoma. A complex intimal flap (orange arrowhead) is present in the dilated aortic root. Aortic rupture may be heralded by sudden hypotension or recurrent acute pain.

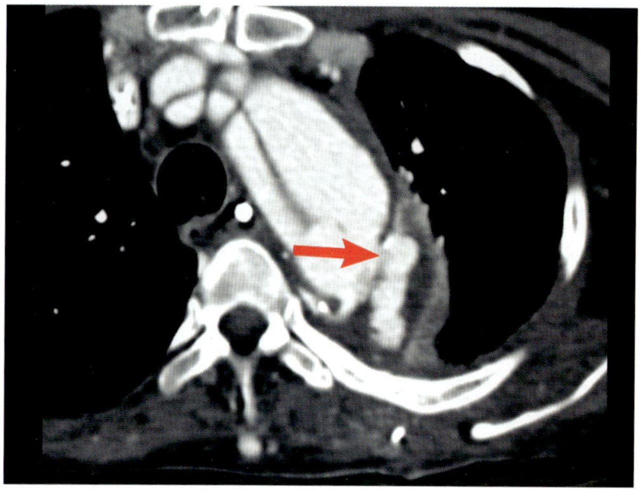

Fig. 51.17: Contrast CT scan in a patient with acute type A aortic dissection complicated by acute rupture of the aortic arch and active mediastinal bleeding (arrow). The dissection flap is visualized in the arch.

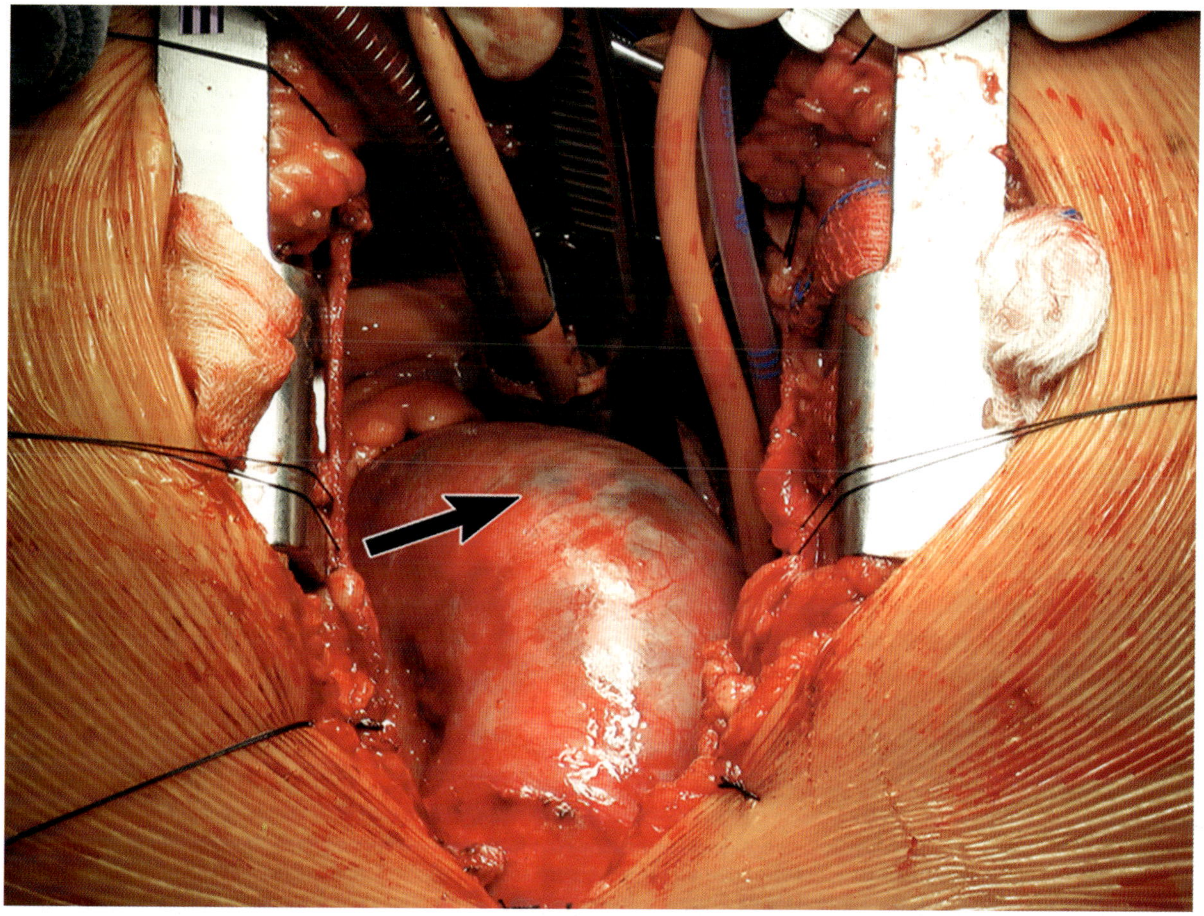

Fig. 51.18: Intraoperative photograph of acute ascending aortic dissection demonstrating a dilated aortic root and ascending aorta. The aorta has a bluish discoloration (black arrow) typical of underlying aortic dissection. (Photograph courtesy of Dr Nicholas Kouchoukos).

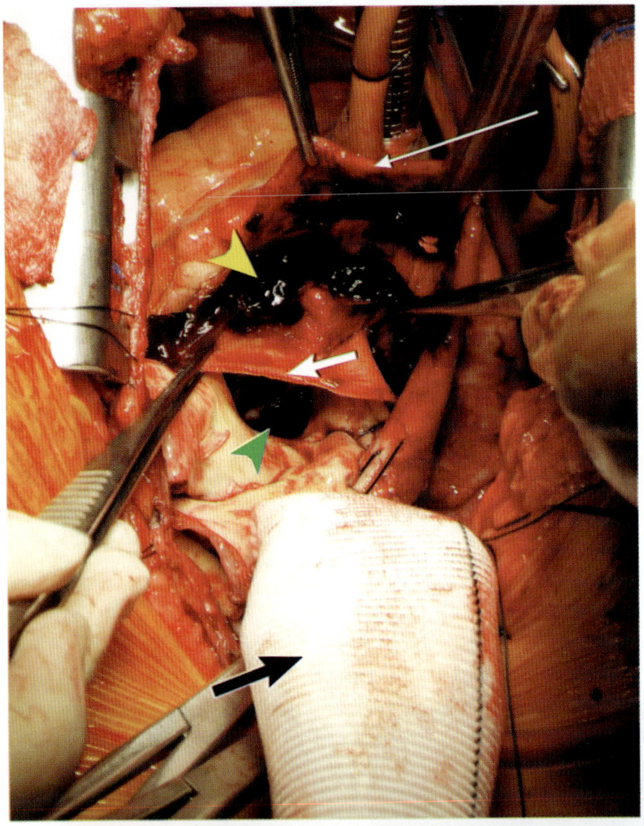

Fig. 51.19: Intraoperative photograph of the aortic root in acute ascending aortic dissection repair. The aortic valve is in the center (green arrowhead). The pickup is on the intimal flap (short white arrow). Forceps elevate the outer wall of the false lumen (long thin white arrow). Thrombus is visualized in the false lumen (yellow arrowhead). The aorta is being prepared for repair using a polyester graft (black arrow). (Photograph courtesy of Dr Nicholas Kouchoukos).

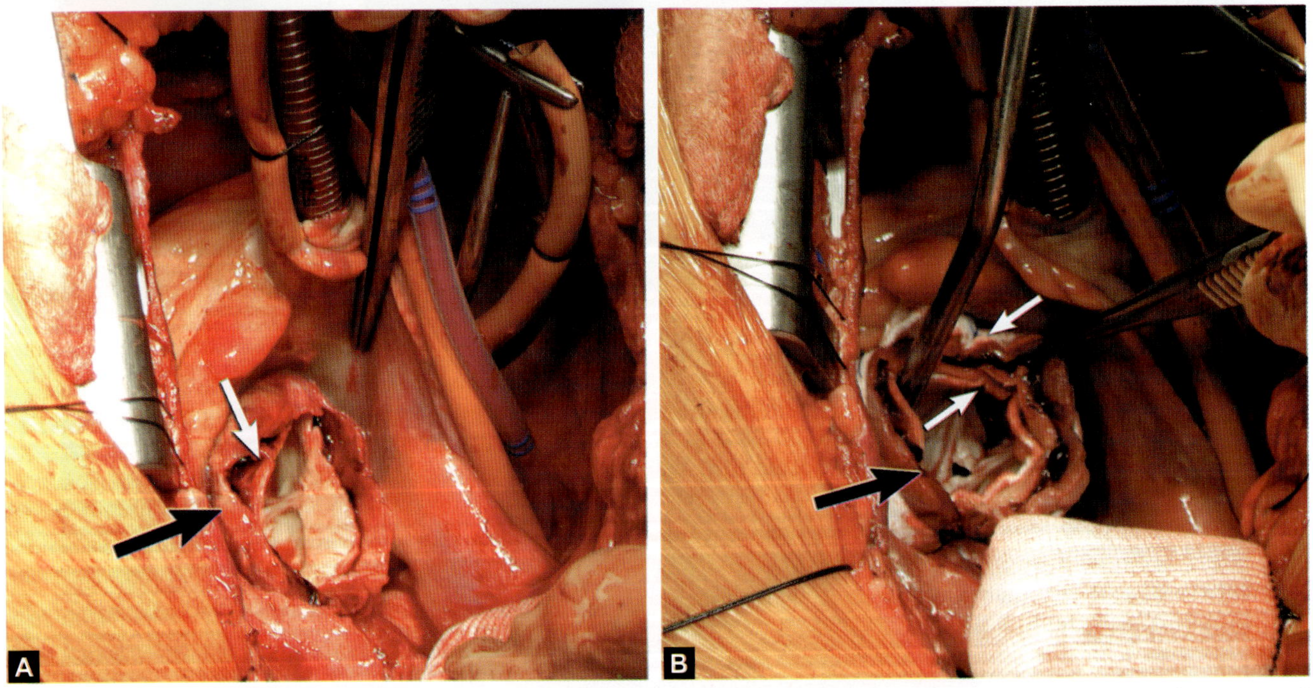

Figs. 51.20A and B: Surgical repair of acute type A aortic dissection. (A) Intraoperative photograph of surgical repair of acute type A aortic dissection. The aorta has been transected above the aortic commissures, and the inner (white arrow) and outer (black arrow) layers are approximated after removal of thrombus from the false lumen; (B) The aortic valve has been suspended by three sutures placed at the top of each commissure (black arrow). A strip of polytetrafluoroethylene felt is placed within the true aortic lumen (white arrow), and another strip is placed outside the aorta (white arrow). A polyester graft will be sutured to the aorta, incorporating the two layers of the aorta and the two strips of felt. (Photograph courtesy of Dr Nicholas Kouchoukos).

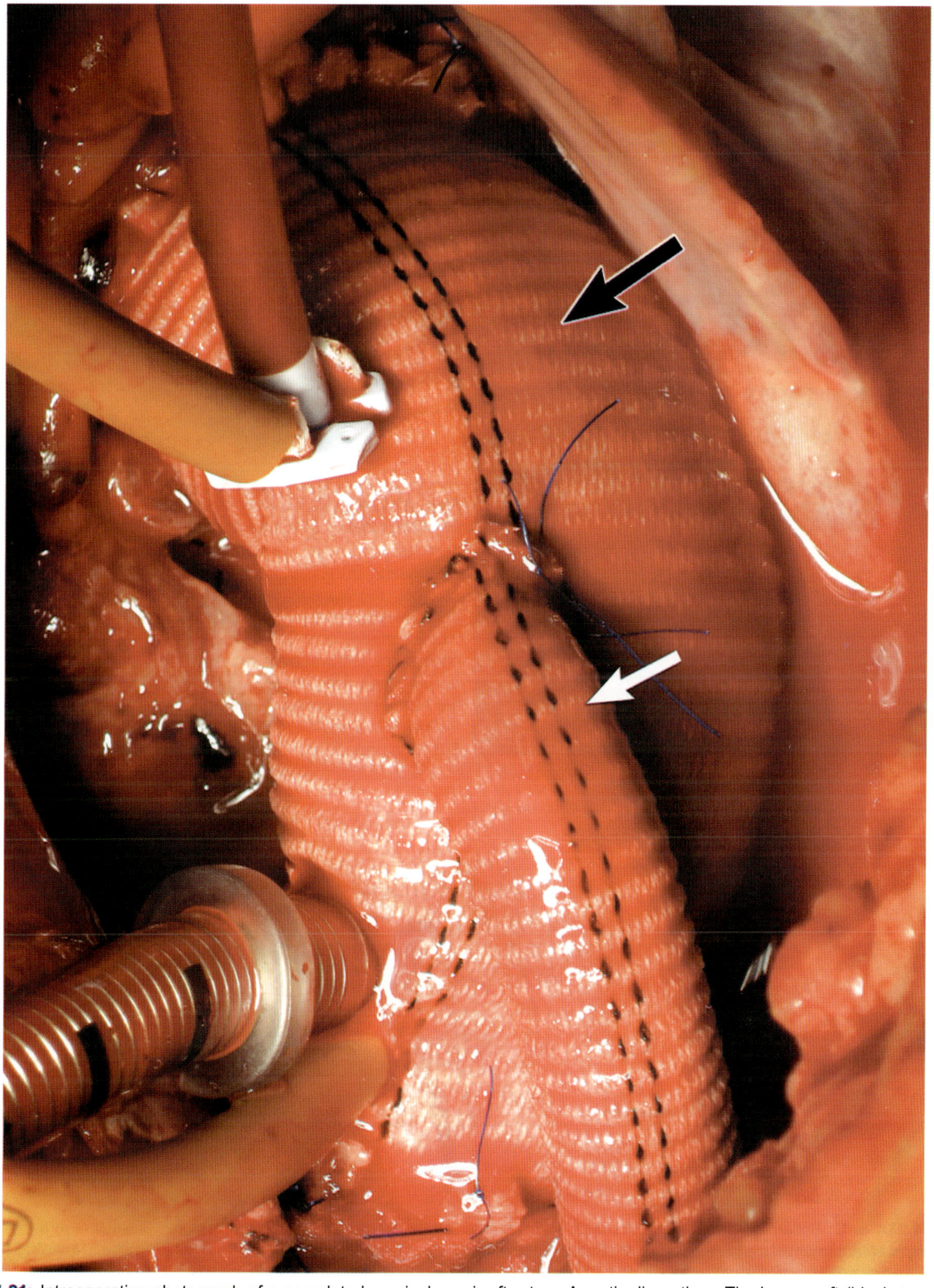

Fig. 51.21: Intraoperative photograph of a completed surgical repair after type A aortic dissection. The large graft (black arrow) has been sutured to the proximal and distal aorta and a separate graft (white arrow) has been placed to the innominate artery which was also dissected. (Photograph courtesy of Dr Nicholas Kouchoukos).

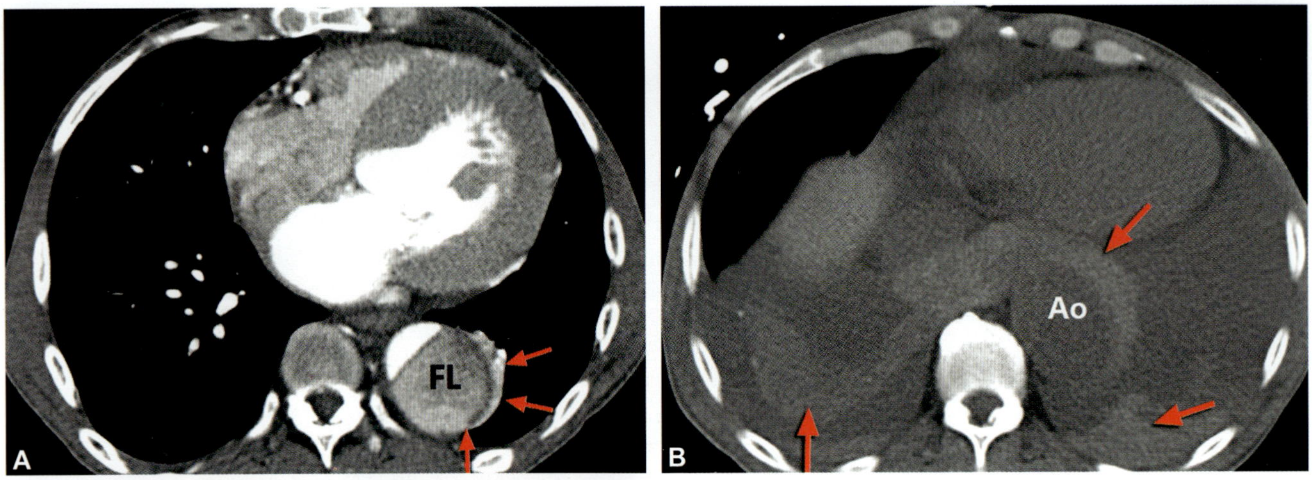

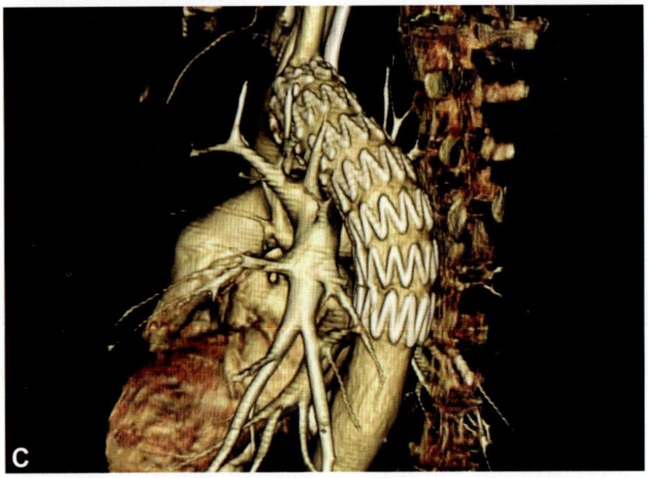

Figs. 51.22A to C: Thoracic endovascular aortic repair (TEVAR) for acute rupture of a type B aortic dissection. (A) Contrast CT demonstrating early leaking of blood (arrows) from the dilated false lumen (FL). The small true lumen is densely opacified with contrast; (B) Noncontrast CT demonstrating acute hemorrhage from the ruptured type B dissection (Ao denotes aorta); (C) Three-dimensional reconstruction of the descending thoracic aorta after emergency endovascular repair of the ruptured aortic dissection. [Reproduced with permission from Braverman AC. Diseases of the Aorta. In: Braunwald's Heart Disease, 10th Edition. Mann DL, Bonow RO, Zipes DP, Libby P, (Eds). Philadelphia, USA: Elsevier; 2014. (In press)].

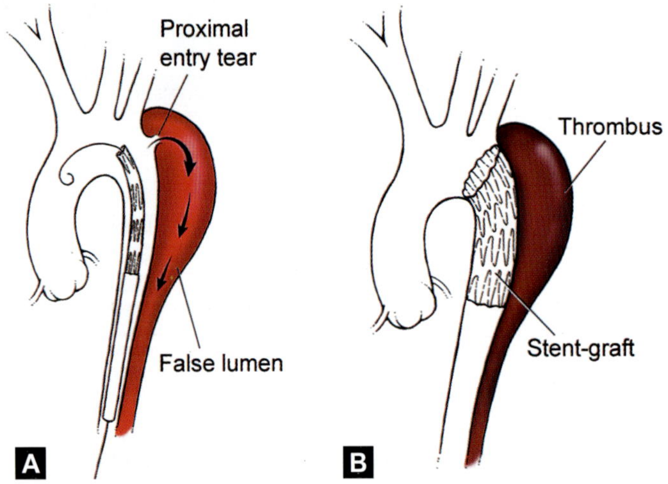

Figs. 51.23A to C: Schematic illustration of thoracic endovascular aneurysm repair (TEVAR) after aortic dissection in the setting of aneurysmal enlargement of the false channel. (A) Endograft is advanced to cover the proximal entry tear into the false channel; (B) Sealing of the entry tear promotes false lumen thrombosis; (C) Remodeling of the aorta occurs with expansion of the true lumen and a thrombosed false lumen. TEVAR may reduce long-term expansion of the false lumen. TEVAR is not currently indicated for stable uncomplicated type B aortic dissection. [Reproduced with permission from Braverman AC. Diseases of the Aorta. In, Braunwald's Heart Disease, 10th Edition. Mann DL, Bonow RO, Zipes DP, Libby P, (Eds). Philadelphia, USA: Elsevier; 2014. (In press)].

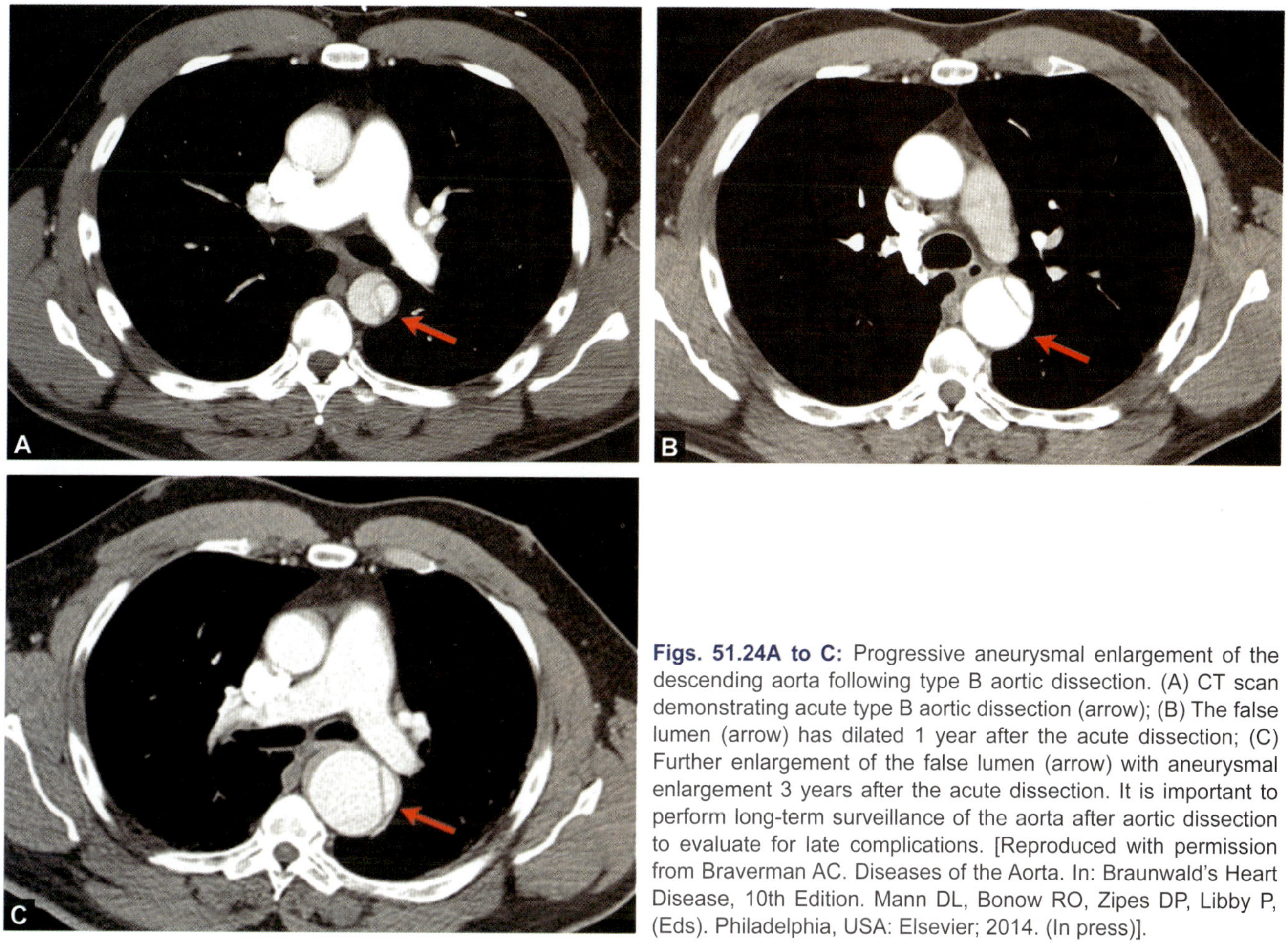

Figs. 51.24A to C: Progressive aneurysmal enlargement of the descending aorta following type B aortic dissection. (A) CT scan demonstrating acute type B aortic dissection (arrow); (B) The false lumen (arrow) has dilated 1 year after the acute dissection; (C) Further enlargement of the false lumen (arrow) with aneurysmal enlargement 3 years after the acute dissection. It is important to perform long-term surveillance of the aorta after aortic dissection to evaluate for late complications. [Reproduced with permission from Braverman AC. Diseases of the Aorta. In: Braunwald's Heart Disease, 10th Edition. Mann DL, Bonow RO, Zipes DP, Libby P, (Eds). Philadelphia, USA: Elsevier; 2014. (In press)].

VIDEO LEGENDS

Video 51.1: Echocardiography videoclip illustrating a dissection flap in a patient with aortic dissection. Color Doppler shows flow only in what in this case is the true lumen.

Video 51.2: Transthoracic echocardiogram demonstrating a dilated aortic root and ascending aorta and acute type A aortic dissection. There is malcoaptation of the aortic valve leaflets due to aortic root and annular dilatation. The intimal flap prolapses across the aortic valve.

Video 51.3: Transthoracic echocardiogram of acute type A aortic dissection with severe aortic regurgitation. Multiple mechanisms are present contributing to aortic regurgitation including dilatation of the aortic root; loss of commissural support of the valve leaflets and intimal flap prolapse across the aortic valve.

Video 51.4: Transesophageal echocardiogram of an acute type B aortic dissection. The mobile intimal flap separates the true lumen (at the top of the image) from the larger false lumen (at the bottom on the image).

REFERENCES

Braverman AC. Acute aortic dissection: clinician update. Circulation. 2010;122(2):184-8.

Braverman AC. Aortic dissection: prompt diagnosis and emergency treatment are critical. Cleve Clin J Med. 2011;78(10): 685-96.

Fattori R, Cao P, De Rango P, et al. Interdisciplinary expert consensus document on management of type B aortic dissection. J Am Coll Cardiol. 2013;61(16):1661-78.

Hagan PG, Nienaber CA, Isselbacher EM, et al. The International Registry of Acute Aortic Dissection (IRAD): new insights into an old disease. JAMA. 2000;283(7):897-903.

Harris KM, Braverman AC, Eagle KA, et al. Acute aortic intramural hematoma: an analysis from the International Registry of Acute Aortic Dissection. Circulation. 2012;126: S91-6.

Hiratzka LF, Bakris GL, Beckman JA, et al. 2010 ACCF/AHA/AATS/ACR/ASA/SCA/SCAI/SIR/STS/SVM Guidelines for the diagnosis and management of patients with thoracic aortic disease. J Am Coll Cardiol. 2010;55(14):e27-e129.

Sundt TM. Intramural hematoma and penetrating atherosclerotic ulcer of the aorta. Ann Thorac Surg. 2007;83(2):S835-41.

Tsai TT, Trimarchi S, Neinaber CA. Acute aortic dissection: perspectives from the International Registry of Acute Aortic Dissection (IRAD). Eur J Vasc Endovasc Surg. 2009;37(2): 149-59.

CHAPTER 52

Renovascular Disease

Ido Weinberg, Michael R Jaff

INTRODUCTION

Atherosclerotic renal artery stenosis (ARAS) is a common finding (Fig. 52.1). ARAS is most prevalent in at-risk populations, including patients with poorly controlled hypertension (HTN), systemic atherosclerosis and most specifically among patients with coronary (18–20%) or peripheral artery disease, where it was found in up to

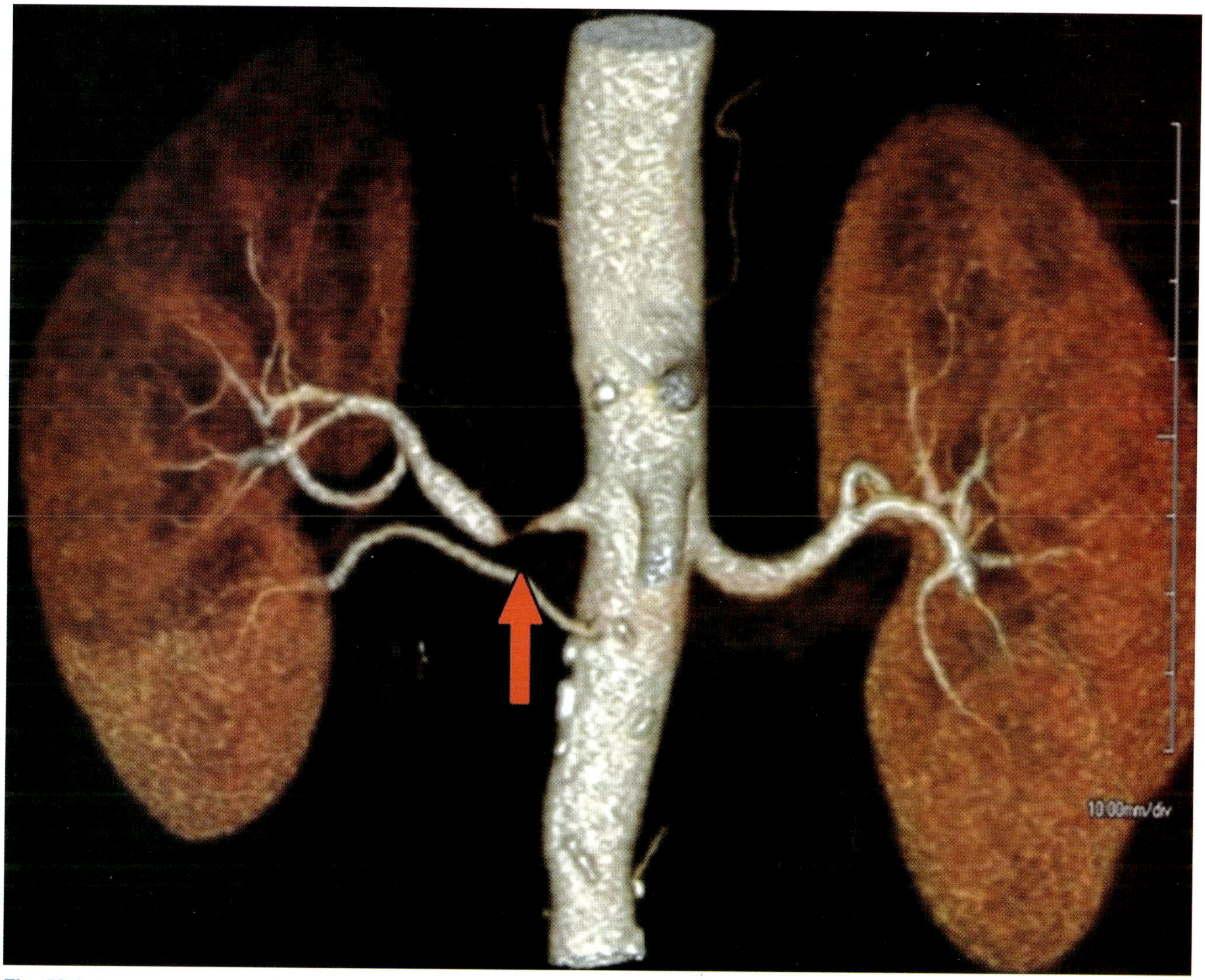

Fig. 52.1: Renal artery stenosis (RAS) demonstrated by computed tomographic angiography (CTA).

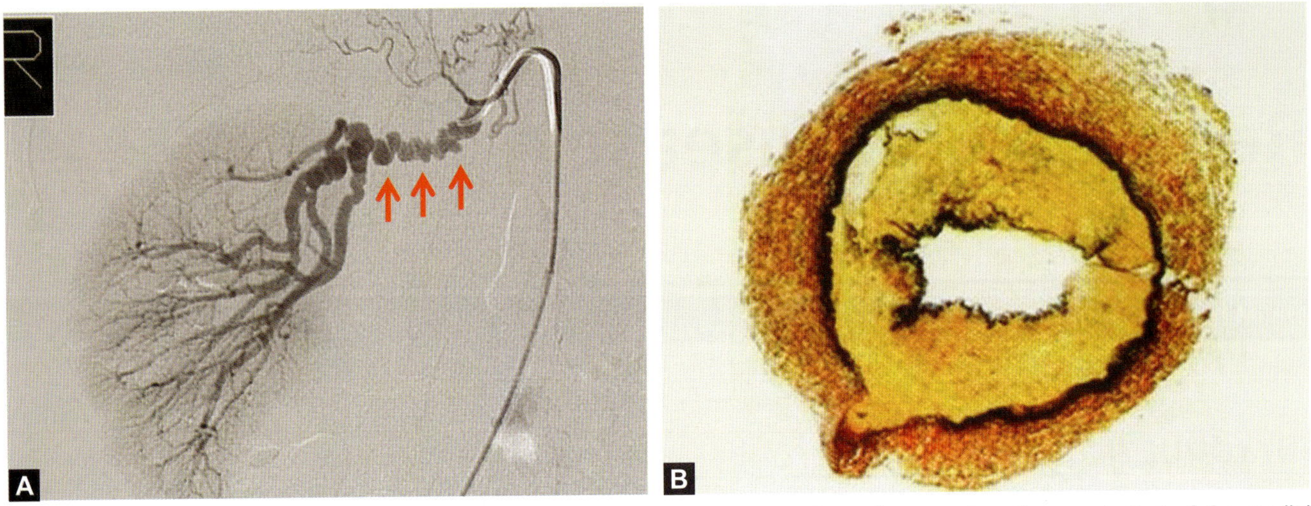

Figs. 52.2A and B: Fibromuscular dysplasia (FMD). (A) Digital subtraction angiography revealing changes typical of the medial fibroplasias variant of FMD; (B) Pathology specimen demonstrating FMD leading to narrowing of the renal arterial lumen.

59% of patients. ARAS has been implicated as a cause for HTN, deteriorating renal function and cardiac disturbance syndromes (recurrent unexplained congestive heart failure, refractory angina and "flash" pulmonary edema).

Renal artery stenosis (RAS) may be due to other etiologies, most notably fibromuscular dysplasia (FMD) (Figs. 52.2A and B).

Hypertension related to underlying RAS should be suspected in individuals who are either young (suggesting a non-atherosclerotic etiology) or older than 55 years at the time of onset of HTN. Resistant HTN, defined as the inability to achieve goal blood pressure of 140/90 mm Hg or lower, despite the use of three anti hypertensive medications at maximum tolerable doses used in appropriate combinations is another important clinical clue for underlying RAS.

DIAGNOSTIC MODALITIES

Renal artery duplex ultrasonography (RADUS) (Figs. 52.3 and 52.4), computed tomographic angiography (CTA) (Figs. 52.5A to C) and magnetic resonance angiography (MRA) (Figs. 52.6A and B) can all be used for both diagnosis and surveillance of renovascular disease. Typically, ARAS presents as aorto-ostial disease, representing plaque from the abdominal aorta draped into the origin of the renal artery. Stenosis is diagnosed by RADUS using peak systolic velocities (PSVs) within the renal artery as well as the ratio of the PSV as measured in the renal artery and comparing this to the PSV in the aorta at the level of the superior mesenteric artery [renal to aortic ratio (RAR)]. Categorization of RAS by RADUS includes 0–59% stenosis, 60–99% stenosis, or occluded. Findings suggestive of a 60–99% stenosis include a PSV > 200 cm with post-stenotic turbulence, a RAR > 3.5, and a parvus et tardus waveform in the distal main renal artery or parenchymal branches. Table 52.1 offers a comparison of the advantages and disadvantages of the various imaging modalities.

An invasive modality that can be used to assess the hemodynamic significance of a RAS is the use of pressure wire (Fig. 52.7). In general, a dopamine-induced drop in mean systolic pressure of at least 20 mm Hg is usually considered clinically significant.

INDICATIONS FOR A PROCEDURE

Optimal medical therapy is the backbone of treatment for ARAS in order to control blood pressure and reduce cardiovascular risk. Current guidelines suggest that intervention for ARAS should be offered only to symptomatic patients. A class IIa recommendation was assigned to treating patients with hemodynamically significant RAS and accelerated, resistant or malignant HTN, HTN with an unexplained unilateral small kidney, and HTN with intolerance to medications. Other indications for intervention include progressive chronic kidney disease over the past 3–6 months with bilateral RAS or a RAS to a solitary functioning kidney, unstable angina, recurrent unexplained congestive heart failure or sudden unexplained pulmonary edema. Importantly, not all patients respond favorably to treatment of ARAS, and identifying patients who will respond

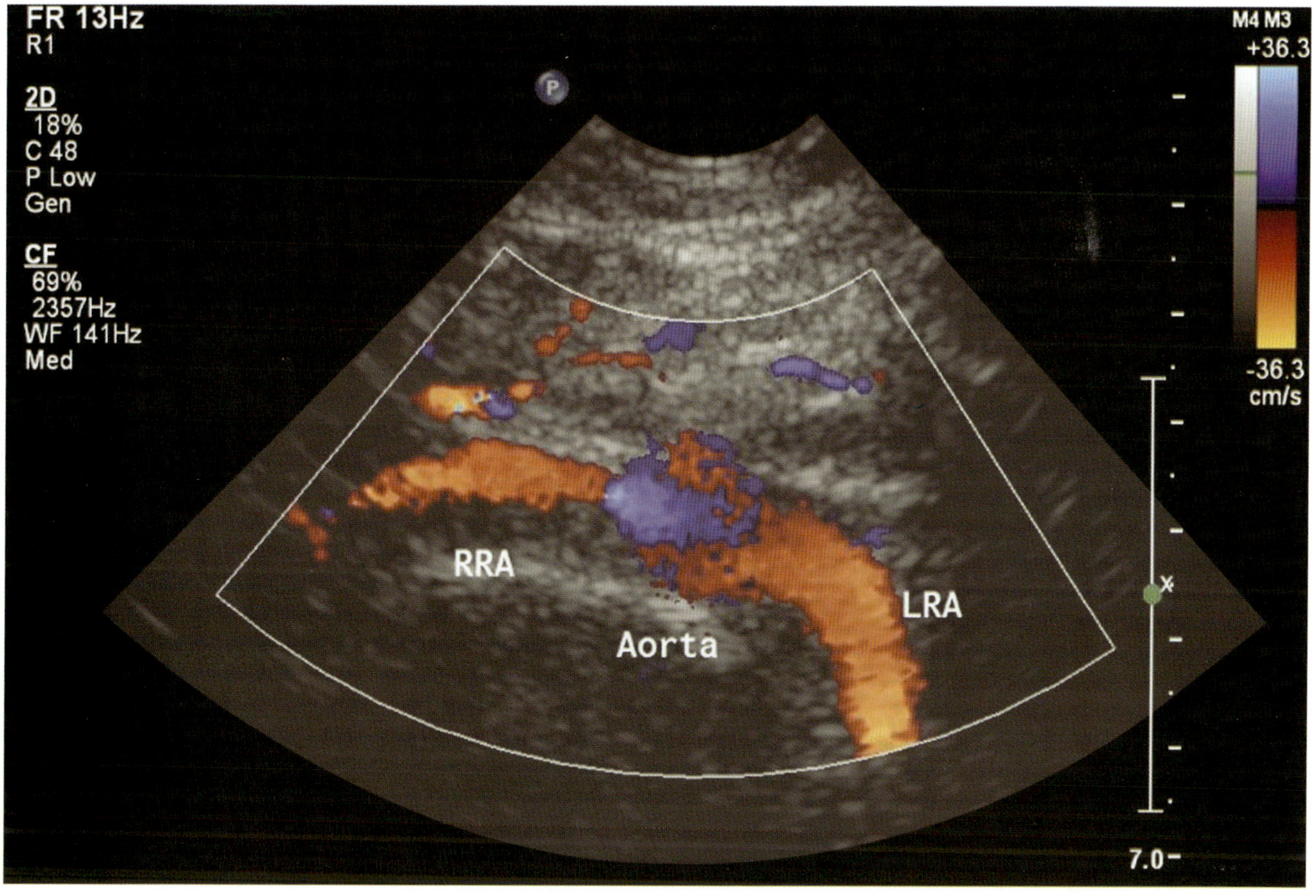

Fig. 52.3: Color flow duplex ultrasound showing the aorta and the two renal arteries from the midline approach. (RRA: Right renal artery; LRA: Left renal artery).

prior to intervention is not straightforward. Aside from identifying hemodynamically significant stenosis, other parameters that are usually considered include degree of HTN, rate of deterioration in renal function, kidney size, cortical thickness, and renal resistive index, among others. Typically, intervention for ARAS includes endovascular renal artery stent revascularization (Figs. 52.8A to D), while patients with FMD do well with percutaneous transluminal balloon angioplasty alone (Figs. 52.8E to G). Furthermore, potential complications must be considered when weighing the benefits and risks of intervention. Local access site complications include hematoma, retroperitoneal hemorrhage, and pseudoaneurysm. Systemic complications include deterioration in renal function (from either contrast-induced acute tubular necrosis or renal atheromatous embolization), renal artery dissection, renal artery occlusion, perforation and death. Finally, it is noteworthy that three contemporary prospective trials examining the efficacy of intervention as compared with medical treatment for ARAS have raised concerns regarding the benefit of intervention. However, despite the prospective, multicenter nature of these trials, they all suffer from inherent flaws that impair our ability to draw conclusions.

RENAL DENERVATION

However, when SYMPLICITY-HTN-3 was published, the delta between the treated arm and sham control arm was insignificant, raising considerable concerns regarding the potential for these technologies to offer significant improvement in control of resistant hypertension.

A novel intervention with potential to become an important management tool for patients with medication-resistant HTN is catheter-based renal artery sympathetic denervation (Figs. 52.9A to E). While the first studies were performed with the SYMPLICITY catheter (Medtronic, Minneapolis, MN, USA), trials with other devices are well under way. In patients with normal appearing renal arteries and resistant HTN, this treatment has shown great promise.

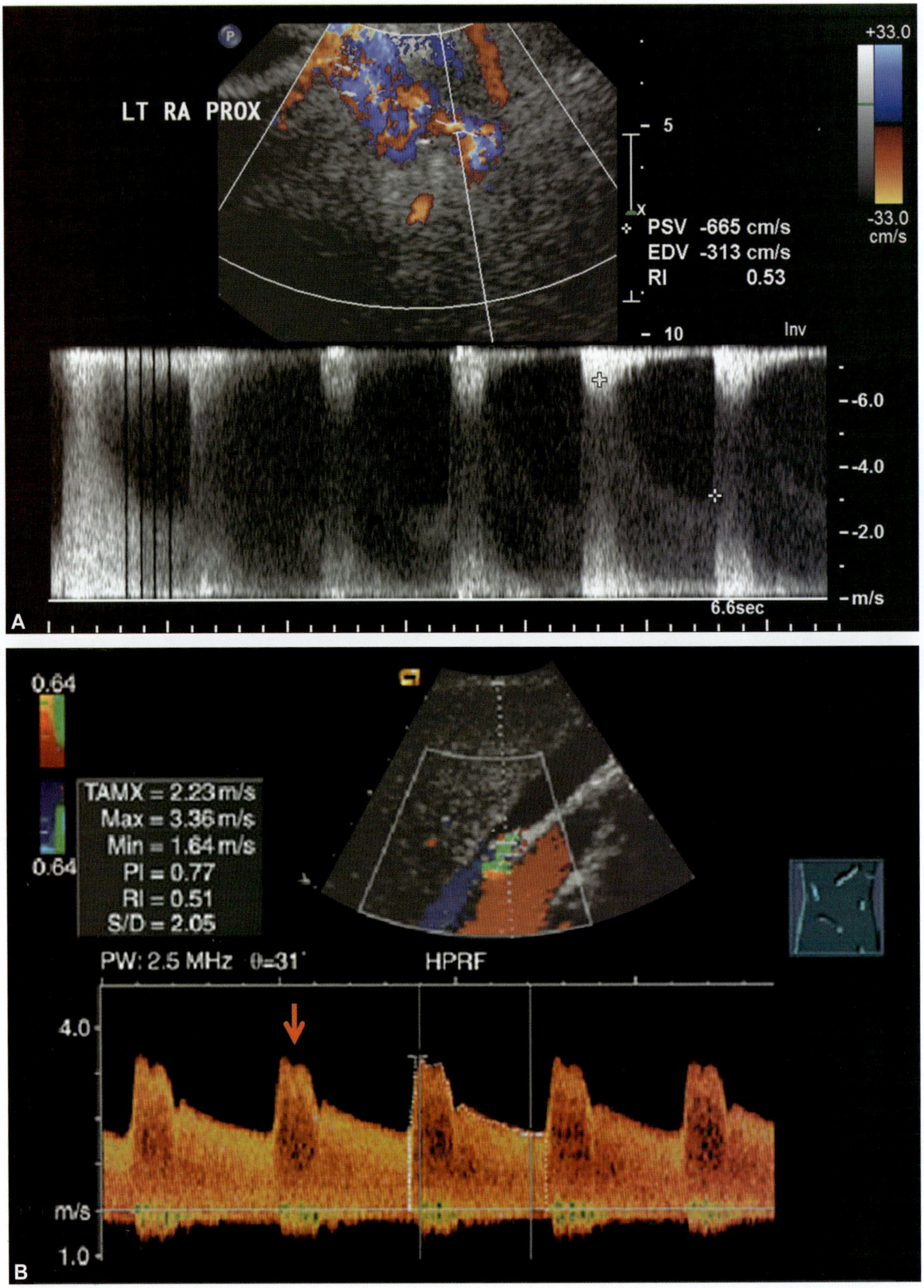

Figs. 52.4A and B: Pulse wave Doppler showing an elevated peak systolic velocity (PSV) (arrow) at the origin of the renal artery.

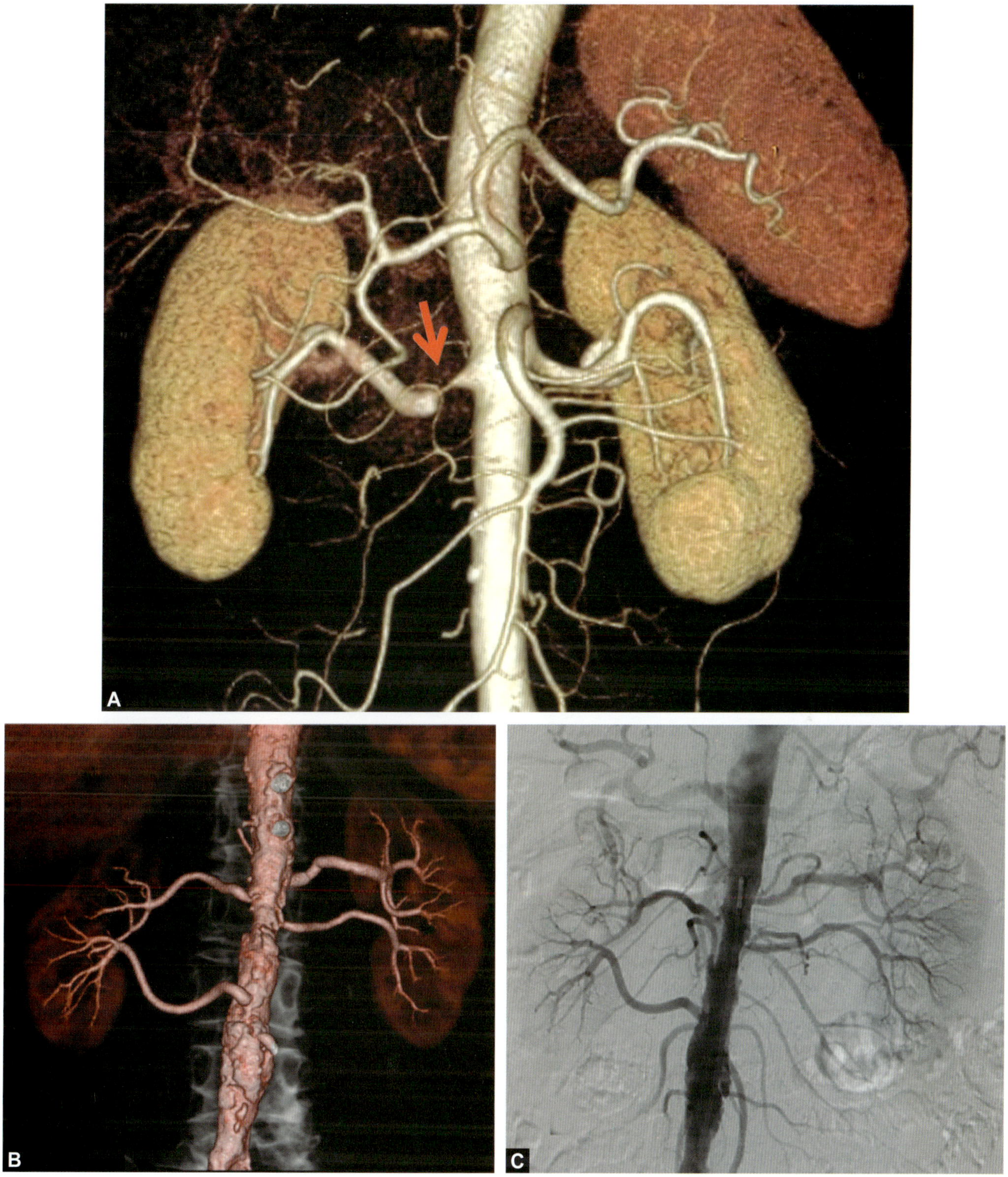

Figs. 52.5A to C: Computed tomographic angiography (CTA) of the renal arteries. (A) A three-dimensional reconstruction of a contrast-enhanced CTA showing right renal artery (RRA) stenosis (arrow); (B and C) CTA revealing multiple renal arteries to each kidney. Note the close correlation with findings with invasive angiography. [Image from Yokoi Y. Angiography for peripheral vascular intervention. In: Forbes TJ (Ed). Angioplasty, Various Techniques and Challenges in the Treatment of Congenital and Acquired Vascular Stenoses. InTech. 2012. pp. 121-68].

Table 52.1: Comparison of the advantages and disadvantages of imaging modalities for atherosclerotic renal artery (ARA) disease. (RADUS: Renal artery duplex ultrasonography; CTA: Computerized tomography angiography; MRA: Magnetic resonance angiography).

	RADUS	*CTA*	*MRA*
Cost	Most inexpensive		
Safe	+	± (radiation, contrast)	± (contrast)
Comfortable for the patient	+	±	– (for some patients)
Accuracy (compared to contrast angiography)	+	+	+
Ability to assess within calcifications	–	–	+
Ability to diagnose in-stent restenosis	+	+	–
Ability to assess distal lesions accurately	±	±	±
Visualization of accessory renal arteries	±	+	+
Visualization of extra renal structures	–	+	+
Common contraindications	None	Contrast allergy, renal dysfunction	Claustrophobia, metallic implants, renal dysfunction

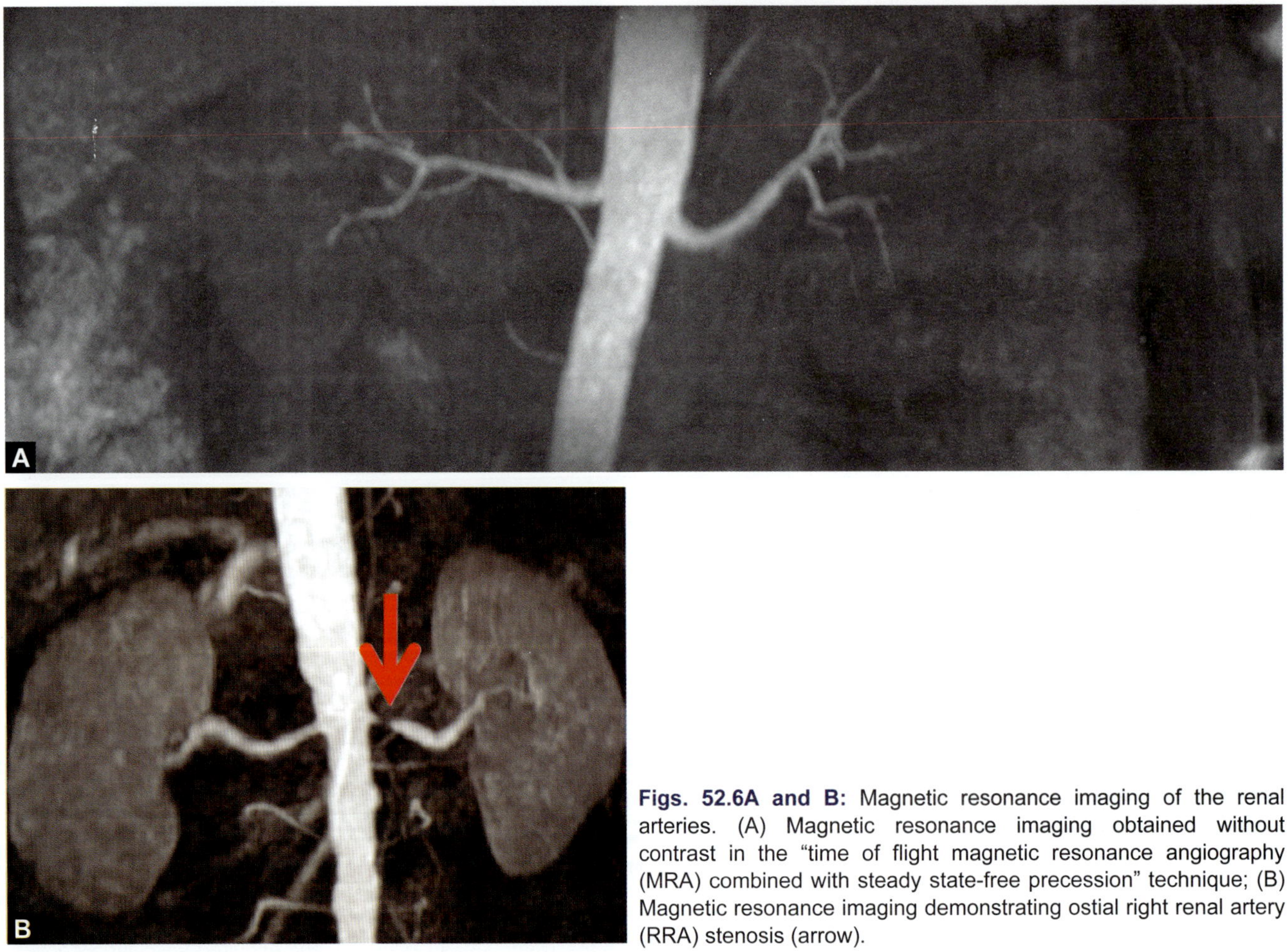

Figs. 52.6A and B: Magnetic resonance imaging of the renal arteries. (A) Magnetic resonance imaging obtained without contrast in the "time of flight magnetic resonance angiography (MRA) combined with steady state-free precession" technique; (B) Magnetic resonance imaging demonstrating ostial right renal artery (RRA) stenosis (arrow).

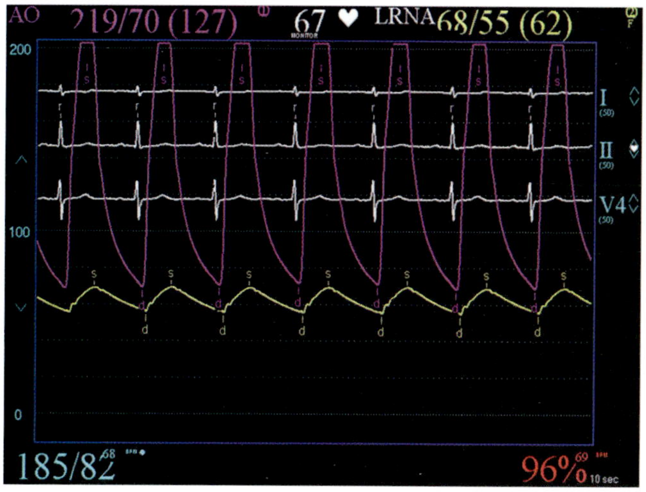

Fig. 52.7: Pressure wire derived measurements across a renal artery lesion consistent with hemodynamically significant renal artery stenosis (RAS).

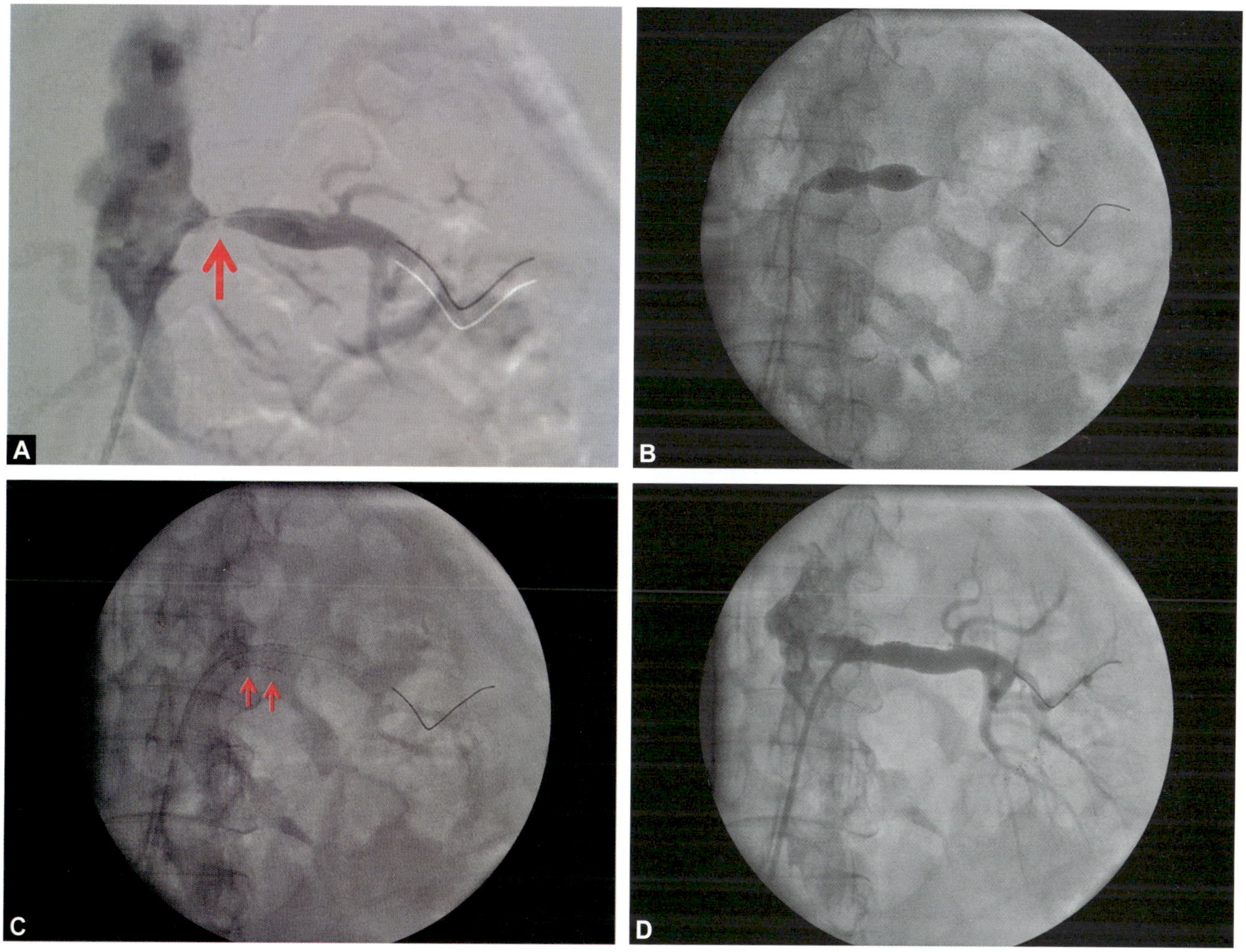

Figs. 52.8A to D: Stenting of renal artery stenosis (RAS). (A) Digital subtraction angiography demonstrating a stenosis (arrow) in the proximal renal artery; (B) Balloon inflation within the stenosis; (C) Stent deployed (arrows) within the proximal renal artery, adequately protruding into the aorta; (D) Final angiogram demonstrating treated stenosis.

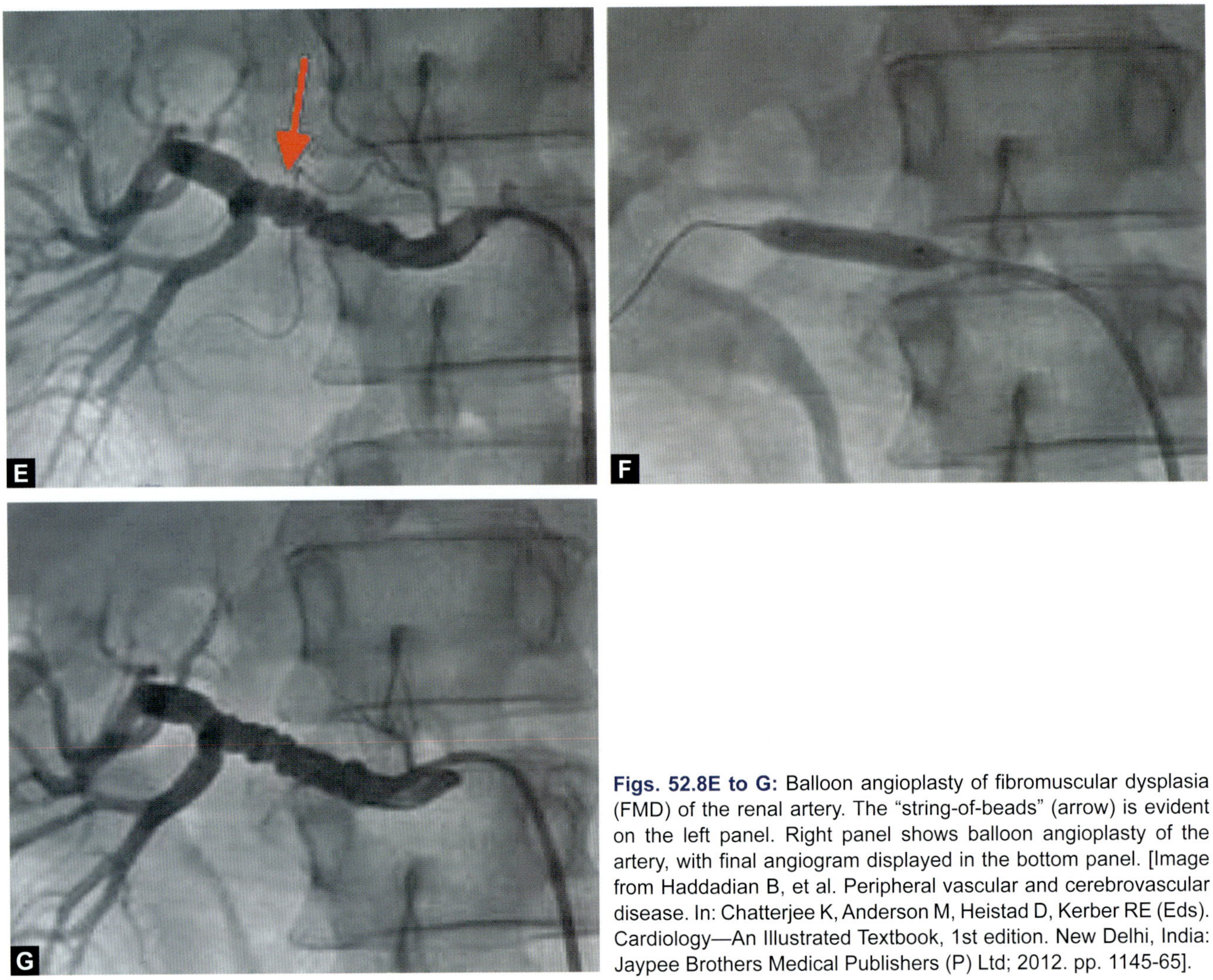

Figs. 52.8E to G: Balloon angioplasty of fibromuscular dysplasia (FMD) of the renal artery. The "string-of-beads" (arrow) is evident on the left panel. Right panel shows balloon angioplasty of the artery, with final angiogram displayed in the bottom panel. [Image from Haddadian B, et al. Peripheral vascular and cerebrovascular disease. In: Chatterjee K, Anderson M, Heistad D, Kerber RE (Eds). Cardiology—An Illustrated Textbook, 1st edition. New Delhi, India: Jaypee Brothers Medical Publishers (P) Ltd; 2012. pp. 1145-65].

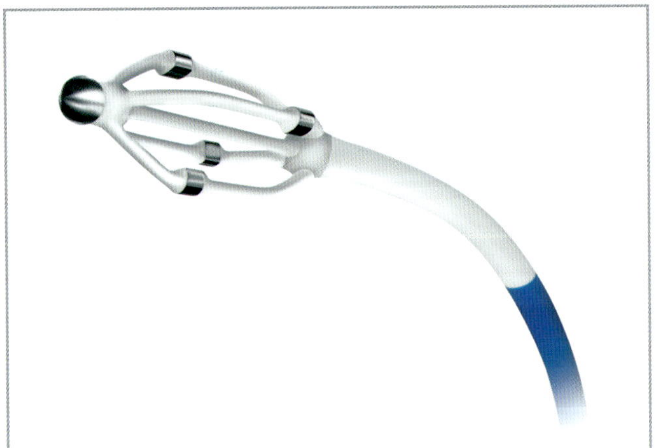

Fig. 52.9A: Renal artery denervation. (A) EnligHTN multi-electrode ablation catheter. (Image provided courtesy of St. Jude Medical).

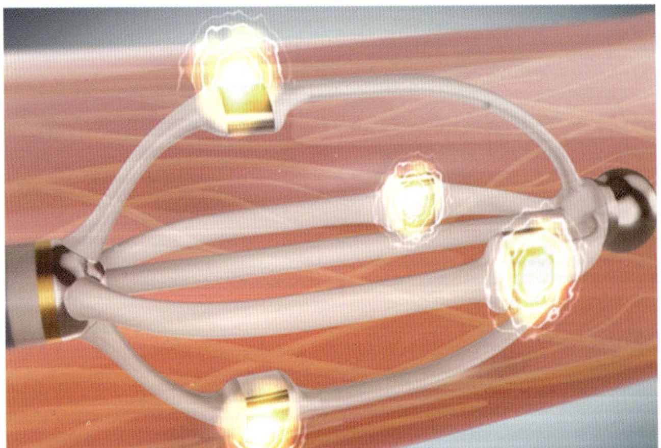

Fig. 52.9B: Illustration of the EnligHTN catheter in the renal artery. (Image provided courtesy of St. Jude Medical).

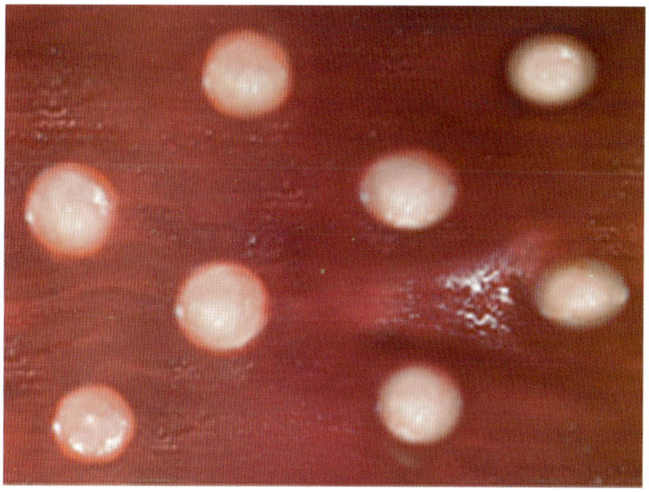

Fig. 52.9C: Pattern of renal artery ablation with the EnligHTN multi-electrode ablation. (Image provided courtesy of St. Jude Medical).

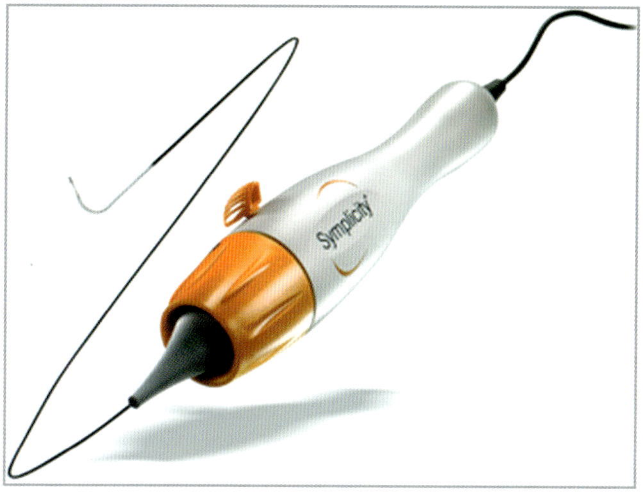

Fig. 52.9D: Medtronic SYMPLICITY ablation catheter. (Image courtesy of Medtronic Inc.).

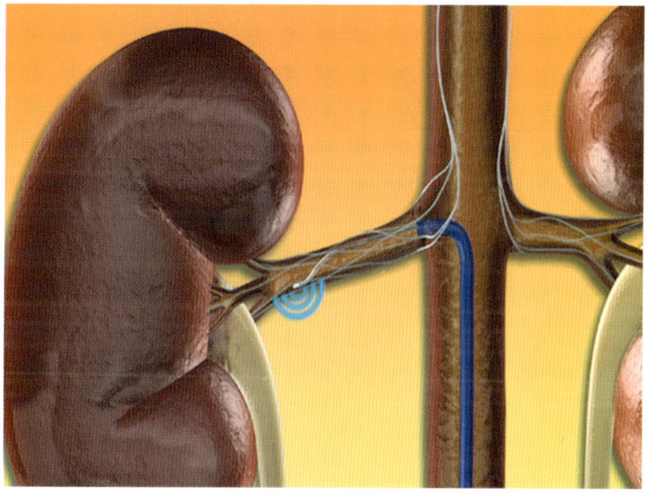

Fig. 52.9E: Renal denervation using the SYMPLICITY catheter. (Image courtesy of Medtronic Inc.).

CONCLUSIONS

Atherosclerotic RAS is prevalent and has potential serious medical consequences. Treatment options are medical and interventional. The key component for clinical efficacy of an interventional procedure most likely resides in proper patient selection. While some indications for intervention remain unequivocal, there is no clinically useful tool to predict which patients will benefit from improved blood pressure control and preservation of renal function.

REFERENCES

Bhatt DL, Kandzari DE, O'Neill WW, et al. SYMPLICITY HTN-3 Investigators. A controlled trial of renal denervation for resistant hypertension. N Engl J Med. 2014 Apr 10;370(15):1393-401.

Davis MI, Filion KB, Zhang D, et al. Effectiveness of renal denervation therapy for resistant hypertension: a systematic review and meta-analysis. J Am Coll Cardiol. 2013;62(3):231-41.

Dworkin LD, Cooper CJ. Clinical practice. Renal-artery stenosis. N Engl J Med. 2009;361(20):1972-8.

Hansen KJ, Edwards MS, Craven TE, et al. Prevalence of renovascular disease in the elderly: a population-based study. J Vasc Surg. 2002;36(3):443-51.

Hirsch AT, Haskal ZJ, Hertzer NR, et al. ACC/AHA 2005 Practice Guidelines for the management of patients with peripheral arterial disease (lower extremity, renal, mesenteric, and abdominal aortic): a collaborative report from the American Association for Vascular Surgery/Society for Vascular Surgery, Society for Cardiovascular Angiography and Interventions, Society for Vascular Medicine and Biology, Society of Interventional Radiology, and the ACC/AHA Task Force on Practice Guidelines (Writing Committee to Develop Guidelines for the Management of Patients With Peripheral Arterial Disease): endorsed by the American Association of Cardiovascular and Pulmonary Rehabilitation; National Heart, Lung, and Blood Institute; Society for Vascular Nursing; TransAtlantic Inter-Society Consensus; and Vascular Disease Foundation. Circulation. 2006;113(11):e463-654.

Jaff MR, Bates M, Sullivan T, et al. Significant reduction in systolic blood pressure following renal artery stenting in patients with uncontrolled hypertension: results from the HERCULES trial. Catheter Cardiovasc Interv. 2012;80(3): 343-50.

Olin JW, Melia M, Young JR, et al. Prevalence of atherosclerotic renal artery stenosis in patients with atherosclerosis elsewhere. Am J Med. 1990;88(1N):46N-51N.

Vasbinder GB, Nelemans PJ, Kessels AG, et al. Diagnostic tests for renal artery stenosis in patients suspected of having renovascular hypertension: a meta-analysis. Ann Intern Med. 2001;135(6):401-11.

CHAPTER

53

Peripheral Venous Insufficiency

Lorena Gonzalez, Carlos F Bechara, George T Pisimisis

VENOUS ANATOMY AND PHYSIOLOGY

There are two venous systems in the lower extremity, a superficial and a deep system, that are joined by venous perforators at various levels and contain numerous valves (Figs. 53.1A to C). The superficial system consists of the great and small saphenous veins—"saphenous" being derived from the Greek word "safaina", which means "evident". The great saphenous vein (GSV) may have significant variation in side branches, including anterior branches and duplication segments. It ascends from the ankle anterior to the medial malleolus, runs a course along the medial aspect of the leg, and joins the common femoral vein at the saphenofemoral junction. The lesser saphenous vein runs a course from the superficial dorsal venous arch behind the lateral malleolus and continues along the midline of the posterior calf to join the popliteal vein.

The deep system veins run in parallel courses to the arteries. At the tibial level, there are two or three vein satellites for each tibial artery that are tributed by muscular sinusoids, forming venous lakes within soleus muscle. Those paired tibial veins merge to form the popliteal vein, which has numerous side-branch collaterals. The collaterals form the deep femoral vein, while the main popliteal vein continues proximally as the femoral vein. At the groin level, the femoral and deep femoral veins merge to form the common femoral vein, situated medial to the femoral artery. The common femoral vein continues as the external iliac vein as it courses underneath and proximal to the inguinal ligament.

Valved venous perforators direct the blood flow from the superficial to the deep venous system of the leg (Fig. 53.2). There are numerous bicuspid thin venous valves that prevent reflux and therefore allow one-way direction of blood flow against gravity from the leg toward the heart. The number of valves decreases from distal leg veins to proximal iliofemoral veins (Fig. 53.3).

The pooled volume of blood and therefore the hydrostatic venous pressure in the lower extremities may increase significantly, when the body switches from reclined to a standing position. Veins dilate to accommodate the increased blood volume and the bicuspid valves close to further decrease reflux. However, even then the hydrostatic pressure generated by the vertical column of blood can exceed 100 cm H_2O at the lower leg in erect posture. Several mechanisms ensure return of the blood back to the heart and prevent venous stasis and overdistension. The first mechanism is the propulsion generated by the arterial inflow, in conjunction to the negative intrathoracic pressure generated during inspiration. Second, at any given time, the valves function in a sequential way to assure unidirectional flow of blood from superficial to deep systems and from the foot back to the heart. Third, as the calf muscles contract, the soleal venous sinusoids empty into the deep veins of the calf and leg (Figs. 53.4A and B). This powerful propulsion of blood with high-velocity stream generates negative pressure (Venturi effect) in the merging deep veins, which in turn siphons blood from those deep veins distally towards the more proximal leg. The expected significant drop in venous pressure with exercise occurring in healthy individuals may be only mild in patients with deep vein incompetence, while even an abnormal elevation is observed in those with proximal venous obstruction.

VARICOSE VEINS

Varicose veins are very common, with a two-year incidence rate of 4–5% according to the Framingham Study, affecting women more commonly than men. Risk factors include age, pregnancy, prolonged standing, prior deep venous thrombosis and genetic predisposition.

Varicose veins can be either primary or secondary. Primary varicose veins are most common and of uncertain

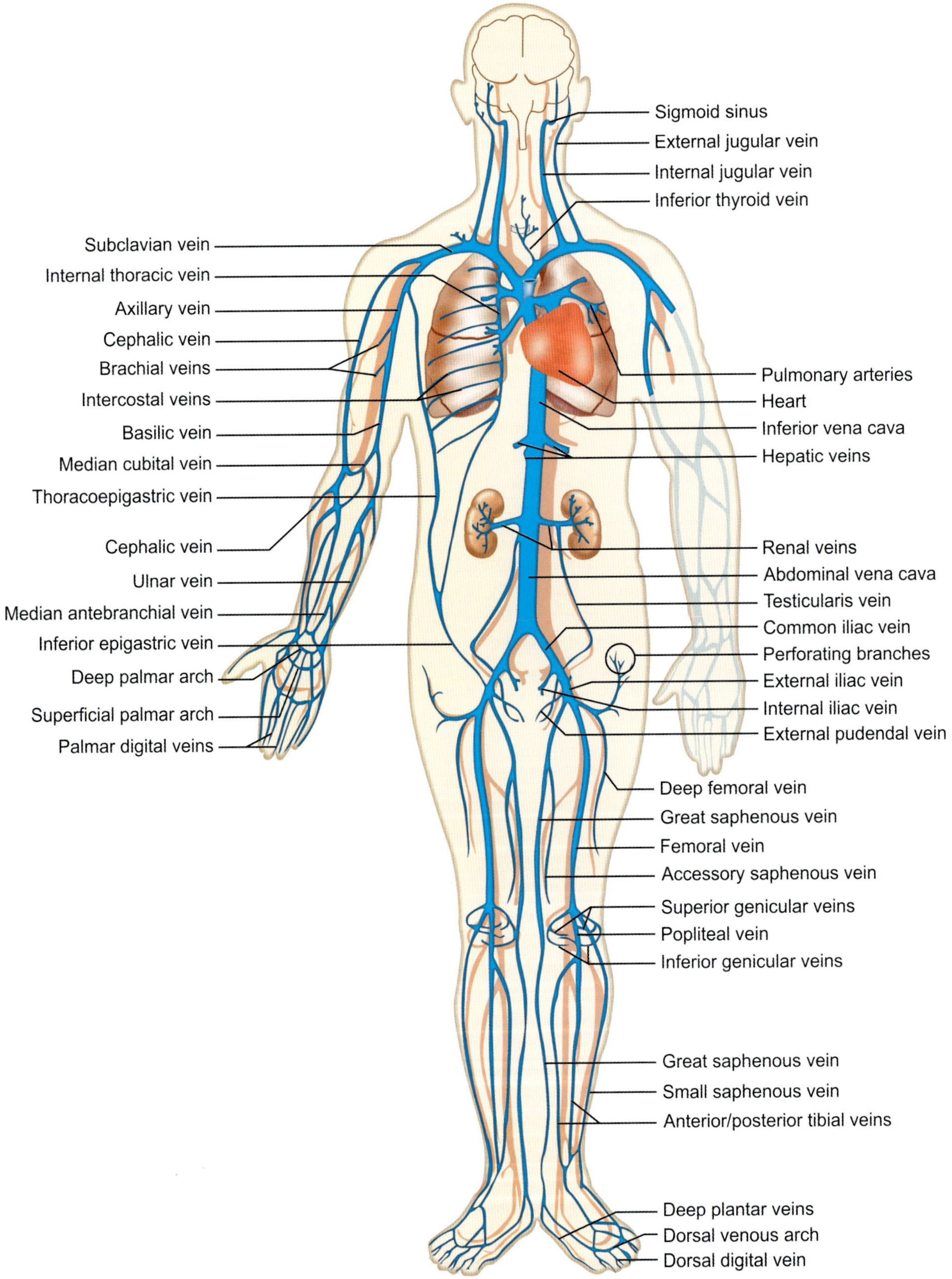

Fig. 53.1A: Venous circulation of the body. (Image created by LadyofHats and posted on Wikipedia Commons).

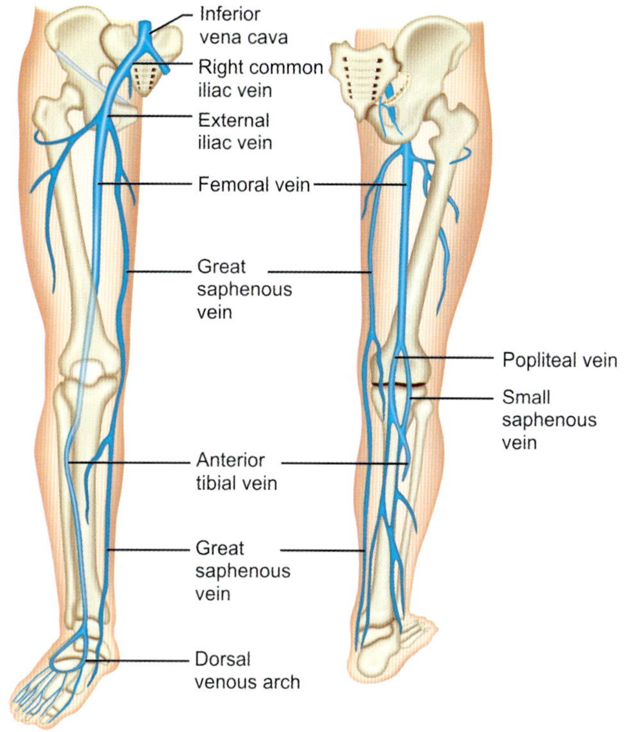

Fig. 53.1B: Veins of the lower extremity.

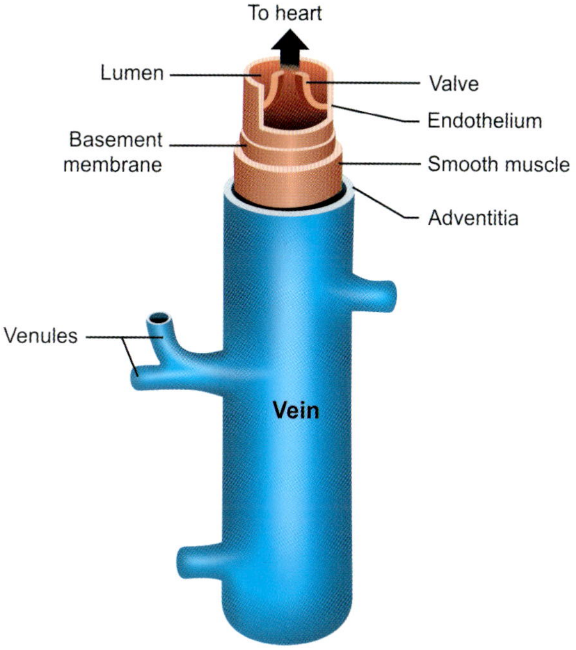

Fig. 53.1C: Structural components of a peripheral vein.

etiology, while secondary varicose veins are related to trauma, deep venous thrombosis, arteriovenous fistula or proximal venous obstruction that lead to valve dysfunction.

Clinical Findings

The clinical presentation of patients with varicose veins is variable (Fig. 53.5) and are classified by clinical, etiologic, anatomic and pathophysiologic criteria (CEAP) based on severity as shown in Table 53.1.

In young patients with extensive varicose veins, Klippel-Trenaunay syndrome should be considered, especially if distribution of the varicose veins involves the lateral leg, a port wine cutaneous malformation (port-wine stain) (Fig. 53.6), and there is limb hypertrophy. In these patients, the deep veins are often anomalous or absent, therefore saphenous vein stripping can be detrimental and limited surgical treatment options are available.

Non-Surgical Treatment

Initial treatment for varicose veins initially pertains to management of venous insufficiency, such as elastic stocking support, periodic leg elevation, avoidance of prolonged sitting or standing posture, and regular exercise. For mild cases, knee-high or thigh-high gradient compression stockings of 15–20 mm Hg should suffice, while more symptomatic patients benefit from 20 mm Hg to 30 mm Hg compression, and in some cases up to 30–40 mm Hg gradient. The compression stockings are not recommended to be worn in the supine position, in order to avoid lower extremity ischemia.

Surgical Treatment

Surgical treatment is indicated for failure of conservative management, persistent pain, venous stasis skin changes, recurrent leg ulcers or bleeding. A "softer" but common indication is cosmetic appearance, especially in female patients.

Preoperative planning includes venous reflux studies to determine the competency of the superficial, deep and perforating veins and the location of those incompetent sites. An older but effective technique for patients with proximal GSV reflux involves high ligation of the GSV at the saphenofemoral junction, followed by stripping of the vein from that level to the knee (Figs. 53.7A and B). More

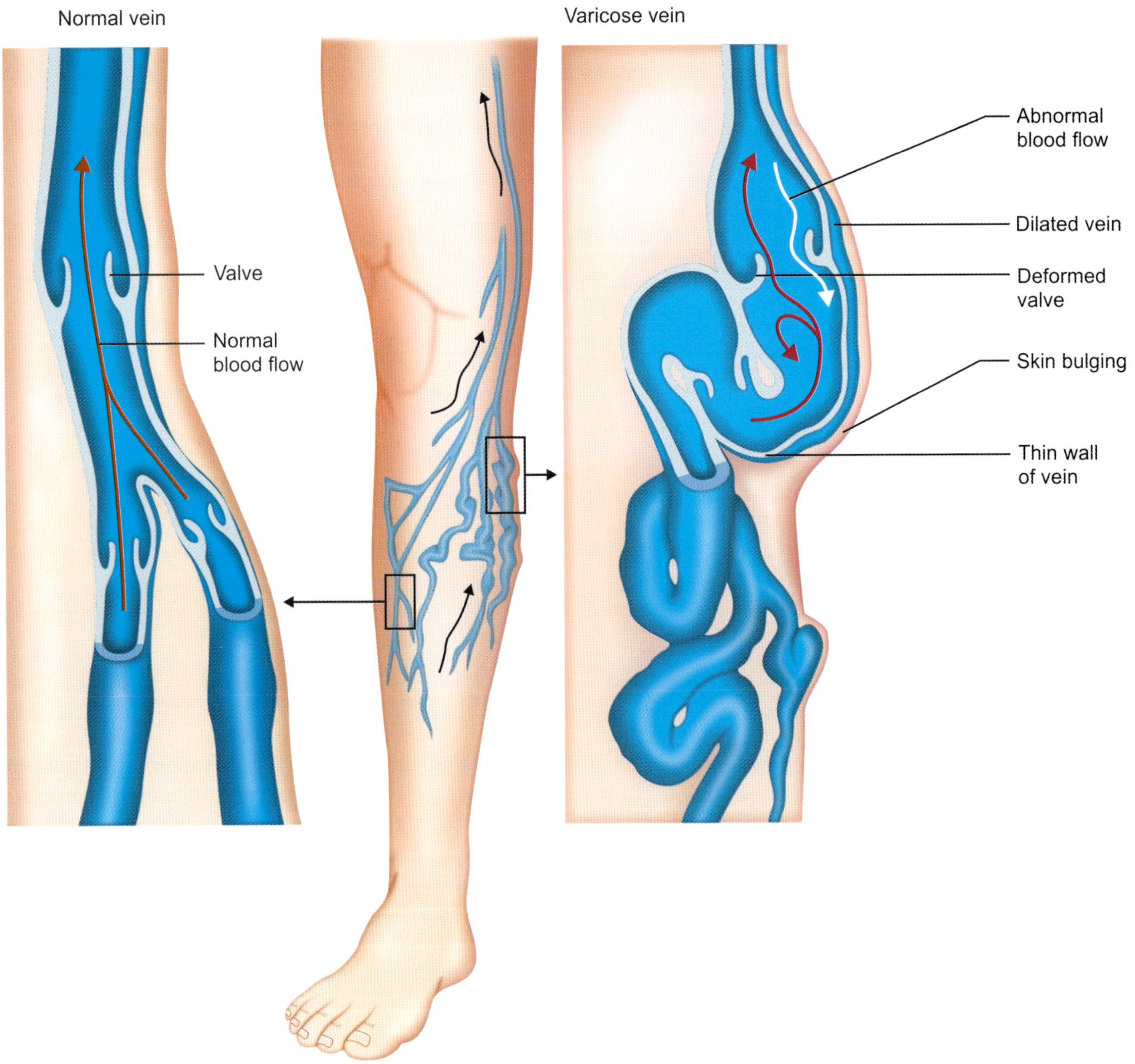

Fig. 53.2: Mechanism of venous flow direction from deep to superficial systems and varicose vein development resulting from valve failure. (Image from the National Heart, Lung and Blood Institute. Image posted on Wikipedia.org).

modern methods can ablate the GSV with endovascular techniques using either radiofrequency ablation (RFA) or endovenous laser treatment (EVLT) (Fig. 53.8A). Isolated clusters of varicose veins can then be removed by the stab-phlebectomy technique that pertains to small 2 mm stab incisions over premarked varicosities, followed by avulsion and removal of the varicosities using dedicated vein hooks (Fig. 53.8B). The leg is then wrapped to avoid hematomas, and long-term compression stockings are typically recommended to decrease risk of recurrence. Persistent small varicosities and spider veins (telangiectasias) can be addressed with sclerotherapy sessions that involve direct injection of sclerosing agent into the varix with eventual fibrotic degeneration. Possible complications include hematoma, infection, saphenous nerve neuropathy, thrombophlebitis, and deep venous thrombosis.

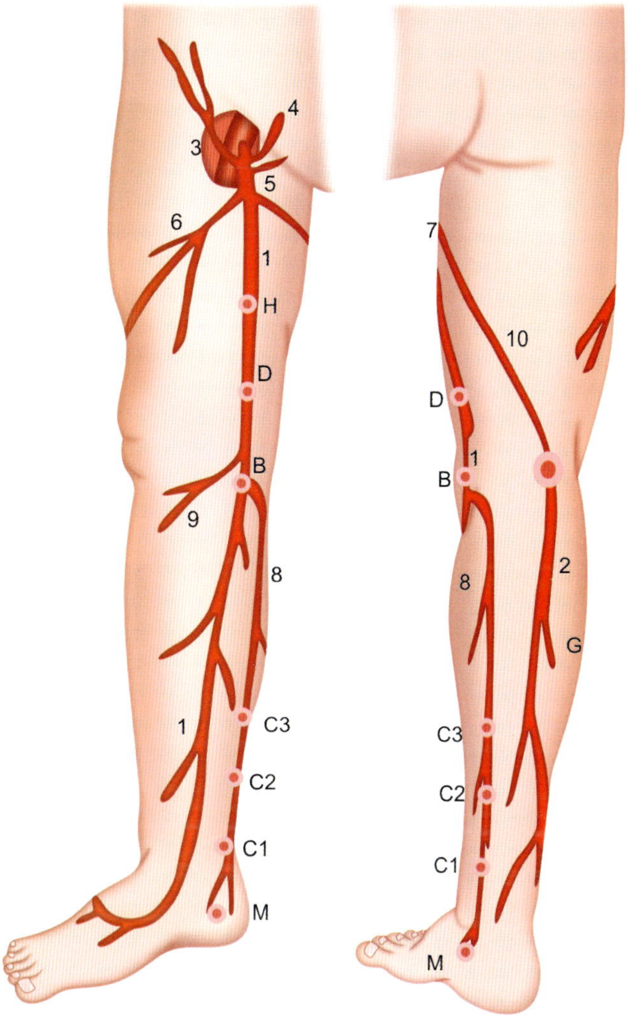

Fig. 53.3: Superficial venous system and perforators of lower limb. Multilevel perforators are located at the level of the adductor canal (H = Hunterian perforator), above the knee (D = Dodd perforator), below the knee (B = Boyd perforator), medial calf (C = Cockett perforators), and below the medial malleolus (M = medial inframalleolar perforator). [Image from Khanna AK. Varicose Veins. In: Khanna AK, Puneet. Manual of Vascular Surgery. New Delhi, India: Jaypee Brothers Medical Publishers (P) Ltd.; 2011].

CHRONIC VENOUS INSUFFICIENCY

Chronic venous insufficiency may involve both superficial and deep systems, but mainly relates to deep system venous reflux. The etiology includes congenital valvular insufficiency, proximal venous obstruction (i.e. May-Thurner syndrome, Figs. 53.9A to C) or previous venous thrombosis (post-thrombotic syndrome). Presentation can range from edema, leg pain upon prolonged standing or sitting, varicose veins, venous stasis pigmentation changes and skin ulceration. In cases of leg pain, heaviness and edema upon ambulation due to proximal venous obstruction, the term *venous claudication* is used. Deep veins are primarily involved; although perforators and superficial veins may also be involved. Occasionally, in cases of deep vein sclerotic obstruction, the superficial veins will dilate and reflux earlier, following a more progressive course.

In areas of significant subcutaneous venous congestion, there is extravasation of plasma, leading to edema. Extravasated red blood cells are lysed and hemosiderin deposits lead to the brown discoloration of the skin. In more severe cases, an inflammatory and proteolytic response by sequestered leucocytes results in cutaneous inflammation, fibrosis and ulceration.

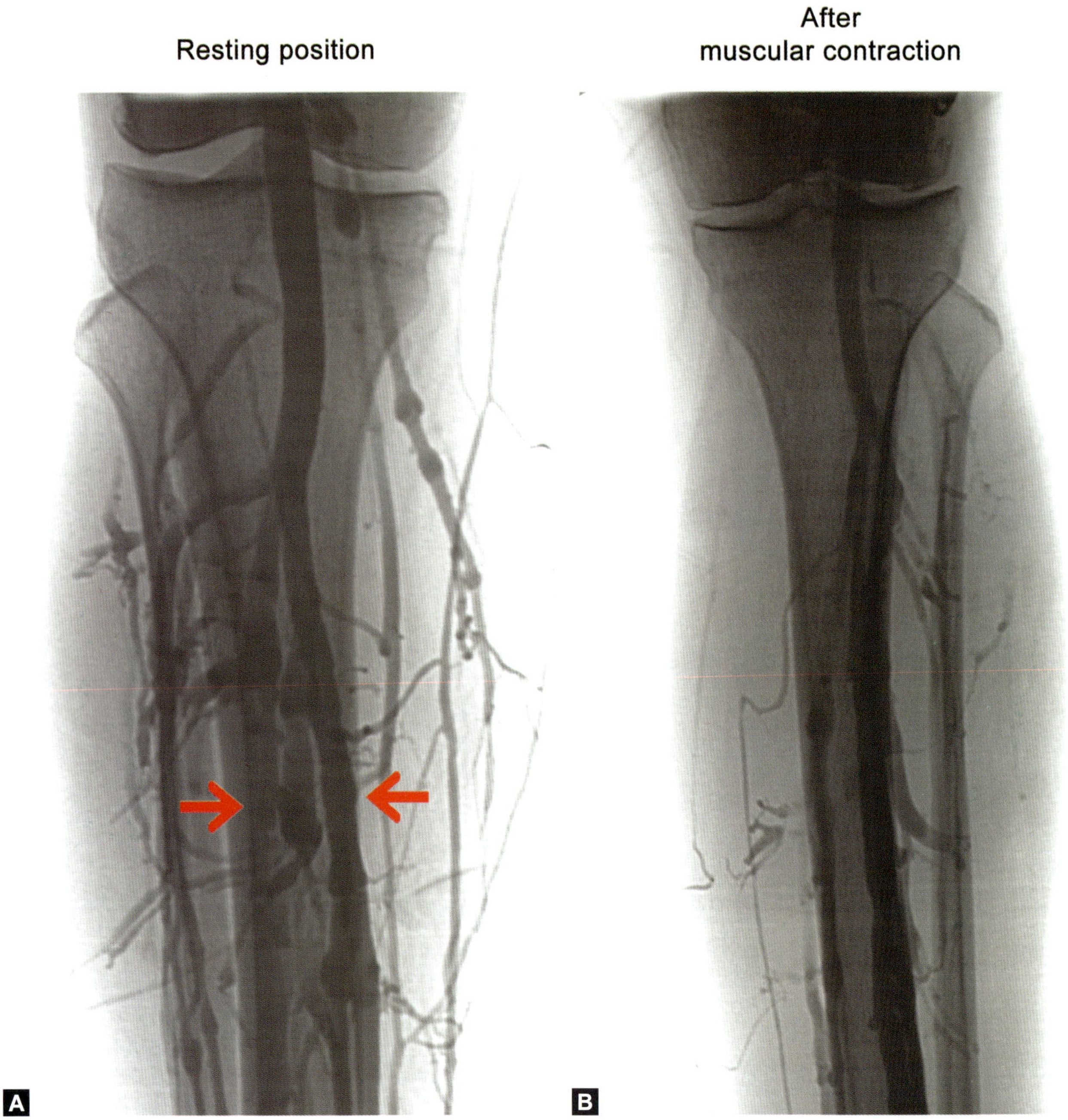

Figs. 53.4A and B: Filling and emptying of the deep venous veins. (A) In a resting position, the deep veins of the calf fill and enlarge (arrows), with the great saphenous vein remaining small, demonstrating normal perforating vein function. (B) Following muscular contraction, there is emptying of the deep veins. [Image from Link D. Late complications of deep venous thrombosis: painful swollen extremities and non-healing ulcers. In: Okuyan E (Ed). Venous Thrombosis—Principles and Practice. Shanghai: InTech; 2012].

Duplex ultrasound has become the main stay of diagnostic imaging. In experienced hands, it can identify location of incompetent valves within the deep system, perforating veins and along with the entire superficial system (Figs. 53.10A and B). Absence of respiratory variation raises suspicion of proximal obstruction. There are additional tests that complement duplex ultrasound, such as air plethysmography, which gives a quantitative assessment of venous reflux, calf muscle pump function, and overall venous function.

Advanced imaging techniques include ascending venography or CT/MR venography to assess for proximal

Table 53.1: Varicose vein CEAP classification schemes. (CEAP: Clinical, etiologic, anatomic and pathophysiologic criteria; CVD: Cardiovascular disease).

Categories of Clinical Classification	
0	No visible or palpable signs of venous disease
1	Telangiectases or reticular veins
2	Varicose veins; distinguished from reticular veins by a diameter of 3 mm or more
3	Edema without skin changes
4	Changes in skin and subcutaneous tissue secondary to CVD
4a	Pigmentation or eczema
4b	Lipodermatosclerosis
5	Healed venous ulcer
6	Active venous ulcer
Etiologic Classification	
Congenital	Apparent at birth or recognized later, e.g. Klippel-Trenaunay syndrome
Primary	Undetermined cause
Secondary	Known cause—post-thrombotic, post-traumatic
Other	No venous etiology identified
Anatomic Classification	
Superficial Veins	
1	Telangiectases/reticular veins
2	Greater (long) saphenous veins: above the knee
3	Greater (long) saphenous veins: below the knee
4	Lesser (short) saphenous vein
5	Non-saphenous
Deep veins	
6	Inferior vena cava
7	Iliac—common
8	Iliac—internal
9	Iliac—external
10	Pelvic—gonadal, broad ligament, other
11	Femoral—common
12	Femoral—deep
13	Femoral—superficial
14	Popliteal
15	Crural—anterior tibial, posterior tibial, peroneal (paired veins)
16	Muscular—gastrocnemial, soleal, other
17	Thigh
18	Calf
Pathophysiologic Classification	
Pr	Reflux (defined as reverse flow with a duration of >0.5 s by duplex ultrasonography)
Po	Obstruction
Pr,o	Reflux and obstruction
Pn	No venous pathophysiology identified

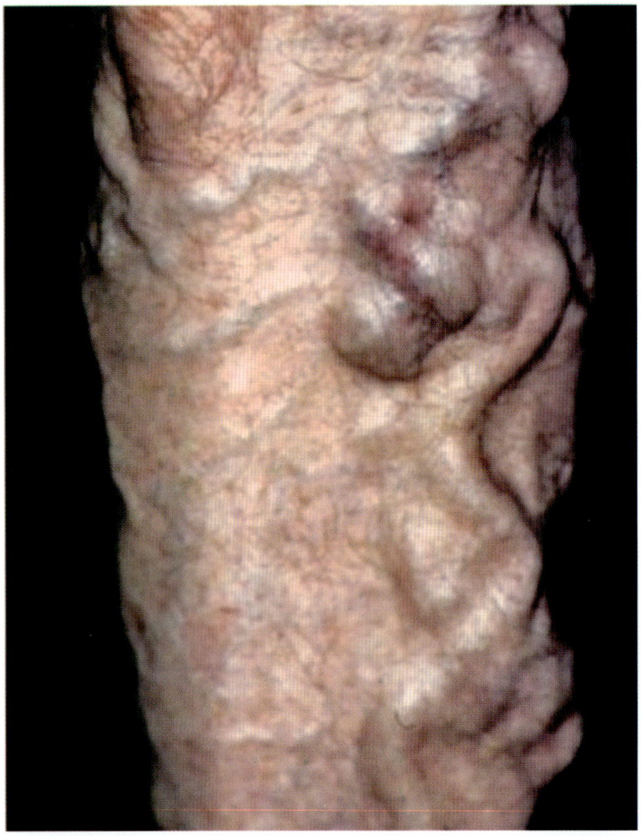

Fig. 53.5: Extensive lower extremity varicosities. [Image from Khanna AK. Varicose Veins. In: Khanna AK, Puneet. Manual of Vascular Surgery. New Delhi, India: Jaypee Brothers Medical Publishers (P) Ltd.; 2011].

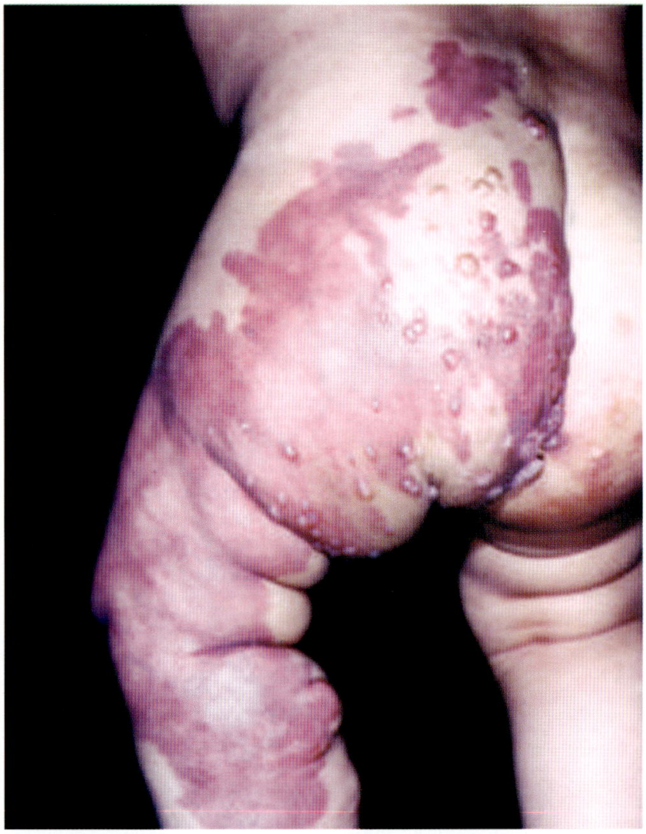

Fig. 53.6: Klippel-Trenaunay syndrome. Child with port-wine stain birthmark. [Image from Gontijo B, Pereira L, Silva C. Vascular malformations. An Bras Dermatol. 2004;79(1):7-25].

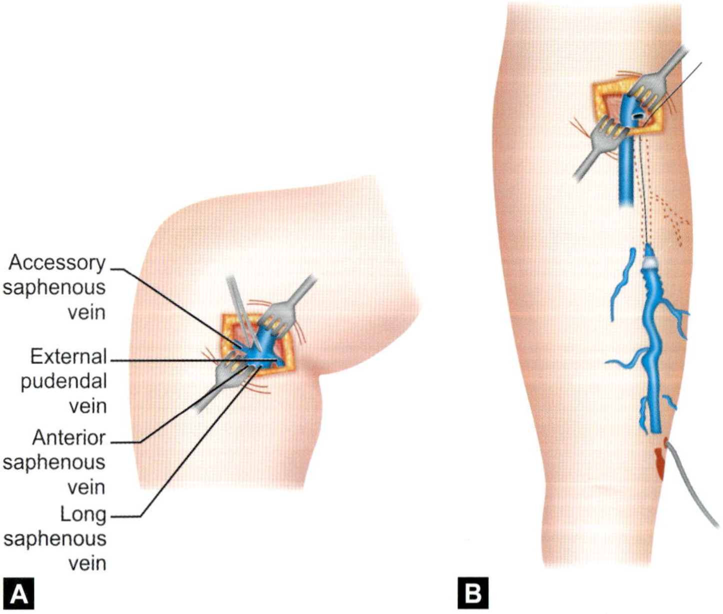

Figs. 53.7A and B: Technique of (A) Saphenofemoral junction exposure, (B) Great saphenous varicose vein stripping. [Image from Bergan JJ, Kistner RL. Atlas of Venous Surgery. Philadelphia: WB Saunders; 1992].

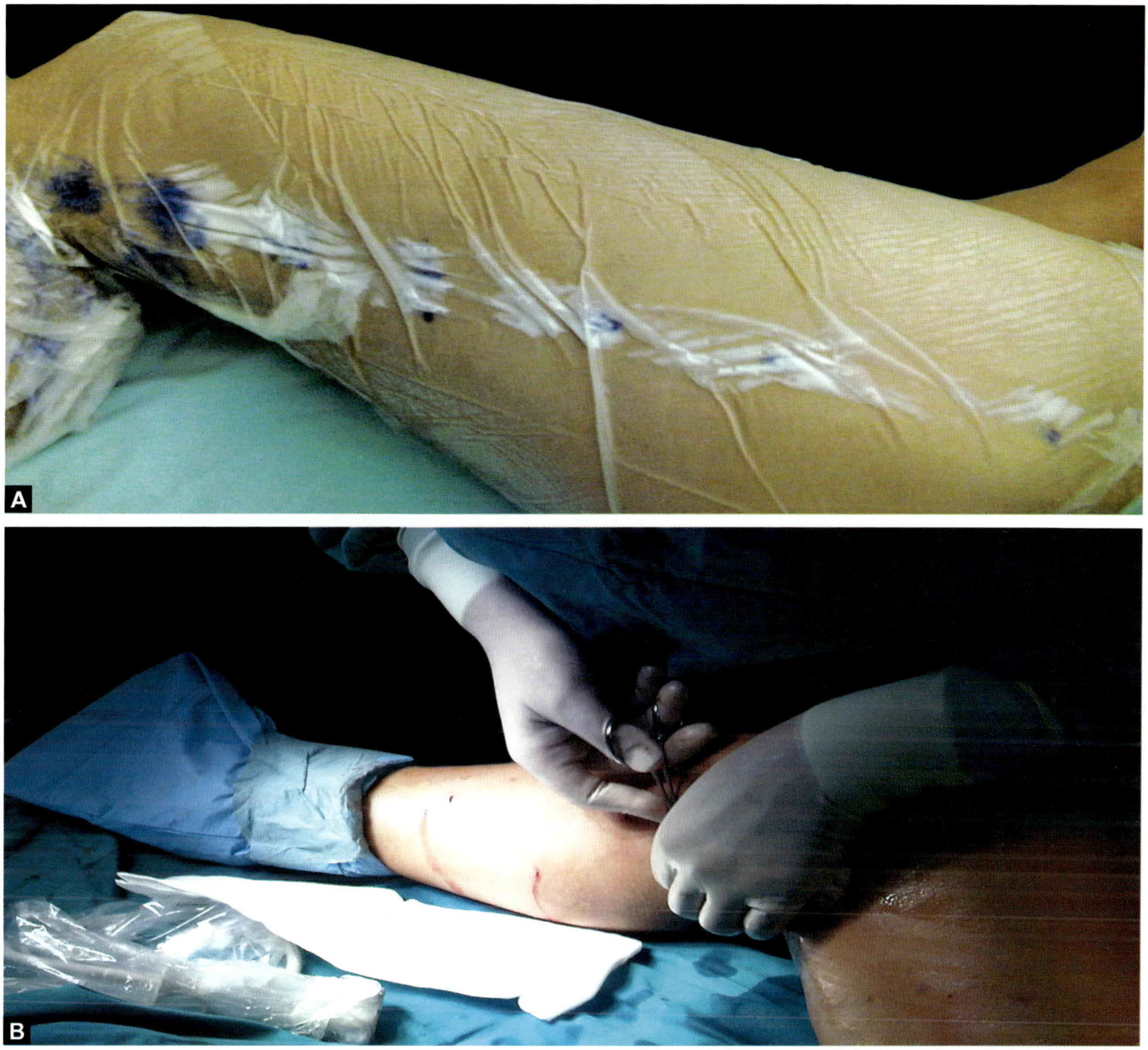

Figs. 53.8A and B: Endovascular laser treatment. (A) Duplex-guided intraoperative marking of the great saphenous vein in preparation for endovascular laser treatment. (B) Stab-phlebectomy performed immediately after the EVLT procedure. [Images from Vaz C Matos A, Pereira MSC, et al. Iatrogenic complications following laser ablation of varicose veins. In: Yamanouchi D (Ed). Vascular Surgery. Shanghai: InTech; 2012].

obstruction (Fig. 53.11). Descending venography involves injection of contrast into the common femoral vein to assess valve competence during normal breathing and Valsalva maneuver.

Treatment

Chronic venous insufficiency management follows the same principles as with varicose veins. Conservative methods with compressing stockings and lifestyle modifications are the cornerstone of treatment (Fig. 53.12).

Surgery is reserved for patients with non-healing ulcers or symptoms refractory to conservative management (Fig. 53.13). The first line of treatment is ablation of the superficial venous system, as long as it is demonstrated to be incompetent. In cases with incompetent perforators, ligation of the perforating veins can help heal or prevent recurrence of ulcerations. Wound complications are

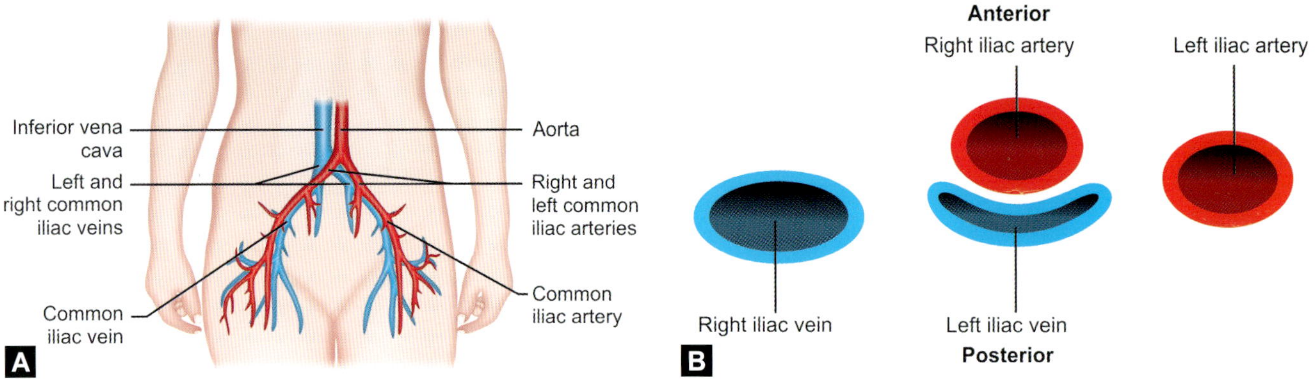

Figs. 53.9A and B: Schematic illustrations of May-Thurner syndrome in which the left common iliac artery compresses the left common iliac vein.

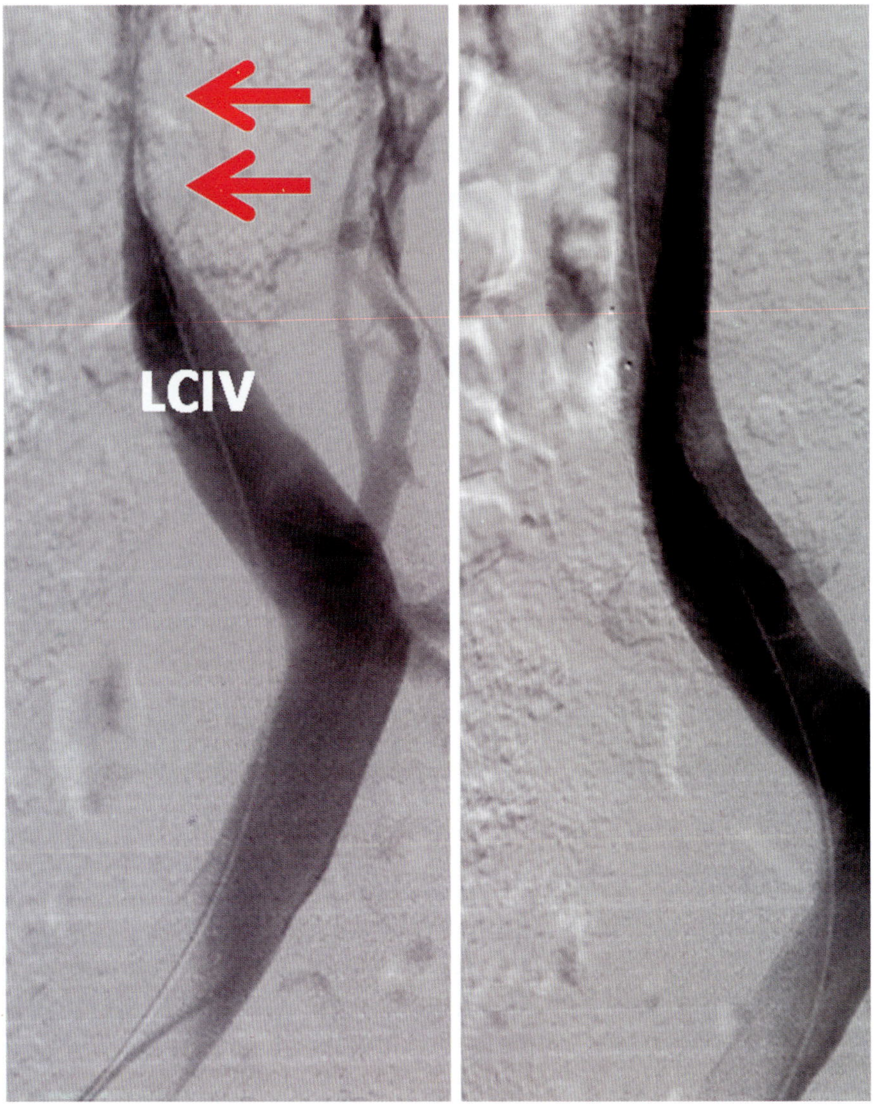

Fig. 53.9C: Venogram demonstrating May-Thurner syndrome. Left panel shows compression (arrows) of the left common iliac vein (LCIV). Right panel shows patency of the vein after stenting. (Image from Cerquozzi S, Pineo GF, Wong J, et al. Iliac vein compression syndrome in an active and healthy young female. Case Rep Med. 2012;2012:786876).

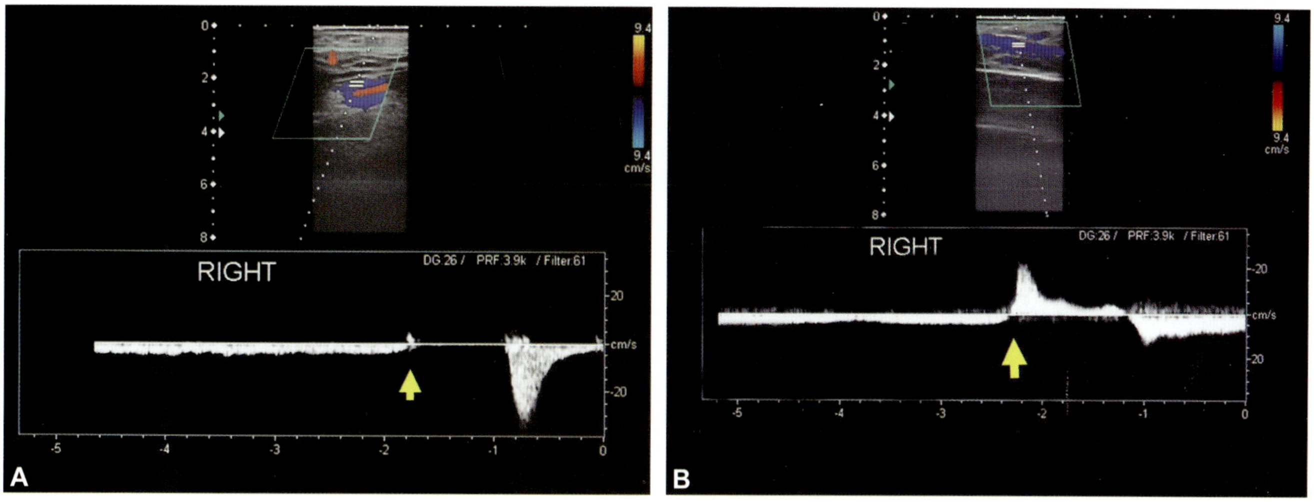

Figs. 53.10A and B: Color and spectral Doppler images of the femoral vein during Valsalva maneuver (arrow). (A) Normal study, and (B) moderate reflux which are indicative of valvular incompetence.

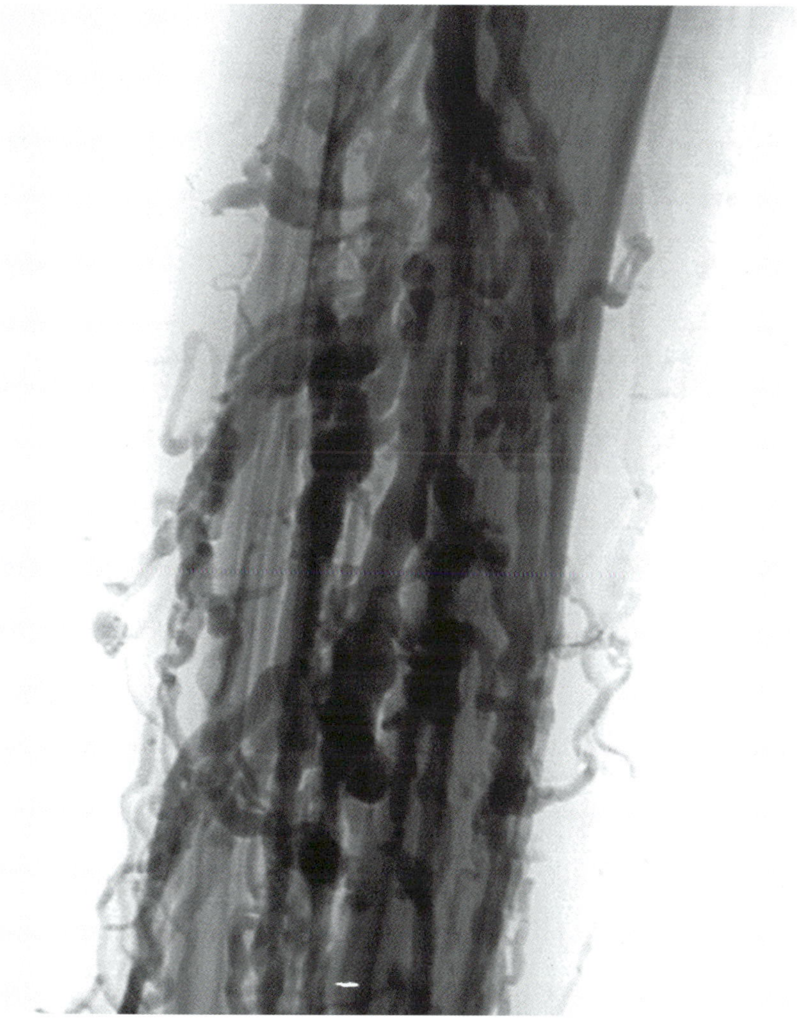

Fig. 53.11: Patient with dilation and tortuosity of subdermal veins due to proximal venous obstruction. [Image from Khanna AK. Varicose veins. In: Khanna AK, Puneet. Manual of Vascular Surgery. New Delhi, India: Jaypee Brothers Medical Publishers (P) Ltd.; 2011].

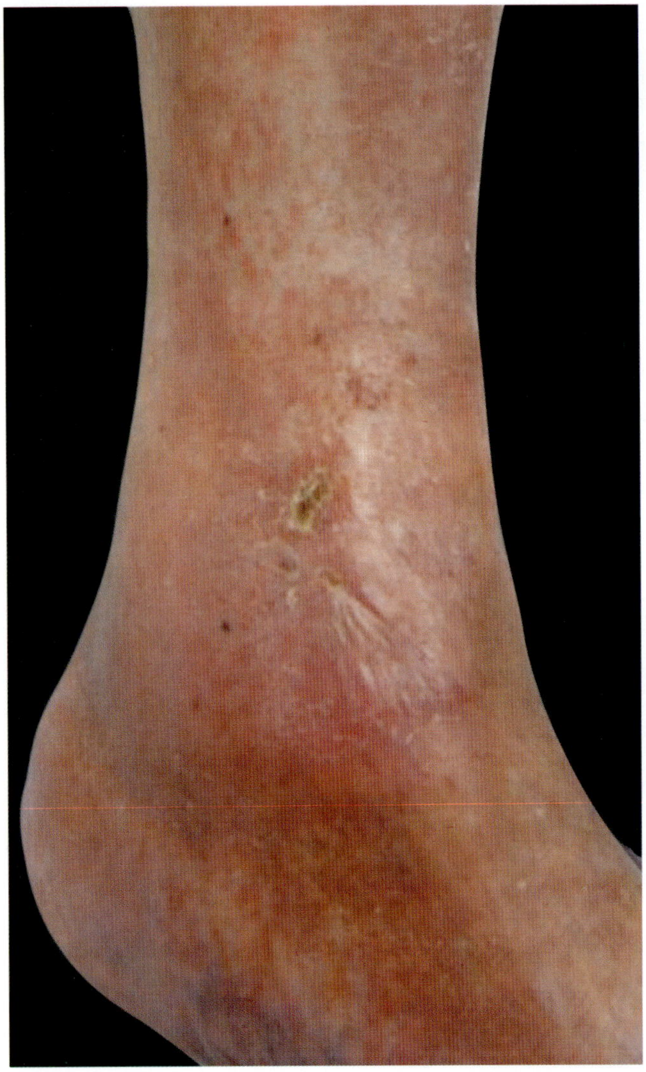

Fig. 53.12: Chronic venous stasis with complete healing of ulcers. [Image from Link D. Late complications of deep venous thrombosis: painful swollen extremities and non-healing ulcers. In: Okuyan E (Ed). Venous Thrombosis—Principles and Practice. Shanghai: InTech; 2012].

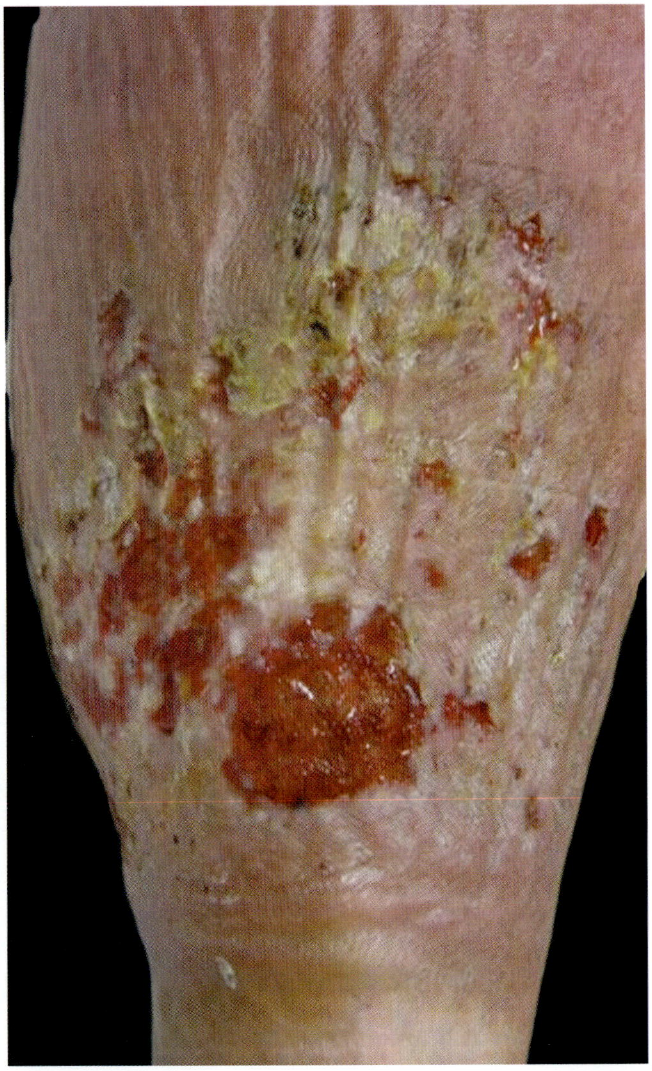

Fig. 53.13: Patient with non-healing venous stasis ulcers despite compression therapy. [Image from Link D. Late complications of deep venous thrombosis: painful swollen extremities and non-healing ulcers. In: Okuyan E (Ed). Venous Thrombosis—Principles and Practice. Shanghai: InTech; 2012].

decreased with the use of modern subfascial endoscopic perforator surgery and endovenous ablation techniques.

Infrequently, venous reconstructive surgery may be used as a last treatment resort. These include valvuloplasty, venous valve transplantation, and GSV transposition (May-Husni procedure) (Fig. 53.14), although the results may not be long lasting.

In cases of proximal venous obstruction, a venous bypass should be considered prior to other surgical procedures, as those other surgical procedures will likely fail unless the obstruction is relieved. Surgical options include the Palma procedure (cross-femoral GSV bypass), iliac bypass with prosthetic graft or endovascular recanalization and stenting angioplasty.

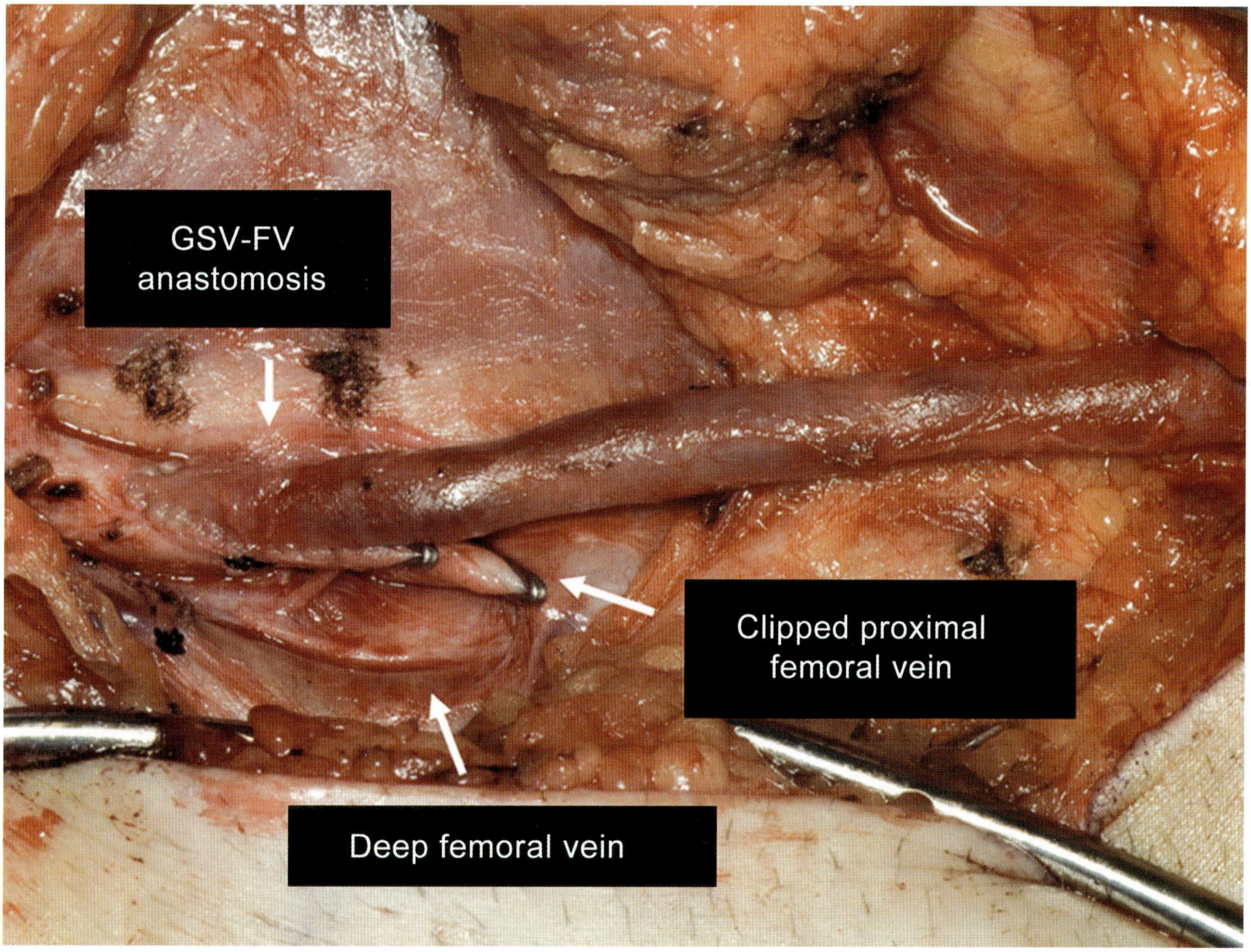

Fig. 53.14: Great saphenous to femoral vein bypass to treat severe deep venous insufficiency.

REFERENCES

Bradbury A, Evans CJ, Allan P, et al. The relationship between lower limb symptoms and superficial and deep venous reflux on duplex ultrasonography: the Edinburgh Vein Study. J Vasc Surg. 2000;32:921-31.

Brand FN, Dannenberg AL, Abbott RD, et al. The epidemiology of varicose veins: the Framingham Study. Am J Prev Med. 1988;4(2):96-101.

Dwerryhouse S, Davies B, Harradine K, et al. Stripping the long saphenous vein reduces the rate of reoperation for recurrent varicose veins: five year results of a randomized trial. J Vasc Surg. 1999;29:589-92.

Caggiati A, Bergan JJ, Gloviczki P, et al. Nomenclature of the veins of the lower limbs: an international interdisciplinary consensus statement. J Vasc Surg. 2002;36:416-22.

Criado E, Farber MA, Marston WA, et al. The role of air plethysmography in the diagnosis of chronic venous insufficiency. J Vasc Surg. 1998;27:660-70.

DePalma RG, Kowallek DL, Barcia TC, et al. Target selection for surgical intervention in severe chronic venous insufficiency: comparison of duplex scanning and phlebography. J Vasc Surg. 2000;32:913-20.

Gloviczki P, Bergan JJ, Rhodes JM, et al. Mid-term results of endoscopic perforator vein interruption for chronic venous insufficiency: lessons learned from the North American subfacial endoscopic perforator surgery registry. The North American Study Group. J Vasc Surg. 1999;29:489-502.

Gohel MS, Barwell JR, Earnshaw JJ, et al. Randomized clinical trial of compression plus surgery versus compression alone in chronic venous ulceration (ESCHAR study): haemodynamic and anatomical changes. Br J Surg. 2005;92:291-7.

Gruss JD, Heimer W. Bypass procedures for venous obstruction. In: Raju S, Villavicencio JL (Eds). Surgical Management of Venous Disease. Baltimore: Williams & Wilkins; 1997.

Heit JA, Rooke TW, Silverstein MD, et al. Trends in the incidence of venous stasis syndrome and venous ulcer: a 25-year population based study. J Vasc Surg. 2001;33:1022-7.

Merchant RF, Pichot O; Closure Study Group. Long-term outcomes of endovenous radiofrequency obliteration of saphenous reflux as a treatment for superficial venous insufficiency. Closure Study Group. J Vasc Surg. 2005;42:502-9.

Puggioni A, Kalra M, Carmo M, et al. Endovenous laser therapy and radiofrequency ablation of the great saphenous vein: analysis of early efficacy and complications. J Vasc Surg. 2005;42:488-93.

Prandoni P, Lensing AW, Cogo A, et al. The long-term clinical course of acute deep venous thrombosis. Ann Intern Med. 1996;125:1-7.

Scultetus AH, Villavicencio JL, Rich NM. Facts and fiction surrounding the discovery of venous valves. J Vasc Surg. 2001; 33:435-41.

Section 8

Miscellaneous Cardiovascular Disease

Chapters

CHAPTER

54

Cardiac Tumors

Eun Young Kim, Yeon Hyeon Choe

INTRODUCTION

Cardiac tumors have a cumulative prevalence of 0.001–0.3%. Primary cardiac neoplasms include both benign and malignant histological types. Secondary cardiac tumors (distant metastases and local invasion from neoplasms in the chest) are approximately 30 times more prevalent than primary cardiac tumors. Three quarters of the primary cardiac tumors are benign, and nearly half of those are myxomas. The majority of primary malignant cardiac tumors are sarcomas, and the more common types are angiosarcomas (30–50%). The clinical presentation is determined mostly by location, size, texture, growth rate, and invasiveness of the tumor.

BENIGN TUMORS

Myxomas

Myxomas (Figs. 54.1 to 54.5, Video 54.1) are the most common benign tumor found in adults. The classic triad of symptoms includes cardiac obstructive symptoms related to the obstruction of blood flow (Figs. 54.6A to D), constitutional symptoms (such as fever, malaise, and weight loss), and embolic events. Thromboembolic events occur in 35% of left-sided myxomas (most commonly to the brain, kidney, spleen, and extremities), and 10% of right-sided myxomas (most commonly to the lung). Myxomas most commonly arise in the left atrium

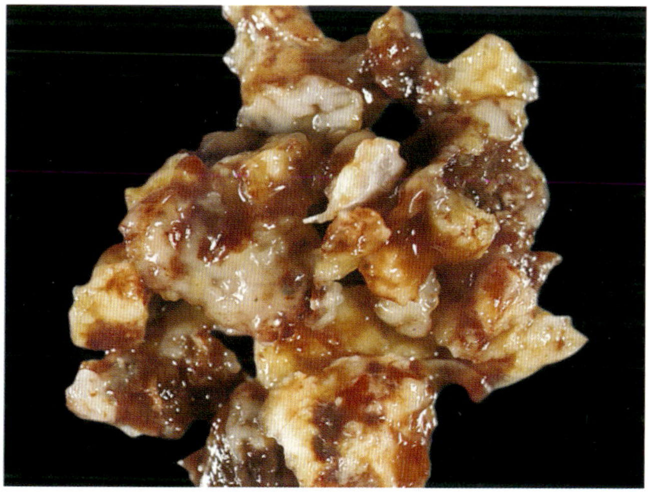

Fig. 54.1: Atrial myxoma. (Image from Armed Forces Institute of Pathology, downloaded from Wikimedia Commons).

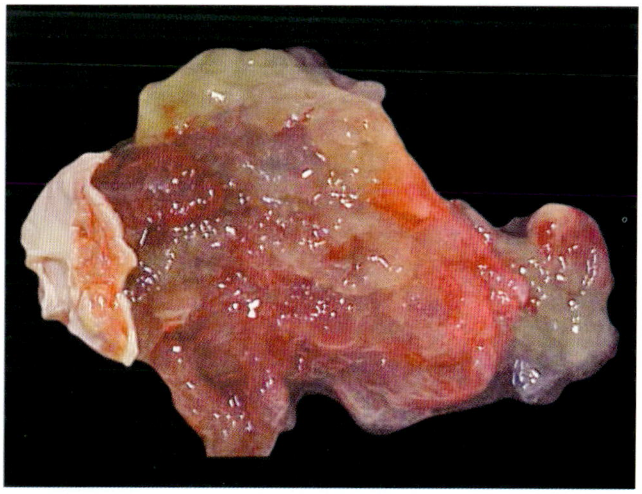

Fig. 54.2: Giant atrial myxoma. [Image from Vilela EP, Moura L, Pepe D, et al. Giant atrial myxoma mimicking severe mitral stenosis in young patient. Arq Bras Cardiol. 2010;95(5):e125-7].

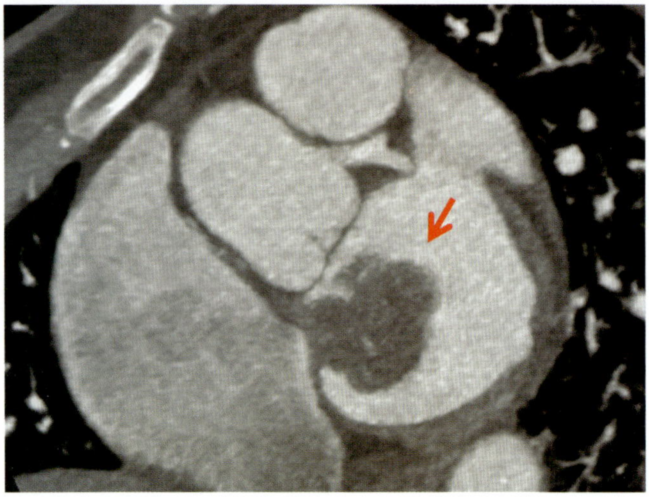

Fig. 54.3: Cardiac computed tomography (CT) image demonstrates a well-defined ovoid intracavitary mass (arrow) in the interatrial septum of left atrium (LA), which typically has lobular contours. These findings are typical of a myxoma, which most commonly occurs in the LA, attached to the interatrial septum.

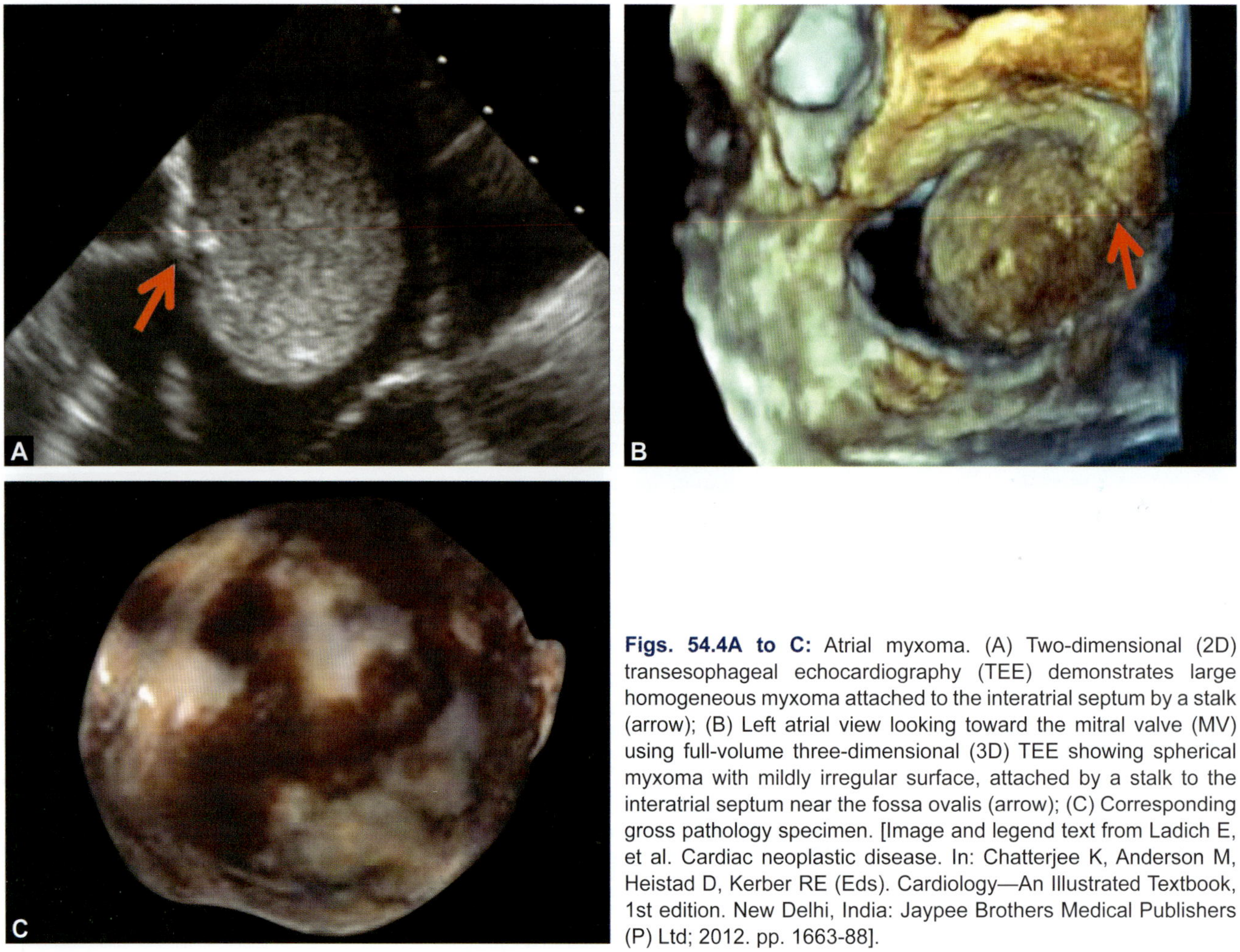

Figs. 54.4A to C: Atrial myxoma. (A) Two-dimensional (2D) transesophageal echocardiography (TEE) demonstrates large homogeneous myxoma attached to the interatrial septum by a stalk (arrow); (B) Left atrial view looking toward the mitral valve (MV) using full-volume three-dimensional (3D) TEE showing spherical myxoma with mildly irregular surface, attached by a stalk to the interatrial septum near the fossa ovalis (arrow); (C) Corresponding gross pathology specimen. [Image and legend text from Ladich E, et al. Cardiac neoplastic disease. In: Chatterjee K, Anderson M, Heistad D, Kerber RE (Eds). Cardiology—An Illustrated Textbook, 1st edition. New Delhi, India: Jaypee Brothers Medical Publishers (P) Ltd; 2012. pp. 1663-88].

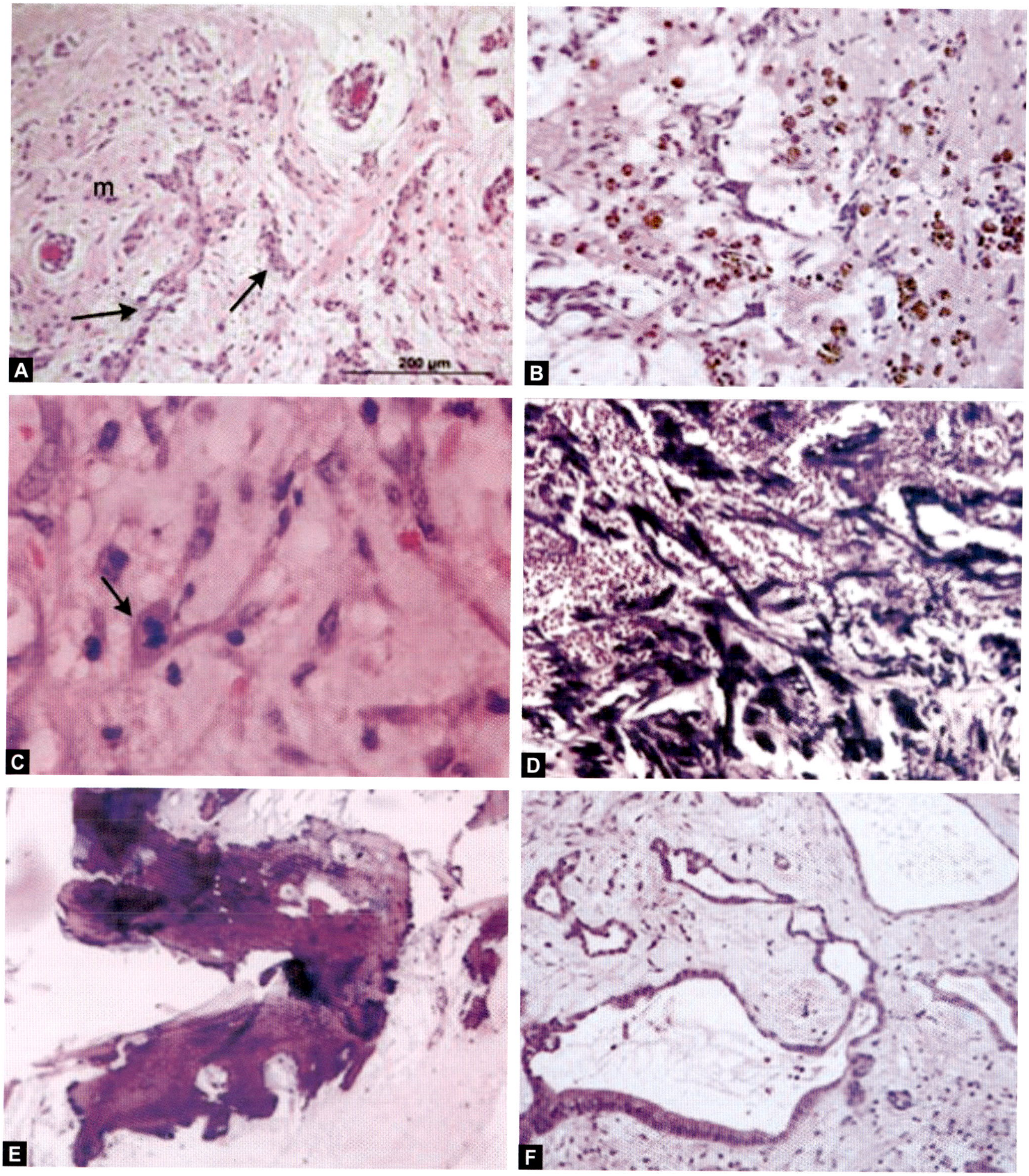

Figs. 54.5A to F: Histologic findings in cardiac myxoma. (A) Histologic appearance of a typical myxoma, showing myxoid matrix (m) and cords of myxoid cells (arrows), which may be single layered, or multiple; (B) Hemosiderin laden macrophages are virtually always present in myxoma; (C) Rarely mitotic figures may be observed (arrow); (D) Gamna-Gandy bodies; (E) Focal calcification and rarely even bone formation within a myxoma is observed; (F) Glandular structures are seen in less than 5% of cases. These are benign and should not be mistaken for metastatic adenocarcinoma.

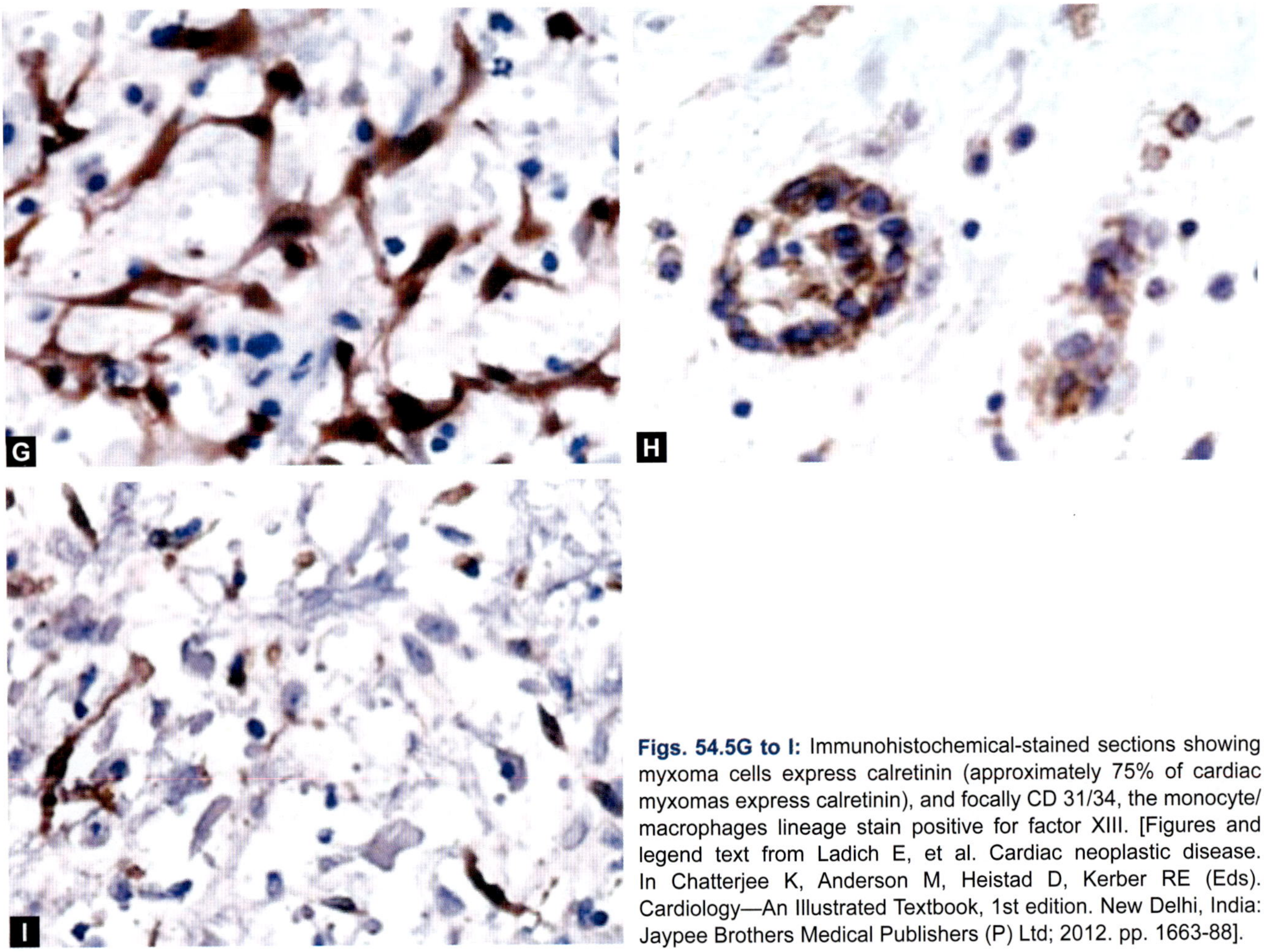

Figs. 54.5G to I: Immunohistochemical-stained sections showing myxoma cells express calretinin (approximately 75% of cardiac myxomas express calretinin), and focally CD 31/34, the monocyte/ macrophages lineage stain positive for factor XIII. [Figures and legend text from Ladich E, et al. Cardiac neoplastic disease. In Chatterjee K, Anderson M, Heistad D, Kerber RE (Eds). Cardiology—An Illustrated Textbook, 1st edition. New Delhi, India: Jaypee Brothers Medical Publishers (P) Ltd; 2012. pp. 1663-88].

(LA) (75% of myxomas), typically on the interatrial septum in the region of the fossa ovalis; rare cases are found in the right atrium (RA) and right ventricle (RV). Familial cardiac myxomas constitute 7% of cardiac myxomas and are characterized by involvement in sites other than the LA, including biatrial and ventricular involvement (Figs. 54.7A to F), and by a high recurrence rate. Familial cardiac myxomas may present as part of a syndrome (Carney's complex) or as non-syndromic familial cardiac myxomas. Carney's complex, as described by Carney JA, is characterized by the association of cutaneous pigmentation, fibromyxoid tumors of the skin, myxomas of the heart, endocrine overactivity, and autosomal dominant inheritance (Figs. 54.8A and B).

Lipomas

Lipomas are the second most common benign neoplasms in adults. Many patients are asymptomatic, and the tumor is found incidentally. They are encapsulated, homogeneous fatty tumors and may arise from the epi/endocardium, from the interatrial septum as broad-based, pedunculated masses protruding into any of the cardiac chambers. These lesions have specific imaging characteristics to demonstrate fatty component; increased echogenicity on echocardiography, homogeneous masses with minus Hounsfield Unit on computed tomography (CT), homogeneous increased signal intensity on the T1- and T2-weighted magnetic resonance (MR) images that decreases with the use of fat-saturated sequences. They do not show enhancement with the administration of a contrast material (Figs. 54.9A to D).

Papillary Fibroelastomas

Papillary fibroelastomas are benign papillomas that mainly affect the cardiac valves (75% of all cardiac valvular tumors). Papillary fibroelastomas are usually not observed

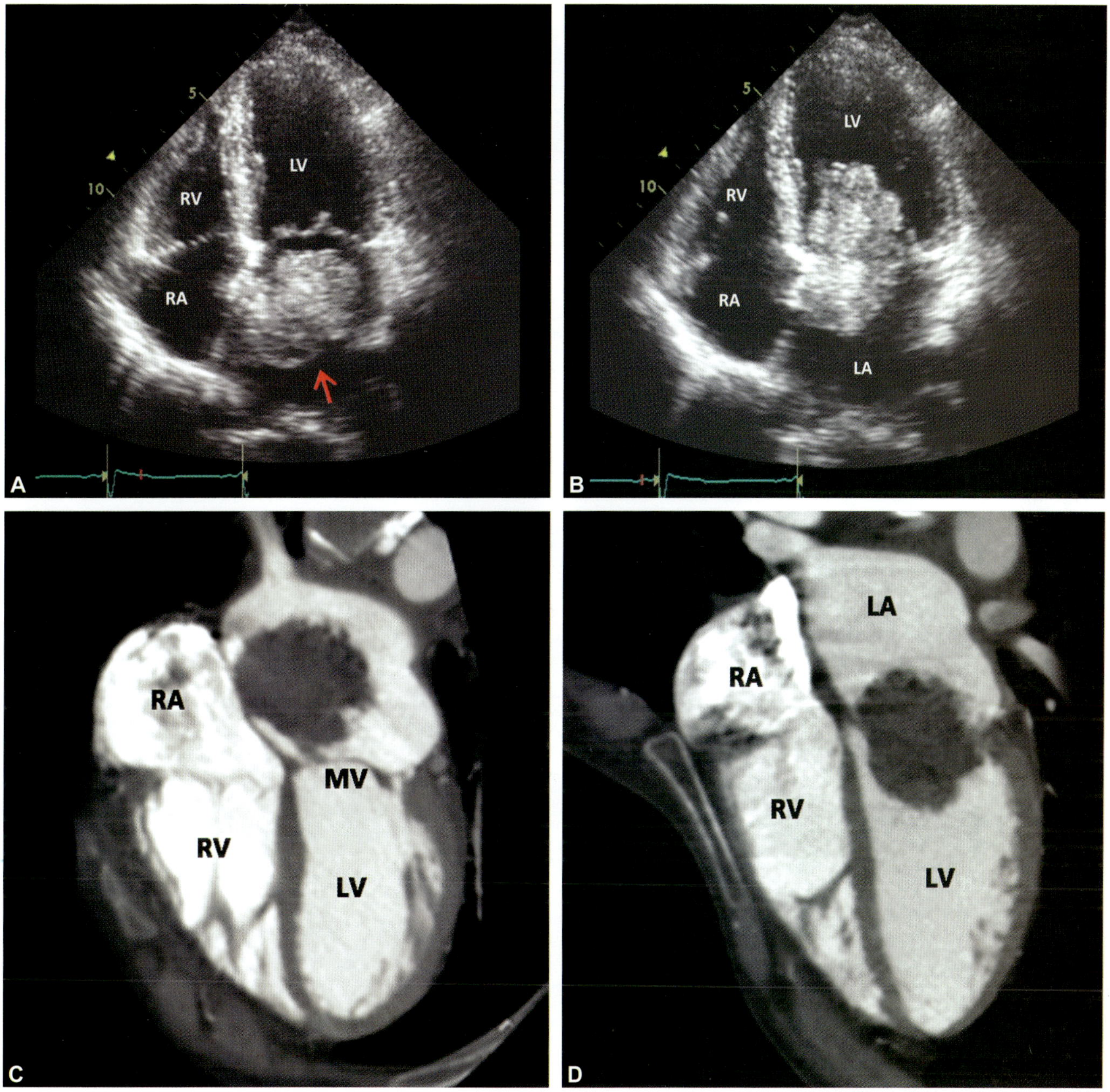

Figs. 54.6A to D: (A and B) Apical four-chamber echocardiography images showing a myxoma in the left atrium (LA). Note that in Figure 54.6B during diastole the mass prolapses through the mitral valve (MV) into left ventricle (LV); (C and D) Cardiac computed tomography (CT) images demonstrating a left atrial myxoma. Figure 54.6C shows the myxoma during ventricular systole. Figure 54.6D shows the myxoma during ventricular diastole, when it prolapses through the MV, obstructing flow. (RA: Right atrium; RV: Right ventricle).

on CT or MR images as they are small and are attached to the moving valves. In sporadic case reports, fibroelastomas have been shown as a well-defined, pedunculated, mobile mass to have intermediate signal intensity on the T1- and T2-weighted images and hyperintense signal intensity on delayed enhancement images caused by the fibroelastic tissue (Figs. 54.10 and 54.11).

Rhabdomyomas

Cardiac rhabdomyomas (Figs. 54.12 to 54.14) are the most common cardiac tumors in infancy and childhood, and are often associated with tuberous sclerosis in up to 50% of cases (Fig. 54.15). Most patients are asymptomatic, and rhabdomyomas generally regress spontaneously.

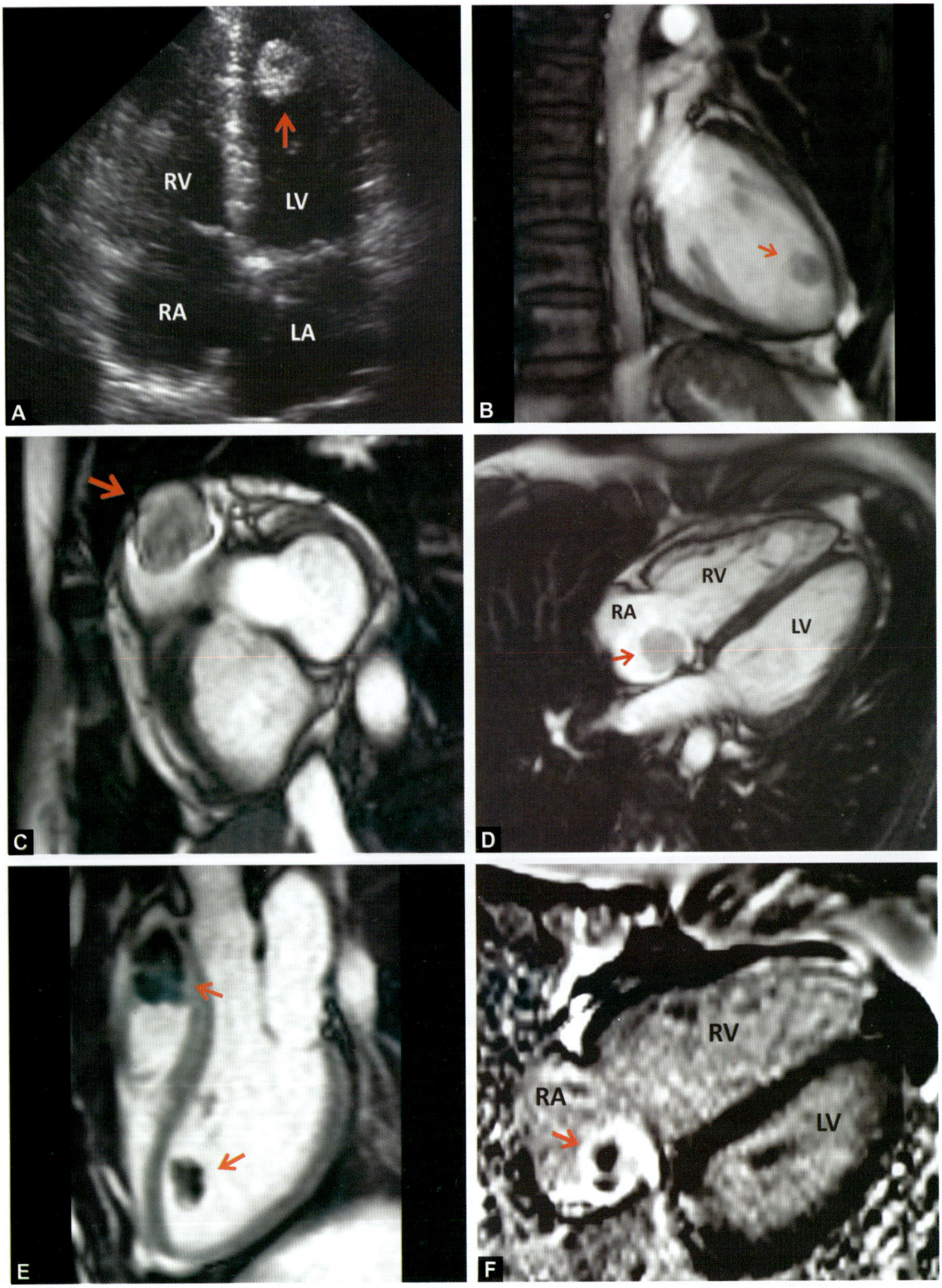

Figs. 54.7A to F: Multiple myxomas. (A) Echocardiography in apical four-chamber view shows a mass in left ventricle (LV) (arrow); (B to D) Cardiac magnetic resonance (MR) cine images show multiple masses (arrows) in the LV (B), right ventricular outflow tract (C), and right atrium (RA) (D). (E and F) Delayed enhancement MR images, obtained 10 minutes after injection of gadolinium, show peripheral enahcement of the masses (arrows). (RA: Right atrium; RV: Right ventricle; LV: Left ventricle).

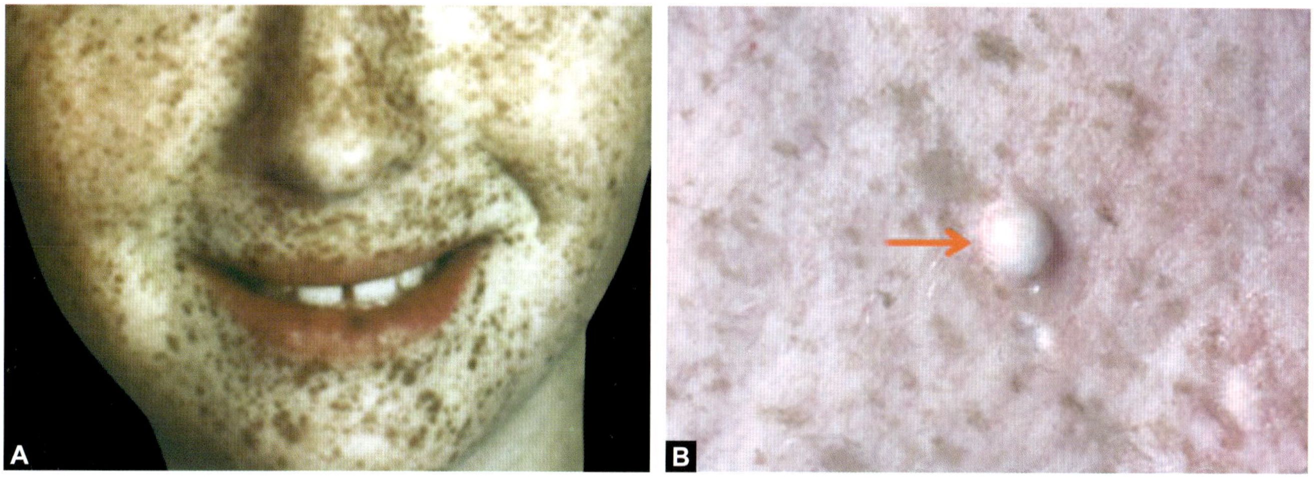

Figs. 54.8A and B: Cutaneous findings in Carney complex. (A) Skin pigmentation. There are numerous non-elevated brown-black spots visible; (B) Skin myxoma (arrow). [Images from Courcoutsakis NA, Tatsi C, Patronas NJ, et al. The complex of myxomas, spotty skin pigmentation and endocrine overactivity (Carney complex): imaging findings with clinical and pathological correlation. Insights Imaging. 2013;4(1):119-33].

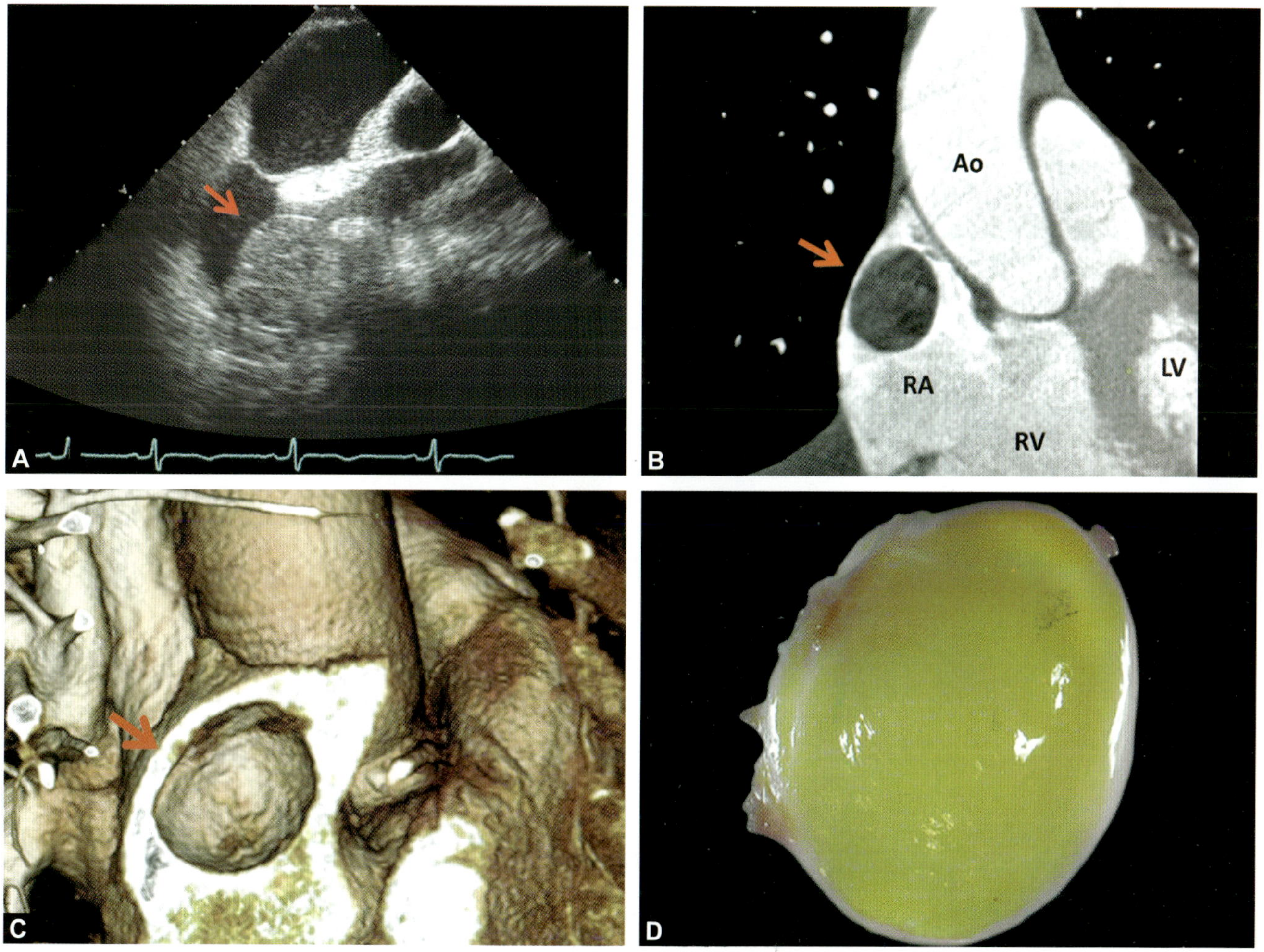

Figs. 54.9A to D: Cardiac lipoma. (A) Echocardiography shows an echogenic mass (arrow) within the right atrium (RA); (B and C) Cardiac computed tomography (CT) images show a homogeneously low-attenuated (minus 50 Hounsfield units) intracavitary mass (arrows); (D) Gross specimen shows fatty nature of the mass. (Ao: Aorta; RV: Right ventricle; LV: Left ventricle; LA: Left atrium).

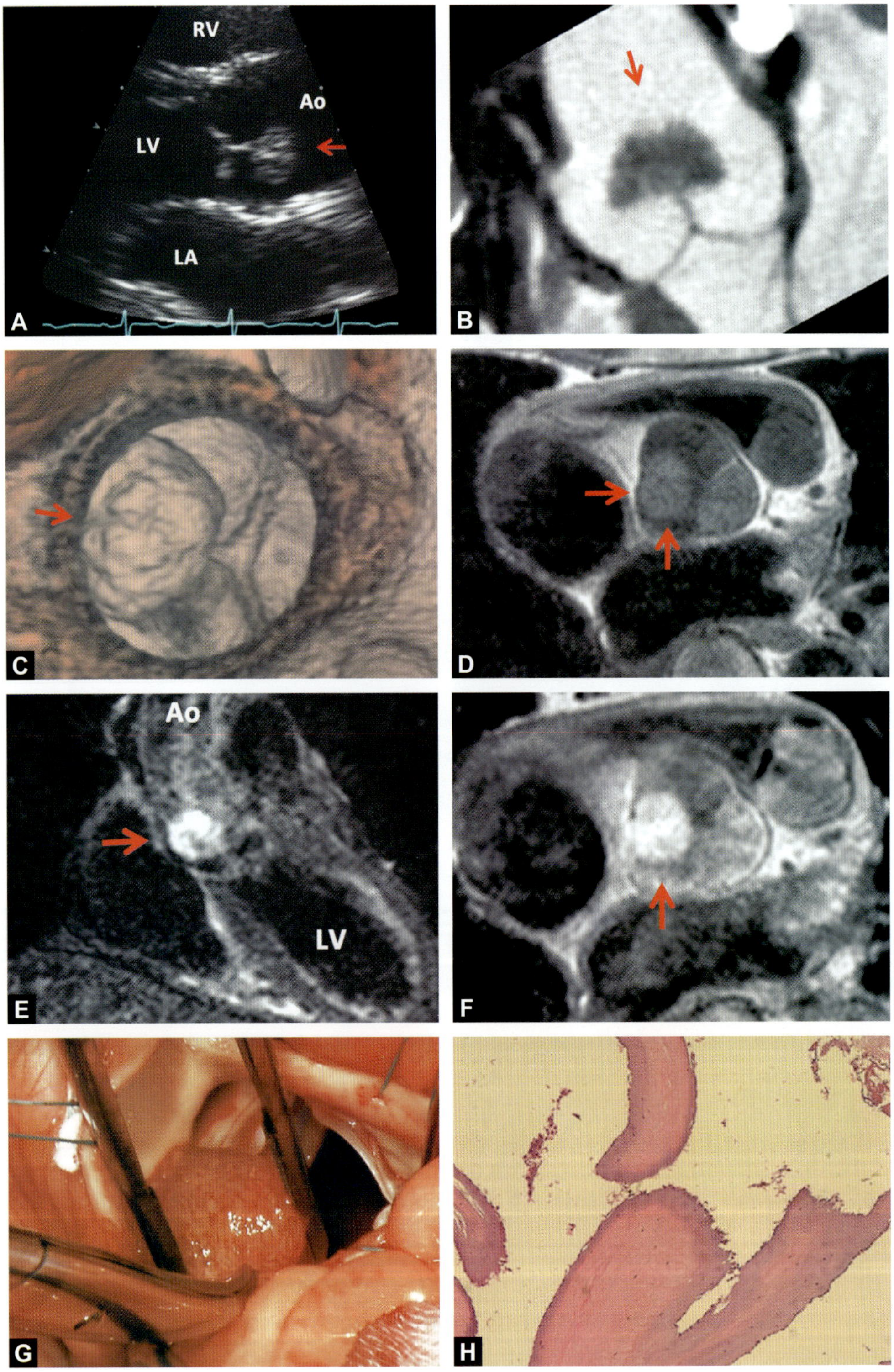

Figs. 54.10A to H: Papillary fibroelastoma. (A) Echocardiography shows a 2 cm-sized mobile mass attached to the aortic valve; (B) Computed tomography (CT) coronal image demonstrates a mass attached to the aortic valve; (C) Color-coded, three-dimensional (3D) reconstructed CT image reveals a well-defined mass involving both of the non-coronary and right coronary cusps; (D to F) Magnetic resonance (MR) images show iso-signal intensity on T1-weighted image (D), high signal intensity on T2-weighted image (E), and hyperenhancement on the postcontrast T1-weighted MR image (F); (G) Intraoperative view shows a lobulated mass involving the right coronary and non-coronary cusp of the aortic valve; (H) Hematoxylin and eosin-stained photograph shows fibrous core and scattered smooth muscle cells within papillary projections (magnification, ×40). (Ao: Aorta; LA: Left atrium; LV: Left ventricle; RV: Right ventricle).

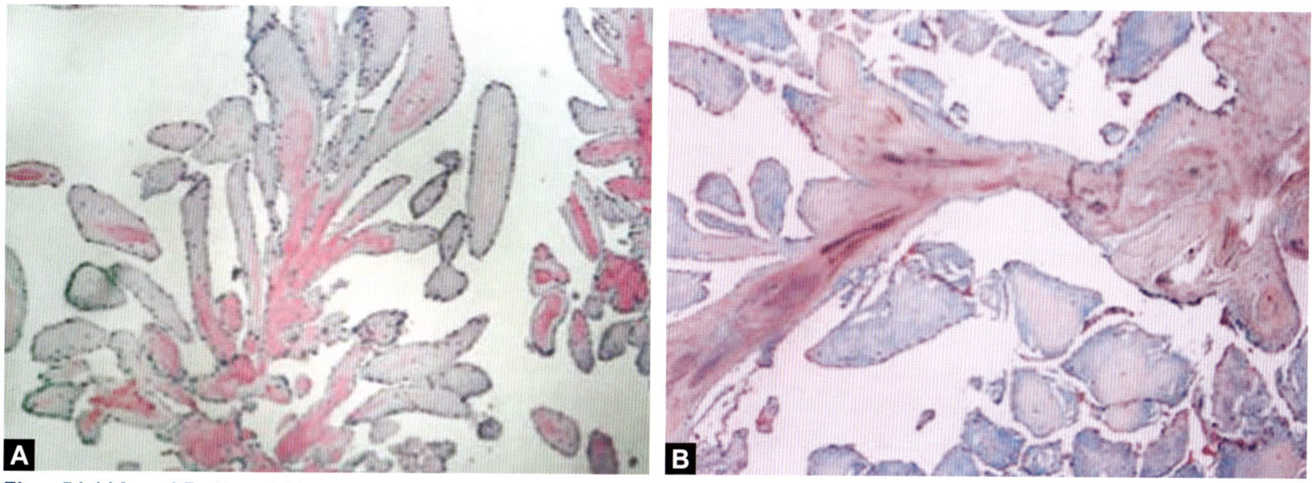

Figs. 54.11A and B: (A and B) Histologic specimen of a papillary fibroelastoma located on the mitral valve (MV). Note the presence of a central stalk made up of collagen (pink area in A) and some elastic fibers (brown black area in B). [Image and legend text from Ladich E, et al. Cardiac neoplastic disease. In: Chatterjee K, Anderson M, Heistad D, Kerber RE (Eds). Cardiology—An Illustrated Textbook, 1st edition. New Delhi, India: Jaypee Brothers Medical Publishers (P) Ltd; 2012. pp. 1663-88].

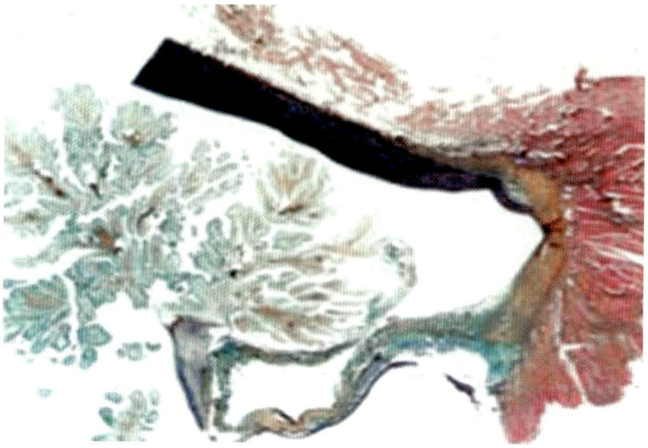

Fig. 54.11C: Papillary fibroelastoma of the aortic valve stained with Movat pentachrome stain. Note the mass consists of multiple papillary fronds that are rich in proteoglycans and collagen. [Image and legend text from Ladich E, et al. Cardiac neoplastic disease. In: Chatterjee K, Anderson M, Heistad D, Kerber RE (Eds). Cardiology—An Illustrated Textbook, 1st edition. New Delhi, India: Jaypee Brothers Medical Publishers (P) Ltd; 2012. pp. 1663-88].

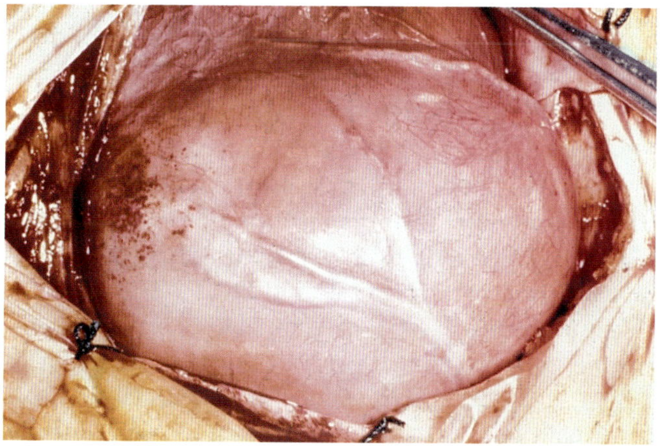

Fig. 54.12: Cardiac rhabdomyoma in the right ventricle (RV) of a 3-year-old girl. (Image from Armed Force Institute of Pathology. Downloaded from Wikimedia Commons).

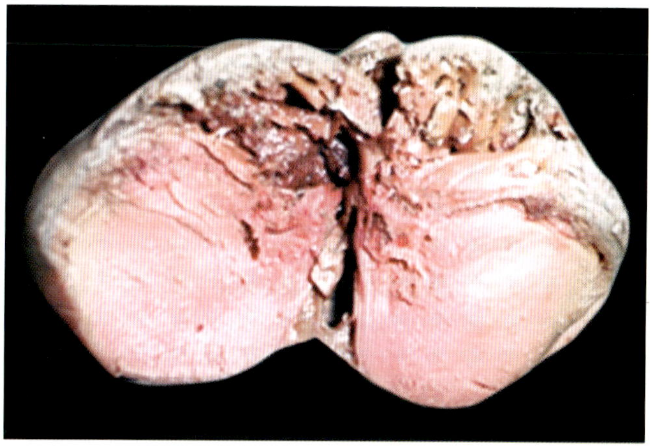

Fig. 54.13: Gross pathology specimen of a cardiac rhabdomyoma. [Image from Chadha V, Kapoor N. History of fetal cardiology. In: Chopra HK, Nanda NC (Eds). Textbook of Cardiology: A Clinical and Historical Perspective, 1st edition. New Delhi, India: Jaypee Brothers Medical Publishers (P) Ltd; 2013. pp. 480-93].

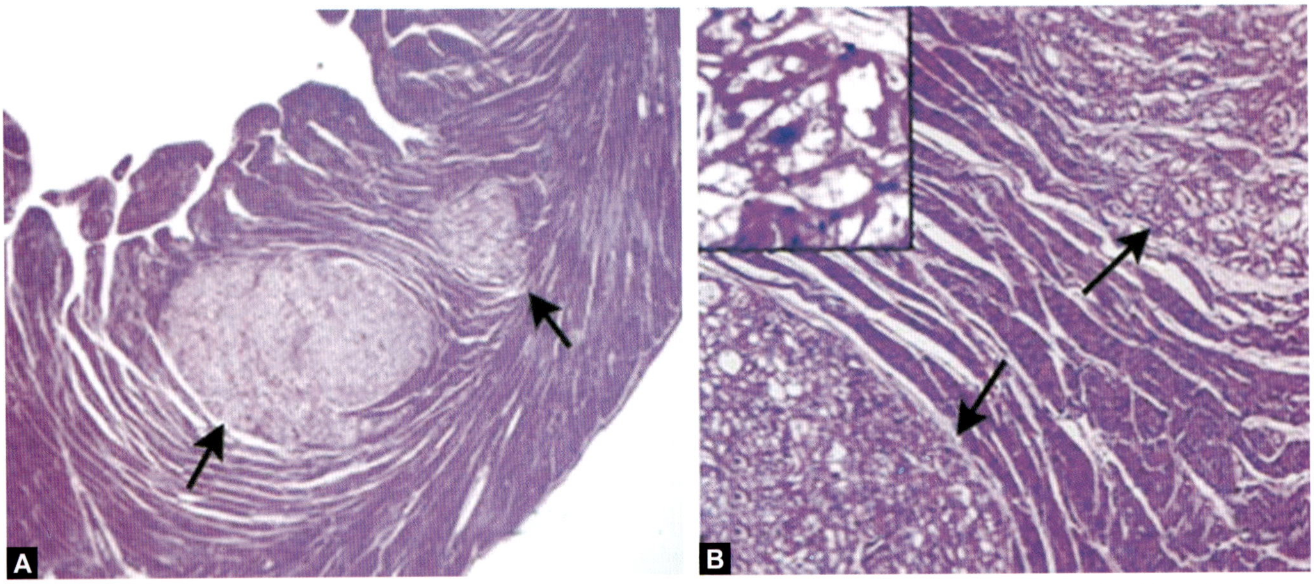

Figs. 54.14A and B: Rhabdomyoma. (A) Histologic section showing two subendocardial rhabdomyomas (arrows); (B) Inset in B shows "spider" cells, several vacuolated tumor cells, and cells with abundant eosinophilic cytoplasm. [Image and legend text from Ladich E, et al. Cardiac neoplastic disease. In: Chatterjee K, Anderson M, Heistad D, Kerber RE (Eds). Cardiology—An Illustrated Textbook, 1st edition. New Delhi, India: Jaypee Brothers Medical Publishers (P) Ltd; 2012. pp. 1663-88].

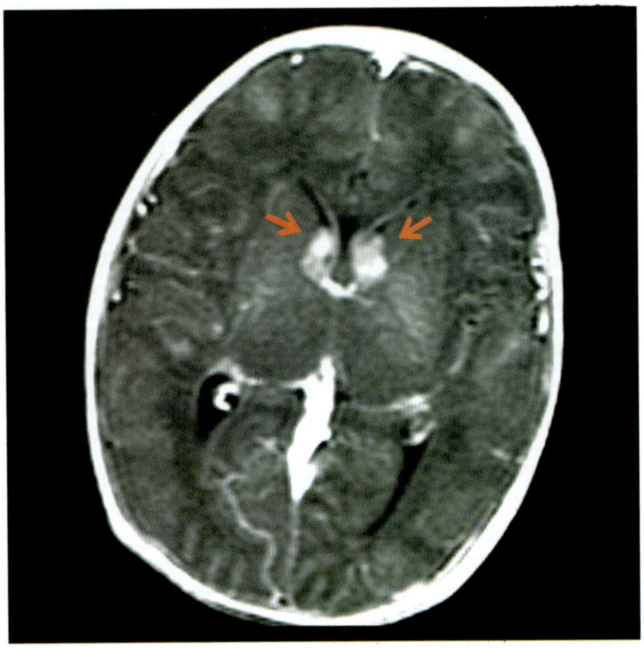

Fig. 54.15: Gadolinium-enhanced T1-weighted magnetic resonance (MR) image shows enhancing nodules (arrows) in both caudate nuclei, indicating the presence of tubers, in a newborn with cardiac rhabdomyoma (*see* Figs. 54.16A and B). [Image from Kim EY, Choe YH, Sung K, et al. Multidetector CT and MR imaging of cardiac tumors. Korean J Radiol. 2009;10(2):164-75].

These tumors originate within the myocardium, typically in the ventricles, and multiple lesions may be present in up to 90% of cases. At echocardiography, tumors are seen as solid hyperechoic masses, usually in the ventricular myocardium or ventricular septum and possibly protruding into and deforming the cardiac chambers. Rhabdomyomas appear isointense to marginally hyperintense as compared with the myocardium as seen on T1-weighted images and hyperintense as seen on T2-weighted images. After contrast administration, the mass shows mild enhancement (Figs. 54.16A and B).

Fibromas

Fibromas (Figs. 54.17A and B) mainly affect infants and children, being the second most common tumors found in this age group. There is an increased risk of cardiac fibromas in patients with Gorlin syndrome, which is characterized by multiple nevoid basal cell carcinomas of the skin, jaw cysts, and bifid ribs. Common clinical manifestations in patients with cardiac fibromas are heart failure, arrhythmias, and sudden death. Cardiac fibromas are usually located within the myocardium and can grow to a size that obliterates the cavity.

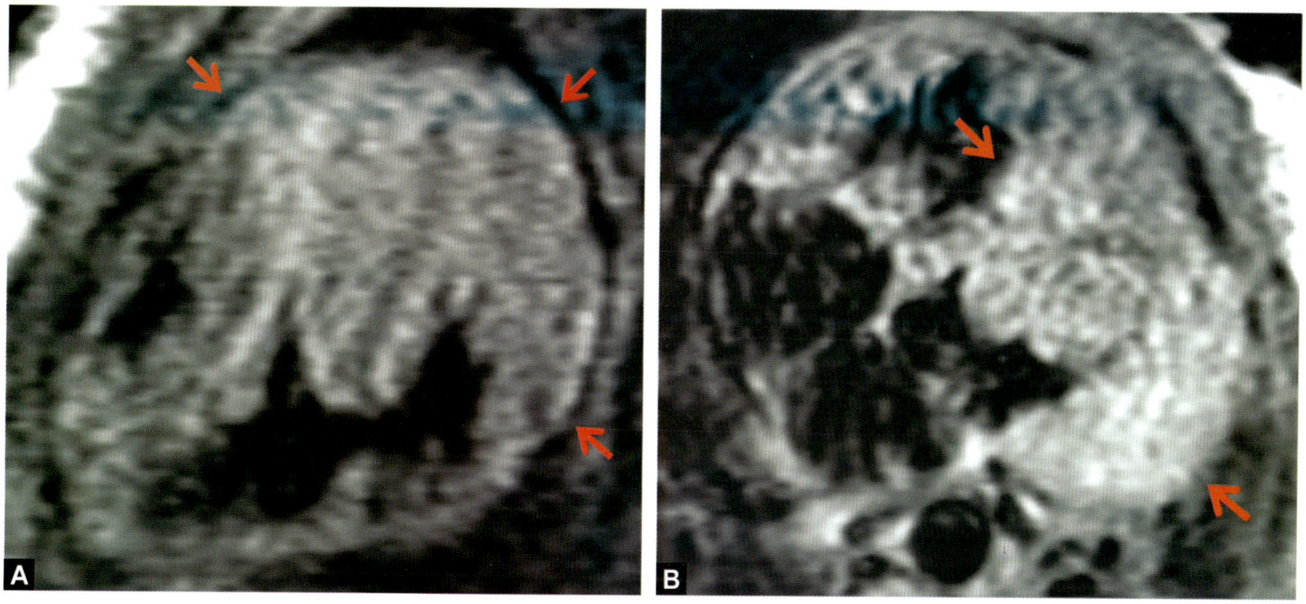

Figs. 54.16A and B: Cardiac rhabdomyoma in a newborn with tuberous sclerosis shown in Figure 54.15. (A) T1-weighted magnetic resonance (MR) image shows isointense mass (arrows) in the left ventricle (LV); (B) Gadolinium-enhanced T1-weighted MR image shows mild enhancement of the mass (arrows). [Image from Kim EY, Choe YH, Sung K, et al. Multidetector CT and MR imaging of cardiac tumors. Korean J Radiol. 2009;10(2):164-75].

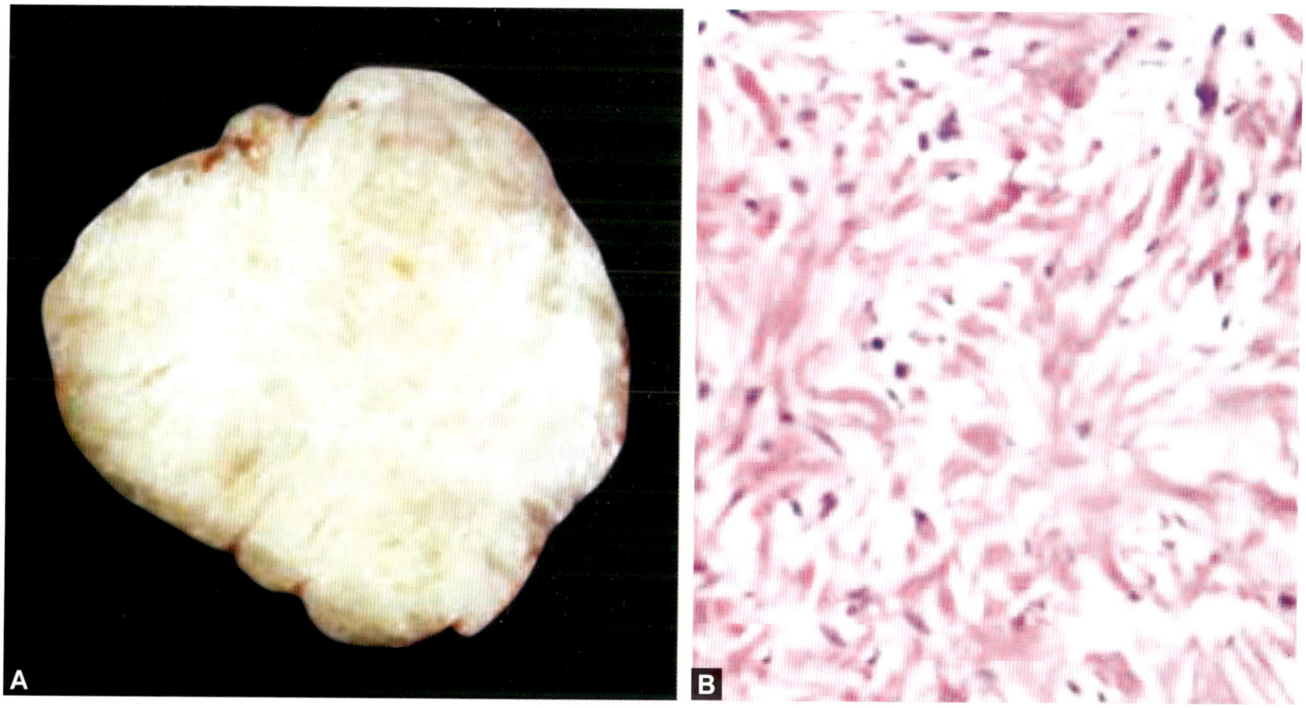

Figs. 54.17A and B: Cardiac fibroma. (A) Cardiac fibroma cut section showing prominent whorled surface; (B) Microscopy showing that the tumor is composed of spindle shape cells with pale cytoplasm and interspersed collagen bundles, forming intersecting bundles. [Images and legend text from Ladich E, et al. Cardiac neoplastic disease. In: Chatterjee K, Anderson M, Heistad D, Kerber RE (Eds). Cardiology—An Illustrated Textbook, 1st edition. New Delhi, India: Jaypee Brothers Medical Publishers (P) Ltd; 2012. pp. 1663-88].

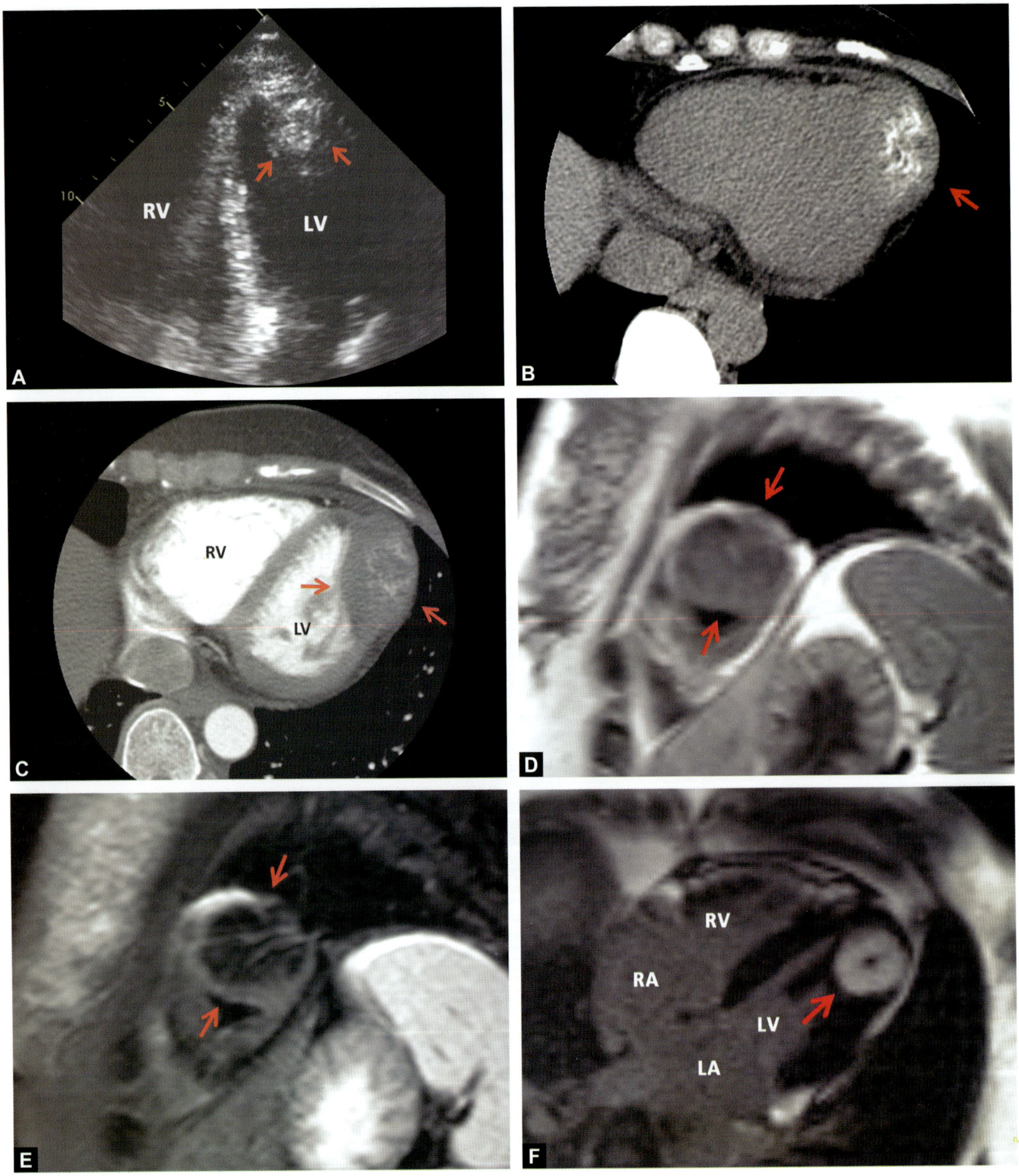

Figs. 54.18A to F: Cardiac fibroma. (A) Echocardiography in apical four-chamber view shows mass in left ventricle (LV); (B and C) Cardiac computed tomography (CT) shows mass in the lateral wall of left ventricular myocardium. Precontrast CT shows calcification within the mass (B); (D to F) On cardiac magnetic resonance (MR), the mass shows low signal intensity on the T1- and T2-weighted images (D and E) and hyperenhancement on the delayed image obtained after 10 minutes later from intravenous injection of gadolinium (F). (LA: Left atrium; RA: Right atrium; RV: Right ventricle).

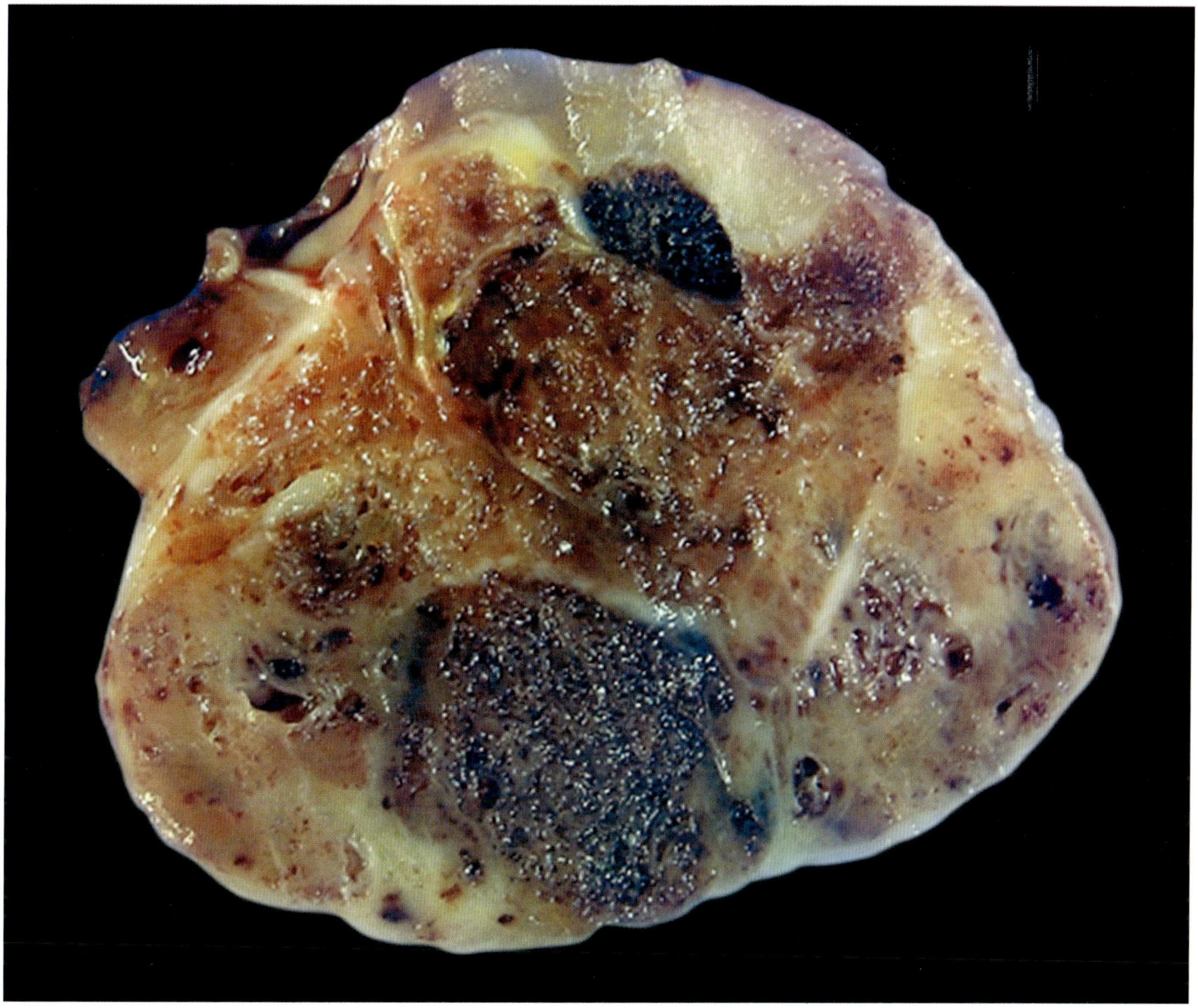

Fig. 54.19: Gross specimen of a cardiac hemangioma with cut section demonstrating trabecular, hemorrhagic, and cystic appearances of the mass.

On CT scan, fibromas often appear as homogeneous mass with calcifications. On MR examination, these tumors are normally homogeneously iso- to hypointense relative to the myocardium on T1- and T2-weighted images due to their dense and fibrous nature. After intravenous administration of gadolinium, cardiac fibromas do not show enhancement during first-pass perfusion, suggesting a low vascularity. However, 10 minutes after contrasts administration, intense late gadolinium enhancement is observed, reflecting an increased extracellular volume of distribution within the ventricular myocardium (Figs. 54.18A to F).

Hemangiomas

Hemangiomas (Fig. 54.19) are benign vascular tumors that comprise approximately 5–10% of benign tumors. They are classified according to the size of their vascular channels into capillary, cavernous, or venous hemangiomas. On MR examination, cardiac hemangiomas show intermediate signal intensity on T1-weighted images, which is comparable to myocardium. On T2-weighted images, bright signal intensity is typically observed. Cardiac hemangiomas enhance intensely and very rapidly after administration of contrast media, indicating a high vascularity (Figs. 54.20A to F).

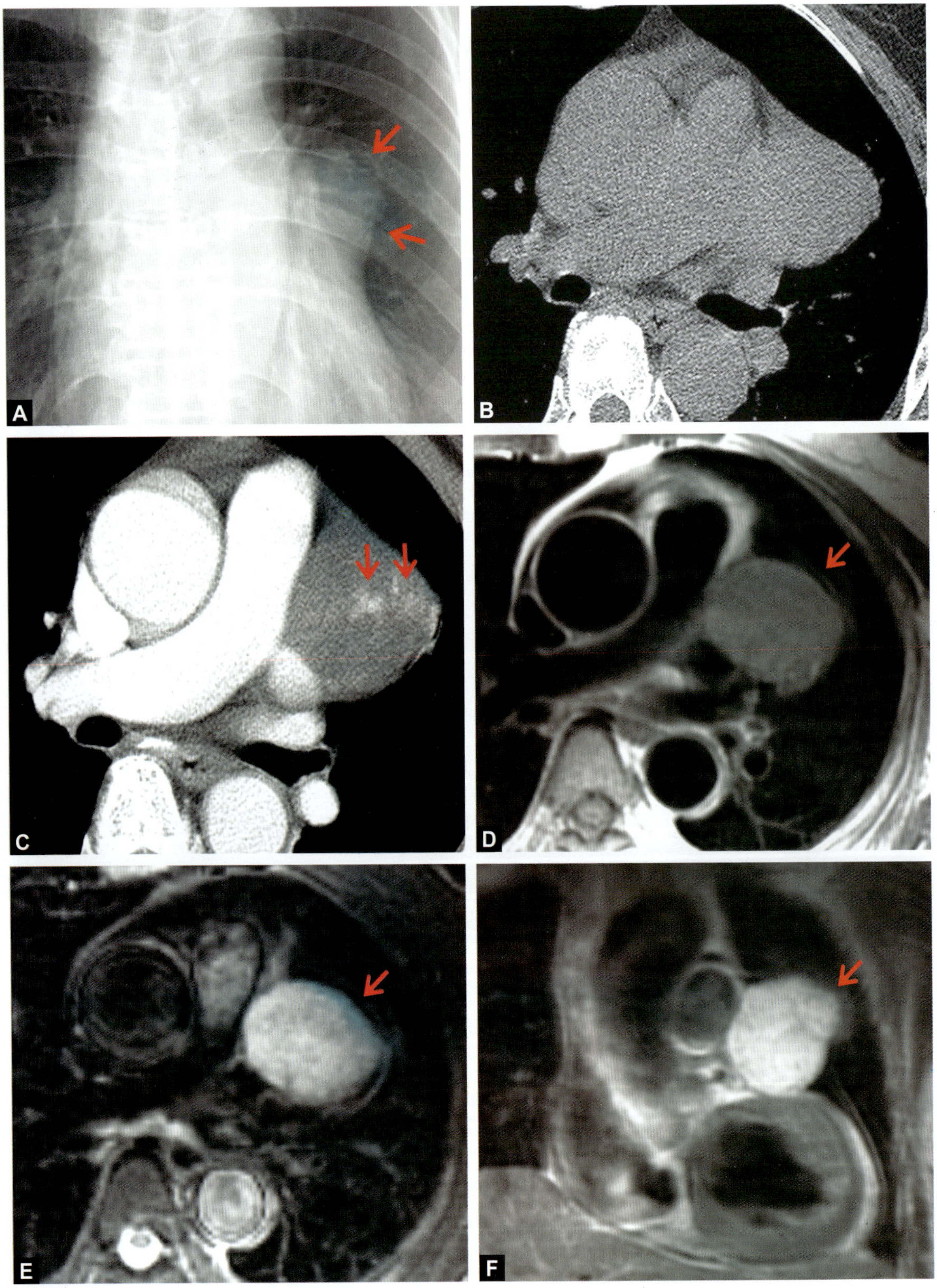

Figs. 54.20A to F: Cavernous hemangioma. (A) Chest radiograph shows enlargement of left upper cardiac border (arrows); (B and C) Precontrast (B) and postcontrast (C) computed tomography (CT) images show a low-attenuation mass with areas of hyperenhancement (arrows) in the left atrial appendage. (D to F) Cardiac magnetic resonance (MR) demonstrates the mass with low signal intensity on T1-weighted imaging (D) and bright signal intensity on T2-weighted imaging, and hyperenhancement on the postcontrast image (F).

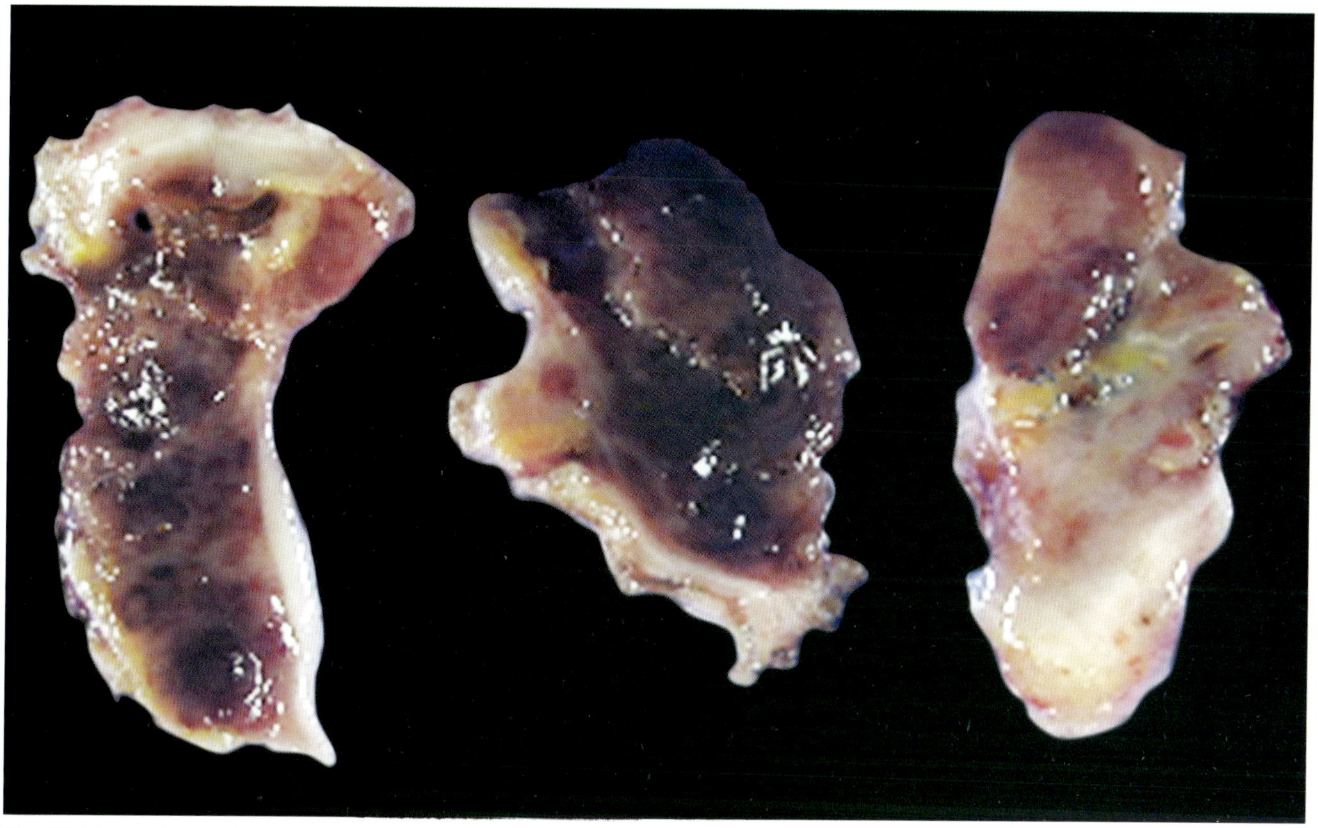

Fig. 54.21: Cardiac angiosarcoma. Gross pathology shows a fragile and hemorrhagic mass.

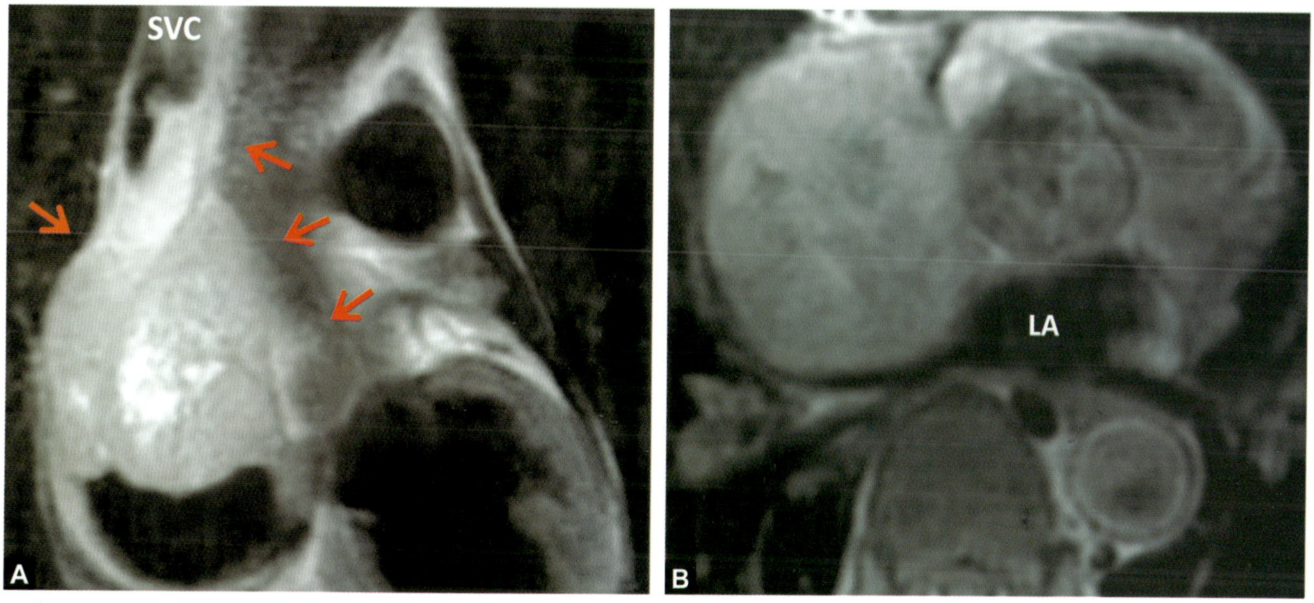

Figs. 54.22A and B: Cardiac angiosarcoma. (A) A postcontrast enhancement magnetic resonance (MR) image shows a large mass (arrows) in the right atrium (RA), extending to the superior vena cava (SVC). High signal intensity indicating vascular structures within the mass (so-called "cauliflower" appearance) is clearly visible. (B) Magnetic resonance imaging also demonstrates that the mass is compressing the left atrium (LA).

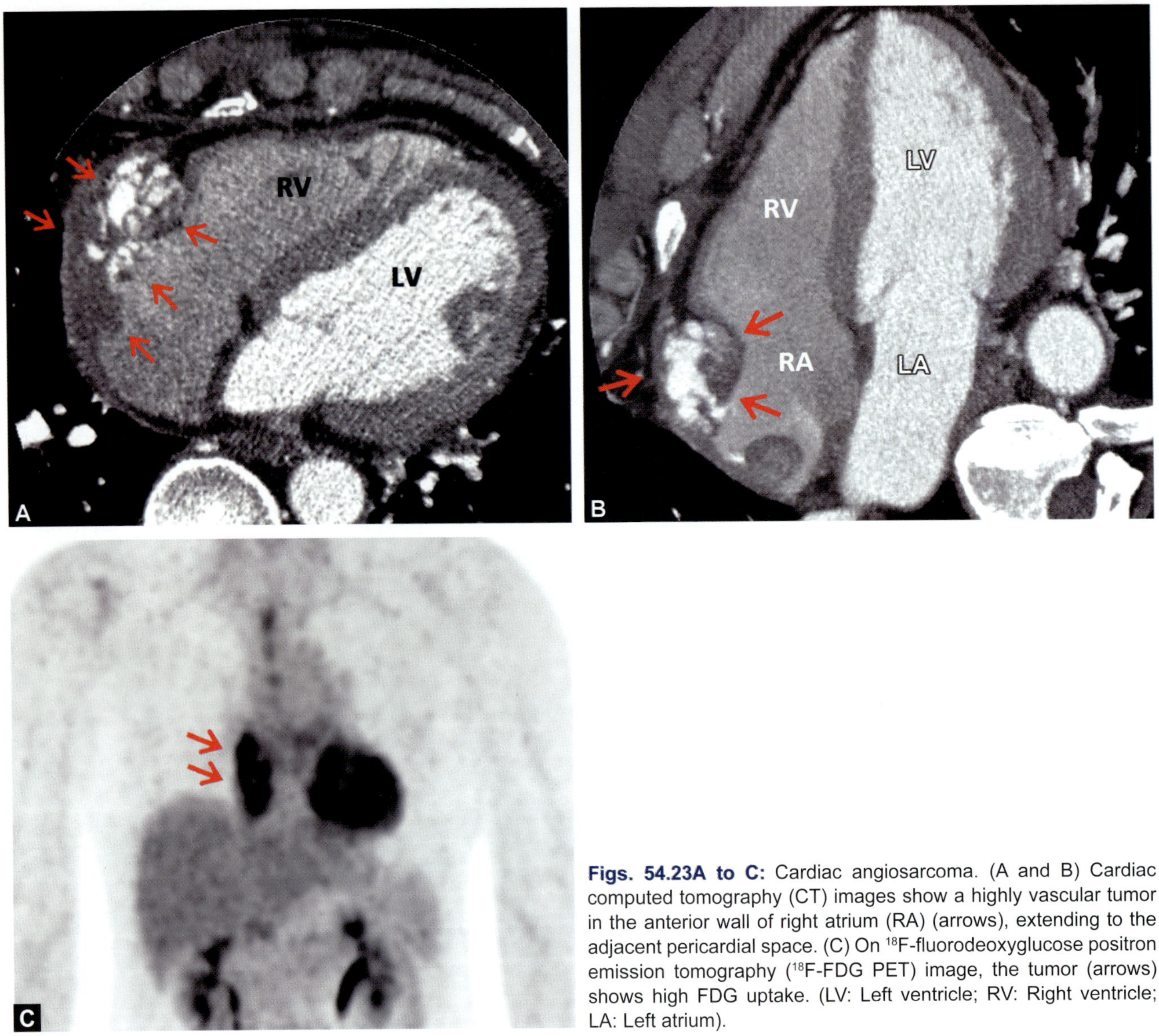

Figs. 54.23A to C: Cardiac angiosarcoma. (A and B) Cardiac computed tomography (CT) images show a highly vascular tumor in the anterior wall of right atrium (RA) (arrows), extending to the adjacent pericardial space. (C) On ^{18}F-fluorodeoxyglucose positron emission tomography (^{18}F-FDG PET) image, the tumor (arrows) shows high FDG uptake. (LV: Left ventricle; RV: Right ventricle; LA: Left atrium).

PRIMARY MALIGNANCIES

Angiosarcomas

The most common cardiac sarcomas are angiosarcomas (Fig. 54.21). Since the tumors tend to occur in the RA and involve the pericardium, they usually cause right-sided heart failure or tamponade. Presentation is late, and there is often the presence of metastases at the time of diagnosis, particularly to the lung.

On MR examination, angiosarcomas are depicted as large, heterogeneous, invasive masses in the RA, frequently with extensive pericardial invasion and hemorrhagic pericardial effusion. Pericardial and extracardiac invasion, valvular destruction, and metastases are frequently seen. They have a marked heterogeneity of signal intensity and hyperintense on MR images due to vascular structures within the tumor, which has been described as a "cauliflower" appearance (Figs. 54.22A and B). On ^{18}F-fluorodeoxyglucose positron emission tomography (^{18}F-FDG PET) imaging, the tumors show high FDG uptake (Figs. 54.23A to C).

Other Cardiac Sarcomas

Although angiosarcomas are the most common cardiac sarcomas, all types of sarcomas, including undifferentiated sarcomas, malignant fibrous histiocytomas, leiomyosar-

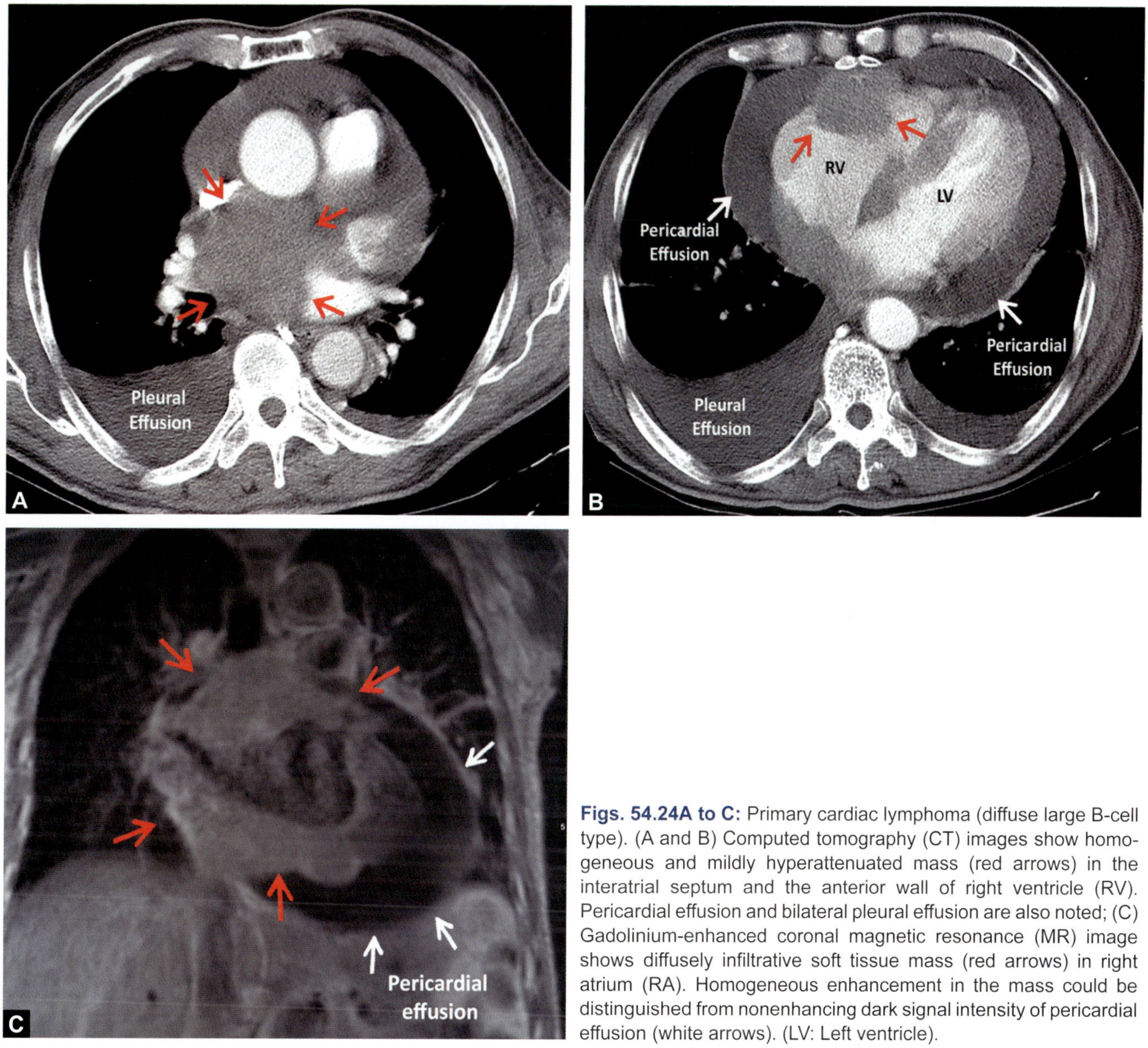

Figs. 54.24A to C: Primary cardiac lymphoma (diffuse large B-cell type). (A and B) Computed tomography (CT) images show homogeneous and mildly hyperattenuated mass (red arrows) in the interatrial septum and the anterior wall of right ventricle (RV). Pericardial effusion and bilateral pleural effusion are also noted; (C) Gadolinium-enhanced coronal magnetic resonance (MR) image shows diffusely infiltrative soft tissue mass (red arrows) in right atrium (RA). Homogeneous enhancement in the mass could be distinguished from nonenhancing dark signal intensity of pericardial effusion (white arrows). (LV: Left ventricle).

comas, osteosarcomas, lymphosarcomas, myxosarcomas, neurogenic sarcomas, malignant melanoma, neurofibrosarcomas, Kaposi's sarcomas, and synovial sarcomas can affect the heart. Although most angiosarcomas occur in the RA, the other sarcomas affect the LA more frequently, which is an important differentiating feature.

Primary Cardiac Lymphomas

Primary cardiac lymphomas are extremely rare (0.15–1%). A diffuse large B-cell lymphoma is the most common type of primary cardiac lymphoma. Most cases of cardiac lymphomas are infiltrative masses involving one or multiple chambers of the heart (Figs. 54.24A to C) and the massive infiltration of lymphoma cells in the myocardium may result in irregular thickening, mimicking hypertrophic cardiomyopathy or infiltrative cardiomyopathy. Due to the high cellularity of the tumor, cardiac lymphomas have hypo- or isoattenuating relative to myocardium on CT and iso- to slightly hypointensity on T1-and T2-weighted MR images.

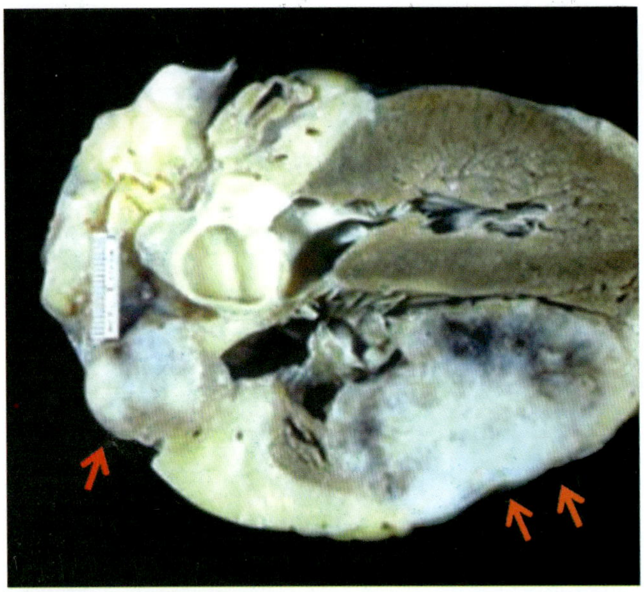

Fig. 54.25: Massive infiltration of the right ventricle (RV) and infiltration of the right atrium (RA) in a patient with widespread metastatic colon cancer. Colon cancer only rarely leads to clinically significant metastasis to the heart, and is not one of the more common cancers that metastasize to the heart. [Image from Ladich E, et al. Cardiac neoplastic disease. In: Chatterjee K, Anderson M, Heistad D, Kerber RE (Eds). Cardiology—An Illustrated Textbook, 1st edition. New Delhi, India: Jaypee Brothers Medical Publishers (P) Ltd; 2012. pp. 1663-88].

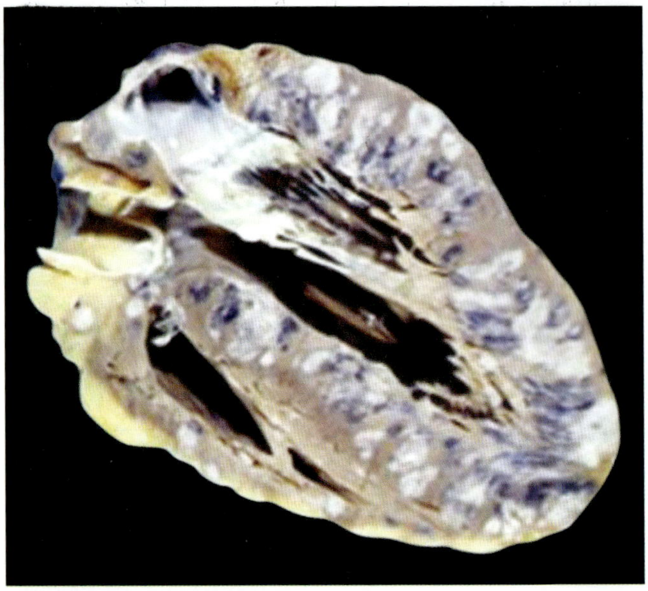

Fig. 54.26: Gross pathology of the heart from a patient with metastatic melanoma. [Image from Ladich E, et al. Cardiac neoplastic disease. In: Chatterjee K, Anderson M, Heistad D, Kerber RE (Eds). Cardiology—An Illustrated Textbook, 1st edition. New Delhi, India: Jaypee Brothers Medical Publishers (P) Ltd; 2012. pp. 1663-88].

METASTASES

Metastases to the heart (Fig. 54.25) are much more common than primary involvement, with a ratio of 30:1. In the presence of a malignant tumor, cardiac metastases are encountered in 10–20% of cases. The tumors that most frequently metastasize to the heart are lung and breast cancers, melanomas (Fig. 54.26) and lymphomas. The epicardium is the most often affected site by metastases, mainly via a retrograde route through the mediastinal lymphatics. Other tumors such as melanomas and sarcomas usually spread hematogenously to the myocardium through the coronary arteries. Figures 54.27A to D demonstrate a case of hematogenous metastasis from hepatocellular carcinoma. Transvenous tumor spread rarely can be seen with an extension of the tumor into the RA through the superior or inferior vena cava or an extension into the LA via the pulmonary veins. Direct tumor extension can occur with malignancies located adjacent to the heart (e.g., thymic, breast, bronchogenic and esophageal malignancy).

The enhancement patterns after the administration of gadolinium may be helpful to differentiate a thrombus from a combined tumor. Tumors would be expected to show heterogeneous enhancement whereas thrombi should not enhance with exception in chronic organized cases.

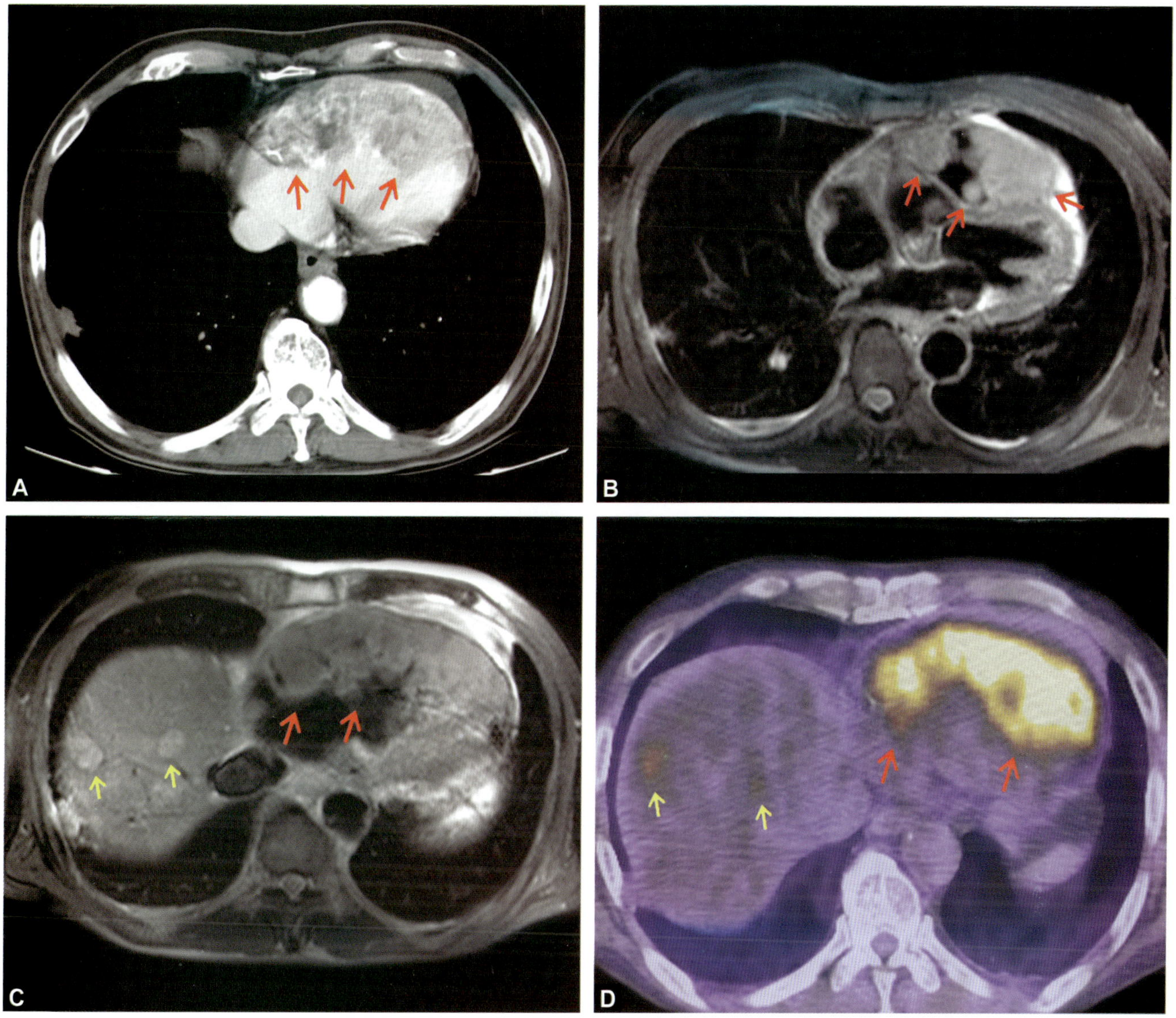

Figs. 54.27A to D: Hematogenous metastases (red arrows) from hepatocellular carcinoma. (A) Computed tomography (CT) image shows irregular thickening of free wall of right ventricle (RV); (B and C) Gadolinium-enhanced magnetic resonance (MR) images show diffuse irregular thickening of right ventricular wall (red arrows) and masses in the liver (yellow arrows); (D) ^{18}F-fluorodeoxyglucose positron emission tomography (18-FDG PET)/CT image shows FDG uptake in the hepatocellular carcinoma (yellow arrows) and cardiac metastases (red arrows).

VIDEO LEGEND

Video 54.1: Magnetic resonance imaging (MRI) demonstrating a left atrial myxoma. (Video courtesy of Scott D Flamm, MD).

REFERENCES

De Cobelli F, Esposito A, Mellone R, et al. Images in cardiovascular medicine. Late enhancement of a left ventricular cardiac fibroma assessed with gadolinium-enhanced cardiovascular magnetic resonance. Circulation. 2005;112(13):e242-3.

Dorsay TA, Ho VB, Rovira MJ, et al. Primary cardiac lymphoma: CT and MR findings. J Comput Assist Tomogr. 1993;17(6):978-81.

Grebenc ML, Rosado-de-Christenson ML, Green CE, et al. Cardiac myxoma: imaging features in 83 patients. Radiographics. 2002;22(3):673-89.

Kim EY, Choe YH, Sung K, et al. Multidetector CT and MR imaging of cardiac tumors. Korean J Radiol. 2009;10(2):164-75.

Sparrow PJ, Kurian JB, Jones TR, et al. MR imaging of cardiac tumors. Radiographics. 2005;25(5):1255-76.

Yahata S, Endo T, Honma H, et al. Sunray appearance on enhanced magnetic resonance image of cardiac angiosarcoma with pericardial obliteration. Am Heart J. 1994;127(2):468-71.

CHAPTER

55

Hyperlipidemia

Yashashwi Pokharel, Salim S Virani

INTRODUCTION

Hypercholesterolemia is one of the most important risk factor for atherosclerosis. Atherosclerosis starts with foam cells, which consist of macrophages filled with lipids, with subsequent formation of a fatty streak that can progress to an atherosclerotic plaque (Figs. 55.1A to G). If untreated, the plaque can increase in size and with time can cause

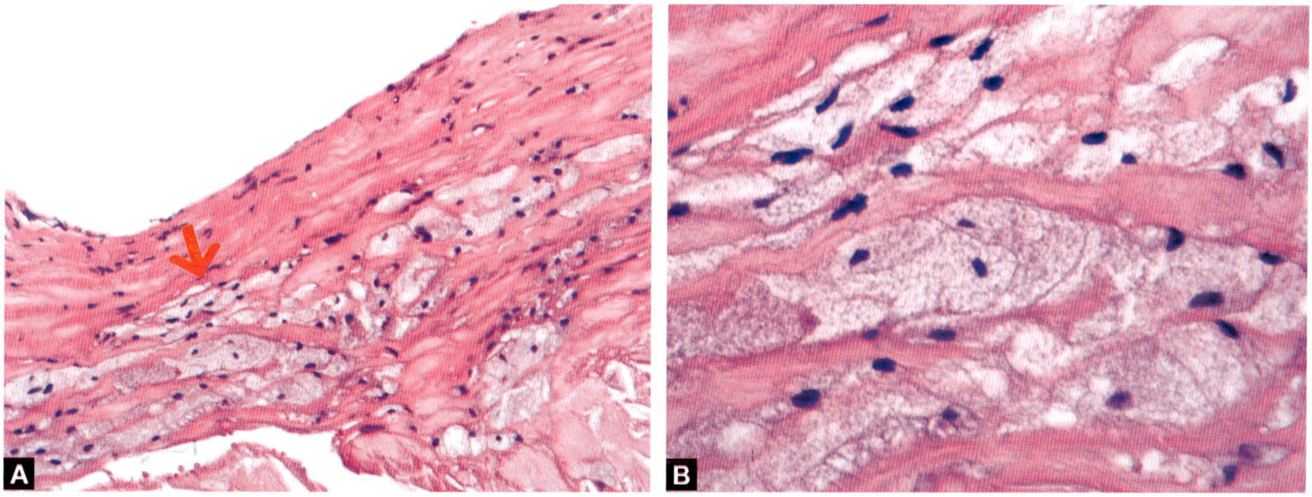

Figs. 55.1A and B: Foam cells and the early formation of an atherosclerotic plaque. Lipid-laden macrophages with abundant foamy cytoplasm and small nuclei. (Image posted by Patho on Wikipedia Commons).

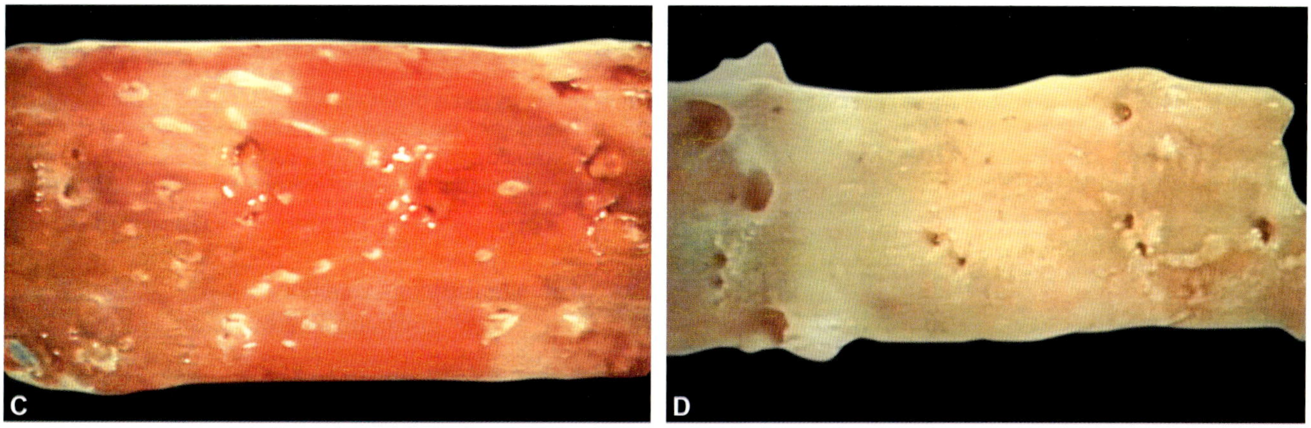

Figs. 55.1C and D: Pathology example of fatty streak, an early stage of atherosclerosis. (Image from Armed Forces Institute of Pathology).

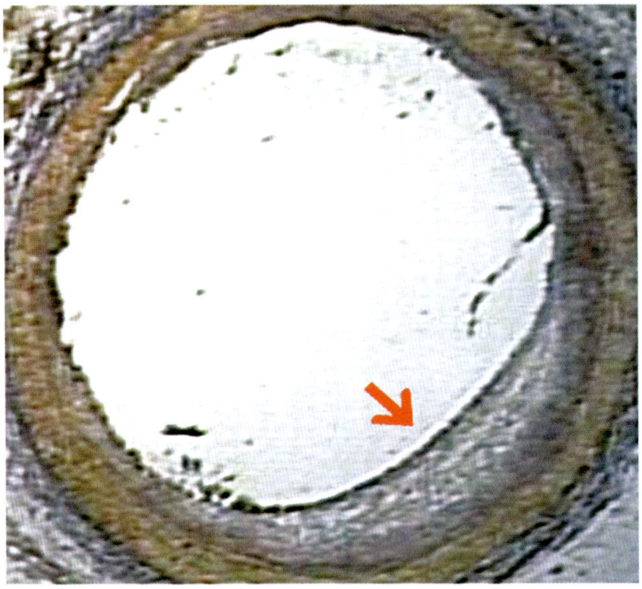

Fig. 55.1E: Histology image of atherosclerosis (arrow) in a coronary artery. (Image from Armed Forces Institute of Pathology).

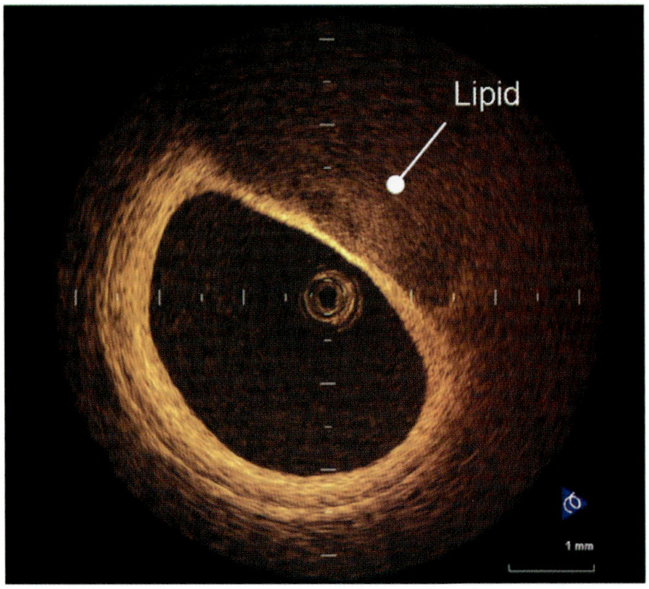

Fig. 55.1F: Optical coherence tomography (OCT) demonstrating a vulnerable plaque consisting of a large lipid pool and thin fibrous cap. (Image from Kubo T, Akasaka T. Identification of vulnerable plaques with optical coherence tomography. In: Pesek K (Ed). Atherosclerotic cardiovascular disease. Shanghai: InTech; 2011).

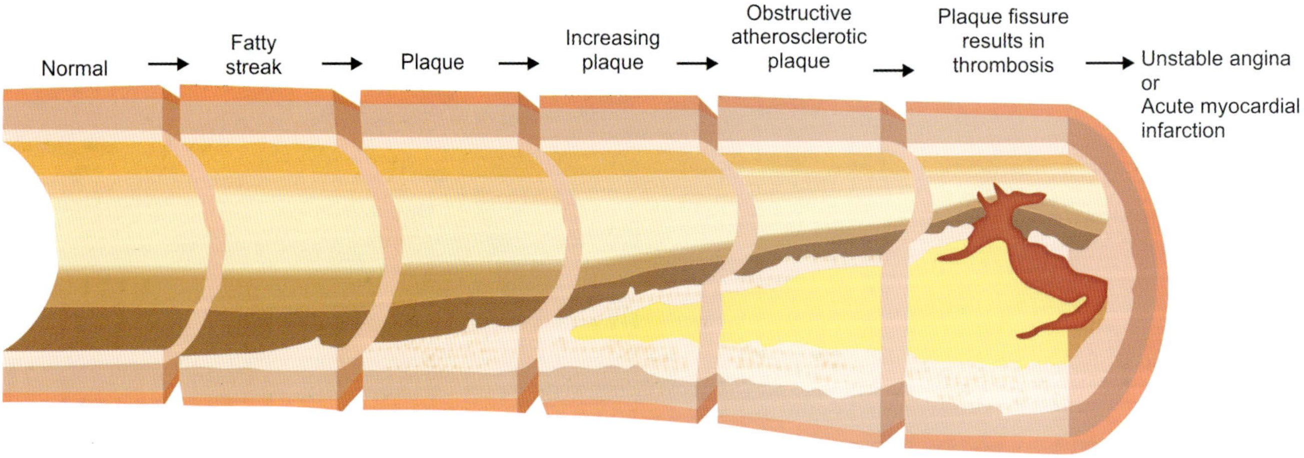

Fig. 55.1G: Schematic of atherosclerosis progression. Endothelial injury facilitates atherogenic lipoproteins to enter the vessel wall that signals inflammatory cells to enter the intima. Fat deposits inside macrophage forming "foam cells" and eventually a fatty streak, which is the first stage of atherosclerosis. An atherosclerotic plaque with a lipid rich core and a thin fibrous cap can form over time. Tissue ischemia can occur after about ≥ 70% or more of the lumen is obstructed, especially if the oxygen demand is increased (for example, during a stress test). The content of the lipid core of the atherosclerotic plaque can predict complications such as formation of ulceration with subsequent thrombosis and tissue infarction. Aggressive lipid lowering, especially with the use of statins can reduce the size of the lipid core of the plaque. Stable plaques have thicker fibrous cap and are calcified.

demand ischemia, or it can become unstable by plaque fissuring or ulceration with thrombosis resulting in tissue infarction.

There are different types of lipoproteins. A lipoprotein is made up of a protein and a lipid portion (Fig. 55.2). The lipid moiety has a hydrophobic core and a hydrophilic surrounding. The core generally consists of lipids such as triglycerides and cholesterol esters. The relative content of the cholesterol esters and the triglycerides vary in different lipoprotein cholesterols. Cholesterol esters are the predominant lipid core in low- and high-density lipoproteins. The core of the lipoprotein particle is

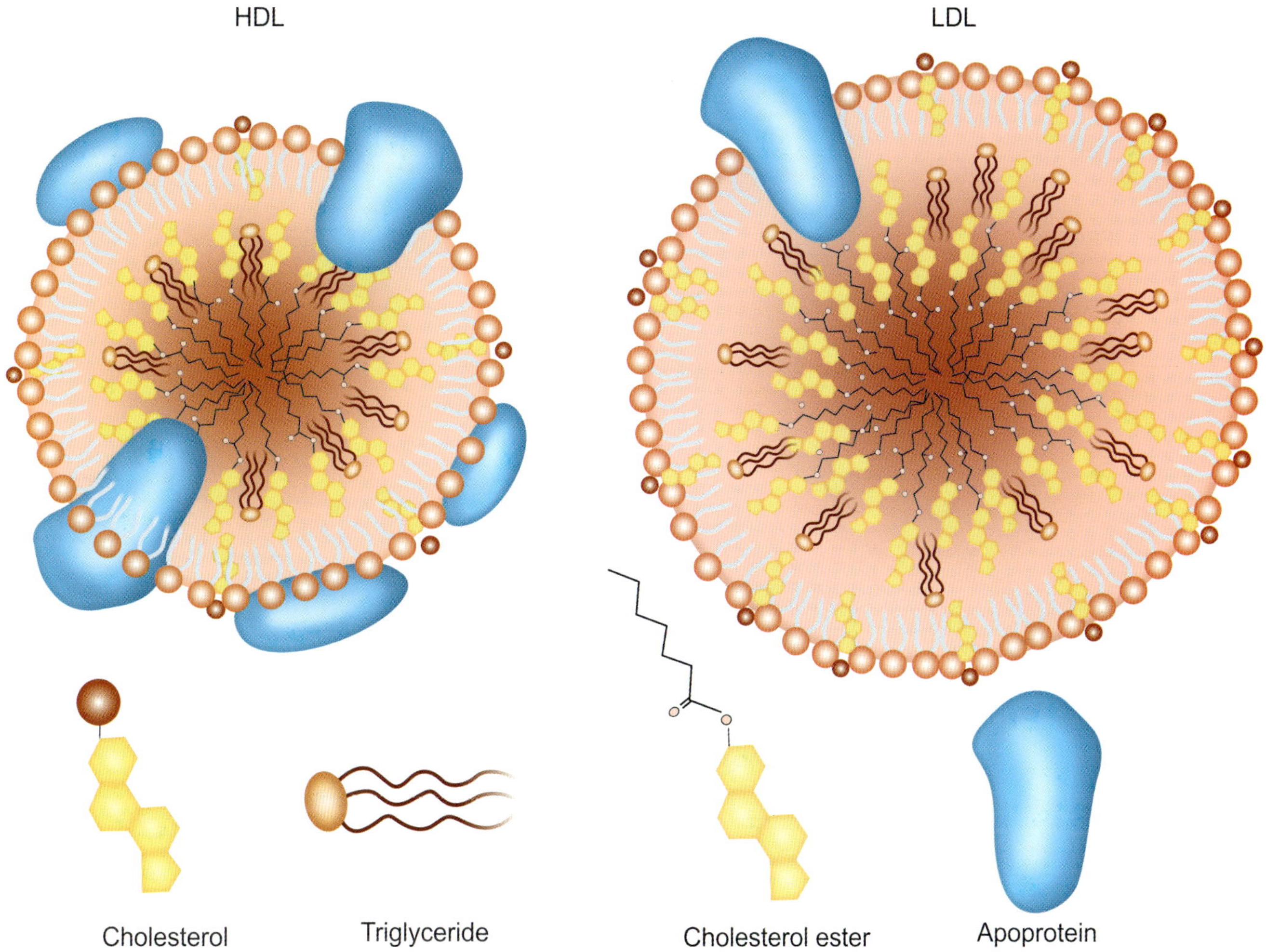

Fig. 55.2: Schematic of a lipoprotein cholesterol particle. (HDL: High-density lipoprotein; LDL: Low-density lipoprotein).

surrounded by phospholipid monolayer. Apoproteins, the protein moiety of lipoprotein, are present on the surface close to the phospholipids. Different lipoproteins contain different apoproteins.

TREATMENT OF HYPERLIPIDEMIA

3-hydroxy-3-methyl-glutaryl-coenzyme-A reductase (HMG-CoA reductase) inhibitors (commonly known as statins) are the cornerstone of cholesterol treatment for both primary and secondary cardiovascular disease prevention (Fig. 55.3). Multiple clinical trials have shown that statins lower cardiovascular events over long-term follow-up. Other lipid lowering medications include bile acid sequestering agents, fibric acid derivatives, nicotinic acid, cholesterol absorption inhibitors like ezetimibe and omega-3 fatty acids.

Heart healthy lifestyle habits are the foundation of cardiovascular disease prevention. According to the current guidelines, statins are the preferred agent for the treatment of hypercholesterolemia. The four different groups that will benefit from treatment with statins are: (1) presence of clinical atherosclerotic cardiovascular disease (ASCVD) as defined by acute coronary syndromes, history of myocardial infarction, stable or unstable angina, coronary or other arterial revascularization, stoke, transient ischemic attacks, or peripheral arterial disease presumed to be of atherosclerotic origin; (2) low-density lipoprotein cholesterol (LDL-C) ≥190 mg/dL; (3) LDL-C 70–189 mg/dL and age 40–75 years with type 1 or 2 diabetes; and (4) LDL-C 70–189 mg/dL and age 40–75 years without diabetes and ASCVD with estimated 10-year ASCVD risk ≥7.5% (Table 55.1). A high-intensity statin is recommended and if it is not tolerated, a moderate-intensity

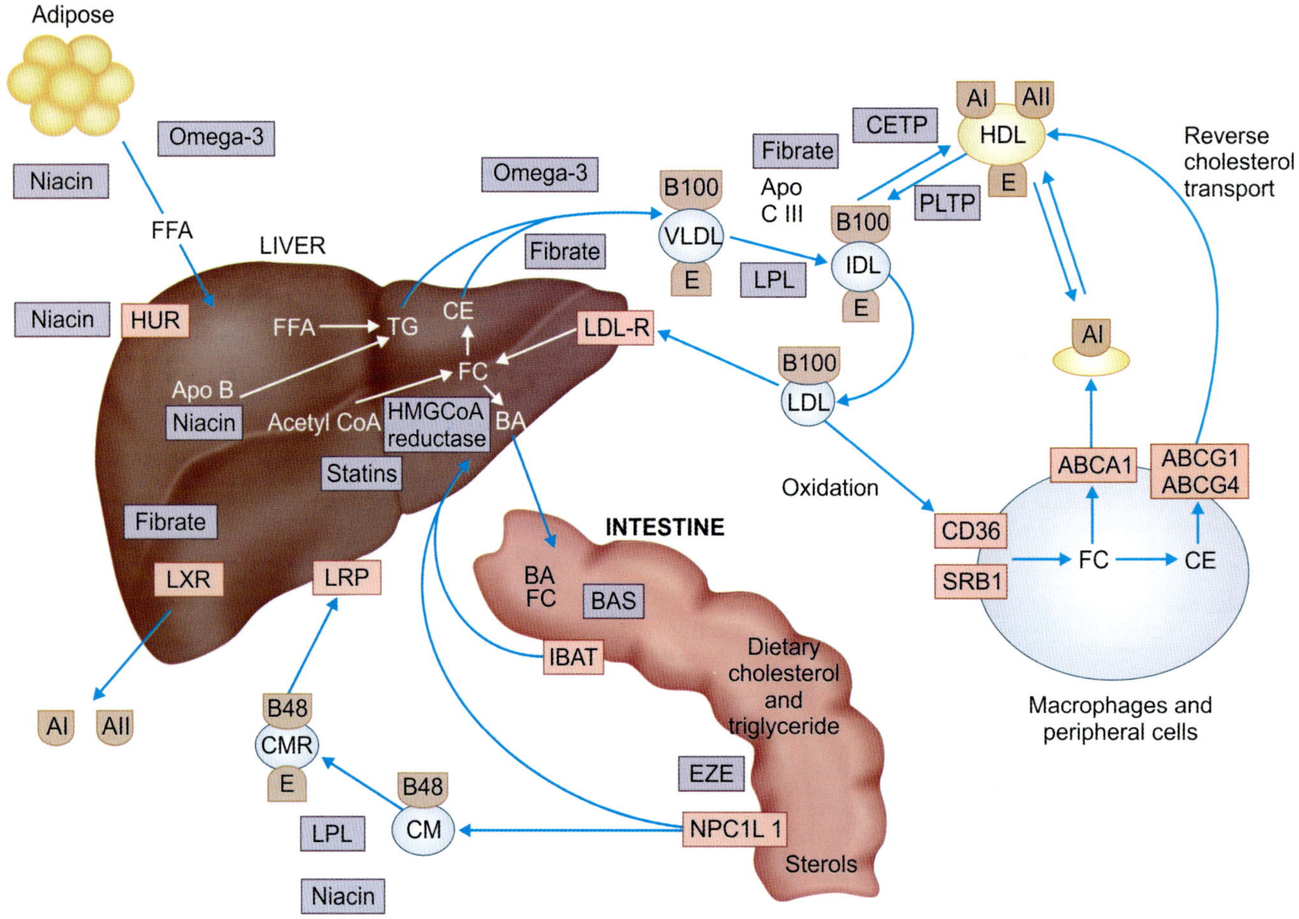

Fig. 55.3: Mechanism of action of various lipid-lowering medications. *Statins* inhibit 3-hydroxy-3-methyl-glutaryl-coenzyme-A reductase (HMG-CoA reductase), which is the rate-limiting step in cholesterol synthesis in liver. This results in reduced intrahepatic free cholesterol (FC) resulting in increased removal of low-density lipoprotein cholesterol (LDL-C) from plasma by upregulation of cell membrane LDL receptor (LDL-R). *Bile-acid sequestering agents (BAS)* interrupt the enterohepatic bile circulation by the intestinal bile acid transporter (IBAT). Cholesterol absorption inhibitors like *ezetimibe (EZE)* prevent absorption of dietary and biliary cholesterol (including plant sterols) via Niemann-Pick C1-Like 1 (NPC1L1) transporter in the intestinal wall. *Dietary sterol/stanols* competitively inhibit the uptake of cholesterol in the intestine. Intestinal inhibition of cholesterol absorption by either of these three agents can be associated with a compensatory increase in hepatic cholesterol synthesis. The mechanism of action of *niacin* is not completely understood. It is proposed that *niacin* inhibits the release of free fatty acids (FFA) from adipose tissue; increases lipoprotein lipase (LPL) activity thereby enhancing removal of chylomicron (CM) triglyceride from plasma; decreases apolipoprotein B (apo B) synthesis resulting in lower levels of very low-density lipoprotein cholesterol (VLDL-C) and intermediate-density lipoprotein cholesterol (IDL-C) and thus plasma triglycerides; and increases high-density cholesterol (HDL-C) through possibly decreased hepatic uptake. *Fibric acid derivatives (fibrates)* lower triglyceride levels by decreasing VLDL-C secretion and increasing catabolism of triglyceride-rich particles via several mechanisms, such as reduced apolipoprotein C-III production which upregulates lipoprotein-lipase-mediated lipolysis and increased cellular FFA uptake as well as increasing FFA catabolism. *Fibrates* increase apolipoprotein A-I and A-II (AI and AII) synthesis via the liver X receptor/retinoid X receptor heterodimer (LXR). The exact mechanism of action of *Omega-3 fatty acids (O-3)* is not fully understood. It likely reduces the rate of VLDL-C by inhibiting release of FFA from adipose tissue; inhibiting FFA synthesis, and increasing apo B degradation. [Image from Robinson JG. Antilipid agents. In: Chatterjee K, Anderson M, Heistad D, Kerber RE (Eds). Cardiology: An Illustrated Textbook. New Delhi, India: Jaypee Brothers Medical Publishers (P) Ltd; 2012].

Table 55.1: Summary of revised guidelines for the treatment of hyperlipidemia in the 2013 ACCF/AHA guidelines. ASCVD = atherosclerotic cardiovascular disease (including acute coronary syndromes, history of myocardial infarction, stable or unstable angina, coronary or other arterial revascularization, stroke, transient ischemic attacks, or peripheral arterial disease presumed to be of atherosclerotic origin). (LDL-C: Low-density lipoprotein cholesterol).

Clinical Factors	***Moderate Intensity Statin (daily dose lowers LDL-C by approximately 30% to < 50%)***	***High Intensity Statin (daily dose lowers LDL-C by approximately ≥ 50%)***
Clinical ASCVD	Clinical ASCVD and age ≤ 75 years but not a candidate for high-intensity statin	Clinical ASCVD and age ≤ 75 years
	Clinical ASCVD and age > 75 years	
LDL-C ≥ 190 mg/dL	LDL-C ≥ 190 mg/dL but not a candidate for high-intensity statin	LDL-C ≥ 190 mg/dL
Diabetes (type 1 or 2) without ASCVD	Diabetes (type 1 or 2) and age 40–75 years with estimated 10-year ASCVD risk < 7.5%	Diabetes (type 1 or 2) and age 40–75 years with estimated 10-year ASCVD risk ≥ 7.5%
Estimated 10-year ASCVD risk alone	≥ 7.5% estimated 10-year ASCVD risk and age 40–75 years (moderate to high intensity statin recommended)	

Table 55.2: HMG-CoA reductase inhibitor mediated reduction in LDL-C (from a meta-analysis of 164 trials independent of pretreatment LDL-C). Except for pitavastatin data are presented for all statins as the absolute reductions in LDL-C (mg/dL), with the percent reductions in LDL-C standardized to a LDL-C of 186 mg/dL given in parenthesis.

Statin	***10 mg/day***	***20 mg/day***	***40 mg/day***	***80 mg/day***
Atorvastatin	†69 (37)	†80 (43)	*91 (49)	*102 (55)
Fluvastatin	29 (15)	39 (21)	50 (27)	†61 (33)
Lovastatin‡	39 (21)	54 (29)	†68 (37)	83 (45)
Pravastatin	37 (20)	45 (24)	†53 (29)	†62 (33)
Rosuvastatin§	†80 (43)	*90 (48)	*99 (53)	108 (58)
Simvastatin	51 (27)	†60 (32)	†69 (37)	78 (42)
Pitavastatin	1 mg (33)	†2 mg (39)	†4 mg (45)	—

Note:

- Corresponding doses with * indicate high-intensity statin and with † indicate moderate-intensity statin therapy. In addition Rosuvastatin 5 mg and Fluvastatin 40 mg twice daily or Fluvastatin XL 80 mg are all also considered moderate-intensity statin therapy
- ‡Maximum dose of 80 mg/day administered as two 40-mg tablets
- §Not approved by the Food and Drug Administration at 80 mg/day
- §Recommended maximum dose in Asians is 20 mg/day
- ¶Pitavastatin was not included in the meta-analysis. Data presented as Pitavastatin dose and percent reductions in LDL-C (in parentheses). Result on the table is based on the drug manufacturer's package insert
- HMG-CoA: 3-hydroxy-3-methyl-glutaryl-coenzyme-A
- LDL-C: Low-density lipoprotein cholesterol

statin should be considered. High- and moderate-intensity statin therapy is defined as the daily statin dose that lowers LDL-C by ≥ 50% and by approximately 30% to <50% respectively. The guideline further considers moderate-intensity statin therapy for individuals with age >75 years with clinical ASCVD, and for patients with diabetes age 40–75 years without ASCVD and estimated 10-year ASCVD risk < 7.5%.

There are seven Food and Drug Administration (FDA) approved statins available for use in the United States. The efficacy of each of these agents and doses corresponding to high- and moderate-intensity statin therapy are listed in Table 55.2. For every doubling of the standard dose, an approximate 6% further decrease in the LDL-C levels can be expected. In general, statins are very well tolerated. Potential adverse effects such as myositis, rhabdomyolysis and abnormalities of liver enzymes are uncommon.

Non-high-density lipoprotein cholesterol (Non-HDL-C) levels reflect the cholesterol content of all atherogenic lipoprotein particles (Fig. 55.4). It is equal to total cholesterol minus high-density lipoprotein cholesterol. It includes

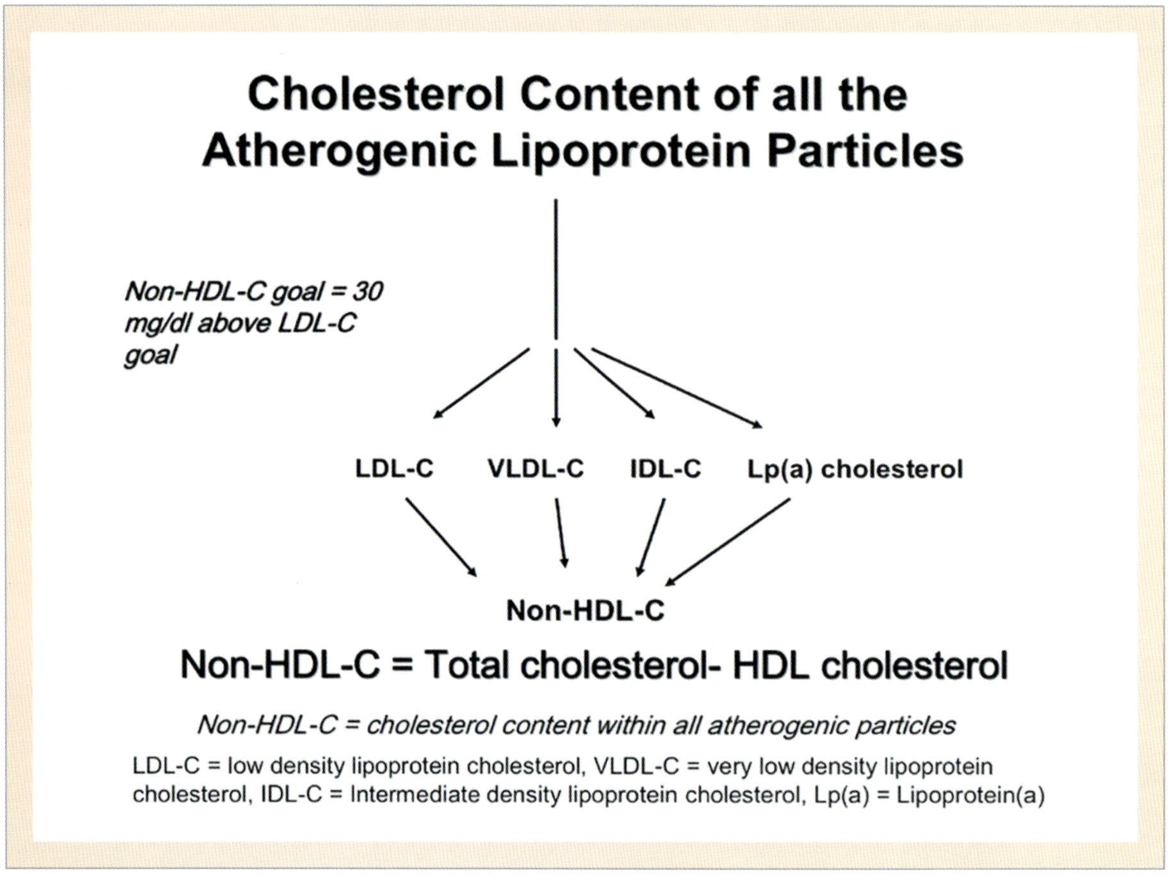

Fig. 55.4: Non-high-density lipoprotein cholesterol. (Image with permission from Virani S. Non-HDL cholesterol as a metric of good quality of care: opportunities and challenges. Tex Heart Ins J. 2011;38;160-2).

LDL-C, very low-density lipoprotein cholesterol (VLDL-C), intermediate-density lipoprotein cholesterol (IDL-C) and lipoprotein(a) [Lp(a)] cholesterol.

FAMILIAL HYPERCHOLESTEROLEMIA

Familial hypercholesterolemia (FH) results from defects in genes for low-density lipoprotein receptor, apolipoprotein (Apo) B, proprotein convertase subtilisin/kexin type 9 (PCSK9) or yet other unidentified defects. Hypercholesterolemia is present since childhood leading to extensive atherosclerosis and premature coronary heart disease. In the overall population, heterozygous FH is present in 1/(300–500) persons, and homozygous FH is present in 1/1,000,000 persons. FH should be suspected if LDL-C ≥ 190 mg/dL or non-HDL-C is ≥ 220 mg/dL in adults ≥ 20 years, and if LDL-C ≥ 160 mg/dL or non-HDL-C is ≥ 190 mg/dL in person < 20 years. All first-degree family members of the affected individual should have lipids level checked. Usually there is positive family history of very high cholesterol levels. Tendon xanthoma is very specific for FH. Other features such as tuberous xanthomas, xanthelasma and arcus corneae, if present, especially in patients with age < 45 years, can indicate FH (Figs. 55.5 to 55.10).

Genetic screening for FH is generally not needed for diagnosis or treatment. Aggressive lipid lowering to achieve LDL-C reduction of at least 50% or more is necessary using 3-hydroxy-3-methyl-glutaryl-coenzyme-A (HMG-CoA) reductase inhibitor (mostly useful only in heterozygous FH), novel agents such as mipomersen and lomitapide, other lipid-lowering medications (e.g. bile acid binding resins, niacin, ezetimibe, plant stanols), LDL apheresis, and therapeutic lifestyle changes. Referral to a lipid specialist should be considered. Liver transplantation and ileal bypass may be considered in some cases of homozygous FH.

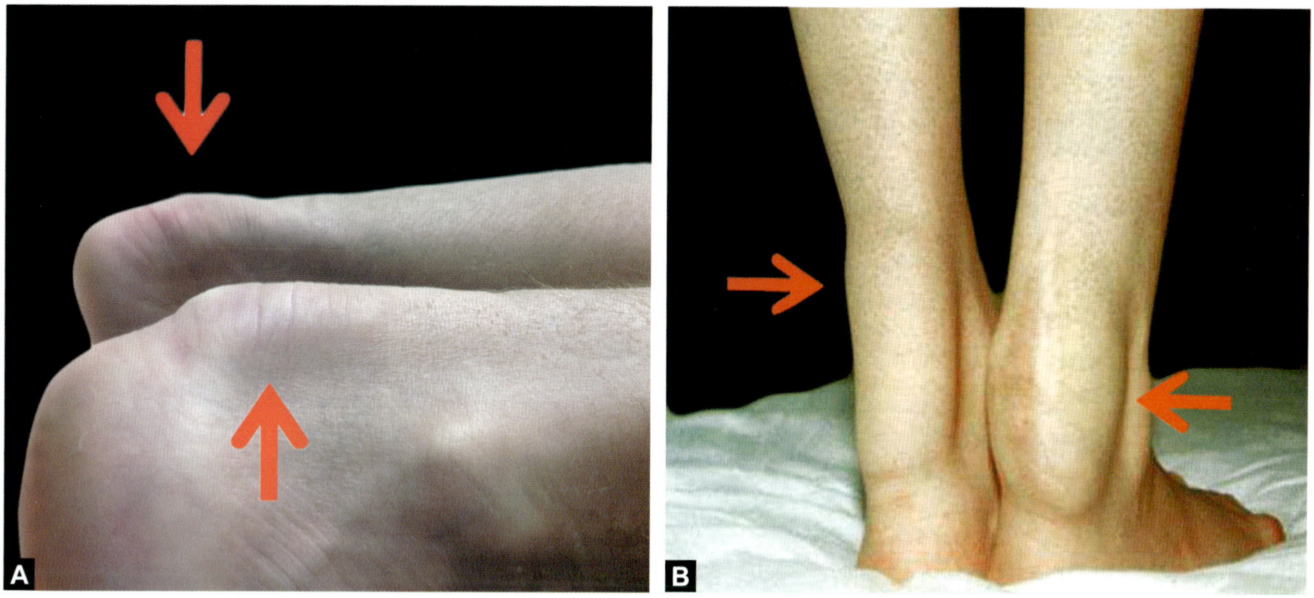

Figs. 55.5A and B: Tendon xanthomas of Achilles tendon in two different patients with familial hypercholesterolemia. Achilles tendon is the most common site for tendon xanthomas. Subtle cases may be missed by inspection, and therefore it is important to palpate the tendons. [Figure 55.5B with permission from Nihal I, Reyhan G. Cerebrotendinous xanthomatosis: description of a case. Afri J Neuro Sci. 2005;24(2):90-5].

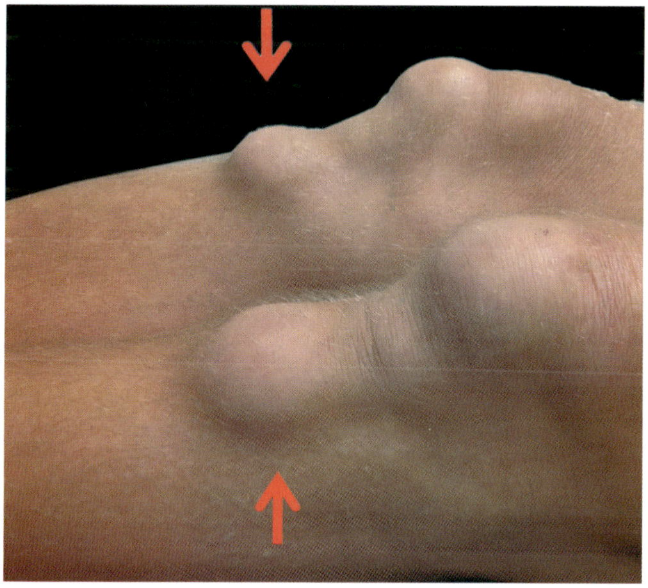

Fig. 55.6A: Patellar tendon xanthomas. Tendon xanthomas results from deposition of cholesterol in tendons, especially tendons that are irritated by frequent movements and friction. Tendon xanthomas are pathognomonic of familial hypercholesterolemia. Cholesterol levels should be checked in anyone with suspected tendon xanthomas.

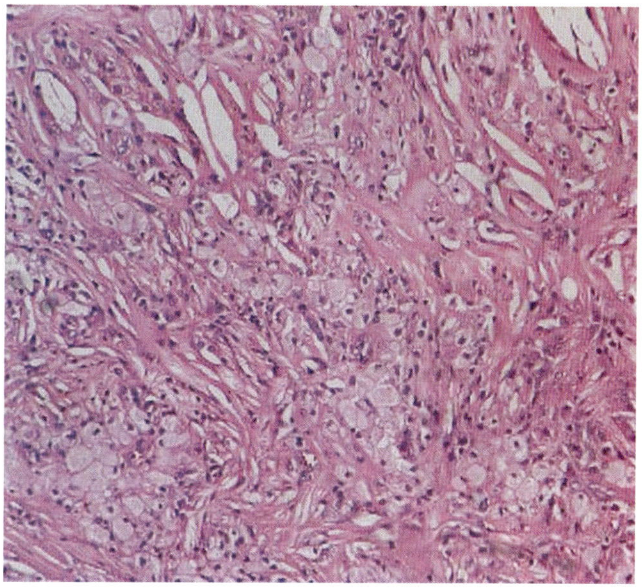

Fig. 55.6B: Histology of a xanthoma. Image demonstrates lipid-laden foam cells with large areas of cholesterol clefts. (Image from Kumar AA, Shantha GPS, Srinivasan Y, et al. Acute myocardial infarction in an 18-year-old South Indian girl with familial hypercholesterolemia: a case report. Cases J. 2008;1:71).

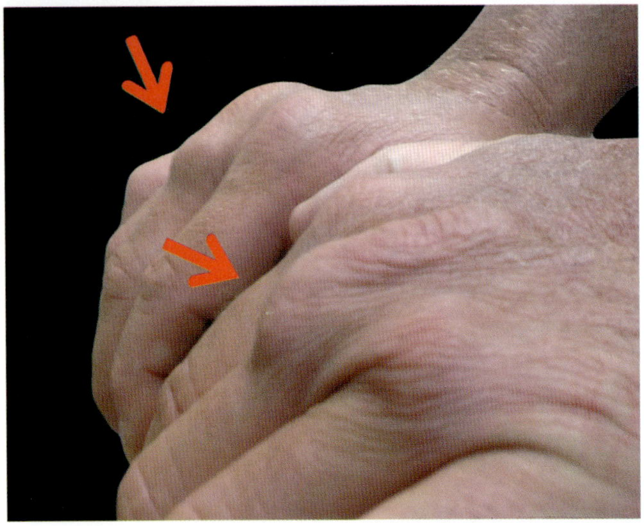

Fig. 55.7: Tendon xanthomas around the tendons of the dorsal surface of hand. Tendon xanthomas are painless, indurated lesions. Other common tendons involved by tendon xanthomas include the plantar tendons of the foot and the triceps tendon. Tendon xanthomas usually do not regress after lowering cholesterol.

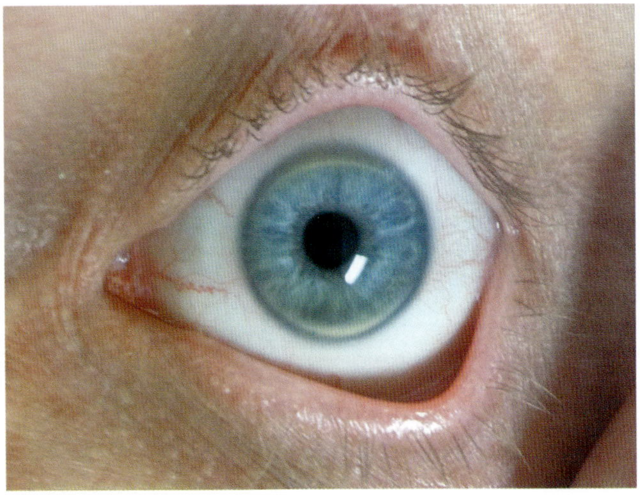

Fig. 55.8A: Incomplete corneal arcus in a patient with familial hypercholesterolemia (FH). Corneal arcus is a gray or white arc present above or below the outer margin of the cornea. It starts as an incomplete arc and finally becomes a complete ring. It is indicative of FH if found under the age of 45 years.

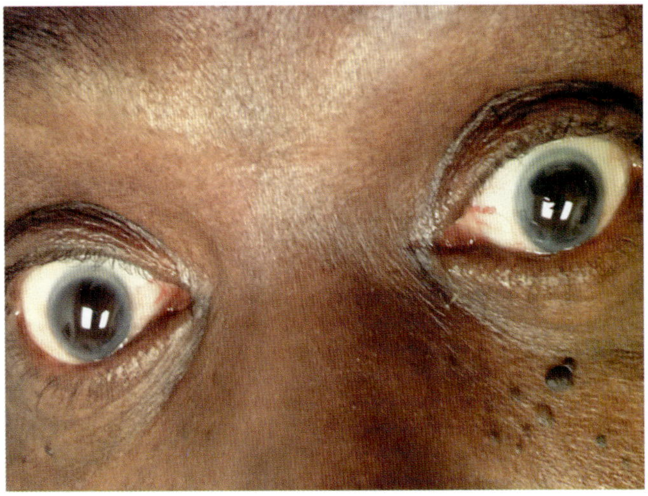

Fig. 55.8B: Complete corneal arcus. Corneal arcus is common in older adults, which could be unrelated to hypercholesterolemia. An average person with hyperlipidemia but without familial hypercholesterolemia does not develop an arc solely because of the cholesterol. Congenital form of corneal arcus also exists.

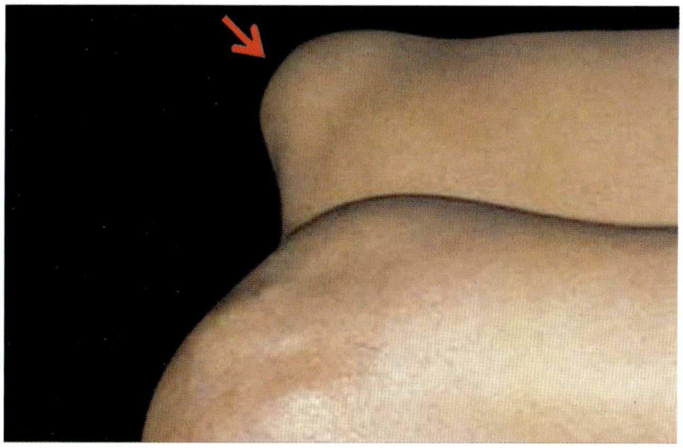

Fig. 55.9: Tuberous xanthomas of the knee joint. Tuberous xanthomas are painless lesions present near joints, especially joints prone to frequent motions and friction. Some of the other common sites for tuberous xanthomas include elbow and knuckles of the hands. In extreme cases, they can be found outside the joints. (Image with permission from Bel S, Garcia-Patos V, Rodriguez L, et al. Cerebrotendinous xanthomatosis. J Am Acad Dermat. 2001; 45:292-5).

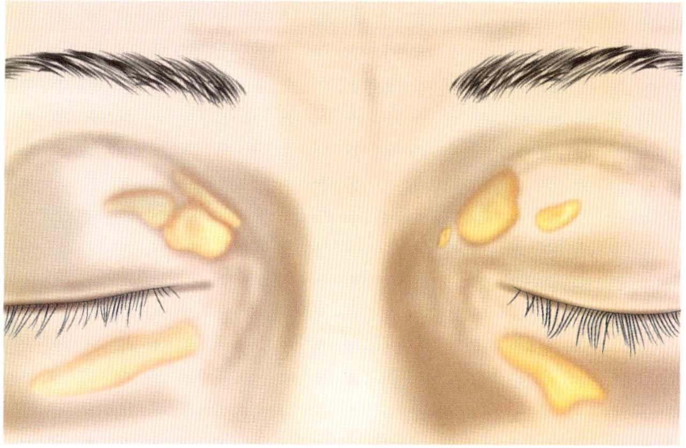

Fig. 55.10: Palpebral xanthelasmas. Xanthelasmas are painless cutaneous deposition of lipids, visible as yellowish sharply demarcated lesions usually present around the eyelids. Cholesterol-related xanthelasmas may regress after lowering the cholesterol level. Although tuberous xanthomas and xanthelasmas are not specific for familial hypercholesterolemia, their presence in a young patient should prompt evaluation by measurement of cholesterol level.

REFERENCES

AstraZenecaus. (2013). CESTOR rosuvastatin calcium. [online] Available from http://www1.astrazeneca-us.com/pi/crestor.pdf [Accessed February, 2014].

Baigent C, Blackwell L, Emberson J, et al. Efficacy and safety of more intensive lowering of LDL cholesterol: a meta-analysis of data from 170,000 participants in 26 randomised trials. Lancet. 2010;376(9753):1670-81.

Goldberg AC, Hopkins PN, Toth PP, et al. Familial hypercholesterolemia: screening, diagnosis and management of pediatric and adult patients: clinical guidance from the National Lipid Association Expert Panel on Familial Hypercholesterolemia. J Clin Lipidol. 2011;5(3):133-40.

Kowa Pharmaceuticals America, Inc. (2013). Livalo (pitavastatin) tablet. [online] Available from http://www.kowapharma.com/documents/LIVALO_PI_CURRENT.pdf [Accessed February, 2014].

Law MR, Wald NJ, Rudnicka AR. Quantifying effect of statins on low density lipoprotein cholesterol, ischaemic heart disease, and stroke: systematic review and meta-analysis. BMJ. 2003;326(7404):1423.

Stone NJ RJ, Lichtenstein AH, Bairey Merz CN, et al. Guideline on the treatment of blood cholesterol to reduce atherosclerotic cardiovascular risk in adults. J Am College Cardiol. 2013;pii: S0735-1097(13)06028-2.

Virani SS. Non-HDL cholesterol as a metric of good quality of care: opportunities and challenges. Texas Heart Institute journal/from the Texas Heart Institute of St Luke's Episcopal Hospital, Texas Children's Hospital. 2011;38(2):160-2.

CHAPTER

56

Physical Findings in Cardiovascular Disease

Glenn N Levine

Although older diagnostic studies, such as electrocardiography and chest X-ray, and newer imaging modalities such as transthoracic echocardiography, transesophageal echocardiography, cardiac computed tomography (CT) scanning, and magnetic resonance imaging are relied upon to make many cardiovascular diagnoses, simple physical examination can often provide important clues as to the cause of a patient's symptoms.

Physical examination of the neck veins (Figs. 56.1 and 56.2) and peripheral pulses are important in the diagnosis of such cardiovascular diseases as congestive heart failure, valvular heart disease, aortic coarctation and peripheral arterial disease. Simple carotid sinus massage (Fig. 56.3) can determine the cause of syncope in a patient with carotid sinus hypersensitivity. Alternating strong and weak pulses suggest pulses alternans (Fig. 56.4) and severe left ventricular dysfunction and heart failure. The finding on physical examination of marked and unexplained neck vein

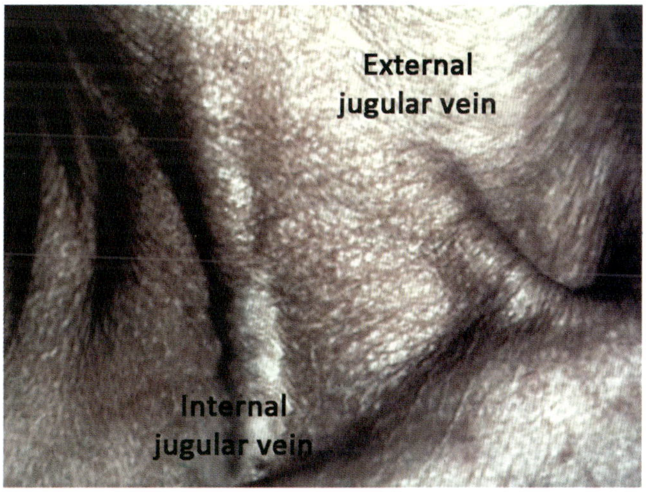

Fig. 56.1: The courses of the external and internal jugular veins. The external jugular vein runs from lateral to the medial side of the neck across the sternocleidomastoid muscle. The internal jugular vein starts at the root of the neck in between the two heads of the sternocleidomastoid muscle runs superiorly toward the angle of the jaw. [Image and legend text from Chatterjee K. Physical examination. In: Chatterjee K, Anderson M, Heistad D, Kerber RE (Eds). Cardiology—An Illustrated Textbook, 1st edition. New Delhi, India: Jaypee Brothers Medical Publishers (P) Ltd.; 2012. pp. 151-73].

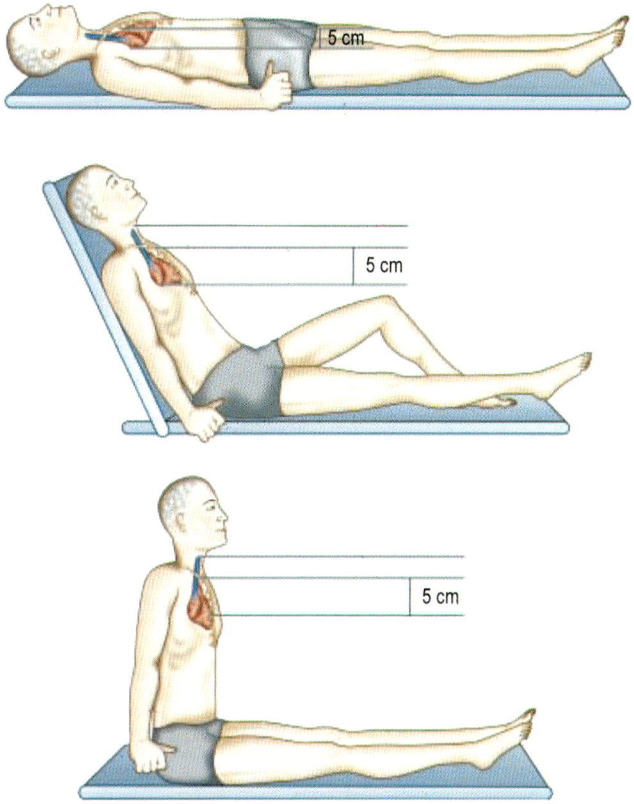

Fig. 56.2: The angle at which the patient is examined may have to be adjusted in order to appreciate and assess jugular venous pressure. Note however, that regardless of the body angle, the distance between the center of the right atrium and the sternal angle is fixed at 5 cm. [Image from Sarkar A. Bedside Cardiology, 1st edition. New Delhi, India: Jaypee Brothers Medical Publishers (P) Ltd.; 2012].

distention and on careful sphygmomanometry of pulses paradoxus (Fig. 56.5) may make the diagnosis of pericardial tamponade well before an echocardiogram is obtained.

Careful examination of the skin (Figs. 56.6 to 56.13) can yield findings associated with many cardiovascular conditions (Tables 56.1 to 56.4). Examination of the extremities

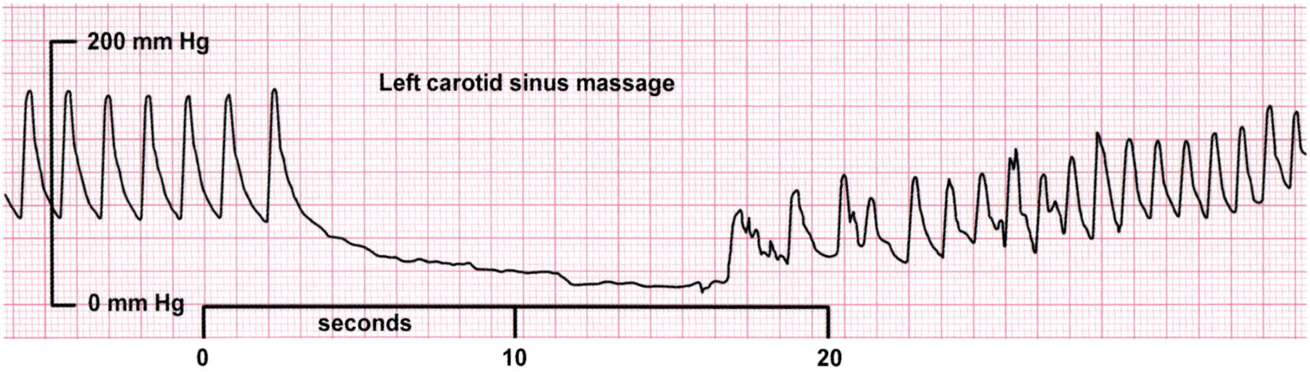

Fig. 56.3: Carotid sinus massage. Intraarterial tracing during carotid sinus massage. Carotid sinus massage results in increased vagal tone. In this case, there is a dramatic response with 12 seconds of asystole occurring. The patient was diagnosed with carotid sinus hypersensitivity. (Image courtesy of Dr Addison Taylor, Baylor College of Medicine).

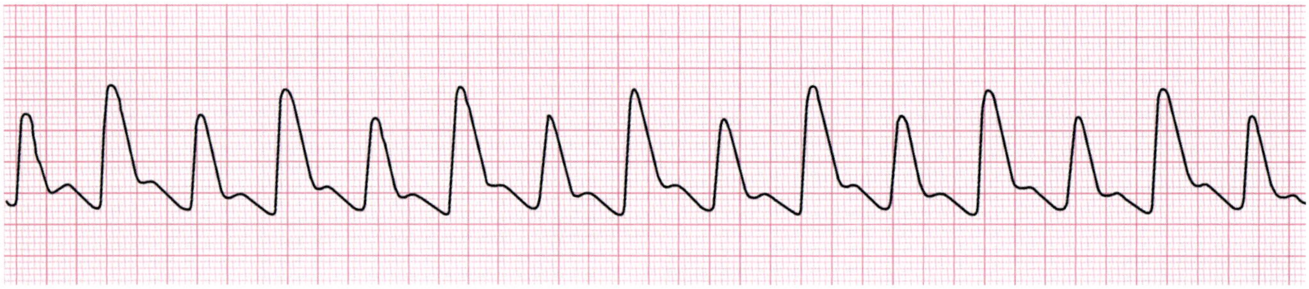

Fig. 56.4: Arterial tracing of pulses alternans. The finding on arterial palpation or during blood pressure measurement by manual sphygmomanometer of alternating stronger and weaker pulse may be a clue that the patient has severe left ventricular systolic dysfunction and heart failure. [Image from Chatterjee K. Physical examination. In: Chatterjee K, Anderson M, Heistad D, Kerber RE (Eds). Cardiology—An Illustrated Textbook, 1st edition. New Delhi, India: Jaypee Brothers Medical Publishers (P) Ltd.; 2012. pp. 151-73].

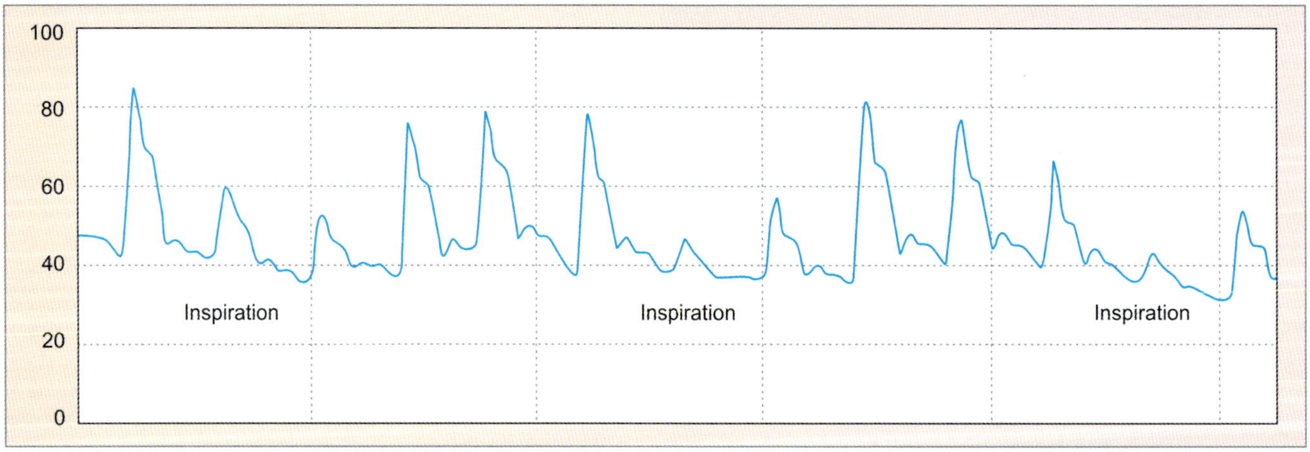

Fig. 56.5: Pulses paradoxus. Arterial line tracing demonstrating the finding of pulses paradoxus in a patient with cardiac tamponade. There is a marked decrease in arterial pressure with inspiration. This finding is appreciated during careful physical examination using a manual sphygmomanometer. [Image adapted from Chatterjee K. Physical examination. In: Chatterjee K, Anderson M, Heistad D, Kerber RE (Eds). Cardiology—An Illustrated Textbook, 1st edition. New Delhi, India: Jaypee Brothers Medical Publishers (P) Ltd.; 2012. pp. 151-73].

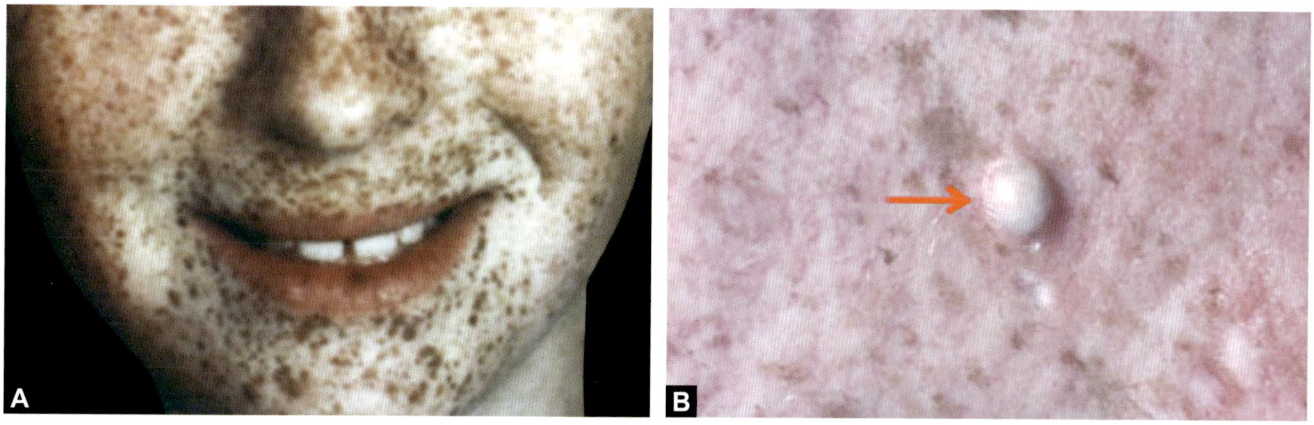

Figs. 56.6A and B: Cutaneous findings in Carney complex. (A) There are numerous nonelevated brown-black spots visible; (B) Skin myxoma (arrow) in a patient with Carney complex. [Images from Courcoutsakis NA, Tatsi C, Patronas NJ, et al. The complex of myxomas, spotty skin pigmentation and endocrine overactivity (Carney complex): imaging findings with clinical and pathological correlation. Insights Imaging. 2013;4(1):119-33].

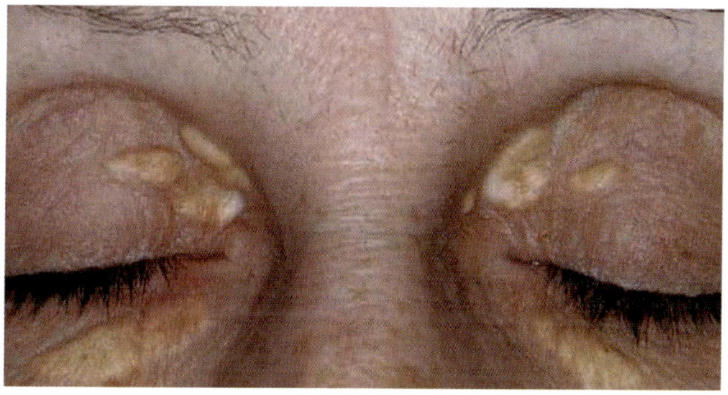

Fig. 56.7: Xanthelasmas—These are yellowish papules and plaques involving the upper and lower eyelids, and should raise concerns that the patient has a form of familial hyperlipidemia. [Image and legend text from Mendiratta V, Malik M. Cardiocutaneous diseases. In: Chopra HK, Nanda NC (Eds). Textbook of Cardiology: A Clinical and Historical Perspective, 1st edition. New Delhi, India: Jaypee Brothers Medical Publishers (P) Ltd.; 2013. pp. 396-407].

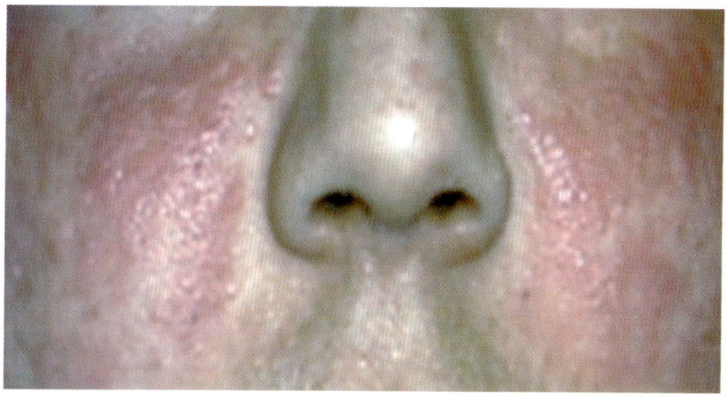

Fig. 56.8: The malar rash in systemic lupus erythematosus (SLE). [Image from Mendiratta V, Malik M. Cardiocutaneous diseases. In: Chopra HK, Nanda NC (Eds). Textbook of Cardiology: A Clinical and Historical Perspective, 1st edition. New Delhi, India: Jaypee Brothers Medical Publishers (P) Ltd.; 2013. pp. 396-407].

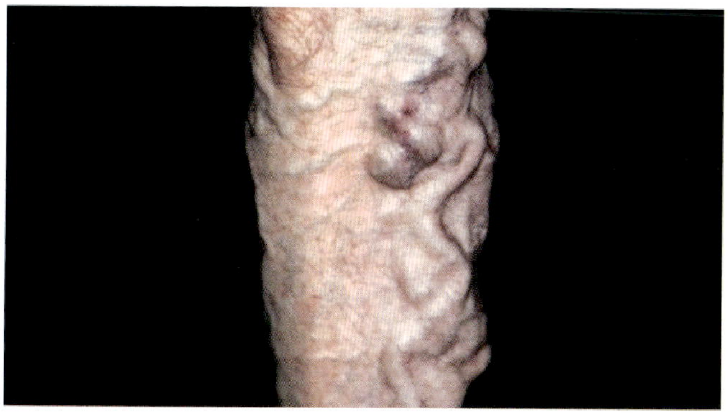

Fig. 56.9: Livedo reticularis. There is mottled cyanotic skin discoloration of the lower extremities in a network pattern. [Image and legend text from Mendiratta V, Malik M. Cardiocutaneous diseases. In: Chopra HK, Nanda NC (Eds). Textbook of Cardiology: A Clinical and Historical Perspective, 1st edition. New Delhi, India: Jaypee Brothers Medical Publishers (P) Ltd.; 2013. pp. 396-407].

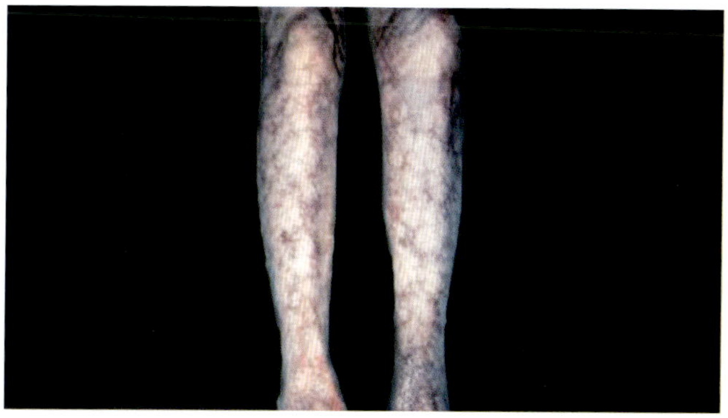

Fig. 56.10: Varicose veins. While most varicose veins have no clear secondary cause, varicose veins may occasionally be due to prior deep vein thrombosis (DVT). [Image from Khanna AK. Varicose veins. In: Khanna AK, Puneet (Eds). Manual of Vascular Surgery, 1st edition. New Delhi, India: Jaypee Brothers Medical Publishers (P) Ltd.; 2010. pp. 267-90].

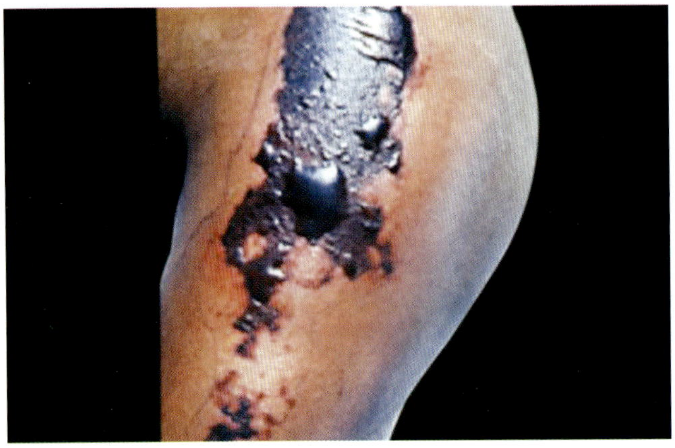

Fig. 56.11: Coumadin-induced skin necrosis. (Image posted by Herbert L Fred, MD and Hendrik A van Dij, Images of memorable cases. Available on cnx.org).

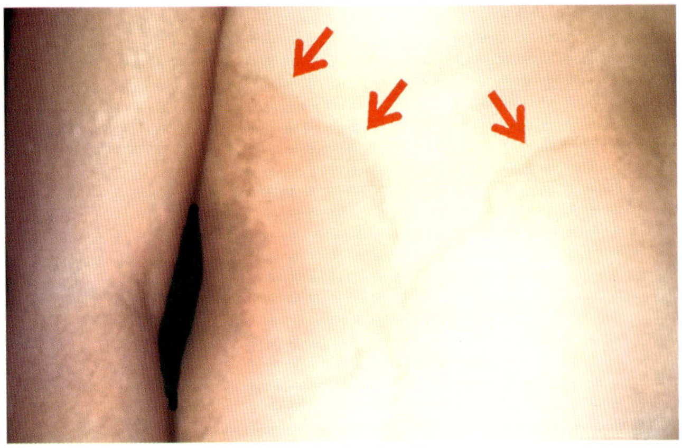

Fig. 56.12: Erythema marginatum (arrows) on the trunk of a patient with rheumatic fever. [Image from Bhalerao JC. Rheumatic fever. In: Bhalerao JC (Ed). Essentials of Clinical Cardiology, 1st edition. New Delhi, India: Jaypee Brothers Medical Publishers (P) Ltd.; 2013. pp. 85-86].

Table 56.1: Autoimmune disorders that can cause cardiovascular disease, and the cutaneous features of the disease. [Table adapted from Mendiratta V, Malik M. Cardiocutaneous diseases. In: Chopra HK, Nanda NC (Eds). Textbook of Cardiology: A Clinical and Historical Perspective. New Delhi, India: Jaypee Brothers Medical Publishers (P) Ltd.; 2013. pp. 396-407].

Disease	*Cardiovascular Morbidity*	*Cutaneous Features*
Antiphospholipid antibody syndrome	Recurrent arterial and venous thromboses	Livedo reticularis, retiform purpura, Raynaud's phenomenon, nailfold and leg ulcers, cutaneous necrosis and splinter hemorrhages
Churg-Strauss vasculitis	Cardiac granulomas and fibrosis, pericarditis, mitral regurgitation (MR) and coronary artery vasculitis	Palpable purpura, infiltrated nodules on scalp or limbs, livedo reticularis, retiform purpura, migratory erythema and Raynaud's phenomenon
Dermatomyositis/polymyositis	Atrioventricular defects, arrhythmias, pericarditis, pericardial effusion and dilated cardiomyopathy	Gottron's papules, Gottron's sign, periungual telangiectasias, dystrophic cuticles, heliotrope rash, confluent macular violaceous erythema, calcinosis cutis and poikiloderma
Neonatal systemic lupus erythematosus (SLE)	Complete heart block, second-degree heart block, dilated cardiomyopathy, myocarditis and valvular defects	Raccoon sign, erythema annulare, vitiligo-like eruption, morphea-like lesions and papules on the feet
Polyarteritis nodosa	Coronary artery vasculitis, hypertension and myocardial infarction (MI)	Dermal or subcutaneous nodules commonly on distal lower extremities, retiform purpura and digital gangrene
Rheumatoid arthritis	Pericarditis, pericardial effusion, aortic regurgitation (AR), MR, aortitis and aneurysmal rupture	Rheumatoid nodules, rheumatoid vasculitis, Felty's syndrome and pyoderma gangrenosum
Scleroderma	Myocardial fibrosis, congestive heart failure (CHF), arrhythmias, pericarditis, primary pulmonary hypertension (PHT) and cor pulmonale	Swelling of skin at initial presentation, skin sclerosis in later stages and Raynaud's phenomenon
Systemic lupus erythematosus	Pericarditis, pericardial effusion, Libman-Sacks endocarditis, atherosclerosis, hypertension, MR and AR	Malar rash, discoid rash, photosensitivity, oral ulcers, Raynaud's phenomenon, livedo reticularis and leg ulcers
Takayasu's arteritis (Pulseless disease and aortic arch syndrome)	Hypertension, AR, pulseness, occlusion of subclavian of carotid arteries and vascular bruits	Erythema nodosum-like lesions, erythema induratum-like lesions, pyoderma gangrenosum and necrotizing vasculitis
Temporal arteritis (Giant cell arteritis)	Aortitis, aortic aneurysms, angina and MI	Prominence of superficial temporal arteries with presence of focal nodules

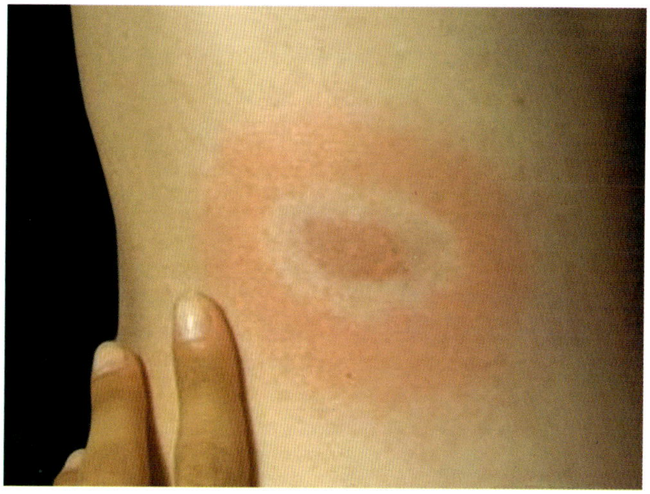

Fig. 56.13: Erythema migrans in a patient with Lyme disease. In its later stage, Lyme disease is associated with a risk of high degree atrioventricular (AV) block. (Image uploaded by Jongarrison on Wikipedia).

Table 56.2: Endocrinological disorders that can cause cardiovascular disease, and the cutaneous features of the disease. [Table adapted from Mendiratta V, Malik M. Cardiocutaneous diseases. In: Chopra HK, Nanda NC (Eds). Textbook of Cardiology: A Clinical and Historical Perspective. New Delhi, India: Jaypee Brothers Medical Publishers (P) Ltd.; 2013. pp. 396-407].

Disease	*Cardiovascular Morbidity*	*Cutaneous Features*
Acromegaly	Left ventricular hypertrophy, CHF and hypertension	Protruding, thickened lower lip, edema of eyelids, large and furrowed tongue, triangular large ears, skin tags and acne
Carcinoid syndrome	Right-sided endocardial fibrosis, pulmonary stenosis (PS), tricuspid incompetence and CHF	Flushing, telangiectasias and periorbital edema
Cushing's syndrome	Hypertension, accelerated atherosclerosis and MI	Truncal obesity, "buffalo hump", "moon facies", skin atrophy, fragility and easy bruisability, telangiectasias, striae, hirsutism and acneiform lesions
Diabetes mellitus	Autonomic disturbances, atherosclerosis, hypertension and CHF	Diabetic dermopathy, delayed wound healing, necrobiosis lipoidica diabeticorum, bullous diabeticorum and xanthelasma
Hyperthyroidism	Palpitations, MR, atrial fibrillation, hypertension, heart failure	Soft, smooth skin facial flushing, palmar erythema, pruritus, pretibial myxedema, silky hair
Hypothyroidism	Mild hypertension, sinus bradycardia, coronary artery disease and pericardial effusion	Dry, cold skin, madarosis, periorbital puffiness, itch and dry hair
Pheochromocytoma	Supraventricular tachycardia, hypertension, orthostatic hypotension and heart failure	Flushing and increased sweating

Table 56.3: Infiltrative disorders that can cause cardiovascular disease, and the cutaneous features of the disease. [Table adapted from Mendiratta V, Malik M. Cardiocutaneous diseases. In: Chopra HK, Nanda NC (Eds). Textbook of Cardiology: A Clinical and Historical Perspective. New Delhi, India: Jaypee Brothers Medical Publishers (P) Ltd.; 2013. pp. 396-407].

Disease	*Cardiovascular Morbidity*	*Cutaneous Features*
Amyloidosis	Congestive heart failure, syncope, arrhythmia, heart block and MI	Smooth, waxy papules or nodules and pinch purpura
Hemochromatosis	Arrhythmias, cardiomyopathy and heart failure	Gray-brown discoloration on face, flexural creases and exposed areas, dry skin, koilonychias and hair loss
Sarcoidosis	Arrhythmias, heart block, cor pulmonale and myocardial fibrosis	Translucent, yellow-brown or red-brown papules showing "apple jelly" appearance, alopecia and nail involvement
Wilson's disease (Hepatolenticular degeneration)	Arrhythmias, cardiomyopathy and autonomic disturbances	Bluish discoloration of nail lunula

may reveal the presence of clubbing (Figs. 56.14 and 56.15); suggestive of cyanotic heart disease. Cyanotic digits (Fig. 56.16) suggest Raynaud's phenomenon or other similar vasoreactive diseases. The finding of abnormally long extremities and arachnodactyly suggest Marfan's syndrome (Fig. 56.17).

Table 56.4: Inherited disorders of collagen and elastin that can cause cardiovascular disease, and the cutaneous features of the disease. [Table adapted from Mendiratta V, Malik M. Cardiocutaneous diseases. In: Chopra HK, Nanda NC (Eds). Textbook of Cardiology: A Clinical and Historical Perspective. New Delhi, India: Jaypee Brothers Medical Publishers (P) Ltd.; 2013. pp. 396-407].

Disease	*Cardiovascular Morbidity*	*Cutaneous Features*
Cutis laxa	Pulmonary stenosis, aortic aneurysms, cardiomegaly and cor pulmonale	Loose, wrinkled "bloodhound" appearance of skin returning slowly to its normal shape after stretching
Ehlers-Danlos syndrome	Tetralogy of Fallot, aortic aneurysms, ASD, MR and spontaneous rupture of large vessels	Hyperextensible, soft, smooth skin with easy bruisability atrophic scars, pseudotumors and elastosis perforans serpiginosa
Marfan syndrome	Dilatation of aortic root, aortic dissection or rupture, MR, AR and mitral valve prolapse	Striae, elastosis perforans serpiginosa, frontal bossing and atrophy of subcutaneous fat
Osteogenesis imperfecta	Aortic regurgitation, MR, and fragility of large blood vessels	Thin, translucent skin with easy bruisability, blue sclera and cutaneous scarring
Pseudoxanthoma elasticum	Intermittent claudication, coronary insufficiency, premature calcification of peripheral arteries, and hypertension	Waxy yellow papules coalescing to form plaques, usually on the neck and flexures; severely affected lax, redundant skin resembling "plucked chicken skin"

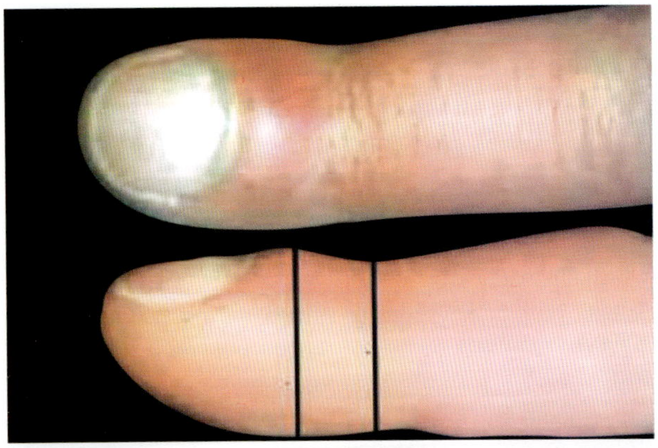

Fig. 56.14: Clubbing—It is more likely due to hypoxia secondary to cyanotic congenital heart disease than to pulmonary hypoxemia. [Image from Sarkar A. Bedside Cardiology, 1st edition. New Delhi, India: Jaypee Brothers Medical Publishers (P) Ltd.; 2012].

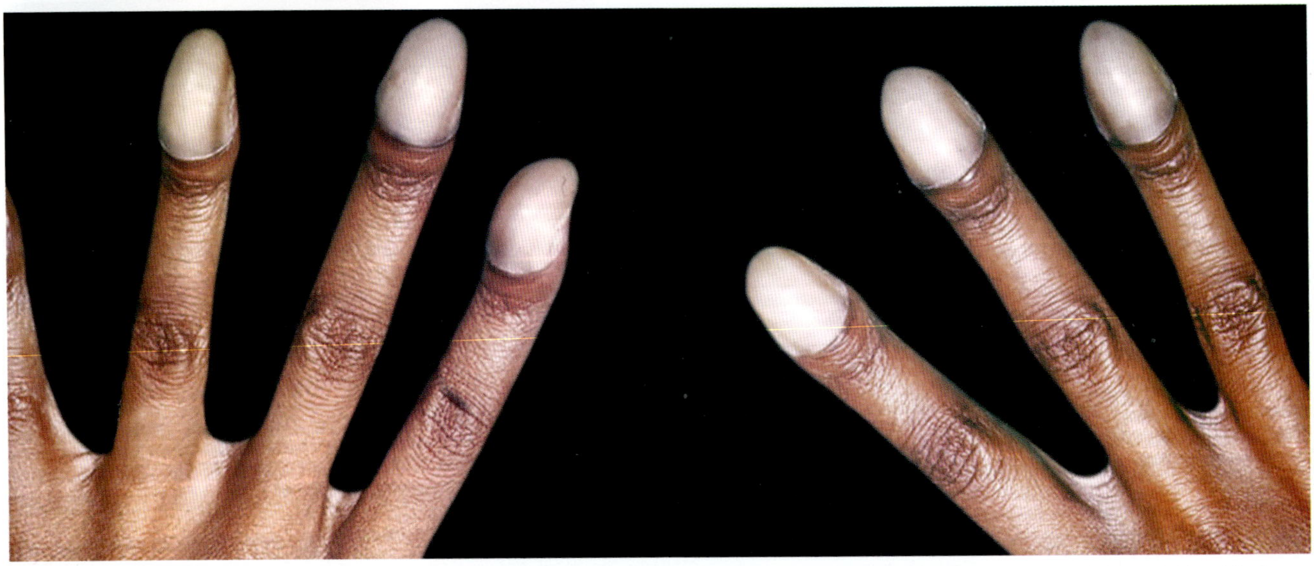

Fig. 56.15: Marked clubbing, suggestive of the presence of cyanotic heart disease. (Image from Herbert L Fred, MD and Hendrik A van Dijk, posted on Wikimedia Commons).

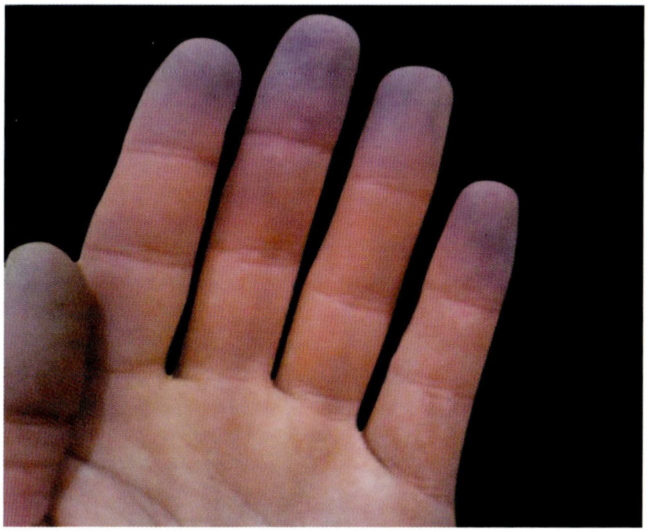

Fig. 56.16: Cyanotic digits in Raynaud's phenomenon.

Cardiac auscultation (Figs. 56.18 to 56.23) may allow presumptive diagnosis of valvular heart disease, congenital heart disease, or abnormalities of ventricular systolic and diastolic function.

Ophthalmological examination (Figs. 56.24 to 56.33) often reveals findings associated with systemic illnesses that can affect the cardiovascular system or may reveal a finding directly caused by cardiovascular pathology.

Numerous physical findings suggest the diagnosis of infective endocarditis, including splinter hemorrhage (Fig. 56.34), Osler's nodes (Figs. 56.35 and 56.36), Janeway lesions (Figs. 56.37 and 56.38), Roth spots (Fig. 56.39), and vascular purpura (Fig. 56.40). Similarly, there are numerous clues detectible on physical examination in a patient with heart failure symptoms that the underlying etiology may be amyloidosis (Figs. 56.41 to 56.44).

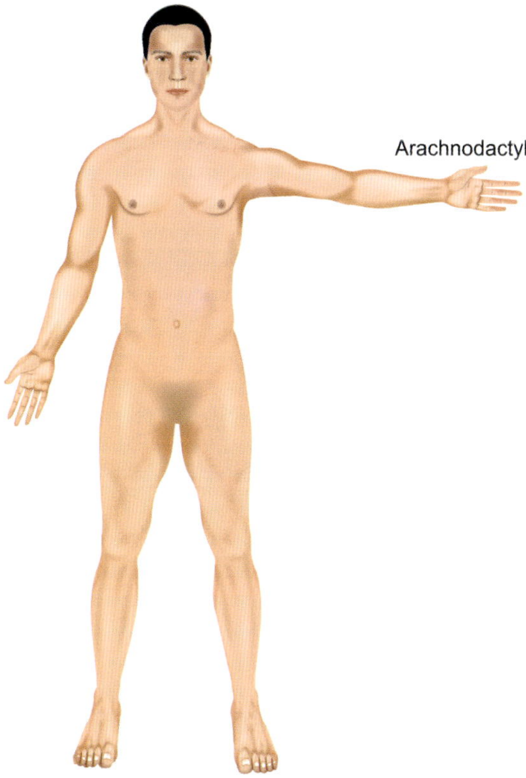

Fig. 56.17: Schematic illustration of the finding of abnormally long extremities and arachnodactyly in Marfan's syndrome.

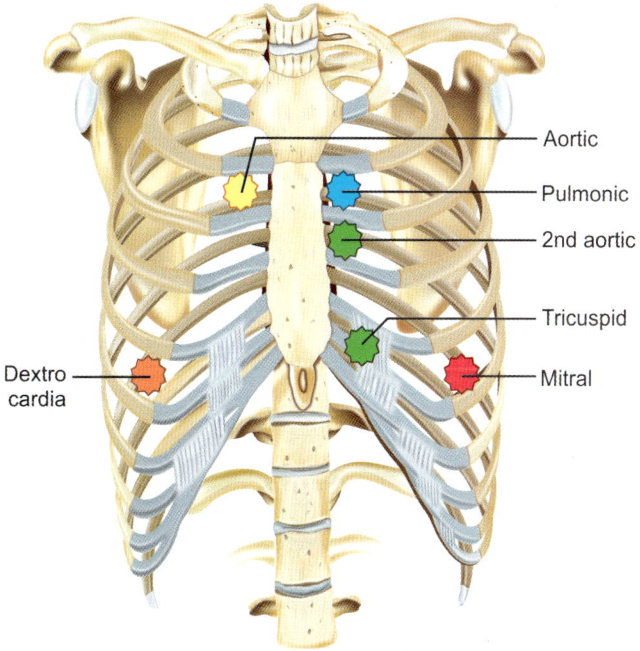

Fig. 56.18: The standard areas for auscultation of normal heart sounds and valvular dysfunction. [Image from Vijayalakshmi IB, Satpathy M. Bedside diagnosis of acyanotic congenital heart disease. In: Vijayalakshmi IB, Rao PS, Chugh R (Eds). Comprehensive Approach to Congenital Heart Disease, 1st edition. New Delhi, India: Jaypee Brothers Medical Publishers (P) Ltd.; 2013. pp. 166-82].

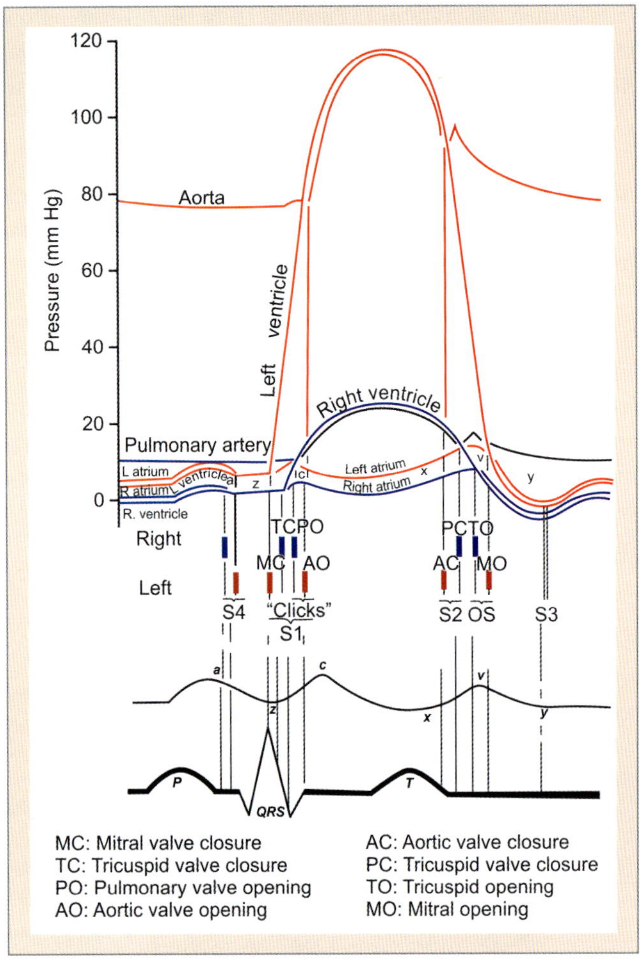

Fig. 56.19: Correlation of hearts sounds to the electrocardiogram (ECG) and pressures and pulsations in the cardiac cycle. [Image from Sarkar A. Bedside Cardiology, 1st edition. New Delhi, India: Jaypee Brothers Medical Publishers (P) Ltd.; 2012].

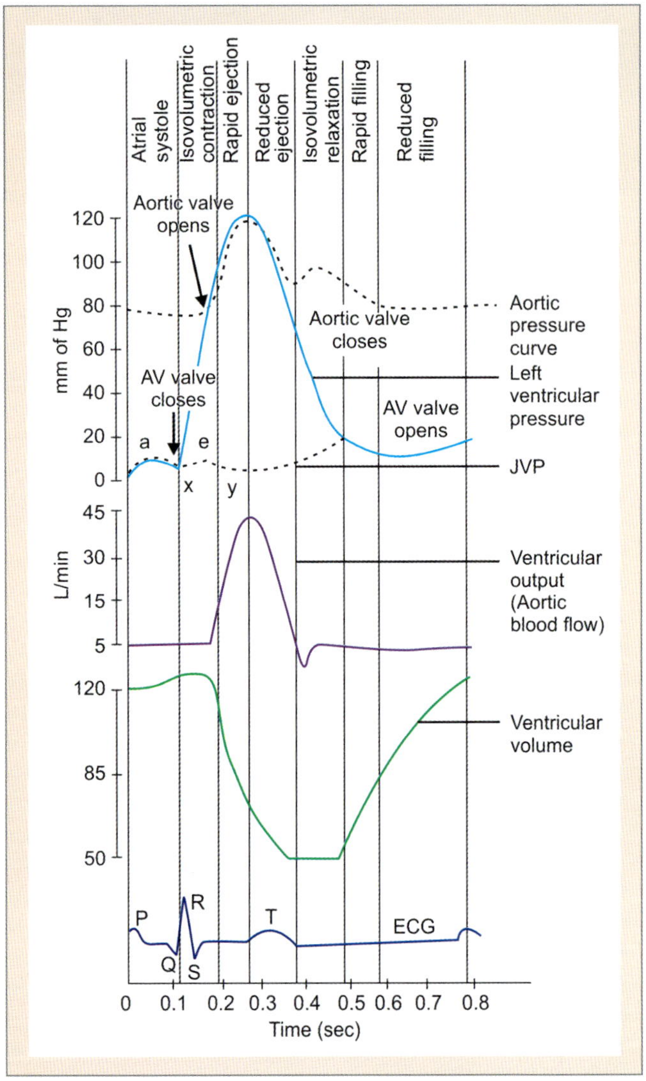

Fig. 56.20: Wiggins diagram, depicting events in the cardiac cycle. [Image from Ashalatha PR. The cardiovascular system. In: Ashalatha PR, Deepa G (Eds). Textbook of Anatomy and Physiology for Nurses, 3rd edition. New Delhi, India: Jaypee Brothers Medical Publishers (P) Ltd.; 2011. pp. 138-77].

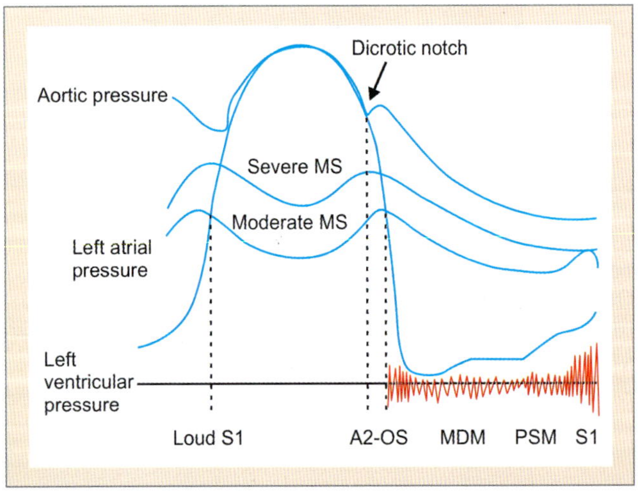

Fig. 56.21: Auscultatory findings in mitral stenosis and physiological correlates. The aortic valve closure-opening snap (A2-OS) interval is shorter in patients with more severe mitral stenosis than in patients with milder mitral stenosis. [Image and legend text adapted from Chatterjee K. Physical examination. In: Chatterjee K, Anderson M, Heistad D, Kerber RE (Eds). Cardiology—An Illustrated Textbook, 1st edition. New Delhi, India: Jaypee Brothers Medical Publishers (P) Ltd.; 2012. pp. 151-73]. (MDM: Mid-diastolic murmur; PSM: Presystolic murmur; MS: Mitral stenosis; S1: First heart sound).

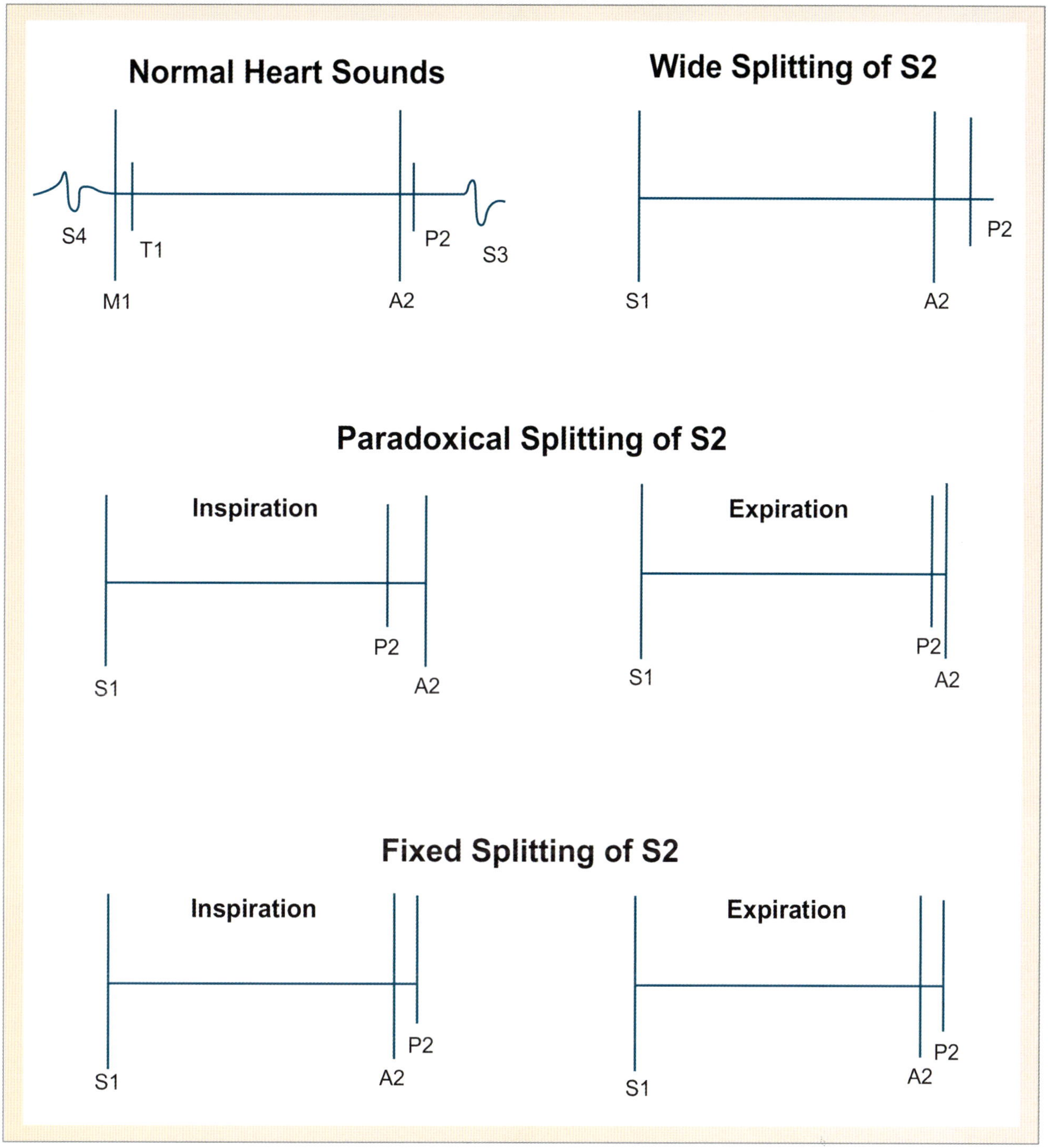

Fig. 56.22: The schematic illustration of normal heart sounds and splitting of S2. S4 is the presystolic low pitch atrial sound. The S1 consists of higher pitch mitral (M1) and tricuspid valve (T1) closure sounds. The S2 consists of higher pitch closure sounds of aortic (A2) and pulmonary (P2) valves. The S3 is a lower pitch early diastolic filling sound. The wide splitting of S2 is defined when the interval between A2 and P2 is longer than normal. The A2 precedes P2 and during inspiration the interval between A2 and P2 widens. The paradoxical splitting is defined when P2 precedes A2 during the expiratory phase of the respiratory cycle and during inspiration the P2-A2 interval shortens. The "fixed splitting" is defined when the A2-P2 interval remains relatively unchanged during expiration and inspiration. [Image and legend text from Chatterjee K. Physical examination. In: Chatterjee K , Anderson M, Heistad D, Kerber RE (Eds). Cardiology—An Illustrated Textbook, 1st edition. New Delhi, India: Jaypee Brothers Medical Publishers (P) Ltd.; 2012. pp. 151-73]. (S4: Fourth heart sound; M1: Mitral valve closure sound; T1: The tricuspid valve closure sound; A2: The aortic valve closure sound; P2: The pulmonary valve closure sound; S3: The third heart sound).

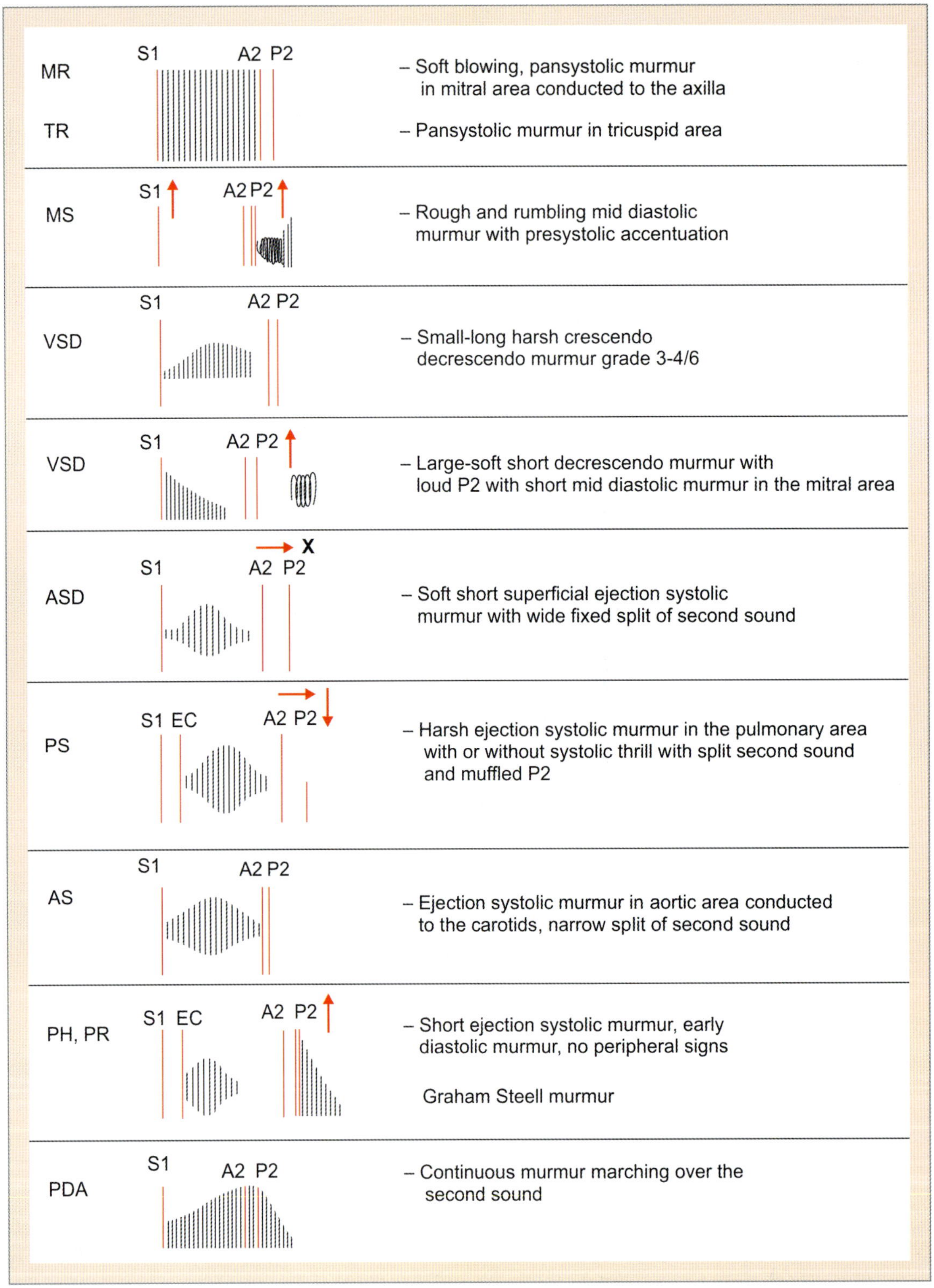

Fig. 56.23: Heart murmurs heard in congenital and acquired heart disease. [Image adapted from Vijayalakshmi IB, Satpathy M. Bedside diagnosis of acyanotic congenital heart disease. In: Vijayalakshmi IB, Rao PS, Chugh R (Eds). Comprehensive Approach to Congenital Heart Disease, 1st edition. New Delhi, India: Jaypee Brothers Medical Publishers (P) Ltd.; 2013. pp. 166-82].

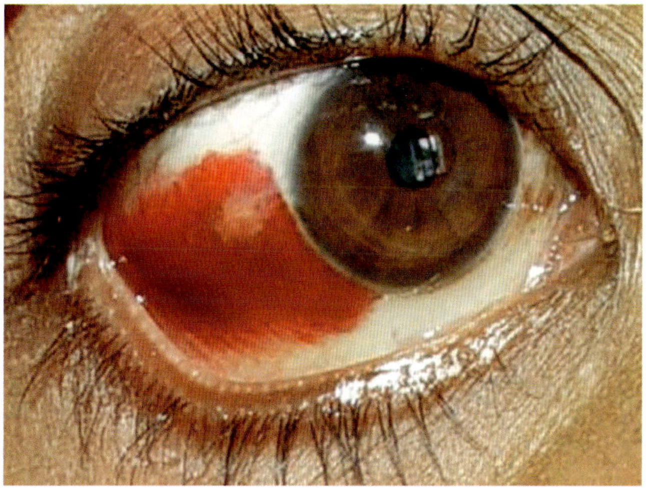

Fig. 56.24: Conjunctival hemorrhage. Causes of conjunctival hemorrhage include blunt trauma and acute conjunctivitis. It is likely that antiplatelet and anticoagulant therapy may contribute to bleeding, though there is still likely an underlying initial cause. No specific treatment is recommended, and spontaneous resolution within a week usually occurs. [Image and legend text adapted from Basak SK. Diseases of conjunctiva. In: Basak SK (Ed). Atlas of Clinical Ophthalmology, 2nd edition. New Delhi, India: Jaypee Brothers Medical Publishers (P) Ltd.; 2013. pp. 43-80].

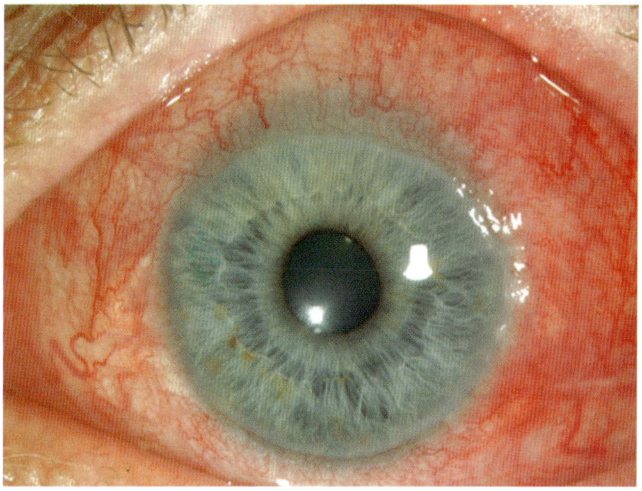

Fig. 56.25: Scleritis in a patient with antiphospholipid syndrome. Antiphospholipid syndrome is an autoimmune disease associated with both venous and arterial thrombosis. Factors in antiphospholipid syndrome include lupus anticoagulant and anticardiolipin antibody. Ocular manifestations that should raise suspicion for the condition in patients with venous or arterial thrombosis include central or branch retinal artery or vein occlusion, anterior uveitis, episcleritis, and scleritis. [Images and figure legend from Wang BZ, Chen CS. Venous thrombosis and the eye. In: Okuyan E (Ed). Venous Thrombosis—Principles and Practice. InTech].

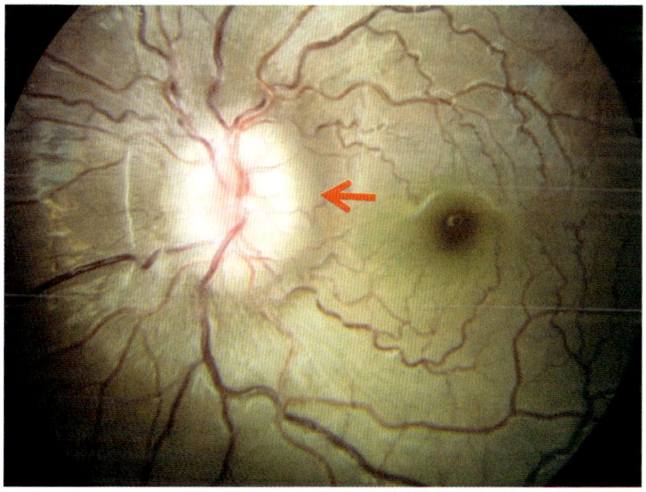

Fig. 56.26: Papilledema. The optic disk may appear hyperemic with a blurred disk margin (arrow). Papilledema is caused by increased intracranial pressure. Cardiovascular conditions that can cause papilledema include malignant hypertension, intracranial aneurysm, subdural hematoma, and venous thrombosis. [Image and legend text adapted from Basak SK. Diseases of conjunctiva. In: Basak SK (Ed). Atlas of Clinical Ophthalmology, 2nd edition. New Delhi, India: Jaypee Brothers Medical Publishers (P) Ltd.; 2013. pp. 43-80].

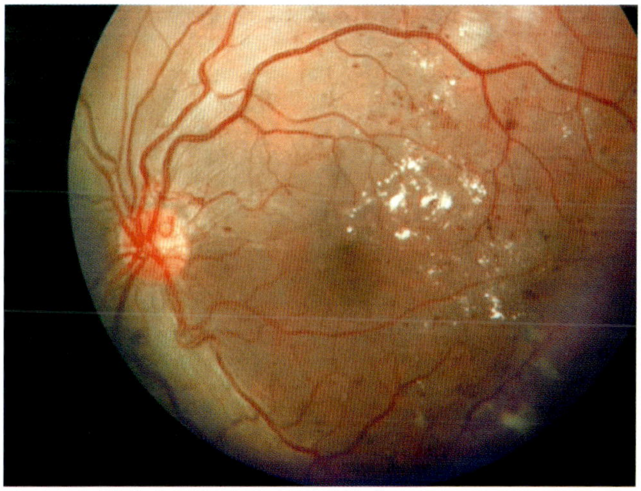

Fig. 56.27: Diabetic retinopathy, with venous dilation, microaneurysms, hard white exudates, and hemorrhages. [Image and legend text adapted from Basak SK. Diseases of conjunctiva. In: Basak SK (Ed). Atlas of Clinical Ophthalmology, 2nd edition. New Delhi, India: Jaypee Brothers Medical Publishers (P) Ltd.; 2013. pp. 43-80].

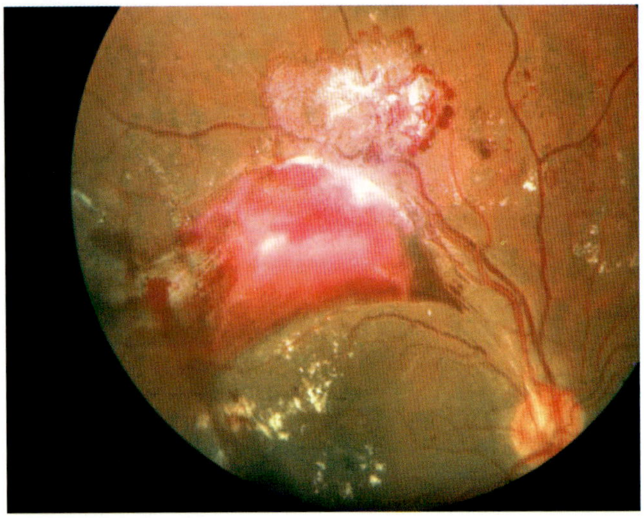

Fig. 56.28: Proliferative diabetic retinopathy, with new vessel formation in the disk and surface of the retina. [Image and legend text adapted from Basak SK. Diseases of conjunctiva. In: Basak SK (Ed). Atlas of Clinical Ophthalmology, 2nd edition. New Delhi, India: Jaypee Brothers Medical Publishers (P) Ltd.; 2013. pp. 43-80].

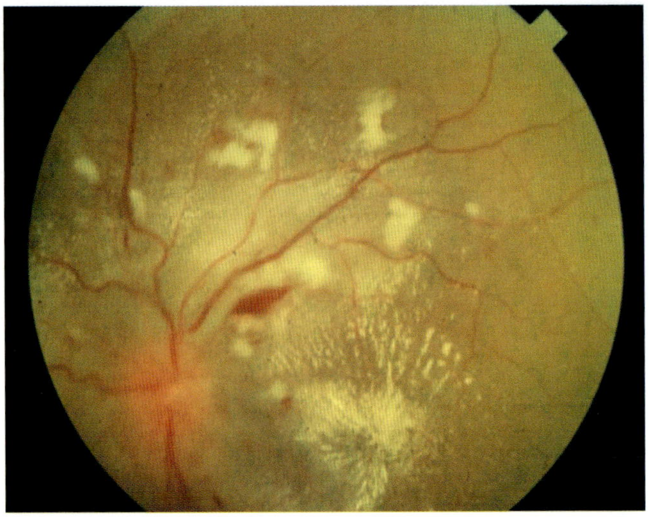

Fig. 56.29: Malignant hypertension. Retinal findings in malignant hypertension can include retinal edema, arterial narrowing, cotton wool patches, superficial hemorrhages, and papilledema. [Image and legend text adapted from Basak SK. Diseases of conjunctiva. In: Basak SK (Ed). Atlas of Clinical Ophthalmology, 2nd edition. New Delhi, India: Jaypee Brothers Medical Publishers (P) Ltd.; 2013. pp. 43-80].

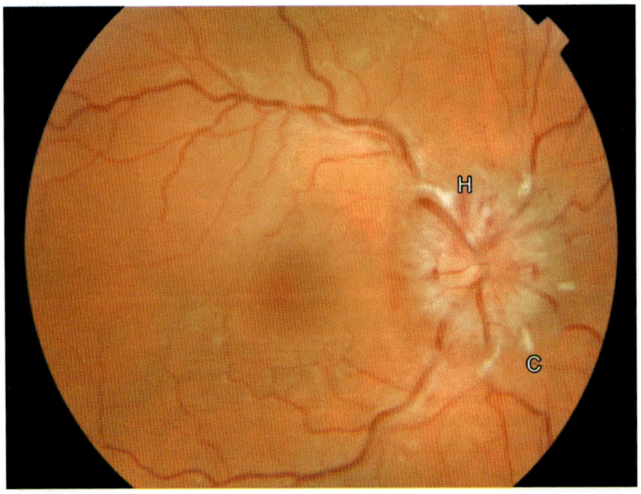

Fig. 56.30: Acute papilledema, with hemorrhage (H) and cotton wool spots (C). The optic disk margin is clearly blurred. [Images and figure legend from Wang BZ, Chen CS. Venous thrombosis and the eye. In: Okuyan E (Ed). Venous Thrombosis—Principles and Practice. InTech].

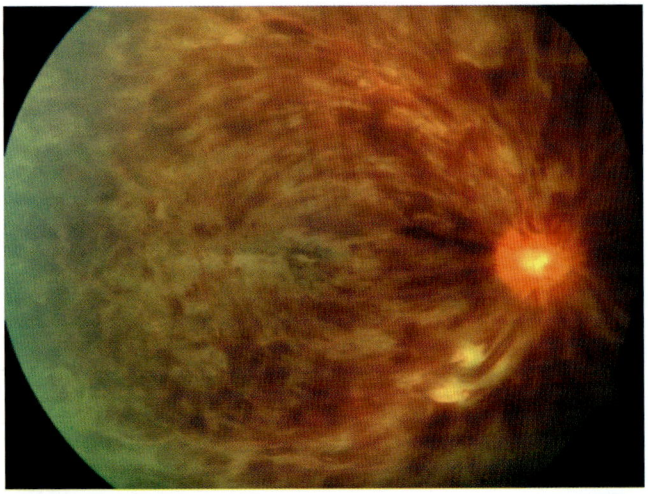

Fig. 56.31: Central retinal vein occlusion. The veins are dilated; there are deep and superficial hemorrhages, cotton wool spots, papilledema and macular edema. Central retinal vein occlusion results in sudden or rapid impairment in vision. Elderly persons with cardiovascular disease, hypertension and atherosclerosis are predisposed to the condition. [Image and legend text adapted from Basak SK. Diseases of conjunctiva. In: Basak SK (Ed). Atlas of Clinical Ophthalmology, 2nd edition. New Delhi, India: Jaypee Brothers Medical Publishers (P) Ltd.; 2013. pp. 43-80].

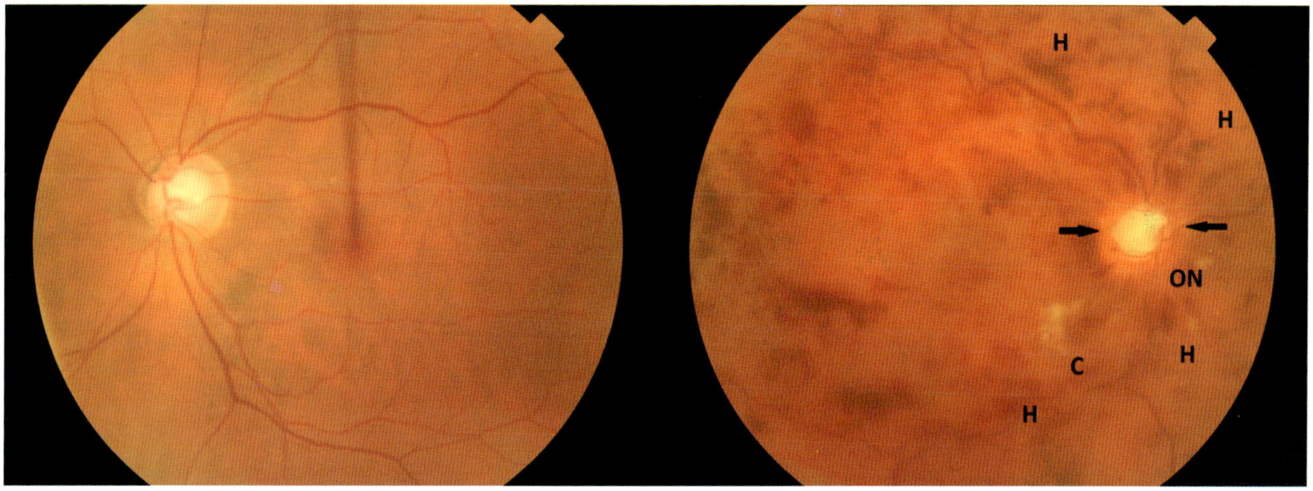

Fig. 56.32: Central retinal vein occlusion. Normal retina (left panel) and one with central retinal vein occlusion (right panel). There are scattered hemorrhages (H), cotton wool spots (C), and optic nerve swelling (ON), which is characterized by indistinct disk margins (arrows). [Images and figure legend from Wang BZ, Chen CS. Venous thrombosis and the eye. In: Okuyan E (Ed). Venous Thrombosis—Principles and Practice. InTech].

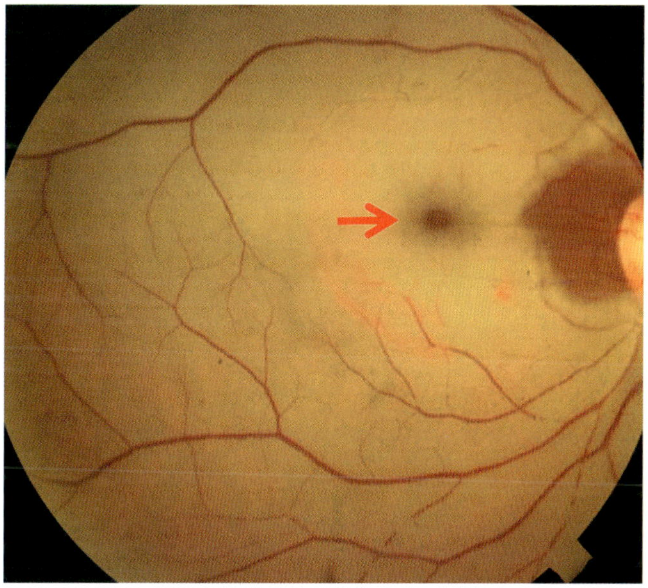

Fig. 56.33: Central retinal artery occlusion with cherry red spot (arrow) at the macula. Symptoms of central retinal artery occlusion are a sudden loss of vision, often described as a "curtain falling in the form of a visual field". Central retinal artery occlusion is the result of embolization of calcium, cholesterol, platelet aggregates and/or thrombus. The origin of the embolus may be from the carotid artery, aorta, or endocardium of the heart. Embolization may occur in patients with atrial fibrillation and left atrial appendage thrombus, or other conditions in which thrombus in a cardiac chamber is present. [Image and legend text adapted from Basak SK. Diseases of conjunctiva. In: Basak SK (Ed). Atlas of Clinical Ophthalmology, 2nd edition. New Delhi, India: Jaypee Brothers Medical Publishers (P) Ltd.; 2013. pp. 43-80].

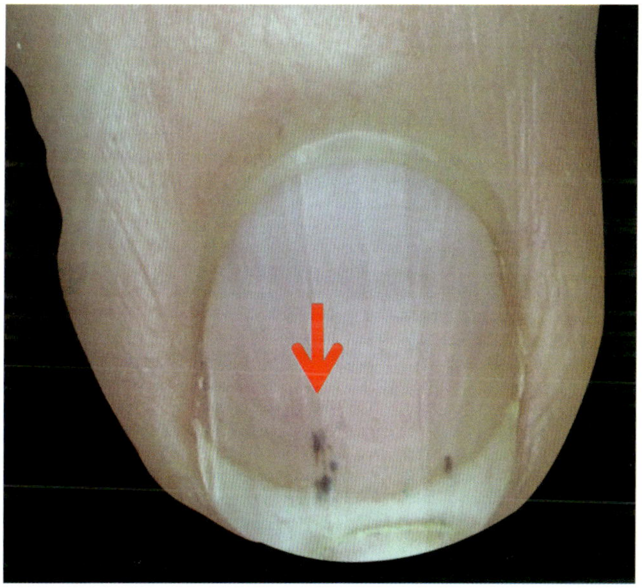

Fig. 56.34: Splinter hemorrhage (arrow) in a patient with infective endocarditis. (Image posted by Splarkla on Wikimedia Commons).

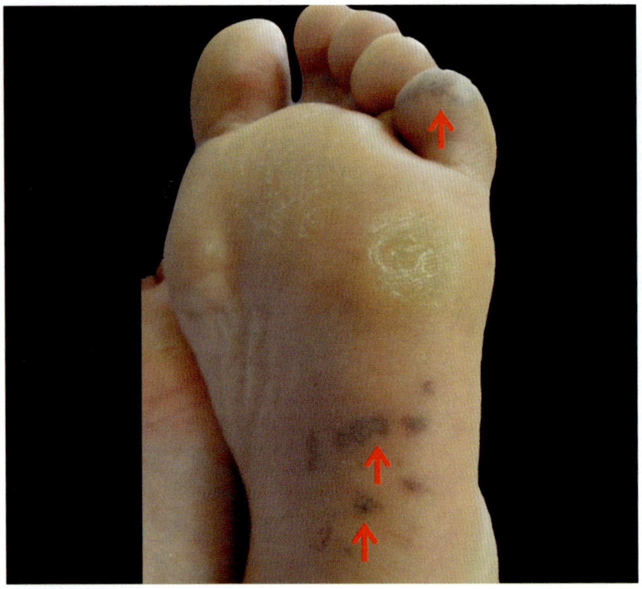

Fig. 56.35: Osler's nodes (arrows), suggestive of the presence of infective endocarditis. [Image reproduced with permission from Park MY, Jeon HK, Shim BJ, et al. Complete Atrioventricular Block due to Infective Endocarditis of Bicuspid Aortic Valve. J Cardiovasc Ultrasound. 2011;19(3):140-3].

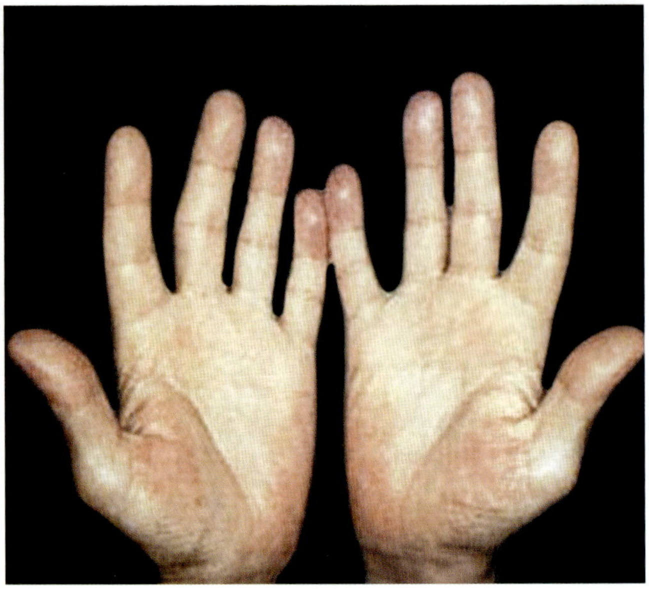

Fig. 56.36: Osler's nodes in a patient with endocarditis.

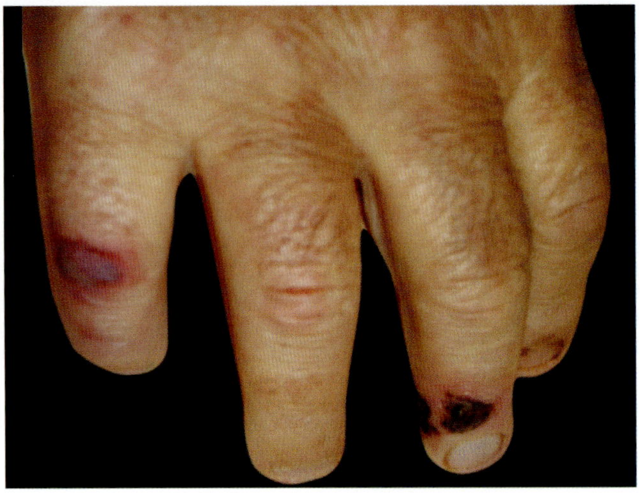

Fig. 56.37: Janeway lesions, another finding suggestive of the presence of infective endocarditis. [Image from Amandine S, et al. Importance of dermatology in infective endocarditis. In: Gaze D (Ed). The Cardiovascular System—Physiology, Diagnosis and Clinical Implication. InTech].

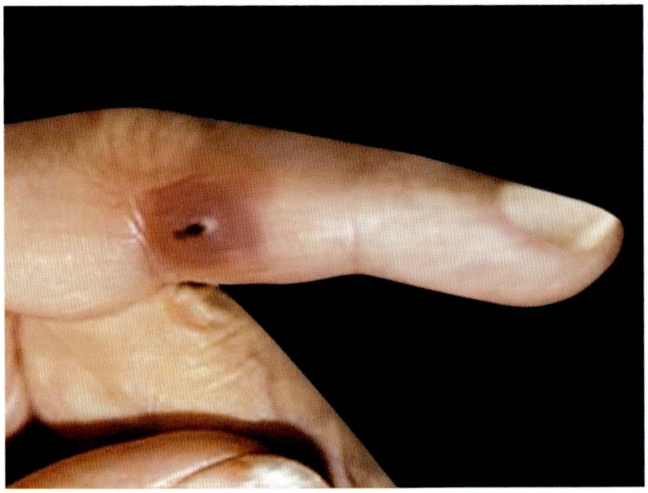

Fig. 56.38: Janeway lesion (usually seen in staphylococcal endocarditis; painless, septic emboli). [Image from Bhalerao JC. Bacterial endocarditis. In: Bhalerao JC (Ed). Essentials of Clinical Cardiology, 1st edition, Jaypee Brothers Medical Publishers; 2013. pp. 113-7].

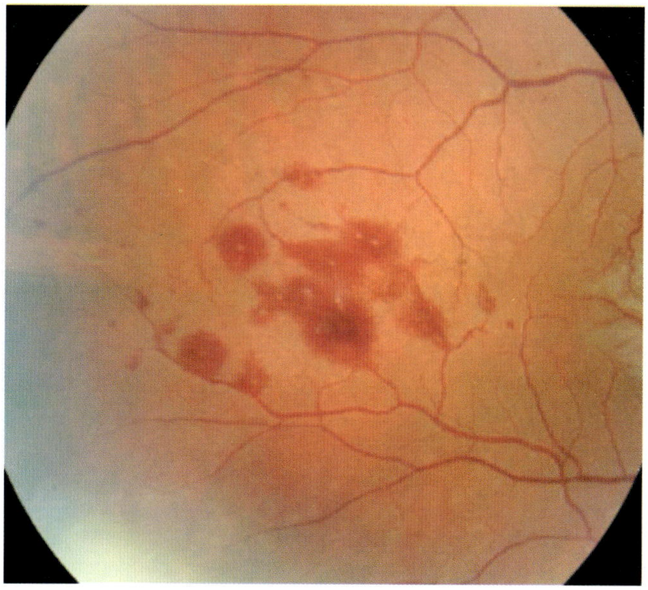

Fig. 56.39: Roth spots in a patient with infective endocarditis. [Image from Sahin O. Ocular complications of endocarditis. In: Breijo-Marquez FR (Ed). Endocarditis. InTech].

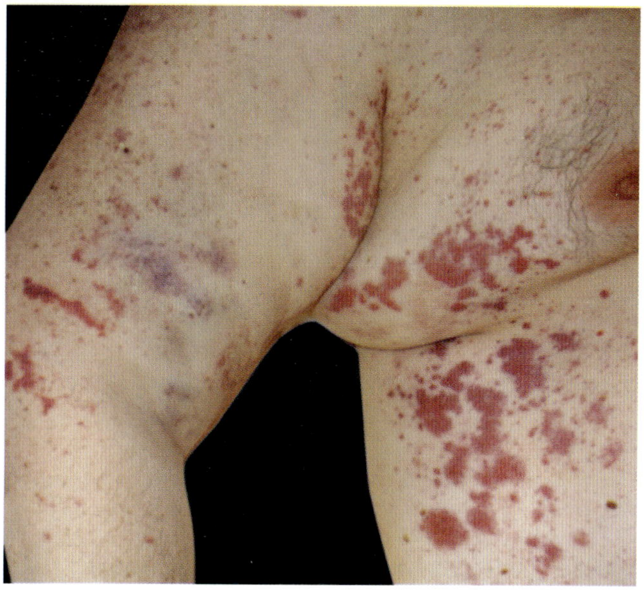

Fig. 56.40: Vascular purpura in a patient with infective endocarditis. [Image from Amandine S, et al. Importance of dermatology in infective endocarditis. In: Gaze D (Ed). The Cardiovascular System—Physiology, Diagnosis and Clinical Implication. InTech].

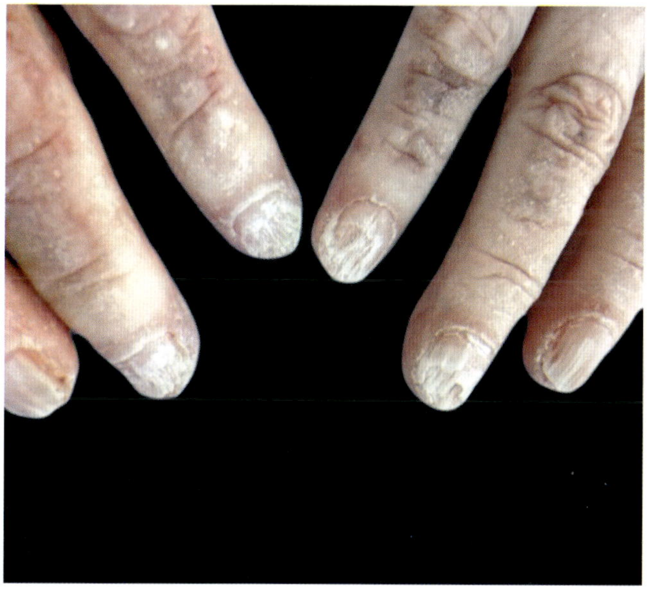

Fig. 56.41: Fingernails of a patient with systemic amyloidosis showing longitudinal ridging and splitting. [Image and legend text from Yamamoto T. Amyloidosis in the skin. In: Guvenc IA (Ed). Amyloidosis—An Insight to Disease of Systems and Novel Therapies. InTech].

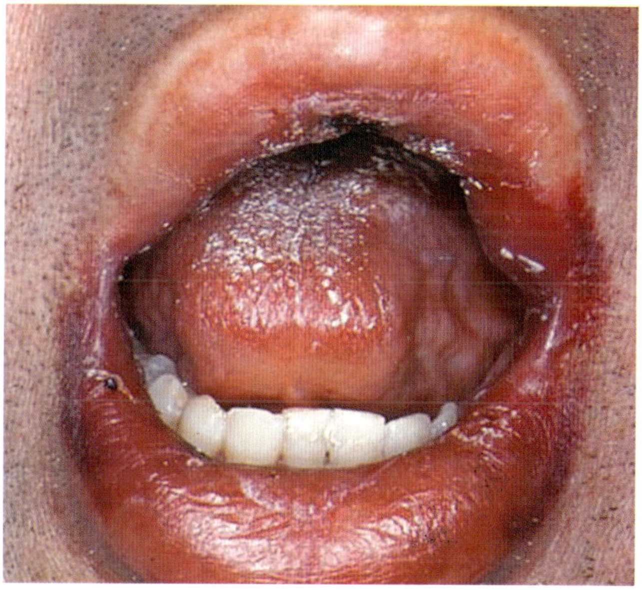

Fig. 56.42: Macroglossia in a patient with systemic amyloidosis. [Image and legend text from Yamamoto T. Amyloidosis in the skin. In: Guvenc IA (Ed). Amyloidosis—An Insight to Disease of Systems and Novel Therapies. InTech].

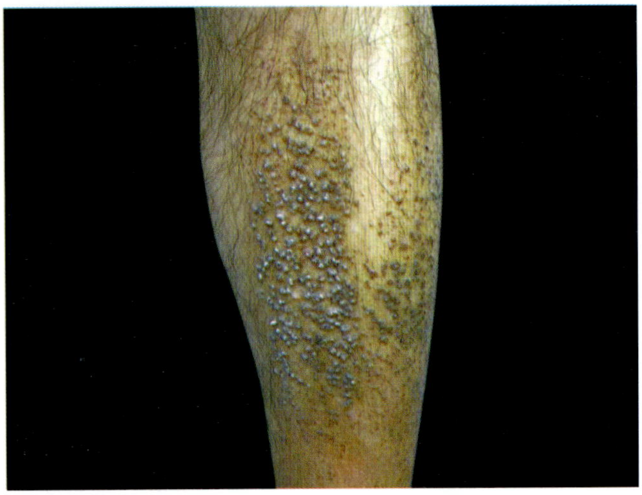

Fig. 56.43: Lichen amyloidosis on the lower leg. [Image and legend text from Yamamoto T. Amyloidosis in the skin. In: Guvenc IA (Ed). Amyloidosis—An Insight to Disease of Systems and Novel Therapies. InTech].

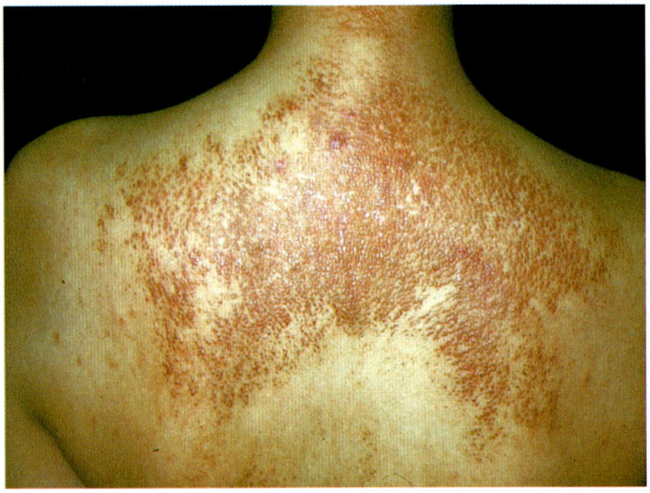

Fig. 56.44: Macular amyloidosis on the upper back. [Image and legend text from Yamamoto T. Amyloidosis in the skin. In: Guvenc IA (Ed). Amyloidosis—An Insight to Disease of Systems and Novel Therapies. InTech].

REFERENCES

Mangione S. Physical Diagnosis Secrets 2nd edition. Mosby Elsevier. Philadelphia PA 2008

Sarkar A. Bedside Cardiology. Jaypee Brothers Medical Publishers (P) Ltd., New Dehli, India, 2012.

Okuyan E. Venous thrombosis Principles and Practice. Intechweb. org. Rijeka, Croatia 2011

Chopra HK, et al. Textbook of Cardiology—A Clinical and Historic Perspective. Jaypee Brothers Medical Publishers(P) Ltd., New Dehli, India, 2013.

CHAPTER

57

Stroke

Sharyl R Martini, Aaron W Grossman, Thomas A Kent

INTRODUCTION

The classic definition of stroke is "a sudden, focal injury of the central nervous system (CNS) due to a vascular cause". This definition was updated by the American Heart Association in 2013. The resulting consensus statement uses the umbrella term "stroke" to encompass: ischemic stroke (also called CNS infarction) (Fig. 57.1), hemorrhagic stroke (intracerebral and subarachnoid hemorrhage) (Fig. 57.2), and cerebral venous sinus thrombosis (Flow chart. 57.1). Ischemic stroke or CNS infarction is due to insufficient blood flow to a region of the brain. Approximately 80% of strokes are ischemic. Hemorrhage into an area of ischemic stroke (known as hemorrhagic transformation; Fig. 57.3) may occur.

Stroke symptoms are related to the part of the brain affected, thus ischemic strokes caused by occlusion of major cerebral arteries (Figs. 57.4 and 57.5) typically result in a classic constellation of symptoms (Table 57.1). Globally insufficient perfusion may result in infarction of the "watershed" territories at the border between major arterial territories (Figs. 57.6A and B). Symptoms due to hemorrhagic strokes and cerebral venous sinus thrombosis are also related to the part of the brain affected, but the symptoms may involve more than one arterial territory. Hemorrhagic strokes and cerebral venous thrombosis typically cause headache, often very severe, and patients may exhibit symptoms and signs of increased intracranial pressure (early onset of somnolence, nausea, vomiting, papilledema).

The ECG in patients with intracerebral processes, classically hemorrhagic stroke, may show diffuse, deep T-wave inversions, often with prolongation of the QT interval (Figs. 57.7A and B). The finding of these deep and diffuse T wave inversions in the setting of a CNS process has been called "cerebral T-waves". These T-wave inversions should not be mistaken as representing cardiac ischemia. Rather, they appear to be abnormalities of cardiac repolarization

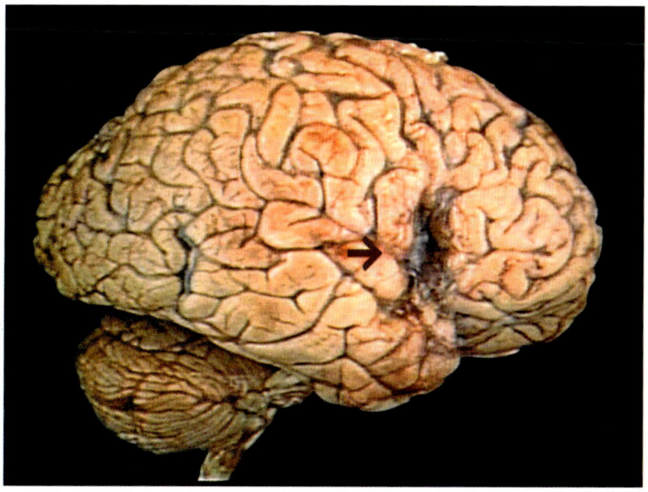

Fig. 57.1: Old cerebral infarction due to ischemic stroke. (Image from Armed Forces Institute of Pathology).

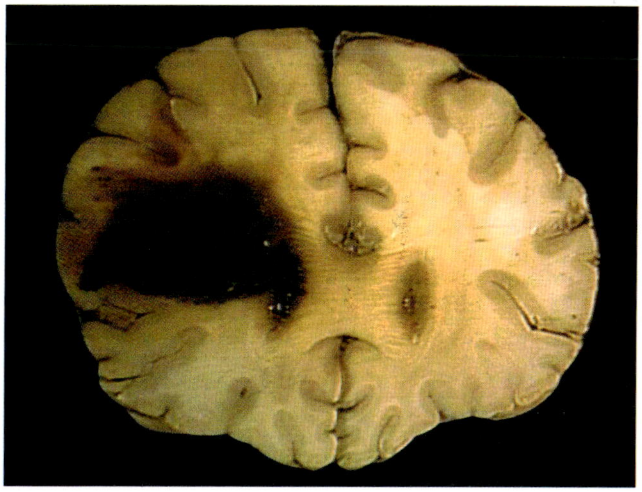

Fig. 57.2: Intracerebral hemorrhage involving the deep white matter. (Image from Armed Forces Institute of Pathology).

Flow chart 57.1: Types and common causes of stroke. Stroke is a term encompassing arterial occlusion (ischemic), arterial rupture (hemorrhagic), and venous occlusion (cerebral venous sinus thrombosis). Major subtypes within each category are indicated with the most common underlying etiology or etiologies listed below.

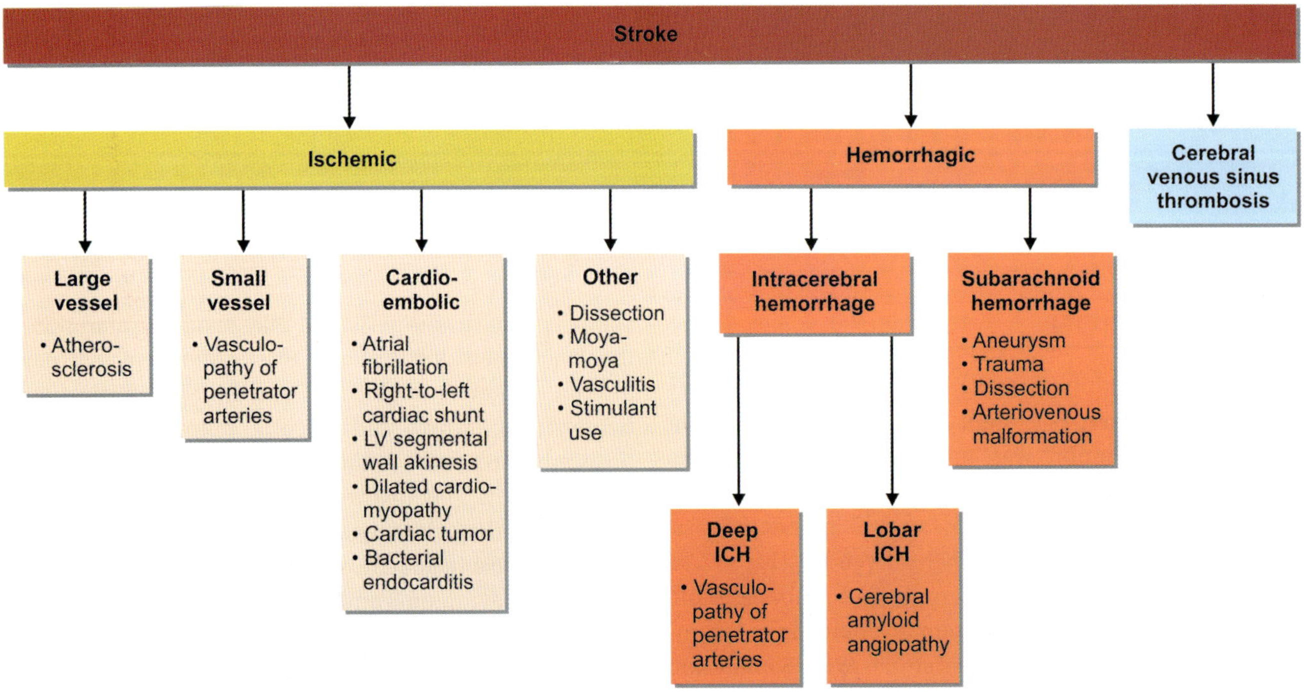

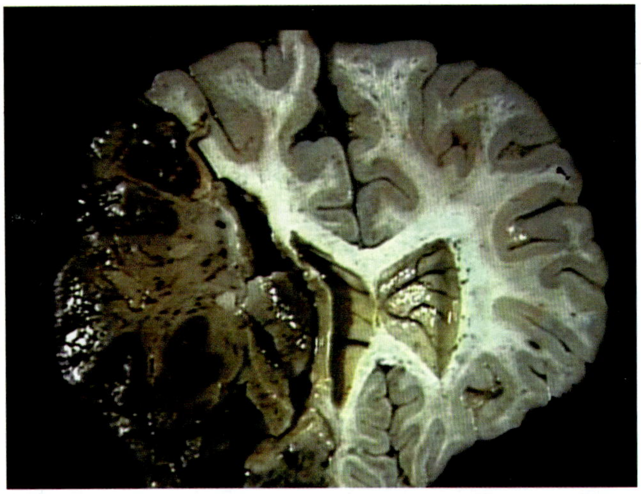

Fig. 57.3: Hemorrhagic transformation of an ischemic stroke. (Image from Armed Forces Institute of Pathology).

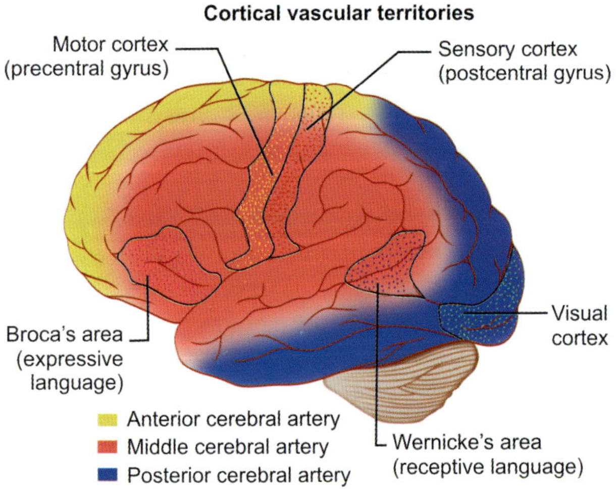

Fig. 57.4: Arterial supply and functional regions of the cerebral cortex. The middle cerebral artery (red) and anterior cerebral artery (yellow) are fed by the ipsilateral carotid; the posterior cerebral artery (blue) is usually fed by the basilar artery. Regions at the border of two territories are the "watershed" zones, which are particularly susceptible to ischemia during low flow states. The motor and sensory cortices control the contralateral hemi-body, the visual cortex controls the contralateral visual field. Language areas are most often found on left side of the brain.

Table 57.1: Ischemic stroke subtypes by occluded artery.

Vessel	*Symptoms*
Bilateral anterior cerebral arteries	Akinetic mutism, apathy
Left middle cerebral artery	Aphasia, R weakness and numbness (face and arm > leg), R hemianopia
Right middle cerebral artery	L weakness and numbness (face and arm > leg), L neglect, L hemianopia
Left or right posterior cerebral artery	Contralateral hemianopia
Top of the basilar	Decreased level of consciousness, cortical blindness

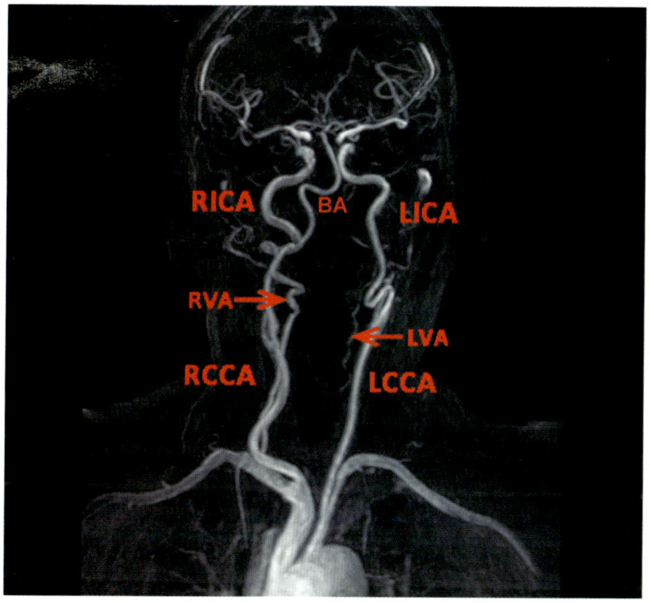

Fig. 57.5A: Magnetic resonance angiogram of cerebral arterial vasculature. The entire cerebral arterial vasculature is visualized from the aortic arch. The right common carotid artery (RCCA) and left common carotid artery (LCCA) give rise to the right internal carotid artery (RICA) and left internal common artery (LICA) respectively. The right vertebral artery (RVA) is dominant and can be seen giving rise to the basilar artery (arrow). The left vertebral artery (LVA) is hypoplastic.

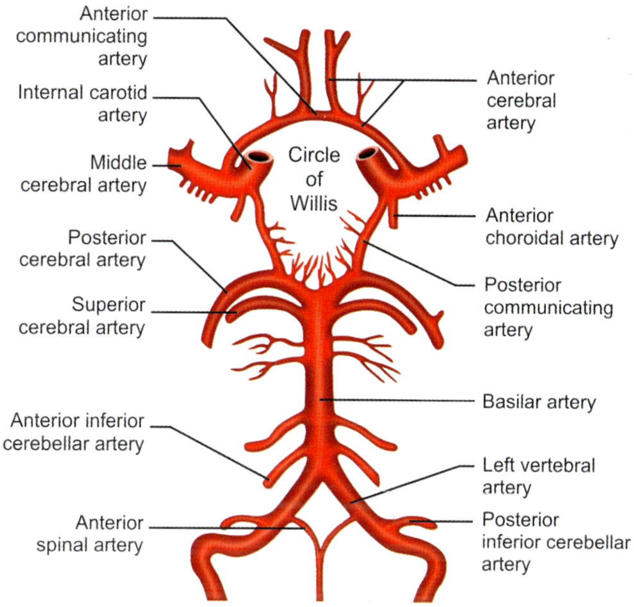

Fig. 57.5B: Schematic illustration of the cerebral circulation and the circle of Willis. [Image from Ashalatha PR. Nervous system. In: Ashalatha PR (Ed). Textbook of Anatomy and Physiology for Nurses. New Delhi, India: Jaypee Brothers Medical Publishers (P) Ltd.].

due to dysfunctional cerebral control of the autonomic nervous system. This abnormality is seen when the insular cortex is affected by ischemic or hemorrhagic strokes, and often occurs in the setting of increased intracranial pressure.

ISCHEMIC STROKE

Unlike hemorrhagic strokes, ischemic strokes are not usually visible on CT scan until 6–24 hours after onset of symptoms. The amount of time until the ischemic stroke can be visualized on CT scan depends on both size and location: small strokes and those in the posterior fossa may not ever be visible by CT. Diffusion-weighted MRI can identify most strokes shortly after symptom onset but is not sensitive enough to completely "rule out" a small stroke. Diffusion-weighted imaging is also not 100% specific for stroke, although stroke is the most common cause of diffusion positivity.

Although there are a number of causative etiologies for acute ischemic stroke, almost all are treated the same way in the first few hours. Tissue plasminogen activator (TPA) is the only FDA-approved treatment for ischemic stroke and should be considered for any stroke presenting

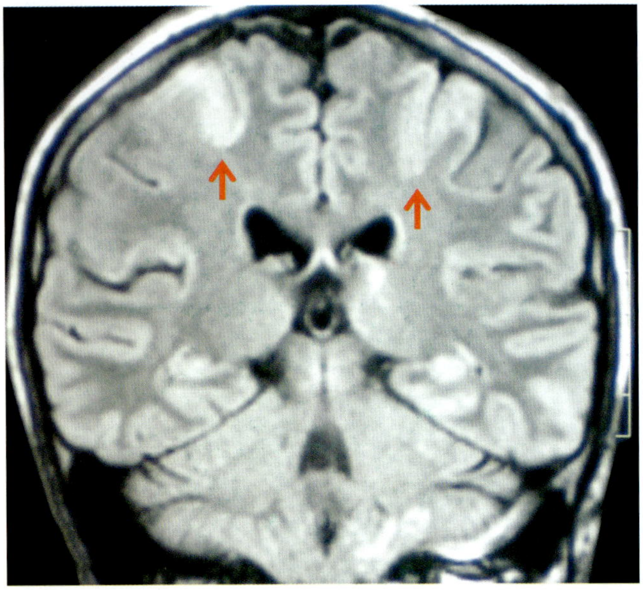

Fig. 57.6A: Watershed ischemic strokes. Coronal MRI of the brain revealing hyperintensities (arrows) in the bilateral watershed areas. Inadequate perfusion can result in watershed infarcts causing "man-in-a-barrel syndrome", including weakness/numbness of bilateral arms and proximal legs with preservation of face, hands and lower legs. A focal stenosis can result in unilateral watershed-type infarcts. [Image from Sanz-Ayan MP, Diaz D, Martinez-Salio A, et al. Neurologic complications in aortic valve surgery and rehabilitation treatment used. In: Motomura N (Ed). Aortic Valve Surgery. Shanghai: InTech; 2011].

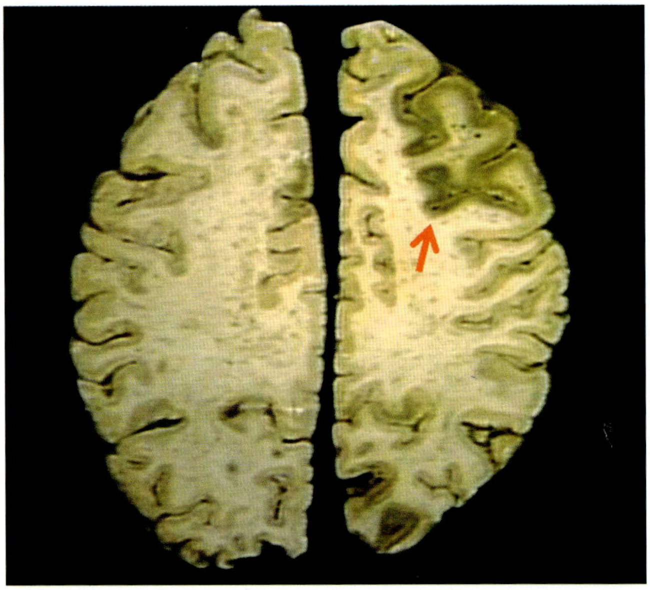

Fig. 57.6B: Gross pathology specimen of watershed infarct. (Image from Armed Forces Institute of Pathology).

within 3 hours (in some cases up to 4.5 hours) from symptom onset. The stroke team or on-call neurologist should be contacted immediately and a non-contrast head CT obtained. Common contraindications to TPA include anticoagulation, thrombocytopenia, and active bleeding. Contraindications may be relative or absolute and should be assessed on a case-by-case basis with the stroke specialist. TPA is not given in cases of bacterial endocarditis or aortic dissection. Intra-arterial TPA and mechanical embolectomy have not been shown to be superior to IV TPA and are not recommended as usual care.

Extensive effort is made to identify the underlying etiology of the ischemic stroke because it influences both acute management and long-term secondary prevention strategy. The three most common mechanisms for ischemic stroke are: (1) large vessel atherosclerosis of vessels leading to the brain, (2) small vessel arteriopathy of penetrating brain arteries, and (3) cardioembolism (Figs. 57.8A to C). Aortic or carotid artery dissection (Figs. 57.9A and B), vasculitis, stimulant use, procoagulant conditions are among other, less common, stroke etiologies and are classified as "other". In a certain percentage of strokes, no etiology can be found despite intensive investigation. These types of strokes are classified as "cryptic".

Ischemic Stroke: Large Vessel Subtype due to Atherosclerosis

Large vessel atherosclerosis may occur in a cerebral artery, at the carotid bifurcation (Figs. 57.10 and 57.11), or at the origin of a vessel off the aorta. Risk factors include hypertension, hyperlipidemia, and diabetes. Strokes due to large vessel atherosclerosis may affect the deep structures, the cortex, or both. Symptoms may wax and wane. Treatment includes an antiplatelet agent and maximal medical management of risk factors plus carotid endarterectomy or carotid stenting if applicable. Stenting of intracranial vessels is rarely performed as it was found in a randomized controlled trial to be inferior to optimal medical management. Dual antiplatelet therapy is often used in patients with severe intracranial stenosis for the first 90 days after stroke, followed by single antiplatelet therapy beyond 90 days.

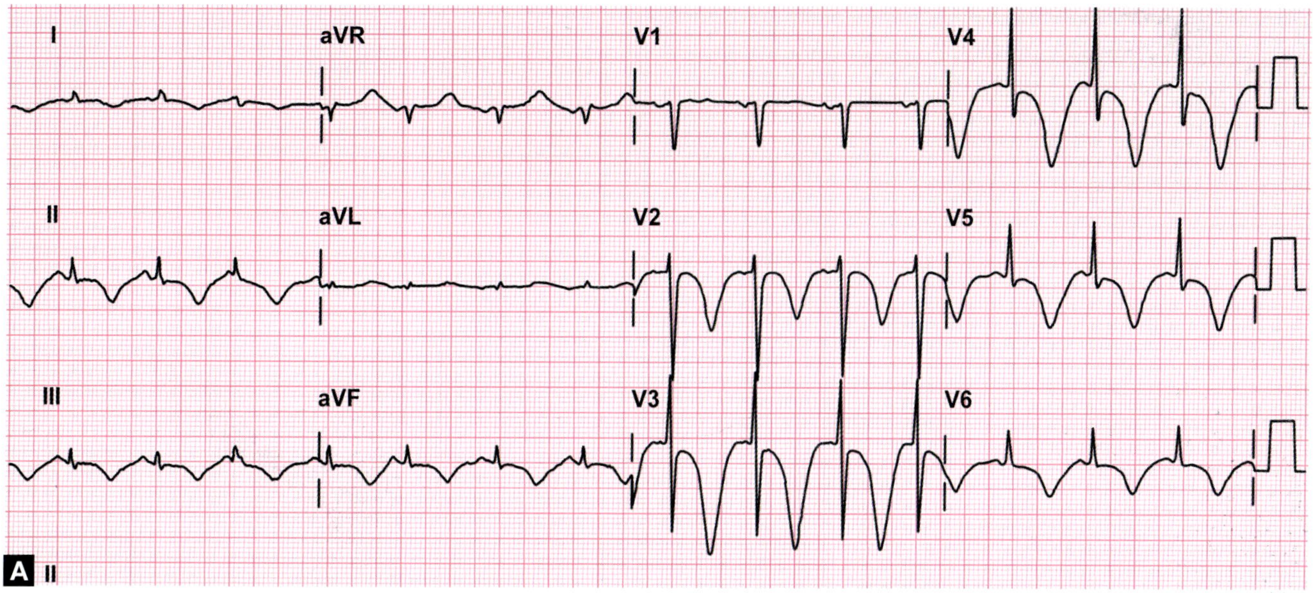

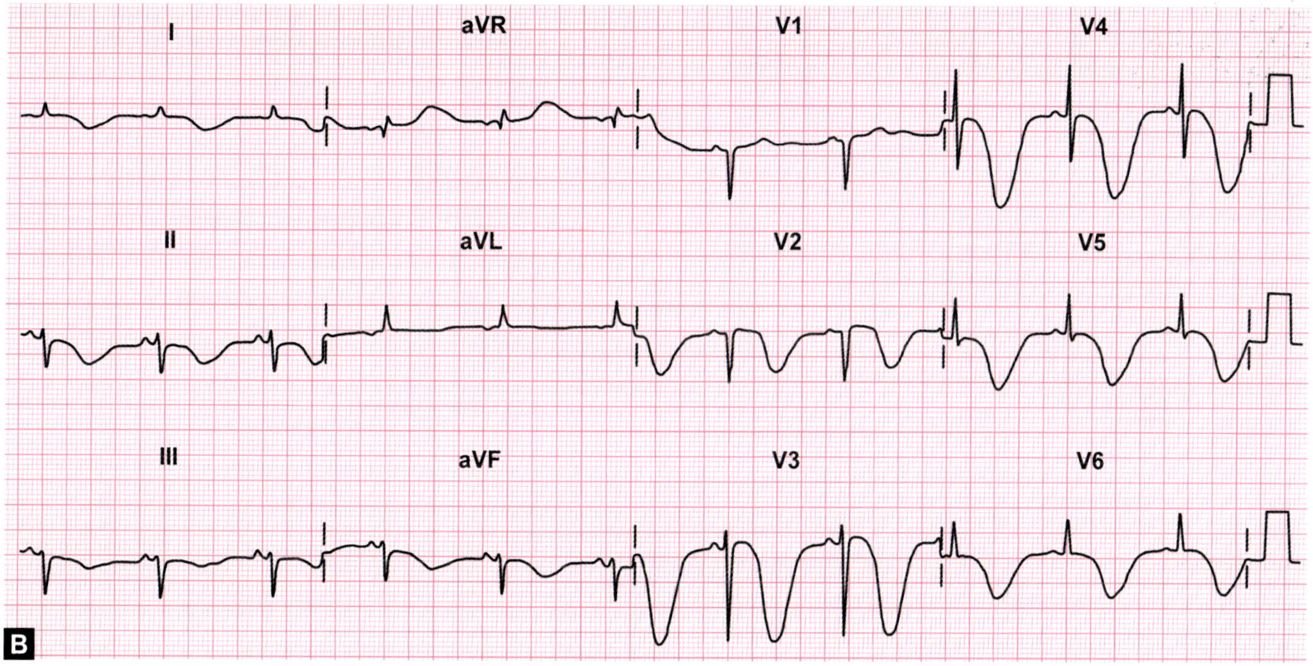

Figs. 57.7A and B: Cerebral T waves. A 12-lead ECG showing the diffuse, deep, T wave inversions that may be seen with intracerebral hemorrhage, subarachnoid hemorrhage and ischemic stroke. Associated abnormalities include prolonged QT interval and U waves. This pattern was presumed to be due to increased intracranial pressure, however, can be seen with smaller strokes affecting the insular cortex in the absence of increased intracranial pressure. The current hypothesis is that dysfunction of the insular cortex—an area of the brain that plays a key role in autonomic control—causes these abnormalities in cardiac repolarization. The findings on the ECG are often referred to as "cerebral T waves" and should not be mistaken as indicating myocardial ischemia. [Figure 57.7A from Wang K. Atlas of Electrocardiography. New Delhi: Jaypee Brothers Medical Publishers (P) Ltd.; 2013. Figure 57.7B courtesy of Dr Ed Burns, posted on www.lifeinthefastlane.com].

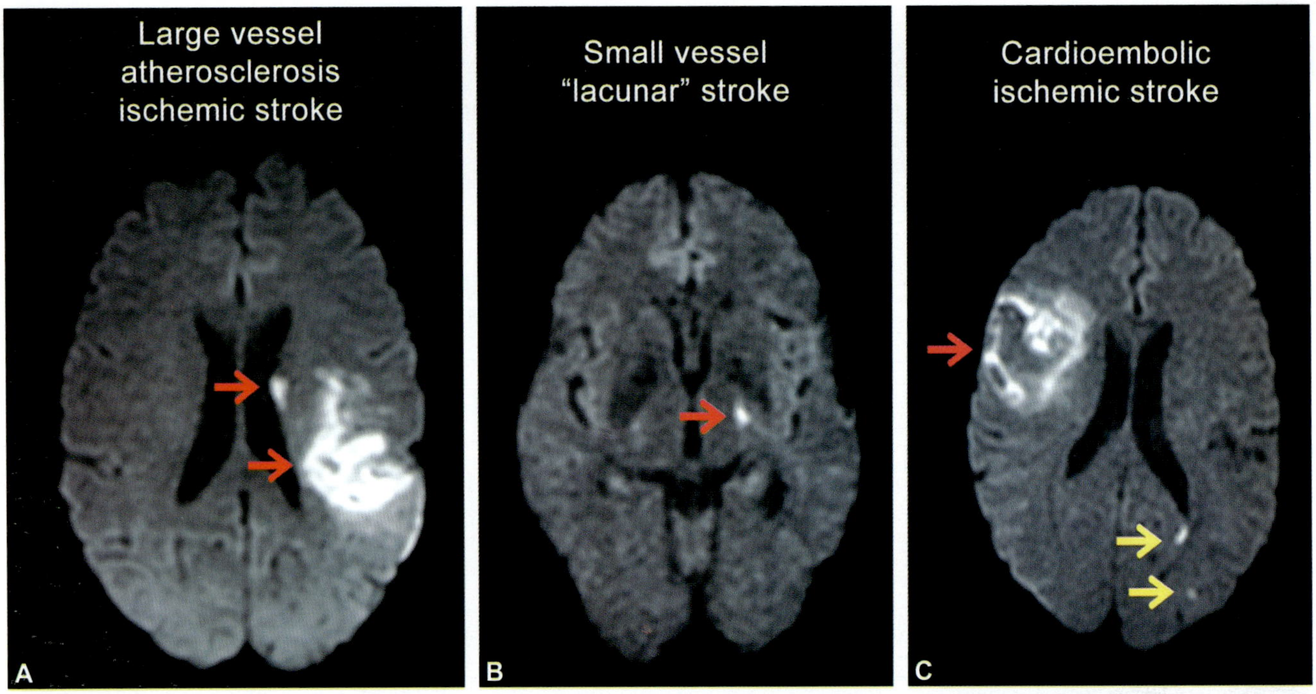

Figs. 57.8A to C: Diffusion weighted MRI of ischemic stroke subtypes. (A) Ischemic stroke due to large vessel atherosclerosis. Axial diffusion-weighted MRI shows multiple strokes (arrows) in the distribution of a single artery, the left middle cerebral artery (MCA). This could result from atherosclerosis of the MCA itself, or embolization from an ipsilateral proximal vessel (such as the carotid) or the heart. (B) Small vessel ("lacunar") ischemic stroke. Axial diffusion-weighted MRI shows a tiny stroke (arrow) resulting from occlusion of a small penetrating artery of the left basal ganglia. Such infarcts may occur as a result of intrinsic small vessel disease, as well as embolism from either a large vessel or cardioembolic source. (C) Cardioembolic ischemic stroke. Axial diffusion-weighted MRI shows a large stroke with areas of hemorrhage in the right MCA distribution (red arrow), as well as punctate areas of infarction in the left PCA distribution (yellow arrows). Because the right MCA is distal to the right brachiocephalic artery and the left vertebral is usually a branch off the aorta, the source of embolus is either the proximal aorta or the heart. (Images 57.8A and B courtesy of Dr. Achala Vagal).

Ischemic Stroke: Lacunar Subtype due to Small Vessel Arteriopathy

Small vessel arteriopathy occurs in the penetrating arteries supplying the basal ganglia, thalamus, and brainstem. Strokes due to small vessel arteriopathy (often called lacunar strokes) are < 2 cm in diameter and occur in these same regions. Small vessel strokes do not cause infarction of the cortex. Symptoms may wax and wane. The main risk factors for cerebral small vessel arteriopathy and lacunar strokes are chronic hypertension and diabetes. Treatment involves an antiplatelet therapy and guideline-directed management of risk factors.

Ischemic Stroke: Cardioembolic Subtype

Cardioembolic stroke occurs when material from the heart lodges in a cerebral vessel, causing occlusion. Strokes due to cardioembolism typically occur at the branch of a major vessel, and may affect the cortical structures, deep structures, or both. The pathognomonic feature of cardioembolic strokes is that they can occur in multiple vascular territories; they are often multiple and of different ages. Symptoms are usually maximal at onset. Spontaneous hemorrhagic conversion is more likely in this ischemic stroke subtype. Risk factors for cardioembolic stroke include atrial fibrillation (Figs. 57.12 to 57.14, Video 57.1), recent myocardial infarction, akinetic segment of the left ventricle (Fig. 57.15, Videos 57.2 to 57.7), acute heart failure, severe cardiomyopathy, bacterial endocarditis (Figs. 57.16 and 57.17, Videos 57.8 to 57.10), valvular disease (Figs. 57.18 and 57.19), and atrial myxoma (Figs. 57.20 and 57.21, Video 57.11). A right-to-left shunt in the setting of a venous source of embolism is considered a cause of stroke (Fig. 57.22), but patent foramen ovale alone (Videos 57.12 and 57.13) is not considered sufficient evidence for cardioembolic etiology because of its

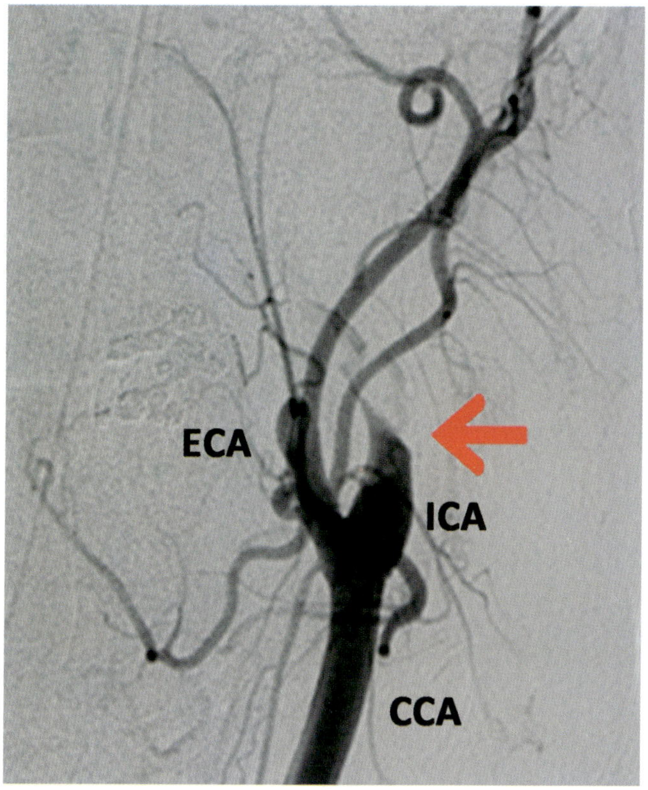

Fig. 57.9A: Carotid angiogram demonstrating dissection of the internal carotid artery (arrow). There is a classic "flame shape" appearance at the area of dissection. More cranial in the image, only external carotid artery branches are filling with contrast. (CCA: Common carotid artery; ECA: External carotid artery; ICA: Internal carotid artery).

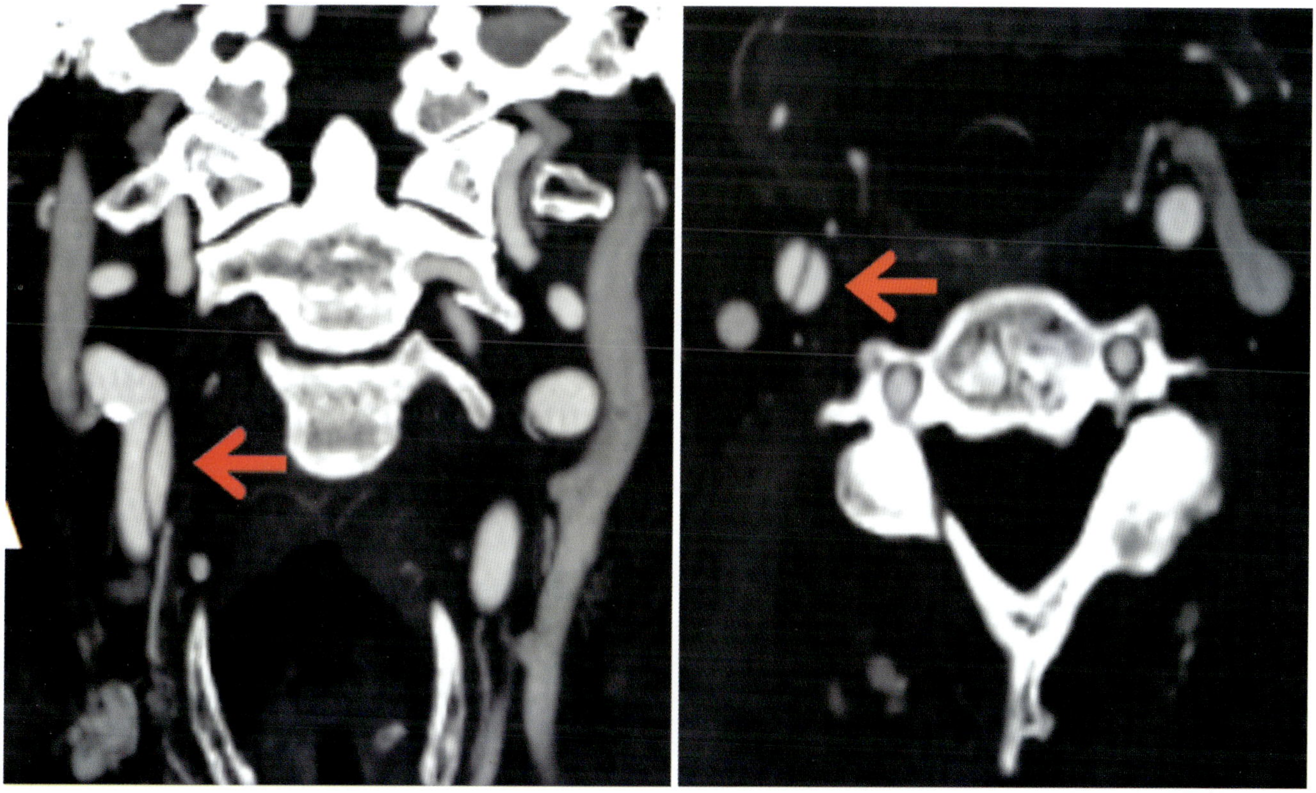

Fig. 57.9B: CT angiogram demonstrating dissection (arrows) of the common carotid artery. (Image courtesy of Gerd Brunner, George Pisimisis, and Vijay Nambi).

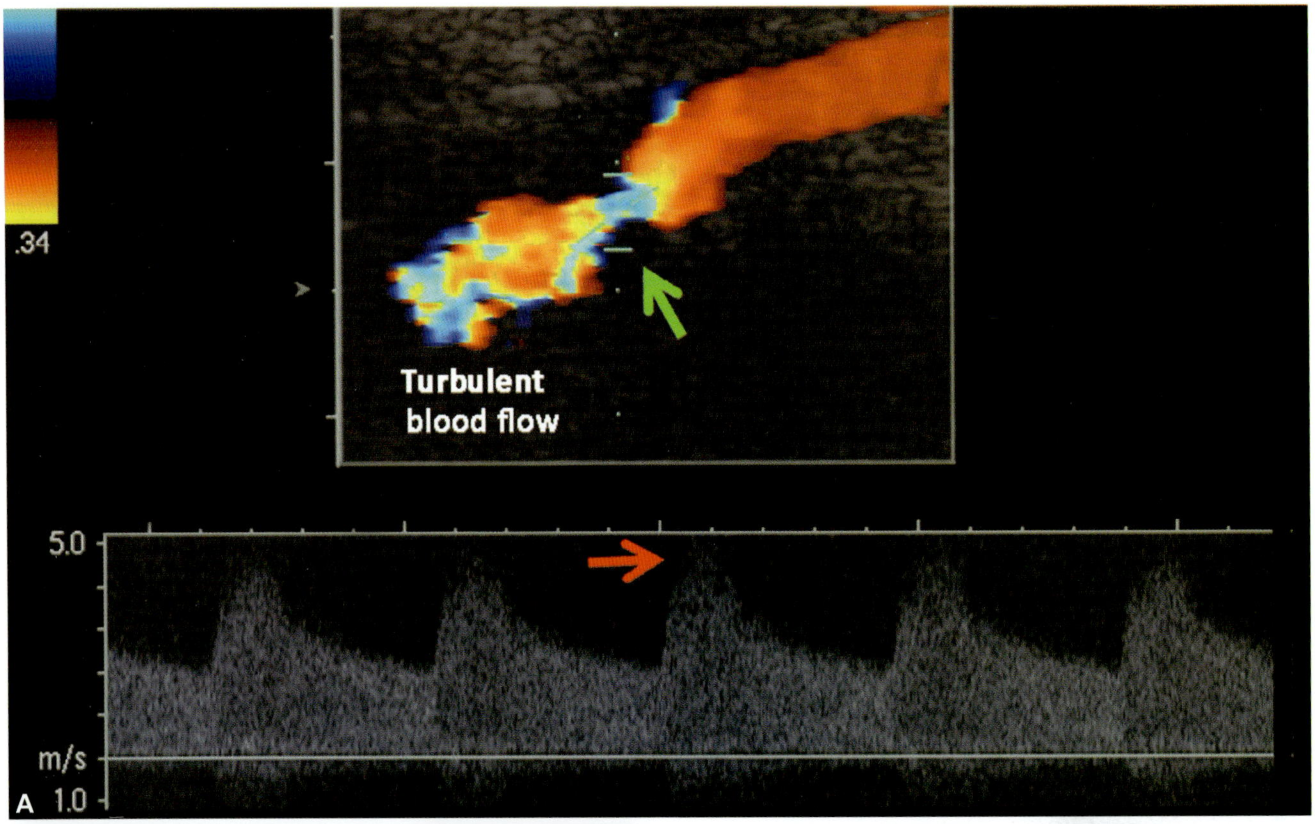

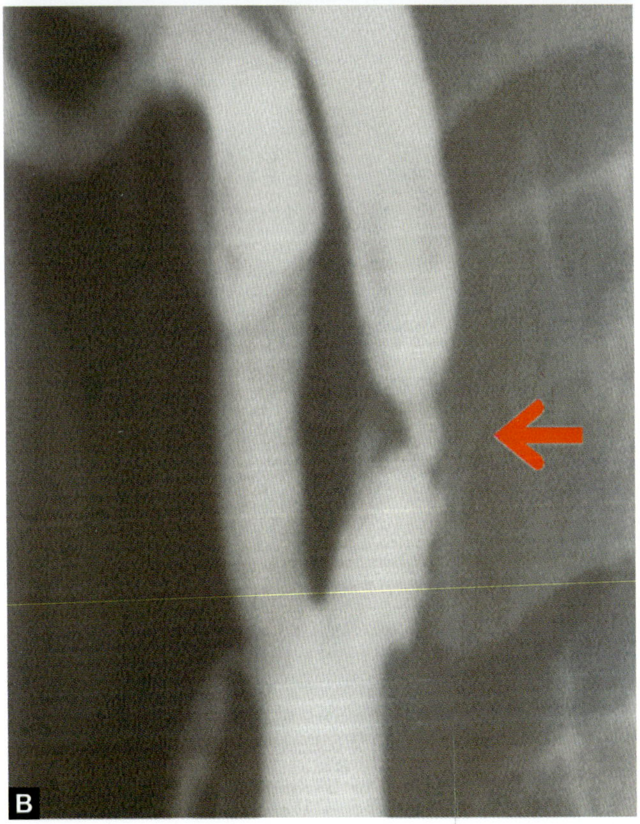

Figs. 57.10A and B: Carotid artery stenosis. (A) Ultrasound of tightly stenotic carotid artery. Highest velocity (red arrow) occurs at the area of stenosis (green arrow), with turbulence distally as indicated by different velocities in close proximity. (B) Angiogram showing tight stenosis of the internal carotid artery (arrow) just past the carotid bifurcation. The irregular plaque contour suggests atherosclerotic disease. (Images 57.10A and B from Arning C, Grzyska U. Color Doppler imaging of cervicocephalic fibromuscular dysplasia. Cardiovascular Ultrasound. 2004;2:7).

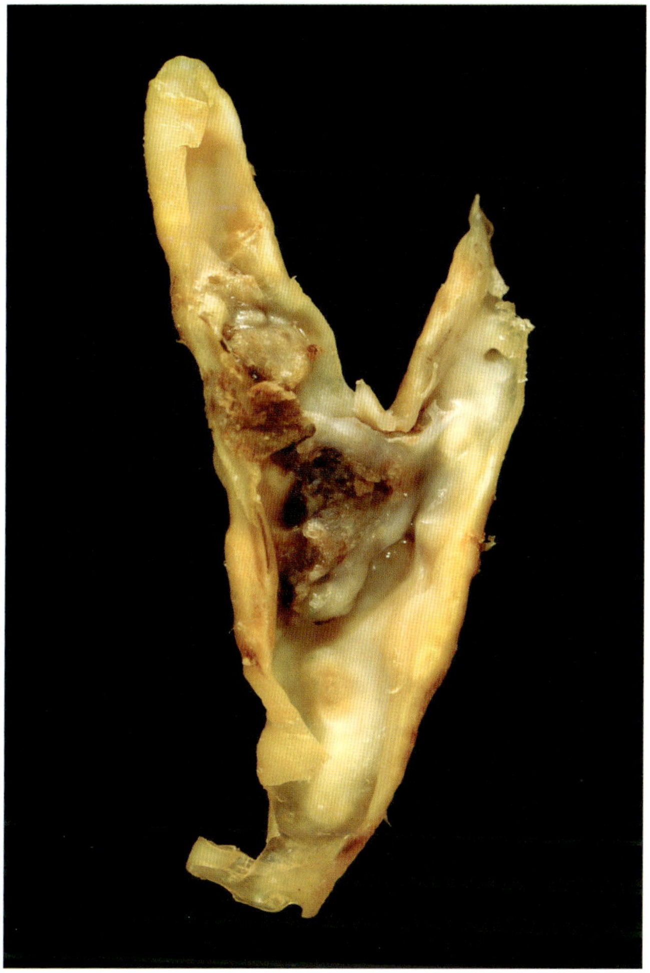

Fig. 57.11: Pathology specimen from an atherosclerotic carotid artery bifurcation revealing plaque and areas of intraplaque hemorrhage. (Image posted by Ed Uthman, MD on Wikimedia Commons).

frequent occurrence in the normal population. Long-term secondary prevention of cardioembolic stroke is oral anticoagulation when not contraindicated. Anticoagulation is usually not initiated in cases of bacterial endocarditis due to an unacceptable bleeding risk.

Severe atheromatous disease of the ascending aorta (Fig. 57.23 and Video 57.14) may also cause strokes in multiple vascular territories, mimicking a cardioembolic etiology. Risk factors for aortic atheroembolic are similar to those for large vessel atherosclerosis. Treatment of severe aortic atheroma includes guideline-directed management of risk factors. Some practitioners may initiate antiplatelet therapy for secondary prevention, while others may initiate oral anticoagulation therapy.

HEMORRHAGIC STROKE

Hemorrhagic stroke is due to spontaneous blood vessel rupture. Hemorrhagic strokes are classified by the location of the rupture, which usually indicates the etiology. The hemorrhage may occur directly into the brain parenchyma (intracerebral hemorrhage, ICH) (Figs. 57.24 and 57.25) or into the subarachnoid space (subarachnoid hemorrhage, SAH) (Fig. 57.26). The term "hemorrhagic stroke" refers to events in which hemorrhage is the primary event, so hemorrhagic transformation of an ischemic stroke (Fig. 57.27) is not considered an ICH. Intracranial bleeds such as subdural hemorrhage (Fig. 57.28) or epidural hemorrhage are not considered strokes, but are important to consider. ICH accounts for about 10% of strokes, and SAH accounts for another 5%. Unlike ischemic strokes, a hemorrhagic stroke is usually visible on CT scan immediately after symptom onset (Figs. 57.29A to C). SAH is usually due to rupture of an intracranial aneurysm (Figs. 57.30A and B), but can be due to other vascular abnormalities or trauma, and is classically associated with the "worst headache of life". The most important risk factors for intracranial aneurysms are hypertension and smoking. Intracerebral hemorrhage in deep locations (i.e. basal ganglia, thalamus, brainstem) is due to small vessel vasculopathy of penetrating arteries commonly associated with chronic hypertension, and is caused by the same vessels involved in ischemic small vessel lacunar stroke. Lobar or cortical ICHs are most commonly due to cerebral amyloid angiopathy. Tumors and arteriovenous malformations are important other causes of hemorrhages in this location.

CEREBRAL VENOUS SINUS THROMBOSIS

Cerebral venous sinus thrombosis accounts for less than 1% of strokes, but is nevertheless important to consider in the differential diagnosis of a patient with stroke-like symptoms, as immediate anticoagulation is an important treatment for this highly lethal condition. Cerebral venous sinus thrombosis is caused by occlusion of one of the major draining veins or dural sinuses (Figs. 57.31 to 57.34). Inadequate perfusion caused by impaired venous drainage can result in ischemia, hemorrhage, or both. Bilateral brain regions are usually affected (frontal lobes, thalami) but cerebral venous sinus thrombosis can be

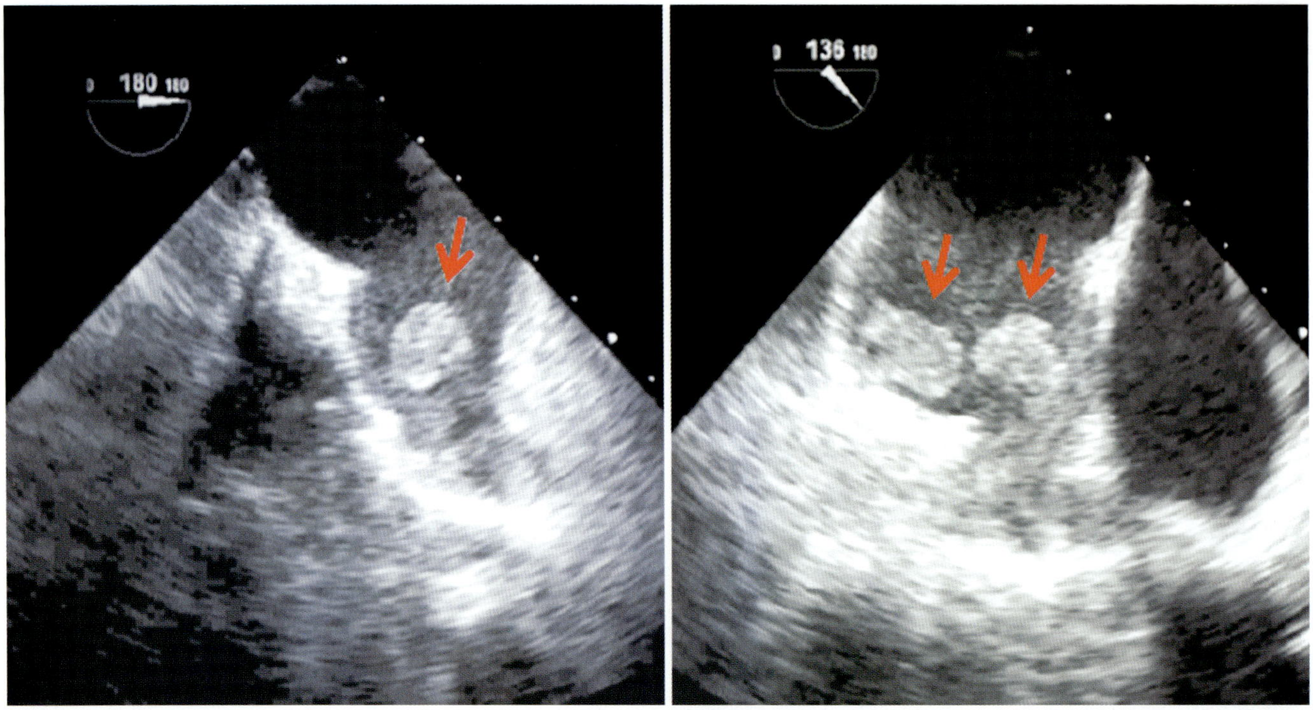

Fig. 57.12: Transesophageal echocardiograms demonstrating mobile thrombi (arrows) in the left atrial appendage. [Image from Jacob SP. Left atrial thrombosis in rheumatic mitral stenosis. In: Harikrishnan S (Ed). Percutaneous Mitral Valvotomy. New Delhi, India: Jaypee Brothers Medical Publishers (P) Ltd.; 2011].

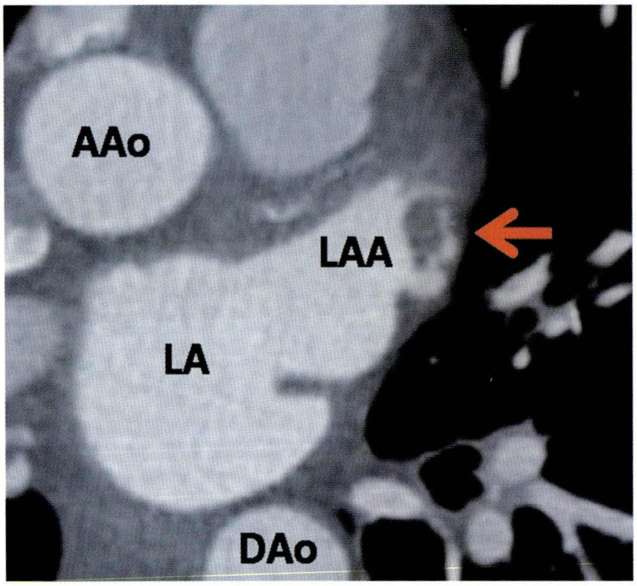

Fig. 57.13: Cardiac CT demonstrating a left atrial appendage (LAA) thrombus (arrow). Left atrial appendage thrombi are a common source of cardioembolic stroke. [Image from Okere IC, Sigurdsson G. Cardiac Computed Tomography. In: Chatterjee K, Anderson M, Heistad D, Kerber RE (Eds). Cardiology: An Illustrated Textbook. Jaypee Brothers Medical Publishers (P). Ltd. 2012]. (AAo: Ascending aorta; Dao: Descending aorta; LA: Left atrium).

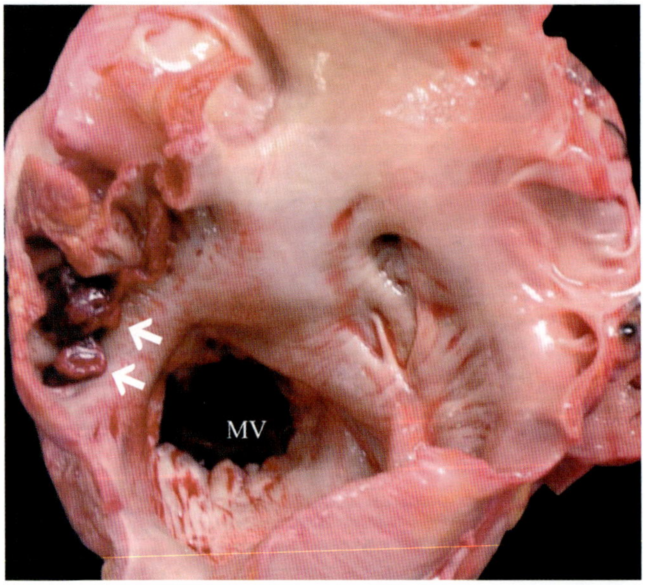

Fig. 57.14: Pathologic specimen showing small left atrial appendage thrombi (arrows), in this case due to amyloidosis. [Image from Feng D, Klarich K, Oh JK. Intracardiac thrombosis, embolism and anticoagulation therapy in patients with cardiac amyloidosis—inspiration from a case observation. In: Güvenç IA (Ed). Amyloidosis: An Insight to Disease of Systems and Novel Therapies. Shanghai: InTech; 2011]. (MV: Mitral valve).

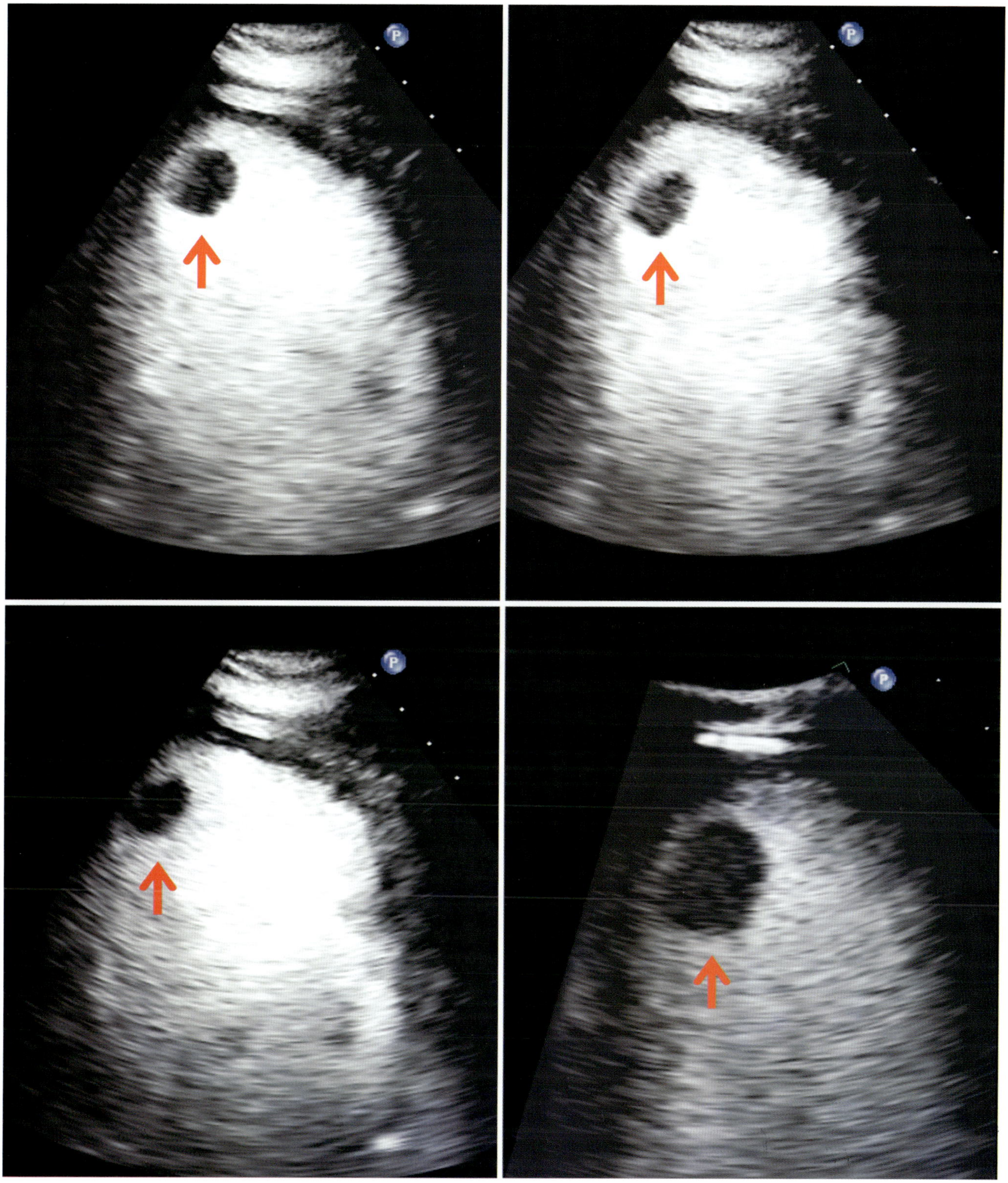

Fig. 57.15: Left ventricular thrombus. Sequential images from contrast-enhanced transthoracic echocardiogram demonstrating a mobile left ventricular apex. The thrombus has formed on the akinetic apex of the left ventricle. Acute myocardial infarction, particularly a large transmural anterior or anteroapical myocardial infarction, is considered a potential source of cardioembolic stroke, even without this dramatic finding. (Image courtesy of Glenn N Levine).

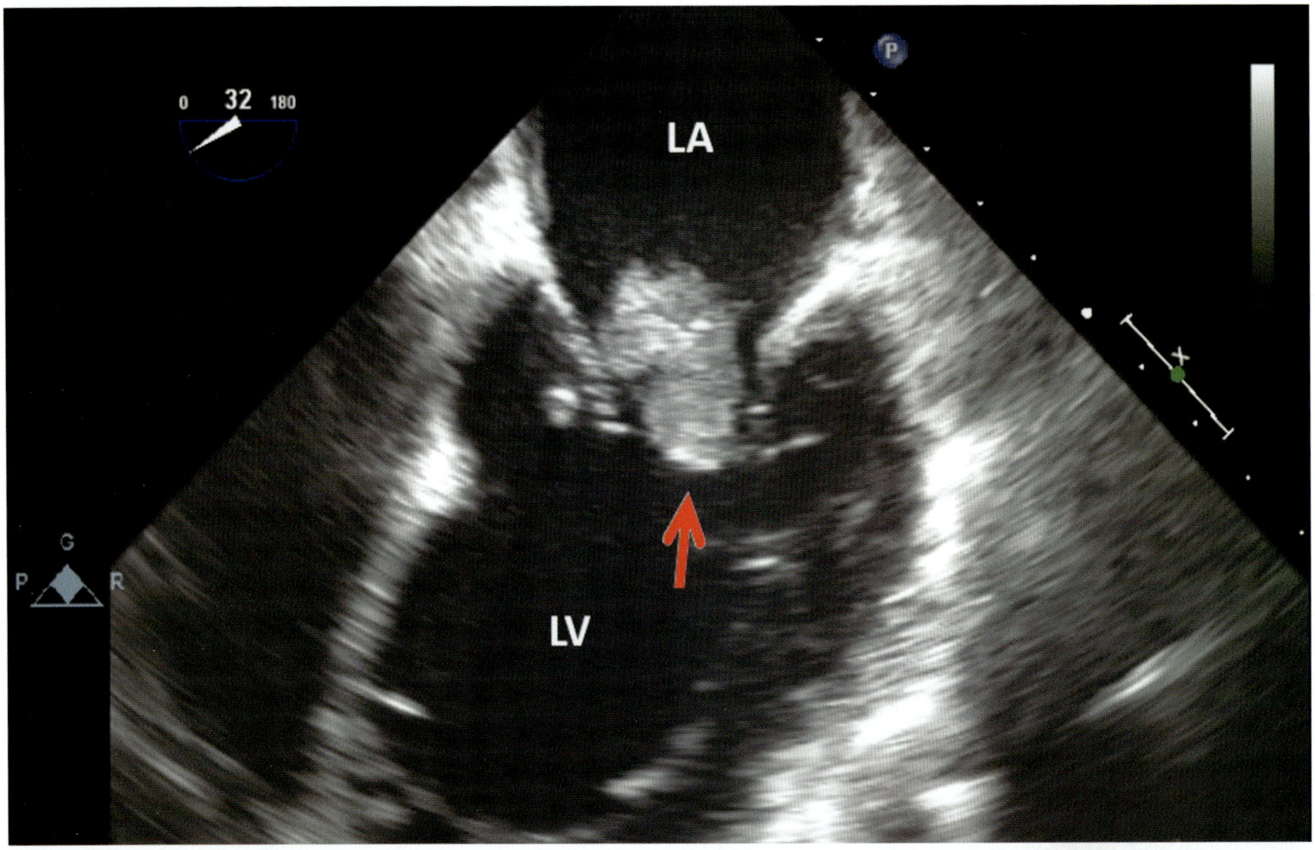

Fig. 57.16: Transesophageal echocardiogram demonstrating a large mitral valve vegetation (arrow) in a patient with bacterial endocarditis. (Image courtesy of Glenn N Levine).

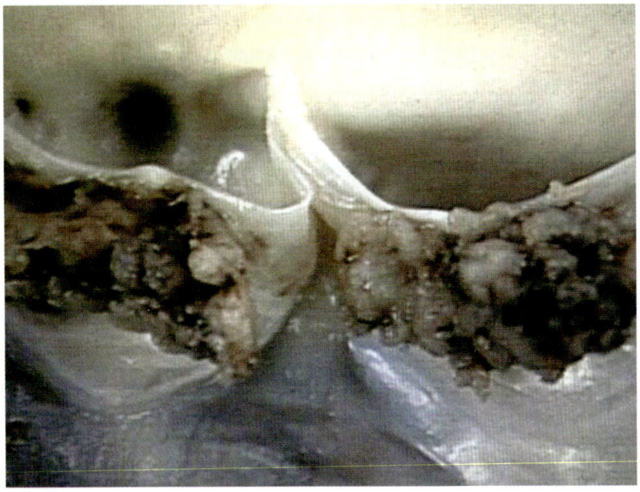

Fig. 57.17: Pathology specimen demonstrating endocarditis on the aortic valve. (Image from Armed Forces Institute of Pathology).

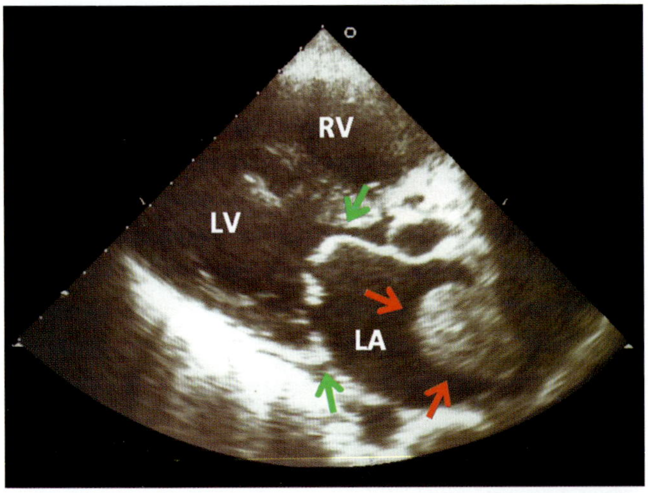

Fig. 57.18: Parasternal long axis transthoracic echo demonstrating a large thrombus (red arrows) in this patient with mitral stenosis (green arrows). (Image from Mocumbi AO. Role of echocardiography in research into neglected cardiovascular disease in Sub-Saharan Africa. In: Gaze DC. The Cardiovascular System — Physiology, Diagnostics and Clinical Implications. Shanghai: InTech; 2011). (RV: Right ventricle; LV: Left ventricle; LA: Left atrium).

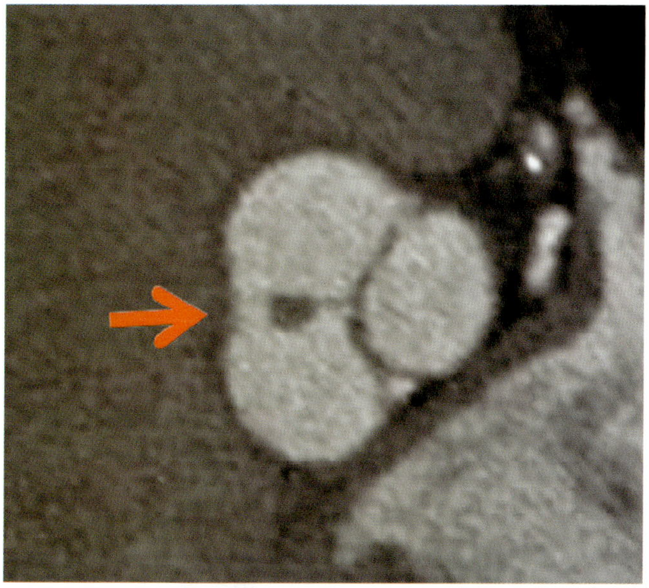

Fig. 57.19: Cardiac CT scan showing a papillary fibroelastoma on the aortic valve. These small tumors are usually asymptomatic, but can embolize and result in a thromboembolic event. [Image from Okere IC, Sigurdsson G. Cardiac computed tomography. In: Chatterjee K, Anderson M, Heistad D, Kerber RE (Eds). Cardiology: An Illustrated Textbook. Jaypee Brothers Medical Publishers (P) Ltd.; 2012].

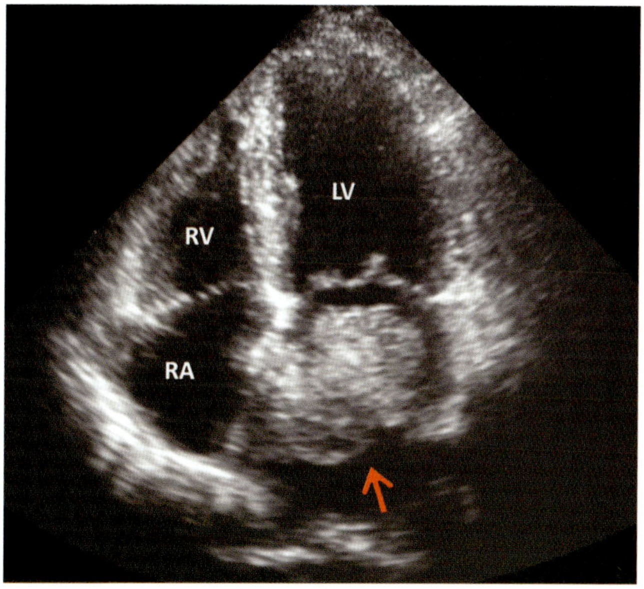

Fig. 57.20: Apical four-chamber echocardiography images showing a myxoma (arrow) in the left atrium. (Image courtesy of Glenn N Levine). (LV: Left ventricle; RA: Right atrium; RV: Right ventricle).

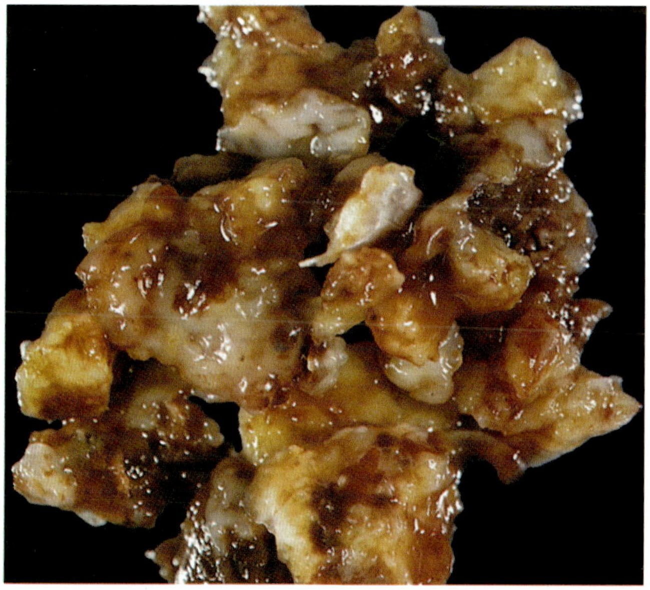

Fig. 57.21: Gross pathology specimen of an atrial myxoma. Note the somewhat gelatinous consistency of the tumor, predisposing part of the tumor to break off and embolize. (Image from Armed Forces Institute of Pathology, downloaded from Wikimedia Commons).

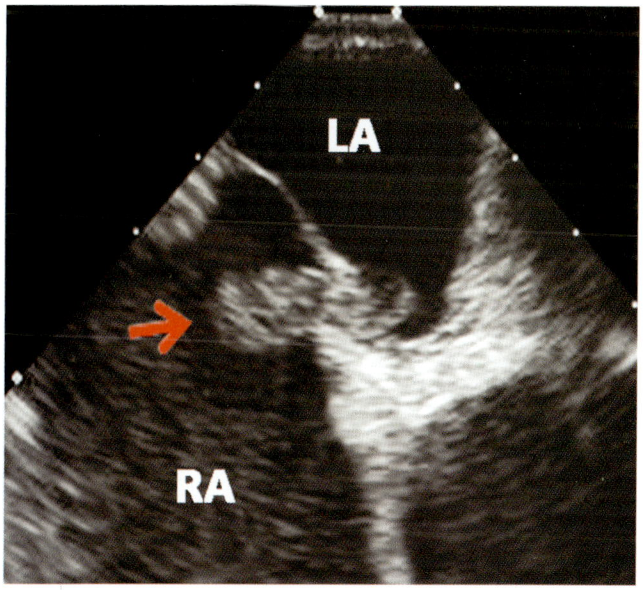

Fig. 57.22: Transesophageal image showing thrombus (arrow) passing through a patent foramen ovale (PFO). Although PFOs themselves are common, they are only considered causative when a clot is directly visualized (as in this case), or a venous source of embolism is found (deep vein thrombosis or pelvic vein thrombosis).

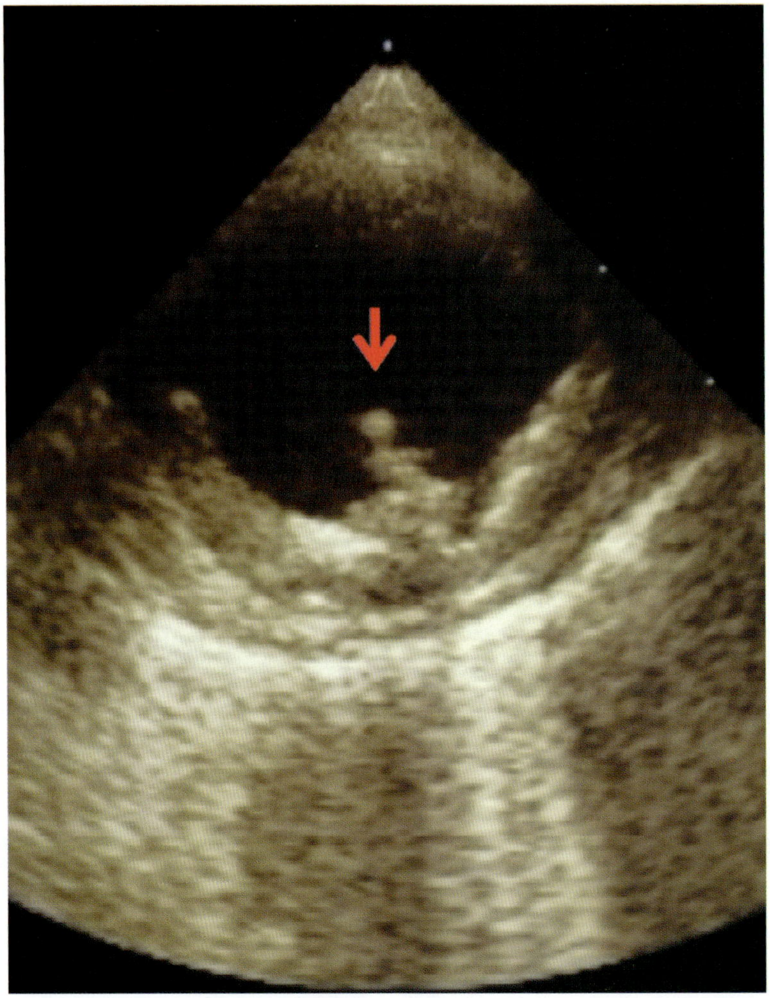

Fig. 57.23: Aortic arch atheroma. Transesophageal echocardiogram showing aortic arch atheroma (arrow). Strokes due to cerebral embolization of aortic debris also occur in multiple vascular distributions. [Image from Royse A, Royse C. Ultrasound assessment of the thoracic aorta in cardiac surgery. In: Bajraktari G (Ed). Echocardiography in Specific Diseases. Shanghai: InTech; 2011].

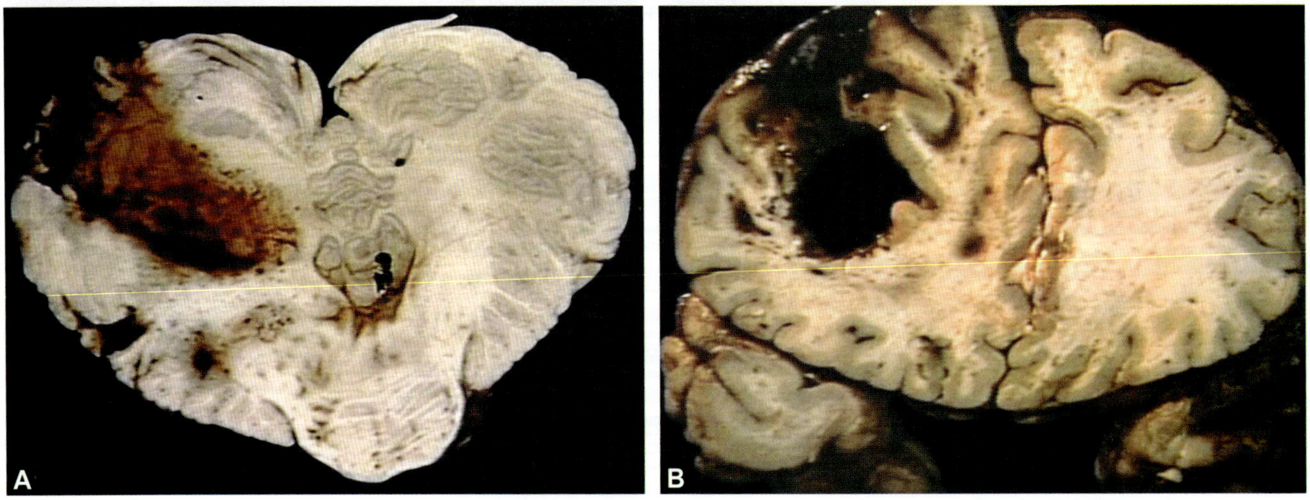

Figs. 57.24A and B: Gross pathology examples of hemorrhagic stroke. (Images from Armed Forces Institute of Pathology).

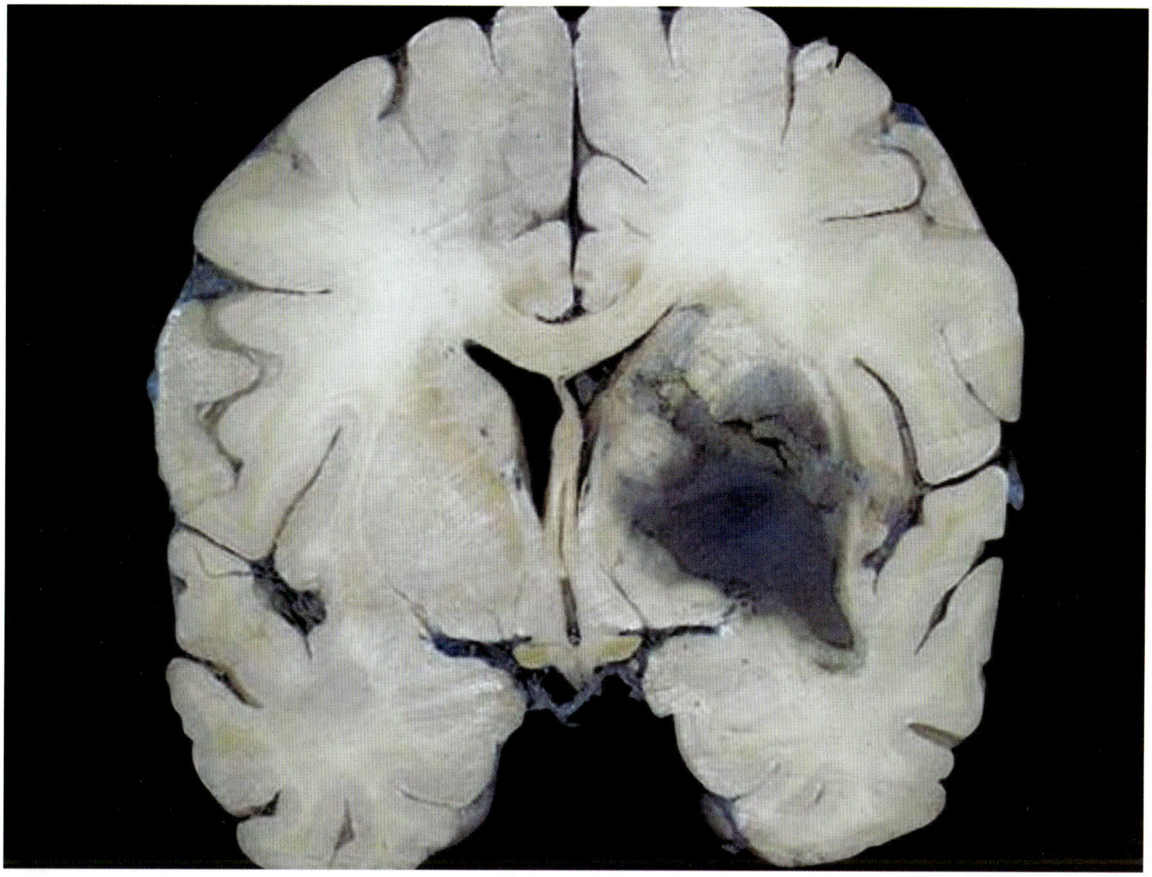

Fig. 57.25: Hemorrhagic stroke due to uncontrolled hypertension involving the right basal ganglia region. [Image from Gupta K, Vasishta RK. Basic neuropathy. In: Gupta AK, Khandelwal N, Chowdhury N (Eds). Diagnostic Radiology: Neuroradiology, including Head and Neck Imaging. New Delhi, India: Jaypee Brothers Medical Publishers (P) Ltd.; 2010].

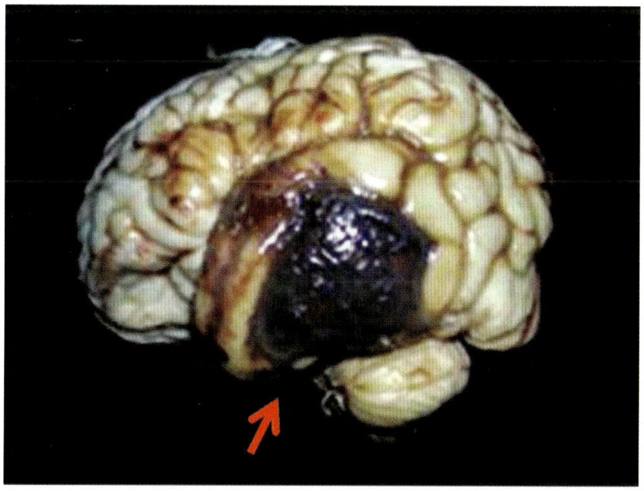

Fig. 57.26: Gross pathology specimen showing a patch of subarachnoid hemorrhage over the left temporal lobe. [Image and legend text from Gupta K, Vasishta RK. Basic neuropathy. In: Gupta AK, Khandelwal N, Chowdhury N (Eds). Diagnostic Radiology: Neuroradiology, including Head and Neck Imaging. New Delhi, India: Jaypee Brothers Medical Publishers (P) Ltd.; 2010].

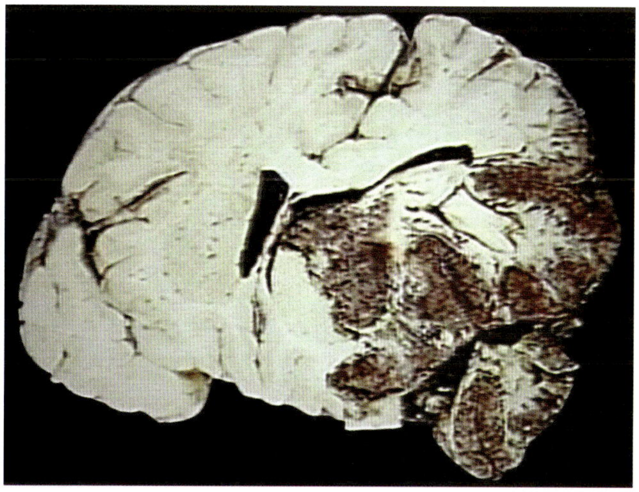

Fig. 57.27: Hemorrhagic transformation of an ischemic stroke. Hemorrhagic transformation of a recent ischemic stroke is not categorized as a hemorrhagic stroke. (Image from Armed Forces Institute of Pathology).

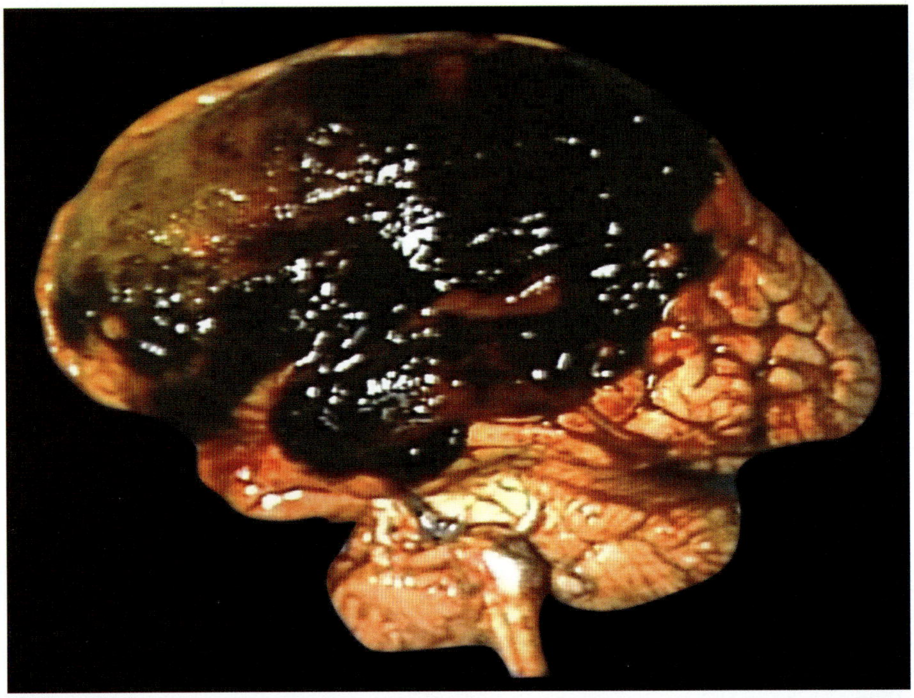

Fig. 57.28: Gross pathology specimen of a subdural hematoma. Subdural hematoma is not considered a stroke, but is still an important entity to be considered in patients with cardiovascular disease who are on antiplatelet or anticoagulant therapy, or have had a recent fall. (Image from Armed Forces Institute of Pathology).

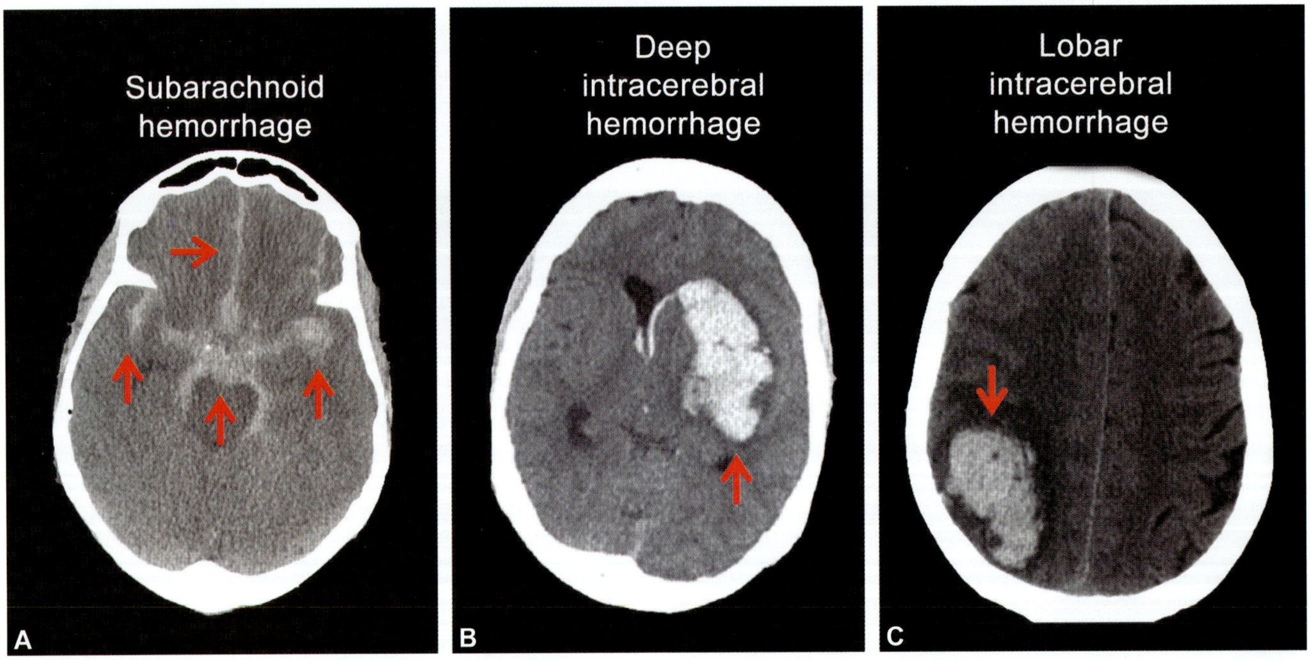

Figs. 57.29A to C: CT imaging of hemorrhagic strokes. (A) Subarachnoid hemorrhage. Axial CT scan of the brain showing diffuse hyperdensity throughout the subarachnoid space (arrows), as seen following rupture of an intracranial aneurysm. (B) Deep intracerebral hemorrhage. Axial CT of the brain demonstrates hyperdensity within the left basal ganglia (arrow), typical of a hypertensive intracerebral hemorrhage. (C) Lobar intracerebral hemorrhage. Axial CT scan of the brain demonstrates a right cortical hyperdensity as would be seen with a lobar hemorrhage due to cerebral amyloid angiopathy (arrow). [Images courtesy of Dr Achala Vagal. Image 57.29B from Adams HP. Stroke: prevention and treatment. In: Chatterjee K, Anderson M, Heistad D, (Eds). Cardiology: An Illustrated Textbook. New Delhi, India: Jaypee Brothers Publishers (P) Ltd.; 2012].

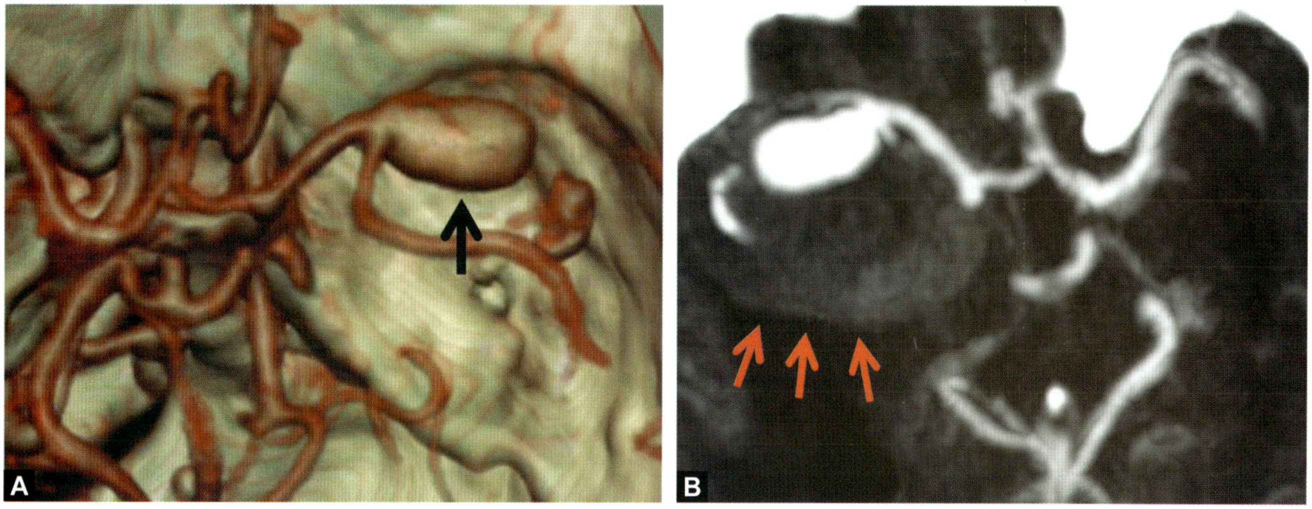

Figs. 57.30A and B: (A) CT volume rendering image showing a large middle cerebral artery aneurysm (black arrow). (B) CT maximum intensity projection (MIP) imaging of the same aneurysm reveals that there is a large thrombosed portion (red arrows) of the aneurysm surrounding the patent central aneurysm. [Images and legend text from Khandelwal N, Gupta V. Imaging of subarachnoid hemorrhage. In: Gupta AK, Khandelwal N, Chowdhury N (Eds). Diagnostic Radiology: Neuroradiology, including Head and Neck Imaging. New Delhi, India: Jaypee Brothers Medical Publishers (P) Ltd.; 2010].

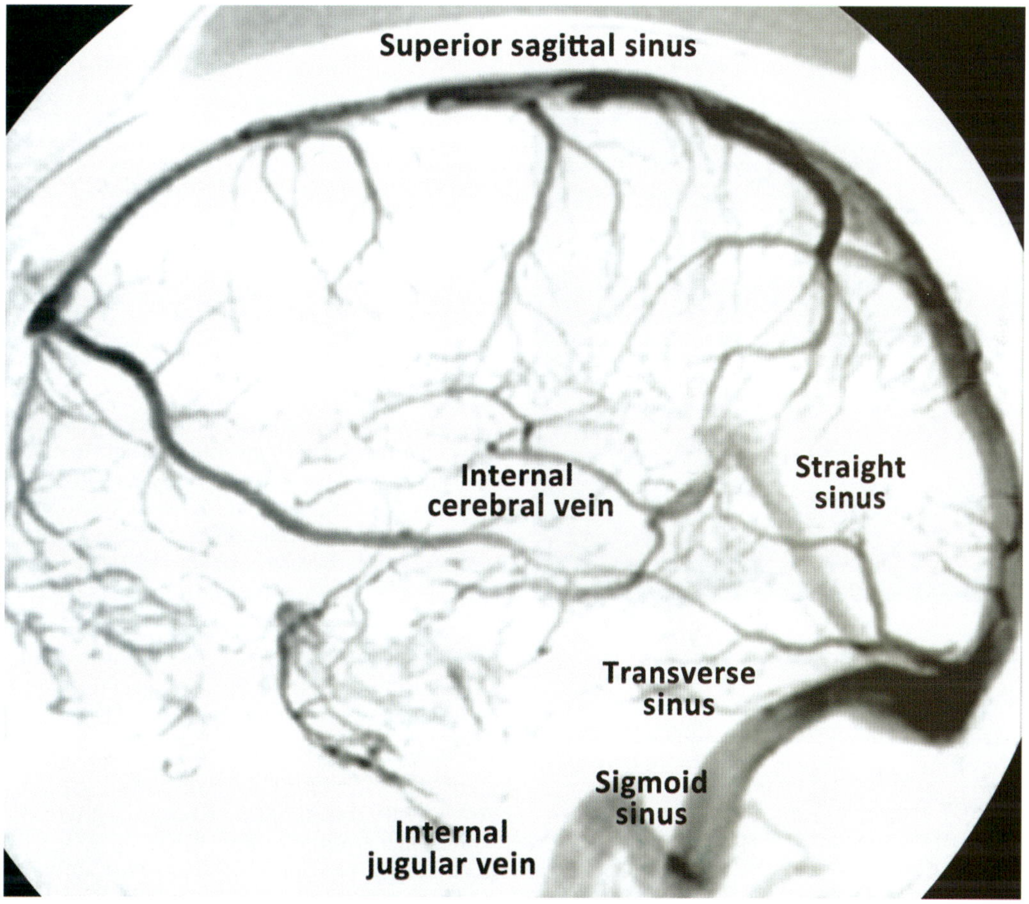

Fig. 57.31: Cerebral vein anatomy. Venous phase cerebral angiogram (lateral view) showing normal venous anatomy. [Image from Gaikwad SB, Kumar A. Normal cerebral angiography. In: Gupta AK, Khandelwal N, Chowdhury N (Eds). Diagnostic Radiology: Neuroradiology, including Head and Neck Imaging. New Delhi, India: Jaypee Brothers Medical Publishers (P) Ltd.; 2010].

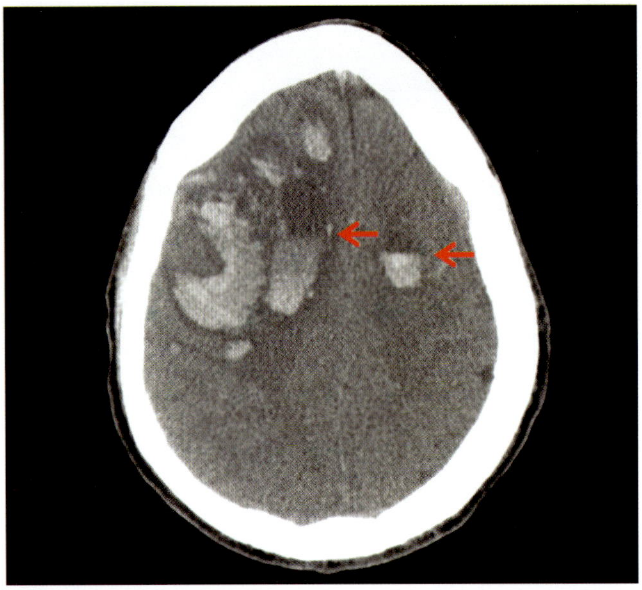

Fig. 57.32: Hemorrhage due to cerebral venous sinus thrombosis. Axial CT of the brain showing bilateral frontal lobe hemorrhages due to occlusion of the superior sagittal sinus. Note the layering of blood in the hemorrhages (arrows) frequently seen when there is limited ability to clot (heparinization, post-tissue plasminogen activator, or disseminated intravascular coagulation).

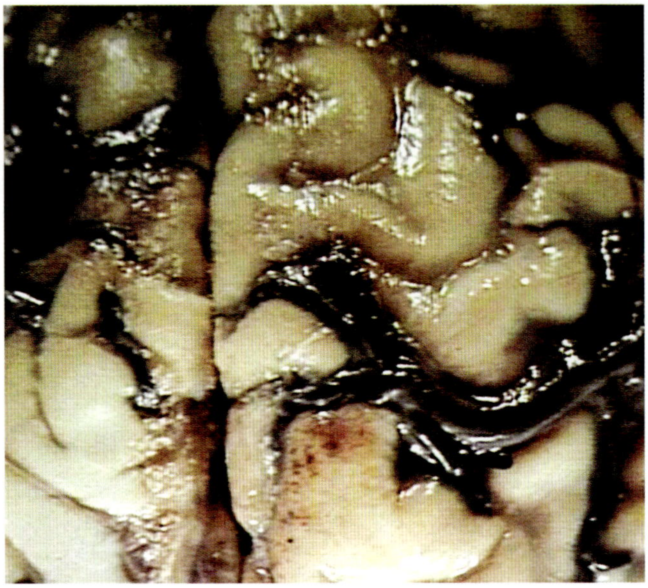

Fig. 57.33: Gross pathology specimen showing cerebral vein thrombosis. (Image from Armed Forces Institute of Pathology).

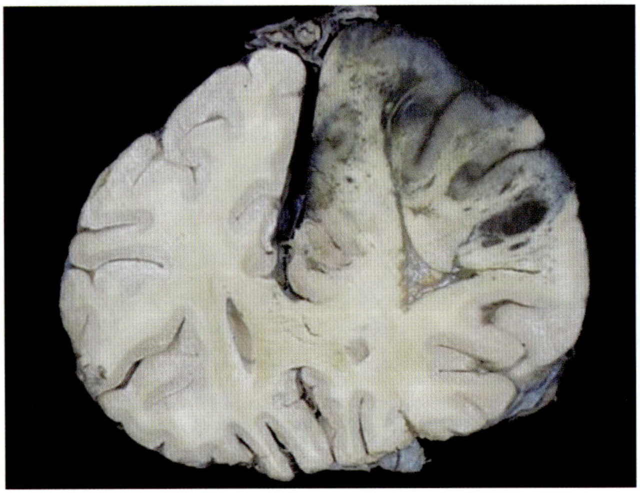

Fig. 57.34: Venous infarcts: thrombosed superior sagittal sinus with hemorrhagic infarct involving the right frontal lobe with midline shift, edema and herniation of cingulate gyrus. [Image and legend text from Gupta K, Vasishta RK. Basic neuropathology. In: Gupta AK, Khandelwal N, Chowdhury N (Eds). Diagnostic Radiology: Neuroradiology, including Head and Neck Imaging. New Delhi, India: Jaypee Brothers Medical Publishers (P) Ltd.; 2010].

unilateral. Symptoms are often gradual in onset, typically include headache, and may involve decreased level of consciousness. Risk factors for the development of cerebral venous sinus thrombosis include dehydration and hypercoagulablity.

VIDEO LEGENDS

Video 57.1: Transesophageal echocardiogram showing thrombus in the left atrial appendage of a patient with atrial fibrillation and recent stroke. (Videos courtesy of Glenn N Levine).

Videos 57.2 to 57.7: Transthoracic echocardiography videos demonstrating left ventricular apical thrombi in patients with an akinetic apex. (Videos courtesy of Glenn N Levine).

Video 57.8: Transthoracic echocardiography showing vegetations on the posterior mitral leaflet.

Video 57.9: Transthoracic echocardiography showing vegetations on a prosthetic mitral valve.

Video 57.10: Transthoracic echocardiography showing mobile vegetations on a prosthetic mitral valve. (Video courtesy of Glenn N Levine).

Video 57.11: Cardiac MRI showing a left atrial myxoma. (Video courtesy of Scott D Flamm).

Video 57.12: Transthoracic echocardiography showing a patent foramen ovale with intermittent right to left flow during an agitated saline ("bubble") study.

Video 57.13: Color Doppler transthoracic echocardiography demonstrating a patent foramen ovale.

Video 57.14: Transthoracic echocardiography study showing mobile atheroma in the aortic arch. (Video courtesy of Glenn N Levine).

REFERENCES

Burch GE, Meyers R, Abildskov JA. A new electrocardiographic pattern observed in cerebrovascular accidents. Circulation. 1954;9:719-23.

Connolly ES Jr, Rabinstein AA, Carhuapoma JR, et al. Guidelines for the management of aneurysmal subarachnoid hemorrhage: a guideline for healthcare professionals from the American Heart Association/American Stroke Association. Stroke. 2012; 43:1711-37.

Furie KL, Kasner SE, Adams RJ, et al. Guidelines for the prevention of stroke in patients with stroke or transient ischemic attack: a guideline for healthcare professionals from the American Heart Association/American Stroke Association. Stroke. 2011; 42:227-76.

Jauch EC, Saver JL, Adams HP Jr, et al. Guidelines for the early management of patients with acute ischemic stroke: a guideline for healthcare professionals from the American Heart Association/American Stroke Association. Stroke. 2013;44: 870-947.

Morgenstern LB, Hemphill JC 3rd, Anderson C, et al. Guidelines for the management of spontaneous intracerebral hemorrhage: a guideline for healthcare professionals from the American Heart Association/American Stroke Association. Stroke. 2010; 41(9):2108-29.

Sacco RL, Kasner SE, Broderick JP, et al. An updated definition of stroke for the 21st century: a statement for healthcare professionals from the American Heart Association/American Stroke Association. Stroke. 2013;44:2064-89.

CHAPTER

58

Venous Thromboembolism

Luis H Eraso, Taki Galanis, Geno J Merli

INTRODUCTION

Venous thromboembolic disease (Figs. 58.1A and B) is the third most common cause of cardiovascular-related deaths after acute coronary syndromes and cerebrovascular disease. The term venous thromboembolism (VTE) usually refers to deep vein thrombosis of the lower extremity (DVT) or pulmonary embolism (PE). However, vein thrombosis may occur in other less usual vascular territories, such as central veins of the brain, neck, upper arm, or mesenteric

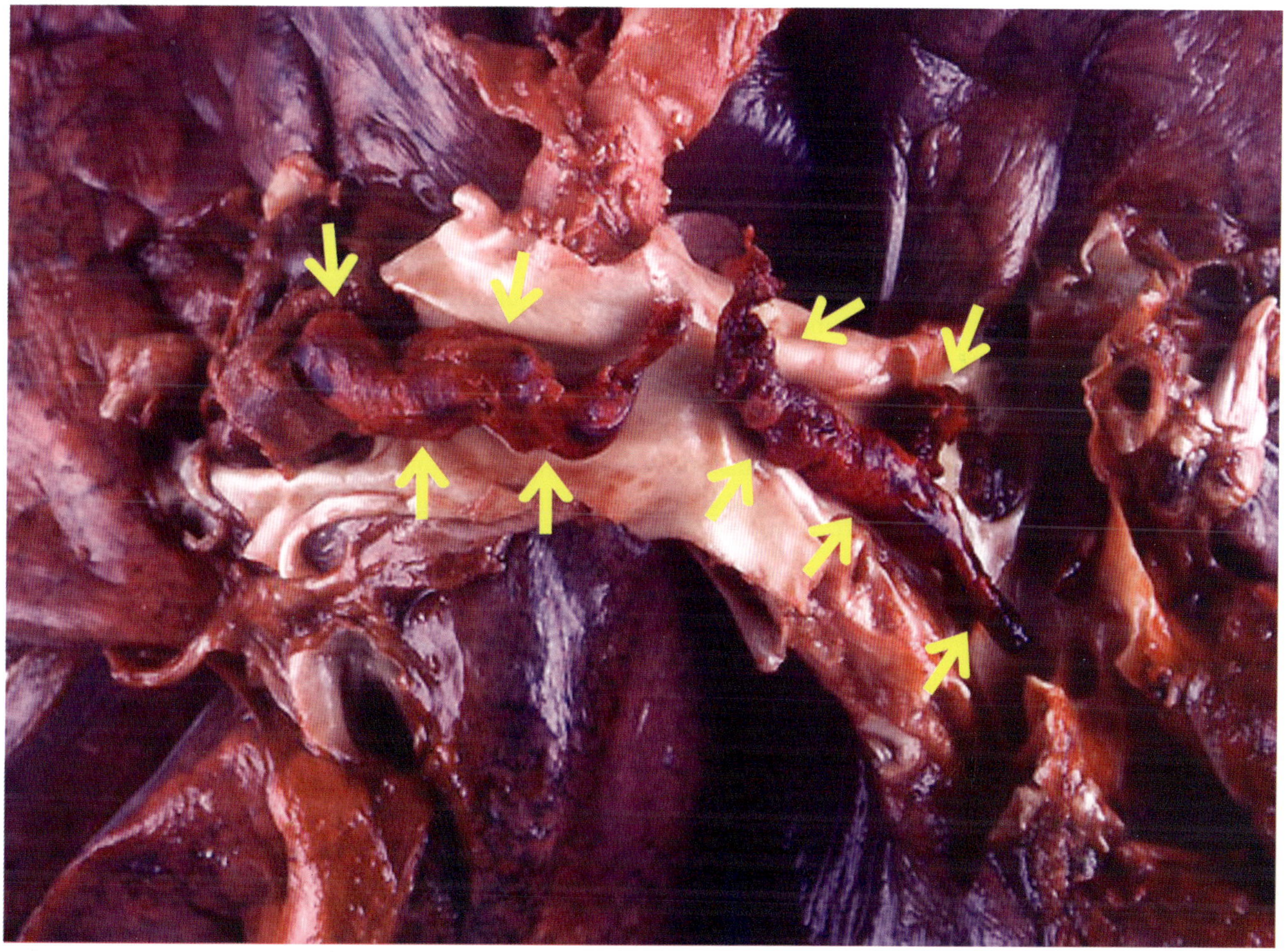

Fig. 58.1A: Autopsy specimen demonstrating massive saddle embolism (arrows). (Image posted by Yale Rosen on Wikimedia Commons).

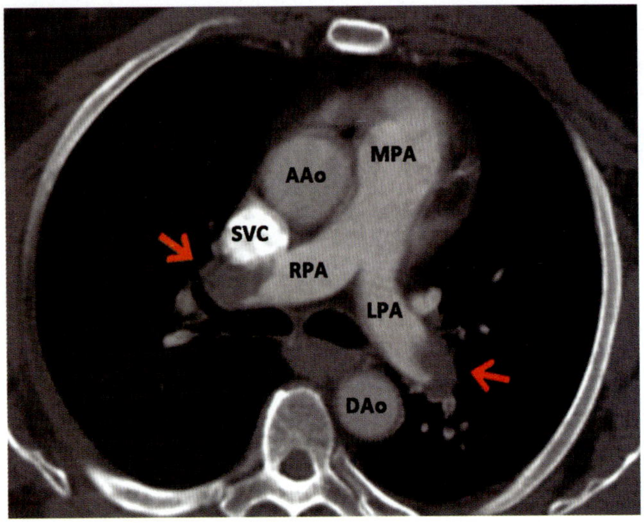

Fig. 58.1B: Contrast-enhanced CT scan showing massive pulmonary emboli (arrows) in both the right pulmonary artery (RPA) and left pulmonary artery (LPA). (Image courtesy Glenn N Levine, MD). (AAo: Ascending aorta; DAo: Descending aorta; MPA: Main pulmonary artery; SVC: Superior vena cava).

veins (Fig. 58.2). The majority of pulmonary embolic events originate in the veins of the lower extremity at the site of venous valvular pockets (Fig. 58.3), which act as microscopic niduses where blood flow disturbances facilitate thrombi growth and propagation in the setting of a triggering factor such as immobility or hypercoagulability. Similar to arterial thrombosis, venous thrombosis entails disruption of vascular coagulation homeostasis (Fig. 58.4), endothelial injury, and acute inflammation. Imbalances between the coagulation and fibrinolysis processes, such as occur in some hypercoagulable states, may predispose to venous thrombosis (Fig. 58.5).

Anatomical characteristics of the crural vein and muscles, particularly the soleal vein, also play a major role in the occurrence, propagation and embolic risk of venous thrombi of the lower extremities (Figs. 58.6A and B). Several retrospective analyses have established the association of pulmonary embolism and soleal vein thrombosis. The soleal muscle contraction depends entirely on the functionality of the ankle joint. Therefore, in the case of prolonged immobility, venous flow stagnation of the soleal vein flow occurs rapidly. The soleal vein has no functioning valves, and in contrast to proximal venous thrombi formed at the valve pockets, soleal vein thrombi form circumferentially within the dilated vein, attached to the wall only by a thin fibrin membrane, making them more prone to rapid propagation and embolism.

DIAGNOSIS OF VENOUS THROMBOEMBOLIC DISEASE

Contemporary diagnosis of VTE is established through application of clinical prediction rules for deep vein thrombosis (Table 58.1) and pulmonary embolism (Table 58.2). Quantification of serum biomarkers of cross-linked fibrin (D-Dimer by ELISA) have a high sensitivity and negative predictive value (> 95%) to rule out the presence of VTE if the threshold levels are 500 μg/L, particularly in patients with a low or intermediate clinical probability assessment. Confirmatory diagnosis requires the use of multimodality imaging derived from clinical probability assessment diagnostic algorithms.

Compression ultrasonography is an accurate method to confirm the diagnosis of DVT and establish treatment. Ultrasonographic noncompressibility of the affected vein in the setting of high probability risk has similar diagnostic accuracy as venography (Figs. 58.7A to C). Abnormal flow detected by Doppler, color Doppler filling defects, or presence of intravascular echogenic material are adjuvant diagnostic tools (Figs. 58.8A and B). Compression ultrasonography is also useful to monitor thrombus resolution and establish the presence of residual vein obstruction (RVO), an important predictor of recurrent thrombotic events and postthrombotic syndrome (PTS). Partial compressibility (< 40%), residual thrombus of greater than 2 mm,

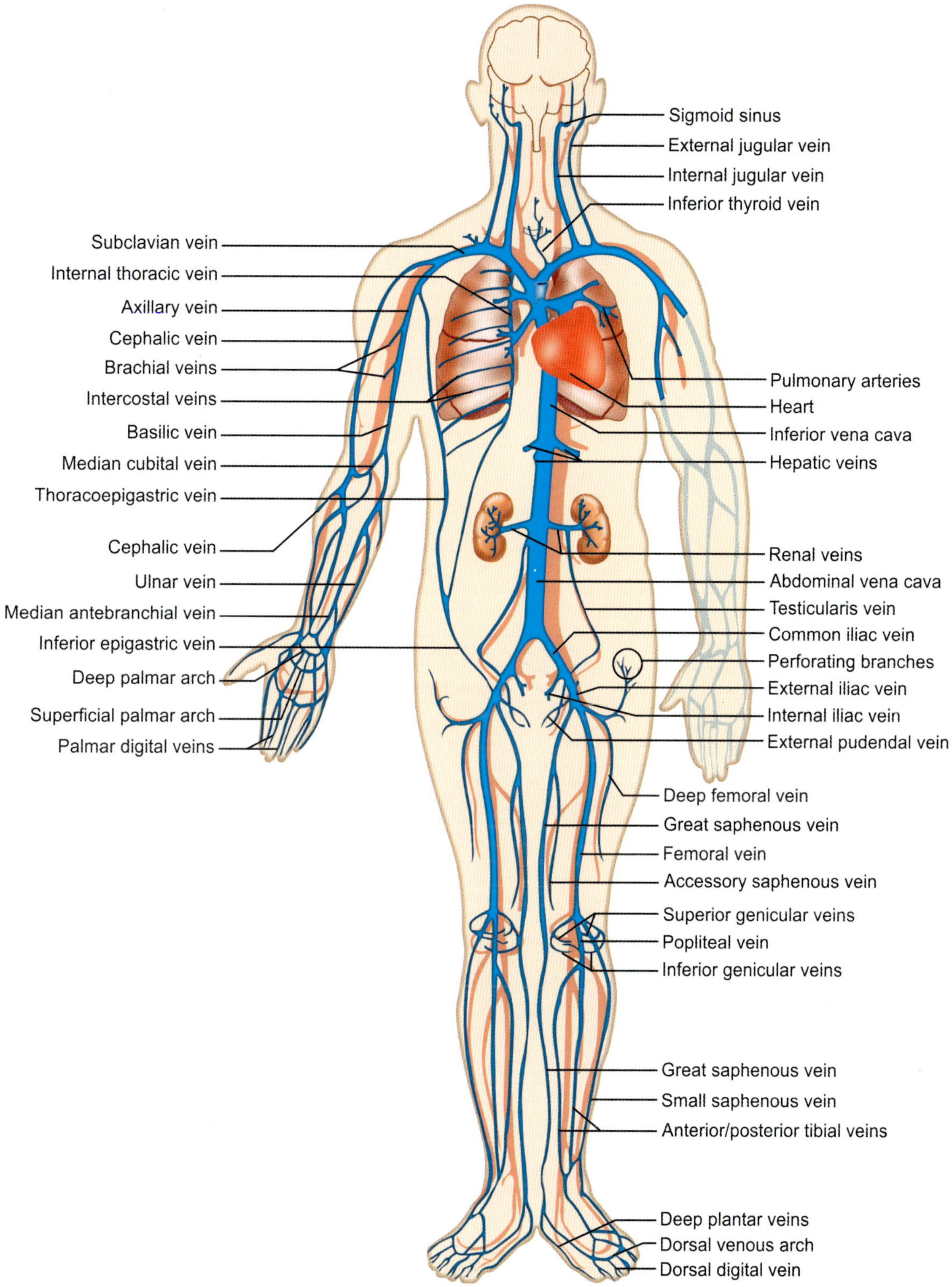

Fig. 58.2: Schematic illustration of the venous system. (Image created and posted by LadyofHats on Wikimedia Commons).

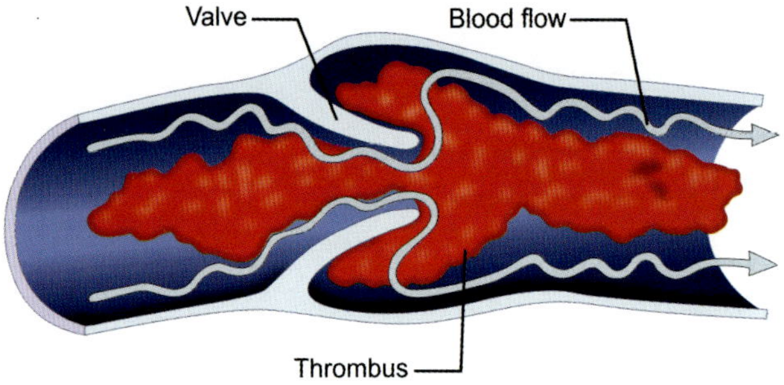

Fig. 58.3: Venous valvular pockets and thrombus formation. The valvular pockets act as a microscopic niduse where blood flow disturbances facilitate thrombi growth and propagation in the setting of a triggering factor such as immobility or hypercoagulability.

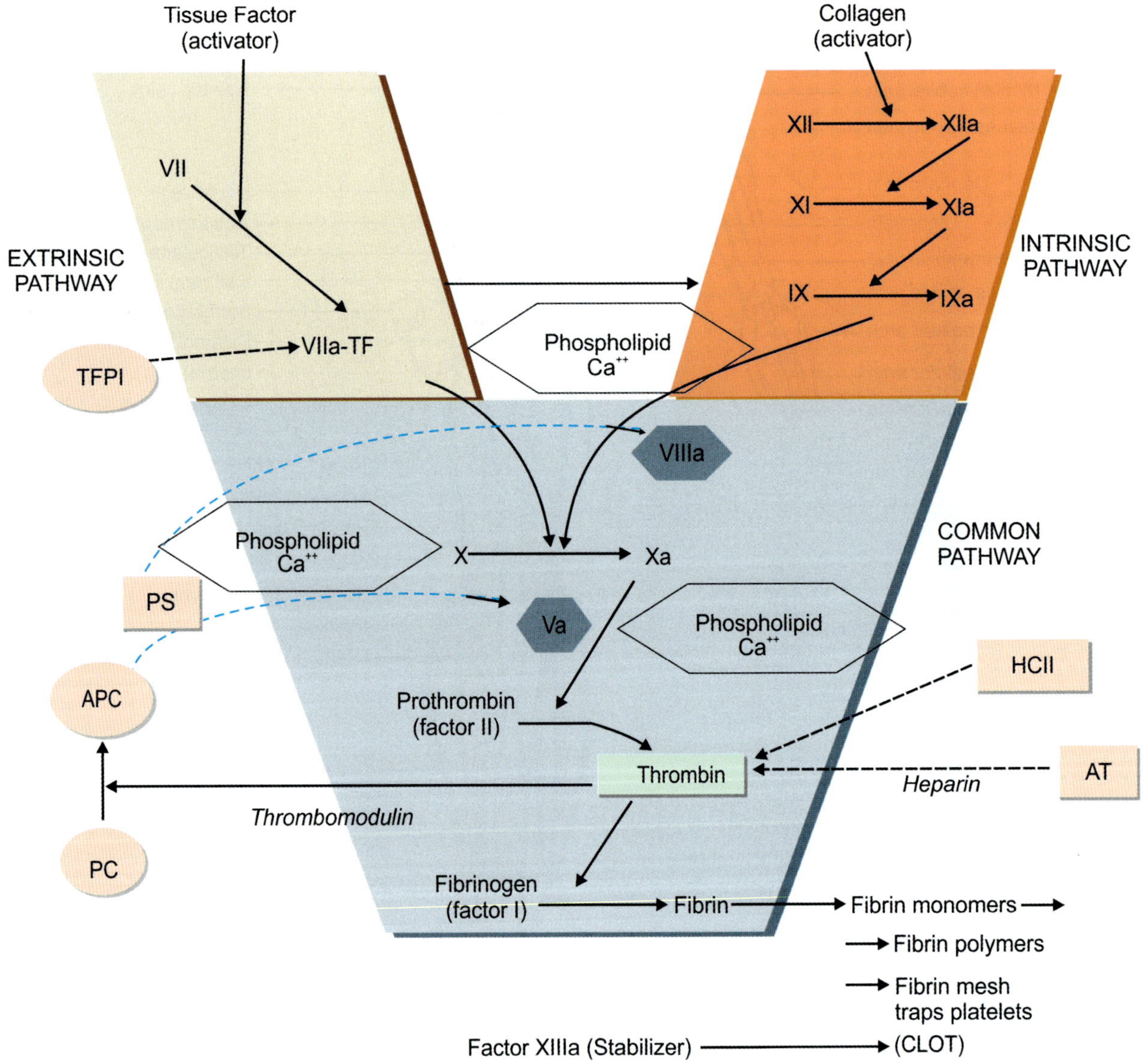

Fig. 58.4: The coagulation process and its control elements. Solid arrows indicate activation; dotted arrows indicate inactivation. [Image and figure text from Jadaon MM. Aetiology of venous thrombosis. In: Okuyan E (Ed). Venous thrombosis—principles and practice. Intechweb.org. CC].

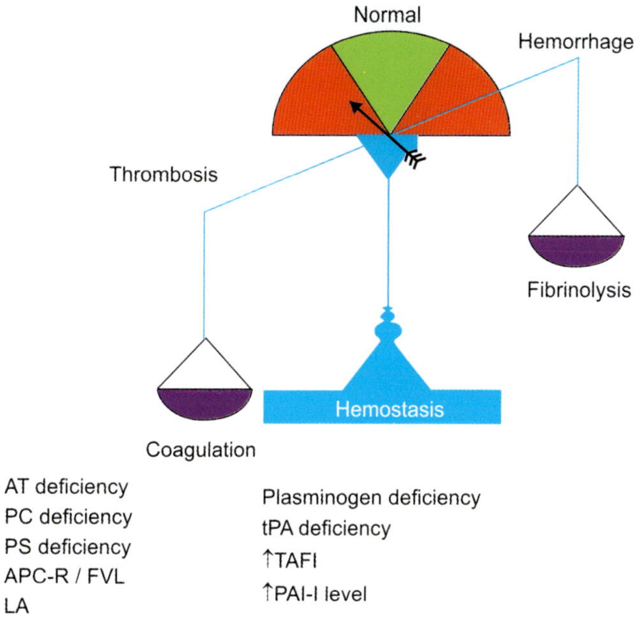

Fig. 58.5: Imbalances between the coagulation and fibrinolysis processes, such as occur in some hypercoagulable states, may predispose to venous thrombosis. [Image adapted from Jadaon MM. Aetiology of venous thrombosis. In: Okuyan E (Ed). Venous thrombosis—principles and practice. Intechweb.org. CC].

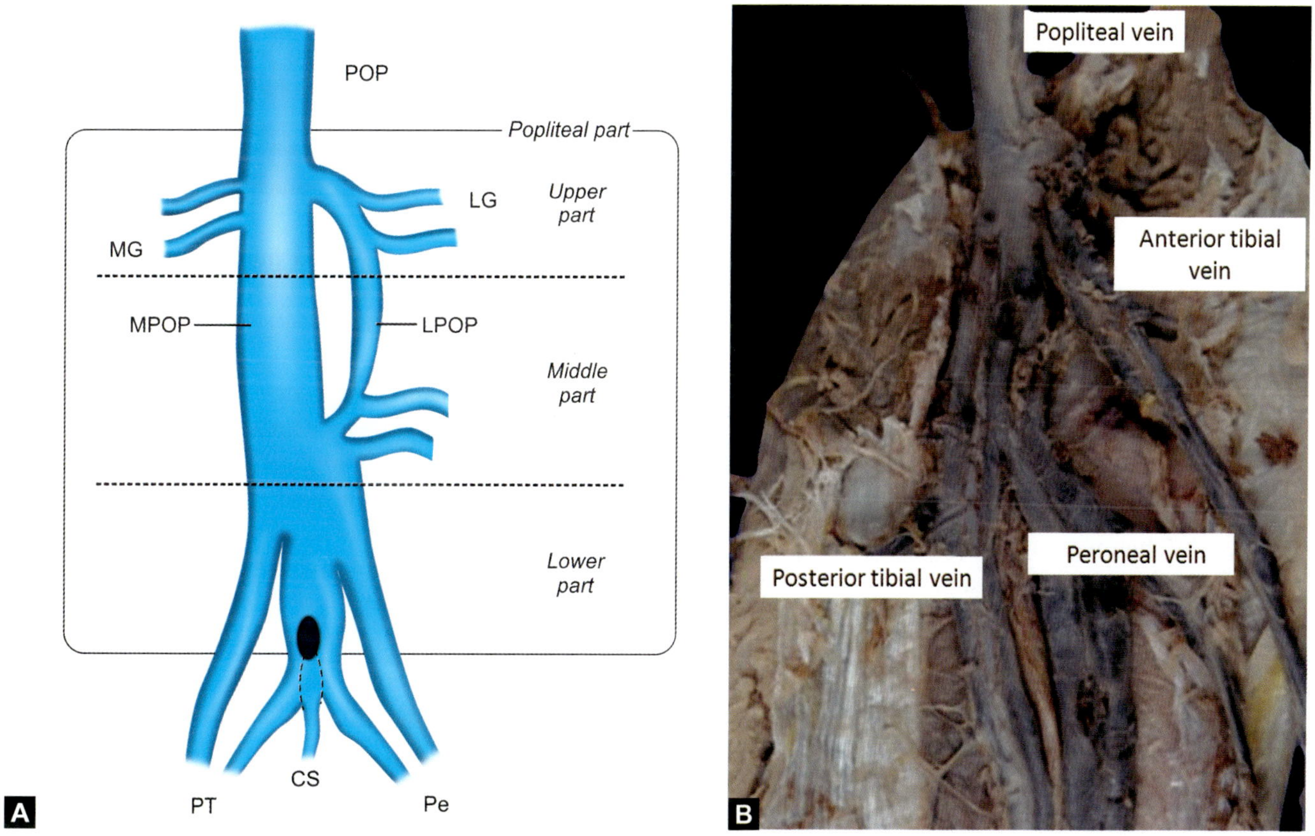

Figs. 58.6A and B: Anatomical scheme (A) and macroscopic photo (B) of crural deep veins and popliteal trunk. [Adapted from Kageyama N, Ro A, Tanifuji T, Fukunaga T. Significance of the soleal vein and its drainage veins in cases of massive pulmonary thromboembolism. Ann Vasc Dis. 2008;1(1):35-39]. (POP: Popliteal vein; MG: Medialis of the gastrocnemius vein; LG: Lateralis of the gastrocnemius vein; MPOP: Medialis of the popliteal vein; LPOP: Lateralis of the popliteal vein; AT: Anterior tibial vein; PT: Posterior tibial vein; CS: Centralis of the soleal vein; Pe: Peroneal vein).

Table 58.1: Clinical probability assessment (Wells score) for lower extremity deep vein thrombosis. A score of 0 or less indicates low probability, 1 or 2 indicates moderate probability, and 3 or more indicates high probability. [Adapted from Guyatt et al. Executive summary: Antithrombotic therapy and prevention of thrombosis, 9th edition: American College of Chest Physicians Evidence-based Clinical Practice Guidelines. Chest. 2012;141 (2 Suppl):7S-47S].

Clinical Findings	*Score*
• Active cancer (treatment ongoing within previous 6 months or palliative)	1
• Paralysis, paresis, or recent plaster immobilization of the lower extremities	1
• Recent immobility > 3 days or major surgery within 3 months requiring anesthesia	1
• Localized tenderness of the deep veins of the leg	1
• Diffuse lower extremity edema	1
• Calf swelling > 3 cm larger than asymptomatic side measured 10 cm below tibial tuberosity	1
• Asymmetric pitting edema limited to the symptomatic low	1
• Collateral superficial veins (not including varicose veins)	1
• Previously documented DVT	1
• Alternative diagnosis as likely as or more likely than DVT	–2

and reduction of vein diameter with a hyperechoic vein wall (hypoplastic vein changes) or presence of echogenic intravascular banding (sinequea) are ultrasonographic findings consistent with residual vein obstruction and disruptive vein healing (Figs. 58.9 and 58.10). Alternative diagnostic imaging for deep vein thrombosis, particularly of the proximal segments such as the iliac vein or inferior vena cava, include CT or MR venography (Fig. 58.11).

Although the chest X-ray is normal, or has nonspecific findings, in the majority of patients with pulmonary embolism, the chest X-ray in a patient with shortness of breath may rarely suggest the diagnosis of pulmonary embolism. The Westermark sign is a finding of focal oligemia, which occurs distal to a pulmonary embolism. Pulmonary infarction and subsequent edema of the infarcted pulmonary tissue may rarely result in the finding of a wedge-shaped opacity in the periphery of the lung (Fig. 58.12), which is called "Hampton's hump".

Echocardiography is not usually performed specifically to assess the patient with suspected pulmonary embolism, but may be performed as part of the evaluation of the patient with dyspnea. Findings on echocardiography

Table 58.2: Clinical probability assessment (Wells score) for pulmonary embolism. A score of 0 or less indicates low probability, 1 or 2 low risks, 2–6 intermediate risk, and more than 7 indicates high risk. Alternative dichotomize prediction rule define a PE unlikely (≤ 4) or likely (≥ 4). [Adapted from Guyatt et al. Executive summary: Antithrombotic therapy and prevention of thrombosis, 9th edition: American College of Chest Physicians Evidence-based Clinical Practice Guidelines. Chest. 2012;141 (2 Suppl):7S-47S].

Clinical Findings	*Score*
Hemoptysis	1
Cancer	1
Previous VTE	1.5
Heart rate > 100	1.5
Recent surgery or immobility	1.5
Clinical signs of deep vein thrombosis	3
Alternative diagnosis unlikely	3

that increase suspicion for pulmonary embolism include an unexplained dilated right ventricle with signs of right ventricular pressure overload (Fig. 58.13A) or a dilated right ventricle with hypokinesis of the RV free wall but spared systolic function at the apex (McConnell's sign) (Fig. 58.13B). Rarely, echocardiography may image an embolus actually passing through the heart (Figs. 58.14A and 58.14B) or in the pulmonary artery (Fig. 58.14C, Videos 58.1 and 58.2).

The diagnosis of suspected pulmonary embolism is usually confirmed by a more advanced imaging modality. Ventilation-perfusion scintigraphy (VQ scan) has been used for decades to assess patients with suspected pulmonary embolism (Figs. 58.15 and 58.16). V/Q scan may still be used in patients who are at high risk of contrast nephropathy from iodinated contrast administration. Although used in the past, pulmonary angiogram (Fig. 58.17) is now only used rarely to diagnose pulmonary embolism. More commonly in current practice, computed tomography (CT) scanning is obtained to confirm a diagnosis of pulmonary embolism (Figs. 58.18 to 58.22).

TREATMENT OF VENOTHROMBOEMBOLIC DISEASE

The standard treatment of VTE is based on the latest American College of Chest Physicians guidelines that entail a phasic anticoagulation therapy approach that matches the pathophysiological phases of thrombus formation, organization and resolution. The following

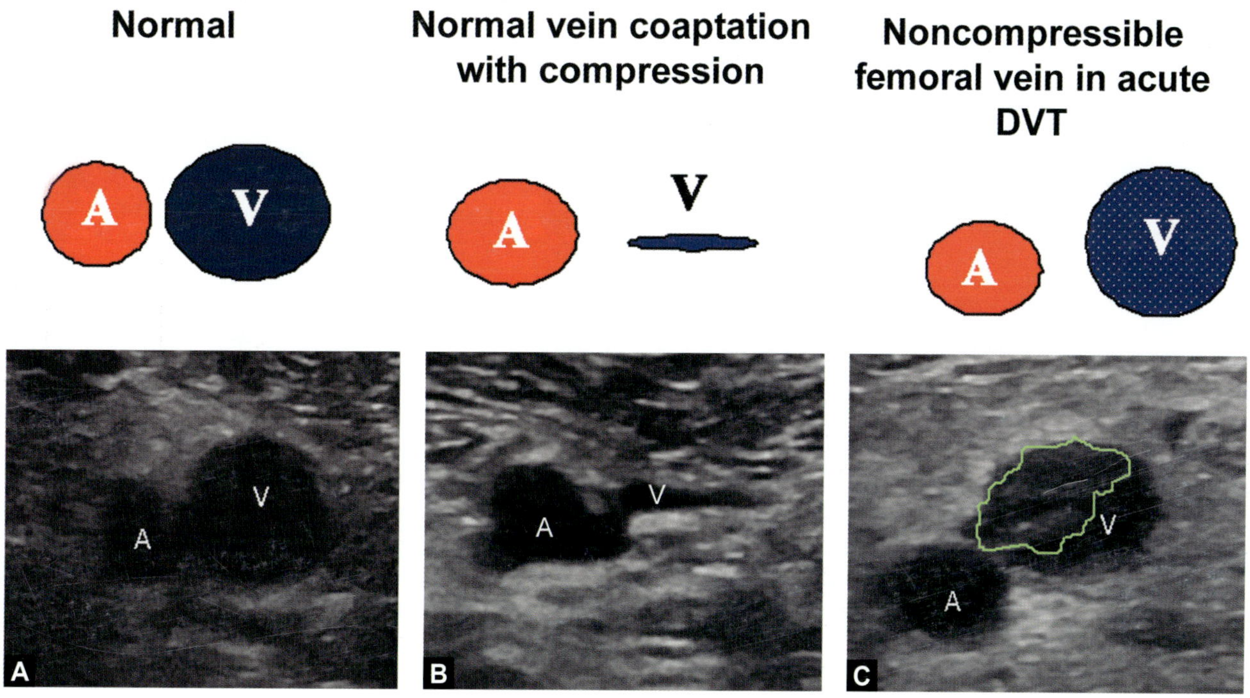

Normal femoral artery (A) and vein (V) on gray scale ultrasound imaging vein (V) diameter is slightly larger than artery (A). A normal anatomic finding at the groin. There is no evidence of intravascular echoic material

Vein (V) compressibility is nearly complete with coaptation of the vein walls less than 0.5 mm. There is no evidence of intravascular echogenic material. Artery (A) diameter is not significantly changed with compression

Noncompressible femoral vein with evidence of intravascular echoic thrombus (green outline), Vein (V) diameter is larger than artery (A), a finding also consistent with acute thrombosis

Figs. 58.7A to C: Deep vein thrombosis diagnosis by compression ultrasonography.

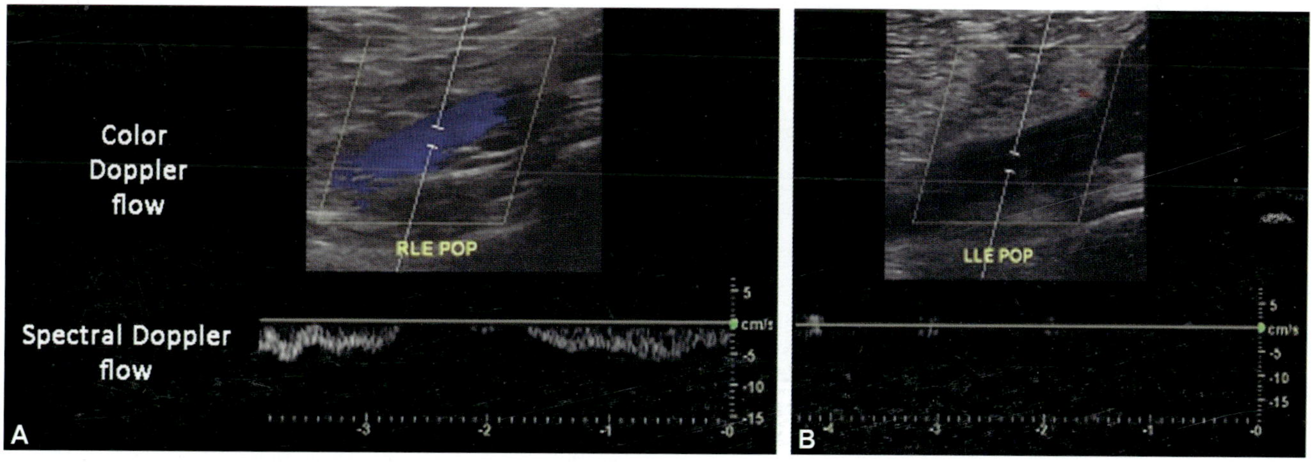

Figs. 58.8A and B: Spectral and color Doppler flow changes observed with vein thrombosis. (A) Normal color Doppler imaging with evidence of phasic spectral Doppler signal (bottom aspect of Figure 58.8A); (B) Absent color Doppler signal and absent spectral Doppler signal (bottom aspect of Figure 58.8B).

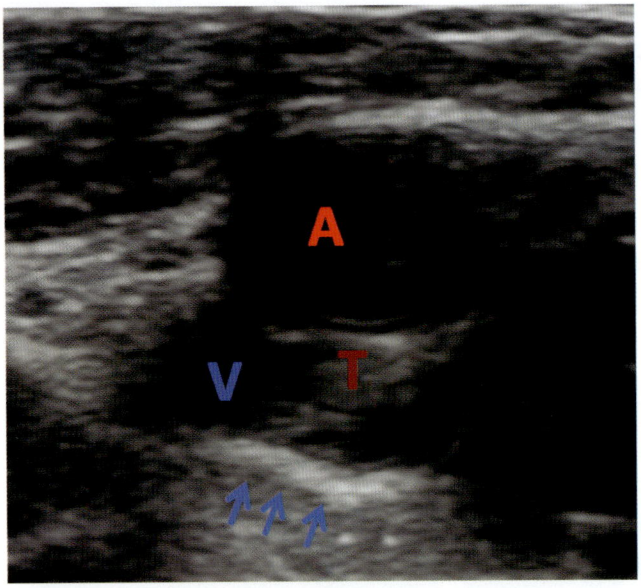

Fig. 58.9: Ultrasonographic imaging of a chronic venous thrombus. There is partial vein (V) compressibility of the vein (V) and residual vein thrombosis (T). Notice the echogenic posterior vein wall (arrows), consistent with vein scaring. (A: Artery).

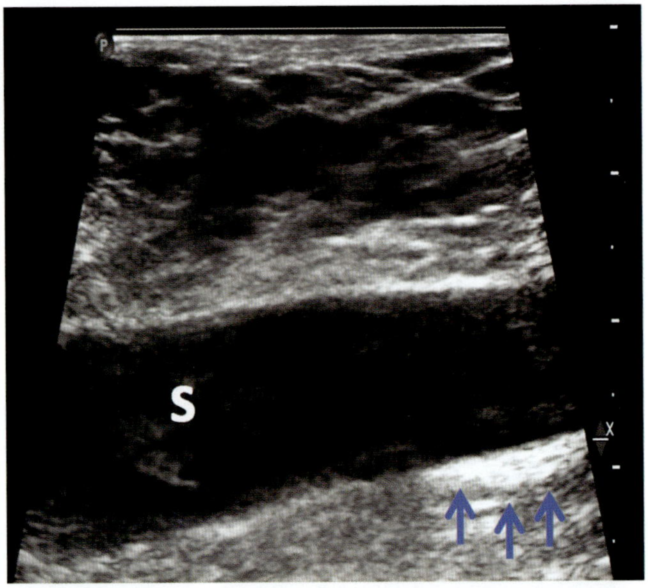

Fig. 58.10: Ultrasonographic imaging of chronic vein thrombosis and residual vein obstruction. Echogenic intravascular banding (S) and posterior vein wall (sharp white shadow) consistent with vein scaring (blue arrows).

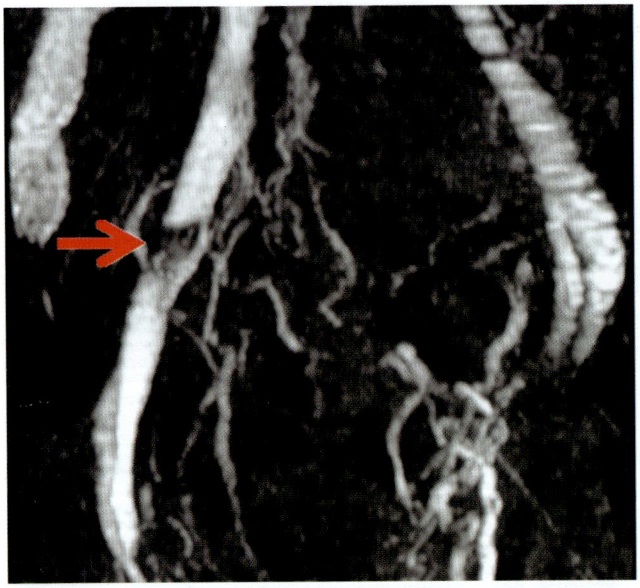

Fig. 58.11: Magnetic resonance venography (MRV) showing thrombosis and flow disturbance (arrow) of the right iliac vein.

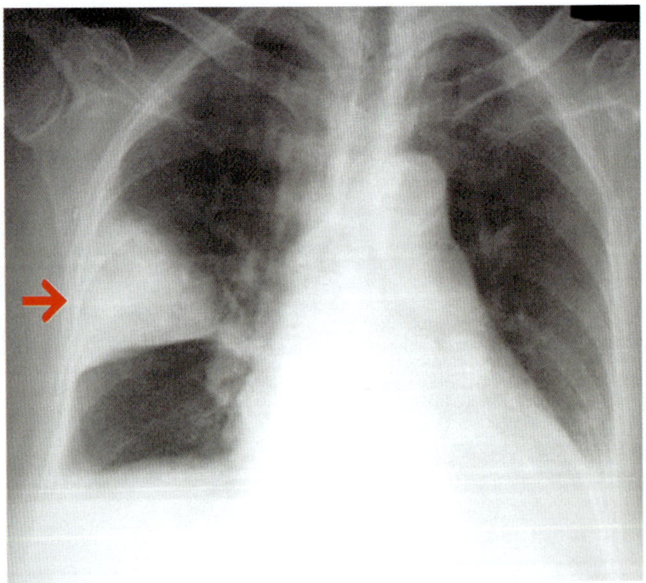

Fig. 58.12: Chest X-ray showing a wedge-shaped defect (Hampton's hump) as a result of pulmonary embolus and subsequent pulmonary infarction. [Image from Hegde M and Vijayalakshmi IB. Vijayalakshmi IB et al (Ed). Comprehensive approach to congenital heart disease. New Delhi, India: Jaypee Brothers Medical Publishers (P) Ltd.].

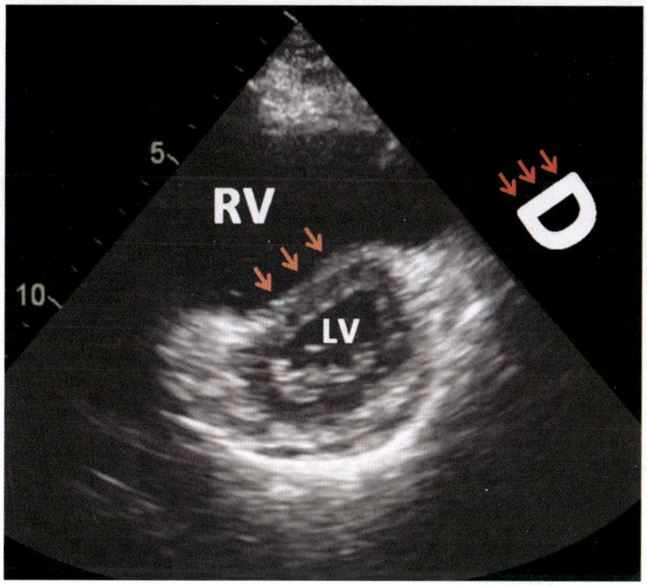

Fig. 58.13A: Short-axis transthoracic echocardiogram in a patient with massive pulmonary embolism showing an enlarged right ventricle (RV) and a flattened interventricular septum (arrows). While the interventricular septum normally bows into the right ventricle, with right ventricular pressure overload, the septum appears flattened, and the left ventricular (LV) walls appear as a "D" shape. [Image modified from Chin CWL. Risk stratification of patients with acute pulmonary embolism. In: Cobanoglu U (Ed). Pulmonary embolism. Intechweb.org. CC].

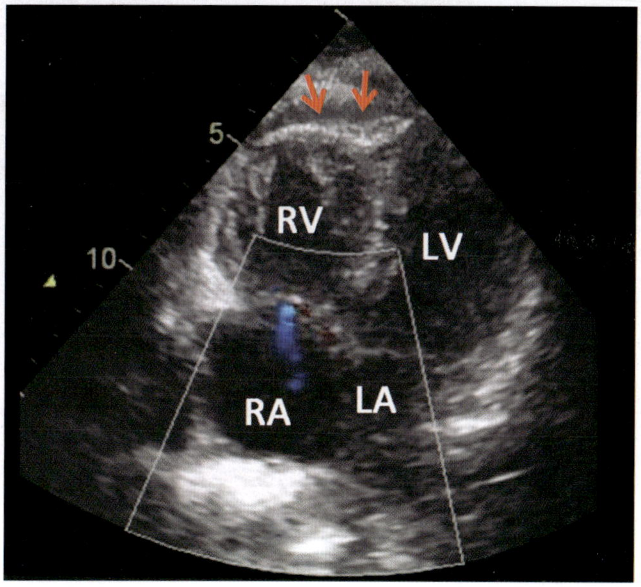

Fig. 58.13B: Apical four-chamber transthoracic echocardiogram demonstrating a markedly dilated right ventricle with hypokinesis of the right ventricle (RV) free wall but preserved systolic function of the apex (arrows). This finding, called the McConnell sign, is suggestive of hemodyanimcally signficant pulmonary embolism. [Image from Chin CWL. Risk stratification of patients with acute pulmonary embolism. In: Cobanoglu U (Ed). Pulmonary embolism. Intechweb.org. CC].

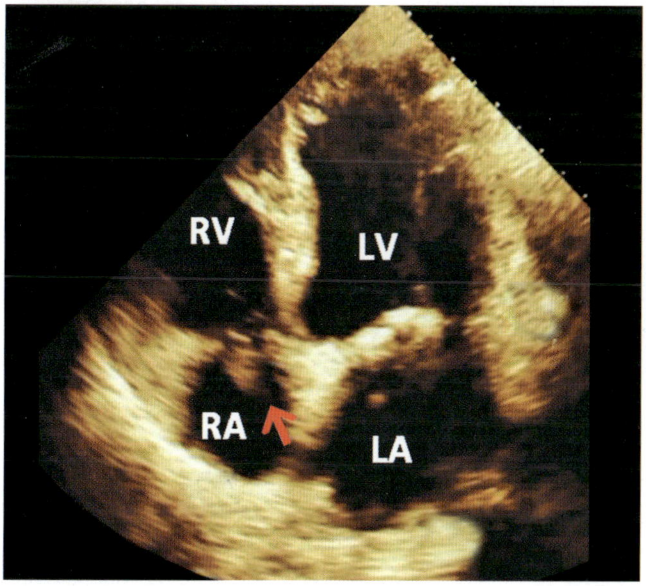

Fig. 58.14A: Three-dimensional echocardiography showing a thrombus (arrow) passing between the right atrium (RA) and right ventricle (RV). [Image from Harris R and Ofili E. Echocardiography in life-threatening conditions. In: Nanda NC (Ed). Comprehensive Textbook of Echocardiography. New Delhi, India: Jaypee Brothers Medical Publishers (P) Ltd.]. (LA: Left atrium; LV: Left ventricle).

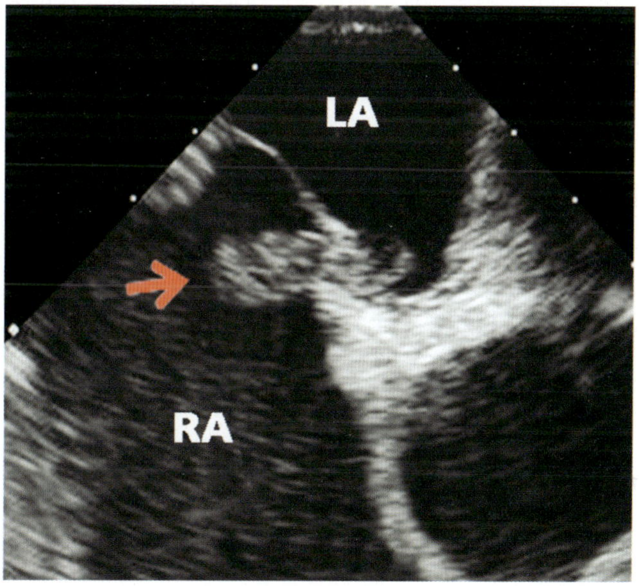

Fig. 58.14B: TEE showing paradoxical embolus. A thrombus is seen (arrow) crossing a patent foramen ovale.

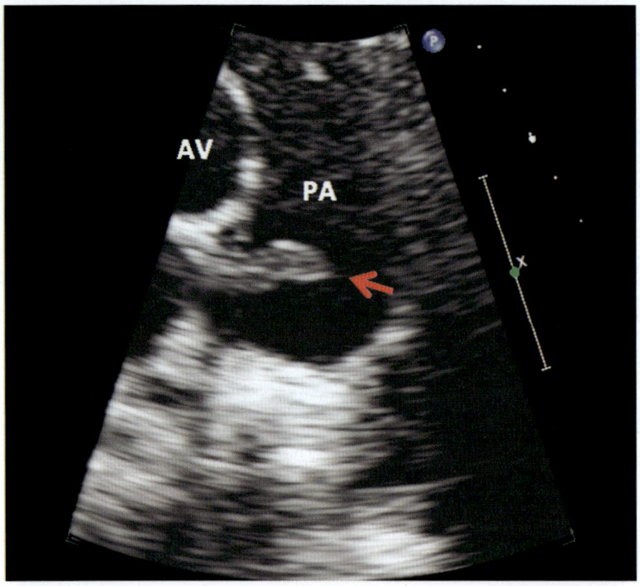

Fig. 58.14C: Parasternal short-axis transthoracic echocardiogram (TTE) showing a thrombus present in the distal main and proximal right pulmonary artery. Videos 58.1 and 58.2 show this in video loops, in which the mobile nature of the thrombus can be better appreciated. (Image courtesy of Glenn N Levine, MD).

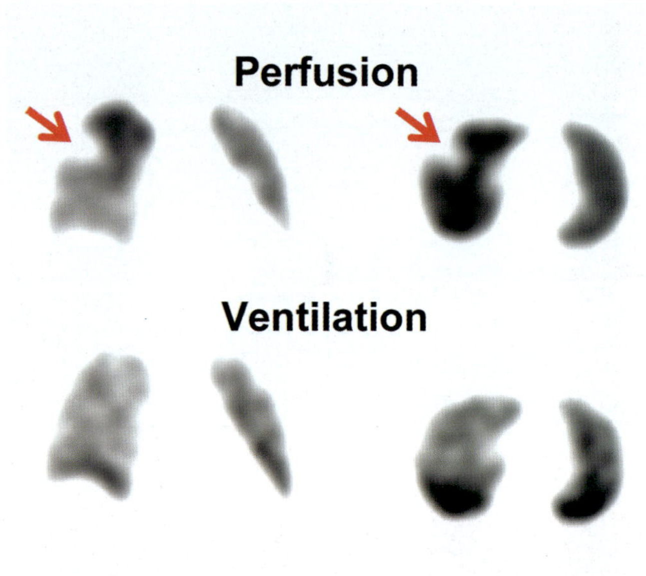

Fig. 58.15: Ventilation-perfusion scan showing a typical wedge-shaped perfusion defect (arrows) with normal ventilation. [Image from Leblanc M. Ventilation perfusion single photon emission tomography (V/Q SPECT in the diagnosis of pulmonary embolism). In: Cobanoglu U (Ed). Pulmonary embolism. Intechweb.org. CC].

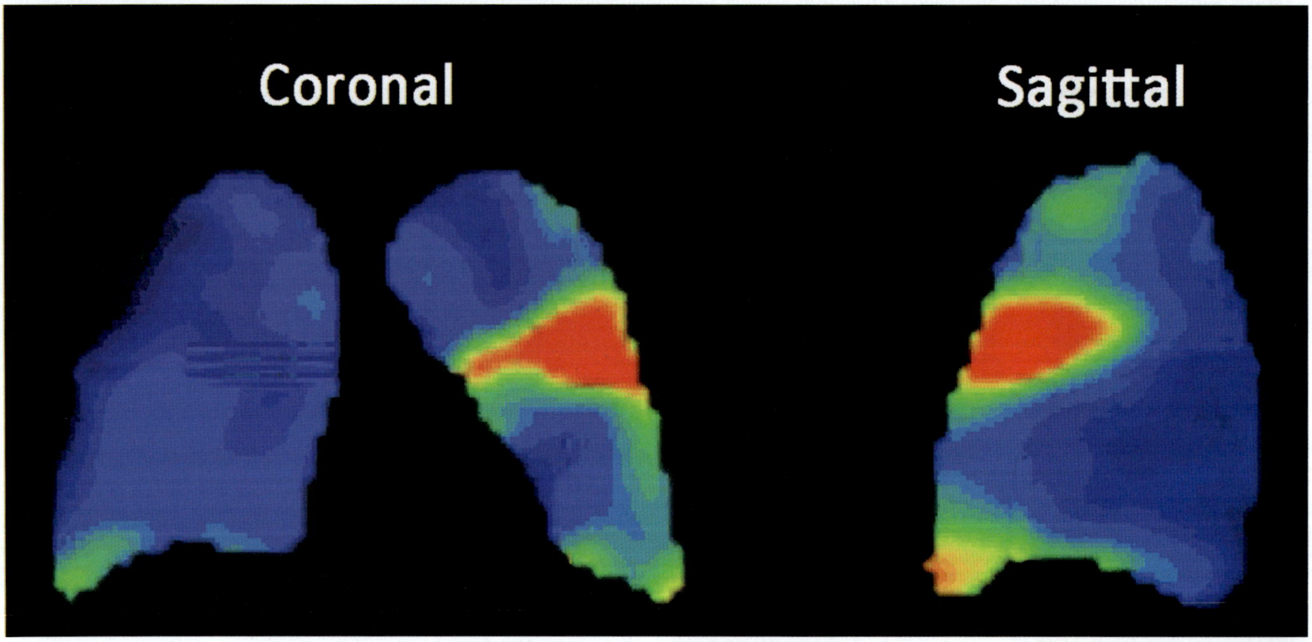

Fig. 58.16: Quantitative evaluation of perfusion and ventilation imaging (V/Q quotient of embolism), displayed in the coronal (left) and sagittal (right) slices. Red indicates the area of complete mismatch, while blue shows normally matched regions. [Image from Leblanc M. Ventilation perfusion single photon emission tomography (V/Q SPECT in the diagnosis of pulmonary embolism). In: Cobanoglu U (Ed). Pulmonary embolism. Intechweb.org. CC].

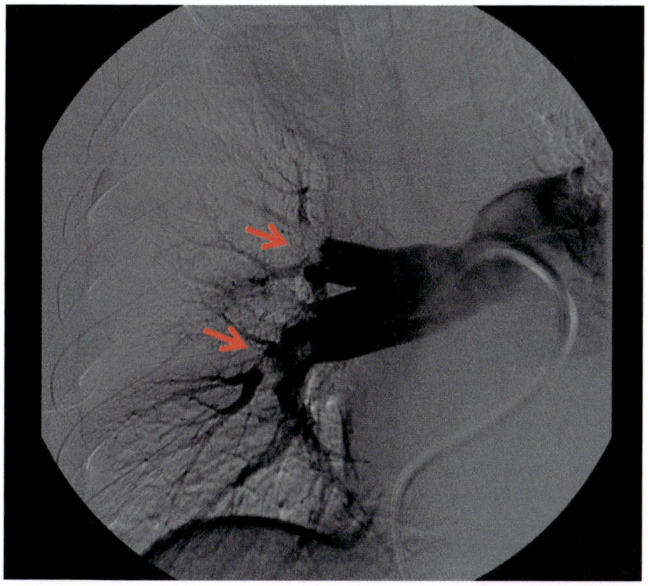

Fig. 58.17: Pulmonary arteriogram demonstrating multiple pulmonary emboli (arrows) to the right lung with markedly decreased perfusion. [Image from Stambo GW. Current endovascular treatments for venous thrombosis. In: Okuyan E (Ed). Venous thrombosis—principles and practice. Intechweb.org. CC].

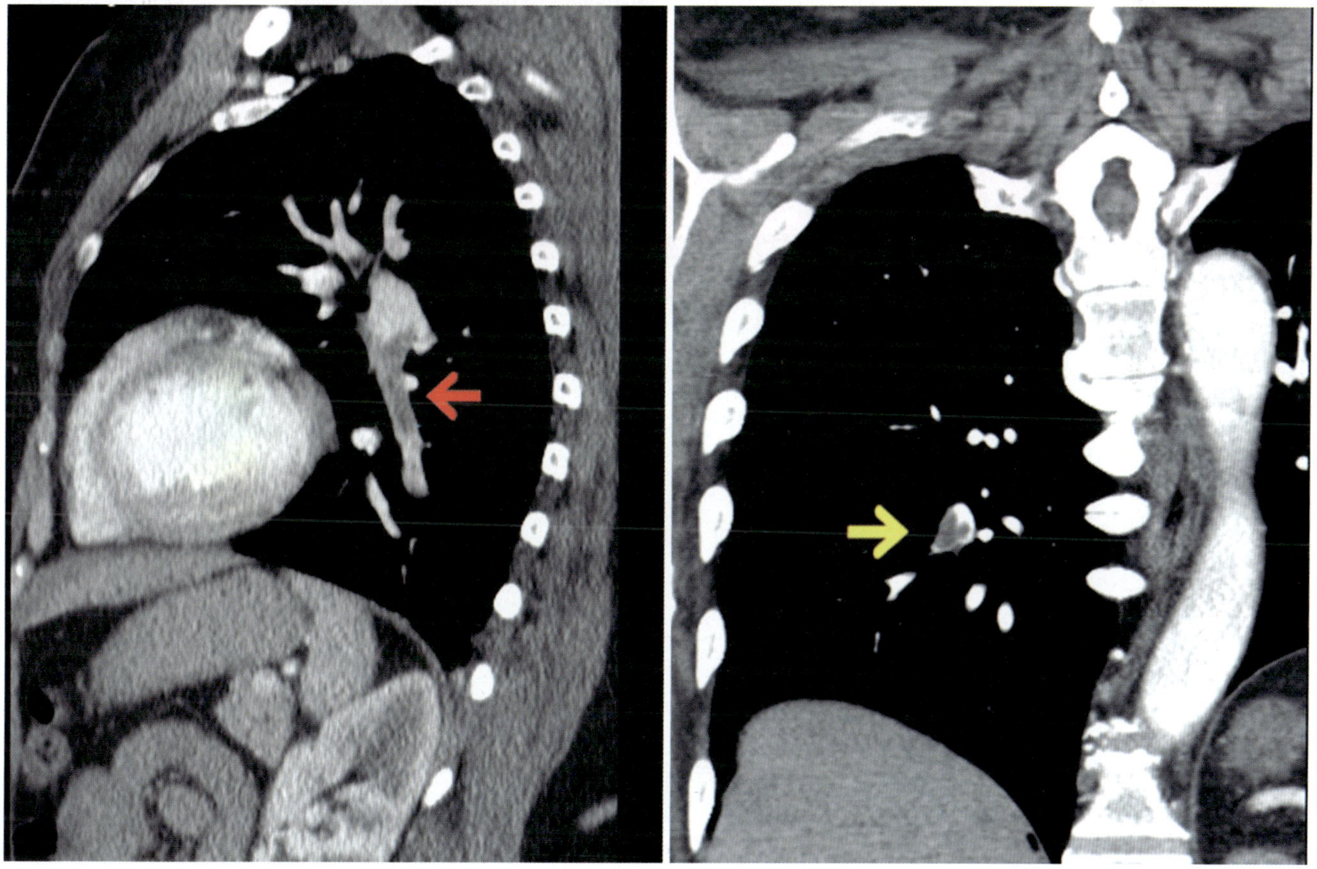

Fig. 58.18: Segmental and subsegmental pulmonary embolism detected by computed tomographic angiography (CTA). MIP (Maximal intense projection) images CT angiogram of the chest with contrast showing perfusion abnormalities (red arrow) of the large segmental left main pulmonary artery extending into the lobar arteries and subsegmental right pulmonary branches (yellow arrow).

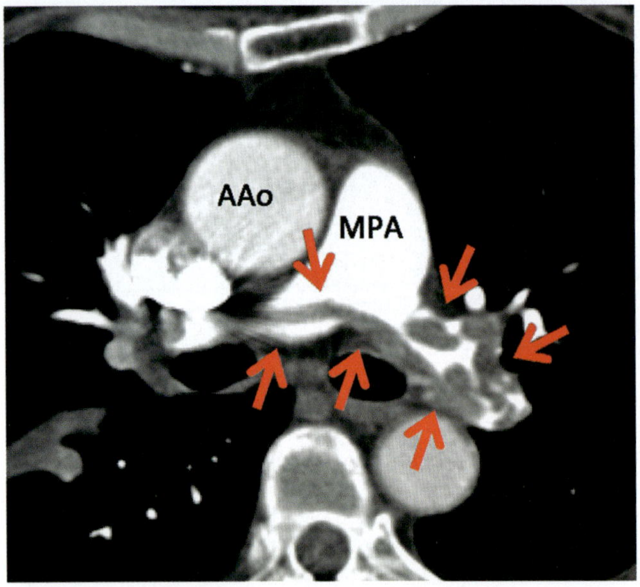

Fig. 58.19: CT image of a massive saddle pulmonary embolism (arrows). [Image from Kim WY et al. Risk stratification of submassive pulmonary embolism: the role of chest computed tomography as an alternative to echocardiography. In: Cobanoglu U (Ed). Pulmonary embolism. Intechweb.org. CC]. (AAo: Ascending aorta; MPA: Main pulmonary artery).

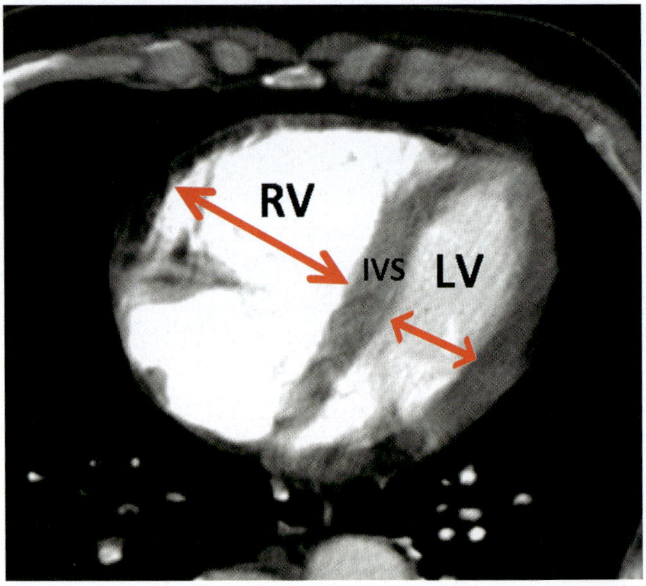

Fig. 58.20: CT scan obtained in a patient with suspected pulmonary embolism showing markedly enlarged right ventricle (RV) in comparison to the left ventricle (LV). Note additionally that the interventricular septum (IVS) is shifted towards the left ventricle. [Image from Kim WY et al. Risk stratification of submassive pulmonary embolism: the role of chest computed tomography as an alternative to echocardiography. In: Cobanoglu U (Ed). Pulmonary embolism. Intechweb.org. CC].

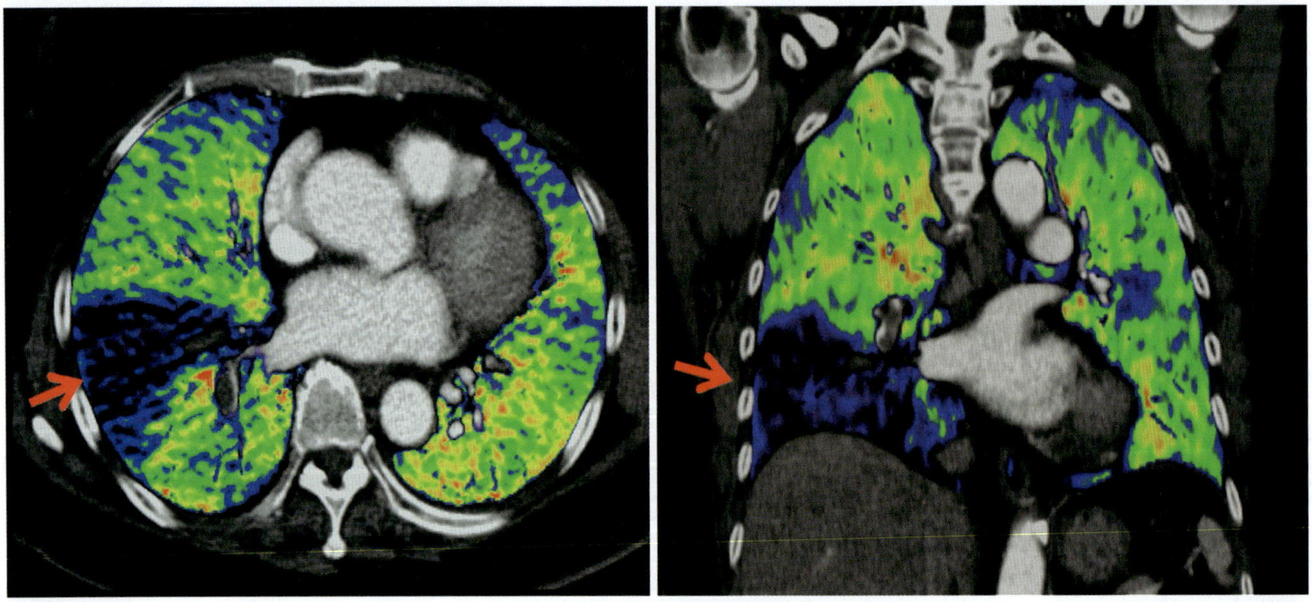

Fig. 58.21: Lung iodine imaging demonstrating wedge-shaped pulmonary perfusion defect (arrows) in the right lower lobe lateral basal segment. [Image from Kim WY et al. Risk stratification of submassive pulmonary embolism: the role of chest computed tomography as an alternative to echocardiography. In: Cobanoglu U (Ed). Pulmonary embolism. Intechweb.org. CC].

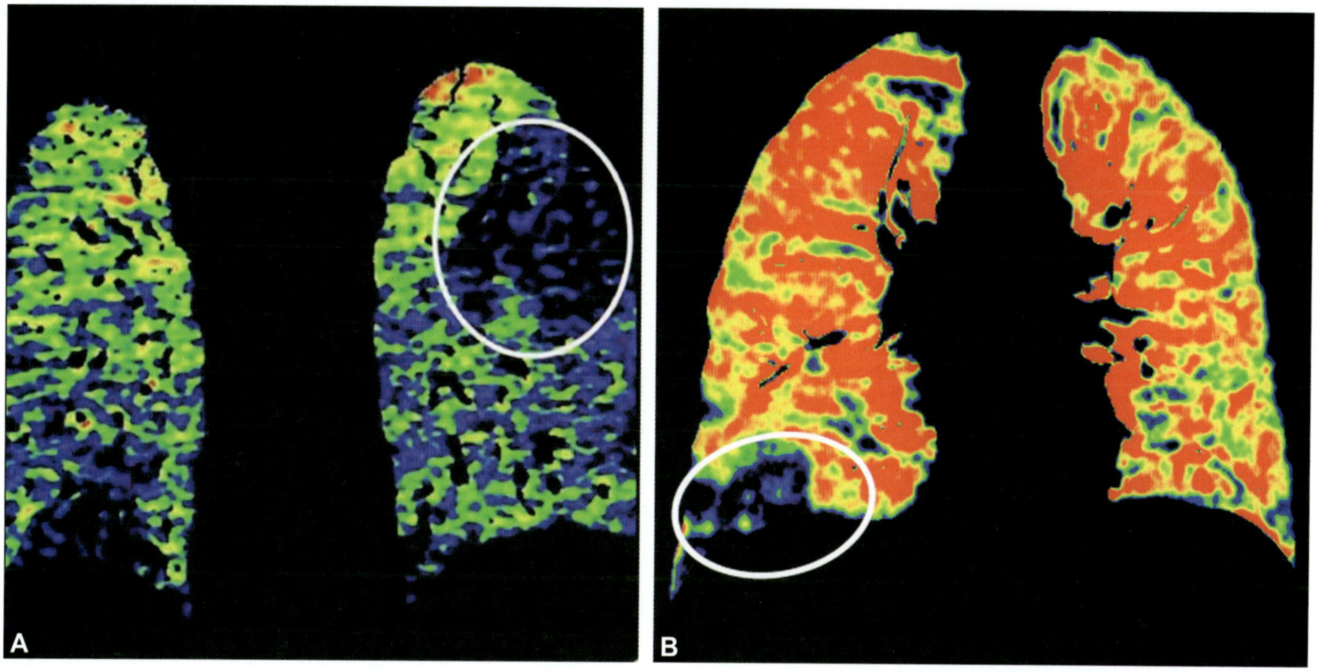

Figs. 58.22A and B: Blood flow imaging (BFI) images demonstrating wedge-shaped perfusion defects in patients with pulmonary emboli. (A) Perfusion defect in the left lung lower lobe dorsal segment; (B) Perfusion defect in the right lung lower lobe dorsal segment. [Images from Zhao YE. Dual source, dual energy computed tomography in pulmonary embolism. In: Cobanoglu U (Ed). Pulmonary embolism. Intechweb.org. CC].

recommendations are based on the 9th iteration of these guidelines. In the initial phase (<5 days from incident event) short-intermediate acting agents such as heparin, low-molecular-weight heparin or the synthetic pentasaccharide Factor Xa inhibitor fondaparinux or rivaroxaban, are preferred to prevent clot progression or embolism. The early maintenance phase, which coincides with the intermediate stage of the disease, extends for three months. This phase is usually treated by oral vitamin K antagonist. After three months, patients continued on anticoagulation in the early maintenance phase enter the long-term secondary prevention phase. A simplified approach can be achieved if low-molecular-weight heparin, fondaparinux or novel factor Xa inhibitors recently approved by the FDA are used to treat VTE in selected populations.

In patients with pulmonary embolism with hemodynamic compromise or large clot burden in the segmental and subsegmental pulmonary arterial vasculature thrombectomy, systemic thrombolysis or catheter directed thrombolysis is used to reduce short-term mortality. Similarly, large clot burden in the proximal and central veins of the lower extremities (Fig. 58.23), or occlusive venous outflow with limb ischemic compromise (phlegmasia cerulea dolmens) may require emergency measures to reduce thrombus size, with catheter directed thrombolysis (CDT) to establish vessel patency (Fig. 58.24), or surgical thrombectomy, along with decompression fasciotomy, if indicated, to reduce short- and long-term limb morbidity caused by acute limb ischemia.

If the risk for bleeding is high and anticoagulation is contraindicated, deployment of a retrievable inferior vena cava filter is an alternative option to reduce the risk of pulmonary embolic events (Figs. 58.25A to D). Several complications with IVC filters have been reported, which include IVC thrombosis (6–30%), insertion site thrombosis (2–28%) and IVC perforation (9–24%). Generally, IVC perforation (Figs. 58.26A and B) is an incidental and asymptomatic finding.

In some cases in which there is external compression of the vein by adjacent structures that results in thrombosis and vein stenosis, such as compression of the left iliac vein by the right iliac artery (May–Thurner syndrome) or compression of the subclavian vein by an accessory rib or hypertrophy of the scalene muscle (thoracic outlet syndrome) (Fig. 58.27), angioplasty and stent placement (Figs. 58.28A and B) may be indicated to ensure proper venous outflow from the affected limb.

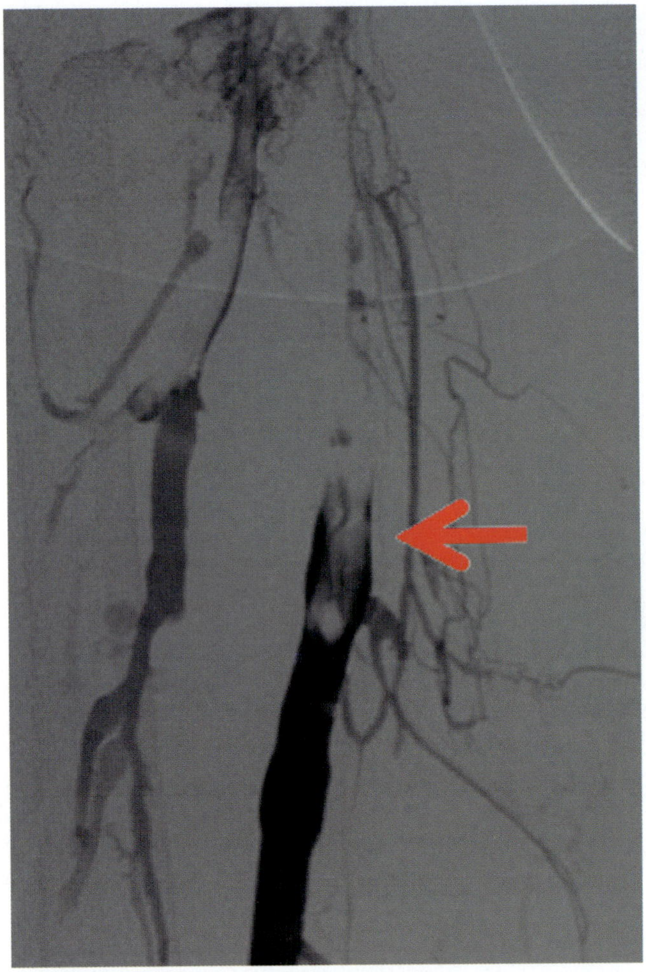

Fig. 58.23: Venogram demonstrating extensive DVT of the left superior femoral vein, extending into the iliac system. [Image from Stambo GW. Current endovascular treatments for venous thrombosis. In: Okuyan E (Ed). Venous thrombosis—principles and practice. Intechweb.org. CC].

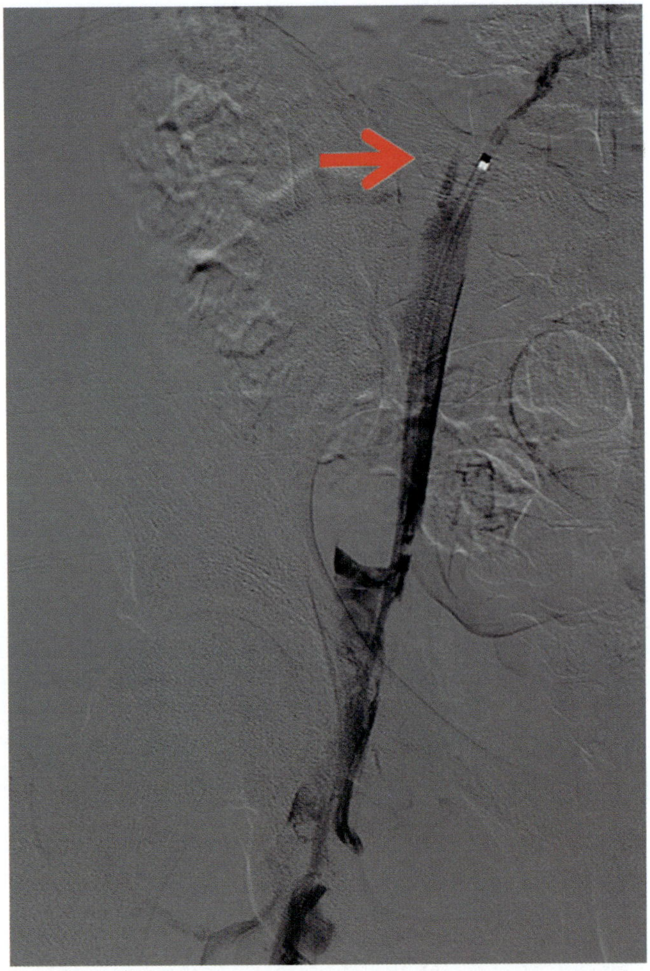

Fig. 58.24: Catheter directed thrombolysis of the left iliac vein. Venogram of catheter directed thrombolysis of left iliac vein thrombosis in a patient with May–Thurner syndrome (left iliac vein compression by right iliac artery).

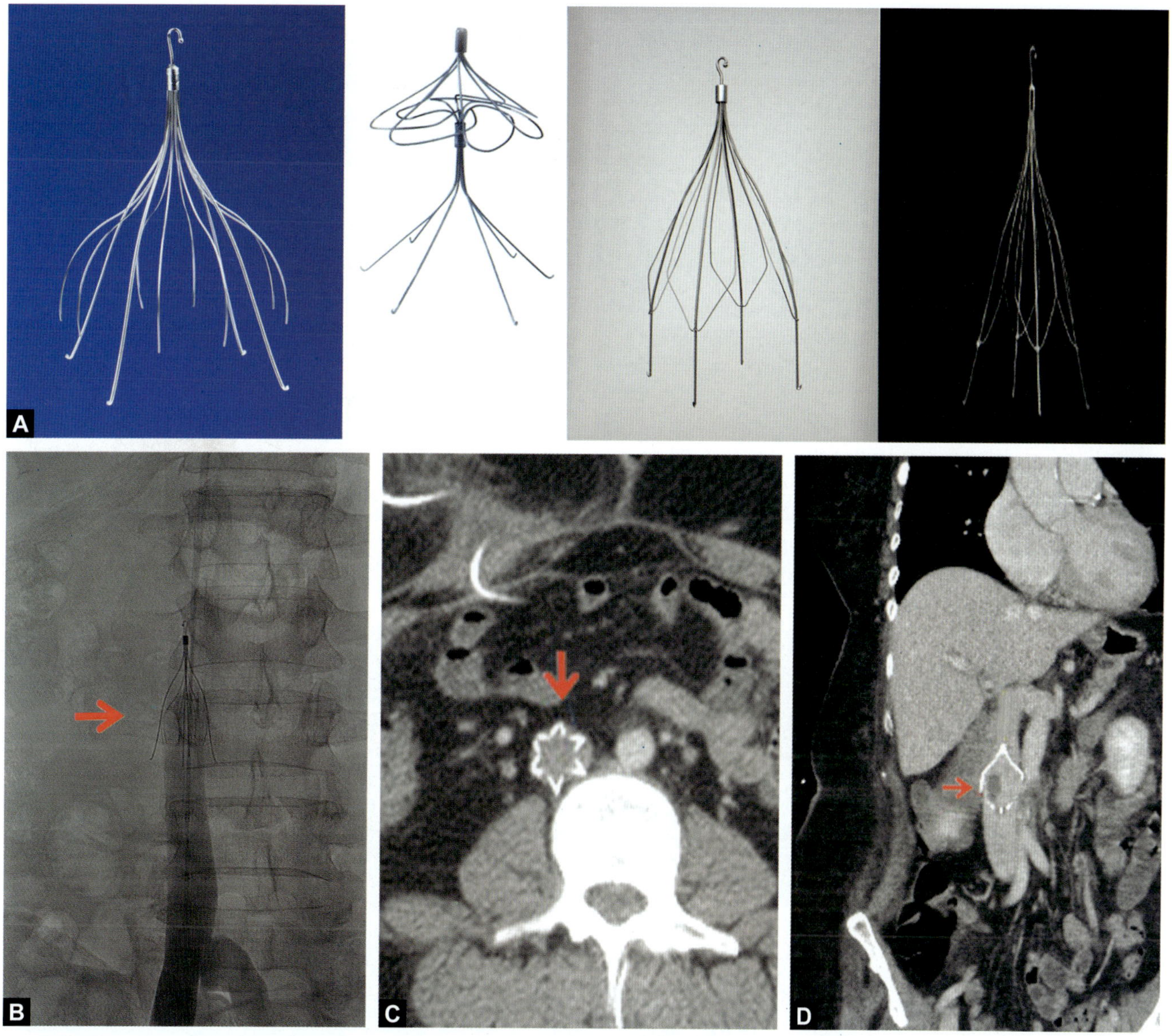

Figs. 58.25A to D: Inferior vena cava (IVC) filters. (A) Examples of IVC filters; (B) Venogram showing a temporary infrarenal filter (arrow) with well positioned intravascular prones with no evidence of angle disruption or tilting. A caudal hook for retrieval can be observed; (C) CT of the abdomen showing star-shaped hyperintense intravascular filter (arrow) in the inferior vena cava; (D) Contrast-enhanced CT scan coronal image illustrating an IVC filter with a deep vein thrombosis (arrow) within the IVC filter.

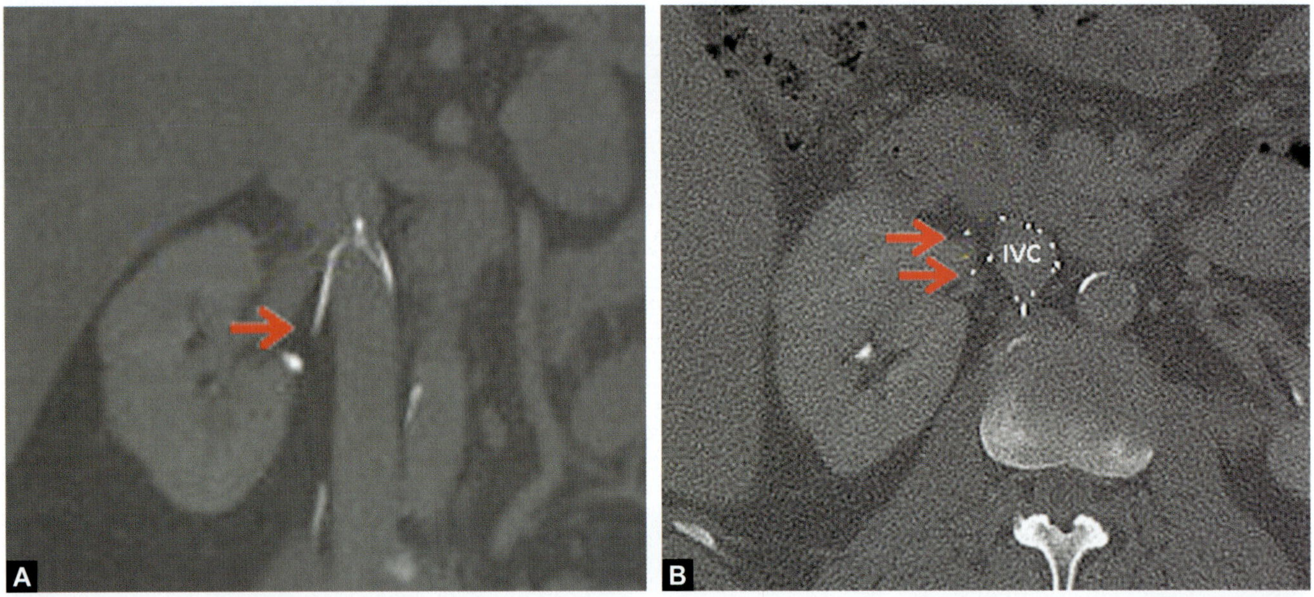

Figs. 58.26A and B: Inferior vena cava (IVC) perforation by an IVC filter. CT images of IVC filter struts (arrows) that have perforated the IVC.

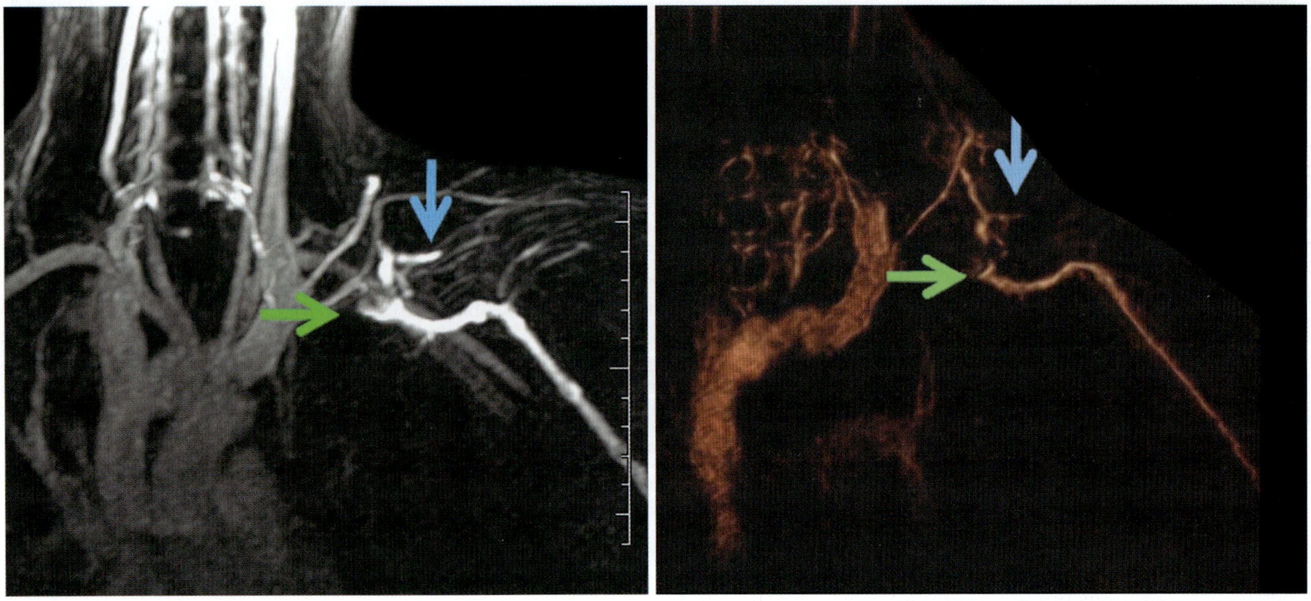

Fig. 58.27: Subclavian vein stenosis and thrombosis caused by thoracic outlet syndrome. Magnetic resonance venography images demonstrating left subclavian vein stenosis and occlusion (green arrows) and reconstitution of venous outflow through collaterals (blue arrows).

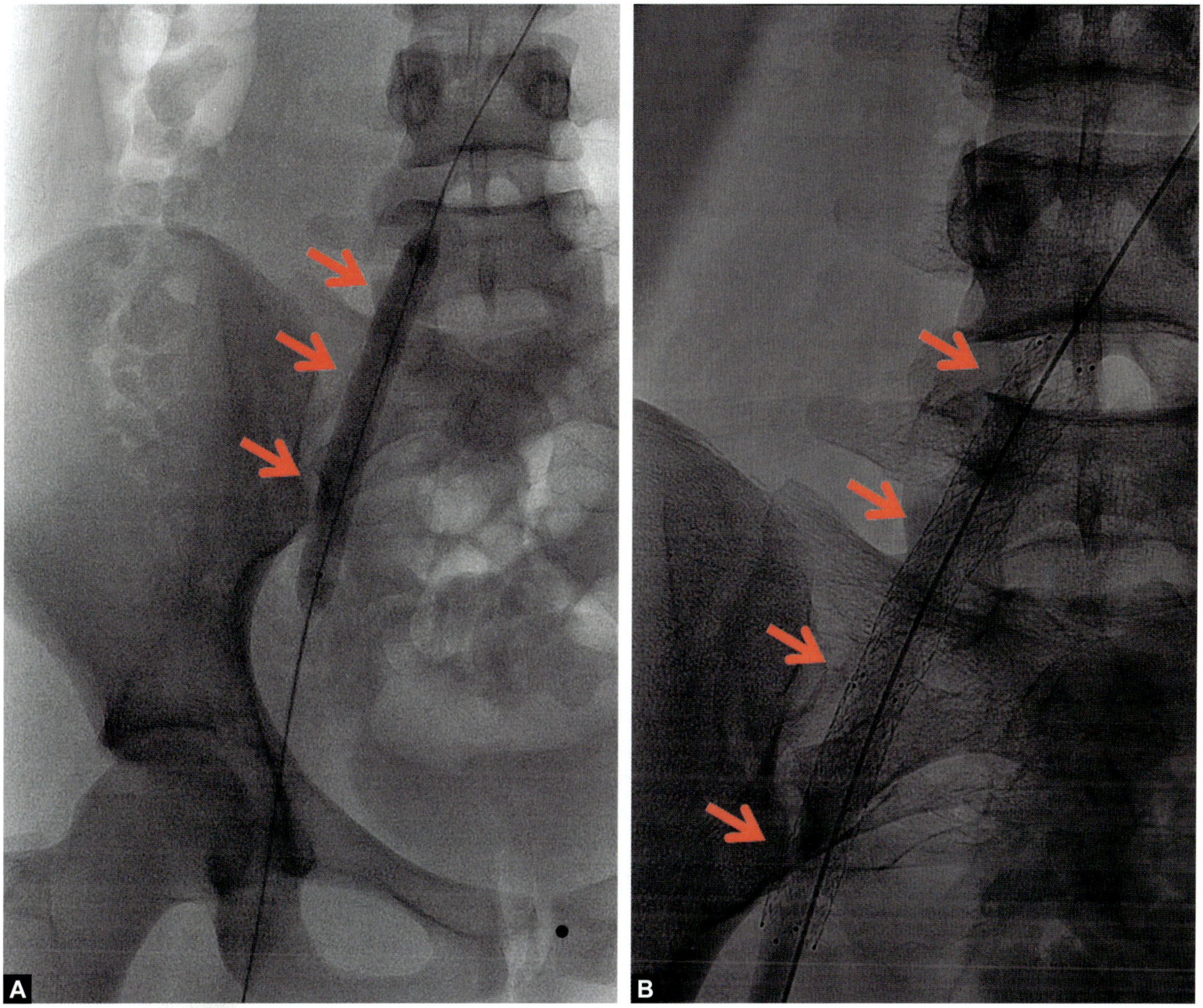

Figs. 58.28A and B: Balloon angioplasty (A) and stenting (B) of a right iliac vein stenosis.

VIDEO LEGENDS

Videos 58.1 and 58.2: Parasternal short-axis TTE imaging showing a thrombus present in the distal main and proximal right pulmonary artery. (Videos courtesy of Glenn N Levine, MD).

REFERENCES

Galanis T, Eraso L, Perez A, et al. Venous thromboembolic disease. ISBN 139781935395737. In: David Paul Slovut, Steven M. Dean, Michael R. Jaff, Peter A. Schneider, (Eds. Comprehensive Review in Vascular and Endovascular Medicine. Vol I.; 2012: 251-84.

Guyatt GH, Akl EA, Crowther M, Gutterman DD, Schuunemann HJ, American College of Chest Physicians Antithrombotic Therapy and Prevention of Thrombosis Panel. Executive summary: Antithrombotic therapy and prevention of thrombosis, 9th edition: American College of Chest Physicians Evidence-based Clinical Practice Guidelines. Chest. 2012;141 (2 Suppl):7S-47S.

Goldhaber SZ, Bounameaux H. Pulmonary embolism and deep vein thrombosis. Lancet. 2012;379(9828):1835-46.

Kageyama N, Ro A, Tanifuji T, et al. Significance of the soleal vein and its drainage veins in cases of massive pulmonary thromboembolism. Ann Vasc Dis. 2008;1(1):35-9.

Wells PS, Ginsberg JS, Anderson DR, et al. Use of a clinical model for safe management of patients with suspected pulmonary embolism. Ann Intern Med. 1998;129(12):997-1005.

Wolberg AS, Aleman MM, Leiderman K, et al. Procoagulant activity in hemostasis and thrombosis: Virchow's triad revisited. Anesth Analg. 2012;114(2):275-85.

Index

Note: Page numbers followed by *f* and *t* indicate figures and tables respectively.

A

B

C

D

E

F

G

H

I

N

O

P

Q

R

S

T

U

V

W

X